HEALTH ALERTS

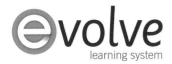
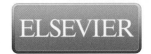
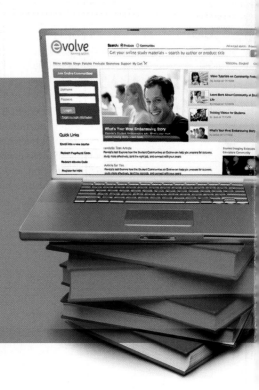

Understanding Pathophysiology

Fifth Edition

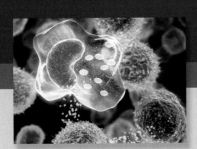

Sue E. Huether, MS, PhD
Professor Emeritus
College of Nursing
University of Utah
Salt Lake City, Utah

Kathryn L. McCance, MS, PhD
Professor
College of Nursing
University of Utah
Salt Lake City, Utah

Section Editors
Valentina L. Brashers, MD
Professor of Nursing and Attending Physician in Internal Medicine
University of Virginia Health System
Charlottesville, Virginia

Neal S. Rote, PhD
Academic Vice-Chair and Director of Research
Department of Obstetrics and Gynecology
University Hospitals of Cleveland;
Professor of Reproductive Biology and Pathology
Case School of Medicine
Case Western Reserve University
Cleveland, Ohio

ELSEVIER

with 1,000 illustrations

3251 Riverport Lane
St. Louis, Missouri 63043

Notices

Knowledge and best practice in this field are constantly changing. As new research and experience broaden our understanding, changes in research methods, professional practices, or medical treatment may become necessary.

Practitioners and researchers must always rely on their own experience and knowledge in evaluating and using any information, methods, compounds, or experiments described herein. In using such information or methods they should be mindful of their own safety and the safety of others, including parties for whom they have a professional responsibility.

With respect to any drug or pharmaceutical products identified, readers are advised to check the most current information provided (i) on procedures featured or (ii) by the manufacturer of each product to be administered, to verify the recommended dose or formula, the method and duration of administration, and contraindications. It is the responsibility of practitioners, relying on their own experience and knowledge of their patients, to make diagnoses, to determine dosages and the best treatment for each individual patient, and to take all appropriate safety precautions.

To the fullest extent of the law, neither the Publisher nor the authors, contributors, or editors, assume any liability for any injury and/or damage to persons or property as a matter of products liability, negligence or otherwise, or from any use or operation of any methods, products, instructions, or ideas contained in the material herein.

Previous editions copyrighted 2008, 2004, 2000, 1996

Library of Congress Cataloging-in-Publication Data
Understanding pathophysiology / [edited by] Sue E. Huether, Kathryn L. McCance;
section editors, Valentina L. Brashers, Neal S. Rote. — 5th ed.
    p. ; cm.
Includes bibliographical references and index.
ISBN 978-0-323-07891-7 (pbk. : alk. paper)
I. Huether, Sue E. II. McCance, Kathryn L.
    [DNLM: 1. Pathology—Nurses' Instruction. 2. Disease—Nurses' Instruction.
    3. Physiology—Nurses' Instruction. QZ 4]
616.07—dc23   2011039731

Vice President and Publisher: Loren S. Wilson
Senior Editor: Sandra Clark
Senior Developmental Editor: Charlene Ketchum
Editorial Assistant: Brooke Kannady
Publishing Services Manager: Jeffrey Patterson
Project Manager: Jeanne Genz
Designer: Paula Catalano
Multimedia Producer: Lisa Godoski

Printed in the United States of America

Last digit is the print number: 9 8 7 6 5 4 3

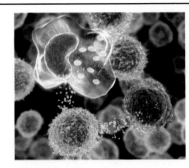

ABOUT THE COVER

Image of white blood cells and inflammation: B lymphocytes (orange) communicate via cytokines with other inflammatory cells, such as T lymphocytes (purple) and monocytes/macrophages (purple in bag), to maintain and amplify the cycle of inflammation.

Jan Belden, MSN, RN-BC, FNP-BC
Pain Management Nurse Practitioner
Loma Linda University Medical Center
Linda, California

Barbara J. Boss, PhD, RN, CFNP, CANP
Director of DNP Program and Professor of
    Nursing
School of Nursing
University of Mississippi Medical Center
Jackson, Mississippi

Kristen Lee Carroll, MD
Associate Professor of Orthopedics
Assistant Professor of Pediatric Neurology
University of Utah Medical Center
Shriner's Intermountain Unit
Salt Lake City, Utah

Margaret F. Clayton, PhD, APRN-BC
Assistant Professor
College of Nursing
University of Utah
Salt Lake City, Utah

**Christy L. Crowther-Radulewicz,
RN, MS, CRNP**
Nurse Practitioner
Anne Arundel Orthopaedic Surgeons
Annapolis, Maryland
Adjunct Faculty
Johns Hopkins School of Nursing
Department of Community-Public Health
Baltimore, Maryland

Curtis DeFriez, MD
Professor
Department of Health Sciences
Weber State University
Ogden, Utah

Angela Deneris, PhD, CNM
Associate Professor, Clinical
University of Utah College of Nursing
Salt Lake City, Utah

Sharon Dudley-Brown, PhD, FNP-BC
Assistant Professor
Schools of Medicine and Nursing
Johns Hopkins University
Baltimore, Maryland

Kristi K. Gott, MSN, RN, CPNP
Pediatric Pulmonary Nurse Practitioner
University of Virginia School of Nursing
Charlottesville, Virginia

Todd C. Grey, MD
Chief Medical Examiner
State of Utah
Associate Clinical Professor of Pathology
University of Utah School of Medicine
Salt Lake City, Utah

Robert E. Jones, MD, FACP, FACE
Professor of Medicine
University of Utah School of Medicine
Salt Lake City, Utah

Lynn B. Jorde, PhD
H.A. and Edna Benning Presidential
    Professor and Chair
Department of Human Genetics
University of Utah School of Medicine
Salt Lake City, Utah

Lynne M. Kerr, MD, PhD
Associate Professor
Pediatric Neurology
Primary Children's Medical Center
Salt Lake City, Utah

Nancy E. Kline, PhD, RN, CPNP, FAAN
Director, Research and Evidence-Based
    Practice
Department of Nursing
Memorial Sloan-Kettering Cancer Center
New York, New York

Gwen Latendresse, PhD, CNM
Assistant Professor
University of Utah College of Nursing
Salt Lake City, Utah

Nancy L. McDaniel, MD
Associate Professor of Pediatrics
University of Virginia
Charlottesville, Virginia

Vinodh Narayanan, MD
Child Neurologist
St. Joseph's Hospital and Medical Center
Professor of Clinical Pediatrics and
    Neurology
University of Arizona College of Medicine
Phoenix, Arizona

**Noreen Heer Nicol, PhD,
RN, FNP, NEA-BC**
Director, Professional Development
The Children's Hospital
Clinical Senior Instructor
University of Colorado
Affiliate Associate Professor
University of Northern Colorado

Patricia Ring, RN, PNP-BC
Pediatric Nephrology Nurse Practitioner
Children's Hospital of Wisconsin
Milwaukee, Wisconsin

Anna L. Schwartz, PhD, FNP, FAAN
Associate Professor, School of Nursing
Idaho State University
Oncology Nurse Practitioner
Wilson Medical
Jackson, Wyoming

Richard A. Sugerman, PhD
Professor of Anatomy
College of Osteopathic Medicine
Western University of Health Sciences
Pomona, California

David Virshup, MD
Professor and Director
Program in Cancer and Stem Cell Biology
Duke-NUS Graduate Medical School
Singapore
Professor of Pediatrics
Duke University School of Medicine
Durham, North Carolina

Jo Voss, PhD, RN, CNS
Associate Professor
South Dakota State University
Rapid City, South Dakota

*The authors would also like to thank the previous edition contributors.

Mandi Counters, RN, MSN, CNRC
Assistant Professor
Mercy College of Health Sciences
Des Moines, Iowa

April N. Hart, RN, MSN, FNP-BC, CNE
Assistant Professor
Bethel College
Mishawaka, Indiana

Stephen D. Krau, PhD, RN, CNE, CT
Associate Professor
Vanderbilt University Medical Center
Nashville, Tennessee

Bruce S. McEwen, PhD
Alfred E. Mirsky Professor
Head, Harold and Margaret Milliken Hatch
    Laboratory of Neuroendocrinology
The Rockefeller University
New York, New York

**Charles Preston Molsbee,
    EdD, MSN, RN, CNE**
Assistant Professor
University of Arkansas
Little Rock, Arkansas

Judith L. Myers, MSN, RN
Assistant Professor of Nursing
Grand View University
Des Moines, Iowa

Louise Suit, EdD, RN, CNS, CAS
Assistant Professor
Regis University
Denver, Colorado

Jo Voss, PhD, RN, CNS
Associate Professor
West River Department of Nursing
South Dakota State University
Rapid City, South Dakota

Kim Lee Webb, RN, MN
Nursing Department Chair
Northern Oklahoma College
Tonkawa, Oklahoma

This edition, like the previous one, has been rigorously updated and revised, with many sections completely rewritten to reflect recent findings. The pace of advances in areas such as immunity, inflammation, cancer, genetics, and cardiovascular disease is astounding. And although some of this progress already has been translated into clinical practice, many challenges remain on just *how* to use this new information to help improve diagnostic and disease management and caring practices. Nonetheless, we believe students should be exposed to these emerging understandings as they unfold and be encouraged to follow these developments throughout their professional lives.

A major goal of this edition of *Understanding Pathophysiology* was to make it even more understandable. Toward that end, we have edited the book to improve clarity by defining more of the terms used, by explaining some concepts more fully, by simplifying the more difficult content, by reorganizing the sequence of some content, and by revising and adding more color illustrations and photos. For example, the chapters on altered cellular and tissue biology, inflammation, and immunity were rewritten entirely for simplification. We believe we have met our challenge without deleting any key information.

Although the primary focus of the text is pathophysiology, we continue to include discussions of the following interconnected topics to highlight their importance for clinical practice:

- A life span approach that includes special sections on aging and separate chapters on children
- Epidemiology and incidence rates showing dramatic, worldwide differences that reflect the importance of environmental and lifestyle factors on disease initiation and progression
- Clinical manifestations and summaries of treatment
- Gender differences that affect epidemiology and pathophysiology
- Molecular biology—mechanisms of normal cell function and how their alteration leads to disease
- Health promotion/risk reduction

ORGANIZATION AND CONTENT: WHAT'S NEW IN THE FIFTH EDITION

The book is organized into two parts: Part One, Basic Concepts of Pathophysiology, and Part Two, Body Systems and Diseases.

Part One: Basic Concepts of Pathophysiology

Part One introduces basic principles and processes. The concepts include descriptions of cellular communication; genes and genetic disease; forms of cell injury; fluid and electrolytes and acid and base balance; immunity and inflammation; mechanisms of infection; stress, coping, and illness; and tumor biology. Knowledge of these principles and processes is essential to gaining a contemporary understanding of the pathophysiology of common diseases.

Significant revisions to Part One include new or updated information on the following topics:

- Updated content on cell communication, membrane transport, fluids and solute transportation (Chapter 1)
- Updated content on oxidative stress, types of cell death, and aging (Chapter 3)
- Extensive entire chapter revisions of mechanisms of human defense—characteristics of innate and adaptive immunity (Chapters 5 and 6)

- Updated and revised content on alterations of immunity and inflammation (Chapter 7)
- Extensive revisions and reorganization of stress and disease (Chapter 8)
- Extensive revisions and reorganization of tumor biology (Chapter 9)
- Extensive entire chapter revisions and reorganization of epidemiology of cancer (Chapter 10)

Part Two: Body Systems and Diseases

Part Two presents the pathophysiology of the most common alterations according to body system. To guarantee readability and comprehension, we have used a logical sequence and uniform approach in presenting the content of the units and chapters. Each unit focuses on a specific organ system and contains chapters related to anatomy and physiology, the pathophysiology of the most common diseases, and common alterations in children. The anatomy and physiology content is presented as a review to enhance the learner's understanding of the structural and functional changes inherent in pathophysiology. A brief summary of normal aging effects is included at the end of these review chapters. The general organization of each disease/disorder discussion includes an introductory paragraph on relevant risk factors and epidemiology, then related pathophysiology, clinical manifestations, and a brief review of evaluation and treatment. Significant revisions to Part Two include new and/or updated information on the following topics:

- The blood-brain barrier (Chapter 12)
- Mechanisms of pain and pain syndromes and sleep disorders including restless legs syndrome (Chapter 13)
- Alterations in levels of arousal, seizure disorders, and delirium. Pathogenesis of degenerative brain diseases, the dementias, motor neuron syndromes, traumatic brain and spinal cord injury, stroke syndromes, and headache (Chapters 14, 15, 16)
- Mechanisms of hormone receptors and hormone action (Chapter 17)
- Thyroid disorders, insulin resistance and inflammatory cytokines, and diabetes mellitus (Chapter 18)
- Platelet function and coagulation; alterations of leukocyte function and myeloid tumors (Chapters 19 and 20)
- Mechanisms of cardiac workload, cardiac muscle remodeling, angiogenesis and growth factors, endothelial function (Chapter 22)
- Mechanisms of atherosclerosis, hypertension, coronary artery disease, heart failure, and shock (Chapter 23)
- Pediatric valvular disorders, heart failure, hypertension, obesity, and heart disease (Chapter 24)
- Clinical manifestations of respiratory disease, acute respiratory distress syndrome, asthma, and respiratory tract infections (Chapter 26)
- Croup, respiratory distress in the newborn, asthma, cystic fibrosis (Chapter 27)
- Urinary tract obstruction, urinary tract infection, glomerulonephritis, acute and chronic kidney injury (Chapter 29)
- Polycystic kidney disease and pediatric glomerular disorders (Chapter 30)
- Female and male reproductive disorders, prostate cancer, breast diseases and mechanisms of breast cancer, male breast cancer, and sexually transmitted infections (Chapter 32)
- Peptic ulcer disease, obesity, liver disease, pancreatitis (Chapter 34)

- Gluten-sensitive enteropathy, necrotizing enterocolitis, and neonatal jaundice (Chapter 35)
- Bone cells, bone remodeling, joint and tendon diseases, osteoporosis, rheumatoid and osteoarthritis (Chapters 36 and 37)
- Congenital and acquired musculoskeletal disorders, and muscular dystrophies in children (Chapter 38)
- Psoriasis, discoid lupus erythematosus, and scleroderma (Chapter 39)
- Acne vulgaris and impetigo (Chapter 40)

Cancer of the various organ systems was updated for all of the chapters.

FEATURES TO PROMOTE LEARNING

A number of features are incorporated into this text that guide and support learning and understanding, including:

- A *Glossary* of more than 850 terms related to pathophysiology
- *Chapter Outlines* including page numbers for easy reference
- *Quick Check* questions strategically placed throughout each chapter to help readers confirm their understanding of the material; answers are included on the textbook's Evolve website
- *Health Alerts* with concise discussions of the latest research
- *Risk Factors* boxes for selected diseases
- End-of-chapter *Did You Understand?* summaries that condense the major concepts of each chapter into an easy-to-review list format
- *Key Terms* set in boldface in text and listed, with page numbers, at the end of each chapter
- Special headings for *Aging* and *Pediatrics* content that highlight discussions of life span alterations

ART PROGRAM

The art program was carefully considered. This edition features more than 100 new and revised illustrations and photographs. The art program received as much attention as the narrative with a total of 900 images. With new biologic understandings many new spectacular figures were designed to help students visually understand sometimes difficult and complex material. Hundreds of high-quality photographs show clinical manifestations, pathologic specimens, and clinical imaging techniques. Numerous micrographs show normal and abnormal cellular structure. The combination of illustrations, algorithms, photographs, and use of color for tables and boxes allows keen understanding of essential information.

TEACHING/LEARNING PACKAGE

For Students

The free **Student Learning Resource**s on Evolve include review questions and answers, numerous animations, answers to the Quick Check questions in the book, algorithm completion exercises, key term/definition matching exercises, critical thinking questions with answers, and WebLinks. These electronic resources enhance learning options for students. Go to http://evolve.elsevier.com/Huether.

The **Study Guide** includes learning objectives, "Memory Check!" anatomy and physiology reviews, concise summaries of key chapter concepts, a practice examination for each chapter, and case studies with critical thinking questions. Answers to the practice examinations and a discussion of each case study can be found in the back of the Study Guide.

For Instructors

The **Instructor's Evolve Resources** are available free to instructors with qualified adoptions of the textbook and include the following: an *Instructor's Manual* with learning objectives, difficult concepts discussions, and critical thinking exercises with answers; a *Test Bank* of approximately 1,400 items (available as text files or in ExamView computerized testing software); a *PowerPoint Presentation* of more than 2,000 lecture slides; an *Image Collection* of approximately 800 key figures from the text; and *Audience Response Questions* for use with i>clicker and other systems.

All of these teaching resources are also available to instructors on the book's Evolve site, along with access to the WebLinks and other student learning resources. Plus the *Evolve Learning System* provides a comprehensive suite of course communication and organization tools that allow you to upload your class calendar and syllabus, post scores and announcements, and more. Go to http://evolve.elsevier.com/Huether.

The newest and most exciting part of the package is **Pathophysiology Online,** a complete set of online modules that provide thoroughly developed lessons on the most important and difficult topics in pathophysiology supplemented with illustrations, animations, interactive activities, interactive algorithms, self-assessment reviews, and exams. Instructors can use it to enhance traditional classroom lecture courses or for distance and online-only courses. Students can use it as a self-guided study tool.

ACKNOWLEDGMENTS

Although we can never really thank our contributors adequately, we would like to try by expressing our enormous gratitude for their generous contributions of time, knowledge, and talent. With today's major emphasis on evidence-based practice, the challenges to read, interpret, synthesize, and clearly communicate are notable. Times are changing, with enormous amounts of published literature in many major fields creating unique opportunities to "get it right"— increase patient-centered quality care, safety, and satisfaction. So quite simply, without our contributors' expertise, we would not have a textbook tending to establish rigorous and robust facts or evidence.

For this edition Tina Brashers, MD, and Neal Rote, PhD, continued to serve as Section Editors and contributing authors. Tina is a distinguished teacher and has received numerous awards for her work with nursing and medical students and faculty. She is nationally known for contributions in promoting and teaching interprofessional collaboration. Tina brings innovation and clarity to the subject of pathophysiology. Her work on *Pathophysiology Online* continues to be intensive and creative, and a significant learning enhancement for students. Thank you Tina for your writing, guidance of authors, review of manuscript, and foresight about the overall scope of this project. Neal has major expertise, passion, and hard-to-find precision in the topics of immunity and human defenses. He is a top-notch and successful researcher and has received numerous awards and recognition for his teaching. Neal has a gift for creating images that bring clarity to the complex content of immunology. Thank you Neal for your persistence in promoting understanding and your continuing devotion to students.

As always we are deeply indebted to Sue Meeks. She has worked with us on this project for 30 years, orchestrating the various stages of manuscript preparation. She single-handedly word-processes the entire revision of the manuscript and continues to amaze us with her sincere level of enthusiasm for attention to detail. We are grateful for the extraordinary effort she devotes to organizing, preparing, and accomplishing the task. Thank you Sue for, well—everything!

The reviewers for this edition provided excellent recommendations for revision and content emphasis and we appreciate their insightful work.

A special thank you to the entire Elsevier team for the production of this book. Charlene Ketchum, our Developmental Editor, was critical. She worked with us day-to-day, always unflappable, reassuring, and focused, with a great sense of humor. Thanks again Charlene. Sandra Clark, our Senior Editor, was responsible for overseeing the entire project. Thank you for your continued vigilance Sandra. Executive Vice President Sally Schrefer has given us years of unwavering support and vision for the future—thanks again, Sally.

Jeanne Genz, the Project Manager for this edition, sounded the alarms early with her 5:30 AM e-mails. Jeanne works all the time. Bright, always courteous, Jeanne was focused, exacting, and a breath of fresh air. Thanks much Jeanne. The smart and colorful book design was done by Paula Catalano. Paula managed to fit numerous elements into a reader-friendly style we hope students find helpful and attractive. Brooke Kannady, our Editorial Assistant, routed materials to authors, contributors, and reviewers. Thank you Brooke for a job well-done. Trudi Elliott from Graphic World handled the file clean-up and scanning of artwork obtained from many resources. Thank you Trudi for your attention to detail.

We are grateful to Ed Reschke and Dennis Kunkel, who granted permission for the use of their remarkable and unique micrographs. We would like to thank the following authors for permission to use some of their outstanding figures: Kevin Patton and Gary Thibodeau, Ivan Damjanov, Alan Stevens and James Lowe, Carol Wells (wife of the late Stanley Erlandsen), Vinay Kumar, and Marilyn Hockenberry. We thank the Department of Dermatology at the University of Utah School of Medicine, which provided numerous photos of skin lesions. Thanks also to Arthur R. Brothman, PhD, University of Utah School of Medicine, for the *N-myc* gene amplification slides used to illustrate the discussion of neuroblastoma and John Hoffman, MD, for the PET scan figure of cancer metastases. Thank you to our many colleagues and friends at the University of Utah College of Nursing, School of Medicine, Eccles Medical Library, and College of Pharmacy for their helpfulness, suggestions, and critiques.

The newly drawn and revised artwork for this edition was completed by George Barile of Accurate Art Inc. Despite our simple and pathetic drawings, George interpreted, redrew, and produced fabulous illustrations. He worked hard on the conceptual arrangements, labels, and colors. Thank you so much George.

A special thanks to Mandi Counters, Mary Dowell, Susan Frazier, and April Hart for their very organized and thorough approach in preparing the instructor materials for the Evolve website. A special thanks to Mandi Counters, Linda Turchin, and Sharon Souter for the excellent revisions to the glossary, review questions, test bank, quick check answers, and other resources on the Evolve website. Thanks to Diane Young for revising the lecture slides on the Instructor's Evolve website. Tina Brashers, Nancy Burruss, Mandi Counters, Joe Gordon, Melissa J. Geist, Kay Gaehle, Stephen D. Krau, Jason Mott, and Kim Webb also updated the interactive online lessons and activities for *Pathophysiology Online*. And thanks as always to Clayton Parkinson for revising the study guide.

Special thanks to faculty and nursing students and other health science students for your letters, e-mail messages, and phone calls. It is because of you, the future clinicians, that we are so motivated to put our best efforts into this work.

Sincerely and with great affection we thank our families, especially Mae, John, Anne, Ray, Mark, Eric, Greg, Sue, Kallie, Rosie, Margot, and Sarah. Always supportive, you make the work possible!

Sue E. Huether
Kathryn L. McCance

The word root "patho" is derived from the Greek word *pathos,* which means suffering. The Greek word root *"logos"* means discourse or more simply, system of formal study, and *"physio"* refers to functions of an organism. Altogether, pathophysiology is the study of the underlying changes in body physiology (molecular, cellular, and organ systems) that result from disease or injury. Important, however, is the inextricable component of suffering.

The science of pathophysiology seeks to provide an understanding of the mechanisms of disease and how and why alterations in body structure and function lead to the signs and symptoms of disease. Understanding pathophysiology guides health care professionals in the planning, selection, and evaluation of therapies and treatments.

Knowledge of human anatomy and physiology and the interrelationship among the various cells and organ systems of the body is an essential foundation for the study of pathophysiology. Review of this subject matter enhances comprehension of pathophysiologic events and processes. Understanding pathophysiology also entails the utilization of principles, concepts, and basic knowledge from other fields of study including pathology, genetics, immunology, and epidemiology. A number of terms are used to focus the discussion of pathophysiology; they may be used interchangeably at times, but that does not necessarily indicate that they have the same meaning. Those terms are reviewed here for the purpose of clarification.

Pathology is the investigation of structural alterations in cells, tissues, and organs, which can help identify the cause of a particular disease. Pathology differs from **pathogenesis,** which is the pattern of tissue changes associated with the *development* of disease. **Etiology** refers to the study of the *cause* of disease. Diseases may be caused by infection, heredity, gene-environment interactions, alterations in immunity, malignancy, malnutrition, degeneration, or trauma. Diseases that have no identifiable cause are termed **idiopathic.** Diseases that occur as a result of medical treatment are termed **iatrogenic.** For example, some antibiotics can injure the kidney and cause renal failure. Diseases that are acquired as a consequence of being in a hospital environment are called **nosocomial.** An infection that develops as a result of a person's immune system being depressed after receiving cancer treatment during a hospital stay would be defined as a nosocomial infection.

Diagnosis is the naming or identification of a disease. A diagnosis is made from an evaluation of the evidence accumulated from the presenting signs and symptoms, health and medical history, physical examination, laboratory tests, and imaging. A **prognosis** is the expected outcome of a disease. **Acute disease** is the sudden appearance of signs and symptoms that last only a short time. **Chronic disease** develops more slowly and the signs and symptoms last for a long time, perhaps for a lifetime. Chronic diseases may have a pattern of remission and exacerbation. **Remissions** are periods when symptoms disappear or diminish significantly. **Exacerbations** are periods when the symptoms become worse or more severe. A **complication** is the onset of a disease in a person who is already coping with another existing disease. For example, a person who has undergone surgery to remove a diseased appendix may develop the complication of a wound infection or pneumonia. **Sequelae** are unwanted outcomes of having a disease or are the result of trauma, such as paralysis resulting from a stroke or severe scarring resulting from a burn.

Clinical manifestations are the signs and symptoms or *evidence* of disease. **Signs** are objective alterations that can be observed or measured by another person, measures of bodily functions such as pulse rate, blood pressure, body temperature, or white blood cell count. Some signs are **local** such as redness or swelling, and other signs are **systemic** such as fever. **Symptoms** are subjective experiences reported by the person with disease, such as pain, nausea, or shortness of breath, and they vary from person to person. The **prodromal period** of a disease is the time during which a person experiences vague symptoms such as fatigue or loss of appetite before the onset of specific signs and symptoms. The term **insidious symptoms** refers to vague or nonspecific feelings and an awareness that there is a change within the body. Some diseases have a **latent period,** a time during which no symptoms are readily apparent in the affected person, but the disease is nevertheless present in the body; an example is the incubation phase of an infection or the early growth phase of a tumor. A **syndrome** is a group of symptoms that occur together and may be caused by several interrelated problems or a specific disease. Severe acute respiratory syndrome (SARS), for example, presents with a set of symptoms that include headache, fever, body aches, an overall feeling of discomfort, and sometimes dry cough and difficulty breathing. A **disorder** is an abnormality of function; this term also can refer to an illness or a particular problem such as a bleeding disorder.

Epidemiology is the study of tracking patterns or disease occurrence and transmission among populations and by geographic areas. **Incidence** of a disease is the number of new cases occurring in a specific time period. **Prevalence** of a disease is the number of existing cases within a population during a specific time period.

Risk factors, also known as **predisposing factors,** increase the probability that disease will occur, but these factors are not the *cause* of disease. Risk factors include heredity, age, gender, race, environment, and lifestyle. A **precipitating factor** is a condition or event that *does* cause a pathologic event or disorder. For example, asthma is precipitated by exposure to an allergen, or angina (pain) is precipitated by exertion.

Pathophysiology is an exciting field of study that is ever changing as new discoveries are made. Understanding pathophysiology empowers health care professionals with the knowledge of how and why disease develops and informs their decision making to ensure optimal health care outcomes. Embedded in the study of pathophysiology is understanding that suffering is a major component.

CONTENTS

PART 2: BODY SYSTEMS AND DISEASES

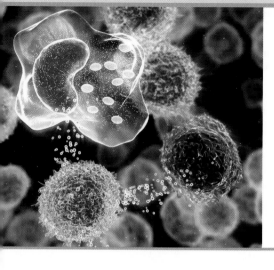

Cellular Biology

Kathryn L. McCance

⊖volve WEBSITE

http://evolve.elsevier.com/Huether/
- Review Questions and Answers
- Animations
- Quick Check Answers

- Key Terms Exercises
- Critical Thinking Questions with Answers
- Algorithm Completion Exercises
- WebLinks

CHAPTER OUTLINE

All body functions depend on the integrity of cells. Therefore an understanding of cellular biology is increasingly necessary to comprehend disease processes. An overwhelming amount of information reveals how cells behave as a multicellular "social" organism. At the heart of it all is cellular communication (cellular "crosstalk")—how messages originate and are transmitted, received, interpreted, and used by the cell. Streamlined conversation between, among, and within cells maintains cellular function. Cells must demonstrate a "chemical fondness" for other cells to maintain the integrity of the entire organism. When they no longer tolerate this fondness, the conversation breaks down, and cells either adapt (sometimes altering function) or become vulnerable to isolation, injury, or disease.

PROKARYOTES AND EUKARYOTES

Living cells generally are divided into eukaryotes and prokaryotes. The cells of higher animals and plants are eukaryotes, as are the single-celled organisms, fungi, protozoa, and most algae. Prokaryotes include cyanobacteria (blue-green algae), bacteria, and rickettsiae. Prokaryotes traditionally were studied as core subjects of molecular biology. Today, emphasis is on the eukaryotic cell; much of its structure and function have no counterpart in bacterial cells.

 Eukaryotes (*eu* = good; *karyon* = nucleus) are larger and have more extensive intracellular anatomy and organization than prokaryotes. Eukaryotic cells have a characteristic set of membrane-bound intracellular compartments, called *organelles,* that includes a well-defined nucleus. The prokaryotes contain no organelles, and their nuclear material is not encased by a nuclear membrane. Prokaryotic cells are characterized by lack of a distinct nucleus.

Besides having structural differences, prokaryotic and eukaryotic cells differ in chemical composition and biochemical activity. The *nuclei* of prokaryotic cells carry genetic information in a single circular chromosome, and they lack a class of proteins called *histones,* which in eukaryotic cells bind with deoxyribonucleic acid (DNA) and are involved in the supercoiling of DNA. Eukaryotic cells have several or many chromosomes. Protein production, or synthesis, in the two classes of cells also differs because of major structural differences in ribonucleic acid (RNA)-protein complexes. Other distinctions include differences in mechanisms of transport across the outer cellular membrane and in enzyme content.

CELLULAR FUNCTIONS

Cells become specialized through the process of differentiation, or maturation, so that some cells eventually perform one kind of function and other cells perform other functions. Cells with a highly developed function, such as movement, often lack some other property, such as hormone production, which is more highly developed in other cells.

The eight chief cellular functions are as follows:
1. *Movement.* Muscle cells can generate forces that produce motion. Muscles that are attached to bones produce limb movements, whereas those muscles that enclose hollow tubes or cavities move or empty contents when they contract (e.g., the colon).
2. *Conductivity.* Conduction as a response to a stimulus is manifested by a wave of excitation, an electrical potential that passes along the surface of the cell to reach its other parts. Conductivity is the chief function of nerve cells.

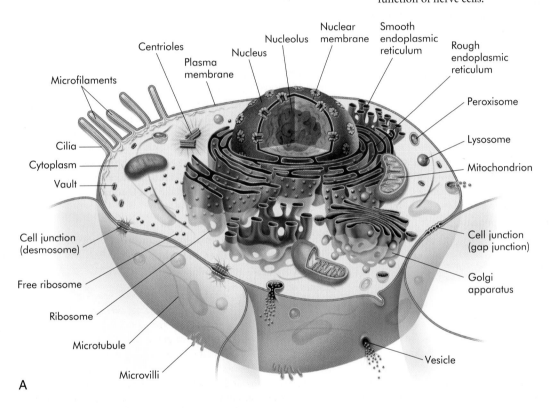

A

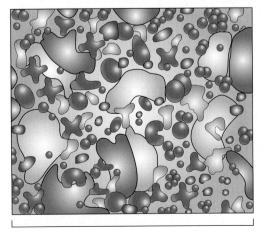

B

100 nm

FIGURE 1-1 Typical Components of a Eukaryotic Cell and Structure of the Cytoplasm. A, Components of a eukaryotic cell. **B,** The drawing is approximately to scale and emphasizes the crowding in the cytoplasm. Only the macromolecules are shown: RNAs are shown in *blue,* ribosomes in *green,* and proteins in *pink.* Enzymes and other macromolecules diffuse relatively slowly in the cytoplasm, in part because they interact with many other macromolecules; small molecules, by contrast, diffuse nearly as rapidly as they do in water. (**B** adapted from Alberts B et al: *Molecular biology of the cell,* ed 5, New York, 2008, Garland.)

3. *Metabolic absorption.* All cells can take in and use nutrients and other substances from their surroundings.
4. *Secretion.* Certain cells, such as mucous gland cells, can synthesize new substances from substances they absorb and then secrete the new substances to serve as needed elsewhere.
5. *Excretion.* All cells can rid themselves of waste products resulting from the metabolic breakdown of nutrients. Membrane-bound sacs (lysosomes) within cells contain enzymes that break down, or digest, large molecules, turning them into waste products that are released from the cell.
6. *Respiration.* Cells absorb oxygen, which is used to transform nutrients into energy in the form of adenosine triphosphate (ATP). Cellular respiration, or oxidation, occurs in organelles called mitochondria.
7. *Reproduction.* Tissue growth occurs as cells enlarge and reproduce themselves. Even without growth, tissue maintenance requires that new cells be produced to replace cells that are lost normally through cellular death. Not all cells are capable of continuous division (see Chapter 3).
8. *Communication.* Communication is vital for cells to survive as a society of cells. Appropriate communication allows the maintenance of a dynamic steady state.

STRUCTURE AND FUNCTION OF CELLULAR COMPONENTS

Figure 1-1, *A*, shows a "typical" eukaryotic cell. It consists of three components: an outer membrane called the plasma membrane, or plasmalemma; a fluid "filling" called cytoplasm (Figure 1-1, *B*); and the "organs" of the cell—the membrane-bound intracellular organelles, among them the nucleus.

Nucleus

The nucleus, which is surrounded by the cytoplasm and generally is located in the center of the cell, is the largest membrane-bound organelle. Two membranes compose the nuclear envelope (Figure 1-2, *A*). The outer membrane is continuous with membranes of the endoplasmic reticulum. The nucleus contains the nucleolus (a small dense structure composed largely of ribonucleic acid), most of the cellular DNA, and the DNA-binding proteins (i.e., the histones) that regulate its activity. The DNA "chain" in eukaryotic cells is so long that it is easily broken. Therefore the histones that bind to DNA cause DNA to fold into chromosomes (Figure 1-2, *C*), which decreases the risk of breakage and is essential for cell division in eukaryotes.

The primary functions of the nucleus are cell division and control of genetic information. Other functions include the replication and repair of DNA and the transcription of the information stored in DNA. Genetic information is transcribed into RNA, which can be processed into messenger, transport, and ribosomal RNAs and introduced into the cytoplasm, where it directs cellular activities. Most of the processing of RNA occurs in the nucleolus. (The role of DNA and RNA in protein synthesis is discussed in Chapter 2.)

Cytoplasmic Organelles

Cytoplasm is an aqueous solution (cytosol) that fills the cytoplasmic matrix—the space between the nuclear envelope and the plasma membrane. The cytosol represents about half the volume of a eukaryotic cell. It contains thousands of enzymes involved in intermediate metabolism and is crowded with ribosomes making proteins (see Figure 1-1, *B*). Newly synthesized proteins remain in the cytosol if they lack a signal for transport to a cell organelle.[1] The organelles

suspended in the cytoplasm are enclosed in biologic membranes, so they can simultaneously carry out functions requiring different biochemical environments. Many of these functions are directed by coded messages carried from the nucleus by RNA. They include synthesis of proteins and hormones and their transport out of the cell, isolation and elimination of waste products from the cell, metabolic processes, breakdown and disposal of cellular debris and foreign proteins (antigens), and maintenance of cellular structure and motility. The cytosol is a storage unit for fat, carbohydrates, and secretory vesicles. Table 1-1 lists the principal cytoplasmic organelles.

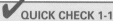

> **QUICK CHECK 1-1**
> 1. Why is the process of differentiation essential to specialization? Give an example.
> 2. Describe at least two cellular functions.

Plasma Membranes

Whether they surround the cell or enclose an intracellular organelle, membranes are exceedingly important to normal physiologic function because they control the composition of the space, or compartment, they enclose. Membranes can include or exclude various molecules, and by controlling the movement of substances from one compartment to another, membranes exert a powerful influence on metabolic pathways. The plasma membrane also has an important role in cell-to-cell recognition. Other functions of the plasma membrane include cellular mobility and the maintenance of cellular shape (Table 1-2).

Membrane Composition

The outer surface of the plasma membrane is not smooth, but dimpled with cavelike indentations known as caveolae ("tiny caves"). Caveolae serve as a storage site for many receptors and provide a route for transport into the cell (see p. 21).

The major chemical components of all membranes are lipids and proteins, but the percentage of each varies among different membranes. Intracellular membranes have a higher percentage of proteins than plasma membranes have, presumably because most enzymatic activity occurs within organelles. Carbohydrates are associated mainly with plasma membranes, where they combine chemically with lipids, forming glycolipids, and with proteins, forming glycoproteins.

Lipids. The basic component of the plasma membrane is a bilayer of lipid molecules—phospholipids, glycolipids, and cholesterol. Lipids are responsible for the structural integrity of the membrane. Each lipid molecule is said to be polar, or amphipathic, which means that one part is hydrophobic (uncharged, or "water hating") and another part is hydrophilic (charged, or "water loving") (Figure 1-3).

The membrane spontaneously organizes itself into two layers because of these two incompatible solubilities. The hydrophobic region (hydrophobic tail) of each lipid molecule is protected from water, whereas the hydrophilic region (hydrophilic head) is immersed in it. The bilayer serves as a barrier to the diffusion of water and hydrophilic substances, while allowing lipid-soluble molecules, such as oxygen (O_2) and carbon dioxide (CO_2), to diffuse through it readily.

Proteins. A protein is made from a chain of amino acids, known as polypeptides. There are 20 types of amino acids in proteins and each type of protein has a unique sequence of amino acids. Thus they are very versatile! Proteins can be classified as integral or peripheral membrane proteins. Integral membrane proteins are embedded in the

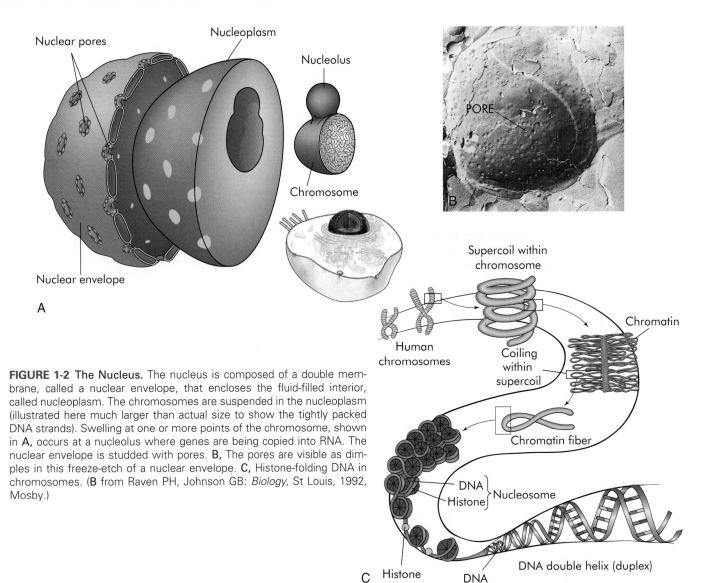

FIGURE 1-2 The Nucleus. The nucleus is composed of a double membrane, called a nuclear envelope, that encloses the fluid-filled interior, called nucleoplasm. The chromosomes are suspended in the nucleoplasm (illustrated here much larger than actual size to show the tightly packed DNA strands). Swelling at one or more points of the chromosome, shown in **A**, occurs at a nucleolus where genes are being copied into RNA. The nuclear envelope is studded with pores. **B,** The pores are visible as dimples in this freeze-etch of a nuclear envelope. **C,** Histone-folding DNA in chromosomes. (B from Raven PH, Johnson GB: *Biology,* St Louis, 1992, Mosby.)

TABLE 1-1	PRINCIPAL CYTOPLASMIC ORGANELLES
ORGANELLE	**CHARACTERISTICS AND DESCRIPTION**
Ribosomes	RNA-protein complexes (nucleoproteins) synthesized in nucleolus and secreted into cytoplasm. Provide sites for cellular protein synthesis.
Endoplasmic reticulum	Network of tubular channels (cisternae) that extend throughout outer nuclear membrane. Specializes in synthesis and transport of protein and lipid components of most organelles.
Golgi complex	Network of smooth membranes and vesicles located near nucleus. Responsible for processing and packaging proteins onto secretory vesicles that break away from the complex and migrate to various intracellular and extracellular destinations, including plasma membrane. Best-known vesicles are those that have coats largely made of the protein *clathrin*. Proteins in the complex bind to the cytoskeleton, generating tension that helps organelle function and keep its stretched shape intact.
Lysosomes	Saclike structures that originate from Golgi complex and contain enzymes for digesting most cellular substances to their basic form, such as amino acids, fatty acids, and sugars. Cellular injury leads to release of lysosomal enzymes that cause cellular self-destruction.
Peroxisomes	Similar to lysosomes but contain several oxidative enzymes (e.g., catalase, urate oxidase) that produce hydrogen peroxide; reactions detoxify various wastes.
Mitochondria	Contain metabolic machinery needed for cellular energy metabolism. Enzymes of respiratory chain (electron-transport chain), found in inner membrane of mitochondria, generate most of cell's ATP (oxidative phosphorylation). Have a role in osmotic regulation, pH control, calcium homeostasis, and cell signaling.
Cytoskeleton	"Bone and muscle" of cell. Composed of a network of protein filaments, including microtubules and actin filaments (microfilaments); forms cell extensions (microvilli, cilia, flagella).
Caveolae	Tiny indentations (caves) that can capture extracellular material and shuttle it inside the cell or across the cell.
Vaults	Cytoplasmic ribonucleoproteins shaped like octagonal barrels. Believed to act as "trucks," shuttling molecules from nucleus to elsewhere in cell.

TABLE 1-2   PLASMA MEMBRANE FUNCTIONS

CELLULAR MECHANISM	MEMBRANE FUNCTIONS
Structure	Usually thicker than membranes of intracellular organelles
	Containment of cellular organelles
	Maintenance of relationship with cytoskeleton, endoplasmic reticulum, and other organelles
	Maintenance of fluid and electrolyte balance
	Outer surfaces of plasma membranes in many cells are not smooth but are dimpled with cavelike indentations called *caveolae;* they are also studded with cilia or even smaller cylindrical projections called *microvilli;* both are capable of movement
Protection	Barrier to toxic molecules and macromolecules (proteins, nucleic acids, polysaccharides)
	Barrier to foreign organisms and cells
Activation of cell	Hormones (regulation of cellular activity)
	Mitogens (cellular division; see Chapter 2)
	Antigens (antibody synthesis; see Chapter 5)
	Growth factors (proliferation and differentiation; see Chapter 9)
Storage	Storage site for many receptors
	Transport
	Diffusion and exchange diffusion
	Endocytosis (pinocytosis, phagocytosis)
	Exocytosis (secretion)
	Active transport
Cell-to-cell interaction	Communication and attachment at junctional complexes
	Symbiotic nutritive relationships
	Release of enzymes and antibodies to extracellular environment
	Relationships with extracellular matrix

Modified from King DW, Fenoglio CM, Lefkowitch JH: *General pathology: principles and dynamics,* Philadelphia, 1983, Lea & Febiger.

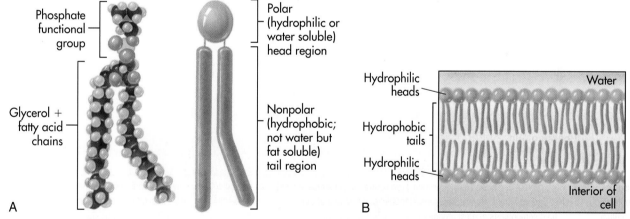

FIGURE 1-3 Structure of a Phospholipid Molecule. A, Each phospholipid molecule consists of a phosphate functional group and two fatty acid chains attached to a glycerol molecule. **B,** The fatty acid chains and glycerol form nonpolar, hydrophobic "tails," and the phosphate functional group forms the polar, hydrophilic "head" of the phospholipid molecule. When placed in water, the hydrophobic tails of the molecule face inward, away from the water, and the hydrophilic head faces outward, toward the water. (From Raven PH, Johnson GB: *Understanding biology,* ed 3, Dubuque, Iowa, 1995, Brown.)

lipid bilayer and linked to either *phosphatidylinositol,* a minor phospholipid, or a fatty acid chain. The integral proteins can be removed from the membrane only by detergents that solubilize (dissolve) the lipid. Peripheral membrane proteins are not embedded in the bilayer but reside at one surface or the other, bound to an integral protein.

Proteins exist in densely folded molecular configurations rather than straight chains, so most hydrophilic units are at the surface of the molecule and most hydrophobic units are inside. Although membrane structure is determined by the lipid bilayer, membrane functions are determined largely by proteins. Proteins act as (1) recognition and binding units (receptors) for substances moving into and out of the cell; (2) pores or transport channels for various electrically charged particles, called *ions* or *electrolytes,* and specific carriers for amino acids and monosaccharides; (3) specific enzymes that drive active pumps to promote concentration of certain ions, particularly potassium (K^+), within the cell while keeping concentrations of other ions, for

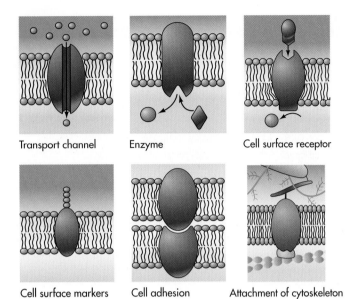

Transport channel

Enzyme

Cell surface receptor

Cell surface markers

Cell adhesion

Attachment of cytoskeleton

FIGURE 1-4 Functions of Plasma Membrane Proteins. The plasma membrane proteins illustrated here show a variety of functions performed by the different types of plasma membranes. (From Raven PH, Johnson GB: *Understanding biology*, ed 3, Dubuque, Iowa, 1995, Brown.)

example, sodium (Na⁺), below concentrations found in the extracellular environment; (4) cell surface markers, such as glycoproteins (proteins attached to carbohydrates), that identify a cell to its neighbor; (5) cell adhesion molecules (CAMs), or proteins that allow cells to hook together and form attachments of the cytoskeleton for maintaining cellular shape; and (6) catalysts of chemical reactions, for example, conversion of lactose to glucose (Figure 1-4).

The interaction of plasma membrane proteins with lipids is complex. The role of proteins in the onset and progression of disease is important because of their enzymatic, transport, and recognition-receptor functions in cellular physiology.

Carbohydrates. The carbohydrates (oligosaccharides) contained within the plasma membrane are generally bound to membrane proteins (glycoproteins) and lipids (glycolipids). Intercellular recognition is an important function of membrane oligosaccharides.

Fluid Mosaic Model

In the 1960s G.L. Nicholson and S.J. Singer proposed the popular fluid mosaic model for biologic membranes (Figure 1-5). The model, which is continually being modified, presents integral proteins as pieces of a mosaic that float singly or as aggregates in the fluid lipid bilayer. The protein molecules (1) transport other molecules into and out of the cell; (2) facilitate (catalyze) membrane reactions; (3) receive messages, thus acting as receptors for extracellular and intracellular signals; and (4) create structural linkages between the external and internal cellular environments. The fluid mosaic model accounts for the flexibility of cellular membranes as well as their self-sealing properties and impermeability to many substances.

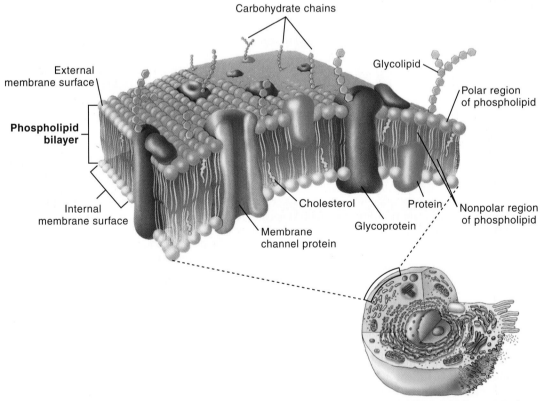

Carbohydrate chains

External membrane surface

Glycolipid

Phospholipid bilayer

Polar region of phospholipid

Internal membrane surface

Cholesterol

Protein

Nonpolar region of phospholipid

Membrane channel protein

Glycoprotein

FIGURE 1-5 Fluid Mosaic Model. Schematic, three-dimensional view of the fluid mosaic model of membrane structure. The lipid bilayer provides the basic structure and serves as a relatively impermeable barrier to most water-soluble molecules.

New revisions of the model now state that most membrane proteins do not have unrestricted lateral movement. Thus some proteins may randomly diffuse, others are confined, and still others are tethered to the cytoskeleton. The degree of a membrane's fluidity depends on temperature. At lower temperatures the lipids are in a gel crystalline state, and at higher temperatures they become highly fluid. These properties are critical for cellular growth, division, and receptor function. Because *some* proteins are free to move within the plasma membranes (like floating icebergs), certain foreign proteins (antigens) may become buried in the bilayer, emerging at the surface only after injury and then attracting antibodies (proteins produced by the immune system), which attack host cells. Antigens and antibodies, which are integral to the immune response, are discussed in Chapter 6. The burial and reemergence of antigens may be one cause of autoimmune disease, described in Chapter 7.

Cells, however, can immobilize specific membrane proteins in a region of the membrane. Confinement may be needed for certain functions to occur. The fluid mosaic model describes the membrane as existing in a state of change and modulation, which allows the cell to protect itself actively against injurious agents. Hormones, bacteria, viruses, drugs, antibodies, chemicals that transmit nerve impulses (neurotransmitters), and other substances attach to the plasma membrane by means of receptor molecules on its outer layer.

The number of receptors present may vary at different times, and the cell can modulate the effects of injurious agents by altering receptor number and pattern.[1] This aspect of the fluid mosaic model has drastically modified previously held concepts concerning the onset of disease.

The concentration of cholesterol in the plasma membrane affects membrane fluidity. Increased concentration means less fluidity on the membrane's hydrophilic outer surface and more fluidity at its hydrophobic core. Cholesterol content changes are factors in some diseases. In cirrhosis of the liver, for example, the cholesterol content of the red blood cell's plasma membrane increases, causing a decrease in membrane fluidity that seriously affects the cell's ability to transport oxygen.

Cellular Receptors

Cellular receptors are protein molecules on the plasma membrane, in the cytoplasm, or in the nucleus that can recognize and bind with specific smaller molecules called ligands (Figure 1-6). Hormones, for example, are ligands. Recognition and binding depend on the chemical configuration of the receptor and its smaller ligand, which must fit together somewhat like pieces of a jigsaw puzzle (see Chapter 17). New data illustrate that activation of a receptor also may depend on differences in *movement* and *binding* of the extracellular face of the receptor.[1]

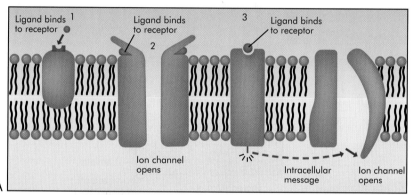

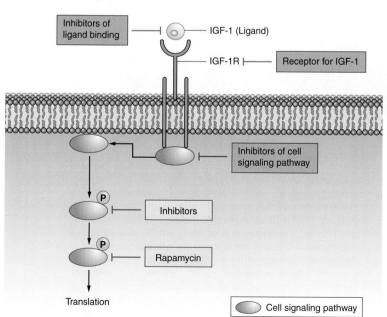

FIGURE 1-6 Cellular Receptors. **(A)** *1,* Plasma membrane receptor for a ligand (here, a hormone molecule) on the surface of an integral protein. A neurotransmitter can exert its effect on a postsynaptic cell by means of two fundamentally different types of receptor proteins: *2,* channel-linked receptors, and *3,* non–channel-linked receptors. Channel-linked receptors are also known as *ligand-gated channels.* **(B)** Example of ligand-receptor interaction. Insulin-like growth factor 1 (IGF-1) is a ligand and binds to the insulin-like growth factor 1 receptor (IGF-1R). With binding at the cell membrane the intracellular signaling pathway is activated, causing translation of new proteins to act as intracellular communicators. This pathway is important for cancer growth. Researchers are developing pharmacologic strategies to reduce signaling at and downstream of the insulin-like growth factor 1 receptor (IGF-1R), hoping this will lead to compounds useful in cancer treatment.

Plasma membrane receptors protrude from or are exposed at the external surface of the membrane and are important for cellular uptake of ligands (see Figure 1-6). The ligands that bind with membrane receptors include hormones, neurotransmitters, antigens, complement components, lipoproteins, infectious agents, drugs, and metabolites. Many new discoveries concerning the specific interactions of cellular receptors with their respective ligands have provided a basis for understanding disease.

Although the chemical nature of ligands and their receptors differs, receptors are classified based on their location and function. Cellular type determines overall cellular function, but plasma membrane receptors determine which ligands a cell will bind with and how the cell will respond to the binding. Specific processes also control intracellular mechanisms.

Receptors for different drugs are found on the plasma membrane, in the cytoplasm, and in the nucleus. Membrane receptors have been found for certain anesthetics, opiates, endorphins, enkephalins, antibiotics, cancer chemotherapeutic agents, digitalis, and other drugs. Membrane receptors for endorphins, which are opiate-like peptides isolated from the pituitary gland, are found in large quantities in pain pathways of the nervous system (see Chapters 12 and 13). With binding, the endorphins (or drugs such as morphine) change the cell's permeability to ions, increase the concentration of molecules that regulate intracellular protein synthesis, and initiate molecular events that modulate pain perception.

Receptors for infectious microorganisms, or antigen receptors, bind bacteria, viruses, and parasites. Antigen receptors on white blood cells (lymphocytes, monocytes, macrophages, granulocytes) recognize and bind with antigenic microorganisms and activate the immune and inflammatory responses (see Chapter 5).

CELL-TO-CELL ADHESIONS

Cells are small and squishy, *not* like bricks. They are enclosed only by a flimsy membrane, yet the cell depends on the integrity of this membrane for its survival. How can cells be formed together strongly, with their membranes intact, to form a muscle that can lift this textbook? Plasma membranes not only serve as the outer boundaries of all cells but also allow groups of cells to be held together robustly, in cell-to-cell adhesions, to form tissues and organs. Once arranged, cells are held together by three different means: (1) cell adhesion molecules in the cell's plasma membrane (see p. 9), (2) the extracellular matrix, and (3) specialized cell junctions.

Extracellular Matrix

Cells can be united by attachment to one another or through the extracellular matrix (also including the basement membrane), which the cells secrete around themselves. The extracellular matrix is an intricate meshwork of fibrous proteins embedded in a watery, gel-like substance

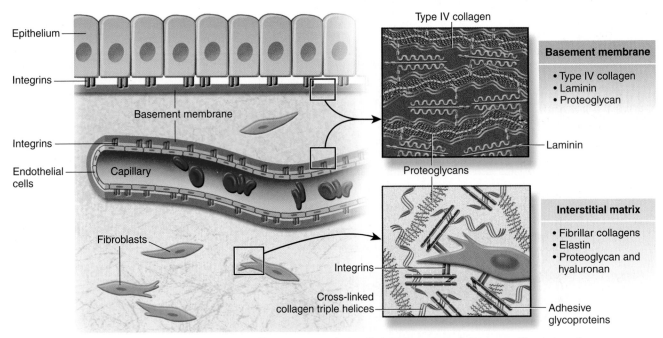

FIGURE 1-7 Extracellular Matrix. Tissues are not just cells but also extracellular space. The extracellular space is an intricate network of macromolecules called the *extracellular matrix (ECM)*. The macromolecules that constitute the ECM are secreted locally (by mostly fibroblasts) and assembled into a meshwork in close association with the surface of the cell that produced them. Two main classes of macromolecules include proteoglycans, which are bound to polysaccharide chains called *glycosaminoglycans,* and fibrous proteins (e.g., collagen, elastin, fibronectin, and laminin), which have structural and adhesive properties. Together the proteoglycan molecules form a gel-like ground substance in which the fibrous proteins are embedded. The gel permits rapid diffusion of nutrients, metabolites, and hormones between the blood and the tissue cells. Matrix proteins modulate cell-matrix interactions including normal tissue remodeling (which can become abnormal, for example, with chronic inflammation). Disruptions of this balance result in serious diseases such as arthritis, tumor growth, and others. (Modified from Kumar V, Abbas A, Fausto N: *Robbins and Cotran pathologic basis of disease,* ed 7, Philadelphia, 2005, Saunders.)

composed of complex carbohydrates (Figure 1-7). The matrix is like glue; however, it provides a pathway for diffusion of nutrients, wastes, and other water-soluble substances between the blood and tissue cells. Interwoven within the matrix are three groups of macromolecules: (1) fibrous structural proteins, including collagen and elastin; (2) adhesive glycoproteins, such as fibronectin; and (3) proteoglycans and hyaluronic acid.

1. Collagen forms cablelike fibers or sheets that provide tensile strength or resistance to longitudinal stress. Collagen breakdown, such as occurs in osteoarthritis, destroys the fibrils that give cartilage its tensile strength.
2. Elastin is a rubber-like protein fiber most abundant in tissues that must be capable of stretching and recoiling, such as found in the lungs.
3. Fibronectin, a large glycoprotein, promotes cell adhesion and cell anchorage. Reduced amounts have been found in certain types of cancerous cells; this allows cancer cells to travel, or metastasize, to other parts of the body. All of these macromolecules occur in intercellular junctions and cell surfaces and may assemble into two different components: interstitial matrix and basement membrane (BM) (see Figure 1-7).

The extracellular matrix is secreted by fibroblasts ("fiber formers") (Figure 1-8), local cells that are present in the matrix. The matrix and the cells within it are known collectively as connective tissue, because they interconnect cells to form tissues and organs. Human connective tissues are enormously varied. They can be hard and dense, like bone; flexible, like tendons or the dermis of the skin; resilient and shock absorbing, like cartilage; or soft and transparent, similar to the jellylike substance that fills the eye. In all these examples, the majority of the tissue is composed of extracellular matrix, and the cells that

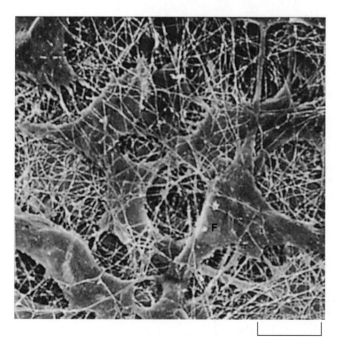

FIGURE 1-8 Fibroblasts in Connective Tissue. This micrograph shows tissue from the cornea of a rat. The extracellular matrix surrounds the fibroblasts **(F)**. (From Nishida T et al: The extracellular matrix of animal connective tissues, *Invest Ophthalmol Vis Sci* 29:1887–1880, 1998.)

0.1 μm

produce the matrix are scattered within it like raisins in a pudding (see Figure 1-8).

The matrix is not just a passive scaffolding for cellular attachment; it also helps regulate the function of the cells with which it interacts. The matrix helps regulate such important functions as cell growth and differentiation.

Specialized Cell Junctions

Cells in direct physical contact with neighboring cells are often interconnected at specialized plasma membrane regions called cell junctions. Cell junctions have two main functions: (1) to hold cells together and (2) to permit small molecules to pass from cell to cell, allowing coordination of the activities of cells that form tissues.

The three main types of cell junctions are (1) desmosomes (also known as macula adherens), (2) tight junctions (also known as zonula occludens), and (3) gap junctions, or adhering junctions (Figure 1-9). Together they form the junctional complex. Desmosomes unite cells either by forming continuous bands or belts of epithelial sheets or by developing button-like points of contact. Desmosomes also act as a system of braces to maintain structural stability. Tight junctions are barriers to diffusion, prevent the movement of substances through transport proteins in the plasma membrane, and prevent the leakage of small molecules between the plasma membranes of adjacent cells. Gap junctions are clusters of communicating tunnels or connexons that allow small ions and molecules to pass directly from the inside of one cell to the inside of another. Connexons are joining proteins that extend outward from each of the adjacent plasma membranes. Cells connected by gap junctions are considered ionically (electrically) and metabolically coupled. Gap junctions coordinate the activities of adjacent cells; for example, they are important for synchronizing contractions of heart muscle cells through ionic coupling and for permitting action potentials to spread rapidly from cell to cell in neural tissues. The reason that gap junctions occur in tissues that are not electrically active is unknown. Although most gap junctions are associated with junctional complexes, they sometimes exist as independent structures.

The junctional complex is a highly permeable part of the plasma membrane. Its permeability is controlled by a process called gating, which depends on concentrations of calcium ions in the cytoplasm. Increased cytoplasmic calcium causes decreased permeability at the junctional complex. Gating enables uninjured cells to protect themselves from injured neighbors. Calcium is released from injured cells.

CELLULAR COMMUNICATION AND SIGNAL TRANSDUCTION

Cells need to communicate with each other to maintain a stable internal environment, or homeostasis; to regulate their growth and division; to oversee their development and organization into tissues; and to coordinate their functions. Cells communicate by using hundreds of kinds of signal molecules, for example, insulin (see Figure 1-6, *B*). Cells communicate in three main ways: (1) they display plasma membrane–bound signaling molecules (receptors) that affect the cell itself and other cells in direct physical contact (Figure 1-10, *A*); (2) they use receptor proteins *inside* the target cell and the signal molecule has to enter the cell to bind to them (Figure 1-10, *B*); and (3) they form protein channels (gap junctions) that directly coordinate the activities of adjacent cells (Figure 1-10, *C*). Alterations in cellular communication affect disease onset and progression. In fact, if a cell cannot perform gap junctional intercellular communication, normal

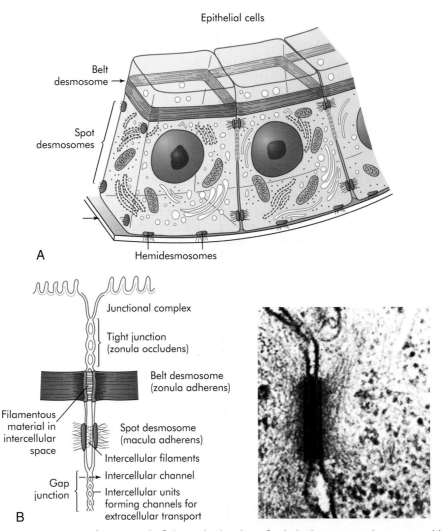

FIGURE 1-9 Junctional Complex. A, Schematic drawing of a belt desmosome between epithelial cells. This junction, also called the *zonula adherens,* encircles each of the interacting cells. The spot desmosomes and hemidesmosomes, like the belt desmosomes, are adhering junctions. This tight junction is an impermeable junction that holds cells together but seals them in such a way that molecules cannot leak between them. The gap junction, as a communicating junction, mediates the passage of small molecules from one interacting cell to the other. **B,** Electron micrograph of desmosomes. (From Raven PH, Johnson GB: *Biology,* St Louis, 1992, Mosby.)

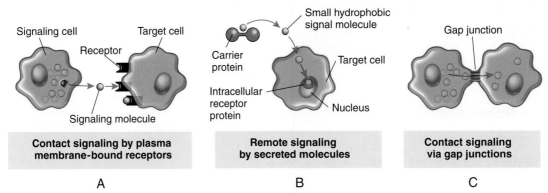

FIGURE 1-10 Cellular Communication. Three primary ways in which cells communicate with one another. (**B** adapted from Alberts B et al: *Molecular biology of the cell,* ed 5, New York, 2008, Garland.)

growth control and cell differentiation is compromised, thereby favoring cancerous tumor development (see Chapter 9). (Communication through gap junctions was discussed earlier, and contact signaling by plasma membrane–bound molecules is discussed on this page and on p. 12.) Secreted chemical signals involve communication locally and at a distance. Primary modes of intercellular signaling are contact-dependent, paracrine, hormonal, neurohormonal, and neurotransmitter. Autocrine stimulation occurs when the secreting cell targets itself (Figure 1-11).

Contact-dependent signaling requires cells to be in close membrane-membrane contact. In paracrine signaling cells secrete local chemical mediators that are quickly taken up, destroyed, or immobilized. Paracrine signaling usually involves different cell types; however, cells also can produce signals to which they alone respond, called autocrine signaling (see Figure 1-11). For example, cancer cells use this form of signaling to stimulate their survival and proliferation. The mediators act only on nearby cells. Hormonal signaling involves specialized endocrine cells that secrete chemicals called hormones; hormones are released by one set of cells and travel through the bloodstream to produce a response in other sets of cells (see Chapter 17). In neurohormonal signaling hormones are released into the blood by neurosecretory neurons. Like endocrine cells, neurosecretory neurons release blood-borne chemical messengers, whereas ordinary neurons secrete short-range neurotransmitters into a small discrete space (i.e., synapse). Neurons communicate directly with the cells they innervate by releasing chemicals or neurotransmitters at specialized junctions called chemical synapses; the neurotransmitter diffuses across the synaptic cleft and acts on the postsynaptic target cell (see Figure 1-11). Many of these same signaling molecules are receptors used in hormonal, neurohormonal, and paracrine signaling. Important differences lie in the speed and selectivity with which the signals are delivered to their targets.[1]

Plasma membrane receptors belong to one of three classes that are defined by the signaling (transduction) mechanism used. Table 1-3 summarizes these classes of receptors. Cells respond to external stimuli by activating a variety of signal transduction pathways, which are communication pathways, or signaling cascades (Figure 1-12, C). Signals are passed between cells when a particular type of molecule is produced by one cell—the signaling cell—and received

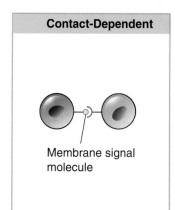

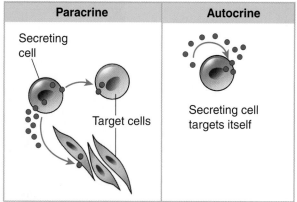

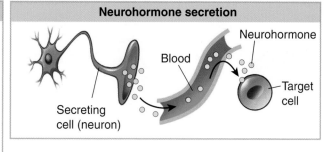

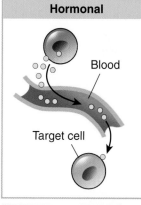

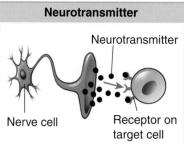

FIGURE 1-11 Primary Modes of Chemical Signaling. Five forms of signaling mediated by secreted molecules. Hormones, paracrines, neurotransmitters, and neurohormones are all intercellular messengers that accomplish communication between cells. Autocrines bind to receptors on the same cell. Not all neurotransmitters act in the strictly synaptic mode shown; some act in a contact-dependent mode as local chemical mediators that influence multiple target cells in the area.

TABLE 1-3   CLASSES OF PLASMA MEMBRANE RECEPTORS

TYPE OF RECEPTOR	DESCRIPTION
Ion channel coupled	Also called *transmitter-gated* ion channels; involve rapid synaptic signaling between electrically excitable cells. Channels open and close briefly in response to neurotransmitters, changing ion permeability of plasma membrane of postsynaptic cell.
Enzyme coupled	Once activated by ligands, function directly as enzymes or associate with enzymes.
G-protein coupled	Indirectly activate or inactivate plasma membrane enzyme or ion channel; interaction mediated by *GTP-binding regulatory protein (G-protein).* May also interact with inositol phospholipids, which are significant in cell signaling, and with molecules involved in *inositol-phospholipid transduction pathway.*

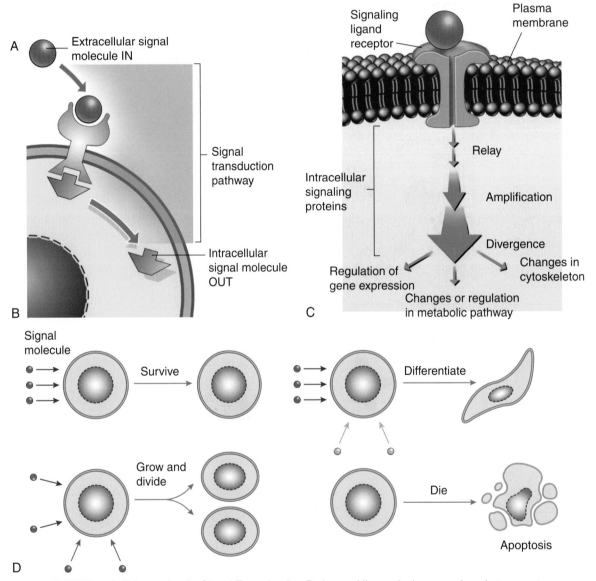

FIGURE 1-12 Schematic of a Signal Transduction Pathway. Like a telephone receiver that converts an electrical signal into a sound signal, a cell converts an extracellular signal, **A,** into an intracellular signal, **B. C,** An extracellular signal molecule (ligand) bonds to a receptor protein located on the plasma membrane, where it is transduced into an intracellular signal. This process initiates a signaling cascade that relays the signal into the cell interior, amplifying and distributing it en route. Amplification is often achieved by stimulating enzymes. Steps in the cascade can be modulated by other events in the cell. **D,** Different cell behaviors rely on multiple extracellular signals.

by another—the target cell—by means of a receptor protein that recognizes and responds specifically to the signal molecule (Figure 1-12, *A* and *B*). In turn, the signaling molecules activate a pathway of intracellular protein kinases that results in various responses, such as grow and reproduce, die, survive, or differentiate (Figure 1-12, *D*).

CELLULAR METABOLISM

All of the chemical tasks of maintaining essential cellular functions are referred to as cellular metabolism. The energy-using process of metabolism is called anabolism (*ana* = upward), and the energy-releasing process is known as catabolism (*kata* = downward). Metabolism provides the cell with the energy it needs to produce cellular structures.

Dietary proteins, fats, and starches (i.e., carbohydrates) are hydrolyzed in the intestinal tract into amino acids, fatty acids, and glucose, respectively. These constituents are then absorbed, circulated, and incorporated into the cell, where they may be used for various vital cellular processes, including the production of ATP. The process by which ATP is produced is one example of a series of reactions called a metabolic pathway. A metabolic pathway involves several steps whose end products are not always detectable. A key feature of cellular metabolism is the directing of biochemical reactions by protein catalysts or enzymes. Each enzyme has a high affinity for a substrate, a specific substance converted to a product of the reaction.

Role of Adenosine Triphosphate

For a cell to function, it must be able to extract and use the chemical energy in organic molecules. When one mole of glucose metabolically breaks down in the presence of oxygen into carbon dioxide and water, 686 kilocalories (kcal) of chemical energy are released. The chemical energy lost by one molecule is transferred to the chemical structure of another molecule by an energy-carrying or energy-transferring molecule, such as ATP. The energy stored in ATP can be used in various energy-requiring reactions and in the process is generally converted to adenosine diphosphate (ADP) and inorganic phosphate (Pi). The energy available as a result of this reaction is about 7 kcal/mol of ATP. The cell uses ATP for muscle contraction and active transport of molecules across cellular membranes. ATP not only stores energy but also *transfers* it from one molecule to another. Energy stored by carbohydrate, lipid, and protein is catabolized and transferred to ATP.

Food and Production of Cellular Energy

Catabolism of the proteins, lipids, and polysaccharides found in food can be divided into the following three phases (Figure 1-13):

Phase 1: Digestion. Large molecules are broken down into smaller subunits: proteins into amino acids, polysaccharides into simple sugars (i.e., monosaccharides), and fats into fatty acids and glycerol. These processes occur outside the cell and are activated by secreted enzymes.

Phase 2: Glycolysis and oxidation. The most important part of phase 2 is glycolysis, the splitting of glucose. Glycolysis produces two molecules of ATP per glucose molecule through oxidation, or the removal and transfer of a pair of electrons. The total process is called *oxidative cellular metabolism* and involves nine biochemical reactions (Figure 1-14).

Phase 3: Citric acid cycle (Krebs cycle, tricarboxylic acid cycle). Most of the ATP is generated during this final phase. It begins with the citric acid cycle and ends with oxidative phosphorylation. About two thirds of the total oxidation of carbon compounds in most cells is accomplished during this phase. The major end products are carbon dioxide (CO_2) and two dinucleotides, reduced nicotinamide adenine dinucleotide (NADH) and the reduced form of flavin adenine dinucleotide ($FADH_2$), that transfer their electrons into the electron-transport chain.

Oxidative Phosphorylation

Oxidative phosphorylation occurs in the mitochondria and is the mechanism by which the energy produced from carbohydrates, fats, and proteins is transferred to ATP. During the breakdown (catabolism) of foods, many reactions involve the removal of electrons from various intermediates. These reactions generally require a coenzyme (a nonprotein carrier molecule), such as nicotinamide adenine dinucleotide (NAD), to transfer the electrons and thus are called transfer reactions.

Molecules of NAD and flavin adenine dinucleotide (FAD) transfer electrons they have gained from the oxidation of substrates to molecular oxygen, O_2. The electrons from reduced NAD and FAD, NADH and $FADH_2$, respectively, are transferred to the electron-transport chain on the inner surfaces of the mitochondria with the release of hydrogen ions. Some carrier molecules are brightly

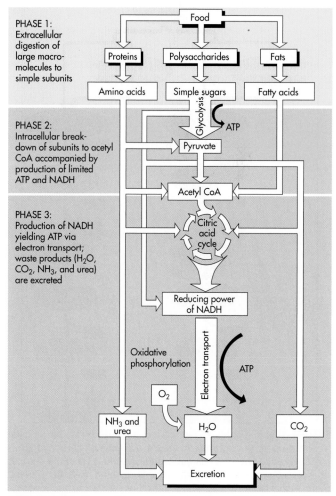

FIGURE 1-13 Three Phases of Catabolism, Which Lead From Food to Waste Products. These reactions produce adenosine triphosphate (ATP), which is used to power other processes in the cell.

colored, iron-containing proteins known as cytochromes that accept a pair of electrons. These electrons eventually combine with molecular oxygen.

If oxygen is not available to the electron-transport chain, ATP will not be formed by the mitochondria. Instead, an anaerobic (without oxygen) metabolic pathway synthesizes ATP. This process, called **substrate phosphorylation** or **anaerobic glycolysis,** is linked to the breakdown (glycolysis) of carbohydrate (see Figure 1-14). Because glycolysis occurs in the cytoplasm of the cell, it provides energy for cells that lack mitochondria. The reactions in anaerobic glycolysis involve the conversion of glucose to pyruvic acid (pyruvate) with the simultaneous production of ATP. With the glycolysis of one molecule of glucose, two ATP molecules and two molecules of pyruvate are liberated. If oxygen is present, the two molecules of pyruvate move into the mitochondria, where they enter the citric acid cycle (Figure 1-15).

If oxygen is absent, pyruvate is converted to lactic acid, which is released into the extracellular fluid. The conversion of pyruvic acid to lactic acid is reversible; therefore once oxygen is restored, lactic acid is quickly converted back to either pyruvic acid or glucose. The anaerobic generation of ATP from glucose through glycolysis is not as efficient as the aerobic generation process. Adding an oxygen-requiring stage to the catabolic process (phase 3; see Figure 1-13) provides cells with a much more powerful method for extracting energy from food molecules.

MEMBRANE TRANSPORT: CELLULAR INTAKE AND OUTPUT

Cells continually incorporate nutrients, fluids, and chemical messengers from the extracellular environment and expel metabolites, or the products of metabolism, and end products of lysosomal digestion. The mechanisms involved depend on the characteristics of the substance to be transported. In **passive transport,** water and small, electrically uncharged molecules move easily through pores in the plasma membrane's lipid bilayer. This process occurs naturally through any semipermeable barrier. It is driven by osmosis, hydrostatic pressure, and diffusion, all of which depend on the laws of physics and do not require life. The process does not require any energy expenditure by the cell.

Other molecules are too large to pass through pores or are ligands bound to receptors on the cell's plasma membrane. Some of these

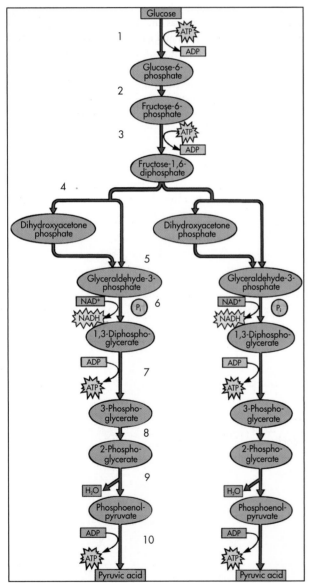

FIGURE 1-14 Glycolysis. Each of the numbered reactions is catalyzed by a different enzyme. At step *4,* a six-carbon carbohydrate is metabolized to two three-carbon carbohydrates, so that the number of molecules at every step after this is doubled. Reactions *5* and *6* are responsible for the net synthesis of adenosine triphosphate (ATP) and reduced nicotinamide adenine dinucleotide (NADH) molecules. (Modified from Thibodeau GA, Patton KT: *Anatomy & physiology,* ed 6, St Louis, 2007, Mosby.)

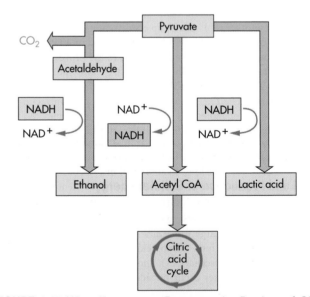

FIGURE 1-15 What Happens to Pyruvate, the Product of Glycolysis? In the presence of oxygen, pyruvate is oxidized to acetyl coenzyme A (CoA) and enters the citric acid cycle. In the absence of oxygen, pyruvate instead is reduced, accepting the electrons extracted during glycolysis and carried by reduced nicotinamide adenine dinucleotide (NADH). When pyruvate is reduced directly, as it is in muscles, the product is lactic acid. When CO_2 is first removed from pyruvate and the remainder is reduced, as it is in yeasts, the resulting product is ethanol.

molecules are moved into and out of the cell by **active transport,** which requires life, biologic activity, and the cell's expenditure of metabolic energy. Unlike passive transport, active transport occurs across only living membranes that (1) use energy generated by cellular metabolism and (2) have receptors that can recognize and bind with the substance to be transported. Large molecules (macromolecules), along with fluids, are transported by endocytosis (taking in) and exocytosis (expelling). Water and electrically charged molecules are transported by protein channels embedded in the plasma membrane. Ligands enter the cell by means of receptor-mediated endocytosis.

Movement of Water and Solutes

Cellular membranes are semipermeable and generally allow passage of water and small particles of dissolved substances called **solutes,** depending on their size, solubility, electrical properties, and concentration on either side of the membrane (also see Chapter 4). Small, lipid-soluble particles, such as oxygen, carbon dioxide, and urea, readily pass through the lipid bilayers of the plasma membrane. Larger, water-soluble particles may pass through pores in the membranes. Although large protein molecules, such as albumin and globulin, pass through membranes by endocytosis, they exert an osmotic effect on the movement of water (see p. 16).

Body fluids are composed of **electrolytes,** which are electrically charged and dissociate into constituent **ions** when placed in solution, and nonelectrolytes, such as glucose, urea, and creatinine, which do not dissociate. Electrolytes account for approximately 95% of the solute molecules in body water. Electrolytes exhibit **polarity** by orienting themselves toward the positive or negative pole. Ions with a positive charge are known as **cations** and migrate toward the negative pole, or cathode, if an electrical current is passed through the electrolyte solution. **Anions** carry a negative charge and migrate toward the positive pole, or anode, in the presence of electrical current. Anions and cations are located in both the intracellular fluid (ICF) and the extracellular fluid (ECF) compartments, although their concentration depends on their location. (Fluid and electrolyte balance between body compartments is discussed in Chapter 4.) For example, sodium (Na^+) is the predominant extracellular cation, and potassium (K^+) is the principal intracellular cation. The difference in ICF and ECF concentrations of these ions is important to the transmission of electrical impulses across the plasma membranes of nerve and muscle cells.

Electrolytes are measured in milliequivalents per liter (mEq/L) or milligrams per deciliter (mg/dl). The term *milliequivalent* indicates the chemical-combining activity of an ion, which depends on the electrical charge, or **valence,** of its ions. In abbreviations, valence is indicated by the number of plus or minus signs. One milliequivalent of any cation can combine chemically with 1 mEq of any anion: one monovalent anion will combine with one monovalent cation. Divalent ions combine more strongly than monovalent ions. To maintain electrochemical balance, one divalent ion will combine with two monovalent ions (e.g., $Ca^{++} + 2Cl^- = CaCl_2$).

Passive Transport: Diffusion, Filtration, and Osmosis

Diffusion. Diffusion is the movement of a solute molecule from an area of greater solute concentration to an area of lesser solute concentration. This difference in concentration is known as a **concentration gradient.** Although particles in a solution move randomly in any direction, if the concentration of particles in one part of the solution is greater than that in another part, the particles distribute themselves evenly throughout the solution. According to the same principle, if the concentration of particles is greater on one side of a *permeable*

membrane than on the other side, the particles diffuse spontaneously from the area of greater concentration to the area of lesser concentration until equilibrium is reached. The higher the concentration on one side, the greater the diffusion rate.

The diffusion rate is influenced by differences of electrical potential across the membrane (see p. XX). Because the pores in the lipid bilayer are often lined with Ca^{++}, other cations (e.g., Na^+ and K^+) diffuse slowly because they are repelled by positive charges in the pores.

The rate of diffusion of a substance depends also on its size (diffusion coefficient) and its lipid solubility (Figure 1-16). Usually, the smaller the molecule and the more soluble it is in oil, the more hydrophobic or nonpolar it is and the more rapidly it will diffuse across the bilayer. Oxygen, carbon dioxide, and steroid hormones are all nonpolar molecules. Water-soluble substances, such as glucose and inorganic ions, diffuse very slowly, whereas uncharged lipophilic ("lipid-loving") molecules, such as fatty acids and steroids, diffuse rapidly. Ions and other polar molecules generally diffuse across cellular membranes more slowly than lipid-soluble substances.

Water readily diffuses through biologic membranes because water molecules are small and uncharged. The dipolar structure of water allows it to cross rapidly the regions of the bilayer containing the lipid head groups. The lipid head groups constitute the two outer regions of the lipid bilayer.

Filtration: hydrostatic pressure. **Filtration** is the movement of water and solutes through a membrane because of a greater pushing pressure (force) on one side of the membrane than on the other side. **Hydrostatic pressure** is the mechanical force of water pushing against

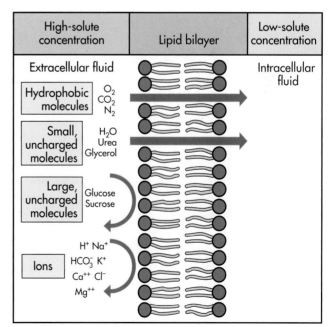

FIGURE 1-16 Passive Diffusion of Solute Molecules Across the Plasma Membrane. Oxygen, nitrogen, water, urea, glycerol, and carbon dioxide can diffuse readily down the concentration gradient. Macromolecules are too large to diffuse through pores in the plasma membrane. Ions may be repelled if the pores contain substances with identical charges. If the pores are lined with cations, for example, other cations will have difficulty diffusing because the positive charges will repel one another. Diffusion can still occur, but it occurs more slowly.

cellular membranes (Figure 1-17, *A*). In the vascular system, hydrostatic pressure is the *blood pressure* generated in vessels when the heart contracts. Blood reaching the capillary bed has a hydrostatic pressure of 25 to 30 mm Hg, which is sufficient force to push water across the thin capillary membranes into the interstitial space. Hydrostatic pressure is partially balanced by osmotic pressure, whereby water moving *out* of the capillaries is partially balanced by osmotic forces that tend to *pull* water *into* the capillaries. Water that is not osmotically attracted back into the capillaries moves into the lymph system (see the discussion of Starling forces in Chapter 4).

Osmosis. Osmosis is the movement of water "down" a concentration gradient—that is, across a semipermeable membrane from a region of higher water concentration to one of lower concentration. For osmosis to occur, (1) the membrane must be more permeable to water than to solutes and (2) the concentration of solutes on one side of the membrane must be greater than that on the other side so that water moves more easily. Osmosis is directly related to both hydrostatic pressure and solute concentration but *not* to particle size or weight. For example, particles of the plasma protein albumin are small but are more concentrated in body fluids than the larger and heavier particles of globulin. Therefore albumin exerts a greater osmotic force than does globulin.

Osmolality controls the distribution and movement of water between body compartments. The terms *osmolality* and *osmolarity* often are used interchangeably in reference to osmotic activity, but they define different measurements. Osmolality measures the number of milliosmoles per kilogram (mOsm/kg) of water, or the concentration of molecules per *weight* of water. Osmolarity measures the number of milliosmoles per liter of solution, or the concentration of molecules per *volume* of solution.

In solutions that contain only dissociable substances, such as sodium and chloride, the difference between the two measurements is negligible. When considering all the different solutes in plasma (e.g., proteins, glucose, lipids), however, the difference between osmolality and osmolarity becomes more significant. Less of plasma's weight is water, and the overall concentration of particles is therefore greater. The osmolality will be greater than the osmolarity because of the smaller proportion of water. Osmolality is thus preferred in human clinical assessment.

The normal osmolality of body fluids is 280 to 294 mOsm/kg. The osmolalities of intracellular and extracellular fluids tend to equalize, providing a measure of body fluid concentration and thus the body's hydration status. Hydration is affected also by hydrostatic pressure, because the movement of water by osmosis can be opposed by an equal amount of hydrostatic pressure. The amount of hydrostatic pressure required to oppose the osmotic movement of water is called the osmotic pressure of the solution. Factors that determine osmotic pressure are the type and thickness of the plasma membrane, the size of the molecules, the concentration of molecules or the concentration gradient, and the solubility of molecules within the membrane.

Effective osmolality is sustained osmotic activity and depends on the concentration of solutes remaining on one side of a permeable membrane. If the solutes penetrate the membrane and equilibrate with the solution on the other side of the membrane, the osmotic effect will be diminished or lost.

Plasma proteins influence osmolality because they have a negative charge (see Figure 1-17, *B*). The principle involved is known as *Gibbs-Donnan equilibrium;* it occurs when the fluid in one compartment contains small, diffusible ions, such as Na^+ and chloride (Cl^-), together with large, nondiffusible, charged particles, such as plasma proteins. Because the body tends to maintain an electrical equilibrium, the nondiffusible protein molecules cause asymmetry in the distribution of small ions. Anions such as Cl^- are thus driven out of the cell or plasma, and cations such as Na^+ are attracted to the cell. The protein-containing compartment maintains a state of electroneutrality, but the osmolality is higher. The overall osmotic effect of colloids, such as plasma proteins, is called the oncotic pressure, or colloid osmotic pressure.

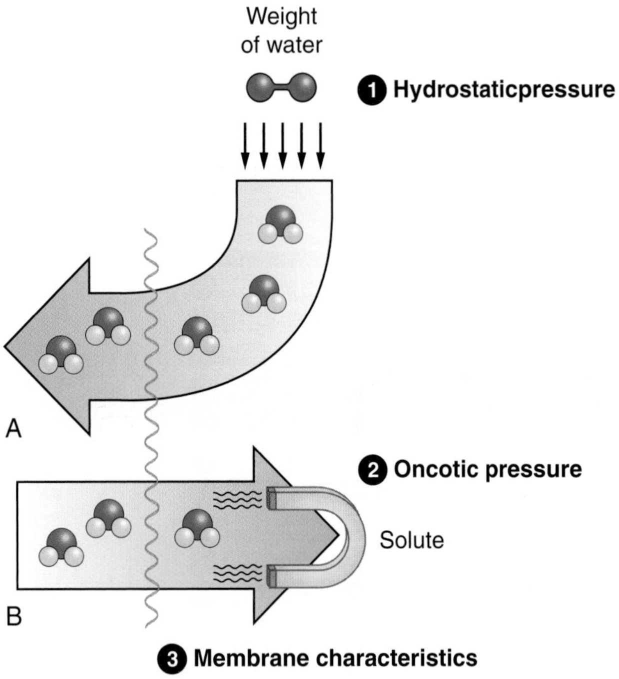

Weight
of water

1 Hydrostaticpressure

A

2 Oncotic pressure

Solute

B

3 Membrane characteristics

FIGURE 1-17 Hydrostatic Pressure and Oncotic Pressure in Plasma. *1,* Hydrostatic pressure in plasma. ***2,*** Oncotic pressure exerted by proteins in the plasma usually tends to *pull* water into the circulatory system. ***3,*** Individuals with low protein levels (e.g., starvation) are unable to maintain a normal oncotic pressure; therefore water is not reabsorbed into the circulation and, instead, causes body edema.

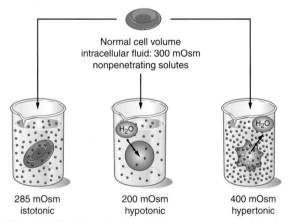

Normal cell volume
intracellular fluid: 300 mOsm
nonpenetrating solutes

285 mOsm
istotonic

200 mOsm
hypotonic

400 mOsm
hypertonic

FIGURE 1-18 Tonicity. Tonicity is important, especially for red blood cell function. (Adapted from Sherwood L: *Human physiology,* ed 7, 2008, Brooks Cole.)

Tonicity describes the effective osmolality of a solution. (The terms *osmolality* and *tonicity* may be used interchangeably.) Solutions have relative degrees of tonicity. An isotonic solution (or isosmotic solution) has the same osmolality or concentration of particles (285 mOsm) as the ICF or ECF. A hypotonic solution has a lower concentration and is thus more dilute than body fluids (Figure 1-18). A hypertonic solution has a concentration of more than 285 to 294 mOsm/kg. The concept of tonicity is important when correcting water and solute imbalances by administering different types of replacement solutions (see Figure 1-18) (see Chapter 4).

> ✔ **QUICK CHECK 1-2**
> 1. What does glycolysis produce?
> 2. Describe the difference between diffusion and osmosis.
> 3. Why do water and small, electrically charged molecules move easily through pores in the plasma membrane?

Mediated and Active Transport

Mediated transport. Mediated transport (passive and active) involves integral or transmembrane proteins with receptors that are highly specific for the substance being transported. Inorganic anions and cations (e.g., Na^+, K^+, Ca^{++}, Cl^-, HCO_3^-) and charged and uncharged organic compounds require specific transport systems to facilitate movement (thus the term *facilitated diffusion*) through different cellular membranes. Mediated transport is much faster than simple diffusion.

A transport protein (*carrier protein*) is a transmembrane or integral protein that binds with and transfers a specific solute molecule across the lipid bilayer. Each transport protein, or transporter, has receptors for a specific solute. When the transporter is saturated—that is, when all receptor sites are occupied by solute molecules—the rate of transport is maximal. Solute binding can be blocked by competitive inhibitors that compete for the same receptor site and may or may not be transported by the transport protein. Noncompetitive inhibitors bind elsewhere but can alter the structure of the transporter.

The polypeptide chain of the transport protein crosses the lipid bilayer multiple times. This chain forms a continuous pathway, enabling solutes to pass across the membrane without directly contacting the hydrophobic interior of the lipid bilayer (Figure 1-19).[1]

Another mechanism of mediated transport is the channel protein. The protein transporter creates a water-filled pore or channel across the bilayer through which specific ions can diffuse. These channels are sometimes called *ion channels* or K^+ *leak channels* (Figure 1-20). The channel is controlled by a gate mechanism that determines which receptor-bound solutes can move into it. Binding stimulates conformational changes in the protein transporter that move the solute through the channel short distances until it reaches the other side of the membrane. Ion channels are responsible for the electrical excitability of nerve and muscle cells and play a critical role in the membrane potential.

Mediated transport systems can move solute molecules singly or two at a time. Two molecules can be moved simultaneously in one direction (a process called symport, for example, sodium-glucose in the digestive tract) or in opposite directions (called antiport, for example, the sodium-potassium pump in all cells), or a single molecule can be moved in one direction (called uniport, for example, glucose) (Figure 1-21).

In passive mediated transport, or facilitated diffusion, the protein transporter moves solute molecules through cellular membranes

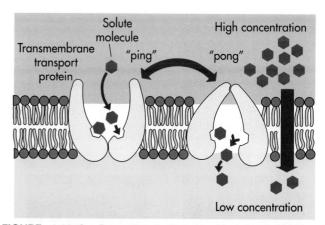

FIGURE 1-19 Conformational Change Model of Mediated Transport (Facilitated Diffusion). The transporter protein has two states: "ping" and "pong." In the ping state, sites for molecules of a specific solute are exposed on the outside of the bilayer. In the pong state, the sites are exposed to the inner side of the bilayer.

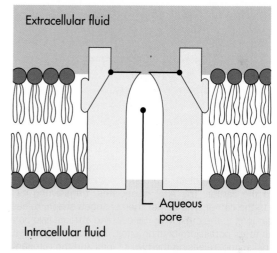

FIGURE 1-20 Channel Mode of Mediated Transport (Facilitated Diffusion). A channel protein forms a water-filled pore across the bilayer through which specific ions can diffuse.

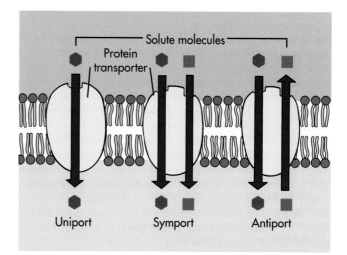

FIGURE 1-21 Mediated Transport. Illustration shows simultaneous movement of a single solute molecule in one direction (uniport), of two different solute molecules in one direction (symport), and of two different solute molecules in opposite directions (antiport).

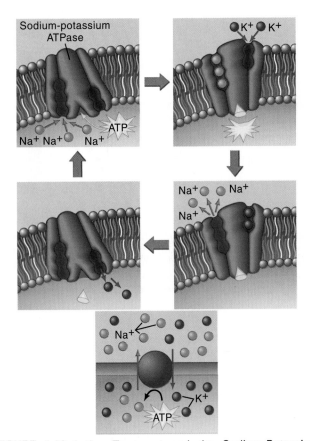

FIGURE 1-22 Active Transport and the Sodium-Potassium Pump. Three Na$^+$ ions bind to sodium-binding sites on the carrier's inner face. At the same time, an energy-containing adenosine triphosphate (ATP) molecule produced by the cell's mitochondria binds to the carrier. The ATP dissociates, transferring its stored energy to the carrier. The carrier then changes shape, releases the three Na$^+$ ions to the outside of the cell, and attracts two potassium (K$^+$) ions to its potassium-binding sites. The carrier then returns to its original shape, releasing the two K$^+$ ions and the remnant of the ATP molecule to the inside of the cell. The carrier is now ready for another pumping cycle. (From Thibodeau GA, Patton KT: *Anatomy & physiology*, ed 6, St Louis, 2007, Mosby.)

pores or protein channels and maintaining the ionic concentration gradients needed for cellular excitation and membrane conductivity (see p. 21). The maintenance of intracellular K$^+$ concentrations is required also for enzyme activity, including enzymes involved in protein synthesis.

Active Transport of Na$^+$ and K$^+$

The active transport system for Na$^+$ and K$^+$ is found in virtually all mammalian cells. The Na$^+$, K$^+$ antiport system (i.e., Na$^+$ moving out of the cell and K$^+$ moving into the cell) uses the direct energy of ATP to transport these cations. The transporter protein is ATPase, which requires Na$^+$, K$^+$, and magnesium (Mg^{++}) ions. The concentration of ATPase in plasma membranes is directly related to Na$^+$, K$^+$ transport activity. Approximately 60% to 70% of the ATP synthesized by cells, especially muscle and nerve cells, is used to maintain the Na$^+$, K$^+$ transport system. Excitable tissues have a high concentration of Na$^+$, K$^+$ ATPase, as do other tissues that transport significant amounts of Na$^+$. For every ATP molecule hydrolyzed, three molecules of Na$^+$ are transported out of the cell, whereas only two molecules of K$^+$ move into the cell. The process leads to an electrical potential and is called *electrogenic*, with the inside of the cell more negative than the outside. Although the exact mechanism for this transport is uncertain, it is possible that ATPase induces the transporter protein to undergo several conformational changes, causing Na$^+$ and K$^+$ to move short distances (see Figure 1-22). The conformational change lowers the affinity for Na$^+$ and K$^+$ to the ATPase transporter, resulting in the release of the cations after transport.

Table 1-4 summarizes the major mechanisms of transport through pores and protein transporters in the plasma membranes. Many disease states are caused or manifested by loss of these membrane transport systems.

Transport by Vesicle Formation
Endocytosis and Exocytosis

The active transport mechanisms by which the cells move large proteins, polynucleotides, or polysaccharides (macromolecules) across

without expending metabolic energy. The direction of movement is the same as in simple diffusion—down the concentration gradient. A well-known passive transport system is that used for glucose in erythrocytes (red blood cells). Glucose is transported by a uniport mechanism and demonstrates saturation kinetics—that is, the transport system is saturated when all the glucose-specific receptors on the membrane are occupied and operating at their maximal capacity.

In **active mediated transport,** or active transport, the protein transporter moves molecules against, or up, the concentration gradient. Unlike passive mediated transport, active mediated transport requires the expenditure of energy. Many, but not all, active mediated transport systems, or pumps, have ATP as their primary energy source. Some use the electrochemical gradient of Na$^+$ across the membrane (Figure 1-22). Energy in the form of ATP, however, is required for activation of the Na$^+$ gradient (Box 1-1).

A "carrier" mechanism in the plasma membrane mediates the transport of ions and nutrients. The best-known pump is the Na$^+$, K$^+$–dependent adenosinetriphosphatase (ATPase) pump. It continuously regulates the cell's volume by controlling leaks through

TABLE 1-4   MAJOR TRANSPORT SYSTEMS IN MAMMALIAN CELLS

SUBSTANCE TRANSPORTED	MECHANISM OF TRANSPORT*	TISSUES
Carbohydrates		
Glucose	Passive: protein channel	Most tissues
Fructose	Active: symport with Na^+	Small intestines and renal tubular cells
	Passive	Intestines and liver
Amino Acids		
Amino acid specific transporters	Coupled channels	Intestines, kidney, and liver
All amino acids except proline	Active: symport with Na^+	Liver
Specific amino acids	Active: group translocation	Small intestine
	Passive	
Other Organic Molecules		
Cholic acid, deoxycholic acid, and taurocholic acid	Active: symport with Na^+	Intestines
Organic anions (e.g., malate, α-ketoglutarate, glutamate)	Antiport with counter–organic anion	Mitochondria of liver cells
ATP-ADP	Antiport transport of nucleotides; can be active	Mitochondria of liver cells
Inorganic Ions		
Na^+	Passive	Distal renal tubular cells
Na^+/H^+	Active antiport, proton pump	Proximal renal tubular cells and small intestines
Na^+/K^+	Active: ATP driven, protein channel	Plasma membrane of most cells
Ca^{++}	Active: ATP driven, antiport with Na^+	All cells, antiporter in red cells
H^+/K^+	Active	Parietal cells of gastric cells secreting H^+
Cl^-/HCO_3^- (perhaps other anions)	Mediated: antiport (anion transporter–band 3 protein)	Erythrocytes and many other cells
Water	Osmosis passive	All tissues

Data from Alberts B et al: *Molecular biology of the cell,* ed 4, New York, 2001, Garland; Devlin TM, editor: *Textbook of biochemistry: with clinical correlations,* ed 3, New York, 1992, Wiley; Raven PH, Johnson GB: *Understanding biology,* ed 3, Dubuque, IA, 1995, Brown.
*NOTE: The known transport systems are listed here; others have been proposed. Most transport systems have been studied in only a few tissues, and their sites of activity may be more limited than indicated.
ADP, Adenosine diphosphate; *ATP,* adenosine triphosphate.

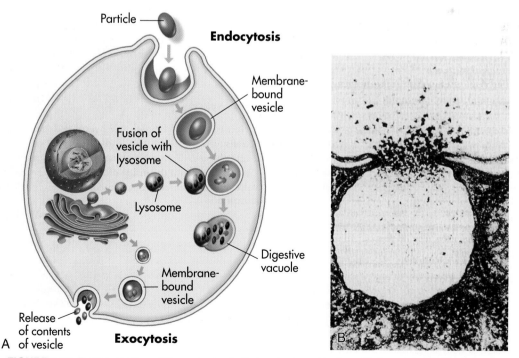

FIGURE 1-23 Endocytosis and Exocytosis. A, Endocytosis and fusion with lysosome and exocytosis. **B,** Electron micrograph of exocytosis. (**B** from Raven PH, Johnson GB: *Biology,* ed 5, New York, 1999, McGraw-Hill.)

BOX 1-2   THE NEW ENDOCYTIC MATRIX

An explosion of new data is disclosing a much more involved role for endocytosis than just a simple way to internalize nutrients and membrane-associated molecules. These new data show that endocytosis not only is a master organizer of signaling pathways but also has a major role in managing signals in time and space. Endocytosis appears to control signaling; therefore it determines the net output of biochemical pathways. This occurs because endocytosis modulates the presence of receptors and their ligands as well as effectors at the plasma membrane or at intermediate stations of the endocytic route. The overall processes and anatomy of these new functions are sometimes called the "endocytic matrix." All of these functions ultimately have a large impact on almost every cellular process, including the nucleus.

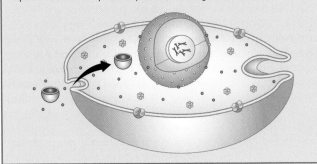

From Scita G, DiFiore PP: The endocytic matrix, *Nature* 463(28): 464–473, 2010.

the plasma membrane are very different from those that mediate small solute and ion transport. Transport of macromolecules involves the sequential formation and fusion of membrane-bound vesicles.

In **endocytosis,** a section of the plasma membrane enfolds substances from outside the cell, invaginates (folds inward), and separates from the plasma membrane, forming a vesicle that moves into the cell (Figure 1-23, *A*). Two types of endocytosis are designated based on the size of the vesicle formed. **Pinocytosis** (cell drinking) involves the ingestion of fluids and solute molecules through formation of small vesicles, and **phagocytosis** (cell eating) involves the ingestion of large particles, such as bacteria, through formation of large vesicles (vacuoles).

Because most cells continually ingest fluid and solutes by pinocytosis, the terms *pinocytosis* and *endocytosis* often are used interchangeably. In pinocytosis, the vesicle containing fluids, solutes, or both fuses with a lysosome, and lysosomal enzymes digest the vesicle's contents for use by the cell. In phagocytosis, the large molecular substances are engulfed by the plasma membrane and enter the cell so that they can be isolated and destroyed by lysosomal enzymes (see Chapter 5). Substances that are not degraded by lysosomes are isolated in residual bodies and released by exocytosis. Both pinocytosis and phagocytosis require metabolic energy and often involve binding of the substance with plasma membrane receptors before membrane invagination and fusion with lysosomes in the cell. New data are revealing that endocytosis has an even larger and more important role than previously known (Box 1-2).

In eukaryotic cells, secretion of macromolecules almost always occurs by exocytosis (see Figure 1-23). **Exocytosis** has two main functions: (1) replacement of portions of the plasma membrane that have been removed by endocytosis and (2) release of molecules synthesized by the cells into the extracellular matrix.

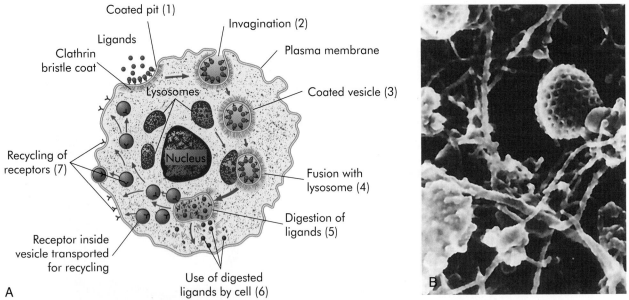

FIGURE 1-24 Ligand Internalization by Means of Receptor-Mediated Endocytosis. A, The ligand attaches to its surface receptor (through the bristle coat or clathrin coat) and, through receptor-mediated endocytosis, enters the cell. The ingested material fuses with a lysosome and is processed by hydrolytic lysosomal enzymes. Processed molecules can then be transferred to other cellular components. **B,** Electron micrograph of a coated pit showing different sizes of filaments of the cytoskeleton (×82,000). (**B** from Erlandsen SL, Magney JE: *Color atlas of histology,* St Louis, 1992, Mosby.)

Receptor-Mediated Endocytosis

Ligand binding to *some* plasma membrane receptors leads to clustering, aggregation, and immobilization of the receptors in specialized areas of the membrane called coated pits (Figure 1-24). The pits, which are coated with bristlelike structures (clathrin), deepen and enfold (invaginate), internalizing ligand-receptor complexes and forming a coated vesicle. The clathrin coat or bristles may be responsible for trapping membrane receptors in coated pits. This internalization process, called receptor-mediated endocytosis (ligand internalization), is rapid and enables the cell to ingest large amounts of specific ligands without ingesting large volumes of extracellular fluid. The cellular uptake of cholesterol, for example, depends on receptor-mediated endocytosis.

Caveolae

The outer surface of the plasma membrane is dimpled with tiny flask-shaped pits (cavelike) called *caveolae.* Caveolae are thought to form from membrane microdomains or lipid rafts. Caveolae are cholesterol-rich domains where protein caveolae are involved in several processes, including clathrin-independent endocytosis, the regulation and transport of cellular cholesterol, and cell communication.[1] Many proteins, including a variety of receptors, cluster in these tiny chambers. Caveolae possibly invaginate and gather cargo proteins from the lipid-rich caveolar membrane.[1] This invagination is in contrast to receptor-mediated endocytosis, which also transports molecules into the cell but with the formation of a vesicle. Caveolae pinch off from the membrane using dynamin, a clathrin-coated protein, and deliver their contents to either an endosome or the plasma membrane on the opposite side of a polarized cell.[1]

Caveolae are not only uptake vehicles but also important sites for signal transduction, a tedious process in which extracellular chemical messages or *signals* are communicated to the cell's interior for execution (see p. 12). For example, strong evidence now exists that plasma membrane estrogen receptors localize in caveolae, and crosstalk with estradiol facilitates several intracellular biologic actions.[1]

Movement of Electrical Impulses: Membrane Potentials

All body cells are electrically polarized, with the inside of the cell more negatively charged than the outside. The difference in electrical charge, or voltage, is known as the resting membrane potential and is about −70 to −85 millivolts. The difference in voltage across the plasma membrane results from the differences in ionic composition of ICF and ECF. Sodium ions are more concentrated in the ECF, and potassium ions are in greater concentration in the ICF. The concentration difference is maintained by the active transport of Na^+ and K^+ (the sodium-potassium pump), which transports sodium outward and potassium inward (Figure 1-25). Because the resting plasma membrane is more permeable to K^+ than to Na^+, K^+ diffuses easily from the ICF to the ECF. Because both sodium and potassium are cations, the net result is an excess of anions inside the cell, resulting in the resting membrane potential.

Nerve and muscle cells are excitable and can change their resting membrane potential in response to electrochemical stimuli. Changes

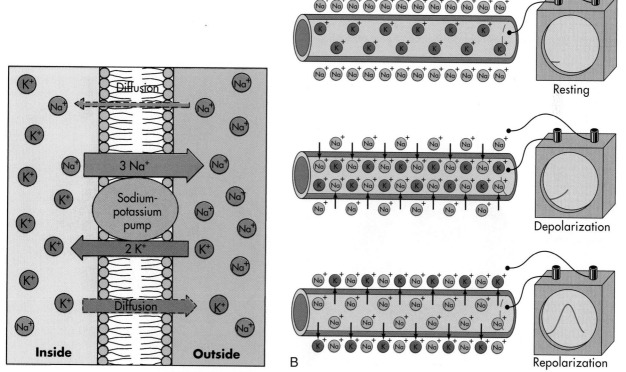

FIGURE 1-25 Sodium-Potassium Pump and Propagation of an Action Potential. A, Concentration difference of sodium (Na^+) and potassium (K^+) intracellularly and extracellularly. The direction of active transport by the sodium-potassium pump is also shown. **B,** The top diagram represents the polarized state of a neuronal membrane when at rest. The lower diagrams represent changes in sodium and potassium membrane permeabilities with depolarization and repolarization. (From Thibodeau GA, Patton KT: *Anatomy & physiology,* ed 6, St Louis, 2007, Mosby.)

in resting membrane potential convey messages from cell to cell. When a nerve or muscle cell receives a stimulus that exceeds the membrane threshold value, a rapid change occurs in the resting membrane potential, known as the **action potential.** The action potential carries signals along the nerve or muscle cell and conveys information from one cell to another. (Nerve impulses are described in Chapter 12.) When a resting cell is stimulated through voltage-regulated channels, the cell membranes become more permeable to sodium, so a net movement of sodium into the cell occurs and the membrane potential decreases, or moves forward, from a negative value (in millivolts) to zero. This decrease is known as **depolarization.** The depolarized cell is more positively charged, and its polarity is neutralized.

To generate an action potential and the resulting depolarization, the **threshold potential** must be reached. Generally this occurs when the cell has depolarized by 15 to 20 millivolts. When the threshold is reached, the cell will continue to depolarize with no further stimulation. The sodium gates open, and sodium rushes into the cell, causing the membrane potential to drop to zero and then become positive (depolarization). The rapid reversal in polarity results in the action potential.

During **repolarization,** the negative polarity of the resting membrane potential is reestablished. As the voltage-gated sodium channels begin to close, voltage-gated potassium channels open. Membrane permeability to sodium decreases and potassium permeability increases, so potassium ions leave the cell. The sodium gates close, and with the loss of potassium the membrane potential becomes more negative. The Na$^+$, K$^+$ pump then returns the membrane to the resting potential by pumping potassium back into the cell and sodium out of the cell.

During most of the action potential, the plasma membrane cannot respond to an additional stimulus. This time is known as the **absolute refractory period** and is related to changes in permeability to sodium. During the latter phase of the action potential, when permeability to potassium increases, a stronger-than-normal stimulus can evoke an action potential; this time is known as the **relative refractory period.**

When the membrane potential is more negative than normal, the cell is in a **hyperpolarized** (less excitable) state. A stronger-than-normal stimulus is then required to reach the threshold potential and generate an action potential. When the membrane potential is more positive than normal, the cell is in a **hypopolarized** (more excitable than normal) **state** and a weaker-than-normal stimulus is required to reach the threshold potential. Changes in the intracellular and extracellular concentrations of ions or a change in membrane permeability can cause these alterations in membrane excitability.

> ✔ **QUICK CHECK 1-3**
> 1. Identify examples of molecules transported in one direction (symport) and opposite directions (antiport).
> 2. If oxygen is no longer available to make ATP, what happens to the transport of Na$^+$?
> 3. Why are caveolae important to the cell?

CELLULAR REPRODUCTION: THE CELL CYCLE

Human cells are subject to wear and tear, and most do not last for the lifetime of the individual. In most tissues, new cells are created as fast as old cells die. Cellular reproduction is therefore necessary for the maintenance of life. Reproduction of gametes (sperm and egg cells) occurs through a process called *meiosis,* described in Chapter 2. The reproduction, or division, of other body cells (somatic cells) involves two sequential phases: **mitosis,** or nuclear division, and **cytokinesis,** or cytoplasmic division. Before a cell can divide, however, it must double

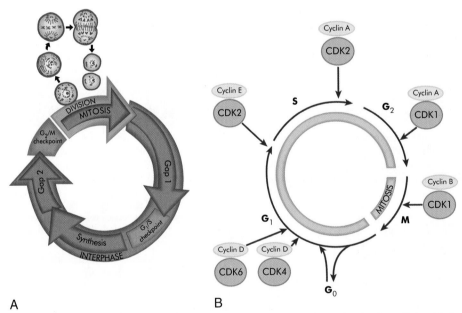

FIGURE 1-26 Interphase and the Phases of Mitosis. **A,** The G$_1$/S checkpoint is to "check" for cell size, nutrients, growth factors, and DNA damage. See text for resting phases. The G$_2$/M checkpoint checks for cell size and DNA replication. **B,** The orderly progression through the phases of the cell cycle is regulated by *cyclins* (so-called because levels rise and fall) and *cyclin-dependent protein kinases* (CDKs) and their inhibitors. When cyclins are complexed with CDKs, cell cycle events are triggered.

its mass and duplicate all its contents. Separation for division occurs during the growth phase, called interphase. The alternation between mitosis and interphase in all tissues with cellular turnover is known as the cell cycle.

The four designated phases of the cell cycle (Figure 1-26) are (1) the S phase (S = synthesis), in which DNA is synthesized in the cell nucleus; (2) the G2 phase (G = gap), in which RNA and protein synthesis occurs, namely, the period between the completion of DNA synthesis and the next phase (M); (3) the M phase (M = mitosis), which includes both nuclear and cytoplasmic division; and (4) the G1 phase, which is the period between the M phase and the start of DNA synthesis.

Phases of Mitosis and Cytokinesis

Interphase (the G_1, S, and G_2 phases) is the longest phase of the cell cycle. During interphase, the chromatin consists of very long, slender rods jumbled together in the nucleus. Late in interphase, strands of chromatin (the substance that gives the nucleus its granular appearance) begin to coil, causing shortening and thickening.

The M phase of the cell cycle, mitosis and cytokinesis, begins with prophase, the first appearance of chromosomes. As the phase proceeds, each chromosome is seen as two identical halves called chromatids, which lie together and are attached by a spindle site called a centromere. (The two chromatids of each chromosome, which are genetically identical, are sometimes called sister chromatids.) The nuclear membrane, which surrounds the nucleus, disappears. Spindle fibers are microtubules formed in the cytoplasm. They radiate from two centrioles located at opposite poles of the cell and pull the chromosomes to opposite sides of the cell, beginning metaphase. Next, the centromeres become aligned in the middle of the spindle, which is called the equatorial plate (or metaphase plate) of the cell. In this stage, chromosomes are easiest to observe microscopically because they are highly condensed and arranged in a relatively organized fashion.

Anaphase begins when the centromeres split and the sister chromatids are pulled apart. The spindle fibers shorten, causing the sister chromatids to be pulled, centromere first, toward opposite sides of the cell. When the sister chromatids are separated, each is considered to be a chromosome. Thus the cell has 92 chromosomes during this stage. By the end of anaphase, there are 46 chromosomes lying at each side of the cell. Barring mitotic errors, each of the 2 groups of 46 chromosomes is identical to the original 46 chromosomes present at the start of the cell cycle.

During telophase, the final stage, a new nuclear membrane is formed around each group of 46 chromosomes, the spindle fibers disappear, and the chromosomes begin to uncoil. Cytokinesis causes the cytoplasm to divide into almost equal parts during this phase. At the end of telophase, two identical diploid cells, called daughter cells, have been formed from the original cell.

Rates of Cellular Division

Although the complete cell cycle lasts 12 to 24 hours, about 1 hour is required for the four stages of mitosis and cytokinesis. All types of cells undergo mitosis during formation of the embryo, but many adult cells, such as nerve cells, lens cells of the eye, and muscle cells, lose their ability to replicate and divide. The cells of other tissues, particularly epithelial cells (e.g., cells of the intestine, lung, or skin), divide continuously and rapidly, completing the entire cell cycle in less than 10 hours.

The difference between cells that divide slowly and cells that divide rapidly is the length of time spent in the G_1 phase of the cell cycle. Once the S phase begins, however, progression through mitosis takes a relatively constant amount of time.

The mechanisms that control cell division depend on genes and protein growth factors. Protein growth factors govern the proliferation of different cell types. Individual cells are members of a complex cellular society in which survival of the entire organism is key—not survival or proliferation of just the individual cells. When a need arises for new cells, as in repair of injured cells, previously nondividing cells must be triggered rapidly to reenter the cell cycle. With continual wear and tear, the cell birth rate and the cell death rate must be kept in balance.

Growth Factors

Growth factors, also called cytokines, are peptides (protein fractions) that transmit signals within and between cells. They have a major role in the regulation of tissue growth and development (Table 1-5). Having nutrients is not enough for a cell to proliferate; it must also receive

TABLE 1-5   EXAMPLES OF GROWTH FACTORS AND THEIR ACTIONS

GROWTH FACTOR	PHYSIOLOGIC ACTIONS
Platelet-derived growth factor (PDGF)	Stimulates proliferation of connective tissue cells and neuroglial cells
Epidermal growth factor (EGF)	Stimulates proliferation of epidermal cells and other cell types
Insulin-like growth factor 1 (IGF-1)	Collaborates with PDGF and EGF; stimulates proliferation of fat cells and connective tissue cells
Vascular endothelial growth factor (VEGF)	Mediates functions of endothelial cells; proliferation, migration, invasion, survival, and permeability
Insulin-like growth factor 2 (IGF-2)	Collaborates with PDGF and EGF; stimulates or inhibits response of most cells to other growth factors; regulates differentiation of some cell types (e.g., cartilage)
Transforming growth factor β (TGBβ; multiple subtypes)	Stimulates or inhibits response of most cells to other growth factors; regulates differentiation of some cell types (e.g., cartilage)
Fibroblast growth factor (FGF; multiple subtypes)	Stimulates proliferation of fibroblasts, endothelial cells, myoblasts, and other multiple subtypes
Interleukin-2 (IL-2)	Stimulates proliferation of T lymphocytes
Nerve growth factor (NGF)	Promotes axon growth and survival of sympathetic and some sensory and central nervous system (CNS) neurons
Hematopoietic cell growth factors (IL-3, GM-CSF, G-CSF, erythropoietin)	Promote proliferation of blood cells

G-CSF, Granulocyte colony-stimulating factor; *GM-CSF*, granulocyte-macrophage colony-stimulating factor.

stimulatory chemical signals (growth factors) from other cells, usually its neighbors or the surrounding supporting tissue called **stroma.** These signals act to overcome intracellular braking mechanisms that tend to restrain cell growth and block progress through the cell cycle (see Figure 1-27).

An example of a brake that regulates cell proliferation is the **retinoblastoma (Rb) protein,** first identified through studies of a rare childhood eye tumor called *retinoblastoma,* in which the Rb protein is missing or defective (see p. 423). The Rb protein is abundant in the nucleus of all vertebrate cells. It binds to gene regulatory proteins, preventing them from stimulating the transcription of genes required for cell proliferation (see Figure 1-27). Extracellular signals, such as growth factors, activate intracellular signaling pathways that inactivate the Rb protein, leading to cell proliferation.

Different types of cells require different growth factors; for example, **platelet-derived growth factor (PDGF)** stimulates the production of connective tissue cells. Table 1-5 summarizes the most significant growth factors. Evidence shows that some growth factors also regulate other cell processes, such as cellular differentiation. In addition to growth factors that stimulate cellular processes, there are factors that inhibit these processes; these factors are not well understood. Cells that are starved of growth factors come to a halt after mitosis and enter the **arrested (resting) (G0) state** of the cell cycle (see p. 22 for cell cycle).[1]

TISSUES

Cells of one or more types are organized into tissues, and different types of tissues compose organs. Finally, organs are integrated to perform complex functions as tracts or systems.

All cells are in contact with a network of extracellular macromolecules known as the **extracellular matrix** (see p. 8). This matrix not only holds cells and tissues together but also provides an organized latticework within which cells can migrate and interact with one another.

Tissue Formation

The process by which differentiated cells create tissues and organs is called **pattern formation.**[5] To form tissues, cells must exhibit intercellular recognition and communication, adhesion, and memory. Specialized cells sense their environment through signals, such as growth factors, from other cells. This type of communication ensures that new cells are produced only when and where they are required. Different cell types have different adhesion molecules in their plasma membranes, sticking selectively to other cells of the same type. They can also adhere to extracellular matrix components. Because cells are tiny and squishy and enclosed by a flimsy membrane, it is remarkable that they form a strong human being. Strength can occur because of the extracellular matrix and the strength of the cytoskeleton with cell-cell adhesions to neighboring cells. Cells have memory because of specialized patterns of gene expression evoked by signals that acted during embryonic development. Memory allows cells to autonomously preserve their distinctive character and pass it on to their progeny.[1]

Types of Tissues

The four basic types of tissues are nerve, epithelial, connective, and muscle. The structure and function of these four types underlie the structure and function of each organ system. Neural tissue is composed of highly specialized cells called *neurons,* which receive and transmit electrical impulses rapidly across junctions called *synapses* (see Figure 11-1). Different types of neurons have special characteristics that depend on their distribution and function within the nervous system. Epithelial, connective, and muscle tissues are summarized in Boxes 1-3, 1-4, and 1-5, respectively.

> ✔ **QUICK CHECK 1-4**
> 1. Why is cell cycle communication so important?
> 2. Discuss the five types of intracellular communication.
> 3. Why is cell-to-cell adhesion so important?
> 4. Why is the extracellular matrix important for tissue cells?

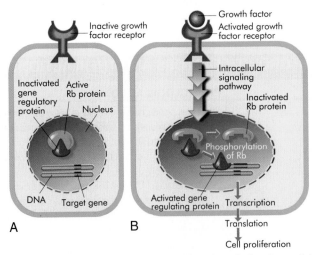

FIGURE 1-27 How Growth Factors Stimulate Cell Proliferation. A, Resting cell. With the absence of growth factors, the retinoblastoma (Rb) protein is not phosphorylated; thus it holds the gene regulatory proteins in an inactive state. The gene regulatory proteins are required to stimulate the transcription of genes needed for cell proliferation. **B,** Proliferating cell. Growth factors bind to the cell surface receptors and activate intracellular signaling pathways, leading to activation of intracellular proteins. These intracellular proteins phosphorylate and thereby inactivate the Rb protein. The gene regulatory proteins are now free to activate the transcription of genes, leading to cell proliferation.

BOX 1-3   CHARACTERISTICS OF EPITHELIAL TISSUES

SIMPLE SQUAMOUS EPITHELIUM

Structure

Single layer of cells

Location

Lining of blood vessels

Lining of pulmonary alveoli (air sacs)

Function

Diffusion and filtration

Separation of blood from fluids in tissues

Separation of air from fluids in tissues

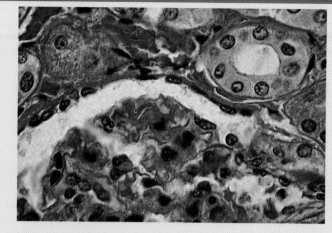

Bowman's capsule (kidney)

Filtration of substances from blood, forming urine

Simple Squamous Epithelial Cell. Photomicrograph of simple squamous epithelial cell in parietal wall of Bowman's capsule in kidney. (From Erlandsen SL, Magney JE: *Color atlas of histology*, St Louis, 1992, Mosby.)

STRATIFIED SQUAMOUS EPITHELIUM

Structure

Two or more layers, depending on location, with cells closest to basement membrane tending to be cuboidal

Location

Epidermis of skin

Linings of mouth, pharynx, esophagus, anus

Function

Protection and secretion

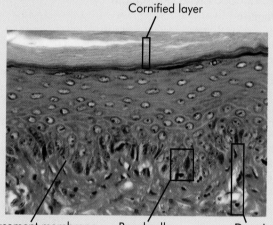

Cornified layer

Basement membrane   Basal cells   Dermis

Cornified Stratified Squamous Epithelium. Diagram of stratified squamous epithelium of skin. (Copyright Ed Reschke. Used with permission.)

TRANSITIONAL EPITHELIUM

Structure

Vary in shape from cuboidal to squamous depending on whether basal cells of bladder are columnar or are composed of many layers; when bladder is full and stretched, the cells flatten and stretch like squamous cells

Location

Linings of urinary bladder and other hollow structures

Function

Stretching that permits expansion of hollow organs

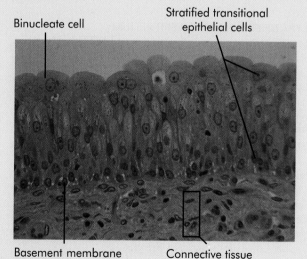

Binucleate cell

Stratified transitional epithelial cells

Basement membrane   Connective tissue

Stratified Squamous Transitional Epithelium. Photomicrograph of stratified squamous transitional epithelium of urinary bladder. (Copyright Ed Reschke. Used with permission.)

Continued

BOX 1-3   CHARACTERISTICS OF EPITHELIAL TISSUES—cont'd

SIMPLE CUBOIDAL EPITHELIUM

Structure
Simple cuboidal cells; rarely stratified (layered)

Location
Glands (e.g., thyroid, sweat, salivary)
Parts of kidney tubule and outer covering
  of ovary

Function
Secretion

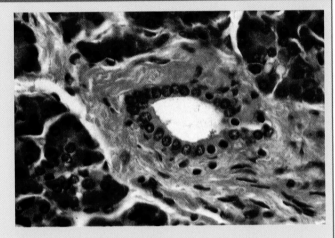

Simple Cuboidal Epithelium. Photomicrograph of simple cuboidal epithelium of pancreatic duct. (From Erlandsen SL, Magney JE: *Color atlas of histology,* St Louis, 1992, Mosby.)

SIMPLE COLUMNAR EPITHELIUM

Structure
Large amounts of cytoplasm and cellular organelles

Location
Lining of digestive tract

Ducts of many glands

Function
Secretion and absorption from
  stomach to anus

CILIATED SIMPLE COLUMNAR EPITHELIUM

Structure
Same as simple columnar epithelium but ciliated

Location
Linings of bronchi of lungs, nasal cavity,
  and oviducts

Function
Secretion, absorption, and
  propulsion of fluids and
  particles

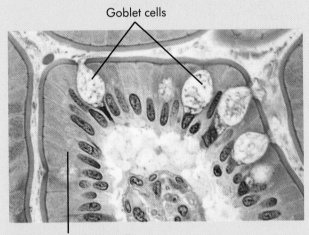

Goblet cells

Columnar epithelial cell

Simple Columnar Epithelium. Photomicrograph of simple columnar epithelium. (Copyright Ed Reschke. Used with permission.)

STRATIFIED COLUMNAR EPITHELIUM

Structure
Small and rounded basement membrane (columnar
  cells do not touch basement membrane)

Location
Linings of epiglottis, part of pharynx, anus, and
  male urethra

Function
Protection

PSEUDOSTRATIFIED CILIATED COLUMNAR EPITHELIUM

Structure
All cells in contact with basement membrane
Nuclei found at different levels within cell, giving
  stratified appearance
Free surface often ciliated

Location
Linings of large ducts of some glands (parotid,
  salivary), male urethra, respiratory passages,
  and eustachian tubes of ears

Function
Transport of substances

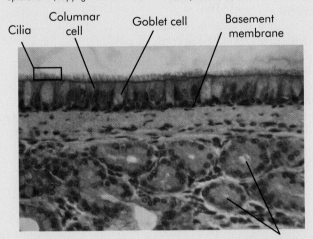

Cilia   Columnar cell   Goblet cell   Basement membrane

Mucous glands

Pseudostratified Ciliated Columnar Epithelium. Photomicrograph of pseudostratified ciliated columnar epithelium of trachea. (Copyright Robert L. Calentine. Used with permission.)

BOX 1-4   CONNECTIVE TISSUES

LOOSE OR AREOLAR TISSUE
Structure
Unorganized; spaces between fibers
Most fibers collagenous, some elastic and reticular
Includes many types of cells (fibroblasts and macrophages most common) and large
   amount of intercellular fluid
Location and Function
Attaches skin to underlying tissue; holds organs in place by filling spaces between
   them; supports blood vessels
Intercellular fluid transports nutrients and waste products
Fluid accumulation causes swelling (edema)

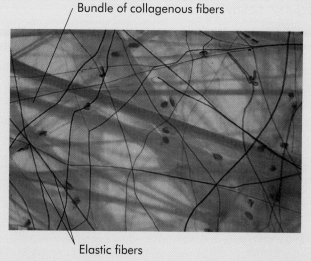

Bundle of collagenous fibers

Elastic fibers

Loose Areolar Connective Tissue. (Copyright Ed Reschke. Used with permission.)

DENSE IRREGULAR TISSUE
Structure
Dense, compact, and areolar tissue, with fewer cells and greater number
   of closely woven collagenous fibers than in loose tissue
Location and Function
Dermis layer of skin; acts as protective barrier

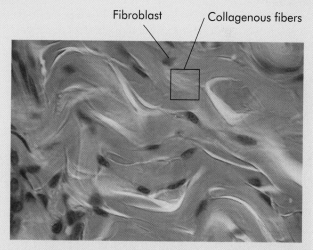

Fibroblast   Collagenous fibers

Dense, Irregular Connective Tissue. (Copyright Ed Reschke. Used with permission.)

DENSE, REGULAR (WHITE FIBROUS) TISSUE
Structure
Collagenous fibers and some elastic fibers, tightly packed into parallel bundles,
   with only fibroblast cells
Location and Function
Forms strong tendons of muscle, ligaments of joints, some fibrous membranes,
   and fascia that surrounds organs and muscles

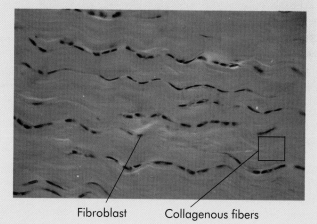

Fibroblast   Collagenous fibers

Dense, Regular (White Fibrous) Connective Tissue. (Copyright Phototake. Used with permission.)

Continued

BOX 1-4 CONNECTIVE TISSUES—cont'd

ELASTIC TISSUE

Structure

Elastic fibers, some collagenous fibers, fibroblasts

Location and Function

Lends strength and elasticity to walls of arteries, trachea, vocal cords, and other structures

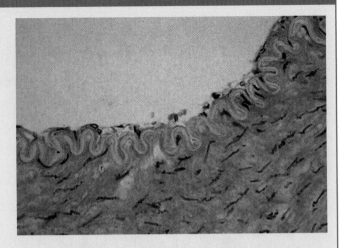

Elastic Connective Tissue. (From Erlandsen SL, Magney JE: *Color atlas of histology*, St Louis, 1992, Mosby.)

ADIPOSE TISSUE

Structure

Fat cells dispersed in loose tissues; each cell containing a large droplet of fat flattens nucleus and forces cytoplasm into a ring around cell's periphery

Location and Function

Stores fat, which provides padding and protection

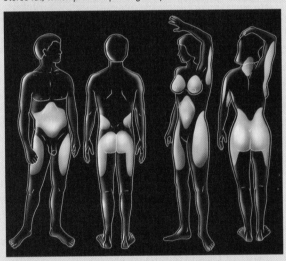

A

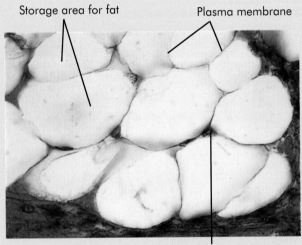

Storage area for fat

Plasma membrane

B

Nucleus of adipose cell

Adipose Tissue. A, Fat storage areas—distribution of fat in male and female bodies. **B,** Photomicrograph of adipose tissue. (**A** from Thibodeau GA, Patton KT: *Anatomy & physiology*, ed 6, St Louis, 2007, Mosby; **B** Copyright Ed Reschke. Used with permission.)

BOX 1-4   CONNECTIVE TISSUES—cont'd

CARTILAGE (HYALINE, ELASTIC, FIBROUS)
Structure
Collagenous fibers embedded in a firm matrix (chondrin); no blood supply
Location and Function
Gives form, support, and flexibility to joints, trachea, nose, ear, vertebral disks, embryonic skeleton, and many internal structures

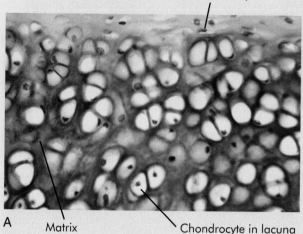

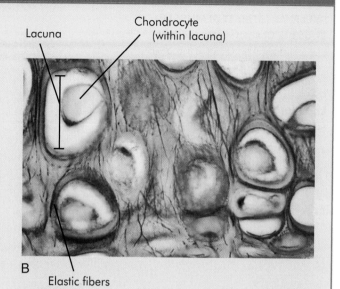

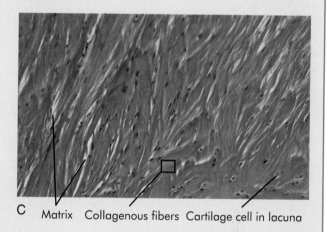

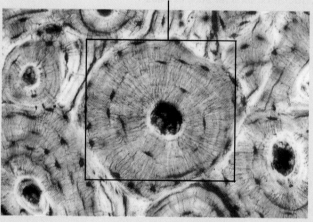

Cartilage. A, Hyaline cartilage. **B,** Elastic cartilage. **C,** Fibrous cartilage. (**A** and **C** copyright Robert L. Calentine; **B** copyright Ed Reshke. Used with permission.)

BONE
Structure
Rigid connective tissue consisting of cells, fibers, ground substances, and minerals
Location and Function
Lends skeleton rigidity and strength

SPECIAL CONNECTIVE TISSUES
Plasma
Structure
Fluid
Location and Function
Serves as matrix for blood cells

Macrophages in Tissue, Reticuloendothelial, or Macrophage System
Structure
Scattered macrophages (phagocytes) called Kupffer's cells (in liver), alveolar macrophages (in lungs), microglia (in central nervous system)
Location and Function
Facilitate inflammatory response and carry out phagocytosis in loose connective, lymphatic, digestive, medullary (bone marrow), splenic, adrenal, and pituitary tissues

Bone. (Copyright Phototake. Used with permission.)

BOX 1-5 MUSCLE TISSUES

SKELETAL (STRIATED) MUSCLE
Structure Characteristics of Cells

Long, cylindrical cells that extend throughout
  length of muscles
Striated myofibrils (proteins)
Many nuclei on periphery

Location

Attached to bones directly or by tendons

Function

Voluntary movement of skeleton;
  maintenance of posture

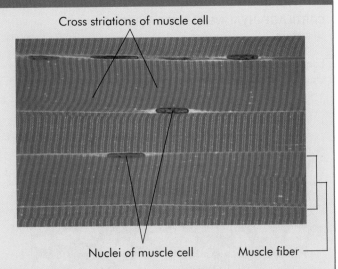

Skeletal (Striated) Muscle. (From Thibodeau GA, Patton KT:
Anatomy & physiology, ed 6, St Louis, 2007, Mosby.)

CARDIAC MUSCLE
Structure Characteristics of Cells

Branching networks throughout muscle tissue
Striated myofibrils

Location

Cells attached end-to-end at intercalated disks;
  tissue forms walls of heart (myocardium)

Function

Involuntary pumping action of
  heart

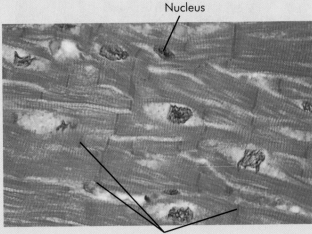

Cardiac Muscle. (Copyright Ed Reschke. Used with permission.)

SMOOTH (VISCERAL) MUSCLE
Structure Characteristics of Cells

Long spindles that taper to a point
Absence of striated myofibrils

Location

Walls of hollow internal structures, such as
  digestive tract and blood vessels (viscera)

Function

Voluntary and involuntary contractions that move substances
  through hollow structures

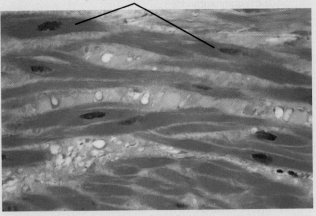

Smooth (Visceral) Muscle. (Copyright Phototake. Used with
permission.)

DID YOU UNDERSTAND?

Cellular Functions

1. Cells become specialized through the process of differentiation or maturation.
2. The eight specialized cellular functions are movement, conductivity, metabolic absorption, secretion, excretion, respiration, reproduction, and communication.

Structure and Function of Cellular Components

1. The eukaryotic cell consists of three general components: the plasma membrane, the cytoplasm, and the intracellular organelles.
2. The nucleus is the largest membrane-bound organelle and is found usually in the cell's center. The chief functions of the nucleus are cell division and control of genetic information.
3. Cytoplasm, or the cytoplasmic matrix, is an aqueous solution (cytosol) that fills the space between the nucleus and the plasma membrane.
4. The organelles are suspended in the cytoplasm and are enclosed in biologic membranes.
5. The endoplasmic reticulum is a network of tubular channels (cisternae) that extend throughout the outer nuclear membrane. It specializes in the synthesis and transport of protein and lipid components of most of the organelles.
6. The Golgi complex is a network of smooth membranes and vesicles located near the nucleus. The Golgi complex is responsible for processing and packaging proteins into secretory vesicles that break away from the Golgi complex and migrate to a variety of intracellular and extracellular destinations, including the plasma membrane.
7. Lysosomes are saclike structures that originate from the Golgi complex and contain digestive enzymes. These enzymes are responsible for digesting most cellular substances to their basic form, such as amino acids, fatty acids, and sugars.
8. Cellular injury leads to a release of the lysosomal enzymes, causing cellular self-digestion.
9. Peroxisomes are similar to lysosomes but contain several enzymes that either produce or use hydrogen peroxide.
10. Mitochondria contain the metabolic machinery necessary for cellular energy metabolism. The enzymes of the respiratory chain (electron-transport chain), found in the inner membrane of the mitochondria, generate most of the cell's ATP.
11. The cytoskeleton is the "bone and muscle" of the cell. The internal skeleton is composed of a network of protein filaments, including microtubules and actin filaments (microfilaments).
12. The plasma membrane encloses the cell and, by controlling the movement of substances across it, exerts a powerful influence on metabolic pathways.
13. Protein receptors (recognition units) on the plasma membrane enable the cell to interact with other cells and with extracellular substances.
14. The plasma membrane is a bilayer of lipids (phospholipids, glycolipids) and cholesterol, which gives the membrane its structural integrity.
15. Membrane functions are determined largely by proteins. These functions include recognition by protein receptors and transport of substances into and out of the cell.
16. The fluid mosaic model accounts for the fluidity of the lipid bilayer and the flexibility, self-sealing properties, and selective impermeability of the plasma membrane. The model has been updated.
17. Cellular receptors are protein molecules on the plasma membrane, in the cytoplasm, or in the nucleus that are capable of recognizing and binding smaller molecules, called *ligands.*
18. The dynamic nature of the fluid plasma membrane enables it to vary the number of receptors on its surface. Altering receptor number and pattern is related to disease states.

19. The ligand-receptor complex initiates a series of protein interactions, causing adenylate cyclase to catalyze the transformation of cellular ATP to messenger molecules that stimulate specific responses within the cell.

Cell-to-Cell Adhesions

1. Cell-to-cell adhesions are formed on plasma membranes, thereby allowing the formation of tissues and organs. Cells are held together by three different means: (1) the extracellular membrane, (2) cell adhesion molecules in the cell's plasma membrane, and (3) specialized cell junctions.
2. The extracellular matrix includes three groups of macromolecules: (1) fibrous structural proteins (collagen and elastin), (2) adhesive glycoproteins, and (3) proteoglycans and hyaluronic acid. The matrix helps regulate cell growth, movement, and differentiation.
3. The three major types of cell junctions are desmosomes, tight junctions, and gap junctions.

Cellular Communication and Signal Transduction

1. Cells communicate in three main ways: (1) they form protein channels (gap junctions); (2) they display receptors that affect intracellular processes or other cells in direct physical contact; and (3) they use receptor proteins *inside* the target cell.
2. Primary modes of intercellular signaling include contact-dependent, paracrine, hormonal, neurohormonal, and neurotransmitter.
3. Signal transduction involves signals or instructions from extracellular chemical messengers that are conveyed to the cell's interior for execution.

Cellular Metabolism

1. The chemical tasks of maintaining essential cellular functions are referred to as *cellular metabolism.* Anabolism is the energy-using process of metabolism, whereas catabolism is the energy-releasing process.
2. Adenosine triphosphate (ATP) functions as an energy-transferring molecule. Energy is stored by molecules of carbohydrate, lipid, and protein, which, when catabolized, transfer energy to ATP.
3. Oxidative phosphorylation occurs in the mitochondria and is the mechanism by which the energy produced from carbohydrates, fats, and proteins is transferred to ATP.

Membrane Transport: Cellular Intake and Output

1. Water and small, electrically uncharged molecules move through pores in the plasma membrane's lipid bilayer in the process called *passive transport.*
2. Passive transport does not require the expenditure of energy; rather, it is driven by the physical effects of osmosis, hydrostatic pressure, and diffusion.
3. Larger molecules and molecular complexes (e.g., ligand-receptor complexes) are moved into the cell by active transport, which requires the cell to expend energy (by means of ATP).
4. The largest molecules (macromolecules) and fluids are transported by the processes of endocytosis (ingestion) and exocytosis (expulsion).
5. Two types of solutes exist in body fluids: electrolytes and nonelectrolytes. Electrolytes are electrically charged and dissociate into constituent ions when placed in solution. Nonelectrolytes do not dissociate when placed in solution.
6. Diffusion is the passive movement of a solute from an area of higher solute concentration to an area of lower solute concentration.
7. Filtration is the measurement of water and solutes through a membrane because of a greater pushing pressure.
8. Hydrostatic pressure is the mechanical force of water pushing against cellular membranes.

DID YOU UNDERSTAND?—cont'd

9. Osmosis is the movement of water across a semipermeable membrane from a region of lower solute concentration to a region of higher solute concentration.

10. The amount of hydrostatic pressure required to oppose the osmotic movement of water is called the *osmotic pressure of the solution*.

11. The overall osmotic effect of colloids, such as plasma proteins, is called the *oncotic pressure* or *colloid osmotic pressure*.

12. Mediated transport can be passive or active. Mediated transport includes the movement of two molecules simultaneously in one direction (symport) or in opposite directions (antiport) or the movement of a single molecule in one direction (uniport).

13. Passive mediated transport is also called *facilitated diffusion*. It does not require the expenditure of metabolic energy.

14. Active mediated transport requires metabolic energy (ATP) to move molecules against the concentration gradient.

15. Active transport occurs also by endocytosis, or vesicle formation, in which the substance to be transported is engulfed by a segment of the plasma membrane, forming a vesicle that moves into the cell.

16. Pinocytosis is a type of endocytosis in which fluids and solute molecules are ingested through formation of small vesicles.

17. Phagocytosis is a type of endocytosis in which large particles, such as bacteria, are ingested through formation of large vesicles, called *vacuoles*.

18. In receptor-mediated endocytosis, the plasma membrane receptors are clustered, along with bristlelike structures, in specialized areas called *coated pits*.

19. Endocytosis occurs when coated pits invaginate, internalizing ligand-receptor complexes in coated vesicles.

20. Inside the cell, lysosomal enzymes process and digest material ingested by endocytosis.

21. Caveolae are cavelike pits, and are involved in transport and cell communication.

22. All body cells are electrically polarized, with the inside of the cell more negatively charged than the outside. The difference in voltage across the plasma membrane is the resting membrane potential.

23. When an excitable (nerve or muscle) cell receives an electrochemical stimulus, cations enter the cell, causing a rapid change in the resting membrane potential known as the *action potential*. The action potential "moves" along the cell's plasma membrane and is transmitted to an adjacent cell. This is how electrochemical signals convey information from cell to cell.

Cellular Reproduction: The Cell Cycle

1. Cellular reproduction in body tissues involves mitosis (nuclear division) and cytokinesis (cytoplasmic division).

2. Only mature cells are capable of division. Maturation occurs during a stage of cellular life called *interphase (growth phase)*.

3. The cell cycle is the reproductive process that begins after interphase in all tissues with cellular turnover. There are four phases of the cell cycle: (1) the S phase, during which DNA synthesis takes place in the cell nucleus; (2) the G_2 phase, the period between the completion of DNA synthesis and the next phase (M); (3) the M phase, which involves both nuclear (mitotic) and cytoplasmic (cytokinetic) division; and (4) the G_1 phase (growth phase), after which the cycle begins again.

4. The M phase (mitosis) involves four stages: prophase, metaphase, anaphase, and telophase.

5. The mechanisms that control cell division depend on "social control genes" and protein growth factors.

Tissues

1. Cells of one or more types are organized into tissues, and different types of tissues compose organs. Organs are organized to function as tracts or systems.

2. Three key factors that maintain the cellular organization of tissues are (a) recognition and cell communication, (b) selective cell-to-cell adhesion, and (c) memory.

3. Tissue cells are linked at cell junctions, which are specialized regions on their plasma membranes called *desmosomes, tight junctions,* and *gap junctions*. Cell junctions attach adjacent cells and allow small molecules to pass between them.

4. The four basic types of tissues are epithelial, muscle, nerve, and connective tissues.

5. Neural tissue is composed of highly specialized cells called neurons that receive and transmit electrical impulses rapidly across junctions called *synapses*.

6. Epithelial tissue covers most internal and external surfaces of the body. The functions of epithelial tissue include protection, absorption, secretion, and excretion.

7. Connective tissue binds various tissues and organs together, supporting them in their locations and serving as storage sites for excess nutrients.

8. Muscle tissue is composed of long, thin, highly contractile cells or fibers called *myocytes*. Muscle tissue that is attached to bones enables voluntary movement. Muscle tissue in internal organs enables involuntary movement, such as the heartbeat.

KEY TERMS

- Absolute refractory period   22
- Action potential   22
- Active mediated transport   18
- Active transport   15
- Amphipathic   3
- Anabolism   13
- Anaphase   23
- Anion   15
- Antiport   17
- Arrested (resting) (G_0) state   24
- Autocrine signaling   11
- Basement membrane   8
- Catabolism   13
- Cation   15
- Caveolae   3
- Caveolin
- Cell adhesion molecule (CAM)   6
- Cell cycle   23
- Cell junction   9
- Cell-to-cell adhesion   8
- Cellular metabolism   13
- Cellular receptor   7
- Centromere   23
- Chemical synapse   11
- Chromatid   23
- Chromatin   23
- Citric acid cycle (Krebs cycle, tricarboxylic acid cycle)   13
- Clathrin   21
- Coated pit   21
- Collagen   9
- Competitive inhibitor   17
- Concentration gradient   15
- Connective tissue   9
- Connexon   9
- Cytokinesis   22
- Cytoplasm   3
- Cytoplasmic matrix   3
- Cytosol   3
- Daughter cell   23
- Depolarization   22
- Desmosome   9
- Differentiation   2
- Diffusion   15
- Digestion   13
- Effective osmolality   16
- Elastin   9
- Electrolyte   15
- Electron-transport chain   13
- Endocytosis   20
- Equatorial plate (metaphase plate)   23
- Eukaryote   1
- Exocytosis   20
- Extracellular matrix   8
- Fibroblast   9
- Fibronectin   9
- Filtration   15
- Fluid mosaic model   6
- G_1 phase   23
- G_2 phase   23
- Gap junction   9
- Gating   9
- Glycolysis   13
- Glycoprotein   6
- Growth factor (cytokine)   23
- Homeostasis   9
- Hormonal signaling   11
- Hydrostatic pressure   15
- Hyperpolarized state   22
- Hypertonic solution   17
- Hypopolarized state   22
- Hypotonic solution   17
- Integral membrane protein   3
- Interphase   23
- Ion   15
- Isotonic solution   17
- Junctional complex   9
- Ligand   7
- M phase   23
- Macromolecule   9
- Mediated transport   17
- Metabolic pathway   13
- Metaphase   23
- Mitosis   22
- Neurohormonal signaling   11
- Neurotransmitter   11
- Nuclear envelope   3
- Nucleolus   3
- Nucleus   3
- Oncotic pressure (colloid osmotic pressure)   16
- Organelle   3
- Osmolality   16
- Osmolarity   16
- Osmosis   16
- Osmotic pressure   16
- Oxidation   13
- Oxidative phosphorylation   13
- Paracrine signaling   11
- Passive mediated transport (facilitated diffusion)   17
- Passive transport   14
- Pattern formation   24
- Peripheral membrane protein   5
- Phagocytosis   20
- Pinocytosis   20
- Plasma membrane (plasmalemma)   3
- Plasma membrane receptor   8
- Platelet-derived growth factor (PDGF)   24
- Polarity   15
- Polypeptide   3
- Prokaryote   2
- Prophase   23
- Protein   3
- Receptor protein   13
- Receptor-mediated endocytosis (ligand internalization)   21
- Relative refractory period   22
- Repolarization   22
- Resting membrane potential   21
- Retinoblastoma (Rb) protein   24
- S phase   23
- Signal transduction pathway   11
- Signaling cell   11
- Solute   15
- Spindle fiber   23
- Stroma   24
- Substrate   13
- Substrate phosphorylation (anaerobic glycolysis)   14
- Symport   17
- Target cell   13
- Telophase   23
- Threshold potential   22
- Tight junction   9
- Tonicity   17
- Transfer reaction   13
- Transport protein (transporter)   17
- Uniport   17
- Valence   15

REFERENCES

1. Alberts B, et al: *Molecular biology of the cell,* ed 5, New York, 2008, Garland.
2. Catt KJ, et al: Hormonal regulation of peptide receptors and target cell responses, *Nature* 280(5718):109–116, 1979.
3. LaPorte SL, et al: Molecular and structural basis of cytokine receptor pleiotrophy in the interleukin-4/13 system, *Cell* 132:259–272, 2008.
4. Kiss AL, et al: Oestrogen-mediated tyrosine phosphorylation of caveolin-1 and its effect on the oestrogen receptor localization: an in vivo study, *Mol Cell Endocrinol* 245(1-2):128–137, 2005.
5. Jorde LB, et al: *Medical genetics,* ed 4, St Louis, 2010, Mosby.

2

Genes and Genetic Diseases

Lynn B. Jorde

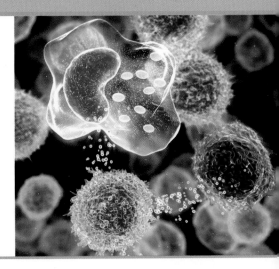

Genetics occupies a central position in the entire study of biology. An understanding of genetics is essential to study human, animal, plant, or microbial life. Genetics is the study of biologic inheritance. In the nineteenth century, microscopic studies of cells led scientists to suspect that the nucleus of the cell contained the important mechanisms of inheritance. Scientists found that chromatin, the substance that gives the nucleus a granular appearance, is observable in nondividing cells. Just before the cell divides, the chromatin condenses to form discrete, dark-staining organelles, which are called **chromosomes.** (Cell division is discussed in Chapter 1.) With the rediscovery of Mendel's important breeding experiments at the turn of the twentieth century, it soon became apparent that the chromosomes contained **genes,** the basic units of inheritance (Figure 2-1).

  The primary constituent of chromatin is **deoxyribonucleic acid (DNA)**. Genes are composed of sequences of DNA. By serving as

the blueprints of proteins in the body, genes ultimately influence all aspects of body structure and function. Estimates suggest that there are approximately 20,000 to 25,000 genes. An error in one of these genes often leads to a recognizable genetic disease.

  To date, more than 20,000 genetic traits and diseases have been identified and cataloged. As infectious diseases continue to be more effectively controlled, the proportion of beds in pediatric hospitals occupied by children with genetic diseases has risen. In addition, many common diseases that primarily affect adults, such as hypertension, coronary heart disease, diabetes, and cancer, are now known to have important genetic components.

  Great progress is being made in the diagnosis of genetic diseases and in the understanding of genetic mechanisms underlying them. With the huge strides being made in molecular genetics, "gene therapy"—the utilization of normal genes to correct genetic disease—has begun.

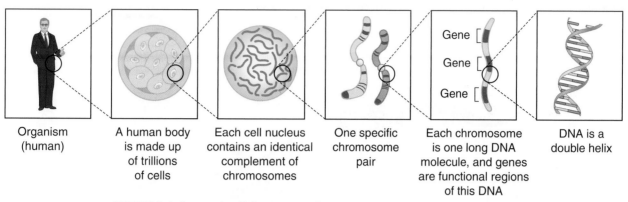

Organism (human)

A human body is made up of trillions of cells

Each cell nucleus contains an identical complement of chromosomes

One specific chromosome pair

Each chromosome is one long DNA molecule, and genes are functional regions of this DNA

DNA is a double helix

FIGURE 2-1 Successive Enlargements from a Human to the Genetic Material.

DNA, RNA, AND PROTEINS: HEREDITY AT THE MOLECULAR LEVEL

Definitions

Composition and Structure of DNA

Genes are composed of DNA, which has three basic components: the five-carbon monosaccharide deoxyribose; a phosphate molecule; and four types of nitrogenous bases. Two of the bases, **cytosine** and **thymine,** are single carbon-nitrogen rings called **pyrimidines.** The other two bases, **adenine** and **guanine,** are double carbon-nitrogen rings called **purines.** The four bases are commonly represented by their first letters: A, C, T, and G.

Watson and Crick demonstrated how these molecules are physically assembled as DNA, proposing the **double-helix model,** in which DNA appears like a twisted ladder with chemical bonds as its rungs (Figure 2-2). The two sides of the ladder consist of deoxyribose and phosphate molecules, united by strong phosphodiester bonds. Projecting from each side of the ladder, at regular intervals, are the nitrogenous bases. The base projecting from one side is bound to the base projecting from the other by a weak hydrogen bond. Therefore the nitrogenous bases form the rungs of the ladder; adenine pairs with thymine, and guanine pairs with cytosine. Each DNA subunit—consisting of one deoxyribose molecule, one phosphate group, and one base—is called a **nucleotide.**

DNA as the Genetic Code

DNA directs the synthesis of all the body's proteins. Proteins are composed of one or more **polypeptides** (intermediate protein compounds), which are in turn consist of sequences of **amino acids.** The body contains 20 different types of amino acids; they are specified by the 4 nitrogenous bases. To specify (code for) 20 different amino acids with only 4 bases, different combinations of bases, occurring in groups of 3, are used. These triplets of bases are known as **codons.** Each codon specifies a single amino acid in a corresponding protein. Because there are 64 (4 × 4 × 4) possible codons but only 20 amino acids, there are many cases in which several codons correspond to the same amino acid.

The genetic code is universal: *all* living organisms use precisely the same DNA codes to specify proteins except for mitochondria, the cytoplasmic organelles in which cellular respiration takes place (see Chapter 1)—they have their own extranuclear DNA. Several codons of mitochondrial DNA encode different amino acids, as compared to the same nuclear DNA codons.

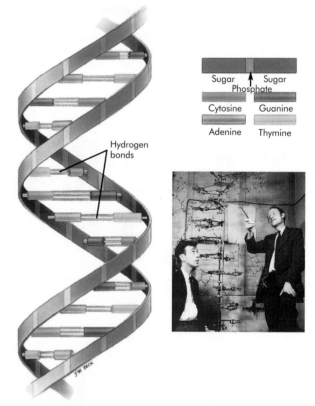

Hydrogen bonds

Sugar   Sugar
Phosphate
Cytosine   Guanine
Adenine   Thymine

FIGURE 2-2 Watson-Crick Model of the DNA Molecule. The DNA structure illustrated here is based on that published by James Watson *(left)* and Francis Crick *(photograph, right)* in 1953. Note that each side of the DNA molecule consists of alternating sugar and phosphate groups. Each sugar group is bonded to the sugar group opposite it by a pair of nitrogenous bases (adenine-thymine or cytosine-guanine). The sequence of these pairs constitutes a genetic code that determines the structure and function of a cell. (From Thibodeau GA, Patton KT: *Anatomy & physiology,* ed 6, St Louis, 2007, Mosby.)

Replication of DNA

DNA replication consists of breaking the weak hydrogen bonds between the bases, leaving a single strand with each base unpaired. The consistent pairing of adenine with thymine and of guanine with cytosine, known as **complementary base pairing,** is the key to accurate replication. The unpaired base attracts a free nucleotide only if

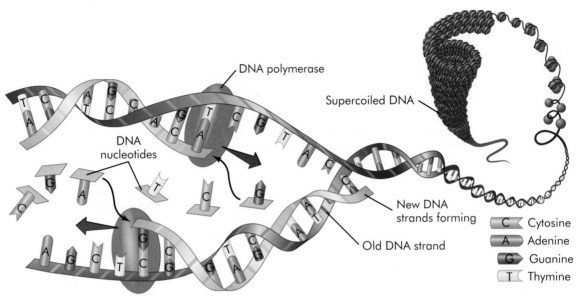

FIGURE 2-3 Replication of DNA. The two chains of the double helix separate, and each chain serves as the template for a new complementary chain. (From Patton KT, Thibodeau GA: *Anatomy & physiology,* ed 7, St Louis, 2010, Mosby.)

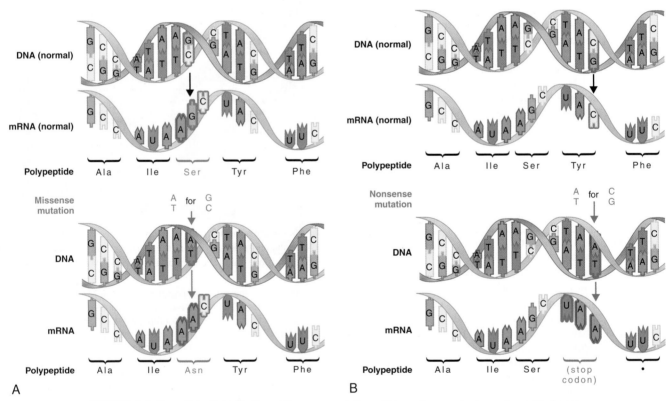

FIGURE 2-4 Base Pair Substitution. Missense mutations **(A)** produce a single amino acid change, whereas nonsense mutations **(B)** produce a stop codon in the mRNA. Stop codons terminate translation of the polypeptide. (From Jorde L et al: *Medical genetics,* ed 4, St Louis, 2010, Mosby.)

the nucleotide has the proper complementary base. When replication is complete, a new double-stranded molecule identical to the original is formed (Figure 2-3). The single strand is said to be a **template,** or molecule on which a complementary molecule is built, and is the basis for synthesizing the new double strand.

Several different proteins are involved in DNA replication. The most important of these proteins is an enzyme known as **DNA polymerase.** This enzyme travels along the single DNA strand, adding the correct nucleotides to the free end of the new strand and checking to make sure that its base is actually complementary to the template base. This mechanism of DNA proofreading substantially enhances the accuracy of DNA replication.

Mutation

A **mutation** is any inherited alteration of genetic material. Mutations may cause disease or be subtle, silent substitutions that do not change amino acids. One type of mutation is the **base pair substitution,** in which one base pair replaces another. This replacement *can* result in a change in the amino acid sequence. However, because of the redundancy of the genetic code, many of these mutations do not change the amino acid sequence and thus have no consequence. Such mutations are called **silent mutations.** Base pair substitutions that alter amino acids consist of two basic types: **missense** mutations, which produce a change (i.e., the "sense") in a single amino acid; and **nonsense** mutations, which produce one of the three stop codons (UAA, UAG, or UGA) in the messenger RNA (mRNA) (Figure 2-4). Missense mutations (Figure 2-4, *A*) produce a single amino acid change, whereas nonsense mutations (Figure 2-4, *B*) produce a stop codon in the mRNA. Stop codons terminate translation of the polypeptide.

The **frameshift mutation** involves the insertion or deletion of one or more base pairs of the DNA molecule. As Figure 2-5 shows, these mutations change the entire "reading frame" of the DNA sequence because the deletion or insertion is not a multiple of three base pairs (the number of base pairs in a codon). Frameshift mutations can thus greatly alter the amino acid sequence. (*In-frame* insertions or deletions, in which a multiple of three bases is inserted or lost, tend to have less severe disease consequences than do frameshift mutations.)

Agents known as **mutagens** increase the frequency of mutations. Examples include radiation and chemicals such as nitrogen mustard, vinyl chloride, alkylating agents, formaldehyde, and sodium nitrite.

Mutations are rare events. The rate of **spontaneous mutations** (those occurring in the absence of exposure to known mutagens) in humans is about 10^{-4} to 10^{-7} per gene per generation. This rate varies from one gene to another. Some DNA sequences have particularly high mutation rates and are known as **mutational hot spots.**

From Genes to Proteins

DNA is formed and replicated in the cell nucleus, but protein synthesis takes place in the cytoplasm. The DNA code is transported from nucleus to cytoplasm, and subsequent protein is formed through two basic processes: transcription and translation. These processes are mediated by **ribonucleic acid (RNA),** which is chemically similar to DNA except that the sugar molecule is ribose rather than deoxyribose, and uracil rather than thymine is one of the four bases. The other bases of RNA, as in DNA, are adenine, cytosine, and guanine. Uracil is structurally similar to thymine, so it also can pair with adenine. Whereas DNA usually occurs as a double strand, RNA usually occurs as a single strand.

Transcription

In **transcription,** RNA is synthesized from a DNA template, forming **messenger RNA (mRNA). RNA polymerase** binds to a **promoter site,** a sequence of DNA that specifies the beginning of a gene. RNA polymerase then separates a portion of the DNA, exposing unattached DNA bases. One DNA strand then provides the template for the sequence of mRNA nucleotides.

The sequence of bases in the mRNA is thus complementary to the template strand, and except for the presence of uracil instead of thymine, the mRNA sequence is identical to the other DNA strand. Transcription continues until a **termination sequence,** codons that act as signals for the termination of protein synthesis, is reached. Then the RNA polymerase detaches from the DNA, and the transcribed mRNA is freed to move out of the nucleus and into the cytoplasm (Figures 2-6 and 2-7).

Gene Splicing

When the mRNA is first transcribed from the DNA template, it reflects exactly the base sequence of the DNA. In eukaryotes, many RNA sequences are removed by nuclear enzymes, and the remaining sequences are spliced together to form the functional mRNA that migrates to the cytoplasm. The excised sequences are called **introns** (intervening sequences), and the sequences that are left to code for proteins are called **exons.**

Translation

In **translation,** RNA directs the synthesis of a polypeptide (see Figure 2-7), interacting with **transfer RNA (tRNA),** a cloverleaf-shaped strand of about 80 nucleotides. The tRNA molecule has a site where an amino acid attaches. The three-nucleotide sequence at the opposite side of the cloverleaf is called the anticodon. It undergoes complementary base

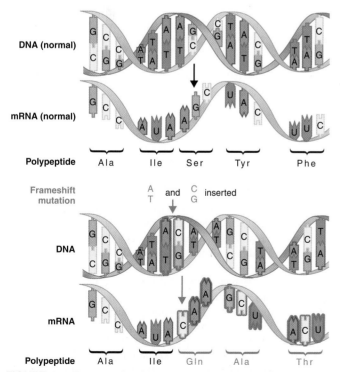

FIGURE 2-5 Frameshift Mutations. Frameshift mutations result from the addition or deletion of a number of bases that is not a multiple of three. This mutation alters all of the codons downstream from the site of insertion or deletion. (From Jorde L et al: *Medical genetics*, ed 4, St Louis, 2010, Mosby.)

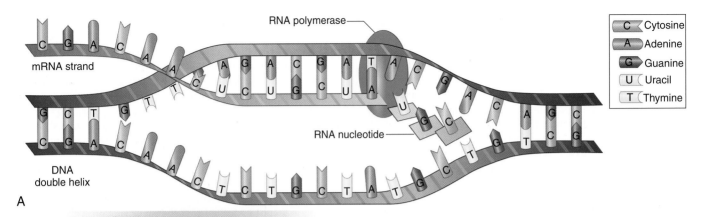

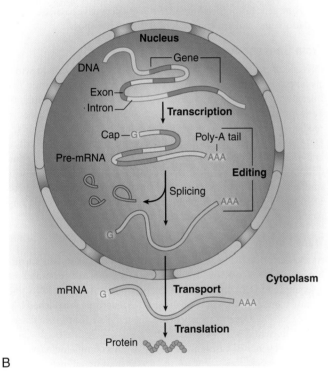

FIGURE 2-6 General Scheme of Ribonucleic Acid (RNA) Transcription. **A,** Transcription of messenger RNA (mRNA). A DNA molecule "unzips" in the region of the gene to be transcribed. RNA nucleotides already present in the nucleus temporarily attach themselves to exposed DNA bases along one strand of the unzipped DNA molecule according to the principle of complementary pairing. As the RNA nucleotides attach to the exposed DNA, they bind to each other and form a chainlike RNA strand called a *messenger RNA (mRNA)* molecule. Notice that the new mRNA strand is an exact copy of the base sequence on the opposite side of the DNA molecule. As in all metabolic processes, the formation of mRNA is controlled by an enzyme—in this case, the enzyme is called *RNA polymerase.* **B,** Editing of an mRNA transcript. (From Patton KT, Thibodeau GA: *Anatomy & physiology,* ed 7, St Louis, 2010, Mosby.)

pairing with an appropriate codon in the mRNA, which specifies the sequence of amino acids through tRNA.

The site of actual protein synthesis is in the **ribosome,** which consists of approximately equal parts of protein and **ribosomal RNA (rRNA).** During translation, the ribosome first binds to an initiation site on the mRNA sequence and then binds to its surface, so that base pairing can occur between tRNA and mRNA. The ribosome then moves along the mRNA sequence, processing each codon and translating an amino acid by way of the interaction of mRNA and tRNA.

The ribosome provides an enzyme that catalyzes the formation of covalent peptide bonds between the adjacent amino acids, resulting in a growing polypeptide. When the ribosome arrives at a termination signal on the mRNA sequence, translation and polypeptide formation cease; the mRNA, ribosome, and polypeptide separate from one another; and the polypeptide is released into the cytoplasm to perform its required function.

CHROMOSOMES

Human cells can be categorized into **gametes** (sperm and egg cells) and **somatic cells,** which include all cells other than gametes. Each somatic cell nucleus has 46 chromosomes in 23 pairs (Figure 2-8). These are **diploid cells,** and the individual's father and mother each donate one chromosome per pair. New somatic cells are formed through **mitosis** and **cytokinesis.** Gametes are **haploid cells:** they have only 1 member of each chromosome pair, for a total of 23 chromosomes. Haploid cells are formed from diploid cells by **meiosis** (Figure 2-9).

In 22 of the 23 chromosome pairs, the 2 members of each pair are virtually identical in microscopic appearance: thus they are **homologous.** These 22 chromosome pairs are homologous in both males and females and are termed **autosomes.** The remaining pair of chromosomes, the sex chromosomes, consists of two homologous X chromosomes in females and a nonhomologous pair, X and Y, in males.

Figure 2-10, *A,* illustrates a **metaphase spread,** which is a photograph of the chromosomes as they appear in the nucleus of a somatic

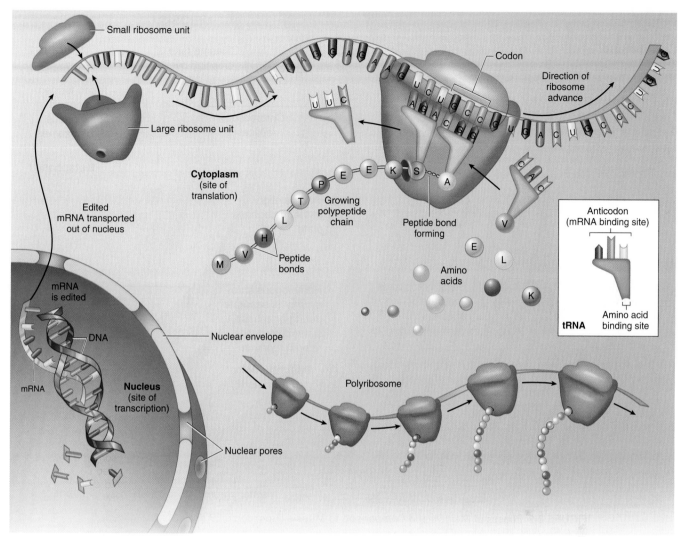

FIGURE 2-7 Protein Synthesis. (From Patton KT, Thibodeau GA: *Anatomy & physiology,* ed 7, St Louis, 2010, Mosby.)

DNA
The structure of DNA is similar to a twisted ladder, with base pairs forming the rungs. **Genes** are composed of DNA segments.

COILED DNA
The DNA in each cell would be about 6 feet long if stretched out. To fit inside the cell, the DNA is tightly coiled.

CHROMOSOMES
One chromosome of every pair is from each parent.

NUCLEUS
Each nucleus of a somatic cell contains 46 chromosomes arranged in 23 pairs.

CELLS
A nucleus resides in most human cells.

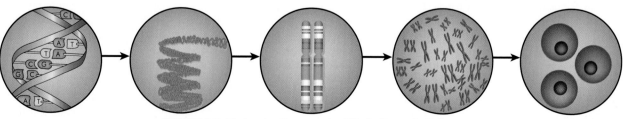

FIGURE 2-8 Molecular Parts to the Whole Somatic Cell.

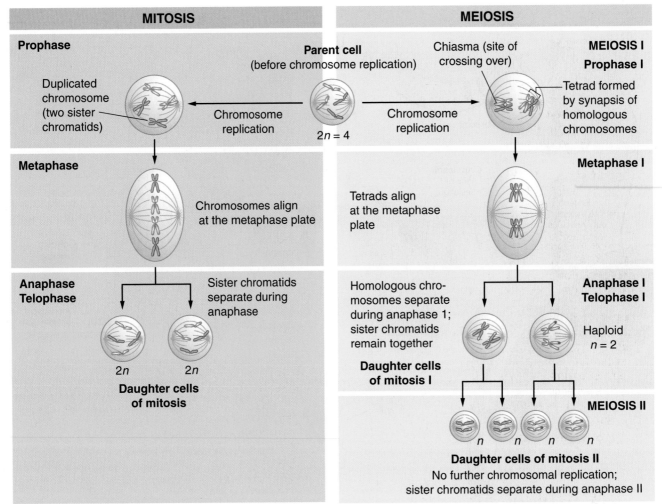

FIGURE 2-9 Phases of Meiosis and Comparison to Mitosis (From Jorde LB et al: *Medical genetics,* ed 4, St Louis, 2010, Mosby.)

cell during metaphase. (Chromosomes are easiest to visualize during this stage of mitosis.) In Figure 2-10, *B*, the chromosomes are arranged according to size, with the homologous chromosomes paired (this is now typically done by a computer). The 22 autosomes are numbered according to length, with chromosome number 1 the longest and chromosome 22 the shortest. A karyotype, or karyogram, is an ordered display of chromosomes. Some natural variation in relative chromosome length can be expected from person to person, so it is not always possible to distinguish each chromosome by its length. Therefore the position of the centromere also is used to classify chromosomes (Figure 2-11).

The chromosomes in Figure 2-10 were stained with Giemsa stain, resulting in distinctive chromosome bands. These form various patterns in the different chromosomes so that each chromosome can be distinguished easily. Using banding techniques, researchers can number chromosomes and study individual variations. Missing or duplicated portions of chromosomes, which often result in serious diseases, also are readily identified. More recently, techniques have been devised that permit each chromosome to be visualized with a different color.

Chromosome Aberrations and Associated Diseases

Chromosome abnormalities are the leading known cause of mental retardation and miscarriage. Estimates indicate that a major chromosome aberration occurs in at least 1 in 12 conceptions. Most of these fetuses do not survive to term; about 50% of all recovered first-trimester spontaneous abortuses have major chromosome aberrations.[1] The number of live births affected by these abnormalities is, however, significant; approximately 1 in 150 has a major diagnosable chromosome abnormality.[1]

Polyploidy

Cells with a multiple of the normal number of chromosomes are euploid cells (Greek *eu* = good or true). Because normal gametes are haploid and most normal somatic cells are diploid, they are both euploid forms. When a euploid cell has more than the diploid number of chromosomes, it is said to be a polyploid cell. Several types of body tissues, including some liver, bronchial, and epithelial tissues, are normally polyploid. A zygote that has three copies of each chromosome, rather than the usual two, has a form of polyploidy called triploidy. Tetraploidy, a condition in which euploid cells have 92 chromosomes,

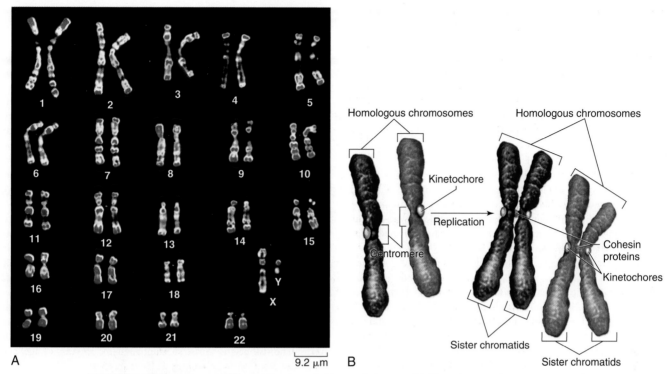

FIGURE 2-10 Karyotype of Chromosomes. A, Human karyotype. **B,** Homologous chromosomes and sister chromatids. (From Raven PH et al: *Biology,* ed 8, New York, 2008, McGraw-Hill.)

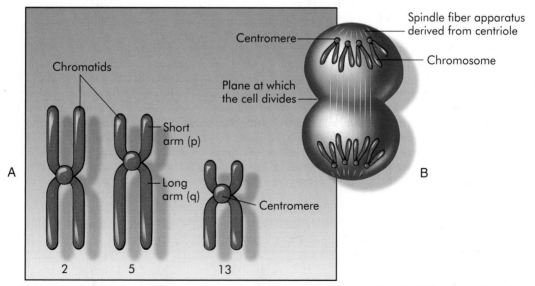

FIGURE 2-11 Structure of Chromosomes. A, Human chromosomes 2, 5, and 13. Each is replicated and consists of two chromatids. Chromosome 2 is a metacentric chromosome because the centromere is close to the middle; chromosome 5 is submetacentric because the centromere is set off from the middle; chromosome 13 is acrocentric because the centromere is at or very near the end. **B,** During mitosis, the centromere divides and the chromosomes move to opposite poles of the cell. At the time of centromere division, the chromatids are designated as chromosomes.

has been observed also. Both of these conditions are incompatible with postnatal survival. Nearly all triploid fetuses are spontaneously aborted or stillborn. The prevalence of triploidy among live births is approximately 1 in 10,000. Tetraploidy has been found primarily in early abortuses, although occasionally affected infants have been born alive. Like triploid infants, however, they do not survive. Triploidy and tetraploidy are relatively common conditions, accounting for approximately 10% of all known miscarriages.[2]

Aneuploidy

A cell that does not contain a multiple of 23 chromosomes is an **aneuploid cell.** A cell containing three copies of one chromosome is said to be trisomic (a condition termed **trisomy**) and is aneuploid. Monosomy, the presence of only one copy of a given chromosome in a diploid cell, is the other common form of aneuploidy. Among the autosomes, monosomy of any chromosome is lethal, but newborns with trisomy of some chromosomes can survive. This difference illustrates an important principle: *in general, loss of chromosome material has more serious consequences than duplication of chromosome material.*

Aneuploidy of the sex chromosomes is less serious than that of the autosomes. Very little genetic material—only about 40 genes—is located on the Y chromosome. For the X chromosome, inactivation of extra chromosomes (see p. 51) largely diminishes their effect. A zygote bearing *no* X chromosome, however, will not survive.

Aneuploidy is usually the result of **nondisjunction,** an error in which homologous chromosomes or sister chromatids fail to separate normally during meiosis or mitosis (Figure 2-12). Nondisjunction produces some gametes that have two copies of a given chromosome and others that have no copies of the chromosome. When such gametes unite with normal haploid gametes, the resulting zygote is monosomic or trisomic for that chromosome. Occasionally, a cell can be monosomic or trisomic for more than one chromosome.

Autosomal aneuploidy. Trisomy can occur for any chromosome, but the only forms seen with an appreciable frequency in live births are trisomies of the thirteenth, eighteenth, or twenty-first chromosomes. Fetuses with most other chromosomal trisomies do not survive to term. Trisomy 16, for example, is the most common trisomy among abortuses, but it is not seen in live births.[3]

Partial trisomy, in which only an extra portion of a chromosome is present in each cell, can occur also. The consequences of partial trisomies are not as severe as those of complete trisomies. Trisomies may occur in only some cells of the body. Individuals thus affected are said to be **chromosomal mosaics,** meaning that the body has two or more different cell lines, each of which has a different karyotype. Mosaics are often formed by early mitotic nondisjunction occurring in one embryo cell but not in others.

The best-known example of aneuploidy in an autosome is trisomy of the twenty-first chromosome, which causes **Down syndrome** (named after J. Langdon Down, who first described the disease in 1866). Down syndrome is seen in approximately 1 in 800 to 1 in 1000 live births[4]; its principal features are shown and outlined in Figure 2-13 and Table 2-1.

The risk of having a child with Down syndrome increases greatly with maternal age. As Figure 2-14 demonstrates, women younger than 30 years have a risk ranging from about 1 in 1000 births to 1 in 2000 births. The risk begins to rise substantially after 35 years of age, and it reaches 3% to 5% for women older than 45 years. This dramatic increase in risk is caused by the age of maternal egg cells, which are held in an arrested state of prophase I from the time they are formed in the female embryo until they are shed in ovulation. Thus an egg cell formed by a 45-year-old woman is itself 45 years old. This long suspended state may allow defects to accumulate in the cellular proteins responsible for meiosis, leading to nondisjunction. The risk of Down syndrome, as well as other trisomies, does not increase with paternal age.[4]

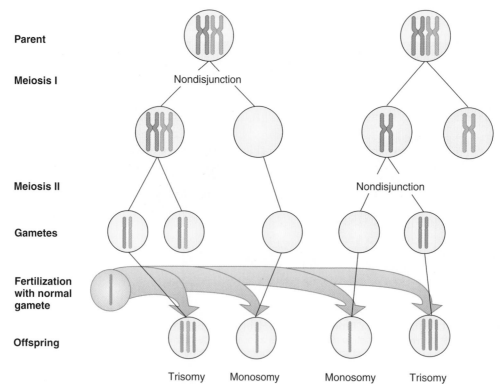

FIGURE 2-12 Nondisjunction. Nondisjunction causes aneuploidy when chromosomes or sister chromatids fail to divide properly. (From Jorde LB et al: *Medical genetics,* ed 4, St Louis, 2010, Mosby.)

Sex chromosome aneuploidy. The incidence of sex chromosome aneuploidies is fairly high. Among live births, about 1 in 500 males and 1 in 900 females have a form of sex chromosome aneuploidy.[5] Because these conditions are generally less severe than autosomal aneuploidies, all forms except complete absence of any X chromosome material allow at least some individuals to survive.

One of the most common sex chromosome aneuploidies, affecting about 1 in 1000 newborn females, is trisomy X. Instead of two X chromosomes, these females have three X chromosomes in each cell. Most of these females have no overt physical abnormalities, although sterility, menstrual irregularity, or mental retardation is sometimes seen. Some females have four X chromosomes, and they are more often mentally retarded. Those with five or more X chromosomes generally have more severe mental retardation and various physical defects.

A condition that leads to somewhat more serious problems is the presence of a single X chromosome and no homologous X or Y chromosome, so that the individual has a total of 45 chromosomes. The

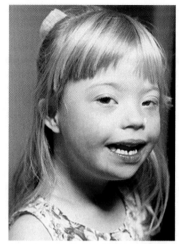

FIGURE 2-13 Child With Down Syndrome. (Courtesy Drs. A. Olney and M. MacDonald, University of Nebraska Medical Center, Omaha.)

TABLE 2-1 CHARACTERISTICS OF VARIOUS CHROMOSOME DISORDERS

DISEASE/DISORDER	FEATURES
Down Syndrome **Trisomy of Chromosome 21**	
IQ	Usually ranges from 20 to 70 (mental retardation)
Male/female findings	Virtually all males are sterile; some females can reproduce
Face	Distinctive: low nasal bridge, epicanthal folds, protruding tongue, low-set ears
Musculoskeletal system	Poor muscle tone (hypotonia), short stature
Systemic disorders	Congenital heart disease (one third to one half of cases), reduced ability to fight respiratory tract infections, increased susceptibility to leukemia—overall reduced survival rate; by age 40 years usually develop symptoms similar to those of Alzheimer disease
Mortality	About 76% of fetuses with Down syndrome abort spontaneously or are stillborn; 20% of infants die before age 10 years; those who live beyond 10 years have life expectancy of about 60 years
Causative factors	97% caused by nondisjunction during formation of one of parent's gametes or during early embryonic development; 3% result from translocations; in 95% of cases, nondisjunction occurs when mother's egg cell is formed; remainder involve paternal nondisjunction; 1% are mosaics—these have a large number of normal cells, and effects of trisomic cells are attenuated and symptoms are generally less severe
Turner Syndrome **(45,X) Monosomy of X Chromosome**	
IQ	Not considered retarded, although some impairment of spatial and mathematical reasoning ability is found
Male/female findings	Found only in females
Musculoskeletal system	Short stature common, characteristic webbing of neck, widely spaced nipples, reduced carrying angle at elbow
Systemic disorders	Coarctation (narrowing) of aorta, edema of feet in newborns, usually sterile and have gonadal streaks rather than ovaries; streaks are sometimes susceptible to cancer
Mortality	About 15-20% of spontaneous abortions with chromosome abnormalities have this karyotype, most common single-chromosome aberration; highly lethal during gestation, only about 0.5% of these conceptions survive to term
Causative factors	75% inherit X chromosome from mother, thus caused by meiotic error in father; frequency low compared with other sex chromosome aneuploidies (1:5000 newborn females); 50% have simple monosomy of X chromosome; remainder have more complex abnormalities; combinations of 45X cells with XX or XY cells common
Klinefelter Syndrome **(47,XXY) XXY Condition**	
IQ	Moderate degree of mental impairment may be present
Male/female findings	Have a male appearance but usually sterile; 50% develop female-like breasts (gynecomastia); occurs in 1:1000 male births
Face	Voice somewhat high pitched
Systemic disorders	Sparse body hair, sterile, testicles small
Causative factors	50% of cases the result of nondisjunction of X chromosomes in mother, frequency rises with increasing maternal age; also involves XXY and XXXY karyotypes with degree of physical and mental impairment increasing with each added X chromosome; mosaicism fairly common with most prevalent combination of XXY and XY cells

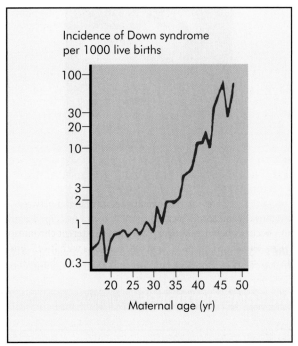

FIGURE 2-14 Down Syndrome Increases With Maternal Age. Rate is per 1000 live births related to maternal age.

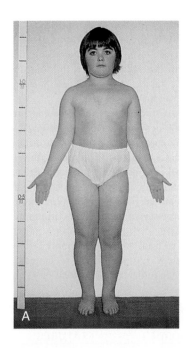

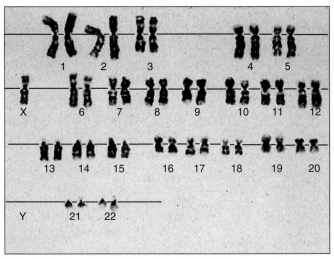

B

FIGURE 2-15 Turner Syndrome. A, A sex chromosome is missing, and the person's chromosomes are 45,X. Characteristic signs are short stature, female genitalia, webbed neck, shieldlike chest with underdeveloped breasts and widely spaced nipples, and imperfectly developed ovaries. **B,** As this karyotype shows, Turner syndrome results from monosomy of sex chromosomes (genotype XO). (From Patton KT, Thibodeau GA: *Anatomy & physiology*, ed 7, St Louis, 2010, Mosby.)

karyotype is usually designated 45,X, and it causes a set of symptoms known as **Turner syndrome** (Figure 2-15; see Table 2-1).

Individuals with at least two X chromosomes and one Y chromosome in each cell (47,XXY karyotype) have a disorder known as **Klinefelter syndrome** (Figure 2-16; see Table 2-1).

Abnormalities of Chromosome Structure

In addition to the loss or gain of whole chromosomes, parts of chromosomes can be lost or duplicated as gametes are formed, and the arrangement of genes on chromosomes can be altered. Unlike aneuploidy and polyploidy, these changes sometimes have no serious consequences for an individual's health. Some of them can even go entirely unnoticed, especially when very small pieces of chromosomes are involved. Nevertheless, abnormalities of chromosome structure can also produce serious disease in individuals or their offspring.

During meiosis and mitosis, chromosomes usually maintain their structural integrity, but **chromosome breakage** occasionally occurs. Mechanisms exist to "heal" these breaks and usually repair them perfectly with no damage to the daughter cell. However, some breaks remain or heal in a way that alters the chromosome's structure. The risk of chromosome breakage increases when harmful agents called **clastogens,** such as ionizing radiation, viral infections, or some chemicals, are present.

Deletions. Broken chromosomes and lost DNA cause **deletions** (Figure 2-17). Usually, a gamete with a deletion unites with a normal gamete to form a zygote. The zygote thus has one chromosome with the normal complement of genes and one with some missing genes. Because many genes can be lost in a deletion, serious consequences result even though one normal chromosome is present. The most often cited example of a disease caused by a chromosomal deletion is the **cri du chat syndrome.** The term literally means "cry of the cat" and describes the characteristic cry of the affected child.

Other symptoms include low birth weight, severe mental retardation, microcephaly (smaller than normal head size), and heart defects. The disease is caused by a deletion of part of the short arm of chromosome 5.

Duplications. A deficiency of genetic material is more harmful than an excess, so **duplications** usually have less serious consequences than deletions. For example, a deletion of a region of chromosome 5 causes cri du chat syndrome, but a duplication of the same region causes mental retardation but less serious physical defects.

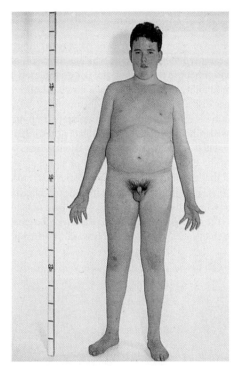

FIGURE 2-16 **Klinefelter Syndrome.** This young man exhibits many characteristics of Klinefelter syndrome: small testes, some development of the breasts, sparse body hair, and long limbs. This syndrome results from the presence of two or more X chromosomes with one Y chromosome (genotypes XXY or XXXY, for example). (From Patton KT, Thibodeau GA: *Anatomy & physiology*, ed 7, St Louis, 2010, Mosby.)

Inversions. An inversion occurs when two breaks take place on a chromosome, followed by the reinsertion of the missing fragment at its original site but in inverted order. Therefore a chromosome symbolized as ABCDEFG might become ABEDCFG after an inversion.

Unlike deletions and duplications, no loss or gain of genetic material occurs, so inversions are "balanced" alterations of chromosome structure, and they often have no apparent physical effect. Some genes are influenced by neighboring genes, however, and this position effect, a change in a gene's expression caused by its position, sometimes results in physical defects in these persons. Inversions can cause serious problems in the offspring of individuals carrying the inversion because the inversion can lead to duplications and deletions in the chromosomes transmitted to the offspring.

Translocations. The interchange of genetic material between nonhomologous chromosomes is called translocation. A reciprocal translocation occurs when breaks take place in two different chromosomes and the material is exchanged (Figure 2-18, *A*). As with inversions, the carrier of a reciprocal translocation is usually normal, but his or her offspring can have duplications and deletions.

A second and clinically more important type of translocation is robertsonian translocation. In this disorder, the long arms of two nonhomologous chromosomes fuse at the centromere, forming a single chromosome. Robertsonian translocations are confined to chromosomes 13, 14, 15, 21, and 22 because the short arms of these chromosomes are very small and contain no essential genetic material. The short arms are usually lost during subsequent cell divisions. Because the carriers of robertsonian translocations lose no important genetic material, they are normal, although they have only 45 chromosomes in each cell. Their offspring, however, may have serious monosomies or trisomies. For example, a common robertsonian translocation involves the fusion of the long arms of chromosomes 21 and 14. An offspring who inherits a gamete carrying the fused chromosome can receive an extra copy of the long arm of chromosome 21 and develop Down syndrome. Robertsonian translocations are responsible for approximately 3% to 5% of Down syndrome cases. Parents who carry a robertsonian translocation involving chromosome 21 have an increased risk for producing multiple offspring with Down syndrome.

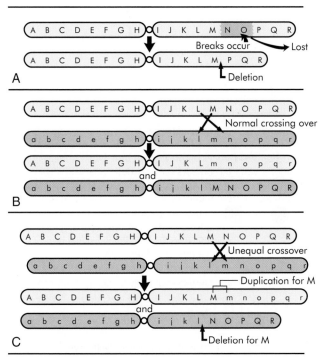

FIGURE 2-17 **Abnormalities of Chromosome Structure.** **A,** Deletion occurs when a chromosome segment is lost. **B,** Normal crossing over. **C,** The generation of duplication and deletion through unequal crossing over.

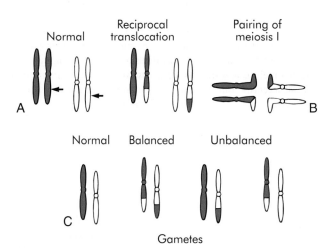

FIGURE 2-18 **Normal and Abnormal Chromosome Translocation.** **A,** Normal chromosomes and reciprocal translocation. **B,** Pairing at meiosis. **C,** Consequences of translocation in gametes; unbalanced gametes result in zygotes that are partially trisomic and partially monosomic and consequently develop abnormally.

Fragile sites. A number of areas on chromosomes develop distinctive breaks and gaps (observable microscopically) when the cells are cultured. Most of these fragile sites do not appear to be related to disease. However, one fragile site, located on the long arm of the X chromosome, is associated with *fragile X syndrome.* The most important feature of this syndrome is mental retardation. With a relatively high population prevalence (affecting approximately 1 in 4000 males and 1 in 8000 females), fragile X syndrome is the second most common genetic cause of mental retardation (after Down syndrome).

In fragile X syndrome, females who inherit the mutation do not necessarily express the disease condition but they can pass it on to descendants who do express it. Ordinarily, a male who inherits a disease gene on the X chromosome expresses the condition, because he has only one X chromosome. An uncommon feature of this disease is that about one third of carrier females are affected, although less severely than males. Unaffected transmitting males have been shown to have more than about 50 repeated DNA sequences near the beginning of the fragile X gene. These "repeats" consist of CGG sequences duplicated many times. Affected males have 230 or more.[6] Increased numbers of these repeated sequences in successive generations can lead to expression of fragile X syndrome. More than a dozen other genetic diseases, including Huntington disease and myotonic dystrophy, also are caused by this mechanism.[7]

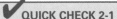

✔ QUICK CHECK 2-1
1. What is the major composition of DNA?
2. Define the terms mutation, autosomes, and sex chromosomes.
3. What is the significance of mRNA?
4. What is the significance of chromosomal translocation?

ELEMENTS OF FORMAL GENETICS

The mechanisms by which an individual's set of paired chromosomes produces traits are the principles of genetic inheritance. Mendel's work with garden peas first defined these principles. Later geneticists have refined Mendel's work to explain patterns of inheritance for traits and diseases that appear in families.

Analysis of traits that occur with defined, predictable patterns has helped geneticists link the pieces of the human gene map. Current research focuses on determining the protein products of each gene and understanding the way they contribute to disease. Eventually, diseases and defects caused by single genes can be traced and therapies to prevent and treat such diseases can be developed.

Traits caused by single genes are called mendelian traits (after Gregor Mendel). Each gene occupies a position along a chromosome known as a **locus.** The genes at a particular locus can have different forms (i.e., they can be composed of different nucleotide sequences) called **alleles.** A locus that has two or more alleles that each occur with an appreciable frequency in a population is said to be **polymorphic** (or a **polymorphism**).

Because humans are diploid organisms, each chromosome is represented twice, with one member of the chromosome pair contributed by the father and one by the mother. At a given locus, an individual has one allele whose origin is paternal and one whose origin is maternal. When the two alleles are identical, the individual is **homozygous** at that locus. When the alleles are not identical, the individual is **heterozygous** at that locus.

Phenotype and Genotype

The composition of genes at a given locus is known as the **genotype.** The outward appearance of an individual, which is the result of both genotype and environment, is the **phenotype.** For example, an infant who is born with an inability to metabolize the amino acid phenylalanine has the single-gene disorder known as phenylketonuria (PKU) and thus has the PKU genotype. If the condition is left untreated, abnormal metabolites of phenylalanine will begin to accumulate in the infant's brain and irreversible mental retardation will occur. Mental retardation is thus one aspect of the PKU phenotype. By imposing dietary restrictions to exclude food that contains phenylalanine, however, retardation can be prevented. Foods high in phenylalanine include proteins found in milk, dairy products, meat, fish, chicken, eggs, beans, and nuts. Although the child still has the PKU genotype, a modification of the environment (in this case, the child's diet) produces an outwardly normal phenotype.

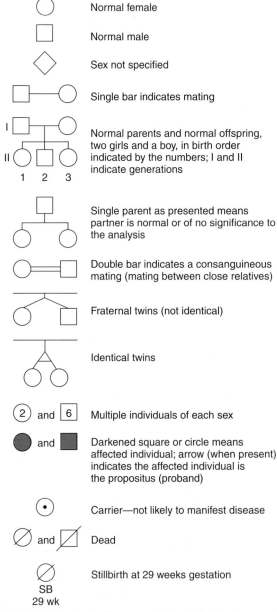

FIGURE 2-19 Symbols Commonly Used in Pedigrees. (From Jorde LB et al: *Medical genetics,* ed 4, St Louis, 2010, Mosby.)

Dominance and Recessiveness

In many loci, the effects of one allele mask those of another when the two are found together in a heterozygote. The allele whose effects are observable is said to be dominant. The allele whose effects are hidden is said to be recessive (from the Latin root for "hiding"). Traditionally, for loci having two alleles, the dominant allele is denoted by an uppercase letter and the recessive allele is denoted by a lowercase letter. When one allele is dominant over another, the heterozygote genotype *Aa* has the same phenotype as the dominant homozygote *AA*. For the recessive allele to be expressed, it must exist in the homozygote form, *aa*. When the heterozygote is distinguishable from both homozygotes, the locus is said to exhibit codominance.

A carrier is an individual who has a disease gene but is phenotypically normal. Many genes for a recessive disease occur in heterozygotes who carry one copy of the gene but do not express the disease. When recessive genes are lethal in the homozygous state, they are eliminated from the population when they occur in homozygotes. By "hiding" in carriers, however, recessive genes for diseases are passed on to the next generation.

TRANSMISSION OF GENETIC DISEASES

The pattern in which a genetic disease is inherited through generations is termed the mode of inheritance. Knowing the mode of inheritance can reveal much about the disease gene itself, and members of families with the disease can be given reliable genetic counseling.

Gregor Mendel systematically studied modes of inheritance and formulated two basic laws of inheritance. His principle of segregation states that homologous genes separate from one another during reproduction and that each reproductive cell carries only one homologous gene. Mendel's second law, the principle of independent assortment, states that the hereditary transmission of one gene does not affect the transmission of another. Mendel discovered these laws in the mid-nineteenth century by performing breeding experiments with garden peas, even though he had no knowledge of chromosomes. Early twentieth-century geneticists found that chromosomal behavior essentially corresponds to Mendel's laws, which now form the basis for the chromosome theory of inheritance.

The known single-gene diseases can be classified into four major modes of inheritance: autosomal dominant, autosomal recessive, X-linked dominant, and X-linked recessive. The first two types involve genes known to occur on the 22 pairs of autosomes. The last two types occur on the X chromosome; very few disease genes occur on the Y chromosome.

The pedigree chart summarizes family relationships and shows which members of a family are affected by a genetic disease (Figure 2-19). Generally, the pedigree begins with one individual in the family, the proband. This individual is usually the first person in the family diagnosed or seen in a clinic.

Autosomal Dominant Inheritance
Characteristics of Pedigrees

Diseases caused by autosomal dominant genes are rare, with the most common occurring in fewer than 1 in 500 individuals. Therefore it is uncommon for two individuals that are both affected by the same autosomal dominant disease to produce offspring together. Figure 2-20, *A*, illustrates this unusual pattern. Affected offspring are usually produced by the union of a normal parent with an affected heterozygous parent. The Punnett square in Figure 2-20, *B*, illustrates this mating. The affected parent can pass either a disease gene or a normal gene to the next generation. On average, half the children will be heterozygous and will express the disease, and half will be normal.

The pedigree in Figure 2-21 shows the transmission of an autosomal dominant gene. Several important characteristics of this pedigree support the conclusion that the trait is caused by an autosomal dominant gene:

1. The two sexes exhibit the trait in approximately equal proportions, and males and females are equally likely to transmit the trait to their offspring.
2. No generations are skipped. If an individual has the trait, one parent must also have it. If neither parent has the trait, none of the children have it (with the exception of new mutations, as discussed later).
3. Affected heterozygous individuals transmit the trait to approximately half their children, and because gamete transmission is subject to chance fluctuations, all or none of the children of an affected parent may have the trait. When large numbers of matings of this type are studied, however, the proportion of affected children closely approaches one half.

Figure 2-20 A

		Affected parent	
		D	d
Affected parent	D	DD Homozygous affected (usually rare)	Dd Heterozygous affected
	d	Dd Heterozygous affected	dd Homozygous normal

A

Figure 2-20 B

		Normal parent	
		d	d
Affected parent	D	Dd Heterozygous affected	Dd Heterozygous affected
	d	dd Homozygous normal	dd Homozygous normal

B

FIGURE 2-20 Punnett Square and Autosomal Dominant Traits. **A,** Punnett square for the mating of two individuals with an autosomal dominant gene. Here both parents are affected by the trait. **B,** Punnett square for the mating of a normal individual with a carrier for an autosomal dominant gene.

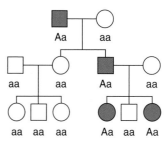

FIGURE 2-21 Pedigree Illustrating the Inheritance Pattern of Postaxial Polydactyly, an Autosomal Dominant Disorder. Affected individuals are represented by shading. (From Jorde LB et al: *Medical genetics,* ed 4, St Louis, 2010, Mosby.)

Recurrence Risks

Parents at risk for producing children with a genetic disease nearly always ask the question, "What is the *chance* that our child will have this disease?" The probability that an individual will develop a genetic disease is termed the recurrence risk. When one parent is affected by an autosomal dominant disease (and is a heterozygote) and the other is unaffected, the recurrence risk for each child is one half.

An important principle is that each birth is an independent event, much like a coin toss. Thus, even though parents may have already had a child with the disease, their recurrence risk remains one half. Even if they have produced several children, all affected (or all unaffected) by the disease, the law of independence dictates that the probability that their next child will have the disease is still one half. Parents' misunderstanding of this principle is a common problem encountered in genetic counseling.

If a child is born with an autosomal dominant disease and there is no history of the disease in the family, the child is probably the product of a new mutation. The gene transmitted by one of the parents has thus undergone a mutation from a normal to a disease-causing allele. The genes at this locus in most of the parent's other germ cells are still normal. In this situation the recurrence risk for the parent's subsequent offspring is not greater than that of the general population. The offspring of the affected child, however, will have a recurrence risk of one half. Because these diseases often reduce the potential for reproduction, many autosomal dominant diseases result from new mutations.

Occasionally, two or more offspring have symptoms of an autosomal dominant disease when there is no family history of the disease. Because mutation is a rare event, it is unlikely that this disease would be a result of multiple mutations in the same family. The mechanism most likely responsible is termed germline mosaicism. During the embryonic development of one of the parents, a mutation occurred that affected all or part of the germline but few or none of the somatic cells of the embryo. Thus the parent carries the mutation in his or her germline but does not actually express the disease. As a result, the unaffected parent can transmit the mutation to multiple offspring. This phenomenon, although relatively rare, can have significant effects on recurrence risks.[8]

Delayed Age of Onset

One of the best-known autosomal dominant diseases is Huntington disease, a neurologic disorder whose main features are progressive dementia and increasingly uncontrollable limb movements (chorea; discussed further in Chapter 14). A key feature of this disease is its delayed age of onset: symptoms usually are not seen until 40 years of age or later. Thus those who develop the disease often have borne children before they are aware that they have the disease-causing mutation. If the disease was present at birth, nearly all affected persons would die

before reaching reproductive age and the occurrence of the disease-causing allele in the population would be much lower. An individual whose parent has the disease has a 50% chance of developing it during middle age. He or she is thus confronted with a torturous question: Should I have children, knowing that there is a 50:50 chance that I may have this disease-causing gene and will pass it to half of my children? A DNA test can now be used to determine whether an individual has inherited the mutation that causes Huntington disease.

Penetrance and Expressivity

The penetrance of a trait is the percentage of individuals with a specific genotype who also exhibit the expected phenotype. Incomplete penetrance means that individuals who have the disease-causing genotype may not exhibit the disease phenotype at all, even though the genotype and the associated disease may be transmitted to the next generation. A pedigree illustrating the transmission of an autosomal dominant mutation with incomplete penetrance is given in Figure 2-22. Retinoblastoma, the most common malignant eye tumor affecting children, typically exhibits incomplete penetrance. About 10% of the individuals who are obligate carriers of the disease-causing mutation (i.e., those who have an affected parent and affected children and therefore must themselves carry the mutation) do not have the disease. The penetrance of the disease-causing genotype is then said to be 90%.

The gene responsible for retinoblastoma has been mapped to the long arm of chromosome 13, and its DNA sequence has been studied extensively. This gene is known as a tumor-suppressor gene: the normal function of its protein product is to regulate the cell cycle so that cells do not divide uncontrollably. When the protein is altered because of a genetic mutation, its tumor-suppressing capacity is lost and a tumor can form[9] (see Chapters 9 and 16).

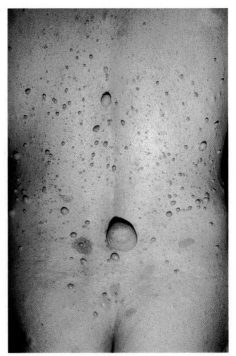

FIGURE 2-23 Neurofibromatosis. Tumors. The most common is sessile or pedunculated. Early tumors are soft, dome-shaped papules or nodules that have a distinctive violaceous hue. Most are benign. (From Habif et al: *Skin disease: diagnosis and treatment,* ed 2, St Louis, 2005, Mosby.)

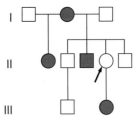

FIGURE 2-22 Pedigree for Retinoblastoma Showing Incomplete Penetrance. Female with marked arrow in line II must be heterozygous, but she does not express the trait.

Expressivity is the extent of variation in phenotype associated with a particular genotype. If the expressivity of a disease is variable, penetrance may be complete but the severity of the disease can vary greatly. A good example of variable expressivity in an autosomal dominant disease is neurofibromatosis type 1, or von Recklinghausen disease. The gene that causes neurofibromatosis has been mapped to the long arm of chromosome 17, and studies of its DNA sequence indicate that, like the retinoblastoma gene, it is a tumor-suppressor gene.[10] The expression of this disease varies from a few harmless café-au-lait (light brown) spots on the skin to numerous neurofibromas, scoliosis, seizures, gliomas, neuromas, malignant peripheral nerve sheath tumors, hypertension, and learning disorders (Figure 2-23).

Several factors cause variable expressivity. Genes at other loci sometimes modify the expression of a disease-causing gene. Environmental factors can influence expression of a disease-causing gene. Finally, different mutations at a locus can cause variation in severity. For example, a mutation that alters only one amino acid of the factor VIII gene usually produces a mild form of hemophilia A, whereas a "stop" codon (premature termination of translation) usually produces a more severe form of this blood coagulation disorder.

Epigenetics and Genomic Imprinting

Although this chapter focuses on DNA sequence variation and its consequence for disease, there is increasing evidence that the same DNA sequence can produce dramatically different phenotypes because of chemical modifications that alter the *expression* of genes (these modifications are collectively termed **epigenetic**). An important example of such a modification is **DNA methylation,** the attachment of a methyl group to a cytosine base that is followed by a guanine base in the DNA sequence (Figure 2-24). These sequences, which are common near many genes, are termed **CpG islands.** When the CpG islands located near a gene become heavily methylated, the gene is less likely to be transcribed into mRNA. In other words, the gene becomes transcriptionally inactive. One study showed that identical (monozygotic) twins accumulate different methylation patterns in the DNA sequences of their somatic cells as they age, causing increasing numbers of phenotypic

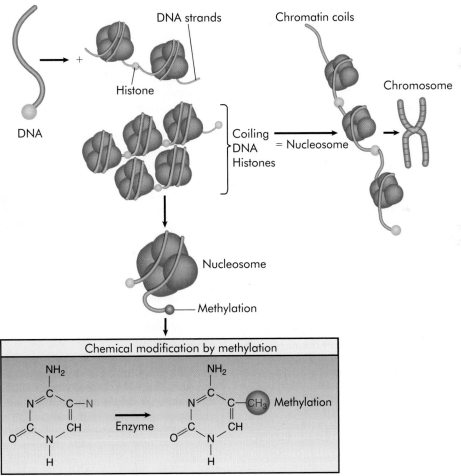

FIGURE 2-24 Epigenetic Modifications. Because DNA is a long molecule, it needs packaging to fit in the tiny nucleus. Packaging involves *coiling* of the DNA in a "left-handed" spiral around spools, made of four pairs of proteins individually known as histones and collectively as the histone octamer. The entire spool is called a nucleosome (also see Figure 1-2). Nucleosomes are organized into chromatin, the repeating building blocks of a chromosome. Histone modifications are correlated with methylation, are reversible, and occur at multiple sites. Methylation occurs at the 5 position of cytosine and provides a "footprint" or signature as a unique epigenetic alteration *(red).* When genes are expressed, chromatin is open or active; however, when chromatin is condensed because of methylation and histone modification, genes are inactivated.

differences.[11] Intriguingly, twins with more differences in their life-styles (e.g., smoking versus nonsmoking) accumulated larger numbers of differences in their methylation patterns. The twins, despite having identical DNA sequences, become more and more different as a result of epigenetic changes, which in turn affect the expression of genes.

Epigenetic alteration of gene activity can have important disease consequences. For example, a major cause of one form of inherited colon cancer (termed hereditary nonpolyposis colorectal cancer [HNPCC]) is the methylation of a gene whose protein product repairs damaged DNA. When this gene becomes inactive, damaged DNA accumulates, eventually resulting in colon tumors. Epigenetic changes are also discussed in Chapters 9 and 10.

Approximately 100 human genes are thought to be methylated differently, depending on which parent transmits the gene. This epigenetic modification, characterized by methylation and other changes, is termed **genomic imprinting**. For each of these genes, one of the parents *imprints* the gene (inactivates it) when it is transmitted to the offspring. An example is the insulin-like growth factor 2 gene *(IGF2)* on chromosome 11, which is transmitted by both parents, but the copy inherited from the mother is normally methylated and inactivated (imprinted). Thus only one copy of *IGF2* is active in normal individuals. However, the maternal imprint is occasionally lost, resulting in two active copies of *IGF2*. This causes excess fetal growth and a condition known as *Beckwith-Weidemann syndrome*.

A second example of genomic imprinting is a deletion of part of the long arm of chromosome 15 (15q11-q13), which, when inherited from the father, causes the offspring to manifest a disease known as *Prader-Willi syndrome* (short stature, obesity, hypogonadism). When the same deletion is inherited from the mother, the offspring develop *Angelman syndrome* (mental retardation, seizures, ataxic gait). The two different phenotypes reflect the fact that different genes are normally active in the maternally and paternally transmitted copies of this region of chromosome 15.

Autosomal Recessive Inheritance
Characteristics of Pedigrees

Like autosomal dominant diseases, diseases caused by autosomal recessive genes are rare in populations, although there can be numerous carriers. The most common lethal recessive disease in white children, cystic fibrosis, occurs in about 1 in 2500 births. Approximately 1 in 25 whites carries a copy of the gene for cystic fibrosis (see Chapter 27). Carriers are phenotypically normal. Some autosomal recessive diseases are characterized by delayed age of onset, incomplete penetrance, and variable expressivity.

Figure 2-25 shows a pedigree for cystic fibrosis. The gene responsible for cystic fibrosis encodes a chloride ion channel in some epithelial cells. Defective transport of chloride ions leads to a salt imbalance that results in secretions of abnormally thick, dehydrated mucus. Some digestive organs, particularly the pancreas, become obstructed, causing malnutrition, and the lungs become clogged with mucus, making them highly susceptible to bacterial infections. Death from lung disease or heart failure occurs before 40 years of age in about one half of persons with cystic fibrosis.

The important criteria for discerning autosomal recessive inheritance include the following:
1. Males and females are affected in equal proportions.
2. Consanguinity (marriage between related individuals) is sometimes present, especially for rare recessive diseases.
3. The disease may be seen in siblings of affected individuals but usually not in their parents.
4. On average, one fourth of the offspring of carrier parents will be affected.

Recurrence Risks

In most cases of recessive disease, both of the parents of affected individuals are heterozygous carriers. On average, one fourth of their offspring will be normal homozygotes, one half will be phenotypically normal carrier heterozygotes, and one fourth will be homozygotes with the disease (Figure 2-26). Thus the recurrence risk for the offspring of carrier parents is 25%. However, in any given family, there are chance fluctuations.

If two parents have a recessive disease, they each must be homozygous for the disease. Therefore all their children also must be affected. This distinguishes recessive from dominant inheritance because two parents both affected by a dominant gene are nearly always both heterozygotes and thus one fourth of their children will be unaffected.

Because carrier parents usually are unaware that they both carry the same recessive allele, they often produce an affected child before becoming aware of their condition. **Carrier detection tests** can identify heterozygotes by measuring the reduced amount of a critical enzyme. This enzyme is totally lacking in a homozygous recessive individual, but a carrier, although phenotypically normal, will typically have half the normal enzyme level. Increasingly, carriers are now detected by direct examination of their DNA to reveal a mutation. Some recessive diseases for which carrier detection tests are now available are PKU, sickle cell disease, cystic fibrosis, Tay-Sachs disease, hemochromatosis, and galactosemia.

Consanguinity

Consanguinity and **inbreeding** are related concepts. **Consanguinity** refers to the mating of two related individuals, and the offspring

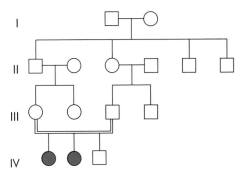

FIGURE 2-25 Pedigree for Cystic Fibrosis. Cystic fibrosis is an autosomal recessive disorder. The double bar denotes a consanguineous mating. Because cystic fibrosis is relatively common in European populations, most cases do not involve consanguinity.

	D	d
D	DD Homozygous normal	Dd Heterozygous carrier
d	Dd Heterozygous carrier	dd Homozygous affected

FIGURE 2-26 Punnett Square for the Mating of Heterozygous Carriers Typical of Most Cases of Recessive Disease.

of such matings are said to be *inbred*. Consanguinity is sometimes an important characteristic of pedigrees for recessive diseases because relatives share a certain proportion of genes received from a common ancestor. The proportion of shared genes depends on the closeness of their biologic relationship. Consanguineous matings produce a significant increase in recessive disorders and are seen most often in pedigrees for rare recessive disorders.

X-Linked Inheritance

Some genetic conditions are caused by mutations in genes located on the sex chromosomes, and this mode of inheritance is termed sex linked. Only a few diseases are known to be inherited as X-linked dominant or Y chromosome traits, so only the more common X-linked recessive diseases are discussed here.

Because females receive two X chromosomes, one from the father and one from the mother, they can be homozygous for a disease allele at a given locus, homozygous for the normal allele at the locus, or heterozygous. Males, having only one X chromosome, are hemizygous for genes on this chromosome. If a male inherits a recessive disease gene on the X chromosome, he will be affected by the disease because the Y chromosome does not carry a normal allele to counteract the effects of the disease gene. Because a single copy of an X-linked recessive gene will cause disease in a male, whereas two copies are required for disease expression in females, more males are affected by X-linked recessive diseases than are females.

X Inactivation

In the late 1950s Mary Lyon proposed that one X chromosome in the somatic cells of females is permanently inactivated, a process termed X inactivation.[12,13] This proposal, the Lyon hypothesis, explains why most gene products coded by the X chromosome are present in equal amounts in males and females, even though males have only one X chromosome and females have two X chromosomes. This phenomenon is called dosage compensation. The inactivated X chromosomes are observable in many interphase cells as highly condensed intranuclear

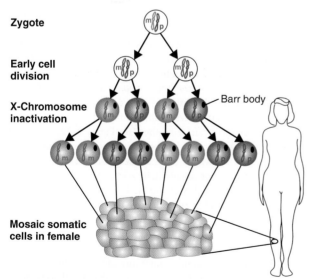

FIGURE 2-27 The X Inactivation Process. The maternal (m) and paternal (p) X chromosomes are both active in the zygote and in early embryonic cells. X inactivation then takes place, resulting in cells having either an active paternal X or an active maternal X. Females are thus X chromosome mosaics, as shown in the tissue sample at the bottom of the page. (From Jorde LB et al: *Medical genetics,* ed 4, St Louis, 2010, Mosby.)

chromatin bodies, termed Barr bodies (after Barr and Bertram, who discovered them in the late 1940s). Normal females have one Barr body in each somatic cell, whereas normal males have no Barr bodies.

X inactivation occurs very early in embryonic development—approximately 7 to 14 days after fertilization. In each somatic cell, one of the two X chromosomes is inactivated. In some cells, the inactivated X chromosome is the one contributed by the father; in other cells it is the one contributed by the mother. Once the X chromosome has been inactivated in a cell, all the descendants of that cell have the same chromosome inactivated (Figure 2-27). Thus inactivation is said to be random but *fixed*.

Some individuals do not have the normal number of X chromosomes in their somatic cells. For example, males with Klinefelter syndrome typically have two X chromosomes and one Y chromosome. These males do have one Barr body in each cell. Females whose cell nuclei have three X chromosomes have two Barr bodies in each cell, and females whose cell nuclei have four X chromosomes have three Barr bodies in each cell. Females with Turner syndrome have only one X chromosome and no Barr bodies. Thus the number of Barr bodies is always one less than the number of X chromosomes in the cell. All but one X chromosome are always inactivated.

Persons with abnormal numbers of X chromosomes, such as those with Turner syndrome or Klinefelter syndrome, are not physically normal. This situation presents a puzzle because they presumably have only one active X chromosome, the same as individuals with normal numbers of chromosomes. This is probably because the distal tips of the short and long arms of the X chromosome, as well as several other regions on the chromosome arm, are not inactivated. Thus X inactivation is also known to be *incomplete*.

Methylation of X chromosome DNA appears to be involved in X inactivation. Inactive X chromosomes can be at least partially reactivated in vitro by administering 5-azacytidine, a demethylating agent.

Sex Determination

The process of sexual differentiation, in which the embryonic gonads become either testes or ovaries, begins during the sixth week of gestation. A key principle of mammalian sex determination is that one copy of the Y chromosome is sufficient to initiate the process of gonadal differentiation that produces a male fetus. The number of X chromosomes does not alter this process. For example, an individual with two X chromosomes and one Y chromosome in each cell is still phenotypically a male. Thus the Y chromosome contains a gene that begins the process of male gonadal development.

This gene, termed *SRY* (for "sex-determining region on the Y"), has been located on the short arm of the Y chromosome.[14] The *SRY* gene lies just outside the pseudoautosomal region (Figure 2-28), which pairs with the distal tip of the short arm of the X chromosome during meiosis and exchanges genetic material with it (crossover), just as autosomes do. The DNA sequences of these regions on the X and Y chromosomes are highly similar. The rest of the X and Y chromosomes, however, do not exchange material and are not similar in DNA sequence.

Other genes that contribute to male differentiation are located on other chromosomes. Thus *SRY* triggers the action of genes on other chromosomes. This concept is supported by the fact that the *SRY* protein product is similar to other proteins known to regulate gene expression.

Occasionally, the crossover between X and Y occurs closer to the centromere than it should, placing the *SRY* gene on the X chromosome after crossover. This variation can result in offspring with an apparently normal XX karyotype but a male phenotype. Such XX males are

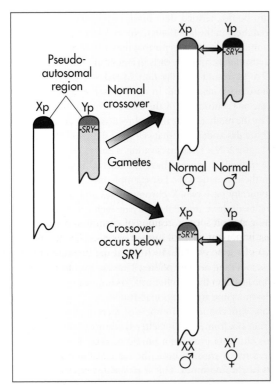

FIGURE 2-28 Distal Short Arms of the X and Y Chromosomes Exchange Material During Meiosis in the Male. The region of the Y chromosome in which this crossover occurs is called the *pseudoautosomal region*. The *SRY* gene, which triggers the process leading to male gonadal differentiation, is located just outside the pseudoautosomal region. Occasionally, the crossover occurs on the centromeric side of the *SRY* gene, causing it to lie on an X chromosome instead of a Y chromosome. An offspring receiving this X chromosome will be an XX male, and an offspring receiving the Y chromosome will be an XY female.

seen in about 1 in 20,000 live births and resemble males with Klinefelter syndrome. Conversely, it is possible to inherit a Y chromosome that has lost the *SRY* gene (the result of either a crossover error or a deletion of the gene). This situation produces an XY female. Such females have gonadal streaks rather than ovaries and have poorly developed secondary sex characteristics.

✔ **QUICK CHECK 2-2**
1. Why is the influence of environment significant to phenotype?
2. Discuss the differences between a dominant and a recessive allele.
3. Why are the concepts of variable expressivity, incomplete penetrance, and delayed age of onset so important in relation to genetic diseases?
4. What is the recurrence risk for autosomal dominant inheritance and recessive inheritance?

Characteristics of Pedigrees

X-linked pedigrees show distinctive modes of inheritance. The most striking characteristic is that females seldom are affected. To express an X-linked recessive trait, a female must be homozygous: either both her parents are affected, or her father is affected and her mother is a carrier. Such matings are rare.

The following are important principles of X-linked recessive inheritance:
1. The trait is seen much more often in males than in females.
2. Because a father can give a son only a Y chromosome, the trait is never transmitted from father to son.
3. The gene can be transmitted through a series of carrier females, causing the appearance of one or more "skipped generations."
4. The gene is passed from an affected father to all his daughters, who, as phenotypically normal carriers, transmit it to approximately half their sons, who are affected.

A relatively common X-linked recessive disorder is Duchenne muscular dystrophy (DMD), which affects approximately 1 in 3500 males. As its name suggests, this disorder is characterized by progressive muscle degeneration. Affected individuals usually are unable to walk by age 10 or 12 years. The disease affects the heart and respiratory muscles, and death caused by respiratory or cardiac failure usually occurs before 20 years of age. Identification of the disease-causing gene (on the short arm of the X chromosome) has greatly increased our understanding of the disorder.[15] The *DMD* gene is the largest gene ever found in humans, spanning more than 2 million DNA bases. It encodes a previously undiscovered muscle protein, termed **dystrophin.** Extensive study of dystrophin indicates that it plays an essential role in maintaining the structural integrity of muscle cells: it may also help to regulate the activity of membrane proteins. When dystrophin is absent, as in DMD, the cell cannot survive, and muscle deterioration ensues. Most cases of DMD are caused by frameshift deletions of portions of the *DMD* gene and thus involve alterations of all the amino acids encoded by the DNA following the deletion.

Recurrence Risks

The most common mating type involving X-linked recessive genes is the combination of a carrier female and a normal male (Figure 2-29, *A*). On average, the carrier mother will transmit the disease-causing allele to half her sons (who are affected) and half her daughters (who are carriers).

The other common mating type is an affected father and a normal mother (Figure 2-29, *B*). In this situation, all the sons will be normal because the father can transmit only his Y chromosome to them. Because all the daughters must receive the father's X chromosome, they will all be heterozygous carriers. Because the sons *must* receive the Y chromosome and the daughters *must* receive the X chromosome with the disease gene, these are precise outcomes and not probabilities. None of the children will be affected.

The final mating pattern, less common than the other two, involves an affected father and a carrier mother (see Figure 2-29, *C*). With this pattern, on average, half the daughters will be heterozygous carriers, and half will be homozygous for the disease allele and thus affected. Half the sons will be normal, and half will be affected. Some X-linked recessive diseases, such as DMD, are fatal or incapacitating before the affected individual reaches reproductive age, and therefore affected fathers are rare.

Sex-Limited and Sex-Influenced Traits

A **sex-limited trait** can occur in only one sex, often because of anatomic differences. Inherited uterine and testicular defects are two obvious examples. A **sex-influenced trait** occurs much more often in one sex than the other. For example, male-pattern baldness occurs in both males and females but is much more common in males. Autosomal dominant breast cancer, which is now much more commonly expressed in females than males, is another example of a sex-influenced trait.

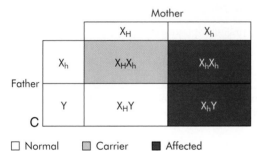

Evaluation of Pedigrees

With complications such as incomplete penetrance, variable expressivity, delayed age of onset, and sex-influenced traits, it is not always possible simply to look at a disease pedigree and determine the mode of inheritance. A sophisticated statistical methodologic approach has evolved to deal with such complications. Incorporated into computer programs, these statistical techniques assess the probability of observing a certain pedigree if a particular mode of inheritance (e.g., autosomal dominant with incomplete penetrance) is in effect.

LINKAGE ANALYSIS AND GENE MAPPING

Locating genes on specific regions of chromosomes has been one of the most important goals of human genetics. The location and identification of a gene can tell much about the function of the gene, the interaction of the gene with other genes, and the likelihood that certain individuals will develop a genetic disease.

Classic Pedigree Analysis

Mendel's second law, the principle of independent assortment, states that an individual's genes will be transmitted to the next generation independently of one another. This law is only partly true, however, because genes located close together on the same chromosome do tend to be transmitted together to the offspring. Thus Mendel's principle of independent assortment holds true for most pairs of genes but not those that occupy the same region of a chromosome. Such loci demonstrate **linkage** and are said to be linked.

During the first meiotic stage, the arms of homologous chromosome pairs intertwine and sometimes exchange portions of their DNA (Figure 2-30) in a process known as **crossover**. During crossover, new combinations of alleles can be formed. For example, two loci on a chromosome have alleles *A* and *a* and alleles *B* and *b*. Alleles *A* and *B* are located together on one member of a chromosome pair, and alleles *a* and *b* are located on the other member. The genotype of this individual is denoted as *AB/ab*.

□ Normal   ▨ Carrier   ■ Affected

FIGURE 2-29 Punnett Square and X-Linked Recessive Traits. A, Punnett square for the mating of a normal male (X_HY) and a female carrier of an X-linked recessive gene (X_HX_h). **B,** Punnett square for the mating of a normal female (X_HX_H) with a male affected by an X-linked recessive disease (X_hY). **C,** Punnett square for the mating of a female who carries an X-linked recessive gene (X_HX_h) with a male who is affected with the disease caused by the gene (X_hY).

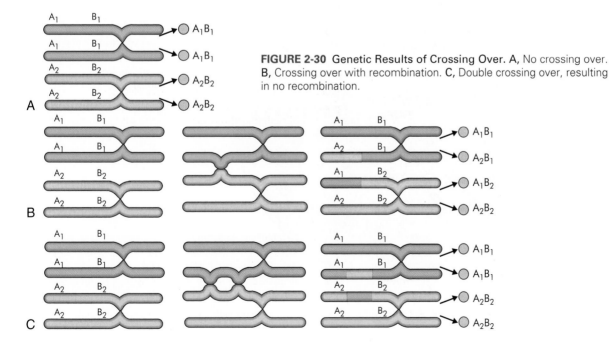

FIGURE 2-30 Genetic Results of Crossing Over. A, No crossing over. **B,** Crossing over with recombination. **C,** Double crossing over, resulting in no recombination.

As Figure 2-30, *A*, shows, the allele pairs *AB* and *ab* would be transmitted together when no crossover occurs. However, when crossover occurs (Figure 2-30, *B*), all four possible pairs of alleles can be transmitted to the offspring: *AB*, *aB*, *Ab*, and *ab*. The process of forming such new arrangements of alleles is called recombination. Crossover does not necessarily lead to recombination, however, because double crossover between two loci can result in no actual recombination of the alleles at the loci (Figure 2-30, *C*).

Once a close linkage has been established between a disease locus and a "marker" locus (a DNA sequence that varies among individuals) and once the alleles of the two loci that are inherited together within a family have been determined, reliable predictions can be made as to whether a member of a family will develop the disease. Linkage has been established between several DNA polymorphisms and each of the two major genes that can cause autosomal dominant breast cancer (about 5% of breast cancer cases are caused by these autosomal dominant genes). Determining this kind of linkage means that it is possible for offspring of an individual with autosomal dominant breast cancer to know whether they also carry the gene and thus could pass it on to their own children. In most cases, specific disease-causing mutations can be identified, allowing direct detection and diagnosis. For some genetic diseases, prophylactic treatment is available if the condition can be diagnosed in time. An example of this is hemochromatosis, a recessive genetic disease in which excess iron is absorbed, causing degeneration of the heart, liver, brain, and other vital organs. Individuals at risk for developing the disease can be determined by testing for a mutation in the hemochromatosis gene and through clinical tests, and preventive therapy (periodic phlebotomy) can be initiated to deplete iron stores and ensure a normal life span.

Complete Human Gene Map: Prospects and Benefits

The major goals of the Human Genome Project were to find the locations of all human genes (the "gene map") and to determine the entire human DNA sequence. These goals have now been accomplished and the genes responsible for most mendelian conditions have been identified (Figure 2-31).[1,16,17] This has greatly increased our understanding of the mechanisms that underlie many diseases, such as retinoblastoma, cystic fibrosis, neurofibromatosis, and Huntington disease. It also has led to more accurate diagnosis of these conditions, and in some cases more effective treatment.

DNA sequencing has become much less expensive and more efficient in recent years. Consequently, dozens of individuals have now been completely sequenced, leading in some cases to the identification of disease-causing genes (see *Health Alert:* Gene Therapy).[18]

HEALTH ALERT

Gene Therapy

More than 6000 individuals are enrolled in more than 1300 protocols. Most of these protocols involve the genetic alteration of cells to combat various types of cancer. Other protocols involve the treatment of inherited diseases, such as β-thalassemia, severe combined immunodeficiency, and retinitis pigmentosa.

Data from Edelstein ML, Abedi MR, Wixon J: Gene therapy clinical trials worldwide to 2007—an update, *J Gene Med* 9:833–842, 2007.

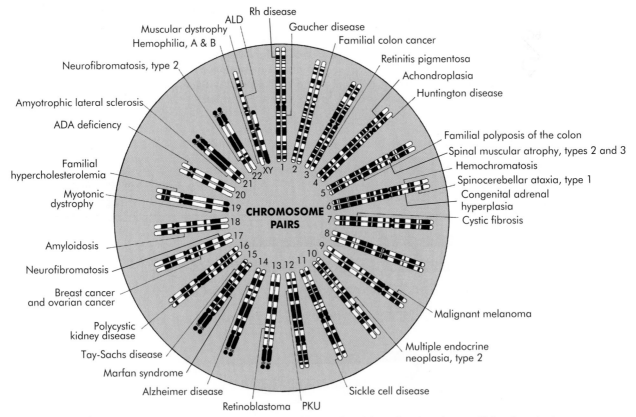

FIGURE 2-31 Example of Diseases: A Gene Map. *ADA,* Adenosine deaminase; *ALD,* adrenoleukodystrophy; *PKU,* phenylketonuria.

MULTIFACTORIAL INHERITANCE

Not all traits are produced by single genes; some traits result from several genes acting together. These are called **polygenic traits.** When environmental factors influence the expression of the trait (as is usually the case), the term **multifactorial inheritance** is used. Many multifactorial and polygenic traits tend to follow a normal distribution in populations (the familiar bell-shaped curve). Figure 2-32 shows how three loci acting together can cause grain color in wheat to vary in a gradual way from white to red, exemplifying multifactorial inheritance. If both alleles at each of the three loci are white alleles, the color is pure white. If most alleles are white but a few are red, the color is somewhat darker; if all are red, the color is dark red.

Other examples of multifactorial traits include height and IQ. Although both height and IQ are determined in part by genes, they are influenced also by environment. For example, the average height of many human populations has increased by 5 to 10 cm in the past 100 years because of improvements in nutrition and health care. Also, IQ scores can be improved by exposing individuals (especially children) to enriched learning environments. Thus both genes and environment contribute to variation in these traits.

A number of diseases do not follow the bell-shaped distribution. Instead they appear to be either present in or absent from an individual. Yet they do not follow the patterns expected of single-gene diseases. Many of these are probably polygenic or multifactorial, but a certain **threshold of liability** must be crossed before the disease is expressed. Below the threshold the individual appears normal; above it, the individual is affected by the disease (Figure 2-33).

One of the best-known examples of such a threshold trait is pyloric stenosis, a disorder characterized by a narrowing or obstruction of the pylorus, the area between the stomach and intestine. Chronic vomiting, constipation, weight loss, and electrolyte imbalance can result from the condition, but it is easily corrected by surgery. The prevalence of pyloric stenosis is about 3 in 1000 live births in whites. This disorder is much more common in males than females, affecting 1 in 200 males and 1 in 1000 females. The apparent reason for this difference is that the threshold of liability is much lower in males than females, as shown in Figure 2-33. Thus fewer defective alleles are required to generate the disorder in males. This situation also means that the offspring of affected females are more likely to have pyloric stenosis because affected females necessarily carry more disease-causing alleles than do most affected males.

A number of other common diseases are thought to correspond to a threshold model. They include cleft lip and cleft palate, neural tube defects (anencephaly, spina bifida), clubfoot (talipes), and some forms of congenital heart disease.

Although recurrence risks can be given with confidence for single-gene diseases (e.g., 50% for autosomal dominants, 25% for autosomal recessives), it is considerably more difficult to do so for multifactorial diseases. The number of genes contributing to the disease is not known, the precise allelic constitution of the parents is not known, and the extent of environmental effects can vary from one population to another. For most multifactorial diseases, **empirical risks** (i.e., those based on direct observation) have been derived. To determine empirical risks, a large sample of families in which one child has developed the disease is examined. The siblings of each child are then surveyed to calculate the percentage who also develop the disease.

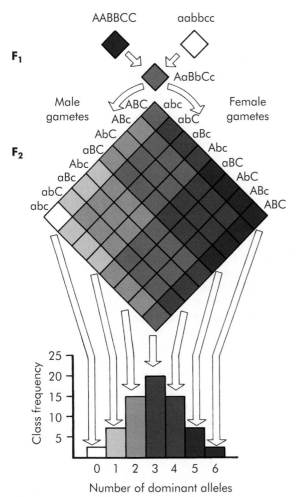

FIGURE 2-32 Multifactorial Inheritance. Analysis of mode of inheritance for grain color in wheat. The trait is controlled by three independently assorted gene loci.

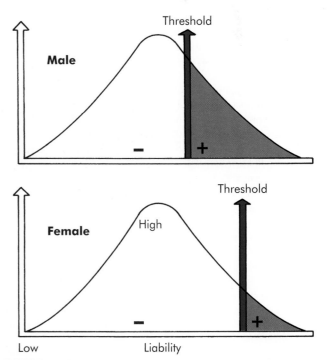

FIGURE 2-33 Threshold of Liability for Pyloric Stenosis in Males and Females.

BOX 2-1 CRITERIA USED TO DEFINE MULTIFACTORIAL DISEASES

1. The recurrence risk becomes higher if more than one family member is affected. For example, the recurrence risk for neural tube defects in a British family increases to 10% if two siblings have been born with the disease. By contrast, the recurrence risk for single-gene diseases remains the same regardless of the number of siblings affected.

2. If the expression of the disease is more severe, the recurrence risk is higher. This is consistent with the liability model; a more severe expression indicates that the individual is at the extreme end of the liability distribution. Relatives of the affected individual are thus at a higher risk for inheriting disease genes. Cleft lip or cleft palate is a condition in which this has been shown to be true.

3. Relatives of probands of the less commonly affected are more likely to develop the disease. As with pyloric stenosis, this occurs because an affected individual of the less susceptible sex is usually at a more extreme position on the liability distribution.

4. Generally, if the population frequency of the disease is f, the risk for offspring and siblings of probands is approximately $\sqrt{f}$. This does not usually hold true for single-gene traits.

5. The recurrence risk for the disease decreases rapidly in more remotely related relatives. Although the recurrence risk for single-gene diseases decreases by 50% with each degree of relationship (e.g., an autosomal dominant disease has a 50% recurrence risk for siblings, 25% for uncle-nephew relationship, 12.5% for first cousins), the risk for multifactorial inheritance decreases much more quickly.

Another difficulty is distinguishing polygenic or multifactorial diseases from single-gene diseases that have incomplete penetrance or variable expressivity. Large data sets and good epidemiologic data often are necessary to make the distinction. Box 2-1 lists criteria that are commonly used to define multifactorial diseases.

The genetics of common disorders such as hypertension, heart disease, and diabetes is complex and often confusing. Nevertheless, the public health impact of these diseases, together with the evidence for hereditary factors in their etiology, demands that genetic studies be pursued. Hundreds of genes that contribute to susceptibility for these diseases have been discovered, and the next decade will undoubtedly witness substantial advancements in our understanding of these disorders.

> ✔ **QUICK CHECK 2-3**
> 1. Define linkage analysis; cite an example.
> 2. Why is "threshold of liability" an important consideration in multifactorial inheritance?
> 3. Discuss the concept of multifactorial inheritance, and include two examples.

DID YOU UNDERSTAND?

DNA, RNA, and Proteins: Heredity at the Molecular Level

1. Genes, the basic units of inheritance, are composed of deoxyribonucleic acid (DNA) and are located on chromosomes.
2. DNA is composed of deoxyribose, a phosphate molecule, and four types of nitrogenous bases. The physical structure of DNA is a double helix.
3. The DNA bases code for amino acids, which in turn make up proteins. The amino acids are specified by triplet codons of nitrogenous bases.
4. DNA replication is based on complementary base pairing, in which a single strand of DNA serves as the template for attracting bases that form a new strand of DNA.
5. DNA polymerase is the primary enzyme involved in replication. It adds bases to the new DNA strand and performs "proofreading" functions.
6. A mutation is an inherited alteration of genetic material (i.e., DNA).
7. Substances that cause mutations are called *mutagens*.
8. The mutation rate in humans varies from locus to locus and ranges from 10^{-4} to 10^{-7} per gene per generation.
9. Transcription and translation, the two basic processes in which proteins are specified by DNA, both involve ribonucleic acid (RNA). RNA is chemically similar to DNA, but it is single stranded, has a ribose sugar molecule, and has uracil rather than thymine as one of its four nitrogenous bases.
10. Transcription is the process by which DNA specifies a sequence of messenger RNA (mRNA).
11. Much of the RNA sequence is spliced from the mRNA before the mRNA leaves the nucleus. The excised sequences are called *introns*, and those that remain to code for proteins are called *exons*.
12. Translation is the process by which RNA directs the synthesis of polypeptides. This process takes place in the ribosomes, which consist of proteins and ribosomal RNA (rRNA).
13. During translation, mRNA interacts with transfer RNA (tRNA), a molecule that has an attachment site for a specific amino acid.

Chromosomes

1. Human cells consist of diploid somatic cells (body cells) and haploid gametes (sperm and egg cells).
2. Humans have 23 pairs of chromosomes. Twenty-two of these pairs are autosomes. The remaining pair consists of the sex chromosomes. Females have two homologous X chromosomes as their sex chromosomes; males have an X and a Y chromosome.
3. A karyotype is an ordered display of chromosomes arranged according to length and the location of the centromere.
4. Various types of stains can be used to make chromosome bands more visible.
5. About 1 in 150 live births has a major diagnosable chromosome abnormality. Chromosome abnormalities are the leading known cause of mental retardation and miscarriage.
6. Polyploidy is a condition in which a euploid cell has some multiple of the normal number of chromosomes. Humans have been observed to have triploidy (three copies of each chromosome) and tetraploidy (four copies of each chromosome); both conditions are lethal.
7. Somatic cells that do not have a multiple of 23 chromosomes are aneuploid. Aneuploidy is usually the result of nondisjunction.
8. Trisomy is a type of aneuploidy in which one chromosome is present in three copies in somatic cells. A partial trisomy is one in which only part of a chromosome is present in three copies.
9. Monosomy is a type of aneuploidy in which one chromosome is present in only one copy in somatic cells.
10. In general, monosomies cause more severe physical defects than do trisomies, illustrating the principle that the loss of chromosome material has more severe consequences than the duplication of chromosome material.

DID YOU UNDERSTAND?—cont'd

11. Down syndrome, a trisomy of chromosome 21, is the best-known disease caused by a chromosome aberration. It affects 1 in 800 live births and is much more likely to occur in the offspring of women older than 35 years.
12. Most aneuploidies of the sex chromosomes have less severe consequences than those of the autosomes.
13. The most commonly observed sex chromosome aneuploidies are the 47,XXX karyotype, 45,X karyotype (Turner syndrome), 47,XXY karyotype (Klinefelter syndrome), and 47,XYY karyotype.
14. Abnormalities of chromosome structure include deletions, duplications, inversions, and translocations.

Elements of Formal Genetics

1. Mendelian traits are caused by single genes, each of which occupies a position, or locus, on a chromosome.
2. Alleles are different forms of genes located at the same locus on a chromosome.
3. At any given locus in a somatic cell, an individual has two genes, one from each parent. An individual may be homozygous or heterozygous for a locus.
4. An individual's genotype is his or her genetic makeup, and the phenotype reflects the interaction of genotype and environment.
5. In a heterozygote, a dominant gene's effects mask those of a recessive gene. The recessive gene is expressed only when it is present in two copies.

Transmission of Genetic Diseases

1. Genetic diseases caused by single genes usually follow autosomal dominant, autosomal recessive, or X-linked recessive modes of inheritance.
2. Pedigree charts are important tools in the analysis of modes of inheritance.
3. Recurrence risks specify the probability that future offspring will inherit a genetic disease. For single-gene diseases, recurrence risks remain the same for each offspring, regardless of the number of affected or unaffected offspring.
4. The recurrence risk for autosomal dominant diseases is usually 50%.
5. Germline mosaicism can alter recurrence risks for genetic diseases because unaffected parents can produce multiple affected offspring. This situation occurs because the germline of one parent is affected by a mutation but the parent's somatic cells are unaffected.
6. Skipped generations are not seen in classic autosomal dominant pedigrees.
7. Males and females are equally likely to exhibit autosomal dominant diseases and to pass them on to their offspring.
8. Many genetic diseases have a delayed age of onset.
9. A gene that is not always expressed phenotypically is said to have incomplete penetrance.
10. Variable expressivity is a characteristic of many genetic diseases.
11. Genomic imprinting, which is associated with methylation, results in differing expression of a disease gene, depending on which parent transmitted the gene.
12. Epigenetics involves changes, such as the methylation of DNA bases, that do not alter the DNA sequence but can alter the expression of genes.
13. Most commonly, parents of children with autosomal recessive diseases are both heterozygous carriers of the disease gene.
14. The recurrence risk for autosomal recessive diseases is 25%.
15. Males and females are equally likely to be affected by autosomal recessive diseases.
16. Consanguinity is sometimes present in families with autosomal recessive diseases, and it becomes more prevalent with rarer recessive diseases.
17. Carrier detection tests for an increasing number of autosomal recessive diseases are available.
18. The frequency of genetic diseases approximately doubles in the offspring of first-cousin matings.
19. In each normal female somatic cell, one of the two X chromosomes is inactivated early in embryogenesis.
20. X inactivation is random, fixed, and incomplete (i.e., only part of the chromosome is actually inactivated). It may involve methylation.
21. Gender is determined embryonically by the presence of the *SRY* gene on the Y chromosome. Embryos that have a Y chromosome (and thus the *SRY* gene) become males, whereas those lacking the Y chromosome become females. When the Y chromosome lacks the *SRY* gene, an XY female can be produced. Similarly, an X chromosome that contains the SRY gene can produce an XX male.
22. X-linked genes are those that are located on the X chromosome. Nearly all known X-linked diseases are caused by X-linked recessive genes.
23. Males are hemizygous for genes on the X chromosome.
24. X-linked recessive diseases are seen much more often in males than in females because males need only one copy of the gene to express the disease.
25. Fathers cannot pass X-linked genes to their sons.
26. Skipped generations often are seen in X-linked recessive disease pedigrees because the gene can be transmitted through carrier females.
27. Recurrence risks for X-linked recessive diseases depend on the carrier and affected status of the mother and father.
28. A sex-limited trait is one that occurs only in one sex (gender).
29. A sex-influenced trait is one that occurs more often in one sex than in the other.

Linkage Analysis and Gene Mapping

1. During meiosis I, crossover occurs and can cause recombinations of alleles located on the same chromosome.
2. The frequency of recombinations can be used to infer the map distance between loci on the same chromosome.
3. A marker locus, when closely linked to a disease-gene locus, can be used to predict whether an individual will develop a genetic disease.
4. A more complete gene map will facilitate marker studies, gene cloning, studies of gene function and interaction, and gene therapy.

Multifactorial Inheritance

1. Traits that result from the combined effects of several loci are polygenic. When environmental factors also influence the trait, it is multifactorial.
2. Many multifactorial traits have a threshold of liability. Once the threshold of liability has been crossed, the disease may be expressed.
3. Empirical risks, based on direct observation of large numbers of families, are used to estimate recurrence risks for multifactorial diseases.
4. Recurrence risks for multifactorial diseases become higher if more than one family member is affected or if the expression of the disease in the proband is more severe.
5. Recurrence risks for multifactorial diseases decrease rapidly for more remote relatives.

KEY TERMS

- Adenine 35
- Allele 46
- Amino acid 35
- Aneuploid cell 42
- Anticodon 37
- Autosome 38
- Barr body 51
- Base pair substitution 37
- Carrier 47
- Carrier detection test 50
- Chromosomal mosaic 42
- Chromosome 34
- Chromosome band 40
- Chromosome breakage 40
- Chromosome theory of inheritance 47
- Clastogen 44
- Codominance 47
- Codon 35
- Complementary base pairing 35
- Consanguinity 50
- CpG islands 49
- Cri du chat syndrome 44
- Crossover 53
- Cytokinesis 38
- Cytosine 35
- Delayed age of onset 48
- Deletion 44
- Deoxyribonucleic acid (DNA) 34
- Diploid cell 38
- DNA methylation 49
- DNA polymerase 37
- Dominant 47
- Dosage compensation 51
- Double-helix model 35
- Down syndrome 42
- Duplication 44
- Dystrophin 52
- Empirical risk 55
- Epigenetic 49
- Euploid cell 40
- Exon 37
- Expressivity 49

- Fragile site 46
- Frameshift mutation 37
- Gamete 38
- Gene 34
- Genomic imprinting 50
- Genotype 46
- Germline mosaicism 48
- Guanine 35
- Haploid cell 38
- Hemizygous 51
- Heterozygote 47
- Heterozygous 46
- Homologous 38
- Homozygote 47
- Homozygous 46
- Inbreeding 50
- Intron 37
- Inversion 45
- Karyotype (karyogram) 40
- Klinefelter syndrome 44
- Linkage 53
- Locus 46
- Meiosis 38
- Messenger RNA (mRNA) 37
- Metaphase spread 38
- Methylation 51
- Missense 37
- Mitosis 38
- Mode of inheritance 47
- Multifactorial inheritance 55
- Mutagen 37
- Mutation 37
- Mutational hot spot 37
- Nondisjunction 42
- Nonsense 37
- Nucleotide 35
- Obligate carrier 48
- Partial trisomy 42
- Pedigree 47
- Penetrance 48
- Phenotype 46
- Polygenic trait 55

- Polymorphic (polymorphism) 46
- Polypeptide 35
- Polyploid cell 40
- Position effect 45
- Principle of independent assortment 47
- Principle of segregation 47
- Proband 47
- Promoter site 37
- Pseudoautosomal 51
- Purine 35
- Pyrimidine 35
- Recessive 47
- Reciprocal translocation 45
- Recombination 54
- Recurrence risk 48
- Ribonucleic acid (RNA) 37
- Ribosomal RNA (rRNA) 38
- Ribosome 38
- RNA polymerase 37
- Robertsonian translocation 45
- Sex-influenced trait 52
- Sex-limited trait 52
- Sex linked (inheritance) 51
- Silent mutation 37
- Somatic cell 38
- Spontaneous mutation 37
- Template 37
- Termination sequence 37
- Tetraploidy 40
- Threshold of liability 55
- Thymine 35
- Transcription 37
- Transfer RNA (tRNA) 37
- Translation 37
- Translocation 45
- Triploidy 40
- Trisomy 42
- Tumor-suppressor gene 48
- Turner syndrome 44
- X inactivation 51

REFERENCES

1. Jorde LB, et al: *Medical genetics*, ed 4, St Louis, 2010, Mosby.
2. Hassold TJ: Chromosome abnormalities in human reproductive wastage, *Trends Genet* 2:105–110, 1986.
3. Hassold T, Hunt PA: To err (meiotically) is human: the genesis of human aneuploidy, *Nat Rev Genet* 2(4):280–291, 2001.
4. Antonarakis SE, Epstein CJ: The challenge of Down syndrome, *Trends Mol Med* 12:473–479, 2006.
5. Graham GE, Allanson JE, Gerritsen JA: Sex chromosome abnormalities. In Rimoin DL, editor: *Emery and Rimoin's principles and practice of medical genetics*, ed 5, London, 2007, Churchill Livingstone.
6. Garber KB, Visootsak J, Warren ST: Fragile X syndrome, *Eur J Hum Genet* 16:666–672, 2008.
7. Orr HT, Zoghbi HY: Trinucleotide repeat disorders, *Annu Rev Neurosci* 30:575–621, 2007.
8. Zlotogora J: Germ line mosaicism, *Hum Genet* 102(4):381–386, 1998.
9. Vogelstein G, Kinzler KW, editors: *The genetic basis of human cancer*, ed 2, New York, 2002, McGraw-Hill.
10. Lee MJ, Stephenson DA: Recent developments in neurofibromatosis type 1, *Curr Opin Neurol* 20:135–141, 2007.
11. Fraga MF, et al: Epigenetic differences arise during the lifetime of monozygotic twins, *Proc Natl Acad Sci U S A* 102:10604–10609, 2005.
12. Lyon MF: X-chromosome inactivation, *Curr Biol* 9(7):R235–R237, 1999.
13. Wutz A, Gribnau J: X inactivation Xplained, *Curr Opin Genet Dev* 17:387–393, 2007.
14. Fleming A, Vilain E: The endless quest for sex determination genes, *Clin Genet* 67(1):15–25, 2005.
15. Emery AEH: Duchenne and other X-linked muscular dystrophies. In Rimoin DL, editor: *Emery and Rimoin's principles and practice of medical genetics*, ed 5, London, 2007, Churchill Livingstone.
16. Collins FS, Morgan M, Patrinos A: The Human Genome Project: lessons from large-scale biology, *Science* 300(5617):286–290, 2003.
17. McKusick VA: A 60-year tale of spots, maps, and genes, *Annu Rev Genom Hum Genet* 7:1–27, 2006.
18. Anonymous: Human genome at ten: the sequence explosion, *Nature* 464:670–671, 2010.

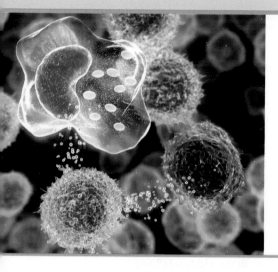

Altered Cellular and Tissue Biology

Kathryn L. McCance and Todd Cameron Grey

evolve WEBSITE

http://evolve.elsevier.com/Huether/

- Review Questions and Answers
- Animations
- Quick Check Answers

- Key Terms Exercises
- Critical Thinking Questions with Answers
- Algorithm Completion Exercises
- WebLinks

CHAPTER OUTLINE

All forms of disease begin with alterations in cells. Injury to cells and their surrounding environment, called the extracellular matrix, leads to tissue and organ injury. Although the normal cell is restricted by a narrow range of structure and function, it can *adapt* to physiologic demands or stress to maintain a steady state called *homeostasis*. **Adaptation** is a reversible, structural, or functional response both to normal or physiologic conditions and to adverse or pathologic conditions. For example, the uterus adapts to pregnancy—a normal physiologic state—by enlarging. Enlargement occurs because of an increase in the size and number of uterine cells. In an adverse condition such as

high blood pressure, myocardial cells are stimulated to enlarge by the increased work of pumping. Like most of the body's adaptive mechanisms, however, cellular adaptations to adverse conditions are usually only temporarily successful. Severe or long-term stressors overwhelm adaptive processes, and cellular injury or death ensues. Altered cellular and tissue biology can result from adaptation, injury, neoplasia, aging, or death (neoplasia is discussed in Chapters 9 to 11).

Injury may be reversible (sublethal) or irreversible (lethal) and is classified broadly as chemical, hypoxic (lack of sufficient oxygen), free radical, intentional, unintentional, immunologic, infection, and inflammatory. Cellular injuries from various causes have different clinical and pathophysiologic manifestations. Cellular death is confirmed by structural changes seen when cells are stained and examined under a microscope.

Cellular aging causes structural and functional changes that eventually may lead to cellular death or a decreased capacity to recover from injury. Mechanisms explaining how and why cells age are not known, and distinguishing between pathologic changes and physiologic changes that occur with aging is often difficult. Aging clearly causes alterations in cellular structure and function, yet growing old is both inevitable and normal.

CELLULAR ADAPTATION

Cells adapt to their environment to escape and protect themselves from injury. An adapted cell is neither normal nor injured—its condition lies somewhere between these two states. Cellular adaptations, however, are a common and central part of many disease states. In the early stages of a successful adaptive response, cells may have enhanced function; thus it is hard to know whether the response is pathologic or an extreme adaptation to an excessive functional demand. The most significant adaptive changes in cells include atrophy (decrease in cell size), hypertrophy (increase in cell size), hyperplasia (increase in cell number), and metaplasia (reversible replacement of one mature cell type by another less mature cell type). Dysplasia (deranged cellular growth) is not considered a true cellular adaptation but rather an atypical hyperplasia. These changes are shown in Figure 3-1.

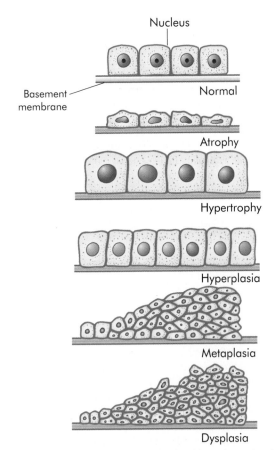

FIGURE 3-1 Adaptive and Dysplastic Alterations in Simple Cuboidal Epithelial Cells.

Atrophy

Atrophy is a decrease or shrinkage in cellular size. If atrophy occurs in a sufficient number of an organ's cells, the entire organ shrinks or becomes atrophic. Atrophy can affect any organ, but it is most common in skeletal muscle, the heart, secondary sex organs, and the brain. Atrophy can be classified as *physiologic* or *pathologic*. **Physiologic atrophy** occurs with early development. For example, the thymus gland undergoes physiologic atrophy during childhood. **Pathologic atrophy** occurs as a result of decreases in workload, pressure, use, blood supply, nutrition, hormonal stimulation, and nervous stimulation (Figure 3-2). Individuals immobilized in bed for a prolonged time exhibit a type of skeletal muscle atrophy called **disuse atrophy**. Aging causes brain cells to become atrophic and endocrine-dependent organs, such as the gonads, to shrink as hormonal stimulation decreases. Whether atrophy is caused by normal physiologic conditions or by pathologic conditions, atrophic cells exhibit the same basic changes.

The atrophic muscle cell contains less endoplasmic reticulum and fewer mitochondria and myofilaments (part of the muscle fiber that controls contraction) than found in the normal cell. In muscular atrophy caused by nerve loss, oxygen consumption and amino acid uptake are immediately reduced. The biochemical changes of atrophy are just beginning to be understood. The mechanisms probably include decreased protein synthesis, increased protein catabolism, or both. The primary pathway of protein catabolism is the **ubiquitin-proteosome pathway** and catabolism involves **proteosomes** (protein degrading complexes). Proteins degraded in this pathway are first conjugated to **ubiquitin** (another small protein) and then degraded by proteosomes. Muscles atrophy can occur because of this pathway. Deregulation of this pathway often leads to abnormal cell growth and is associated with cancer and other diseases.

Atrophy as a result of chronic malnutrition is often accompanied by a "self-eating" process called *autophagy* that creates **autophagic vacuoles** (see p. 88). These vacuoles are membrane-bound vesicles

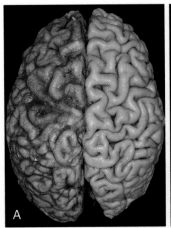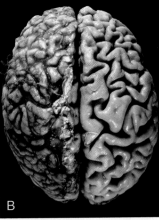

FIGURE 3-2 Atrophy. A, Normal brain of a young adult. **B,** Atrophy of the brain in an 82-year-old male with atherosclerotic cerebrovascular disease, resulting in reduced blood supply. Note that loss of brain substance narrows the gyri and widens the sulci. The meninges have been stripped from the right half of each specimen to reveal the surface of the brain. (From Kumar V et al: Cellular responses to stress and toxic insults: adaptation, injury, and death. In Kumar V et al, editors: *Robbins and Cotran pathologic basis of disease,* ed 8, St Louis, 2010, Saunders.)

within the cell that contain cellular debris and hydrolytic enzymes, which function to break down substances to the simplest units of fat, carbohydrate, or protein. The level of hydrolytic enzymes rises rapidly in atrophy. The enzymes are isolated in autophagic vacuoles to prevent uncontrolled cellular destruction. Thus the vacuoles form as needed to protect uninjured organelles from the injured organelles and are eventually engulfed and destroyed by lysosomes. Certain contents of the autophagic vacuole may resist destruction by lysosomal enzymes and persist in membrane-bound residual bodies. An example of this is granules that contain lipofuscin, the yellow-brown age pigment. Lipofuscin accumulates primarily in liver cells, myocardial cells, and atrophic cells.

Hypertrophy

Hypertrophy is an increase in the size of cells and consequently in the size of the affected organ (Figure 3-3). The cells of the heart and kidneys are particularly prone to enlargement. The increased cellular size is associated with an increased accumulation of protein in the cellular components (plasma membrane, endoplasmic reticulum, myofilaments, mitochondria) and *not* with an increase in cellular fluid. Hypertrophy can be *physiologic* or *pathologic* and is caused by specific hormone stimulation or by increased functional demand. The triggers for hypertrophy include two types of signals: (1) mechanical signals, such as stretch, and (2) trophic signals, such as growth factors, hormones, and vasoactive agents. For example, in skeletal muscles, physiologic hypertrophy occurs in response to heavy work. Muscular hypertrophy tends to diminish if the excessive workload diminishes. When a diseased kidney is removed, the remaining kidney adapts to the increased workload with an increase in both the size and the number of cells. The major contributing factor to this renal enlargement is hypertrophy. Another example of normal or physiologic hypertrophy is the increased growth of the uterus and mammary glands in response to pregnancy. A pathologic example is pathophysiologic hypertrophy in the heart secondary to hypertension or diseased heart valves.

Hyperplasia

Hyperplasia is an increase in the number of cells resulting from an increased rate of cellular division. Hyperplasia, as a response to injury, occurs when the injury has been severe and prolonged enough to have caused cell death. Loss of epithelial cells and cells of the liver and kidney triggers deoxyribonucleic acid (DNA) synthesis and mitotic division. Increased cell growth is a multistep process involving the production of growth factors, which stimulate the remaining cells to synthesize new cell components and, ultimately, to divide. Hyperplasia and hypertrophy often occur together, and both take place if the cells can synthesize DNA; however, in *nondividing cells* (e.g., myocardial fibers) only hypertrophy occurs.

Two types of normal, or physiologic, hyperplasia are (1) compensatory and (2) hormonal. Compensatory hyperplasia is an adaptive mechanism that enables certain organs to regenerate. For example, removal of part of the liver leads to hyperplasia of the remaining liver cells (hepatocytes) to compensate for the loss. Even with removal of 70% of the liver, regeneration is complete in about 2 weeks. Several growth factors and cytokines (chemical messengers) are induced and play critical roles in liver regeneration.[1]

Some cells—such as nerve, skeletal muscle, and myocardial cells and the lens cells of the eye—are classically known *not* to regenerate. Additional skeletal muscle cells, however, can be made by the fusion of myoblasts.[2] Much new research also is being done with the peripheral nervous system (PNS). PNS nerve regeneration enables severed limbs to be reattached and continue growing. Significant compensatory hyperplasia occurs in epidermal and intestinal epithelia, hepatocytes, bone marrow cells, and fibroblasts, and some hyperplasia is noted in bone, cartilage, and smooth muscle cells. Another example of compensatory hyperplasia is the callus, or thickening, of the skin as a result of hyperplasia of epidermal cells in response to a mechanical stimulus.

Hormonal hyperplasia occurs chiefly in estrogen-dependent organs, such as the uterus and breast. After ovulation, for example, estrogen stimulates the endometrium to grow and thicken in preparation for receiving the fertilized ovum. If pregnancy occurs, hormonal hyperplasia, as well as hypertrophy, enables the uterus to enlarge. (Hormone function is described in Chapters 18 and 32.)

Pathologic hyperplasia is the abnormal proliferation of normal cells, usually in response to excessive hormonal stimulation or growth factors on target cells (Figure 3-4). The most common example is pathologic hyperplasia of the endometrium (caused by an imbalance between estrogen and progesterone secretion, with oversecretion of estrogen) (see Chapter 32). Pathologic endometrial hyperplasia, which

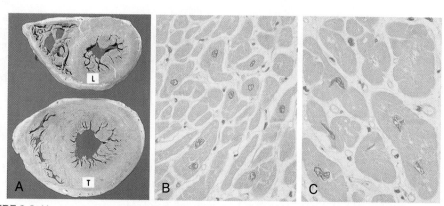

FIGURE 3-3 Hypertrophy of Cardiac Muscle in Response to Valve Disease. **A,** Transverse slices of a normal heart and a heart with hypertrophy of the left ventricle (L, normal thickness of left ventricular wall; T, thickened wall from heart in which severe narrowing of aortic valve caused resistance to systolic ventricular emptying). **B,** Histology of cardiac muscle from the normal heart. **C,** Histology of cardiac muscle from a hypertrophied heart. (From Stevens A, Lowe J: *Pathology: illustrated review in color,* ed 2, Edinburgh, 2000, Mosby.)

causes excessive menstrual bleeding, is under the influence of regular growth-inhibition controls. If these controls fail, hyperplastic endometrial cells can undergo malignant transformation.

Dysplasia: Not a True Adaptive Change

Dysplasia refers to abnormal changes in the size, shape, and organization of mature cells. Dysplasia is not considered a true adaptive process but is related to hyperplasia and is often called atypical hyperplasia. Dysplastic changes often are encountered in epithelial tissue of the cervix and respiratory tract, where they are strongly associated with common neoplastic growths and often are found adjacent to cancerous cells. Importantly, however, the term *dysplasia* does *not* indicate cancer and may not progress to cancer. Dysplasia is often classified as mild, moderate, or severe; yet, because this classification scheme is somewhat subjective, it has prompted some to recommend the use

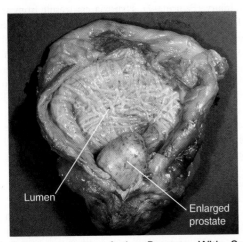

FIGURE 3-4 Hyperplasia of the Prostate With Secondary Thickening of the Obstructed Urinary Bladder. The enlarged prostate is seen protruding into the lumen of the bladder, which appears trabeculated. These "trabeculae" result from hypertrophy and hyperplasia of smooth muscle cells that occur in response to increased intravesical pressure caused by urinary obstruction. (From Damjanov I: *Pathology for the health professions*, ed 3, St Louis, 2006, Saunders.)

of either "low grade" or "high grade" instead. If the inciting stimulus is removed, dysplastic changes often are reversible. (Dysplasia is discussed further in Chapter 9.)

Metaplasia

Metaplasia is the reversible replacement of one mature cell type by another, sometimes less differentiated, cell type. It is thought to develop from a reprogramming of stem cells that exist on most epithelia or of undifferentiated mesenchymal (tissue from embryonic mesoderm) cells present in connective tissue. These precursor cells mature along a new pathway because of signals generated by growth factors in the cell's environment. The best example of metaplasia is replacement of normal columnar ciliated epithelial cells of the bronchial (airway) lining by stratified squamous epithelial cells (Figure 3-5). The newly formed cells do not secrete mucus or have cilia, causing loss of a vital protective mechanism. Bronchial metaplasia can be reversed if the inducing stimulus, usually cigarette smoking, is removed. With prolonged exposure to the inducing stimulus, however, dysplasia and cancerous transformation can occur.

CELLULAR INJURY

Most diseases begin with cell injury. Cellular injury occurs if the cell is unable to maintain homeostasis—a normal or adaptive steady state—in the face of injurious stimuli. Injured cells may recover (reversible injury) or die (irreversible injury). Injurious stimuli include chemical agents, lack of sufficient oxygen (hypoxia), free radicals, infectious agents, physical and mechanical factors, immunologic reactions, genetic factors, and nutritional imbalances. Types of injuries and their responses are summarized in Table 3-1 and Figure 3-6.

The extent of cellular injury depends on the type, state (including level of cell differentiation and increased susceptibility to fully differentiated cells), and adaptive processes of the cell, as well as the type, severity, and duration of the injurious stimulus. Two individuals exposed to an identical stimulus may incur varying degrees of cellular injury. Modifying factors, such as nutritional status, can profoundly influence the extent of injury. The precise "point of no return" that

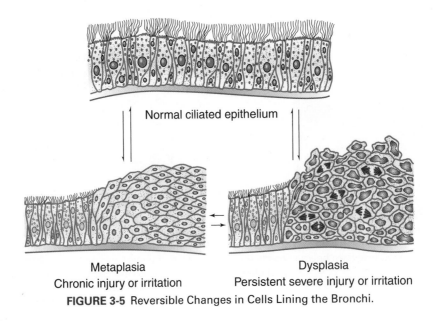

Normal ciliated epithelium

Metaplasia
Chronic injury or irritation

Dysplasia
Persistent severe injury or irritation

FIGURE 3-5 Reversible Changes in Cells Lining the Bronchi.

TABLE 3-1   TYPES OF PROGRESSIVE CELL INJURY AND RESPONSES

TYPE	RESPONSES
Adaptation	Atrophy, hypertrophy, hyperplasia, metaplasia
Active cell injury	Immediate response of "entire" cell
Reversible	Loss of ATP, cellular swelling, detachment of ribosomes, autophagy of lysosomes
Irreversible	"Point of no return" structurally when severe vacuolization of mitochondria occurs and Ca++ moves into cell
Necrosis	Common type of cell death with severe cell swelling and breakdown of organelles
Apoptosis, or programmed cell death	Cellular self-destruction for elimination of unwanted cell populations
Autophagy	Eating of self, cytoplasmic vesicles engulf cytoplasm and organelles, recycling factory
Chronic cell injury (subcellular alterations)	Persistent stimuli response may involve only specific organelles or cytoskeleton (e.g., phagocytosis of bacteria)
Accumulations or infiltrations	Water, pigments, lipids, glycogen, proteins
Pathologic calcification	Dystrophic and metastatic calcification

ATP, Adenosine triphosphate; *Ca++,* calcium.

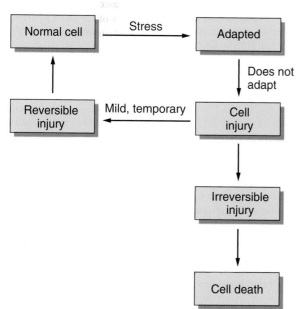

FIGURE 3-6 Stages of Cellular Adaptation, Injury, and Death. The normal cell responds to physiologic and pathologic stresses by adapting (atrophy, hypertrophy, hyperplasia, metaplasia). Cell injury occurs if the adaptive responses are exceeded or compromised by injurious agents, stress, and mutations. The injury is reversible if it is mild or transient, but if the stimulus persists the cell suffers irreversible injury and eventually death.

leads to cellular death is a biochemical puzzle, and the exact mechanisms responsible for the transition from reversible to irreversible cellular damage are being debated.

General Mechanisms of Cell Injury

Common biochemical themes are important to understanding cell injury and cell death regardless of the injuring agent. These include ATP (adenosine triphosphate) depletion, mitochondrial damage, oxygen and oxygen-derived free radicals, membrane damage (depletion of ATP), protein folding defects, DNA damage defects, and calcium level alterations (Table 3-2). Examples of common forms of cell injury are (1) hypoxic injury, (2) free radicals and reactive oxygen species injury, and (3) chemical injury.

Hypoxic Injury

Hypoxia, or lack of sufficient oxygen, is the single most common cause of cellular injury (Figure 3-7). Hypoxia can result from a reduced amount of oxygen in the air, loss of hemoglobin or decreased efficacy of hemoglobin, decreased production of red blood cells, diseases of the respiratory and cardiovascular systems, and poisoning of the oxidative enzymes (cytochromes) within the cells. Hypoxia can induce

TABLE 3-2   COMMON THEMES IN CELL INJURY AND CELL DEATH

THEME	COMMENTS
ATP depletion	Loss of mitochondrial ATP and decreased ATP synthesis; results include cellular swelling, decreased protein synthesis, decreased membrane transport, and lipogenesis, all changes that contribute to loss of integrity of plasma membrane
Reactive oxygen species (ROS)	Lack of oxygen is key in progression of cell injury in ischemia (reduced blood supply); activated oxygen species (ROS, O_2^-, H_2O_2, $OH \cdot$) cause destruction of cell membranes and cell structure
Ca++ entry	Normally intracellular cytosolic calcium concentrations are very low; ischemia and certain chemicals cause an increase in cytosolic Ca++ concentrations; sustained levels of Ca++ continue to increase with damage to plasma membrane; Ca++ causes intracellular damage by activating a number of enzymes
Mitochondrial damage	Can be damaged by increases in cytosolic Ca++, ROS; two outcomes of mitochondrial damage are loss of membrane potential, which causes depletion of ATP and eventual death or necrosis of cell, and activation of another type of cell death (apoptosis) (see p. 87)
Membrane damage	Early loss of selective membrane permeability found in all forms of cell injury, lysosomal membrane damage with release of enzymes causing cellular digestion
Protein misfolding, DNA damage	Proteins may misfold, triggering *unfolded protein response* that activates corrective responses; if overwhelmed, response activates cell suicide program or apoptosis; DNA damage (genotoxic stress) also can activate apoptosis (see p. 87)

ATP, Adenosine triphosphate; *Ca++,* calcium.

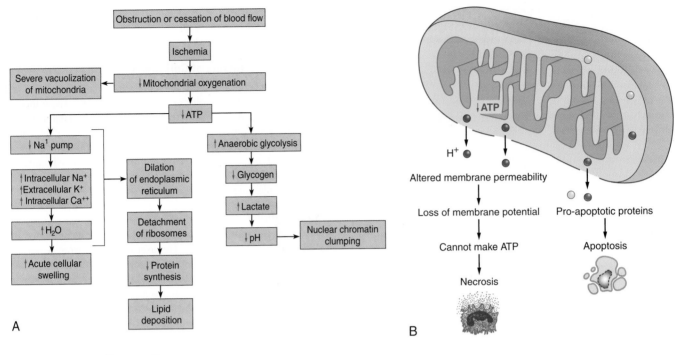

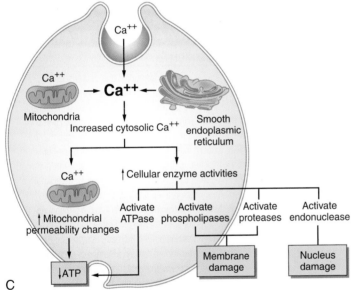

FIGURE 3-7 Hypoxic Injury Induced by Ischemia. A, Consequences of decreased oxygen delivery or ischemia with decreased ATP. The structural and physiologic changes are reversible if oxygen is delivered quickly. Significant decreases in ATP result in cell death, mostly by necrosis. **B,** Mitochondrial damage can result in changes in membrane permeability, loss of membrane potential, and decreased ATP. Between the outer and inner membranes of the mitochondria are proteins that can activate the cell's suicide pathways, called apoptosis. **C,** Calcium ions are critical mediators of cell injury. Calcium ions are usually maintained at low concentrations in the cell's cytoplasm; thus ischemia and certain toxins can initially cause an increase in the release of Ca^{++} from intracellular stores and later an increased movement (influx) across the plasma membrane.

inflammation and inflamed lesions can become hypoxic (Figure 3-8).[3] The cellular mechanisms involved in hypoxia and inflammation are emerging and include activation of immune responses and oxygen-sensing compounds called *ptolyl hydroxylases (PHDs)* and *hypoxia–inducible transcription factor (HIF)*. Hypoxia induced signaling involves complicated cross-talk between hypoxia and inflammation linking hypoxia and inflammation to inflammatory bowel disease, certain cancers, and infections.[3]

The most common cause of hypoxia is ischemia (reduced blood supply). Ischemic injury often is caused by the gradual narrowing of arteries (arteriosclerosis) and complete blockage by blood clots (thrombosis). Progressive hypoxia caused by gradual arterial obstruction is better tolerated than the acute anoxia (total lack of oxygen) caused by a sudden obstruction, as with an embolus (a blood clot or other plug in the circulation). An acute obstruction in a coronary artery can cause myocardial cell death (infarction) within minutes if

the blood supply is not restored, whereas the gradual onset of ischemia usually results in myocardial adaptation. Myocardial infarction and stroke, which are common causes of death in the United States, generally result from atherosclerosis (a type of arteriosclerosis) and consequent ischemic injury. (Vascular obstruction is discussed in Chapter 23.)

Cellular responses to hypoxic injury caused by ischemia have been demonstrated in studies of the heart muscle. Within 1 minute after blood supply to the myocardium is interrupted, the heart becomes pale and has difficulty contracting normally. Within 3 to 5 minutes, the ischemic portion of the myocardium ceases to contract because of a rapid decrease in mitochondrial phosphorylation, causing insufficient ATP production. Lack of ATP leads to increased anaerobic metabolism, which generates ATP from glycogen when there is insufficient oxygen. When glycogen stores are depleted, even anaerobic metabolism ceases.

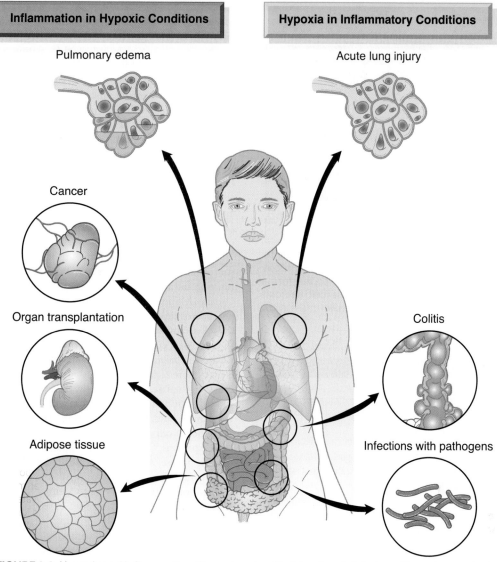

Inflammation in Hypoxic Conditions

Hypoxia in Inflammatory Conditions

Pulmonary edema

Acute lung injury

Cancer

Organ transplantation

Adipose tissue

Colitis

Infections with pathogens

FIGURE 3-8 Hypoxia and Inflammation. Shown is a simplified drawing of clinical conditions characterized by tissue hypoxia that causes inflammatory changes *(left)* and inflammatory diseases that ultimately lead to hypoxia *(right)*. These diseases and conditions are discussed in more detail in their respective chapters. (Adapted from Eltzschig HK, Carmeliet P: Hypoxia and inflammation, *N Engl J Med* 364:656-665, 2011.)

A reduction in ATP levels causes the plasma membrane's sodium-potassium (Na^+-K^+) pump and sodium-calcium exchange mechanism to fail, which leads to an intracellular accumulation of sodium and calcium and diffusion of potassium out of the cell. Sodium and water then can enter the cell freely, and cellular swelling, as well as early dilation of the endoplasmic reticulum, results. Dilation causes the ribosomes to detach from the rough endoplasmic reticulum, reducing protein synthesis. With continued hypoxia, the entire cell becomes markedly swollen, with increased concentrations of sodium, water, and chloride and decreased concentrations of potassium. These disruptions are reversible if oxygen is restored. If oxygen is not restored, however, **vacuolation** (formation of vacuoles) occurs within the cytoplasm and swelling of lysosomes and marked mitochondrial swelling result from damage to the outer membrane. Continued hypoxic injury with accumulation of calcium subsequently activates multiple enzyme systems resulting in membrane damage, cytoskeleton disruption, DNA and chromatin degradation, ATP depletion, and eventual cell death (see Figures 3-7, *C*, and 3-20). Structurally, with plasma membrane damage, extracellular calcium readily moves into the cell and intracellular calcium stores are released. Increased intracellular calcium levels activate cell enzymes (caspases) that promote cell death by apoptosis (see Figures 3-23 and 3-30). If ischemia persists, irreversible injury is associated structurally with severe swelling of the mitochondria, severe damage to plasma membranes, and swelling of lysosomes.

Restoration of oxygen, however, can cause additional injury called **reperfusion injury** (Figure 3-9). Reperfusion injury results from the generation of highly reactive oxygen intermediates (oxidative stress), including hydroxyl radical (OH^-), superoxide radical (O_2^-), and hydrogen peroxide (H_2O_2) (see p. 67). These radicals can all cause further membrane damage and mitochondrial calcium overload. The white blood cells (neutrophils) are especially affected with reperfusion injury, including neutrophil adhesion to the endothelium. Antioxidant treatment not only reverses neutrophil adhesion but also can reverse neutrophil-mediated heart injury. Other potential and current treatments may include blockage of inflammatory mediators and inhibition of certain cell death pathways.

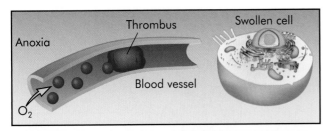

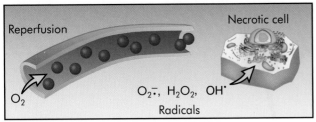

FIGURE 3-9 Reperfusion Injury. Without oxygen, or anoxia, the cells display hypoxic injury and become swollen. With reoxygenation, reperfusion injury increases because of the formation of reactive oxygen radicals that can cause cell necrosis. (Redrawn from Damjanov I: *Pathology for the health professions,* ed 3, St Louis, 2006, Saunders.)

HEALTH ALERT

Whole Food Antioxidants

Nutrient antioxidants—vitamin C, vitamin E, and β-carotene (a precursor to vitamin A)—work by inactivating free radicals. Especially important is the prevention of oxidative damage to mitochondrial DNA. Vitamin C, found in citrus fruits, broccoli, and potatoes, is probably the most notable of the antioxidant nutrients. A water-soluble vitamin, it is the first line of defense, scavenging free radicals before they enter cell membranes. Vitamin C promotes wound healing, growth, and tissue repair. It also enhances the effect of vitamin E. It is known to lower the risk of cataracts and heart disease. Most of the protective antioxidant effects of vitamin E, which is fat soluble and available in unprocessed oils, wheat germ, hazelnuts, almonds, egg yolk, and butter, occur within the lipid-rich cell membrane. It is an anticoagulant and important in the formation of blood cells. It also helps to utilize vitamin K, and it reduces the risk of cataracts. β-Carotene, found in carrots, dark green and yellow-orange vegetables and fruits, leafy vegetables, sweet potatoes, tomatoes, spinach, squash, and broccoli, is converted to vitamin A in the small intestine and *may* be associated with reduced risk of cancer, cataracts, and heart disease.

✔ QUICK CHECK 3-1
1. When does a cell become irreversibly injured?
2. Why are oxidative free radicals damaging to cells?
3. How do cells become markedly swollen with hypoxic injury?

Free Radicals and Reactive Oxygen Species—Oxidative Stress

An important mechanism of cellular injury is injury induced by free radicals, especially by reactive oxygen species (ROS); this form of injury is called oxidative stress. Oxidative stress occurs when *excess* ROS overwhelm endogenous antioxidant systems. A free radical is an electrically uncharged atom or group of atoms that has an unpaired electron. Having one unpaired electron makes the molecule unstable; the molecule becomes stabilized either by donating or by accepting an electron from another molecule. When the attacked molecule loses its electron, it becomes a free radical. Therefore it is capable of injurious chemical bond formation with proteins, lipids, and carbohydrates—key molecules in membranes and nucleic acids. Free radicals are difficult to control and initiate chain reactions. They are *highly* reactive because they have low chemical specificity, meaning they can react with most molecules in their proximity.

Free radicals may be initiated within cells by (1) absorption of extreme energy sources (e.g., ultraviolet light, radiation); (2) activation of endogenous reactions by systems involved in electron and oxygen transport; for example, reduction of oxygen to water (redox reactions); all biologic membranes contain redox systems important for cell defense (e.g., inflammation, iron uptake, growth and proliferation, and signal transduction) (Figure 3-10); and (3) enzymatic metabolism of exogenous chemicals or drugs (e.g., CCl_3^-, a product of carbon tetrachloride [CCl_4]). Table 3-3 describes the most significant free radicals.

During normal metabolism, the mitochondria are the greatest source and target of ROS. These ROS contribute to mitochondria dysfunction and are related to many human diseases and the aging process. Usually ROS are reduced by intracellular antioxidant enzymes, including superoxide dismutase (SOD), glutathione peroxidase, and catalase, as well as antioxidant molecules such as glutathione and vitamin E. In pathologic conditions, however, the large numbers of ROS overwhelm the balance by antioxidants. This inefficiency of antioxidants is even more serious in mitochondria because mitochondria in most cells lack catalase.[4] Consequently, the excessive production of hydrogen peroxide and eventually hydroxyl radical (OH•) in mitochondria will damage lipid, proteins, and **mitochondrial DNA (mDNA)**, resulting either in cell death by necrosis or in a specific type of cell suicide called *apoptosis*.[4-7] Mitochondrial oxidative stress has been implicated in heart disease, Alzheimer disease, Parkinson disease, prion diseases, and amyotrophic lateral sclerosis (ALS), as well as aging itself.[8-11] Currently, investigators are trying to identify the polypeptides (i.e., proteomes) directly involved in diseases associated with mitochondrial dysfunction.

Free radicals cause several damaging effects by (1) **lipid peroxidation,** which is the destruction of polyunsaturated lipids (the same process by which fats become rancid), leading to membrane damage and increased permeability; (2) protein alterations, causing fragmentation of polypeptide chains; (3) DNA fragmentation, causing decreased protein synthesis; and (4) mitochondrial damage, causing the liberation of calcium into the cytosol (see p. 83 and Fig. 3-7, *C*). Because of the increased understanding of free radicals, a growing number of diseases and disorders have been linked either directly or indirectly to these reactive species (Box 3-1).

It is fortunate that the body can sometimes eliminate free radicals. The oxygen free radical superoxide may spontaneously decay into oxygen and hydrogen peroxide. Table 3-4 summarizes other methods that contribute to inactivation or termination of free radicals. The toxicity of certain drugs and chemicals can be attributed either to conversion of these chemicals to free radicals or to the formation of oxygen-derived metabolites (see the following discussion).

Chemical Injury
Mechanisms

About 4 billion pounds of toxic chemicals are released per year in the United States. Of these, approximately 72 million pounds are known carcinogens (see Chapter 10). Only a very small proportion of the 100,000 chemicals in use for commercial purposes have been tested for health effects. Individual sensitivities to chemicals vary because of

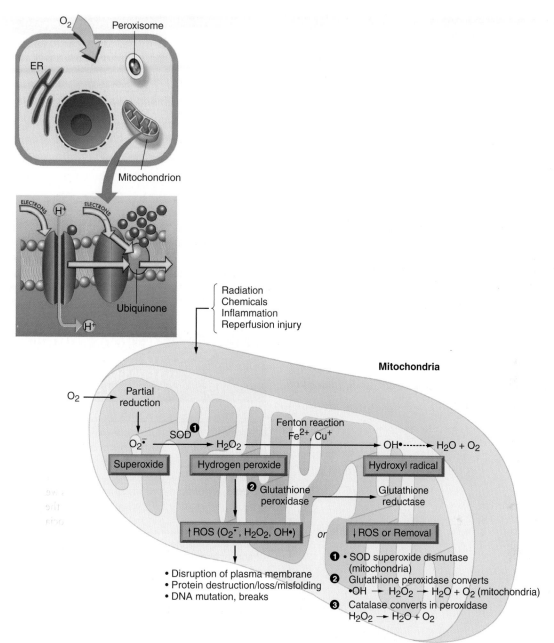

FIGURE 3-10 Generation of Reactive Oxygen Species and Antioxidant Mechanisms in Biologic Systems. Free radicals are generated within cells in several ways, including from normal respiration; absorption of radiant energy; activation of leukocytes during inflammation; metabolism of chemicals or drugs; transition metals, such as iron (Fe^{+++}) or copper (Cu^+), where the metals donate or accept electrons as in the Fenton reaction; nitric oxide (NO) generated by endothelial cells (not shown); and reperfusion injury. Ubiquinone (coenzyme Q), a lipophilic molecule, transfers electrons in the inner membrane of mitochondria, ultimately enabling their interaction with oxygen (O_2) and hydrogen (H_2) to yield water (H_2O). In so doing, the transport allows free energy change and the synthesis of 1 mole of adenosine triphosphate (ATP). With the transport of electrons, free radicals are generated within the mitochondria. Reactive oxygen species (O_2^-, H_2O_2, OH·) act as physiologic modulators of some mitochondrial functions but may also cause cell damage. O_2 is converted to superoxide (O_2^-) by oxidative enzymes in the mitochondria, endoplasmic reticulum (ER), plasma membrane, peroxisomes, and cytosol. O_2 is converted to H_2O_2 by superoxide dismutase (SOD) and further to OH· by the Cu/Fe Fenton reaction. Superoxide catalyzes the reduction of Fe^{++} to Fe^{+++}, thus increasing OH· formation by the Fenton reaction. H_2O_2 is also derived from oxidases in peroxisomes. The three reactive oxygen species (H_2O_2, OH·, and O_2^-) cause free radical damage to lipids (peroxidation of the membrane), proteins (ion pump damage), and DNA (impaired protein synthesis). The major antioxidant enzymes include SOD, catalase, and glutathione peroxidase.

TABLE 3-3 BIOLOGICALLY RELEVANT FREE RADICALS

Reactive oxygen species (ROS) Superoxide O_2^- $O_2 \xrightarrow{\text{Oxidase}} O_2^-$	Generated either (1) directly during autoxidation in mitochondria or (2) enzymatically by enzymes in cytoplasm, such as xanthine oxidase or cytochrome P-450; once produced, it can be inactivated spontaneously or more rapidly by enzyme superoxide dismutase (SOD): $O_2^- + O_2^- + -H_2^- \xrightarrow{\text{SOD}} H_2O_2 + O_2$
Hydrogen peroxide (H_2O_2) $O_2^- + O_2^- + -H \xrightarrow{\text{SOD}} H_2O_2 + O_2$ *Or* Oxidases present in peroxisomes $O_2 \text{ peroxisome } O_2^- \xrightarrow{\text{SOD}} H_2O_2$	Generated by SOD or directly by oxidases in intracellular peroxisomes; NOTE: SOD is considered an antioxidant because it converts superoxide to H_2O_2; catalase (another antioxidant) can then decompose H_2O_2 to $O_2 + H_2O\cdot$)
Hydroxyl radicals (OH^-) $H_2O \rightarrow H\cdot + OH\cdot$ *Or* $Fe^{++} + H_2O_2 \rightarrow Fe^{++} + OH\cdot + OH^-$ *Or* $H_2O_2 + O_2^- \rightarrow OH\cdot + OH^- + O_2$	Generated by hydrolysis of water caused by ionizing radiation or by interaction with metals—especially iron (Fe) and copper (Cu); iron is important in toxic oxygen injury because it is required for maximal oxidative cell damage
Nitric oxide (NO) $NO\cdot + O_2^- \rightarrow ONOO^- + H^+$	NO by itself is an important mediator that can act as a free radical; it can be converted to another radical—peroxynitrite anion ($ONOO^-$), as well as NO_2^- and CO_3^-

Data from Cotran RS, Kumar V, Collins T: *Robbins pathologic basis of disease,* ed 6, Philadelphia, 1999, Saunders.

BOX 3-1 DISEASES AND DISORDERS LINKED TO OXYGEN-DERIVED FREE RADICALS

Deterioration noted in aging
   Atherosclerosis
   Ischemic brain injury
   Alzheimer disease
Neurotoxins
Cancer
Cardiac myopathy
Chronic granulomatous disease
Diabetes mellitus
Eye disorders
   Macular degeneration
   Cataracts
Inflammatory disorders
Iron overload
Lung disorders
   Asbestosis
   Oxygen toxicity
   Emphysema
Nutritional deficiencies
Radiation injury
Reperfusion injury
Rheumatoid arthritis
Skin disorders
Toxic states
   Xenobiotics (CCl_4, paraquat, cigarette smoke, etc.)
   Metal irons (Ni, Cu, Fe, etc.)

Adapted from Knight JA: Review: free radicals, antioxidants, and the immune system, *Ann Clin Lab Sci* 30(2):145, 2000.

TABLE 3-4 METHODS CONTRIBUTING TO INACTIVATION OR TERMINATION OF FREE RADICALS

METHOD	PROCESS
Antioxidants	Endogenous or exogenous; either blocks synthesis or inactivates (e.g., scavenges) free radicals; includes vitamin E, vitamin C, cysteine, glutathione, albumin, ceruloplasmin, transferrin, γ-lipoacid, others
Enzymes	Superoxide dismutase,* which converts superoxide to H_2O_2; catalase* (in peroxisomes) decomposes H_2O_2; glutathione peroxidase* decomposes $OH\cdot$ and H_2O_2

*These enzymes are important in modulating the cellular destructive effects of free radicals, also released in inflammation.

Humans are constantly exposed to a variety of compounds termed *xenobiotics* (Greek *xenos*, "foreign;" *bios*, "life") that include toxic, mutagenic, and carcinogenic chemicals (Figure 3-11). Some of these chemicals are found in the human diet. Most xenobiotics are transported in the blood by lipoproteins and penetrate lipid membranes. These chemicals can react with cellular macromolecules, such as proteins and DNA, or can react directly with cell structures to cause cell damage.[12] The body has two defense systems for counteracting these effects: (1) detoxification enzymes and (2) antioxidant systems (see p. 67). Detoxification enzymes are located predominantly in the liver and provide clearance of compounds through the portal circulation, thereby preventing the potentially carcinogenic agent(s) from entering the body through the gastrointestinal tract and portal circulation. These enzymes also occur in the skin epithelia and can be induced in other extrahepatic tissue, such as the lung.

Chemical Agents Including Drugs

Numerous chemical agents cause cellular injury. Because chemical injury remains a constant problem in clinical settings, it is a major limitation to drug therapy. The site of injury is frequently the liver, where many chemicals and drugs are metabolized (Figure 3-12).

age (timing of exposure), genetics, and complex interactions among various pollutants. For example, combinations of chemicals may not be just additive (1 + 2 = 3) but rather synergistic (1 + 2 = 5). Chemicals can act at the site of entry or at other sites following transport in the circulation.

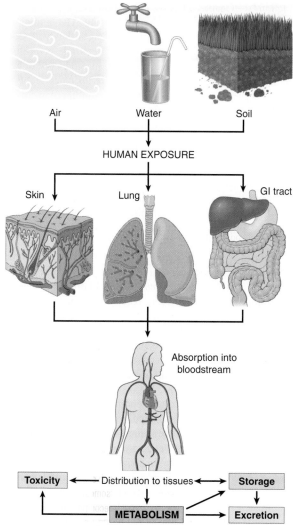

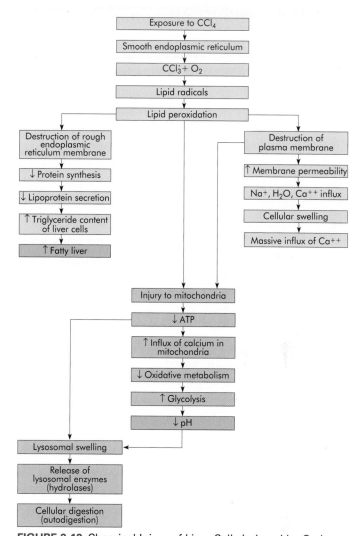

FIGURE 3-11 Human Exposure to Pollutants. Pollutants contained in air, water, and soil are absorbed through the lungs, gastrointestinal tract, and skin. In the body they may act at the site of absorption but are generally transported through the bloodstream to various organs where they can be stored or metabolized. Metabolism of xenobiotics may result in the formation of water-soluble compounds that are excreted, or a toxic metabolite may be created by activation of the agent. (From Kumar V et al, editors: *Robbins and Cotran pathologic basis of disease*, ed 8, St Louis, 2010, Saunders.)

FIGURE 3-12 Chemical Injury of Liver Cells Induced by Carbon Tetrachloride (CCl₄) Poisoning. Light blue boxes are mechanisms unique to chemical injury, purple boxes involve hypoxic injury, and green boxes are clinical manifestations.

The mechanisms by which drug actions, chemicals, and toxins produce injury include (1) direct damage, also called on-target toxicity; (2) exaggerated response at the target, including overdose; (3) biologic activation to toxic metabolites, including free radicals; (4) hypersensitivity and related immunologic reactions; and (5) rare toxicities.[13] These mechanisms are not mutually exclusive; thus several may be operating concurrently.

Direct damage is when chemicals and drugs injure cells by combining *directly* with critical molecular substances. For example, cyanide is highly toxic (e.g., poison) because it inhibits mitochondrial cytochrome oxidase and hence blocks electron transport. Many chemotherapeutic drugs, known as antineoplastic agents, induce cell damage by direct cytotoxic effects. Exaggerated pharmacologic responses at the target include tumors caused by industrial chemicals and estrogens,

and the birth defect attributed to thalidomide.[13] Importantly, another example includes common drugs of abuse (Table 3-5). Drug abuse can involve mind-altering substances beyond therapeutic or social norms (Table 3-6). Drug addiction and overdose are serious public health issues.

Most toxic chemicals are not biologically active in their parent (native) form but must be converted to reactive metabolites, which then act on target molecules. This conversion is usually performed by the cytochrome P-450 oxidase enzymes in the smooth endoplasmic reticulum of the liver and other organs. These toxic metabolites cause membrane damage and cell injury mostly from formation of *free radicals* and subsequent membrane damage called lipid peroxidation. For example, acetaminophen (paracetamol) is converted to a toxic metabolite in the liver, causing cell injury (Figure 3-13). Acetaminophen is one of the most common causes of poisoning world-wide.[14] Hypersensitivity reactions are a common drug toxicity and range from mild skin rashes to immune-mediated organ failure.[13] One type of hypersensitivity reaction is the delayed-onset reaction, which occurs after multiple doses of a drug are administered. Some protein drugs and large polypeptide drugs (e.g., insulin) can directly stimulate antibody

TABLE 3-5 COMMON DRUGS OF ABUSE

CLASS	MOLECULAR TARGET	EXAMPLE
Opioid narcotics	Mu opioid receptor (agonist)	Heroin, hydromorphone (Dilaudid)
		Oxycodone (Percodan, Percocet, OxyContin)
		Methadone (Dolophine)
		Meperidine (Demerol)
Sedative-hypnotics	$GABA_A$ receptor (agonist)	Barbiturates
		Ethanol
		Methaqualone (Quaalude)
		Glutethimide (Doriden)
		Ethchlorvynol (Placidyl)
Psychomotor stimulants	Dopamine transporter (antagonist)	Cocaine
		Amphetamines
	Serotonin receptors (toxicity)	3,4-Methylenedioxy-methamphetamine (MDMA, ecstasy)
Phencyclidine-like drugs	NMDA glutamate receptor channel (antagonist)	Phencyclidine (PCP, angel dust)
		Ketamine
Cannabinoids	CB_1 cannabinoid receptors (agonist)	Marijuana
		Hashish
Hallucinogens	Serotonin 5-HT_2 receptors (agonist)	Lysergic acid diethylamide (LSD)
		Mescaline
		Psilocybin

From Kumar V et al: Cellular responses to stress and toxic insults: adaptation, injury, and death. In Kumar V et al, editors: *Robbins and Cotran pathologic basis of disease*, ed 8, St Louis, 2010, Saunders; Hyman SE: A 28 year old man addicted to cocaine, *JAMA* 286:2586, 2001.
CB_1, Cannabinoid receptor; *GABA*, γ-Aminobutyric acid; *5-HT$_2$*, 5-hydroxytryptamine; *NMDA*, *N*-methyl-D-aspartate.

production (see Chapter 7). Most drugs, however, act as haptens and bind covalently to serum or cell-bound proteins. The binding makes the protein immunogenic, stimulating antidrug antibody production, T-cell responses against the drug, or both. For example, penicillin itself is not antigenic but its metabolic degradation products can become antigenic and cause an allergic reaction. Rare toxicities simply mean infrequent occurrences described by the other four mechanisms. These toxicities reflect individual genetic predispositions that affect drug or chemical metabolism, disposition, and immune responses.

Chronic exposure to air pollutants, insecticides, and herbicides can cause cellular injury. Carbon monoxide, carbon tetrachloride, and social drugs, such as alcohol, can significantly alter cellular function and injure cellular structures. Accidental or suicidal poisonings by chemical agents cause numerous deaths. The injurious effects of some agents—lead, carbon monoxide, ethyl alcohol, mercury—are common cellular injuries. Acetaminophen and common drugs of abuse were discussed earlier (see p. 69).

Lead. Lead is a heavy metal that persists in the environment. Despite efforts to reduce exposure through government regulation, lead toxicity is still a primary hazard for children.[15] Compared to adults, children absorb lead more readily through the intestines. If nutrition is compromised, especially if dietary intake of iron, calcium, zinc, and vitamin D is insufficient, lead's toxic effects are enhanced.[16,17] Particularly worrisome is lead exposure during pregnancy because the developing fetal nervous system is especially vulnerable; lead exposure can result in learning disorders, hyperactivity, and attention problems.[15]

Lead-based paint has a sweet taste and is often ingested by children. Common sources of lead are included in Table 3-7.

The organ systems primarily affected by lead ingestion include the nervous system, the hematopoietic system (tissues that produce blood cells), and the kidneys of the urologic system. Lead affects many different biologic activities, many of which may be related to the function of calcium.[15] Lead is able to *increase* intracellular calcium concentrations. Lead inhibits several enzymes involved in hemoglobin synthesis and causes anemia as a result of lysis of red blood cells (hemolysis). Other

TABLE 3-6 SOCIAL OR STREET DRUGS AND THEIR EFFECTS

TYPE OF DRUG	DESCRIPTION AND EFFECTS
Marijuana (pot)	*Active substance:* Δ9-Tetrahydrocannabinol (THC), found in resin of *Cannabis sativa* plant
	With smoking (e.g., "joints"), about 50% is absorbed through lungs; when ingested only 10% is absorbed; with heavy use the following adverse effects have been reported: alterations of sensory perception; cognitive and psychomotor impairment (e.g., inability to judge time, speed, distance); smoking 3 or 4 joints/day is similar to smoking 20 cigarettes/day; it increases heart rate and blood pressure; increases susceptibility to laryngitis, pharyngitis, bronchitis; causes cough and hoarseness; may contribute to lung cancer; data from animal studies only indicate reproductive changes include reduced fertility, decreased sperm motility, and decreased levels of circulatory testosterone; fetal abnormalities include low birth weight; increased frequency of infectious illness is thought to be result of depressed cell-mediated and humoral immunity; beneficial effects include decreased nausea secondary to cancer chemotherapy and decreased pain in certain chronic conditions
Methamphetamine (Meth)	An amine derivation of amphetamine ($C_{10}H_{15}N$) used as crystalline hydrochloride
	CNS stimulant; in large doses causes irritability, aggressive (violent) behavior, anxiety, excitement, auditory hallucinations, and paranoia (delusions and psychosis); mood changes are common and abuser can swiftly change from friendly to hostile; paranoiac swings can result in suspiciousness, hyperactive behavior, and dramatic mood swings
	Appeals to abusers because body's metabolism is increased and produces euphoria, alertness, and perception of increased energy
	Stages:
	Low intensity: User is not psychologically addicted and uses methamphetamine by swallowing or snorting
	Binge and high intensity: User has psychologic addiction and smokes or injects to achieve a faster, stronger high
	Tweaking: Most dangerous stage; user is continually under the influence, not sleeping for 3-15 days, extremely irritated, and paranoid

TABLE 3-6   SOCIAL OR STREET DRUGS AND THEIR EFFECTS—cont'd

TYPE OF DRUG	DESCRIPTION AND EFFECTS
Cocaine and crack	Extracted from leaves of cocoa plant and sold as a water-soluble powder (cocaine hydrochloride) liberally diluted with talcum powder or other white powders; extraction of pure alkaloid from cocaine hydrochloride is "free-base" called *crack* because it "cracks" when heated
	Crack is more potent than cocaine; cocaine is widely used as an anesthetic, usually in procedures involving oral cavity; it is a potent CNS stimulant, blocking reuptake of neurotransmitters norepinephrine, dopamine, and serotonin; also increases synthesis of norepinephrine and dopamine; dopamine induces sense of euphoria, and norepinephrine causes adrenergic potentiation, including hypertension, tachycardia, and vasoconstriction; cocaine can therefore cause severe coronary artery narrowing and ischemia; reason cocaine increases thrombus formation is unclear; other cardiovascular effects include dysrhythmias, sudden death, dilated cardiomyopathy, rupture of descending aorta (i.e., secondary to hypertension); effects on fetus include premature labor, retarded fetal development, stillbirth, hyperirritability
Heroin	Opiate closely related to morphine, methadone, and codeine
	Highly addictive, and withdrawal causes intense fear ("I'll die without it"); sold "cut" with similar-looking white powder; dissolved in water it is often highly contaminated; feeling of tranquility and sedation lasts only a few hours and thus encourages repeated intravenous or subcutaneous injections; acts on the receptors enkephalins, endorphins, and dynorphins, which are widely distributed throughout body with high affinity to CNS; effects can include infectious complications, especially *Staphylococcus aureus*, granulomas of lung, septic embolism, and pulmonary edema—in addition, viral infections from casual exchange of needles and HIV; sudden death is related to overdosage secondary to respiratory depression, decreased cardiac output, and severe pulmonary edema

Data from Cotran RS, Kumar V, Colllins T: *Robbins pathologic basis of disease,* ed 7, Philadelphia, 2005, Saunders; Nahas G, Sutin K, Bennett WM: Review of marijuana and medicine, *N Engl J Med* 343(7):514, 2000.
CNS, Central nervous system; *HIV,* human immunodeficiency virus.

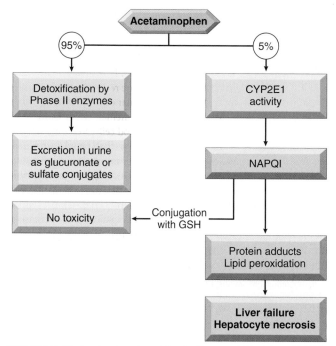

FIGURE 3-13 Acetaminophen Metabolism and Toxicity. *CYP2E1,* a cytochrome; *NAPQI,* toxic byproduct; *GSH,* glutathione.

TABLE 3-7   COMMON SOURCES OF LEAD EXPOSURE

EXPOSURE	SOURCE
Environmental	Lead paint, soil, or dust near roadways or lead-painted homes; plastic window blinds; plumbing materials (from pipes or solder); pottery glazes and ceramic ware; lead-core candle wicks; leaded gasoline; water (pipes)
Occupational	Lead mining and refining, plumbing and pipe fitting, auto repair, glass manufacturing, battery manufacturing and recycling, printing shop, construction work, plastic manufacturing, gas station attendant, firing-range attendant
Hobbies	Glazed pottery making, target shooting at firing ranges, lead soldering, preparing fishing sinkers, stained-glass making, painting, car or boat repair
Other	Gasoline sniffing, costume jewelry, cosmetics, contaminated herbal products

Data from Sanborn MD et al: Identifying and managing adverse environmental health effects, 3, lead exposure, *CMAJ* 166(10):1287–1292, 2002.

manifestations of brain involvement include convulsions and delirium and, with peripheral nerve involvement, wrist, finger, and sometimes foot paralysis. Renal lesions can cause tubular dysfunction resulting in glycosuria (glucose in the urine), aminoaciduria (amino acids in the urine), and hyperphosphaturia (excess phosphate in the urine). Gastrointestinal symptoms are less severe and include nausea, loss of appetite, weight loss, and abdominal cramping.

Carbon Monoxide. Gaseous substances can be classified according to their ability to asphyxiate (interrupt respiration) or irritate. Toxic asphyxiants, such as carbon monoxide, hydrogen cyanide, and hydrogen sulfide, directly interfere with cellular respiration.

Carbon monoxide (CO) is an odorless, colorless, and undetectable gas unless it is mixed with a visible or odorous pollutant. It is produced by the incomplete combustion of fuels such as gasoline. Although CO is a chemical agent, the ultimate injury it produces is a hypoxic injury—namely, oxygen deprivation. Normally, oxygen molecules are carried to tissues bound to hemoglobin in red blood cells (see Chapter 26). Because CO's affinity for hemoglobin is 300 times greater than that of oxygen, it quickly binds with the hemoglobin, preventing oxygen molecules from doing so. Minute amounts of CO can produce a significant percentage of carboxyhemoglobin (carbon monoxide bound with hemoglobin).

Symptoms related to CO poisoning include headache, giddiness, tinnitus (ringing in the ears), nausea, weakness, and vomiting. At risk for carbon monoxide exposure are those who (1) breathe air polluted by gasoline engines or defective furnaces; (2) work in occupations such as coal mining, fire fighting, welding, or engine repair; and (3) smoke cigarettes, cigars, or pipes. The fetus is especially at risk from the effects of carbon monoxide because fetal carboxyhemoglobin levels are likely to be 10% to 15% more than maternal levels.

Ethanol. Alcohol (ethanol) is the primary choice among mood-altering drugs available in the United States. It is estimated there are more than 10 million chronic alcoholics in the United States. Alcohol contributes to more than 100,000 deaths annually with 50% of these deaths from drunk driving accidents, alcohol-related homicides, and suicides.[18] A blood concentration of 80 mg/dl is the legal definition for drunk driving in the United States. This level of alcohol in an average person may be reached after consumption of three drinks (3 12-oz bottles of beer, 15 oz of wine, and 4 to 5 oz of distilled liquor). The effects of alcohol vary by age, gender, and percent body fat; the rate of metabolism affects the blood alcohol level. Because alcohol is not only a psychoactive drug but also a food, it is considered part of the basic food supply in many societies. A large intake of alcohol has enormous effects on nutritional status. Liver and nutritional disorders are the most serious consequences of alcohol abuse. Major nutritional deficiencies include magnesium, vitamin B_6, thiamine, and phosphorus. Folic acid deficiency is a common problem in chronic alcoholic populations. Ethanol alters folic acid (folate) homeostasis by decreasing intestinal absorption of folate, increasing liver retention of folate, and increasing the loss of folate through urinary and fecal excretion.[19] Folic acid deficiency becomes especially serious in pregnant women who consume alcohol and may contribute to fetal alcohol syndrome (see p. 73).

Most of the alcohol in blood is metabolized to acetaldehyde in the liver by three enzyme systems: alcohol dehydrogenase (ADH), the microsomal ethanol oxidizing system (MEOS), and catalase (Figure 3-14). The major pathway involves ADH, an enzyme located in the cytosol of hepatocytes. The microsomal ethanol oxidizing system (MEOS) depends on cytochrome P-450, an enzyme needed for cellular oxidation. Activation of MEOS requires a high ethanol concentration and thus is thought to be important in the accelerated ethanol metabolism (i.e., tolerance) noted in persons with chronic alcoholism. Acetaldehyde has many toxic tissue effects and is responsible for some of the acute effects of alcohol and for development of oral cancers.[18]

The major effects of acute alcoholism involve the central nervous system (CNS). After alcohol is ingested, it is absorbed, unaltered, in the stomach and small intestine. Fatty foods and milk slow absorption. Alcohol then is distributed to all tissues and fluids of the body in direct proportion to the blood concentration.

Individuals differ in their capability to metabolize alcohol. Genetic differences in metabolism of liver alcohol, including aldehyde dehydrogenases, have been identified.[20] These genetic polymorphisms may account for ethnic and gender differences in ethanol metabolism. Persons with chronic alcoholism develop tolerance because of production of enzymes, leading to an increased rate of metabolism (e.g., P-450).

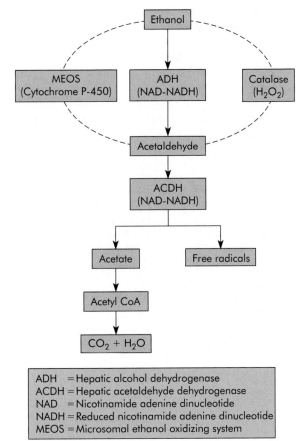

FIGURE 3-14 Major Pathways of ADH Metabolism of Alcohol in the Liver.

Since 1997 studies have consistently validated the so-called *J-* or *U-shaped* inverse association between alcohol and cardiovascular disease. Consistent epidemiologic studies show that people who daily consume light-to-moderate (*not* excessive) amounts of alcohol reduce their risk of coronary heart disease (CHD) as compared to nondrinkers. The suggested mechanisms for cardioprotection include increase in levels of high density lipoprotein–cholesterol (HDL-C), prevention of clot formation, reduction in platelet aggregation, and increase in clot degradation (fibrinolysis). Alcohol also may increase insulin sensitivity.[21] Limited data suggest that the level for optimal benefit may be slightly lower for women; therefore the American Heart Association recommends no more than two drinks per day for men and one drink per day for women. Individuals who do not consume alcohol should not be encouraged to start drinking.[22]

Acute alcoholism affects mainly the CNS but may induce reversible hepatic and gastric changes.[23,24] The hepatic changes, initiated by acetaldehyde, include inflammation, deposition of fat, enlargement of the liver, interruption of microtubular transport of proteins and their secretion, increase in intracellular water, depression of fatty acid oxidation in the mitochondria, increased membrane rigidity, and acute liver cell necrosis (see Chapter 34). In the CNS alcohol is, itself, a depressant, initially affecting subcortical structures (probably the brain stem reticular formation).[23,24] Consequently, motor and intellectual activity becomes disoriented. At higher blood alcohol levels, medullary centers become depressed, affecting respiration. Much investigation now concerns the relationship of alcohol and snoring and obstructive sleep apnea (cessation of breathing).[25,26]

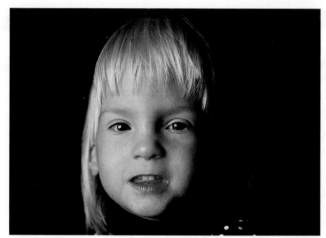

FIGURE 3-15 Fetal Alcohol Syndrome. When alcohol enters the fetal blood, the potential result can cause tragic congenital abnormalities, such as microcephaly ("small head"), low birth weight, and cardiovascular defects, as well as developmental disabilities, such as physical and mental retardation, and even death. Note the small head, thinned upper lip, small eye openings (palpebral fissures), epicanthal folds, and receded upper jaw (retrognathia) typical of fetal alcohol syndrome. (From Fortinash KM, Holoday Worret PA: *Psychiatric mental health nursing*, ed 3, St Louis, 2004, Mosby.)

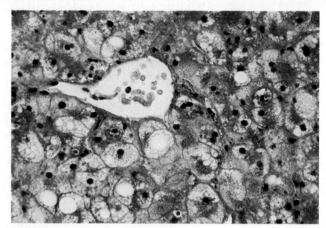

FIGURE 3-16 Alcoholic Hepatitis. Chicken-wire fibrosis extending between hepatocytes (Mallory trichrome stain). (From Damjanov I, Linder J, editors: *Anderson's pathology*, ed 10, St Louis, 1996, Mosby.)

Chronic alcoholism causes structural alterations in practically all organs and tissues in the body because most tissues contain enzymes capable of ethanol oxidation or nonoxidative metabolism. The most significant activity, however, occurs in the liver.[27] The following alterations occur in the liver: fatty liver, alcoholic hepatitis, and cirrhosis. Cirrhosis is associated with portal hypertension and an increased risk for hepatocellular carcinoma.[18] Acute gastritis is a direct toxic effect and chronic use can lead to acute and chronic pancreatitis. Cellular damage is increased by reactive oxygen species (ROS) and oxidative stress (see p. 66). Activation of proinflammatory cytokines from neutrophils and lymphocytes mediates liver damage.[27] Oxidative stress is associated with cell membrane phospholipid depletion, which alters the fluidity and function of cell membranes as well as intercellular transport. Chronic alcoholism is related to several disorders, including injury to the myocardium (alcoholic cardiomyopathy), increased tendency to hypertension, and regressive changes in skeletal muscle (see Chapter 34).

Ethanol is implicated in the onset of a variety of immune defects, including effects on the production of cytokines involved in inflammatory responses (tumor necrosis factor, interleukin-1, interleukin-6).[23,24] The deleterious effects of prenatal alcohol exposure can cause mental retardation and neurobehavioral disorders, as well as fetal alcohol syndrome. Fetal alcohol syndrome includes growth retardation, facial anomalies, cognitive impairment, and ocular malformations (Figure 3-15). Alcohol crosses the placenta, reaching the fetus rapidly.[28] Research has demonstrated an unimpeded bidirectional movement of alcohol between the fetus and the mother. The fetus may completely depend on maternal hepatic detoxification because the activity of alcohol dehydrogenase (ADH) in fetal liver is less than 10% of that in the adult liver.[28] Additionally, the amniotic fluid acts as a reservoir for alcohol, prolonging fetal exposure.[28] The specific mechanisms of injury are unknown; however, acetaldehyde can alter fetal development by disrupting differentiation and

growth; DNA and protein synthesis; modification of carbohydrates, proteins, and fats; and the flow of nutrients across the placenta.[28,29] Alcohol also may cause fetal disturbances, even preconceptual effects, epigenetically.[30]

Whatever the cause, persons with chronic alcoholism have a significantly shortened life span related mainly to damage to the liver, stomach, brain, and heart. Alcohol is a well-known cause of hepatic injury, terminating in cirrhosis (Figure 3-16) (see Chapter 34), yet moderate amounts (e.g., 20 to 30 g/day or 250 ml of wine) of alcohol may decrease the incidence of coronary heart disease.

Mercury. Mercury has been used medically and commercially for centuries. Today people are exposed to mercury from two major sources: fish consumption and dental amalgams. Although no cases of mercury toxicity have been reported secondary to vaccination, thimerosal was removed from all vaccines in 2001, with the exception of inactivated influenza vaccines.[31] The use of mercury as a preservative in vaccines has been greatly decreased or eliminated. Table 3-8 summarizes these sources and their health effects.

✔ QUICK CHECK 3-2

1. Discuss the possible mechanisms of cell injury related to chronic alcoholism.
2. What are some of the systemic effects of methamphetamine, cocaine, marijuana, and heroin use?

Unintentional and Intentional Injuries

Unintentional and intentional injuries are an important health problem in the United States. In 2007 there were 182,479 deaths, an injury death rate of 59.30/100,000.[32] Death from injury is significantly more common for men than women; the overall rate for men is 84.38/100,000 versus 34.31/100,000 for women. Significant racial differences are noted in the death rate, with whites at 59.59/100,000, blacks at 65.15/100,000, and other racial groups at a combined rate of 35.12/100,000. There also is a bimodal age distribution for injury-related deaths, with peaks in the young adult and elderly groups. Unintentional injury is the leading cause of death for people between the ages of 1 and 34 years; intentional injury (suicide, homicide) ranks between the second and fourth leading cause of death in this age

TABLE 3-8 MAJOR SOURCES OF MERCURY EXPOSURE AND HEALTH EFFECTS

SOURCE	COMMENTS
Dental amalgams	Amalgams consist of 50% mercury combined with other metals
	Controversial whether amalgams can release mercury vapors into mouth and when fillings are removed cause transient elevations
	Health concerns from claims that mercury vapor can cause or worsen degenerative diseases (e.g., Alzheimer disease); however, several epidemiologic studies have failed to provide evidence
	Difficult problem is that mercury can inhibit biochemical process in vitro without same effects in vivo
Fish consumption	Consumption of fish and sea mammals is major source of exposure to methyl mercury
	Faroe Islands study showed methyl mercury exposure from whale consumption
	U.S. study showed methyl mercury levels slightly higher than EPA guideline
	FDA recommends pregnant women, nursing mothers, and young children avoid eating fish with high mercury content (>1 parts per million [ppm]), such as shark, swordfish, tile fish, king mackerel, and whale meat
Vaccines	Thimerosal, a preservative in many multidose vials of vaccines, contains ethyl mercury
	Single-dose vials do not require preservatives
	Several vaccines containing thimerosal were given to infants until 1999
	It is presumed that mercury children receive in vaccines containing thimerosal is excreted with no accumulation during 2-month periods between vaccinations
	Since 2001 no vaccines contain thimerosal except inactivated influenza vaccines
	Earlier toxicology studies and a 2007 study found no adverse effects or no support for a causal relationship between thimerosal and neuropyschotic functioning

Data from Centers for Disease Control and Prevention, 2004. Available at www.cdc.gov/nip/vacsafeconcerns/thimerosal/flags-thimerosal.htm#4; Clarkson TW, Magos L, Myers GI: The toxicology of mercury—current exposures and clinical manifestations, *N Engl J Med* 349(18):1731–1737, 2003; Thompson WW et al: Early thimerosal exposure and neuropsychological outcomes at 7 to 10 years, *N Eng J Med* 357(13):1281–1292, 2007.

BOX 3-2 CLASSIFICATION OF PREVENTABLE ADVERSE EVENTS IN PRIMARY CARE

Diagnosis: Misdiagnosis, missed diagnosis, delayed diagnosis
a. Related to symptoms
b. Related to prevention

Treatment
Drug: Incorrect drug, incorrect dose, delayed administration, omitted administration
Nondrug: Inappropriate, delayed, omitted, procedural complication
Preventive services: Inappropriate, delayed, omitted, procedural complication

Process Errors
Clinical factors: Clinical judgment, procedural skills error
Communication factors: Clinician-client, clinician, or healthcare personnel
Administration factors: Clinician, pharmacy, ancillary providers (physical therapy, occupational therapy, etc.), office setting
Other: Personal and family issues of clinicians and staff, insurance company regulations, government regulations, funding and employers, physical size and location of practice, general healthcare system

Data from Elder N, Dovey S: Classification of medical errors and preventable adverse events in primary care: a synthesis of the literature, *J Fam Pract* 51(1):1079, 2002.

group. The 1999 report published by the Institute of Medicine (IOM) indicated that between 44,000 and 98,000 unnecessary deaths per year occurred in hospitals alone as a result of errors by healthcare professionals (see *Health Alert:* Unintentional Injury Errors in Healthcare). Box 3-2 lists classifications of preventable events in primary care,[33] and Box 3-3 contains recommendations to avoid medical errors. Despite disagreements over the reported statistics, an accurate account is a tremendous challenge.[34] Statistics on nonfatal injuries are harder to document accurately, but they are known to be a significant cause of morbidity and disability and to cost society billions of dollars annually. The more common terms used to describe and classify unintentional and intentional injuries and brief descriptions of important features of these injuries are discussed in Table 3-9.

Asphyxial Injuries

Asphyxial injuries are caused by a failure of cells to receive or use oxygen. Deprivation of oxygen may be partial (hypoxia) or total (anoxia). Asphyxial injuries can be grouped into four general categories: suffocation, strangulation, chemical, and drowning.

Suffocation. Suffocation, or oxygen failing to reach the blood, can result from a lack of oxygen in the environment (entrapment in an enclosed space or filling of the environment with a suffocating gas) or blockage of the external airways. Classic examples of these types of asphyxial injuries are a child who is trapped in an abandoned refrigerator or a person who commits suicide by putting a plastic bag over his or her head. A reduction in the ambient oxygen level to 16% (normal is 21%) is immediately dangerous. If the level is below 5%, death can ensue within a matter of minutes. The diagnosis of these types of asphyxial injuries depends on obtaining an accurate and thorough history because there will be no specific physical findings.

Diagnosis and treatment in choking asphyxiation (obstruction of the internal airways) depend on locating and removing the obstructing material. Injury or disease also may cause swelling of the soft tissues of the airway leading to partial or complete obstruction and subsequent asphyxiation. Suffocation also may result from compression of the chest or abdomen (mechanical or compressional asphyxia), preventing normal respiratory movements. Usual signs and symptoms include florid facial congestion and petechiae (pinpoint hemorrhages) of the eyes and face.

Strangulation. Strangulation is caused by compression and closure of the blood vessels and air passages resulting from external pressure on the neck. This causes cerebral hypoxia or anoxia secondary to the alteration or cessation of blood flow to and from the brain. It is important

HEALTH ALERT

Unintentional Injury Errors in Healthcare

Errors in healthcare are an unintended event; no matter how trivial or commonplace, they are errors that could or did harm individuals. Medical errors are one of the leading causes of death and injury in the United States. Medical errors occur because the medical plan fails or is the wrong plan. A 1999 report by the Institute of Medicine (IOM) estimates that as many as 44,000 to 98,000 people in the United States die in hospitals each year as the result of medical errors. These data mean that more people die from medical errors than from motor vehicle accidents, breast cancer, or AIDS. Although these statistics have been challenged, the IOM report noted that many of the errors in healthcare result from a culture and system that are fragmented and solving this major problem will require extensive foundation or infrastructure building. Errors involve medicines, surgery, diagnosis, equipment, and laboratory reports. They can occur anywhere in the healthcare system, including hospitals, clinics, outpatient surgery centers, physicians' and nurse practitioners' offices, pharmacies, and an individual's home. Errors can happen during the most routine of plans, such as when an individual is prescribed a low-salt diet and is given a high-salt meal. Research indicated that most mistakes were not due to clinicians' negligence but rather from inherent shortcomings in the healthcare system. Yet errors can occur when clinicians and their clients have trouble communicating.

Although the literature about errors in healthcare has grown substantially over the last decade, we do not yet have a compelling analysis of the epidemiology of error. More is known about errors in hospitals than in other healthcare delivery settings. Medication-related error has been studied for several reasons: (1) it is the most common type of error, (2) substantial numbers of people are affected, and (3) it accounts for a large increase in healthcare costs. Medication errors are methodologically easier to study because the drug prescribing process provides documentation of medical decisions, administration of drugs is recorded, supplying drugs are documented, and deaths attributable to medication errors are recorded on death certificates. According to the Agency for Healthcare Research and Quality (AHRQ) the rate for potential adverse drug events was three times higher in children and much higher for babies in neonatal intensive care units. New data show bar-code technology with an electronic medication administration record (eMAR) substantially reduces transcription and medication administration errors. This technology also reduces potential drug-related adverse events. Bar-code eMAR is a combination of technologies that ensures the correct medication is administered to the right patient at the right dose and time. When nurses use these technologies, medication orders appear electronically in the individual's chart after pharmacist approval. Electronic alerts are sent to nurses if the medication is overdue and before administering the medication. Nurses are required to scan the bar code on the individual's wristband and then on the medication. A warning is issued if the bar codes do not match or it is the wrong time for administration of the medication.

Other errors, in addition to medication errors, include surgical injuries and wrong-site surgery; preventable suicides, restraint-related injuries, or death; hospital-acquired or other treatment-related infections; falls; burns; pressure ulcers; and mistaken identity. Studies of errors outside the hospital have begun.

The IOM report has galvanized a national movement to improve client safety and eliminate healthcare errors. "Errors and excess mortality can be eliminated but only if concern and attention is shifted away from individuals and toward the error-prone systems in which clinicians work" (Leape, 2000).

Data from Agency for Healthcare Research and Quality (AHRQ): *20 tips to help prevent medical errors* (Pub No. 00-P038), Washington, DC, 2000, U.S. Department of Health and Human Services; Agency for Healthcare Research and Quality (AHRQ): *Advancing patient safety* (Pub No. 09(10)-0084), Washington, DC, 2009, U.S. Department of Health and Human Services; Elder N, Dovey S: Classification of medical errors and preventable adverse events in primary care: a synthesis of the literature, *J Fam Pract* 51(1):1079, 2002; Kohn LT, Corrigan JM, Donaldson M, editors: *To err is human: building a safer health system,* Washington, DC, 1999, Institute of Medicine; Leape L: Institute of Medicine medical error figures are not exaggerated, *J Am Med Assoc* 284(1), 2000. Data from AHRQ: *AHRQ study shows using bar-code technology with eMar reduces medication administration and transcription errors,* Rockville, Md, press release May 5, 2010, Author. Available at www.ahrq.gov/news/press.pr2010/emarpr.htm; Poon EG et al: Effect of bar-code technology on the safety of medication administration, *N Engl J Med* 362(18):1698–1707, 2010.

to remember that the amount of force needed to close the jugular veins (2 kg [4.5 lb]) or carotid arteries (5 kg [11 lb]) is significantly less than that required to crush the trachea (15 kg [33 lb]). It is the alteration of cerebral blood flow in most types of strangulation that causes injury or death—not the lack of airflow. With complete blockage of the carotid arteries, unconsciousness can occur within 10 to 15 seconds.

A noose is placed around the neck, and the weight of the body is used to cause constriction of the noose and compression of the neck in **hanging strangulations.** The body does not need to be completely suspended to produce severe injury or death. Depending on the type of ligature used, there usually is a distinct mark on the neck—an inverted V with the base of the V pointing toward the point of suspension. Internal injuries of the neck are actually quite rare in hangings, and only in judicial hangings, in which the body is weighted and dropped, is significant soft tissue or cervical spinal trauma seen. Petechiae of the eyes or face may be seen, but they are rare.

In **ligature strangulation,** the mark on the neck is horizontal without the inverted V pattern seen in hangings. Petechiae may be more common because intermittent opening and closure of the blood vessels may occur as a result of the victim's struggles. Internal injuries of the neck are rare.

Variable amounts of external trauma on the neck are found with contusions and abrasions in **manual strangulation** caused either by the assailant or by the victim clawing at his or her own neck in an attempt to remove the assailant's hands. Internal damage can be quite severe, with bruising of deep structures and even fractures of the hyoid bone and tracheal and cricoid cartilages. Petechiae are common.

Chemical Asphyxiants. Chemical asphyxiants either prevent the delivery of oxygen to the tissues or block its utilization. Carbon monoxide is the most common chemical asphyxiant (see p. 71). Cyanide acts as an asphyxiant by combining with the ferric iron atom in cytochrome oxidase, thereby blocking the intracellular use of oxygen. A victim of cyanide poisoning will have the same cherry-red appearance as a carbon monoxide intoxication victim because cyanide blocks the use of circulating oxyhemoglobin. An odor of bitter almonds also may be detected. (The ability to smell cyanide is a genetic trait that is absent in a significant portion of the general population.) Hydrogen sulfide (sewer gas) is a chemical asphyxiant in which victims of hydrogen cyanide poisoning may have brown-tinged blood in addition to the nonspecific signs of asphyxiation.

Drowning. Drowning is an alteration of oxygen delivery to tissues resulting from the inhalation of fluid, usually water. In 2007 there were 4086 drowning deaths in the United States. Although research in the 1940s and 1950s indicated that changes in blood electrolyte levels and volume as a result of absorption of fluid from the lungs may be an

TABLE 3-9 UNINTENTIONAL AND INTENTIONAL INJURIES

TYPE OF INJURY	DESCRIPTION
BLUNT-FORCE INJURIES	Mechanical injury to body resulting in tearing, shearing, or crushing; most common type of injury seen in healthcare settings; caused by blows or impacts; motor vehicle accidents and falls most common cause
	Contusion (bruise): Bleeding into skin or underlying tissues; initial color will be red-purple, then blue-black, then yellow-brown or green (see Figure 3-20); duration of bruise depends on extent, location, and degree of vascularization; bruising of soft tissue may be confined to deeper structures; *hematoma* is collection of blood in soft tissue; *subdural hematoma* is blood between inner surface of dura mater and surface of brain; can result from blows, falls, or sudden acceleration/deceleration of head as occurs in *shaken baby syndrome; epidural hematoma* is collection of blood between inner surface of skull and dura; is most often associated with a skull fracture
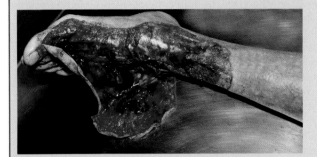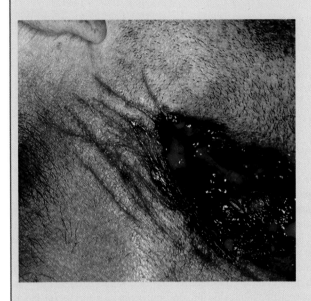	**Laceration:** Tear or rip resulting when tensile strength of skin or tissue is exceeded; is ragged and irregular with abraded edges; an extreme example is *avulsion,* where a wide area of tissue is pulled away; lacerations of internal organs are common in blunt-force injuries; lacerations of liver, spleen, kidneys, and bowel occur from blows to abdomen; thoracic aorta may be lacerated in sudden deceleration accidents; severe blows or impacts to chest may rupture heart with lacerations of atria or ventricles
	Fracture: Blunt-force blows or impacts can cause bone to break or shatter (see Chapter 37)
SHARP-FORCE INJURIES	Cutting and piercing injuries accounted for 2734 deaths in 2007; men have a higher rate (1.37/100,000) than women (0.44/100,000); differences by race are whites 0.71/100,000, blacks 2.12/100,000, and other groups 0.80/100,000
	Incised wound: Is a wound that is *longer* than it is *deep;* wound can be straight or jagged with sharp, distinct edges without abrasion; usually produces significant external bleeding with little internal hemorrhage; are noted in sharp-force injury suicides; in addition to a deep, lethal cut, there will be superficial incisions in same area called *hesitation marks*
	Stab wound: Is a penetrating sharp force injury that is *deeper* than it is *long;* if a sharp instrument is used, depths of wound are clean and distinct but can be abraded if object is inserted deeply and wider portion (e.g., hilt of a knife) impacts skin; depending on size and location of wound, external bleeding may be surprisingly small; after an initial spurt of blood, even if a major vessel or heart is struck, wound may be almost completely closed by tissue pressure, thus allowing only a trickle of visible blood despite copious internal bleeding
	Puncture wound: Instruments or objects with sharp points but without sharp edges produce puncture wounds; classic example is wound of foot after stepping on a nail; wounds are prone to infection, have abrasion of edges, and can be very deep
	Chopping wound: Heavy, edged instruments (axes, hatchets, propeller blades) produce wounds with a combination of sharp- and blunt-force characteristics

TABLE 3-9 UNINTENTIONAL AND INTENTIONAL INJURIES—cont'd

TYPE OF INJURY	DESCRIPTION
GUNSHOT WOUNDS	Accounted for more than 31,224 deaths in the United States in 2007; men more likely to die than women (18.16 vs. 2.73/100,000); black men between ages of 15 and 24 have greatest death rate (86.95/100,000); gunshot wounds are either penetrating (bullet remains in body) or perforating (bullet exits body); bullet also can fragment; most important factors or appearances are whether it is an entrance or exit wound and range of fire
	Entrance wound: All wounds share some common features; overall appearance is most affected by range of fire
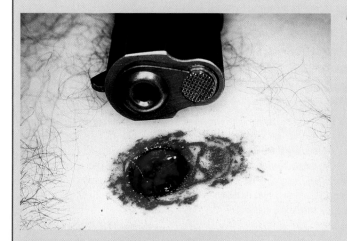	*Contact range entrance wound:* Distinctive type of wound when gun is held so muzzle rests on or presses into skin surface; there is searing of edges of wound from flame and soot or smoke on edges of wound in addition to hole; hard contact wounds of head cause severe tearing and disruption of tissue (because of thin layer of skin and muscle overlying bone); wound is gaping and jagged, known as *blow back;* can produce a patterned abrasion that mirrors weapon used
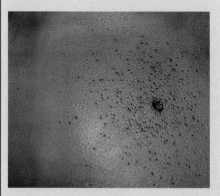	*Intermediate (distance) range entrance wound:* Surrounded by gunpowder tattooing or stippling; *tattooing* results from fragments of burning or unburned pieces of gunpowder exiting barrel and forcefully striking skin; *stippling* results when gunpowder abrades but does not penetrate skin
	Indeterminate range entrance wound: Occurs when flame, soot, or gunpowder does not reach skin surface but bullet does; *indeterminate* is used rather than *distant* because appearance may be same regardless of distance; for example, if an individual is shot at close range through multiple layers of clothing the wound may look the same as if the shooting occurred at a distance
	Exit wound: Has the same appearance regardless of range of fire; most important factors are speed of projectile and degree of deformation; size cannot be used to determine if hole is an exit or entrance wound; usually has clean edges that can often be reapproximated to cover defect; skin is one of toughest structures for a bullet to penetrate; thus it is not uncommon for a bullet to pass entirely through body but stopped just beneath skin on "exit" side
	Wounding potential of bullets: Most damage done by a bullet is a result of amount of energy transferred to tissue impacted; speed of bullet has much greater effect than increased size; some bullets are designed to expand or fragment when striking an object, for example, *hollow-point* ammunition; lethality of a wound depends on what structures are damaged; wounds of brain may not be lethal; however, they are usually immediately incapacitating and lead to significant long-term disability; a person with a "lethal" injury (wound of heart or aorta) also may not be immediately incapacitated

BOX 3-3 RECOMMENDATIONS TO AVOID MEDICAL ERRORS

What can you do? Be Involved in Your Healthcare.

1. *The single most important way you can help prevent errors is to be an active member of your healthcare team.* That means taking part in every decision about your healthcare. Research shows that patients who are more involved with their care tend to get better results.

Medicines

2. Make sure your healthcare providers know everything you are taking, including prescription and over-the-counter medicines and dietary supplements such as vitamins and herbs. At least once a year, take all of your medications and supplements to an appointment with your healthcare provider. "Brown bagging" your medications can help you and your provider talk about them and determine if there are any problems. This action also can help your provider keep your records up to date, which can help you obtain better quality care.

3. Make sure you inform your healthcare providers about any allergies and adverse reactions you have shown to medications. This can help you avoid exposure to a medication that can harm you.

4. When your healthcare provider writes you a prescription, make sure you can read it. If you cannot read your provider's handwriting, your pharmacist might not be able to either.

5. Ask for information about your medicines in terms you can understand—both when your medications are prescribed and when you receive them. What is the purpose of the medicine? How am I supposed to take it and for how long? What side effects are likely? What should I do if side effects occur? Is this medicine safe to take with other medicines or dietary supplements I am taking? What food, drink, or activities should I avoid while taking this medicine?

6. When you pick up your medicine from the pharmacy ask, "Is this the medicine my provider prescribed?" A study conducted by the Massachusetts College of Pharmacy and Allied Health Sciences found that 88% of medicine errors involved the wrong drug or the wrong dose.

7. If you have any questions about the directions on your medicine label, ask. Medicine labels can be hard to understand. For example, ask if "four doses daily" means taking a dose every 6 hours around the clock or just during regular waking hours.

8. Ask your pharmacist for the best device to measure your liquid medicine. Also ask questions if you are not sure how to use it. Research shows that many people do not understand the right way to measure liquid medicines. For example, many use household teaspoons, which often do not hold a true teaspoon of liquid. Special devices, like marked syringes, help to measure the right dose. Being told how to use the devices helps even more.

9. Ask for written information about the side effects your medicine could cause. If you know the possible side effects of a medication, you will be better prepared if a side effect occurs; alternatively, if you have an unexpected reaction, you can report the problem immediately and get help before the condition worsens. A study found that written information about medicines can help patients recognize problem side effects and then communicate that information to their healthcare provider or pharmacist.

Hospital Stays

10. *If you have a choice, choose a hospital in which many patients have the same procedure or surgery you need.* Research shows that patients tend to have better results when they are treated in hospitals that have a great deal of experience with their condition.

11. If you are in a hospital, consider asking all healthcare workers who have direct contact with you whether they have washed their hands. Handwashing is an important way to prevent the spread of infections in hospitals. However, it is not done regularly or thoroughly enough. A recent study found that when patients checked whether healthcare workers washed their hands, the workers washed their hands more often and used more soap.

12. When you are being discharged from the hospital, ask your healthcare provider to explain the treatment plan you will use at home. This includes learning about your medicines and determining when you can resume your regular activities. Recent studies show that healthcare providers often overestimate their patients' understanding of discharge instructions.

Surgery

13. If you are having surgery, make sure you, your healthcare provider, and your surgeon all agree and are clear on exactly what will be done. Performing surgery at the wrong site (for example, operating on the left knee instead of the right) is rare—but even once is too often. The good news is that wrong-site surgery is 100% preventable. The American Academy of Orthopaedic Surgeons urges its members to sign their initials directly on the operative site before the surgery.

Other Steps You Can Take

14. *Speak up if you have questions or concerns.* You have a right to question anyone who is involved with your care.

15. Make sure that someone, such as your personal healthcare provider, is in charge of your care. This is especially important if you have many health problems or are in a hospital.

16. Make sure that all health professionals involved in your care have important health information about you. Do not assume that everyone has the necessary information about your care.

17. Ask a family member or friend to stay with you and to be your advocate (someone who can help get things done and speak for you if you cannot). Even if you do not need help now, you might need it later.

18. *Know that "more" is not always better.* It is a good idea to find out why a test or treatment is needed and how it can help you. You could be better off without it.

19. If you have a test, do not assume that "no news is good news." Ask about the results.

20. *Learn about your condition and treatments by asking your healthcare provider and nurse and by using other reliable sources.* For example, treatment recommendations based on the latest scientific evidence are available from the National Guidelines Clearinghouse at www.guideline.gov. Ask your provider if your treatment is based on the latest evidence.

Data from Agency for Healthcare Research and Quality: *20 tips to help prevent medical errors* (Pub No. 00-PO30), Rockville, Md, 2000, Author; Bates DW et al: *JAMA* 274(1):29–34, 1995; Bates DW et al: *JAMA* 277(4):307–311, 1997; Centers for Disease Control and Prevention, National Center for Health Statistics: *Natl Vital Stats Rep 47* 191:27, 1999; Institute of Medicine: *To err is human: building a safer health system,* Washington, DC, 1999, National Academy Press.

TABLE 3-10   MECHANISMS OF CELLULAR INJURY

MECHANISM	CHARACTERISTICS	EXAMPLES
Genetic Factors	Alter cell's nucleus and plasma membrane's structure, shape, receptors, or transport mechanisms	Sickle cell anemia, Huntington disease, muscular dystrophy, abetalipoproteinemia, familial hypercholesterolemia
Epigenetic Factors	Induction of mitotically heritable alterations in gene expression without changing DNA	Gene silencing in cancer
Nutritional Imbalances	Pathophysiologic cellular effects develop when nutrients are not consumed in diet and transported to body's cells *or* when excessive amounts of nutrients are consumed and transported	Protein deficiency, protein-calorie malnutrition, glucose deficiency, lipid deficiency (hypolipidemia), hyperlipidemia (increased lipoproteins in blood causing deposits of fat in heart, liver, and muscle), vitamin deficiencies
Physical Agents		
Temperature extremes	*Hypothermic injury* results from chilling or freezing of cells, creating high intracellular sodium concentrations; abrupt drops in temperature lead to vasoconstriction and increased viscosity of blood, causing ischemic injury, infarction, and necrosis; reactive oxygen species (ROS) are important in this process	Frostbite
	Hyperthermic injury is caused by excessive heat and varies in severity according to nature, intensity, and extent of heat	Burns, burn blisters, heat cramps usually from vigorous exercise with water and salt loss; heat exhaustion with salt and water loss causes heme contraction; heat stroke is life-threatening with a clinical rectal temperature of 106° F
	Tissue injury caused by compressive waves of air or fluid impinging on body, followed by sudden wave of decreased pressure; changes may collapse thorax, rupture internal solid organs, and cause widespread hemorrhage: carbon dioxide and nitrogen that are normally dissolved in blood precipitate from solution and form small bubbles (gas emboli), causing hypoxic injury and pain	Blast injury (air or immersion), decompression sickness (caisson disease or "the bends"); recently reported in a few individuals with subdural hematomas after riding high-speed roller coasters
Ionizing radiation	Refers to any form of radiation that can remove orbital electrons from atoms; source is usually environment and medical use; damage is to DNA molecule, causing chromosomal aberrations, chromosomal instability, and damage to membranes and enzymes; also induces growth factors and extracellular matrix remodeling; uncertainty exists regarding effects of low levels of radiation	X-rays, γ-rays, and α- and β-particles cause skin redness, skin damage, chromosomal damage, cancer
Illumination	Fluorescent lighting and halogen lamps create harmful oxidative stresses; ultraviolet light has been linked to skin cancer	Eyestrain, obscured vision, cataracts, headaches, melanoma
Mechanical stresses	Injury is caused by physical impact or irritation; they may be overt or cumulative	Faulty occupational biomechanics, leading to overexertion disorders
Noise	Can be caused by acute loud noise or cumulative effects of various intensities, frequencies, and duration of noise; considered a public health threat	Hearing impairment or loss; tinnitus, temporary threshold shift (TTS), or loss can occur as a complication of critical illness, from mechanical trauma, ototoxic medications, infections, vascular disorders, and noise

important factor in some drownings, the major mechanism of injury is hypoxemia (low blood oxygen levels). Even in freshwater drownings, where large amounts of water can pass through the alveolar-capillary interface, there is no evidence that increases in blood volume cause significant electrolyte disturbances or hemolysis, or that the amount of fluid loading is beyond the compensatory capabilities of the kidneys and heart. Airway obstruction is the more important pathologic abnormality, underscored by the fact that in as many as 15% of drownings little or no water enters the lungs because of vagal nerve–mediated laryngospasms. This phenomenon is called dry-lung drowning.

No matter what mechanism is involved, cerebral hypoxia leads to unconsciousness in a matter of minutes. Whether this progresses to death depends on a number of factors, including the age and the health of the individual. One of the most important factors is the temperature of the water. Irreversible injury develops much more rapidly in warm water than it does in cold water. Submersion times of up to 1 hour with subsequent survival have been reported in children who were submerged in very cold water. Complete submersion is not necessary for a person to drown. An incapacitated or helpless individual (epileptic, alcoholic, infant) may drown in water that is only a few inches deep.

It is important to remember that no specific or diagnostic findings *prove* that a person recovered from the water is actually a drowning victim. In cases where water has entered the lung, there may be large amounts of foam exiting the nose and mouth, although this also can be seen in certain types of drug overdoses. A body recovered from water with signs of prolonged immersion could just as easily be a victim of some other type of injury with the immersion acting to obscure the actual cause of death. When working with a living victim recovered from water, it is essential to keep in mind that an underlying condition may have led to the person's becoming incapacitated and submerged—a condition that also may need to be treated or corrected while correcting hypoxemia and dealing with its sequelae.

Infectious Injury

The pathogenicity (virulence) of microorganisms lies in their ability to survive and proliferate in the human body, where they injure cells and tissues. The disease-producing potential of a microorganism depends on its ability to (1) invade and destroy cells, (2) produce toxins, and (3) produce damaging hypersensitivity reactions. (See Chapter 7 for a description of infection and infectious organisms.)

Immunologic and Inflammatory Injury

Cellular membranes are injured by direct contact with cellular and chemical components of the immune and inflammatory responses, such as phagocytic cells (lymphocytes, macrophages) and substances such as histamine, antibodies, lymphokines, complement, and proteases (see Chapter 5). Complement is responsible for many of the membrane alterations that occur during immunologic injury.

Membrane alterations are associated with a rapid leakage of potassium (K^+) out of the cell and a rapid influx of water. Antibodies can interfere with membrane function by binding with and occupying receptor molecules on the plasma membrane. Antibodies also can block or destroy cellular junctions, interfering with intercellular communication. Other mechanisms of cellular injury are genetic factors, nutritional imbalances, and physical agents. These are summarized in Table 3-10.

MANIFESTATIONS OF CELLULAR INJURY: ACCUMULATIONS

An important manifestation of cell injury is the intracellular accumulation of abnormal amounts of various substances and the resultant metabolic disturbances. Cellular accumulations, also known as infiltrations, not only result from sublethal, sustained injury by cells but also result from normal (but inefficient) cell function. Two categories of substances can produce accumulations: (1) a *normal cellular substance* (such as excess water, proteins, lipids, and carbohydrates) or (2) an *abnormal substance,* either endogenous (such as a product of abnormal metabolism or synthesis) or exogenous (such as infectious agents or a mineral). These products can accumulate transiently or permanently and can be toxic or harmless. Most accumulations are attributed to four types of mechanisms, all abnormal (Figure 3-17). Abnormal accumulations of these substances can occur in the cytoplasm (often in the lysosomes) or in the nucleus if (1) the normal, endogenous substance is produced in excess or at an increased rate, thus abnormal metabolism; (2) an abnormal substance, often the result of a mutated gene, accumulates because of defects in protein folding, transport, or abnormal degradation; (3) an endogenous substance (normal or abnormal) is not effectively catabolized, usually because of lack of a vital lysosomal enzyme; or (4) harmful exogenous materials, such as heavy metals, mineral dusts, or microorganisms, accumulate because of inhalation, ingestion, or infection.

In all storage diseases, the cells attempt to digest, or catabolize, the "stored" substances. As a result, excessive amounts of metabolites (products of catabolism) accumulate in the cells and are expelled into the extracellular matrix, where they are consumed by phagocytic cells called *macrophages* (see Chapter 5). Some of these scavenger cells circulate throughout the body, whereas others remain fixed in certain tissues, such as the liver or spleen. As more and more macrophages

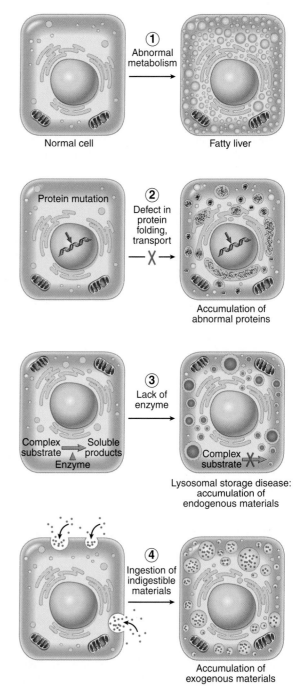

FIGURE 3-17 Mechanisms of Intracellular Accumulations. (From Kumar V et al: Cellular responses to stress and toxic insults: adaptation, injury, and death. In Kumar V et al, editors: *Robbins and Cotran pathologic basis of disease,* ed 8, St Louis, 2010, Saunders.)

and other phagocytes migrate to tissues that are producing excessive metabolites, the affected tissues begin to swell. This is the mechanism that causes enlargement of the liver (hepatomegaly) or the spleen (splenomegaly) as a clinical manifestation of many storage diseases.

Water

Cellular swelling, the most common degenerative change, is caused by the shift of extracellular water into the cells. In hypoxic injury, movement of fluid and ions into the cell is associated with acute failure of metabolism and loss of ATP production. Normally, the pump that

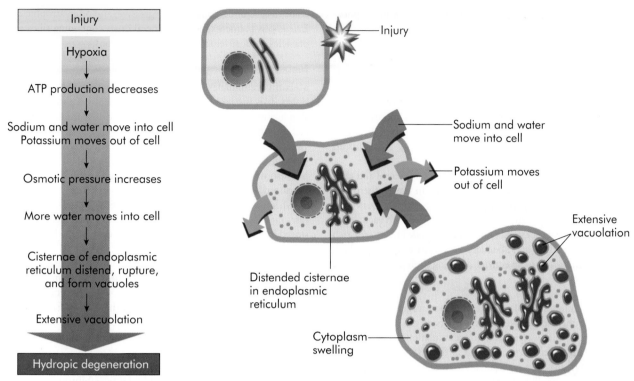

FIGURE 3-18 The Process of Oncosis (Formerly Referred to as "Hydropic Degeneration"). *ATP,* Adenosine triphosphate.

transports sodium ions out of the cell is maintained by the presence of ATP and adenosinetriphosphatase (ATPase), the active transport enzyme. In metabolic failure caused by hypoxia, reduced levels of ATP and ATPase permit sodium to accumulate in the cell while potassium diffuses outward. The increased intracellular sodium concentration increases osmotic pressure, drawing more water into the cell. The cisternae of the endoplasmic reticulum become distended, rupture, and then unite to form large vacuoles that isolate the water from the cytoplasm, a process called *vacuolation*. Progressive vacuolation results in cytoplasmic swelling called **oncosis** (which has replaced the old term *hydropic [water] degeneration*) or **vacuolar degeneration** (Figure 3-18). If cellular swelling affects all the cells in an organ, the organ increases in weight and becomes distended and pale.

Cellular swelling is reversible and is considered sublethal. It is, in fact, an early manifestation of almost all types of cellular injury, including severe or lethal cell injury. It is also associated with high fever, hypokalemia (abnormally low concentrations of potassium in the blood; see Chapter 4), and certain infections.

Lipids and Carbohydrates

Certain metabolic disorders result in the abnormal intracellular accumulation of carbohydrates and lipids. These substances may accumulate throughout the body but are found primarily in the spleen, liver, and CNS. Accumulations in cells of the CNS can cause neurologic dysfunction and severe mental retardation. Lipids accumulate in Tay-Sachs disease, Niemann-Pick disease, and Gaucher disease, whereas in the diseases known as mucopolysaccharidoses, carbohydrates are in excess. The mucopolysaccharidoses are progressive disorders that usually involve multiple organs, including liver, spleen, heart, and blood vessels. The accumulated mucopolysaccharides are found in reticuloendothelial cells, endothelial cells, intimal smooth muscle cells, and fibroblasts throughout the body. These carbohydrate

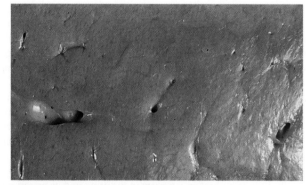

FIGURE 3-19 Fatty Liver. The liver appears yellow. (From Damjanov I, Linder J: *Pathology: a color atlas,* St Louis, 2000, Mosby.)

accumulations can cause clouding of the cornea, joint stiffness, and mental retardation.

Although lipids sometimes accumulate in heart and kidney cells, the most common site of intracellular lipid accumulation, or **fatty change,** is liver cells. Because hepatic metabolism and secretion of lipids are crucial to proper body function, imbalances and deficiencies in these processes lead to major pathologic changes. Lipid accumulation in liver cells causes fatty liver, or fatty change (Figure 3-19). As lipids fill the cells, vacuolation pushes the nucleus and other organelles aside. The liver's outward appearance is yellow and greasy. Alcohol abuse is one of the most common causes of fatty liver (see Chapter 34).

Lipid accumulation in liver cells occurs after cellular injury instigates one or more of the following mechanisms:
1. Increased movement of free fatty acids into the liver (starvation, for example, increases the metabolism of triglycerides in adipose tissue, releasing fatty acids that subsequently enter liver cells)

2. Failure of the metabolic process that converts fatty acids to phospholipids, resulting in the preferential conversion of fatty acids to triglycerides
3. Increased synthesis of triglycerides from fatty acids (increases in an enzyme, α-glycerophosphatase, can accelerate triglyceride synthesis)
4. Decreased synthesis of apoproteins (lipid-acceptor proteins)
5. Failure of lipids to bind with apoproteins and form lipoproteins
6. Failure of mechanisms that transport lipoproteins out of the cell
7. Direct damage to the endoplasmic reticulum by free radicals released by alcohol's toxic effects

Many pathologic states show accumulation of cholesterol and cholesterol esters. These states include atherosclerosis, in which atherosclerotic plaques, smooth muscle cells, and macrophages within the intimal layer of the aorta and large arteries are filled with lipid-rich vacuoles of cholesterol and cholesterol esters. Other states include cholesterol-rich deposits in the gallbladder and Niemann-Pick disease (type C), which involve genetic mutations of an enzyme affecting cholesterol transport.

Glycogen

Intracellular accumulations of glycogen are seen in genetic disorders called *glycogen storage diseases* and in disorders of glucose and glycogen metabolism. As with water and lipid accumulation, glycogen accumulation results in excessive vacuolation of the cytoplasm. The most common cause of glycogen accumulation is the disorder of glucose metabolism, diabetes mellitus (see Chapter 18).

Proteins

Proteins provide cellular structure and constitute most of the cell's dry weight. They are synthesized on ribosomes in the cytoplasm from the essential amino acids lysine, threonine, leucine, isoleucine, methionine, tryptophan, valine, phenylalanine, and histidine. Protein accumulation probably damages cells in two ways. First, metabolites, produced when the cell attempts to digest some proteins, are enzymes that when released from lysosomes can damage cellular organelles. Second, excessive amounts of protein in the cytoplasm push against cellular organelles, disrupting organelle function and intracellular communication.

Protein excess accumulates primarily in the epithelial cells of the renal convoluted tubule and in the antibody-forming plasma cells (B lymphocytes) of the immune system. Several types of renal disorders cause excessive excretion of protein molecules in the urine (proteinuria). Normally, little or no protein is present in the urine, and its presence in significant amounts indicates cellular injury and altered cellular function.

Accumulations of protein in B lymphocytes can occur during active synthesis of antibodies during the immune response. The excess aggregates of protein are called *Russell bodies* (see Chapter 5). Russell bodies have been identified in multiple myeloma (plasma cell tumor) (see Chapter 20).

Mutations in protein can slow protein folding, resulting in the accumulation of partially folded intermediates. An example is α_1-antitrypsin deficiency, which can cause emphysema. Certain types of cell injury are associated with the accumulation of cytoskeleton proteins. For example, the *neurofibrillary tangle* found in the brain in Alzheimer disease contains these types of proteins.

Pigments

Pigment accumulations may be normal or abnormal, endogenous (produced within the body) or exogenous (produced outside the body). Endogenous pigments are derived, for example, from amino acids (e.g., tyrosine, tryptophan). They include melanin and the blood proteins porphyrins, hemoglobin, and hemosiderin. Lipid-rich pigments, such as lipofuscin (the aging pigment), give a yellow-brown color to cells undergoing slow, regressive, and often atrophic changes. Exogenous pigments include mineral dusts containing silica and iron particles, lead, silver salts, and dyes for tattoos.

Melanin

Melanin accumulates in epithelial cells (keratinocytes) of the skin and retina. It is an extremely important pigment because it protects the skin against long exposure to sunlight and is considered an essential factor in the prevention of skin cancer (see Chapters 10 and 39). Ultraviolet light (e.g., sunlight) stimulates the synthesis of melanin, which probably absorbs ultraviolet rays during subsequent exposure. Melanin also may protect the skin by trapping the injurious free radicals produced by the action of ultraviolet light on skin.

Melanin is a brown-black pigment derived from the amino acid *tyrosine*. It is synthesized by epidermal cells called *melanocytes* and is stored in membrane-bound cytoplasmic vesicles called *melanosomes*.

Melanin also can accumulate in melanophores (melanin-containing pigment cells), macrophages, or other phagocytic cells in the dermis. Presumably these cells acquire the melanin from nearby melanocytes or from pigment that has been extruded from dying epidermal cells. This is the mechanism that causes freckles. Melanin also occurs in the benign form of pigmented moles called *nevi* (see Chapter 39). Malignant melanoma is a cancerous skin tumor that contains melanin.

A decrease in melanin production occurs in the inherited disorder of melanin metabolism called *albinism*. Albinism is often diffuse, involving all the skin, the eyes, and the hair. Albinism is also related to phenylalanine metabolism. In classic types, the person with albinism is unable to convert tyrosine to DOPA (3,4-dihydroxyphenylalanine), an intermediate in melanin biosynthesis. Melanin-producing cells are present in normal numbers, but they are unable to make melanin. Individuals with albinism are very sensitive to sunlight and quickly become sunburned. They are also at high risk for skin cancer.

Hemoproteins

Hemoproteins are among the most essential of the normal endogenous pigments. They include hemoglobin and the oxidative enzymes, the cytochromes. Central to an understanding of disorders involving these pigments is knowledge of iron uptake, metabolism, excretion, and storage (see Chapter 19). Hemoprotein accumulations in cells are caused by excessive storage of iron, which is transferred to the cells from the bloodstream. Iron enters the blood from three primary sources: (1) tissue stores, (2) the intestinal mucosa, and (3) macrophages that remove and destroy dead or defective red blood cells. The amount of iron in blood plasma depends also on the metabolism of the major iron transport protein, *transferrin*.

Iron is stored in tissue cells in two forms: as ferritin and, when increased levels of iron are present, as hemosiderin. Hemosiderin is a yellow-brown pigment derived from hemoglobin. With pathologic states, excesses of iron cause hemosiderin to accumulate within cells, often in areas of bruising and hemorrhage and in the lungs and spleen after congestion caused by heart failure. With local hemorrhage, the skin first appears red-blue and then lysis of the escaped red blood cells occurs, causing the hemoglobin to be transformed to hemosiderin. The color changes noted in bruising reflect this transformation (Figure 3-20).

Hemosiderosis is a condition in which excess iron is stored as hemosiderin in the cells of many organs and tissues. This condition is common in individuals who have received repeated blood transfusions or prolonged parenteral administration of iron. Hemosiderosis is associated also with increased absorption of dietary iron, conditions in which iron storage and transport are impaired, and hemolytic anemia. Excessive alcohol (wine) ingestion also can lead to hemosiderosis. Normally, absorption of excessive dietary iron is prevented by an iron absorption process in the intestines. Failure of this process can lead to total body iron accumulations in the range of 60 to 80 g, compared with normal iron stores of 4.5 to 5 g. Excessive accumulations of iron, such as occur in hemochromatosis (a genetic disorder of iron metabolism and the most severe example of iron overload), are associated with liver and pancreatic cell damage.

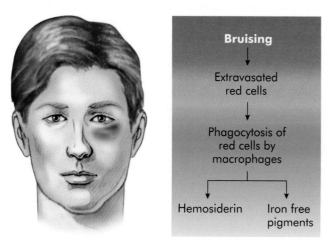

FIGURE 3-20 Hemosiderin Accumulation Is Noted as the Color Changes in a "Black Eye."

Bilirubin is a normal, yellow-to-green pigment of bile derived from the porphyrin structure of hemoglobin. Excess bilirubin within cells and tissues causes jaundice (icterus), or yellowing of the skin. Jaundice occurs when the bilirubin level exceeds 1.5 to 2 mg/dl of plasma, compared with the normal values of 0.4 to 1 mg/dl. Hyperbilirubinemia occurs with (1) destruction of red blood cells (erythrocytes), such as in hemolytic jaundice; (2) diseases affecting the metabolism and excretion of bilirubin in the liver; and (3) diseases that cause obstruction of the common bile duct, such as gallstones or pancreatic tumors. Certain drugs (specifically chlorpromazine and other phenothiazine derivatives), estrogenic hormones, and halothane (an anesthetic) can cause the obstruction of normal bile flow through the liver.

Because unconjugated bilirubin is lipid soluble, it can injure the lipid components of the plasma membrane. Albumin, a plasma protein, provides significant protection by binding unconjugated bilirubin in plasma. Unconjugated bilirubin causes two cellular outcomes: uncoupling of oxidative phosphorylation and a loss of cellular proteins. These two changes could cause structural injury to the various membranes of the cell.

Calcium

Calcium salts accumulate in both injured and dead tissues (Figure 3-21). An important mechanism of cellular calcification is the influx of extracellular calcium in injured mitochondria (see p. 64). Another mechanism that causes calcium accumulation in alveoli (gas-exchange airways of the lungs), gastric epithelium, and renal tubules is the excretion of acid at these sites, leading to the local production of hydroxyl ions. Hydroxyl ions result in precipitation of calcium hydroxide,

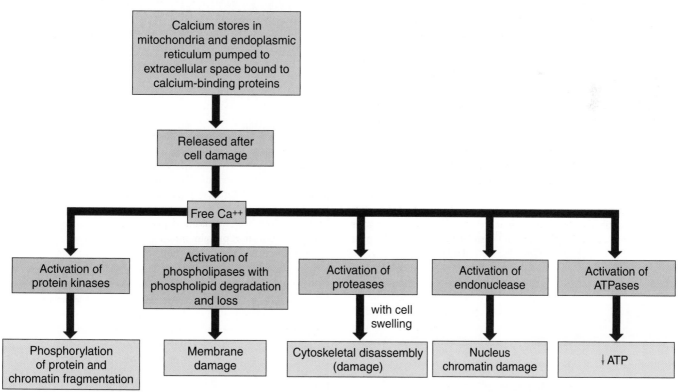

FIGURE 3-21 Free Cytosolic Calcium: A Destructive Agent. Normally, calcium is removed from the cytosol by adenosine triphosphate (ATP)-dependent calcium pumps. In normal cells, calcium is bound to buffering proteins, such as calbindin or paralbumin, and is contained in the endoplasmic reticulum and the mitochondria. If there is abnormal permeability of calcium-ion channels, direct damage to membranes, or depletion of ATP (i.e., hypoxic injury), calcium increases in the cytosol. If the free calcium cannot be buffered or pumped out of cells, uncontrolled enzyme activation takes place, causing further damage. Uncontrolled entry of calcium into the cytosol is an important final common pathway in many causes of cell death.

$Ca(OH)_2$, and hydroxyapatite, $(Ca_3[PO_4]_2)_3 \cdot Ca(OH)_2$, a mixed salt. Damage occurs when calcium salts cluster and harden, interfering with normal cellular structure and function.

Pathologic calcification can be dystrophic or metastatic. **Dystrophic calcification** occurs in dying and dead tissues, chronic tuberculosis of the lungs and lymph nodes, advanced atherosclerosis (narrowing of arteries as a result of plaque accumulation), and heart valve injury (Figure 3-22). Calcification of the heart valves interferes with their opening and closing, causing heart murmurs (see Chapter 23). Calcification of the coronary arteries predisposes them to severe narrowing and thrombosis, which can lead to myocardial infarction. Another site of dystrophic calcification is the center of tumors. Over time, the center is deprived of its oxygen supply, dies, and becomes calcified. The calcium salts appear as gritty, clumped granules that can become hard as stone. When several layers clump together, they resemble grains of sand and are called **psammoma bodies.**

Metastatic calcification consists of mineral deposits that occur in undamaged normal tissues as the result of hypercalcemia (excess calcium in the blood; see Chapter 4). Conditions that cause hypercalcemia include hyperparathyroidism, toxic levels of vitamin D, hyperthyroidism, idiopathic hypercalcemia of infancy, Addison disease (adrenocortical insufficiency), systemic sarcoidosis, milk-alkali syndrome, and the increased bone demineralization that results from bone tumors, leukemia, and disseminated cancers. Hypercalcemia also may occur in advanced renal failure with phosphate retention, resulting in hyperparathyroidism.

Urate

In humans, uric acid (**urate**) is the major end product of purine catabolism because of the absence of the enzyme urate oxidase. Serum urate concentration is, in general, stable: approximately 5 mg/dl in postpubertal males and 4.1 mg/dl in postpubertal females. Disturbances in maintaining serum urate levels result in hyperuricemia and the deposition of sodium urate crystals in the tissues, leading to painful disorders collectively called *gout*. These disorders include acute arthritis, chronic gouty arthritis, tophi (firm, nodular, subcutaneous deposits of urate crystals surrounded by fibrosis), and nephritis (inflammation of the nephron). Chronic hyperuricemia results in the deposition of urate in tissues, cell injury, and inflammation. Because urate crystals are not degraded by lysosomal enzymes, they persist in dead cells.

Systemic Manifestations

Systemic manifestations of cellular injury include a general sense of fatigue and malaise, a loss of well-being, and altered appetite. Fever is often present because of biochemicals produced during the inflammatory response. Table 3-11 summarizes the most significant systemic manifestations of cellular injury.

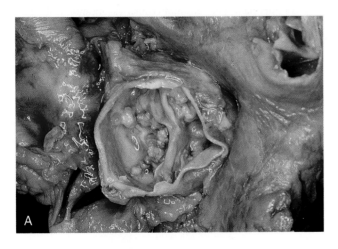

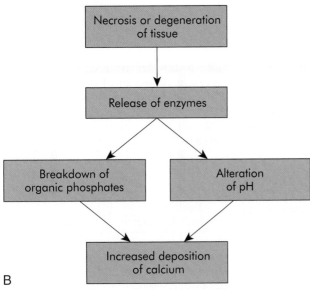

FIGURE 3-22 Aortic Valve Calcification. A, This calcified aortic valve is an example of dystrophic calcification. **B,** This algorithm shows the dystrophic mechanism of calcification. (**A** from Damjanov I: *Pathology for the health professions,* ed 3, St Louis, 2006, Saunders.)

TABLE 3-11	SYSTEMIC MANIFESTATIONS OF CELLULAR INJURY
MANIFESTATION	**CAUSE**
Fever	Release of endogenous pyrogens (interleukin-1, tumor necrosis factor-α, prostaglandins) from bacteria or macrophages; acute inflammatory response
Increased heart rate	Increase in oxidative metabolic processes resulting from fever
Increase in leukocytes (leukocytosis)	Increase in total number of white blood cells because of infection; normal is 5000-9000/mm³ (increase is directly related to severity of infection)
Pain	Various mechanisms, such as release of bradykinins, obstruction, pressure
Presence of cellular enzymes	Release of enzymes from cells of tissue* in extracellular fluid
Lactate dehydrogenase (LDH) (LDH isoenzymes)	Release from red blood cells, liver, kidney, skeletal muscle
Creatine kinase (CK) (CK isoenzymes)	Release from skeletal muscle, brain, heart
Aspartate aminotransferase (AST/SGOT)	Release from heart, liver, skeletal muscle, kidney, pancreas
Alanine aminotransferase (ALT/SGPT)	Release from liver, kidney, heart
Alkaline phosphatase (ALP)	Release from liver, bone
Amylase	Release from pancreas
Aldolase	Release from skeletal muscle, heart

*The rapidity of enzyme transfer is a function of the weight of the enzyme and the concentration gradient across the cellular membrane. The specific metabolic and excretory rates of the enzymes determine how long levels of enzymes remain elevated.

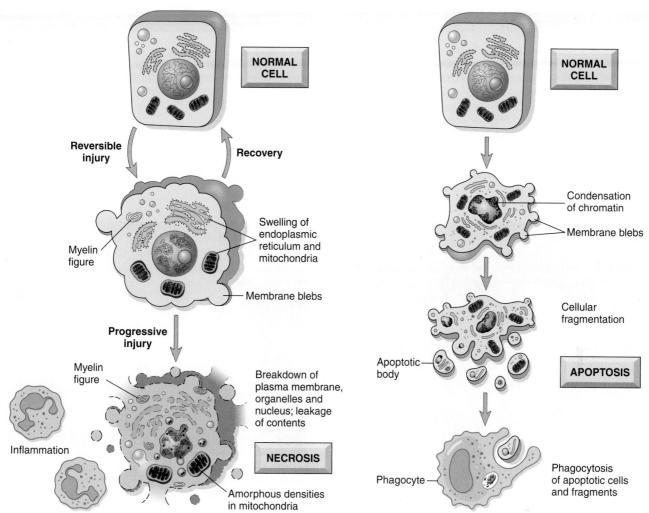

FIGURE 3-23 Schematic Illustration of the Morphologic Changes in Cell Injury Culminating in Necrosis or Apoptosis. Myelin figures come from degenerating cellular membranes and are noted within the cytoplasm or extracellularly. (From Kumar V et al: Cellular responses to stress and toxic insults: adaptation, injury, and death. In Kumar V et al, editors: *Robbins and Cotran pathologic basis of disease,* ed 8, St Louis, 2010, Saunders.)

CELLULAR DEATH

Cell death has historically been classified as necrosis and apoptosis. Necrosis is characterized by rapid loss of the plasma membrane structure, organelle swelling, mitochondrial dysfunction, and the lack of typical features of apoptosis.[35] Apoptosis is known as a regulated or programmed cell process characterized by the "dropping off" of cellular fragments called apoptotic bodies. Until recently, necrosis was only considered passive or accidental cell death occurring after severe and sudden injury. It is the main outcome in several common injuries including ischemia, exposure to toxins, certain infections, and trauma. It is now understood that under certain conditions, such as activation of death proteases, necrosis has been proposed to be regulated or programmed in a well-orchestrated way as a back-up for apoptosis (apoptosis may progress to necrosis).[36-37] Hence the new term programmed necrosis or necroptosis. Historically, programmed cell death only referred to apoptosis. Figure 3-23 illustrates the structural changes in cell injury resulting in necrosis or apoptosis. Table 3-12 compares the unique features of necrosis and apoptosis. Other forms of cell loss include autophagy (self-eating) (see p. 89).

Necrosis

Cellular death eventually leads to cellular dissolution, or necrosis. Necrosis is the sum of cellular changes after local cell death and the process of cellular self-digestion, known as autodigestion or autolysis (see Figure 3-23). Cells die long before any necrotic changes are noted by light microscopy.[37] The structural signs that indicate irreversible injury and progression to necrosis are dense clumping and progressive disruption both of genetic material and of plasma and organelle membranes. In later stages of necrosis, most organelles are disrupted, and karyolysis (nuclear dissolution and lysis of chromatin from the action of hydrolytic enzymes) is under way. In some cells the nucleus shrinks and becomes a small, dense mass of genetic material (pyknosis). The pyknotic nucleus eventually dissolves (by karyolysis) as a result of the action of hydrolytic lysosomal enzymes on DNA. Karyorrhexis means fragmentation of the nucleus into smaller particles or "nuclear dust" (see Figure 3-29).

Although necrosis still refers to death induced by nonspecific trauma or injury (e.g., cell stress or the heat shock response), with the very recent identification of molecular mechanisms regulating the

TABLE 3-12   FEATURES OF NECROSIS AND APOPTOSIS

FEATURE	NECROSIS	APOPTOSIS
Cell size	Enlarged (swelling)	Reduced (shrinkage)
Nucleus	Pyknosis → karyorrhexis → karyolysis	Fragmentation into nucleosome-size fragments
Plasma membrane	Disrupted	Intact; altered structure, especially orientation of lipids
Cellular contents	Enzymatic digestion; may leak out of cell	Intact; may be released in apoptotic bodies
Adjacent inflammation	Frequent	No
Physiologic or pathologic role	Invariably pathologic (culmination of irreversible cell injury)	Often physiologic, means of eliminating unwanted cells; may be pathologic after some forms of cell injury, especially DNA damage

From Kumar V et al: Cellular responses to stress and toxic insults: adaptation, injury, and death. In Kumar V et al, editors: *Robbins and Cotran pathologic basis of disease*, ed 8, St Louis, 2010, Saunders.

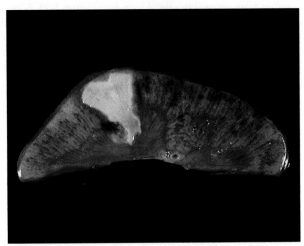

FIGURE 3-24 Coagulative Necrosis. A wedge-shaped kidney infarct (yellow). (From Kumar V et al: Cellular responses to stress and toxic insults: adaptation, injury, and death. In Kumar V et al, editors: *Robbins and Cotran pathologic basis of disease*, ed 8, St Louis, 2010, Saunders.)

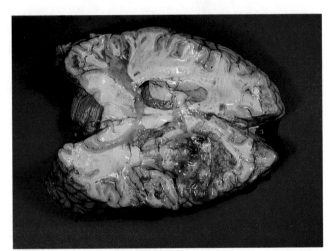

FIGURE 3-25 Liquefactive Necrosis of the Brain. The area of infarction is softened as a result of liquefaction necrosis. (From Damjanov I: *Pathology for the health professions*, ed 3, St Louis, 2006, Saunders.)

process of necrosis, the study of necrosis has experienced a new twist. Unlike apoptosis, necrosis has been viewed as passive with cell death occurring in a disorganized and unregulated manner. Recently, some molecular regulators governing programmed necrosis have been identified and demonstrated to be interconnected by a large network of signaling pathways.[36] Emerging evidence suggests that programmed necrosis is associated with pathologic diseases and provides innate immune response to viral infection.[36]

Different types of necroses tend to occur in different organs or tissues and sometimes can indicate the mechanism or cause of cellular injury. The four major types of necroses are coagulative, liquefactive, caseous, and fatty. Another type, gangrenous necrosis, is *not* a distinctive type of cell death but refers instead to larger areas of tissue death. These necroses are summarized as follows:

1. **Coagulative necrosis.** Occurs primarily in the kidneys, heart, and adrenal glands; commonly results from hypoxia caused by severe ischemia or hypoxia caused by chemical injury, especially ingestion of mercuric chloride. Coagulation is caused by protein denaturation, which causes the protein albumin to change from a gelatinous, transparent state to a firm, opaque state (Figure 3-24).

2. **Liquefactive necrosis.** Commonly results from ischemic injury to neurons and glial cells in the brain (Figure 3-25). Dead brain tissue is readily affected by liquefactive necrosis because brain cells are rich in digestive hydrolytic enzymes and lipids and the brain contains little connective tissue. Cells are digested by their own hydrolases, so the tissue becomes soft, liquefies, and segregates from healthy tissue, forming cysts. This can be caused by bacterial infection, especially *Staphylococci, Streptococci,* and *Escherichia coli.*

3. **Caseous necrosis.** Usually results from tuberculous pulmonary infection, especially by *Mycobacterium tuberculosis* (Figure 3-26). It is a combination of coagulative and liquefactive necroses. The dead cells disintegrate, but the debris is not completely digested by the hydrolases. Tissues resemble clumped cheese in that they are soft and granular. A granulomatous inflammatory wall encloses areas of caseous necrosis.

4. **Fat necrosis.** Fat necrosis is cellular dissolution caused by powerful enzymes, called lipases, that occur in the breast, pancreas, and other abdominal structures (Figure 3-27). Lipases break down triglycerides, releasing free fatty acids that then combine with calcium, magnesium, and sodium ions, creating soaps (saponification). The necrotic tissue appears opaque and chalk-white.

5. **Gangrenous necrosis.** Refers to death of tissue and results from severe hypoxic injury, commonly occurring because of arteriosclerosis, or blockage, of major arteries, particularly those in the lower leg (Figure 3-28). With hypoxia and subsequent bacterial invasion, the tissues can undergo necrosis. Dry gangrene is usually the result of coagulative necrosis. The skin becomes very dry and shrinks, resulting in wrinkles, and its color changes to dark brown or black.

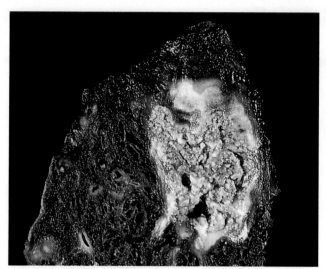

FIGURE 3-26 Caseous Necrosis. Tuberculosis of the lung, with a large area of caseous necrosis containing yellow-white and cheesy debris. (From Kumar V et al: Cellular responses to stress and toxic insults: adaptation, injury, and death. In Kumar V et al, editors: *Robbins and Cotran pathologic basis of disease,* ed 8, St Louis, 2010, Saunders.)

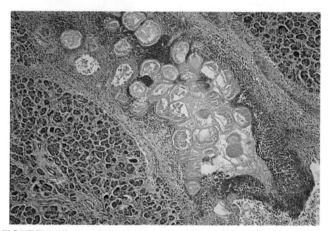

FIGURE 3-27 Fat Necrosis of Pancreas. Interlobular adipocytes are necrotic; acute inflammatory cells surround these. (From Damjanov I, Linder J, editors: *Anderson's pathology,* ed 10, St Louis, 1996, Mosby.)

Wet gangrene develops when neutrophils invade the site, causing liquefactive necrosis. This usually occurs in internal organs, causing the site to become cold, swollen, and black. A foul odor is present, and if systemic symptoms become severe, death can ensue.

6. **Gas gangrene.** Refers to a special type of gangrene caused by infection of injured tissue by one of many species of *Clostridium*. These anaerobic bacteria produce hydrolytic enzymes and toxins that destroy connective tissue and cellular membranes and cause bubbles of gas to form in muscle cells. This can be fatal if enzymes lyse the membranes of red blood cells, destroying their oxygen-carrying capacity. Death is caused by shock.

Apoptosis

Apoptosis ("dropping off") is an important distinct type of cell death that differs from necrosis in several ways (see Figures 3-23, 3-29, and Table 3-12). Apoptosis is an active process of cellular self-destruction called programmed cell death and is implicated in both normal and pathologic tissue changes. Cells need to die; otherwise, endless proliferation would lead to gigantic bodies. The average adult may create 10 billion new cells every day—and destroy the same number.[39]

Normal physiologic death by apoptosis occurs during the following processes:

- Embryogenesis
- Involution of hormone-dependent tissue after hormone withdrawal (such as involution of the lactating breast after weaning)
- Cell loss in proliferating cell populations (such as immature lymphocytes in the bone marrow or thymus that do not express appropriate receptors)
- Elimination of possibly harmful lymphocytes that may be self-reactive and cause cell death after performing useful functions (for example, neutrophils after an acute inflammatory reaction)

Death by apoptosis causes loss of cells in many pathologic states including (1) severe cell injury, (2) accumulation of misfolded proteins, (3) infections, and (4) obstruction in tissue ducts. When cell injury exceeds repair mechanisms, the cell triggers apoptosis. DNA can be damaged either by direct assault or by production of free radicals. Accumulation of misfolded proteins may result from genetic mutations or free radicals. Excessive accumulation of misfolded proteins in the endoplasmic reticulum (ER) leads to a condition known as endoplasmic stress (ER stress). ER stress results in apoptotic cell death and this mechanism has been linked to several degenerative diseases of the CNS and other organs. Infections, particularly viral (e.g., adenovirus and human immunodeficiency virus [HIV]), lead to

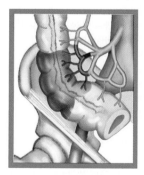
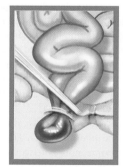
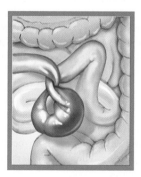
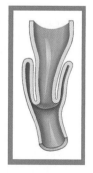
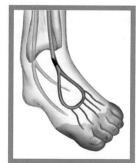

Thrombosis or embolism   Strangulated hernia   Volvulus   Intussusception   Gangrene

FIGURE 3-28 Gangrene, a Complication of Necrosis. In certain circumstances, necrotic tissue will be invaded by putrefactive organisms that are both saccharolytic and proteolytic. Foul-smelling gases are produced, and the tissue becomes green or black as a result of breakdown of hemoglobin. Obstruction of the blood supply to the bowel almost inevitably is followed by gangrene.

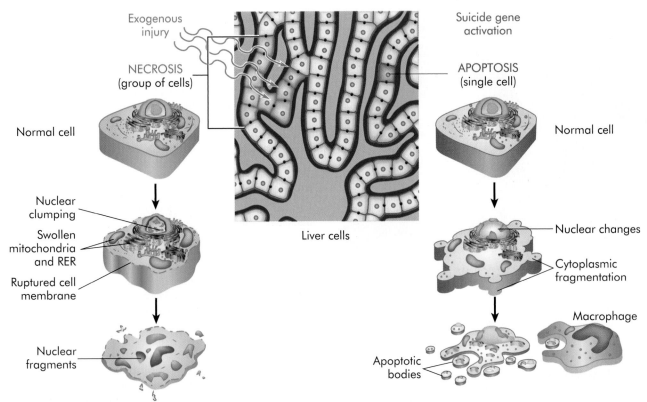

FIGURE 3-29 Necrosis and Apoptosis in Liver Cells. Necrosis is caused by exogenous injury whereby cells are swollen and have nuclear changes in ruptured cell membrane. Apoptosis is single cell death. It is genetically programmed (suicide genes) and depends on energy. Apoptotic bodies contain part of the nucleus and cytoplasmic organelles, which are ultimately engulfed by macrophages or adjacent cells. *RER,* Rough endoplasmic reticulum. (Redrawn from Damjanov I: *Pathology for the health professions,* ed 3, St Louis, 2006, Saunders.)

apoptosis. The virus may directly induce apoptosis, or cell death can occur indirectly as a result of the host immune response. Cytotoxic T lymphocytes respond to viral infections by inducing apoptosis and, therefore, eliminating the infectious cells. The tissue damage caused by this process is the same both for cell death in *tumors* and for rejection of *tissue transplants.* In organs with duct obstruction, including the pancreas, kidney, and parotid gland, the pathologic atrophy is caused by apoptosis.

Excessive or insufficient apoptosis is known as *dysregulated apoptosis.* A low rate of apoptosis can permit the survival of abnormal cells, for example, mutated cells that can increase cancer risk. Defective apoptosis may not eliminate lymphocytes that react against host tissue (self-antigens), leading to autoimmune disorders. Excessive apoptosis is known to occur in several neurodegenerative diseases, from ischemic injury (such as myocardial infarction and stroke), and from death of virus-infected cells (such as seen in many viral infections).

Apoptosis depends on a tightly regulated cellular program for its initiation and execution.[39] This death program involves enzymes that divide other proteins—proteases, which are activated by proteolytic activity in response to signals that induce apoptosis. These proteases are called *caspases,* a family of aspartic acid–specific proteases. The activated suicide caspases cleave and, thereby, activate other members of the family, resulting in an amplifying "suicide" cascade. The activated caspases then cleave other key proteins in the cell, killing the cell quickly and neatly. The two different pathways that converge on caspase activation are called the *mitochondrial pathway* and

the *death receptor pathway* (Figure 3-30). Cells that die by apoptosis release chemical factors that recruit phagocytes that quickly engulf the remains of the dead cell, thus reducing chances of inflammation. With necrosis, cell death is not tidy because cells that die as a result of acute injury swell, burst, and spill their contents all over their neighbors, causing a likely damaging inflammatory response.

Autophagy

The Greek term **autophagy** means "eating of self." Autophagy, as a "recycling factory," is a self-destructive process and a survival mechanism. When cells are starved or nutrient deprived, the autophagic process institutes cannibalization and recycles the digested contents.[18,41] Autophagy can maintain cellular metabolism under starvation conditions and remove damaged organelles under stress conditions, improving the survival of cells. Autophagy begins with a membrane, also known as a *phagophore* (although controversial), likely derived from the lipid bilayer from either the endoplasmic reticulum or the Golgi apparatus (Figure 3-31).[41] This phagophore expands and engulfs intracellular cargo—organelles, ribosomes, proteins—forming a double membrane *autophagosome.* The cargo-laden autophagosome fuses with the lysosome, now called an *autophagolysosome,* which promotes the degradation of the autophagosome by lysosomal acid proteases. Lysosomal transporters export amino acids and other by-products of degradation out of the cytoplasm where they can be reused for the synthesis of macromolecules and for metabolism.[42] ATP is generated and cellular damage reduced during autophagy that removes nonfunctional proteins and organelles.[41] Autophagy is considered a mechanism

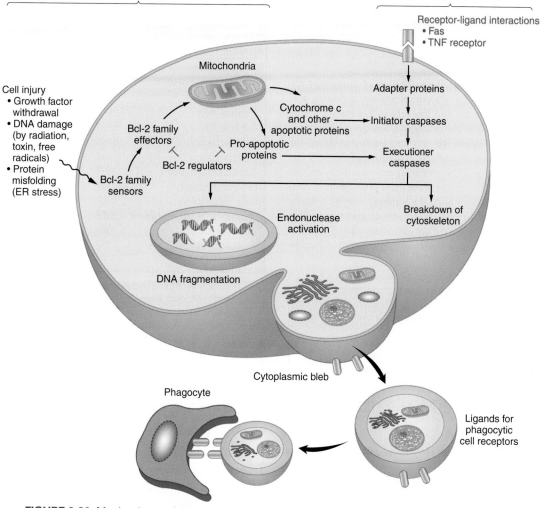

FIGURE 3-30 **Mechanisms of Apoptosis.** The two pathways of apoptosis differ in their induction and regulation, and both culminate in the activation of "executioner" caspases. The induction of apoptosis by the mitochondrial pathway involves the Bcl-2 family, which causes leakage of mitochondrial proteins. The regulators of the death receptor pathway involve the proteases, called caspases. (From Kumar V, Abbas A, Fausto N: *Robbins and Cotran pathologic basis of disease,* ed 8, Philadelphia, 2007, Saunders.)

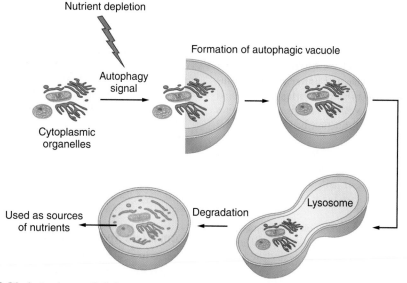

FIGURE 3-31 **Autophagy.** Cellular stresses, such as nutrient deprivation, activate autophagy genes that create vacuoles in which cellular organelles are sequestered and then degraded following fusion of the vesicles with lysosomes. The digested materials are recycled to provide nutrients for the cell.

of cell loss in various diseases, including degenerative diseases of the nervous system and muscle, and there is pathologic evidence in these disorders of damaged cells containing an abundance of autophagic vacuoles.[18]

Investigators are excited about the utilization of autophagy for therapeutic strategies. Autophagy is a critical garbage collecting and recycling process in healthy cells, and this process becomes less efficient and less discriminating as the cell ages. Consequently, harmful agents accumulate in cells, damaging cells and leading to aging: for example, failure to clear protein products in neurons of the CNS can cause dementia; failure to clear ROS-producing mitochondria can lead to nuclear DNA mutations and cancer. Thus these processes may even partially define aging. Therefore normal autophagy may potentially rejuvenate an organism and prevent cancer development as well as other degenerative diseases.[46] In addition, autophagy may be the last immune defense against infectious microorganisms that penetrate intracellularly.[43]

✔ **QUICK CHECK 3-4**
1. Why is an increase in the concentration of intracellular calcium injurious?
2. Compare and contrast necrosis and apoptosis.
3. Why is apoptosis significant?
4. Define autophagy.

AGING & ALTERED CELLULAR AND TISSUE BIOLOGY

Aging is usually defined as a normal physiologic process that is both universal and inevitable. The basic mechanisms of aging depend on the irreversible and universal processes at the cellular and molecular levels. Understanding aging requires the separation of irreversible processes from potentially reversible mechanisms (i.e., those that result from disease or age-related debilities)—a very difficult task!

Aging traditionally has not been considered a disease because it is "normal"; disease is usually considered "abnormal." Conceptually, this distinction seems clear until the concept of injury or damage is introduced; some pathologists have defined disease as the result of injury. Aging has been defined as the time-dependent loss of structure and function that proceeds slowly and in such small increments that it appears to be the result of the accumulation of small, imperceptible injuries—a gradual result of "wear and tear." Historical theories of aging are summarized in Table 3-13.

Injuries may result from unavoidable and universal microinsults caused by continuous bombardment by ultraviolet light, toxins and chemicals, countless mechanical insults, and reactions to metabolites (Figure 3-32).[44] In this context, the distinction between aging and disease is unclear. For example, some degree of atrophy of the brain is considered normal in old age until it proceeds far enough to cause clinically significant disability and is then called a *disease*. Likewise, most human beings have atherosclerosis, and the plaques progress with age, but at what point in this progression is atherosclerosis considered abnormal?

Cellular aging is the result of increasing molecular disorder or *entropy*. Molecular disorder is caused by random targeted events (i.e., stochastic) that affect cellular renewal and repair. The loss of molecular order ultimately exceeds repair and turnover capacity and, thus, increases vulnerability to pathologic processes or age-associated disease.[45] Table 3-14 includes emerging data on the biology of aging.

TABLE 3-13 THEORIES OF AGING

THEORY	YEAR	PROPONENT
Waste product theory	1923	Carrell & Ebeling
Wear-and-tear theory	1924	Pearl
Rate of living theory*	1928	Pearl
Endocrine theory	1947	Korenchevsky & Jones
Free radical theory†	1955	Harman
Collagen theory‡	1957	Verzar
Metabolic theory*	1957; 1961	Carlson et al; Johnson et al
Somatic mutation theory	1959	Sziliard
Error-catastrophe theory	1963; 1970	Orgel
Cross-linking theory‡	1968	Bjorksten
Programmed senescence theory	1969	Hayflick
Immunologic theory	1969	Walform
Evolution theory	1977	Kirkwood
Mitochondrial theory	1980	Miguel & Fleming

Data from Schneider EL: Theories of aging: a perspective. In Warner HR et al, editors: *Modern biological theories of aging,* New York, 1987, Raven; Melov S: Mitochondrial oxidative stress: physiologic consequences and potential for a role in aging, *Ann N Y Acad Sci* 908: 219–225, 2000; Biesalsk HK: Free radical theory of aging, *Curr Opin Clin Nutr Metab Care* 5(1):5–10, 2002.
*May represent the same theory.
†Current emphasis on mitochondrial oxidative stress and genetic variability for antioxidant protection.
‡May represent the same theory.

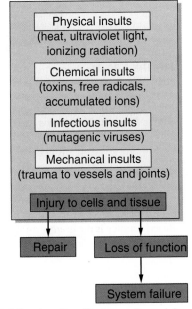

FIGURE 3-32 Microinsults. (Redrawn from Johnson HA, editor: *Is aging physiological or pathological? Relations between normal aging and a disease,* New York, 1985, Raven.)

Normal Life Span and Life Expectancy

The **maximal life span** of humans is between 80 and 100 years and does not vary significantly among populations. However, in primitive societies few individuals reach the maximal life span; most die in infancy or the early years. In societies with improved sanitation, housing, nutrition, and healthcare, many persons do attain the

TABLE 3-14   BIOLOGY OF AGING

EMERGING FOCUS	COMMENTS
Endocrine regulation through signaling pathways	Insulin-like growth factor 1 (IGF-1) signaling pathways have a role in certain tissues to regulate life span; IGF-1 is necessary for homeostasis, growth, and survival
	Reduced insulin signaling (rodents and mammals) causes glucose intolerance and hyperinsulinemia, type 2 diabetes mellitus, and shortened life span
	Main factors affected by insulin-like signaling are transcription factors such as forkhead box 0 (FOXO); FOXO controls gene expression that regulates cell cycle, apoptosis, DNA repair, metabolism, and resistance to oxidative stress
Nuclear architecture and genomic instability	Cells vary in size and shape, yet all seem to age
	DNA-protein complexes, or chromatin, stabilize genome and determine gene expression; thus *maintenance of chromatin dictates nuclear architecture*
	DNA damage may lead to changes in gene expression to promote aging; however, *epigenetic balance hypothesis* is proposed to explain gene expression changes that occur as a result of chromatic modification
	Oxidative stress may lead to DNA damage that accelerates aging; confusing, however, is that aging could *directly* affect chromatin structure through some unknown mechanism that *then* leads to DNA damage
Decline in cell renewal by adult stem cells	Aging might be associated with a decline in replication directed by adult stem cells
	Data suggest that as we grow older our stem cells age as a result of mechanisms that suppress development of cancer (e.g., senescence, apoptosis)
	Stem cell aging may occur with accumulating DNA damage or other nuclear support mechanisms, or both
	Telomeres, like plastic ends of shoelaces, form the end of chromosomes; they are short, repeated sequences of DNA that are important for ensuring complete replication of chromosome ends and protect the end from degradation
	Thus as cells age, their telomeres shorten, causing cell cycle arrest and an inability to generate new cells to replace damaged cells
Accumulation of cellular damage related to disease and aging	Accumulation of metabolic and genetic damage can exceed repair mechanisms
	One group of particularly toxic products are *reactive oxygen species (ROS)*
	These free radicals cause modifications of proteins, lipids, and nucleic acids
	Increased oxidative damage (stress) could result from repeated environmental exposures, for example, ionizing radiation, mitochondrial dysfunction, or reduction of antioxidant defense mechanisms with age
	Autophagy (see p. 88) also may slow and become less discriminating; consequently, harmful agents accumulate in cells, damage cells, and increase aging
	Effect of calorie restriction on longevity appears to be modulated by a family of proteins called *sirtuins;* sirtuins are thought to promote gene expression of products that increase longevity; these products include proteins that increase metabolic activity, reduce apoptosis, stimulate protein folding, and inhibit damaging effects of ROS
	One product, *resveratrol* (found in grapes, mulberries, peanuts, and especially red wine), may protect against aging cells by acting as an antioxidant, antimutagen, and anti-inflammatory

From Haigis MC, Sinclair DA: *Annu Rev Pathol Mech Dis* 5:253–295, 2010; Hopkiss AR: *Biogerontol* 9(1):49–55, 2008; Kumar A, Sharma SS: *Biochem Biophys Res Comm* 394:360–365, 2010; Kumar V et al: Cellular responses to stress and toxic insults: adaptation, injury, and death. In Kumar V et al, editors: *Robbins and Cotran pathologic basis of disease*, ed 8, St Louis, 2010, Saunders.

maximal life span. Although the maximal life span has not changed significantly over time, life expectancy has increased, but *not* for all Americans (see *Health Alert:* Decline in Life Expectancy in Some U.S. Counties). Life expectancy is the *average* number of years of life remaining at a given age.

Degenerative Extracellular Changes

Extracellular factors that affect the aging process include the binding of collagen; the increase in the effects of free radicals on cells; the structural alterations of fascia, tendons, ligaments, bones, and joints; and the development of peripheral vascular disease, particularly arteriosclerosis (see Chapter 23).

Aging affects the extracellular matrix with increased cross-linking (e.g., aging collagen becomes more insoluble, chemically stable but rigid, resulting in decreased cell permeability), decreased synthesis, and increased degradation of collagen. The extracellular matrix determines the tissue's physical properties.[1] These changes, together with the disappearance of elastin and changes in proteoglycans and plasma proteins, cause disorders of the ground substance that result in dehydration and wrinkling of the skin (see Chapter 39).

Other age-related defects in the extracellular matrix include skeletal muscle alterations (e.g., atrophy, decreased tone, loss of contractility), cataracts, diverticula, hernias, and rupture of intervertebral disks.

Free radicals of oxygen that result from oxidative cellular metabolism, *oxidative stress* (e.g., respiratory chain, phagocytosis, prostaglandin synthesis), damage tissues during the aging process. The oxygen radicals produced include superoxide radical, hydroxyl radical, and hydrogen peroxide (see p. 66). These oxygen products are extremely reactive and can damage nucleic acids, destroy polysaccharides, oxidize proteins, peroxidize unsaturated fatty acids, and kill and lyse cells. Oxidant effects on target cells can lead to malignant transformation, presumably through DNA damage. That progressive and cumulative damage from oxygen radicals may lead to harmful alterations in cellular function is consistent with those alterations of aging. This hypothesis is founded on the wear-and-tear theory of aging, which states that damages accumulate with time, decreasing the organism's ability to maintain a steady state. Because these oxygen-reactive species not only can permanently damage cells but also may lead to cell death, there is new support for their role in the aging process.

HEALTH ALERT

Decline in Life Expectancy in Some U.S. Counties

Continuing rise in life expectancy for *all* Americans is not happening. Long-term analysis of county trends has revealed startling data.

Between 1961 and 1999, *average* life expectancy in the United States increased from 73.5 to 79.6 years for women and from 66.9 to 74.1 years for men. However, the differences in mortality by county between the most disadvantaged populations and those with the most advantages began to *widen* in the early 1980s. Life expectancy between 1961 and 1999 in the male advantaged population (best-off group) rose from 70.5 to 78.7 years and from 76.9 to 83.0 years for females. In the female disadvantaged populations (worst-off group) starting in the early 1980s, life expectancy remained relatively stable (68.7 years in 1961, 74.5 years in 1983, and only 75.5 years in 1999). The worst-off men had a decline, rising again in the 1990s.

The gains made, particularly for cardiovascular disease, began to plateau in the 1980s because of rising mortality from lung cancer, chronic obstructive pulmonary disease, and diabetes. A major contributor, which peaked later for women than men, is smoking. Smoking is thought to be a significant contributor for women, as well as overweight, obesity, and hypertension. The worst-off counties also showed an increase in HIV/AIDS deaths and homicide in men.

Statistically significant declines for women occurred in 180 of 3141 counties and in 11 counties for men. In addition, 783 counties for women and 48 for men declined but this was not statistically significant. Life expectancy was worse in all Southwestern Virginia counties with a drop over the 16-year period of about 6 years in women and 2.5 years in men. The greatest improvements occurred in Western desert counties, where life expectancy rose almost 5 years for women and about 7 years for men.

The life expectancy "gap" is *increasing* between rich and poor and high and low educational attainment. This increase is occurring despite the gap between men and women and between blacks and whites. In addition, other indices include geography and community assets.

The analysis of county data demonstrates that the 1980s and 1990s were the beginning of the era of increased inequalities in mortality in the United States. Dividing the United States to eight "Americas," it is now evident that disparities in mortality affect millions of Americans. The gap is enormous. The eight Americas' analysis revealed the highest levels of life expectancy on record were for U.S.-born Asian females (America 1), which was 3 years higher than that for females in Japan. The next highest group was low-income, white rural populations in Minnesota, the Dakotas, Iowa, Montana, and Nebraska (America 2), with a life expectancy of 76.2 years for males and 81.8 years for females. Blacks living in high-risk urban areas (America 8) had the lowest life expectancy, being almost four times more likely than the America 1 (Asian) group to die before the age of 60 years and between 3.8 and 4.7 times more likely to die before age 45! The excess young and middle-aged deaths in America 8 were observed to be caused by injuries, cardiovascular disease, liver cirrhosis, diabetes, HIV, and homicide.

In summary, large disparities in life expectancy exist across America because of differences in chronic diseases and injuries with known risk factors, including using alcohol or tobacco, being overweight or obese, and having elevated blood pressure, high cholesterol levels, and uncontrolled glucose levels.

Data from Ezzati M et al: The reversal of fortunes: trends in county mortality and cross-country mortality disparances in the United States, *PLOS Med* 5(4):e66 doi:10.1371/journal.pmed.0050066; Murray CJL et al: Eight Americas: investigating mortality disparities across races, counties, and race-counties in the United States, *PLOS Med* 3(9):e260 doi:10.1371/journal.pmed.0030260.
AIDS, Acquired immunodeficiency syndrome; *HIV,* Human immunodeficiency virus.

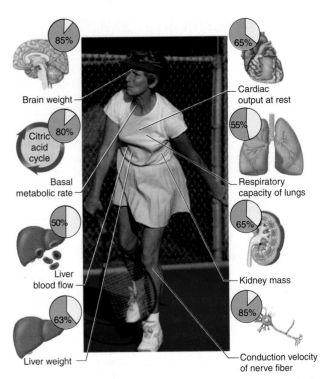

FIGURE 3-33 Some Biological Changes Associated With Aging. Insets show proportion of remaining functions in the organs of a person in late adulthood compared with a 20-year-old.

Of much interest is the relationship between aging and the disappearance or alteration of extracellular substances important for vessel integrity. With aging, lipid, calcium, and plasma proteins are deposited in vessel walls. These depositions cause serious basement membrane thickening and alterations in smooth muscle functioning, resulting in arteriosclerosis (a progressive disease that causes such problems as stroke, myocardial infarction, renal disease, and peripheral vascular disease).

Cellular Aging

Cellular changes characteristic of aging include atrophy, decreased function, and loss of cells, possibly caused by apoptosis (Figure 3-33). Loss of cellular function from any of these causes initiates the compensatory mechanisms of hypertrophy and hyperplasia of the remaining cells, which can lead to metaplasia, dysplasia, and neoplasia. All of these changes can alter receptor placement and function, nutrient pathways, secretion of cellular products, and neuroendocrine control mechanisms. In the aged cell, DNA, RNA, cellular proteins, and membranes are most susceptible to injurious stimuli. DNA is particularly vulnerable to such injuries as breaks, deletions, and additions. Lack of DNA repair increases the cell's susceptibility to mutations that may be lethal or may promote the development of neoplasia (see Chapter 9).

Mitochondria are the organelles responsible for the generation of most of the energy used by eukaryotic cells. Mitochondrial DNA (mtDNA) encodes some of the proteins of the electron transfer chain, the system necessary for the conversion of adenosine diphosphate (ADP) to ATP. Mutations in mtDNA can deprive the cell of ATP, and mutations are correlated with the aging process. The most common age-related mtDNA mutation in humans is a large rearrangement called the *4977 deletion,* or *common deletion,* and is found in humans older than 40 years. It is a deletion that removes all or part of 7 of the 13 protein-encoding mtDNA genes and 5 of the 22 tRNA genes. Individual cells containing this deletion have a condition known as *heteroplasmy*. Heteroplasmy levels rise with aging and are tissue-dependent.[46-48]

The production of ROS under physiologic conditions is associated with activity of the respiratory chain in aerobic ATP production. Therefore on its own accord, increased mitochondrial activity can cause "oxidative stress" in cells. The production of ROS is markedly increased in many pathologic conditions in which the respiratory chain is impaired. Because mtDNA, which is essential for normal oxidative phosphorylation, is located in proximity to the ROS-generating respiratory chain, it is more oxidatively damaged than is nuclear DNA. Cumulative damage of mtDNA is implicated in the aging process as well as in the progression of such common diseases as diabetes, cancer, and heart failure.

Tissue and Systemic Aging

It is probably safe to say that every physiologic process functions less efficiently with increasing age. The most characteristic tissue change with age is a progressive stiffness or rigidity that affects many systems, including the arterial, pulmonary, and musculoskeletal systems. A consequence of blood vessel and organ stiffness is a progressive increase in peripheral resistance to blood flow. The movement of intracellular and extracellular substances also decreases with age, as does the diffusion capacity of the lung. Blood flow through organs also decreases.

Changes in the endocrine and immune systems include thymus atrophy. Although this occurs at puberty, causing a decreased immune response to T-dependent antigens (foreign proteins), increased numbers of autoantibodies and immune complexes (antibodies that are bound to antigens) and an overall decrease in the immunologic tolerance for the host's own cells further diminish the effectiveness of the immune system later in life. In women the reproductive system loses ova, and in men spermatogenesis decreases. Responsiveness to hormones decreases in the breast and endometrium.

The stomach experiences decreases in the rate of emptying and secretion of hormones and hydrochloric acid. Muscular atrophy diminishes mobility by decreasing motor tone and contractility. Sarcopenia, loss of muscle mass and strength, can occur into old age. The skin of the aged individual is affected by atrophy and wrinkling of the epidermis and alterations in underlying dermis, fat, and muscle.

Total body changes include a decrease in height; a reduction in circumference of the neck, thighs, and arms; widening of the pelvis; and lengthening of the nose and ears. Several of these changes are the result of tissue atrophy and of decreased bone mass caused by osteoporosis and osteoarthritis. Although reduced growth hormone production and efficacy, reflected in diminished levels of insulin-like growth factor 1, is a current hypothesis for explaining decreased bone and lean body mass, recent research has found advancing age rather than declining levels of these hormones as a major determinant.[49]

Body composition changes with age. With middle age, there is an increase in body weight (men gain until 50 years of age and women until 70 years) and fat mass, followed by a decrease in stature, weight, fat-free mass (FFM) (includes all minerals, proteins, and water plus all other constituents except lipids), and body cell mass at older ages. As fat increases, total body water decreases. Increased body fat and centralized fat distribution (abdominal) are associated with non–insulin-dependent diabetes (type 2 diabetes mellitus) and heart disease. Total body potassium levels also decrease because of decreased cellular mass. An increased sodium/potassium ratio suggests that the decreased cellular mass is accompanied by an increased extracellular fluid compartment.

Although some of these alterations are probably inherent in aging, others represent consequences of the process. Advanced age increases susceptibility to disease, and death occurs after an injury or insult because of diminished cellular, tissue, and organic function.

Frailty

Frailty is a common clinical syndrome in older adults, leaving a person vulnerable to falls, functional decline, disability, disease, and death. Recently investigators hypothesized that the clinical manifestations of frailty include a cycle of negative energy balance, sarcopenia, and diminished strength and tolerance for exertion.[50,51] (For research and clinical purposes the criteria indicating compromised energetics include low grip strength, slowed waking speed, low physical activity, and unintentional weight loss).[51] The syndrome is complex, involving oxidative stress, dysregulation of inflammatory cytokines and hormones, malnutrition, physical inactivity, and muscle apoptosis (see review).[51] Additionally, the clinical condition of frailty includes decreased lean body mass (sarcopenia), osteopenia, cognitive impairment, and anemia.[52] Several physiologic gender differences may explain differing levels of frailty: (1) higher baseline levels of muscle mass for men may be protective *against* frailty, (2) testosterone and growth hormone can provide advantages in muscle mass maintenance, (3) cortisol is more dysregulated in older women than older men, (4) alterations in immune function and immune responsiveness to sex steroids make men more vulnerable to sepsis and infection and women vulnerable to chronic inflammatory conditions and muscle mass loss, and (5) lower levels of activity and caloric intake may influence greater susceptibility to frailty in women.[53]

SOMATIC DEATH

Somatic death is death of the entire person. Unlike the changes that follow cellular death in a live body, postmortem change is diffuse and does not involve components of the inflammatory response. Within minutes after death, postmortem changes appear, eliminating any difficulty in determining that death has occurred. The most notable manifestations are complete cessation of respiration and circulation. The surface of the skin usually becomes pale and yellowish; however, the lifelike color of the cheeks and lips may persist after death that is caused by carbon monoxide poisoning, drowning, or chloroform poisoning.[53]

Body temperature falls gradually immediately after death and then more rapidly (approximately 1.0° to 1.5° F/hr) until, after 24 hours, body temperature equals that of the environment.[55] After death caused by certain infective diseases, body temperature may continue to rise for a short time. Postmortem reduction of body temperature is called algor mortis.

Blood pressure within the retinal vessels decreases, causing muscle tension to decrease and the pupils to dilate. The face, nose, and chin become sharp or peaked-looking as blood and fluids drain from the head.[53] Gravity causes blood to settle in the most dependent, or lowest, tissues, which develop a purple discoloration called livor mortis. Incisions made at this time usually fail to cause bleeding. The skin loses its elasticity and transparency.

Within 6 hours after death, acidic compounds accumulate within the muscles because of the breakdown of carbohydrates and depletion of ATP. This interferes with ATP-dependent detachment of myosin from actin (contractile proteins), and muscle stiffening, or rigor mortis, develops. The smaller muscles are usually affected first, particularly the muscles of the jaw. Within 12 to 14 hours, rigor mortis usually affects the entire body.

Signs of putrefaction are generally obvious about 24 to 48 hours after death. Rigor mortis gradually diminishes, and the body becomes flaccid at 36 to 62 hours. Putrefactive changes vary depending on the temperature of the environment. The most visible is greenish discoloration of the skin, particularly on the abdomen. The discoloration is thought to be related to the diffusion of hemolyzed blood into the tissues and the production of sulfhemoglobin.[55] Slippage or loosening of the skin from underlying tissues occurs at the same time. After

this, swelling or bloating of the body and liquefactive changes occur, sometimes causing opening of the body cavities. At a microscopic level, putrefactive changes are associated with the release of enzymes and lytic dissolution called **postmortem autolysis.**

✔ **QUICK CHECK 3-5**

1. Why are microinsults important to aging?
2. What are the body composition changes that occur with aging?
3. Define frailty and possible endocrine-immune system involvement.

DID YOU UNDERSTAND?

Cellular Adaptation

1. Cellular adaptation is a reversible, structural, or functional response both to normal or physiologic conditions and to adverse or pathologic conditions. Cells can adapt to physiologic demands or stress to maintain a steady state called homeostasis.
2. The most significant adaptive changes include atrophy, hypertrophy, hyperplasia, and metaplasia.
3. Atrophy is a decrease in cellular size caused by aging, disuse, or reduced/absent blood supply, hormonal stimulation, or neural stimulation. The amounts of endoplasmic reticulum, mitochondria, and microfilaments decrease. The mechanisms of atrophy probably include decreased protein synthesis, increased protein catabolism, or both.
4. Hypertrophy is an increase in the size of cells caused by increased work demands or hormonal stimulation. The amounts of protein in the plasma membrane, endoplasmic reticulum, microfilaments, and mitochondria increase.
5. Hyperplasia is an increase in the number of cells caused by an increased rate of cellular division. Normal hyperplasia is stimulated by hormones or the need to replace lost tissues.
6. Metaplasia is the reversible replacement of one mature cell type by another less mature cell type.
7. Dysplasia, or atypical hyperplasia, is an abnormal change in the size, shape, and organization of mature tissue cells. It is considered an atypical rather than a true adaptational change.

Cellular Injury

1. Cellular injury occurs if the cell is unable to maintain homeostasis. Injured cells may recover (reversible injury) or die (irreversible injury). Injury is caused by lack of oxygen (hypoxia), free radicals, caustic or toxic chemicals, infectious agents, inflammatory and immune responses, genetic factors, insufficient nutrients, or physical trauma from many causes.
2. Four biochemical themes are important to cell injury: (a) ATP depletion, resulting in mitochondrial damage; (b) accumulation of oxygen and oxygen-derived free radicals, causing membrane damage; (c) protein folding defects; and (d) increased intracellular calcium concentration and loss of calcium steady state.
3. The sequence of events leading to cell death is commonly decreased ATP production, failure of active transport mechanisms (the sodium-potassium pump), cellular swelling, detachment of ribosomes from the endoplasmic reticulum, cessation of protein synthesis, mitochondrial swelling as a result of calcium accumulation, vacuolation, leakage of digestive enzymes from lysosomes, autodigestion of intracellular structures, lysis of the plasma membrane, and death.
4. The initial insult in hypoxic injury is usually ischemia (the cessation of blood flow into vessels that supply the cell with oxygen and nutrients).

5. Free radicals cause cellular injury because they have an unpaired electron that makes the molecule unstable. To stabilize itself, the molecule either donates or accepts an electron from another molecule. Therefore it forms injurious chemical bonds with proteins, lipids, and carbohydrates—key molecules in membranes and nucleic acids.
6. The damaging effects of free radicals, especially activated oxygen species such as O_2^-, $OH\cdot$, and H_2O_2, called oxidative stress, include (a) peroxidation of lipids, (b) alteration of ion pumps and transport mechanisms, (c) fragmentation of DNA, and (d) damage to mitochondria, releasing calcium into the cytosol.
7. Restoration of oxygen, however, can cause additional injury, called reperfusion injury. Reperfusion injury results from the generation of highly reactive oxygen intermediates increasing cellular oxidative stress and damage.
8. The initial insult in chemical injury is damage or destruction of the plasma membrane. Examples of chemical agents that cause cellular injury are carbon tetrachloride, lead, carbon monoxide, and ethyl alcohol.
9. Unintentional and intentional injuries are an important health problem in the United States. Death as a result of these injuries is more common for men than women and higher among blacks than whites and other racial groups.
10. Injuries by blunt force are the result of the application of mechanical energy to the body, resulting in tearing, shearing, or crushing of tissues. The most common types of blunt-force injuries include motor vehicle accidents and falls.
11. A contusion is bleeding into the skin or underlying tissues as a consequence of a blow. A collection of blood in soft tissues or an enclosed space may be referred to as a hematoma.
12. An abrasion (scrape) results from removal of the superficial layers of the skin caused by friction between the skin and injuring object. Abrasions and contusions may have a patterned appearance that mirrors the shape and features of the injuring object.
13. A laceration is a tear or rip resulting when the tensile strength of the skin or tissue is exceeded.
14. An incised wound is a cut that is longer than it is deep. A stab wound is a penetrating sharp-force injury that is deeper than it is long.
15. Gunshot wounds may be either penetrating (bullet retained in the body) or perforating (bullet exits the body). The most important factors determining the appearance of a gunshot injury are whether it is an entrance or an exit wound and the range of fire.
16. Asphyxial injuries are caused by a failure of cells to receive or utilize oxygen. These injuries can be grouped into four general categories: suffocation, strangulation, chemical, and drowning.
17. Activation of inflammation and immunity, which occurs after cellular injury or infection, involves powerful biochemicals and proteins capable of damaging normal (uninjured and uninfected) cells.

DID YOU UNDERSTAND?—cont'd

18. Genetic disorders injure cells by altering the nucleus and the plasma membrane's structure, shape, receptors, or transport mechanisms.

19. Deprivation of essential nutrients (proteins, carbohydrates, lipids, vitamins) can cause cellular injury by altering cellular structure and function, particularly of transport mechanisms, chromosomes, the nucleus, and DNA.

20. Injurious physical agents include temperature extremes, changes in atmospheric pressure, ionizing radiation, illumination, mechanical stresses (e.g., repetitive body movements), and noise.

21. Errors in healthcare are a leading cause of injury or death in the United States. Errors involve medicines, surgery, diagnosis, equipment, and laboratory reports. They can occur anywhere in the healthcare system including hospitals, clinics, outpatient surgery centers, physicians' offices, pharmacies, and the individual's home.

Manifestations of Cellular Injury

1. An important manifestation of cell injury is the resultant metabolic disturbances of intracellular accumulation (infiltration) of abnormal amounts of various substances. Two categories of accumulations are (a) normal cellular substances, such as water, proteins, lipids, and carbohydrate excesses; and (b) abnormal substances, either endogenous (e.g., from abnormal metabolism) or exogenous (e.g., a virus).

2. Most accumulations are attributed to four types of mechanisms, all abnormal: (a) An endogenous substance is produced in excess or at an increased rate; (b) an abnormal substance, often the result of a mutated gene, accumulates; (c) an endogenous substance is not effectively catabolized; and (d) a harmful exogenous substance accumulates because of inhalation, ingestion, or infection.

3. Accumulations harm cells by "crowding" the organelles and by causing excessive (and sometimes harmful) metabolites to be produced during their catabolism. The metabolites are released into the cytoplasm or expelled into the extracellular matrix.

4. Cellular swelling, the accumulation of excessive water in the cell, is caused by the failure of transport mechanisms and is a sign of many types of cellular injury. Oncosis is a type of cellular death resulting from cellular swelling.

5. Accumulations of organic substances—lipids, carbohydrates, glycogen, proteins, pigments—are caused by disorders in which (a) cellular uptake of the substance exceeds the cell's capacity to catabolize (digest) or use it or (b) cellular anabolism (synthesis) of the substance exceeds the cell's capacity to use or secrete it.

6. Dystrophic calcification (accumulation of calcium salts) is always a sign of pathologic change because it occurs only in injured or dead cells. Metastatic calcification, however, can occur in uninjured cells in individuals with hypercalcemia.

7. Disturbances in urate metabolism can result in hyperuricemia and deposition of sodium urate crystals in tissue—leading to a painful disorder called gout.

8. Systemic manifestations of cellular injury include fever, leukocytosis, increased heart rate, pain, and serum elevations of enzymes in the plasma.

Cellular Death

1. Cellular death has historically been classified as necrosis and apoptosis. Necrosis is characterized by rapid loss of the plasma membrane structure, organelle swelling, mitochondrial dysfunction, and the lack of features of apoptosis. Apoptosis is known as regulated or programmed cell death

and is characterized by "dropping off" of cellular fragments, called apoptotic bodies. It is now understood that under certain conditions necrosis is regulated or programmed, hence the new term "programmed necrosis" or necroptosis.

2. There are four major types of necroses: coagulative, liquefactive, caseous, and fat necroses. Different types of necroses occur in different tissues.

3. Structural signs that indicate irreversible injury and progression to necrosis are the dense clumping and disruption of genetic material and the disruption of the plasma and organelle membranes.

4. Apoptosis, a distinct type of sublethal injury, is a process of selective cellular self-destruction that occurs in both normal and pathologic tissue changes.

5. Death by apoptosis causes loss of cells in many pathologic states including (a) severe cell injury, (b) accumulation of misfolded proteins, (c) infections, and (d) obstruction in tissue ducts.

6. Excessive accumulation of misfolded proteins in the endoplasmic reticulum (ER) leads to a condition known as endoplasmic stress. ER stress results in apoptotic cell death and this mechanism has been linked to several degenerative diseases of the CNS and other organs.

7. Excessive or insufficient apoptosis is known as dysregulated apoptosis.

8. Autophagy means "eating of self" and as a recycling factory it is a self-destructive process and a survival mechanism. When cells are starved or nutrient deprived, the autophagic process institutes cannibalization and recycles the digested contents. Autophagy can maintain cellular metabolism under starvation conditions and remove damaged organelles under stress conditions, improving the survival of cells. Autophagy declines and becomes less efficient as the cell ages, thus contributing to the aging process.

9. Gangrenous necrosis, or gangrene, is tissue necrosis caused by hypoxia and the subsequent bacterial invasion.

Aging and Altered Cellular and Tissue Biology

1. It is difficult to determine the physiologic (normal) from the pathologic changes of aging. Cellular aging is the result of increasing molecular disorder or entropy.

2. Humans have an inherent maximal life span (80 to 100 years) that is dictated by currently unknown intrinsic mechanisms.

3. Although the maximal life span has not changed significantly over time, the average life span, or life expectancy, has increased, but not for all Americans. Life expectancy is the average number of years of life remaining at a given age.

4. The physiologic mechanisms of aging apparently are associated with (a) cellular changes produced by genetic and environmental/life-style factors, (b) changes in cellular regulatory or control mechanisms, and (c) degenerative extracellular and vascular alterations.

5. Frailty is a common clinical syndrome in older adults, leaving a person vulnerable to falls, functional decline, disability, disease, and death.

Somatic Death

1. Somatic death is death of the entire organism. Postmortem change is diffuse and does not involve the inflammatory response.

2. Manifestations of somatic death include cessation of respiration and circulation, gradual lowering of body temperature, pupil dilation, loss of elasticity and transparency in the skin, muscle stiffening (rigor mortis), and skin discoloration (livor mortis). Signs of putrefaction are obvious about 24 to 48 hours after death.

KEY TERMS

- Abrasion 94
- Adaptation 59
- Aging 90
- Algor mortis 93
- Anoxia 64
- Apoptosis 87
- Asphyxial injury 74
- Atrophy 60
- Autolysis 85
- Autophagic vacuole 60
- Autophagy 88
- Bilirubin 83
- Blunt force 76
- Carbon monoxide (CO) 71
- Carboxyhemoglobin 72
- Caseous necrosis 86
- Caspase 88
- Cellular accumulation (infiltration) 80
- Cellular swelling 80
- Chemical asphyxiant 75
- Choking asphyxiation 74
- Chopping wound 76
- Coagulative necrosis 86
- Compensatory hyperplasia 61
- Contusion (bruise) 76
- Cyanide 75
- Cytochrome 82
- Disuse atrophy 60
- Drowning 75
- Dry-lung drowning 79
- Dysplasia (atypical hyperplasia) 62
- Dystrophic calcification 84
- Endoplasmic stress (ER stress) 87

- Ethanol 72
- Exit wound 77
- Fat necrosis 86
- Fat-free mass (FFM) 93
- Fatty change 81
- Fetal alcohol syndrome 73
- Frailty 93
- Free radical 66
- Gangrenous necrosis 86
- Gas gangrene 87
- Hanging strangulation 75
- Hemoprotein 82
- Hemosiderin 82
- Hemosiderosis 82
- Hormonal hyperplasia 61
- Hydrogen sulfide 75
- Hyperplasia 61
- Hypertrophy 61
- Hypoxia 63
- Incised wound 76
- Irreversible injury 62
- Ischemia 64
- Karyolysis 85
- Karyorrhexis 85
- Laceration 76
- Lead 70
- Life expectancy 91
- Ligature strangulation 75
- Lipid peroxidation 66
- Lipofuscin 61
- Liquefactive necrosis 86
- Livor mortis 93
- Manual strangulation 75

- Maximal life span 90
- Melanin 82
- Mesenchymal (tissue from embryonic mesoderm) cells 62
- Metaplasia 62
- Metastatic calcification 84
- Mitochondrial DNA (mDNA) 66
- Necrosis 85
- Oncosis (vacuolar degeneration) 81
- Oxidative stress 66
- Pathologic atrophy 60
- Pathologic hyperplasia 61
- Physiologic atrophy 60
- Postmortem autolysis 94
- Postmortem change 93
- Programmed necrosis (necroptosis) 85
- Proteosome 60
- Psammoma body 84
- Puncture wound 76
- Pyknosis 85
- Reperfusion injury 65
- Reversible injury 62
- Rigor mortis 93
- Sarcopenia 93
- Somatic death 93
- Stab wound 76
- Strangulation 74
- Suffocation 74
- Ubiquitin 60
- Ubiquitin-proteosome pathway 60
- Urate 84
- Vacuolation 65
- Xenobiotic 68

REFERENCES

1. Fausto A, Campbell JS, Riehle KJ: Liver regeneration, *Heptalogy* 43:S45–S53, 2006.
2. Kraus RS: Evolutionary conservation in myoblast fusion, *Nat Genet* 39:704–705, 2007.
3. Eltzschig HK, Carmeliet P: Hypoxia and inflammation, *N Engl J Med* 364(7):656–665, 2011.
4. Bai J, Cederbaum AI: Mitochondrial catalase and oxidative injury, *Biol Signals Recept* 10(3-4):189–199, 2001.
5. Lee HC, Wei YH: Mitochondrial biogenesis and mitochondrial DNA maintenance of mammalian cells under oxidative stress, *Int J Biochem Cell Biol* 37(4):822–834, 2005.
6. Bayir H, Kagan VE: Bench to bedside review: mitochondrial injury, oxidative stress and apoptosis—there is nothing more practical than a good theory, *Crit Care* 12:206, 2008:doi.10.1186/cc6779.
7. Samper E, Nicholls DG, Melov S: Mitochondrial oxidative stress causes chromosomal instability of mouse embryonic fibroblasts, *Aging Cell* 2(5):277–285, 2003.
8. Robb EL, Page MM, Stuart JA: Mitochondria, cellular stress resistance, somatic cell depletion and lifespan, *Curr Aging Sci* 2(1):12–27, 2009:review.
9. Young KJ, Bennett JP: The mitochondrial secret(ase) of Alzheimer's disease, *J Alzheimers Dis* 20(suppl 2):S381–S400, 2010.
10. Zhang K: Integration of ER stress, oxidative stress and the inflammatory response in health and disease, *Int J Exp Med* 3(1):33–40, 2010.
11. Lenaz G, et al: Role of mitochondria in oxidative stress and aging, *Ann N Y Acad Sci* 959:99–213, 2002.
12. Jones DP, Delong MJ: Detoxification and protective functions of nutrients. In Stipanuk M, editor: *Biochemical and physiological aspects of nutrition*, Philadelphia, 2000, Saunders.
13. Liebler DC, Guengerich FP: Elucidating mechanisms of drug-induced toxicity, *Nature* 4:410–420, 2005.
14. Gunnell D, Murray V, Hawton K: Use of paracetamol (acetaminophen) for suicide and nonfatal poisoning: worldwide patterns of use and misuse, *Suicide Life Threat Behav* 30:313–326, 2000.
15. Murata K, et al: Lead toxicity: does the critical level of lead resulting in adverse effects differ between adults and children? *J Occup Health* 51(1):1–12, 2009.
16. Marshall L, et al: Identifying and managing adverse environmental health effects. 1. Taking an exposure history, *CMAJ* 166(8):1049–1055, 2002.
17. Weir E: Identifying and managing adverse environmental health effects: a new series, *Can Med Assoc J* 166(8):1041–1043, 2002.
18. Kumar V, et al: Environmental and nutritional diseases. In Kumar V, et al, editors: *Robbins and Cotran pathologic basis of disease*, ed 8, St Louis, 2010, Saunders/Elsevier.
19. Romanoff R, et al: Acute ethanol exposure inhibits renal folate transport, but repeated exposure upregulates folate transport proteins in rats and human cells, *J Nutr* 137:1260–1265, 2007.
20. Hines LM, et al: Alcoholism: the dissection for endophenotypes, *Dialogues Clin Neurosci* 7(2):153–163, 2005.
21. O'Keefe JH, Bybee KA, Lavie CJ: Alcohol and cardiovascular health: the razor-sharp double-edged sword, *Am J Coll Cardiol* 50(11):1009–1014, 2007.

22. Costanzo S, et al: Cardiovascular and overall mortality risk in relation to alcohol consumption in patients with cardiovascular disease, *Circulation* 121:1951–1959, 2010.

23. Molina PE, et al: Mechanisms of alcohol-induced tissue injury, *Alcohol Clin Exp Res* 27(3):563–575, 2003.

24. Jaeschke H, et al: Mechanisms of hepatotoxicity, *Toxicol Sci* 65(2):166–176, 2002.

25. Traviss KA, et al: Lifestyle-related weight gain in obese men with newly diagnosed obstructive sleep apnea, *J Am Diet Assoc* 102(5):703–706, 2002.

26. Young T, Peppard PE, Gottlieb DJ: Epidemiology of obstructive sleep apnea: a population health perspective, *Am J Respir Crit Care Med* 165(9):1217–1239, 2002.

27. Leiber CS: Metabolism of alcohol, *Clin Liver Dis* 9(1):1–35, 2005.

28. Vaux KK, Chambers C: *Fetal alcohol syndrome*, 2009. Available at emedicine.medscape.com/article/974016-overview.

29. Gutierrez C, et al: An experimental study on the effects of ethanol and folic acid deficiency, alone or in combination, on pregnant Swiss mice, *Pathology* 39(5):495–503, 2007.

30. Haycock PC: Fetal alcohol spectrum disorders: the epigenetic perspective, *Biol Reprod* 81(4):607–617, 2009.

31. Schecter R, Grether JK: Continuing increases in autism reported to California's developmental services system: mercury in retrograde, *Arch Gen Psych* 65(1):19–24, 2008.

32. Centers for Disease Control and Prevention, National Center for Injury Prevention and Control: *Injury statistics website*, Washington, DC, 2007, Author. Available at http://webapp.cdc.gov/cgi-bin/broker.exe.

33. Elder N, Dovey S: Classification of medical errors and preventable adverse events in primary care: a synthesis of the literature, *J Family Pract* 51(1):1079, 2002.

34. Kopec D, et al: The state of the art in the reduction of medical errors, *Stud Health Technol Inform* 121:126–137, 2006.

35. Hitomi J, et al: Identification of a molecular signaling network that regulates a cellular necrotic cell death pathway by a genome wide siRNA screen, *Cell* 135(7):1311–1323, 2008.

36. Cho YS, et al: Physiological consequences of programmed necrosis, an alternative form of cell demise, *Mol Cell*, March 31, 2010:Epub ahead of print.

37. Moquin D, Chan F: The molecular regulation of programmed necrotic cell injury, *Trends Biochem Sci* 35(8):434–441, 2010.

38. Majno G, Joris I: Apoptosis, oncosis, and necrosis: an overview of cell death, *Am J Pathol* 146(1):3–15, 1995.

39. Raloff J: Coming to terms with death: accurate descriptions of a cell's demise may offer clues to diseases and treatments, *Sci News* 159:378–380, 2001.

40. Wyllie AH, Kerr JFR, Currie AR: Cell death: the significance of apoptosis, *Int Rev Cytol* 68:251–306, 1980.

41. Glick D, Barth S, MacLeod KF: Autophagy: cellular and molecular mechanisms, *J Pathol* 221(1):3–12, 2010.

42. Mizushima N: Autophagy: process and function, *Genes Dev* 21(22):2861–2873, 2007:review.

43. Levine B, Mizushima N, Virgin HW: Autophagy in immunity and inflammation, *Nature* 469:323–335, 2011.

44. Johnson HA: Is aging physiological or pathological? In Johnson HA, editor: *Relation between normal aging and disease*, New York, 1985, Raven.

45. Hayflick L: Biological aging is no longer an unsolved problem, *Ann N Y Acad Sci* 1100:1–13, 2007:review.

46. Butow RA, Avadhani NG: Mitochondrial signaling: the retrograde response, *Mol Cell* 14(1):1–15, 2004.

47. Maassen JA, et al: Mitochondrial diabetes: molecular mechanisms and clinical presentation, *Diabetes* 52(suppl 1):S103–S109, 2004.

48. Samules DC: Mitochondrial DNA repeats constrain the life span of mammals, *Trends Genet* 20(5):226–229, 2004.

49. O'Connor KG, et al: Serum levels of insulin-like growth factor-I are related to age and not to body composition in healthy women and men, *J Gerontol A Biol Sci Med Sci* 53(3):M176–M182, 1998.

50. Fried LP, et al: Frailty in older adults: evidence for a phenotype, *J Gerontol A Biol Sci Med Sci* 56(3):M146–M156, 2001.

51. Walston JD: Frailty Clinics in Geriatric Medicine 27(1), 2011:Saunders.

52. Gillick M: Pinning down frailty, *J Gerontol A Biol Sci Med Sci* 56(3):M134–M135, 2001.

53. Shennan T: *Postmortems and morbid anatomy*, ed 3, Baltimore, 1935, William Wood.

54. Minckler J, Anstall HB, Minckler TM: *Pathobiology: an introduction*, St Louis, 1971, Mosby.

55. Riley MW: Foreword: the gender paradox. In Ory MG, Warner HR, editors: *Gender, health, and longevity: multidisciplinary perspectives*, New York, 1990, Springer.

CHAPTER

4

Fluids and Electrolytes, Acids and Bases

Sue E. Huether

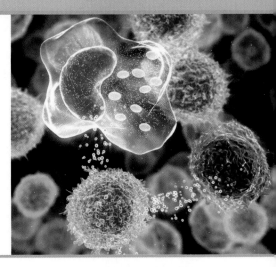

evolve WEBSITE

http://evolve.elsevier.com/Huether/
- Review Questions and Answers
- Animations
- Quick Check Answers

- Key Terms Exercises
- Critical Thinking Questions with Answers
- Algorithm Completion Exercises
- WebLinks

CHAPTER OUTLINE

The cells of the body live in a fluid environment with electrolyte and acid-base concentrations maintained within a narrow range. Changes in electrolyte concentration affect the electrical activity of nerve and muscle cells and cause shifts of fluid from one compartment to another. Alterations in acid-base balance disrupt cellular functions. Fluid fluctuations also affect blood volume and cellular function. Disturbances in these functions are common and can be life-threatening. Understanding how alterations occur and how the body compensates or corrects the disturbance is important for comprehending many pathophysiologic conditions.

DISTRIBUTION OF BODY FLUIDS

The sum of fluids within all body compartments constitutes **total body water (TBW)**—about 60% of body weight in adults (Table 4-1). The volume of TBW is usually expressed as a percentage of body weight in

kilograms. One liter of water weighs 2.2 lb (1 kg). The rest of the body weight is composed of fat and fat-free solids, particularly bone.

Body fluids are distributed among functional compartments, or spaces, and provide a transport medium for cellular and tissue function. Intracellular fluid (ICF) comprises all the fluid within cells, about two thirds of TBW. Extracellular fluid (ECF) is all the fluid outside the cells (about one third of TBW) and is divided into smaller compartments. The two main ECF compartments are the interstitial fluid (the space between cells and outside the blood vessels) and the intravascular fluid (blood plasma) (Table 4-2). The total volume of body water for a 70-kg person is about 42 liters. Other ECF compartments include lymph and transcellular fluids, such as synovial, intestinal, and cerebrospinal fluid; sweat; urine; and pleural, peritoneal, pericardial, and intraocular fluids.

Although the amount of fluid within the various compartments is relatively constant, solutes (e.g., salts) and water are exchanged between

TABLE 4-1	TOTAL BODY WATER (%) IN RELATION TO BODY WEIGHT*				
BODY BUILD	ADULT MALE	ADULT FEMALE	CHILD (1-10 yr)	INFANT (1 mo to 1 yr)	NEWBORN (up to 1 mo)
Normal	60	50	65	70	70-80
Lean	70	60	50-60	80	
Obese	50	42	50	60	

*NOTE: Total body water is a percentage of body weight.

TABLE 4-2	DISTRIBUTION OF BODY WATER (70-KG MAN)	
FLUID COMPARTMENT	% OF BODY WEIGHT	VOLUME (L)
Intracellular fluid (ICF)	40	28
Extracellular fluid (ECF)	20	14
Interstitial	15	11
Intravascular	5	3
Total body water (TBW)	60	42

TABLE 4-3	NORMAL WATER GAINS AND LOSSES (70-KG MAN)		
	DAILY INTAKE (mL)		DAILY OUTPUT (mL)
Drinking	1400-1800	Urine	1400-1800
Water in food	700-1000	Stool	100
Water of oxidation	300-400	Skin	300-500
		Lungs	600-800
TOTAL	2400-3200	TOTAL	2400-3200

compartments to maintain their unique compositions. The percentage of TBW varies with the amount of body fat and age. Because fat is water repelling (hydrophobic), very little water is contained in adipose (fat) cells. Individuals with more body fat have proportionately less TBW and tend to be more susceptible to dehydration.

Maturation and the Distribution of Body Fluids

The distribution and the amount of TBW change with age (see the *Pediatric* and *Aging* boxes), and although daily fluid intake may fluctuate widely, the body regulates water volume within a relatively narrow range. Water obtained by drinking, water ingested in food, and water derived from oxidative metabolism are the primary sources of body water. Normally, the largest amounts of water are lost through renal excretion, with lesser amounts lost through the stool and through vaporization from the skin and lungs (insensible water loss) (Table 4-3).

Water Movement Between Plasma and Interstitial Fluid

The distribution of water and the movement of nutrients and waste products between the capillary and interstitial spaces occur as a result of changes in hydrostatic pressure (pushes water) and osmotic (oncotic) pressure (pulls water) at the arterial and venous ends of the capillary. Water, sodium, and glucose readily move across the capillary membrane. The plasma proteins do not cross the capillary membrane and maintain effective osmolality by generating plasma oncotic pressure (particularly albumin).

As plasma flows from the arterial to the venous end of the capillary, four forces determine if fluid moves out of the capillary and into the interstitial space (filtration) or if fluid moves back into the capillary from the interstitial space (reabsorption):

1. Capillary hydrostatic pressure (blood pressure) facilitates the outward movement of water from the capillary to the interstitial space.
2. Capillary (plasma) oncotic pressure osmotically attracts water from the interstitial space back into the capillary.
3. Interstitial hydrostatic pressure facilitates the inward movement of water from the interstitial space into the capillary.
4. Interstitial oncotic pressure osmotically attracts water from the capillary into the interstitial space.

PEDIATRIC CONSIDERATIONS
Distribution of Body Fluids

Newborn Infants
At birth TBW represents about 75% to 80% of body weight and decreases to about 67% during the first year of life. Physiologic loss of body water amounting to 5% of body weight occurs as an infant adjusts to a new environment. Infants are particularly susceptible to significant changes in TBW because of a high metabolic rate and greater body surface area, as compared to adults. Consequently, they have a greater fluid intake and output in relation to their body size. Renal mechanisms of fluid and electrolyte conservation may not be mature enough to counter abnormal losses related to vomiting or diarrhea, thereby allowing dehydration to occur. Symptoms of dehydration include increased thirst, decreased urine output, decreased body weight, decreased skin elasticity, sunken fontanels, absent tears, dry mucous membranes, increased heart rate, and irritability.

Children and Adolescents
TBW slowly decreases to 60% to 65% of body weight. At adolescence the percentage of TBW approaches adult levels and differences according to gender appear. Males have a greater percentage of body water because of increased muscle mass, and females have more body fat because of the influence of estrogen and thus less water.

The movement of fluid back and forth across the capillary wall is called net filtration and is best described as Starling forces:

Net filtration =
(Forces favoring filtration) − (Forces opposing filtration)
Forces favoring filtration =
Capillary hydrostatic pressure and interstitial oncotic pressure
Forces opposing filtration =
Capillary oncotic pressure and interstitial hydrostatic pressure

At the arterial end of the capillary, hydrostatic pressure exceeds capillary oncotic pressure and fluid moves into the interstitial space (filtration). At the venous end of the capillary, capillary oncotic pressure exceeds capillary hydrostatic pressure and fluids are attracted back

GERIATRIC CONSIDERATIONS
Distribution of Body Fluids

The further decline in the percentage of TBW in the elderly is in part the result of a decreased free fat mass and decreased muscle mass, as well as a reduced ability to regulate sodium and water balance. Kidneys are less efficient in producing either a concentrated or dilute urine, and sodium-conserving responses are sluggish. Thirst perception also may decline and loss of cognitive function can influence access to beverages. Healthy older adults can adequately maintain their hydration status. When disease is present, a decrease in TBW, dehydration and hypernatremia can become life-threatening.

Data from Luckey AE, Parsa CJ: Fluid and electrolytes in the aged, *Arch Surg* 138(10):1055-1060, 2003; Schols JM et al: Preventing and treating dehydration in the elderly during periods of illness and warm weather, *J Nutr Health Aging* 13(2):150-157, 2009; Schlanger LE, Bailey JL, Sands JM: Electrolytes in the aging, *Adv Chronic Kidney Dis* 17(4):308-319, 2010.

into the circulation (reabsorption). Interstitial hydrostatic pressure promotes the movement of about 10% of the interstitial fluid along with small amounts of protein into the lymphatics, which then returns to the circulation. Because albumin does not normally cross the capillary membrane, interstitial oncotic pressure is normally minimal. Figure 4-1 illustrates net filtration.

Water Movement Between ICF and ECF

Water moves between ICF and ECF compartments primarily as a function of osmotic forces (see Chapter 1 for definitions). Water moves freely by diffusion through the lipid bilayer cell membrane and through **aquaporins,** a family of water channel proteins that provide permeability to water.[1] Sodium is responsible for the ECF osmotic balance, and potassium maintains the ICF osmotic balance. The osmotic force of ICF proteins and other nondiffusible substances is balanced by the active transport of ions out of the cell. Water crosses cell membranes freely, so the osmolality of TBW is normally at equilibrium. Normally the ICF is not subject to rapid changes in osmolality, but when ECF osmolality changes, water moves from one compartment to another until osmotic equilibrium is reestablished (see Figure 4-7, p. 104).

ALTERATIONS IN WATER MOVEMENT

Edema

Edema is excessive accumulation of fluid within the interstitial spaces. The forces favoring fluid movement from the capillaries or lymphatic channels into the tissues are increased capillary hydrostatic pressure, decreased plasma oncotic pressure, increased capillary membrane permeability, and lymphatic channel obstruction[2] (Figure 4-2).

PATHOPHYSIOLOGY Hydrostatic pressure increases as a result of venous obstruction or salt and water retention. Venous obstruction causes hydrostatic pressure to increase behind the obstruction, pushing fluid from the capillaries into the interstitial spaces. Thrombophlebitis (inflammation of veins), hepatic obstruction, tight clothing around the extremities, and prolonged standing are common causes of venous obstruction. Congestive heart failure, renal failure, and cirrhosis of the liver are associated with excessive salt and water retention, which cause plasma volume overload, increased capillary hydrostatic pressure, and edema.

Lost or diminished plasma albumin production (e.g., from liver disease or protein malnutrition) contributes to decreased plasma

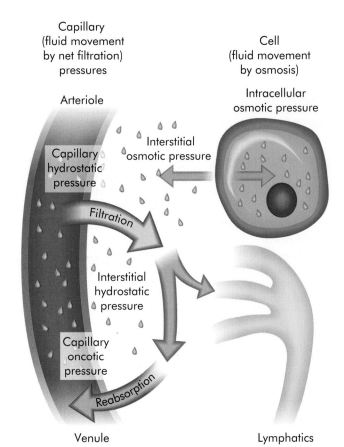

FIGURE 4-1 Net Filtration—Fluid Movement Between Plasma and Interstitial Space. The movement of fluid between the vascular, interstitial spaces and the lymphatics is the result of net filtration of fluid across the semipermeable capillary membrane. *Capillary hydrostatic pressure* is the primary force for fluid movement out of the arteriolar end of the capillary and into the interstitial space. At the venous end, *capillary oncotic pressure* (from plasma proteins) attracts water back into the vascular space. *Interstitial hydrostatic pressure* promotes the movement of fluid and proteins into the lymphatics. *Osmotic pressure* accounts for the movement of fluid between the interstitial space and the intracellular space. Normally, intracellular and extracellular fluid osmotic pressures are equal (280 to 294 mOsm) and water is equally distributed between the interstitial and intracellular compartments.

oncotic pressure. Plasma proteins are lost in glomerular diseases of the kidney, serous drainage from open wounds, hemorrhage, burns, and cirrhosis of the liver. The decreased oncotic attraction of fluid within the capillary causes filtered capillary fluid to remain in the interstitial space, resulting in edema.

Capillaries become more permeable with inflammation and immune responses, especially with trauma such as burns or crushing injuries, neoplastic disease, and allergic reactions. Proteins escape from the vascular space and produce edema through decreased capillary oncotic pressure and interstitial fluid protein accumulation.

The lymphatic system normally absorbs interstitial fluid and a small amount of proteins. When lymphatic channels are blocked or surgically removed, proteins and fluid accumulate in the interstitial space, causing **lymphedema.**[3] For example, lymphedema of the arm or leg occurs after surgical removal of axillary or femoral lymph nodes, respectively, for treatment of carcinoma. Inflammation or tumors may cause lymphatic obstruction, leading to edema of the involved tissues.[4]

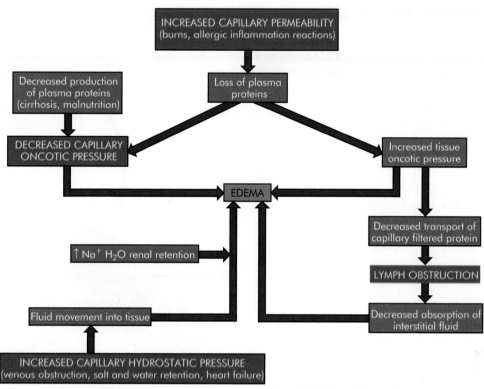

FIGURE 4-2 Mechanisms of Edema Formation. *H_2O,* Water; *Na^+,* sodium ion.

CLINICAL MANIFESTATIONS   Edema may be localized or generalized. *Localized edema* is usually limited to a site of trauma, as in a sprained finger. Another kind of localized edema occurs within particular organ systems and includes cerebral edema, pulmonary edema, pleural effusion (fluid accumulation in the pleural space), pericardial effusion (fluid accumulation within the membrane around the heart), and ascites (accumulation of fluid in the peritoneal space). *Generalized edema* is manifested by a more uniform distribution of fluid in interstitial spaces. Dependent edema, in which fluid accumulates in gravity-dependent areas of the body, might signal more generalized edema. Dependent edema appears in the feet and legs when standing and in the sacral area and buttocks when supine (lying on back). It can be identified by pressing on tissues overlying bony prominences. A pit left in the skin indicates edema (hence the term *pitting edema*) (Figure 4-3).

Edema usually is associated with weight gain, swelling and puffiness, tight-fitting clothes and shoes, limited movement of affected joints, and symptoms associated with the underlying pathologic condition. Fluid accumulations increase the distance required for nutrients and waste products to move between capillaries and tissues. Blood flow may be impaired also. Therefore wounds heal more slowly, and with prolonged edema the risks of infection and pressure sores over bony prominences increase. Edema of specific organs, such as the brain, lung, or larynx, can be life-threatening.

As edematous fluid accumulates, it is trapped in a "third space" (i.e., the interstitial space, pleural space, pericardial space) and is unavailable for metabolic processes or perfusion. Dehydration can develop as a result of this sequestering. Such sequestration occurs with severe burns, where large amounts of vascular fluid are lost to the interstitial spaces, reducing plasma volume and causing shock (see Chapter 23).

EVALUATION AND TREATMENT   Specific conditions causing edema require diagnosis. Edema may be treated symptomatically until

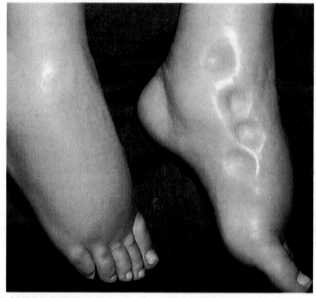

FIGURE 4-3 Pitting Edema. (From Patton KT, Thibodeau GA: *Anatomy & physiology,* ed 7, St Louis, 2010, Mosby.)

the underlying disorder is corrected. Supportive measures include elevating edematous limbs, using compression stockings, avoiding prolonged standing, restricting salt intake, and taking diuretics.

> ✔ **QUICK CHECK 4-1**
> 1. How does an increase in capillary hydrostatic pressure cause edema?
> 2. How does a decrease in capillary oncotic pressure cause edema?

TABLE 4-4	REPRESENTATIVE DISTRIBUTION OF ELECTROLYTES IN BODY COMPARTMENTS	
ELECTROLYTES	**ECF (mEq/L)**	**ICF (mEq/L)**
Cations		
Sodium	142	12
Potassium	4.2	150
Calcium	5	0
Magnesium	2	24
TOTAL	153.2	186
Anions		
Bicarbonate	24	12
Chloride	103	4
Phosphate	2	100
Proteins	16	65
Other anions	8	6
TOTAL	153	187

ECF, Extracellular fluid; *ICF,* intracellular fluid.

SODIUM, CHLORIDE, AND WATER BALANCE

The kidneys and hormones have a central role in maintaining sodium and water balance. Because water follows the osmotic gradients established by changes in salt concentration, sodium and water balance are intimately related. Sodium is regulated by renal effects of aldosterone (see Figure 17-17, p. 442). Water balance is regulated primarily by antidiuretic hormone (ADH; also known as *vasopressin*).

Sodium and Chloride Balance

Sodium (Na+) accounts for 90% of the ECF cations (positively charged ions). (The distribution of electrolytes in body compartments is summarized in Table 4-4.) Along with its constituent anions (negatively charged ions) chloride and bicarbonate, sodium regulates extracellular osmotic forces and therefore regulates water balance. Sodium is important in other functions, including maintenance of neuromuscular irritability for conduction of nerve impulses (in conjunction with potassium and calcium), regulation of acid-base balance (using sodium bicarbonate and sodium phosphate), participation in cellular chemical reactions, and transport of substances across the cellular membrane.

The kidney, in conjunction with neural and hormonal mediators, maintains normal serum sodium concentration within a narrow range (135 to 145 mEq/L) primarily through renal tubular reabsorption. Hormonal regulation of sodium (and potassium) balance is mediated by aldosterone, a mineralocorticoid synthesized and secreted from the adrenal cortex as a component of the renin-angiotensin-aldosterone system (see Chapters 17 and 28). Aldosterone secretion is influenced both by circulating blood volume and blood pressure and by plasma concentrations of sodium and potassium.

When circulating blood volume or blood pressure is reduced, or sodium levels are depressed or potassium levels are increased, renin, an enzyme secreted by the juxtaglomerular cells of the kidney, is released. Renin stimulates the formation of angiotensin I, an inactive polypeptide. Angiotensin-converting enzyme (ACE) in pulmonary vessels converts angiotensin I to angiotensin II, which stimulates the secretion of aldosterone and also causes vasoconstriction. The aldosterone then promotes renal sodium and water reabsorption and excretion

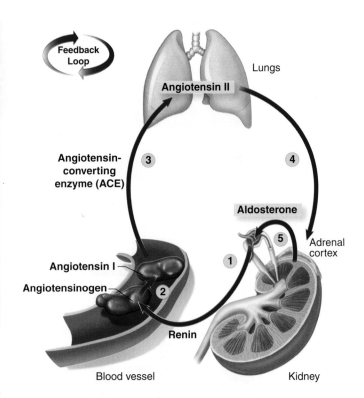

FIGURE 4-4 The Renin-Angiotensin-Aldosterone System. *(1)* Renal juxtaglomerular cells sense decrease in blood pressure and release renin; *(2)* renin activates angiotensinogen to angiotensin I; *(3)* angiotensin I is converted to angiotensin II via angiotensin-converting enzyme (ACE) in the lung capillaries; *(4)* angiotensin II promotes vasoconstriction and stimulates aldosterone secretion from the adrenal cortex, resulting in renal sodium and water retention, potassium excretion, and an increase in blood pressure; *(5)* aldosterone causes increased reabsorption of sodium and water retention. (From Patton KT, Thibodeau GA: *Anatomy & physiology,* ed 7, St Louis, 2010, Mosby.)

of potassium, increasing blood volume (Figure 4-4). Vasoconstriction elevates the systemic blood pressure and restores renal perfusion (blood flow). This restoration inhibits the further release of renin.

Natriuretic peptides are hormones, including atrial natriuretic hormone (ANH), produced by the myocardial atria; brain natriuretic peptide (BNP) is produced by the myocardial ventricles and urodilatin (an ANP analogue) is synthesized within the kidney. Natriuretic peptides are released when there is an increase in transmural atrial pressure (increased volume), which may occur with congestive heart failure or when there is an increase in mean arterial pressure[5] (Figure 4-5). They are natural antagonists to the renin-angiotensin-aldosterone system. Natriuretic peptides cause vasodilation and increase sodium and water excretion, decreasing blood pressure. Natriuretic peptides are sometimes called a "third factor" in sodium regulation. (Increased glomerular filtration rate is thus the first factor and aldosterone the second factor.)

Chloride (Cl^-) is the major anion in the ECF and provides electroneutrality, particularly in relation to sodium. Chloride transport is generally passive and follows the active transport of sodium so that increases or decreases in chloride concentration are proportional to changes in sodium concentration. Chloride concentration tends to vary inversely with changes in the concentration of bicarbonate (HCO_3^-), the other major anion.

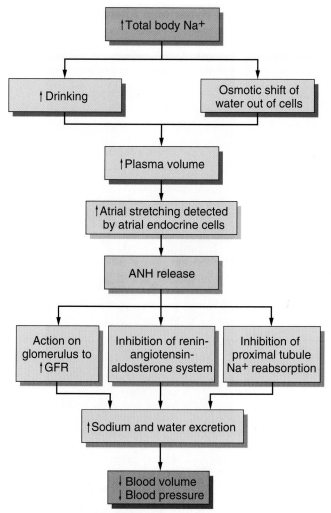

FIGURE 4-5 The Atrial Natriuretic Hormone (ANH) System. *GFR,* Glomerular filtration rate; *Na+,* sodium ion.

Water Balance

Water balance is regulated by the secretion of ADH (also known as vasopressin).[6] ADH is secreted when plasma osmolality increases or circulating blood volume decreases and blood pressure drops (Figure 4-6). Increased plasma osmolality occurs with water deficit or sodium excess in relation to total body water. The increased osmolality stimulates hypothalamic **osmoreceptors.** In addition to causing thirst, these osmoreceptors signal the posterior pituitary gland to release ADH. Thirst stimulates water drinking and ADH increases water reabsorption into the plasma from the distal tubules and collecting ducts of the kidney (see Chapter 28). The reabsorbed water decreases plasma osmolality, returning it toward normal, and urine concentration increases.

With fluid loss (dehydration) from vomiting, diarrhea, or excessive sweating, a decrease in blood volume and blood pressure often occurs. **Volume-sensitive receptors** and **baroreceptors** (nerve endings that are sensitive to changes in volume and pressure) also stimulate the release of ADH from the pituitary gland and stimulate thirst. The volume receptors are located in the right and left atria and thoracic vessels; baroreceptors are found in the aorta, pulmonary arteries, and carotid sinus. ADH secretion also occurs when atrial pressure drops, as occurs with decreased blood volume. The reabsorption of water mediated by ADH then promotes the restoration of plasma volume and blood pressure (Figure 4-6).

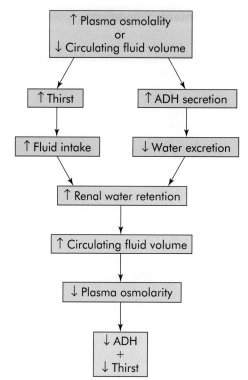

FIGURE 4-6 The Antidiuretic Hormone (ADH) System.

TABLE 4-5	WATER AND SOLUTE IMBALANCES
TONICITY	**MECHANISM**
Isotonic (isoosmolar) imbalance	Gain or loss of ECF* resulting in concentration equivalent to 0.9% sodium chloride (salt) solution (normal saline); no shrinking or swelling of cells
Hypertonic (hyperosmolar) imbalance	Imbalances that result in ECF concentration >0.9% salt solution (i.e., water loss or solute gain); cells shrink in hypertonic fluid
Hypotonic (hypoosmolar) imbalance	Imbalance that results in ECF <0.9% salt solution (i.e., water gain or solute loss); cells swell in hypotonic fluid

ECF, Extracellular fluid.

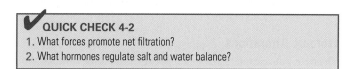

✔ **QUICK CHECK 4-2**
1. What forces promote net filtration?
2. What hormones regulate salt and water balance?

ALTERATIONS IN SODIUM, WATER, AND CHLORIDE BALANCE

Alterations in sodium and water balance are closely related. Water imbalances may develop with gains or losses of salt. Likewise, sodium imbalances occur with alterations in body water volume. Generally, these alterations can be classified as changes in tonicity—the change in the concentration of solutes in relation to water (see Chapter 1). Alterations can therefore be classified as isotonic, hypertonic, or hypotonic (Table 4-5 and Figure 4-7).

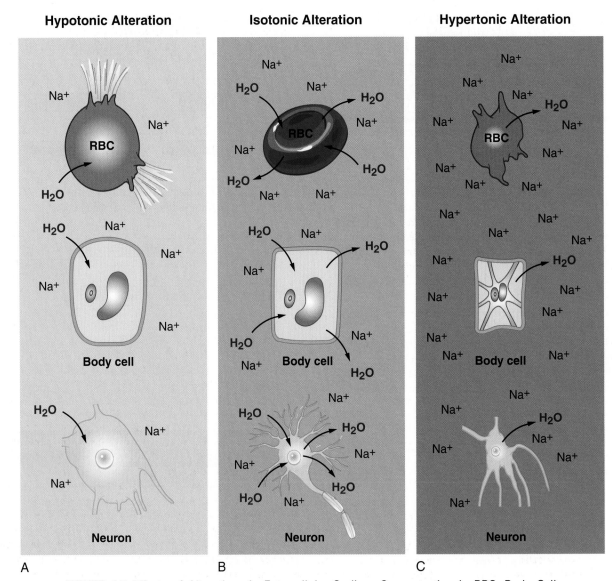

FIGURE 4-7 Effects of Alterations in Extracellular Sodium Concentration in RBC, Body Cell, and Neuron. A, Hypotonic Alteration: Decrease in ECF sodium (Na) concentration (hyponatremia) results in ICF osmotic attraction of water with swelling and potential bursting of cells. B, Isotonic Alteration: Normal concentration of sodium in the ECF and no change in shifts of fluid in or out of cells. C, Hypertonic Alteration: An increase in ECF sodium concentration (hypernatremia) results in osmotic attraction of water out of cells with cell shrinkage. *RBC,* Red blood cell.

Isotonic Alterations

The term isotonic refers to a solution that has the same concentration of solutes as the plasma. Isotonic alterations occur when TBW changes are accompanied by proportional changes in the concentrations of electrolytes (see Figure 4-7).

Isotonic fluid loss causes hypovolemia. For example, if an individual loses pure plasma or ECF, fluid volume is depleted but the concentration and type of electrolytes and the osmolality remain in the normal range (280 to 294 mOsm). Causes include hemorrhage, severe wound drainage, excessive diaphoresis (sweating), and inadequate fluid intake. There is loss of extracellular fluid volume with weight loss, dryness of skin and mucous membranes, decreased urine output, and symptoms of hypovolemia. Indicators of hypovolemia include a rapid heart rate, flattened neck veins, and normal or decreased blood pressure. In severe states, hypovolemic shock can occur (see Chapter 23). Isotonic solutions of electrolytes and glucose are given orally, intravenously or in some cases subcutaneously (hypodermoclysis).

Isotonic fluid excess causes hypervolemia. Common causes include excessive administration of intravenous fluids, hypersecretion of aldosterone, or the effects of drugs such as cortisone (which causes renal reabsorption of sodium and water). As plasma volume expands, hypervolemia develops with weight gain. The diluting effect of excess plasma volume leads to decreased hematocrit and decreased plasma protein concentration. The neck veins may distend, and the blood pressure increases. Increased capillary hydrostatic pressure leads to edema formation. Ultimately, pulmonary edema and heart failure may develop. Diuretics are commonly used for treatment.

Hypertonic Alterations

Hypertonic fluid alterations develop when the osmolality of the ECF is elevated above normal (greater than 294 mOsm). The most common causes are increased concentration of ECF sodium (hypernatremia) or deficit of ECF water. In both instances, ECF hypertonicity attracts water from the intracellular space, causing ICF dehydration (see Figure 4-7).

Hypernatremia

PATHOPHYSIOLOGY Hypernatremia occurs when serum sodium levels exceed 145 mEq/L. Increased levels of serum sodium may be caused by retention or infusion of sodium or by decreased intake or increased loss of water.[7] Because sodium is largely in the ECF, increases in sodium concentration cause intracellular dehydration. The movement of water to the ECF may cause hypervolemia, or with an accompanying water loss both ICF and ECF dehydration may occur. Hyperosmolality is a common result of hypernatremia.

Increased sodium retention commonly occurs as a result of oversecretion of aldosterone (as in primary hyperaldosteronism) or oversecretion of adrenocorticotropic hormone (ACTH), which also causes increased secretion of aldosterone (as in Cushing syndrome).[8] Less commonly there may be inappropriate administration of hypertonic saline solution (e.g., as sodium bicarbonate for treatment of acidosis during cardiac arrest). High amounts of dietary sodium rarely cause hypernatremia in a healthy individual because the sodium is eliminated by the kidneys.

Increased sodium concentration caused by water loss or decreased intake of water is associated with fever or respiratory tract infections, which increase the respiratory rate and enhance water loss from the lungs. Diabetes insipidus (deficiency of ADH), diabetes mellitus (hyperglycemia), polyuria (frequent urination), profuse sweating, and diarrhea also cause water loss in relation to sodium. Infants with severe diarrhea are particularly vulnerable. Insufficient water intake can cause hypernatremia, particularly in individuals who are comatose, confused, or immobilized or are receiving gastric feedings. Infants are particularly at risk because they cannot communicate thirst.

Because chloride follows sodium, hyperchloremia (elevation of serum chloride concentration above 105 mEq/L) often accompanies hypernatremia, as well as plasma bicarbonate deficits as in metabolic acidosis (see p. 111). There are no specific symptoms or treatment for chloride excess.

HEALTH ALERT

Breast-Feeding and Hypernatremia

Hypernatremic dehydration (serum sodium >150 mEq/L) is an uncommon but serious complication of breast-fed infants, particularly those born by cesarean section. At risk are babies older than 48 hours who have lost greater than 10% of body weight and have not regained original birthweight by day 10. The most common presenting symptom is nonhemolytic jaundice. Nonmetabolic symptoms include apnea or bradycardia, or both. Higher breast milk sodium levels also are found. Babies with significant weight loss require maternal support to establish successful breast-feeding; daily monitoring of weight and supplemental fluids.

Data from Konetzny G et al: Prevention of hypernatraemic dehydration in breastfed newborn infants by daily weighing, *Eur J Pediatr* 168(7):815–818, 2009; Kusuma S et al: Hydration status of exclusively and partially breastfed near-term newborns in the first week of life, *J Hum Lact* 25(3):280–286, 2009; Shroff R et al: Life-threatening hypernatraemic dehydration in breastfed babies, *Arch Dis Child* 91(12):1025–1026, 2006.

Clinical manifestations. When there is excessive sodium intake or decreased sodium loss, water is redistributed to the extracellular space, resulting in hypervolemia, and intracellular dehydration ensues. Clinical manifestations include weight gain, bounding pulse, and increased blood pressure. Central nervous system symptoms are the most serious and are related to alterations in membrane potentials and shrinking of brain cells. Symptoms include muscle twitching and hyperreflexia (hyperactive reflexes), confusion, coma, convulsions, and cerebral hemorrhage from stretching of veins.

Evaluation and treatment. The treatment of hypernatremia is to give oral fluids or isotonic salt-free fluid (5% dextrose in water) until the serum sodium level returns to normal. Fluid replacement must be given slowly to prevent cerebral edema. Hypervolemia or hypovolemia requires treatment of the underlying clinical condition.

Water Deficit

PATHOPHYSIOLOGY Dehydration refers to water deficit but also is commonly used to indicate both sodium and water loss (isotonic or isoosmolar dehydration).[9] Pure water deficits (hyperosmolar or hypertonic dehydration) are rare because most people have access to water. Individuals who are comatose or paralyzed continue to have insensible water losses through the skin and lungs with a minimal obligatory formation of urine. Hyperventilation caused by fever also may precipitate water deficit. The most common cause of water loss is increased renal clearance of free water as a result of impaired tubular function or inability to concentrate the urine, as occurs in diabetes insipidus (decreased ADH) (see Chapter 18).

CLINICAL MANIFESTATIONS Marked water deficit is manifested by symptoms of dehydration, such as headache, thirst, dry skin and mucous membranes, elevated temperature, weight loss, and decreased or concentrated urine (with the exception of diabetes insipidus). Skin turgor may be normal or decreased. Symptoms of hypovolemia include tachycardia, weak pulses, and postural hypotension (a decrease in blood pressure with movement from lying or sitting to standing).

EVALUATION AND TREATMENT An elevated hematocrit and increased serum sodium concentration are associated with moderate water loss in addition to clinical signs and symptoms. The magnitude of dehydration is determined from evaluation of the plasma and urine osmolality.

Treatment is to give water and stop fluid loss. Fluid replacement must be administered slowly enough to prevent rapid movement of water into brain cells, which causes cerebral edema, seizures, brain injury, and death. When intravenous replacement is required, 5% dextrose in water should be used because pure water lyses red blood cells.

Hypotonic Alterations

Hypotonic fluid imbalances occur when the osmolality of the ECF is less than normal (i.e., less than 280 mOsm) (see Figure 4-7). The most common causes are sodium deficit or water excess. Either leads to *intracellular overhydration* (cellular edema) and cell swelling. When there is a sodium deficit, the osmotic pressure of the ECF decreases and water moves into the cell where the osmotic pressure is greater. The plasma volume then decreases, leading to symptoms of hypovolemia. With water excess, increases in both the ICF and ECF volume occur, causing symptoms of hypervolemia and water intoxication with cerebral and pulmonary edema.

Hyponatremia

PATHOPHYSIOLOGY Hyponatremia develops when the serum sodium concentration falls below 135 mEq/L. It occurs frequently among hospitalized elderly individuals. This occurs when there is loss of sodium, inadequate intake of sodium, or dilution of sodium by water excess.[10] Sodium depletion usually causes hypoosmolality with movement of water into cells. Pure sodium depletion is usually caused by vomiting, diarrhea, suctioning of gastrointestinal secretions, and burns or renal losses from use of diuretics. Inadequate intake of dietary sodium is rare but possible in individuals on low-sodium diets, particularly when diuretics are taken. Dilutional hyponatremia occurs when there is replacement of fluid loss with intravenous 5% dextrose in water. The glucose is metabolized to carbon dioxide and water, leaving a hypotonic solution with a diluting effect. Excessive sweating may stimulate thirst and intake of large amounts of water, which dilute sodium. During acute oliguric renal failure, severe congestive heart failure, or cirrhosis renal excretion of water is impaired. Both TBW and sodium levels are increased, but TBW exceeds the increase in sodium concentration, producing hypervolemia and hyponatremia.

Hypochloremia, a low level of serum chloride (less than 97 mEq/L), usually occurs with hyponatremia or an elevated bicarbonate concentration, as in metabolic alkalosis (see p. 112). Sodium deficit related to restricted intake, use of diuretics, and vomiting is accompanied by chloride deficiency. Cystic fibrosis is characterized by hypochloremia (see Chapter 27). Treatment of the underlying cause is required.

CLINICAL MANIFESTATIONS A decrease in sodium concentration changes the cell's ability to depolarize and repolarize normally, altering the action potential in neurons and muscle (see Chapter 1). Neurologic changes characteristic of hyponatremia include lethargy, confusion, apprehension, depressed reflexes, seizures, and coma. Muscle twitching and weakness are common. Pure sodium losses may be accompanied by loss of ECF, causing hypovolemia with symptoms of hypotension, tachycardia, and decreased urine output. Dilutional hyponatremia is accompanied by weight gain, edema, ascites, and jugular vein distention. Cerebral edema can be a life-threatening complication of hypervolemic hyponatremia.

EVALUATION AND TREATMENT The cause of hyponatremia must be determined and treatment planned accordingly. Hypertonic saline solutions are used cautiously with severe symptoms, such as seizures and must be given slowly to prevent osmotic demyelination syndrome in the brain. Restriction of water intake is required in most cases of dilutional hyponatremia because body sodium levels may be normal or increased even though serum sodium levels are low. Serum sodium concentration must be monitored.[11]

Water Excess

PATHOPHYSIOLOGY When the body is functioning normally, it is almost impossible to produce an excess of TBW because water balance is regulated by the kidneys. Some individuals with psychogenic disorders develop water intoxication from compulsive water drinking. Acute renal failure, severe congestive heart failure, and cirrhosis can precipitate water excess during intravenous infusion of 5% dextrose in water. Decreased urine formation from renal disease or decreased renal blood flow contributes to water excess. The overall effect is dilution of the ECF, with water moving to the intracellular space by osmosis. The syndrome of inappropriate secretion of ADH (SIADH), also known as vasopressin dysregulation, also enhances water retention[12] (see Chapter 18). Water excess is usually accompanied by hyponatremia.

CLINICAL MANIFESTATIONS The symptoms of water excess are related to the rate at which water loading has occurred. Acute excesses cause cerebral edema with confusion and convulsions. Weakness, nausea, muscle twitching, headache, and weight gain are common symptoms of chronic water accumulation.

EVALUATION AND TREATMENT The cause and acuity of water excess must be determined. Serum and urine osmolalities are decreased because water will be in excess of sodium. Urine sodium level will be reduced. The hematocrit is reduced from the dilutional effect of water excess.

Fluid restriction for 24 hours is effective treatment if there are no convulsions. Small amounts of intravenous hypertonic sodium chloride (i.e., 3% sodium chloride) can be given when neurologic manifestations are severe.[13]

> ✔ **QUICK CHECK 4-3**
> 1. What causes isotonic imbalance?
> 2. Give two examples of hypertonic alterations, and explain the mechanisms of action for each.
> 3. What is a hypotonic imbalance? Give two examples.

ALTERATIONS IN POTASSIUM AND OTHER ELECTROLYTES

Potassium

Potassium (K^+) is the major intracellular electrolyte and is essential for normal cellular functions. Total body potassium content is about 4000 mEq, with most of it (98%) located in the cells. The ICF concentration of potassium is 150 to 160 mEq/L; the ECF potassium concentration is 3.5 to 5.0 mEq/L. The difference in concentration is maintained by a sodium-potassium adenosinetriphosphatase active transport system (Na^+, K^+ ATPase pump) (see Chapter 1).

As the predominant ICF ion, potassium exerts a major influence on the regulation of ICF osmolality and fluid balance as well as on intracellular electrical neutrality in relation to hydrogen (H^+) and sodium. Potassium is required for glycogen and glucose deposition in liver and skeletal muscle cells. It also maintains the resting membrane potential, as reflected in the transmission and conduction of nerve impulses, the maintenance of normal cardiac rhythms, and the contraction of skeletal muscle and smooth muscle.

Dietary potassium moves rapidly into cells after ingestion. However, the distribution of potassium between intracellular and extracellular fluids is influenced by several factors. Insulin, aldosterone, epinephrine, and alkalosis facilitate the shift of potassium into cells. Insulin deficiency, aldosterone deficiency, acidosis, cell lysis, and strenuous exercise facilitate the shift of potassium out of cells. Glucagon blocks entry of potassium into cells, and glucocorticoids promote potassium excretion. Potassium also will move out of cells along with water when there is increased ECF osmolarity.

Although potassium is found in most body fluids, the kidney is the most efficient regulator of potassium balance. Potassium is freely filtered by the renal glomerulus, and 90% is reabsorbed by the proximal tubule and loop of Henle. In the distal tubules, principal cells secrete potassium and intercalated cells reabsorb potassium. These cells determine the amount of potassium excreted from the body. The gut may also sense the amount of K^+ ingested and stimulate renal K^+ excretion.[14]

The potassium concentration in the distal tubular cells is determined primarily by the plasma concentration in the peritubular capillaries. When plasma potassium concentration increases from increased dietary intake or shifts of potassium from the ICF to the ECF occur, potassium is secreted into the urine by the distal tubules.[15] Decreased levels of plasma potassium result in decreased distal tubular secretion, although approximately 5 to 15 mEq per day will continue to be lost. Changes in the rate of filtrate (urine) flow through the distal tubule also influence the concentration gradient for potassium secretion. When the flow rate is high, as with the use of diuretics, potassium concentration in the distal tubular urine is lower, leading to the secretion of potassium into the urine.

Changes in pH and thus in hydrogen ion concentration also affect potassium balance. During acute acidosis, hydrogen ions accumulate in the ICF and potassium shifts out of the cell to the ECF to maintain a balance of cations across the cell membrane. This occurs in part because of a decrease in sodium-potassium ATPase pump activity. Decreased ICF potassium results in decreased secretion of potassium by the distal tubular cells, contributing to hyperkalemia. In acute alkalosis, intracellular fluid levels of hydrogen diminish and potassium shifts into the cell; in addition, the distal tubular cells increase their secretion of potassium, further contributing to hypokalemia.

Besides conserving sodium, aldosterone also regulates potassium concentration. Elevated plasma potassium concentration causes the release of renin by renal juxtaglomerular cells and the adrenal secretion of aldosterone through the renin-angiotensin-aldosterone system. Aldosterone then stimulates the release of potassium into the urine by the distal renal tubules. Aldosterone also increases the secretion of potassium from sweat glands.

Insulin helps regulate plasma potassium levels by stimulating the sodium-potassium ATPase pump, thus promoting the movement of potassium into liver and muscle cells, particularly after eating. Insulin can also be used to treat hyperkalemia. Dangerously low levels of plasma potassium can result when insulin is given while potassium levels are depressed. Potassium balance is especially significant in the treatment of conditions requiring insulin administration, such as insulin-dependent diabetes mellitus.

Potassium adaptation is the ability of the body to adapt to increased levels of potassium intake over time. A sudden increase in potassium may be fatal, but if the intake of potassium is slowly increased by amounts of more than 120 mEq per day, the kidney can increase the urinary excretion of potassium and maintain potassium balance.

Hypokalemia

PATHOPHYSIOLOGY   Potassium deficiency, or **hypokalemia**, develops when the serum potassium concentration falls below 3.5 mEq/L. Because cellular and total body stores of potassium are difficult to measure, changes in potassium balance are described, although not always accurately, by the plasma concentration. Generally, lowered serum potassium level indicates loss of total body potassium. With potassium loss from the ECF, the concentration gradient change favors movement of potassium from the cell to the ECF. The ICF/ECF concentration ratio is maintained, but the amount of total body potassium is depleted.

Factors contributing to the development of hypokalemia include reduced intake of potassium, increased entry of potassium into cells, and increased losses of body potassium. Dietary deficiency of potassium is rare but may occur in elderly individuals with both low protein intake and inadequate intake of fruits and vegetables and in individuals with alcoholism or anorexia nervosa. Reduced potassium intake generally becomes a problem when combined with other causes of potassium depletion.

ECF hypokalemia can develop without losses of total body potassium. For example, potassium shifts from the ECF to the ICF in exchange for hydrogen to maintain plasma acid-base balance during respiratory or metabolic alkalosis. Insulin promotes cellular uptake of potassium and insulin administration may cause an ECF potassium deficit.

Potassium shifts from the ICF to the ECF in conditions such as diabetic ketoacidosis, in which the increased hydrogen ion concentration in the ECF causes H^+ to shift into the cell in exchange for potassium. A normal level of potassium is maintained in the plasma, but potassium continues to be lost in the urine, causing a deficit in the amount of total body potassium. Severe, even fatal, hypokalemia may occur if insulin is administered without also providing potassium supplements. Thus total body potassium depletion becomes evident when insulin treatment and rehydration therapy are initiated. Potassium replacement is instituted cautiously to prevent hyperkalemia.

Losses of potassium from body stores are usually caused by gastrointestinal and renal disorders. Diarrhea, intestinal drainage tubes or fistulae, and laxative abuse also result in hypokalemia. Normally, only 5 to 10 mEq of potassium and 100 to 150 ml of water are excreted in the stool each day. With diarrhea, fluid and electrolyte losses can be voluminous, with several liters of fluid and 100 to 200 mEq of potassium lost per day. Vomiting or continuous nasogastric suctioning often is associated with potassium depletion, partly because of the potassium lost from the gastric fluid but principally because of renal compensation for volume depletion and the metabolic alkalosis (elevated bicarbonate levels) that occurs from sodium, chloride, and hydrogen ion losses. The loss of fluid and sodium stimulates the secretion of aldosterone, which in turn causes renal losses of potassium.

Renal potassium losses occur with increased secretion of potassium by the distal tubule. Use of potassium-wasting diuretics, excessive aldosterone secretion, increased distal tubular flow rate, and low plasma magnesium concentration all may contribute to urinary losses of potassium. The elevated flow of bicarbonate at the distal tubule during alkalosis also contributes to renal excretion of potassium because the increased tubular lumen electronegativity attracts potassium. Many diuretics inhibit the reabsorption of sodium chloride, causing the diuretic effect. The distal tubular flow rate then increases, promoting potassium excretion. If sodium loss is severe, the compensating aldosterone secretion may further deplete potassium stores. Primary hyperaldosteronism with excessive secretion of aldosterone from an adrenal adenoma (tumor) also causes potassium wasting. Many kidney diseases reduce the ability to conserve sodium. The disordered sodium reabsorption produces a diuretic effect, and the increased distal tubule flow rate favors the secretion of potassium. Magnesium deficits increase renal potassium secretion and promote hypokalemia. Several antibiotics are known to cause hypokalemia by increasing the rate of potassium excretion. Rare hereditary defects in potassium transport (e.g., Bartter and Gitelman syndromes) also can cause hypokalemia.

CLINICAL MANIFESTATIONS   Mild losses of potassium are usually asymptomatic. Severe loss of potassium, however, results in neuromuscular and cardiac manifestations. Neuromuscular excitability decreases, causing skeletal muscle weakness, smooth muscle atony, cardiac dysrhythmias, glucose intolerance and impaired urinary concentrating ability.[16]

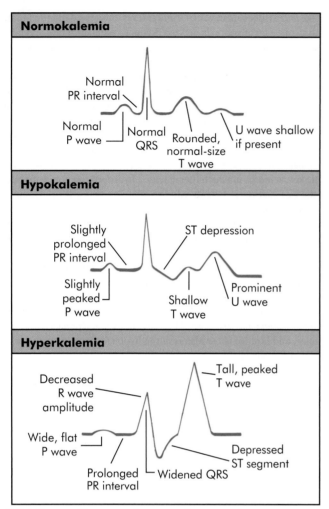

FIGURE 4-8 Electrocardiogram Changes With Potassium Imbalance.

TABLE 4-6	CLINICAL MANIFESTATIONS OF POTASSIUM LEVEL ALTERATIONS	
ORGAN SYSTEM	**HYPOKALEMIA**	**HYPERKALEMIA**
Cardiovascular	Dysrhythmias	Dysrhythmias
	ECG changes (flattened T waves, U waves, ST depression, peaked P wave, prolonged QT interval)	ECG changes (peaked T waves, prolonged PR interval, absent P wave with widened QRS complex)
	Cardiac arrest	Bradycardia
	Weak, irregular pulse rate	Heart block
	Postural hypotension	Cardiac arrest
Nervous	Lethargy	Anxiety
	Fatigue	Tingling
	Confusion	Numbness
	Paresthesias	
Gastrointestinal	Nausea and vomiting	Nausea and vomiting
	Decreased motility	Diarrhea
	Distention	Colicky pain
	Decreased bowel sounds	
	Ileus	
Kidney	Water loss	Oliguria
	Thirst	Kidney damage
	Inability to concentrate urine	
	Kidney damage	
Skeletal and smooth muscle	Weakness	Early: hyperactive muscles
	Flaccid paralysis	
	Respiratory arrest	Late: weakness and flaccid paralysis
	Constipation	
	Bladder dysfunction	

Symptoms occur in relation to the rate of potassium depletion. Because the body can accommodate slow losses of potassium, the decrease in ECF concentration may allow potassium to shift from the intracellular space, restoring the potassium concentration gradient toward normal, with less severe neuromuscular changes. With acute and severe losses of potassium, changes in neuromuscular excitability are more profound. Skeletal muscle weakness occurs initially in the larger muscles of the legs and arms and ultimately affects the diaphragm and depresses ventilation. Paralysis and respiratory arrest can occur. Loss of smooth muscle tone is manifested by constipation, intestinal distention, anorexia, nausea, vomiting, and paralytic ileus (paralysis of the intestinal muscles).

The cardiac effects of hypokalemia are related also to changes in membrane excitability. Because potassium contributes to the repolarization phase of the action potential, hypokalemia delays ventricular repolarization. Various dysrhythmias may occur, including sinus bradycardia, atrioventricular block, and paroxysmal atrial tachycardia. The characteristic changes in the electrocardiogram (ECG) reflect delayed repolarization. For instance, the amplitude of the T wave decreases, the amplitude of the U wave increases, and the ST segment is depressed (Figure 4-8). In severe states of hypokalemia, P waves peak and the QT interval is prolonged. Hypokalemia also increases the risk of digitalis toxicity.

A wide range of metabolic dysfunctions may result from potassium deficiency (Table 4-6). Carbohydrate metabolism is affected because hypokalemia depresses insulin secretion and alters hepatic and skeletal muscle glycogen synthesis. Renal function is impaired, with a decreased ability to concentrate urine. Polyuria (increased urine) and polydipsia (increased thirst) are associated with decreased responsiveness to ADH. Long-term potassium deficits lasting more than 1 month may damage renal tissue, with interstitial fibrosis and tubular atrophy.

EVALUATION AND TREATMENT The diagnosis of hypokalemia is significantly related to the medical history and the identification of disorders associated with potassium loss or shifts of extracellular potassium to the intracellular space. Treatment involves an estimation of total body potassium losses and correction of acid-base imbalances. Further losses of potassium should be prevented and the individual should be encouraged to eat foods rich in potassium. The maximal rate of oral replacement is 40 to 80 mEq/day if renal function is normal. A maximal safe rate of intravenous replacement is 20 mEq/hr. Because potassium is irritating to blood vessels, a maximal concentration of 40 mEq/L should be used. Serum potassium values are monitored until normokalemia is achieved.

Hyperkalemia

PATHOPHYSIOLOGY Elevation of ECF potassium concentration above 5.5 mEq/L constitutes **hyperkalemia**.[17] Because of efficient renal excretion, increases in total body potassium level are relatively rare. Acute increases in serum potassium level are handled quickly through increased cellular uptake and renal excretion of body potassium excesses.

Potassium excesses may be caused by increased intake, a shift of potassium from cells to the ECF, decreased renal excretion, or drugs that decrease renal potassium excretion (i.e., ACE inhibitors, angiotensin receptor blockers, and aldosterone antagonists). If renal function is normal, slow, long-term increases in potassium intake are usually well tolerated through potassium adaptation, although short-term potassium loading can exceed renal excretion rates. Dietary excesses of potassium are uncommon but accidental ingestion of potassium salt substitutes can cause toxicity. Use of stored whole blood and intravenous boluses of potassium penicillin G or replacement potassium can precipitate hyperkalemia, particularly with impaired renal function. Potassium moves from the ICF to the ECF with cell trauma or a change in cell membrane permeability, acidosis, insulin deficiency, or cell hypoxia. Burns, massive crushing injuries, and extensive surgeries can cause loss of potassium to the ECF as a result of cell trauma. If renal function is sustained, potassium is excreted. As cell repair begins, hypokalemia develops without an adequate replacement of potassium.

In acidosis, ECF hydrogen ions shift into the cells in exchange for ICF potassium and sodium; hyperkalemia and acidosis therefore often occur simultaneously. Because insulin promotes cellular entry of potassium, insulin deficits, which occur with such conditions as diabetic ketoacidosis, are accompanied by hyperkalemia. Hypoxia can lead to hyperkalemia by diminishing the efficiency of cell membrane active transport, resulting in the potassium escaping to the ECF. Digitalis overdose may cause hyperkalemia by inhibiting the Na^+, K^+ ATPase pump, which maintains increased intracellular potassium and extracellular sodium (see Chapter 1).

Decreased renal excretion of potassium commonly is associated with hyperkalemia. Renal failure that results in oliguria (urine output of 30 ml/hr or less) is accompanied by elevations of serum potassium level. The severity of hyperkalemia is related to the amount of potassium intake, the degree of acidosis, and the rate of renal cell damage. Decreases in the secretion or renal effects of aldosterone also can cause decreases in the urinary excretion of potassium. For example, Addison disease (a disease of adrenal cortical insufficiency) results in decreased production and secretion of aldosterone (and other steroids) and thus contributes to hyperkalemia.

CLINICAL MANIFESTATIONS   Symptoms vary with the severity of hyperkalemia. During mild attacks, increased neuromuscular irritability may be manifested as restlessness, intestinal cramping, and diarrhea. Severe hyperkalemia causes muscle weakness, loss of muscle tone, and paralysis.[18] Hyperkalemia causes decreased cardiac conduction and more rapid repolarization of heart muscle. In mild states of hyperkalemia, the more rapid repolarization is reflected in the ECG as narrow and taller T waves with a shortened QT interval. Severe hyperkalemia depresses the ST segment, prolongs the PR interval, and widens the QRS complex because of decreased conduction velocity (see Figure 4-8). Bradydysrhythmias and delayed conduction are common in hyperkalemia; severe hyperkalemia can cause ventricular fibrillation or cardiac arrest.

As with hypokalemia, changes in the ratio of intracellular to extracellular potassium concentration contribute to the symptoms of hyperkalemia (see Table 4-6). The neuromuscular effects of hyperkalemia are related to the increase in rate of repolarization and the presence of other contributing factors, such as acidosis and calcium balance. Long-term increases in ECF potassium

concentration result in shifts of potassium into the cell, because the tendency is to maintain a normal ratio of ICF to ECF potassium concentrations. Acute elevations of extracellular potassium concentration affect neuromuscular irritability as this ratio is disrupted. Increases in extracellular fluid calcium concentration can override the neuromuscular effects of hyperkalemia because calcium is also a cation.

EVALUATION AND TREATMENT   Hyperkalemia should be investigated when there is a history of renal disease, massive trauma, insulin deficiency, Addison disease, use of potassium salt substitutes, or metabolic acidosis. The acuity of the onset of symptoms may be related to the underlying cause.

Management of hyperkalemia is related to treating the contributing causes and correcting the potassium excess. Calcium gluconate can be administered to restore normal neuromuscular irritability when serum potassium levels are dangerously high. Administration of glucose (which readily stimulates insulin secretion) or administration of both glucose and insulin for diabetic individuals facilitates cellular entry of potassium. Sodium bicarbonate corrects metabolic acidosis and lowers serum potassium concentration. Oral or rectal administration of cation exchange resins, which exchange sodium for potassium in the intestine, can be effective. Dialysis effectively removes potassium when renal failure has occurred.

> **QUICK CHECK 4-4**
> 1. What role does potassium play in the body? What metabolic dysfunctions occur in potassium deficiency? In potassium excess?
> 2. Explain how a person can have normal total body potassium levels but still exhibit hypokalemia.
> 3. What is the most prominent ECG change associated with hyperkalemia? With hypokalemia?

Other Electrolytes—Calcium, Magnesium, and Phosphate

The specifics of balance for the other body electrolytes—calcium (Ca^{++}), phosphate (P^+), and magnesium (Mg^{++})—are summarized in Table 4-7. Parathyroid hormone and vitamin D are important for the regulation of these minerals[19] (see Chapter 17).

ACID-BASE BALANCE

Acid-base balance must be regulated within a narrow range for the body to function normally. Slight changes in amounts of hydrogen can significantly alter biologic processes in cells and tissues.[20] Hydrogen ion is needed to maintain membrane integrity and the speed of metabolic enzyme reactions. Most pathologic conditions disturb acid-base balance, producing circumstances possibly more harmful than the disease process itself.

Hydrogen Ion and pH

The concentration of hydrogen ions in body fluids is very small—approximately 0.0000001 mg/L. This number may be expressed as 10^{-7} mg/L, is indicated as pH 7.0. The symbol *pH* represents the acidity or alkalinity of a solution. As the pH changes 1 unit (e.g., from pH 7.0 to pH 6.0), the [H^+] ([H^+] = hydrogen ion concentration) changes tenfold. The greater the [H^+], the more acidic the solution and the lower the pH. The lower the [H^+], the more alkaline or basic the solution and the higher the pH. In biologic fluids, a pH of less than 7.4 is

TABLE 4-7 ALTERATIONS IN OTHER BODY ELECTROLYTES

PARAMETER	CALCIUM	PHOSPHATE	MAGNESIUM
Normal values	Serum: 8.8-10.5 mg/dl (total), 4.5-5.6 mg/dl (ionized); 99% in bone as hydroxyapatite; remainder in plasma and body cells with 50% bound to plasma proteins; 40% free or ionized; ionized form most important physiologically	Serum: 2.5-5.0 mg/dl, but may be as high as 6.0-7.0 mg/dl in infants and young children; mainly in bone with some in ICF and ECF; exists as phospholipids, phosphate esters, and inorganic phosphate (ionized form)	Serum: 1.8-3.0 mEq/L; 40%-60% stored in bone, 33% bound to plasma proteins; primary intracellular divalent cation
Function	Needed for fundamental metabolic processes; major cation for structure of bone and teeth; enzymatic cofactor for blood clotting; required for hormone secretion and function of cell receptors; directly related to plasma membrane stability and permeability, as well as transmission of nerve impulses and contraction of muscles	Intracellular and extracellular anion buffer in regulation of acid-base balance; provides energy for muscle contraction (as ATP)	Cofactor in intracellular enzymatic reactions and causes neuromuscular excitability; often interacts with calcium and potassium in reactions at cellular level and has important role in smooth muscle contraction and relaxation
Excess	**Hypercalcemia** (serum concentrations >10-12 mg/dl)	**Hyperphosphatemia** (serum concentrations >4.7 mg/dl)	**Hypermagnesemia** (serum concentrations >3.0 mEq/L)
Causes	Hyperparathyroidism; bone metastases with calcium resorption from breast, prostate, renal, and cervical cancer; sarcoidosis; excess vitamin D; many tumors that produce PTH	Acute or chronic renal failure with significant loss of glomerular filtration; treatment of metastatic tumors with chemotherapy that releases large amounts of phosphate into serum; long-term use of laxatives or enemas containing phosphates; hypoparathyroidism	Usually renal insufficiency or failure; also excessive intake of magnesium-containing antacids, adrenal insufficiency
Effects	Many nonspecific; fatigue, weakness, lethargy, anorexia, nausea, constipation; impaired renal function, kidney stones; dysrhythmias, bradycardia, cardiac arrest; bone pain, osteoporosis	Symptoms primarily related to low serum calcium levels (caused by high phosphate levels) similar to results of hypocalcemia; when prolonged, calcification of soft tissues in lungs, kidneys, joints	Skeletal smooth muscle contraction; excess nerve function; loss of deep tendon reflexes; nausea and vomiting; muscle weakness; hypotension; bradycardia; respiratory distress
Deficit	**Hypocalcemia** (serum calcium concentration <8.5 mg/dl)	**Hypophosphatemia** (serum phosphate concentration <2.0 mg/dl)	**Hypomagnesemia** (serum magnesium concentration <1.5 mEq/L)
Causes	Related to inadequate intestinal absorption, deposition of ionized calcium into bone or soft tissue, blood administration, or decreases in PTH and vitamin D; nutritional deficiencies occur with inadequate sources of dairy products or green leafy vegetables	Most commonly by intestinal malabsorption related to vitamin D deficiency, use of magnesium- and aluminum-containing antacids, long-term alcohol abuse, and malabsorption syndromes; respiratory alkalosis; increased renal excretion of phosphate associated with hyperparathyroidism	Malnutrition, malabsorption syndromes, alcoholism, urinary losses (renal tubular dysfunction, loop diuretics)
Effects	Increased neuromuscular excitability; tingling, muscle spasm (particularly in hands, feet, and facial muscles), intestinal cramping, hyperactive bowel sounds; severe cases show convulsions and tetany; prolonged QT interval, cardiac arrest	Conditions related to reduced capacity for oxygen transport by red blood cells and disturbed energy metabolism; leukocyte and platelet dysfunction; deranged nerve and muscle function; in severe cases, irritability, confusion, numbness, coma, convulsions; possibly respiratory failure (because of muscle weakness), cardiomyopathies, bone resorption (leading to rickets or osteomalacia)	Behavioral changes, irritability, increased reflexes, muscle cramps, ataxia, nystagmus, tetany, convulsions, tachycardia, hypotension

ATP, Adenosine triphosphate; *PTH,* parathyroid hormone.

defined as acidic and a pH greater than 7.4 is defined as alkaline or basic (Table 4-8).

Body acids are formed as end products of protein, carbohydrate, and fat metabolism. This must be balanced by the amount of basic substances in the body to maintain normal pH. The lungs, kidneys, and bones are the major organs involved in regulating acid-base balance. The systems work together to regulate short- and long-term changes in acid-base status.

Body acids exist in two forms: **volatile** (can be eliminated as CO_2 gas) and **nonvolatile** (can be eliminated by the kidney). The volatile acid is carbonic acid (H_2CO_3), a *weak acid* (i.e., it does not release its hydrogen easily). In the presence of the enzyme carbonic anhydrase,

it readily dissociates into carbon dioxide (CO_2) and water (H_2O). The carbon dioxide is then eliminated by pulmonary ventilation.

Sulfuric, phosphoric, and other organic acids are nonvolatile *strong acids* (i.e., they readily release their hydrogens). Nonvolatile acids are secreted into the urine by the renal tubules in amounts of about 60 to 100 mEq of hydrogen per day or about 1 mEq per kilogram of body weight.

Buffer Systems

Buffering occurs in response to changes in acid-base status. **Buffers** can absorb excessive hydrogen ion (H^+) (acid) or hydroxyl ion (OH^-) (base) and prevent a significant change in pH. The buffer systems are located in both the ICF and the ECF compartments, and they function at different rates (Table 4-9). The most important plasma buffer systems are carbonic acid–bicarbonate and the protein hemoglobin (Figure 4-9). Phosphate and protein are the most important intracellular buffers. Ammonia and phosphate are important renal buffers.

Carbonic Acid–Bicarbonate Buffering

The carbonic acid–bicarbonate buffer pair *operates in both the lung and the kidney* and is a major extracellular buffer. The lungs can decrease the amount of carbonic acid by blowing off carbon dioxide and leaving water. The kidneys can reabsorb bicarbonate or regenerate new bicarbonate from carbon dioxide and water. The relationship between bicarbonate and carbonic acid is usually expressed as a ratio. Normal bicarbonate level is about 24 mEq/L, and normal carbonic acid level is about 1.2 mEq/L (when the arterial CO_2 partial pressure [$Paco_2$] is 40 mm Hg), producing a 20:1 ratio and the normal pH of 7.4. These two systems are very effective together because the lungs can adjust acid concentration rapidly and bicarbonate is easily reabsorbed or regenerated by the kidneys.

Renal and respiratory adjustments to primary changes in pH are known as compensation. The respiratory system compensates for changes in pH by increasing or decreasing the concentration of carbon dioxide by changing ventilation. The renal system compensates by producing more acidic or more alkaline urine. Correction occurs when the values for both components of the buffer pair (carbonic acid and bicarbonate) return to normal levels.

TABLE 4-8 PH OF BODY FLUIDS

BODY FLUID	pH	FACTORS AFFECTING pH
Gastric juices	1.0-3.0	Hydrochloric acid production
Urine	5.0-6.0	H^+ ion excretion from waste products
Arterial blood	7.35-7.45	pH is slightly higher because there is less carbonic acid (H_2CO_3)
Venous blood	7.37	pH is slightly lower because there is more carbonic acid
Cerebrospinal fluid	7.32	Decreased bicarbonate and higher carbon dioxide content decrease pH
Pancreatic fluid	7.8-8.0	Contains bicarbonate produced by exocrine cells

Protein Buffering

Both intracellular and extracellular proteins have negative charges and can serve as buffers for hydrogen, but because most proteins are inside cells, they are primarily an intracellular buffer system. Hemoglobin (Hb) is an excellent intracellular blood buffer because it can bind with hydrogen ion (H^+) (forming HHb) and carbon dioxide (forming $HHbCO_2$). Hemoglobin bound to hydrogen ion becomes a weak acid. Hemoglobin not saturated with oxygen (venous blood) is a better buffer than hemoglobin saturated with oxygen (arterial blood). The pH control mechanism is illustrated in Figure 4-9.

Renal Buffering

The distal tubule of the kidney regulates acid-base balance by secreting hydrogen into the urine and reabsorbing bicarbonate. Dibasic phosphate ($HPO_4^=$) and ammonia (NH_3) are two important renal buffers. The renal buffering of hydrogen ions requires the use of carbon dioxide (CO_2) and water (H_2O) to form carbonic acid (H_2CO_3). The enzyme carbonic anhydrase catalyzes the reaction. The hydrogen is then secreted from the tubular cell and buffered in the lumen by phosphate and ammonia (i.e., forms $H_2PO_3^-$ and NH_4^+). The remaining bicarbonate is reabsorbed. The end effect is the addition of new bicarbonate to the plasma, which contributes to the alkalinity of the plasma because the hydrogen ion is excreted from the body (see Figure 28-13, p. 734).

Acid-Base Imbalances

Pathophysiologic changes in the concentration of hydrogen ion in the blood lead to acid-base imbalances.[20,21] In acidemia the pH of arterial blood is less than 7.4. A systemic increase in hydrogen ion concentration or loss of base is termed acidosis. In alkalemia the pH of arterial blood is greater than 7.4. A systemic decrease in hydrogen ion concentration or excess of base is termed alkalosis. These changes may be caused by metabolic or respiratory processes. Figure 4-10 summarizes the relationship among pH, the partial pressure of carbon dioxide, and the concentration of bicarbonate during different primary acid-base states.

Metabolic Acidosis

In metabolic acidosis the concentrations of non–carbonic acids increase or bicarbonate is lost from extracellular fluid or cannot be regenerated by the kidney (Table 4-10). This can occur either quickly, as in lactic acidosis caused by poor perfusion or hypoxemia, or slowly

TABLE 4-9 BUFFER SYSTEMS

BUFFER PAIRS	BUFFER SYSTEM	CHEMICAL REACTION	RATE
HCO_3^-/H_2CO_3	Bicarbonate	$H^+ + HCO_3^- \gtrless H_2O + CO_2$	Instantaneously
Hb^-/HHb	Hemoglobin	$HHb \rightleftharpoons H^+ + Hb^-$	Instantaneously
$HPO_4^=/H_2PO_4^-$	Phosphate	$H_2PO_4^- + H^+ + HPO_4^=$	Instantaneously
Pr^-/HPr	Plasma proteins	$HPr \rightleftharpoons H^+ + Pr^-$	Instantaneously

ORGANS	PHYSIOLOGIC MECHANISM		RATE
Lungs	Regulates retention or elimination of CO_2 and therefore H_2CO_3 concentration		Minutes to hours
Ionic shifts	Exchange of intracellular potassium and sodium for hydrogen		2-4 hours
Kidneys	Bicarbonate reabsorption and regeneration, ammonia formation, phosphate buffering		Hours to days
Bone	Exchanges of calcium and phosphate and release of carbonate		Hours to days

CO_2, Carbon dioxide; *Hb^-,* hemoglobin; *HCO_3^-,* bicarbonate; *H_2CO_3,* carbonic acid; *HHb,* hydrogenated hemoglobin; *$HPO_4^=$,* dibasic phosphate; *$H_2PO_4^-$,* monobasic phosphate; *HPr,* hydrogenated protein; *Pr^-,* protein.

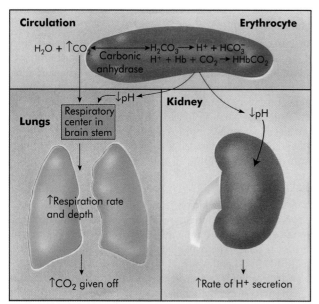

FIGURE 4-9 Integration of pH Control Mechanisms. Elevated carbon dioxide (CO_2) levels result in increased formation of carbonic acid (H_2CO_3) in red blood cells. The resulting increase in hydrogen ions (H^+), coupled with elevated CO_2 levels, results in $HHbCO_2$ and an increase in respiratory rate and secretion of H^+ by the kidneys, thus helping to regulate the pH of body fluids. (From Patton KT, Thibodeau GA: *Anatomy & physiology,* ed 7, St Louis, 2010, Mosby.)

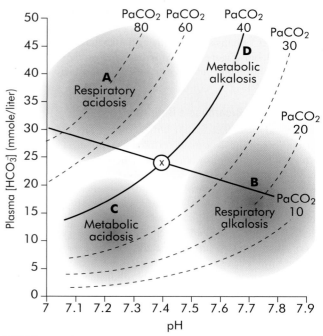

FIGURE 4-10 Davenport Diagram: Classic Working Diagram for Studying Primary Uncompensated Acid-Base Imbalance. The point $\otimes$ represents a normal pH value (7.4) and normal values for the partial pressure of arterial carbon dioxide ($Paco_2$ = 40 mm Hg) and the bicarbonate concentration (HCO_3^- = 24 mEq/L). Note that as the $Paco_2$ increases toward 60 mm Hg *(A)* the pH decreases (respiratory acidosis), and that as it decreases toward 20 mm Hg *(B)* the pH increases (respiratory alkalosis). Metabolic acidosis develops as the concentration of HCO_3^- decreases *(C),* and metabolic alkalosis develops as the concentration of HCO_3^- increases *(D).*

over an extended time, as in renal failure or diabetic ketoacidosis (see Chapter 18).[22]

The buffering systems normally compensate for excess acid and maintain arterial pH within normal range. When acidosis is severe, buffers become depleted and cannot compensate, and the ratio of the concentrations of bicarbonate to carbonic acid decreases to less than 20:1 (Figure 4-11). The specific type of acidosis can be determined by examining the serum anion gap (see Table 4-10).

Metabolic acidosis is manifested by changes in the function of the neurologic, respiratory, gastrointestinal, and cardiovascular systems. Early symptoms include headache and lethargy, which progress to coma in severe acidosis. The respiratory system's efforts to compensate for the increase in metabolic acids result in what are termed *Kussmaul respirations* (a form of hyperventilation), which are deep and rapid. This represents the body's attempt to increase pH by expelling carbon dioxide, which decreases carbonic acid concentration. Other symptoms include anorexia, nausea, vomiting, diarrhea, and abdominal discomfort. Death can result in the most severe and prolonged cases preceded by dysrhythmias and hypotension. The underlying condition must be diagnosed to establish effective treatment.

Metabolic Alkalosis

When excessive loss of metabolic acids occurs, bicarbonate concentration increases, causing metabolic alkalosis.[23] When acid loss is caused by vomiting, renal compensation is not very effective because loss of chloride (an anion) in hydrochloric (HCl) acid stimulates renal retention of bicarbonate (an anion), known as hypochloremic metabolic alkalosis. Hyperaldosteronism also can lead to alkalosis as a result of sodium bicarbonate retention and loss of hydrogen and potassium. Diuretics may produce a mild alkalosis because they promote greater excretion of sodium, potassium, and chloride than of bicarbonate (Figure 4-12).

TABLE 4-10	**CAUSES OF METABOLIC ACIDOSIS**
INCREASED NON–CARBONIC ACIDS (ELEVATED ANION GAP*)	**BICARBONATE LOSS OR HYPERCHLOREMIC ACIDOSIS (NORMAL ANION GAP)**
Increased H^+ load	Diarrhea
Ketoacidosis (e.g., diabetes mellitus, starvation)	Ureterosigmoidoscopy
Lactic acidosis (e.g., shock, hypoxemia)	
Ingestion (e.g., ammonium chloride, ethylene glycol, methanol, salicylates, paraldehyde)	
Decreased renal H^+ excretion	Renal HCO_3^- loss
Proximal renal tubule acidosis	Decreased renal H^+ secretion
Distal renal tubule acidosis	

*Anion gap refers to anions not usually measured in laboratory reports (e.g., sulfate, phosphate, and lactate). The anions usually measured are chloride (Cl^-) and bicarbonate (HCO_3^-). When the sum of the concentrations of measured anions (e.g., chloride and bicarbonate) is subtracted from the sum of the concentrations of measured cations (e.g., sodium and potassium), there is a "gap" of approximately 10 to 12 mEq/L; this is the normal anion gap. An elevated anion gap provides clues to the cause of the acidosis (i.e., to the addition of endogenously or exogenously generated acids). In a normal anion gap acidosis chloride is retained to replace lost bicarbonate.

H^+, Hydrogen ion.

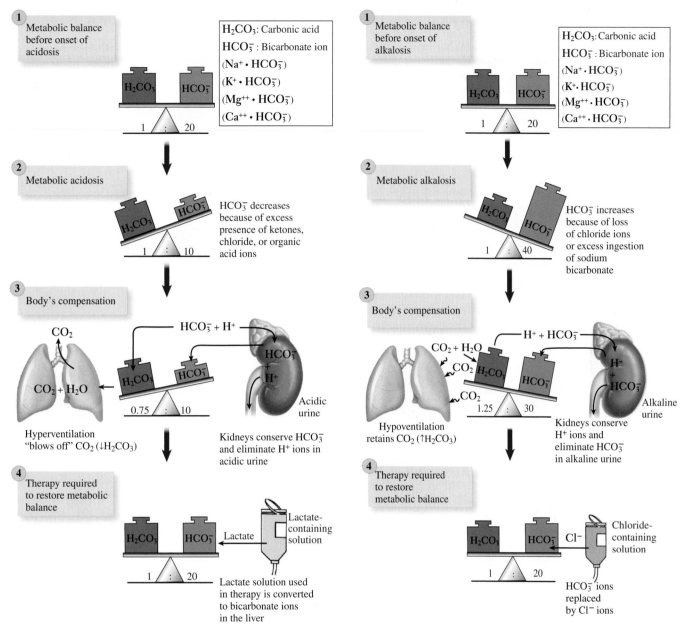

FIGURE 4-11 Metabolic Acidosis. (From Patton KT, Thibodeau GA: *Anatomy & physiology,* ed 7, St Louis, 2010, Mosby.)

FIGURE 4-12 Metabolic Alkalosis. (From Patton KT, Thibodeau GA: *Anatomy & physiology,* ed 7, St Louis, 2010, Mosby.)

Some common signs and symptoms of metabolic alkalosis are weakness, muscle cramps, hyperactive reflexes, tetany, confusion, convulsions, and atrial tachycardia. Respirations may be shallow and slow ventilation as the lungs attempt to compensate by increasing carbon dioxide retention. The manifestations vary with the cause and severity of the alkalosis. The symptoms of hyperactive reflexes and tetany occur because alkalosis increases binding of Ca^{++} to plasma proteins, thus decreasing ionized calcium concentration. The decreased ionized calcium concentration causes excitable cells to become hypopolarized, initiating an action potential more easily and causing muscle contraction.

Treatments are related to the underlying cause of the condition. With hypochloremic alkalosis or contraction alkalosis with volume depletion, a sodium chloride solution is required for correction because chloride must be replaced before bicarbonate can be excreted by the kidney.

Respiratory Acidosis

Respiratory acidosis occurs when there is alveolar hypoventilation, resulting in an excess of carbon dioxide in the blood (**hypercapnia**). The arterial carbon dioxide tension (or pressure) ($Paco_2$) is >45 mm Hg and the pH is less than normal. A decrease in alveolar ventilation in relation to the metabolic production of carbon dioxide produces respiratory acidosis by an increase in the concentration of carbonic acid.[24] Respiratory acidosis can be acute or chronic. Common causes include depression of the respiratory center (e.g., from drugs or head injury), paralysis of the respiratory muscles, disorders of the chest wall (e.g., kyphoscoliosis or broken ribs), and disorders of the lung parenchyma (e.g., pneumonia, pulmonary edema, emphysema, asthma, bronchitis). Renal compensation occurs by elimination of hydrogen ion and retention of bicarbonate (Figure 4-13).

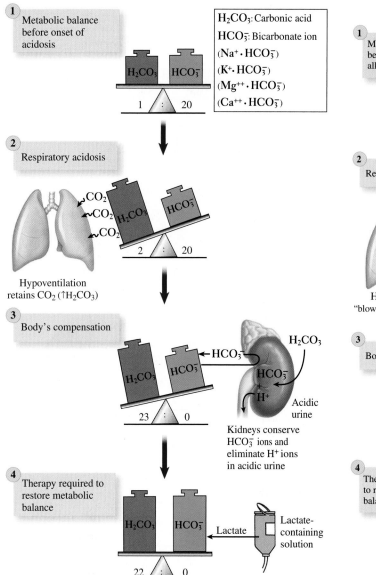

FIGURE 4-13 Respiratory Acidosis. (From Patton KT, Thibodeau GA: *Anatomy & physiology,* ed 7, St Louis, 2010, Mosby.)

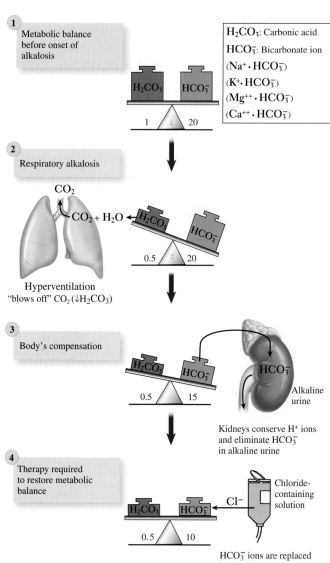

FIGURE 4-14 Respiratory Alkalosis. (From Patton KT, Thibodeau GA: *Anatomy & physiology,* ed 7, St Louis, 2010, Mosby.)

The signs and symptoms seen often include headache, blurred vision, breathlessness, restlessness, and apprehension followed by lethargy, disorientation, muscle twitching, tremors, convulsions, and coma. Respiratory rate is rapid at first and gradually becomes depressed as the respiratory center adapts to increasing levels of carbon dioxide. The skin may be warm and flushed because the elevated carbon dioxide concentration causes vasodilation. The restoration of adequate alveolar ventilation removes the excess CO_2 ($\downarrow H_2CO_3$).

Respiratory Alkalosis

Respiratory alkalosis occurs when there is alveolar hyperventilation (deep, rapid respirations). Excessive reduction in plasma carbon dioxide levels (hypocapnia) decrease carbonic acid concentration.[25,26] The $Paco_2$ is <35 mm Hg and the pH is greater than normal. Respiratory alkalosis can be chronic or acute. Hypoxemia (caused by pulmonary disease, congestive heart failure, or high altitudes), hypermetabolic states (e.g., fever, anemia, thyrotoxicosis), early salicylate intoxication, hysteria, cirrhosis, and gram-negative sepsis stimulate

hyperventilation. Improper use of mechanical ventilators also can cause iatrogenic (treatment-related) respiratory alkalosis, and secondary alkalosis may develop as a result of hyperventilation stimulated by metabolic or respiratory acidosis. The kidneys compensate by decreasing hydrogen excretion and bicarbonate reabsorption (Figure 4-14).

The central and peripheral nervous systems are stimulated by respiratory alkalosis, causing dizziness, confusion, tingling of extremities (paresthesias), convulsions, and coma. Cerebral vasoconstriction reduces cerebral blood flow. Carpopedal spasm (spasm of muscles in the fingers and toes), tetany, and other symptoms of hypocalcemia (see Table 4-7, p. 110) are similar to those of metabolic alkalosis. The underlying disturbance must be treated, particularly hypoxemia.

> ✓ **QUICK CHECK 4-5**
> 1. What two chemicals are altered in metabolic acid-base disturbances?
> 2. How do alterations in carbon dioxide concentration influence acid-base status?

DID YOU UNDERSTAND?

Distribution of Body Fluids

1. Body fluids are distributed among functional compartments and are classified as intracellular fluid (ICF) and extracellular fluid (ECF).
2. The sum of all fluids is the total body water (TBW), which varies with age and amount of body fat.
3. Water moves between the ICF and ECF compartments principally by osmosis.
4. Water moves between the plasma and interstitial fluid by osmosis (pulling of water) and hydrostatic pressure (pushing of water), which occur across the capillary membrane.
5. Movement across the capillary wall is called *net filtration* and is described according to Starling law (the balance between hydrostatic and osmotic forces).

Alterations in Water Movement

1. Edema is a problem of fluid distribution that results in accumulation of fluid within the interstitial spaces.
2. The pathophysiologic process that leads to edema is related to an increase in forces favoring fluid filtration from the capillaries or lymphatic channels into the tissues.
3. Edema is caused by arterial dilation, venous or lymphatic obstruction, increased vascular volume, or increased capillary permeability.
4. Edema may be localized or generalized and usually is associated with weight gain, swelling and puffiness, tighter-fitting clothes and shoes, and limited movement of the affected area.

Sodium, Chloride, and Water Balance

1. There is an intimate relationship between the balance of sodium and water levels; chloride levels are generally proportional to changes in sodium levels.
2. Water balance is regulated by the sensation of thirst and by antidiuretic hormone (ADH), which is secreted in response to an increase in plasma osmolality or a decrease in circulating blood volume.
3. Sodium balance is regulated by aldosterone, which increases reabsorption of sodium from the urine into the blood by the distal tubule of the kidney.
4. Renin and angiotensin are enzymes that promote secretion of aldosterone and thus regulate sodium and water balance.
5. Atrial natriuretic hormone is involved in decreasing tubular reabsorption and promoting urinary excretion of sodium.

Alterations in Sodium, Water, and Chloride Balance

1. Alterations in water balance may be classified as isotonic, hypertonic, or hypotonic.
2. Isotonic alterations occur when changes in TBW are accompanied by proportional changes in electrolytes.
3. Hypertonic alterations develop when the osmolality of the ECF is elevated above normal, usually because of an increased concentration of ECF sodium or a deficit of ECF water.
4. Hypernatremia (sodium levels more than 145 mEq/L) may be caused by an acute increase in sodium level or a loss of water.
5. Water deficit, or hypertonic dehydration, is rare but can be caused by lack of access to water, pure water losses, hyperventilation, arid climates, and increased renal elimination of water.
6. Hyperchloremia is caused by an excess of sodium or a deficit of bicarbonate.
7. Hypotonic alterations occur when the osmolality of the ECF is less than normal.
8. Hyponatremia (serum sodium concentration less than 135 mEq/L) usually causes movement of water into cells.
9. Hyponatremia may be caused by sodium loss, inadequate sodium intake, or dilution of the body's sodium level with excess water.
10. Water excess is rare but can be caused by compulsive water ingestion, decreased urine formation, or the syndrome of inappropriate secretion of ADH (SIADH).
11. Hypochloremia usually is the result of hyponatremia or elevated bicarbonate concentrations.

Alterations in Potassium and Other Electrolytes

1. Potassium is the predominant ICF ion; it regulates ICF osmolality, maintains the resting membrane potential, and is required for deposition of glycogen in liver and skeletal muscle cells.
2. Potassium balance is regulated by the kidney, by aldosterone and insulin secretion, and by changes in pH.
3. Potassium adaptation allows the body to accommodate slowly to increased levels of potassium intake.
4. Hypokalemia (serum potassium concentration less than 3.5 mEq/L) indicates loss of total body potassium, although ECF hypokalemia can develop without losses of total body potassium, and plasma potassium levels may be normal or elevated when total body potassium is depleted.
5. Hypokalemia may be caused by reduced potassium intake, a shift of potassium from the ECF to the ICF, increased aldosterone secretion, and increased renal excretion.
6. Hyperkalemia (potassium levels that are more than 5.5 mEq/L) may be caused by increased potassium intake, a shift of potassium from the ICF to the ECF, or decreased renal excretion.
7. Calcium is an ion necessary for bone and teeth formation, blood coagulation, hormone secretion and cell receptor function, and membrane stability.
8. Phosphate acts as a buffer in acid-base regulation and provides energy for muscle contraction.
9. Calcium and phosphate concentrations are rigidly controlled by parathyroid hormone (PTH), vitamin D, and calcitonin.
10. Hypocalcemia (serum calcium concentration less than 8.5 mg/dl) is related to inadequate intestinal absorption, deposition of calcium into bone or soft tissue, blood administration, or decreased PTH and vitamin D levels.
11. Hypercalcemia (serum calcium concentration more than 12 mg/dl) can be caused by a number of diseases, including hyperparathyroidism, bone metastases, sarcoidosis, and excess vitamin D.
12. Hypophosphatemia is usually caused by intestinal malabsorption and increased renal excretion of phosphate.
13. Hyperphosphatemia develops with acute or chronic renal failure when there is significant loss of glomerular filtration.
14. Magnesium is a major intracellular cation and is regulated principally by PTH.
15. Magnesium functions in enzymatic reactions and often interacts with calcium at the cellular level.
16. Hypomagnesemia (serum magnesium concentrations less than 1.5 mEq/L) may be caused by malabsorption syndromes.
17. Hypermagnesemia (serum magnesium concentrations more than 2.5 mEq/L) is rare and usually is caused by renal failure.

Acid-Base Balance

1. Hydrogen ions, which maintain membrane integrity and the speed of enzymatic reactions, must be concentrated within a narrow range if the body is to function normally.
2. Hydrogen ion concentration, $[H^+]$, is expressed as pH, which represents the negative logarithm (i.e., 10^{-7}) of hydrogen ions in solution (i.e., 0.0000001 mg/L).
3. Different body fluids have different pH values.
4. The renal and respiratory systems, together with the body's buffer systems, are the principal regulators of acid-base balance.

DID YOU UNDERSTAND?—cont'd

5. Buffers are substances that can absorb excessive acid or base without a significant change in pH.
6. Buffers exist as acid-base pairs; the principal plasma buffers are carbonic acid–bicarbonate, protein (hemoglobin), and phosphate.
7. The lungs and kidneys act to compensate for changes in pH by increasing or decreasing ventilation and by producing more acidic or more alkaline urine.
8. Correction is a process different from compensation; correction occurs when the values for both components of the buffer pair return to normal.
9. Acid-base imbalances are caused by changes in the concentration of hydrogen ion in the blood; an increase causes acidosis, and a decrease causes alkalosis.
10. An abnormal increase or decrease in bicarbonate concentration causes metabolic alkalosis or metabolic acidosis; changes in the rate of alveolar ventilation and removal of carbon dioxide produce respiratory acidosis or respiratory alkalosis.
11. Metabolic acidosis is caused by an increase in the levels of non–carbonic acids or by loss of bicarbonate from the extracellular fluid.
12. Metabolic alkalosis occurs with an increase in bicarbonate concentration, which is usually caused by loss of metabolic acids from conditions such as vomiting or gastrointestinal suctioning or by excessive bicarbonate intake, hyperaldosteronism, and diuretic therapy, which increase plasma bicarbonate concentration.
13. Respiratory acidosis occurs with decreased alveolar ventilation, which in turn causes hypercapnia (an increase in carbon dioxide concentration) and increased carbonic acid concentration.
14. Respiratory alkalosis occurs with alveolar hyperventilation and excessive reduction of carbon dioxide level, or hypocapnia with decreases in carbonic acid concentration.

KEY TERMS

- Acidemia 111
- Acidosis 111
- Aldosterone 102
- Alkalemia 111
- Alkalosis 111
- Angiotensin I 102
- Anion gap 112
- Aquaporin 100
- Baroreceptor 103
- Buffer 110
- Buffering 110
- Capillary hydrostatic pressure (blood pressure) 99
- Capillary (plasma) oncotic pressure 99
- Carbonic acid–bicarbonate buffer 111
- Chloride (Cl⁻) 102
- Compensation 111
- Correction 111
- Dehydration 105
- Dilutional hyponatremia 106
- Edema 100
- Extracellular fluid (ECF) 98
- Hypercapnia 113
- Hyperchloremia 105
- Hyperkalemia 108
- Hypernatremia 105
- Hypocapnia 114
- Hypochloremia 106
- Hypochloremic metabolic alkalosis 112
- Hypokalemia 107
- Hyponatremia 106
- Interstitial fluid 99
- Interstitial hydrostatic pressure 99
- Interstitial oncotic pressure 99
- Intracellular fluid (ICF) 98
- Intravascular fluid 98
- Isotonic fluid excess 104
- Isotonic fluid loss 104
- Lymphedema 100
- Metabolic acidosis 111
- Metabolic alkalosis 112
- Natriuretic peptide 102
- Net filtration 99
- Nonvolatile 110
- Osmoreceptor 103
- Potassium (K+) 106
- Potassium adaptation 107
- Pure water deficit 105
- Renin 102
- Renin-angiotensin-aldosterone system 102
- Respiratory acidosis 113
- Respiratory alkalosis 114
- Sodium (Na+) 102
- Starling forces 99
- Total body water (TBW) 98
- Volatile 110
- Volume-sensitive receptor 103
- Water intoxication 106

REFERENCES

1. Ishibashi K, et al: The evolutionary aspects of aquaporin family, *Am J Physiol Regal Integr Comp Physiol* 300(3):R566–R576, 2011.
2. O'Brien JC, Chennubhotla SA, Chennubhotla RV: Treatment of edema, *Am Fam Physician* 17(11):2111–2117, 2005.
3. Linnitt N: Lymphoedema: recognition, assessment and management, *Br J Community Nurs* 10(3):S20–S26, 2005.
4. Olszewski WL, Ambujam PJ, Zaleska M, et al: Where do lymph and tissue fluid accumulate in lymphedema of the lower limbs caused by obliteration of lymphatic collectors? *Lymphology* 42(3):105–111, 2009.
5. Lee CY, Burnett JC Jr: Natriuretic peptides and therapeutic applications, *Heart Fail Rev* 12(2):131–142, 2007.
6. Boone M, Deen PM: Physiology and pathophysiology of the vasopressin-regulated renal water reabsorption, *Pflugers Arch* 456(6):1005–1024, 2008.
7. Agrawal V, et al: Hyponatremia and hypernatremia: disorders of water balance, *J Assoc Physicians India* 56:956–964, 2008.
8. Bagshaw SM, Townsend DR, McDermid RC: Disorders of sodium and water balance in hospitalized patients, *Can J Anaesth* 56(2):151–167, 2009.
9. Thomas DR, et al: Dehydration council: understanding clinical dehydration and its treatment, *J Am Med Dir Assoc* 9(5):292–301, 2008.
10. Overgaard-Steensen C: Initial approach to the hyponatremic patient, *Acta Anesthesiol Scand* 55(2):139–148, 2011.
11. Vaidya C, Ho W, Freda B: Management of hyponatremia: providing treatment and avoiding harm, *Cleve Clin J Med* 77(10):715–726, 2010.
12. Multz AS: Vasopressin dysregulation and hyponatremia in hospitalized patients, *J Intensive Care Med* 22(4):216–223, 2007.
13. Vaidya C, Ho EW, Freda BJ: Management of hyponatremia: providing treatment and avoiding harm, *Cleve Clin J Med* 77(10):715–726, 2010.
14. Youn JH, McDonough AA: Recent advances in understanding integrative control of potassium homeostasis, *Annu Rev Physiol* 71:381–401, 2009.
15. Wang WH, Giebisch G: Regulation of potassium (K) handling in the renal collecting duct, *Pflugers Arch* 458(1):157–168, 2009.
16. Palmer BF: A physiologic-based approach to the evaluation of a patient with hypokalemia, *Am J Kidney Dis* 56(6):1184–1190, 2010.
17. Lim S: Approach to hyperkalemia, *Acta Med Indones* 39(2):99–103, 2007.
18. Weisberg LS: Management of severe hyperkalemia, *Crit Care Med* 36(12):L3246–L3251, 2008.

19. Moe SM: Disorders involving calcium, phosphorus and magnesium, *Prim Care* 35(2):215–237, 2008.
20. Palmer BF: Approach to fluid and electrolyte disorders and acid-base problems, *Prim Care* 35(2):195–213, 2008.
21. Edwards SL: Pathophysiology of acid base balance: the theory practice relationship, *Intensive Crit Care Nurs* 24(1):28–38, 2008.
22. Kraut JA, Madias NE: Metabolic acidosis: pathophysiology, diagnosis and management, *Nat Rev Nephrol* 6(5):274–285, 2010.
23. Khanna A, Kurtzman NA: Metabolic alkalosis, *J Nephrol* 19(Suppl 9):S86–S96, 2006.
24. Epstein SK, Singh N: Respiratory acidosis, *Respir Care* 46(4):366–383, 2001.
25. Foster GT, Vaziri ND, Sassoon CS: Respiratory alkalosis, *Respir Care* 46(4):384–391, 2001.
26. Madias NE: Renal acidification responses to respiratory acid base disorders, *J Nephrol* 16(Suppl 16):S85–S91, 2010.

Innate Immunity: Inflammation and Wound Healing

Neal S. Rote

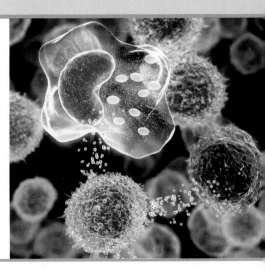

ⓔvolve WEBSITE

CHAPTER OUTLINE

The human body is continually exposed to a large variety of conditions that result in damage, such as sunlight, pollutants, agents that can cause physical trauma, and infectious agents (viruses, bacteria, fungi, parasites). Damage can also arise from within, such as cancers. The damage may be at the level of a single cell, which can be easily repaired, or may be at the level of multiple cells or tissues or organs, which can result in disease and potentially the death of the individual. To protect us from these conditions, the body has developed a highly sophisticated, multilevel system of interactive defense mechanisms.

HUMAN DEFENSE MECHANISMS

The human body has developed several means of protecting itself from injury and infection. Innate immunity, also known as natural or native immunity, includes natural barriers (physical, mechanical, and biochemical) and inflammation. Innate barriers form the first line of defense at the body's surfaces and are in place at birth to prevent damage by substances in the environment and thwart infection by pathogenic microorganisms.[1] Surface barriers may also harbor a group of microorganisms known as the "normal flora" that can protect us from pathogens. If the surface barriers are breached, the second line of defense, the inflammatory response,[2] is activated to protect the body from further injury, prevent infection of the injured tissue, and promote healing. The inflammatory response is a rapid activation of biochemical and cellular mechanisms that are relatively nonspecific, with similar responses being initiated against a wide variety of causes of tissue damage. The third line of defense, adaptive immunity (also known as acquired or specific immunity), is induced in a relatively slower and more specific process and targets particular invading microorganisms for the purpose of eradicating them. Adaptive immunity also involves "memory," which results in a more rapid response during future exposure to the same microorganism (Table 5-1). The focus of this chapter is innate immunity: barriers, the inflammatory response, and wound healing. Adaptive immunity is the focus of Chapter 6.

TABLE 5-1   OVERVIEW OF HUMAN DEFENSES

CHARACTERISTICS	BARRIERS	INNATE IMMUNITY	ADAPTIVE (ACQUIRED) IMMUNITY
Level of defense	First line of defense against infection and tissue injury	Second line of defense; occurs as response to tissue injury or infection	Third line of defense; initiated when innate immune system signals cells of adaptive immunity
Timing of defense	Constant	Immediate response	Delay between primary exposure to antigen and maximal response; immediate against secondary exposure to antigen
Specificity	Broadly specific	Broadly specific	Response is very specific toward "antigen"
Cells	Epithelial cells	Mast cells, granulocytes (neutrophils, eosinophils, basophils), monocytes/macrophages, natural killer (NK) cells, platelets, endothelial cells	T lymphocytes, B lymphocytes, macrophages, dendritic cells
Memory	No memory involved	No memory involved	Specific immunologic memory by T and B lymphocytes
Active molecules	Defensins, cathelicidins, collectins, lactoferrin, bacterial toxins	Complement, clotting factors, kinins, cytokines	Antibodies, complement, cytokines
Protection	Protection includes anatomic barriers (i.e., skin and mucous membranes), cells and secretory molecules (e.g., lysozymes, low pH of stomach and urine), and ciliary activity	Protection includes vascular responses, cellular components (e.g., mast cells, neutrophils, macrophages), secretory molecules or cytokines, and activation of plasma protein systems	Protection includes activated T and B lymphocytes, cytokines, and antibodies

INNATE IMMUNITY

First Line of Defense: Physical and Biochemical Barriers and Normal Flora

Physical Barriers

The physical barriers that cover the external parts of the human body offer considerable protection from damage and infection. These barriers are composed of tightly associated epithelial cells of the skin and of the linings of the gastrointestinal, genitourinary, and respiratory tracts (Figure 5-1). When pathogens attempt to penetrate this physical barrier, they may be removed by mechanical means—sloughed off with dead skin cells as they are routinely replaced, expelled by coughing or sneezing, vomited from the stomach, or flushed from the urinary tract by urine. Epithelial cells of the upper respiratory tract also produce mucus and have hair-like cilia that trap and move pathogens upward to be expelled by coughing or sneezing. Additionally, the low temperature, such as on the skin, and low pH, such as of the skin and stomach, generally inhibit microorganisms, most of which routinely require temperatures near 37° C (98.6° F) and pH near neutral for efficient growth.

Epithelial Cell–Derived Chemicals

Epithelial cells secrete several substances that protect against infection, including mucus, perspiration (or sweat), saliva, tears, and earwax. These can trap potential invaders and contain substances that will kill microorganisms. Perspiration, tears, and saliva contain an enzyme (lysozyme) that attacks the cell walls of gram-positive bacteria. Sebaceous glands in the skin also secrete fatty acids and lactic acid that kill bacteria and fungi. These glandular secretions create an acidic (pH 3 to 5) and inhospitable environment for most bacteria.

Epithelial cell secretions also contain small-molecular-weight antimicrobial peptides that kill or inhibit the growth of certain disease-causing bacteria, fungi, and viruses.[3] These are generally positively charged polypeptides of approximately 15 to 95 amino acids. More than a thousand antimicrobial peptides have been found, but the best studied are cathelicidins and defensins, which are differentiated based on their three-dimensional chemical structures.

Several cathelicidins have been discovered in other species, but only one is currently known to function in humans. Bacteria have cholesterol-free cell membranes into which cathelicidin can insert and disrupt the membrane, killing the bacteria. Cathelicidin is produced by epithelial cells of the skin, gut, urinary tract, and respiratory tract, and is stored in neutrophils, mast cells, and monocytes and can be released during inflammation.

In contrast, many different human defensins have been identified thus far. Defensin molecules can be further subdivided into α (at least 6 identified in humans) and β types (at least 6 identified, but perhaps up to 40 different molecules). The α-defensins often require activation by proteolytic enzymes, whereas the β-defensins are synthesized in active forms. Given the similarity in their chemical charges, defensins may kill bacteria in the same way as cathelicidin. The α-defensins are particularly rich in the granules of neutrophils and may contribute to the killing of bacteria by those cells. They are also found in Paneth cells lining the small intestine, where they protect against a variety of disease-causing microorganisms. The β-defensins are found in a variety of epithelial cells lining the respiratory, urinary, and intestinal tracts, as well as in the skin.[4] In addition to antibacterial properties, β-defensins may also help protect epithelial surfaces from infection with adenovirus (one of the causes of the common cold) and human immunodeficiency virus (HIV). Both classes of antimicrobial peptides also can activate cells of the next levels of defense: innate and acquired immunity.

The lung also produces and secretes a family of glycoproteins, collectins, which includes surfactant proteins A through D and mannose-binding lectin. Collectins react with carbohydrates on the surface of a wide array of pathogenic microorganisms and help cells of the innate immune system (macrophages) to recognize and kill the microorganism. Mannose-binding lectin (MBL) is a powerful activator of a plasma protein system (complement) resulting in damage to bacteria or increased recognition by macrophages.

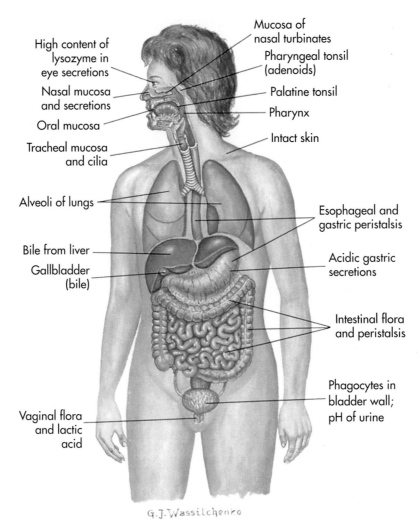

High content of lysozyme in eye secretions

Nasal mucosa and secretions

Oral mucosa

Tracheal mucosa and cilia

Alveoli of lungs

Bile from liver

Gallbladder (bile)

Vaginal flora and lactic acid

Mucosa of nasal turbinates

Pharyngeal tonsil (adenoids)

Palatine tonsil

Pharynx

Intact skin

Esophageal and gastric peristalsis

Acidic gastric secretions

Intestinal flora and peristalsis

Phagocytes in bladder wall; pH of urine

G.J.Wassilchenko

FIGURE 5-1 The Closed Barrier. The digestive, respiratory, and genitourinary tracts and skin form closed barriers between the internal organs and the environment. (From Grimes DE: *Infectious diseases,* St Louis, 1991, Mosby.)

Normal Flora

A spectrum of nonpathogenic microorganisms, collectively called the normal flora, resides on the body's surfaces. Each surface is colonized by a combination of mostly bacteria and occasionally fungi that is unique to the particular location, including the skin and the mucous membranes of the eyes, upper and lower gastrointestinal tracts, urethra, and vagina. Although frequently referred to as *commensal* (to the benefit of one organism without affecting the other) organisms, the relationship with humans may be more *mutualistic* (to the benefit of both organisms).[5]

Using the colon for an example, at birth the lower gut is relatively sterile, but colonization with bacteria begins quickly, with the number, diversity, and concentration increasing progressively during the first year of life. The environment of the intestine provides the needed temperature and nutrients for the growth of many bacterial species. To the benefit of humans, many of these microorganisms help digest fatty acids, large polysaccharides, and other dietary substances; produce biotin and vitamin K; and assist in the absorption of various ions, such as calcium, iron, and magnesium.

These bacteria contribute to our innate protection against pathogenic microorganisms in the colon.[6] They compete with pathogens for nutrients and block attachment to the epithelium. Members of the normal flora also produce chemicals (ammonia, phenols, indoles,

and other toxic materials) and toxic proteins *(bacteriocins)* that inhibit colonization by pathogenic microorganisms. Prolonged treatment with broad-spectrum antibiotics can alter the normal intestinal flora, decreasing its protective activity, and lead to an overgrowth of pathogenic microorganisms, such as the yeast *Candida albicans* or the bacteria *Clostridium difficile* (overgrowth can cause pseudomembranous colitis, an infection of the colon). Additionally, the normal flora of the gut help train the adaptive immune system by inducing growth of gut-associated lymphoid tissue (where cells of the adaptive immune system reside) and the development of both local and systemic adaptive immune systems.[7]

The bacterium *Lactobacillus* is a major constituent of the normal vaginal flora in healthy women. This microorganism produces chemicals (hydrogen peroxide, lactic acid, and other molecules) that help prevent infections of the vagina and urinary tract by other bacteria and yeast. Diminished colonization with lactobacilli (e.g., as a result of prolonged antibiotic treatment) increases the risk for urologic or vaginal infections, such as vaginosis.

It should be noted that some members of the normal bacterial flora are opportunistic; opportunistic microorganisms can cause disease if the individual's defenses are compromised. These organisms are normally controlled by the innate and acquired immune systems and contribute to our defenses. For example, *Pseudomonas aeruginosa* is a member of the normal flora of the skin and produces a toxin that protects against infections with staphylococcal and other bacteria. However, severe burns compromise the integrity of the skin and may lead to life-threatening systemic pseudomonal infections.

QUICK CHECK 5-1

1. How do physical and mechanical barriers contribute to defense mechanisms?
2. What are antimicrobial peptides?
3. What two types of defensins contribute to the biochemical barrier?
4. What is the normal bacterial flora? What is its role in defense?
5. What are opportunistic microorganisms?

Second Line of Defense: Inflammation

The innate immune system is programmed to respond to damage to the body, whether the damaged tissue is septic or sterile.[8] That response rapidly initiates an interactive system of humoral (soluble in the blood) and cellular systems, called inflammation.

Inflammation is the first response to injury. The inflammatory response (1) occurs in tissues with a blood supply (vascularized); (2) is activated *rapidly* (within seconds) after damage occurs; (3) depends on the activity of both *cellular and chemical components;* and (4) is *nonspecific,* meaning that it takes place in approximately the same way regardless of the type of stimulus or whether exposure to the same stimulus has occurred in the past.

Virtually any injury to vascularized tissues will activate inflammation. The classic symptoms of acute inflammation include redness (erythema), heat, swelling, pain, and loss of function. Microscopic inflammatory changes occur within seconds in the microcirculation (arterioles, capillaries, and venules) near the site of an injury and include the following processes (Figure 5-2):

1. Vasodilation (increased size of the blood vessels), which causes slower blood velocity and increases blood flow to the injured site
2. Increased vascular permeability (the blood vessels become porous from contraction of endothelial cells) and leakage of fluid out of the vessel (exudation), causing swelling (edema) at the site of injury; as plasma moves outward, blood in the microcirculation becomes more viscous and flows more slowly, and the increased blood flow and increasing concentration of red cells at the site of inflammation cause locally increased redness (erythema) and warmth
3. White blood cell adherence to the inner walls of vessels and their migration through enlarged junctions between the endothelial cells lining the vessels into the surrounding tissue

Each of the characteristic changes associated with inflammation is the direct result of the activation and interactions of a host of chemicals and cellular components found in the blood and tissues. The vascular changes deliver leukocytes (particularly neutrophils), plasma proteins, and other biochemical mediators to the site of injury, where they act in concert. Some of these chemical mediators activate pain fibers. The tissue injury, pain, and swelling contribute to loss of function. Figure 5-3 summarizes the process of inflammation.

There are several benefits of inflammation, including the following:

1. Prevents infection and further damage by contaminating microorganisms through the influx of plasma to dilute toxins produced by bacteria and released from dying cells, the influx and activation of plasma protein systems that help contain and destroy bacteria

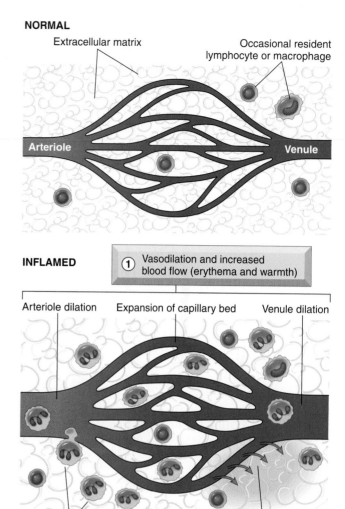

NORMAL

Extracellular matrix

Occasional resident lymphocyte or macrophage

Arteriole

Venule

INFLAMED

① Vasodilation and increased blood flow (erythema and warmth)

Arteriole dilation   Expansion of capillary bed   Venule dilation

③ Leukocyte (neutrophil) recruitment and migration

② Leakage of plasma proteins → edema

FIGURE 5-2 The Major Local Changes in the Process of Inflammation. Compared to the normal circulation, inflammation is characterized by *(1)* dilation of the blood vessels and increased blood flow, leading to erythema and warmth; *(2)* increased vascular permeability with leakage of plasma from the vessels, leading to edema; and *(3)* movement of leukocytes from the vessels into the site of injury. (From Kumar V et al: *Robbins and Cotran pathological basis of disease,* ed 8, Philadelphia, 2009, Saunders.)

(e.g., complement system, clotting system), and the influx of cells (e.g., neutrophils, macrophages) that destroy cellular debris and infectious agents
2. Limits and control the inflammatory process through the influx of plasma protein systems (e.g., clotting system), plasma enzymes, and cells (e.g., eosinophils) that prevent the inflammatory response from spreading to areas of healthy tissue
3. Interacts with components of the adaptive immune system to elicit a more specific response to contaminating pathogen(s) through the influx of macrophages and lymphocytes
4. Prepares the area of injury for healing through removal of bacterial products, dead cells, and other products of inflammation (e.g., by way of channels through the epithelium or drainage by lymphatic vessels) and initiation of mechanisms of healing and repair

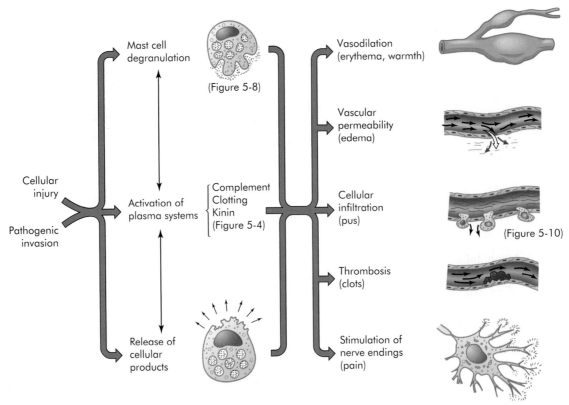

FIGURE 5-3 Acute Inflammatory Response. Inflammation is usually initiated by cellular injury and may be complicated by infection. Mast cell degranulation, the activation of three plasma systems, and the release of subcellular components from the damaged cells occur as a consequence. These systems are interdependent, so that induction of one (e.g., mast cell degranulation) can result in the induction of the other two. The result is the development of the characteristic microscopic and clinical hallmarks of inflammation. The figure numbers refer to additional figures in which more detailed information may be found on that portion of the response.

Fluid and debris that accumulate at an inflamed site are drained by lymphatic vessels. This process also facilitates the development of acquired immunity because microbial antigens in lymphatic fluid pass through the lymph nodes, where they encounter lymphocytes.

> ✔ **QUICK CHECK 5-2**
> 1. Why is innate immunity and inflammation described as "non-specific"?
> 2. How are the five classic superficial symptoms of inflammation related to the process of inflammation?
> 3. Describe the basic steps in acute inflammation.
> 4. What are the benefits of inflammation?

Plasma Protein Systems and Inflammation

Three key plasma protein systems are essential to an effective inflammatory response (Figure 5-4). These are the complement system, the clotting system, and the kinin system. Although each system has a unique role in inflammation, they have many similarities. Each system consists of multiple proteins in the blood. They are normally in inactive forms; several are enzymes that circulate in inactive forms as proenzymes. Each system contains a few proteins that can be activated during inflammation. Activation of these first components results in

sequential activation of other components of the system, leading to a biologic function that helps protect the individual. This sequential activation is referred to as a *cascade*. Thus, we occasionally refer to the complement cascade, the clotting cascade, or the kinin cascade. In some cases, activation of a particular protein in the system may require that it be enzymatically cut into two pieces of different size. Usually the larger fragment continues the cascade by activating the next component, and the smaller fragment frequently has potent biologic activities to promote inflammation.

Complement System

The complement system consists of a large number of proteins (sometimes called complement factors) that together constitute about 10% of the total circulating serum protein. The complement system is extremely important because activation produces factors that can destroy pathogens directly or can activate or increase the activity of many other components of the inflammatory and adaptive immune response.[9] Factors produced during activation of the complement system are among the body's most potent defenders against bacterial infection.

The most important function of the complement cascade is activation of C3 and C5, which results in a variety of molecules that are (1) opsonins, (2) chemotactic factors, or (3) anaphylatoxins.

Opsonins coat the surface of bacteria and increase their susceptibility to being phagocytized (eaten) and killed by inflammatory cells, such as neutrophils and macrophages. **Chemotactic factors** diffuse from a site of inflammation and attract phagocytic cells to that site. **Anaphylatoxins** induce rapid degranulation of mast cells (i.e., release of histamine that induces vasodilation and increased capillary permeability), a major cellular component of inflammation. The most potent complement products are C3b (opsonin), C3a (anaphylatoxin), and

C5a (anaphylatoxin, chemotactic factor).[10] Activation of complement components C5b through C9 (membrane attack complex, or MAC) results in a complex that creates pores in the outer membranes of cells or bacteria. The pores disrupt the cell's membrane and permit water to enter, causing the cell to burst and die or at least prevent its reproduction.

Three major pathways control the activation of complement (see Figure 5-4). The **classical pathway** is primarily activated by antibodies,

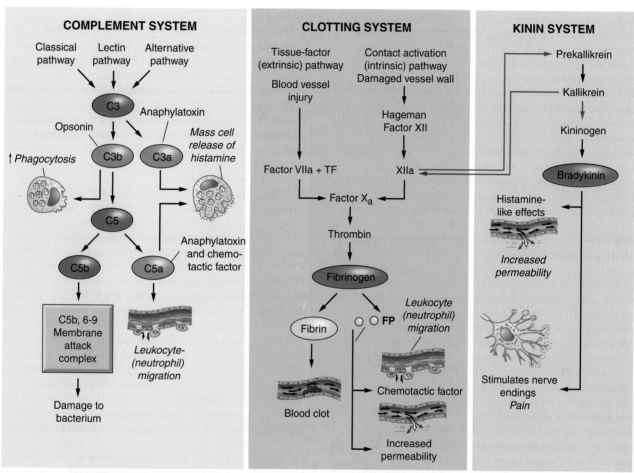

FIGURE 5-4 Plasma Protein Systems in Inflammation: Complement, Clotting, and Kinin Systems. Each plasma protein system consists of a family of proteins that are activated in sequence to create potent biologic effects. The **complement system** can be activated by three mechanisms, each of which results in proteolytic activation of C3. The fragments of C3 activation, C3a and C3b, are major components of inflammation. C3a is a potent anaphylatoxin, which induces degranulation of mast cells. C3b can bind to the surface or cells, such as bacteria, and either serve as an opsonin for phagocytosis or proteolytically activate the next component of the complement cascade, C5. The smaller fragment of C5 activation is C5a, a powerful anaphylatoxin, and is also chemotactic for neutrophils, attracting them to the site of inflammation. The larger fragment, C5b, activates the components of the membrane attack complex (C5-C9), which damage the bacterial membrane and kill the bacteria. The **clotting system** can be activated by the tissue factor (extrinsic) pathway and the contact activation (intrinsic) pathway. All routes of clotting initiation lead to activation of factor X and thrombin. Thrombin is an enzyme that proteolytically activates fibrinogen to form fibrin and small fibrinopeptides (FPs). Fibrin polymerizes to form a clot, and the FPs are highly active as chemotactic factors and causing increased vascular permeability. The XIIa produced by the clotting system can also be activated by kallikrein of the **kinin system** (red arrow). Prekallikrein is enzymatically converted to kininogen, which activates bradykinin. Bradykinin functions similar to histamine and increases vascular permeability. Bradykinin can also stimulate nerve endings to cause pain. *TF,* tissue factor; *FPs,* Fibrinopeptides.

which are proteins of the acquired immune system. Antibodies must first bind to their targets, called antigens (molecules that stimulate the production of antibodies). Antigens can be proteins or carbohydrates from bacteria or other infectious agents. Antibodies activate the first component of complement, C1, which leads to activation of other complement components, leading to activation of C3 and C5. Thus, antibodies of the acquired immune response can use the complement system to kill bacteria and activate inflammation.

The **alternative pathway** is activated by several substances found on the surface of infectious organisms (e.g., lipopolysaccharides [endotoxin] on the bacterial surface or yeast cell wall carbohydrates [zymosan]). This pathway uses unique proteins (factor B, factor D, and properdin) to form a complex that activates C3. C3 activation leads to C5 activation and convergence with the classical pathway. Thus, the complement system can be directly activated by certain infectious organisms without antibody being present.

The **lectin pathway** is similar to the classical pathway but is independent of antibody. It is activated by several plasma proteins, particularly mannose-binding lectin (MBL). MBL is similar to C1 and binds to bacterial polysaccharides containing the carbohydrate mannose. Thus, infectious agents that do not activate the alternative pathway may be susceptible to complement through the lectin pathway.

In summary, the complement cascade can be activated by at least three different means, and its products have four functions: (1) opsonization, (2) anaphylatoxic activity resulting in mast cell degranulation, (3) leukocyte chemotaxis, and (4) cell lysis.

Clotting System

The **clotting (coagulation) system** is a group of plasma proteins that, when activated sequentially, form a blood clot. A **blood clot** is a meshwork of protein (fibrin) strands that stabilizes the platelet plug and traps other cells, such as erythrocytes, phagocytes, and microorganisms.[11] Clots (1) plug damaged vessels and stop bleeding, (2) trap microorganisms and prevent their spread to adjacent tissues, and (3) provide a framework for future repair and healing. Specific details and illustrations of the clotting system are presented in Chapter 19 and only the relationship between clotting and inflammation is presented here.

The clotting system can be activated by many substances that are released during tissue injury and infection, including collagen, proteinases, kallikrein, and plasmin, as well as by bacterial products such as endotoxins. Like the complement cascade, the coagulation cascade can be activated through different pathways that converge and result in the formation of a clot (see Figure 5-4). These pathways are the tissue factor (extrinsic) pathway and the contact activation (intrinsic) pathway. The **tissue factor (extrinsic) pathway** is activated when there is tissue injury and membrane-bound or soluble **tissue factor (TF)** (also called **tissue thromboplastin**), a substance released by damaged endothelial cells in blood vessels, reacts with activated factor VII (VIIa). The **contact activation (intrinsic) pathway** is activated when there is an abnormal vessel wall and Hageman factor (factor XII) in plasma contacts negatively charged subendothelial substances. Kallikrein and kininogen can also activate factor XII. The clotting pathways converge at factor X. Activation of factor X begins a common pathway leading to activation of fibrin that polymerizes to form a fibrin clot.

As with the complement cascade, activation of the clotting cascade produces fragments known as fibrinopeptides (FPs) A and B that enhance the inflammatory response.[12] Fibrinopeptides are released from fibrinogen when fibrin is produced. Both fibrinopeptides (especially fibrinopeptide B) are chemotactic for neutrophils and increase vascular permeability by enhancing the effects of bradykinin (formed from the kinin system).

Kinin System

The third plasma protein system, the **kinin system** (see Figure 5-4), interacts closely with the coagulation system. Both the clotting and kinin systems can be initiated through activation of **Hageman factor (factor XII)** to factor XIIa.[13] Another name for factor XIIa is *prekallikrein* activator because it enzymatically activates the first component of the kinin system, prekallikrein. The final product of the kinin system is a small-molecular-weight molecule, **bradykinin,** which is produced from a larger precursor molecule, kininogen. Bradykinin causes dilation of blood vessels, acts with prostaglandins to induce pain, causes smooth muscle cell contraction, and increases vascular permeability.

Control and Interaction of Plasma Protein Systems

The three plasma protein systems are highly interactive so that activation of one results in production of a large number of very potent, biologically active substances that further activate the other systems. Very tight regulation of these processes is essential for the following two reasons.

1. The inflammatory process is critical for an individual's survival; thus efficient activation must be guaranteed regardless of the cause of tissue injury. Interaction among the plasma systems results in activation of the entire inflammatory response regardless of which system is activated initially.

2. The biochemical mediators generated during these processes are so potent and potentially detrimental to the individual that their actions must be strictly confined to injured or infected tissues.

Therefore, multiple mechanisms are available to either activate or inactivate (regulate) these plasma protein systems. For instance, the plasma that enters the tissues during inflammation (edema) contains enzymes that destroy mediators of inflammation. **Carboxypeptidase** inactivates the anaphylatoxic activities of C3a and C5a, and kininases that degrade kinins. **Histaminase** degrades histamine and kallikrein and down-regulates the inflammatory response.

The formation of clots also activates a **fibrinolytic system** that is designed to limit the size of the clot and remove the clot after bleeding has ceased. Thrombin of the clotting system activates **plasminogen** in the blood to form the enzyme plasmin. The primary activity of **plasmin** is to degrade fibrin polymers in clots. However, plasmin can also activate the complement cascade through components C1, C3, and C5 and the kinin cascade by activating factor XII and producing prekallikrein activator.

Another example of a common regulator is **C1 esterase inhibitor (C1 inh)**.[14] C1 inh inhibits complement activation through C1 (classical pathway), MASP-2 (lectin pathway), and C3b (alternative pathway). It is also a major inhibitor of the clotting and kinin pathway components (e.g., kallikrein, factor XIIa). A genetic defect in C1 inh (**C1 inh deficiency**) results in **hereditary angioedema**, which is a self-limiting edema of cutaneous and mucosal layers resulting from stress, illness, or relative minor or unapparent trauma. The disease is characterized by hyperactivation of all three plasma protein systems, although excessive production of bradykinin appears to be the principal cause of increased vascular permeability.

> ✔ **QUICK CHECK 5-3**
> 1. What are the three most important products of the complement system?
> 2. How is the coagulation cascade activated? How is it related to the plasma kinin cascade?
> 3. What factors control the plasma protein systems of inflammation?

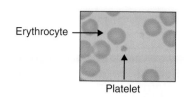

Erythrocyte

Platelet

LEUKOCYTES

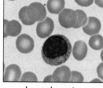

Lymphocyte

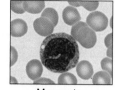

Monocyte

Granulocytes

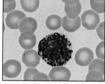

Basophil

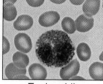

Eosinophil

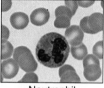

Neutrophil

FIGURE 5-5 Cellular Components of the Blood. Cells in the blood can be classified as red blood cells (erythrocytes), cellular fragments (platelets), or white blood cells (leukocytes). Leukocytes consist of lymphocytes, monocytes, and granulocytes (neutrophils, eosinophils, basophils). (Erythrocyte plate from Goldman L, Ausiello DA, editors: *Cecil medicine*, ed 23, Philadelphia, 2007, Saunders; rest of plates from McPherson RA, Pincus MR, editors: *Henry's clinical diagnosis and management by laboratory methods*, ed 21, Philadelphia, 2006, Saunders.)

Cellular Components of Inflammation

Inflammation is a process in vascular tissue; thus the cellular components of the response can be found in the blood or in tissue surrounding the blood vessels. The blood vessels are lined with endothelial cells, which under normal conditions actively maintain normal blood flow. During inflammation, however, the vascular endothelium becomes a principal coordinator of blood clotting and the passage of cells and fluid into the tissue. The tissues close to the vessels contain mast cells, which are probably the most important activators of inflammation. The tissue also contains dendritic cells, which connect the innate and acquired immune responses. The most complex mixture of cells is found in the blood (Figure 5-5). Blood cells are divided into erythrocytes (red blood cells), platelets, and leukocytes (white blood cells). Leukocytes are subdivided into granulocytes, monocytes, and lymphocytes. Granulocytes are the most common leukocytes and are classified by the type of stains needed to visualize enzyme-containing granules in their cytoplasm: basophils, eosinophils, and neutrophils. Monocytes are precursors of macrophages that are found in the tissue. Various forms of lymphocytes participate in the innate immune response (natural killer [NK] cells) and the acquired immune response (B and T cells).

Cells of both innate and acquired immune systems respond to molecules produced at a site of cellular damage and are recruited to that site to augment the protective response.[8] The molecules originate from destroyed or damaged cells, contaminating microbes, activation of the plasma protein systems, or secretions by other cells of the innate or acquired immune systems. Each cell has a set of cell-surface receptors that specifically bind these molecules, resulting in activation of intracellular signaling pathways and activation of the cell itself. Activation may result in the cell gaining a function critical to the inflammatory response or induction of the release of additional cellular products that increase inflammation, or both. Most of these inflammatory cells and protein systems, along with the substances they produce, act at the site of tissue injury to confine the extent of damage, kill microorganisms, and remove the cellular debris in preparation for healing: tissue regeneration (a process known as resolution) or repair.

Cellular Receptors

As will be discussed in Chapter 6, B and T lymphocytes of the acquired immune system have evolved surface receptors (i.e., the T-cell receptor, or TCR, and the B-cell receptor, or BCR) that bind a large spectrum of antigens. Cells involved in innate resistance have evolved a different set of receptors that recognize a much more limited array of specific molecules. These are referred to as **pattern recognition receptors (PRRs)**.[15] PRRs recognize two types of molecular *patterns*: molecules that are expressed by infectious agents, either found on their surface or released as soluble molecules (**pathogen-associated molecular patterns, or PAMPs**); or products of cellular damage (**damage-associated molecular patterns, or DAMPs**). Thus cells of the innate immune system can respond to both sterile (through DAMPs) or septic (through PAMPs and DAMPs) tissue damage.

PRRs are generally expressed on cells in tissues at the body's surface (i.e., skin, respiratory tract, gastrointestinal tract, genitourinary tract) where they monitor the environment for products of cellular damage and potentially infectious microorganisms. Classes of cellular PRRs primarily differ in the specificity of ligands they bind: toll-like receptors (microbial substances), complement receptors (components of the complement system), scavenger receptors (changes on the surface of the damaged cell), and glucan and mannose receptors (carbohydrates expressed on the surface of some microorganisms). Although most PRRs are on the cell surface, some are in the cytoplasm or secreted.[16] An example of a secreted PRR is mannose-binding lectin of the lectin pathway of complement activation.

A major class of cell-surface PRRs is **Toll-like receptors (TLRs)**, which primarily recognize a large variety of PAMPs located on the microorganism's cell wall or surface (e.g., bacterial lipopolysaccharide [LPS], peptidoglycans, lipoproteins, yeast zymosan, viral coat proteins), other surface structures (e.g., bacterial flagellin), or microbial nucleic acid (e.g., bacterial DNA, viral double-stranded RNA). Ten different TLRs have been described in humans. They are expressed on the surface of many cells that have direct and early contact with potential pathogenic microorganisms, including mucosal epithelial cells, mast cells, neutrophils, macrophages, dendritic cells, and some subpopulations of lymphocytes.

In addition to PRRs, other receptors recognize molecules produced by activation of plasma protein systems. For instance, **complement receptors** are found on many cells of the innate and acquired immune responses (e.g., granulocytes, monocytes/macrophages, lymphocytes, mast cells, erythrocytes, platelets), as well as some epithelial cells. They recognize several fragments produced through activation of the complement system, particularly C3a, C5a, and C3b.

Cellular Products

Many different kinds of cells must cooperate during effective protective responses, both innate and acquired. That cooperation is achieved by the secretion of a variety of molecules (primarily proteins, but also some lipids) that affect other cells (Figure 5-6). These factors are referred to as **cytokines**.[8] Cytokines can be either

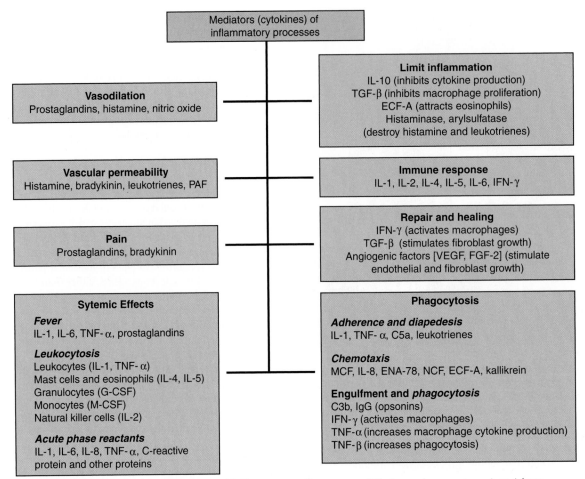

FIGURE 5-6 Principal Mediators of Inflammatory Processes. *C3b,* Large fragment produced from complement component C3; *C5a,* small fragment produced from complement component C5; *ECF-A,* eosinophil chemotactic factor of anaphylaxis; *FGF,* fibroblast growth factor; *IFN,* interferon; *IgG,* immunoglobulin G (predominant class of antibody in the blood); *IL,* interleukin; *MCF,* monocyte chemotactic factor; *NCF,* neutrophil chemotactic factor; *PAF,* platelet-activating factor; *TGF,* T-cell growth factor; *TNF,* tumor necrosis factor; *VEGF,* vascular endothelial growth factor.

proinflammatory or anti-inflammatory in nature, depending on whether they tend to induce or inhibit the inflammatory response. Cytokines usually diffuse over short distances, bind to the appropriate target cells, and affect the function of the target cell. Some effects occur over long distances, such as the induction of fever by some cytokines (i.e., endogenous pyrogens) that are produced at an inflammatory site. Cytokines affect other cells through specific cell-surface receptors and activation of intracellular signaling pathways. The affected cell may become activated and produce other cytokines to further enhance the response.

To date more than 100 different cytokines have been discovered.[17] The majority of important cytokines are classified as interleukins or interferons. **Interleukins (ILs)** are produced predominantly by macrophages and lymphocytes in response to stimulation of PRRs or by other cytokines. More than 30 interleukins have been identified. Their effects include the following:

1. Alteration of adhesion molecule expression on many types of cells
2. Attraction of leukocytes to a site of inflammation (chemotaxis)
3. Induction of proliferation and maturation of leukocytes in the bone marrow
4. General enhancement or suppression of inflammation.

Perhaps the most important proinflammatory ILs are interleukin-1 and interleukin-6, which cooperate closely with another cytokine, tumor necrosis factor-alpha.[18] **Interleukin-1 (IL-1)** is produced mainly by macrophages.[19] It activates monocytes, other macrophages, and lymphocytes, thereby enhancing both the innate and acquired immunity, and acts as a growth factor for many cells. It has several effects on neutrophils, including induction of proliferation (resulting in an increase in the number of circulating neutrophils), attraction to an inflammatory site (chemotaxis), and increased cellular respiration and lysosomal enzyme activity (both effects resulting in increased cellular killing of bacteria).[20] IL-1 is an endogenous pyrogen (i.e., fever-causing cytokine) that reacts with receptors on cells of the hypothalamus and affects the body's thermostat, resulting in fever.

Interleukin-6 (IL-6) is produced by macrophages, lymphocytes, fibroblasts, and other cells.[18] IL-6 directly induces hepatocytes (liver cells) to produce many of the proteins needed in inflammation (acute-phase reactants, discussed later in this chapter). IL-6 also stimulates growth and differentiation of blood cells in the bone marrow and the growth of fibroblasts (required for wound healing).

Tumor necrosis factor-alpha (TNF-α) is secreted by macrophages and other cells (e.g., mast cells) in response to stimulation of TLRs.

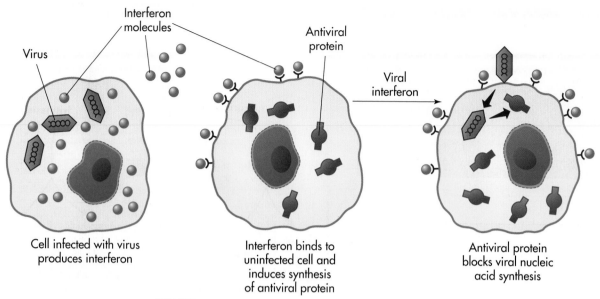

FIGURE 5-7 The Action of Interferon. See text for details.

TNF-α induces a multitude of proinflammatory effects, particularly on the vascular endothelium and macrophages. When secreted in large amounts, TNF-α has systemic effects that include the following:

1. Inducing fever by acting as an endogenous pyrogen
2. Causing increased synthesis of inflammation-related serum proteins by the liver
3. Causing muscle wasting (cachexia) and intravascular thrombosis in cases of severe infection and cancer

Very high levels of TNF-α can be lethal and are probably responsible for fatalities from shock caused by gram-negative bacterial infections.

Some cytokines are anti-inflammatory and diminish the inflammatory response. The most important are interleukin-10 and transforming growth factor-beta (TGF-β). **Interleukin-10 (IL-10)** is primarily produced by lymphocytes and suppresses the growth of lymphocytes and the production of proinflammatory cytokines by macrophages, leading to down-regulation of both inflammatory and acquired immune responses. **Transforming growth factors,** including **transforming growth factor-beta (TGF-β),** are produced by many types of cells in response to inflammation and induce cell division and differentiation of other cell types, such as immature blood cells. **Interferons (IFNs)** are members of a family of cytokines that protect against viral infections. The principal interferons are IFN-α, IFN-β, and IFN-γ. Macrophages and cells that become infected with viruses produce and secrete both IFN-α and IFN-β, which bind to specific receptors on neighboring cells and induce those cells to produce antiviral proteins (Figure 5-7). Thus, IFN-α and IFN-β protect the surrounding cells from infection and limit the spread of the virus. IFN-γ is produced by lymphocytes; it activates macrophages, resulting in increased capacity to kill infectious agents (including viruses and bacteria), and enhances the development of acquired immune responses against viruses.

Chemokines are members of a special family of low-molecular-weight (8 to 12 kilodaltons [kDa]) peptide cytokines that primarily attract leukocytes to sites of inflammation. Chemokines are synthesized by many cell types, including macrophages, fibroblasts, and endothelial cells, in response to proinflammatory cytokines, such as TNF-α. To date, more than 50 different human chemokines have been described. Examples include those that primarily attract macrophages

(e.g., monocyte/macrophage chemotactic proteins [MCP-1, MCP-2, and MCP-3], macrophage inflammatory proteins [MIP-1α and MIP-1β]) or attract neutrophils (e.g., interleukin 8 [IL-8]).

Mast Cells and Basophils

The mast cell is probably the most important cellular activator of the inflammatory response.[21] **Mast cells** are filled with granules and located in the loose connective tissues close to blood vessels near the body's outer surfaces (i.e., in the skin and lining the gastrointestinal and respiratory tracts). **Basophils** are found in the blood and probably function in the same way as tissue mast cells.[22] A great number of stimuli activate mast cells to release potent soluble inducers of inflammation. These are released by (1) **degranulation** (the release of the contents of mast cell granules) and (2) *synthesis* (the new production and release of mediators in response to a stimulus) (Figure 5-8).

Degranulation. In response to a stimulus, biologically active molecules are released from the mast cell granules within seconds and exert their effects immediately. These molecules include histamine and chemotactic factors.

Histamine is a small-molecular-weight molecule with potent effects on many other cells, particularly those that control the circulation. Histamine, along with serotonin (found in many cells, but not human mast cells), is called a vasoactive amine. These molecules cause temporary, rapid constriction of smooth muscle and dilation of the postcapillary venules, which results in increased blood flow into the microcirculation. Histamine also causes increased vascular permeability resulting from retraction of endothelial cells lining the capillaries and increased adherence of leukocytes to the endothelium. Histamine affects cells by binding to histamine H1 and H2 receptors on the target cell surface (Figure 5-9).[23] Antihistamines are drugs that block the binding of histamine to its receptors, resulting in decreased inflammation.

Mast cell granules also contain chemotactic factors, two of which are **neutrophil chemotactic factor (NCF)** and **eosinophil chemotactic factor of anaphylaxis (ECF-A).**[24] Neutrophils are the predominant cell needed to kill bacteria in the early stages of inflammation. Eosinophils help regulate the inflammatory response. Both cells are discussed in more detail later in this chapter.

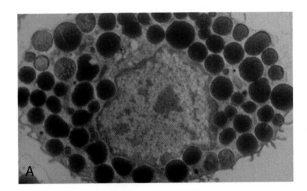

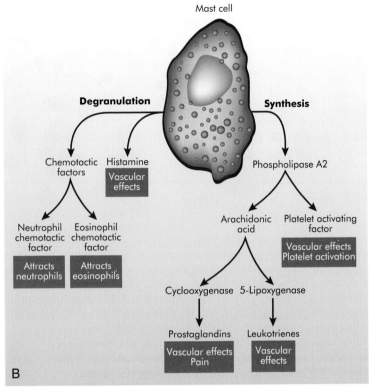

FIGURE 5-8 Mast Cell and Mast Cell Degranulation and Synthesis of Biologic Mediators During Inflammation. (A) Colorized photomicrograph of mast cell; dense red granules contain histamine and other biologically active substances. Among these are histamine, which is a major initiator of vascular changes, and a variety of chemotactic factors. **(B)** Mast cell degranulation (left) and synthesis (right). Histamine and biologically active substances are released immediately after stimulation of mast cells. Other substances are synthesized in response to mast cell stimulation. These include lipid-based molecules that originate from plasma membrane phospholipids as a result of the action of phospholipase A2. These include platelet-activating factor and a variety of prostaglandins and leukotrienes. (*A* from Patton KT and Thibodeau GA: *Anatomy & physiology,* ed 7, St Louis, 2010, Mosby.)

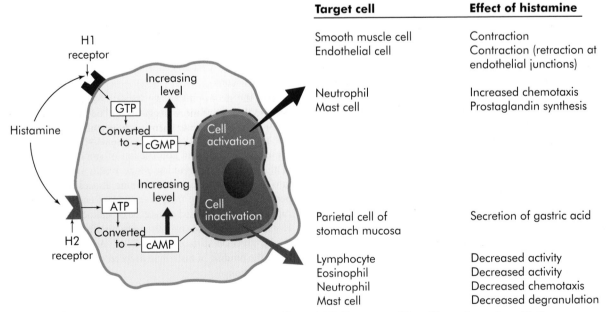

Target cell	Effect of histamine
Smooth muscle cell	Contraction
Endothelial cell	Contraction (retraction at endothelial junctions)
Neutrophil	Increased chemotaxis
Mast cell	Prostaglandin synthesis
Parietal cell of stomach mucosa	Secretion of gastric acid
Lymphocyte	Decreased activity
Eosinophil	Decreased activity
Neutrophil	Decreased chemotaxis
Mast cell	Decreased degranulation

FIGURE 5-9 Effects of Histamine Through H1 and H2 Receptors. The effects depend on (1) the density and affinity of H1 or H2 receptors on the target cell and (2) the identity of the target cell. *ATP,* Adenosine triphosphate; *cAMP,* cyclic adenosine monophosphate; *cGMP,* cyclic guanosine monophosphate; *GTP,* guanosine triphosphate.

Synthesis of Mediators. Activated mast cells begin new synthesis of other mediators of inflammation, which are released later than those in the granules. These include leukotrienes, prostaglandins, and platelet-activating factor, which are produced from lipids (arachidonic acid) in the plasma membrane. **Leukotrienes (slow-reacting substances of anaphylaxis [SRS-A])** are sulfur-containing lipids that produce histamine-like effects: smooth muscle contraction and increased vascular permeability. Leukotrienes appear to be important in the later stages of the inflammatory response because they stimulate slower and more prolonged responses than do histamines.

Prostaglandins cause increased vascular permeability, neutrophil chemotaxis, and pain by direct effects on nerves. They are long-chain, unsaturated fatty acids produced by the action of the enzyme cyclooxygenase on arachidonic acid from membrane phospholipids; prostaglandins are classified into groups (E, D, A, F, and B) according to their structure. Prostaglandins E_1 and E_2 cause increased vascular permeability and smooth muscle contraction. Aspirin and some other nonsteroidal anti-inflammatory drugs (NSAIDs) block the synthesis of prostaglandins of the E series and other arachidonic acid derivatives, thereby inhibiting inflammation.[25]

Platelet-activating factor (PAF) is produced by removal of a fatty acid from the plasma membrane phospholipid by phospholipase A2. Although mast cells are a major source of PAF, this molecule also can be produced during inflammation by neutrophils, monocytes, endothelial cells, and platelets. The biologic activity of PAF is virtually identical to that of leukotrienes, namely, causing endothelial cell retraction to increase vascular permeability, leukocyte adhesion to endothelial cells, and platelet activation.

Thus, at a site of tissue damage all the hallmarks of inflammation can be caused by mast cell products. Histamine causes dilation of the blood vessels and slows the circulation in nearby vessels. Histamine also causes endothelial cells to change their shapes and open intercellular junctions, which allows fluid to leak from the blood into the surrounding tissues. Increased blood flow and vasodilation result in increased redness and warmth, and increased vascular permeability results in local swelling from increased fluid in the tissues. Lipid-derived mediators are released later and continue the inflammatory process through histamine-like effects and cause pain.

Endothelium

The vessel walls consist of a layer of endothelial cells that adhere to an underlying matrix of connective tissue. The matrix contains a variety of proteins, including collagen, fibronectin, and laminins. Circulating cells and platelets and components of plasma protein systems continually contact endothelial cells lining the blood vessels. **Endothelial cells** regulate circulating components of the inflammatory system and maintain normal blood flow by preventing spontaneous activation of platelets and members of the clotting system. Endothelial cells produce **nitric oxide (NO)** from arginine and **prostacyclin (PGI_2)** from arachidonic acid. Both NO and PGI_2 maintain blood flow and pressure and inhibit platelet activation. PGI_2 and NO are synergistic. NO is released continually to relax vascular smooth muscle and suppress the effects of low levels of cytokines, thus maintaining vascular tone. PGI_2 production varies a great deal and is increased when additional regulation is needed.

Damage to the endothelial cell lining of the vessel exposes the subendothelial connective tissue matrix, which is prothrombogenic and initiates platelet activation and formation of clots (the contact activation [intrinsic] clotting pathway). Proinflammatory cytokines affect the endothelium, resulting in adherence of leukocytes to the vessel surface, invasion of leukocytes into the tissue, and efflux of plasma from the vessel.[17]

Platelets

Platelets are cytoplasmic fragments formed from *megakaryocytes*. They circulate in the bloodstream until vascular injury occurs. After injury, platelets are activated by many products of tissue destruction and inflammation, including collagen, thrombin, and platelet-activating factor.[26] Activation results in (1) their interaction with components of the coagulation cascade to stop bleeding[11] and (2) degranulation, releasing biochemical mediators such as serotonin, which has vascular effects similar to those of histamine. Platelets also release growth factors that promote wound healing. (Platelet function is described in detail in Chapter 19.)

Phagocytes

Neutrophils. The **neutrophil, or polymorphonuclear neutrophil (PMN)**, is a member of the granulocytic series of white blood cells and is named for the characteristic staining pattern of its granules as well as its multilobed nucleus. Neutrophils are the predominant phagocytes in the early inflammatory site, arriving within 6 to 12 hours after the initial injury. Several inflammatory mediators (e.g., some bacterial proteins, complement fragments C3a and C5a, and mast cell neutrophil chemotactic factor) specifically and rapidly attract neutrophils from the circulation and activate them.

Because the neutrophil is a mature cell that is incapable of division and sensitive to acidic environments, it is short lived at the inflammatory site and becomes a component of the purulent exudate, or pus, which is removed from the body through the epithelium or drained from the infected site via the lymphatic system. (The lymphatic system is described in Chapter 22.) The primary roles of the neutrophil are removal of debris and dead cells in sterile lesions, such as burns, and destruction of bacteria in nonsterile lesions.

Monocytes and Macrophages. **Monocytes** (the immature form of this white blood cell in the blood) and **macrophages** (the mature cell in the tissues) have fewer and larger lysosomes in their cytoplasm than do granulocytes. Monocytes are the largest normal blood cells and have a nucleus that is often indented or horseshoe shaped. Monocytes are produced in the bone marrow, enter the circulation, and migrate to the inflammatory site, where they develop into macrophages. Monocytes also appear to be the precursors of macrophages that are fixed in tissues (tissue macrophages), including Kupffer's cells in the liver, alveolar macrophages in the lungs, and microglia in the brain. Macrophages are generally larger and are more active as phagocytes than their monocytic precursors.

Macrophages enter the site after 24 hours, or later, and gradually replace the neutrophils. They migrate to the site after neutrophils because they move more sluggishly and because many of the chemotactic factors that attract them, such as macrophage chemotactic factor, must first be released by neutrophils.[27] Macrophages are better suited than neutrophils to long-term defense against infectious agents because macrophages can survive and divide in the acidic inflammatory site.[28] Macrophages orchestrate the wound healing process by cleaning up the site of injury by phagocytosis, promoting angiogenesis, releasing cytokines and growth factors that promote epithelial cell division, activating fibroblasts, and promoting the synthesis of extracellular matrix and collagen formation.[29]

Several bacteria are resistant to killing by granulocytes and can even survive inside macrophages. Microorganisms, such as *Mycobacterium tuberculosis* (tuberculosis), *Mycobacterium leprae* (leprosy), *Salmonella typhi* (typhoid fever), *Brucella abortus* (brucellosis), and *Listeria monocytogenes* (listeriosis), can remain dormant or multiply inside the phagolysosomes of macrophages. The bactericidal activity of macrophages can increase markedly with the help of inflammatory cytokines produced by cells of the acquired immune system

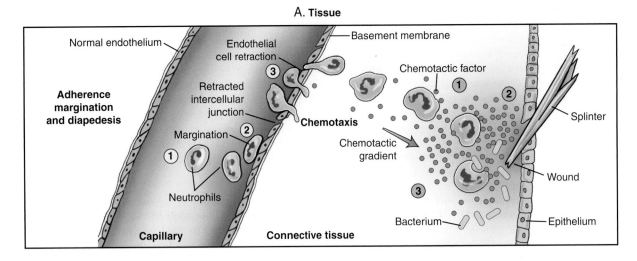

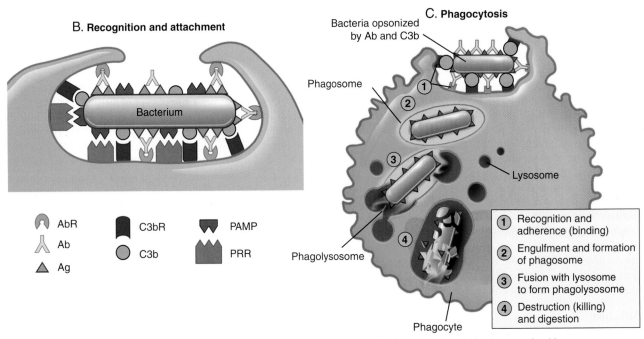

FIGURE 5-10 **Process of Phagocytosis.** The process that results in phagocytosis is characterized by three interrelated steps: adherence and diapedesis, tissue invasion by chemotaxis, and phagocytosis. **A,** *Adherence, margination, diapedesis,* and *chemotaxis.* The primary phagocyte in the blood is the neutrophil, which usually moves freely within the vessel *(1).* At sites of inflammation, the neutrophil progressively develops increased adherence to the endothelium, leading to accumulation along the vessel wall (margination or pavementing) *(2).* At sites of endothelial cell retraction the neutrophil exits the blood by means of diapedesis *(3).* *Chemotaxis.* In the tissues, the neutrophil detects chemotactic factor gradients through surface receptors *(1)* and migrates towards higher concentrations of the factors *(2).* The high concentration of chemotactic factors at the site of inflammation immobilizes the neutrophil *(3).* **B,** *Specific receptors for recognition and attachment.* **C,** *Phagocytosis.* Opsonized microorganisms bind to the surface of a phagocyte through specific receptors *(1).* The microorganism is ingested into a phagocytic vacuole, or phagosome *(2).* Lysosomes fuse with the phagosome, resulting in the formation of a phagolysosome *(3).* During this process the microorganism is exposed to products of the lysosomes, including a variety of enzymes and products of the hexose-monophosphate shunt (e.g., H_2O_2, O_2^-). The microorganism is killed and digested *(4).* *Ab,* Antibody; *AbR,* antibody receptor; *C3b,* complement component C3b; *C3bR,* complement C3b receptor; *PAMP,* pathogen-associated molecular pattern; *PRR,* pattern recognition receptor.

(subsets of T lymphocytes) or cells activated through Toll-like receptors. Macrophages have cell-surface receptors for these cytokines and are further activated to become more effective killers of infectious microorganisms.

Eosinophils. Although **eosinophils** are only mildly phagocytic, they have two specific functions: (1) they serve as the body's primary defense against parasites, and (2) they help regulate vascular mediators released from mast cells.[24] The role of eosinophils in resistance to parasites occurs in collaboration with specific antibodies produced by the acquired immune system (discussed later in this chapter).

The second function, regulation of mast cell–derived inflammatory mediators, is a critical function of eosinophils and helps limit and control inflammation. Mast cells produce eosinophil chemotactic factor-A (ECF-A), which attracts eosinophils to the site of inflammation. Eosinophil lysosomes contain several enzymes that degrade vasoactive molecules, thereby controlling the vascular effects of inflammation. These enzymes include histaminase, which mediates the degradation of histamine, and arylsulfatase B, which degrades some of the lipid-derived mediators produced by mast cells.

Dendritic Cells and T Lymphocytes. **Dendritic cells** provide one of the major links between the innate and acquired immune responses.[30] They are primary phagocytic cells located in the peripheral organs and skin, where molecules released from infectious agents are encountered, recognized through PRRs, and internalized through phagocytosis. Dendritic cells then migrate through the lymphatic vessels to lymphoid tissue, such as lymph nodes, and interact with **T lymphocytes** to generate an acquired immune response.[31] Through the production of a family of cytokines, they guide development of a subset of T cells (helper cells) that coordinate the development of functional B and T cells (discussed in Chapter 6). T lymphocytes are active during the proliferative phase of wound healing (see p. 135).[32,33]

Phagocytosis. **Phagocytosis** is the process by which a cell ingests and disposes of foreign material, including microorganisms. Cells that perform this process are called **phagocytes.** The two most important phagocytes are neutrophils and macrophages. Both cells are circulating in the blood and must first leave the circulation and migrate to the site of inflammation before initiating phagocytosis (Figure 5-10). Many products of inflammation affect expression of surface molecules involved in cell-to-cell adherence. Both leukocytes and endothelial cells begin expressing molecules that increase adhesion, or stickiness, causing the leukocytes to adhere more avidly to the endothelial cells in the walls of the capillaries and venules in a process called **margination,** or **pavementing.** Leukocyte-endothelial interactions lead to diapedesis, or emigration of the cells through the inter-endothelial junctions that have loosened in response to inflammatory mediators.[34]

Once inside the tissue, leukocytes undergo a process of directed migration, called **chemotaxis,** by which they are attracted to the inflammatory site by chemotactic factors (Figure 5-11). The primary chemotactic factors include many bacterial products, neutrophil chemotactic factor produced by mast cells, complement fragments C3a and C5a, and products of the clotting and kinin systems.

At the inflammatory site, the process of phagocytosis involves five steps: (1) recognition and adherence of the phagocyte to its target, (2) engulfment (ingestion or endocytosis), (3) formation of a phagosome, (4) fusion of the phagosome with lysosomal granules within the phagocyte, and (5) destruction of the target. Throughout the process, both the target and digestive enzymes are isolated within membrane-bound vesicles. Isolation protects the phagocyte itself from the harmful effects of the target microorganisms, as well as its own enzymes.

Most phagocytes can trap and engulf bacteria using PRRs, although the process is relatively slow. **Opsonization** greatly enhances adherence by acting as a glue to tighten the affinity of adherence between the phagocyte and the target cell. The most efficient opsonins are antibodies and C3b produced by the complement system. Antibodies are made against antigens on the surface of bacteria and are highly specific to that particular microorganism. Certain bacterial and fungal polysaccharide coatings activate the alternative and lectin pathways of complement activation, which deposits C3b on the bacterial surface and

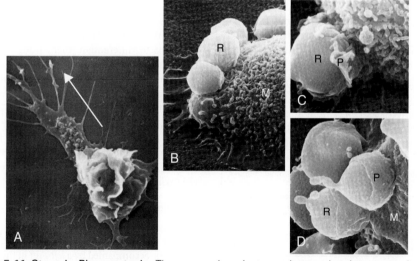

FIGURE 5-11 Steps in Phagocytosis. These scanning electron micrographs show examples of the progressive steps in phagocytosis. **A,** A leukocyte undergoes chemotactic movement (in direction of arrow) by extending a filopodium (upper left) from the trailing body of the cell. **B,** Engulfment of red blood cells by a macrophage *(M)* that attaches to the red blood cells *(R).* **C,** An extension of the macrophage membrane *(P; pseudopod)* starts to enclose the red cell. **D,** The red blood cells are almost totally engulfed by the macrophage. (**A** from Kumar V et al: *Robbins and Cotran pathologic basis of disease, professional edition,* ed 8, Philadelphia, 2009, Saunders; **B-D** modified from King DW, Fenoglio CM, Lefkowitch JH: *General pathology: principles and dynamics,* Philadelphia, 1983, Lea & Febiger.)

increases phagocytosis. The surface of phagocytes contains a variety of specific receptors that will strongly bind to opsonins. These include complement receptors that bind to C3b and Fc receptors that bind to a site on antibody molecules.

Engulfment (endocytosis) is carried out by small pseudopods that extend from the plasma membrane and surround the adherent microorganism, forming an intracellular phagocytic vacuole, or phagosome (see Figures 5-10 and 5-11). After the formation of the phagosome, lysosomes converge, fuse with the phagosome, and discharge their contents, creating a phagolysosome. Destruction of the bacterium takes place within the phagolysosome and is accomplished by both oxygen-dependent and oxygen-independent mechanisms.

Oxygen-dependent killing mechanisms result from the production of toxic oxygen species. Phagocytosis is accompanied by a burst of oxygen uptake by the phagocyte; this is termed the *respiratory burst* and results from a shift in much of the cell's glucose metabolism to the hexose-monophosphate shunt, which produces nicotinamide adenine dinucleotide phosphate (NADPH). A membrane-associated enzyme, NADPH oxidase uses NADPH to generate superoxide (O_2^-), hydrogen peroxide (H_2O_2), and other reactive oxygen species that can be highly damaging to bacteria. Hydrogen peroxide also can collaborate with the lysosomal enzyme *myeloperoxidase* and halide anions (Cl^- and Br^-) to form acids that kill bacteria and fungi.

Oxygen-independent mechanisms of microbial killing include (1) the acidic pH (3.5 to 4.0) of the phagolysosome, (2) cationic proteins that bind to and damage target cell membranes, (3) enzymatic attack of the microorganism's cell wall by lysozyme and other enzymes, and (4) inhibition of bacterial growth by lactoferrin binding of iron.

When a phagocyte dies at an inflammatory site, it frequently lyses (breaks open) and releases its cytoplasmic contents, including the lysosomal enzymes, into the tissue. They can digest the connective tissue matrix, causing much of the tissue destruction associated with inflammation. The destructive effects of many enzymes released by dying phagocytes are minimized by natural inhibitors found in the blood, such as α1-antitrypsin, a plasma protein produced by the liver. An inherited deficiency of α_1-antitrypsin often leads to chronic lung damage and emphysema as a result of inflammation. (The pulmonary effects of α_1-antitrypsin deficiency are described in Chapter 25.) Released lysosomal products also may contribute to inflammation by increasing vascular permeability, attracting additional monocytes, and activating the complement and kinin systems.

> ✔ **QUICK CHECK 5-4**
> 1. What are pattern recognition receptors?
> 2. What are cytokines? How do cytokines promote inflammation?
> 3. What products do the mast cells release during inflammation, and what are their effects?
> 4. What phagocytic cell types are involved in the acute inflammatory response? What is the role of each?
> 5. What are the four steps in the process of phagocytosis?

ACUTE AND CHRONIC INFLAMMATION

Inflammation can be divided into phases of acute and chronic inflammation. The acute inflammatory response is self-limiting—that is, it continues only until the threat to the host is eliminated. This usually takes 8 to 10 days from onset to healing. If the acute inflammatory response proves inadequate, a chronic inflammation may develop and persist for weeks or months. If a continued response is necessary, inflammation may progress to a granulomatous response that is designed to contain the infection or damaged site so it no longer poses any harm to the individual. The characteristics of the early (i.e., acute) inflammatory response differ from those of the later (i.e., chronic) response, and each phase involves different biochemical mediators and cells that function together. Depending on the successful containment of tissue damage and infection, the acute and chronic phases may lead to healing without progression to the next phase.

Local Manifestations of Acute Inflammation

The cells and plasma protein systems of the inflammatory response interact to produce all the characteristics of inflammation, whether local or systemic (discussed in the next section), as well as determine the duration of inflammation, either acute or chronic. All the local characteristics of acute inflammation (i.e., swelling, pain, heat, and redness [erythema]) result from vascular changes and the subsequent leakage of circulating components into the tissue. The symptoms of acute inflammation were previously described on page 121 and can be reviewed in Figure 5-3.

The exudate of inflammation varies in composition, depending on the stage of the inflammatory response and, to some extent, the injurious stimulus. In early or mild inflammation, the exudate is watery (serous exudate) with very few plasma proteins or leukocytes. An example of serous exudate is the fluid in a blister. In more severe or advanced inflammation, the exudate may be thick and clotted (fibrinous exudate), such as in the lungs of individuals with pneumonia. If a large number of leukocytes accumulate, as in persistent bacterial infections, the exudate consists of pus and is called a purulent (suppurative) exudate. Purulent exudate is characteristic of walled-off lesions (cysts or abscesses). If bleeding occurs, the exudate is filled with erythrocytes and is described as a hemorrhagic exudate.

Systemic Manifestations of Acute Inflammation

The three primary systemic changes associated with the acute inflammatory response are fever, leukocytosis (a transient increase in the levels of circulating leukocytes), and increased levels of circulating plasma proteins.

Fever

Fever is partially induced by specific cytokines (e.g., IL-1, released from neutrophils and macrophages). These are known as endogenous pyrogens to differentiate them from pathogen-produced *exogenous pyrogens*. Pyrogens act directly on the hypothalamus, the portion of the brain that controls the body's thermostat (see Figure 13-5). (Mechanisms of temperature regulation and fever are discussed in Chapter 13.) A fever can be beneficial because some microorganisms (e.g., syphilis, gonococcal urethritis) are highly sensitive to small increases in body temperature. On the other hand, fever may have harmful side effects because it may enhance the host's susceptibility to the effects of endotoxins associated with gram-negative bacterial infections (bacterial toxins are described in Chapter 7).

Leukocytosis

Leukocytosis is an increase in the number of circulating white blood cells (greater than $11,000/ml^3$ in adults). During many infections, leukocytosis may be accompanied by a *left shift* in the ratio of immature to mature neutrophils, so that the more immature forms of neutrophils, such as band cells, metamyelocytes, and occasionally myelocytes, are present in relatively greater than normal proportions. (Chapter 19 contains a more complete discussion of the development and maturation of blood cells.) Production of immature leukocytes increases primarily from proliferation and release of granulocyte and monocyte precursors in the bone marrow, which is stimulated by several products of inflammation.

TABLE 5-2	CIRCULATING LEVELS OF ACUTE-PHASE REACTANTS DURING INFLAMMATION	
FUNCTION	**INCREASED**	**DECREASED**
Coagulation components	Fibrinogen	None
	Prothrombin	
	Factor VIII	
	Plasminogen	
Protease inhibitors	α_1-Antitrypsin	Inter-α-antitrypsin
	α_1-Antichymotrypsin	
Transport proteins	Haptoglobin	Transferrin
	Hemopexin	
	Ceruloplasmin	
	Ferritin	
Complement components	C1s, C2, C3, C4, C5, C9, factor B, C1 inhibitor	Properdin
Miscellaneous proteins	α_1-Acid glycoprotein	Albumin
	Fibronectin	Prealbumin
	Serum amyloid A (SAA)	α_1-Lipoprotein
	C-reactive protein (CRP)	β-Lipoprotein

Plasma Protein Synthesis

The synthesis of many plasma proteins, mostly products of the liver, is increased during inflammation. These proteins, which can be either proinflammatory or anti-inflammatory in nature, are referred to as **acute-phase reactants** (Table 5-2). Acute-phase reactants reach maximal circulating levels within 10 to 40 hours after the start of inflammation. IL-1 is indirectly responsible for the synthesis of acute-phase reactants through the induction of IL-6, which directly stimulates liver cells to synthesize most of these proteins.

Common laboratory tests for inflammation measure levels of acute-phase reactants. For example, an increase in blood levels of acute-phase reactants, primarily fibrinogen, is associated with an increased adhesion among erythrocytes and a corresponding increase in the sedimentation rate. The erythrocyte sedimentation rate is a measurement of the rate at which red blood cells sediment in a tube over a prescribed time span (usually an hour). Although increased erythrocyte sedimentation is a nonspecific reaction, it is considered a good indicator of an acute inflammatory response.

Chronic Inflammation

Superficially, the difference between acute and chronic inflammation is duration; **chronic inflammation** lasts 2 weeks or longer, regardless of cause. Chronic inflammation is sometimes preceded by an unsuccessful acute inflammatory response (Figure 5-12). For example, if bacterial contamination or foreign objects (e.g., dirt, wood splinter, and glass) persist in a wound, an acute response may be prolonged

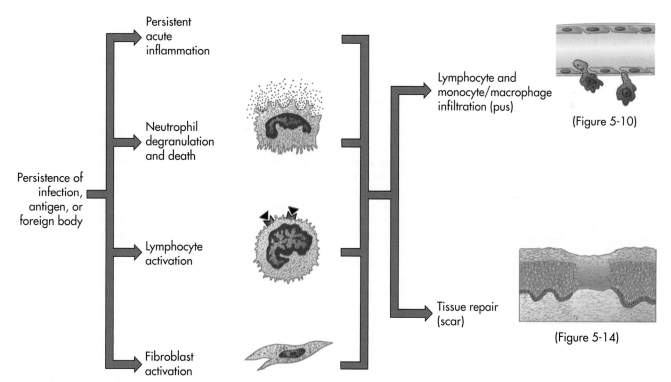

FIGURE 5-12 The Chronic Inflammatory Response. Inflammation usually becomes chronic because of the persistence of an infection, an antigen, or a foreign body in the wound. Chronic inflammation is characterized by the persistence of many of the processes of acute inflammation. In addition, large amounts of neutrophil degranulation and death, the activation of lymphocytes, and the concurrent activation of fibroblasts result in the release of mediators that induce the infiltration of more lymphocytes and monocytes/macrophages and the beginning of wound healing and tissue repair. For more detailed information on each portion of the response, see the figures referenced in this illustration.

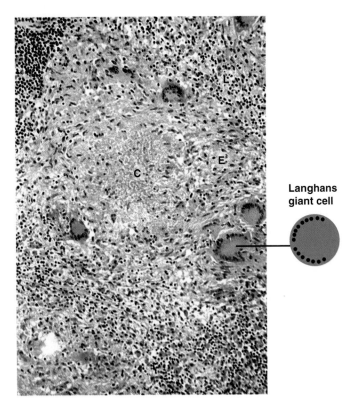

Langhans giant cell

FIGURE 5-13 Tuberculous Granuloma. A central area of amorphous caseous necrosis *(C)* is surrounded by a zone of lymphocytes *(L)* and enlarged epithelioid cells *(E).* Activated macrophages frequently fuse to form multinucleated cells (Langhans giant cells). In tuberculoid granulomas the nuclei of the giant cells move to the cellular margins in a horseshoe-like formation.

beyond 2 weeks.[35] Pus formation, suppuration (purulent discharge), and incomplete wound healing may characterize this type of chronic inflammation.

Chronic inflammation can occur also as a distinct process without previous acute inflammation. Some microorganisms (e.g., mycobacteria that cause tuberculosis) have cell walls with a very high lipid and wax content, making them relatively insensitive to breakdown by phagocytes. Other microorganisms (e.g., those that cause leprosy, syphilis, and brucellosis) can survive within the macrophage and avoid removal by the acute inflammatory response. Other microorganisms produce toxins that damage tissue and cause persistent inflammation even after the organism is killed. Finally, chemicals, particulate matter, or physical irritants (e.g., inhaled dusts, wood splinters, and suture material) can cause a prolonged inflammatory response.

Chronic inflammation is characterized by a dense infiltration of lymphocytes and macrophages. If macrophages are unable to protect the host from tissue damage, the body attempts to wall off and isolate the infected area, thus forming a **granuloma** (Figure 5-13). For example, infections caused by some bacteria (*Listeria* sp., *Brucella* sp.), fungi (histoplasmosis, coccidioidomycosis), and parasites (leishmaniasis, schistosomiasis, toxoplasmosis) can result in granuloma formation. The process of granuloma formation begins when some macrophages differentiate into large **epithelioid cells,** which specialize in taking up debris and other small particles. Other macrophages fuse into multinucleated **giant cells,** which are active phagocytes that can engulf very large particles—larger than can be engulfed by a single macrophage. These two types of differentiated macrophages form the center of the

granuloma, which is surrounded by a wall of lymphocytes. The granuloma itself is often encapsulated by fibrous deposits of collagen and may become cartilaginous or possibly calcified by deposits of calcium carbonate and calcium phosphate.

The classic granuloma associated with tuberculosis is characterized by a wall of epithelioid cells surrounding a center of dead and decaying tissue (caseous necrosis) and mycobacteria. Decay of cells within the granuloma results in the release of acids and the enzymatic contents of lysosomes from dead phagocytes. In this inhospitable environment, the cellular debris is broken down into its basic constituents, and a clear fluid remains (liquefaction necrosis). Eventually, this fluid diffuses out and leaves a hollow, thick-walled structure in the tissue that may remain for the life of the individual.

> ✔ **QUICK CHECK 5-5**
> 1. Describe how acute inflammation differs from chronic inflammation. What characteristics do they share?
> 2. List the types of exudate produced in inflammation.

WOUND HEALING

Tissue injury is followed by a period of healing that begins during acute inflammation. The most favorable outcome is a return to normal structure and function, and may take up to 2 years for some tissue injury. The repaired tissues may be close to normal if damage is minor, no complications occur, and destroyed tissues are capable of **regeneration** (Figure 5-14). This restoration is called **resolution.** Resolution may not be possible if extensive damage is present, the tissue is not capable of regeneration, infection results in abscess or granuloma formation, or fibrin persists in the lesion. In those cases, repair takes place instead of resolution. **Repair** is the replacement of destroyed tissue with scar tissue. **Scar** tissue is composed primarily of collagen that fills in the lesion and restores strength but cannot carry out the physiologic functions of destroyed tissue.

Wound healing involves processes that (1) fill in, (2) seal, and (3) shrink the wound. These characteristics of healing vary in importance and duration among different types of wounds. A clean incision, such as a paper cut or a sutured surgical wound, heals primarily through the process of collagen synthesis. Because this type of wound has minimal tissue loss and close apposition of the wound edges, very little sealing (**epithelialization**) and shrinkage (**contraction**) are required. Wounds that heal under conditions of minimal tissue loss are said to heal by **primary intention** (see Figure 5-14).

Other wounds do not heal as easily. Healing of an open wound, such as a stage IV pressure ulcer (decubitus ulcer), requires a great deal of tissue replacement so that epithelialization, scar formation, and contraction take longer and healing occurs through **secondary intention** (see Figure 5-14). Healing by either primary or secondary intention may occur at different rates for different types of tissue injury.

Epidermal wounds that heal by secondary intention and unsutured internal lesions are not completely restored by healing. At best, repaired tissue regains 80% of its original tensile strength. Only epithelial, hepatic (liver), and bone marrow cells are capable of the complete mitotic regeneration of the normal tissue known as *compensatory hyperplasia.* In fibrous connective tissue, such as joints and ligaments, normal healing results in replacement of the original tissue with new tissue that does not have exactly the same structure or function as that of the original. Some tissues heal without replacement of cells. For example, damage resulting from myocardial infarction heals with a scar composed of fibrous tissue rather than with cardiac muscle.

HEALING BY PRIMARY INTENTION   HEALING BY SECONDARY INTENTION

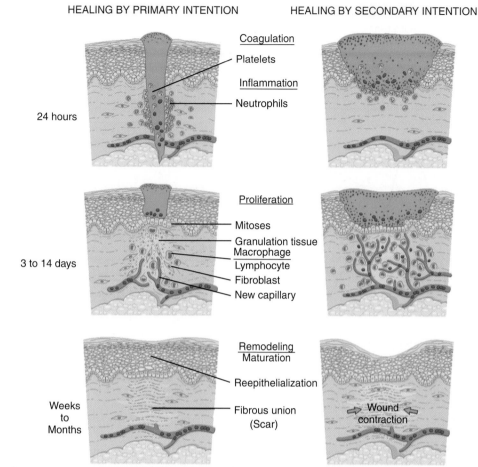

FIGURE 5-14 Wound Healing by Primary and Secondary Intention and Phases of Wound Healing. Phases of wound healing (coagulation, inflammation, proliferation, remodeling, and maturation) and steps in wound healing by primary intention *(left)* and secondary intention *(right)*. Note large amounts of granulation tissue and wound contraction in healing by secondary intention. (From Roberts JR, Hedges J: *Clinical procedures in emergency medicine,* ed 5, Philadelphia, 2009, Saunders.)

Wound healing occurs in three overlapping phases: inflammation, proliferation and new tissue formation, and remodeling and maturation.

Phase I: Inflammation

The early phase of wound healing begins during acute inflammation and usually lasts for 1 to 2 days. The **inflammatory phase** includes coagulation and the infiltration of cells that participate in wound healing, including platelets, neutrophils, and macrophages (Figure 5-15). The fibrin mesh of the blood clot acts as a scaffold for cells that participate in healing. Platelets contribute to clot formation and, as they degranulate, release growth factors. Neutrophils clear the wound of debris and bacteria and are later replaced by macrophages. Macrophages are essential to wound healing because they are phagocytic, release wound healing mediators and growth factors, recruit fibroblasts, and help promote angiogenesis during the proliferative phase of wound healing.

Phase II: Proliferation and New Tissue Formation

The proliferative phase begins 3 to 4 days after the injury and continues for as long as 2 weeks. The wound is sealed and the fibrin clot is replaced by normal tissue or scar tissue during this phase. The **proliferative phase** is characterized by macrophage recruitment of fibroblasts (connective tissue cells) and fibroblast proliferation, followed by fibroblast collagen synthesis, epithelialization, contraction of the wound, and cellular differentiation.

Macrophages invade the dissolving clot and clear away debris and dead cells and orchestrate the wound healing process.[29] Macrophages secrete the following biochemical mediators that promote healing:

1. **Transforming growth factor-beta (TGF-β)** stimulates fibroblasts entering the lesion to synthesize and secrete the collagen precursor procollagen.
2. **Angiogenesis factors,** such as vascular endothelial growth factor (VEGF) and fibroblast growth factor-2 (FGF-2), stimulate vascular endothelial cells to form capillary buds that grow into the lesion; decreased pH and decreased wound oxygen tension also promote angiogenesis.
3. **Matrix metalloproteinases (MMPs)** degrade and remodel extracellular matrix proteins (e.g., collagen and fibrin) at the site of injury.

Granulation tissue grows into the wound from surrounding healthy connective tissue. Granulation tissue is filled with new capillaries (angiogenesis) derived from capillaries in the surrounding tissue, giving the granulation tissue a red, granular appearance. New lymphatic vessels also grow into the granulation tissue by a similar process.

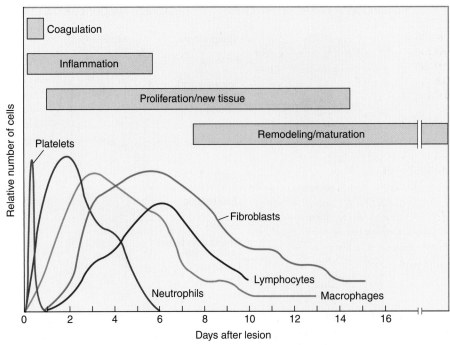

FIGURE 5-15 Time Course of Cells Infiltrating a Wound. Neutrophils and macrophages are the predominant cells that infiltrate a wound during inflammation. Lymphocytes appear later and peak at day 7. Fibroblasts are the predominant cells during the proliferative and remodeling phases of the healing process. (Adapted From Townsend CM et al, editors: *Satiston textbook of surgery,* ed 18, St Louis, 2007, Elsevier.)

During this process the healing wound must be protected. Epithelialization is the process by which epithelial cells grow into the wound from surrounding healthy tissue. Epithelial cells migrate under the clot or scab using MMPs to unravel collagen. Migrating epithelial cells contact similar cells from all sides of the wound and seal it, thereby halting migration and proliferation. The epithelial cells remain active, undergoing differentiation to give rise to the various epidermal layers (see Chapter 39. Epithelialization of a skin wound can be hastened if the wound is kept moist, preventing the fibrin clot from becoming a scab.

Fibroblasts are important cells during healing because they secrete collagen and other connective tissue proteins. Fibroblasts are stimulated by macrophage-derived TGF-β to proliferate, enter the lesion, and deposit connective tissue proteins in débrided areas about 6 days after the fibroblasts have entered the lesion. **Collagen** is the most abundant protein in the body. It contains high concentrations of the amino acids glycine, proline, and lysine, many of which are enzymatically modified. Modification of proline and lysine requires several cofactors that are absolutely necessary for proper collagen polymerization and function. These include iron, ascorbic acid (vitamin C), and molecular oxygen (O_2); absence of any of these results in impaired wound healing. As healing progresses, collagen molecules are cross-linked by intermolecular covalent bonds to form collagen fibrils that are further cross-linked to form collagen fibers. The complete process takes several months.

The granulation tissue contains **myofibroblasts,** specialized cells responsible for wound contraction. Myofibroblasts have features of both smooth muscle cells and fibroblasts. They appear microscopically similar to fibroblasts but differ in that their cytoplasm contains bundles of parallel fibers similar to those found in smooth muscle cells. **Wound contraction** occurs as extensions from the plasma membrane of myofibroblasts establish connections between neighboring cells,

contract their fibers, and exert tension on the neighboring cells while anchoring themselves to the wound bed. Wound contraction is necessary for closure of all wounds, especially those that heal by secondary intention. Contraction is noticeable 6 to 12 days after injury.

Phase III: Remodeling and Maturation

Tissue remodeling and maturation begins several weeks after injury and is normally complete within 2 years. During this phase, there is continuation of cellular differentiation, scar formation, and scar remodeling.[36] The fibroblast is the major cell of tissue remodeling with the deposition of collagen into an organized matrix. Tissue regeneration and wound contraction continue in the remodeling and maturation phase—a phase for recovering normal tissue structure that can persist for years. For wounds that heal by scarring, scar tissue is remodeled and capillaries disappear, leaving the scar avascular. Within 2 to 3 weeks after maturation has begun, the scar tissue has gained about two thirds of its eventual maximal strength.

Dysfunctional Wound Healing

Dysfunctional wound healing and impaired epithelialization may occur during any phase of the healing process. The cause of dysfunctional wound healing includes ischemia, excessive bleeding, excessive fibrin deposition, a predisposing disorder such as diabetes mellitus, wound infection, inadequate nutrients, numerous drugs, and tobacco smoke.[37]

Oxygen-deprived (ischemic) tissue is susceptible to infection, which prolongs inflammation and delays healing. *Ischemia* reduces energy production and impairs collagen synthesis and the tensile strength of regenerating connective tissue.

Healing is prolonged if there is *excessive bleeding.* Large clots increase the amount of space that granulation tissue must fill and serve as mechanical barriers to oxygen diffusion. Accumulated blood is an excellent culture medium for bacteria and promotes infection, thereby prolonging inflammation by increasing exudation and pus formation. Decreased blood volume also inhibits inflammation because of vessel constriction rather than the dilation required to deliver inflammatory cells to the site of injury.

Excessive fibrin deposition is detrimental to healing. Fibrin released in response to injury must eventually be reabsorbed to prevent organization into fibrous adhesions. Adhesions formed in the pleural, pericardial, or abdominal cavities can bind organs together by fibrous bands and distort or strangulate the affected organ.

Persons with *diabetes* are at risk for prolonged wound healing. Wounds are often ischemic because of the potential for small-vessel diseases that impair the microcirculation and alter (glycosylated) hemoglobin, which has an increased affinity for oxygen and thus does not readily release oxygen in tissues. Consequences of hyperglycemia also include suppression of macrophages and increased risk for wound infection.

Wound infection is caused by the infiltration of pathogens. Pathogens damage cells, stimulate the release of inflammatory mediators, consume nutrients, and delay wound healing.

Optimal *nutrition* is important during all phases of healing because metabolic needs increase. Leukocytes need glucose to produce the adenosine triphosphate (5′-ATP) needed for chemotaxis, phagocytosis, and intercellular killing; therefore the wounds of persons with diabetes who receive insufficient insulin heal poorly. Hypoproteinemia impairs fibroblast proliferation and collagen synthesis. Prolonged lack of vitamins A and C results in poorly formed connective tissue and greatly impaired healing because they are cofactors required for collagen synthesis.[38] Other nutrients, including iron, zinc, manganese, and copper, are also required as cofactors for collagen synthesis. Malnutrition increases risk for wound infection, delays healing, and reduces wound tensile strength.[39]

Medications, including antineoplastic (anticancer) agents, nonsteroidal anti-inflammatory drugs (NSAIDs), and steroids, delay wound healing. Antineoplastic agents slow cell division and inhibit angiogenesis. Although NSAIDs inhibit prostaglandin production and suppress acute inflammation and relieve pain, they also can delay wound healing, particularly bone formation, and may contribute to the formation of excessive scarring.[40] Steroids prevent macrophages from migrating to the site of injury and inhibit release of collagenase and plasminogen activator. Steroids also inhibit fibroblast migration into the wound during the proliferative phase and delay epithelialization. Toxic agents in *tobacco smoke* (i.e., nicotine, carbon monoxide, and hydrogen cyanide) delay wound healing and increase the risk for wound infection.[41]

Dysfunctional collagen synthesis may involve excessive production of collagen, causing surface overhealing, leading to a hypertrophic scar or keloid.[42] A **hypertrophic scar** is raised but remains within the original boundaries of the wound and tends to regress over time (Figure 5-16, *A*). A **keloid** is a raised scar that extends beyond the original boundaries of the wound, invades surrounding tissue, and is likely to recur after surgical removal (Figure 5-16, *B*). A familial tendency to keloid formation has been observed, with a greater incidence in blacks than whites.

Wound Disruption

A potential complication of wounds that are sutured closed is **dehiscence,** in which the wound pulls apart at the suture line. Dehiscence generally occurs 5 to 12 days after suturing, when collagen synthesis is at its peak. Approximately half of dehiscence occurrences are associated with wound infection, but they also may be the result of sutures

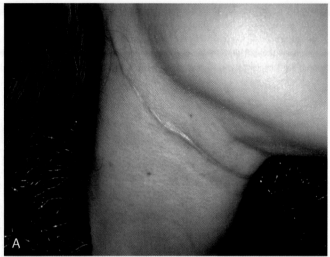
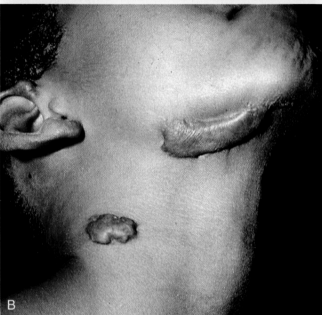

FIGURE 5-16 Hypertrophic Scar and Keloid Scar Formation. Hypertrophic scar (**A**) and keloid scar (**B**) caused by excessive synthesis of collagen at suture sites. (**A** from Flint PW et al: *Cummings otolaryngology: head & neck surgery,* ed 5, Philadelphia, 2010, Mosby; **B** from Damjanov I, Linder J: *Anderson's pathology,* ed 10, St Louis, 1996, Mosby.)

breaking because of excessive strain. Obesity increases the risk for dehiscence because adipose tissue is difficult to suture. Wound dehiscence usually is heralded by increased serous drainage from the wound and a patient's perception that "something gave way." Prompt surgical attention is required.

Impaired Contraction

Wound contraction, although necessary for healing, may become pathologic when contraction is excessive, resulting in a deformity or **contracture of scar tissue.** Burns of the skin are especially susceptible to contracture development, particularly at joints. Internal contractures include duodenal strictures caused by dysfunctional healing of a peptic ulcer; esophageal strictures caused by chemical burns, such as lye ingestion; or abdominal adhesions caused by surgery, infection, or radiation. Contracture may occur in cirrhosis of the liver, constricting vascular flow and contributing to the development of portal hypertension and esophageal varices. Proper positioning, range-of-motion exercises, and surgery are among the physical means used to overcome myofibroblast pull and prevent skin contractures. Surgery is performed to release internal contractures.

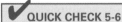

> **QUICK CHECK 5-6**
> 1. How does regeneration of tissue differ from repair of tissue?
> 2. What does it mean to heal by primary intention?
> 3. What is the role of fibroblasts in wound healing?
> 4. Describe various ways wound healing may be dysfunctional.

PEDIATRIC CONSIDERATIONS

Age-Related Factors Affecting Innate Immunity in the Newborn Child

- Newborns have transiently depressed inflammatory responses.
- Neutrophils are incapable of chemotaxis, lacking fluidity in the plasma membrane.
- Complement levels are diminished, especially components of the alternative pathways (e.g., factor B), particularly in premature newborns.
- Monocyte/macrophage numbers are normal but chemotaxis of monocytes is delayed.

- There is a tendency for infections associated with chemotactic defects, for example, cutaneous abscesses caused by staphylococci and cutaneous candidiasis.
- There are diminished oxidative and bacterial responses in those stressed by in utero infection or respiratory insufficiency.
- There is a tendency to develop severe overwhelming sepsis and meningitis when infected by bacteria against which no maternal antibodies are present.

GERIATRIC CONSIDERATIONS

Age-Related Factors Affecting Innate Immunity in the Elderly

- Normal numbers of cells of innate immunity but possible diminished function (e.g., decreased phagocytic activity)
- Increased incidence of chronic inflammation, possibly related to increased production of proinflammatory mediators
- At risk for impaired healing—often associated with chronic illness (e.g., diabetes mellitus, peripheral vascular disease, or cardiovascular disease)

- Use of medications that may interfere with healing (e.g., anti-inflammatory steroids)
- Loss of subcutaneous fat, diminishing layers of protection against injury
- Atrophied epidermis, including underlying capillaries, which decreases perfusion and increases risk of hypoxia in wound bed

Data from Freund A et al: Inflammatory networks during cellular senescence: causes and consequences, *Trends Mol Med* 16(5):238–246, 2010; Gist S et al: Wound care in the geriatric client, *Clin Interv Aging* 4:269–287, 2009; Jaul E: Non-healing wounds: the geriatric approach, *Arch Gerontol Geriatr* 49(2):224–246, 2009; Shaw AC et al: Aging of the innate immune system, *Curr Opin Immunol* 22(4):507–513, 2010.

DID YOU UNDERSTAND?

Human Defense Mechanisms
1. There are three layers of human defense: barriers; innate immunity, which includes the inflammatory response; and adaptive (acquired) immunity.

Physical and Mechanical Barriers
1. Physical and mechanical barriers are the first lines of defense that prevent damage to the individual and prevent invasion by pathogens; these include the skin and mucous membranes.

Biochemical Barriers
1. Antibacterial peptides in mucous secretions, perspiration, saliva, tears, and other secretions provide a biochemical barrier against pathogenic microorganisms.
2. The normal bacterial flora provides protection by releasing chemicals that prevent colonization by pathogens.

The Inflammatory Process
1. Inflammation is a rapid and nonspecific protective response to cellular injury from any cause. It can occur only in vascularized tissue.
2. The macroscopic hallmarks of inflammation are redness, swelling, heat, pain, and loss of function of the inflamed tissues.
3. The microscopic hallmark of inflammation is an accumulation of fluid and cells at the inflammatory site.

Plasma Protein Systems
1. Inflammation is mediated by three key plasma protein systems: the complement system, the clotting system, and the kinin system. The components of all three systems are a series of inactive proteins that are activated sequentially.
2. The complement system can be activated by antigen-antibody reactions (through the classical pathway) or by other products, especially bacterial polysaccharides (through the lectin pathway or the alternative pathway), resulting in the production of biologically active fragments and destruction of cells.
3. The most biologically potent products of the complement system are C3b (opsonin), C3a (anaphylatoxin), and C5a (anaphylatoxin, chemotactic factor).
4. The clotting system stops bleeding, localizes microorganisms, and provides a meshwork for repair and healing.
5. Bradykinin is the most important product of the kinin system and causes vascular permeability, smooth muscle contraction, and pain.

Cellular Components of Inflammation
1. Many different types of cells are involved in the inflammatory process including mast cells, endothelial cells, platelets, phagocytes (neutrophils, eosinophils, monocytes and macrophages, dendritic cells), natural killer (NK) cells, and lymphocytes.

DID YOU UNDERSTAND?—cont'd

2. Most cells express plasma membrane pattern recognition receptors (PRRs) that recognize molecules produced by infectious microorganisms (pathogen-associated molecular patterns, or PAMPs), or products of cellular damage (damage-associated molecular patterns, or DAMPs).

Cellular Products

1. The cells of the innate immune system secrete many biochemical mediators (cytokines) that are responsible for activating other cells; these cytokines include interleukins, chemokines, interferons, and other molecules.
2. The most important proinflammatory cytokines are interleukin-1 (IL-1), interleukin-6 (IL-6), and tumor necrosis factor-alpha (TNF-α).
3. Interferons are produced by cells that are infected by viruses. Once released from infected cells, interferons can stimulate neighboring healthy cells to produce substances that prevent viral infection.
4. Chemokines are synthesized by a number of different cells and induce leukocyte chemotaxis.

Mast Cell

1. The most important activator of the inflammatory response is the mast cell, which initiates inflammation by releasing biochemical mediators (histamine, chemotactic factors) from preformed cytoplasmic granules and synthesizing other mediators (prostaglandins, leukotrienes) in response to a stimulus.
2. Histamine is the major vasoactive amine released from mast cells. It causes dilation of capillaries and retraction of endothelial cells lining the capillaries, which increases vascular permeability.

Endothelium and Platelets

1. The endothelial cells lining the circulatory system (vascular endothelium) normally regulate circulating components of the inflammatory system and maintain normal blood flow by preventing spontaneous activation of platelets and members of the clotting system.
2. During inflammation the endothelium expresses receptors that help leukocytes leave the vessel and retract to allow fluid to pass into the tissues.
3. Platelets interact with the coagulation cascade to stop bleeding and release a number of mediators that promote and control inflammation.

Phagocytes

1. The polymorphonuclear neutrophil (PMN), the predominant phagocytic cell in the early inflammatory response, exits the circulation by diapedesis through the retracted endothelial cell junctions and moves to the inflammatory site by chemotaxis.
2. Eosinophils release products that control the inflammatory response and are the principal cell that kills parasitic organisms.
3. The macrophage, the predominant phagocytic cell in the late inflammatory response, is highly phagocytic, responsive to cytokines, and promotes wound healing.
4. Dendritic cells connect the innate and acquired immune systems by collecting antigens at the site of inflammation and transporting them to sites, such as the lymph nodes, where immunocompetent B and T cells reside.
5. Phagocytosis is a multistep cellular process for the elimination of pathogens and foreign debris. The steps include recognition and attachment, engulfment, formation of a phagosome and phagolysosome, and destruction of pathogens or foreign debris. Phagocytic cells engulf microorganisms and enclose them in phagocytic vacuoles (phagolysosomes), within which toxic products (especially metabolites of oxygen) and degradative lysosomal enzymes kill and digest the microorganisms.

6. Opsonins, such as antibody and complement component C3b, coat microorganisms and make them more susceptible to phagocytosis by binding them more tightly to the phagocyte.

Local Manifestations of Acute Inflammation

1. Local manifestations of inflammation are the result of the vascular changes associated with the inflammatory process, including vasodilation and increased capillary permeability. The symptoms include redness, heat, swelling, and pain.

Systemic Manifestations of Acute Inflammation

1. The principal systemic effects of inflammation are fever and increases in levels of circulating leukocytes (leukocytosis) and plasma proteins (acute-phase reactants).

Chronic Inflammation

1. Chronic inflammation can be a continuation of acute inflammation that lasts 2 weeks or longer. It also can occur as a distinct process without much preceding acute inflammation.
2. Chronic inflammation is characterized by a dense infiltration of lymphocytes and macrophages. The body may wall off and isolate the infection to protect against tissue damage by formation of a granuloma.

Wound Healing

1. Resolution (regeneration) is the return of tissue to nearly normal structure and function. Repair is healing by scar tissue formation.
2. Damaged tissue proceeds to resolution (restoration of the original tissue structure and function) if little tissue has been lost or injured tissue is capable of regeneration. This is called healing by primary intention.
3. Tissues that sustained extensive damage or those incapable of regeneration heal by the process of repair resulting in the formation of a scar. This is called healing by secondary intention.
4. Resolution and repair occur in two separate phases: the reconstructive phase in which the wound begins to heal and the maturation phase in which the healed wound is remodeled.
5. Dysfunctional wound healing can be related to ischemia, excessive bleeding, excessive fibrin deposition, a predisposing disorder (such as diabetes mellitus), wound infection, inadequate nutrients, numerous drugs, or altered collagen synthesis.
6. Dehiscence is a disruption in which the wound pulls apart at the suture line.
7. A contracture is a deformity caused by the excessive shortening of collagen in scar tissue.

PEDIATRIC CONSIDERATIONS: Age-Related Factors Affecting Innate Immunity in the Newborn Child

1. Neonates often have transiently depressed inflammatory function, particularly neutrophil chemotaxis and alternative complement pathway activity.

GERIATRIC CONSIDERATIONS: Age-Related Factors Affecting Innate Immunity in the Elderly

1. Elderly persons are at risk for impaired wound healing, usually because of chronic illnesses.

KEY TERMS

- Abscess 132
- Acute inflammation 132
- Acute-phase reactant 133
- Adaptive immunity 118
- Alternative pathway 124
- Anaphylatoxin 123
- Angiogenesis factor 135
- Antimicrobial peptide 119
- α_1-Antitrypsin 132
- Basophil 127
- Blood clot 124
- Bradykinin 124
- C1 esterase inhibitor (C1-inh) 124
- C1-inh deficiency 124
- Carboxypeptidase 124
- Cathelicidin 119
- Chemokine 127
- Chemotactic factor 123
- Chemotaxis 131
- Chronic inflammation 133
- Classical pathway 123
- Clotting (coagulation) system 124
- Collagen 136
- Collectin 119
- Complement receptor 125
- Complement system 122
- Contact activation (intrinsic) pathway 124
- Contraction 134
- Contracture of scar tissue 137
- Cyst 132
- Cytokine 125
- Damage-associated molecular pattern (DAMP) 125
- Defensin 119
- Degranulation 127
- Dehiscence 137
- Dendritic cell 131
- Diapedesis 131
- Endogenous pyrogen 132
- Endothelial cell 129
- Eosinophil 131
- Eosinophil chemotactic factor of anaphylaxis (ECF-A) 127

- Epithelialization 134
- Epithelioid cell 134
- Exudate 132
- Fc receptor 132
- Fever 132
- Fibrinolytic system 124
- Fibrinous exudate 132
- Fibroblast 136
- Giant cell 134
- Granulation tissue 135
- Granuloma 134
- Hageman factor (factor XII) 124
- Hemorrhagic exudate 132
- Hereditary angioedema 124
- Hexose-monophosphate shunt 132
- Histaminase 124
- Histamine 127
- Hypertrophic scar 137
- Inflammation 121
- Inflammatory phase 135
- Inflammatory response 118
- Innate immunity 118
- Interferon (IFN) 127
- Interleukin (IL) 126
- Interleukin-1 (IL-1) 126
- Interleukin-6 (IL-6) 126
- Interleukin-10 (IL-10) 127
- Keloid 137
- Kinin system 124
- Lectin pathway 124
- Leukocytosis 132
- Leukotriene (slow-reacting substance of anaphylaxis [SRS-A]) 129
- Lymphocyte 125
- Lysozyme 119
- Macrophage 129
- Mannose-binding lectin (MBL) 119
- Margination (pavementing) 131
- Mast cell 127
- Matrix metalloproteinase (MMP) 135
- Monocyte 129
- Myofibroblast 136
- Neutrophil (polymorphonuclear neutrophil [PMN]) 129

- Neutrophil chemotactic factor (NCF) 127
- Nitric oxide (NO) 129
- Normal flora 120
- Opportunistic microorganism 120
- Opsonin 123
- Opsonization 131
- Pathogen-associated molecular pattern (PAMP) 125
- Pattern recognition receptor (PRR) 125
- Phagocyte 131
- Phagocytosis 131
- Phagolysosome 132
- Phagosome 132
- Plasma protein system 122
- Plasmin 124
- Plasminogen 124
- Platelet 129
- Platelet-activating factor (PAF) 129
- Primary intention 134
- Proliferative phase 135
- Prostacyclin (PGI$_2$) 129
- Prostaglandin 129
- Purulent (suppurative) exudate 132
- Pyrogen 132
- Regeneration 134
- Repair 134
- Resolution 134
- Scar tissue 134
- Secondary intention 134
- Serous exudate 132
- T lymphocyte 131
- Tissue factor (extrinsic) pathway 124
- Tissue factor (TF; tissue thromboplastin) 124
- Toll-like receptor (TLR) 125
- Transforming growth factor 127
- Transforming growth factor-beta (TGF-β) 127
- Tumor necrosis factor-alpha (TNF-α) 126
- Wound contraction 136

REFERENCES

1. Turvey SE, Broide DH: Innate immunity, *J Allergy Clin Immunol* 125(2):S24–S32, 2010.
2. Rock KL, et al: The sterile inflammatory response, *Annu Rev Immunol* 28(1):321–342, 2010.
3. Guani-Guerr E, et al: Antimicrobial peptides: general overview and clinical implications in human health and disease, *Clin Immunol* 135(1):1–11, 2010.
4. Stowell SR, et al: Innate immune lectins kill bacteria expressing blood group antigen, *Nat Med* 16(3):295–302, 2010.
5. Lebeer S, Vanderleyden J, De Keersmaecker SCJ: Host interactions of probiotic bacterial surface molecules: comparison with commensals and pathogens, *Nat Rev Microbiol* 8(3):171–184, 2010.
6. Clarke TB, et al: Recognition of peptidoglycan from the microbiota by Nod1 enhances systemic innate immunity, *Nat Med* 16(2):228–232, 2010.
7. Hand T, Belkaid Y: Microbial control of regulatory and effector T cell responses in the gut, *Curr Opin Immunol* 22(1):63–72, 2010.
8. Medzhitov R: Inflammation: new adventures of an old flame, *Cell* 140(6):771–776, 2010.
9. Dunkelberger JR, Song W-C: Complement and its role in innate and adaptive immune responses, *Cell Res* 20(1):34–50, 2010.
10. Sacks SH: Complement fragments C3a and C5a: the salt and pepper of the immune response, *Eur J Immunol* 40(3):668–670, 2010.
11. Levi M, van der Poll T: Inflammation and coagulation, *Crit Care Med* 38(suppl 2):S26–S34, 2010.
12. Levi M: The coagulation response in sepsis and inflammation, *Hämostaseologie* 30(1):10–16, 2010.

13. Stavrou E, Schmaier AH: Factor X II: what does it contribute to our understanding of the physiology and pathophysiology of hemostasis & thrombosis? *Thromb Res* 125(3):210–215, 2010.

14. Chinen J, Shearer WT: Advances in basic and clinical immunology in 2009, *J Allergy Clin Immunol* 125(3):563–568, 2010.

15. Takeuchi O, Akira S: Pattern recognition receptors and inflammation, *Cell* 140(6):805–820, 2010.

16. Blasius AL, Beutler B: Intracellular Toll-like receptors, *Immunity* 32(3):305–315, 2010.

17. Commins SP, Borish L, Steinke JW: Immunologic messenger molecules: cytokines, interferons, and chemokines, *J Allergy Clin Immunol* 125(2):S53–S72, 2010.

18. Nishimoto N: Interleukin-6 as a therapeutic target in candidate inflammatory diseases, *Clin Pharm Ther* 87(4):483–487, 2010.

19. Dinarello CA: IL-1: discoveries, controversies and future directions, *Eur J Immunol* 40(3):595–653, 2010.

20. Mills KHG, Dunne A: IL-1, master mediator or initiator of inflammation? *Nat Med* 15(12):1363–1364, 2009.

21. Moon TC, et al: Advances in mast cell biology: new understanding of heterogeneity and function, *Mucosal Immunol* 3(2):111–128, 2010.

22. Sokol CL, Medzhitov R: Emerging functions of basophils in protective and allergic immune responses, *Mucosal Immunol* 3(2):129–137, 2010.

23. Jutel M, Akdis M, Akdis CA: Histamine, histamine receptors and their role in immune pathology, *Clin Exp Allergy* 39(12):1786–1800, 2009.

24. Stone KD, Prussin C, Metcalfe DD: IgE, mast cells, basophils, and eosinophils, *J Allergy Clin Immunol* 125(2):S73–S80, 2010.

25. Dinarello CA: Anti-inflammatory agents: present and future, *Cell* 140(6):935–950, 2010.

26. Semple JW, Freedman J: Platelets and innate immunity, *Cell Mol Life Sci* 67(4):499–511, 2010.

27. Soehnlein O, Lindborn L, Weber C: Mechanisms underlying neutrophil-mediated monocyte recruitment, *Blood* 114(21):4613–4623, 2009.

28. Soehnlein O, Lindborn L: Phagocyte partnership during the onset and resolution of inflammation, *Nat Rev Immunol* 10(6):427–439, 2010.

29. Rodero MP, Khosrotehrani K: Skin wound healing modulation by macrophages, *Int J Clin Exp Pathol* 3(7):643–653, 2010.

30. Novak N, et al: Dendritic cells: bridging innate and adaptive immunity in atopic dermatitis, *J Allergy Clin Immunol* 125(1):50–59, 2010.

31. Jung S: Dendritic cells: a question of upbringing, *Immunity* 32(4):502–504, 2010.

32. Havran WL, Jameson JM: Epidermal T cells and wound healing, *J Immunol* 184(10):5423–5428, 2010.

33. Toulon A, et al: A role for human skin-resident T cells in wound healing, *J Exp Med* 206(4):743–750, 2009.

34. Muller WA: Mechanisms of transendothelial migration of leukocytes, *Circ Res* 105(3):223–230, 2009.

35. Nathan C, Ding A: Nonresolving inflammation, *Cell* 140(6):871–882, 2010.

36. Teller P, White TK: The physiology of wound healing: injury through maturation, *Surg Clin North Am* 89(3):599–610, 2009.

37. Guo S, Dipietro LA: Factors affecting wound healing, *J Dent Res* 89(3):219–229, 2010.

38. Olmedo JM, et al: Scurvy: a disease almost forgotten, *Int J Dermatol* 245(8):909–913, 2006.

39. Kavalukas SL, Barbul A: Nutrition and wound healing: an update, *Plast Reconstr Surg* 127(Suppl 1):38S–43S, 2011.

40. Vuolteenaho K, Moilanen T, Moilanen E: Non-steroidal anti-inflammatory drugs, cyclooxygenase-2 and the bone healing process, *Basic Clin Pharmacol Toxicol* 102(1):10–14, 2008.

41. Kean J: The effects of smoking on the wound healing process, *J Wound Care* 19(1):5–8, 2010.

42. Juckett G, Hartman-Adams H: Management of keloids and hypertrophic scars, *Am Fam Physician* 80(3):253–260, 2009.

Adaptive Immunity

Neal S. Rote

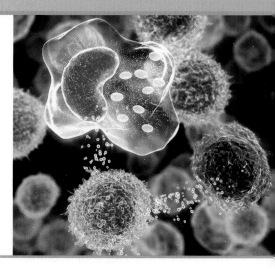

CHAPTER OUTLINE

The third line of defense in the human body is adaptive (acquired) immunity, often called the immune response or immunity. Once external barriers have been compromised and inflammation (innate immunity, see Chapter 5) has been activated, the adaptive immune response is called into action.

It develops more slowly than the inflammatory response and is specific (compared to inflammation that is nonspecific) and has memory. Adaptive immunity serves two purposes: destroying infectious microorganisms that are resistant to inflammation and providing long-term highly effective protection against future exposure to the same microorganism.

Genetic or acquired deficiencies in components of the innate or adaptive immune systems may prevent an effective protective response. Many of these defects are discussed in Chapter 7.

THIRD LINE OF DEFENSE: ADAPTIVE IMMUNITY

The third line of defense is adaptive (acquired) immunity, often called the immune response.[1] It is *inducible* (must recognize the pathogen as foreign or "nonself") and thus develops more slowly than the inflammatory response. The immune response is also

specific (among many pathogens a unique pathogen is identified and eliminated) and has memory, conferring a permanent or long-term protection against specific microorganisms. Many components of innate resistance are necessary for the development of the adaptive immune response. Conversely, products of the adaptive immune response activate components of innate resistance. Thus, both systems are essential for complete protection against infectious disease.

The immune system is capable of identifying substances that are foreign, or *nonself*. In general, substances that react with molecules of the immune system (antibodies, receptors on B and T cells) are called antigens. Antigens are on infectious agents (e.g., viruses, bacteria, fungi, or parasites), on noninfectious substances from the environment (e.g., pollens, foods, or bee venoms), or on drugs, vaccines, transfusions, and transplanted tissues (Table 6-1).

The products of the adaptive immune response include a type of serum protein—immunoglobulins (Ig) or antibodies—and a type of blood cell—lymphocytes (Figure 6-1). Before birth, humans produce a large population of T lymphocytes (T cells, T indicates thymus) and B lymphocytes (B cells, B indicates bone marrow derived) that have the capacity to recognize almost any foreign antigen found

TABLE 6-1 CLINICAL USE OF ANTIGEN OR ANTIBODY

	USE OF ANTIGEN OR ANTIBODY			
ANTIGEN SOURCE	PROTECTION: COMBAT ACTIVE DISEASE	PROTECTION: VACCINATION	DIAGNOSIS	THERAPY
Infectious agents	Neutralize or destroy pathogenic microorganisms (e.g., antibody response against viral infections)	Induce safe and protective immune response (e.g., recommended childhood vaccines)	Measure circulating antigen from infectious agent or antibody (e.g., diagnosis of hepatitis B infection)	Passive treatment with antibody to treat or prevent infection (e.g., administration of antibody against hepatitis A)
Cancers	Prevent tumor growth or spread (e.g., immune surveillance to prevent early cancers)	Prevent cancer growth or spread (e.g., vaccination with cancer antigens)	Measure circulating antigen (e.g., circulating PSA for diagnosis of prostate cancer)	Immunotherapy (e.g., treatment of cancer with antibodies against cancer antigens)
Environmental substances	Prevent entrance into body (e.g., secretory IgA limits systemic exposure to potential allergens)	No clear example	Measure circulating antigen or antibody (e.g., diagnosis of allergy by measuring circulating IgE)	Immunotherapy (e.g., administration of antigen for desensitization of individuals with severe allergies)
Self-antigens	Immune system tolerance to self-antigens, which may be altered by an infectious agent leading to autoimmune disease (see Chapter 7)	Some cases of vaccination alter tolerance to self-antigens, leading to autoimmune disease	Measure circulating antibody against self-antigen for diagnosis of autoimmune disease (see Chapter 7)	Oral administration of self-antigens to diminish production of autoimmune disease associated autoantibodies

PSA, Prostate-specific antigen.

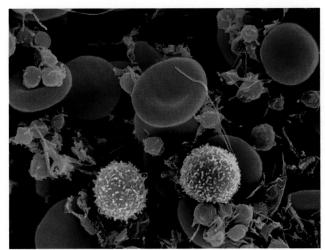

FIGURE 6-1 Lymphocytes. A scanning electron micrograph showing lymphocytes (yellow, like cotton candy), red blood cells, and platelets. (Copyright Dennis Kunkel Microscopy, Inc.)

in the environment. Each individual T or B cell, however, specifically recognizes only one particular antigen, but the sum of the population of lymphocyte specificities may represent millions of foreign antigens. This process is called the generation of *clonal diversity* and occurs in specialized (primary) lymphoid organs (see Figure 6-3). While passing through these organs, the lymphocytes mature and undergo changes that commit them to either B or T cells. Lymphocytes are released from these organs into the circulation as immature cells that react with antigens (**immunocompetent**). These cells migrate to other (secondary) lymphoid organs in the body in preparation for exposure to antigens (Figure 6-2).

The lymphocytes remain dormant until antigen initiates the second phase of the immune response, *clonal selection* (see Figure 6-3). This process involves a complex interaction among cells, discussed further in the section titled Immune Response: Collaboration of B Cells and T Cells.

Humoral and Cellular Immunity

Adaptive immunity or the immune response has two components: antibodies and T cells, both of which protect against infection (Figure 6-3).[2] Antibodies are proteins that are produced by B cells, circulate in the blood, and bind to antigens on infectious agents. This interaction can result in direct inactivation of the microorganism or activation of a variety of inflammatory mediators that will destroy the pathogen. Antibodies are primarily responsible for protection against many bacteria and viruses. This arm of the immune response is termed **humoral immunity.**

T cells are a subset of lymphocytes that undergo differentiation during an immune response and develop into several subpopulations of *effector T cells* that have an effect on many other cells. Some develop into **T-cytotoxic (Tc) cells** that attack and kill targets directly. Targets for Tc cells include cells infected by viruses, as well as cells that have become cancerous. Others may develop into T cells that can stimulate the activities of other leukocytes through cell-to-cell contact or through the secretion of cytokines. This arm of the immune response is termed **cellular,** or cell-mediated, **immunity.**

The success of an acquired immune response depends on the functions of both the humoral and cellular responses, as well as the appropriate interactions between them. The collaboration between B cells and a subset of T cells (T-helper cells, Th cells) is essential for almost all antibody responses to antigens. Additionally, both arms produce specialized subpopulations of **memory cells,** which are capable of *remembering* the specific antigen and responding more rapidly and efficiently against future infections.

Active and Passive Immunity

Adaptive immunity can be either active or passive, depending on whether the antibodies or T cells are produced by the individual in response to antigens or are administered directly to the individual. **Active acquired immunity (active immunity)** is produced by an individual either after natural exposure to antigens or after immunization, whereas **passive acquired immunity (passive immunity)** does not involve the host's immune response at all. Rather, passive immunity occurs when preformed antibodies or T cells are transferred from

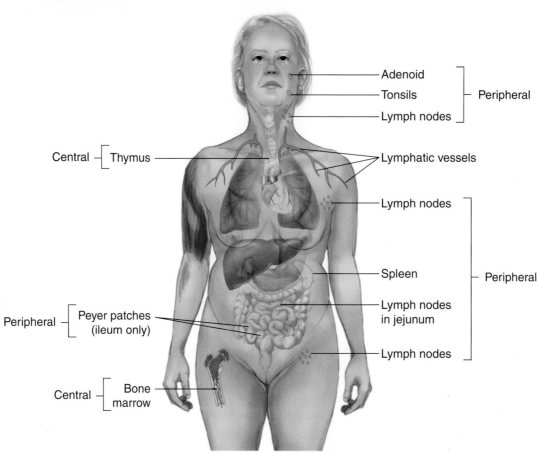

FIGURE 6-2 Lymphoid Tissues: Sites of B Cell and T Cell Differentiation. Immature lymphocytes migrate through central (primary) lymphoid tissues: the bone marrow (central lymphoid tissue for B lymphocytes) and the thymus (central lymphoid tissue for T lymphocytes). Mature lymphocytes later reside in the T and B lymphocyte–rich areas of the peripheral (secondary) lymphoid tissues.

a donor to the recipient. This can occur naturally, as during pregnancy when maternal antibodies cross the placenta to the fetus, or artificially, as when antibodies are injected to fight against a specific disease.[3,4] For instance, unvaccinated individuals who are exposed to particular infectious agents (e.g., hepatitis A virus, rabies virus) often will be given immune globulins, which are prepared from individuals who already have antibodies against that particular pathogen. Whereas active acquired immunity is long lived, passive immunity is only temporary because the donor's antibodies or T cells are eventually destroyed.

ANTIGENS AND IMMUNOGENS

Although the terms *antigen* and *immunogen* are commonly used as synonyms, there are important differences between the two. Whereas an **antigen,** a molecule or molecular fragment (i.e., proteins or carbohydrates), can *bind with* antibodies or antigen receptors on B and T cells, a molecule that will *induce* an immune response is an **immunogen.** Thus all immunogens are antigens but not all antigens are immunogens and some clinically important conditions arise when particular antigens are not immunogenic. For example, urushiol is a toxin found in poison ivy and is a very small antigen (called a hapten) but not immunogenic. Several of these types of conditions will be discussed in Chapter 7.

Certain criteria influence the degree to which an antigen is immunogenic. These include (1) foreignness to the host, (2) adequate size, and (3) being present in a sufficient quantity. These criteria are important for development of vaccines, which must be highly immunogenic to produce protective immune responses against pathogenic microorganisms.

Foremost among the criteria for immunogenicity is the antigen's foreignness. A *self-antigen* that fulfills all the criteria listed previously *except* foreignness does not normally elicit an immune response. Thus, most individuals are *tolerant* to their own antigens. Some pathogens are successful because they develop the capacity to mimic self-antigens and avoid inducing an immune response. In Chapter 7 we discuss specific diseases resulting from a breakdown of tolerance that leads to an individual's immune system attacking its own antigens (autoimmune diseases).

Molecular size also contributes to an antigen's immunogenicity. In general, large molecules (those bigger than 10,000 daltons), such as proteins, polysaccharides, and nucleic acids, are most immunogenic. Many low-molecular-weight molecules can function as **haptens,** antigens that are too small to be immunogens by themselves but become immunogenic after combining with larger molecules that function as carriers for the hapten. For example, the antigens of poison ivy are haptens, but they initiate allergic responses in individuals after binding to large-molecular-weight proteins in the skin. Antigens that induce an allergic response are also called **allergens.**

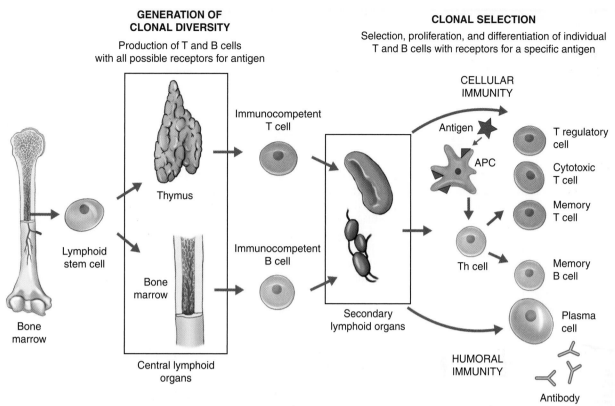

GENERATION OF CLONAL DIVERSITY

Production of T and B cells with all possible receptors for antigen

CLONAL SELECTION

Selection, proliferation, and differentiation of individual T and B cells with receptors for a specific antigen

FIGURE 6-3 Overview of the Immune Response. The immune response can be separated into two phases: the *generation of clonal diversity* and *clonal selection.* During the generation of clonal diversity, lymphoid stem cells from the bone marrow migrate to the central lymphoid organs (the thymus or regions of the bone marrow), where they undergo a series of cellular division and differentiation stages resulting in either immunocompetent T cells from the thymus or immunocompetent B cells from the bone marrow. These cells are still naïve in that they have never encountered foreign antigen. The immunocompetent cells enter the circulation and migrate to the secondary lymphoid organs (e.g., spleen and lymph nodes), where they establish residence in B and T cell–rich areas. The clonal selection phase is initiated by exposure to foreign antigen. The antigen is usually processed by antigen-presenting cells (APCs) for presentation to T-helper cells (Th cells). The intercellular cooperation among APCs, Th cells, and immunocompetent T and B cells results in a second stage of cellular proliferation and differentiation. Because antigen has "selected" those T and B cells with compatible antigen receptors, only a small population of T and B cells undergo this process at one time. The result is an active cellular immunity or humoral immunity, or both. Cellular immunity is mediated by a population of *effector* T cells that can kill targets (T-cytotoxic cells) or regulate the immune response (T-regulatory cells), as well as a population of memory cells (T-memory cells) that can respond more quickly to a second challenge with the same antigen. Humoral immunity is mediated by a population of soluble proteins (antibodies) produced by plasma cells and by a population of memory B cells that can produce more antibody rapidly to a second challenge with the same antigen.

Finally, antigens that are present in extremely small or large quantities may be unable to elicit an immune response. In many cases, high or low extremes of antigen quantities may induce a state of tolerance rather than immunity.

Even if an antigen fulfills all these criteria, the quality and intensity of the immune response may still be affected by a variety of additional factors. For example, the route of antigen entry or administration is critical to the immunogenicity of some antigens. This has important clinical implications. The most common routes for clinical administration of antigens are intravenous, intraperitoneal, subcutaneous, intranasal, and oral. Each route preferentially stimulates a different set of lymphocyte-containing (lymphoid) tissues and therefore results in the induction of different types of cell-mediated or humoral immune responses. For some vaccines, the route may affect the protectiveness of the immune response so that the individual is protected if immunized by one route, but may be less protected if administered through a different route (e.g., oral versus injected polio vaccines, discussed later in this chapter under Secretory Immune System). Immunogenicity of an antigen also may be altered by being delivered along with substances that stimulate the immune response; these substances are known as adjuvants. Finally, the genetic makeup of the individual can play a critical role in the immune system's ability to respond to many antigens. Some individuals appear to be unable to respond to immunization with a particular antigen, whereas they respond well to other antigens. For instance, a small percentage of the population may fail to produce a measurable immune response to a common vaccine, despite multiple injections. An individual's immune response can also be affected by age, nutritional status, genetic background, and reproductive status, as well as exposure to traumatic injury, concurrent disease, or the use of immunosuppressive medications.

HUMORAL IMMUNE RESPONSE

Antibodies

An antibody, or immunoglobulin (Ig), is a serum glycoprotein produced by plasma cells that mature from lymphocytes, called B lymphocytes (B cells), in response to an antigen.[5] Although B cells develop in the bone marrow of humans, a discrete organ (bursa of Fabricius) for B cell maturation was originally discovered in chickens, resulting in the term B cell. The term immunoglobulin (Ig) is generally used for all antibodies, whereas the term antibody is mostly used to denote one particular set of immunoglobulins known to have specificity for a particular antigen. There are five classes of immunoglobulins (IgG, IgA, IgM, IgE, and IgD), which are characterized by differences in structure and function (Table 6-2 and Figure 6-4). Within two of the immunoglobulin classes are several distinct subclasses: four subclasses of IgG and two subclasses of IgA.

Classes of Immunoglobulins

IgG is the most abundant class of immunoglobulins, constituting 80% to 85% of the immunoglobulins in the blood and accounting for most of the protective activity against infections. As a result of selective transport across the placenta, maternal IgG is the major class of antibody found in blood of the fetus and newborn. Four subclasses of IgG have been described: IgG1, IgG2, IgG3, and IgG4.

IgA has two subclasses: IgA1 and IgA2. IgA1 is found predominantly in the blood, whereas IgA2 is the predominant class found in body secretions (secretory IgA). Secretory IgA is a *dimer* (a molecule consisting of two identical smaller molecules) of two IgA molecules held together through a J chain and secretory piece. The secretory piece is attached to IgA inside mucosal epithelial cells to protect these immunoglobulins against degradation by enzymes also found in secretions.

IgM is the largest immunoglobulin and usually exists as a pentamer (a molecule consisting of five identical smaller molecules) that is stabilized by a J chain. It is the first antibody produced during the initial, or

TABLE 6-2   PROPERTIES OF IMMUNOGLOBULINS

CLASS	SUBCLASS	ADULT SERUM LEVELS (mg/dl)	PRESENT IN SECRETIONS	COMPLEMENT ACTIVATION	OPSONIN	AGGLUTININ	MAST CELL ACTIVATION	PLACENTAL TRANSFER
IgG	IgG1	800–900	+	++	++	+	–	+++
	IgG2	280–300	+	+	–	+	–	+
	IgG3	90–100	+	+++	++	+	–	+++
	IgG4	50	–	–	–	+	+	++
IgM		120–150	+	++++	–	++++	–	–
IgA	IgA1	280–300	+	–	–	+	–	–
	IgA2	50	+	–	–	+	–	–
	sIgA	5	++++	–	–	+	–	–
IgD		3	–	–	–	–	–	–
IgE		0.03	+	–	–	–	+++	–

sIgA, Secretory immunoglobulin A; – indicates lack of activity; + to ++++ indicate relative activity or concentration.

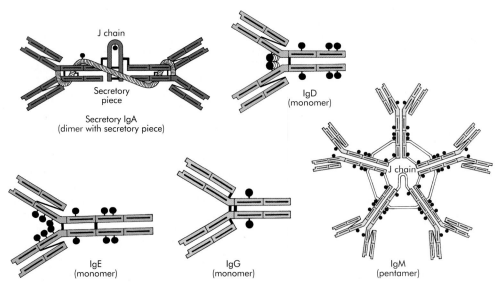

FIGURE 6-4 Structure of Different Immunoglobulins. Secretory IgA, IgD, IgE, IgG, and IgM. The black circles attached to each molecule represent carbohydrate residues.

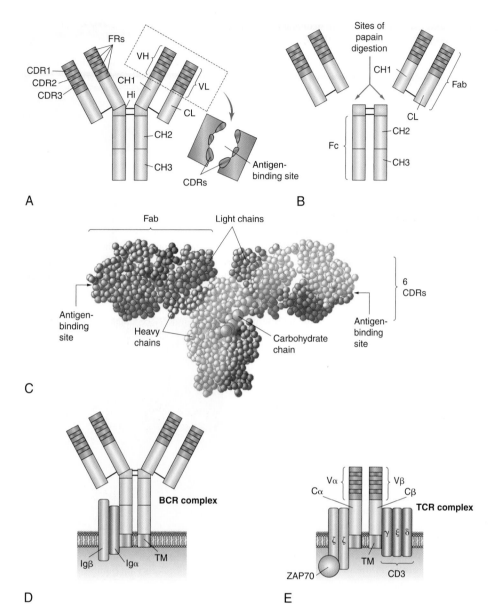

FIGURE 6-5 Molecular Structure of an Antibody and Other Antigen-Binding Molecules. Antigen-binding molecules include antibody and cell-surface receptors. **A,** The typical antibody molecule consists of two identical heavy chains and two identical light chains connected by interchain disulfide bonds (— between chains in the figure). Each heavy chain is divided into three regions with relatively constant amino acid sequences (CH1, CH2, and CH3) and a region with a variable amino acid sequence (VH). Each light chain is divided into a constant region (CL) and a variable region (VL). The hinge region (Hi) provides flexibility in some classes of antibody. Within each variable region are three highly variable complementary-determining regions (CDR1, CDR2, CDR3) separated by relatively constant framework regions (FRs). **B,** Fragmentation of the antibody molecule by limited digestion with the enzyme papain has identified three important portions of the molecule: an Fc fragment (crystalline fragment that binds complement and Fc receptors) and two identical Fab fragments (antigen-binding fragments). **C,** A molecular model of a typical antibody molecule; the light chains are the strands of red spheres (each represents an individual amino acid). As the antibody folds, the CDRs are placed in proximity to form the antigen-binding site. **D,** The antigen receptor on the surface of B cells (BCR complex) is a monomeric antibody with a structure similar to that of circulating antibody, with an additional transmembrane region (TM) that anchors the molecule to the cell surface. The active BCR complex contains molecules (Igα and Igβ) that are responsible for intracellular signaling after the receptor has bound antigen. **E,** The T cell receptor (TCR) consists of an α and a β chain joined by a disulfide bond. Each chain consists of a constant region (Cα and Cβ) and a variable region (Vα and Vβ). Each variable region contains CDRs and FRs in a structure similar to that of antibody. The active TCR is associated with several molecules that are responsible for intracellular signaling. These include CD3, which is a complex of γ (gamma), ε (epsilon), and δ (delta) subunits and a complex of two ζ (zeta) molecules. The ζ molecules are attached to a cytoplasmic protein kinase (ZAP70) that is critical to intracellular signaling.

primary, response to antigens. IgM is synthesized early in neonatal life, and its synthesis may be increased as a response to infection in utero.

IgD is found in low concentrations in the blood. Its primary function is as an antigen receptor on the surface of early B cells.

IgE is normally at low concentrations in the circulation. It has very specialized functions as a mediator of many common allergic responses (see Chapter 7) and in the defense against parasitic infections.

Molecular Structure

The parts of an antibody molecule were named based on studies using the enzyme papain to digest IgG. Three fragments resulted, two of which were identical (Figure 6-5). The two identical fragments retained the ability to bind antigen and were termed antigen-binding fragments (Fab).[5] The third fragment crystallized and was termed the crystalline fragment (Fc). The Fab portions contain the recognition sites (receptors) for antigens and confer the molecule's specificity toward a particular antigen. The Fc portion is responsible for most of the biologic functions of antibodies.

An immunoglobulin molecule consists of four polypeptide chains: two identical light (L) chains and two identical heavy (H) chains. The class of antibody is determined by which heavy chain is used: gamma (γ, IgG), mu (μ, IgM), alpha (α, IgA), epsilon (ε, IgE), or delta (δ, IgD). The light chains of an antibody molecule are of either the kappa (κ) or the lambda (λ) type. The light and heavy chains are held together by noncovalent bonds and covalent disulfide linkages. A set of disulfide linkages between the heavy chains occurs in the hinge region and, in some instances, lends a degree of flexibility at that site. An individual plasma cell produces only one type of H chain and one type of L chain at a time; for instance, one plasma cell may produce only IgGκ, whereas other plasma cells will be producing other classes of antibody or the same class with the λ light chain.

Each L and H chain is further subdivided structurally into constant (C) and variable (V) regions. The constant regions have relatively stable amino acid sequences within a particular immunoglobulin class or subclass. Thus, the amino acid sequence of the constant region of one IgG1 should be almost identical with the sequence of the same region of another IgG1, even if they react with different antigens. Conversely, among different antibodies, the sequences of the variable regions are characterized by a large number of amino acid differences. Therefore, two IgG1 molecules against different antigens will have many differences in the amino acid sequence of their variable regions. The amino acid differences are clustered into three areas in the variable region. These three areas were once called *hypervariable regions* but are now called complementary-determining regions (CDRs) (see Figure 6-5, *A*). The four regions surrounding the CDRs have relatively stable amino acid sequences and are called framework regions (FRs).

Antigen-Antibody Binding

Because antigens are relative small, a large molecule (e.g., protein, polysaccharide, nucleic acid) usually contains multiple and diverse antigens. The precise area of the molecule that is recognized by an antibody is called its antigenic determinant, or epitope (Figure 6-6). The matching portion on the antibody is sometimes referred to as the antigen-binding site, or paratope. The size of an antigenic determinant is generally only a few amino acids or sugar residues.

The antigen-binding site is formed by folding of an antibody molecule so that the CDRs of the variable regions of both the heavy (V_H) and the light (V_L) chains are moved into close proximity, resulting in an antigen-binding site that is lined by the three CDRs of the heavy chain and the three CDRs of the light chain (see Figure 6-5, *C*).[5] The antibody's specificity toward a particular antigen is determined by the

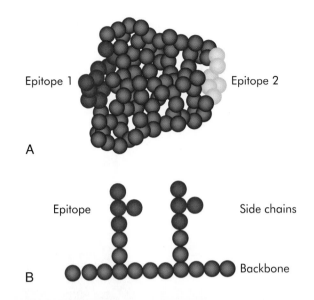

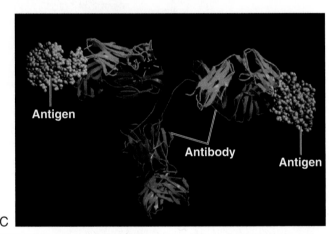

FIGURE 6-6 **Antigenic Determinants (Epitopes).** Generic examples of epitopes on protein (**A**) and polysaccharide (**B**) molecules are shown. In **A**, an antigenic protein may have multiple different epitopes (epitopes 1 and 2) that react with different antibodies. Each sphere represents an amino acid with the red spheres representing epitope 1 and the yellow spheres representing epitope 2. Individual epitopes may consist of eight or nine amino acids. In **B**, a polysaccharide is constructed of a backbone with branched side chains. Each sphere represents an individual carbohydrate with the red spheres representing the carbohydrates that form the epitope. In this example, two identical epitopes are shown that would bind two identical antibodies. In **C**, this ribbon model of an antibody shows the heavy chains in blue and the light chains in red. Green represents antigen molecules bound to each antigen-binding site. (*C* from Patton KT, Thibodeau GA: *Anatomy & physiology,* ed 7, St Louis, 2010, Mosby.)

chemical nature of the particular amino acids in the CDRs and the shape of the binding site (see Figure 6-5, *A*). The antigen that will bind most strongly must have complementary chemistry and topography with the binding site formed by the antibody. The antigen fits into this binding site with the specificity of a key into a lock and is held there by noncovalent chemical interactions.

Because the heavy and light chains are identical within the same antibody molecule, the two binding sites are also identical and have specificity for the same antigen. The number of functional binding

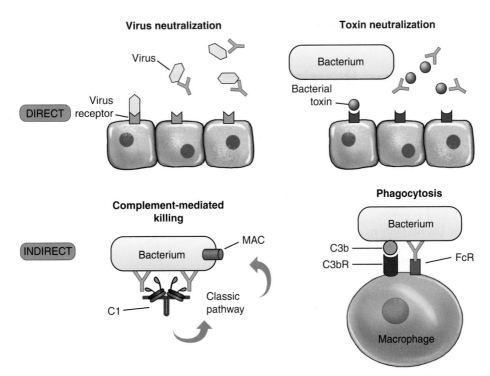

Virus neutralization

Toxin neutralization

DIRECT

INDIRECT

Complement-mediated killing

Phagocytosis

FIGURE 6-7 Direct and Indirect Functions of Antibody. Protective activities of antibodies can be direct (through the action of antibody alone) or indirect (requiring activation of other components of the innate immune response, usually through the Fc region). *Direct* means include neutralization of viruses or bacterial toxins before they bind to receptors on the surface of the host's cells. *Indirect* means include activation of the classical complement pathway through C1, resulting in formation of the membrane-attack complex (MAC), or increased phagocytosis of bacteria opsonized with antibody and complement components bound to appropriate surface receptors (FcR and C3bR).

sites on a molecule is called its valence. Most antibody classes (i.e., IgG, IgE, IgD, and circulating IgA) have a valence of 2, but secretory IgA has a valence of 4. IgM, being a pentamer, has a theoretic valence of 10, but it can simultaneously use only about five binding sites because antigen binding to one site blocks antigen binding to another site.

Function of Antibodies

The chief function of antibodies is to protect against infection. The mechanism can be either direct or indirect (Figure 6-7). Directly, antibodies can affect infectious agents or their toxic products by neutralization (inactivating or blocking the binding of antigens to receptors), agglutination (clumping insoluble particles that are in suspension), or precipitation (making a soluble antigen into an insoluble precipitate). Indirectly, antibodies activate components of innate resistance, including complement and phagocytes. Antibodies are generally a mixed population of classes, specificities, and capacity to provide the functions previously listed. It is now a common procedure to clone the "best" antibodies (monoclonal antibodies) for use in diagnostic tests and for therapy (Box 6-1).

Direct effects. Many pathogens initiate infection by attaching to specific receptors on cells. For instance, viruses that cause the common cold or the influenza virus must attach to specific receptors on respiratory epithelial cells. Some bacteria, such as *Neisseria gonorrhoeae* that causes gonorrhea, must attach to specific sites on urogenital epithelial cells. Antibodies may protect the host by covering sites on the microorganism that are needed for attachment, thereby preventing infection. Many viral infections can be prevented by vaccination with inactivated or attenuated (weakened) viruses to induce neutralizing antibody production at the site of the entrance of the virus into the body.

BOX 6-1 MONOCLONAL ANTIBODIES

Most humoral immune responses are polyclonal—that is, a mixture of antibodies produced from multiple B lymphocytes. Most antigenic molecules have multiple antigenic determinants, each of which induces a different group of antibodies. Thus, a polyclonal response is a mixture of antibody classes, specificities, and function, some of which are more protective than others.

Monoclonal antibody is produced in the laboratory from one B cell that has been cloned; thus all the antibody is of the same class, specificity, and function. The advantages of monoclonal antibodies are that (1) a single antibody of known antigenic specificity is generated rather than a mixture of different antibodies; (2) monoclonal antibodies have a single, constant binding affinity; (3) monoclonal antibodies can be diluted to a constant titer (concentration in fluid) because the actual antibody concentration is known; and (4) the antibody can be easily purified. Thus, a highly concentrated antibody with optimal function has been used to develop extremely specific and sensitive laboratory tests (e.g., home and laboratory pregnancy tests) and therapies (e.g., for certain infectious diseases or several experimental therapies for cancer).

Some bacteria secrete toxins that harm individuals. For instance, specific bacterial toxins cause the symptoms of tetanus or diphtheria. Most toxins are proteins that bind to surface molecules on cells and damage those cells. Protective antibodies can bind to the toxins, prevent their interaction with host cells, and neutralize their biologic effects. Detection of the presence of an antibody response against a specific toxin (antibodies referred to as *antitoxins*) can aid in the diagnosis of diseases. For example, laboratory tests that detect antistreptolysin O can be useful in diagnosing group A streptococcal infections.

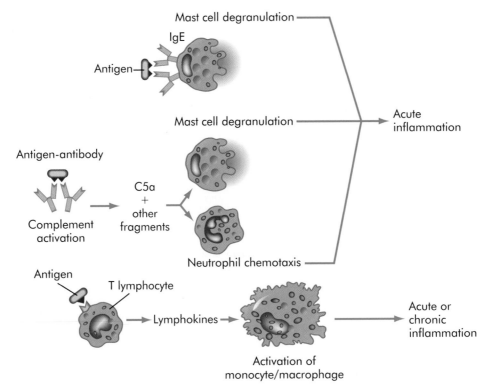

FIGURE 6-8 Immunologic Mechanisms That Activate the Inflammatory Response. Immunologic factors may activate inflammation through three mechanisms: (1) IgE can bind to the surface of a mast cell and, after binding antigen, induce the cell's degranulation; (2) antigen and antibody can activate the complement system, releasing anaphylatoxins and chemotactic factors, especially C5a, that result in mast cell degranulation and neutrophil chemotaxis; and (3) antigen may also react with T lymphocytes, resulting in the production of lymphokines that may contribute to the development of either acute or chronic inflammation.

Indirect effects. Antibodies are protective by interacting with or activating components of inflammation (Figure 6-8). The Fc portion is responsible for opsonic activity leading to enhanced phagocytosis and activation of the complement system that may lead to destruction of the pathogen or increased opsonic activity through deposition of C3b.

IgE. IgE is a special class of antibody that protects the individual from infection with large parasites. However, when IgE is produced against relatively innocuous environmental antigens, it is also the primary cause of common allergies (e.g., hay fever, dust allergies, bee stings). The role of IgE in allergies is discussed in Chapter 7.

Large multicellular parasites usually invade mucosal tissues. Many antigens from the parasites induce IgE, as well as other antibody classes. IgG, IgM, and IgA bind to the surface of parasites, activate complement, generate chemotactic factors for neutrophils and macrophages, and serve as opsonins for those phagocytic cells. This response, however, does not greatly damage parasites. The only inflammatory cell that can adequately damage a parasite is the eosinophil because of the special contents of its granules, particularly major basic protein.[6] Thus, IgE is designed to specifically initiate an inflammatory reaction that preferentially attracts eosinophils to the site of parasitic infection (Figure 6-9).

Mast cells in the tissues have Fc receptors that specifically and with high affinity bind IgE. IgEs against antigens of the parasite are rapidly bound to the mast cell surface. Soluble parasite antigens with multiple antigenic determinants diffuse to neighboring mast cells and simultaneously bind to multiple IgE molecules. This reaction initiates mast cell degranulation and secretion of eosinophil chemotactic factor of

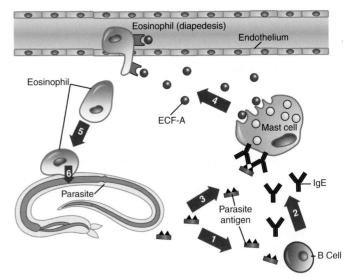

FIGURE 6-9 IgE Function. *(1)* Soluble antigens from a parasitic infection cause production of IgE antibody by B cells. *(2)* Secreted IgE binds to IgE-specific receptors on the mast cell. *(3)* Additional soluble parasite antigen cross-links the IgE on the mast cell surface, *(4)* leading to mast cell degranulation and release of many proinflammatory products, including eosinophil chemotactic factor of anaphylaxis (ECF-A). *(5)* ECF-A attracts eosinophils from the circulation. *(6)* The eosinophil attaches to the surface of the parasite and releases potent lysosomal enzymes that damage microorganisms.

anaphylaxis (ECF-A). ECF-A is specifically chemotactic for eosino-phils, resulting in eosinophil migration from the circulation into the tissues as well as increased expression of surface receptors for IgG and complement component C3b.[7] The eosinophil attaches to the surface of the parasite through these receptors and attempts phagocytosis.

Because of the extremely large size of typical parasites, engulfment is unsuccessful. The eosinophilic granules move to the cell membrane in contact with the parasite and undergo normal degranulation, releasing major basic protein and other antimicrobial peptides onto the para-site's surface. Being highly cationic, major basic protein acts almost

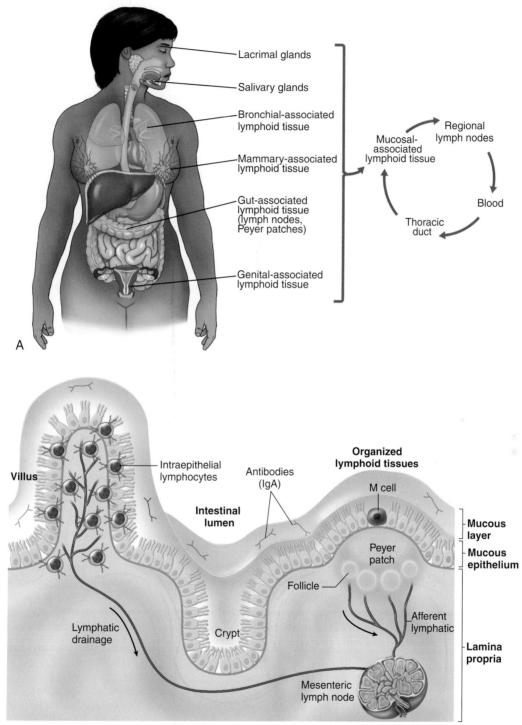

FIGURE 6-10 Secretory Immune System. A, Lymphocytes from the mucosal-associated lymphoid tissues circulate throughout the body in a pattern separate from other lymphocytes. For example, lymphocytes from the gut-associated lymphoid tissue circulate through the regional lymph nodes, the thoracic duct, and the blood and return to other mucosal-associated lymphoid tissues rather than to lymphoid tissue of the systemic immune system. **B,** Lymphoid tissue associated with mucous mem-branes is called mucosal-associated lymphoid tissue (MALT).

like sodium hydroxide and causes extensive damage to the parasite. The parasite will die if an adequate number of eosinophils are involved.

Secretory Immune System

The entire body is protected by the systemic immune system. Another, partially independent, immune system protects the external surfaces of the body. This system is called the secretory (mucosal) immune system (Figure 6-10).[2] Antibodies in bodily secretions such as tears, sweat, saliva, mucus, and breast milk provide local protection against infectious microorganisms. Pathogens can infect the body's surfaces and possibly penetrate to cause systemic disease. Alternatively, the microorganisms may reside in the membranes without causing disease and be a source of infection for other individuals. Thus, an individual may become a carrier for a particular infectious organism. For instance, in the 1950s two vaccines were developed to prevent infection with polio virus, which enters through the gastrointestinal tract. The Sabin vaccine was administered orally as an attenuated (i.e., inactivated so as to render relatively harmless) live virus. This route caused a transient, limited infection and induced effective systemic and secretory immunity that prevented both the disease and the establishment of a carrier state. The Salk vaccine, on the other hand, consisted of killed viruses administered by injection in the skin. It induced adequate systemic protection but did not generally prevent an intestinal carrier state. Thus, recipients of the Salk vaccine were protected from disease but could still shed the virus and infect others.

IgA is the dominant secretory immunoglobulin, although IgM and IgG also are present in secretions. The primary role of IgA is to prevent the attachment and invasion of pathogens through mucosal membranes, such as those of the gastrointestinal, pulmonary, and genitourinary tracts. Antibodies in secretions are produced by plasma cells of the secretory (mucosal) immune system.

The B cells of the secretory immune system follow a different pattern of migration through the body than cells of the systemic immune system, residing in a different group of lymphoid tissues including the lacrimal and salivary glands and the lymphoid tissues of the breasts, bronchi, intestines, and genitourinary tract. The lymphoid tissues of the secretory immune system are connected; thus many foreign antigens in a mother's gastrointestinal tract (e.g., polio virus) induce secretion of specific IgAs, IgMs, and IgGs into the breast milk.[8] Antibodies in the milk may protect the nursing newborn against these infectious disease agents. Although colostral antibodies (i.e., found in colostrum of breast milk) provide the newborn with passive immunity against gastrointestinal infections, they do not provide systemic immunity because they do not cross the newborn's gut into the bloodstream after the first 24 hours of life. Maternal antibodies that pass across the placenta into the fetus before birth provide passive systemic immunity.

CELL-MEDIATED IMMUNITY

T Lymphocytes

Most lymphocytes are members of the acquired immune system. The B cells and plasma cells produce antibodies, whereas T lymphocytes (T cells) represent a large spectrum of cell types and functions. These cell types include broadly T-cytotoxic (Tc) cells that attack antigens directly and destroy cells that bear foreign antigens; regulatory cells, primarily T-helper (Th) cells, that control both cell-mediated and humoral immune responses (including *lymphokine-producing cells* that secrete cytokines that activate other cells, such as macrophages); and memory cells that remember an antigen that has been previously seen by the immune system and induce a secondary immune response that is much quicker than the initial (primary) immune response. T cells are particularly important in protection against viruses, tumors, and pathogens that are resistant to killing by normal neutrophils and macrophages. They are also absolutely essential for the development of most humoral responses. Because *both* B cell and T cell functions produce the effective immune response, the mechanisms governing these functions will be discussed in the following section.

IMMUNE RESPONSE: COLLABORATION OF B CELLS AND T CELLS

Generation of Clonal Diversity

The immune response occurs in two phases: generation of clonal diversity and clonal selection (Table 6-3 and see Figure 6-3). Before birth, humans produce a large population of T cells and B cells that have the capacity to recognize almost any foreign antigen found in the environment (generation of clonal diversity). This process mostly occurs in specialized lymphoid organs (the primary [central] lymphoid organs): the thymus for T cells and the bone marrow for B cells. The result is the differentiation of lymphoid stem cells into B and T lymphocytes with the ability to react against almost any antigen that will be encountered throughout life. It is estimated that B and T cells can collectively recognize more than 10^8 different antigenic determinants. Lymphocytes are released from these organs into the circulation as mature cells that have the capacity to react with antigens (*immunocompetent*) and migrate to other (secondary) lymphoid organs in the body.

Development of B Lymphocytes

In birds, an organ called the bursa of Fabricius is responsible for the maturation of B (bursal-derived) lymphocytes. Humans have no discrete bursa, but the bone marrow makes up the human bursal equivalent and serves as the primary lymphoid organ for B cell development.

TABLE 6-3	GENERATION OF CLONAL DIVERSITY VS. CLONAL SELECTION	
	GENERATION OF CLONAL DIVERSITY	**CLONAL SELECTION**
Purpose?	To produce large numbers of T and B lymphocytes with maximum diversity of antigen receptors	Select, expand, and differentiate clones of T and B cells against specific antigen
When does it occur?	Primarily in fetus	Primarily after birth and throughout life
Where does it occur?	Central lymphoid organs: thymus for T cells, bone marrow for B cells	Peripheral lymphoid organs, including lymph nodes, spleen, and other lymphoid tissues
Is foreign antigen involved?	No	Yes, antigen determines which clones of cells will be selected
What hormones or cytokines are involved?	Thymic hormones, IL-7, others	Many cytokines produced by Th cells and APCs
Final product?	Immunocompetent T and B cells that can react with antigen, but have not seen antigen, and migrate to secondary lymphoid organs	Plasma cells that produce antibody, effector T cells that help (Th cells), kill targets (Tc cells), or regulate immune responses (Treg cells); memory B and T cells

APCs, Antigen-presenting cells; *Tc cells,* T-cytotoxic cells; *Th cells,* T-helper cells; *Treg cells,* T-regulatory cells.

Lymphocytes destined to become B cells circulate through the bursal equivalent, where they are exposed to hormones that, without the presence of antigens, induce proliferation and differentiation into B cells. Each B cell, however, responds to only one specific antigen. They exit the bone marrow and establish residence in other lymphoid organs (secondary lymphoid organs) as immunocompetent B cells.

Development of T Lymphocytes

The process of T cell proliferation and differentiation is similar to that for B cells. The primary lymphoid organ for T cell development is the thymus. Lymphoid stem cells journey through the thymus, where, under the pressure and guidance of thymic hormones (thymosin, thymopoietin, thymostimulin, and several other hormones produced by the epithelium), the cytokine IL-7, and without the presence of antigens, they are driven to undergo cell division and simultaneously produce receptors (T cell receptors [TCRs]) against the diversity of antigens the individual will encounter throughout life.[9] They exit the thymus through the blood vessels and lymphatics as mature (immunocompetent) T cells with antigen-specific receptors on the cell surface and establish residence in secondary lymphoid organs.

QUICK CHECK 6-2

1. What are the major functions of antibodies?
2. What is the difference between the secretory and systemic immune systems?
3. What are the different types of T cells, and what function does each have?

Clonal Selection

Antigens initiate the second phase of the immune response, clonal selection. This process involves a complex interaction among cells in the secondary lymphoid organs (see Figure 6-3). To initiate an effective immune response, most antigens must be *processed:* because they cannot react directly with cells of the immune system the antigens must be shown or *presented* to the immune cells in a specific manner. This is the job of antigen-processing (antigen-presenting) cells (usually dendritic cells, macrophages, or similar cells), generally referred to as APCs. The interaction among APCs, subpopulations of T cells that facilitate immune responses (T-helper [Th] cells), and immunocompetent B or T cells results in differentiation of B cells into active antibody-producing cells (plasma cells) and T cells into effector cells,

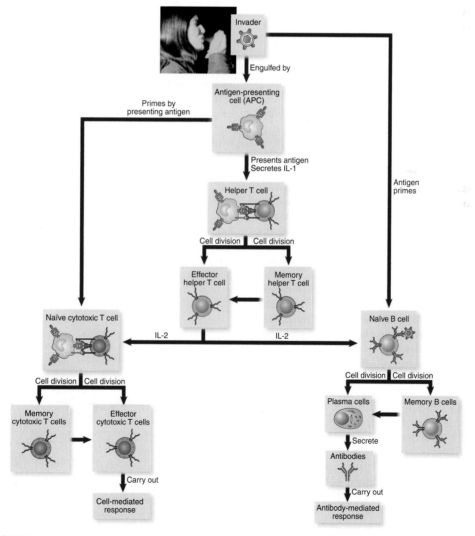

FIGURE 6-11 Summary of Adaptive Immunity This simplified flowchart summarizes an example of adaptive immune responses when exposed to a microbial antigen. (From Patton KT, Thibodeau GA: *Anatomy & physiology,* ed 7, St Louis, 2010, Mosby.)

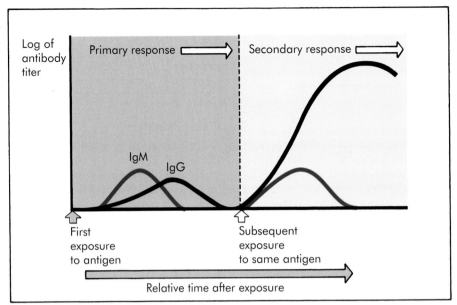

FIGURE 6-12 Primary and Secondary Immune Responses. The initial administration of antigen induces a primary response during which IgM is initially produced, followed by IgG. Another administration of the antigen induces the secondary response in which IgM is transiently produced and larger amounts of IgG are produced over a longer period of time.

such as T-cytotoxic cells. Both lines also develop into memory cells that respond even faster when that antigen enters the body again. Thus, activation of the immune system produces a specific and long-lasting protection against specific antigens (Figure 6-11). Defects in any aspect of cellular collaboration will lead to defects in cell-mediated immunity, humoral immunity, or both and, depending on the particular defect, the individual's death (Chapter 7).

Primary and Secondary Immune Responses

The immune response to antigens has classically been divided into two phases—the primary and secondary responses—that are most easily demonstrated by measuring concentrations of circulating antibodies over time (Figure 6-12). After a single initial exposure to most antigens, there is a latent period, or lag phase, during which antigen processing and B cell differentiation and proliferation occur. After approximately 5 to 7 days, IgM antibody is detected in the circulation. The lag phase is the time necessary for the process of clonal selection. This is the primary immune response, characterized typically by initial production of IgM followed by production of IgG against the same antigen. The quantity of IgG may be about equal to or less than the amount of IgM. The amount of antibody in a serum sample is frequently referred to as the titer; a higher titer indicates more antibodies. If no further exposure to the antigen occurs, the circulating antibody is catabolized (broken down) and measurable quantities fall. The individual's immune system, however, has been primed.

A second challenge by the same antigen results in the secondary immune response, which is characterized by the more rapid production of a larger amount of antibody than the primary response. The rapidity of the secondary immune response is the result of memory cells that do not require further differentiation. IgM may be transiently produced in the secondary response, but IgG production is increased considerably, making it the predominant antibody class. If the antigenic challenge is in the form of a vaccine (e.g., polio) or occurs through natural infection (e.g., rubella), the level of protective IgG may remain elevated for decades.

Cellular Interactions in the Immune Response

Clonal selection generally occurs in lymphoid organs called the secondary (peripheral) lymphoid organs, in which antigens selectively react with B or T cells. The secondary lymphoid organs include the spleen, lymph nodes, adenoids, tonsils, Peyer patches (intestines), and the appendix. Under the control of a variety of cytokines and complex cellular interactions, the selected B or T cells further proliferate and differentiate into plasma cells that produce antibodies, T cells that can attack cellular targets, or B or T memory cells that will respond more quickly to a second exposure to the same antigen.

B cell receptor for antigen. During differentiation into effector cells both T cells and B cells must react directly with antigens through antigen-specific receptors on the cell surface. The B cell receptor (BCR) is a complex of antibody bound to the cell surface and other molecules involved in intracellular signaling (see Figure 6-5, *D*). Its role is to recognize an antigen and communicate that information to the cell's nucleus.

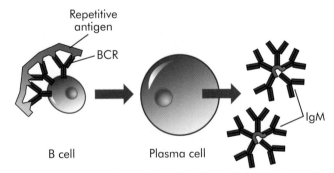

FIGURE 6-13 Activation of a B Cell by a T Cell–Independent Antigen. Molecules containing repeating identical antigenic determinants may interact simultaneously with several receptors on the surface of the B cell and induce the proliferation and production of immunoglobulins. Because Th2 cells do not participate, class switch does not occur and the resultant antibody response is IgM.

The BCRs in immunocompetent cells are membrane-associated IgM and IgD immunoglobulins that have identical specificities. The IgM is a monomer rather than the pentamer primarily found in the blood. After having reacted with antigens and undergoing differentiation, the BCR on the developing plasma cell may change to other classes of antibody.

Although most antigens require B cells to interact with Th cells, a few antigens can bypass the need for cellular interactions and can directly stimulate B cell maturation and proliferation. These are called *T cell–independent antigens* (Figure 6-13). They are mostly bacterial products that are large and are likely to have repeating identical antigenic determinants that bind and cross-link several B cell receptors. The accumulated intracellular signal is adequate to induce differentiation into a plasma cell but is not adequate to induce a change in the class of antibody that will be produced. Therefore, T cell–independent

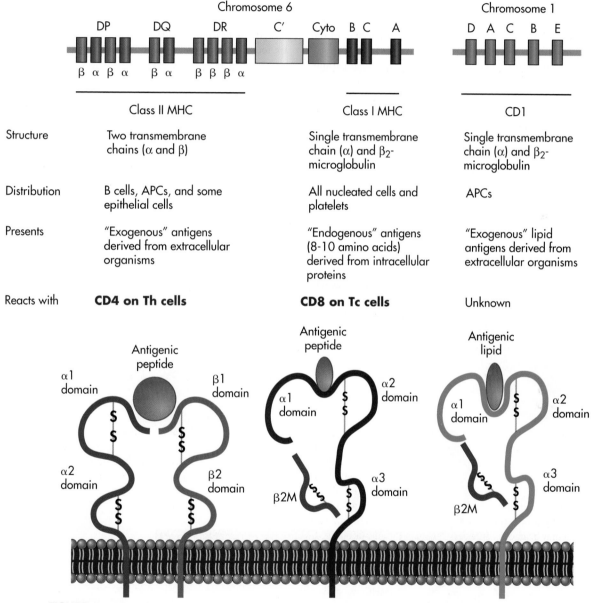

FIGURE 6-14 Antigen-Presenting Molecules. Two sets of molecules are primarily responsible for antigen presentation: MHC class I and MHC class II. The MHC molecules are encoded from the major histocompatibility complex on chromosome 6. This region contains information for the α chains of three principal class I molecules, called HLA-A, HLA-B, and HLA-C. These will be discussed in more detail in Chapter 7. Each of the MHC class I α chains forms a complex with β_2-microglobulin, which is encoded by a gene on chromosome 15. The MHC class I molecules present small peptide antigens (eight or nine amino acids in length) in a pocket formed by the α1 and α2 domains of the α chain. The conformation of the molecule is stabilized by β_2-microglobulin as well as by intrachain disulfide bonds. The α and β chains of class II molecules are also encoded in the MHC region. The principal class II molecules are HLA-DR, HLA-DP, and HLA-DQ. The MHC class II molecules present peptide antigens in a pocket formed by the α1 domain of the α chain and the β1 domain of the β chain. Both MHC class I and class II molecules are anchored to the plasma membrane by hydrophobic regions on the ends of the α and β chains.

antigens usually induce relatively pure IgM primary and secondary immune responses. All other antigens must be processed and presented to Th cells before an antibody response can occur.

Antigen processing and presentation. In most cases several steps involving cellular interactions must occur to produce a protective humoral or cellular immune response. Antigens that enter the bloodstream or lymphatics encounter a variety of phagocytic cells, including dendritic cells and macrophages, that phagocytose, break up (process), and present antigenic fragments.[10] Although these cells are the principal APCs, almost every cell can present antigens to some degree.

Antigen-presenting molecules. Processed antigens must be presented on the APC surface by specialized molecules, molecules of the major histocompatibility complex (MHC) (Figure 6-14). MHC molecules are discussed in more detail in Chapter 7. Major histocompatibility complex (MHC) molecules are glycoproteins found on the surface of all human cells except red blood cells. They are divided into two general classes, class I and class II, based on their molecular structure, distribution among cell populations, and function in antigen presentation. MHC class I molecules are composed of a large alpha (α) chain along with a smaller chain called β2-microglobulin. MHC class II molecules are composed of α and β chains that differ from the ones used for MHC class I. The α and β chains of the MHC molecules are encoded from different genetic loci located as a large complex of genes on human chromosome 6 (β2-microglobulin is found on a different chromosome).

MHC class I molecules present antigens that are *endogenous*—antigens originating within the cell. Examples of endogenous antigens include antigens from viruses that infect cells and use the normal cellular protein-synthesizing machinery to produce viral proteins and antigens that are uniquely produced by cancerous cells. Antigens presented by MHC class I molecules are primarily recognized by T-cytotoxic cells. Because MHC class I molecules are expressed on all cells, except red blood cells, any change in that cell caused by viral infection or malignancy may result in foreign antigens being presented.

MHC class II molecules present *exogenous antigens*—antigens that originate from outside the body (Figure 6-15). These antigens are found primarily on infectious microorganisms that must initially undergo phagocytosis. MHC class II molecules are co-expressed with MHC class I on a limited number of cells that have APC function, including macrophages, dendritic cells, and B lymphocytes. A dendritic cell is an antigen-presenting leukocyte that is found in the skin, mucosa, and lymphoid tissues and that initiates a primary immune response (Figure 6-16). Antigen presented by MHC class II molecules is preferentially recognized by T-helper cells.

Thus, the term antigen processing relates to the process by which large exogenous and endogenous antigens are cut up by enzymes into small antigenic fragments that are linked with the appropriate MHC molecules.

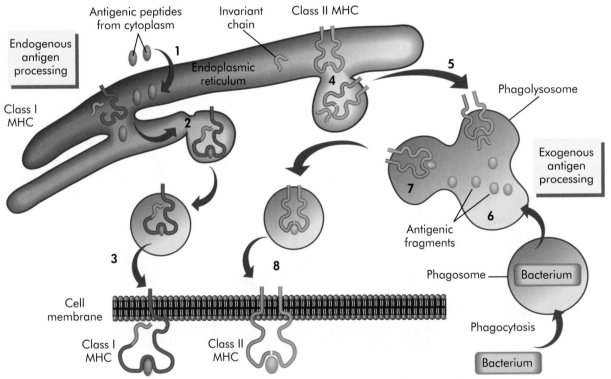

FIGURE 6-15 Antigen Processing. Antigen processing and presentation are required for initiation of most immune responses. Foreign antigen may be either endogenous (cytoplasmic protein) or exogenous (e.g., bacterium). Endogenous antigenic peptides are transported into the endoplasmic reticulum (ER) *(1)*, where the MHC molecules are being assembled. In the ER, antigenic peptides bind to the α chains of the MHC class I molecule *(2)*, and the complex is transported to the cell surface *(3)*. The α and β chains of the MHC class II molecules are also being assembled in the endoplasmic reticulum *(4)*, but the antigen-binding site is blocked by a small molecule (invariant chain) to prevent interactions with endogenous antigenic peptides. The MHC class II–invariant chain complex is transported to phagolysosomes *(5)* where exogenous antigenic fragments have been produced as a result of phagocytosis *(6)*. In the phagolysosomes, the invariant chain is digested and replaced by exogenous antigenic peptides *(7)*, after which the MHC class II–antigen complex is inserted into the cell membrane *(8)*.

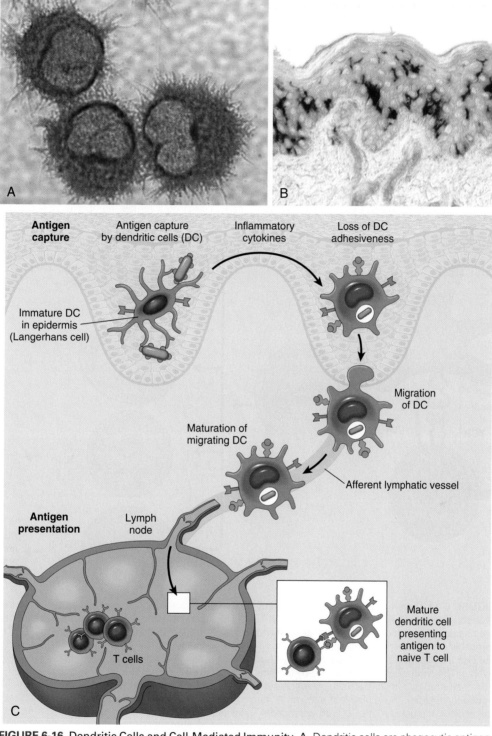

FIGURE 6-16 **Dendritic Cells and Cell-Mediated Immunity. A,** Dendritic cells are phagocytic antigen-presenting cells (APCs) found in the skin, mucosa, and lymphoid tissues. **B,** Dendritic cells (Langerhans cells) are marked by the blue stain in the epidermis. **C,** Dendritic cells capturing microbial antigens from epithelia and transporting them to regional lymph nodes. The T cells are then activated to proliferate and to differentiate into effector and memory cells, which migrate to sites of infection and promote various functions in cell-mediated immunity. (**A** and **B** from Patton KT, Thibodeau GA: *Anatomy & physiology,* ed 7, St Louis, 2010, Mosby; **C** from Kumar V, Abbas A, Fausto N: *Robbins and Cotran pathologic basis of disease,* ed 7, Philadelphia, 2005, Saunders.)

T cell receptor for antigen. T lymphocytes recognize processed antigens using a receptor that is similar to the B cell receptor. The **T cell receptor (TCR)** complex is composed of an antibody-like protein (TCR) and a group of accessory proteins that are involved in signaling to the nucleus (see Figure 6-5, *E*). Although the components of the TCR resemble antibody, they are encoded by different genes. All of the TCRs on a single T cell are identical in structure and specificity.

CD molecules. Cellular cooperation to produce an immune response requires a large array of accessory molecules. Many accessory molecules are part of a nomenclature that uses the prefix CD (cluster of differentiation) followed by a number (e.g., CD1 or CD2). The list of

CD molecules is constantly increasing (currently in excess of 250). We will focus on a small number of highly important examples to illustrate the immensely complicated, but highly effective, interactions that take place to produce a protective immune response.

T-helper lymphocytes. Regardless of whether an antigen primarily induces a cellular or humoral immune response, APCs usually must present antigens to T-helper cells (Th cells). This extremely important role involves three distinct steps: (1) the Th cell directly interacts with the APC through a variety of antigen-specific and antigen-independent mechanisms; (2) the Th cell undergoes a differentiation process during which a variety of cytokine genes are activated; and (3) depending on the pattern of cytokines expressed, the mature Th cell interacts

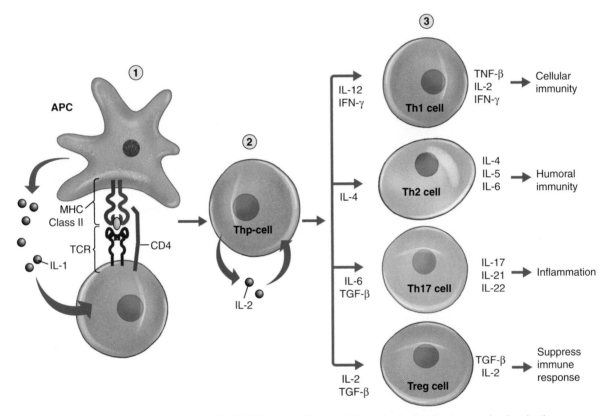

FIGURE 6-17 Development of T Cell Subsets. The most important step in clonal selection is the production of populations of T-helper (Th) cells (Th1, Th2, and Th17) and T-regulatory (Treg) cells that are necessary for the development of cellular and humoral immune responses. In this model, APCs *(1)* (probably multiple populations) may influence whether a precursor Th cell (Thp cell) *(2)* will differentiate into a Th1, Th2, Th17, or Treg cell *(3).* Differentiation of the Thp cell is initiated by three signaling events. The antigen signal is produced by the interaction of the T cell receptor (TCR) and CD4 with antigen presented by MHC class II molecules. A set of co-stimulatory signals is produced from interactions between adhesion molecules (not shown). A third signal is produced by the interactions of cytokines (particularly interleukin-1 [IL-1]) with appropriate cytokine receptors (IL-1R) on the Thp cell. The Thp cell up-regulates IL-2 production and expression of the IL-2 receptor (IL-2R), which acts in an autocrine fashion to accelerate Thp cell differentiation and proliferation. Commitment to a particular phenotype results from the relative concentrations of other cytokines. IL-12 and IFN-γ produced by some populations of APCs favor differentiation into the Th1 cell phenotype; IL-4, which is produced by a variety of cells, favors differentiation into the Th2 cell phenotype; IL-6 and TGF-β (T cell growth factor) facilitate differentiation into Th17 cells; IL-2 and TGF-β induce differentiation into Treg cells. The Th1 cell is characterized by the production of cytokines that assist in the differentiation of T-cytotoxic (Tc) cells, leading to cellular immunity, whereas the Th2 cell produces cytokines that favor B cell differentiation and humoral immunity. Th1 and Th2 cells affect each other through the production of inhibitory cytokines: IFN-γ will inhibit development of Th2 cells, and IL-4 will inhibit the development of Th1 cells. Th17 cells produce cytokines that affect phagocytes and increase inflammation. Treg cells produce immunosuppressive cytokines that prevent the immune response from being excessive. *APC,* Antigen-presenting cell; *IFN,* interferon; *MHC,* major histocompatibility complex; *TGF,* transforming growth factor.

with either immunocompetent B or T cells to cause their differentiation into either plasma cells or effector T cells, respectively.

When T cells develop in the thymus, two different populations are produced. T cells that are destined to become Th cells emerge from the thymus with a characteristic cell-surface protein, called **CD4** (CD4-positive cells). Cells destined to become Tc cells have a different cell-surface protein, called **CD8** (CD8-positive cells). The role of CD4 and CD8 is to help the interaction between T cells and APCs by reacting with antigen-presenting molecules. Interaction is restricted because CD4 can only interact with MHC class II molecules, whereas CD8 reacts only with MHC class I molecules. Thus CD4-positive Th cells are restricted to interactions with cells presenting antigens by MHC class II molecules.

Other intercellular signals are required for maturation of Th cells: interaction of cell-surface adhesion molecules (not discussed further here) and exposure to specific cytokines.[11] At this early stage of cell differentiation, the Th cell needs IL-1 secreted by the APC (Figure 6-17).[12] Afterwards the Th cell produces IL-2, which is secreted and acts in an autocrine (self-stimulating) fashion to induce further maturation and proliferation of the Th cell. Without IL-2 production, the Th cell cannot efficiently mature into a functional helper cell.

At this point, Th cells undergo differentiation into either Th1, Th2, or Th17 cells.[13] These subsets have different functions: **Th1 cells** appear to provide more help in developing cell-mediated immunity, **Th2 cells** provide more help for humoral immunity, and **Th17 cells** activate macrophages.[14] The Th subsets differ considerably in the spectrum of cytokines they produce. Additionally, Th1 and Th2 cells may suppress each other so that the immune response may favor either antibody formation, with suppression of a cell-mediated response, or the opposite. For example, antigens derived from viral or bacterial pathogens and those derived from cancer cells seem to induce a greater number of Th1 cells relative to Th2 cells, whereas antigens derived from multicellular parasites and allergens may result in production of more Th2 cells. Many antigens (e.g., tetanus vaccine), however, will produce excellent humoral and cell-mediated responses simultaneously. Th cells are necessary for development of most humoral and cellular immune responses; therefore the virus that causes acquired immune deficiency syndrome (AIDS) results in life-threatening infections because it specifically infects and destroys Th cells.

T cell clonal selection: the cellular immune response. For T cells to mature, another set of cellular interactions is required. Because T-cytotoxic (Tc) cells express CD8, rather than CD4, they must react with antigens presented by MHC class I molecules on the surface of antigen-presenting cells or other target cells (Figure 6-18).[15] Differentiation of Tc cells also requires IL-2 produced by Th1 cells.

Superantigens. Certain diseases are produced by a group of molecules called **superantigens (SAGs)**. SAGs bind to the portion of the TCR outside of its normal antigen-specific binding site, as well as to MHC class II molecules outside of their antigen-presentation sites (Figure 6-19). Thus, SAGs are not digested and processed by an APC to be presented to an immune cell. This binding, which is independent of antigen recognition, provides a signal for Th cell activation, proliferation, and cytokine production. The normal antigen-specific recognition between Th cells and APCs results in activation of relatively few cells—only those cells with specific TCRs against that antigen. SAGs activate a large population of Th cells, regardless of antigen specificity, and induce excessive production of cytokines, including IL-2, interferon gamma (IFN-γ), and tumor necrosis factor-alpha (TNF-α). The overproduction of inflammatory cytokines results in symptoms of a systemic inflammatory reaction, including fever, low blood pressure, and, potentially, fatal shock. Some examples of SAGs are the bacterial

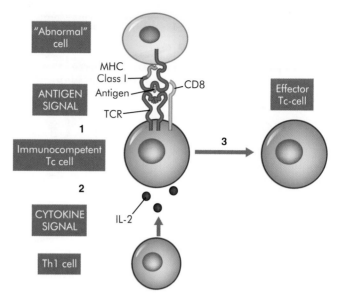

FIGURE 6-18 Tc Cell Clonal Selection. The immunocompetent Tc cell can react with antigen but cannot yet kill target cells. During clonal selection, this cell reacts with antigen presented by MHC class I molecules on the surface of a virally infected or cancerous *abnormal* cell. *(1)* The antigen–MHC class I complex is recognized simultaneously by the T cell receptor (TCR), which binds to antigen, and CD8, which binds to the MHC class I molecule. *(2)* A separate signal is provided by cytokines, particularly IL-2 from Th1 cells. *(3)* In response to these signals, the Tc cell develops into an effector Tc cell with the ability to kill abnormal cells.

toxins produced by *Staphylococcus aureus* and *Streptococcus pyogenes* (SAGs that cause toxic shock syndrome and food poisoning).

B cell clonal selection: the humoral immune response. A further sequence of cellular interactions is required to produce an effective antibody response. The immunocompetent B cell is also an APC and expresses surface IgM and IgD B cell receptors (BCRs) (Figure 6-20). Unlike the T cell receptor that can only *see* processed and presented antigens, the BCR can react with soluble antigens that have not been processed. Antigen binding to the BCR activates the B cell, resulting in internalization and processing of the antigen and presentation of antigen fragments by MHC class II molecules. The antigen presented on the B cell surface is recognized by a Th2 cell through the TCR and CD4.[16] The intercellular bridges created through antigen and other intercellular adhesion molecules induce the Th2 cell to secrete cytokines (particularly IL-4) that cause B cell proliferation and maturation into plasma cells.

A major component of B cell maturation is **class switch**, the process that results in the change in antibody production from one class to another (e.g., IgM to IgG during the primary immune response). Before exposure to antigens and Th2 cells, the B cell produces IgM and IgD, which are used as cell membrane receptors. During the clonal selection process, a B cell proliferates and develops into antibody-secreting plasma cells, and each B cell has the option of becoming a secretor of IgM or changing the class of antibody to a secreted form of IgG, IgA, or IgE. Class switch occurs at the genetic level with the variable region of the antibody heavy chain being combined with a different constant region of the heavy chain. Because the variable region is conserved and the light chain remains unchanged the antigenic specificity of the antibody also remains unchanged. The particular constant region chosen by each cell during class switch appears to be, at least

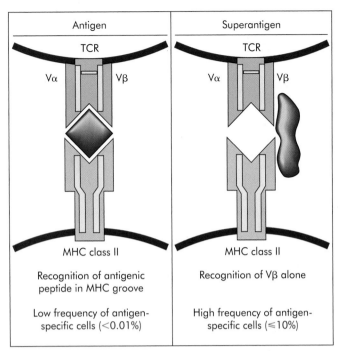

FIGURE 6-19 Superantigens. The T cell receptor (TCR) and major histocompatibility complex (MHC) class II molecule are normally held together by processed antigen. Superantigens, such as some bacterial exotoxins, bind directly to the variable region of the TCR β chain and the MHC class II molecule. Each superantigen activates sets of Vβ chains independently of the antigen specificity of the TCR.

partially, under the control of specific Th2 cytokines. For instance, IL-4 and IL-13 appear to preferentially stimulate switch to IgE secretion, and transforming growth factor-beta (TGF-β) and IL-5 appear to play major roles in class switch to IgA secretion. Thus, during clonal selection, a B cell may produce a population of plasma cells that are capable of producing many different classes of antibodies against the same antigen.

Memory cells. During the clonal selection process, both B cells and T cells differentiate into sets of long-lived **memory cells.**[17] Memory cells remain inactive until subsequent exposure to the same antigen. Upon reexposure, these memory cells do not require much further differentiation and will therefore rapidly become new plasma cells or effector T cells without the cellular interactions described previously.[18]

T Lymphocyte Functions
T-Cytotoxic Lymphocytes
T-cytotoxic (Tc) cells are responsible for the cell-mediated destruction of tumor cells or cells infected with viruses. The Tc cell must directly adhere to the target cell through antigen presented by MHC class I molecules and CD8 (Figure 6-21). Because of the broad cellular distribution of MHC class I molecules, Tc cells can recognize antigens on the surface of almost any type of cell that has been infected by a virus or has become cancerous.[19] After attachment to a target cell, killing occurs by induction of apoptosis.[20]

Various other cells kill targets in a fashion similar to Tc lymphocytes. Prominent among these cells are natural killer cells.[21] **Natural killer (NK) cells** are a special group of lymphoid cells that are similar to T cells but lack antigen-specific receptors. Instead, they express a variety of cell-surface receptors that identify protein changes on the surface of cells infected with viruses or that have become cancerous. After attachment, the NK cell kills its target in a manner similar to that

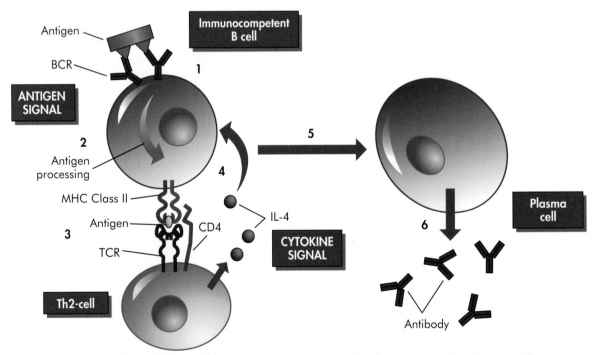

FIGURE 6-20 Bc Cell Clonal Selection. Immunocompetent B cells undergo proliferation and differentiation into antibody-secreting plasma cells. Multiple signals are necessary *(1).* The B cell itself can directly bind soluble antigen through the B cell receptor (BCR) and act as an antigen processing cell. Antigen is internalized, processed *(2),* and presented *(3)* to the TCR on a Th2 cell by MHC class II molecules *(4).* A cytokine signal is provided by the Th2 cell cytokines (e.g., IL-4) that react with the B cell *(5).* The B cell differentiates into plasma cells that secrete antibody *(6).*

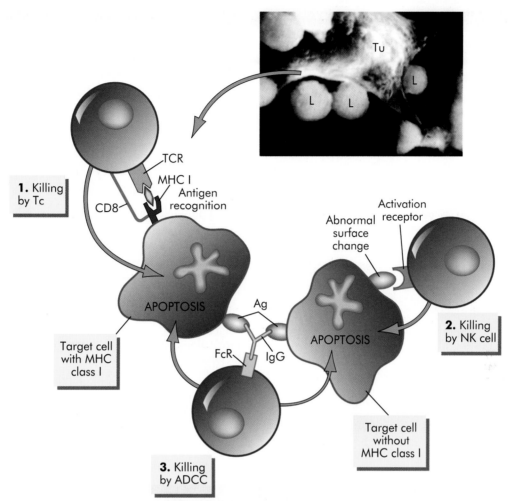

FIGURE 6-21 Cellular Killing Mechanisms. Several cells have the capacity to kill abnormal (e.g., virally infected, cancerous) target cells. *(1)* T-cytotoxic (Tc) cells recognized endogenous antigen presented by MHC class I molecules. The Tc cell mobilizes multiple killing mechanisms that induce apoptosis of the target cell. *(2)* Natural killer (NK) cells identify and kill target cells through receptors that recognize abnormal surface changes. NK cells specifically kill targets that do not express surface MHC class I molecules. *(3)* Several cells, including macrophages and NK cells, can kill by antibody-dependent cellular cytotoxicity (ADCC). IgG antibodies bind to foreign antigen on the target cell, and cells involved in ADCC bind IgG through Fc receptors (FcR) and initiate killing. The insert is a scanning electron microscopic view of Tc cells *(L)* attacking a much larger tumor cell *(Tu)*. (Insert from Thibodeau GA, Patton KT: *Anatomy & physiology*, ed 6, St Louis, 2007, Mosby.)

of Tc cells. NK cells also have receptors for MHC class I. However, NK cells lack CD8; therefore binding to MHC class I molecules results in inactivation of the NK cell. Thus, NK cells primarily kill target cells that have suppressed the expression of MHC class I, as do some tumors.

NK cells, as well as some macrophages, can specifically kill targets through use of antibodies.[22] These cells also express Fc receptors for IgG. If antigens on a pathogen or abnormal cell bind IgG, the NK cell can attach through Fc receptors and activate its normal killing mechanisms. This is referred to as **antibody-dependent cellular cytotoxicity (ADCC).**

T Cells That Activate Macrophages

During inflammation Th17 cells may produce cytokines that activate macrophages. The cytokines (particularly IFN-γ) stimulate the macrophage to become a more efficient phagocyte and increase production of proteolytic enzymes and other antimicrobial substances (see Chapter 5).

T-Regulatory Lymphocytes

T-regulatory (Treg) cells are a group of T cells that control the immune response, usually suppressing the response.[23] This population of Treg cells express CD4, as do Th cells, and bind to antigens presented by MHC class I molecules. Unlike Th cells, however, Treg cells express CD17. However, their differentiation is controlled by a different group of cytokines, primarily TGF-β and IL-2. Treg cells produce very high levels of TGF-β and IL-10, an immunosuppressive cytokine, which generally decrease Th1 and Th2 activity by suppressing antigen recognition and Th cell proliferation.[24]

✔ **QUICK CHECK 6-3**

1. What are antigen-presenting cells?
2. Define BCR and TCR.
3. What is the role of T-helper cells?
4. Why are cytokines important to the immune response?

PEDIATRIC CONSIDERATIONS

Age-Related Factors Affecting Mechanisms of Self-Defense in the Newborn Child

- Normal human newborns are immunologically immature; they have deficient antibody production, phagocytic activity, and complement activity, especially components of alternative pathways (e.g., factor B).
- The newborn cannot produce all classes of antibody; IgM is produced by the newborn (develops in the last trimester) to in utero infections (e.g., cytomegalovirus, rubella virus, and *Toxoplasma gondii*); only limited amounts of IgA are produced in the newborn; IgG production begins after birth and rises steadily throughout the first year of life.
- Maternal antibodies provide protection within the newborn's circulation (see figure below).
- Deficits in specific maternal transplacental antibody may lead to a tendency to develop severe, overwhelming sepsis and meningitis in the newborn.

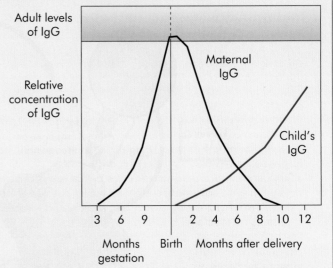

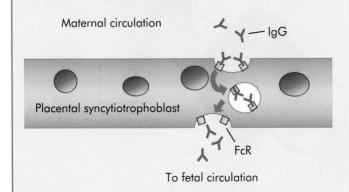

Antibody Levels in Umbilical Cord Blood and in Neonatal Circulation. Early in gestation, maternal IgG begins active transport across the placenta and enters the fetal circulation. At birth, the fetal circulation may contain nearly adult levels of IgG, which is almost exclusively from the maternal source. The fetal immune system has the capacity to produce IgM and small amounts of IgA before birth (not shown). After delivery, maternal IgG is rapidly destroyed and neonatal IgG production increases.

GERIATRIC CONSIDERATIONS

Age-Related Factors Affecting Mechanisms of Self-Defense in the Elderly

- Immune function decreases with age; diminished T cell function and reduced antibody responses to antigenic challenge occur with age.
- The thymus reaches maximum size at sexual maturity and then undergoes involution until it is a vestigial remnant by middle age; by 45 to 50 years of age, the thymus is only 15% of its maximum size.
- With age there is a decrease in thymic hormone production and the organ's ability to mediate T cell differentiation.

DID YOU UNDERSTAND?

Third Line of Defense: Adaptive Immunity

1. Adaptive immunity is a state of protection, primarily against infectious agents, that differs from inflammation by being slower to develop, being more specific, and having memory that makes it much longer lived.
2. The adaptive immune response is most often initiated by cells of the innate system. These cells process and present portions of invading pathogens (i.e., antigens) to lymphocytes in peripheral lymphoid tissue.
3. The adaptive immune response is mediated by two different types of lymphocytes—B lymphocytes and T lymphocytes. Each has distinct functions. B cells are responsible for humoral immunity that is mediated by circulating antibodies (immunoglobulins), whereas T cells are responsible for cell-mediated immunity, in which they kill targets directly or stimulate the activity of other leukocytes.
4. Adaptive immunity can be either active or passive depending on whether immune response components originated in the host or came from a donor.

Antigens and Immunogens

1. Antigens are molecules that bind and react with components of the immune response, such as antibodies and receptors on B and T cells. Most antigens can induce an immune response, and these antigens are called immunogens.
2. All immunogens are antigens but not all antigens are immunogens.
3. Some pathogens are successful because they mimic self-antigens but avoid inducing an immune response.
4. Large molecules, such as proteins, polysaccharides, and nucleic acids, are most immunogenic. Thus molecular size is an important factor for antigen immunogenicity.
5. Haptens are antigens too small to be immunogens by themselves but become immunogenic after combining with larger molecules.
6. The antigenic determinant, or epitope, is the precise chemical structure with which an antibody or B cell/T cell receptor reacts.

DID YOU UNDERSTAND?—cont'd

7. Self-antigens are antigens on an individual's own cells. The individual's immune system does not normally recognize self-antigens as immunogenic, a condition known as tolerance.

8. The response to antigen can be divided into two phases: the primary and secondary responses. The primary response of humoral immunity is usually dominated by IgM, with lesser amounts of IgG. The secondary immune response has a more rapid production of a larger amount of antibodies, predominantly IgG.

Humoral Immune Response

1. The humoral immune response consists of molecules (antibodies) produced by B cells. B cells are lymphocytes.

2. Antibodies are plasma glycoproteins that can be classified by chemical structure and biologic activity as IgG, IgM, IgA, IgE, or IgD.

3. A typical antibody molecule is constructed of two identical heavy chains and two identical light chains (either κ or λ) and has two Fab portions that bind antigen and an Fc portion that interacts with complement or receptors on cells.

4. The protective effects of antibodies may be direct or indirect.

5. Direct effects result from the binding of antibodies directly to a harmful antigen or infectious agent. These include inhibition of processes that are necessary for infection, such as the reaction of an infectious agent with a particular cell in the body or neutralization of harmful bacterial toxins.

6. Indirect effects result from activation of inflammation by antibodies through the Fc portion of the molecule. These include opsonization to increase phagocytosis, destruction of the infectious agent through activation of complement, and widespread activation of inflammation through the production of biologically active complement components, such as C5a.

7. IgE is a special class of antibody that helps defend against parasitic infections.

8. Antibodies of the systemic immune system function internally, in the bloodstream and tissues. Antibodies of the secretory, or mucosal, immune system (primarily secretory IgA) function externally, in the secretions of mucous membranes.

Cell-Mediated Immunity

1. T cells are responsible for the cell-mediated immune response. T cells are lymphocytes.

2. There are several types of mature T cells: T-cytotoxic cells (Tc), T-helper cells (Th), T-regulatory cells (Treg), and memory cells.

Immune Response: B Cells and T Cells Together

1. The production of B and T lymphocytes with receptors against millions of antigens that possibly will be encountered in an individual's lifetime occurs in the fetus in the primary lymphoid organs: the thymus for T cells and portions of the bone marrow for B cells. This diversity is called clonal diversity.

2. Immunocompetent T and B cells migrate from the primary lymphoid organs into the circulation and secondary lymphoid organs to await antigen.

3. Induction of an immune response, or clonal selection, begins when antigen enters the individual's body.

4. Most antigens must first interact with antigen-presenting cells (APCs) (e.g., macrophages). Dendritic cells present in the skin, mucosa, and lymphoid tissues also present antigen.

5. Antigen is processed in the APCs and presented on the cell surface by molecules of the MHC. The particular MHC molecule (class I or class II) that presents antigen determines which cell will respond to that antigen. Th cells require that the antigen be presented in a complex with MHC class II molecules. Tc cells require that the antigen be presented by MHC class I molecules.

6. The T cell sees the presented antigen through the T cell receptor (TCR) and accessory molecules: CD4 or CD8. CD4 is found on Th cells and reacts specifically with MHC class II. CD8 is found on Tc cells and reacts specifically with MHC class I.

7. Th cells consist of Th1 cells, which help Tc cells respond to antigen; Th2 cells, which help B cells develop into plasma cells; and Th17 cells, which help activate macrophages.

8. Tc cells bind to and kill cellular targets such as cells infected with viruses or cancer cells.

9. The natural killer (NK) cell has some characteristics of the Tc cells and is important for killing target cells in which viral infection or malignancy has resulted in the loss of cellular MHC molecules.

PEDIATRIC CONSIDERATIONS: Age-Related Factors
Affecting Mechanisms of Self-Defense in the Newborn Child

1. Neonates often have transiently depressed inflammatory function, particularly neutrophil chemotaxis and alternative complement pathway activity.

2. The T cell–independent immune response is adequate in the fetus and neonate, but the T cell–dependent immune response develops slowly during the first 6 months of life.

3. Maternal IgG antibodies are transported across the placenta into the fetal blood and protect the neonate for the first 6 months, after which they are replaced by the child's own antibodies.

GERIATRIC CONSIDERATIONS: Age-Related Factors
Affecting Mechanisms of Self-Defense in the Elderly

1. Elderly persons are at risk for impaired wound healing, usually because of chronic illnesses.

2. T cell function and antibody production are somewhat deficient in elderly persons. Elderly individuals also tend to have increased levels of circulating autoantibodies (antibodies against self-antigens).

KEY TERMS

- Active acquired immunity (active immunity) 143
- Adaptive (acquired) immunity 142
- Agglutination 149
- Allergen 144
- Antibody 142
- Antibody-dependent cellular cytotoxicity (ADCC) 161
- Antigen 142
- Antigen-binding fragment (Fab) 148
- Antigen-binding site (paratope) 148
- Antigen processing 153
- Antigen processing (antigen-presenting) cell (APC) 153
- Antigenic determinant (epitope) 148
- B cell receptor (BCR) 154
- B lymphocyte (B cell) 146
- CD molecule 158
- CD4 159
- CD8 159
- Cellular immunity 143
- Class switch 159
- Clonal selection 153
- Complementary-determining region (CDR) 148
- Crystalline fragment (Fc) 148
- Dendritic cell 156
- Generation of clonal diversity 152
- Hapten 144
- Human bursal equivalent 152
- Humoral immunity 143
- Immune response 142
- Immunity 142
- Immunocompetent 143
- Immunogen 144
- Immunoglobulin (Ig) 142
- Lymphocyte 142
- Lymphoid stem cell 152
- Major histocompatibility complex (MHC) 156
- Memory cell 143
- Natural killer (NK) cell 160
- Neutralization 149
- Passive acquired immunity (passive immunity) 143
- Plasma cell 146
- Precipitation 149
- Primary immune response 154
- Primary (central) lymphoid organ 152
- Regulatory cell 152
- Secondary immune response 154
- Secondary (peripheral) lymphoid organ 154
- Secretory (mucosal) immune system 152
- Secretory immunoglobulin 152
- Superantigen (SAG) 159
- Systemic immune system 152
- T cell receptor (TCR) 153
- T-cytotoxic (Tc) cell 143
- T-helper (Th) cell 153
- T lymphocyte (T cell) 152
- T-regulatory (Treg) cell 161
- Th1 cell 159
- Th2 cell 159
- Th17 cell 159
- Titer 154

REFERENCES

1. Bonilla FA, Oettgen HC: Adaptive immunity, *J Allergy Clin Immunol* 125(2):S33–S40, 2010.
2. Chaplin DD: Overview of the immune response, *J Allergy Clin Immunol* 125(2):S3–S23, 2010.
3. Chan AC, Carter PJ: Therapeutic antibodies for autoimmunity and inflammation, *Nat Rev Immunol* 10(5):301–316, 2010.
4. Beck A, et al: Strategies and challenges for the next generation of therapeutic antibodies, *Nat Rev Immunol* 10(5):345–352, 2010.
5. Schroeder HW Jr, Cavacini L: Structure and function of immunoglobulins, *J Allergy Clin Immunol* 125(2 suppl 2):S41–S52, 2010.
6. Abraham SN, St. John AL: Mast cell-orchestrated immunity to pathogens, *Nat Rev Immunol* 10(6):440–452, 2010.
7. Cadman ET, Lawrence RA: Granulocytes: effector cells or immunomodulators in the immune response to helminth infection? *Parasite Immunol* 32(1):1–19, 2010.
8. Brandtzaeg P: The mucosal immune system and its integration with the mammary glands, *J Pediatr* 156(2 suppl 1):S8–S15, 2010.
9. He R, Geha RS: Thymic stromal lymphopoietin, *Ann N Y Acad Sci* 1183(1):13–24, 2010.
10. Sadegh-Nasseri S, et al: Suboptimal engagement of the T-cell receptor by a variety of peptide-MHC ligands triggers T-cell anergy, *Immunol* 129(1):1–7, 2010.
11. Gascoigne NR, et al: Co-receptors and recognition of self at the immunological synapse, *Curr Top Microbiol Immunol* 340(1):171–189, 2010.
12. Sims JE, Smith DE: The IL-1 family: regulators of immunity, *Nat Rev Immunol* 10(2):89–102, 2010.
13. Damsker JM, Hansen AM, Caspi RR: Th1 and Th17 cells: adversaries and collaborators, *Ann N Y Acad Sci* 1183(1):211–221, 2010.
14. Zhu J, Paul WE: Heterogeneity and plasticity of T helper cells, *Cell Res* 20(1):4–12, 2010.
15. Reichardt P, Dombach B, Gunzer M: APC, T cells, and the immune synapse, *Curr Top Microbiol Immunol* 340(1):229–249, 2010.
16. Paul WE, Zhu J: How are T$_H$2-type immune responses initiated and amplified? *Nat Rev Immunol* 10(4):225–235, 2010.
17. Belz GT, Masson F: Interleukin-2 tickles T cell memory, *Immunity* 32(1):7–9, 2010.
18. Jameson SC, Masopust D: Diversity in T cell memory: an embarrassment of riches, *Immunity* 31(6):859–871, 2009.
19. Whiteside TL: Immune responses to malignancies, *J Allergy Clin Immunol* 125(2):S272–283, 2010.
20. Zitvogel L, Kepp O, Kroemer G: Decoding cell death signals in inflammation and immunity, *Cell* 140(6):798–804, 2010.
21. Moretta A, et al: NK cells at the interface between innate and adaptive immunity, *Cell Death Differ* 15(2):226–283, 2008.
22. Ramirez K, Kee BL: Multiple hats for natural killers, *Curr Opin Immunol* 22(2):193–198, 2010.
23. Littman DR, Rudensky AY: Th17 and regulatory T cells in mediating and restraining inflammation, *Cell* 140(6):845–858, 2010.
24. Saraiva M, O'Garra A: The regulation of IL-10 production by immune cells, *Nat Rev Immunol* 10(3):170–181, 2010.

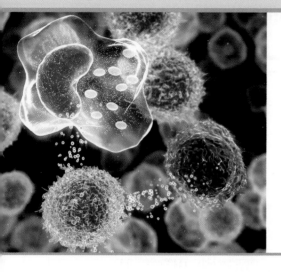

Infection and Defects in Mechanisms of Defense

Neal S. Rote

evolve WEBSITE

http://evolve.elsevier.com/Huether/
- Review Questions and Answers
- Animations
- Quick Check Answers
- Key Terms Exercises

- Critical Thinking Questions with Answers
- Algorithm Completion Exercises
- WebLinks

CHAPTER OUTLINE

The defensive system protecting the body from infection is a finely tuned network. Sometimes infectious agents can inhibit or escape defense mechanisms or the system may break down, leading to inadequate or inappropriate activation of the defenses. An inadequate response (commonly called an immune deficiency) may range from relatively mild defects to life-threatening severity. Inappropriate responses (hypersensitivity reactions) may be (1) exaggerated against noninfectious environmental substances (allergy); (2) misdirected against the body's own cells (autoimmunity); or (3) directed against beneficial foreign tissues, such as transfusions or transplants (alloimmunity). Several of these inappropriate responses can be serious or life-threatening.

INFECTION

Modern healthcare has shown great progress in preventing and treating infectious diseases. In developed countries, sanitary living conditions, clean water, uncontaminated food, vaccinations, and antimicrobial medications make death from infectious disease most common only among those with debilitating diseases or immunosuppression. In the United States, heart disease and malignancies greatly surpass infectious disease as major causes of death.[1] However, many deaths related to cancer are the result of secondary infections because the immune system can be severely depressed both by the cancer itself and by many of the treatments used to fight the cancer. Influenza/pneumonia (eighth leading cause) and sepsis (eleventh leading cause) accounted for more than 89,000 deaths (3.6% of the total number of deaths).

Infectious disease remains a significant threat to life in many parts of the world, including India, Africa, and Southeast Asia, although the advent of sanitary living conditions, clean water, uncontaminated food, vaccinations, and antimicrobial medications has improved the health of many. As a result of these initiatives smallpox has been eradicated from the globe (the last reported case was in 1975 in Somalia); measles has nearly been eliminated in the Western Hemisphere; and many diseases, such as measles (decreased by 78% since 2000)[2] and polio (declined by more than 99% since 1988),[3] are decreasing in prevalence worldwide. Although vaccines and antimicrobials have altered the prevalence of some infectious diseases, mutant strains of bacteria and viruses have emerged with resistance to protection provided by drug therapy. The emergence of new diseases—such as West Nile virus, severe acute respiratory syndrome (SARS), Lyme disease, and *Hantavirus*—and the development of drug-resistant tuberculosis are examples of the current intense challenges in the struggle to prevent and control infectious disease. Some tropical diseases are emerging for the first time in the United States (see *Health Alert:* Increase in United States of "Tropical Diseases").

HEALTH ALERT

Increase in United States of "Tropical Diseases"

There was a time when vector-borne tropical diseases were contained, particularly by active insect control programs. Recently, diseases such as malaria, dengue hemorrhagic fever, yellow fever, and African trypanosomiasis are reemerging in areas of Africa and the Americas where they had been eliminated or unreported. Although in recent history the United States has been relatively free of most of these diseases, it should not be forgotten that in 1793 a yellow fever outbreak in Philadelphia killed 2000 of the city's 55,000 inhabitants and forced the U.S. government to abandon the city until the outbreak ceased. The conditions necessary for resurgence of outbreaks still exist; the necessary vectors are still available, the population density and socioeconomic conditions are favorable, and the population generally does not have existing immunity to these disease-causing agents. The effects of global warming on the spread of these diseases can only be speculated.

In early 2010 the CDC reported the results of their study of 28 cases of locally-acquired dengue hemorrhagic fever in Key West, Florida. The dengue virus is transmitted by mosquitoes and yearly causes 50 to 100 million infections worldwide and 25,000 deaths. These were the first cases of locally acquired disease in the United States since 1945. A survey of mosquito breeding pools discovered the virus in at least two sites. The report surmised, while acknowledging that other factors could play a role, the increased incidence of dengue fever resulted from increased travel to localities where the disease was endemic, return of infected travelers, and transmission of the virus to the vector pool. The development of dengue vaccines is in progress.

Data from Miller N: Recent progress in dengue vaccine research and development, *Curr Opin Mol Ther* 12(1):31–38, 2010; Randolph SE, Rogers DJ: The arrival, establishment and spread of exotic diseases: patterns and predictions, *Nat Rev Microbiol* 8(5):361–371, 2010; Trout A et al: Locally acquired dengue—Key West, Florida, 2009–2010, *MMWR Morb Mortal Wkly Rep* 59(19):577–581, 2010.

Microorganisms and Humans: A Dynamic Relationship

For many microorganisms, the human body is a very hospitable site to grow and flourish. The microorganisms are provided with nutrients and appropriate conditions of temperature and humidity. In many cases a mutual relationship exists in which humans and the microorganisms benefit (Box 7-1). For instance, the human gut is colonized by a large variety of microorganisms that make up normal human flora. The normal flora of different body areas are summarized in Table 7-1. Bacteria in the GI tract are provided with nutrients from ingested food, and in exchange they produce (1) enzymes that facilitate the digestion and utilization of many molecules in the human diet, (2) antibacterial factors that prevent colonization by pathogenic microorganisms (see Chapter 5), and (3) usable metabolites (e.g., vitamin K, B vitamins). This relationship normally is maintained through the physical integrity of the skin and mucosal epithelium and other mechanisms that

---

BOX 7-1 THE MANY RELATIONSHIPS BETWEEN HUMANS AND MICROORGANISMS

Symbiosis: Benefits only the human; no harm to the microorganism
Mutualism: Benefits the human and the microorganism
Commensalism: Benefits only the microorganism; no harm to the human
Pathogenicity: Benefits the microorganism; harms the human (*Opportunism* is the situation that occurs when benign microorganisms become pathogenic because of decreased human host resistance.)

TABLE 7-1 NORMAL INDIGENOUS FLORA OF THE HUMAN BODY

LOCATION	MICROORGANISMS
Skin	Predominantly gram-positive cocci and rods *Staphylococcus epidermidis,* corynebacteria, mycobacteria, and streptococci are primary inhabitants; *Staphylococcus aureus* in some people; also yeasts (*Candida, Pityrosporum*) in some areas of skin Numerous transient microorganisms may become temporary residents In moist areas, gram-negative bacteria Around sebaceous glands, *Propionibacteria* and *Brevibacteria* Mite *Demodex folliculorum* lives in hair follicles and sebaceous glands around face
Nose	Predominantly gram-positive cocci and rods, especially *S. epidermidis* Some people are nasal carriers of pathogenic bacteria, including *S. aureus,* β-hemolytic streptococci, and *Corynebacterium diphtheriae*
Mouth	Complex of bacteria that includes several species of streptococci, *Actinomyces,* lactobacilli, and *Haemophilus* Anaerobic bacteria and spirochetes colonize gingival crevices
Pharynx	Similar to flora in mouth plus staphylococci, *Neisseria,* and diphtheroids Some asymptomatic persons also harbor pathogens pneumococcus, *Haemophilus influenzae, Neisseria meningitidis,* and *C. diphtheria*
Distal intestine	Enterobacteria, streptococci, lactobacilli, anaerobic bacteria, and *C. albicans*
Colon	Bacteroides, lactobacilli, clostridia, *Salmonella, Shigella, Klebsiella, Proteus, Pseudomonas,* enterococci, and other streptococci, bacilli, and *Escherichia coli*
Distal urethra	Typical bacteria found on skin, especially *S. epidermidis* and diphtheroids; also lactobacilli and nonpathogenic streptococci
Vagina	Birth to 1 month: similar to adult 1 month to puberty: *S. epidermidis,* diphtheroids, *E. coli,* and streptococci Puberty to menopause: *Lactobacillus acidophilus,* diphtheroids, staphylococci, streptococci, and variety of anaerobes Postmenopause: similar to prepubescence

From Grimes DE: *Infectious diseases, Mosby's Clinical Nursing Series,* St Louis, 1991, Mosby.

guarantee that the immune and inflammatory systems do not attack these symbiotes. If those systems are compromised, many microorganisms will leave their normal sites and cause infection. Individuals with deficiencies in their immune system become easily infected with opportunistic microorganisms—those that normally would not cause disease but seize the opportunity provided by the person's decreased immune or inflammatory responses.

True pathogens have devised means to circumvent the normal controls provided by the host's main defensive barriers: the inflammatory system and the immune system. Several factors influence the capacity of a pathogen to cause disease.

- *Communicability:* Ability to spread from one individual to others and cause disease—for example, measles and pertussis spread very easily; human immunodeficiency virus (HIV) is of lower communicability
- *Immunogenicity:* Ability of pathogens to induce an immune response
- *Infectivity:* Ability of the pathogen to invade and multiply in the host
- *Mechanism of action:* Manner in which the microorganism damages tissue
- *Pathogenicity:* Ability of an agent to produce disease—success depends on communicability, infectivity, extent of tissue damage, and virulence
- *Portal of entry:* Route by which a pathogenic microorganism infects the host: direct contact, inhalation, ingestion, or bites of an animal or insect
- *Toxigenicity:* Ability to produce soluble toxins or endotoxins, factors that greatly influence the pathogen's degree of virulence
- *Virulence:* Capacity of a pathogen to cause severe disease—for example, measles virus is of low virulence; rabies virus is highly virulent

Infectivity is facilitated by the ability of pathogens to attach to cell surfaces, release enzymes that dissolve protective barriers, escape the action of phagocytes, or resist the effect of low pH. After penetrating protective barriers, pathogens then spread through the lymph and blood for invasion of tissues and organs, where they multiply and cause disease. In humans the route of entrance of many pathogenic microorganisms also becomes the site of shedding of new infectious agents to other individuals, completing a cycle of infection.

Classes of Infectious Microorganisms

Infectious disease can be caused by microorganisms that range in size from 20 nanometers (nm) (poliovirus) to 10 meters (m) (tapeworm). Classes of pathogenic microorganisms and their characteristics are summarized in Table 7-2. Some mechanisms of tissue damage caused by microorganisms are summarized in Table 7-3.

TABLE 7-2   CLASSES OF ORGANISMS INFECTIOUS TO HUMANS

CLASS	SIZE	SITE OF REPRODUCTION	EXAMPLE
Virus	20-300 nm	Intracellular	Poliomyelitis
Chlamydiae	200-1000 nm	Intracellular	Urethritis
Rickettsiae	300-1200 nm	Intracellular	Rocky Mountain spotted fever
Mycoplasma	125-350 nm	Extracellular	Atypical pneumonia
Bacteria	0.8-15 mcg	Skin	Staphylococcal wound infection
		Mucous membranes	Cholera
		Extracellular	Streptococcal pneumonia
		Intracellular	Tuberculosis
Fungi	2-200 mcg	Skin	Tinea pedis (athlete's foot)
		Mucous membranes	Candidiasis (e.g., thrush)
		Extracellular	Sporotrichosis
		Intracellular	Histoplasmosis
Protozoa	1-50 mm	Mucosal	Giardiasis
		Extracellular	Sleeping sickness
Helminths	3 mm to 10 m	Intracellular	Trichinosis
		Extracellular	Filariasis

TABLE 7-3   EXAMPLES OF MICROORGANISMS THAT CAUSE TISSUE DAMAGE

PATHOGENS THAT DIRECTLY CAUSE TISSUE DAMAGE

Produce Exotoxin

Streptococcus pyogenes	Tonsillitis, scarlet fever
Staphylococcus aureus	Boils, toxic shock syndrome, food poisoning
Corynebacterium diphtheriae	Diphtheria
Clostridium tetani	Tetanus
Vibrio cholerae	Cholera

Produce Endotoxin

Escherichia coli	Gram-negative sepsis
Haemophilus influenzae	Meningitis, pneumonia
Salmonella typhi	Typhoid
Shigella	Bacillary dysentery
Pseudomonas aeruginosa	Wound infection
Yersinia pestis	Plague

Cause Direct Damage With Invasion

Variola	Smallpox
Varicella-zoster	Chickenpox, shingles
Hepatitis B virus	Hepatitis
Poliovirus	Poliomyelitis
Measles virus	Measles, subacute sclerosing panencephalitis
Influenza virus	Influenza
Herpes simplex virus	Cold sores

PATHOGENS THAT INDIRECTLY CAUSE TISSUE DAMAGE

Produce Immune Complexes

Hepatitis B virus	Kidney disease
S. pyogenes	Glomerulonephritis
Treponema pallidum	Kidney damage in secondary syphilis
Most acute infections	Transient renal deposits

Cause Cell-Mediated Immunity

Mycobacterium tuberculosis	Tuberculosis
Mycobacterium leprae	Tuberculoid leprosy
Lymphocytic choriomeningitis virus	Aseptic meningitis
Borrelia burgdorferi	Lyme arthritis
Herpes simplex virus	Herpes stromal keratitis

Data modified from Janeway CA et al: *Immunobiology: the system in health and disease,* ed 5, New York, 2001, Garland.

TABLE 7-4 **EXAMPLES OF MECHANISMS USED BY PATHOGENS TO RESIST THE IMMUNE SYSTEM**

MECHANISMS	EFFECT ON IMMUNITY	EXAMPLE OF SPECIFIC MICROORGANISMS
Destroy or Block Component of Immune System		
Produce toxins	Kills phagocyte or interferes with chemotaxis	*Staphylococcus*
	Prevents phagocytosis by inhibiting fusion between phagosome and lysosomal granules	*Streptococcus*
		Mycobacterium tuberculosis
Produce antioxidants (e.g., catalase, superoxide dismutase)	Prevents killing by O_2-dependent mechanisms	*Mycobacterium* sp.
	Promotes bacterial attachment	*Salmonella typhi*
Produce protease to digest IgA		*Neisseria gonorrhoeae* (urinary tract infection), *Haemophilus influenzae*, and *Streptococcus pneumoniae* (pneumonia)
Produce surface molecules that mimic Fc receptors and bind antibody	Prevents activation of complement system	*Staphylococcus*
	Prevents antibody functioning as opsonin	Herpes simplex virus
Mimic Self-Antigens		
Produce surface antigens (e.g., M protein, red blood cell antigens) that are similar to self-antigens	Pathogen resembles individual's own tissue; in some individuals, antibodies can be formed against self-antigen, leading to hypersensitivity disease (e.g., antibody to M protein also reacts with cardiac tissue, causing rheumatic heart disease; antibody to red blood cell antigens can cause anemia)	Group A *Streptococcus* (M protein) *Mycoplasma pneumoniae* (red cell antigens)
Change Antigenic Profile		
Undergo mutation of antigens or activate genes that change surface molecules	Immune response delayed because of failure to recognize new antigen	Influenza HIV Some parasites

---

Pathogenic Defense Mechanisms

Our multiple layers of defense against infection were described in Chapters 5 and 6. True pathogens have devised ways of circumventing these barriers.[4] For example, some bacteria produce thick capsules of carbohydrate or protein that are antiphagocytic, preventing efficient phagocytosis.[5] Others defend themselves by producing toxins that destroy neutrophils. Because the primary immune response may take a week to develop adequately, some pathogens proliferate at rates that surpass the development of a protective response. Table 7-4 contains examples of microorganisms that defeat the immune system or cause it to attack the host.

Viral pathogens bypass many defense mechanisms by hiding within cells and away from normal inflammatory or immune responses.[6] Because some viral agents must leave the infected cell in order to spread, the immune response blocks spread and eventually cures the infection; therefore the disease is described as self-limiting. Other viruses (e.g., measles, herpes) are inaccessible to antibodies after initial infection because they do not circulate in the bloodstream but instead remain inside infected cells, spreading by direct cell-to-cell contact. Antibodies that block a virus from attaching to a target cell (neutralizing antibodies) are most effective in preventing the initial infection. Other viruses, such as polio and influenza, are distributed through the blood, are more susceptible to the effects of circulating antibodies, and can be controlled by antibodies even after the initial infection. Most antiviral drugs help control the virus rather than destroy it (i.e., by preventing its replication). Because the virus replicates inside the host cell, it is difficult to kill a specific virus without also damaging the host cell.

Some viruses can elude the immune response by undergoing *antigenic variation*.[7] The virus can change its appearance by altering surface antigens. Influenza infection provides an example of how this occurs.[8] The influenza virus undergoes yearly **antigenic drift** resulting from mutations in key surface antigens, hemagglutinin (H antigen) and neuraminidase (N antigen), allowing the emergence of new strains of influenza virus. Thus immunity against the previous year's viruses is no longer completely protective, creating the need for new vaccines every year. **Antigenic shifts** are major changes in antigenicity that occur from recombination of genes for H and N among different strains of viruses and can result in major worldwide pandemics. Other pathogens, such as some parasitic microorganisms, use a similar approach and change surface antigens by gene switching. A parasite (i.e., African trypanosomes) may carry thousands of genes for different surface molecules that the parasite can either activate or deactivate at frequent intervals. Consequently, the immune system is always trying to catch up by generating new antibodies and T cells against the new antigens.

Infection and Injury
Bacterial Disease

Bacteria are prokaryocytes (lacking a discrete nucleus) and are relatively small. They can be aerobic or anaerobic and motile or immotile. Spherical bacteria are called cocci, rodlike forms are called bacilli, and spiral forms are termed *spirochetes*. Gram stain and acid-fast stain are important for differentiating gram-positive or gram-negative types of bacteria. Examples of human diseases caused by specific bacteria are listed in Table 7-5. The general structure of bacteria is reviewed in Figure 7-1.

Bacterial survival and growth depend on the effectiveness of the body's defense mechanisms and on the bacterium's ability to resist these defenses. Many pathogens have devised ways of preventing destruction by the inflammatory and immune systems. The thick capsules of carbohydrate or protein on encapsulated bacteria are

TABLE 7-5   EXAMPLES OF COMMON BACTERIAL INFECTIONS

MICROORGANISM	GRAM STAIN	RESPIRATORY PATHWAY	INTRACELLULAR OR EXTRACELLULAR
Respiratory Infections			
Upper Respiratory Tract Infections			
Corynebacterium diphtheriae (diphtheria)	Gram +	Facultative anaerobic	Extracellular
Haemophilus influenzae	Gram −	Facultative anaerobic	Extracellular
Streptococcus pyogenes (group A)	Gram +	Facultative anaerobic	Extracellular
Otitis Media			
Haemophilus influenzae	Gram −	Facultative anaerobic	Extracellular
Streptococcus pneumoniae	Gram +	Facultative anaerobic	Extracellular
Lower Respiratory Tract Infections			
Bacillus anthracis (pulmonary anthrax)	Gram +	Facultative anaerobic	Extracellular
Bordetella pertussis (whooping cough)	Gram −	Aerobic	Extracellular
Chlamydia pneumoniae	Not stainable	Aerobic	Obligate intracellular
Escherichia coli	Gram −	Facultative anaerobic	Extracellular
Haemophilus influenzae	Gram −	Facultative anaerobic	Extracellular
Legionella pneumophila	Gram −	Aerobic	Facultative intracellular
Mycobacterium tuberculosis	Gram + (weakly)	Aerobic	Extracellular
Mycoplasma pneumoniae	Not stainable	Aerobic	Extracellular
Neisseria meningitidis (develops into meningitis)	Gram −	Aerobic	Extracellular
Pseudomonas aeruginosa	Gram −	Aerobic	Extracellular
Streptococcus agalactiae (group B; develops to meningitis)	Gram +	Facultative anaerobic	Extracellular
Streptococcus pneumoniae	Gram +	Facultative anaerobic	Extracellular
Yersinia pestis (plague)	Gram −	Facultative anaerobic	Extracellular
Gastrointestinal Infections			
Inflammatory Gastrointestinal Infections			
Bacillus anthracis (gastrointestinal anthrax)	Gram +	Facultative anaerobic	Extracellular
Clostridium difficile	Gram +	Anaerobic	Extracellular
Escherichia coli O157:H7	Gram −	Facultative anaerobic	Extracellular
Vibrio cholerae	Gram −	Facultative anaerobic	Extracellular
Invasive Gastrointestinal Infections			
Brucella abortus (brucellosis, undulant fever, leading to sepsis, heart infection)	Gram −	Aerobic	Intracellular
Helicobacter pylori (gastritis and peptic ulcers)	Gram −	Microaerophilic	Extracellular
Listeria monocytogenes (leading to sepsis and meningitis)	Gram +	Aerobic	Intracellular
Salmonella typhi (typhoid fever)	Gram −	Anaerobic	Extracellular
Shigella sonnei	Gram −	Facultative anaerobic	Extracellular
Food Poisoning			
Bacillus cereus	Gram +	Facultative anaerobic	Extracellular
Clostridium botulinum	Gram +	Anaerobic	Extracellular
Clostridium perfringens	Gram +	Anaerobic	Extracellular
Staphylococcus aureus	Gram +	Facultative anaerobic	Extracellular
Sexually Transmitted Infections			
Chlamydia trachomatis (pelvic inflammatory disease)	Not stainable	Aerobic	Intracellular
Neisseria gonorrhoeae (urethritis)	Gram −	Aerobic	Facultative intracellular
Treponema pallidum (spirochete; syphilis)	Gram −	Aerobic	Extracellular
Skin and Wound Infections			
Bacillus anthracis (cutaneous anthrax)	Gram +	Facultative anaerobic	Extracellular
Borrelia burgdorferi (Lyme disease; spirochete)	Gram −	Aerobic	Extracellular
Clostridium tetani (tetanus)	Gram +	Anaerobic	Extracellular
Clostridium perfringens (gas gangrene)	Gram +	Anaerobic	Extracellular
Mycobaterium leprae (leprosy)	Gram + (weakly)	Aerobic	Extracellular

Continued

TABLE 7-5 EXAMPLES OF COMMON BACTERIAL INFECTIONS—cont'd

MICROORGANISM	GRAM STAIN	RESPIRATORY PATHWAY	INTRACELLULAR OR EXTRACELLULAR
Pseudomonas aeruginosa	Gram –	Aerobic	Extracellular
Rickettsia prowazekii (rickettsia; typhus)	Gram –	Aerobic	Obligate intracellular
Staphylococcus aureus	Gram +	Facultative anaerobic	Extracellular
Streptococcus pyogenes (group A)	Gram +	Facultative anaerobic	Extracellular
Eye Infections			
Chlamydia trachomatis (conjunctivitis)	Not stainable	Aerobic	Obligate intracellular
Haemophilus aegyptius (pink eye)	Gram –	Facultative anaerobic	Extracellular
Zoonotic Infections			
Bacillus anthracis (anthrax)	Gram +	Facultative anaerobic	Extracellular
Brucella abortus (brucellosis, also called undulant fever)	Gram –	Aerobic	Intracellular
Borrelia burgdorferi (spirochete; Lyme disease)	Gram –	Aerobic	Extracellular
Listeria monocytogenes	Gram +	Aerobic	Intracellular
Rickettsia rickettsii (rickettsia; Rocky Mountain spotted fever)	Gram –	Aerobic	Obligate intracellular
Rickettsia prowazekii (rickettsia; typhus)	Gram –	Aerobic	Obligate intracellular
Yersinia pestis (plague)	Gram –	Facultative anaerobic	Extracellular
Nosocomial Infections			
Enterococcus faecalis	Gram +	Facultative anaerobic	Extracellular
Enterococcus faecium	Gram +	Facultative anaerobic	Extracellular
Escherichia coli (cystitis)	Gram –	Facultative anaerobic	Extracellular
Pseudomonas aeruginosa	Gram –	Obligate anaerobic	Extracellular
Staphylococcus aureus	Gram +	Facultative anaerobic	Extracellular
Staphylococcus epidermidis	Gram +	Facultative anaerobic	Extracellular

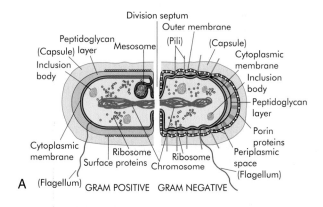

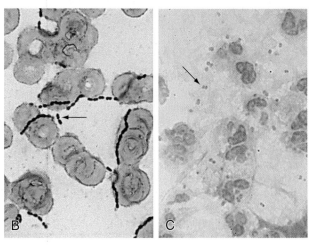

FIGURE 7-1 General Structure of Bacteria. A, The structure of the bacterial cell wall determines its staining characteristics with gram stain. A gram-positive bacterium has a thick layer of peptidoglycan *(left)*. A gram-negative bacterium has a thick peptidoglycan layer and an outer membrane *(right)*. **B,** Example of a gram-positive (darkly stained microorganisms, *arrow*) group A *Streptococcus*. This microorganism consists of cocci that frequently form chains. **C,** Example of a gram-negative (pink microorganisms, *arrow*) *Neisseria meningitides* in cerebrospinal fluid. *Neisseria* form complexes of two cocci (diplococci). (From Murray PR et al: *Medical microbiology,* ed 4, St Louis, 2002, Mosby.)

antiphagocytic, preventing efficient opsonization and phagocytosis. Such coatings include the polysaccharide covering of the pneumococcus and the waxy capsule surrounding the tubercle bacillus. The long M protein on the cell wall of the streptococcus suppresses complement activation.

Other bacteria survive and proliferate in the body by producing exotoxins and endotoxins that injure cells and tissues. **Exotoxins** are proteins released during bacterial growth. They are usually enzymes and have highly specific effects on host cells; they include cytotoxins, neurotoxins, pneumotoxins, enterotoxins, and hemolysins. Exotoxins can damage cell membranes, activate second messengers, and inhibit protein synthesis. Exotoxins are immunogenic and elicit the production of antibodies known as **antitoxins**. Consequently, vaccines are available for many of the exotoxins (i.e., tetanus, diphtheria, and pertussis). Some strains of toxin-producing group A streptococci cause destructive skin infections (e.g., flesh-eating bacteria syndrome, or necrotizing fasciitis) and pneumonia that may result in an individual's death within 2 days.

Endotoxins (lipopolysaccharides [LPSs]) are contained in the cell walls of gram-negative bacteria and are released during lysis, or destruction, of the bacteria. Endotoxin may be released also from the membrane of the bacteria during bacterial growth or during treatment with antibiotics, which therefore cannot prevent the toxic effects of the endotoxin. Bacteria that produce endotoxins are called pyrogenic bacteria because they activate the inflammatory process and produce fever. The innermost part of the lipopolysaccharide, lipid A, consists of polysaccharide and fatty acids and is responsible for the substance's toxic effects.

Inflammation is the body's initial response to the presence of the bacteria. Vascular permeability is increased, allowing blood-borne substances (i.e., the complement system) involved in bacterial destruction to access the site of infection. Endotoxins increase capillary permeability further by activating the anaphylatoxins (C5a and C3a) of the complement cascade.[9] Capillary permeability may increase sufficiently to permit the escape of large volumes of plasma, contributing to hypotension and, in severe cases, cardiovascular shock (see Chapter 23). Endotoxin also can activate the coagulation cascade, leading to the syndrome of disseminated (or diffuse) intravascular coagulation (see Chapter 20).

Bacteremia is the presence of bacteria in the blood, whereas **septicemia** is growth of bacteria in the blood and is caused by a failure of the body's defense mechanisms. The usual cause is proliferation of gram-negative bacteria, although a few gram-positive bacteria and fungi can also proliferate. Symptoms of gram-negative septic shock are produced by endotoxins. Once in the blood, endotoxins cause the release of vasoactive peptides and cytokines that affect blood vessels by producing vasodilation, which reduces blood pressure, causes decreased oxygen delivery, and produces subsequent cardiovascular shock (see Chapter 23). Sepsis is diagnosed from evaluation of blood cultures.

Endotoxic shock is a complication of sepsis and can be fatal to the individual. The cytokine tumor necrosis factor-alpha (TNF-α) plays a pivotal role in the pathogenesis of endotoxic shock. TNF-α is produced by activated macrophages on exposure to endotoxin from gram-negative bacterial infections. It is sometimes called cachectin because of its role in promoting cachexia in individuals with cancer. (Types of shock are discussed in Chapter 23.)

Viral Disease

Viral diseases are the most common afflictions of humans and include a variety of diseases ranging from the common cold and the "cold sore" of herpes simplex to several types of cancers and acquired immune deficiency syndrome (AIDS). Viruses are very simple microorganisms consisting of nucleic acid (the viral genome) protected from the environment by a layer or layers of proteins. They are sensitive to many environmental factors and have a short life span outside the cell.

Viral replication. Virions (viral particles) do not possess any of the metabolic organelles found in prokaryotes (e.g., bacteria) or eukaryotes (e.g., human cells). Thus viruses have no metabolism. Unlike bacteria, viruses are incapable of independent reproduction. Their replication depends totally on their ability to infect a permissive host cell—a cell that cannot resist viral invasion and replication. The replication cycle of most viruses can be divided into six distinct phases: adsorption, penetration, uncoating, replication, assembly, and release. Infection with a virus begins with a virion binding to a specific receptor on the plasma membrane of a host cell (Figure 7-2). The specificity of this virus-receptor interaction dictates the range of host cells that a particular virus will infect and therefore the clinical symptoms, which reflect the alteration of the function of the infected cells. For example, the influenza virus binds to a receptor on respiratory epithelial cells, causing symptoms of an upper respiratory tract infection. Once bound, the virion penetrates the plasma membrane by one of several means: by receptor-mediated endocytosis, by viral envelope fusion with the plasma membrane, or by directly crossing the plasma membrane.

Viruses contain their genetic information in either deoxyribonucleic acid (DNA) or ribonucleic acid (RNA). The viral genetic material is protected by a protein coat that must be removed in the cytoplasm of the infected host cell (uncoating). The viral genetic material may be processed by one of several paths, depending on the particular virus. Generally, all RNA viruses, except influenza and retroviruses, replicate their genetic material in the cytoplasm of the infected cell, and all DNA viruses, except poxviruses, require the DNA to enter the nucleus and use the cell's DNA polymerases to replicate. Poxviruses provide their own DNA polymerase and replicate their DNA in the cytoplasm of the infected cell. Retroviruses generally convert their RNA genetic information to DNA using an enzyme contained in the virion—reverse transcriptase.

After infection, viruses usually make multiple copies of their genetic material and produce the necessary viral proteins for replication. New

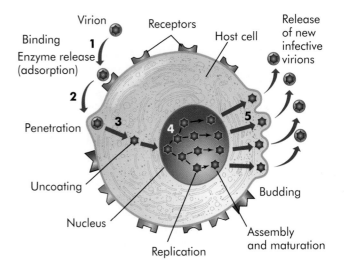

FIGURE 7-2 Stages of Viral Infection of a Host Cell. The virion *(1)* becomes attached to the cell's plasma membrane by absorption; *(2)* releases enzymes that weaken the membrane and allow it to penetrate the cell; *(3)* uncoats itself; *(4)* replicates; and *(5)* matures and escapes from the cell by budding from the plasma membrane. The infection then can spread to other host cells.

virions are assembled in the host cell's cytoplasm and are released from the cell for transmission of the viral infection to other host cells. This cycle is referred to as the productive or lytic cycle because a large number of progeny are produced, and the result is often the destruction of the host cell.

Some viruses will not be productive initially but instead initiate a latency phase, during which the host cell is transformed. During this phase, the viral DNA may be integrated into the DNA of the host cell and become a permanent passenger in that cell and its progeny. In response to stimuli, such as stress, hormonal changes, or disease, the virus may exit latency and enter a productive cycle.

Cellular effects of viruses. Besides assuming control of the host cell's metabolic machinery, viral infection can injure cells. In some viral infections, cellular destruction results from large quantities of virus being released from the cell's plasma membrane. Alteration of the plasma membrane by the expression of new antigens as a result of viral infection can incite an immune response against the individual's infected cells (e.g., hepatitis B virus). Once inside the cell, virions have many harmful effects, including the following:
1. Cessation of DNA, RNA, and protein synthesis (e.g., herpesvirus)
2. Disruption of lysosomal membranes, resulting in release of digestive lysosomal enzymes that can kill the cell (e.g., herpesvirus)

TABLE 7-6 EXAMPLES OF HUMAN DISEASES CAUSED BY SPECIFIC VIRUSES

BALTIMORE CLASSIFICATION	FAMILY	VIRUS	ENVELOPE	MAIN ROUTE OF TRANSMISSION	DISEASE
dsDNA	Adenoviruses	Adenovirus	No	Droplet contact	Acute febrile pharyngitis
	Herpesviruses	Herpes simplex type 1 (HSV-1)	Yes	Direct contact with saliva or lesions	Lesions in mouth, pharynx, conjunctivitis
		Herpes simplex type 2 (HSV-2)	Yes	Sexually, contact with lesions during birth	Sores on labia, meningitis in children
		Herpes simplex type 8 (HSV-8)	Yes	Sexually?, body fluids	Kaposi sarcoma
		Epstein-Barr virus (EBV)	Yes	Saliva	Mononucleosis, Burkitt lymphoma
		Cytomegalovirus (CMV)	Yes	Body fluids, mother's milk, transplacental	Mononucleosis, congenital infection
		Varicella-zoster virus (VZV)	Yes	Droplet contact	Chickenpox, shingles
ssDNA	Papovaviruses	Papillomavirus	No	Direct contact	Warts, cervical carcinoma
dsRNA	Reoviruses	Rotavirus	No	Fecal-oral	Severe diarrhea
ssRNA+	Picornaviruses	Coxsackievirus	No	Fecal-oral, droplet contact	Nonspecific febrile illness, conjunctivitis, meningitis
		Hepatitis A virus	No	Fecal-oral	Acute hepatitis
		Poliovirus	No	Fecal-oral	Poliomyelitis
		Rhinovirus	No	Droplet contact	Common cold
	Flaviviruses	Hepatitis C virus	Yes	Blood, sexually	Acute or chronic hepatitis, hepatocellular carcinoma
		Yellow fever virus	Yes	Mosquito vector	Yellow fever
		Dengue virus	Yes	Mosquito vector	Dengue fever
		West Nile virus	Yes	Mosquito vector	Meningitis, encephalitis
	Togaviruses	Rubella virus	Yes	Droplet contact, transplacental	Acute or congenital rubella
	Coronaviruses	SARS	Yes	Droplets in aerosol or direct contact	Severe respiratory disease
	Caliciviruses	Norovirus	No	Fecal-oral	Gastroenteritis
ssRNA−	Orthomyxoviruses	Influenza virus	Yes	Droplet contact	Influenza
	Paramyxoviruses	Measles virus	Yes	Droplet contact	Measles
		Mumps virus	Yes	Droplet contact	Mumps
		Parainfluenza virus	Yes	Droplet contact	Croup, pneumonia, common cold
		Respiratory syncytial virus (RSV)	Yes	Droplet contact, hand-to-mouth	Pneumonia, influenza-like syndrome
	Rhabdoviruses	Rabies virus	Yes	Animal bite, droplet contact	Rabies
	Bunyaviruses	Hantavirus	Yes	Aerosolized animal fecal material	Viral hemorrhagic fever
	Filoviruses	Ebola virus	Yes	Direct contact with body fluids	Viral hemorrhagic fever
		Marburg virus	Yes	Direct contact with body fluids	Viral hemorrhagic fever
	Arenavirus	Lassa virus	Yes	Aerosolized animal fecal material	Viral hemorrhagic fever
ssRNA+ with RT	Retroviruses	HIV	Yes	Sexually, blood products	AIDS
dsDNA with RT	Hepadnaviruses	Hepatitis B virus	Yes	All body fluids	Acute or chronic hepatitis, hepatocellular carcinoma

AIDS, Acquired immunodeficiency syndrome; *DNA,* deoxyribonucleic acid; *ds,* double-stranded; *HIV,* human immunodeficiency virus; *RNA,* ribonucleic acid; *RT,* reverse transcriptase; *SARS,* severe acute respiratory syndrome; *ss,* single-stranded.

3. Fusion of host cells, producing multinucleated giant cells (e.g., respiratory syncytial virus)
4. Alteration of the antigenic properties, or identity, of the infected cell, causing the individual's immune system to attack the cell as if it were foreign (e.g., hepatitis B virus)
5. Transformation of host cells into cancerous cells, resulting in uninhibited and unregulated growth (e.g., human papillomavirus)
6. Promotion of secondary bacterial infection in tissues damaged by viruses

Examples of human diseases caused by specific viruses are listed in Table 7-6.

Viral pathogens bypass many defense mechanisms by developing intracellularly, thus hiding within cells and away from normal inflammatory or immune responses. In many cases, however, because viral agents must spread from cell to cell, the developing immune response eventually cures the infection; therefore the disease is usually self-limiting in that it resolves without the need for medications. Some viruses will persist, and a state of unapparent infection may result. In persistent infections, cellular injury may be minimal, and the virus persists until it is activated to replicate (e.g., the cold sores of herpesvirus infection). Immunity may limit recurrent outbreaks and protect the individual from an acute exacerbation only or may be sufficiently strong to prevent disease.

Fungal Disease

Fungi are relatively large microorganisms with thick walls that have two basic structures: single-celled yeasts (spheres) or multicelled molds (filaments or hyphae) (Figure 7-3). Some fungi can exist in either form and are called **dimorphic fungi.** The cell walls of fungi are rigid and multilayered. The wall is composed of polysaccharides different from the peptidoglycans of bacteria. The lack of peptidoglycans

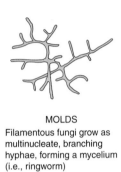

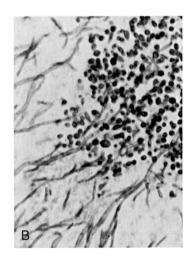

MOLDS
Filamentous fungi grow as multinucleate, branching hyphae, forming a mycelium (i.e., ringworm)

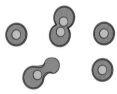
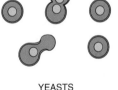

YEASTS
Yeasts grow as ovoid or spherical; single cells multiply by budding and division (i.e., *Histoplasma*)

A

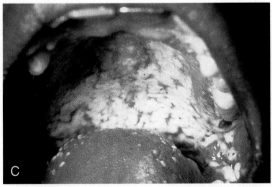

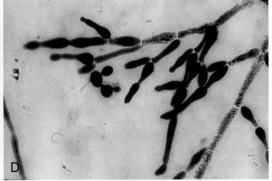

FIGURE 7-3 Morphology of Fungi. **(A)** Fungi may be either mold or yeast forms, or dimorphic. **(B)** Photograph showing *Candida albicans* with both the mycelial and the yeast forms. **(C)** Oral infection with *C. albicans* (candidiasis, i.e., thrush). **(D)** Gram stain of sputum showing that clinical isolates of *C. albicans* present as chains of elongated budding yeasts (× 1000). (A from Mims CA et al: *Medical microbiology,* ed 3, London, 2004, Mosby; B from Townsend C et al: *Sabiston textbook of surgery,* ed 18, Philadelphia, 2008, Saunders; C from Mandell G, Bennett J, Dolin R: *Principles and practice of infectious diseases,* ed 6, Philadelphia, 2005, Churchill Livingstone; D from McPherson R, Pincus M: *Henry's clinical diagnosis and management by laboratory methods,* ed 21, Philadelphia, 2006, Saunders.)

TABLE 7-7 COMMON PATHOGENIC FUNGI

PRIMARY SITE OF INFECTION	FUNGUS	DISEASE (PRIMARY)	SYMPTOMS
Superficial (no tissue invasion, little inflammation)	*Malassezia furfur*	Tinea versicolor, seborrheic dermatitis, dandruff	Red rash on body
Cutaneous (no tissue invasion, inflammatory response)	Dermatophytes	Tinea pedis (athlete's foot)	Scaling, fissures, pruritus
	Trichophyton mentagrophytes	Tinea cruris (jock itch)	Rash, pruritus
	Trichophyton rubrum	Tinea corporis (ringworm)	Lesion, raised border, scaling
	Microsporum canis		
	Candida albicans	Cutaneous candidiasis	Lesions in most areas of skin, mucous membranes, thrush, vaginal infection
Subcutaneous (tissue invasion)	*Sporothrix schenckii*	Sporotrichosis	Ulcers or abscesses on skin and other organ systems
Systemic (dimorphic; causes disease in healthy individuals)	*Stachybotrys chartarum* or "black mold"	Black mold disease	Rash, headaches, nausea, pain
	Coccidioides immitis	Coccidioidomycosis	Valley fever, flulike symptoms
	Histoplasma capsulatum	Histoplasmosis	Lung, flulike symptoms, disseminates to multiple organs, eye
	Blastomyces dermatitidis	Blastomycosis	Flulike symptoms, chest pains
Systemic (opportunistic)	*Aspergillus fumigatus, Aspergillus flavus*	Aspergillosis	Invasive to lungs and other organs
	Pneumocystis jiroveci	Pneumocystis pneumonia (PCP)	Pneumonia
	Cryptococcus neoformans	Cryptococcosis	Pneumonia-like illness, skin lesions, disseminates to brain, meningitis
	Candidia albicans	Systemic candidiasis	Sepsis, endocarditis, meningitis

allows fungi to resist the action of bacterial cell wall inhibitors such as penicillin and cephalosporin. In contrast to bacteria, the cytosols of fungi contain organelles: mitochondria, ribosomes, Golgi apparatus, microtubules, microvesicles, endoplasmic reticulum, and nuclei. Molds are aerobic, and yeasts are facultative anaerobes, which adapt to, but do not require, anaerobic conditions. They usually reproduce by simple division or budding.

Pathologic fungi cause disease by adapting to the host environment. Fungi that colonize the skin can digest keratin. Other fungi can grow with wide temperature variations in lower oxygen environments. Still other fungi have the capacity to suppress host immune defenses. Phagocytes and T lymphocytes are important in controlling fungi. Low white blood cell counts promote fungal infection and infection control is particularly important for individuals who are immunosuppressed.

Diseases caused by fungi are called **mycoses.** Mycoses can be superficial, deep, or opportunistic. Superficial mycoses occur on or near skin or mucous membranes and usually produce mild and superficial disease. Fungi that invade the skin, hair, or nails are known as **dermatophytes.** The diseases they produce are called *tineas* (ringworm), for example, tinea capitis (scalp), tinea pedis (feet), and tinea cruris (groin). Superficial dermatophytes grow in a ringlike, erythematous patch with a raised border. Itching (pruritus) often is intense, and cracking of tissue can occur and lead to secondary bacterial infection. Infections of the scalp are accompanied by scaling and hair loss. (Chapter 39 discusses the various skin disorders caused by fungi.)

Deep infections involving internal organs can be life-threatening and are most common in association with other diseases or as an opportunistic infection in immunosuppressed individuals. Fungi causing deep infection enter the body through inhalation or through open wounds. Filamentous forms can multiply extracellularly, but the spherical yeasts multiply within cells, including white blood cells. Some fungi are a part of the normal body flora and become pathologic only when immunity is compromised, allowing exaggerated growth and translocation. For example, *Candida albicans* is normally found in the mouth, gastrointestinal tract, and vagina of normal individuals. Changes in pH and use of antibiotics that destroy bacteria that normally inhibit *Candida* growth permit rapid proliferation and overgrowth, which can lead to superficial or deep infection. Common pathologic fungi are summarized in Table 7-7.

Fungi are diagnosed by microscopic observation of specimens treated with potassium hydroxide and stained to enhance visualization of spheres and filaments. Specimens also can be cultured. Skin tests are available for species of *Aspergillus*. No vaccines are available to prevent fungal disease effectively and techniques to prevent infection are important.[10] Many of the antifungal drugs (e.g., amphotericin B, ketoconazole, fluconazole) used to treat deep or systemic infections are toxic to the host because the fungal cell composition is similar to the host cell.

Parasitic Disease

Parasitic microorganisms establish symbiosis with another species in which the parasite benefits at the expense of the other species. Parasites range from unicellular protozoan to large worms. Parasitic worms (helminths) include intestinal and tissue nematodes (e.g., hookworm, roundworm), flukes (e.g., liver fluke, lung fluke), and tapeworms. A protozoan is a eukaryotic, unicellular microorganism with a nucleus and cytoplasm. Pathogenic protozoa include malaria (*Plasmodium*), amoebae (e.g., *Entamoeba histolytica*, which causes amoebic dysentery), and flagellates (e.g., *Giardia lamblia*, which causes diarrhea; *Trypanosoma*, which causes sleeping sickness). Although less common in the United States, parasites and protozoa are common causes of infections worldwide, with a significant effect on the mortality and morbidity of individuals in developing countries. Important parasites of humans are listed in Table 7-8.

Parasitic and protozoal infections are rarely transmitted from human to human. The predominant means is through vectors in which the microorganism spends part of its life cycle. Examples include the transmission of malaria (*Plasmodium* spp.) by mosquitoes, trypanosomes (*Trypanosoma cruzi*, which causes Chagas disease in

TABLE 7-8   EXAMPLES OF PARASITES THAT ARE IMPORTANT IN HUMANS

CATEGORY	SUBGROUP	SPECIES	DISEASE	ORGANS AFFECTED/SYMPTOMS
Protozoa	Ameboid	*Entamoeba histolytica*	Amebiasis	Dysentary, liver abscess
	Flagellate	*Giardia lamblia*	Giardiasis*	Diarrhea
		Trichomonas vaginalis	Trichomoniasis	Inflammation of reproductive organs
		Trypanosoma cruzi, T. brucei	Chagas disease: African sleeping sickness	Generalized, blood and lymph nodes, progressing to cardiac and CNS
	Ciliate	*Balantidium coli*	Balantidiasis	Small intestines, invasion of colon, diarrhea
	Sporozoa (nonmotile)	*Cryptosporidium parvum, C. hominis*	Cryptosporidiosis*	Intestine, diarrhea
		Plasmodium spp.	Malaria	Blood, liver
		Toxoplasma gondii	Toxoplasmosis*	Intestine, eyes, blood, heart, liver
Helminths	Flukes (trematodes)	*Fasciola hepatica*	Fasciolosis	Liver destruction
		Schistosoma mansoni	Schistosomiasis	Blood, diarrhea, bladder, generalized symptoms
	Tapeworms (cestodes)	*Taenia solium*	Pork tapeworm	Encysts in muscle, brain, liver
	Roundworms (nematodes)	*Ascaris lumbricoides*	Ascariasis	Intestinal obstruction, bile duct obstruction
		Necator americanus (hookworm)	Hookworm disease	Intestinal parasite
		Trichinella spiralis	Trichinosis*	Intestine, diarrhea, muscle, CNS, death
		Wuchereria bancrofti	Filariasis, elephantiasis	Lymphatics
		Enterobius vermicularis (pinworm)	Pinworm infection	Intestines
		Onchocerca volvulus	Onchocerciasis	Blindness, dermatitis

*Most common in the United States.

South America; *Trypanosoma brucei*, which causes sleeping sickness in Africa) by the tsetse fly, and *Leishmania* spp. by sand fleas. Many of the protozoal infectious agents (e.g., *E. histolytica*, *G. lamblia*) are encountered in contaminated water or food and transmission is by ingestion.

The initial attachment depends on whether the microorganism is injected into the bloodstream by a vector or whether entrance is through the gastrointestinal tract. Microorganisms in the bloodstream frequently have surface lectins that react with carbohydrates on specific cells. Malarial parasites attach to erythrocytes that express Duffy blood group antigens. Thus Duffy-negative individuals are resistant to malaria. *T. cruzi* can infect both CD4- and CD8-positive T cells through a T cell surface receptor. Several parasites express surface glycoproteins that facilitate preferential entrance into monocytes/macrophages using various receptors. *Leishmania* expresses a surface glycoprotein (gp63) that binds complement components (e.g., C3b) and uses the macrophage complement receptors to gain entrance to the macrophage.

Tissue damage may result directly by parasitic infestation in the tissue or be secondary to the individual's immune and inflammatory responses. The particular process depends a great deal on the burden of parasites infesting the site and the sensitivity of the particular site to damage. Large infestations may lead to physical loss of function in a tissue or organ. For instance, a large number of intestinal parasites (e.g., the roundworm *Ascaris lumbricoides*, tapeworms, *Giardia* spp.) compete for and prevent uptake of nutrients, leading to various forms of malabsorption, blocked uptake of fats, or anemia from malabsorption of vitamin B_{12} or from large amounts of blood loss. Filarial parasites (e.g., *Wuchereria bancrofti* and *Brugia malayi*, which causes elephantiasis) block the lymphatics and cause accumulation of lymph in tissues. The larvae of tapeworms (e.g., *Taenia solium*) encyst in and prevent normal function of organs (e.g., muscle, liver, eye), which is particularly dangerous in the human brain.

Toxins released from the parasite may cause significant irreversible organ damage. Proteolytic enzymes from *E. histolytica* are very cytolytic, leading to ulceration of intestinal walls, bloody diarrhea, amoebic dysentery, dehydration, and death in infants and young children. *T. cruzi* secretes a neurotoxin that affects the anatomic nervous system, a small-molecular-weight toxin that causes fever, and proteases and phospholipases, leading to tissue destruction.

The infected individual's immune and inflammatory responses result in considerable pathology. Schistosomiasis results in the deposition of eggs in organs (e.g., liver), which leads to formation of granulomas and tissue destruction through fibrosis. Some parasitic products (*T. brucei*, malarial parasites) activate macrophages to overproduce cytokines, which leads to exacerbated inflammation.

Clinical Manifestations of Infection

The progression from infection to infectious disease follows predictable stages (infection, incubation, symptoms, shedding of the microorganism). Clinical manifestations of infectious disease vary, depending on the pathogen and the organ system affected. Manifestations can arise directly from the infecting microorganism or its products; however, the majority of the clinical symptoms result from the host's inflammatory and immune responses. Infectious diseases typically begin with the nonspecific or general symptoms of fatigue, malaise, weakness, and loss of concentration. Generalized aching and loss of appetite are common complaints. However, the hallmark of most infectious diseases is fever.

Fever resulting from cytokines has been discussed in Chapter 5. Exogenous pyrogens produced by an infectious agent may not cause fever directly but induce the production of endogenous pyrogens during inflammation. Endogenous pyrogens include interleukin-1 (IL-1), interleukin-6 (IL-6), interferon, tumor necrosis factor-alpha (TNF-α), and other cytokines. It is generally accepted that fever has a beneficial effect against infection, although the mechanisms have not been fully established.

Countermeasures Against Pathogenic Defenses

The body's innate and acquired responses against microorganisms are numerous and involve an interaction between the immune and inflammatory systems. Pathogenic microorganisms, however, have developed

TABLE 7-9	REDUCTION IN VACCINE-PREVENTABLE DISEASES IN THE UNITED STATES		
DISEASE	**BASELINE 20TH CENTURY ANNUAL CASES***	**2009 CASES**	**% REDUCTION**
Diphtheria	175,885	0	100
Measles	503,282	61	99.9
Mumps	152,209	982	99.4
Pertussis	147,271	13,506	90.8
Smallpox	48,164	0	100
Polio	16,316	0	100
Rubella	47,745	4	99.9
Tetanus	1,314	14	98.9
Haemophilus influenzae type b, invasive	20,000	25	99.9

From Centers for Disease Control and Prevention: *MMWR Morb Mortal Wkly Rep* 48(12):243–248, 1999; *Morb Mortal Wkly Rep* 58(11):289–291, 2008; 2009 data from Provisional cases of selected notifiable diseases, *MMWR Morb Mortal Wkly Rep* 58(51,52):1446–1456, 2010.
*Average number of reported cases over multiple years before initiation of vaccine.

TABLE 7-10	CHEMICALS OR ANTIMICROBIALS IDENTIFIED THAT PREVENT GROWTH OF OR DESTROY MICROORGANISMS
MECHANISM OF ACTION	**AGENT**
Inhibits synthesis of cell wall	Penicillins, cephalosporins, monobactams, carbapenems, vancomycin, bacitracin, cycloserine, fosfomycin
Damages cytoplasmic membrane	Polymyxins, polyene antifungals, imidazoles
Alters metabolism of nucleic acid	Quinolones, rifampin, nitrofurans, nitroimidazoles
Inhibits protein synthesis	Aminoglycosides, tetracyclines, chloramphenicol, macrolides, clindamycin, spectinomycin, sulfonamides
Alters energy metabolism	Trimethoprim, dapsone, isoniazid

Modified from Ellner PD, Neu HCP: *Understanding infectious disease,* St Louis, 1992, Mosby.

means of circumventing the individual's protective defenses. Therefore prophylactic or interventive procedures have been developed either to prevent the pathogen from initiating disease (vaccines) or to destroy the pathogen once the disease process has started (antimicrobials). Most vaccine development has focused on preventing the most severe and common infections (Table 7-9). With the initial success of antibiotic therapy, there was no perceived need for vaccination against many common and non–life-threatening infections. The increasing problem of antibiotic-resistant pathogens, however, has forced a reappraisal of that strategy, and a greater emphasis now is being placed on the development of new vaccines.[11]

Antimicrobials

Since initiation of the widespread use of penicillin during World War II, antibiotics have shown the greatest impact on successful resistance to infection. Antibiotics are natural products of fungi, bacteria, and related microorganisms that affect the growth of other microorganisms. Some antibacterial antibiotics are bactericidal (kill the microorganism), whereas others are bacteriostatic (inhibit growth until the microorganism is destroyed by the individual's own protective mechanisms). The mechanisms of action of most antibiotics are (1) inhibition of the function or production of the cell wall, (2) prevention of protein synthesis, (3) blockage of DNA replication, or (4) interference with folic acid metabolism (Table 7-10). Because viruses use the enzymes of the host's cells, there has been far less success in developing antiviral antibiotics.

Immediately after antibiotics became widely used, microorganisms mutated and developed resistance.[12] By 1944 an adequate supply of penicillin allowed its widespread use to treat infections. In 1946 a hospital in Britain reported that 14% of all *Staphylococcus aureus* infections were penicillin resistant. By 1950 the same hospital reported an increase to 59% and to greater than 89% in the 1990s. Over the past few decades healthcare providers have observed increasing incidences of drug-resistant malaria, tuberculosis,

gonorrhea, salmonellosis, shigellosis, and staphylococcal infections. *Streptococcus pneumoniae*, which causes pneumonia, meningitis, and acute otitis media (middle ear infection), was once routinely susceptible to penicillin. Since the 1980s, however, the incidence of penicillin-resistant microorganisms has risen to greater than 30% in some populations.

Antibiotic resistance is usually a result of genetic mutations that can be transmitted directly to neighboring microorganisms by plasmid exchange. Microorganisms commonly develop the capacity to inactivate antibiotics. Penicillin resistance, for example, results from the production of an enzyme (β-lactamase) that breaks down the structure of the antibiotic. Other forms of resistance result from modification of the target molecule. Azidothymidine (AZT) is a family of antivirals that suppresses the enzymatic activity of reverse transcriptase, a viral-specific enzyme responsible for the replication of viral RNA and production of a DNA copy. HIV frequently mutates and produces an AZT-resistant reverse transcriptase. A third mechanism of resistance is mediated by multidrug transporters in the microorganism's membrane. These transporters affect the rate of intracellular accumulation of the antimicrobial by preventing entrance or, more commonly, by increasing active efflux of the antibiotic. Antibiotic-resistant strains of *M. tuberculosis* are protected from aminoglycosides and tetracycline by a multidrug pump that increases efflux.

A rapid emergence of multiple antibiotic–resistant bacteria has been observed. These microorganisms are resistant to almost all currently available antibiotics. For example, *Streptococcus pneumoniae*, which initially was only resistant to penicillin, is now resistant to multiple antibiotics. In some areas, more than 20% of tuberculosis cases are caused by multiple antibiotic–resistant *M. tuberculosis*. **Methicillin-resistant *Staphylococcus aureus* (MRSA)** incorporates several different mechanisms of resistance and has become a major health problem in hospitals. Also, the incidence of drug-resistant malaria, pneumococcal disease, salmonellosis, shigellosis, and staphylococcal infections has increased dramatically (see *Health Alert:* The Continued Rise of Antibiotic-Resistant Microorganisms).

Why have multiple antibiotic–resistant microorganisms appeared? Lack of compliance concerning the necessity of completing the

HEALTH ALERT

The Continued Rise of Antibiotic-Resistant Microorganisms

The existence of antibiotic-resistant pathogenic bacteria was observed soon after the advent of antibiotic therapy during World War II. In most cases alternative antibiotics were readily available. Many common pathogenic bacteria and yeast have since developed resistance to multiple antibiotics: *Mycobacterium tuberculosis, Enterococcus, Clostridium difficile, Streptococcus pneumoniae, Klebsiella pneumoniae, Pseudomonas aeruginosa, Candida,* and others. A major example has been *Staphylococcus aureus. S. aureus* is part of the normal bacterial flora present in healthy individuals; about 30% of healthy individuals have asymptomatic colonization in the nostrils. Penicillin-resistant *S. aureus* was reported in the 1950s and methicillin-resistant *S. aureus* (MRSA) organisms were reported in the early 1960s. Currently, the prevalence of MRSA with resistance to other antibiotics (multidrug resistant) is increasing. In the past MRSA was observed primarily in hospitals and nursing homes in persons whose defenses had been compromised. Now it is becoming the primary microorganism found in community-acquired infections, primarily skin infections such as cellulitis and abscesses, of healthy individuals. Community-acquired MRSA has not yet developed multiple antibiotic resistance.

The situation may be about to become considerably worse. Very recently strains of multiple antibiotic-resistant *Neisseria gonorrhoeae* have emerged. The incidence of gonorrhea has been relatively stable in the United States with more than 260,000 new cases of gonorrhea reported for 2009, which may be considerably underestimated. In 2007 27% of isolates were resistant to a large variety of antibiotics, and the CDC had recommended cephalosporins as the only class of antibiotics for treating gonorrhea. Recently investigators from Australia and England have identified strains that are resistant to cefiximine and ceftriaxone, widely used cephalosporins.

Data from DeLeo FR: Community-associated methicillin-resistant *Staphylococcus aureus, Lancet* 375(9725):1557–1568, 2010; Centers for Disease Control and Prevention (CDC): Provisional cases of selected notifiable diseases, *MMWR Morb Mortal Wkly Rep* 58(51,52):1446–1456, 2010; Centers for Disease Control and Prevention (CDC): Update to CDC's sexually transmitted diseases treatment guidelines, 2006: fluoroquinolones no longer recommended for treatment of gonococcal infections, *MMWR Morb Mortal Wkly Rep* 56(14):332–336, 2007.

therapeutic regimen with antibiotics allows the selective resurgence of microorganisms that are more relatively resistant to the antibiotic. Overuse of antibiotics can lead to the destruction of the normal flora, allowing the selective overgrowth of antibiotic-resistant strains or pathogens that had previously been controlled. For example, after treatment with the antibiotic clindamycin, the normal intestinal flora can become compromised, allowing the overgrowth of *Clostridium difficile* and the development of pseudomembranous colitis (a bacterial infection of the intestines). *C. difficile* infections are often acquired in hospitals or other healthcare institutions with a long-term patient population and the number of deaths is rising steadily; reported deaths rose from 793 in 1999 to 6372 deaths in 2007, with 92% of the deaths occurring in individuals age 65 years or older.[1]

Vaccines

Vaccines are biologic preparations of weakened or dead pathogens that when administered stimulate production of antibodies or cellular immunity against the pathogen without causing disease. The purpose of vaccination is to induce long-lasting protective immune responses under conditions that will not result in disease in a healthy recipient of the vaccine. The primary immune response from vaccination is generally short lived; therefore booster injections are used to push the immune response through multiple secondary responses that result in large numbers of memory cells and sustained protective levels of antibody or T cells, or both.

Mass vaccination programs have been tremendously successful and have led to major changes in the health of the world's population. In the early 1950s an estimated 50 million cases of smallpox occurred each year, with about 15 million deaths. The World Health Organization (WHO) conducted a smallpox immunization campaign from 1967 to 1977 that resulted in the global eradication of smallpox by 1979.[13] Many vaccines are used in the United States to protect against pathogens. The Centers for Disease Control and Prevention (CDC) provides updated vaccine schedules at their website: www.cdc.gov/vaccines/recs/schedules/default.htm.

Development of a successful vaccine is costly and depends on several factors. These include identification of the protective immune response and the appropriate antigen to induce that response. For instance, individuals with ongoing HIV infection produce a great deal of antibody against several HIV antigens. But, for development of a successful vaccine, we must first understand which antibody will protect against an initial infection.

Once a good candidate antigen is identified, it must be developed into an effective, cost-efficient, stable, and safe vaccine. For instance, most vaccines against viral infection (measles, mumps, rubella, varicella [chickenpox]) contain live viruses that are weakened (**attenuated virus**) so they continue to express appropriate antigens but establish only a limited and easily controlled infection. For most common vaccines against viral infections, limited replication of the virus appears to afford better long-term protection than using viral antigen. One current exception is the hepatitis B vaccine, which uses a recombinant viral protein. The hepatitis A vaccine is an inactivated (killed) virus and normally should not cause an infection.

Even attenuated viruses can establish life-threatening infections in individuals whose immune systems are congenitally deficient or suppressed. The risk of infection by the vaccine strain of virus is extremely small, but it may affect the choice of recommended vaccines.[14] For instance, the Sabin vaccine was an attenuated virus that was administered orally. It provided systemic protection and induced a secretory immune response to prevent growth of the poliovirus in the intestinal tract. Being a live virus, the vaccine could cause polio in some children who had unsuspected immune deficiencies (about 1 case in 2.4 million doses). The Salk vaccine was a completely inactivated virus administered by injection. It induced protective systemic immunity but did not provide adequate secretory immunity. Therefore even if the individual was protected from systemic infection by poliovirus, the virus could transiently infect the individual's intestinal mucosa, be shed, and spread to others. When polio was epidemic, the oral vaccine was preferred. Vaccination has been extremely effective: 2525 cases of paralytic polio were reported in the United States in 1960, 61 cases were reported in 1965, and no cases of polio have been reported since 1979. In 1994 the disease polio was declared officially eradicated in all the Americas. The goal of the World Health Organization is to eradicate polio worldwide in the next few years. However, the live attenuated vaccine itself caused about eight cases of paralytic polio per year in the United States in individuals with inadequate immune systems. As a result, the current recommendation of the Centers for Disease Control and Prevention is vaccination with the killed virus.

Some common bacterial vaccines are killed microorganisms or extracts of bacterial antigens. The vaccine against pneumococcal pneumonia consists of a mixture of capsular polysaccharides from 10 strains of *Streptococcus pneumoniae*. Of the more than 90 known strains of this microorganism, only these 10 cause the most severe illnesses. However, the capsular vaccine is not very immunogenic in young children. A *conjugated* vaccine is available that contains capsular polysaccharides from seven strains that are conjugated to carrier proteins in order to increase immunogenicity. A similar vaccine is available for *Haemophilus influenzae* type b (Hib).

Some bacterial pathogens are not invasive, but do colonize mucosal membranes or wounds and release potent toxins that act locally or systemically. These include the bacteria that cause diphtheria, cholera, and tetanus. Vaccination against systemic toxins (e.g., diphtheria, tetanus) has been achieved using toxoids—purified toxins that have been chemically detoxified without loss of immunogenicity. Pertussis (whooping cough) vaccine has been changed from a killed whole-cell vaccine to cellular extract (acellular) vaccine that contains the pertussis toxoid and additional bacterial antigens. This change has dramatically reduced adverse side effects (fever, local inflammatory reactions, and others).

With so many available vaccines there has been an effort to combine vaccines in order to minimize the number of required injections. One of the first licensed vaccine mixtures was DPT, which now usually contains diphtheria (D) and tetanus (T) toxoids and acellular pertussis vaccine (aP). More recent mixtures include DTaP with inactivated poliovirus, either with Hib conjugate to tetanus toxoid or with hepatitis B vaccine.

A common problem is compliance of the susceptible population in vaccination programs. Even with successful development of a vaccine, however, a certain percentage of the population will be genetically unresponsive to vaccination and therefore will not produce a protective immune response. With most vaccines, the percentage of unresponsive individuals is low, and they will benefit from successful immunization of the rest of the population. Depending on the microorganism, a certain percentage of the population (usually about 85%) should be immunized in order to achieve protection of the total population. This is referred to as herd immunity. If this level of immunization is not achieved, outbreaks of infection can occur. For instance, an effective measles (rubeola) vaccine was made available in 1963 and resulted in a dramatic decrease in the number of measles cases. Many parents became complacent and did not obtain measles vaccination for their preschool children. As a result, a large increase in the number of cases and deaths in 1989 and 1990 occurred, which initiated a reemphasis on complete immunization before children could start school.[15] More recently resistance to immunization with measles has increased, and in early 2008 the number of measles cases in the United States increased by about fourfold. In several European countries immunization programs have been disrupted by antivaccine groups. As a result the incidence of pertussis (whooping cough) increased by 10 to 100 times compared with neighboring countries that maintained a high incidence of immunization.

The reluctance to vaccinate has generally been based on potential vaccine dangers. As with any medicine, complications can arise. In the case of vaccines, these include pain and redness at the injection site, fever, allergic reactions to vaccine ingredients, infection associated with attenuated viruses in immune-deficient individuals, and others. Some dangers do exist, although extremely rarely. For instance, a rotavirus vaccine approved more than a decade ago was found to increase the risk for a life-threatening bowel obstruction resulting from twisting of the intestines, and the vaccine was recalled.[16] More commonly the reluctance is based on inadequate information. A commonly discussed fear is related to the presence of the preservative thimerosal in vaccines. Thimerosal is a mercury-containing compound that has been used as a preservative since the 1930s. Although no cases of mercury toxicity have been reported secondary to vaccination, thimerosal was removed from all vaccines in 2001, with the exception of some inactivated influenza vaccines.[17] In 2003 groups in northern Nigeria claimed that the oral polio vaccine was unsafe and were tainted with antifertility drugs (estradiol), HIV, and cancer-causing agents. The reasoning appeared to be secondary to mounting distrust of Western nations because of conflicts in the Middle East. The effect was suspension of polio immunization for almost 1 year in two states and reduction of immunization in three other states.[18] The incidence of polio rose dramatically and more than 27,000 cases of paralysis resulted. By 2006 Nigeria accounted for 51% of the global polio cases, and this region acted as a reservoir for the dissemination of polio to previously polio-free areas in neighboring countries.[19] After renewal of immunization programs the number of cases of polio in Nigeria has since dropped by more than 90% to only 388 new cases in 2009.[20]

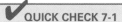

QUICK CHECK 7-1
1. How do antigenic changes in viral pathogens promote disease?
2. What are three mechanisms pathogens use to block the immune system?
3. What is the difference between an endotoxin and an exotoxin?

DEFICIENCIES IN IMMUNITY

An immune deficiency is the failure of the immune or inflammatory response to function normally, resulting in increased susceptibility to infections. Primary (congenital) immune deficiency is caused by a genetic defect, whereas secondary (acquired) immune deficiency is caused by another condition, such as cancer, infection, or normal physiologic changes, such as aging. Acquired forms of immune deficiency are far more common than the congenital forms.

Initial Clinical Presentation

The clinical hallmark of immune deficiency is a tendency to develop unusual or recurrent, severe infections. Preschool and school-age children normally may have 6 to 12 infections per year, and adults may have 2 to 4 infections per year. Most of these are not severe and are limited to viral infections of the upper respiratory tract, recurrent streptococcal pharyngitis, or mild otitis media (middle ear infections).

Potential immune deficiencies should be considered if the individual has experienced severe, documented bouts of pneumonia, otitis media, sinusitis (sinus infection), bronchitis, septicemia (blood infection), or meningitis or infections with opportunistic microorganisms that normally are not pathogenic (e.g., *Pneumocystis carinii*). Infections are generally recurrent with only short intervals of relative health, and multiple simultaneous infections are common. Individuals with immune deficiencies often have eight or more ear infections, two or more serious sinus infections, and two or more pneumonias, recurrent abscesses, or persistent fungal infections (particularly thrush) within a year. Recurrent internal infections, such as meningitis, osteomyelitis, or sepsis, are common. Prolonged antibiotic use is commonly ineffective by oral or injected routes and may necessitate intravenous administration. A familial history of immune deficiency may be found in some types of primary deficiency.

The type of recurrent infections may indicate the type of immune defect.[21] Deficiencies in T cell immune responses are suggested when recurrent infections are caused by certain viruses (e.g., varicella, vaccinia, herpes, cytomegalovirus), fungi and yeasts (e.g., *Candida*, *Histoplasma*), or certain atypical microorganisms (e.g., *P. carinii*). B cell deficiencies and phagocyte deficiencies, however, are suggested if the individual has documented, recurrent infections with microorganisms that require opsonization (e.g., encapsulated bacteria) or with viruses against which humoral immunity is normally effective (e.g., rubella). Some complement deficiencies resemble defects in antibody or phagocyte function, but others are associated with disseminated infections with bacteria of the genus *Neisseria* (*Neisseria meningitides* and *Neisseria gonorrhoeae*).

Primary (Congenital) Immune Deficiencies

Most primary immune deficiencies are the result of a single gene defect (Table 7-11). Generally, the mutations are sporadic and not inherited: a family history exists in only about 25% of individuals. The sporadic mutations occur before birth, but the onset of symptoms may be early or later, depending on the particular syndrome.[21] In some instances, symptoms of immune deficiency appear within the first 2 years of life. Other immune deficiencies are progressive, with the onset of symptoms appearing in the second or third decade of life.

Many immune deficiencies also are associated with other characteristic defects, some of which appear to be unrelated to the immune system yet may be life-threatening by themselves. Examples are given in the following discussion. These associated symptoms can be useful diagnostically and can clarify the pathophysiology of the disease.

Individually, primary immune deficiencies are rare. For instance, only 30 to 50 new cases of severe combined immunodeficiency (SCID) are diagnosed in the United States yearly. However, more than 70 different deficiencies have been identified. Together, primary immune deficiencies are more common than cystic fibrosis, hemophilia, childhood leukemia, or many other well-known diseases. The distribution between genders is about even, although some specific diseases have a male or female predominance. The three most commonly diagnosed deficiencies are common variable immune deficiency (34%), selective immunoglobulin A (IgA) deficiency (24%), and IgG subclass deficiency (17%).

Primary immune deficiencies are classified into five groups, based on which principal component of the immune or inflammatory systems is defective: defects of B lymphocytes, T lymphocytes, both B and T lymphocytes (combined), phagocytes, or complement.

TABLE 7-11   EXAMPLES OF PRIMARY IMMUNE DEFICIENCIES

CLASSIFICATION	EXAMPLE	IMMUNE DEFICIENCY	OUTCOME
B Lymphocyte Deficiencies			
Defective development of B cells in central lymphoid organ (bone marrow)	Bruton agammaglobulinemia	Lack of B cells, little or no antibody production	Recurrent, life-threatening bacterial infections
Defect in class-switch	Selective IgA deficiency	Little or no production of IgA, with normal production of other classes of antibody	Mild infections of gastrointestinal and respiratory tracts
T Lymphocyte Deficiencies			
Defective development of T cells in central lymphoid organ (thymus)	DiGeorge syndrome	Lack of T cells	Recurrent, life-threatening fungal and viral infections
Defect in development of cellular immunity against specific antigen	Chronic mucocutaneous candidiasis	Lack of T cell response to *Candida*	Recurrent and disseminated infections with fungus *Candida albicans*
Combined Immune Deficiencies			
Defective development of both B and T cells	Severe combined immunodeficiencies (SCIDs)	Lack of both T and B cells, little or no antibody production or cellular immunity	Recurrent, life-threatening infections with variety of microorganisms
Defects in cooperation among B cells, T cells, and antigen-presenting cells	Bare lymphocyte syndrome	No antigen presentation because of lack of MHC class I or MHC class II molecules on cell surface	Recurrent, life-threatening infections with variety of microorganisms
Large variety of defects that affect function of B or T cells	Wiskott-Aldrich syndrome	Cytoskeletal defect resulting in selective decrease in IgM production	Recurrent infections with select groups of microorganisms; in this example bacteria with polysaccharide capsules
Complement Deficiencies			
Defective production of one early component of complement system	C3 deficiency	Little or no C3 produced	Recurrent, life-threatening bacterial infections
Defective production of component of membrane attack complex	C6 deficiency	Little or no C6 produced	Recurrent disseminated infections with *Neisseria gonorrhoeae* or *N. meningitidis*
Phagocyte Deficiencies			
Defects in production of neutrophils	Severe congenital neutropenia	Lack of neutrophils	Recurrent, life-threatening bacterial infections
Defects in bacterial killing	Chronic granulomatous disease	Lack of production of oxygen products (e.g., hydrogen peroxide)	Recurrent infections with bacteria that are sensitive to killing by oxygen-dependent mechanisms

B Lymphocyte Deficiencies

B lymphocyte deficiencies result from defects in antibody production.[21] Because T cell immunity rarely depends on competent B cell responses, T cell immune responses are not affected in pure B lymphocyte deficiencies. The results are lower levels of circulating immunoglobulins (hypogammaglobulinemia) or occasionally totally or nearly absent immunoglobulins (agammaglobulinemia).[22]

Some defects may involve a particular class of antibody, such as selective IgA deficiency. This occurs in 1 in 700 to 1 in 400 individuals. Individuals with this deficiency produce other classes of immunoglobulins but not IgA. This suggests a failure to class-switch to IgA and mature into IgA-producing plasma cells. Many individuals are asymptomatic, although others have a history of severe, recurring sinus, pulmonary, and gastrointestinal infections. Individuals with IgA deficiency often have chronic intestinal candidiasis (infection with *C. albicans*). Complications of IgA deficiency include severe allergic disease and autoimmune diseases. Studies of these individuals show that secretory IgA normally may prevent the uptake of allergens from the environment. Therefore IgA deficiency may lead to increased allergen uptake and a more intense challenge to the immune system because of prolonged exposure to environmental antigens.

Bruton agammaglobulinemia is caused by blocked development of mature B cells in bursal-equivalent tissue. There are few or no circulating B cells, although T cell number and function are normal, resulting in repeated infections, such as otitis media, streptococcal sore throat, and conjunctivitis, and more serious conditions, such as septicemia.

T Lymphocyte Deficiencies

T lymphocyte deficiencies are defects in the development and function of cell-mediated immunity.[21] Because Th cells are obligatory in the development of many B lymphocyte responses, antibody production is often diminished, although the B cells are fully capable of producing an adequate antibody response. Immunodeficiency of T cell function contributes to failure to thrive (severely diminished rate of growth), oral infections (e.g., candidiasis), chronic diarrhea, pneumonia, and skin rashes.

Some immune deficiencies are characterized by a defect in the capacity to produce an immune response against a particular antigen. In chronic mucocutaneous candidiasis, the T lymphocytes cannot respond to a specific infectious agent, *C. albicans*. These individuals usually have mild to extremely severe recurrent *Candida* infections involving the mucous membranes and skin.

DiGeorge syndrome (congenital thymic aplasia or hypoplasia and diminished parathyroid gland development) is caused by the lack or partial lack of the thymus, resulting in greatly decreased T cell numbers and function. The cause is defective development of several tissues originating from the third and fourth pharyngeal pouches during embryonic development. Lack of the parathyroid gland causes an inability to regulate calcium concentration. Low blood calcium levels cause the development of tetany or involuntary rigid muscular contraction. DiGeorge syndrome is frequently associated with abnormal development of facial features that are controlled by the same embryonic pouches; these include low-set ears, fish-shaped mouth, and other altered features (Figure 7-4).

Combined Deficiencies

Combined deficiencies result from defects that directly affect the development of both T and B lymphocytes.[21] Some combined deficiencies result in major defects in both the T and B cell immune

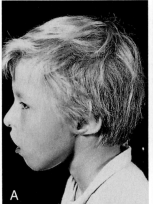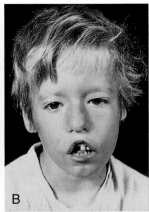

FIGURE 7-4 Facial Anomalies Associated With DiGeorge Syndrome. Note the wide-set eyes, low-set ears, and shortened structure of the upper lip. (From Male D et al: *Immunology*, ed 7, St Louis, 2006, Mosby.)

responses, whereas others are partial and more adversely affect T cells than B cells. The most severe disorders are called severe combined immunodeficiencies (SCIDs). Most individuals with SCIDs have few detectable lymphocytes in the circulation and secondary lymphoid organs (spleen, lymph nodes). The thymus usually is underdeveloped because of the absence of T cells. Immunoglobulin levels, especially IgM and IgA, are absent or greatly reduced. Several forms of SCID are caused by autosomal recessive enzymatic defects that result in the accumulation of toxic metabolites to which rapidly dividing cells, such as lymphocytes, are especially sensitive. For instance, deficiency of adenosine deaminase (ADA deficiency) results in the accumulation of toxic purines.

Even if nearly adequate numbers of B and T cells are produced, their cooperation may be defective. The bare lymphocyte syndrome is an immune deficiency characterized by an inability of lymphocytes and macrophages to produce major histocompatibility complex (MHC) class I or class II molecules. Without MHC molecules, antigen presentation and intercellular cooperation cannot occur effectively. Children with this deficiency develop serious, life-threatening infections and usually die before the age of 5 years.

Some combined immune deficiencies result in depressed development of a small portion of the immune system. For instance, an individual can be unable to produce a certain class of antibody, as in Wiskott-Aldrich syndrome (an X-linked recessive disorder), where IgM antibody production is greatly depressed. Antibody responses against antigens that elicit primarily an IgM response, such as polysaccharide antigens from bacterial cell walls (e.g., of *P. aeruginosa*, *S. pneumoniae*, *Haemophilus influenzae*, and other microorganisms with polysaccharide outer capsules), are deficient. In addition, there are defects in platelets presumably because of the absence of certain glycoproteins. Clinical manifestations include bleeding because of decreases in circulating platelets, eczema, and recurrent infections (e.g., otitis media, pneumonia, herpes simplex, cytomegalovirus).

Complement Deficiencies

Many complement deficiencies have been described.[21] C3 deficiency is the most severe defect. C3 unites all pathways of complement activation, and complement component C3b is a major opsonin. Persons with C3 deficiency are at risk for recurrent life-threatening infections with encapsulated bacteria (e.g., *Haemophilus influenzae* and *Streptococcus pneumoniae*) at an early age. Deficiencies of terminal components of the complement cascade (C5, C6, C7, C8, or C9 deficiencies) are associated with increased infections with only one group of bacteria—those of the genus *Neisseria* (*Neisseria meningitides* or *N. gonorrhoeae*). *Neisseria* usually cause localized infections (meningitis or gonorrhea), but those with terminal pathway defects have more than an 8000-fold increased risk for systemic infections with atypical strains of these microorganisms.

Phagocytic Deficiencies

Phagocytic deficiencies usually result in recurrent infections with the same group of microorganisms (encapsulated bacteria) associated with antibody and complement deficiencies.[21] A variety of defects in the destruction of microorganisms have been described. Chronic granulomatous disease (CGD) is a severe defect in the myeloperoxidase-hydrogen peroxide system. A major means of bacterial destruction uses the enzyme myeloperoxidase, halides (e.g., chloride ion), and hydrogen peroxide (H_2O_2). As a result of phagocytosis, neutrophils and other phagocytes switch much of their glucose metabolism to the hexose-monophosphate shunt. A by-product of this pathway is the conversion of molecular oxygen by nicotinamide adenine dinucleotide phosphate (NADPH) oxidase into highly reactive oxygen derivatives, including hydrogen peroxide. Mutations in NADPH oxidase result in deficient production of hydrogen peroxide and other oxygen products. Thus affected individuals have adequate myeloperoxidase and halide but lack the necessary hydrogen peroxide, resulting in recurrent severe pneumonias; tumor-like granulomata in lungs, skin, and bones; and other infections with some normal, relatively innocuous microorganisms, such as *Staphylococcus aureus*, *Serratia marcescens*, *Aspergillus* spp., and others.

Secondary (Acquired) Immune Deficiencies

Secondary, or acquired, immune and inflammatory deficiencies are far more common than primary deficiencies. These deficiencies are not related to genetic defects but are complications of other physiologic or pathophysiologic conditions.[23] Some conditions that are known to be associated with acquired deficiencies are summarized in Box 7-2.

Although secondary deficiencies are common, many are not clinically relevant. In many cases, the degree of the immune deficiency is relatively minor and without any apparent increased susceptibility to infection. Alternatively, the immune system may be substantially suppressed, but only for a short duration, thus minimizing the incidence of clinically relevant infections. Some secondary immune deficiencies (e.g., AIDS), however, are extremely severe and may result in recurrent life-threatening infections.

Evaluation and Care of Those With Immune Deficiency

Routine care of individuals with primary or secondary immune deficiencies must be tempered with the knowledge that the immune system may be totally ineffective. It is unsafe to administer conventional immunizing agents or blood products to many of these individuals because of the risk of causing an uncontrolled infection. Uncontrolled infection is a particular problem when attenuated vaccines that contain live but weakened microorganisms are used (e.g., live polio vaccine; vaccines against measles, mumps, and rubella).

The most common presenting symptom of immune deficiencies is recurrent severe infections. Significant information on the specific immune deficiency can be obtained by noting certain characteristics

---

BOX 7-2 SOME CONDITIONS KNOWN TO BE ASSOCIATED WITH ACQUIRED IMMUNE DEFICIENCIES

Normal Physiologic Conditions
Pregnancy
Infancy
Aging

Psychologic Stress
Emotional trauma
Eating disorders

Dietary Insufficiencies
Malnutrition caused by insufficient intake of large categories of nutrients, such as protein or calories
Insufficient intake of specific nutrients, such as vitamins, iron, or zinc
Infections
Congenital infections, such as rubella, cytomegalovirus, hepatitis B
Acquired infections, such as AIDS

Malignancies
Malignancies of lymphoid tissues, such as Hodgkin disease, acute or chronic leukemia, or myeloma
Malignancies of nonlymphoid tissues, such as sarcomas and carcinomas

Physical Trauma
Burns

Medical Treatments
Stress caused by surgery
Anesthesia
Immunosuppressive treatment with corticosteroids or antilymphocyte antibodies
Splenectomy
Cancer treatment with cytotoxic drugs or ionizing radiation

Other Diseases or Genetic Syndromes
Diabetes
Alcoholic cirrhosis
Sickle cell disease
Systemic lupus erythematosus (SLE)
Chromosome abnormalities, such as trisomy 21

---

of the individual, including age, gender, family history, the presence of any associated anomalies, the types of infections (bacterial, viral, or fungal, and the specific microorganisms involved), and risk factors associated with secondary immune deficiencies.[21] A variety of laboratory tests are available to evaluate specific immune deficiencies (Table 7-12). A review of clinical characteristics can help select the appropriate tests.[24] A basic screening test is a complete blood count (CBC) with a differential. The CBC provides information on the numbers of red blood cells, white blood cells, and platelets, and the differential indicates the quantities of lymphocytes, granulocytes, and monocytes in the blood. Quantitative determination of immunoglobulins (IgG, IgM, IgA) is a screening test for antibody production, and an assay for total complement (total hemolytic complement, CH_{50}) is useful if a complement defect is suspected. Further testing is described in Table 7-12.

TABLE 7-12	**LABORATORY EVALUATION OF IMMUNE DEFICIENCIES**	
FUNCTION TESTED	**LABORATORY TEST**	**SIGNIFICANCE OF TEST**
Tests of Humoral Immune Function		
Antibody production	Total immunoglobulin levels, including IgG, IgM, and IgA	Decrease or absence of total antibody production or of specific classes of antibody, which is associated with many B cell and combined deficiencies
	Levels of isohemagglutinins	Production of specific IgM antibodies, which is decreased in some combined deficiencies; not useful with persons who are blood type AB and do not have naturally occurring isohemagglutinins
	Levels of antibodies against vaccines—especially diphtheria and tetanus toxoids	Production of specific IgG antibodies, which is decreased when B cells are deficient or class-switch is blocked
B cell numbers	Numbers of lymphocytes with surface immunoglobulin	Production of circulating B cells, which is decreased in many severe B cell or combined deficiencies
Antibody subclasses	Level-specific subclasses, particularly IgG1, IgG2, and IgG3	Decrease or absence of a particular subclass, which is characteristic of several immune deficiencies
Tests of Cellular Immune Function		
Delayed hypersensitivity skin test	Skin test reaction against previously encountered antigens, especially *Candida albicans* or tetanus toxoid	Defects in antigen-responsive T cells and skin test cellular interactions (e.g., lymphokine activity and macrophage function)
T cell numbers	Numbers of T cells expressing characteristic membrane antigens (CD3 or CD11)	Defects in production of circulating T cells
T cell proliferation in vitro	Proliferative response to nonspecific mitogens (e.g., phytohemagglutinin)	General T cell defects in response to nonspecific stimulation (mitogens)
	Proliferative response to antigens (e.g., tetanus toxoid)	Defects in response of T cells to specific antigens
T cell subpopulations	Quantify percentage of T cells with specific markers for total T cells (CD3), Th cells (CD4), Tc cells (CD8)	Decrease in numbers of CD4 cells, which is related to AIDS progression

Replacement Therapies for Immune Deficiencies

Many immune deficiencies can be successfully treated by replacing the missing component of the immune system. Individuals with B cell deficiencies that cause hypogammaglobulinemia or agammaglobulinemia usually are treated by administration of gamma globulins, which are antibody-rich fractions prepared from plasma pooled from large numbers of donors. Administration of gamma globulin temporarily replaces the individual's antibodies. Antibodies from these preparations are removed slowly from the person's blood, with half of the antibodies being removed by 3 to 4 weeks. Thus individuals must be treated repeatedly to maintain a protective level of antibodies in the blood.

Defects in lymphoid cell development in the primary lymphoid organs (e.g., SCID, Wiskott-Aldrich syndrome, leukocyte adhesion defect) can sometimes be treated by replacement of stem cells through transplantation of bone marrow, umbilical cord cells, or other cell populations that are rich in stem cells.[25] Thymic defects (e.g., DiGeorge syndrome, ataxia-telangiectasia, or chronic mucocutaneous candidiasis) may be treated by transplantation of fetal thymus tissue or thymic epithelial cells (the cells that produce the thymic hormones). However, in most cases improvement is only temporary.

Enzymatic defects that cause SCID (e.g., adenosine deaminase deficiency) have been treated successfully with transfusions of glycerol frozen-packed erythrocytes. The donor erythrocytes contain the needed enzyme and can, at least temporarily, provide sufficient enzyme for normal lymphocyte function. The first successful gene therapy was performed in ADA deficiency, resulting in reconstitution of the immune systems.[26] This procedure is being used experimentally to treat X-linked SCID, ADA-deficient SCID, and X-linked chronic granulomatous disease.

Individuals with immune deficiencies are at risk for graft-versus-host disease (GVHD). This occurs if T cells in a transplanted graft (e.g., transfused blood, bone marrow transplants) are mature and therefore capable of cell-mediated immunity against the recipient's human leukocyte antigen (HLA).[27] The primary targets for GVHD are the skin (e.g., rash, loss or increase of pigment, thickening of skin), liver (e.g., damage to bile duct, hepatomegaly), mouth (e.g., dry mouth, ulcers, infections), eyes (e.g., burning, irritation, dryness), and gastrointestinal tract (e.g., severe diarrhea), and the disease may lead to death from infections. GVHD is less of a problem when the recipient is immunocompetent—that is, has an immune system that can control the donor's lymphocytes. If, however, the recipient's immune system is deficient, the grafted T cells remain unchecked and attack the recipient's tissues. Most cases of GVHD should be prevented by the current practices of irradiating blood to destroy white blood cells before transfusion or removing mature T cells from tissue used to treat individuals with immune deficiencies.

Steroids are commonly used to suppress GVHD in recipients of bone marrow transplants to treat certain malignancies or primary immune deficiencies. In cases where steroids are ineffective, promising new data support the use of mesenchymal stem cells (MSCs).[27,28] Stem cells are relatively undifferentiated cells and can be obtained from a variety of sources (e.g., embryos, bone marrow, adult tissues). MSCs are present in all adult tissues.[29] These particular stem cells undergo differentiation into other cell types and, more importantly, have potent immunosuppressive properties. Several recent clinical trials have demonstrated complete suppression of GVHD in a large number of recipients of MSCs.

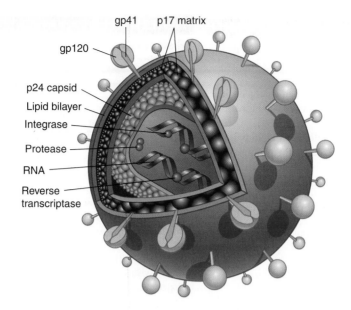

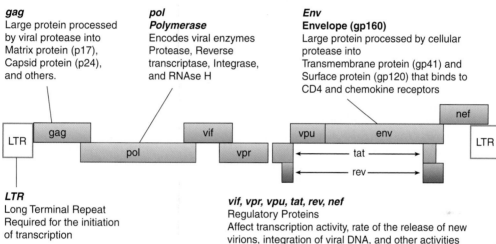

gag
Large protein processed
by viral protease into
Matrix protein (p17),
Capsid protein (p24),
and others.

pol
Polymerase
Encodes viral enzymes
Protease, Reverse
transcriptase, Integrase,
and RNAse H

Env
Envelope (gp160)
Large protein processed by cellular
protease into
Transmembrane protein (gp41) and
Surface protein (gp120) that binds to
CD4 and chemokine receptors

LTR
Long Terminal Repeat
Required for the initiation
of transcription

vif, vpr, vpu, tat, rev, nef
Regulatory Proteins
Affect transcription activity, rate of the release of new
virions, integration of viral DNA, and other activities

FIGURE 7-5 The Structure and Genetic Map of HIV-1. The HIV-1 virion consists of a core of two identical strands of viral RNA molecules of viral enzymes (reverse transcriptase [RT], protease [PR], integrase [IN]) encoated in a core capsid structure consisting primarily of the structural viral protein p24. The capsid is further encased in a matrix consisting primarily of viral protein p17. The outer surface is an envelope consisting of the plasma membrane of the cell from which the virus budded (lipid bilayer) and two viral glycoproteins: a transmembrane glycoprotein, gp41, and a noncovalently attached surface protein, gp120. The HIV-1 genome contains regions that encode the structural proteins *(gag)*, the viral enzymes *(pol)*, and the envelope proteins *(env)*. The genome of complex retroviruses, like HIV-1, often contains a variety of small regions that regulate expression of the virus. (Modified from Kumar V et al: *Robbins and Cotran pathologic basis of disease*, ed 8, Philadelphia, 2009, Saunders.)

Acquired Immunodeficiency Syndrome (AIDS)

Acquired immunodeficiency syndrome is a secondary immune deficiency that develops in response to viral infection. The human immunodeficiency virus (HIV) infects and destroys the Th cell, which is necessary for the development of both plasma cells and cytotoxic T cells. Therefore HIV suppresses the immune response against itself and secondarily creates a generalized immune deficiency by suppressing the development of immune responses against other pathogens and opportunistic microorganisms, leading to the development of acquired immunodeficiency syndrome (AIDS).

Despite major efforts by healthcare agencies around the world, the number of cases and deaths from HIV infection and AIDS (HIV/AIDS) remains a major health concern. The WHO estimated that in 2008 33.4 million people were living with HIV/AIDS worldwide and 2.7 million were newly infected.[30] Approximately 3 million deaths occur each year from AIDS. Since 1980 it is estimated that more than 24 million individuals have died from AIDS worldwide.

The majority of cases are still in sub-Saharan Africa, but the epidemic is worldwide, and the number of new cases is increasing rapidly, particularly in Asia. As an example of the prevalence of HIV/AIDS, in sub-Saharan Africa approximately 1.3 million pregnant women are HIV infected.[30]

In the United States the spread of HIV/AIDS remains somewhat stable. The Centers for Disease Control and Prevention (CDC) estimated in 2008 (the most recent data) that approximately 56,300 people were newly infected with HIV and about 38,000 were diagnosed with AIDS.[31] Deaths related to HIV/AIDS continue at about 18,000 per year. The cumulative number of HIV/AIDS-related deaths in the United States is in excess of 600,000, and more than 470,000 individuals are currently living with AIDS.

Before the implementation of massive public health campaigns and the use of antiviral drugs in the United States, the progression from HIV infection to AIDS and death was unrelenting. In 1995 AIDS became the number one killer of individuals between the ages of 25 and 44 years. With the advent of effective therapy to stabilize progression of the disease in the mid-1990s, HIV infection has become a chronic disease in the United States, with many fewer deaths.

Epidemiology of AIDS

HIV is a blood-borne pathogen with the typical routes of transmission: blood or blood products, intravenous drug abuse, both heterosexual and homosexual activity, and maternal-child transmission before or during birth. Although the disease first gained attention in the United States related to sexual transmission between males, the most common route worldwide is through heterosexual activity (see *Health Alert: Risk of HIV Transmission Associated With Sexual Practices*). Worldwide, women constitute more than half of those living with HIV/AIDS. In the United States, as in the rest of the world, the predominant means of transmission to women is through heterosexual contact, and the incidence of HIV/AIDS is increasing faster in women than men, particularly in the adolescent age groups. Hundreds of thousands of cases of HIV/AIDS have been reported in children who contracted the virus from their mothers across the placenta, through contact with infected blood during delivery, or through the milk during breast-feeding.

Pathogenesis of AIDS

HIV is a member of a family of viruses called retroviruses, which carry genetic information in the form of RNA rather than DNA (Figure 7-5). Retroviruses use a viral enzyme, reverse transcriptase, to convert RNA into double-stranded DNA. Using a second viral enzyme, an integrase, the new DNA is inserted into the infected cell's genetic material, where it may remain dormant. If the cell is activated, translation of the viral information may be initiated, resulting in the formation of new virions, lysis and death of the infected cell, and shedding of infectious HIV particles. During that process the viral protease is essential in processing proteins needed from the viral internal structure (capsid). If, however, the cell remains relatively dormant, the viral genetic material may remain latent for years and is probably present for the life of the individual.

The primary surface receptor on HIV is the envelope protein gp120, which binds to the molecule CD4 on the surface of Th cells. Several other necessary co-receptors, particularly the chemokine receptor CCR5, have been identified on target cells. Thus the major immunologic finding in AIDS is the striking decrease in the number of CD4-positive (CD4+) Th cells (Figure 7-6).

Clinical Manifestations of AIDS

Depletion of CD4+ cells has a profound effect on the immune system, causing a severely diminished response to a wide array of infectious pathogens and malignant tumors (Box 7-3). At the time of diagnosis, the individual may present with one of several different conditions: serologically negative (no detectable antibody), serologically positive

---

HEALTH ALERT

Risk of HIV Transmission Associated With Sexual Practices

High Risk (in descending order of risk)
Receptive anal intercourse with ejaculation (no condom)
Receptive vaginal intercourse with ejaculation (no condom)
Insertive anal intercourse (no condom)
Insertive vaginal intercourse (no condom)
Receptive anal intercourse with withdrawal before ejaculation
Insertive anal intercourse with withdrawal before ejaculation
Receptive vaginal intercourse (with spermicidal foam but no condom)
Insertive vaginal intercourse (with spermicidal foam but no condom)
Receptive anal or vaginal intercourse (with a condom)*
Insertive anal or vaginal intercourse (with a condom)*

Some Risk (in descending order of risk)
Oral sex with men with ejaculation
Oral sex with women
Oral sex with men with preejaculation fluid (precum)
Oral sex with men, no ejaculation or precum
Oral sex with men (with a condom)

Some Risk (depending on situation, intactness of mucous membranes, etc.)
Mutual masturbation with external or internal touching
Sharing sex toys
Anal or vaginal fisting

No Risk
Masturbating with another person without touching one another
Hugging/massage/dry kissing
Frottage (rubbing genitals while remaining clothed)
Masturbating alone
Abstinence

Unresolved Issues
The role of precum in transmission
The protection offered by covering female genitals with a dental dam during oral sex on the women
The risk of transmission from wet kissing

Data from Grimes DE, Grimes RM: *HIV infection: progression and management. Mosby's clinical nursing series*, St Louis, 1994, Mosby; modified from Schram NR: Refusing safer sex, *Focus* 5(7):3–4, 1990.
*Risk lower if no ejaculation or if spermicidal foam is used.

(positive for antibody against HIV proteins) but asymptomatic, early stages of HIV disease, or AIDS (Figure 7-7).

The presence of circulating antibody against the HIV protein p24 followed by more complex tests for antibodies against additional HIV proteins (e.g., Western blot analysis) or for HIV DNA (e.g., polymerase chain reaction) indicates infection by the virus, although many of these individuals are asymptomatic.[22] Antibody appears rather rapidly after infection through blood products, usually within 4 to 7 weeks. After sexual transmission, however, the individual can be infected yet seronegative for 6 to 14 months or longer. The period between infection and the appearance of antibody is referred to as the window period. Although a person does not have antibody against HIV, he or she may have virus growing, have virus in the blood and body fluids, and be infectious to others.

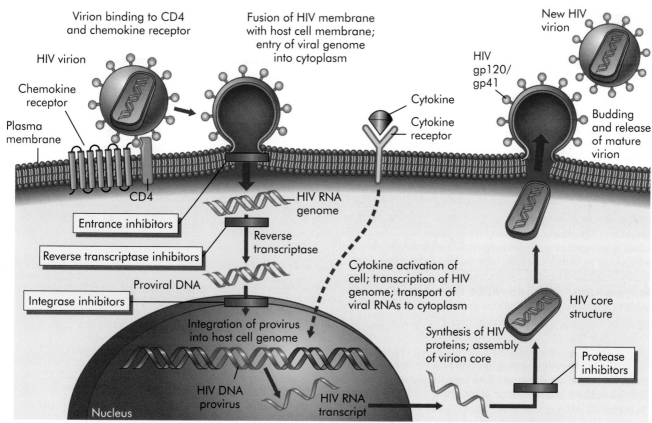

FIGURE 7-6 Life Cycle and Possible Sites of Therapeutic Intervention of Human Immunodeficiency Virus (HIV). The HIV virion consists of a core of two identical strands of viral RNA encoated in a protein structure with viral proteins gp41 and gp120 on its surface (envelope). HIV infection begins when a virion binds to CD4 and chemokine co-receptors on a susceptible cell and follows the process described here. The provirus may remain latent in the cell's DNA until it is activated (e.g., by cytokines). The HIV life cycle is susceptible to blockage at several sites (see the text for further information), including entrance inhibitors, reverse transcriptase inhibitors, integrase inhibitors, and protease inhibitors. (Modified from Kumar V, Abbas A, Fausto N: *Robbins and Cotran pathologic basis of disease,* ed 7, Philadelphia, 2005, Saunders.)

BOX 7-3   AIDS-DEFINING OPPORTUNISTIC INFECTIONS AND NEOPLASMS FOUND IN INDIVIDUALS WITH HIV INFECTION

Infections

Protozoal and Helminthic Infections

Cryptosporidiosis or isosporiasis (enteritis)

Pneumocystosis (pneumonia or disseminated infection)

Toxoplasmosis (pneumonia or CNS infection)

Fungal Infections

Candidiasis (esophageal, tracheal, or pulmonary)

Coccidioidomycosis (disseminated)

Cryptococcosis (CNS infection)

Histoplasmosis (disseminated)

Bacterial Infections

Mycobacteriosis ("atypical," e.g., *Mycobacterium avium-intracellulare,* disseminated or extrapulmonary; *M. tuberculosis,* disseminated or extrapulmonary)

Nocardiosis (pneumonia, meningitis, disseminated)

Salmonella infections (disseminated)

Viral Infections

Cytomegalovirus (pulmonary, intestinal, retinitis, or CNS)

Herpes simplex virus (localized or disseminated)

Progressive multifocal leukoencephalopathy

Varicella-zoster virus (localized or disseminated)

Neoplasms

Invasive cancer of the uterine cervix

Kaposi sarcoma

Non-Hodgkin lymphomas (Burkitt, immunoblastic)

Primary lymphoma of brain

From Kumar V et al: *Robbins and Cotran pathologic basis of disease,* ed 8, Philadelphia, 2009, Saunders.
CNS, Central nervous system.

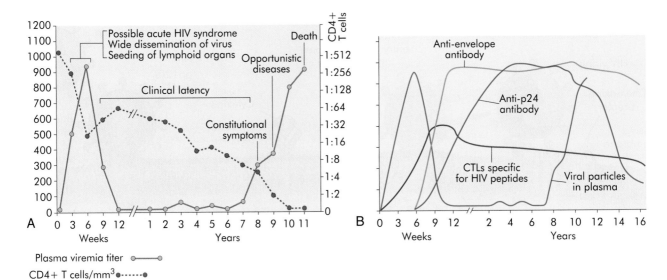

Plasma viremia titer o———o

CD4+ T cells/mm³ •·····•

FIGURE 7-7 Typical Progression from HIV Infection to AIDS in Untreated Persons. **A,** Clinical progression begins within weeks after infection; the person may experience symptoms of acute HIV syndrome. During this early period, the virus progressively infects T cells and other cells and spreads to the lymphoid organs, with a sharp decrease in the number of circulating CD4+ T cells. During a period of clinical latency, the virus replicates and T cell destruction continues, although the person is generally asymptomatic. The individual may develop HIV-related disease (constitutional symptoms)—a variety of symptoms of acute viral infection that do not involve opportunistic infections or malignancies. When the number of CD4+ cells is critically suppressed, the individual becomes susceptible to a variety of opportunistic infections and cancers with a diagnosis of AIDS. The length of time for progression from HIV infection to AIDS may vary considerably from person to person. **B,** Laboratory tests are changing throughout infection. Antibody and Tc cell (cytotoxic T lymphocytes [CTLs]) levels change during the progression to AIDS. During the initial phase antibodies against HIV-1 are not yet detectable (window period), but viral products, including proteins and RNA, and infectious virus may be detectable in the blood a few weeks after infection. Most antibodies against HIV are not detectable in the early phase. During the latent phase of infection antibody levels against p24 and other viral proteins, as well as HIV-specific CTLs, increase, and then remain constant until the development of AIDS. (**A** redrawn from Fauci AS, Lane HC: Human immunodeficiency virus disease: AIDS and related conditions. In Fauci AS et al, editors: *Harrison's principles of internal medicine,* ed 14, New York, 1997, McGraw-Hill; **B** from Kumar V, Abbas A, Fausto N: *Robbins and Cotran pathologic basis of disease,* ed 7, Philadelphia, 2005, Saunders.)

Those with the early stages of HIV disease (early-stage disease) usually initially present with relatively mild and nonspecific symptoms resembling influenza, such as headaches, fever, or fatigue.[23] These symptoms disappear after 1 to 6 weeks, and although individuals appear to be in clinical latency the virus is actively proliferating in lymph nodes.

The currently accepted definition of AIDS relies on both laboratory tests and clinical symptoms. If the individual is positive for antibodies against HIV, the diagnosis of AIDS is made in association with various clinical symptoms (Figure 7-8; also see Box 7-3). The symptoms include atypical or opportunistic infections and cancers, as well as indications of debilitating chronic disease (e.g., wasting syndrome, recurrent fevers). Most commonly, new cases of AIDS are diagnosed initially by decreased CD4+ T cell numbers. Individuals who are not HIV infected typically have 800 to 1000 CD4+ cells per cubic millimeter of blood, with a range from 600/mm³ to 1200/mm³. A diagnosis of AIDS can be made if the CD4+ T cell numbers decrease to less than 200/mm³. The average time from infection to development of AIDS has been estimated at just over 10 years. Some estimates are that approximately 99% of untreated HIV-infected individuals would eventually progress to AIDS.

Treatment and Prevention of AIDS

Approved AIDS medications are classified by mechanism of action: nucleoside and nonnucleoside inhibitors of reverse transcriptase (**reverse transcriptase inhibitors**), inhibitors of the viral protease (**protease inhibitors**), inhibitors of cell fusion (cell fusion inhibitors), inhibitors of viral entrance into the target cell (**entrance inhibitors**), and inhibitors of the viral integrase (**integrase inhibitors**).[22] The current regimen for treatment of HIV infection is a combination of drugs, termed **highly active antiretroviral therapy (HAART)**. HAART protocols require a combination of three synergist drugs from two different classes (see Figure 7-6). The clinical benefits of HAART are profound. Death from AIDS-related diseases has been reduced significantly since the introduction of HAART.[26] However, resistant variants to these drugs have been identified. Drug therapy for AIDS is not curative because HIV incorporates into the genetic material of the host and may never be removed by antimicrobial therapy. Therefore drug administration to control the virus may have to continue for the lifetime of the individual. Additionally, HIV may persist in regions where the antiviral drugs are not as effective, such as the CNS.

Vaccine development is probably the most effective means of preventing HIV infection and may be useful in treating preexisting

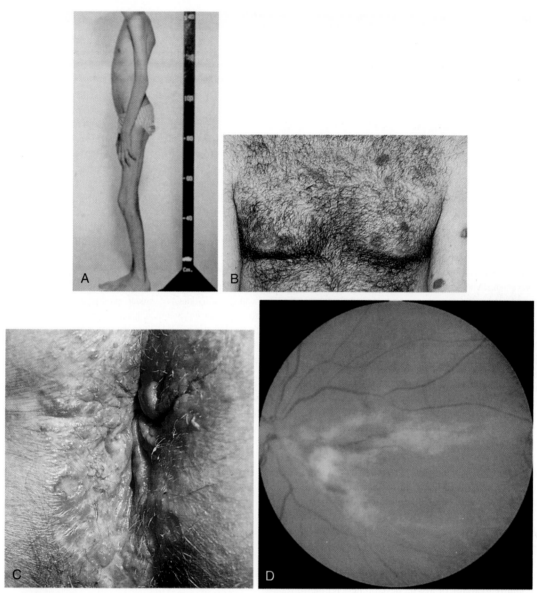

FIGURE 7-8 Clinical Symptoms of AIDS. A, Severe weight loss and anorexia. **B,** Kaposi sarcoma lesions. **C,** Perianal lesions of herpes simplex infection. **D,** Deterioration of vision from cytomegalovirus retinitis leading to areas of infection, which can lead to blindness. (**A** and **D** from Taylor PK: *Diagnostic picture tests in sexually transmitted diseases,* London, 1995, Mosby; **B** and **C** from Morse SA, Ballard RC, Holmes KK et al, editors: *Atlas of sexually transmitted diseases and AIDS,* ed 3, Edinburgh, 2003, Mosby.)

infection. Most of the common viral vaccines (e.g., rubella, mumps, influenza) induce protective antibodies that block the initial infection. Only one vaccine (rabies) is used after the infection has occurred.[32] The rabies vaccine is successful because the rabies virus proliferates and spreads very slowly. The ability of an HIV vaccine to either successfully prevent or treat HIV infection is questionable for several reasons. First, the AIDS virus is genetically and antigenically variable, like the influenza virus, so that a vaccine created against one variant may not provide protection against another variant. Second, although individuals with AIDS have high levels of circulating antibodies against the virus, these antibodies do not appear to be protective. Therefore even if a circulating antibody response can be induced by vaccination, that response might not be effective. A vaccine may have to induce both circulating and secretory (to prevent initial infection of the mucosal T cell) antibody and Tc cells (see *Health Alert: AIDS Vaccine Trials*).

Pediatric AIDS and Central Nervous System Involvement

HIV can be transmitted from mother to child during pregnancy, at the time of delivery, or through breast-feeding. The clinical diagnosis of HIV infection in young children born of HIV-infected mothers is very often a difficult task because the presence of maternal antibodies may result in a misleading false-positive test for antibodies against HIV for as long as 18 months after birth.[33] Testing for antibody against HIV can be performed recurrently from birth until 18 months; if the test results become negative and remain so after 12 months, the child can be considered uninfected.

The 2008 revised surveillance case definition for HIV infection in children younger than 18 months recommends testing for HIV or viral components in two separate specimens, not including cord blood. These include detection of HIV nucleic acid or p24 antigen, or direct isolation of HIV in viral cultures.

AIDS Vaccine Trials

Very soon after the discovery in 1983 of the virus that causes AIDS, knowledgeable scientists and public officials predicted that an effective vaccine would be marketed within a few years. The prediction was not viewed as overly optimistic because vaccines had been produced against many other viral diseases, and the technology was available to swiftly purify, test, and manufacture viral antigens. In 2011, more than 25 years after the discovery of HIV, optimism about producing vaccine protection against AIDS continues to vacillate.

The goal of an AIDS vaccine is to either prevent the initial infection or enhance the immune response of an infected individual to reduce viral load, or both. Several recent trails of promising AIDS vaccines failed to protect recipients. The STEP Study was a trial of vaccine V520, produced by Merck. The immunization protocol was very complex and elicited a T cell immune response against several HIV antigens, including products of HIV *env, gag, pol,* and *nef* genes expressed in an altered adenovirus—a common cold virus. The trial was prematurely terminated in September of 2007 because the initial analysis indicated that the vaccine neither prevented HIV infection nor lowered viral load in the blood of those who became infected; in fact, the vaccine was suspected of increasing the risk for HIV infection in some recipients.

The most recent trial, however, has fostered a new, but cautious, optimism. More than 16,000 men and women in Thailand were immunized with HIV vaccines or with placebo. The efficacy of vaccination in reducing initial infection

with HIV was 31.2%, which was regarded as modest. This is the first positive effect reported for an HIV vaccine. However, considerable caution was advised in interpreting the long-term significance of these observations. The HIV vaccine protocol consisted of four priming injections with a canarypox virus that was altered to prevent infection of humans and genetically engineered to express versions of HIV *gag, pol,* and *env* proteins (ALVAC-HIV vaccine), followed by two booster injections with a vaccine containing recombinant gp120 subunits (AIDS-VAX B/E vaccine). The effects of the priming-booster protocol were surprising because neither vaccine appeared to be beneficial when tested separately. The ALVAC-HIV vaccine, after recurrent testing, was considered of inadequate immunogenicity, and the AIDSVAX B/E vaccine was not efficacious in two previous clinical trials. Additionally, the test population was considered low to medium risk for contracting HIV and was primarily heterosexual. Another drawback was that the HIV strains used to produce the vaccine were common in Thailand, Europe, and the Americas, but far less common in Africa. Thus the efficacy of this protocol is unknown in the African population, in individuals at high risk for contracting HIV infection through intravenous drug abuse, or in men who have sex with men. Regardless of those limitations, this trial was the first indication that an HIV vaccine could affect the rate of initial infection. With further refinements and implementation of our expanding knowledge about HIV, future vaccine efforts may approach the goal of preventing global HIV infection and AIDS.

Data from Johnston MI, Fauci AS: *N Engl J Med* 359(9):888–890, 2008; Editorial: HIV vaccine trials and tribulations, *Lancet Infect Dis* 9(11):651, 2009; Dolin R: HIV vaccine trial results—an opening for further research, *N Engl J Med* 361(23):2279–2280, 2009; Rerks-Ngarm S et al: Vaccination with ALVAC and AIDSVAX to prevent HIV-1 infection in Thailand, *N Engl J Med* 361(23):2209–2220, 2009; Bansal GP, Malaspina A, Flores J: Future paths for HIV vaccine research: exploiting results from recent clinical trials and current scientific advances, *Curr Opin Mol Ther* 12(1):39–46, 2010.

HIV infection of babies is generally more aggressive than in adults; on average an untreated child will die by his or her second birthday. Neurologic involvement occurs more commonly in children than in adults and results from CNS involvement, rather than effects on peripheral portions of the nervous system. HIV encephalopathy occurs with varying degrees of severity and is a clinical component in the diagnosis of AIDS in children. Most HIV-infected newborns appear normal, but may progressively develop signs of CNS involvement. These usually appear as failure to attain, or loss of, developmental milestones or loss of intellectual ability, verified by standard developmental scale or neuropsychologic tests; acquired symmetric motor deficits, seen in children older than age 1 month; impaired brain growth or acquired microcephaly, demonstrated by head circumference measurements; or brain atrophy, demonstrated by computed tomography (CT) or magnetic resonance imaging (MRI) with serial imaging and required in children younger than 2 years of age.

It may be difficult to completely differentiate the effect of HIV infection on the CNS from other risk factors, including prenatal drug exposure, prematurity, chronic illness, and a chaotic social atmosphere. The pathogenesis of HIV encephalopathy in children is poorly understood, but the presence of inflammatory mediators may be a contributing factor.

Because HIV infection in infants progresses very rapidly, treatment must begin at the diagnosis of infection. In older children the criteria for treatment are similar to those used in adults. A growing number of investigational protocols are available for treatment of children with HIV. In general, treatment is focused on the preservation and maintenance of the immune system, aggressive response to opportunistic infections, support and relief of symptomatic occurrences, and administration of HAART.

> **✔ QUICK CHECK 7-2**
> 1. Why is the development of recurrent or unusual infections the clinical hallmark of immunodeficiency?
> 2. Compare and contrast the most common infections in individuals with defects in cell-mediated immune response and those with defects in humoral immune response.
> 3. What are the new treatments for HIV?

HYPERSENSITIVITY: ALLERGY, AUTOIMMUNITY, AND ALLOIMMUNITY

Allergy, autoimmunity, and alloimmunity are classified as *hypersensitivity reactions.* Hypersensitivity is an altered immunologic response to an antigen that results in disease or damage to the individual. Allergy, autoimmunity, and alloimmunity (also termed *isoimmunity*) can be most easily understood in relationship to the source of the antigen against which the hypersensitivity response is directed (Table 7-13). Allergy refers to a hypersensitivity to environmental antigens. These can include medicines, natural products (e.g., pollens, bee stings), infectious agents, and any other antigen that is not naturally found in the individual.

Autoimmunity is a disturbance in the immunologic tolerance of self-antigens. The immune system normally does not strongly recognize the individual's own antigens. Healthy individuals of all ages, but particularly the elderly, may produce low quantities of antibodies against their own antigens (*autoantibodies*) without developing overt autoimmune disease. Therefore the presence of low quantities of autoantibodies does not necessarily indicate a disease state. Autoimmune

TABLE 7-13   RELATIVE INCIDENCE AND EXAMPLES OF HYPERSENSITIVITY DISEASES*

	MECHANISM			
TARGET ANTIGEN	**TYPE I (IGE MEDIATED)**	**TYPE II (TISSUE SPECIFIC)**	**TYPE III (IMMUNE COMPLEX MEDIATED)**	**TYPE IV (CELL MEDIATED)**
Allergy	++++	+	+	++
Environmental antigens	Hay fever	Hemolysis in drug allergies	Gluten (wheat) allergy	Poison ivy allergy
Autoimmunity	+	++	+++	++
Self-antigens	May contribute to some type III reactions	Autoimmune thrombocytopenia	Systemic lupus erythematosus	Hashimoto thyroiditis
Alloimmunity	+	++	+	++
Another person's antigens	May contribute to some type III reactions	Hemolytic disease of the newborn	Individuals who do not make their own IgA may have an anaphylactic response against IgA in human immune globulin	Graft rejection

*The frequency of each reaction is indicated in a range from rare (+) to very common (++++). An example of each reaction is given.

TABLE 7-14   EXAMPLES OF AUTOIMMUNE DISORDERS

SYSTEM DISEASE	ORGAN OR TISSUE	PROBABLE SELF-ANTIGEN
Endocrine System		
Hyperthyroidism (Graves disease)	Thyroid gland	Receptors for thyroid-stimulating hormone on plasma membrane of thyroid cells
Hashimoto hypothyroidism	Thyroid gland	Thyroid cell-surface antigens, thyroglobulin
Insulin-dependent diabetes	Pancreas	Islet cells, insulin, insulin receptors on pancreatic cells
Addison disease	Adrenal gland	Surface antigens on steroid-producing cells; microsomal antigens
Male infertility	Testis	Surface antigens on spermatozoa
Skin		
Pemphigus vulgaris	Skin	Intercellular substances in stratified squamous epithelium
Bullous pemphigoid	Skin	Basement membrane
Vitiligo	Skin	Surface antigens on melanocytes (melanin-producing cells)
Neuromuscular Tissue		
Multiple sclerosis	Neural tissue	Surface antigens of nerve cells
Myasthenia gravis	Neuromuscular junction	Acetylcholine receptors; striations of skeletal and cardiac muscle
Rheumatic fever	Heart	Cardiac tissue antigens that cross-react with group A streptococcal antigen
Cardiomyopathy	Heart	Cardiac muscle
Gastrointestinal System		
Ulcerative colitis	Colon	Mucosal cells
Pernicious anemia	Stomach	Surface antigens of parietal cells; intrinsic factor
Primary biliary cirrhosis	Liver	Cells of bile duct
Chronic active hepatitis	Liver	Surface antigens of hepatocytes, nuclei, microsomes, smooth muscle
Eye		
Sjögren syndrome	Lacrimal gland	Antigens of lacrimal gland, salivary gland, thyroid, and nuclei of cells
Connective Tissue		
Ankylosing spondylitis	Joints	Sacroiliac and spinal apophyseal joint
Rheumatoid arthritis	Joints	Collagen, IgG
Systemic lupus erythematosus	Multiple sites	Numerous antigens in nuclei, organelles, and extracellular matrix
Renal System		
Immune complex glomerulonephritis	Kidney	Numerous immune complexes
Goodpasture syndrome	Kidney	Glomerular basement membrane
Hematologic System		
Idiopathic neutropenia	Neutrophil	Surface antigens on polymorphonuclear neutrophils
Idiopathic lymphopenia	Lymphocytes	Surface antigens on lymphocytes
Autoimmune hemolytic anemia	Erythrocytes	Surface antigens on erythrocytes
Autoimmune thrombocytopenic purpura	Platelets	Surface antigens on platelets
Respiratory System		
Goodpasture syndrome	Lung	Septal membrane of alveolus

diseases occur when the immune system reacts against self-antigens to such a degree that autoantibodies or autoreactive T cells damage the individual's tissues. Many clinical disorders are associated with autoimmunity and are generally referred to as autoimmune diseases (Table 7-14).

Alloimmune diseases occur when the immune system of one individual produces an immunologic reaction against tissues of another individual. Alloimmunity can be observed during immunologic reactions against transfusions, transplanted tissue, or the fetus during pregnancy.

The mechanism that initiates the onset of hypersensitivity, whether allergy, autoimmunity, or alloimmunity, is not completely understood. It is generally accepted that genetic, infectious, and possibly environmental factors contribute to development of hypersensitivity reactions.

Mechanisms of Hypersensitivity

Diseases caused by hypersensitivity reactions can be characterized also by the particular immune mechanism that results in the disease (Table 7-15). These mechanisms are apparent in most hypersensitivity reactions and have been divided into four distinct types: *type I* (IgE-mediated reactions), *type II* (tissue-specific reactions), *type III* (immune complex–mediated reactions), and *type IV* (cell-mediated reactions). This classification is artificial and seldom is a particular disease associated with only a single mechanism. The four mechanisms are interrelated, and in most hypersensitivity reactions several mechanisms can be functioning simultaneously or sequentially.

As with all immune responses, hypersensitivity reactions require sensitization against a particular antigen that results in a primary immune response. Disease symptoms appear after an adequate secondary immune response occurs. Hypersensitivity reactions are immediate or delayed, depending on the time required to elicit clinical symptoms after reexposure to the antigen. Reactions that occur within minutes to a few hours after exposure to antigen are termed immediate hypersensitivity reactions. Delayed hypersensitivity reactions may take several hours to appear and are at maximal severity days after reexposure to the antigen. Generally, immediate reactions are caused by antibody, whereas delayed reactions are caused by cells (e.g., T cells, NK cells, macrophages).

The most rapid and severe immediate hypersensitivity reaction is anaphylaxis. Anaphylaxis occurs within minutes of reexposure to the antigen and can be either systemic (generalized) or cutaneous (localized).[34] Symptoms of systemic anaphylaxis include pruritus, erythema, vomiting, abdominal cramps, diarrhea, and breathing difficulties. Severe anaphylactic reactions may include contraction of bronchial smooth muscle, edema of the throat, breathing difficulties, decreased blood pressure, shock, and death. An example of systemic anaphylaxis

is an allergic reaction to bee stings. Cutaneous anaphylaxis results in local symptoms, such as pain, swelling, and redness, which occur at the site of exposure to an antigen (e.g., a painful local reaction to an injected vaccine or drug).

Type I: IgE-Mediated Hypersensitivity Reactions

Type I reactions are mediated by antigen-specific IgE and the products of tissue mast cells (Figure 7-9). Most common allergic reactions are type I reactions. In addition, most type I reactions occur against environmental antigens and are therefore allergic. Because of this strong association, many healthcare professionals use the term *allergy* to indicate only IgE-mediated reactions. However, IgE can contribute to some autoimmune and alloimmune diseases, and many common allergies (e.g., poison ivy) are not mediated by IgE.

IgE has a relatively short life span in the blood because it rapidly binds to Fc receptors on mast cells.[35] Unlike Fc receptors on phagocytes, which bind IgG that has previously reacted with antigen, the Fc receptors on mast cells specifically bind IgE that has not previously interacted with antigen. After a large amount of IgE has bound to the mast cells, an individual is considered *sensitized*. Further exposure of a sensitized individual to the allergen results in degranulation of the mast cell and the release of mast cell products (see Chapter 5).

Mechanisms of IgE-mediated hypersensitivity. The most potent mediator of IgE-mediated hypersensitivity is histamine, which affects several key target cells. Acting through H1 receptors, histamine contracts bronchial smooth muscles (bronchial constriction), increases vascular permeability (edema), and causes vasodilation (increased blood flow) (see Chapter 5). The interaction of histamine with H2 receptors results in increased gastric acid secretion. Some type I allergic responses can be controlled by blocking histamine receptors with antihistamines.

Clinical manifestations of IgE-mediated hypersensitivity. The clinical manifestations of type I reactions are attributable mostly to the biologic effects of histamine. The tissues most commonly affected by type I responses contain large numbers of mast cells and are sensitive to the effects of histamine released from them. These tissues are found in the gastrointestinal tract, the skin, and the respiratory tract (Figure 7-10 and Table 7-16).

Gastrointestinal allergy is caused primarily by allergens that enter through the mouth—usually foods or medicines. Symptoms include vomiting, diarrhea, or abdominal pain. Foods most often implicated in gastrointestinal allergies are milk, chocolate, citrus fruits, eggs, wheat, nuts, peanut butter, and fish. The most common food allergy in adults is a reaction to shellfish, which may initiate an anaphylactic

TABLE 7-15   IMMUNOLOGIC MECHANISMS OF TISSUE DESTRUCTION

TYPE	NAME	RATE OF DEVELOPMENT	CLASS OF ANTIBODY INVOLVED	PRINCIPAL EFFECTOR CELLS INVOLVED	PARTICIPATION OF COMPLEMENT	EXAMPLES OF DISORDERS
I	IgE-mediated reaction	Immediate	IgE	Mast cells	No	Seasonal allergic rhinitis Asthma
II	Tissue-specific reaction	Immediate	IgG IgM	Macrophages in tissues	Frequently	Autoimmune thrombocytopenic purpura, Graves disease, autoimmune hemolytic anemia
III	Immune complex–mediated reaction	Immediate	IgG IgM	Neutrophils	Yes	Systemic lupus erythematosus
IV	Cell-mediated reaction	Delayed	None	Lymphocytes Macrophages	No	Contact sensitivity to poison ivy and metals (jewelry)

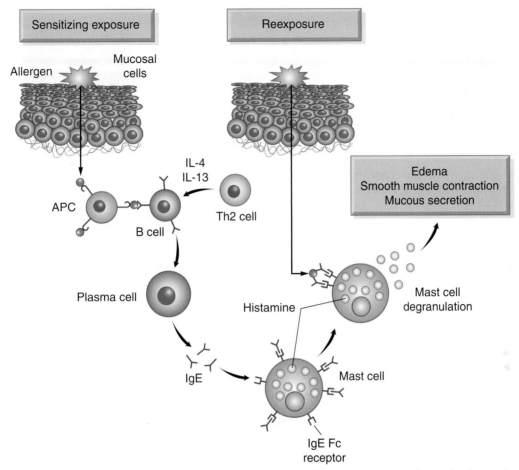

FIGURE 7-9 Mechanism of Type I, IgE-Mediated Reactions. First exposure to an allergen leads to antigen processing and presentation of antigen by an antigen-presenting cell (APC) to B lymphocytes, which is under the direction of T-helper 2 (Th2) cells. Th2 cells produce specific cytokines (e.g., IL-4, IL-13, and others) that favor maturation of the B lymphocytes into plasma cells that secrete IgE. The IgE is adsorbed to the surface of the mast cell by binding with IgE-specific Fc receptors. When an adequate amount of IgE is bound the mast cell is sensitized. During a reexposure, the allergen cross-links the surface-bound IgE and causes degranulation of the mast cell. Contents of the mast cell granules, primarily histamine, induce local edema, smooth muscle contraction, mucous secretion, and other characteristics of an acute inflammatory reaction. (See Chapter 5 for more details on the role of mast cells in inflammation.)

response and death.[36] When food is the source of an allergen, the active immunogen may be an unidentifiable product of food breakdown by digestive enzymes. Sometimes the allergen is a drug, an additive, or a preservative in the food. For example, cows treated for mastitis with penicillin yield milk containing trace amounts of this antibiotic. Thus hypersensitivity apparently caused by milk proteins may instead be the result of an allergy to penicillin.

Urticaria, or hives, is a dermal (skin) manifestation of allergic reactions (see Figure 7-10). The underlying mechanism is the localized release of histamine and increased vascular permeability, resulting in limited areas of edema. Urticaria is characterized by white fluid-filled blisters (wheals) surrounded by areas of redness (flares). This **wheal and flare reaction** is usually accompanied by pruritus. Not all urticarial symptoms are caused by immunologic reactions. Some, termed *nonimmunologic urticaria,* result from exposure to cold temperatures, emotional stress, medications, systemic diseases, or malignancies (e.g., lymphomas).

Effects of allergens on the mucosa of the eyes, nose, and respiratory tract include conjunctivitis (inflammation of the membranes lining the eyelids) (see Figure 7-10), rhinitis (inflammation of the mucous membranes of the nose),[37] and asthma (constriction of the bronchi).[38]

Symptoms are caused by vasodilation, hypersecretion of mucus, edema, and swelling of the respiratory mucosa. Because the mucous membranes lining the respiratory tract are continuous, they are all adversely affected. The degree to which each is affected determines the symptoms of the disease.

The central problem in allergic diseases of the lung is obstruction of the large and small airways (bronchi) of the lower respiratory tract by bronchospasm (constriction of smooth muscle in airway walls), edema, and thick secretions. This leads to ventilatory insufficiency, wheezing, and difficult or labored breathing (see Chapter 26).[39]

Certain individuals are genetically predisposed to develop allergies and are called **atopic**.[40] In families in which one parent has an allergy, allergies develop in about 40% of the offspring. If both parents have allergies, the incidence may be as high as 80%. Atopic individuals tend to produce higher quantities of IgE and have more Fc receptors for IgE on their mast cells. The airways and the skin of atopic individuals have increased responsiveness to a wide variety of both specific and nonspecific stimuli.

Evaluation and treatment of IgE hypersensitivity. Allergic reactions can be life-threatening; therefore it is essential that severely allergic individuals be informed of the specific allergen against which they are

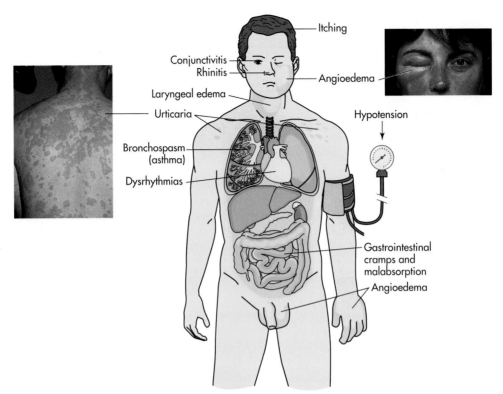

FIGURE 7-10 Type I Hypersensitivity Reactions. Manifestations of allergic reactions as a result of type I hypersensitivity include pruritus, angioedema (swelling caused by exudation), edema of the larynx, urticaria (hives), bronchospasm (constriction of airways in the lungs), hypotension (low blood pressure), and dysrhythmias (irregular heartbeat) because of anaphylactic shock, and gastrointestinal cramping caused by inflammation of the gastrointestinal mucosa. Photographic inserts show a diffuse allergic-like eye and skin reaction on an individual. The skin lesions have raised edges and develop within minutes or hours, with resolution occurring after about 12 hours. (From Roitt I, Brostoff J, Male D: *Immunology,* ed 6, St Louis, 2001, Mosby.)

TABLE 7-16 CAUSES OF CLINICAL ALLERGIC REACTIONS

TYPICAL ALLERGEN	MECHANISM OF HYPERSENSITIVITY	CLINICAL MANIFESTATION
Ingestants		
Foods	Type I	Gastrointestinal allergy
Drugs	Types I, II, III	Urticaria, immediate drug reaction, hemolytic anemia, serum sickness
Inhalants		
Pollens, dust, molds	Type I	Allergic rhinitis, bronchial asthma
Aspergillus fumigatus	Types I, III	Allergic bronchopulmonary aspergillosis
Thermophilic actinomycetes*	Types III, IV	Extrinsic allergic alveolitis
Injectants		
Drugs	Types I, II, III	Immediate drug reaction, hemolytic anemia, serum sickness
Bee venom	Type I	Anaphylaxis
Vaccines	Type III	Localized Arthus reaction
Serum	Types I, III	Anaphylaxis, serum sickness
Contactants		
Poison ivy, metals	Type IV	Contact dermatitis

Modified from Bellanti JA: *Immunology III,* Philadelphia, 1985, Saunders.
*An order of fungi that grows best at high temperatures (between 45° and 80° C [113° and 176° F]).

sensitized and instructed to avoid contact with that material. Several tests are available to evaluate allergic individuals.[41] These include food challenges, skin tests with allergens, and laboratory tests for total IgE and allergen-specific IgE.

Clinical desensitization to allergens can be achieved in some individuals.[42] Minute quantities of the allergen to which the person is sensitive are injected in increasing doses over a prolonged period. This procedure may reduce the severity of the allergic reaction in the treated individual. However, this form of therapy is associated with a risk of systemic anaphylaxis, which can be severe and life-threatening.

Type II: Tissue-Specific Hypersensitivity Reactions

Type II hypersensitivities are generally reactions against a specific cell or tissue. Cells express a variety of antigens on their surfaces, some of which are called tissue-specific antigens because they are expressed on the plasma membranes of only certain cells. Platelets, for example, have groups of antigens that are found on no other cells of the body. The symptoms of many type II diseases are determined by which tissue or organ expresses the particular antigen. Environmental antigens (e.g., drugs or their metabolites) may bind to the plasma membranes of specific cells (especially erythrocytes and platelets) and function as targets of type II reactions. The five general mechanisms by which type II hypersensitivity reactions can affect cells are shown in Figure 7-11. All of these mechanisms begin with antibody binding to tissue-specific antigens or antigens that have attached to particular tissues.

In the first mechanism, *the cell may be destroyed by antibody and complement.* The antibody (IgM or IgG) reacts with an antigen on the surface of the cell, causing activation of the complement cascade through the classical pathway. Formation of the membrane attack complex (C5-9) damages the membrane and may result in lysis of the cell (see Figure 7-11, *A*). For example, erythrocytes are destroyed by complement-mediated lysis in individuals with autoimmune hemolytic anemia (see Chapters 20 and 21) or as a result of an alloimmune reaction to mismatched transfused blood cells.

In the second mechanism, *antibody may cause cell destruction through phagocytosis by macrophages.* The antibody may additionally activate complement, resulting in the deposition of C3b on the cell surface. Receptors on the macrophage recognize and bind opsonins (e.g., antibody or C3b) and increase phagocytosis of the target cell (see Figure 7-11, *B*; phagocytosis is illustrated in Chapter 5). For example, antibodies against platelet-specific antigens or against red blood cell antigens of the Rh system cause their removal by phagocytosis in the spleen.

The third mechanism involves *toxic products produced by neutrophils.* Soluble antigens such as medications, molecules released from infectious agents, or molecules released from an individual's own cells may enter the circulation. In some instances, the antigens are deposited on the surface of tissues, where they bind antibody (see Figure 7-11, *C*). The antibody may activate complement, resulting in the release of C3a and C5a, which are chemotactic for neutrophils, and the deposition of complement component C3b. Neutrophils are attracted, bind to the tissues through receptors for the Fc portion of antibody (Fc receptor) or for C3b, and release their granules onto the healthy tissue. The components of neutrophil granules, as well as the toxic oxygen products produced by these cells, will damage the tissue.

The fourth mechanism is antibody-dependent cell-mediated cytotoxicity (ADCC) (see Figure 7-11, *D*). This mechanism involves natural killer (NK) cells. Antibody on the target cell is recognized by Fc receptors on the NK cells, which release toxic substances that destroy the target cell.

The fifth mechanism does not destroy the target cell but rather *causes the cell to malfunction.* The antibody is usually directed against antigenic determinants associated with specific cell-surface receptors (see Figure 7-11, *E*). The antibody changes the function of the receptor by preventing interactions with their normal ligands, replacing the ligand and inappropriately stimulating the receptor, or destroying the receptor. For example, in the hyperthyroidism (excessive thyroid activity) of Graves disease, autoantibody binds to and activates receptors for thyroid-stimulating hormone (TSH) (a pituitary hormone that controls the production of the hormone thyroxine by the thyroid).[43] In this way, the antibody stimulates the thyroid cells to produce thyroxine. Under normal conditions, the increasing levels of thyroxine in the blood would signal the pituitary to decrease TSH production, which would result in less stimulation of the TSH receptor in the thyroid and a concomitant decrease in thyroxine production. Increasing amounts of thyroxine in the blood have no effect on antibody levels, and thyroxine production continues to increase despite decreasing amounts of TSH (see Chapter 18).

Type III: Immune Complex–Mediated Hypersensitivity Reactions

Mechanisms of type III hypersensitivity. Most type III hypersensitivity diseases are caused by antigen-antibody (immune) complexes that are formed in the circulation and deposited later in vessel walls or other tissues (Figure 7-12). The primary difference between type II and type III mechanisms is that in type II hypersensitivity antibody binds to antigen on the cell surface, whereas in type III antibody binds to soluble antigen that was released into the blood or body fluids, and the complex is then deposited in the tissues. Type III reactions are not organ specific, and symptoms are mostly unrelated to the particular antigenic target of the antibody. The harmful effects of immune complex deposition are caused by complement activation, particularly through the generation of chemotactic factors for neutrophils. The neutrophils bind to antibody and C3b contained in the complexes and attempt to ingest the immune complexes. They are often unsuccessful because the complexes are bound to large areas of tissue. During the attempted phagocytosis, large quantities of lysosomal enzymes are released into the inflammatory site instead of into phagolysosomes. The attraction of neutrophils and the subsequent release of lysosomal enzymes cause most of the resulting tissue damage.

Immune complex disease. Two prototypic models of type III hypersensitivity help explain the variety of diseases in this category. Serum sickness is a model of systemic type III hypersensitivities, and the Arthus reaction is a model of localized or cutaneous reactions.

Serum sickness–type reactions are caused by the formation of immune complexes in the blood and their subsequent generalized deposition in target tissues. Typically affected tissues are the blood vessels, joints, and kidneys.[44] Symptoms include fever, enlarged lymph nodes, rash, and pain at sites of inflammation. Serum sickness was initially described as a complication of therapeutic administration of horse serum that contained antibody against tetanus toxin. Foreign serum generally is not administered to individuals today, although serum sickness reactions can be caused by the repeated intravenous administration of other antigens, such as drugs, and the characteristics of serum sickness are observed in systemic type III autoimmune diseases.

A form of serum sickness is Raynaud phenomenon, a condition caused by the temperature-dependent deposition of immune complexes in the capillary beds of the peripheral circulation. Certain immune complexes precipitate at temperatures below normal body temperature, particularly in the tips of the fingers, toes, and nose, and

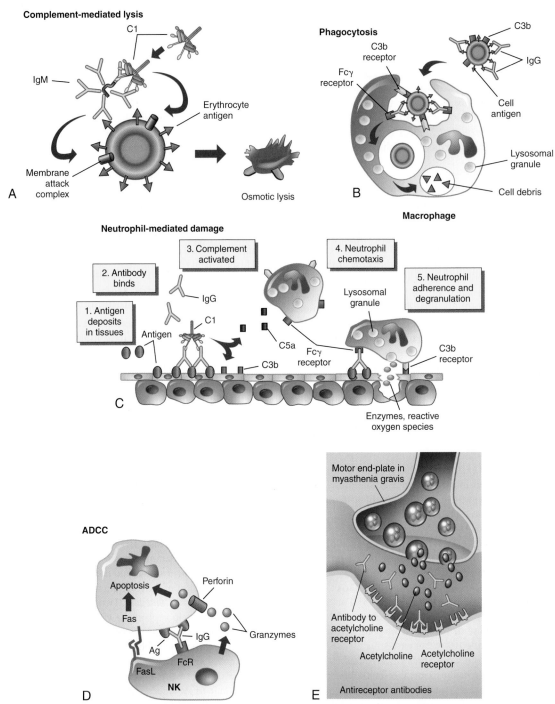

FIGURE 7-11 Mechanisms of Type II, Tissue-Specific Reactions. Antigens on the target cell bind with antibody and are destroyed or prevented from functioning by one of the following mechanisms: **(A)** complement-mediated lysis (an erythrocyte target is illustrated here); **(B)** clearance (phagocytosis) by macrophages in the tissue; **(C)** neutrophil-mediated immune destruction; **(D)** antibody-dependent cell-mediated cytotoxicity (ADCC) (apoptosis of target cells is induced by natural killer [NK] cells by two mechanisms: by the release of granzymes and perforin, which is a molecule that creates pores in the plasma membrane, and enzymes [granzymes] that enter the target through the perforin pores; by the interactions of Fas ligand [FasL; a molecule similar to TNF-α] on the surface of NK cells with Fas [the receptor for FasL] on the surface of target cells); or **(E)** modulation or blocking of the normal function of receptors by antireceptor antibody. This example of mechanism **(E)** depicts myasthenia gravis in which acetylcholine receptor antibodies block acetylcholine from attaching to its receptors on the motor end-plates of skeletal muscle, thereby impairing neuromuscular transmission and causing muscle weakness. *C1,* Complement component C1; *C3b,* complement fragment produced from C3, which acts as an opsonin; *C5a,* complement fragment produced from C5, which acts as a chemotactic factor for neutrophils; *Fcγ receptor,* cellular receptor for the Fc portion of IgG; *FcR,* Fc receptor.

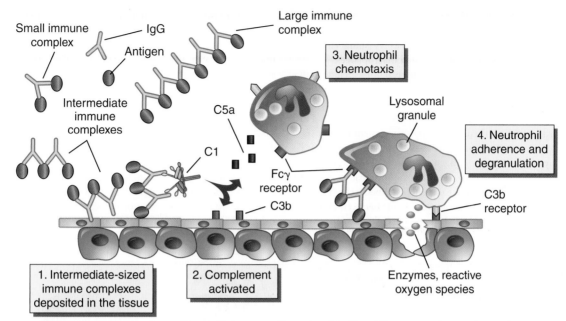

FIGURE 7-12 Mechanism of Type III, Immune Complex–Mediated Reactions. Immune complexes form in the blood from circulating antigen and antibody. Both small and large immune complexes are removed successfully from the circulation and do not cause tissue damage. Intermediate-sized complexes are deposited in certain target tissues in which the circulation is slow or filtration of the blood occurs. The complexes activate the complement cascade through C1 and generate fragments including C5a and C3b. C5a is chemotactic for neutrophils, which migrate into the inflamed area and attach to the IgG and C3b in the immune complexes. The neutrophils attempt unsuccessfully to phagocytose the tissue and in the process release a variety of degradative enzymes that destroy the healthy tissues. Fcγ receptor is the cellular receptor for the Fc portion of IgG.

are called **cryoglobulins.** The precipitates block the circulation and cause localized pallor and numbness, followed by cyanosis (a bluish tinge resulting from oxygen deprivation) and eventually gangrene if the circulation is not restored.

An **Arthus reaction** is caused by repeated local exposure to an antigen that reacts with preformed antibody and forms immune complexes in the walls of the local blood vessels. Symptoms of an Arthus reaction begin within 1 hour of exposure and peak 6 to 12 hours later. The lesions are characterized by a typical inflammatory reaction, with increased vascular permeability, an accumulation of neutrophils, edema, hemorrhage, clotting, and tissue damage.

Arthus reactions may be observed after injection, ingestion, or inhalation of allergens. Skin reactions can follow subcutaneous or intradermal inoculation with drugs, fungal extracts, or antigens used in skin tests. Gastrointestinal reactions, such as gluten-sensitive enteropathy (celiac disease), follow ingestion of antigen, usually gluten from wheat products (see Chapter 35).[45] Allergic alveolitis (farmer lung, pigeon breeder disease) is an Arthus-like acute hemorrhagic inflammation of the air sacs (alveoli) of the lungs resulting from inhalation of fungal antigens, usually particles from moldy hay or pigeon feces (see Chapter 26).[46]

Type IV: Cell-Mediated Hypersensitivity Reactions

Whereas types I, II, and III hypersensitivity reactions are mediated by antibody, type IV reactions are mediated by T lymphocytes and do not involve antibody (Figure 7-13). Type IV mechanisms occur through either cytotoxic T lymphocytes (Tc cells) or cytokine-producing Th1 cells. Tc cells attack and destroy cellular targets directly. Th1 cells

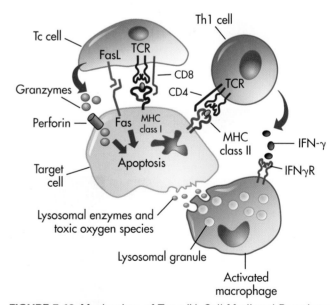

FIGURE 7-13 Mechanism of Type IV, Cell-Mediated Reactions. Antigens from target cells stimulate T cells to differentiate into T-cytotoxic cells *(Tc cells)*, which have direct cytotoxic activity, and T-helper cells *(Th1 cells)* involved in delayed hypersensitivity. The Th1 cells produce lymphokines (especially interferon-γ [*IFNγ*]) that activate the macrophage through specific receptors (e.g., IFNγ receptor [*IFNγR*]). The macrophages can attach to targets and release enzymes and reactive oxygen species that are responsible for most of the tissue destruction.

produce cytokines that recruit and activate phagocytic cells, especially macrophages. Destruction of the tissue is usually caused by direct killing by Tc cells or the release of soluble factors, such as lysosomal enzymes and toxic reactive oxygen species, from activated macrophages.

Clinical examples of type IV hypersensitivity reactions include graft rejection, the skin test for tuberculosis, and allergic reactions resulting from contact with such substances as poison ivy and metals. A type IV component also may be present in many autoimmune diseases. For example, T cells against type II collagen (a protein present in joint tissues) contribute to the destruction of joints in rheumatoid arthritis; T cells against a thyroid cell-surface antigen contribute to the destruction of the thyroid in autoimmune thyroiditis (Hashimoto disease); and T cells against an antigen on the surface of pancreatic beta cells (the cell that normally produces insulin) are responsible for beta-cell destruction in insulin-dependent (type 1) diabetes mellitus.

In 1891 Ehrlich was the first to thoroughly describe a type IV hypersensitivity reaction in the skin, leading to the development of a diagnostic skin test for tuberculosis. The reaction follows an intradermal injection of tuberculin antigen into a suitably sensitized individual and is called a delayed hypersensitivity skin test because of its slow onset—24 to 72 hours to reach maximal intensity. The reaction site is infiltrated with T lymphocytes and macrophages, resulting in a clear hard center (induration) and a reddish surrounding area (erythema).

Allergic type IV reactions are elicited by some environmental antigens that are haptens (Chapter 5) and become immunogenic after binding to larger (carrier) proteins in the individual.[47] In allergic contact dermatitis, the carrier protein is in the skin.[48] The best-known example is poison ivy (Figure 7-14). The antigen is a plant catechol, urushiol, which reacts with normal skin proteins and evokes a cell-mediated immune response. Skin reactions to industrial chemicals,

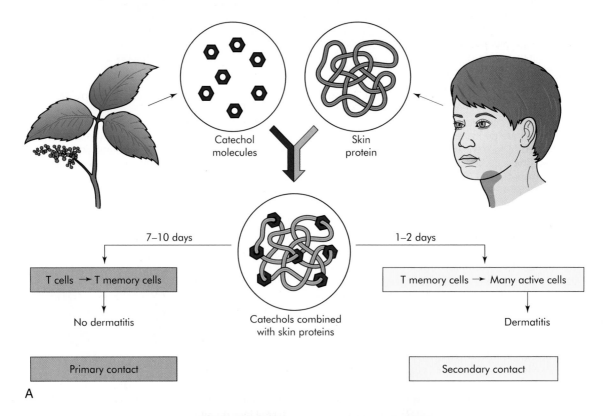

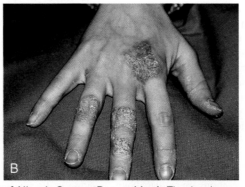

FIGURE 7-14 Development of Allergic Contact Dermatitis. A, The development of allergy to poison ivy. The first (primary) contact with allergen sensitizes (produces reactive T cells) the individual but does not produce a rash (dermatitis). Secondary contact activates a type IV cell-mediated reaction that causes dermatitis. **B,** Contact dermatitis caused by a delayed hypersensitivity reaction leading to vesicles and scaling at the sites of contact. (From Damjanov I, Linder J: *Anderson's pathology,* ed 10, St Louis, 1996, Mosby.)

cosmetics, detergents, clothing, food, metals, and topical medicines (such as penicillin) are elicited by the same mechanism. Contact dermatitis consists of lesions only at the site of contact with the allergen, such as a metal allergy to jewelry.

✔ **QUICK CHECK 7-3**

1. Distinguish among the four types of hypersensitivity mechanisms.
2. What is the mechanism of anaphylaxis?
3. What are some clinical examples of type IV hypersensitivity?

Antigenic Targets of Hypersensitivity Reactions
Allergy

Allergens. Environmental antigens that cause allergic responses are called allergens. It is not known why some antigens are allergens and others are not. Typical allergens include pollens (e.g., ragweed), molds and fungi (e.g., *Penicillium notatum*), foods (e.g., milk, eggs, fish), animals (e.g., cat dander, dog dander), cigarette smoke, and components of house dust (e.g., fecal pellets of house mites). Often the allergen is contained within a particle that is too large to be phagocytosed or is surrounded by a protective nonallergenic coat. The actual allergen is released after enzymatic breakdown (e.g., by lysozyme in secretions) of the larger particle.

Allergic disease: bee sting allergy. Allergies are the most common hypersensitivity diseases. The majority of allergies are type I reactions that lead to annoying symptoms, including rhinitis, sneezing, and other relatively mild reactions. In some individuals, however, these reactions can be excessive and life-threatening (anaphylaxis). Anaphylactic reactions have been described against peanuts and other nuts, shellfish, fish, milk, eggs, and some medications.

Bee venoms contain a mixture of enzymes and other proteins that may serve as allergens. About 1% of children may have an anaphylactic reaction to bee venom. Within minutes they may develop excessive swelling (edema) at the bee sting site, followed by generalized hives, pruritus, and swelling in areas distal from the sting (e.g., eyes, lips), and other systemic symptoms including flushing, sweating, dizziness, and headache. The most severe symptoms may include gastrointestinal (e.g., stomach cramps, vomiting), respiratory (e.g., tightness in the throat, wheezing, difficulty breathing), and vascular (e.g., low blood pressure, shock) reactions. Severe respiratory and vascular reactions may lead to death.

For an individual with known bee sting hypersensitivity, life-style changes include avoidance of stinging or biting insects. If a child has experienced a previous anaphylactic reaction, the chance of having another is about 60%. The primary life-threatening symptoms result from contraction of respiratory smooth muscle. Autonomic nervous system mediators, such as epinephrine, bind to specific receptors on smooth muscle and reverse the effects of histamine, resulting in muscle relaxation. Thus most individuals carry self-injectable epinephrine. The administration of antihistamines will have little effect because histamine has already bound H1 receptors and initiated severe bronchial smooth muscle contraction. Long-term protection may be afforded by desensitization in most individuals.

Autoimmunity

It is fairly well established that most autoimmune diseases originate from a genetic predisposition to mount a hypersensitivity reaction to an environmental stimulus.[49] Some autoimmune diseases can be familial and attributed to the presence of a very small number of susceptibility genes; affected family members may not all develop the same disease, but several members may have different disorders characterized by a variety of hypersensitivity reactions, including autoimmune and allergic. Although most autoimmune diseases appear as isolated events without a positive family history, susceptibility for developing such diseases appears to be linked to a combination of multiple genes.

Breakdown of tolerance. An individual is usually tolerant to his or her own antigens. Tolerance is a state of immunologic control so that the individual does not make a detrimental immune response against his or her own cells and tissues. Autoimmune disease results from a breakdown of this tolerance.

Although many theories exist concerning the initial cause of autoimmune diseases,[50] only one example is known: acute rheumatic fever. In a small number of individuals with group A streptococcal sore throats, the M proteins in the bacterial capsule mimic *(antigenic mimicry)* normal heart antigens and induce antibodies that also react with proteins in the heart valve, damaging the valve.[51] Thus rheumatic fever is a type II autoimmune hypersensitivity. Additionally, some streptococcal skin or throat infections release bacterial antigens into the blood that form circulating immune complexes. The complexes may deposit in the kidneys and initiate an immune complex-mediated glomerulonephritis (inflammation of the kidney). Thus streptococcal antigens (an environmental antigen) may also cause a type III allergic hypersensitivity (poststreptococcal glomerulonephritis).

Autoimmune disease: systemic lupus erythematosus. Systemic lupus erythematosus (SLE) is the most common, complex, and serious of the autoimmune disorders.[52] SLE is characterized by the production of a large variety of antibodies (autoantibodies) against self-antigens, including nucleic acids, erythrocytes, coagulation proteins, phospholipids, lymphocytes, platelets, and many other self-components. The most characteristic autoantibodies are against nucleic acids (e.g., single-stranded DNA, double-stranded DNA), histones, ribonucleoproteins, and other nuclear materials. Approximately 98% of persons with SLE have detectable antibodies against nuclear antigens.[53] The blood normally contains many of these products of cellular turnover and breakdown. Excessive levels of autoantibodies react with the circulating antigen and form circulating immune complexes. The deposition of circulating DNA/anti-DNA complexes in the kidneys can cause severe kidney inflammation. Similar reactions can occur in the brain, heart, spleen, lung, gastrointestinal tract, peritoneum, and skin. Thus some of the symptoms of SLE result from a type III hypersensitivity reaction. Other symptoms, such as destruction of red blood cells (anemia), lymphocytes (lymphopenia), and other cells, may be type II hypersensitivity reactions.

SLE, like most autoimmune diseases, occurs more often in women (approximately a 10:1 predominance of females), especially in the 20- to 40-year-old age group. Blacks are affected more often than whites (about an eightfold increased risk). A genetic predisposition for the disease has been implicated on the basis of increased incidence in twins and the existence of autoimmune disease in the families of individuals with SLE.

Clinical manifestations of SLE include arthralgias or arthritis (90% of individuals), vasculitis and rash (70% to 80% of individuals), renal disease (40% to 50% of individuals), hematologic abnormalities (50% of individuals, with anemia being the most common complication), and cardiovascular diseases (30% to 50% of individuals). (See Discoid lupus erythematosus in Chapter 39.) As with most autoimmune diseases, SLE is characterized by frequent remissions and exacerbations. Because the signs and symptoms affect almost every body system and tend to vacillate, SLE is extremely difficult to diagnose. This has led to the development of a list of 11 common clinical findings.[54] The serial or simultaneous presence of at least four of these findings indicates that the individual has SLE. The findings are as follows:

1. Facial rash confined to the cheeks (malar rash)
2. Discoid rash (raised patches, scaling)
3. Photosensitivity (development of skin rash as a result of exposure to sunlight)
4. Oral or nasopharyngeal ulcers
5. Nonerosive arthritis of at least two peripheral joints
6. Serositis (inflammation of membranes of lung [pleurisy] or heart [pericarditis])
7. Renal disorder (proteinuria of 0.5 g/day or cellular casts)
8. Neurologic disorders (seizures or psychosis)
9. Hematologic disorders (hemolytic anemia, leukopenia, lymphopenia, or thrombocytopenia)
10. Immunologic disorders (positive lupus erythematosus [LE] cell preparation, anti–double-stranded DNA, anti-Smith [Sm] antigen, false-positive serologic test for syphilis, or antiphospholipid antibodies [anticardiolipin antibody or lupus anticoagulant])
11. Presence of antinuclear antibody (ANA)

There is no cure for SLE or most other autoimmune diseases. The goals of treatment are to control symptoms and prevent further damage by suppressing the autoimmune response. Nonsteroidal anti-inflammatory drugs, such as aspirin, ibuprofen, or naproxen, reduce inflammation and relieve pain. Corticosteroids are often prescribed for more serious active disease. Immunosuppressive drugs (e.g., methotrexate, azathioprine, or cyclophosphamide) are used to treat severe symptoms involving internal organs. Ultraviolet light can worsen symptoms (known as flares), and protection from sun exposure is helpful. Prolonged use of certain drugs can cause transient SLE-like symptoms, and the medication history is important for differential diagnosis. Improved outcomes may be available in the future with the continued advances in medical research and the use of stem cell treatments.

Other therapeutic approaches have been used for SLE and other autoimmune diseases. Several decades ago preparations of intravenous immune globulin (IVIg), which was routinely used to replenish antibodies in persons with hypogammaglobulinemia, were administered to children with autoimmune thrombocytopenia (an autoimmune disease in which platelets were destroyed by an autoantibody).[55] IVIg therapy resulted in a rebound of platelet levels and temporary resolution of the thrombocytopenia. IVIg is currently being used for a variety of autoimmune diseases, including SLE. More recently, monoclonal antibodies and other reagents have specifically targeted B and T cells that are participating in autoimmune responses.[56,57] This approach has been somewhat successful in SLE, rheumatoid arthritis, and other autoimmune diseases.

Alloimmunity

Alloantigens. Genetic diversity is the norm in humans. Diversity is also observed among self-antigens, so that two individuals may have different antigens on their tissues and, therefore, be able to establish an immune response against each other's tissues. Some self-antigens, such as the ABO blood group, have limited diversity with very few different antigens being expressed in the population, whereas others, such as the HLA system, have tremendous diversity.

Alloimmune disease: transfusion reactions. Red blood cells (erythrocytes) express several important surface antigens, known collectively as the blood group antigens, which can be targets of alloimmune reactions. More than 80 different red cell antigens are grouped into several dozen blood group systems. The most important of these, because they provoke the strongest humoral alloimmune response, are the ABO and Rh systems.

ABO system. The ABO blood group consists of two major carbohydrate antigens, labeled A and B (Figure 7-15), that are expressed on virtually all cells. These are co-dominant so that both A and B can be simultaneously expressed, resulting in an individual having any one of four different blood types. The erythrocytes of persons with blood type A have the type A carbohydrate antigen (i.e., carry the A antigen), those with blood type B carry the B antigen, those with blood type AB carry both A and B antigens, and those of blood type O carry neither the A nor the B antigen. A person with type A blood also has circulating antibodies to the B carbohydrate antigen. If this person receives blood from a type AB or B individual, a severe transfusion reaction occurs, and the transfused erythrocytes are destroyed by agglutination or complement-mediated lysis. Similarly, a type B individual (whose blood contains anti-A antibodies) cannot receive blood from a type A or AB donor. Type O individuals, who have neither antigen but have both anti-A and anti-B antibodies, cannot accept blood from any of the other three types. These naturally occurring antibodies, called isohemagglutinins, are IgM immunoglobulins and are induced early in life against similar antigens expressed on naturally occurring bacteria in the intestinal tract.

Because individuals with type O blood lack both types of antigens, they are considered universal donors, meaning that anyone can accept their red blood cells. Similarly, type AB individuals are considered universal recipients because they lack both anti-A and anti-B antibodies and can be transfused with any ABO blood type. Agglutination and lysis cause harmful transfusion reactions that can be prevented only by complete and careful ABO matching between donor and recipient.

Rh system. The Rh blood group is a group of antigens expressed only on red blood cells. This is most diverse group of red cell antigens, consisting of at least 45 separate antigens, although only one is considered of major importance: the D antigen. Individuals who express the D antigen on their red cells are Rh-positive, whereas individuals who do not express the D antigen are Rh-negative. When discussing the gene for the Rh antigen, the letter *d* is used to indicate lack of D. Rh-positive individuals can have either a *DD* or *Dd* genotype, whereas Rh-negative individuals have the *dd* genotype. About 85% of North Americans are Rh-positive. Rh-negative individuals can make an IgG antibody to the D antigen (anti-D) if exposed to Rh-positive erythrocytes.

A disease called *hemolytic disease of the newborn* was most commonly caused by IgG anti-D alloantibody produced by Rh-negative mothers against erythrocytes of their Rh-positive fetuses (see Chapter 21). The mother's antibody crossed the placenta and destroyed the red blood cells of the fetus. The occurrence of this particular form of the disease has decreased dramatically because of the use of prophylactic anti-D immunoglobulin (i.e., RhoGAM). By mechanisms that are still not completely understood, administration of anti-D antibody within a few days of exposure to RhD-positive erythrocytes completely prevents sensitization against the D antigen.[58] Because hemolytic disease of the newborn related to the D antigen has been controlled, alloantibodies against the other Rh antigens have become more important. In general, these alloantibodies are associated with a less severe hemolytic disease.

Alloimmune disease: transplant rejection

Major histocompatibility complex. Molecules of the major histocompatibility complex (MHC) were discussed in Chapter 5 as antigen-presenting molecules. MHC molecules are also a major target of transplant rejection. As a result of studies of transplantation, the human MHC molecules are also referred to as human leukocyte antigens (HLAs) and the different MHC genetic loci are commonly called HLA-A, HLA-B, HLA-C, HLA-DR, HLA-DQ, and HLA-DP (Figure 7-16). Additional genes for complement components (e.g., C4, factor B)

Blood Type

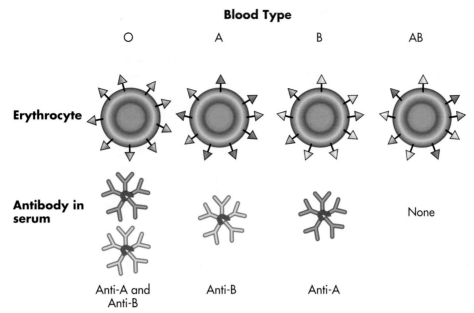

FIGURE 7-15 ABO Blood Types. This figure shows the relationship of antigens and antibodies associated with the ABO blood groups. The surfaces of erythrocytes of individuals with blood group O have a core carbohydrate that is present on cells of all ABO blood groups (H antigen). The sera of blood group O individuals contain IgM antibodies against both A and B carbohydrates. In individuals of the blood group A, some of the H antigens have been modified into A antigens. The sera of these individuals have IgM antibodies against the B antigen. In individuals with blood group B, some of the H antigens have been modified into B antigens. These individuals have IgM antibodies against the A antigen in their sera. In individuals of the blood group AB, some of the H antigens have been modified into both the A and B antigens. These individuals do not have antibody to either A or B antigens.

Chromosome 6: Site of genes that encode HLA antigens

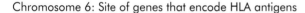

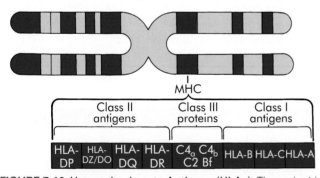

FIGURE 7-16 Human Leukocyte Antigens (HLAs). The major histocompatibility complex (MHC) is located on chromosome 6 and contains genes that code for class I antigens, class II antigens, and class III proteins (i.e., complement proteins and cytokines). (From Mudge-Grout C: *Immunologic disorders,* St Louis, 1992, Mosby.)

are also contained in the MHC region and are referred to as class III loci. The class I (HLA-A, -B, and -C) and class II MHC loci (HLA-DR, -DQ, and -DP) are the most genetically diverse (polymorphic) of any human genetic loci. Within the human population, the number of possible different alleles (i.e., forms of the gene) expressed by each locus is astounding. For example, more than 300 different HLA-A antigens are expressed in the population. These numbers are based on the polymorphism of observed DNA sequences and may not reflect differences in function.

Clearly, not every allele is expressed in the same individual. Humans have two copies of each MHC locus (one inherited from each parent)

that are co-dominant so that molecules encoded by each parent's genes are expressed on the cell surface. Within an individual, each locus will express only one allele. For instance, each person will have at most two different HLA-A proteins (one from each parent). However, with the tremendous number of possible alleles that can be expressed throughout the population, it is likely that any two unrelated individuals will have different MHC antigens and would reject organs transplanted from one to another.

Transplantation. The diversity of MHC molecules becomes clinically relevant during organ transplantation.[25] The recipient of a transplant can mount an immune response against the foreign MHC antigens on the donor tissue, resulting in rejection. To minimize the chance of tissue rejection, the donor and recipient are often tissue-typed beforehand to identify differences in HLA antigens. Because of the large number of different alleles, it is highly unlikely that a perfect match can be found between someone who needs a transplant and a potential donor from the general population. The more similar two individuals are in their HLA tissue type, the more likely a transplant from one to the other will be successful. Clearly, the most successful transplants would be between identical twins because they are identical genetically.

The specific combination of alleles at the six major HLA loci on one chromosome (A, B, C, DR, DQ, and DP) is termed a haplotype. Each individual has two HLA haplotypes, one from the paternal chromosome 6 and another from the maternal chromosome (Figure 7-17). Each parent passes on one set of HLA antigens to each of his or her offspring, meaning that children usually share half their HLA antigens with each parent. Odds dictate that children will share one haplotype with half their siblings and either no haplotypes or both haplotypes with a quarter of their siblings. Thus the chance of finding a match among siblings is much higher (25%) than the general population.

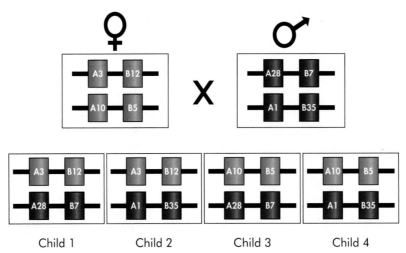

FIGURE 7-17 Inheritance of HLA. HLA alleles are inherited in a co-dominant fashion; both maternal and paternal antigens are expressed. Specific HLA alleles are commonly given numbers to indicate different antigens. In this example, the mother has linked genes for HLA-A3 and HLA-B12 on one chromosome 6 and genes for HLA-A10 and HLA-B5 on the second chromosome 6. The father has HLA-A28 and HLA-B7 on one chromosome and HLA-A1 and HLA-B35 on the second chromosome. The children from this pairing may have one of four possible combinations of maternal and paternal HLA.

Transplant rejection. Transplant rejection may be classified as hyperacute, acute, or chronic, depending on the amount of time that elapses between transplantation and rejection.[25] **Hyperacute rejection** is immediate and rare. When the circulation is reestablished to the grafted area, the graft may immediately turn white (the so-called *white graft*) instead of a normal pink color. Hyperacute rejection usually occurs because of preexisting antibody (type II reaction) to antigens on the vascular endothelial cells in the grafted tissue.

Acute rejection is a cell-mediated immune response that occurs within days to months after transplantation. This type of rejection occurs when the recipient develops an immune response against unmatched HLA antigens after transplantation. A biopsy of the rejected organ usually shows an infiltration of lymphocytes and macrophages characteristic of a type IV reaction.

Chronic rejection may occur after a period of months or years of normal function. It is characterized by slow, progressive organ failure. Chronic rejection may result from a weak cell-mediated (type IV) reaction against minor histocompatibility antigens on the grafted tissue.

> ✔ **QUICK CHECK 7-4**
> 1. Why do certain drugs become immunogenic to the host?
> 2. Why is SLE considered an autoimmune disease?
> 3. Define the different types of graft rejection.

DID YOU UNDERSTAND?

Infection

1. Bacteria injure cells by producing exotoxins or endotoxins. Exotoxins are enzymes that can damage the plasma membranes of host cells or can inactivate enzymes critical to protein synthesis, and endotoxins activate the inflammatory response and produce fever.
2. Septicemia is the proliferation of bacteria in the blood. Endotoxins released by blood-borne bacteria cause the release of vasoactive enzymes that increase the permeability of blood vessels. Leakage from vessels causes hypotension that can result in septic shock.
3. Viruses enter host cells and use the metabolic processes of host cells to proliferate.
4. Viruses that have invaded host cells may decrease protein synthesis, disrupt lysosomal membranes, form inclusion bodies where synthesis of viral nucleic acids is occurring, fuse with host cells to produce giant cells, alter antigenic properties of the host cell, and transform host cells into cancerous cells.
5. Diseases caused by fungi are called mycoses, and they occur in two forms: yeasts (spheres) and molds (filaments or hyphae).
6. Dermatophytes are fungi that infect skin, hair, and nails with diseases such as ringworm and athlete's foot.
7. Fungi release toxins and enzymes that are damaging to tissue.
8. Parasitic microorganisms range from unicellular protozoa to large worms. Although less common in the United States, parasites and protozoa are common causes of infection worldwide.
9. Parasitic and protozoal infections are rarely transmitted from human to human. Infection mainly spreads through vectors (e.g., by mosquito bites) or through contaminated water or food.
10. The most effective means to prevent infection is vaccination; the administration of an antigen specific for the infectious agent in order to induce a long-term and protective secondary immune response.

Deficiencies in Immunity

1. Immunodeficiency is the failure of mechanisms of self-defense to function in their normal capacity.
2. Immunodeficiencies are either congenital (primary) or acquired (secondary). Congenital immunodeficiencies are caused by genetic defects that disrupt lymphocyte development, whereas acquired immunodeficiencies are secondary to disease or other physiologic alterations.

DID YOU UNDERSTAND?—cont'd

3. The clinical hallmark of immunodeficiency is a propensity to unusual or recurrent severe infections. The type of infection usually reflects the immune system defect.
4. The most common infections in individuals with defects of cell-mediated immune response are fungal and viral, whereas infections in individuals with defects of the humoral immune response or complement function are primarily bacterial.
5. Severe combined immunodeficiency (SCID) is a total lack of T cell function and a severe (either partial or total) lack of B cell function.
6. DiGeorge syndrome (congenital thymic aplasia or hypoplasia) is characterized by complete or partial lack of the thymus (resulting in depressed T cell immunity), frequently associated with diminished or parathyroid gland activity (resulting in hypocalcemia) and cardiac anomalies.
7. Defects in B cell function are diverse, ranging from a complete lack of the human bursal equivalent, the lymphoid organs required for B cell maturation (as in Bruton agammaglobulinemia), to deficiencies in a single class of immunoglobulins (e.g., selective IgA deficiency).
8. Acquired immunodeficiencies are caused by superimposed conditions, such as malnutrition, medical therapies, physical or psychologic trauma, or infections.
9. Immunodeficiency syndromes usually are treated by replacement therapy. Deficient antibody production is treated by replacement of missing immunoglobulins with commercial gamma-globulin preparations. Lymphocyte deficiencies are treated by the replacement of host lymphocytes with transplants of bone marrow, fetal liver, or fetal thymus from a donor.
10. AIDS is an acquired dysfunction of the immune system caused by a retrovirus (HIV) that infects and destroys CD4+ lymphocytes (T-helper cells).

Hypersensitivity: Allergy, Autoimmunity, and Alloimmunity

1. Hypersensitivity is an inappropriate immune response misdirected against the host's own tissues (autoimmunity) or directed against beneficial foreign tissues, such as transfusions or transplants (alloimmunity); or it can be exaggerated responses against environmental antigens (allergy).
2. Mechanisms of hypersensitivity are classified as type I (IgE-mediated) reactions, type II (tissue-specific) reactions, type III (immune complex–mediated) reactions, and type IV (cell-mediated) reactions.
3. Hypersensitivity reactions can be immediate (developing within seconds or hours) or delayed (developing within hours or days).
4. Anaphylaxis, the most rapid immediate hypersensitivity reaction, is an explosive reaction that occurs within minutes of reexposure to the antigen and can lead to cardiovascular shock.
5. Allergens are antigens that cause allergic responses.
6. Type I (IgE-mediated) reactions occur after antigen reacts with IgE on mast cells, leading to mast cell degranulation and the release of histamine and other inflammatory substances.
7. Type II (tissue-specific) reactions are caused by four possible mechanisms: complement-mediated lysis, opsonization and phagocytosis, antibody-dependent cell-mediated cytotoxicity, and modulation of cellular function.
8. Type III (immune complex–mediated) reactions are caused by the formation of immune complexes that are deposited in target tissues, where they activate the complement cascade, generating chemotactic fragments that attract neutrophils into the inflammatory site.
9. Immune complex disease can be a systemic reaction, such as serum sickness (e.g., Raynaud phenomenon), or localized, such as the Arthus reaction.
10. Type IV (cell-mediated) reactions are caused by specifically sensitized T cells, which either kill target cells directly or release lymphokines that activate other cells, such as macrophages.
11. Allergies can be mediated by any of the four mechanisms of hypersensitivity.
12. Clinical manifestations of allergic reactions are usually confined to the areas of initial intake or contact with the allergen. Ingested allergens induce gastrointestinal symptoms, airborne allergens induce respiratory or skin manifestations, and contact allergens induce allergic responses at the site of contact.
13. Atopic individuals are genetically predisposed to the development of allergies.
14. Alloimmunity is the immune system's reaction against antigens on the tissues of other members of the same species.
15. Alloimmune disorders include transient neonatal disease, in which the maternal immune system becomes sensitized against antigens expressed by the fetus, and transplant rejection and transfusion reactions, in which the immune system of the recipient of an organ transplant or blood transfusion reacts against foreign antigens on the donor's cells.

KEY TERMS

- ABO blood group 198
- Acquired immunodeficiency syndrome (AIDS) 183
- Acute rejection 200
- Adenosine deaminase (ADA) deficiency 180
- Agammaglobulinemia 180
- Allergen 197
- Allergy 188
- Alloimmune disease 190
- Alloimmunity 190
- Anaphylaxis 190
- Antibody-dependent cell-mediated cytotoxicity (ADCC) 193
- Antigenic drift 168
- Antigenic shift 168
- Antitoxin 171
- Arthus reaction 195
- Atopic 191
- Attenuated virus 177
- Autoimmune disease 190
- Autoimmunity 188
- Bacteremia 171
- Bare lymphocyte syndrome 180
- Blood group antigen 198
- B lymphocyte deficiency 180
- Bruton agammaglobulinemia 180
- C3 deficiency 180
- Chronic granulomatous disease (CGD) 181
- Chronic mucocutaneous candidiasis 180
- Chronic rejection 200
- Combined deficiency 180
- Communicability 167
- Complement deficiency 180
- Contact dermatitis 196
- Cryoglobulins 195
- Delayed hypersensitivity reaction 190
- Delayed hypersensitivity skin test 196
- Dermatophyte 174
- Desensitization 193
- DiGeorge syndrome 180
- Dimorphic fungus (pl., fungi) 173
- Endotoxic shock 171
- Endotoxin (lipopolysaccharide [LPS]) 171
- Entrance inhibitor 186
- Erythema 196
- Exotoxin 171
- Graft-versus-host disease (GVHD) 182
- Herd immunity 178
- Highly active antiretroviral therapy (HAART) 186
- Human immunodeficiency virus (HIV) 183

■ KEY TERMS—cont'd

- Human leukocyte antigen (HLA)   198
- Hyperacute rejection   200
- Hypersensitivity   188
- Hypogammaglobulinemia   180
- Immediate hypersensitivity reaction   190
- Immune deficiency   178
- Immunogenicity   167
- Induration   196
- Infectivity   167
- Integrase inhibitor   186
- Isohemagglutinin   198
- Major histocompatibility complex (MHC)   198
- Mesenchymal stem cell (MSC)   182
- Methicillin-resistant *Staphylococcus aureus* (MRSA)   176
- Mycosis (*pl.,* mycoses)   174

- Parasitic microorganisms   174
- Pathogenecity   167
- Phagocytic deficiency   181
- Portal of entry   167
- Primary (congenital) immune deficiency   178
- Protease   184
- Protease inhibitor   186
- Raynaud phenomenon   193
- Reverse transcriptase   184
- Reverse transcriptase inhibitor   186
- Rh blood group   198
- Secondary (acquired) immune deficiency   178
- Selective IgA deficiency   180
- Septicemia   171
- Serum sickness   193

- Severe combined immunodeficiency (SCID)   180
- Systemic lupus erythematosus (SLE)   197
- Tissue-specific antigen   193
- T lymphocyte deficiency   180
- Tolerance   197
- Toxogenicity   167
- Toxoid   178
- Universal donor   198
- Universal recipient   198
- Urticaria (hives)   191
- Vaccination   177
- Vaccine   177
- Virulence   167
- Wheal and flare reaction   191
- Wiskott-Aldrich syndrome   180

REFERENCES

1. Kochanek KD, et al: Deaths: preliminary data for 2009, *National vital statistics reports web release,* vol 59, no. 4, Hyattsville, Md, 2011, National Center for Health Statistics.
2. World Health Organization (WHO): *Fact sheet no. 286: measles,* updated Dec 2009. Available at www.who.int/mediacentre/factsheets/fs286/en/index.html.
3. World Health Organization (WHO): *Fact sheet no. 286: poliomyelitis,* updated Jan 2009. Available at www.who.int/mediacentre/factsheets/fs114/en/index.html.
4. Lemichez E, et al: Breaking the wall: targeting of the endothelium by pathogenic bacteria, *Nat Rev Microbiol* 8(2):93–104, 2010.
5. Diacovich L, Gorvel J-P: Bacterial manipulation of innate immunity to promote infection, *Nat Rev Microbiol* 8(2):117–128, 2010.
6. Lambotin M, et al: A look behind closed doors: interaction of persistent viruses with dendritic cells, *Nat Rev Microbiol* 8(5):350–360, 2010.
7. Donaldson EF, et al: Viral shape-shifting: norovirus evasion of the human immune system, *Nat Rev Microbiol* 8(3):231–241, 2010.
8. Moss RB, et al: Targeting pandemic influenza: a primer on influenza antivirals and drug resistance, *J Antimicrob Chemother* 65(6):1086–1093, 2010.
9. Opal SM: Endotoxins and other sepsis triggers. In Ronco C, Piccinni P, Rosner MH, editors: *Endotoxemia and endotoxin shock: disease, diagnosis and therapy, contributions to nephrology,* vol 167, Basel, Switzerland, 2010, Karger, pp 14–24.
10. Agency for Healthcare Research and Quality: *Fungal infections.* In *Guidelines for prevention and treatment of opportunistic infections among HIV-exposed and HIV-infected children,* updated Aug 24, 2009. Available at http://guidelines.gov/content.aspx?id=14841.
11. Cohen R: The need for prudent use of antibiotics and routine use of vaccines, *Clin Microbiol Infect* 15(suppl 3):21–23, 2009.
12. Hawkey PM: The growing burden of antimicrobial resistance, *J Antimicrob Chemother* 62(suppl 1):i1–i9, 2008.
13. World Health Organization (WHO): *Fact sheet: smallpox.* Available at www.who.int/mediacentre/factsheets/smallpox/en/index.html.
14. De Jesus NH: Epidemics to eradication: the modern history of poliomyelitis, *Virol J* 4(7):70–88, 2007.
15. Feikin DR, et al: Individual and community risks of measles and pertussis associated with personal exemptions to immunization, *JAMA* 284(24):3145–3150, 2000.
16. Centers for Disease Control and Prevention (CDC): Intussusception among recipients of rotavirus vaccine—United States, 1998-1999, *MMWR Morb Mortal Wkly Rep* 48(27):577–581, 1999.
17. Schecter R, Grether JK: Continuing increases in autism reported to California's developmental services system: mercury in retrograde, *Arch Gen Psych* 65(1):19–24, 2008.

18. Jegede AS: What led to the Nigerian boycott of the polio vaccination campaign? *PLOS Med* 4(3):417–422, 2007.
19. Jenkins HE, et al: Effectiveness of immunization against paralytic poliomyelitis in Nigeria, *N Eng J Med* 359(16):1666–1674, 2008.
20. Centers for Disease Control and Prevention (CDC): Progress toward poliomyelitis eradication—Nigeria, January 2009–June 2010, *MMWR Morb Mortal Wkly Rep* 59(26):802–807, 2010.
21. Notarangelo LD: Primary immunodeficiencies, *J Allergy Clin Immunol* 125(2):S182–S194, 2010.
22. Vale AM, Schroeder HW Jr: Clinical consequences of defects in B-cell development, *J Allergy Clin Immunol* 125(4):778–787, 2010.
23. Chinen J, Shearer WT: Secondary immunodeficiencies, including HIV infection, *J Allergy Clin Immunol* 125(2):S195–S203, 2010.
24. Oliveira JB, Fleisher TA: Laboratory evaluation of primary immunodeficiencies, *J Allergy Clin Immunol* 125(2):S297–S305, 2010.
25. Chinen J, Buckley RH: Transplantation immunology: solid organ and bone marrow, *J Allergy Clin Immunol* 125(2):S324–S335, 2010.
26. Panel on Antiretroviral Guidelines for Adults and Adolescents: *Guidelines for the use of antiretroviral agents in HIV-1-infected adults and adolescents,* pp 1–161, Washington DC, 2001, Department of Health and Human Services. Available at www.aidsinfo.nih.gov/ContentFiles/AdultandAdolescentGL.pdf. Accessed Aug 13, 2010.
27. Buckley RH: B-cell function in severe combined immunodeficiency after stem cell or gene therapy: a review, *J Allergy Clin Immunol* 125(4):790–797, 2010.
28. Brignier AC, Gerwirtz AM: Embryonic and adult stem cell therapy, *J Allergy Clin Immunol* 125(2):S336–S344, 2010.
29. Toubai T, et al: Mesenchymal stem cells for treatment and prevention of graft-versus-host disease after allogeneic hematopoietic cell transplantation, *Curr Stem Cell Res Therapy* 4(4):252–259, 2009.
30. World Health Organization (WHO): *Towards universal access: scaling up priority HIV/AIDS interventions in the health sector: progress report 2009,* Geneva, Switzerland, 2009, Author.
31. Centers for Disease Control and Prevention (CDC): *HIV surveillance report,* 2008, vol 20, June 2010. Accessed Aug 13, 2010. Available at: www.cdc.gov/hiv/topics/surveillance/resources/reports/.
32. Johnson N, Cunningham AF, Fooks AR: The immune response to rabies virus infection and vaccination, *Vaccine* 28(23):3896–3901, 2010.
33. Schneider E, et al: Revised surveillance case definitions for HIV infection among adults, adolescents, and children aged <18 months and for HIV infection and AIDS among children aged 18 months to <13 years—United States, 2008, *MMWR Morb Mortal Wkly Rep* 57(RR10):1–8, 2008.
34. Simons FER: Anaphylaxis, *J Allergy Clin Immunol* 125(2):S161–S181, 2010.
35. Stone KD, Prussin C, Metcalfe DD: IgE, mast cells, basophils, and eosinophils, *J Allergy Clin Immunol* 125(2):S73–S80, 2010.

36. Sicherer SH, Sampson HA: Food allergy, *J Allergy Clin Immunol* 125(2):S116–S125, 2010.
37. Dykewicz MS, Hamilos DL: Rhinitis and sinusitis, *J Allergy Clin Immunol* 125(2):S103–S115, 2010.
38. Lemanske RF Jr, Busse WW: Asthma: clinical expression and molecular mechanisms, *J Allergy Clin Immunol* 125(2):S95–S102, 2010.
39. Peden D, Reed CE: Environmental and occupational allergies, *J Allergy Clin Immunol* 125(2):S150–S160, 2010.
40. Holloway JW, Yang IA, Holgate ST: Genetics of allergic disease, *J Allergy Clin Immunol* 125(2):S81–S94, 2010.
41. Hamilton RG: Clinical laboratory assessment of immediate-type hypersensitivity, *J Allergy Clin Immunol* 125(2):S284–S296, 2010.
42. Frew AJ: Allergen immunotherapy, *J Allergy Clin Immunol* 125(2):S306–S313, 2010.
43. Michels AW, Eisenbarth GS: Immunologic endocrine disorders, *J Allergy Clin Immunol* 125(2):S226–S237, 2010.
44. Langford CA: Vasculitis, *J Allergy Clin Immunol* 125(2):S216–S225, 2010.
45. Atkins D, Furuta GT: Mucosal immunology, eosinophilic esophagitis, and other intestinal inflammatory diseases, *J Allergy Clin Immunol* 125(2):S255–S261, 2010.
46. Greenberger PA, Grammer LC: Pulmonary disorders, including vocal cord dysfunction, *J Allergy Clin Immunol* 125(2):S248–S254, 2010.
47. Khan DA, Solensky R: Drug allergy, *J Allergy Clin Immunol* 125(2):S126–S137, 2010.
48. Fonacier LS, Dreskin SC, Leung DYM: Allergic skin diseases, *J Allergy Clin Immunol* 125(2):S138–S149, 2010.
49. Zenewicz LA, et al: Unraveling the genetics of autoimmunity, *Cell* 140(6):791–797, 2010.
50. Sfriso P, et al: Infections and autoimmunity: the multifaceted relationship, *J Leukoc Biol* 87(3):385–395, 2010.
51. Cunningham MW: Pathogenesis of group A streptococcal infections, *Clin Microbiol Rev* 13(3):470–511, 2000.
52. Joseph A, et al: Immunologic rheumatic disorders, *J Allergy Clin Immunol* 125(2):S204–S215, 2010.
53. Castro C, Gourley M: Diagnostic testing and interpretation of tests for autoimmunity, *J Allergy Clin Immunol* 125(2):S238–S247, 2010.
54. Ginzler E, Tayar J: *Systemic lupus erythematosus*, updated June 2008, American College of Rheumatology. Available at www.rheumatology.org/practice/clinical/patients/diseases_and_conditions/lupus.asp.
55. Lux A, et al: The pro and anti-inflammatory activities of immunoglobulin G, *Ann Rheum Dis* 69(suppl 1):i92–i96, 2010.
56. Lee S, Ballow M: Monoclonal antibodies and fusion proteins and their complications: targeting B cells in autoimmune diseases, *J Allergy Clin Immunol* 125(2):S814–S820, 2010.
57. Steward-Tharp SM, et al: New insights into T cell biology and T cell-directed therapy for autoimmunity, inflammation, and immunosuppression, *Ann N Y Acad Sci* 1183(1):123–148, 2010.
58. Brinc D, Lazarus AH: Mechanisms of anti-D action in prevention of hemolytic disease of the fetus and newborn, *Hematol* 2009(1):185–191, 2009.

8

Stress and Disease

*Margaret F. Clayton, Kathryn L. McCance, and Beth A. Forshee** *

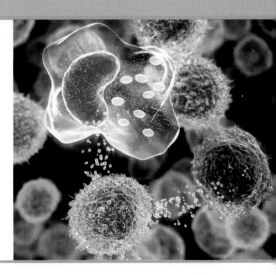

evolve WEBSITE

http://evolve.elsevier.com/Huether/
- Review Questions and Answers
- Animations
- Quick Check Answers

- Key Terms Exercises
- Critical Thinking Questions with Answers
- Algorithm Completion Exercises
- WebLinks

CHAPTER OUTLINE

Modern society is full of stress. Stress experiences involve daily hassles (e.g., fast-paced scheduling, the pressure to remain in constant contact through social media or cell phones, or both), major life events (e.g., loss of family member, loss of job), abuse, and trauma (Figure 8-1). Americans have become accustomed to an accelerated way of life with chronic stress by adopting behaviors (e.g., smoking, drinking, drug abuse, sleep disturbances) that may result in the so-called *stress-related disorders*. In general, stress begins with a stimulus that the brain perceives as stressful and in turn promotes adaptation- and survival-related physiologic responses. These responses can become dysregulated and cause pathophysiologic consequences.[1,2] Another way to think about this is that acute stress is considered to enhance immunity whereas chronic stress is now considered to suppress immunity.[2]

HISTORICAL BACKGROUND AND GENERAL CONCEPTS

Walter B. Cannon used the term *stress* in both a physiologic and a psychologic sense as early as 1914.[3] He applied the engineering concept of stress and strain in a physiologic context and believed that emotional stimuli were also capable of causing stress. In 1946 Hans Selye

popularized these same findings, viewing stress as a biologic phenomenon.[4] During Selye's original attempts to discover a new sex hormone by injecting crude ovarian extracts into rats, he discovered the biologic syndrome of stress.[4] He repeatedly found that three structural changes occurred: (1) enlargement of the cortex of the adrenal gland, (2) atrophy of the thymus gland and other lymphoid structures, and (3) development of bleeding ulcers in the stomach and duodenal lining. Selye soon discovered that these manifestations were not specific to injected ovarian extracts but also occurred after exposure of the rats to other noxious stimuli, such as cold, surgical injury, and restraint. He called these stimuli **stressors.** Selye concluded that this triad or syndrome of manifestations represented a nonspecific response to noxious stimuli, naming it the **general adaptation syndrome (GAS).**

Three successive stages of the GAS were identified: (1) the **alarm stage** or reaction, in which the central nervous system (CNS) is aroused and the body's defenses are mobilized (e.g., "fight or flight") (Figure 8-2); (2) the **stage of resistance or adaptation,** during which mobilization contributes to "fight or flight;" and (3) the **stage of exhaustion,** where continuous stress causes the progressive breakdown of compensatory mechanisms (acquired adaptations) and homeostasis. Exhaustion marks the onset of certain diseases **(diseases of adaptation).**

Interactions among the sympathetic branch of the autonomic nervous system (ANS) and the hypothalamus, pituitary, and adrenal glands (HPA axis, see Figure 8-4) produce the nonspecific physiologic

*Beth A. Forshee, RN, PhD, contributed to this chapter in the previous edition.

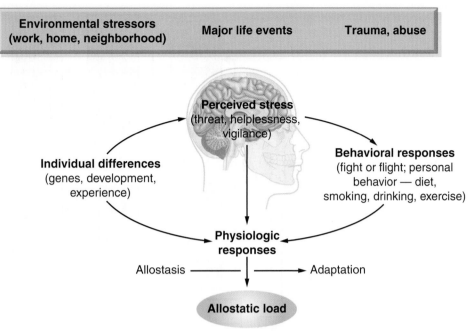

FIGURE 8-1 Physiologic and Behavioral Stress Responses. Stress processes arise from bidirectional communication patterns between the brain and other physiologic systems (autonomic, immune, neural, and endocrine). Importantly, these bidirectional mechanisms are protective, promoting short-term adaptation (allostasis). Chronic stress mechanisms, however, can lead to long-term dysregulation and promote behavioral responses and physiologic responses that lead to stress-induced disorders/diseases (allostatic load), compromising health. (From McEwen BS: Central effects of stress hormones in health and disease: understanding the protective and damaging effects of stress and stress mediators, *Eur J Pharmacol* 583[2–3]:174–185, 2008.)

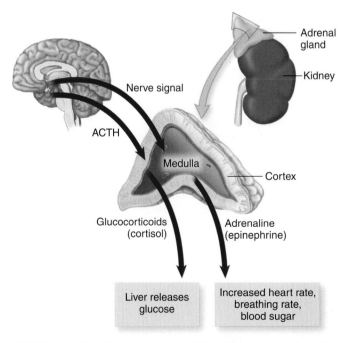

FIGURE 8-2 The Alarm Reaction. The alarm reaction includes increased secretion of glucocorticoids (cortisol) by the adrenal cortex and increased secretion of epinephrine and small amounts of norepinephrine from the adrenal medulla. The response to the release of cortisol and sympathetic nerve activation is summarized in Figure 8-3. *ACTH,* Adrenocorticotropic hormone. (From Thibodeau GA, Patton KT: *Anatomy & physiology,* ed 7, St Louis, 2010, Mosby.)

responses identified by Selye. The alarm phase begins when a stressor activates the hypothalamus and sympathetic nervous system (see Figures 8-2 and 8-3). The resistance or adaptation phase begins with the actions of the adrenal hormones cortisol, norepinephrine, and epinephrine. Exhaustion (also known as allostatic overload; discussed later) occurs if stress continues and adaptation is not successful, ultimately causing impairment of the immune response, heart failure, and kidney failure leading to death.

Physiologic stress is a chemical or physical disturbance produced by a change, either in the external environment or within the body itself, that elicits a response to counteract the disturbance (i.e., begins the GAS). Selye identified three components of physiologic stress: (1) the exogenous or endogenous stressor initiating the disturbance, (2) the chemical or physical disturbance produced by the stressor, and (3) the body's counteracting (adaptational) response to the disturbance.

Although Selye's identification of the GAS is regarded as tremendously important and the cornerstone of stress research, the idea that stress is a purely physiologic response is oversimplified. In the mid-1950s, studies showed that activation of the adrenal cortex occurred in humans in response to psychologic stressors,[5] in monkeys with conditioned emotional responses,[6] and in humans subjected to a stressful interview technique.[7] Mason later demonstrated that occurrence of the GAS depended on psychologic factors surrounding the stressors.[8] He also showed that factors, such as degrees of discomfort, unpleasantness, or suddenness of the stress, could account for the presence or absence of physiologic stress responses.[8]

Research conducted since the 1970s has shown the remarkable sensitivity of the CNS and endocrine systems to emotional, psychologic, and social influences. Psychologic stressors can elicit a reactive or

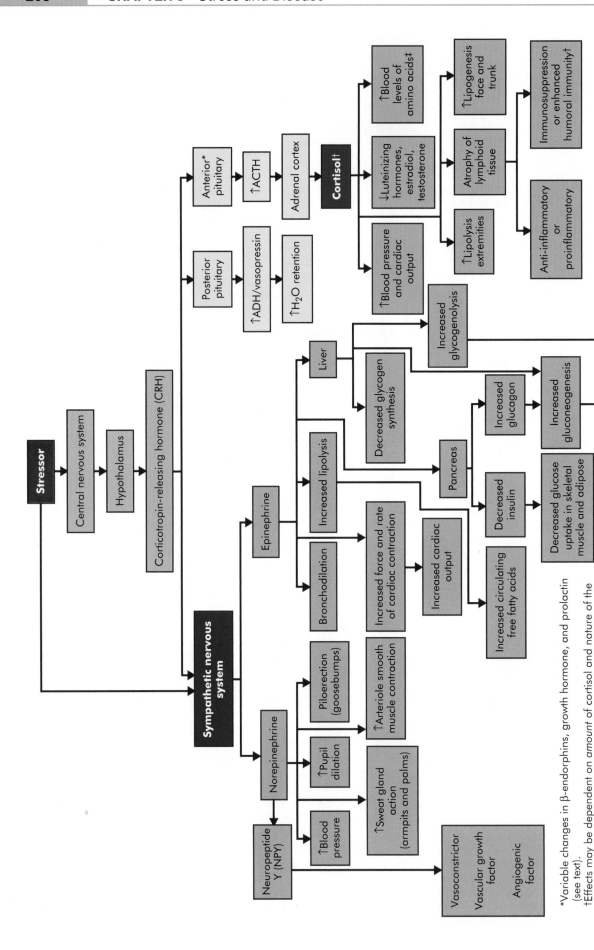

FIGURE 8-3 The Stress Response.

*Variable changes in β-endorphins, growth hormone, and prolactin (see text).

†Effects may be dependent on *amount* of cortisol and nature of the stressor.

‡Caused by protein catabolism in muscle, adipose tissue, skin, bones, lymphoid tissue.

ADH, Antidiuretic hormone; *ACTH*, adrenocorticotropic hormone.

anticipatory stress response. The reactive response is a physiologic response derived from psychologic stressors. For example, the stress of an examination may produce an increased heart rate and dry mouth. Although there is no physical stressor, the psychologic stress of an examination elicits a reactive physiologic response. Anticipatory responses occur when physiologic responses develop in anticipation of disruption of the optimal steady state, also known as homeostasis. Anticipatory responses can be generated by fears (such as a fear of predators) or memories.[9] In a conditioned response, a person learns that specific events are associated with danger. Anticipation of experiencing these events produces a physiologic stress response. For example, a child who is abused by a parent may experience a physiologic stress response in anticipation of further abuse when that parent enters the room. Another well-known example of a conditioned response is the development of post-traumatic stress disorder (PSTD) experienced by military personnel and survivors of natural disasters.

Today there is evidence implicating stress both as a precipitating factor for some diseases and conditions and as a contributor to worsening symptoms and outcomes in other diseases, such as atherosclerosis, irritable bowel syndrome, ulcers, asthma, autoimmune disorders, anxiety, delayed wound healing, chronic pain and fatigue syndromes, reproductive dysfunction, diabetes, and depression.[10-12] In addition, evidence published since 2000 generally supports a role for stress in human immunodeficiency virus (HIV) progression.[13]

The concept that stress may influence immunity and resistance to disease has been considered and investigated since the 1950s. Research in the 1970s determined that life changes or emotions resulting from life changes and occurring over a prolonged time were associated with decreased immune function. More recently, studies have been conducted to investigate the interactions among social, psychologic, and biologic factors and their role in causing and prolonging or shortening the course of disease. What is emerging from the various disciplines involved—molecular biology, immunology, neurology, endocrinology, and behavioral science—is a more holistic and complex model that involves biochemical relationships of the central nervous system (CNS), autonomic nervous system (ANS), endocrine system, and immune system. More simply, these relationships are often cited together as the hypothalamic-pituitary-adrenal (HPA) axis (Figure 8-4). In sequence, the hypothalamus secretes corticotropin-releasing hormone (CRH), which binds to specific receptors on pituitary cells that, in turn, produce adrenocorticotropic hormone (ACTH). ACTH is then transported through the blood to the adrenal glands located on the top of the kidneys. After binding to specific receptors on the adrenal glands, the glucocorticoid hormones (primarily cortisol) are released. Cortisol initiates a series of metabolic changes (discussed in the section Glucocorticoids: Cortisol), but overall these hormones are thought to enhance immunity during acute stress and to suppress immunity during chronic stress because of prolonged exposure and increased concentration.[2]

Psychoneuroimmunology (PNI) is the study of how the consciousness *(psycho)*, the brain and spinal cord *(neuro)*, and the body's defenses against infection and abnormal cell division *(immunology)* interact. Psychoneuroimmunology assumes that all immune-mediated diseases result from interrelationships among psychosocial, emotional, genetic, neurologic, endocrine, immunologic, and behavioral factors.[14,15] The immune system is integrated with other physiologic processes and is sensitive to changes in CNS and endocrine functioning, such as those that accompany psychologic states. Stressors can elicit the stress response or stress system through the action of the nervous and endocrine systems. Stressors include infection, noise, decreased oxygen supply, pain, malnutrition, heat, cold, trauma, prolonged exertion, radiation, responses to life events (including anxiety,

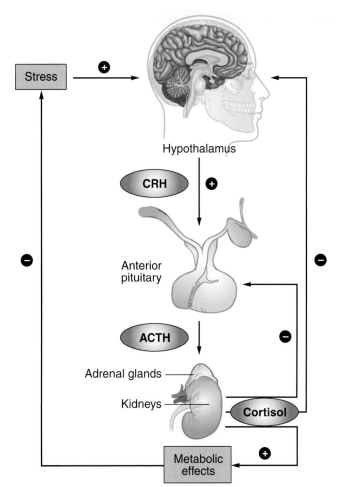

FIGURE 8-4 Hypothalamic-Pituitary-Adrenal (HPA) Axis. The response to stress begins in the brain. The hypothalamus is the control center in the brain for many hormones including corticotropin-releasing hormone (CRH).

depression, anger, fear, loss, and excitement), obesity, advanced age, drugs, disease, surgery, and medical treatment.

Although the field of PNI is relatively new it has elicited strenuous scientific debate, especially with respect to the causal role of personality in cancer mortality and morbidity.[16] For example, mouse models suggest a strong link between stress and breast cancer progression, yet this effect has not been consistently found in humans.[16,17] What is certain, however, is that hormones released by the stress response influence many metabolic systems and corresponding physiologic events, even if the mechanisms and subsequent physiologic events are yet to be fully understood. Further, sufficient data now exist to conclude that immune modulation by psychosocial stressors or interventions is directly related to health outcomes.[1,11,18-31] Along with a greater understanding of the relationship between the human stress response and disease, new strategies for treatment of stress-related disorders are emerging.

STRESS OVERVIEW: MULTIPLE MEDIATORS AND SYSTEMS

Psychologic stress may cause or worsen several diseases or disorders including anxiety, depression, insomnia, chronic pain and fatigue syndromes, obesity, metabolic syndrome, essential hypertension, type 2

TABLE 8-1 EXAMPLES OF STRESS-RELATED DISEASES AND CONDITIONS

TARGET ORGAN OR SYSTEM	DISEASE OR CONDITION	TARGET ORGAN OR SYSTEM	DISEASE OR CONDITION
Cardiovascular system	Coronary artery disease Hypertension Stroke Disturbances of heart rhythm	Gastrointestinal system	Ulcer Irritable bowel syndrome Diarrhea Nausea and vomiting Ulcerative colitis
Muscle	Tension headaches Muscle contraction backache	Genitourinary system	Diuresis Impotence Frigidity
Connective tissues	Rheumatoid arthritis (autoimmune disease) Related inflammatory diseases of connective tissue	Skin	Eczema Neurodermatitis Acne
Pulmonary system	Asthma (hypersensitivity reaction) Hay fever (hypersensitivity reactions)	Endocrine system	Type 2 diabetes mellitus Amenorrhea
Immune system	Immunosuppression or deficiency Autoimmune diseases	Central nervous system	Fatigue and lethargy Type A behavior Overeating Depression Insomnia

diabetes, atherosclerosis and its cardiovascular consequences, osteoporosis, and autoimmune inflammatory and allergic disorders.[11] Some of these disorders are the leading causes of death in the United States (Table 8-1). Effects of stress on inflammatory and immune processes influence coronary artery disease, depression, autoimmune disorders, and, possibly, virally-mediated cancers. These activated inflammatory reactions increase what is called the "sickness syndrome," a collection of nonspecific symptoms caused by excessive levels of inflammatory cytokines during infectious or inflammatory illness. Additionally, stress disrupts the biologic process of sleep and the long-term functions of growth and reproduction.[11]

Chronic inflammation, which can be stimulated by stress, may be important in the functional decline that leads to frailty, disability, and untimely death.[23] As evidence mounts concerning the important role that stress plays in many disease processes, research has focused on the mechanisms responsible for these mind-body interactions.

The term *stress* was used persistently and widely in the past in specialties, such as biology, health sciences, and social sciences, despite a lack of agreement about its definition. Currently, stress is usually defined as a *transactional* or *interactional concept*. Transactionally, stress is viewed as the state of affairs that arises when a person appraises and reacts to a situation. In general, a person experiences stress when a demand exceeds that person's coping abilities, resulting in reactions such as disturbances of cognition, emotion, and behavior (e.g., smoking, drinking, loss of sleep) that can adversely affect well-being.

The physiology involved in meeting the demands and challenges of daily life is an emerging topic of research. Some refer to these challenges as "stressors" and to the chronically stressed person as being "stressed out." The physiology is complex, involving mechanisms of both protection and injury. As previously mentioned, glucocorticoids from the adrenal cortex, in response to ACTH from the pituitary gland (see Figure 8-4), comprise the major stress hormones along with the catecholamines epinephrine and norepinephrine. Other central hormones/mediators also play a role, including the proinflammatory and anti-inflammatory cytokines that are regulated by glucocorticoids and catecholamines (Figure 8-5).[1]

Catecholamines can increase proinflammatory cytokine production, causing, for example, increased heart rate and blood pressure. Glucocorticoids are known to inhibit this proinflammatory production; however, inhibition depends on dose and cell or tissue type.[24] Therefore glucocorticoids can also promote inflammation depending on dose and cell type.[25] The increased understanding of these effects suggests the possibility that chronic and dysfunctional HPA axis stimulation (as may occur during chronic inflammation) increases inflammation in the brain and other tissue, possibly contributing to other diseases including osteoporosis, metabolic disease (e.g., diabetes, obesity), and cardiovascular disease.[26] Additionally, these interactions are nonlinear (see Figure 8-5) and are very complex.

The parasympathetic system also plays a role in opposing the sympathetic (catecholamine) responses and has anti-inflammatory effects.[25] Allostasis is considered an adaptive physiologic response to stressful events (e.g., fight or flight).[32] Chronic or disregulated **allostasis** (long-term or chronic exaggerated responses to stress) can lead to disease (see Figure 8-1). Allostatic load is the individualized cumulative amounts of stressors that exist in our lives and that influence our physiologic responses. Allostatic load includes our genetic makeup, life-style (including damaging health behaviors), daily events, and sometimes, dramatic events such as disasters.[32] Over time this load exacts a toll on our bodies (i.e., "wear and tear"). Because the brain is a key player in deciding what is stressful, the brain is influential in determining when we have reached allostatic overload. Moreover, these responses are individualized—that is, what would be considered normal for one person may be considered extremely stressful for another.[33] In response to acute and chronic stress some regions of the brain (hippocampus, amygdala, and prefrontal cortex) may respond by undergoing structural remodeling that can alter behavioral and physiologic responses, such as cognitive impairment and depression.[32] Key systems involved in **allostatic overload** (exaggerated pathophysiologic responses to stress) include the concentrations of cortisol, catecholamines of the sympathetic nervous system, and proinflammatory cytokines as well as a decline in parasympathetic activity. A prevalent example is sleep deprivation from being "stressed out."[1] Sleep deprivation has

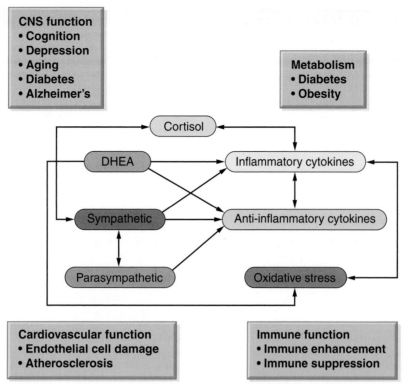

FIGURE 8-5 Stress Interactions Are Nonlinear and Complex. Nonlinearity means that when one mediator is increased or decreased, the subsequent compensatory changes in other mediators depend on time and level of change, causing multiple interacting variables. The inevitable consequences from adapting to daily life over time include changes in behavioral responses. For example, these changes include sleeping patterns, smoking, alcohol consumption, physical activity, and social interactions. These behavioral patterns are a part of the allostatic overload with chronic elevations in cortisol level, sympathetic activity, and levels of proinflammatory cytokines, and a decrease in parasympathetic activity. (From McEwen BS: Central effects of stress hormones in health and disease: understanding the protective and damaging effects of stress and stress mediators, *Eur J Pharmacol* 583[2–3]:174–185, 2008.)

significant damaging effects including elevated evening cortisol concentration; elevated insulin and blood glucose levels; increased blood pressure; reduced parasympathetic activity; increased levels of proinflammatory cytokines; and increased secretion of the hormone ghrelin (primarily by cells of the stomach and pancreas), which increases appetite. Altogether these alterations can lead to increased caloric intake, depressed mood, cognitive problems, and a host of other responses from insomnia.[28]

QUICK CHECK 8-1
1. Define the HPA axis.
2. Discuss the diseases/disorders affected by stress.
3. Briefly describe the three stages of the general adaptation syndrome.
4. Define allostatic load and allostatic overload.

THE STRESS RESPONSE

Neuroendocrine Regulation

The sympathetic nervous system is aroused during the **stress response**, releasing norepinephrine (adrenergic stimulation) and causing the medulla of the adrenal gland to release catecholamines (80% epinephrine and 20% norepinephrine) into the bloodstream. Sympathetic

nerves also contain nonadrenergic mediators that amplify or antagonize the effects of these catecholamines. Simultaneously, hypothalamic CRH stimulates the pituitary gland to release a variety of hormones, including antidiuretic hormone (ADH) from the posterior pituitary gland and prolactin, growth hormone, and adrenocorticotropic hormone (ACTH) from the anterior pituitary gland. ACTH stimulates the cortex of the adrenal gland to release glucocorticoids, mainly cortisol (see Figure 8-3).

Catecholamines

Circulating catecholamines essentially mimic direct sympathetic stimulation. Catecholamines cannot cross the blood-brain barrier and are synthesized locally in the brain. The physiologic effects of the catecholamines on organs and tissues are summarized in Table 8-2. Norepinephrine regulates blood pressure, promotes arousal, and increases vigilance, anxiety, and other protective emotional responses.

Epinephrine in the liver and skeletal muscles is rapidly metabolized. Epinephrine influences cardiac action by enhancing myocardial contractility (inotropic effect), increasing heart rate (chronotropic effect), and increasing venous return to the heart, ultimately increasing both cardiac output and blood pressure. Epinephrine dilates blood vessels supplying skeletal muscles, allowing for greater oxygenation. Metabolically, it causes transient hyperglycemia (high blood sugar), reduces

TABLE 8-2   PHYSIOLOGIC EFFECTS OF CATECHOLAMINES*

ORGAN/TISSUE	PROCESS OR RESULT
Brain	Increased blood flow; increased glucose metabolism
Cardiovascular system	Increased rate and force of contraction
	Peripheral vasoconstriction
Pulmonary system	Bronchodilation
Skeletal muscle	Increased glycogenolysis
	Increased contraction
	Increased dilation of muscle vasculature
	Decreased glucose uptake and utilization (decreases insulin release)
Liver	Increased glucose production
	Increased glycogenolysis
Adipose tissue	Increased lipolysis
	Decreased glucose uptake
Skin	Decreased blood flow
Gastrointestinal and genitourinary tracts	Decreased protein synthesis
	Decreased smooth muscle contraction
	Increased renin release
	Increased gastrointestinal sphincter tone
Lymphoid tissue	Acute and chronic stress inhibits several components of innate immunity, particularly decreasing natural killer cells
Macrophages	Inhibit and stimulate macrophage activity
	Depends on availability of type 1/proinflammatory cytokines, presence or absence of antigenic stressors, and peripheral corticotropin-releasing hormone (CRH)

Data from Elenkov IJ, Chrousos GP: *Ann N Y Acad Sci* 966:290–303, 2002; Granner DK: Hormones of the adrenal medulla. In Murray RK et al, editors: *Harper's biochemistry,* ed 25, New York, 2000, McGraw-Hill.

*Some of these responses require glucocorticoids (e.g., cortisol) for maximal activity (see text for explanation).

glucose uptake in the muscles and other organs, and decreases insulin release from the pancreas, thus preventing glucose uptake by peripheral tissue and preserving it for the CNS. Epinephrine also mobilizes free fatty acids and cholesterol.

The catecholamines stimulate two major classes of receptors: α-adrenergic receptors (α_1 and α_2) and β-adrenergic receptors (β_1 and β_2). Table 12-7 summarizes the actions of the two subclasses of adrenergic receptors. (A discussion of receptors can be found in Chapters 1, 17, and 22.) Epinephrine binds with and activates both α and β receptors whereas norepinephrine binds primarily with α receptors.

Glucocorticoids: Cortisol

During stress ACTH activates the adrenal cortex, increasing secretion of glucocorticoid hormones, primarily cortisol (see Figure 8-3). (Cortisol is known outside the body as *hydrocortisone.*) These steroid molecules reach *all* tissues, including the brain, easily penetrate cell membranes, and react with numerous intracellular glucocorticoid receptors. Because they spare almost no tissue or organ and influence a large proportion of the human genome, they exert significant diverse biologic actions![11] Glucocorticoids regulate many functions of the CNS, including arousal, cognition, mood, sleep, metabolism,

HEALTH ALERT

Psychosocial Stress and Progression to Coronary Heart Disease

The link between stress and coronary heart disease was proposed as early as the 1970s; however, it was only recently that conclusive evidence and proposed mechanisms for development of the disease were identified. Much work continues to focus on elucidating the interaction between stress and cardiovascular disease.

One of the primary risk factors for coronary heart disease is hypertension. A new designation of prehypertension was recently created and found to be a good predictor for future cardiovascular events. Prehypertension is defined as a systolic blood pressure of 120 to 139 mm Hg or a diastolic blood pressure of 80 to 90 mm Hg. Individuals with prehypertension are much more likely to develop frank hypertension and, eventually, coronary heart disease.

Studies show that persons with a highly reactive personality type who experience high levels of anxiety with stress are much more likely to progress from prehypertension to hypertension and then to develop cardiac disease, specifically coronary heart disease, than those who have better coping abilities. Further long-term psychologic stress, such as experienced in a strained marriage or an unhappy work environment, not only was shown to accelerate the progression of hypertension and coronary heart disease but also is correlated with higher mortality rates from coronary heart disease.

Trait anger, defined as a stable personality trait characterized by frequency, intensity, and duration of anger, also was shown to be a factor in the development of coronary heart disease at higher rates than the general population. Individuals with trait anger also experienced more strokes. Hostile individuals with advanced cardiovascular disease may be particularly susceptible to stress-induced increases in sympathetic activity and inflammation.

One popular mechanism for the interaction between psychosocial stress and cardiovascular disease suggests that stress triggers an inflammatory response that, over time, increases the chances of developing coronary heart disease. The primary mechanisms proposed are chronically elevated cortisol levels and dysregulation of the circadian rhythm for cortisol release. Further, chronic stress alters hypothalamic-pituitary-adrenal (HPA) function, resulting in an abnormal stress response pattern. This alteration in HPA activity was found in persons with coronary heart disease along with increased inflammatory markers. The elevation in inflammatory markers seen with chronic stress is important because these markers were shown to interact with lipids, specifically low-density lipoproteins, to increase the production of atherosclerotic plaques.

Because coronary heart disease is one of the major causes of death in industrialized countries, development of successful interventional programs is of high priority. Programs in which dietary changes, exercise, stress management, and positive support systems are implemented continue to show positive results for slowing the progression of heart disease and decreasing the risk factors for disease development. Further, individuals in these programs report decreased levels of depression and stress as well as overall improvement in mental health.

Data from Brydon L et al: *J Psychosom Res* 68(2):109–116, 2010; Davidson KW: *Cleve Clin J Med* 75(suppl 2):S15–S19, 2008; Nijm J et al: *J Int Med* 262(3):375–384, 2007; Player MS et al: *Ann Fam Med* 5(5):403–411, 2007; Shamaei-Tousi A et al: *Cell Stress Chaperones* 12(4):384–392, 2007; Steptoe A, Brydon L: *Neurosci Biobehav Rev* 33:63–70, 2009; Vizza J et al: *J Cardiopulm Rehabil Prev* 27(6):376–383, 2007.

maintenance of cardiovascular tone, the immune and inflammatory reaction, and growth and reproduction. Thus glucocorticoids dramatically affect human pathophysiology and, consequently, longevity.[1,11] The feedback mechanisms of the HPA axis sense and determine the circulating glucocorticoid levels, while other tissues passively accept the actions of circulating glucocorticoids.[11] Thus discrepancy in the glucocorticoid sensing network between the HPA axis and peripheral tissues could possibly produce peripheral tissue *hypercortisolism* or *hypocortisolism*.[11] For example, both high HPA axis reactivity to stress and increased peripheral tissue sensitivity to glucocorticoids have been shown to be associated with severity of coronary artery disease (see *Health Alert:* Psychosocial Stress and Progression to Coronary Heart Disease).[29] Chronic dysregulation of the HPA axis, especially elevated levels of cortisol, has been linked to a wide variety of disorders including obesity, sleep deprivation, lipid abnormalities, hypertension, diabetes, atherosclerosis, loss of bone density, hippocampal atrophy, and cognitive impairment.[33]

Cortisol mobilizes substances needed for cellular metabolism and stimulates gluconeogenesis, or the formation of glucose from noncarbohydrate sources, such as amino acids or free fatty acids in the liver. In addition, cortisol enhances the elevation of blood glucose levels that is promoted by other hormones, such as epinephrine, glucagon, and growth hormone. Cortisol also inhibits the uptake and oxidation of glucose by many body cells. Overall, cortisol's actions on carbohydrate metabolism result in increased blood glucose levels, thereby energizing the body to combat the stressor. The effects of cortisol are summarized in Table 8-3.

Cortisol also affects protein metabolism. It has an anabolic effect; that is, it increases the rate of synthesis of proteins and ribonucleic acid (RNA) in liver. This is countered by its catabolic effect on protein stores in other tissues. Protein catabolism acts to increase levels of circulating amino acids; therefore chronic exposure to excess cortisol can severely deplete protein stores in muscle, bone, connective tissue, and skin. Finally, cortisol promotes gastric secretion in the stomach and intestines, potentially causing gastric ulcers. This could account for the gastrointestinal ulceration observed by Selye. This is in opposition to norepinephrine, which reduces gastric secretion.

Overall, glucocorticoids have an important role in the homeostasis of the CNS.[1,11] These hormones regulate memory, cognition, mood, and sleep. They also influence brain anatomy by reducing hippocampal volume, enlarging ventricles, and causing reversible cortical atrophy.[1,11]

Glucocorticoids contribute to the development of metabolic syndrome and the pathogenesis of obesity (see *Health Alert:* Glucocorticoids, Insulin, Inflammation, and Obesity). They can directly cause insulin resistance and influence genetic variations that predispose to obesity. Glucocorticoids also may affect fetal programming of the HPA axis by causing an adverse intrauterine environment because of alterations in cortisol secretion during pregnancy.[30]

TABLE 8-3 PHYSIOLOGIC EFFECTS OF CORTISOL

FUNCTIONS AFFECTED	PHYSIOLOGIC EFFECTS
Carbohydrate and lipid metabolism	Diminishes peripheral uptake and utilization of glucose; promotes gluconeogenesis in liver metabolism cells; enhances gluconeogenic response to other hormones; promotes lipolysis in adipose tissue
Protein metabolism	Increases protein synthesis in liver and decreases protein synthesis (including immunoglobulin synthesis) in muscle, lymphoid tissue, adipose tissue, skin, and bone; increases plasma level of amino acids; stimulates deamination in liver
Anti-inflammatory effects (systemic effects)	High levels of cortisol used in drug therapy suppress inflammatory response; inhibit proinflammatory activity of many growth factors and cytokines; however, over time some individuals may develop tolerance to glucocorticoids, causing an increased susceptibility to both inflammatory and autoimmune disease
Proinflammatory effects (possible local effects)	Cortisol levels released during stress response may increase proinflammatory effects
Lipid metabolism	Lipolysis in extremities and lipogenesis in face and trunk
Immune effects	*Treatment* levels of glucocorticoids are immunosuppressive; thus they are valuable agents used in numerous diseases/conditions; T cell or innate immune system is particularly affected by these larger doses of glucocorticoids with suppression of Th1 function or innate immunity; *stress* can cause a different pattern of immune response; these nontherapeutic levels can suppress innate (Th1) and increase adaptive (Th2) immunity—the so-called Th2 shift; several factors influence this complex physiology and include long-term adaptations, reproductive hormones (i.e., overall, androgens suppress and estrogens stimulate immune responses), defects of hypothalamic-pituitary-adrenal axis, histamine-generated responses, and acute versus chronic stress; thus stress seems to cause a Th2 shift *systemically* whereas *locally*, under certain conditions, it can induce proinflammatory activities and by these mechanisms may influence onset or course of infections, autoimmune/inflammatory, allergic, and neoplastic disease
Digestive function	Promotes gastric secretion
Urinary function	Enhances excretion of calcium
Connective tissue function	Decreases proliferation of fibroblasts in connective tissue (thus delaying healing)
Muscle function	Maintains normal contractility and maximal work output for skeletal and cardiac muscle
Bone function	Decreases bone formation
Vascular system/myocardial function	Maintains normal blood pressure; permits increased responsiveness of arterioles to constrictive action of adrenergic stimulation; optimizes myocardial performance
Central nervous system function	Somehow modulates perceptual and emotional functioning, essential for normal arousal and initiation of daytime activity
Possible synergism with estrogen in pregnancy?	Suppresses maternal immune system to prevent rejection of fetus?

HEALTH ALERT

Glucocorticoids, Insulin, Inflammation, and Obesity

The signs and symptoms of Cushing syndrome (e.g., excess glucocorticoids [GCs]) include truncal obesity, relatively thin extremities, a "moon face," and a "buffalo [neck] hump." In such individuals the possibility of associated hypertension is high as well as increased risk of infection and metabolic syndrome or frank type 2 diabetes. In addition, the likelihood of an elevated ratio of intraabdominal subcutaneous fat mass to nonabdominal fat mass is high because the glucocorticoids mediate the redistribution of stored calories into the abdominal region. The specific increase in abdominal fat stores is a consequence of elevated levels of glucocorticoids combined with increased insulin action. However, the increased levels of glucocorticoids need not be present in the circulation; instead, they can be generated locally in fat by conversion of inactive cortisone to active cortisol through the action of the isoenzyme 11β-hydroxysteroid dehydrogenase (11β-HSD) type 1. This conversion is referred to as "pre-receptor" metabolism of cortisol. The active steroid is secreted directly to the liver through the portal vein. In vitro insulin synthesis and secretion from the pancreas are inhibited by the glucocorticoids. However, increasing levels of glucocorticoids in vivo are associated with increasing insulin secretion, possibly because of an anti-insulin effect on the liver, which appears to be vulnerable to the negative effects of glucocorticoids on insulin action. Hepatic insulin resistance is strongly associated with abdominal obesity.

Recent data reveal that the plasma concentration of inflammatory mediators, such as tumor necrosis factor-alpha (TNF-α) and interleukin-6 (IL-6), is increased in the insulin-resistant states of obesity and type 2 diabetes. Two mechanisms might be involved in the pathogenesis of inflammation: (1) glucose and macronutrient intake (i.e., which can be mediated through chronic stress) causes oxidative stress; and (2) the increased concentrations of TNF-α and IL-6 associated with obesity and type 2 diabetes might interfere with insulin signal transduction. This interference might promote inflammation. Chronic overnutrition (obesity) might thus be a proinflammatory state with oxidative stress.

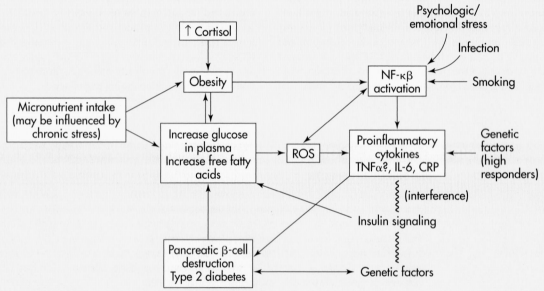

Stress, Inflammation, Obesity, and Type 2 Diabetes. The induction of reactive oxygen species (ROS) generation and inflammation through the proinflammatory transcription factor, NF-κβ, activates most proinflammatory genes. Macronutrient intake, obesity, free fatty acids, infection, smoking, psychologic stress, and genetic factors increase the production of ROS. Interference with insulin signaling (insulin resistance) leads to hyperglycemia and proinflammatory changes. Proinflammatory changes increase levels of TNF-α and IL-6, and also lead to the inhibition of insulin signaling and insulin resistance. Inflammation in pancreatic β cells leads to β cell dysfunction, which in combination with insulin resistance leads to type 2 diabetes. *CRP,* C-reactive protein.

Data from Dallman MF et al: *Endocrinology* 145(6):2633–2638, 2004; Dandona P, Aljada A, Brandyopadhyay A: *Trends Immunol* 25(1):4–7, 2004; Kim SP et al: *Diabetes* 52:2453–2460, 2003; Masuzaki H et al: *Science* 94:2166–2170, 2001; Padgett DA, Glaser R: *Trends Immunol* 24(8):444–448, 2003; Strack AM et al: *Am J Physiol* 268:R142–R149, 1995; Thakore JH et al: *Biol Psychiatry* 47:1140–1142, 1998; Wagen Knecht LE et al: *Diabetes* 52:2490–2496, 2003; Spencer SJ, Tilbrook A: *Stress* 14(3), 2011.

Cortisol secretion during stress exerts beneficial effects by inhibiting initial inflammatory effects, for example, vasodilation and increased capillary permeability.[26] Cortisol also promotes resolution and repair. These actions are mainly accomplished by facilitating the effects of glucocorticoid receptor (GR), namely, the transcription of genetic material (through DNA binding) within leukocytes.[26] Because GR is so widely expressed, glucocorticoids influence virtually all immune cells. The adaptiveness or destructiveness of cortisol-induced effects may depend on the intensity, type, and duration of the stressor; the tissue involved; and the subsequent concentration and length of cortisol exposure. Finally, glucocorticoids have been shown to induce T cell apoptosis.[26]

Stress hormones, especially glucocorticoids (cortisol), have been used therapeutically as powerful anti-inflammatory/immunosuppressive agents for years. The synthetic forms of glucocorticoid hormones (exogenous types of anti-inflammatory glucocorticoids administered for a pharmaceutical reaction) are poorly metabolized when compared to endogenous glucocorticoids, leading to a longer half-life and no circadian rhythm for these compounds. Moreover, these synthetic compounds bind with different targets so each has a unique effect.[25]

Paradoxically, elevated levels of glucocorticoids and catecholamines (epinephrine and norepinephrine), both endogenous and exogenously administered, may decrease innate immunity and increase autoimmune (adaptive) responses. These effects can accentuate inflammation in general and potentially increase neuronal death (e.g., in stroke victims).[25] This may help explain the seemingly contradictory stress response of immunosuppression and increased risk of infection (decreased innate immunity) with a heightened antibody response and autoimmune disease (increased adaptive immunity).

Initially, immune responses are regulated by cells of *innate immunity* called antigen-presenting cells (APCs), such as monocytes/macrophages (see Chapter 6), dendritic cells, and other phagocytic cells, and by Th1 and Th2 lymphocytes (cells involved in *adaptive immunity*). These cells secrete chemical messengers, called *cytokines,* that regulate innate and adaptive immune responses. Antigen-presenting cells also release cytokines that induce T cells to differentiate into Th1 cells. Th1 cells and APC cytokines work together to stimulate the activity of cytotoxic T cells, natural killer (NK) cells, and activated macrophages—the major components of innate immunity.

Cytokines secreted by Th2 cells also act to inhibit Th1 cells and can promote adaptive immunity by stimulating growth and activation of mast cells and eosinophils, as well as the differentiation of B cell immunoglobulins. Thus these cytokines are considered to be the major *anti-inflammatory cytokines* (Figure 8-6).[31] The decrease in Th1 activity and increase in Th2 activity is sometimes called a **Th1 to Th2 shift.**

Corticotropin-releasing hormone (CRH) influences the immune system indirectly by the activation of cortisol (glucocorticoids) and catecholamines (see Figure 8-4). CRH is secreted by the hypothalamus and also peripherally at inflammatory sites (called peripheral or immune CRH).[34,35] **Peripheral (immune) CRH** is proinflammatory, causing an increase in vasodilation and vascular permeability. Therefore it appears that mast cells are the target of peripheral CRH. Mast cells release histamine, which is a well-known mediator of acute inflammation and allergic reactions (see Figure 8-6). Histamine induces acute inflammation and allergic reactions while suppressing

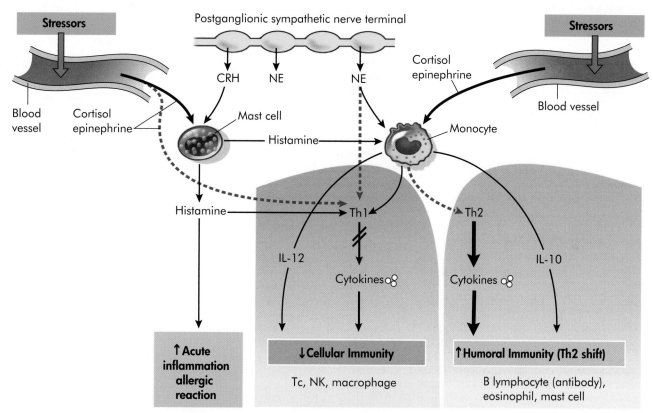

FIGURE 8-6 Effect of Corticotropin-Releasing Hormone (CRH)–Mast Cell–Histamine Axis, Cortisol, and Catecholamines on the Th1/Th2 Balance—Innate and Adaptive Immunity. Adaptive immunity provides protection against multicellular parasites, extracellular bacteria, some viruses, soluble toxins, and allergens. Innate immunity provides protection against intracellular bacteria, fungi, protozoa, and several viruses. Type 1 cytokines or proinflammatory cytokines include IL-12, interferon-gamma (IFN-γ), and tumor necrosis factor-alpha (TNF-α). Type 2 cytokines or anti-inflammatory cytokines include IL-10 and IL-4. Solid lines *(black)* represent stimulation, whereas dashed lines *(blue)* represent inhibition (i.e., Th1 and Th2 are mutually inhibitory, IL-12 and IFN-γ inhibit Th2, and vice versa; IL-4 and IL-10 inhibit Th1 responses). Stress and CRH modulate inflammatory/immune and allergic responses by stimulating cortisol (glucocorticoid), catecholamines, and peripheral (immune) CRH secretion and by changing the production of regulatory cytokines and histamines. *CRH* (peripheral, immune), corticotropin-releasing hormone; *NE,* norepinephrine; *Th,* helper T cell; *IL,* interleukin; *Tc,* cytotoxic T cell; *NK,* natural killer cell; *dashed lines,* decreased (inhibited); *solid lines,* increased (stimulation). (Redrawn from Elenkov IJ, Chrousos GP: Stress hormones, Th1/Th2 patterns, pro/anti-inflammatory cytokines and susceptibility to disease, *Trends Endocrinol Metab* 10[9]:359–368, 1999.)

Th1 activity (decreasing innate immunity) and promoting Th2 activity (increasing adaptive immunity).[36-39]

Locally, stress can exert proinflammatory or anti-inflammatory effects. Moreover, some evidence indicates that stress is not a uniform, nonspecific reaction.[40] Different types of stressors might have variable effects on the immune response. Thus stress may *systemically* cause a decrease in innate immunity and enhance adaptive immunity, whereas *locally,* under certain conditions, it can induce proinflammatory activities that may influence the onset and cause of infection, autoimmune/inflammatory, and allergic responses. In summary, stress can activate an excessive immune response and, through cortisol and the catecholamines, suppress Th1 responses while enhancing Th2 responses.

Parasympathetic System

The parasympathetic system balances the sympathetic nervous system and thus also influences adaptation or maladaptation to stressful events. The parasympathetic system generally opposes the sympathetic system; for example, the parasympathetic nervous system slows the heart rate. The parasympathetic system also has anti-inflammatory effects. Under conditions of allostatic overload, the parasympathetic system may decrease its containment of the sympathetic system, resulting in increased or prolonged inflammatory responses.[32] Researchers evaluate the relative balance of the parasympathetic and sympathetic nervous systems using a technique known as *heart rate variability* (the measurement of R wave variability from heartbeat to heartbeat).

Other Hormones

The immune system is integrated with other physiologic processes and is sensitive to changes in CNS and endocrine functioning, such as those that accompany psychologic states.[41,42] Stressors can elicit the stress response through the action of the nervous and endocrine systems, specifically corticotropin-releasing hormone (CRH) from the hypothalamus, the sympathetic nervous system, the pituitary gland, and the adrenal gland (see Figure 8-3). CRH is also released peripherally at inflammatory sites and called peripheral or immune CRH. The processes of growth and reproduction as well as the synthesis of thyroid hormone are suppressed during stress and may conserve energy during stress. Neuropeptide Y (NPY), a sympathetic neurotransmitter, has recently been shown to be a stress mediator. Because NPY is a growth factor for many cells, it is implicated in atherosclerosis and tissue remodeling. Other hormones that influence the stress response are listed in Table 8-4.

TABLE 8-4   OTHER HORMONES THAT INFLUENCE THE STRESS RESPONSE

HORMONE	SOURCE	ACTION
β-Endorphins (endogenous opiates)	Pituitary and hypothalamus	Activates endorphin (opiate) receptors on peripheral sensory nerves, leading to pain relief or analgesia Hemorrhage increases levels to inhibit blood pressure or delay compensatory changes that would increase blood pressure[1]
Growth hormone (GH, somatotropin)	Anterior pituitary gland	Affects protein, lipid, and carbohydrate metabolism Counters effects of insulin Involved in tissue repair May participate in growth and function of immune system[2] Levels increase after variety of stressful stimuli (cardiac catheterization, electroshock therapy, gastroscopy, surgery, fever, physical exercise) Increased levels associated with psychologic stimuli (taking examinations, viewing violent or sexually arousing films, certain psychologic performance tests) Prolonged stress (chronic stress) suppresses growth hormone
Prolactin	Anterior pituitary gland; numerous extrapituitary tissue sites[12]	Increases in response to many stressful stimuli (including procedures such as gastroscopy, proctoscopy, pelvic examination, and surgery)[3] Requires more intense stimuli than those leading to increases in catecholamine or cortisol levels Levels show little change after exercise
Oxytocin	Hypothalamus	Promotes bonding and social attachment In animals associated with reduced hypothalamic-pituitary-adrenal (HPA) activation levels and reduced anxiety[4]
Testosterone	Leydig cells in testes	Regulates male secondary sex characteristics and libido Levels decrease after stressful stimuli (anesthesia, surgery, marathon running, mountain climbing)[5] Decreased by psychologic stimuli; however, some data indicate that psychologic stress associated with competition (e.g., pistol shooting) increases both testosterone and cortisol levels, especially in athletes older than 45 years[6] Markedly reduced in individuals with respiratory failure, burns, and congestive heart failure[7] Decreased levels occur during aging and are associated with lower cortisol responsiveness to stress-induced inflammation[8]
Estrogen	Ovaries	Works in concert with oxytocin, exerting calming effect during stressful situations[9]
Melatonin	Produced by pineal gland	Increases during stress response; release is suppressed by light and increased in dark; receptors have been identified on lymphoid cells, possibly higher density of receptors on T cells than B cells; suppression of lymphocyte function by trauma was reversed by melatonin[10]

TABLE 8-4 OTHER HORMONES THAT INFLUENCE THE STRESS RESPONSE—cont'd

HORMONE	SOURCE	ACTION
Somatostatin (SOM)	Produced by sensory nerve terminals found in and released from lymphoid cells and hypothalamus	Natural killer (NK) function and immunoglobulin synthesis decreased by SOM; growth hormone secretion decreased by SOM
Vasoactive intestinal peptide (VIP)	Found in neurons of CNS and in peripheral nerves	VIP increases during stress; VIP-containing nerves are located in both primary and secondary lymphoid tissues, around blood vessels, and in gastrointestinal tract; VIP receptors are on both T and B cells; VIP may influence lymphocyte maturation; cytokine production by T cells is modified by VIP; B cell and antibody production is influenced by VIP
Calcitonin gene–related peptide (CGRP)	Found in spinal cord motor neurons and in sensory neurons near dendritic cells of skin and in primary and secondary lymphoid tissues	CGRP receptors are present on T and B lymphocytes; thus it is likely that CGRP can modulate immune function; CGRP may enhance acute inflammatory response because it is vasodilator; maturation of immune B lymphocytes is inhibited by CGRP; IL-1 is inhibited by CGRP, which is important for activation of T cells; it has been shown to interfere with lymphocyte activation
Neuropeptide Y (NPY)	Present in neurons of CNS and in neurons throughout body; colocalized in nerve terminals in lymphatic tissues with norepinephrine	Lymphocytes have receptors for NPY and thus may modulate their function;[11] several lines of evidence suggest that NPY is neurotransmitter and neurohormone involved in stress response; increased levels of NPY occur in plasma in response to severe or prolonged stress; may be responsible for stress-induced regional vasoconstriction (splanchnic, coronary, and cerebral); may also increase platelet aggregation[2]
Substance P (SP)	Produced by neuropeptide classified as tachykinin (increases heart rate subsequent to lowering blood pressure) found in brain, as well as nerves innervating secondary lymphoid tissues	SP increases in response to stress; receptors for SP are found on membrane of both T and B cells, mononuclear phagocytic cells, and mast cells; proinflammatory activity induces release of histamine from mast cells during stress response; causes smooth muscle contraction, causes macrophages and T cells to release cytokines, and increases antibody production

1. Amico JA et al: Anxiety and stress responses in female oxytocin deficient mice (review), *J Neuroendocrinol* 16(4):319–324, 2004.
2. Rabin BS: The nervous system—immune system connection. In *Stress, immune function, and health: the connection*, New York, 1999, Wiley-Liss.
3. Rohleder N et al: Age and sex steroid-related changes in glucocorticoid sensitivity of proinflammatory cytokine production after psychosocial stress, *J Neuroimmunol* 126(1–2):69–77, 2002.
4. Marucha PT, Kiecolt-Glaser JK, Favaghi M: Mucosal wound healing is impaired by examination stress, *Psychosom Med* 60(3):362–365, 1998.
5. Chesnokova V, Melmed S: Mini review: neuro-immmuno-endocrine modulation of the hypothalamic-pituitary-adrenal axis (HPA) by gp130 signaling molecules (review), *Endocrinology* 143(5):1571–1574, 2002.
6. Guezennec CY et al: Effect of competition stress on tests used to assess testosterone administration in athletes, *Int J Sports Med* 16(6):368–372, 1995.
7. Bauer-Wu SM: Psychoneuroimmunology. Part I: Physiology, *Clin J Oncol Nurs* 6(3):167–170, 2002.
8. Bauer-Wu SM: Psychoneuroimmunology. Part II: Mind-body interventions, *Clin J Oncol Nurs* 6(4):243–246, 2002.
9. Repka-Ramirez MS, Baraniuk JN: Histamine in health and disease, *Clin Allergy Immunol* 17:1–17, 2002.
10. Maestroni GJ: MLT and the immune-hematopoietic system, *Adv Exp Med Biol* 460:396, 1999.
11. Petito JM, Huang Z, McCarthy DB: Molecular cloning of NPY-Y1 receptor cDNA from rat splenic lymphocytes: evidence of low levels of mRNA expression and [125I]NPY binding sites, *J Neuroimmunol* 54:81, 1994.
12. Cacioppo JT et al: Autonomic, neuroendocrine, and immune responses to psychological stress: the reactivity hypothesis, *Ann N Y Acad Sci* 840:664–673, 1998.

Role of the Immune System

Several conditions with variable pathophysiologic characteristics appear to have a common origin[15,43] relating to chronic inflammatory processes. These conditions include cardiovascular disease, osteoporosis, arthritis, type 2 diabetes mellitus, chronic obstructive pulmonary disease (COPD), other diseases associated with aging, and some cancers; all are characterized by the prolonged presence of proinflammatory cytokines.[15,43] (Inflammation is discussed in Chapter 5.)

It is important to remember that inflammation is associated with impairment of normal tissue function. Although inflammation is a normal response and considered beneficial, an excessive inflammatory response can damage tissue. Stress and negative emotions are associated directly with the production of increased levels of proinflammatory cytokines, providing a possible link between stress, immune function, and disease.[44-46] More recent research is focused on the regulatory interactions between the immune system (including cell-derived cytokines) and the nervous and endocrine systems.

The immune, nervous, and endocrine systems communicate through similar pathways using hormones, neurotransmitters, neuropeptides, and immune cell products.[26] The complexity of this system can be daunting. Various components of immune system responses can be affected by neuroendocrine-produced factors involved in the stress reaction. Conversely, immune cell–derived cytokines and other products affect neurocrine and endocrine cells.[41,47,48] Several pathways regulate communication among these systems (Figure 8-7).

The stress response directly influences the immune system through hypothalamic and pituitary peptides and through products of the sympathetic branch of the ANS. Immune cells have surface receptors for ACTH, CRH, endorphins, norepinephrine, growth hormone, steroids, and other products of the stress response.[42] There is direct innervation

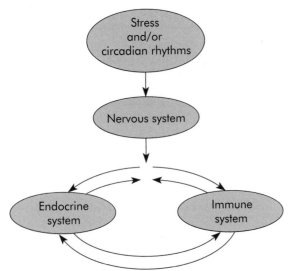

FIGURE 8-7 Nervous System/Endocrine System/Immune System Interactions. Interconnections or pathways of communication among the immune, nervous, and endocrine systems.

of the thymus, spleen, lymph nodes, and bone marrow.[47] Cholinergic, adrenergic, and peptidergic nerve terminals are present in the lymphoid organs and tissues. Endogenous opiates are released during stress and have concentration-dependent, enhancing, and suppressive effects on various immune cells (see Table 8-4).[47,49-52]

The pineal gland regulates immune response and mediates the apparent effects of circadian rhythm on immunity. When melatonin production is blocked (by continuous light or by pharmacologic means), the immune response is suppressed, whereas administration of melatonin reverses these effects.[53] This immunomodulation pathway may effect immune changes found with sleep disturbance and dysregulated circadian rhythm,[54] which are common among acutely ill and stressed persons.

The hypothalamic-pituitary-adrenal (HPA) axis may produce indirect effects on the CNS that modulate immune responses. The result is profound with prolonged severe stress,[41] including enlargement of the adrenal gland with simultaneous involution of the thymus and lymph nodes. Increased levels of circulating glucocorticosteroids (GCSs) may be an important mechanism in stress-related immune structure alterations and in suppression of the immune response.[41] The GCS level increases are attributable to pituitary ACTH production—a result of increased hypothalamic CRH. A number of stress factors initiate CRH production, including high levels of interleukin-1 (IL-1) and interleukin-6 (IL-6). Production of IL-1 by activated macrophages and monocytes is inhibited by GCSs, suggesting a feedback loop with IL-1, CRH, ACTH, and GCS secretion.[47,55]

Lymphocytes also produce ACTH and endorphins in small amounts, which probably influences immune response in an autocrine (same cell stimulation) or paracrine (cell to cell) manner in ongoing immune responses.[47,56] The T cell growth factor IL-2 can up-regulate pituitary ACTH. Immune-derived cytokines have significant influence on neuroendocrine function, with evidence for direct and indirect cytokine effects on nervous and adrenal cell functions. Thus the immune system has an adaptive role as a *signal* organ to alert other systems of internally threatening stimuli (e.g., infection, tissue damage, tumor cells). The release of immune inflammatory mediators (IL-6, tumor necrosis factor-beta [TNF-β], interferon) is triggered by bacterial or viral infections, cancer, tissue injury, and other stressors that in turn initiate a stress response through the HPA pathway. Enhanced

systemic production of these cytokines also induces other CNS and behavior changes during an acute infectious episode.[57-60]

Neuropeptides and hormones have a significant effect on the immune response. Whether this impact on immune function is suppressive or potentiating depends on the type of factor secreted (some factors enhance, some suppress, and some both enhance and suppress), the concentration and length of exposure, the target cell, and the specific immune function studies.[57] Neuropeptides and neuroendocrine hormones may directly control biochemical events affecting cell proliferation, differentiation, and function or may indirectly control immune cell behavior by affecting the production or activity of cytokines.[47,48]

In summary, stress-induced immune changes affect many immune cell functions, including decreased natural killer cell and T cell cytotoxicity and impaired B cell function.[61] These impairments in immune function may have health consequences for stressed individuals, including increased risk of infection and some types of cancer.[62,63]

STRESS, PERSONALITY, COPING, AND ILLNESS

Extreme physiologic stressors, such as severe burn injury, represent a predictable stimulus for stress responses. A less severe and defined event or situation, however, can be a stressor for one person and not for another. Many stressors, such as fasting or temperature changes, do not necessarily cause a physiologic stress response if psychologic factors are minimized. Stress itself is not an independent entity but a system of interdependent processes moderated by the nature, intensity, and duration of the stressor and the perception, appraisal, and coping efficacy of the affected individual, all of which in turn mediate the psychologic and physiologic response to stress. Further, adjustment to repetitive stressors is known to be individualized, based on a person's appraisal of a situation.[64] Illustrating the influence of an individualized stress appraisal on physiologic processes, a meta-analysis of the relationships between stressors and immunity found that a higher perception of stress was associated with reduced Tc cell cytotoxicity, although not with levels of circulating T-helper or Tc lymphocytes.[65]

Psychosocial distress may be predictive of psychologic, social, and physical health outcomes (see *Health Alert:* Acute Emotional Stress and Adverse Heart Effects). In psychologic distress, the individual feels a general state of unpleasant arousal after life events that manifests as physiologic, emotional, cognitive, and behavior changes.[66] Periods of depression and emotional upheaval often are associated with adverse life events and place the affected individual at risk for immunologic deficits, increasing the risk of ill health.[41] Adverse life events having the most negative effect on immunity are characterized as uncontrollable, undesirable, and overtaxing the individual's ability to cope.[67,68] A meta-analysis of studies shows a relationship between depression and reduction in lymphocyte proliferation and NK cell activity.[69] Multiple moderating factors may be important in immune modulation in depressed individuals, including comorbidities such as alcoholism. Examples of triggering circumstances include bereavement, academic pressures, and marital conflict. Aging also may increase psychosocial distress and is associated with immune changes (see *Health Alert:* Partner's Survival and Spouse's Hospitalizations and/or Death).[70,71]

Personality characteristics also are associated with individual differences in appraisal and response to stressors.[42] Specific personality characteristics, such as academic achievement, motivation, and aggression, are correlated with immunologic alterations. For example, aggression is positively associated with changes in T and B cell numbers in male military personnel.[72]

Stressful life events and mood have been reported as important factors preceding the onset or exacerbation of symptoms in acquired

Acute Emotional Stress and Adverse Heart Effects

Myocardial Ischemia
- Individuals with coronary heart disease may develop myocardial ischemia during mental or acute emotional stress even though their exercise or chemical nuclear test results are negative.
- Systemic vascular resistance increases during periods of mental or acute emotional stress with concomitant increased myocardial oxygen demand.

Left Ventricular Dysfunction
- More evidence for left ventricular dysfunction exists in older women.
- After acute emotional stress or trauma, there is an increase in sudden chest pain and shortness of breath.
- Left ventricular dysfunction is more common in the cardiac apex.
- Alterations are possibly a result of increased levels of catecholamines.

Ventricular Dysrhythmias
- Intense or unusual acute stress precipitates about 20% of serious ventricular dysrhythmias or sudden cardiac death.
- Altered brain activity may lead to changes in ventricular repolarization and electrical instability of the cardiac muscle.

Data from Critchley HD et al: *Brain* 128(pt 1):75–85, 2005; Ramachandruni S et al: *J Am Coll Cardiol* 47(5):987–991, 2006; Soufer R: *Circulation* 110(13):1710–1713, 2004; Wittstein IS et al: *N Engl J Med* 352(6):539–548, 2005; Ziegelstein RC: *JAMA* 298(3):324–329, 2007.

Partner's Survival and Spouse's Hospitalizations and/or Death

A Harvard study shows that a spouse's chances of dying increase not only when the partner dies but also when that partner becomes seriously ill. The 9-year follow-up study consisted of 518,240 elderly couples. Mortality after the partner's hospitalization varied according to the spouse's diagnosis. For elderly people whose spouse had been hospitalized, the short-term risk of dying approaches that of an elderly person after his or her spouse's death. A wife's hospitalization increased her husband's chances of dying within 1 month by 35%; a husband's hospitalization increased his wife's chances of dying by 44%. Likewise, a wife's death increased her partner's 1-month mortality risk by 53%, and a husband's death raised his partner's risk by 61%. The researchers commented that a spouse's illness or death can increase a partner's mortality by causing severe stress and removing a primary source of emotional, psychologic, practical, and financial support.

Data from Christakis NA, Allison PD: Mortality after the hospitalization of a spouse, *N Engl J Med* 354(7):719–730, 2006.

immunodeficiency syndrome (AIDS) infection, diabetes, and multiple sclerosis.[73-75] In addition, the interaction with healthcare providers in a clinical setting, the diagnosis of a major illness, and the process of undergoing various clinical procedures (e.g., blood sampling, injections, examinations, surgical procedures) may represent significant negative life events to many individuals (Figure 8-8). These additional stresses may interfere with the efficacy of the medical intervention. Identifying and reducing stress in the clinical setting have particular applicability for both preventing disease and managing illness.

In the past decade, evidence has accumulated linking severe psychosocial stress resulting from negative life events to a chronic syndrome with mental and physical consequences. Post-traumatic stress disorder (PTSD) has been described in many populations.[76-78] The influence of repetitive but episodic stress on cancer survivors demonstrates a connection between events such as mammography and activation of the HPA axis. Early research with breast cancer survivors by Cordova and colleagues[79] demonstrated a link between sympathetic activity and HPA axis activation, noting that some women reported symptoms of post-traumatic stress disorder (heart palpitations, panic, shakiness, nausea) when they thought about cancer recurrence or when they found themselves near the hospital where they received initial treatment.[79] Further, Ma and colleagues[80] reported that the threat of cancer recurrence (using a simulated mammography event as a stressor to elicit thoughts of cancer recurrence) elicited greater alterations in heart rate variability when compared to another simulated controlled stressor. These studies suggest activation of the autonomic nervous system to events, such as mammography, that occur repeatedly throughout breast cancer survivorship, although the timing of onset of these autonomic activation responses to a stressor is unclear.

These additional stresses may affect the course of illness as well as interfere with the efficacy of the medical intervention. Identifying and reducing stress in the clinical setting have particular applicability in both disease prevention and illness management. In addition to medical procedures, patient-provider communication also provides an important area for future research. Recent studies of cancer communication and patient-provider interaction have demonstrated a link between communication events and emotional outcomes, such as uncertainty and mood state in breast cancer survivors.[81,82] Although a logical extension, it remains to be seen if these emotional outcomes impact physiology-based health outcomes caused by activation of the HPA axis and subsequent immune processes.

Coping

Coping is the process of managing stressful challenges that tax the individual's resources.[83] A beneficial influence during stress has been shown with adaptive coping strategies, especially if they are problem focused and involve social support.[83,84] Adverse consequences of stress may be minimized by coping styles. Coping styles that have been associated with altered immunity include repression, denial, escape-avoidance, and concealment.[42] Repression was associated with lower monocyte counts, higher eosinophil counts, higher serum glucose levels, and more self-reported medication reactions in medical outpatients[85] and with higher Epstein-Barr virus (EBV) antibody titers in students.[86] Further, a prospective long-term study found increased markers of accelerated human immunodeficiency virus (HIV) infection in gay men who concealed their homosexual identity.[56]

Coping responses may be adaptive or maladaptive. Maladaptive coping can result in a change in behavior contributing to potentially adverse health effects (e.g., increased smoking, change in eating habits). Serious disturbances of the sleep-wake cycle are observed in many people under stress and in many clinical settings. Recent work has shown that sleep disturbance may exacerbate the pathophysiologic status of some individuals.[87-89] Investigators have reported that sleep deprivation and circadian disruption, even in young otherwise healthy individuals, have detrimental influences on respiratory and immune system function. Even partial sleep deprivation was associated with reduced NK cell activity in healthy subjects, and only recently have seriously ill individuals been assessed for adequacy and structure of sleep during recovery.[87]

Adaptive coping strategies, especially those that are problem focused and those that encourage seeking social support, are considered beneficial during stressful experiences. The extent to which an individual responds to distress, using effective positive coping strategies, determines the degree of successful moderation of the stress challenge.

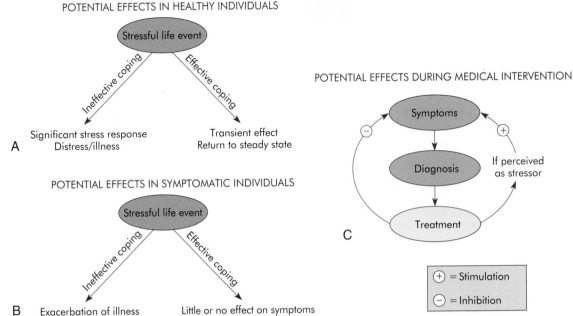

FIGURE 8-8 Health Outcome Determination in Stressful Life Situations Is Moderated by Numerous Factors. Whether a life-challenged individual experiences distress or illness depends on the subject's appraisal of the event and the coping strategies used during the stressful period. Models **(A)** and **(B)** reflect possible outcomes in stressed healthy and symptomatic individuals. Model **(C)** illustrates the dynamic clinical setting in which the diagnosis of a serious illness and subsequent medical interventions may be perceived as stressful challenges and have potentially detrimental influences on physical outcome.

Mediating factors that may influence stress susceptibility or resilience include age, socioeconomic status, gender, social support, religious or spiritual factors, personality, self-esteem, genetics, past experiences, and current health status. Evidence suggests that effective intervention may result in greater stress resilience and improved psychologic and physiologic outcomes.[90] For example, women with recurrent metastatic breast cancer who were provided weekly group counseling in addition to routine medical treatment lived an average of 19 months longer than control subjects, suggesting a mediating influence of additional support for these women.[57,84]

The importance of social support for seriously ill individuals has focused attention also on the health of caregivers. Significant stress manifested as depression, anxiety, and fatigue has been noted in family caregivers of those with cancer, Alzheimer disease, and burn trauma.[91] Enhanced social support has been shown to improve measures of immune function.[84,92-95]

Interventions to potentially prevent or manage stress-related psychologic or physical problems include both short- and long-term coping strategies. Educational components are specific to the individual's problems. Relaxation techniques may include meditation, mindfulness, imagery, massage, and biofeedback. These approaches may be used on an individual or group basis. Incorporation of these approaches into clinical training facilitates their use in the clinical arena. Future research should focus on the efficacy of such approaches with various populations.

In summary, it is clear that the mind and body are connected through a multitude of complex physical and emotional interactions. Understanding the complexity of these interactions is a challenge for many researchers. Areas of promise include investigating relationships between the potential for illness with respect to stressors, as well as developing effective stress management techniques and approaches.

GERIATRIC CONSIDERATIONS
Aging & The Stress-Age Syndrome

With aging, sometimes a set of neurohormonal and immune alterations, as well as tissue and cellular changes, develops. These changes have been defined as stress-age syndrome and include the following:

- Alterations in the excitability of structures of the limbic system and hypothalamus
- Increase of the blood concentrations of catecholamines, ADH, ACTH, and cortisol
- Decrease of the concentrations of testosterone, thyroxine, and others
- Alterations of opioid peptides
- Immunodepression and pattern of chronic inflammation
- Alterations in lipoproteins
- Hypercoagulation of the blood
- Free radical damage of cells

Some of the alterations are adaptational, whereas others are potentially damaging. These stress-related alterations of aging can influence the course of developing stress reactions and lower adaptive reserve and coping capacity.

Data from Frolkis VV: Stress-age syndrome, *Mech Ageing Dev* 69(1–2):93–107, 1993.
ACTH, Adrenocorticotropic hormone; *ADH*, antidiuretic hormone.

✔ QUICK CHECK 8-2
1. Define psychoneuroimmunology.
2. How does the immune system participate in stress-related diseases?
3. Why are stress-related diseases a problem?
4. Why do stress-related diseases occur?
5. What intervention or prevention activities reduce stress-related diseases?

DID YOU UNDERSTAND?

Concepts of Stress

1. Modern society is full of stress. Stress experiences involve daily hassles (fast-paced scheduling, the pressure to remain in constant contact through social media or cell phones, or both), major life events (loss of family member, loss of job), abuse, and trauma.

2. Hans Selye identified three structural changes in rats subjected repeatedly to noxious stimuli (stressors): (a) enlargement of the cortex of the adrenal gland, (b) atrophy of the thymus gland and other lymphoid tissues, and (c) ulceration of the gastrointestinal tract.

3. Selye believed that the three changes were caused by a nonspecific physiologic response to any long-term stressor. He called this response the general adaptation syndrome (GAS).

4. The GAS occurs in three stages: (a) the alarm stage, (b) the stage of resistance or adaptation, and (c) the stage of exhaustion or allostatic overload. Diseases of adaptation develop if the stage of resistance or adaptation does not restore homeostasis. Although important, this approach is now thought to be greatly oversimplified.

5. Selye identified three components of physiologic stress: (a) the stressor, (b) the physiologic or chemical disturbance produced by the stressor, and (c) the body's adaptational response to the stressor.

6. Other investigators have shown that the physiologic stress response also occurs in response to psychologic or emotional stress.

7. Psychologic stressors can be anticipatory and triggered by expectations of an upcoming stressor or can be reactive to a stressor. Both of these psychologic stressors are capable of eliciting a physiologic stress response.

The Stress Response

1. The stress response involves the nervous system (sympathetic branch of the autonomic nervous system), the endocrine system (pituitary and adrenal glands), and the immune system. More simply, these relationships are often cited together as the hypothalamic-pituitary-adrenal (HPA) axis.

2. The stress response is initiated when a stressor is present in the body or perceived by the mind. Psychologic stress may cause or worsen several diseases or disorders including anxiety, depression, insomnia, chronic pain and fatigue syndromes, obesity, metabolic syndrome, essential hypertension, type 2 diabetes, atherosclerosis and its cardiovascular consequences, osteoporosis, and autoimmune inflammatory and allergic disorders.

3. Effects of stress on inflammatory and immune processes influence coronary artery disease, depression, autoimmune disorders, and, possibly, virally-mediated cancers.

4. The physiology involved in meeting the demands and challenges of daily life is an emerging topic of research. Some refer to these challenges as "stressors" and to the chronically stressed person as being "stressed out." The physiology is complex, involving mechanisms of both protection and injury. Glucocorticoids from the adrenal cortex, in response to ACTH from the pituitary gland, comprise the major stress hormones along with the catecholamines epinephrine and norepineprine.

5. The neuroendocrine response to stress consists of sympathetic stimulation of the adrenal medulla to secrete catecholamines (norepinephrine, epinephrine, neuropeptide Y) and stressor-induced stimulation of the pituitary to secrete ACTH, which in turn stimulates the adrenal cortex to secrete steroid hormones, particularly cortisol.

6. In general, catecholamines prepare the body to act, and cortisol mobilizes energy (glucose) and other substances needed for action. The parasympathetic system balances or restrains the sympathetic system, resulting in anti-inflammatory effects.

7. Epinephrine exerts its chief effects on the cardiovascular system. Epinephrine increases cardiac output and increases blood flow to the heart, brain, and skeletal muscles by dilating vessels that supply these organs. It also dilates the airways, thereby increasing delivery of oxygen to the bloodstream.

8. Norepinephrine's chief effects complement those of epinephrine. Norepinephrine constricts blood vessels of the viscera and skin; this has the effect of shifting blood flow to the vessels dilated by epinephrine. Norepinephrine also increases mental alertness.

9. The glucocorticoid molecules reach *all* tissues, including the brain, easily penetrate cell membranes, and react with numerous intracellular glucocorticoid receptors. Because they spare almost no tissue or organ and influence a large proportion of the human genome, they exert significant diverse biologic actions. Cortisol's chief effects involve metabolic processes. By inhibiting the use of metabolic substances while promoting their formation, cortisol mobilizes glucose, amino acids, lipids, and fatty acids and delivers them to the bloodstream.

10. Overall, glucocorticoids have an important role in the homeostasis of the CNS. These hormones regulate memory, cognition, mood, and sleep.

11. Glucocorticoids contribute to the development of metabolic syndrome and the pathogenesis of obesity. They can directly cause insulin resistance and influence genetic variations that predispose to obesity.

12. Cortisol secretion during stress exerts beneficial effects by inhibiting initial inflammatory effects, for example, vasodilation and increased capillary permeability. Cortisol also promotes resolution and repair. Paradoxically, elevated levels of glucocorticoids and catecholamines (epinephrine and norepinephrine), administered both endogenously and exogenously, can decrease innate immunity and increase autoimmune (adaptive) responses. These effects can accentuate inflammation in general and potentially increase neuronal death (e.g., in stroke victims).

13. Other hormones are affected by the stress response, for example, increased circulating levels of β-endorphins, growth hormone, prolactin, oxytocin, the steroid sex hormones, and antidiuretic hormone.

Stress, Personality, Coping, and Illness

1. Stress is a system of interdependent processes that are moderated by the nature, intensity, and duration of the stressor and the coping efficacy of the affected individual, all of which in turn mediate the psychologic and physiologic response to stress.

2. Personality characteristics are associated with individual differences in appraisal and response to stressors.

3. Coping styles associated with altered immunity include repression, denial, escape-avoidance, and concealment.

4. Many studies have linked psychologic distress with altered immune function, and there is now evidence that strengthens the association of stress with the potential for illness in humans.

GERIATRIC CONSIDERATIONS: Aging & The Stress-Age Syndrome

1. With aging, often a set of neurohormonal and immune alterations, including tissue and cellular changes, occur. These changes are collectively called stress-age syndromes.

2. The changes are numerous, with some being adaptative whereas others are potentially damaging.

KEY TERMS

- Adrenocorticotropic hormone (ACTH) 207
- Alarm stage 204
- Allostasis 208
- Allostatic overload 208
- Anticipatory response 207
- Coping 217
- Corticotropin-releasing hormone (CRH) 207
- Diseases of adaptation 204
- General adaptation syndrome (GAS) 204
- Homeostasis 207
- Hypothalamic-pituitary-adrenal (HPA) axis 207
- Neuropeptide Y (NPY) 214
- Peripheral (immune) CRH 213
- Physiologic stress 205
- Psychoneuroimmunology (PNI) 207
- Reactive response 207
- Stage of exhaustion 204
- Stage of resistance or adaptation 204
- Stress response 209
- Stressor 204
- Th1 to Th2 shift 213

REFERENCES

1. McEwen BS: Central effects of stress hormones in health and disease: understanding the protective and damaging effects of stress and stress mediators, *Eur J Pharmacol* 583(2-3):174–185, 2008.
2. Dhabhar FS, McEwen BS: Enhancing versus suppressive effects of stress hormones on skin immune function, *Proc Natl Acad Sci U S A* 96(3):1059–1064, 1999.
3. Cannon WB, Bringer CAL, Fritz R: Experimental hyperthyroidism, *Am J Physiol* 36:363, 1914.
4. Selye H: The general adaptation syndrome and the diseases of adaptation, *J Clin Endocrinol* 6:117–230, 1946.
5. Hill SR, et al: Studies on adrenocortical and psychological responses to stress in man, *Arch Intern Med* 97:269, 1956.
6. Mason JW, Brady JV: Plasma 17-hydroxycorticosteroid changes related to reserpine effects on emotional behaviors, *Science* 124:983, 1956.
7. Hetzel BS, et al: Changes in urinary 17-hydroxycorticosteroid excretion during stressful life experiences in man, *J Clin Endocrinol Metab* 15(9):1057–1068, 1955.
8. Mason JW: Organization of psychoendocrine mechanisms: a review and reconsideration of research. In Greenfield NS, Steinbach RA, editors: *Handbook of psychophysiology*, New York, 1972, Holt, Rinehart, & Winston.
9. Herman JP, et al: Central mechanisms of stress integration: hierarchical circuitry controlling hypothalamo-pituitary-adrenocortical responsiveness, *Front Neuroendocrinol* 24(3):151–158, 2003.
10. Kiecolt-Glaser JK, et al: Psychoneuroimmunology: psychological influences on immune function and health, *J Consult Clin Psychol* 70(3):537–547, 2002.
11. Chrousos GP, Kino T: Glucocorticoid signaling in the cell: expanding clinical complications to complex human behavioral and somatic disorders, *Ann N Y Acad Sci* 1179:153–166, 2009.
12. Liu LY, et al: School examinations enhance airway inflammation to antigen challenge, *Am J Respir Crit Care Med* 165(8):1062–1067, 2002.
13. Vedhara K, Irwin M, editors: *Human pyschoimmunology*, Oxford, England, 2005, Oxford University Press.
14. Bauer-Wu SM: Psychoneuroimmunology. Part I: Physiology, *Clin J Oncol Nurs* 6(3):167–170, 2002.
15. Bauer-Wu SM: Psychoneuroimmunology. Part II: Mind-body interventions, *Clin J Oncol Nurs* 6(4):243–246, 2002.
16. Ranchor AV, Sanderman R, Coyne JC: Invited commentary: personality as a causal factor in cancer risk and mortality—time to retire a hypothesis? *Am J Epidemiol* 172(4):386–388, 2010.
17. Sloan EK, et al: The sympathetic nervous system induces a metastatic switch in primary breast cancer, *Cancer Res* 70(18):7042–7052, 2010.
18. Cacioppo JT, et al: Autonomic, neuroendocrine, and immune responses to psychological stress: the reactivity hypothesis, *Ann N Y Acad Sci* 840:664–673, 1998.
19. Calcagni E, Elenkov I: Stress system activity, innate and T helper cytokines, and susceptibility to immune-related diseases (review), *Ann N Y Acad Sci* 1069:62–76, 2006.
20. Maier SF, Watkins LR: Cytokines for psychologists: implications of bidirectional immune-to-brain communication for understanding behavior, mood, and cognition, *Psychol Rev* 105(1):83–107, 1998.
21. Charmandari E, Tsigos C, Chrousos G: Endocrinology of the stress response (review), *Annu Rev Physiol* 67:259–284, 2005.
22. Carrillo-Vico A, et al: A review of the multiple actions of melatonin on the immune system (review), *Endocrine* 27(2):189–200, 2005.
23. Bruunsgard H, Pedersen BK: Age-related inflammatory cytokines and disease, *Immunol Allergy Clin North Am* 23(1):15–39, 2003.
24. MacPherson A, Dinkel K, Sapolsky R: Glucocorticoids worsen excitotoxin-induced expression of proiinflammatory cytokines in hippocampal cultures, *Exp Neurol* 194(2):376–383, 2005.
25. Sorrells SF, et al: The stressed CNS: when glucocorticoids aggravate inflammation (review), *Neuron* 64(1):33–39, 2009.
26. Coutinho AE, Chapman KE: The anti-inflammatory and immunosuppressive effects of glucocorticoids, recent developments and mechanistic insights, *Mol Cell Endocrinol*, 335(1):2–13, 2011.
27. Thayer JF, Lane RD: A model of neurovisceral integration in emotion regulation and dysregulation, *J Affective Dis* 61:201–216, 2000.
28. McEwen BS: Sleep deprivation as neurobiologic and physiologic stressor, allostasis and allostatic load, *Metabolism* 55:S20–S23, 2006.
29. Alevizaki M, et al: High anticipatory stress plasma cortisol levels and sensitivity to glucocorticoids predict severity of coronary artery disease in subjects undergoing coronary angiography, *Metabolism* 56:222–226, 2007.
30. Kajantie E, et al: Body size at birth predicts hypothalamic-pituitary-adrenal axis response to psychosocial stress at 60 to 70 years, *J Clin Endocrinol Metab* 92(11):4094–4100, 2007.
31. Elenkov IJ, et al: Cytokine dysregulation, inflammation, and well-being, *Neuroimmunomodulation* 12(5):255–269, 2005.
32. McEwen BS: Protective and damaging effects of stress mediators: central role of the brain, *Dialogues Clin Neurosci* 8(4):283–297, 2006.
33. Seeman T, et al: Socio-economic differentials in peripheral biology: cumulative allostatic load, *Ann N Y Acad Sci* 1186:223–239, 2010.
34. Calcagni E, Elenkov I: Stress system activity, innate and T helper cytokines, and susceptibility to immune-related diseases (review), *Ann N Y Acad Sci* 1069:62–76, 2006.
35. Lagier B, et al: Different modulation by histamine of IL-4 and interferon-gamma (IFN-gamma) release according to the phenotype of human Th0, Th1, and Th2 clones, *Clin Exp Immunol* 108(3):545–551, 1997.
36. Rocklin RE, editor: *Histamine and H_2 antagonists in inflammation and immunodeficiency*, New York, 1990, Marcel Dekker.
37. Molina PE: Stress-specific opioid modulation of haemodynamic counter-regulation, *Clin Exp Pharmacol Physiol* 29(3):248–253, 2002.
38. Jochem J, Josko J, Gwozdz B: Endogenous opioid peptides system in haemorrhagic shock—central cardiovascular regulation, *Med Sci Monit* 7(3):545–549, 2001.
39. Molina PE: Opiate modulation of hemodynamic, hormonal, and cytokine responses to hemorrhage, *Shock* 15(6):471–478, 2001.
40. Burguera B, et al: Dual and selective actions of glucocorticoid upon basal and stimulated growth hormone release in man, *Neuroendocrinology* 51(1):51–58, 1990.
41. Shelby J, Ku WW, Nielson HC: Neurohormone and neuropeptide regulation of the post-traumatic immune response. In Faist E, editor: *Host defense alterations of trauma, shock, and sepsis: multi-organ failure/immunotherapy of sepsis*, Berlin, 1996, Pabst.

42. Sundar SK, et al: Brain IL-1–induced immunosuppression occurs through activation of both pituitary-adrenal axis and sympathetic nervous system by corticotropin-releasing factor, *J Neurosci* 10(11):3701–3706, 1990.

43. Frolkis VV: Stress-age syndrome, *Mech Ageing Dev* 69(1–2):93–107, 1993.

44. Hirokawa K: Reversing and restoring immune functions, *Mech Ageing Dev* 93(1–3):119–124, 1997.

45. Kopnisky KL, Stoff DM, Rausch DM: Workshop report: the effects of psychological variables on the progression of HIV-1 disease, *Brain Behav Immun* 18(3):246–261, 2004.

46. Wellen KE, Hotamisligil GS: Inflammation, stress, and diabetes, *J Clin Invest* 115(5):1111–1119, 2005.

47. Reiche EMV, Nunes SOV, Morimoto HK: Stress, depression, the immune system, and cancer (review), *Lancet Oncol* 5(10):617–625, 2004.

48. Coyle PK: The neuroimmunology of multiple sclerosis, *Adv Neuroimmunol* 6(2):143–154, 1996.

49. Granger DA, Booth A, Johnson DR: Human aggression and enumerative measures of immunity, *Psychosom Med* 62(4):583–590, 2000.

50. Folkman S, Lazarus RS: The relationship between coping and emotion: implications for theory and research, *Soc Sci Med* 26(3):309–317, 1988.

51. Baron RS, et al: Social support and immune function among spouses of cancer patients, *J Pers Soc Psychol* 59(2):344–352, 1990.

52. Fawzy FI, et al: Malignant melanoma: effects of an early structured psychiatric intervention, coping, and affective state on recurrence and survival 6 years later, *Arch Gen Psychiatry* 50(9):681–689, 1993.

53. Spiegel D, et al: Effects of psychosocial treatment in prolonging cancer survival may be mediated by neuroimmune pathways, *Ann N Y Acad Sci* 840:674–683, 1998.

54. Jamner LD, Schwartz GE, Leigh H: The relationship between repressive and defensive coping styles and monocyte, eosinophil, and serum glucose levels: support for the opioid peptide hypothesis of regression, *Psychosom Med* 50(6):567–575, 1988.

55. Esterling B, et al: Emotional repression, stress disclosure responses, and Epstein-Barr viral capsid antigen titers, *Psychosom Med* 52(4):397–410, 1990.

56. Cole SW, et al: Accelerated course of human immunodeficiency virus infection in gay men who conceal their homosexual identity, *Psychosom Med* 58(3):219–231, 1996.

57. Spiegel D: Psychosocial aspects of breast cancer treatment, *Semin Oncol* 24(1 suppl 1):S1–36, S1–47, 1997.

58. Busbridge NJ, Grossman AB: Stress and the single cytokine: interleukin modulation of the pituitary-adrenal axis, *Mol Cell Endocrinol* 82(2–3):C209–C214, 1991.

59. Hori T, et al: Immune cytokines and regulation of body temperature, food intake, and cellular immunity, *Brain Res Bull* 27(3–4):309–313, 1991.

60. Navarra P, et al: Interleukins-1 and -6 stimulate the release of corticotropin-releasing hormone-41 from rat hypothalamus in vitro via the eicosanoid cyclooxygenase pathway, *Endocrinology* 128(1):37–44, 1991.

61. Kiecolt-Glaser JK, et al: Psychoneuroimmunology: psychological influences on immune function and health, *J Consult Clin Psychol* 70(3):537–547, 2002.

62. Imia K, et al: Natural cytotoxic activity of peripheral-blood lymphocytes and cancer incidence: an 11-year follow-up study of a general population, *Lancet* 356(9244):1795–1799, 2000.

63. Teicher MH, et al: Developmental neurobiology of childhood stress and trauma, *Psych Clin North Am* 25(2):297–426, 2002:vii–viii.

64. McEwen BS: Protective and damaging effects of stress mediators, *N Engl J Med* 338(3):171–179, 1998.

65. Segerstrom SC, Miller GE: Psychological stress and the human immune system: a meta-analytic study of 30 years of inquiry, *Psychol Bull* 130(4):601–630, 2004.

66. Thoits PA: Dimensions of life events that influence psychological distress: an evaluation and synthesis of the literature. In Kaplan HB, editor: *Psychosocial stress: trends in theory and research*, Orlando, Fla, 1983, Academic Press.

67. Irwin M, et al: Impaired natural killer activity during bereavement, *Brain Behav Immun* 1:98, 1988.

68. Kiecolt-Glaser J, et al: Modulation of cellular immunity in medical students, *J Behav Med* 9(1):5–21, 1986.

69. Irwin M: Immune correlates of depression, *Adv Exp Med Biol* 461:1–24, 1999.

70. Frolkis VV: Stress-age syndrome, *Mech Ageing Dev* 69(1–2):93–107, 1993.

71. Hirokawa K: Reversing and restoring immune functions, *Mech Ageing Dev* 93(1–3):119–124, 1997.

72. Granger DA, Booth A, Johnson DR: Human aggression and enumerative measures of immunity, *Psychosomc Med* 62(4):583–590, 2000.

73. Solomon GF, Kemeny ME, Temoshok L: Psychoneuroimmunologic aspects of human immunodeficiency virus infection. In Alder R, Felten DL, Cohen N, editors: *Psychoneuroimmunology*, ed 2, New York, 1991, Academic Press.

74. Surwit RS, Schneider MS: Role of stress in the etiology and treatment of diabetes mellitus, *Psychosom Med* 55(4):380–393, 1993.

75. Coyle PK: The neuroimmunology of multiple sclerosis, *Adv Neuroimmunol* 6(2):143–154, 1996.

76. Bremner JD, et al: Neural correlates of memories of childhood sexual abuse in women with and without posttraumatic stress disorder, *Am J Psychiatry* 156(11):1787–1795, 1999.

77. Clohessy S, Ehlers A: PTSD symptoms, response to intrusive memories and coping in ambulance service workers, *Br J Clin Psychol* 38(pt 3):251–265, 1999.

78. Donnelly CL, Amaya-Jackson L, March JS: Psychopharmacology of pediatric posttraumatic stress disorder, *J Child Adolesc Psychopharmacol* 9(3):203–220, 1999.

79. Cordova MJ, et al: Frequency and correlates of posttraumatic-stress-disorder-like symptoms after treatment for breast cancer, *J Consult Clin Psychol* 63(6):981–986, 1995.

80. Ma Z, Faber A, Dube L: Exploring women's psychoneuroendocrine responses to cancer threat: insights from a computer-based guided imagery task, *Can J Nurs Res* 39(1):98–115, 2007.

81. Porter LS, et al: Cortisol levels and responses to mammography screening in breast cancer survivors: a pilot study, *Psychosom Med* 65(5):842–848, 2003.

82. Clayton MF, Dudley WN, Musters A: Communication with breast cancer survivors, *Health Commun* 23(3):207–221, 2008.

83. Folkman S, Lazarus RS: The relationship between coping and emotion: implications for theory and research, *Soc Sci Med* 26(3):309–317, 1988.

84. Spiegel D, et al: Effects of psychosocial treatment in prolonging cancer survival may be mediated by neuroimmune pathways, *Ann N Y Acad Sci* 840:674–683, 1998.

85. Jamner LD, Schwartz GE, Leigh H: The relationship between repressive and defensive coping styles and monocyte, eosinophil, and serum glucose levels: support for the opioid peptide hypothesis of regression, *Psychosom Med* 50(6):567–575, 1988.

86. Esterling B, et al: Emotional repression, stress disclosure responses, and Epstein-Barr viral capsid antigen titers, *Psychosom Med* 52(4):397–410, 1990.

87. Irwin M, et al: Partial sleep deprivation reduces natural killer cell activity in humans, *Psychosom Med* 56(6):493–498, 1994.

88. Pollmacher T, et al: Influence of host defense activation on sleep in humans, *Adv Neuroimmunol* 5(2):155–169, 1995.

89. White D, et al: Sleep deprivation and the control of ventilation, *Am Rev Respir Dis* 128(6):984–986, 1983.

90. Lazar JS: Mind-body medicine in primary care. Implications and applications, *Prim Care* 23(1):169–182, 1996.

91. Pinquart M, Sörensen S: Differences between caregivers and noncaregivers in psychological health and physical health: a meta-analysis, *Psychol Aging* 18(2):250–267, 2003.

92. Baron RS, et al: Social support and immune function among spouses of cancer patients, *J Pers Soc Psychol* 59(2):344–352, 1990.

93. Fawzy FI, et al: Malignant melanoma. Effects of an early structured psychiatric intervention, coping, and affective state on recurrence and survival 6 years later, *Arch Gen Psychiatry* 50(9):681–689, 1993.

94. Kiecolt-Glaser J, et al: Chronic stress and immunity in family caregivers of Alzheimers disease victims, *Psychosom Med* 49(5):523–535, 1987.

95. Shelby J, et al: Severe burn injury: effects on psychologic and immunologic function in noninjured close relatives, *J Burn Care Rehabil* 13(1):58–63, 1992.

Biology, Clinical Manifestations, and Treatment of Cancer

David M. Virshup

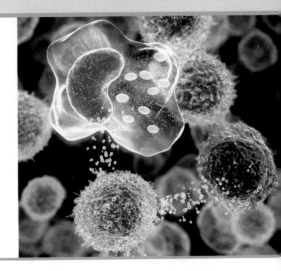

CHAPTER OUTLINE

Cancer is a leading cause of suffering and death in the developed world. The incidence of cancer increases markedly with advancing age and is strongly affected by gender, life-style, ethnicity, infection, inflammation, and genetics. Because of intensive research, we now understand that cancer is a collection of more than 100 different diseases, each caused by a specific and often unique accumulation of genetic and epigenetic alterations. Environment, heredity, and behavior interact to modify the risk of developing cancer and the response to treatment. Improvements in treatment strategies and supportive care, coupled with new, often individualized therapies based on advances in our fundamental understanding of the basic pathophysiology of malignancy, have contributed to an increasing number of effective options for these diverse, often lethal, disorders collectively called cancer.

CANCER TERMINOLOGY AND CHARACTERISTICS

Any discussion of cancer must start with a definition of what it is and what it is not. Although most readers may have an intuitive understanding of this disorder, composing an exact definition that encompasses this broad category is more challenging. A definition from 1922 may summarize cancer as well as any:

> *The most generally accepted definition of a tumor is that it is a tissue overgrowth which is independent of the laws governing the remainder of the body. It is usual to add as a qualifying phrase to separate tumors from reparative processes, such as bone callus, that the neoplasm overgrowth serves no useful purpose to the organism.*[1]

The term cancer derives from the Greek word for crab, *karkinoma*, which the physician Hippocrates used to describe the appendage-like projections extending from tumors. The word tumor originally referred to any swelling that is caused by inflammation, but is now generally reserved for describing a new growth, or neoplasm. Not all tumors or neoplasms, however, are cancer. The term cancer refers to a *malignant* tumor and is not used to refer to *benign* growths such as lipomas or hypertrophy of an organ. Yet it is important to recognize that benign neoplasms also can be life-threatening if they enlarge in critical locations. For example, a benign meningioma at the base of the skull may cause symptoms by compressing adjacent normal brain tissue. The definitions of benign versus malignant are presented in the following text and in Table 9-1.

TABLE 9-1	CHARACTERISTICS OF BENIGN VERSUS MALIGNANT TUMORS
BENIGN TUMORS	**MALIGNANT TUMORS**
Grow slowly	Grow rapidly
Have a well-defined capsule	Are not encapsulated
Are not invasive	Invade local structures and tissues
Are well differentiated; look like tissue from which they arise	Are poorly differentiated; may not be able to determine tissue of origin
Have a low mitotic index; dividing cells are rare	Have a high mitotic index; many dividing cells
Do not metastasize	Can spread distantly, often through blood vessels and lymphatics

Tumor Classification and Nomenclature

The careful evaluation of each cancer is important for many reasons. Different cancers will have different causes, different rates and patterns of progression, and different responses to treatment. The classification starts with knowing the tissue and organ of origin, the extent of distribution to other sites, and the microscopic and immunohistochemical appearance of the lesion. Increasingly, it also includes a detailed description of the critical genetic changes in the cancer.

Benign and Malignant

Benign tumors, which are not referred to as cancers, are made of fairly well-differentiated cells and well-organized stroma, the surrounding capsule of connective tissue. They retain recognizable tissue structure and do not invade beyond their capsule, nor do they spread to regional lymph nodes or distant locations. Mitotic cells are very rarely present during microscopic analysis. Benign tumors are generally named according to the tissues from which they arise, and include the suffix "-oma." For example, a benign tumor of the smooth muscle of the uterus is a *leiomyoma*, and a benign tumor of fat cells is a *lipoma*. Benign tumors will usually have a subset of the genetic lesions found in advanced cancers.

Malignant tumors are distinguished from benign tumors by more rapid growth rates and specific microscopic alterations, including loss of differentiation and absence of normal tissue organization (Figure 9-1). One of the microscopic hallmarks of cancer cells is anaplasia, the loss of cellular differentiation. Malignant cells are also pleomorphic, with marked variability of size and shape. They often have large darkly stained nuclei and mitotic cells are common. Malignant tumors may have a substantial amount of stroma, but it is disorganized, with loss of normal tissue structure. Malignant tumors lack a capsule and grow to invade nearby blood vessels, lymphatics, and surrounding structures. The most important and most deadly characteristic of malignant tumors is their ability to spread far beyond the tissue of origin, a process known as *metastasis*.

In general, cancers are named according to the cell type from which they originate. Cancers arising in epithelial tissue are called carcinomas, and if they arise from or form ductal or glandular structures are named adenocarcinomas. Hence, a malignant tumor arising from breast glandular tissue is a mammary adenocarcinoma. Cancers arising from mesenchymal tissue (including connective tissue, muscle, and bone) usually have the suffix sarcoma. For example, malignant cancers of skeletal muscle are known as rhabdomyosarcomas. Cancers of lymphatic tissue are called lymphomas, whereas cancers of blood-forming cells are called leukemias. However, many cancers, such as Hodgkin disease and Ewing sarcoma, are named for historical reasons that do not follow this nomenclature convention.

Carcinoma in Situ

Cancers develop incrementally, as they accumulate specific genetic lesions. Careful surveillance for cancer often detects abnormal growths in epithelial tissues that have atypical cells and increased proliferation rate compared with normal surrounding tissues. These early stage growths are localized to the epithelium but have not penetrated the local basement membrane or invaded the surrounding stroma (Figure 9-2). Based on these characteristics, they are not malignant but are often called carcinoma in situ (CIS). CIS is commonly found in a number of sites, including the cervix, skin, oral cavity, esophagus, and bronchus. In glandular epithelium, in situ lesions occur in the stomach, endometrium, breast, and large bowel. In the breast, ductal carcinoma in situ (DCIS) can fill the mammary ducts but has not progressed to local tissue invasion.[2] CIS lesions can have one of the following three fates: they can remain stable for a long time, they can progress to invasive and metastatic cancers, or they can regress and disappear. CIS can vary from low-grade to high-grade dysplasia, with the high-grade lesions having the highest likelihood of becoming invasive cancers. Knowing how to best treat low-grade CIS lesions is challenging, because the proportion that progress to cancer versus the proportion that will never cause clinical problems is usually not known. Although most persons prefer removal of any CIS as opposed to "watchful waiting," this topic continues to be a source of great debate.

Classification of Tumors—Classic Histology and Modern Genetics

Because our knowledge about the molecular alterations in cancer can influence the choices of therapy, it becomes increasingly important for clinicians to accurately molecularly classify each cancer (Box 9-1). The classification, and hence the treatment decisions, of cancers was originally based on gross and light microscopic appearance, and is now commonly accompanied by immunohistochemical analysis of protein expression. Increasingly, this is supplemented by a more extensive molecular analysis of the tumors. Sometimes a single gene is examined (for example, to determine if there is a characteristic chromosomal translocation diagnostic of chronic myelogenous leukemia [CML]), and sometimes a panel of genes and proteins are examined (e.g., in breast cancer) to determine if the tumor expresses estrogen receptor, progesterone receptor, and the epidermal growth factor (EGF) receptor HER2, or if there are mutations in specific genes that include response to therapy. In a research setting, and increasingly in clinical settings, gene expression and mutation analysis can be measured using polymerase chain reaction (PCR), microarray, or advanced DNA sequencing technology, so that the status of a large number of genes can be assessed. These analyses can be used to classify tumors more precisely and may predict the most effective therapy. This detailed analysis of each tumor is a form of personalized medicine that offers therapy based on a very detailed knowledge of each individual's characteristics and their specific cancer.[3] This enhanced molecular characterization subdivides cancers into therapeutically and prognostically relevant smaller groups. As an example, breast cancers can now be subclassified into over four types (luminal A, luminal B, basal-like, and others) based on their expression of specific markers, such as estrogen receptor, HER2/Neu, and other specific genes and proteins.

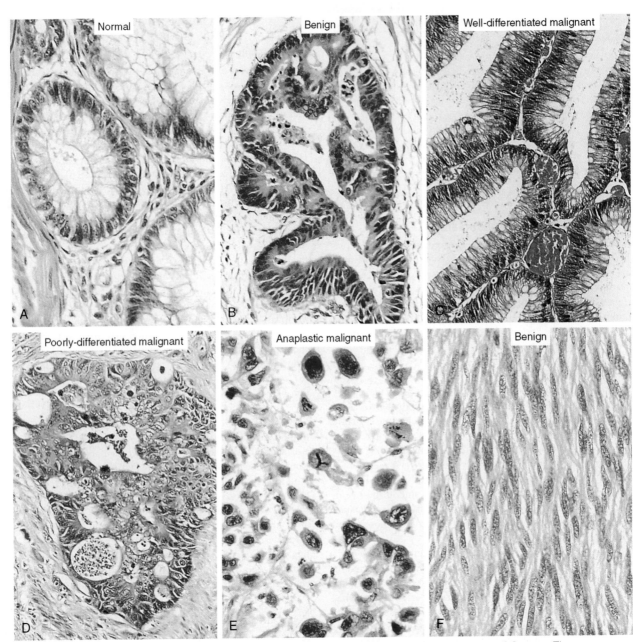

FIGURE 9-1 Loss of Cellular and Tissue Differentiation During the Development of Cancer. The cells of a benign neoplasm (**B**) resemble those of the normal colonic epithelium (**A**), in that they are columnar and have an orderly arrangement. Loss of some degree of differentiation is evident in that the neoplastic cells do not show much mucin vacuolization. Cells of the well-differentiated malignant neoplasm (**C**) of the colon have a haphazard arrangement, and although gland lumina are formed they are architecturally abnormal and irregular. Nuclei vary in shape and size, especially when compared with (**A**). Cells in the poorly-differentiated malignant neoplasm (**D**) have an even more haphazard arrangement, with very poor formation of gland lumina. Nuclei show greater variation in shape and size compared with the well-differentiated malignant neoplasm in (**C**). Cells in anaplastic malignant neoplasms (**E**) bear no relation to the normal epithelium, with no recognizable gland formation. Tremendous variation is found in the size of cells and their nuclei, with very intense staining (hyperchromatic nuclei). Not knowing the site of origin makes it impossible to classify this tumor by microscopic appearance alone. Well-differentiated tumors often resemble their cell of origin, as shown in the example of a benign tumor of smooth muscles (**F**). (From Stevens A, Lowe J: *Pathology,* ed 2, London, 2000, Mosby.)

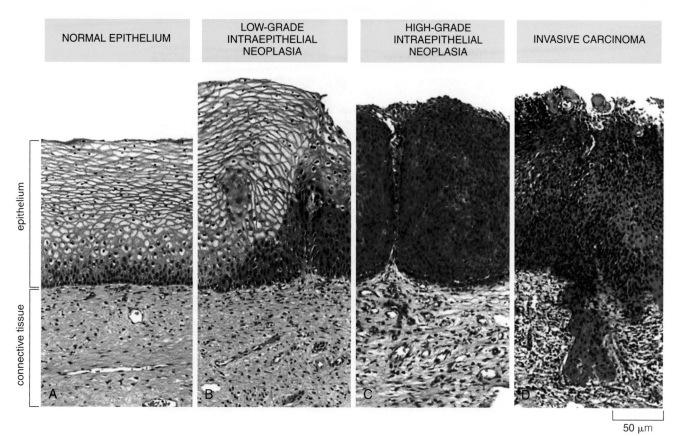

| NORMAL EPITHELIUM | LOW-GRADE INTRAEPITHELIAL NEOPLASIA | HIGH-GRADE INTRAEPITHELIAL NEOPLASIA | INVASIVE CARCINOMA |

50 µm

FIGURE 9-2 Progression from Normal to Neoplasm in the Uterine Cervix. A sequence of cellular and tissue changes progressing from low-grade to high-grade intraepithelial neoplasms (also called carcinoma in situ) and then to invasive cancer is seen often in the development of cancer. In this example of the early stages of cervical neoplastic changes, the presence of anaplastic cells and loss of normal tissue architecture signify the development of cancer. The high rate of cell division and the presence of local mutagens and inflammatory mediators all contribute to the accumulation of genetic abnormalities that lead to cancer. (From Alberts B et al: *Molecular biology of the cell*, ed 5, New York, 2008, Garland.)

BOX 9-1   TYPES OF GENETIC LESIONS IN CANCER

1. Point mutations
2. Subtle alterations (insertions, deletions)
3. Chromosome changes (aneuploidy and loss of heterozygosity)
4. Amplifications
5. Gene silencing (DNA methylation, histone modification, microRNAs)
6. Exogenous sequences (tumor viruses)

Each subtype has a different response to therapy and a different prognosis (Figure 9-3).

Tumor Markers

During surveillance or diagnosis of cancer as well as following therapy, specific biochemical markers of tumors have proven to be helpful. These tumor markers are substances produced by both benign and malignant cells that are either present in or on tumor cells or found in blood, spinal fluid, or urine (Table 9-2). Some tumor markers have been known for many decades. For diseases associated with a tumor marker, there is indeed a "blood test for cancer." Tumor markers include hormones, enzymes, genes, antigens, and antibodies. Liver and germ cell tumors secrete a protein known as *alpha fetoprotein (AFP)* into the blood, and prostate tumors secrete *prostate specific antigen (PSA)* into the blood. If the tumor marker itself has biologic activity, then it can cause symptoms, a phenomenon known as a **paraneoplastic syndrome** (see Table 9-7). For example, the adrenal medulla normally secretes the catecholamine epinephrine (adrenaline). Benign tumors of the adrenal medulla (pheochromocytoma) can produce catecholamines (e.g., adrenaline) in vast excess, leading to rapid pulse rate, high blood pressure, diaphoresis (i.e., sweating), and tremors. Detection of elevated blood or urine levels of catecholamines helps to confirm the diagnosis, and treatment of the disease relieves the symptoms. Tumor markers can be used in three ways: (1) to screen and identify individuals at high risk for cancer; (2) to help diagnose the specific type of tumor in individuals with clinical manifestations relating to their tumor, as in adrenal tumors or enlarged liver or prostate; and (3) to follow the clinical course of a tumor. For example, a falling PSA level after radiation or surgical therapy for prostate cancer indicates successful treatment, and a later rise in the PSA level may indicate a recurrence.

There are several significant problems in using tumor marker assays to screen populations of healthy individuals for cancer. Testing large populations will always detect a few normal individuals with test results at the high end of the normal distribution (the "false positives"), which can lead to expensive and invasive additional tests, and unnecessary concern. Similarly, some individuals with disease will

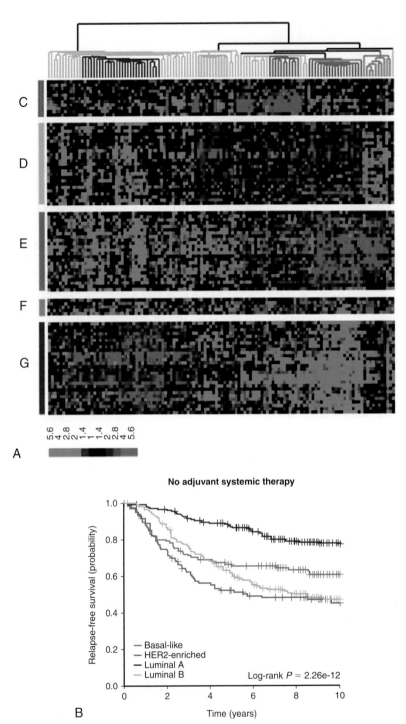

FIGURE 9-3 Molecular Markers Aid in Cancer Classification and Treatment Choices. A, Cancers can be classified based on gene expression patterns. In this breast cancer study, gene expression was measured in tumors from 115 patients. Each row is a different gene, and each column is a different patient sample. Red denotes high gene expression; green signifies low gene expression. Using this molecular subtyping method, breast cancer can be subdivided into at least four molecular subtypes—luminal A, luminal B, HER2, and basal. The group on the far right is normal breast tissue. **B,** Molecular classification predicts overall survival. In this group of women, breast cancer molecular subtypes were determined by gene expression profiles in a group of women with similar stage tumors, as in **(A).** The molecular subtype is a good predictor of response to chemotherapy and survival. This molecular subtyping method can help select the best therapy for women. (**A** from Sorlie T et al: Repeated observation of breast tumor subtypes in independent gene expression data sets, *Proc Natl Acad Sci U S A* 100[14]:8418–8423, 2003; **B** from Parker JS et al: Supervised risk predictor of breast cancer based on intrinsic subtypes, *J Clin Oncol* 27[8]:1160–1167, 2009.)

have test results in the normal range ("false negatives"). Furthermore, some nonmalignant conditions also can produce tumor markers. The presence of an elevated tumor marker therefore may suggest a specific diagnosis, but it is not used alone as a definitive diagnostic test. Identification of ideal sensitive and specific tumor markers that are elevated early in the course of common cancers remains a high priority because the early detection of cancer often improves the treatment outcome.

✔ **QUICK CHECK 9-1**
1. Identify the major differences between benign and malignant tumors.
2. Why is molecular characterization of tumors so important?
3. Discuss the importance of tumor markers.

TABLE 9-2 EXAMPLES OF TUMOR MARKERS

MARKER NAME	NATURE	TYPE OF TUMOR
Alpha fetoprotein (AFP)	70-kDa protein	Hepatic, germ cell
Carcinoembryonic antigen (CEA)	200-kDa glycoprotein	GI, pancreas, lung, breast, etc.
β-Human chorionic gonadotropin (β-HCG)	Glycopeptide hormone	Germ cell
Prostate-specific antigen (PSA)	33-kDa glycoprotein	Prostate
Catecholamines	Epinephrine and precursors	Pheochromocytoma (adrenal medulla)
Homovanillic acid/ vanillylmandelic acid (HVA/VMA)	Catecholamine metabolites	Neuroblastoma
Urinary Bence Jones protein	Ig light chain	Multiple myeloma
Adrenocorticotropic hormone (ACTH)	Peptide hormone	Pituitary adenomas

GI, Gastrointestinal; *Ig,* immunoglobulin; *kDa,* kilodalton(s).

THE BIOLOGY OF CANCER CELLS

Cancer Cells in the Laboratory

Cancer cells behave differently than normal cells in several important ways. The microscopic differences were described previously in this chapter and the genetic differences will be described next. There are also differences in cancer cell behavior that can be analyzed in the laboratory. Cancer cells are sometimes described as **transformed cells,** because they can be created from normal cells. Once transformed, cancer cells display distinct growth properties in the laboratory. They often have markedly decreased requirements for external growth factors. Transformed cells, unlike normal cells, lack **contact inhibition** and continue to crowd, eventually piling up on each other (Figure 9-4). Normal cells usually will not grow unless they are attached to a firm surface (such as a petri dish). However, cancer cells are often **anchorage independent;** that is, they continue to divide even when suspended in a soft agar gel. Normal cells have a limited life span in the laboratory; they may divide in a petri dish 10 or 50 times, but then they cease growing. Cancer cells usually are **immortal** in that they seem to have an unlimited life span and will continue to divide for years under appropriate laboratory conditions. One of the most commonly used laboratory cell lines, HeLa cells, was derived from a cervical cancer specimen obtained in 1951 that continues to grow and divide in laboratories around the world.[4] Cancerous cells can be assayed in mice as well; normal human cells injected into a special type of mouse (genetically engineered to lack an immune system to prevent rejection of human cells) will not grow. However, transformed cells from humans can continue to grow, invade normal tissues, and even metastasize in these mice.

The Genetic Basis of Cancer
Cancer-Causing Mutations in Genes

Before the advent of modern molecular biology, many different causes of cancer were postulated, based on epidemiologic studies as well as investigations of specific carcinogens and viruses. We now understand that the stepwise accumulation of a small set of changes in the deoxyribonucleic acid (DNA) and chromosomes of the cancer cell cause it to become cancerous (Figure 9-5). As our knowledge of cancer biology

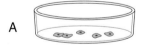

A
Noncancerous cells are anchorage dependent and only proliferate when attached to a surface.

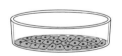

When these cells form a complete monolayer, they stop dividing due to contact inhibition.

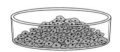

Cancer cells do not exhibit contact inhibition, and continue to divide, piling up on each other.

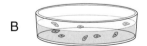

B
Normal cells suspended in soft agar cannot attach and therefore cannot proliferate.

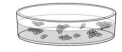

Cancer cells are anchorage independent and can proliferate suspended in soft agar.

FIGURE 9-4 Cancerous Cells Show Abnormal Growth in the Laboratory. Cancer cells, unlike most normal cells **(A),** usually continue to grow and accumulate on top of one another after they have formed a confluent monolayer in culture (loss of contact inhibition) and **(B)** can grow without being attached to a surface, called anchorage independence.

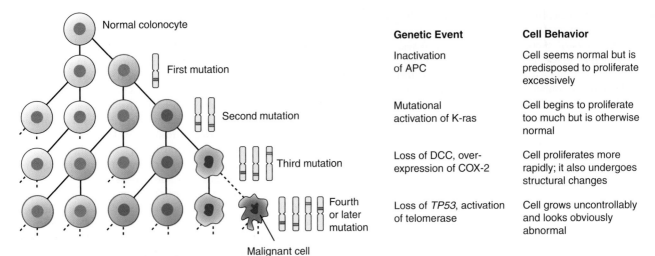

	Genetic Event	Cell Behavior
	Inactivation of APC	Cell seems normal but is predisposed to proliferate excessively
	Mutational activation of K-ras	Cell begins to proliferate too much but is otherwise normal
	Loss of DCC, over-expression of COX-2	Cell proliferates more rapidly; it also undergoes structural changes
	Loss of *TP53*, activation of telomerase	Cell grows uncontrollably and looks obviously abnormal

FIGURE 9-5 Clonal Proliferation Model of Neoplastic Progression in the Colon. During clonal proliferation, progressively altered populations of colon cells (colonocytes) arise over time. As genetic and epigenetic changes occur, different subclones (indicated by different color cells) coexist for a time. Clones that grow the fastest out-compete other clones, producing even more malignant, and abnormal-appearing, growths. The sequential accumulation of mutations has been well studied in the progression from a normal colon cell to a benign intestinal polyp to a malignant colon cancer. One of the earliest mutations in colon cancer is loss of the tumor-suppressor gene *APC*. Additional mutations (often in the oncogene *RAS*), activation of COX-2, and loss of the tumor suppressors *DCC* and *TP53* occur as the lesion progresses from a benign polyp to an invasive carcinoma. *APC*, Adenomatous polyposis coli; *COX-2*, cyclooxygenase-2; *DCC*, deleted in colon cancer; *TP53*, p53 gene. (Modified from Mendelsohn I et al: *The molecular basis of cancer,* ed 2, Philadelphia, 2001, Saunders; and Kumar V, Cotran RS, Robbins SL: *Basic pathology,* ed 6, Philadelphia, 1997, Saunders.)

continues to increase so too does our understanding of the many ways that heritable changes in cells can contribute to cancer. These changes include small and large DNA mutations that alter genes, chromosomes, and non–coding RNAs, as well as epigenetic changes, because of altered chemical modifications of DNA and histones (also see Chapters 2 and 10). Although the word *mutation* is used extensively here, it can also refer to heritable changes in gene and non–coding RNA expression (epigenetics) that do not involve changes in DNA sequence (see p. 233).

Cancer is predominantly a disease of aging. Perhaps the most revealing epidemiologic data are presented in Figure 9-6. The incidence of most cancers, that is, the fraction of individuals in each age group who develop cancer, increases dramatically with age. The best explanation for these epidemiologic data is that each individual acquires a number of genetic "hits" or mutations over time. When sufficient mutations have occurred, cancer develops. These epidemiologic data are consistent with the observation of mutations in early and advanced cancers and with data obtained from the study of experimental cancers created in the laboratory—the accumulation of four to seven specific hits over time is required to cause a full-blown cancer.[5]

Clonal selection. As a cell accumulates specific mutations, it can acquire, step by step, the characteristics of a cancer cell, for example, anchorage-independent growth, lack of contact inhibition, and immortality.[6] That mutant cell may then have a selective advantage over its neighbors; its progeny can accumulate faster than its nonmutant neighbors. This is referred to as clonal proliferation or clonal expansion (see Figure 9-5). As a clone with mutations proliferates, it may become an early stage tumor, for example, a carcinoma in situ or a benign colonic polyp. Additional random heritable changes occur in these proliferating cells, and some of these mutations favor progression to more advanced tumors.

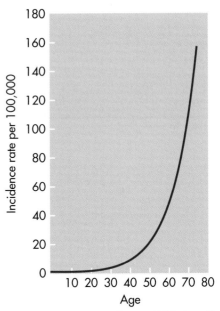

FIGURE 9-6 Marked Increases in Cancer With Age. The incidence of cancer increases exponentially with advancing age. For example, this graph depicts the number of cases of colon cancer diagnosed per 100,000 women in England and Wales in 1 year. Similar data are seen for other cancers, and in men as well. These data suggest that stepwise accumulation of genetic and epigenetic alterations over time increases the risk of developing cancer. The slope of the curve predicts that five to seven mutations must accumulate before full-blown cancer develops. (Modified from Armitage P, Doll R: The age distribution of cancer and a multi-stage theory of carcinogenesis, *Br J Cancer* 91[12]:1983–1989 [reprinted in 2004]; Alberts B et al: *Molecular biology of the cell,* ed 4, New York, 2002, Garland.)

TABLE 9-3   COMPARISON OF CANCER GENE TYPES

GENE TYPE	NORMAL FUNCTION	MUTATION EFFECT
Caretaker	DNA and chromosome stability	Chromosome instability and increased rates of mutation
Dominant oncogenes*	Encode proteins that promote growth (e.g., growth factors)	Overexpression or amplification causes gain of function
Tumor suppressors (recessive oncogenes)	Encode proteins that inhibit proliferation and prevent or repair mutations	Requires loss of function of both alleles to increase cancer risk

*Nonmutant state referred to as proto-oncogene.

The process of tumor development is a form of darwinian evolution; cells with a heritable change that confers a survival advantage out-compete their neighbors. The progressive accumulation of distinct advantageous (from the point of view of the cancer cell, not the individual!) mutations leads step by step from normal cells to fully malignant cancers.

Oncogenes and Tumor-Suppressor Genes: Accelerators and Brakes

Passengers and drivers. The previous discussion refers to the heritable changes in cells as being key in the development of cancer. New technologies that provide massive amounts of information about chromosome and gene structure allow us to see multiple alterations in cancer cells. These methods include massively parallel high-throughput DNA sequencing (the process by which the sequence of nucleotides along a strand of DNA is determined), high-density single-nucleotide polymorphism (SNP), and chromosome copy number analysis (CNA). These approaches confirm that there are a small number of very common genetic alterations in cancer and a very large number of alterations that individually are rare.[7] It is clear that some mutations can contribute to cancer progression (e.g., mutations in *p53* or *RAS*). These mutations are driver mutations; they drive the progression of cancer. Conversely, not all mutations in cancer contribute to the malignant phenotype. Some are just random events, and are referred to as passenger mutations; they are just along for the ride. The increasing amount of cancer genome analysis data poses the following question: how do we determine which mutations are drivers and which are passengers?

What are the driver mutations? To understand how genetic mutations cause cancer, first it is important to distinguish between oncogenes and tumor-suppressor genes. Table 9-3 compares the two types of cancer genes. Oncogenes are mutant genes that in their normal nonmutant state direct synthesis of proteins that positively regulate (accelerate) proliferation. Conversely, tumor-suppressor genes encode proteins that in their normal state negatively regulate (halt, or "put the brakes on") proliferation. Hence, they also have been referred to as anti-oncogenes.

In its normal, nonmutant state, an oncogene is referred to as a proto-oncogene. An example of a proto-oncogene would be a growth factor (e.g., epidermal growth factor) or a growth factor receptor (e.g., epidermal growth factor receptor). Other positive regulators of proliferation are in the signal transduction pathway that transmits the signal from the growth factor receptor to the cell nucleus. Normally, RAS is a proto-oncogene (Figure 9-7).

QUICK CHECK 9-2
1. What are the characteristics of cancer cells in the laboratory?
2. What are the heritable changes in cells that contribute to cancer development?
3. Define oncogene, proto-oncogene, and tumor-suppressor gene.

What Types of Changes in Genes Actually Occur in Cancer?

The activation and inactivation of various genes is key in the development of cancer. The following three types of DNA changes occur in cancer: small DNA changes, large DNA changes, and epigenetic changes.

Mutation of normal genes into oncogenes

Point mutations. Several types of genetic events can activate oncogenes (Figure 9-8). Perhaps the most common events are small-scale changes in DNA, such as point mutations, the alteration of one or a few nucleotide base pairs (see Chapter 2). This type of mutation can have profound effects on the activity of proteins. A point mutation in the *RAS* gene converts it from a regulated proto-oncogene to an unregulated oncogene, an accelerator of cellular proliferation. Activating point mutations in *RAS* are found in many cancers, especially pancreatic and colorectal cancer. Specialized tests, such as direct DNA sequencing, can detect such point mutations in clinical samples.

Chromosome translocations and copy number variation. Chromosome translocations are large changes in chromosome structure in which a piece of one chromosome is translocated to another chromosome. Translocations can activate oncogenes in one of two distinct mechanisms. First, a translocation can cause excess and inappropriate production of a proliferation factor. One of the best examples is the t(8;14) translocation found in many Burkitt lymphomas; t(8;14) designates a chromosome that has a piece of chromosome 8 fused to a piece of chromosome 14 (see Chapter 20). Burkitt lymphoma is an aggressive cancer of B lymphocytes. The *MYC* proto-oncogene found on chromosome 8 is normally activated at low levels in proliferating lymphocytes and is deactivated in mature lymphocytes. The MYC protein is part of the positive signal for cell proliferation. If accidental formation of the t(8;14) translocation occurs, the *MYC* gene is aberrantly placed under the control of a B cell immunoglobulin gene *(IG)* present on chromosome 14. The *IG* gene is very active in maturing B lymphocytes. The t(8;14) translocation alters the control of *MYC*; its normal low level is switched to high levels, as directed by an *IG* gene promoter. MYC protein, when inappropriately high, drives proliferation and blocks differentiation. Hence, the t(8;14) translocation causes cancer of maturing B cells (see Figure 9-8, *C*).

Second, chromosome translocations can lead to production of novel proteins with growth-promoting properties. In a different type of leukemia, chronic myeloid leukemia (CML), a specific chromosome translocation is almost always present. This translocation, t(9;22), was first identified in association with CML in Philadelphia in 1960 and so is often referred to as the Philadelphia chromosome.[8] This translocation fuses two chromosomes in the middle of two different genes: *BCR* on chromosome 9 and *ABL* on chromosome 22. The result is production of a BCR-ABL fusion protein containing the first half of BCR and the second half of ABL. BCR-ABL is a misregulated protein tyrosine kinase that promotes growth of myeloid cells. Imatinib, a drug that specifically targets this tyrosine kinase, represents the first successful chemotherapy targeted against the product of a specific oncogenic mutation. Imatinib and related tyrosine kinase inhibitors (TKIs) are highly effective in the treatment of CML and, because of their specificity, lack the toxic side effects noted with nonspecific anticancer drugs.[9] However, imatinib is not effective in cancers that do not have

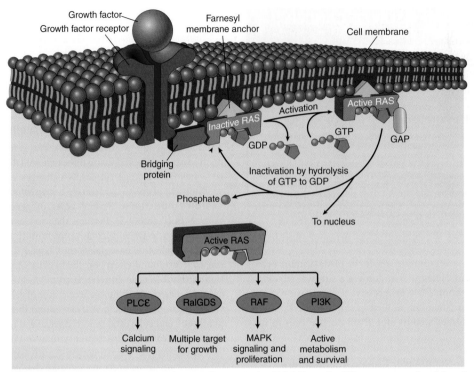

FIGURE 9-7 Many Growth Factors Signal Through the RAS Protein. When a normal cell is stimulated through a growth factor receptor, inactive (GDP-bound) RAS is activated to a GTP-bound state. Activated RAS sends growth signals to the nucleus through cytoplasmic kinases, starting with the activation of kinase RAF. The mutant RAS protein is permanently activated because of its inability to hydrolyze GTP, leading to continual stimulation of the cell without any external trigger. *GAP*, GTPase-activating protein; *GDP*, guanosine diphosphate; *GTP*, guanosine triphosphate; *MAPK*, mitogen-activated protein kinase. (From Kumar V, Cotran RS, Robbins SL: *Basic pathology,* ed 7, Philadelphia, 2003, Saunders; Downward J: *Nat Rev Cancer* 3[1]:11–22, 2003.)

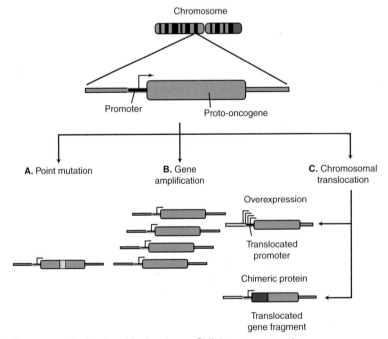

FIGURE 9-8 Oncogene Activation Mechanisms. Cellular genes may become cancerous oncogenes as a result of **(A)** point mutations that alter one or a few nucleotide base pairs, causing the production of a protein that is activated as a result of the altered sequence (e.g., RAS); **(B)** amplification of the cellular gene, resulting in higher levels of protein expression (e.g., MYCN in neuroblastoma); or **(C)** chromosomal translocations that either (1) lead to the juxtaposition of a strong promoter, causing increased protein expression (MYC in Burkitt lymphoma), or (2) produce a novel fusion protein that is derived from gene fragments normally present on different chromosomes (BCR-ABL in chronic myeloid leukemia). (From Haber DA: *Molecular genetics of cancer.* In *ACP medicine,* Danbury, Conn, 2004, WebMD.)

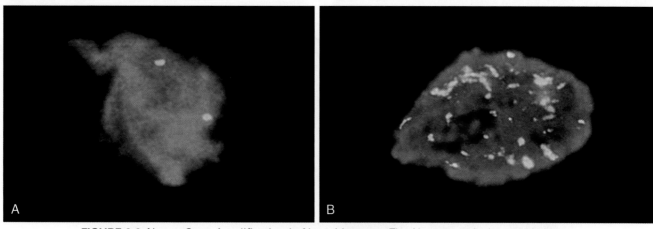

FIGURE 9-9 N-myc Gene Amplification in Neuroblastoma. The *N-myc* gene is detected in human neuroblastoma cells using a technique called FISH (fluorescent in situ hybridization). **(A)** A single pair of *N-myc* genes are detected in normal cells and in low-grade neuroblastoma. **(B)** Multiple, amplified copies of the *N-myc* gene are detected in some cases of neuroblastoma. Amplification of the *N-myc* gene is strongly associated with a poor prognosis in childhood neuroblastoma. (Courtesy Arthur R. Brothman, PhD, FACMG, University of Utah School of Medicine, Salt Lake City, Utah.)

the t(9;22) translocation or related mutations. In modern personalized cancer therapy, knowledge of the specific genetic alteration can dictate the optimal drugs for the individual.

Just as single nucleotides can be gained or lost, larger regions of DNA encompassing entire genes can be gained or lost, a phenomenon known as copy number variation (CNV).[10] CNV can be inherited and accounts for a significant fraction of human genetic diversity. CNV also can occur in the course of cancer development, where it can amplify oncogenes or delete tumor-suppressor genes.

Gene amplification. A type of chromosome structural abnormality that can activate oncogenes is gene amplification (see Figures 9-8, *B*, and 9-9). Amplifications are the result of duplication of a region of a chromosome over and over again, so that instead of the normal two copies of a gene, tens or even hundreds of copies are present (see Chapter 2). Gene amplification results in increased expression of an oncogene, or in some cases drug resistance genes. The *N-MYC* oncogene is amplified in 25% of childhood neuroblastoma cases and confers a poor prognosis.[11] The epidermal growth factor receptor *ERBB2* is amplified in 20% of breast cancers.[12] Individuals whose cancers have *ERBB2* amplification respond well to drugs specifically targeted to this oncogene.[13]

Tumor-suppressor genes. Tumor-suppressor genes are genes whose major function is to negatively regulate cell growth and prevent mutations. Tumor suppressors may normally slow the cell cycle, inhibit proliferation resulting from growth signals, or stop cell division when cells are damaged. Examples of several tumor suppressors are provided in (Table 9-4). One of the first discovered tumor-suppressor genes, the retinoblastoma (RB) gene, normally strongly inhibits the cell division cycle (see Chapter 1). When it is inactivated, the cell division cycle can proceed unchecked. *RB* is mutated in childhood retinoblastoma, and in many lung, breast, and bone cancers as well.

Whereas oncogenes are *activated* in cancers, tumor suppressors must be *inactivated* to allow cancer to occur (see Table 9-4 and Figure 9-10). A single genetic event can activate an oncogene because it can act in a dominant manner in the cell. However, we have two copies, or alleles, of each gene, one from each parent. It therefore takes two hits to inactivate the two alleles of a tumor-suppressor gene. The first

TABLE 9-4	SOME FAMILIAL CANCER SYNDROMES CAUSED BY TUMOR-SUPPRESSOR GENE FUNCTION LOSS
SYNDROME	**GENE**
Retinoblastoma	*RB1*
Li-Fraumeni syndrome	*p53 (TP53)*
Familial melanoma	*p16^{INK4a} (CDKN2A)*
Neurofibromatosis	*Neurofibromin (NF1)*
Familial adenomatous polyps	*APC*
Breast cancer	*BRCA1*

allele of a tumor suppressor is often inactivated by point mutations. For example, the *RB* gene may be inactivated on one chromosome by a point mutation (e.g., the copy inherited from the father). Because the other copy of the retinoblastoma gene (in this example, the one from the mother) is intact, a functional RB protein can still be made and, therefore, the cell division cycle can be regulated appropriately. If the remaining gene is mutated or silenced, then all RB function is lost and another step toward cancer occurs (see Chapter 1).

✔ **QUICK CHECK 9-3**
1. Describe the differences between point mutations, chromosomal translocations, and gene amplification.
2. Biologically, why do tumor-suppressor genes have to be inactivated to cause cancer?

Loss of heterozygosity. For the function of a tumor suppressor to be lost, both chromosomal copies (alleles) of the gene must be inactivated. This is because they act in a recessive manner at the level of the cell. Although it may seem intuitive that simple inactivating mutations might disrupt both alleles, in fact this is not what usually happens.[14] Instead, the first allele (in the preceding example, the paternal copy) is

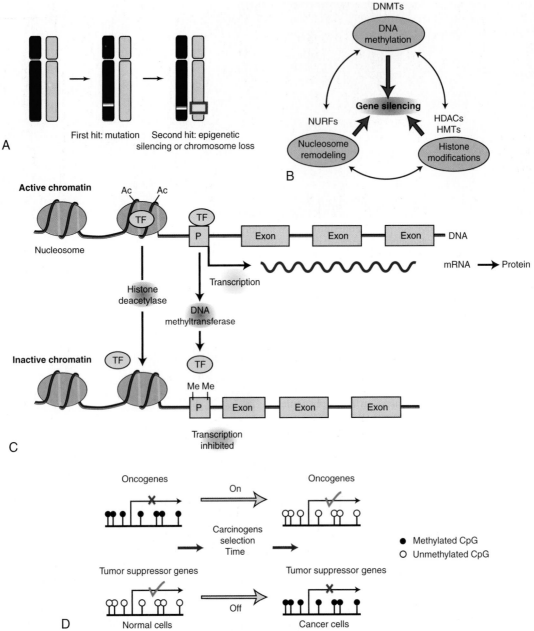

FIGURE 9-10 Silencing Tumor-Suppressor Genes. Tumor-suppressor genes can be deactivated by a variety of mechanisms. **(A)** In this example, the first hit is a point mutation in a tumor-suppressor gene (white box), followed by either epigenetic silencing or chromosome loss of the second allele (red box). **(B)** Genes can normally be silenced by a variety of interacting processes including DNA methylation, histone modification, nucleosomal remodeling, and microRNA changes (not shown). A number of cellular enzymes contribute to these modifications, including DNA methyltransferases *(DNMTs)*, histone deacetylases *(HDACs)*, histone methyltransferases *(HMTs)*, and complex nucleosomal remodeling factors *(NURFs)*. Gene silencing is essential for normal development and differentiation. **(C)** Histone modification and promoter methylation regulate gene expression. Genes are transcribed when chromatin is modified by addition of acetyl *(Ac)* groups to specific lysine groups in histones. Gene expression can be turned off when specific acetyl groups are removed (by HDACs) or when the CpG-rich promoter regions of genes are modified by direct DNA methylation (by DNA methyltransferase). In addition, small endogenous RNA molecules (microRNAs or miRNA) can bind to mRNA and reduce gene expression. **(D)** Changes in promoter methylation turn cancer genes off and on. Oncogenes can be turned on by promoter hypomethylation, and tumor-suppressor genes can be turned off by promoter hypermethylation. Each of these changes can produce selective growth and survival advantages for the cancer cell. *TF,* Transcription factor; *Me,* methylation. (**B** adapted from Jones PA, Baylin SB: The epigenomics of cancer, *Cell* 128:683–692, 2007; **C** from Gluckman PD et al: *N Engl J Med* 359[1]:66, 2008; **D** from Shames DS, Minna JF, Gazdar AF: *Curr Mol Med* 7:85–102, 2007.)

inactivated by simple mutation, but the second allele (in this example, the maternal copy) is lost because entire regions of the maternal chromosome are epigenetically silenced or a piece of the chromosome is simply lost (see Figure 9-10, *A*). Because humans have two chromosomes, one from each parent, they are always *heterozygous* for nearby multiple genetic markers; loss of one copy (allele) of a specific chromosome region in a tumor is referred to as loss of heterozygosity, or LOH. Loss of heterozygosity, like silencing, can unmask inactivating mutations in recessive tumor-suppressor genes. For example, the *RB* gene resides on chromosome 13, in a region referred to as q14 (13q14). Most individuals with *RB* mutations have a subtle mutation in one allele and have lost the other copy allele of *RB* through loss of the 13q14 chromosome region on the other chromosome.

Turning off genes without mutation

Epigenetic silencing. Abnormal gene silencing is emerging as a major factor in cancer progression. Gene expression can be regulated in a heritable manner (i.e., passed from a parent to a child or from a single cell to its progeny) by an "epigenetic" mechanism called silencing. Inheritance of silencing occurs during cell division and does not require mutations or changes in DNA sequence (also see Chapters 2 and 10). More simply, the same DNA sequence can produce dramatically different phenotypes depending on chemical modifications that alter the *expression* of genes. Epigenetic silencing is caused by reversible chemical modification (methylation [addition of a methyl group] or acetylation [addition of an acetyl group]) of histones and related chromatin components, as well as methylation of cytosine residues in DNA (known as DNA methylation) (see Figure 9-10, Figure 2-24 [p. 49], and Chapter 10). Whole regions of chromosomes are normally shut off by silencing, so that the pattern of gene expression is different than that seen in other cells with the same genes. In this way, the progeny of liver cells remain liver cells, and skin cells remain skin cells. Notably, *global* changes in epigenetic silencing can turn these cells back into stem cells.[15]

Changes in gene silencing contribute to the development of cancer.[16] Many cancers have increased methylation of DNA in the promoter region of tumor-suppressor genes, often near gene promoter regions (see Chapters 2 and 10). They also have associated changes in the modification of histones in the chromatin, often correlated with methylation of DNA. These changes in chromatin-modifying genes alter the promoter regions of genes, leading to their silencing. The boundaries of the normally silenced regions can also spread in cancer cells, thereby inactivating previously active genes. In either case, silencing can shut off critical tumor-suppressor genes in the absence of mutations in the gene. Early in the development of cancer, these changes in gene expression can lead to a selective advantage for affected cells, perhaps leading to their immortalization and clonal expansion. Silencing of tumor suppressors may be a faster way to create cancer cells than mutational or genetic loss of tumor suppressors.[17] Conversely, loss of silencing can contribute to inappropriate expression of oncogenes. Chemotherapeutic drugs that can regulate gene silencing, including histone deacetylase (HDAC) inhibitors and 5-azacytidine (which reverses the effects of DNA methyltransferases [DNMTs]), have proven effective in reactivating silenced tumor-suppressor genes and are being evaluated for the treatment of selected cancers (see Figure 9-10).[18]

MicroRNAs, oncomirs, and non–coding RNAs. Changes in gene regulation can affect not just single genes, but also entire networks of signaling. Gene expression networks can be regulated by changes in microRNAs (miRNAs, or miRs) and other non–coding RNAs (ncRNAs). miRNAs are short (approximately 22 nucleotides) RNAs derived from introns of protein coding genes or transcribed as independent genes from regions of the genome previously believed to have no function (erroneously called junk DNA). The human genome encodes more than 1000 miRs. miRs regulate diverse signaling pathways; the miRs that stimulate cancer development and progression are termed oncomirs. miRs decrease the stability and expression of other genes by pairing with mRNA in a process that involves the RNA-induced silencing complex, or RISC. A single miR can have multiple mRNA targets. Changes in miR abundance can therefore affect the expression of many genes, making miRs both powerful regulators and challenging subjects to study.[19] Beyond miRs, longer RNAs without apparent protein coding capacity also are implicated in cellular regulation with an emerging appreciation of their role in cancer.[20]

miRs can play both positive and negative roles in cancer. The importance of miRs in cancer was first shown in chronic lymphocytic leukemia (CLL), where a chromosome region encoding miR15 and miR16 was found to be deleted in a large number of individuals. Decreased expression of these two miRs is seen in many cases of CLL, as well as in prostate and several other cancers, and results in increased expression of a number of oncogenes. Conversely, increased expression of a cluster of miRs (17-18-19-20-92) is seen in some lymphomas and solid tumors, causing the decreased expression of a number of tumor-suppressor genes. miR expression can be easily assessed with microarray technology, leading to the realization that substantial changes in miR expression are seen in many cancers.

Guardians of the Genome

The previous discussion of mutations leads naturally to the question of how mutations occur in the first place. The integrity of genetic information can be compromised at several points: during each round of DNA synthesis, during each mitosis when chromosomes are segregated to daughter cells, and when external mutagens (e.g., chemicals and radiation) alter or disrupt DNA. Multiple mechanisms have evolved to protect and repair the genome. These repair mechanisms are directed by caretaker genes, genes that are responsible for the maintenance of genomic integrity. Caretaker genes encode proteins that are involved in repairing damaged DNA, such as occurs with errors in DNA replication, mutations caused by ultraviolet or ionizing radiation, and mutations caused by chemicals and drugs. Loss of function of caretaker genes leads to increased mutation rates. If DNA damage is severe, the cell undergoes programmed cell death, or apoptosis, rather than simply dividing with damaged DNA.

Inherited mutations can disrupt the caretaker genes that protect the integrity of the genome. Examples include the disorder xeroderma pigmentosum (XP); affected individuals have defects in the repair of ultraviolet light–induced DNA damage and should avoid direct sunlight exposure. They have a very high incidence of skin cancer. Hereditary nonpolyposis colorectal cancer (HNPCC) results from an inherited defect in repairing DNA base pair mismatches that occur occasionally during DNA replication. Affected individuals have an increased rate of small insertions and deletions in DNA, leading to a high rate of colon and other cancers. Finally, there are inherited mutations that threaten the integrity of entire chromosomes. Bloom syndrome, caused by mutations in a DNA helicase, and Fanconi aplastic anemia, caused by loss of function of a multiprotein complex required for repair of DNA double-strand breaks,[21] are autosomal recessive disorders in which affected individuals demonstrate marked chromosomal instability. Chromosome breaks, aberrant fusions, and chromosome loss are common. As a consequence, these individuals have a high risk of developing cancer at an early age.

The rate of individual gene mutation is probably too low to account for the acquisition of many new mutations during the evolution of a malignant cancer clone. In addition to abnormal epigenetic silencing, chromosome instability (often referred to as CIN) also appears to be increased in malignant cells (also see Chapter 10). The underlying mechanism of this instability is not clear but may be caused by malfunctions in the cellular machinery that regulates chromosome segregation at mitosis.[22] Chromosome instability results in a high rate of chromosome loss, as well as loss of heterozygosity and chromosome amplification. Each of these events can accelerate the loss of tumor-suppressor genes and the overexpression of oncogenes.

Genetics and Cancer-Prone Families

Genetic events are the primary basis of carcinogenesis. Most of the genetic and epigenetic alterations that cause cancer occur within the somatic tissues during the lifetime of the individual. As previously discussed, the *frequency* of genetic changes can be increased by exposure to mutagens, that is, agents causing mutations, and by defects in DNA repair. Because these genetic events occur in somatic cells as opposed to germ cells, they are not transmitted to future generations. Even though they are genetic events they are not inherited! It is possible, however, for cancer-predisposing mutations to occur in germline cells (cells that produce gametes). Mutations present in germline cells result in the transmission of cancer-causing genes from one generation to the next, producing families with a high incidence of specific cancers[23] (Figure 9-11). These inherited mutations that predispose to cancer are almost invariably in tumor-suppressor genes (see Table 9-4).

Although rare, such "cancer families" demonstrate that inheritance of a mutated gene can cause cancer. Inheritance of one mutant allele in these families predisposes a person to a specific form of cancer. Individuals who inherit the germline mutant allele will inevitably suffer loss of the normal allele by loss of heterozygosity (LOH) or epigenetic silencing (see Figure 9-10) in some cells and eventually develop the tumor. Examples of human cancers that can be inherited are retinoblastoma, a childhood cancer of the eye that can be caused by germline mutations in one allele of the *RB* gene; Wilms tumor, a childhood cancer of the kidney *(WT1)*; neurofibromatosis *(NF1)*;

inherited breast cancer *(BRCA1)*; and familial polyposis coli or adenomas of the colon *(APC)*. A specific tumor-suppressor gene has been found in each of these cancers. In many cases, these tumor-suppressor genes also are inactivated in sporadic (as opposed to inherited) cancers. For example, inherited mutations in the *APC* gene are rare and account for only a few percent of all colon cancers. However, 85% of sporadic colon cancers also have acquired mutations of *APC*, which occurred over time in the individual. Characterization of cancer-causing genes and other genetic factors helps identify individuals prone to developing cancer and contributes to our understanding of sporadic cancers. Individuals known to carry mutations in tumor-suppressor genes (for example, women with a germline *BRCA1* mutation) are offered targeted cancer screening to facilitate early cancer detection and therapy.[24]

Types of Genes Misregulated in Cancer

We now understand that a handful of genetic hits are required for the evolution of full-blown cancer. There also are a small number of specific pathways that must be altered in order for cancer to develop. There may be more than one way to alter a pathway, but for each tumor only a single mutation in each pathway is needed. These pathways regulate immortality, cell cycle progression, and apoptosis (Figure 9-12) and will now be described in more detail.[6,25]

Alterations in Progrowth and Antigrowth Signals

Cancer cells must have mutations that enable them to attain self-sufficiency and proliferate in the absence of external growth signals, the phenomenon seen in the laboratory as growth factor independence. To achieve this, some cancers acquire the ability to secrete their own growth factors (for example, platelet-derived growth factor [PDGF]) to stimulate their own growth, a process known as autocrine stimulation (also see Chapter 1). Other cancers have an increase in growth factor receptors, which are often receptor tyrosine kinases. For example, in some breast cancers the epidermal growth factor (EGF) receptor 2 (ERBB2), also known as HER2/neu, is up-regulated and this sends growth signals into the cell even when growth factors are at very low levels. Inhibitors of HER2 and other EGF receptor tyrosine kinases can block this pathway and are effective in treating selected breast and lung cancers.[13] Alternatively, the signal cascade from the cell-surface receptor to the nucleus may be mutated in the "on" position. Up to

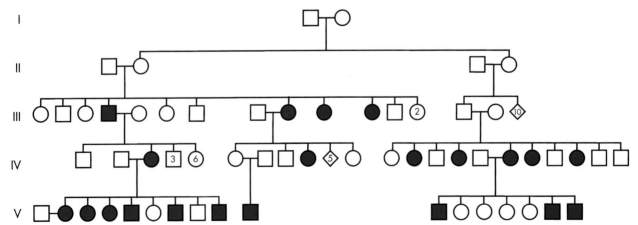

FIGURE 9-11 A Familial Colon Cancer Pedigree. Darkened symbols represent individuals diagnosed with colon cancer. One of the individuals in the first generation must have carried a mutation in the *APC* gene. *Squares,* Males; *circles,* females; *filled circles,* diagnosed with colon cancer. (From Jorde LB et al: *Medical genetics,* ed 3, St Louis, 2003, Mosby.)

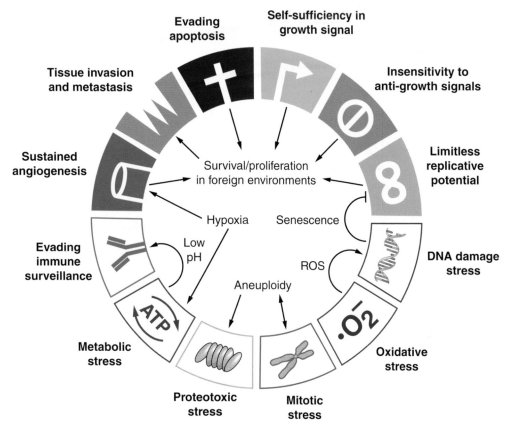

FIGURE 9-12 The Hallmarks of Cancer. Cancers acquire alterations in specific pathways during their evolution. The six key pathways that must be altered are shown at the top of the circle, and supporting pathways are shown at the bottom of the circle. Mutation in key genes often alters several pathways; for example, *p53* mutations alter both angiogenesis and evasion of apoptosis. ⌒ = Inhibits. (From Luo J, Solimini NL, Elledge SJ: Principles of cancer therapy: oncogene and non-oncogene addiction, *Cell* 136:823–837, 2009.)

one third of all cancers have an activating mutation in the gene for an intracellular signaling protein called RAS. This mutant RAS stimulates cell growth even when external growth factors are absent (see Figure 9-7).[26]

Cells also usually receive diverse "antigrowth" signals from their normal milieu. Contact with other cells, with basement membranes, and with soluble factors all normally signal cells to stop proliferating. These mechanisms can halt unregulated cell growth. In addition, this normal antigrowth signal must be inactivated or ignored. Common mutations that subvert the antigrowth signal include inactivation of the tumor-suppressor *retinoblastoma* (RB) or, conversely, activation of the protein kinases that drive the cell cycle, the *cyclin-dependent kinases* (CDKs) (see Chapter 1). Next, cells normally have a mechanism that causes self-destruction when growth is excessive and cell cycle checkpoints have been ignored. This self-destruct mechanism, called apoptosis, is triggered by diverse stimuli, including normal development and excessive growth (see Chapter 3). Advanced cancers develop ways to evade apoptosis. The most common mutations conferring resistance to apoptosis occur in the p53 tumor-suppressor gene *(TP53)*.

Angiogenesis

If cancers are to grow larger than a millimeter in diameter, they need their own blood supply to deliver oxygen and nutrients. However, new blood vessel growth in adults is normally limited to areas of wound healing and to the uterus during the proliferative phase of the menstrual cycle.

Tiny cancers lack the ability to grow new blood vessels and may never grow larger than a grain of sand. More advanced cancers can, however, secrete multiple factors that stimulate new blood vessel growth (called neovascularization or angiogenesis). These angiogenic factors, such as *vascular endothelial growth factor (VEGF)*, *platelet-derived growth factor (PDGF)*, and *basic fibroblast growth factor (bFGF)*, recruit new vascular endothelial cells and initiate the proliferation of existing blood vessel cells, allowing small cancers to become large cancers. Therapies directed against new vessel growth are in clinical use; these agents include bevacizumab, a monoclonal antibody that inhibits VEGF; erlotinib, sorafenib, and sunitinib, inhibitors of the VEGF and PDGF receptor tyrosine kinases; and thalidomide, which decreases vascular proliferation (Figure 9-13).[27]

> ✓ **QUICK CHECK 9-5**
> 1. Distinguish between mutations in somatic cells versus in germ cells.
> 2. What type of cell pathways are altered to cause cancer?
> 3. Why is angiogenesis important to cancer development?

Telomeres and Unlimited Replicative Potential

A hallmark of cancer cells is their immortality. Usually the only cells in the body that are "immortal" are germ cells (those that generate sperm and eggs) and stem cells. Other cells in the body are not immortal and

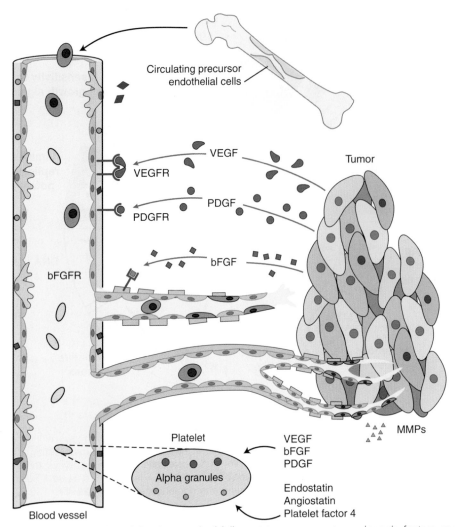

FIGURE 9-13 Tumor-Induced Angiogenesis. Malignant tumors secrete angiogenic factors and tissue-remodeling matrix metalloproteinases *(MMPs)* that actively induce formation of new blood vessels. New blood vessels are formed from both local endothelial cells and circulating precursor cells recruited from the bone marrow. Circulating platelets can also release regulatory proteins into the tumor. *bFGF* and *bFGFR*, Basic fibroblast growth factor and its receptor, respectively; *MMPs*, matrix metalloproteases; *PDGF* and *PDGFR*, platelet-derived growth factor and its receptor, respectively; *VEGF* and *VEGFR*, vascular endothelial growth factor and its receptor, respectively. (Adapted from Folkman J: Angiogenesis: an organizing principle for drug discovery? *Nat Rev Drug Discov* 6[4]:273–286, 2007.)

can divide only a limited number of times (known as the Hayflick limit) before they either cease dividing or die. One major block to unlimited cell division (i.e., immortality) is the size of a specialized structure called the *telomere*. Telomeres are protective ends, or caps, on each chromosome and are placed and maintained by a specialized enzyme called telomerase (Figure 9-14). As one might expect, telomerase is usually active only in germ cells (in ovaries and testes) and in stem cells. All other cells of the body lack telomerase. Therefore, when non–germ cells begin to proliferate abnormally, their telomere caps become smaller and smaller with each cell division. Short telomeres normally signal the cell to cease cell division (senescence). If the telomeres become critically small, the chromosomes become unstable and fragment, and then the cells die. When they reach a critical age, cancer cells somehow activate telomerase to restore and maintain their telomeres, thereby allowing them to continue dividing. Because telomerase is specifically activated in cancer cells, and potentially in cancer stem cells, it is an attractive therapeutic target.[28]

Cancer Metabolism

Cancer cells live in a distinct milieu from normal cells and have different nutritional requirements from nonproliferating cells. The successful cancer cell divides rapidly, with the consequent requirement for the building blocks of new cells. Cancers often must grow in a hypoxic and acidic environment. Cancers also are parasites, able to selectively extract nutrients from the bloodstream without any evolutionary pressure for balanced metabolism. Nonmalignant cells in the presence of adequate oxygen normally generate adenosine triphosphate (ATP) by mitochondrial oxidative phosphorylation (OXPHOS), generating 36 ATP molecules from each glucose molecule that is broken down to water and carbon dioxide. Only in the absence of sufficient oxygen do normal cells perform anaerobic glycolysis, generating only two ATP molecules per molecule of glucose, with lactic acid as a byproduct. However, even in the presence of oxygen, cancer cells perform glycolysis, not OXPHOS[29] (Figure 9-15). Although this aerobic glycolysis was originally postulated to be caused by some form of cancer-specific

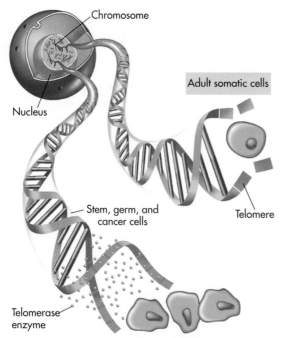

FIGURE 9-14 Control of Immortality: Telomeres and Telomerase
Normal adult somatic cells cannot divide indefinitely because the ends of their chromosomes are capped by telomeres. In the absence of the telomerase enzyme, telomeres become progressively shorter with each division until, when they are critically short, they signal to the cell to stop dividing. In germ cells, adult stem cells, and cancer cells the telomerase gene is "switched on," producing an enzyme that rebuilds the telomeres. Thus, like germ cells, the cancer cell becomes immortal and able to divide indefinitely without losing its telomeres.

mitochondrial dysfunction, it is now apparent that this is instead a highly regulated and beneficial adaptation for cancer cells. This shift from OXPHOS to glycolysis allows lactate and its metabolites to be used for the more efficient production of lipids and other molecular building blocks needed for rapid cell growth. Furthermore, many cancer genes promote this switch to aerobic glycolysis. Alterations in a number of cancer genes, including receptor tyrosine kinases, *AKT*, *PTEN*, *TP53*, and *MYC*, inhibit OXPHOS and promote the activity of glycolytic and related metabolic pathways that support the rapid growth of cancers.[29,30]

Clinically the high glucose utilization of a cancer can be exploited for its detection. ^{18}F-Fluorodeoxyglucose (FDG) is incorporated into cells in the same way as glucose, with two key differences. Because it is missing a key hydroxyl group it cannot be broken down by glycolysis and, thus, FDG accumulates in cells. Because it is tagged with ^{18}F, it can be imaged by positron emission tomography (a PET scan). Small metastatic tumor masses that are consuming huge amounts of glucose can readily be detected with this imaging method (Figure 9-16).

Oncogene Addiction

As described earlier in this chapter, there are a number of common driver mutations in cancer. Cancers that arise because of these mutations often depend on these mutant genes and proteins for their continued growth and survival. If the mutations and abnormal proteins can be returned to their normal states, the cancers often stop growing and even regress. The cancers are addicted to their mutant cancer genes, a concept known as oncogene addiction. This also provides a key example of how targeted cancer therapy can work—for example, if the oncogene is a protein kinase (e.g., BCR-ABL, EGFR, HER2, or BRAF) that can be inhibited by a drug, then the cancer can be deprived of the function of the oncogene. Treating the addiction treats the cancer.[31]

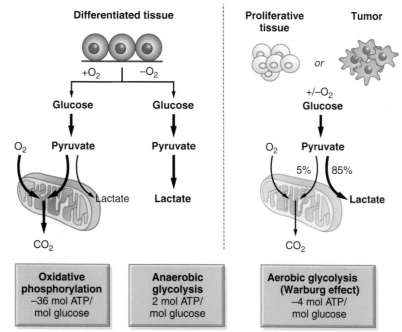

FIGURE 9-15 Cancers Have Altered Metabolism. Normal tissues use oxidative phosphorylation (OXPHOS) to turn glucose into CO_2 and energy (in the form of ATP). Cancers take a different approach; even in the presence of oxygen, they do not use OXPHOS. Instead, they consume large quantities of glucose to make cellular building blocks, supporting rapid proliferation. (From Van der Heiden MG, Cantley LC, Thompson CB: Understanding the Warburg effect: the metabolic requirements of cell proliferation, *Science* 324:1029–1033, 2009.)

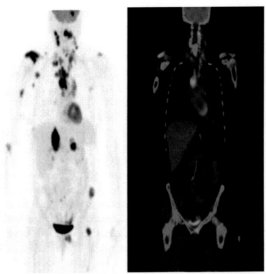

FIGURE 9-16 The Intense Glucose Requirement of Cancer Aids in Diagnosis. This 54-year-old woman had a non–small cell lung cancer (NSCLC) surgically removed. Five years later, these images were obtained. The positron emission tomography (PET) scan using ¹⁸F-deoxyglucose shows metastatic lesions in the brain, right shoulder, and mediastinal and cervical lymph nodes as well as the liver, left pelvis, and proximal femur. *(Left)* PET whole-body image. *(Right)* Representative coronal image from the whole-body FDG-PET/CT–fused image of the same patient. The fused image consists of the CT image with the metabolic information superimposed in color. The pattern of distribution is most likely from the primary tumor to the large mediastinal lymph nodes, followed by lymphatic spread to cervical lymph nodes. Blood-borne dissemination produced the bone, brain, and liver metastases. Normally, only the heart, brain, and bladder show a strong signal on PET scan. *CT,* Computed tomography; *FDG,* fluorodeoxyglucose. (Images courtesy John Hoffman, MD, Huntsman Cancer Institute, Salt Lake City, Utah.)

Cancer Stem Cells

Many tissues, most notably the skin, intestines, and blood-forming cells, continuously renew themselves. The human gut sheds and replaces hundreds of grams of cells each day. This ongoing proliferation of these tissues with a high turnover rate depends on their regeneration from a small fraction of cells known as **adult stem cells.** Adult stem cells have two essential characteristics: first, they self-renew (that is, some fraction of the cell divisions creates new stem cells); second, they are **multipotent,** or have the ability to differentiate into multiple different cell types. In the bone marrow, it is estimated that only 0.05% (1 in 20,000) of the blood-forming cells are stem cells, yet this small pool of stem cells can be stimulated to divide and to repopulate all the mature bone marrow–derived cells in approximately 2 weeks after bone marrow transplantation. As few as 10 stem cells are sufficient to entirely repopulate the entire bone marrow of a mouse in bone marrow transplantation experiments.

Many cancers, like normal tissues, are heterogeneous, with differences in cell shape, size, behavior, and protein expression. There are two models to explain this heterogeneity within tumors. In the clonal evolution model, all the cancer cells divide regularly, and heterogeneity arises from proliferation, mutation, epigenetic changes, differences in local environment, and natural differentiation of cells. In this model, most of these cells are still robust cancer cells, capable of forming complex tumors in experimental animals. In contrast, in the cancer stem cell model, heterogeneity arises because there is a rare cancer stem cell whose offspring do not have stem cell properties, but undergo a limited number of divisions while generating heterogeneity through epigenetic and environmental alterations. However, similar to the adult tissue stem cells, only the cancer stem cell, if transplanted, is postulated to be capable of forming complex and heterogeneous tumors. The typical cancer stem cell experiment separates cancer cells into different pools depending on some measurable characteristic such as cell-surface proteins, and then assays how many cells must be injected into an experimental mouse to form a cancer. In some cases, these tumor-initiating cells are very rare, with only 1 in 10,000 human colon cancer cells able to re-form a complex and heterogeneous colon cancer in mice (Figure 9-17).[32] However,

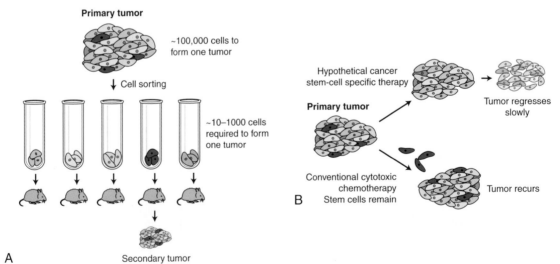

FIGURE 9-17 The Concept of Cancer Stem Cells. (A) Only rare cells within a cancer can initiate cancer regrowth. In laboratory experiments it takes as many as 100,000 breast cancer cells injected into a mouse mammary fat pad to form a new cancer. If the breast cancer cells are sorted, one rare subtype (shown here in red) is much more proficient at forming new cancers. **(B)** Conventional chemotherapy can destroy the bulk of a cancer. However, if the cancer stem cells *(red cells)* are not destroyed, the cancer may regrow. If therapies can be devised that kill the cancer stem cells, then durable long-term responses may be achieved.

these tumor-initiating cells are not always rare; in human melanomas, one in four cells can initiate a complex tumor in the appropriate mouse model.[33] This is an experimentally difficult area of research, because human cancers are examined in mice where there are multiple barriers to transplantation, including immune responses, as well as species differences in the various growth factors, cytokines, and microenvironment that can all influence the results. Therefore most progress is likely to be made by studying cancer stem cells arising in mouse tumors rather than human tumors.

Enthusiasm for the cancer stem cell model arises, in part, from its therapeutic potential. Most of the drugs now used in treating cancer can kill a large fraction of cancer cells but may not touch the cancer stem cell. If less than 1 in 100,000 cells in a cancer is responsible for perpetuating a cancer, then perhaps we should be looking for drugs that target those rare cells instead of using more toxic drugs that initially shrink tumors but do not kill the cancer stem cells.

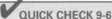

QUICK CHECK 9-6
1. Define telomeres, telomerase, and senescence.
2. What is meant by the clonal evolution model and the stem cell model?
3. Define heterogeneity of tumors.

Stroma-Cancer Interactions

Normal tissues contain a complex mixture of cell types, including specialized cells, fibroblasts, vascular cells, immune cells, and a supporting extracellular matrix. Cancers disrupt this environment, and in turn recruit local and distant cells to assist in cancer progression. Although the immune cells frequently found in tumors were once thought to be futile attempts at an antitumor response, instead it appears that cancers actively recruit an immune and stromal response to assist in remodeling of tissues, formation of new blood vessels, and promotion of metastasis[34] (Figure 9-18). The tumor-associated inflammatory

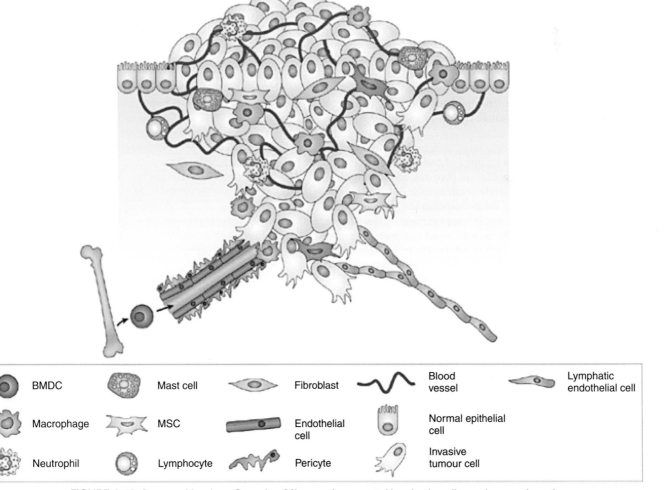

FIGURE 9-18 Cancers Live in a Complex Microenvironment. Neoplastic cells produce angiogenic factors (cytokines and chemokines) that are mitogenic or chemoattractants, or both, for numerous types of stromal cells, including fibroblasts, bone marrow–derived cells *(BMDCs)*, macrophages, mesenchymal stem cells *(MSCs)*, and other inflammatory and immune cells. In return, these activated stroma cells secrete additional proteolytic enzymes and growth factors that stimulate the cancer cells and promote new blood vessel growth. This stromal reaction, which in the normal situation promotes wound healing, now stimulates tumor growth and promotes metastatic dissemination. (From Joyce JA, Pollard JW: Microenvironmental regulation of metastasis, *Nat Rev Cancer* 9:239–252, 2009.)

cells and fibroblasts are stimulated by the cancer cells and the ensuing stromal disruption, and, in turn, these otherwise normal cells secrete a broad range of factors that promote proliferation, angiogenesis, and cancer cell motility. The cancers also may release signals that actively recruit circulating bone marrow–derived mesenchymal stem cells to populate the tumor stroma, subverting a process that normally functions in wound healing.

One of the key cells that promote tumor survival and metastasis is the tumor-associated macrophage, or TAM. These specialized macrophages are recruited to tumors secreting the chemoattractant CSF1. The TAMs in turn secrete factors such as epidermal growth factor (EGF), Wnts, and proteases, further stimulating tumor growth and facilitating tumor invasion of blood vessels. In both animal models and humans, TAMs appear critical for tumor growth and metastasis, and therapies targeting the nonmalignant TAMs are effective at slowing cancer progression.[34,35]

Inflammation, Immunity, and Cancer

Chronic inflammation has been recognized for close to 150 years as being an important factor in the development of cancer.[36] Epidemiologic studies strongly support the conclusion that the active immune response in chronic inflammation predisposes to cancer. Individuals who have suffered with ulcerative colitis for 10 years or more have up to a 30-fold increase in the risk of developing colon cancer. Chronic viral hepatitis caused by hepatitis B virus (HBV) or hepatitis C virus (HCV) infection markedly increases the risk of liver cancer. One large study found a 66% increase in risk of lung cancer among women with chronic asthma, an inflammatory disease of the airways. Table 9-5 details the various inflammatory conditions and infectious agents associated with cancer.

Inflammation and cancer have much in common.[37] In both cancer and inflammation (e.g., after injury and during infection), inflammatory cells, including neutrophils, lymphocytes, and macrophages, migrate to the site of injury and release cytokines and growth and survival factors that stimulate local cell proliferation and new blood vessel growth to promote wound healing by tissue remodeling (see Chapter 5). These factors combine in chronic inflammation to promote continued proliferation. In addition, inflammatory cells release compounds such as reactive oxygen species (ROS) and other reactive molecules that can promote mutations and block the cellular response to DNA damage. Notably, an increased abundance of the enzyme cyclooxygenase-2 (COX-2), which generates prostaglandins during acute inflammation, has been associated with colon and some other cancers. Meta-analysis of multiple clinical studies have concluded that long-term high-dose use of nonsteroidal anti-inflammatory drugs (NSAIDs), such as aspirin, that inhibit COX-2 can reduce the risk of colon cancer by as much as 20% (see Chapter 5).[38]

The Immune System Protects Us Against Viral-Associated Cancers

There is a popular belief that damage to the immune system predisposes to common cancers. This idea arose decades ago as our understanding of the genetic basis of cancer and the details of the immune response against infectious disease developed. Modern data support a more nuanced conclusion. Although the immune system is indeed important in protecting us against cancers caused by specific viral infections (detailed later), it has mixed results when faced with the most common cancers.[39] Individuals taking chronic powerful immunosuppressive drugs, such as those given for kidney, heart, or liver transplant, have a much higher risk of developing viral-associated cancers, with a 10-fold increased risk of non-Hodgkin lymphoma (caused by Epstein-Barr

TABLE 9-5	CHRONIC INFLAMMATORY CONDITIONS AND INFECTIOUS AGENTS ASSOCIATED WITH NEOPLASMS
INFLAMMATORY CONDITION	**ASSOCIATED NEOPLASM(S)**
Asbestosis, silicosis	Mesothelioma, lung carcinoma
Bronchitis	Lung carcinoma
Cystitis, bladder inflammation	Bladder carcinoma
Gingivitis, lichen planus	Oral squamous cell carcinoma
Inflammatory bowel disease, Crohn disease, chronic ulcerative colitis	Colorectal carcinoma
Lichen sclerosus	Vulvar squamous cell carcinoma
Chronic pancreatitis, hereditary pancreatitis	Pancreatic carcinoma
Reflux esophagitis, Barrett esophagus	Esophageal carcinoma
Sialadenitis	Salivary gland carcinoma
Sjögren syndrome, Hashimoto thyroiditis	MALT lymphoma
Skin inflammation	Melanoma
INFECTIOUS AGENT (NONVIRAL)	**ASSOCIATED NEOPLASM(S)**
Helicobacter pylori	Gastric adenocarcinoma, MALT
Chronic bacterial cholecystitis	Gallbladder cancer
Schistosomiasis	Bladder, liver, rectal carcinoma; follicular lymphoma of spleen
Liver flukes	Cholangiocarcinoma
INFECTIOUS AGENT (VIRAL)	**ASSOCIATED NEOPLASM(S)**
Human immunodeficiency virus type 1 (HIV-1)	Non-Hodgkin lymphoma, squamous cell carcinomas, Kaposi sarcoma
Hepatitis B and hepatitis C	Hepatocellular carcinoma
Epstein-Barr virus	B cell non-Hodgkin lymphoma, Burkitt lymphoma, nasopharyngeal carcinoma
KSHV/HHV8 and immunodeficiency	Kaposi sarcoma
HPV-16, -18, -31, others	Cervical, anogenital
HTLV-1	Adult T cell leukemia/lymphoma

From Kuper H, Adami HO, Trichopoulos D: Infections as a major preventable cause of human cancer, *J Intern Med* 248(3):171–183, 2000.

virus) and up to 1000-fold increased risk of Kaposi sarcoma (caused by human herpesvirus 8 [HHV8]) (additional information about viruses and cancer is found under Viral Causes of Cancer). The same immunosuppressed individuals, however, have only a slight increase in the risk of common cancers such as lung and colon cancer (and this could well be because of increased inflammation at those sites).[4,40,41]

In fact, there are many complex interactions between elements of the immune system and tumors (see Figure 9-18). Tumors activate surrounding stromal and inflammatory cells, including tumor-infiltrating lymphocytes and macrophages, to secrete multiple cytokines that support tumor growth and dissemination. In parallel, various cells of the immune system can exert antitumor effects through factors such as tumor necrosis factor (TNF)-related apoptosis-inducing ligand (TRAIL), interleukin-10 (IL-10), and IL-12. The double-edged effects of the immune cells, both promoting and inhibiting proliferation, may explain why it has been so difficult to harness the immune system to fight cancer.

Viral Causes of Cancer

As noted, a number of viruses have been associated with human cancer.[42,43] An even broader spectrum of viruses have been associated with cancer in animals. In humans, *hepatitis B and C viruses (HBV, HCV), Epstein-Barr virus (EBV), Kaposi sarcoma herpesvirus (KSHV)* (also known as *HHV8*), and *human papillomavirus (HPV)* are associated with about 15% of all human cancers worldwide. Cancer of the cervix and hepatocellular carcinoma account for approximately 80% of the cases of virus-linked cancer. The initial infection with hepatitis B or C is not associated with cancer; instead, it is acquisition of a chronic viral hepatitis that markedly increases cancer risk (also see Inflammation, Immunity, and Cancer). Chronic hepatitis B infections are common in parts of Asia and Sub-Saharan Africa and confer up to a 200-fold increased risk of developing liver cancer. Chronic hepatitis C infections have become increasingly recognized in Western countries. Up to 80% of liver cancer cases worldwide are associated with chronic hepatitis caused either by HBV or by HCV. In both cases, it appears that a lifetime of chronic liver inflammation predisposes to the development of hepatocellular carcinoma. Widespread use of the HBV vaccine is expected to significantly decrease the incidence of chronic hepatitis B and hence hepatocellular carcinoma. Unfortunately, a vaccine for HCV is not yet available.

Virtually all cervical cancer is caused by infection with specific subtypes of HPV, which infects basal skin cells and commonly causes warts. There are more than 100 HPV subtypes, but only a few (HPV16, -18, -31, -45, and a few others) are associated with cervical, anogenital, and penile cancer (see Chapters 10 and 32). The initial HPV infection does not cause cancer. HPV only causes cancer when the viral DNA becomes accidentally integrated into the genomic DNA of the infected basal cell of the cervix and directs the persistent production of viral oncogenes. Early oncogenic HPV infection is readily detected by the Papanicolaou (Pap) test, an examination of cervical epithelial scrapings. Early detection of cellular atypia in a Pap test alerts healthcare providers to the possibility of cervical carcinoma in situ, which can be effectively treated. Vaccines protecting against the common oncogenic HPV subtypes were approved for clinical use beginning in 2006; if these vaccines are administered to young women before an initial HPV infection, this is likely to prevent many cases of cervical cancer.[44]

EBV and HHV8 are members of the Herpesviridae family.[42] EBV, the cause of infectious mononucleosis, infects B lymphocytes and stimulates their proliferation. In individuals who are immunosuppressed because of HIV infection or because of drugs given for an organ transplant, persistent EBV infection can lead to the development of B cell lymphomas. Development of B cell lymphomas in persons with organ transplants is known as **post-transplant lymphoproliferative disorder (PTLD)**.[45] One effective therapy for PTLD is, if possible, to decrease or stop the administration of immunosuppressant drugs and allow the immune system to attack the virus. EBV infection also is associated with Burkitt lymphoma in areas of endemic malaria and with nasopharyngeal carcinoma, a cancer endemic in Chinese populations in Southeast Asia.[46] HHV8 is linked to the development of Kaposi sarcoma, a cancer that was once seen primarily in older men but now occurs in a markedly more virulent form in immunocompromised individuals, especially those with acquired immunodeficiency syndrome (AIDS). HHV8 also has been linked to several rare lymphomas.

Human T cell leukemia-lymphoma virus (HTLV) is an oncogenic retrovirus linked to the development of adult T cell leukemia and lymphoma (ATLL).[43] HTLV is transmitted vertically (that is, inherited by children from infected parents) and horizontally (e.g., by breast-feeding, sexual intercourse, blood transfusions, and exposure to infected needles). Infection with HTLV may be asymptomatic, and only a small fraction of infected individuals develop ATLL, often many years after acquiring the virus.

In all of these cases, it is clear that infection by an oncogenic virus is far from sufficient to cause cancer. For example, in some industrialized regions, Epstein-Barr virus can infect 90% of the adolescent and young adult population, yet only a very small percentage of these individuals develop EBV-related cancer. For each of these infections, important cofactors (immunosuppression, cirrhosis, toxins) increase the risk that an infection will develop into cancer.

Bacterial Cause of Cancer

Helicobacter pylori (H. pylori) is a bacterium that infects more than half of the world's population. Chronic infection with *H. pylori* is an important cause of peptic ulcer disease and is strongly associated with gastric carcinoma, a leading cause of cancer deaths worldwide. It is also associated with a less common cancer, gastric mucosa–associated lymphoid tissue (MALT) lymphomas. *H. pylori* infection is often acquired in childhood and disproportionately affects lower socioeconomic classes. Although most infections are asymptomatic, prolonged chronic inflammation can lead to atrophic gastritis that can, in a small fraction of individuals, progress to dysplastic changes and finally frank gastric adenocarcinoma. *H. pylori* infection can both directly and indirectly produce genetic and epigenetic changes in infected stomachs, including mutations in *p53* and alterations in the methylation of specific genes.[47,48] Eradication of *H. pylori* from infected individuals before the development of dysplasia may prevent the development of cancer.[49] However, there is no expert consensus on the value of population screening and treatment strategies. The MALT lymphomas associated with chronic *H. pylori* infections may depend on chronic inflammation and antigenic stimulation associated with infections, and therefore treatment with antibiotics may be useful even in cases of early lymphoma.

> ✔ **QUICK CHECK 9-7**
> 1. Why is the stroma important for cancer growth and invasion?
> 2. Identify cancers that are the result of chronic inflammation.
> 3. Why does inflammation fuel cancer development/invasion?
> 4. Identify common viruses that can cause cancer.

CANCER INVASION AND METASTASIS

Metastasis is the spread of cancer cells from the site of the original tumor to distant tissues and organs through the body. Metastasis is a defining characteristic of cancer, contributes significantly to the pain and suffering from cancer, and is the major cause of death from cancer. Cancer that has not metastasized can often be cured by a combination of surgery, chemotherapy, and radiation. These same therapies are frequently ineffective against cancer that has metastasized. For example, in appropriately treated women with low-stage breast cancer, the 5-year survival rate is often greater than 90%. Tragically, less than 30% of women with metastatic breast cancer are alive 5 years after diagnosis. A growing body of basic and clinical research is defining the biologic principles of metastasis, with the hope that this improved understanding will lead to novel diagnostic approaches and better therapies to prevent and treat metastatic cancers.[50]

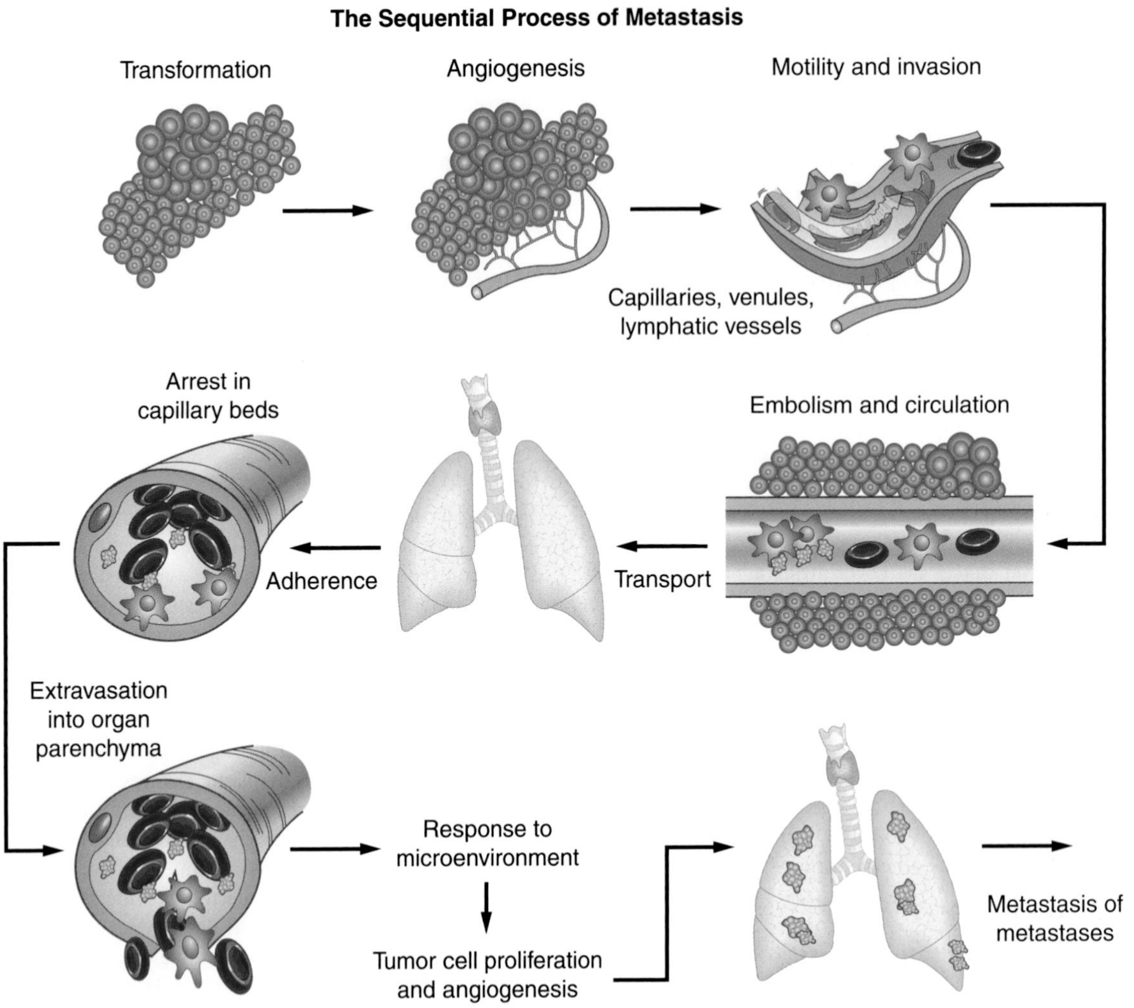

The Sequential Process of Metastasis

FIGURE 9-19 Cancer Metastasis Requires a Complex Series of Events. Cancer cells must gain access to blood and lymphatic vessels, survive the trip to distant locations, move back into the tissues, and initiate a new tumor. Because each of these steps is required, the successful metastatic cell is rare compared with the huge numbers of cancer cells at the primary site. Consequently, metastasis usually only occurs late in cancer evolution. (From Talmadge JE, Fidler IJ: AACR centennial series: the biology of cancer metastasis: historical perspective, *Cancer Res* 70:5649–5669, 2010.)

Invasion, or local spread, is a prerequisite for metastasis and is the first step in the metastatic process. In its earliest stages local invasion may occur by direct tumor extension. Eventually, however, cells migrate away from the primary tumor and invade the surrounding tissues. Mechanisms important in local invasion include recruitment of macrophages and other cell types to the primary tumor, where they promote digestion of connective tissue capsules and other structural barriers by secreted proteases; changes in cell-to-cell adhesion, often by changes in the expression of cell adhesion molecules such as cadherins and integrins, making the cancer cells more slippery and mobile; and increased motility of individual tumor cells[51] (Figure 9-19). To transition from local to distant metastasis, the cancer cells must also be able to invade local blood and lymphatic vessels, a task facilitated by stimulation of neoangiogenesis and lymphangiogenesis by factors such as VEGF. Finally, a successful metastatic cell must be able to survive in the circulation, attach in an appropriate new microenvironment, and multiply to produce an entire new tumor, similar to the characteristics of a cancer stem cell. Different cancers have different patterns of spread, determined by a combination of factors. Cancers often spread first to regional lymph nodes through the lymphatics and then to distant organs through the bloodstream. A cancer's ability to establish a metastatic lesion in a new location requires that the cancer both attach to specific receptors and survive in the specific environment. Because metastasis requires successful completion of each and every step, there may be many opportunities to interrupt this potentially lethal pathway.

Very Few Cells in a Cancer Have the Ability to Metastasize

Metastasis is a highly inefficient process. A landmark clinical review examined a group of women with advanced ovarian cancer.[52] These unfortunate women had accumulated a large amount of peritoneal fluid filled with malignant ovarian cancer cells (malignant ascites). To relieve the pressure caused by the ascites, the fluid was surgically shunted into the venous circulation. This palliative procedure relieved the abdominal pressure but had the side effect of moving billions of ovarian cancer cells an hour directly into the bloodstream. Despite this direct injection of billions of cancer cells into the circulation, these women unexpectedly had no increased number of metastases when they died. The conclusion from this clinical study is that most cancer cells cannot successfully cause metastases, a conclusion that has been supported by many other clinical and laboratory studies. The reason lies both in the seed and in the soil. Cancer cells (the seeds) must surmount multiple physical and physiologic barriers in order to spread, survive, and proliferate in distant locations, and the destination (the soil) must be receptive to the growth of the cancer. It has been suggested that the metastatic cell must, like a decathlon champion, be successful in every event to allow a cancer to spread.

How do cancer cells develop the ability to metastasize? The same heritable changes that occur to cause the primary cancer, including gene mutations, deletions, translocations, epigenetic silencing, and changes in miRNA expression, all work to provide genetic heterogeneity in the tumor cells as they proliferate. As this diversity increases, this increases the number of cells in the cancer mass with new abilities that can facilitate metastasis.

CLINICAL MANIFESTATIONS AND TREATMENT OF CANCER

Clinical Manifestations of Cancer
Diagnosis and Staging
Cancer can be discovered in many ways: after screening tests, from routine exams, and after investigation of symptoms (see *Health Alert: Screening Mammograms: Far from Perfect*). The symptoms a cancer produces are as diverse as the types of cancer. The location of the cancer can determine symptoms by physical pressure, obstruction, and

---

HEALTH ALERT

Screening Mammograms: Far From Perfect

Screening mammograms illustrate many of the difficulties faced by population-based screening tests. The goal of screening tests is early and accurate detection of a treatable disease. We want screening tests not to miss disease (to have a low false-negative rate), but we do not want a lot of false alarms (we want a low false-positive rate). We also do not want to detect as abnormal, conditions that do not need treatment (overdiagnosis). Several large studies suggest that screening mammograms can prevent 15% to 20% of deaths from breast cancer when they are routinely performed in women ages 50 and older. However, these data are confounded by parallel advances in medical care and self-examination and so other studies question how much of the improvement is due to mammography (for example see Autier). Screening mammograms may be valuable in younger women with higher than average risk of breast cancer, for example, those with positive family histories. However, current screening methods remain controversial.

The mammogram is not an ideal screening test. Screening women 50 and older by routine mammography might reduce the relative risk of dying from breast cancer by 15% to 20%, but because most women die of other diseases, the absolute reduction in risk of death from all causes is much lower, as low as 0.05% (i.e., 1 in 2000). Even this calculated benefit from screening mammograms is not reliable. In the combined Canadian National Breast Cancer studies following almost 90,000 women ages 40 to 59, mammography did not decrease deaths from breast cancer when added to routine physical and breast exams. Recent studies continue to provide conflicting data. Screening mammograms also can miss 25% or more of breast cancers (the false-negative rate). In a subset of the same Canadian studies, screening of approximately 32,000 women identified 45 cancers, but missed another 39 that were found clinically within the next 12 months. Screening mammograms also have a remarkably high false-positive rate: in the United States, 9 out of 10 suspicious mammograms interpreted as abnormal (sometimes with computer-aided diagnosis) are eventually determined to be noncancerous. Screening tens of thousands of healthy women annually delivers radiation that,

itself, increases the risk of breast cancer, especially if screening starts at younger ages. In addition, screening mammograms lead to significant **overdiagnosis** and **overtreatment**—they detect DCIS (ductal carcinoma in situ), a condition that might, but often does not, become a malignant disease. The problem with finding DCIS is that because some women with DCIS progress to cancer, once it is found it is usually treated with lumpectomy and radiation therapy. The added unnecessary radiation therapy may cause additional health problems. This accumulation of findings, summarized in a recent Cochrane meta-analysis, found that screening 2000 women over 10 years can prevent 1 breast cancer fatality but at the same time unnecessarily turn 10 healthy women with DCIS into cancer patients. The same authors have generated a fair amount of controversy by concluding: "It is thus not clear whether screening does more good than harm." Women considering screening mammography should be aware that the experts disagree on its value.

What should be recommended? Because the more common the disease the more effective the screening becomes, it makes sense to recommend screening to women 50 and older, especially those with risk factors such as strong family histories of breast and ovarian cancer. Screening has the least benefit and the greatest risks among women younger than age 50 with a negative family history. Based on these data, the United States Preventive Services Task Force recommends that routine screening mammograms should begin at age 50 rather than age 40. Good life-style choices, careful regular breast exams by experienced healthcare providers, and improved analysis of targeted mammograms to reduce false-positive rates might do more to reduce breast cancer deaths than routine screening of the general population. From a public health perspective, the resources allocated to screening mammography might be better spent teaching primary prevention strategies, delivering proven therapies to women without insurance, and performing more research on the root causes and early detection of breast cancer. Women need to understand the limited benefits and the often understated harms of screening mammography to make truly informed choices.

Data from Tabár L, et al: Swedish Two-County Trial: Impact of mammographic screening on breast cancer mortality during 3 decades, *Radiology* (2011). Epub ahead of print; Autier P, et al: Breast cancer mortality in neighbouring European countries with different levels of screening but similar access to treatment: trend analysis of WHO mortality database. *BMJ* 343:d4411, 2011; Miller AB et al: Canadian National Breast Screening Study-2: 13-year results of a randomized trial in women aged 50-59 years, *J Natl Cancer Inst* 92:1490–1499, 2000; Miller AB et al: The Canadian National Breast Screening Study-1: breast cancer mortality after 11 to 16 years of follow-up. A randomized screening trial of mammography in women age 40 to 49 years, *Ann Intern Med* 137:305–312, 2002; Fenton JJ, et al for the Breast Cancer Surveillance Consortium: Effectiveness of computer-aided detection in community mammography practice, *Journal of the National Cancer Institute* pp. 10.1093/jnci/djr206, 2011; Baines CJ, et al: Impact of menstrual phase on false-negative mammograms in the Canadian National Breast Screening Study, *Cancer* 80:720–724, 1997; Elmore JG et al: International variation in screening mammography interpretations in community-based programs, *JNCI, J Natl Cancer Inst* 95:1384, 2003; Berrington de González A, Reeves G: Mammographic screening before age 50 years in the UK: comparison of the radiation risks with the mortality benefits, *Br J Cancer* 93:590–596, 2005; Gøtzsche PC, Nielsen M: Screening for breast cancer with mammography, *Cochrane Database Syst Rev* (Online), CD001877:2006; Fletcher SW, Elmore JG: Clinical practice. Mammographic screening for breast cancer, *N Engl J Med* 348:1672–1680, 2003; Qaseem A, et al: Screening mammography for women 40 to 49 years of age: a clinical practice guideline from the American College of Physicians, *Ann Intern Med* 146:511–515, 2007.

loss of normal function, or a cancer can cause problems far away from its source by pressing on nerves or secreting bioactive compounds. Whatever the initial complaint, once the diagnosis is suspected and a tumor has been identified, it is essential that tumor tissue be obtained to establish a definitive diagnosis and correctly classify the disease. Various methods of obtaining tissue are described in Table 9-6.

Once tissue is obtained, it is examined microscopically by the pathologist for the histologic hallmarks of cancer detailed in the beginning of this chapter. The classification of the cancer can be further facilitated by a variety of clinically available tests, including immunohistochemical stains, flow cytometry, electron microscopy, chromosome analysis, and nucleic acid–based molecular studies.

If the diagnosis of cancer is established, it is critical to determine if the cancer has spread, known as the **stage of the cancer.** Staging

initially involves determining the size of the tumor, the degree to which it has locally invaded, and the extent to which it has spread (metastasized) (Figure 9-20). Specific molecular tests are increasingly used in staging as well. Diverse schemes are used for staging different tumors. In general, a four-stage system is used, with carcinoma in situ regarded as a special case. Cancer confined to the organ of origin is stage 1; cancer that is locally invasive is stage 2; cancer that has spread to regional structures, such as lymph nodes, is stage 3; and cancer that has spread to distant sites, such as a liver cancer spreading to lung or a prostate cancer spreading to bone, is stage 4. One common scheme for standardizing staging is the World Health Organization's TNM system: *T* indicates tumor spread, *N* indicates node involvement, and *M* indicates the presence of distant metastasis (see Figure 9-20). The prognosis generally worsens with increasing tumor size, lymph node involvement, and metastasis. Staging also may alter the choice of therapy, with more aggressive therapy being delivered to more invasive disease.

Paraneoplastic Syndromes

Paraneoplastic syndromes are symptom complexes that are triggered by a cancer but are not caused by direct local effects of the tumor mass. They are most commonly caused by biologic substances released from the tumor (e.g., hormones) or by an immune response triggered by the tumor.[53] For example, a small fraction of carcinoid tumors release hormones, including serotonin, into the bloodstream that cause flushing, diarrhea, wheezing, and rapid heartbeat. A number of cancers trigger an antibody response that attacks the nervous system, causing a variety of neurologic disorders that can precede other symptoms of cancer by months.[54]

Although infrequent, paraneoplastic syndromes are significant because they may be the earliest symptom of an unknown cancer and, in affected individuals, can be serious, often irreversible, and sometimes life-threatening. Table 9-7 presents the classifications of paraneoplastic syndromes.

TABLE 9-6	OBTAINING TISSUE— THE BIOPSY	
PROCEDURE	**PURPOSE**	**EXAMPLE**
Excisional biopsy	Complete removal, usually with margin of normal tissue	Full resection (e.g., mastectomy, partial colectomy)
Incisional biopsy	Removal of portion of lesion	Lymph node biopsy, muscle mass biopsy
Core needle biopsy	Often performed with direct vision, or guided with ultrasound or CT	Needle biopsy of prostate or liver mass
Fine needle aspirate	Obtains dissociated cells for cytologic study but does not preserve tissue structure	Thyroid, breast mass
Exfoliative cytology	Cells shed from surface (e.g., from cervix, sputum [lung], or urine)	Brushings from lung or colon endoscopy

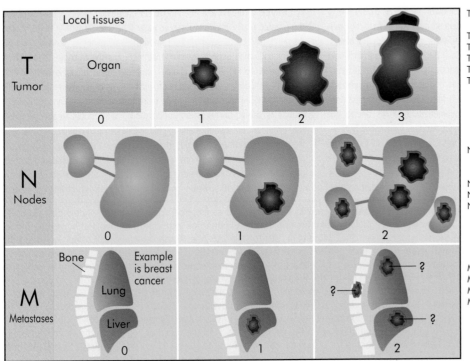

FIGURE 9-20 Tumor Staging by the TNM System. Example of staging for breast cancer. (See figure for explanation of the abbreviations.)

TABLE 9-7   PARANEOPLASTIC SYNDROMES

CLINICAL SYNDROMES	MAJOR FORMS OF UNDERLYING CANCER	CAUSAL MECHANISM
Endocrinopathies		
Cushing syndrome	Small cell carcinoma of lung	ACTH or ACTH-like substance
	Pancreatic carcinoma	
	Neural tumors	
Syndrome of inappropriate antidiuretic hormone (SIAH) secretion	Small cell carcinoma of lung; intracranial neoplasms	Antidiuretic hormone or atrial natriuretic hormones
Hypercalcemia	Squamous cell carcinoma of lung	PTHRP, TGF-α, TNF, IL-1
	Breast carcinoma	
	Renal carcinoma	
	Adult T cell leukemia/lymphoma	
	Ovarian carcinoma	
Hypoglycemia	Fibrosarcoma	Insulin or insulin-like substance
	Other mesenchymal sarcomas	
	Hepatocellular carcinoma	
Carcinoid syndrome	Bronchial adenoma (carcinoid)	Serotonin, bradykinin
	Pancreatic carcinoma	
	Gastric carcinoma	
Polycythemia	Renal carcinoma	Erythropoietin
	Cerebellar hemangioma	
	Hepatocellular carcinoma	
Nerve and Muscle Syndromes		
Myasthenia	Bronchogenic carcinoma	Immunologic
Disorders of central and peripheral nervous systems	Breast carcinoma	
Dermatologic Disorders		
Acanthosis nigricans	Gastric carcinoma	Immunologic; secretion of epidermal growth factor
	Lung carcinoma	
	Uterine carcinoma	
Dermatomyositis	Bronchogenic, breast carcinoma	Immunologic
Osseous, Articular, and Soft Tissue Changes		
Hypertrophic osteoarthropathy and clubbing of fingers	Bronchogenic carcinoma	Unknown
Vascular and Hematologic Changes		
Venous thrombosis (Trousseau phenomenon)	Pancreatic carcinoma	Tumor products (mucins that activate clotting)
	Bronchogenic carcinoma	
	Other cancers	
Nonbacterial thrombotic endocarditis	Advanced cancers	Hypercoagulability
Anemia	Thymic neoplasms	Unknown
Others		
Nephrotic syndrome	Various cancers	Tumor antigens, immune complexes

From Kumar V, Abbas AK, Fausto N: *Pathologic basis of disease*, ed 7, Philadelphia, 2005, Saunders.
ACTH, Adrenocorticotropic hormone; *IL*, interleukin; *PTHRP*, parathyroid hormone–related protein *TGF*, transforming growth factor; *TNF*, tumor necrosis factor.

Pain

Pain is one of the most feared complications of advanced cancer. Although pain can be one of the presenting symptoms of cancer, most commonly there is little or no pain during the early stages of malignant disease. Significant pain, however, occurs in a large fraction of those individuals who are terminally ill with cancer. Pain is strongly influenced by fear, anxiety, sleep loss, fatigue, and overall physical deterioration. It occurs through an interaction among physiologic, cultural, and psychologic components. (The neurophysiology of pain is discussed in Chapter 13.)

Cancer-associated pain can arise from a variety of direct and indirect mechanisms. Direct pressure, obstruction, invasion of a sensitive structure, stretching of visceral surfaces, tissue destruction, infection, and inflammation all can cause pain. Pain can occur at the site of the primary tumor or can result from a distant metastatic lesion. Furthermore, pain may be referred away from the involved site and manifest, for example, as back pain.

Specific sites are more prone to cancer-associated pain. Bone metastases, common in advanced breast and prostate cancer, can cause significant pain because of periosteal irritation, medullary pressure, vertebral collapse, and pathologic fractures. Brain tumors (primary or metastatic) can, depending on the location, cause headache, seizures, or neurologic deficits. Pain in the abdomen may be caused by bowel obstruction, or inflammation and infection. Hepatic malignancies can stretch the liver, resulting in a dull pain or a feeling of fullness over the right upper abdominal quadrant. Mucosal surfaces can develop painful ulcerative lesions from the cancer, chemotherapy, and radiation or leukopenia (or both).

The diagnosis and treatment of pain is one of the primary responsibilities of the medical team. The individual's perception and, hence, reporting of pain can vary widely and be affected by such factors as age and cultural background. The first priority of treatment is to control pain rapidly and completely as judged by the individual. The second priority is to prevent recurrence of pain. Objective measurements of pain are increasingly being included along with the reporting of more traditional vital signs. Many institutions are using specialized pain management teams that are trained to recognize different types of acute and chronic pain, as well as the individual's response to that pain. Many modalities are available to treat pain, ranging from combinations of NSAIDs and narcotics to palliative surgery and radiation therapy. Individual-controlled analgesia provides many benefits, not the least of which is regaining some control over one's own body. Although cancer pain is a complex problem arising from multiple sources, individuals should be assured that suffering is not inevitable and that relief is attainable.[55]

Fatigue

Fatigue is the most frequently reported symptom of cancer and cancer treatment. The exact mechanisms that produce fatigue are poorly understood.[56] Suggested causes include sleep disturbances, various biochemical changes secondary to disease and treatment, numerous psychosocial factors, level of activity, nutritional status, and other environmental and physical factors.[57]

The physiologic understanding of fatigue probably includes mechanisms for decreased muscle contractility. Overall, studies of muscle function suggest that some individuals with cancer may lose portions of muscle function needed to perform normal physical activities. Other areas of research include muscle function consequences from metabolic products of cancer treatment and associated muscle loss from circulating cytokines (e.g., tumor necrosis factor [TNF] and interleukin-1 [IL-1]). Similar to pain, fatigue is a subjective clinical manifestation. Fatigue is described by individuals with cancer as tiredness, weakness, lack of energy, exhaustion, lethargy, inability to concentrate, depression, sleepiness, boredom, lack of motivation, and decreased mental status. Some of these symptoms have been termed "chemo brain," or mild cognitive impairment. The changes in cognitive function can be caused by the cancer itself or by the stress associated with the diagnosis of cancer, however, because symptoms similar to "chemo brain" also occur in individuals who have not received chemotherapy.[58]

Cachexia

The syndrome of cachexia includes a constellation of symptoms including anorexia, early satiety (filling), weight loss, anemia, asthenia (marked weakness), taste alterations, and altered protein, lipid, and carbohydrate metabolism (Figure 9-21). Cachexia is the most severe form of malnutrition associated with cancer and results in wasting, emaciation, and decreased quality of life.[59] Cachexia occurs even with seemingly adequate caloric intake because metabolic disturbances,

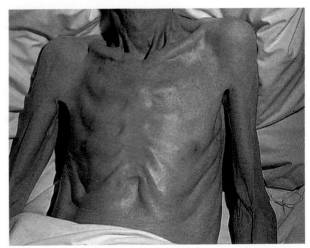

FIGURE 9-21 Cachexia. This severe form of malnutrition results in wasting and extensive loss of adipose tissue. (From Kamal A, Brockelhurst JC: *Color atlas of geriatric medicine,* ed 2, St Louis, 1991, Mosby.)

including insulin resistance, hypertriglyceridemia, muscle wasting, and general increased derangement of metabolism, lead to significant inefficiency of energy usage. Anorexia, or loss of appetite, frequently worsens the weight loss associated with this abnormal metabolic state. Anorexia itself can be caused by pain, depression, chemotherapy, and/or radiotherapy. Alterations in taste, making foods seem bland or distasteful, by these same causes also can account for the anorexia present in individuals with cancer.

Altered carbohydrate metabolism causes a syndrome resembling diabetes mellitus. Individuals show hyperinsulinemia, insulin resistance, hyperglycemia, and abnormal glucose tolerance test results. These disturbances cause increased gluconeogenesis, which produces glucose from amino acids. In starvation, protein usually is spared to protect vital structures; however, in cancer, protein and fatty acids are used to meet energy needs.

An unusual and frustrating component of cancer care is the person's early satiety, or a sense of being full after only a few mouthfuls of food. Cytokines, including TNF-α, IL-6, and interferon-γ, appear to cause the metabolic alterations associated with tissue loss in cancer wasting. Tumor metabolites may also contribute to a cachectic state. For example, a factor found in the urine of some individuals with cancer induces the catabolism of muscle. This factor, originally called proteolysis-inducing factor, is a partial fragment of an antimicrobial peptide, dermcidin, normally expressed in the skin.[60] (Cytokines are discussed in detail in Chapter 6.)

Anemia

Anemia is commonly associated with malignancy, with 20% of persons diagnosed with cancer having hemoglobin concentrations less than 9 g/dl (normal value = 15 g/dl). Mechanisms that cause anemia in persons with cancer include chronic bleeding (resulting in iron deficiency), severe malnutrition, cytotoxic chemotherapy, and malignancy in blood-forming organs. Chronic bleeding and iron deficiency can accompany colorectal or genitourinary malignancy. Iron also is malabsorbed in persons with gastric, pancreatic, or upper intestinal cancer. Often there is a defect in the reutilization of iron because of lack of transfer of iron from the storage pool to blood cell precursors. This defect may be caused by increased secretion of IL-6 and hepcidin.[61] Defects in erythropoietin production and shortened duration of red cell survival have also been documented. In addition, anorexia can cause both iron and folate deficiency. Megaloblastic (large red cell) anemias also may develop after methotrexate treatment.

Administration of erythropoietin, which stimulates production of erythrocytes, has been effective in correcting anemia in persons with cancer; fewer red blood cell transfusions were required in most of the studied subjects. In addition, anemias occurring after chemotherapy or radiotherapy have been treated successfully with erythropoietin. However, recent studies have shown that aggressive use of erythropoietin increases the risk of blood clots and can decrease cancer survival.[62,63]

Leukopenia and Thrombocytopenia

Direct tumor invasion of the bone marrow causes both leukopenia (a decreased total white blood cell count) and thrombocytopenia (a decreased number of platelets). More commonly, many chemotherapeutic drugs are toxic to the bone marrow, often causing granulocytopenia and thrombocytopenia. Granulocytopenia also can result from radiation therapy if it encompasses significant areas of the bone marrow. The duration of granulocytopenia and hence the risk of serious infection can be lessened by treatment with recombinant human granulocyte colony-stimulating factor (rhG-CSF, filgrastim).[64] rhG-CSF stimulates white blood cell precursors in the marrow to proliferate and differentiate rapidly. Thrombocytopenia is a major cause of hemorrhage in persons with cancer and is often treated with platelet transfusions. Thrombocytopenia also is an accompanying disorder of disseminated intravascular coagulation that occurs in persons with acute promyelocytic leukemia (see Chapter 20) and severe infections.

Infection

Infection is the most significant cause of complications and death in persons with malignant disease. When the absolute granulocyte count falls below 500 cells per microliter, the risk of serious microbial (bacterial and fungal) infection increases. Persons with cancer also have debility with advanced disease, and immunosuppression from the underlying cancer and the radiotherapy and chemotherapy used to treat it. (Factors that predispose persons with cancer to infection are summarized in Table 9-8.) Surgery also can lower resistance to infection because removal of large quantities of tissue, together with hemorrhage, dead spaces, and poor tissue perfusion, can create favorable sites for infection. Hospital-related (nosocomial) infections increase because of indwelling medical devices, inadequate wound care, and the introduction of microorganisms from visitors and other individuals.

TABLE 9-8 FACTORS PREDISPOSING INDIVIDUALS WITH CANCER TO INFECTION

FACTOR	BASIS
Age	Many common malignancies occur mostly in older age.
	Immunologic functions decline with age.
	General debility reduces immunocompetence.
	Immobility predisposes to infection.
	Far-advanced cancer often results in immobility and general debility that worsens with age.
	Elderly persons are predisposed to nutritional inadequacies.
	Malnutrition impairs immunocompetence.
Tumor	Nutritional derangements can result.
	Sites and circumstances favorable to growth of microorganisms (obstruction, serous or blood effusion, ulceration) can be created.
	Far-advanced disease predisposes individuals to debility and immobility.
	Humoral or cellular immune defects may result.
	Metastasis to bone marrow may cause leukopenia or other defects in immunity.
Leukemias	Inadequate granulocyte production (impaired phagocytosis) results.
	Thrombocytopenia (bleeding, breaks in skin integrity) can occur.
	Late effect: Chronic lung disease from *Pneumocystis carinii* pneumonia can develop during therapy.
Lymphomas and other mononuclear phagocyte malignancies	Humoral and cellular immune defects (anergy, altered immunoglobulin production) result.
	Late effect: Splenectomy in children can cause increased susceptibility to infection.
Surgical treatment	Invasive procedure interrupts first lines of defense.
	Radical nature of surgery (removal of large blocks of tissue in lengthy procedures) causes hemorrhage, decreased tissue perfusion, creation of dead spaces, devitalization of tissues.
	Procedure may be "dirty" surgery (bowel, infected or contaminated areas).
	Surgery patients are often older and at poor risk.
	Long preoperative hospitalization often precedes surgery.
	Patients may have received previous adrenocorticosteroid therapy.
	Patients may have infections at sites remote from operative area.
	Nutritional derangements (especially important in head and neck surgery) may result.
	Lymph node dissection may predispose patient to local infection and impair containment to area.
	Gynecologic surgery may result in fistulae.
	Lung surgery may cause bronchopleural fistulae.
	Debility and immobility may result.

Data from Donovan MI, Girton SF: *Cancer care nursing,* ed 2, New York, 1984, Appleton-Century-Crofts; Murphy GP, Lawrence W, Lenhard RE: *Clinical oncology,* ed 2, New York, 1994, American Cancer Society.

Gastrointestinal Tract

The entire gastrointestinal (GI) tract relies on rapidly growing cells to produce an effective barrier to trauma and infection and to provide an absorptive surface for nutrients. Both chemotherapy and radiation therapy may cause a decreased cell turnover, thereby leading to oral ulcers (stomatitis), malabsorption, and diarrhea. The disruption of barrier defenses also increases the risk for infection, especially invasion by a person's own GI flora. Therapy-induced nausea, thought to be caused by an agent's direct action upon the central nervous system's vomiting centers, historically has been a major obstacle in therapy.

Aggressive antinausea (antiemetic) therapy, including the centrally acting serotonin 5-hydroxytryptamine (5-HT3) antagonists (such as ondansetron or dolasetron), has allowed better tolerance of highly emetogenic protocols. Other popular antiemetics include steroids and phenothiazines. Synthetic cannabinoids, the active ingredients in marijuana, increase appetite in addition to having antinausea properties. Analgesia often includes opiate agents, vital in treating severe cases of mucosal lesions. Supplemental nutrition through enteral or parenteral routes may be needed to combat malnutrition. Good oral hygiene may help prevent complications arising from mucosal membrane breakdown.

Hair and Skin

Alopecia (hair loss) results from chemotherapy effects on hair follicles. Alopecia is usually temporary, although hair may regrow with a different texture initially. Not all chemotherapeutic agents cause alopecia. Decreased renewal rates of the epidermal layers in the skin may lead to skin breakdown and dryness, altering the normal barrier protection against infection. Radiation therapy may cause skin erythema (redness) and contribute to breakdown.

Treatment of Cancer

The diagnosis of cancer has a profound effect on individuals and their families. Responses range from depression to resigned fatalism to an aggressive no-holds-barred pursuit of therapy. The choice of therapy should be based on full consideration by the individual, the family, and the medical team of the individual's diagnosis, prognosis, and therapeutic options. Many types of cancer can be effectively treated with chemotherapy, radiotherapy, surgery, and combinations of these modalities. Caregivers must recognize that many individuals seek additional nonscience-based explanations and therapies and often use alternative therapies, either concurrently or sequentially. Alternative therapies can be biologically harmless or harmful; rarely is there any evidence these approaches are medically effective and in the worst cases they can be expensive, delay the use of effective therapies, and produce toxic side effects. A challenge for the medical team is to provide the same level of psychosocial comfort and support that alternative therapies can provide, while also providing scientifically rational evidence-based therapies.

Chemotherapy

The era of modern chemotherapy began with the observation in World War II that mustard gas exposure caused suppression of the bone marrow. Related compounds, such as nitrogen mustard and cyclophosphamide, were then tested and produced clinical responses in hematologic malignancies, including lymphomas. Also in the late 1940s, based on the remarkable clinical observation that the vitamin folic acid could *increase* leukemia growth, antifolate drugs were developed (leading ultimately to methotrexate) that produced remissions in previously untreatable leukemias.[65]

All chemotherapeutic agents take advantage of specific vulnerabilities in target cancer cells. Antimetabolites, such as methotrexate and L-asparaginase, block normal growth pathways in all cells, but leukemia and other cancer cells are exquisitely sensitive to folic acid and asparagine deprivation, whereas nonmalignant cells are far less sensitive. Similarly, some cancer cells are highly sensitive to DNA-damaging agents, such as cyclophosphamide and anthracyclines, because of the oncogenic mutations that accelerate the cell cycle and DNA synthesis. Cellular checkpoints prevent normal cells treated with microtubule-directed drugs, such as vincristine and the taxanes, from undergoing mitosis, whereas cancer cells treated with these agents lack normal checkpoints, continue through mitosis, and undergo mitotic catastrophe (see Chapter 1).

Single chemotherapeutic agents often shrink cancers, but these drugs given alone rarely, if ever, provide a cure. Hence, chemotherapy drugs are usually given in combinations designed to attack a cancer from many different weaknesses at the same time and to limit the dose and therefore the toxicity of any single agent. Cancers contain a very large number of cells, and commonly a small fraction of those cells may be resistant to a particular drug. However, those cells are likely to be sensitive to the second or third drug in a chemotherapy cocktail. Scheduling of drug administration is also very important, with many studies showing cancers are more likely to develop drug resistance if there are significant delays between planned courses of chemotherapy.

The newest highly targeted agents used to treat cancer exploit specific vulnerabilities uncovered by molecular analysis in specific diseases (Table 9-9). These new drugs are still used in combination with conventional chemotherapy and to be effective they must be used in diseases in which the molecular target is present. For example, imatinib is highly effect in treating CML and gastrointestinal stromal tumor (GIST) but ineffective in virtually all other cancers. Fortunately, because these drugs are so tightly targeted they have much less toxicity than conventional chemotherapies that have targets in virtually all cells.

Chemotherapy can be used for several distinct purposes. Induction chemotherapy seeks to cause shrinkage or disappearance of tumors. In Hodgkin disease, for example, chemotherapy alone can be used in some cases to cure the disease. In other settings, chemotherapy may shrink the tumor and improve symptoms without ultimately providing a cure. Adjuvant chemotherapy is given after surgical excision of

TABLE 9-9 EXAMPLES OF MOLECULAR-ERA ANTICANCER DRUGS

DRUG (TRADE NAME)	TYPE OF DRUG	MOLECULAR TARGET	DISEASE
Imatinib (Gleevec)	Small molecule TKI	BCR-ABL tyrosine kinase, FGF receptor tyrosine kinase	Chronic myeloid leukemia (CML), gastrointestinal stromal tumor (GIST)
Erlotinib (Tarceva)	Small molecule TKI	EGF receptor tyrosine kinase	Subset of lung cancer
Trastuzumab (Herceptin)	Monoclonal antibody	HER2 receptor tyrosine kinase	HER2-positive breast cancer
Bevacizumab (Avastin)	Monoclonal antibody	VEGF receptor	Advanced colorectal cancer
Rituximab	Monoclonal antibody	CD20 antigen on B lymphocytes	B cell malignancies

EGF, Endothelial growth factor; *FGF*, fibroblast growth factor; *HER2*, human epidermal growth factor receptor 2; *TKI*, tyrosine kinase inhibitor; *VEGF*, vascular endothelial growth factor.

a cancer with the goal of eliminating micrometastases. Neoadjuvant chemotherapy is given before localized (surgical or radiation) treatment of a cancer. As with induction chemotherapy, the effectiveness, or lack thereof, of neoadjuvant therapy can be measured (for example, with follow-up scans). Neoadjuvant therapy can shrink a cancer so that surgery may spare more normal tissue. For example, in the bone cancer *osteogenic sarcoma*, neoadjuvant therapy often converts a large tumor mass into a much smaller mass, allowing the surgeon to perform a limb-sparing excision rather than an amputation.

Radiation Therapy

Radiation therapy is used to kill cancer cells while minimizing damage to normal structures. Ionizing radiation damages cells by imparting enough energy to cause molecular damage, especially to DNA. The damage may be lethal, in which the cell is killed by radiation; potentially lethal, in which the cell is so severely affected by radiation that modifications in its environment will cause it to die; or sublethal, in which the cell can subsequently repair itself. Cellular compartments with rapidly renewing cells are, in general, more radiosensitive. Effective cell killing by radiation also requires good local delivery of oxygen, something not always present in large cancers. Radiation produces slow changes in most cancers and irreversible changes in normal tissues as well. Because of these irreversible changes, each tissue has a maximum lifetime dose of radiation it can tolerate. Radiation is well suited to treat localized disease in areas that are hard to reach surgically, for example, in the brain and pelvis. A number of radiation delivery methods are available, with external beam being the most common. Radiation sources, such as small ^{125}I-labeled capsules (also called seeds), can also be temporarily placed into body cavities, a delivery method termed brachytherapy. Brachytherapy is useful in the treatment of cervical, prostate, and head and neck cancers.

Surgery

Surgery plays many roles in the care of individuals with cancer. The multiple approaches to obtaining tissue for diagnosis have been discussed. Surgery is often the definitive treatment of cancers that do not spread beyond the limits of surgical excision. It is also indicated for the relief of symptoms, for instance, those caused by tumor mass obstruction. In selected high-risk diseases, surgery plays a role in the prevention of cancer. For example, individuals with familial adenomatous polyposis because of germline mutations of the *APC* gene have close to a 100% lifetime risk of colon cancer, so a prophylactic colectomy is indicated. Similarly, women with *BRCA1/2* mutations have a markedly increased risk of breast and ovarian cancer, and often choose prophylactic mastectomy or bilateral salpingo-oophorectomy (removal of ovaries and fallopian tubes), or both.[66]

Key principles apply specifically to cancer surgery, including obtaining adequate surgical margins during a resection to prevent local recurrences, placing needle tracks and biopsy incision scars (that may be contaminated with cancer cells) carefully so they can be removed in subsequent incisions, avoiding the spread of cancer cells during surgical procedures through careful technique, and paying attention to obtaining adequate tissue specimens during biopsies so that the pathologist can be confident of the diagnosis. Additionally, the surgeon provides critical staging information by inspection, sampling, and removal of local and region lymph nodes during procedures.

> ✔ **QUICK CHECK 9-8**
> 1. Define local spread and metastasis.
> 2. Describe the major clinical manifestations of cancer.
> 3. What are the most common treatments of cancer?

DID YOU UNDERSTAND?

Cancer Terminology and Characteristics

1. Benign tumors are usually encapsulated and well differentiated and do not spread to distant locations.
2. Malignant tumors, compared with benign tumors, have more rapid growth rates, specific microscopic alterations (anaplasia, loss of differentiation), absence of normal tissue organization, and no capsule; they invade blood vessels and lymphatics and have distant metastases.
3. Carcinomas arise from epithelial tissue, and leukemias are cancers of blood-forming cells. CIS refers to noninvasive epithelial tumors of glandular or squamous cell origin. Localized cancer is considered low stage, whereas cancers that have spread regionally or distantly are termed *stage 3* and *stage 4*, respectively.
4. The classification, and hence the treatment decisions, of cancers was originally based on gross and light microscopic appearance, and is now commonly accompanied by immunohistochemical analysis of protein expression. Increasingly, this is supplemented by a more extensive molecular analysis of the tumors.
5. Tumor markers are substances (i.e., hormones, enzymes, genes, antigens, antibodies) found in cancer cells and in blood, spinal fluid, or urine. They are used to screen and identify individuals at high risk for cancer, to help diagnose specific types of tumors, and to follow the clinical course of cancer.

The Biology of Cancer Cells

1. Cancer cell behavior is a major topic of laboratory study. Based on these studies cancer cells are identified as transformed cells and lack contact inhibition. Cancer cells are described as anchorage independent; that is, they continue to divide even when suspended in a petri dish.
2. Cancer cells are immortal.
3. Genetic events are the primary basis of carcinogenesis. The stepwise accumulation of a small set of changes in the deoxyribonucleic acid (DNA) and chromosomes of the cancer cell cause it to become cancerous.
4. Heritable changes in cells can contribute to cancer. These changes include small and large DNA mutations that alter genes, chromosomes, and non–coding RNAs, as well as epigenetic changes because of altered chemical modifications of DNA and histones.
5. The incidence of cancer increases with age. An explanation for this increase is the individual acquires a number of genetic hits or mutations with time. Mutations activate growth-promotion pathways, block antigrowth signals, prevent apoptosis, stimulate telomerase and new blood vessel growth, and allow tissue invasion and distant metastasis.
6. From sophisticated molecular analyses it has been determined that some mutations are more important for cancer progression. These mutations can be called driver mutations. Passenger mutations are random mutations that presumably do not contribute to cancer progression.
7. Key genetic mechanisms have a role in human carcinogenesis: (a) activation of proto-oncogenes, resulting in hyperactivity of growth-related gene products (such genes are called *oncogenes*); (b) mutation of genes, resulting in loss or inactivity of gene products that normally would inhibit growth (such genes are called *tumor-suppressor genes*); and (c) mutation of caretaker genes that normally prevent mutations.
8. Caretaker genes are responsible for maintaining genomic integrity. Inherited mutations can disrupt caretaker genes and cause chromosome instability.

DID YOU UNDERSTAND?—cont'd

9. Because each person has two chromosomes, one from each parent, a person is always *heterozygous* for nearby multiple genetic markers; loss of one copy (allele) of a specific chromosome region in a tumor is referred to as loss of heterozygosity, or LOH.

10. Abnormal gene silencing is emerging as a major factor in cancer progression. Gene expression can be regulated in a heritable manner (i.e., passed from a parent to a child or from a single cell to its progeny) by an "epigenetic" mechanism called silencing. Inheritance occurs during cell division and does not require mutations or changes in DNA sequence.

11. Changes in gene regulation can affect not just single genes, but entire networks of signaling. Gene expression networks can be regulated by changes in microRNAs (miRNAs or miRs) and other non–coding RNAs (ncRNAs).

12. Most of the genetic and epigenetic alterations that cause cancer occur within the somatic tissues during the lifetime of the individual.

13. In rare families, cancer is inherited in an autosomal dominant fashion as a result of mutations in tumor-suppressor genes such as *p53, RB,* and *BRCA1.*

14. Like many normal adult tissues, cancers can contain rare stem cells. To fully eradicate a cancer, it may be necessary to target the cancer stem cell.

15. Advanced cancers can secrete multiple factors that stimulate new blood vessel growth (called neovascularization or angiogenesis). Active inflammation predisposes to cancer by stimulating a wound-healing response that includes proliferation and new blood vessel growth.

16. When they reach a critical age, cancer cells somehow activate telomerase to restore and maintain their telomeres, thereby allowing cancer cells to divide repeatedly or become immortal.

17. The successful cancer cell divides rapidly, with the consequent requirement for the building blocks of new cells; cancer cell division often occurs in a hypoxic and acidic environment. Many cancer genes also encourage aerobic glycolysis and promote high glucose utilization of a cancer.

18. Stroma-cancer interactions actively recruit an immune and stromal response to assist in remodeling of tissues, formation of new blood vessels, and promotion of metastasis.

19. In both cancer and inflammation (e.g., after injury and during infection), inflammatory cells, including neutrophils, lymphocytes, and macrophages, migrate to the site of injury and release cytokines and growth and survival factors that stimulate local cell proliferation and new blood vessel growth to promote wound healing by tissue remodeling. These factors combine in chronic inflammation to promote continued proliferation.

20. Defects in the immune system increase the risk of viral-associated cancers but have a minimal effect on the risk of other cancers.

Cancer Invasion and Metastasis

1. Metastasis is the major cause of death from cancer.

2. Metastasis is a complex process that requires cells to have many new abilities, including the ability to invade, survive, and proliferate in a new environment.

Clinical Manifestations and Treatment of Cancer

1. The diagnosis of cancer requires a biopsy and examination of tumor tissue by a pathologist. Cancer classification is established by a variety of tests.

2. Tumor staging involves the size of the tumor, the degree to which it has locally invaded, and the extent to which it has spread. A standard scheme for staging is the T (tumor spread), N (node involvement), and M (metastasis) system.

3. Paraneoplastic syndromes are rare symptom complexes, often caused by biologically active substances released from a tumor or by an immune response triggered by a tumor, that manifest as symptoms not directly caused by the local effects of the cancer.

4. Clinical manifestations of cancer include pain, cachexia, anemia, leukopenia, thrombocytopenia, and infection.

5. Pain is generally associated with the late stages of cancer. It can be caused by pressure, obstruction, invasion of a structure sensitive to pain, stretching, tissue destruction, and inflammation.

6. Fatigue is the most frequently reported symptom of cancer and cancer treatment.

7. Cachexia (loss of appetite, early satiety, weakness, inability to maintain weight, taste alterations, altered metabolism) leads to protein-calorie malnutrition and progressive wasting.

8. Anemia associated with cancer usually occurs because of malnutrition, chronic bleeding and resultant iron deficiency, chemotherapy, radiation, and malignancies in the blood-forming organs.

9. Leukopenia is usually a result of chemotherapy (which is toxic to bone marrow) or radiation (which kills circulating leukocytes).

10. Thrombocytopenia is usually the result of chemotherapy or malignancy in the bone marrow.

11. Infection may be caused by leukopenia, immunosuppression, or debility associated with advanced disease. It is the most significant cause of complications and death.

12. The gastrointestinal tract relies on rapidly growing cells to provide an absorptive surface for nutrients. Both chemotherapy and radiation therapy may cause decreased cell turnover, thereby leading to oral ulcers (stomatitis), malabsorption, and diarrhea.

13. Alopecia (hair loss) results from chemotherapy effects on hair follicles. Alopecia is usually temporary, although hair may initially regrow with a different texture. Not all chemotherapeutic agents cause alopecia. Decreased renewal rates of the epidermal layers in the skin may lead to skin breakdown and dryness, altering the normal barrier protection against infection.

14. Cancer is treated with surgery, radiation therapy, chemotherapy, and combinations of these modalities.

15. The theoretic basis of chemotherapy is the vulnerability of tumor cells in various stages of the cell cycle.

16. Modern chemotherapy uses combinations of drugs with different targets and different toxicities.

17. A new generation of specific targeted drugs attacks targets identified by the molecular analysis of cancers.

18. Ionizing radiation causes cell damage; therefore the goal of radiation therapy is to damage the tumor without causing excessive toxicity or damage to nondiseased structures.

19. Surgical therapy is used for nonmetastatic disease (in which cure is possible by removing the tumor) and as a palliative measure to alleviate symptoms.

KEY TERMS

- Adenocarcinoma 223
- Adjuvant chemotherapy 248
- Adult stem cell 238
- Anaplasia 223
- Anchorage independent 227
- Angiogenesis 235
- Angiogenic factor 235
- Apoptosis 235
- Autocrine stimulation 234
- Benign tumor 223
- Brachytherapy 249
- Cachexia 246
- Cancer 222
- Carcinoma 223
- Carcinoma in situ (CIS) 223
- Caretaker gene 233
- Chromosome instability 233
- Chromosome translocation 229
- Clonal expansion 228
- Clonal proliferation 228
- Contact inhibition 227
- Copy number variation (CNV) 231
- DNA methylation 233
- Epigenetic change 228
- Epigenetics 228
- Epigenetic silencing 233
- Gene amplification 231
- Human T cell leukemia-lymphoma virus (HTLV) 241
- Immortal 227
- Induction chemotherapy 248
- Inheritance 233
- Leukemia 223
- Loss of heterozygosity (LOH) 233
- Lymphoma 223
- Malignant tumor 223
- Metastasis 241
- MicroRNA (miRNA, miR) 233
- Multipotent 238
- Mutagen 234
- Neoadjuvant chemotherapy 249
- Neoplasm 222
- Neovascularization 235
- Non–coding RNA 228
- Oncogene 229
- Oncogene addiction 237
- Oncomir 233
- p53 tumor-suppressor gene (TP53) 235
- Paraneoplastic syndrome 225
- Personalized medicine 223
- Pleomorphic 223
- Point mutation 229
- Post-transplant lymphoproliferative disorder (PTLD) 241
- Proto-oncogene 229
- RAS 235
- Receptor tyrosine kinase 234
- Retinoblastoma gene (RB) 231
- Sarcoma 223
- Silencing 233
- Stage of cancer 244
- Stroma 223
- Telomerase 236
- Telomere 236
- Transformed cell 227
- Tumor 222
- Tumor marker 225
- Tumor-suppressor gene 229

REFERENCES

1. Kern SE: Progressive genetic abnormalities in human neoplasia. In Mendelsohn J, et al: *The molecular basis of cancer*, Philadelphia, 2001, Saunders.
2. Allegra CJ, et al: National Institutes of Health State-of-the-Science Conference statement: diagnosis and management of ductal carcinoma in situ September 22–24, 2009, *J Natl Cancer Inst* 102:161–169, 2010.
3. van't Veer LJ, Bernards R: Enabling personalized cancer medicine through analysis of gene-expression patterns, *Nature* 452(7187):564–570, 2008.
4. Skloot R: *Immortal life of Henrietta Lacks*, New York, 2010, Crown Publishing Group, Division of Random House, Inc.
5. Armitage P, Doll R: The age distribution of cancer and a multi-stage theory of carcinogenesis, *Br J Cancer* 91(12):1983–1989, 2004.
6. Luo J, Solimini NL, Elledge SJ: Principles of cancer therapy: oncogene and non-oncogene addiction, *Cell* 136:823–837, 2009.
7. Stratton MR, Campbell PJ, Futreal PA: The cancer genome, *Nature* 458:719–724, 2009.
8. Nowell P, Hungerford D: A minute chromosome in human granulocytic leukemia, *Science* 132:1497, 1960.
9. Druker BJ: Translation of the Philadelphia chromosome into therapy for CML, *Blood* 112:4808–4817, 2008.
10. Hastings PJ, et al: Mechanisms of change in gene copy number, *Nat Rev Genet* 10:551–564, 2009.
11. Brodeur GM, et al: Amplification of *N-myc* in untreated human neuroblastomas correlates with advanced disease stage, *Science* 224(4653):1121–1124, 1984.
12. Berns EM, et al: Prevalence of amplification of the oncogenes *c-myc*, HER2/neu, and int-2 in one thousand human breast tumors: correlation with steroid receptors, *Eur J Cancer* 28(2–3):697–700, 1992.
13. Ciardiello F, Tortora G: EGFR antagonists in cancer treatment, *N Engl J Med* 358(11):1160–1174, 2008.
14. Cavenee WK, et al: Expression of recessive alleles by chromosomal mechanisms in retinoblastoma, *Nature* 305(5937):779–784, 1983.
15. Takahashi K, Yamanaka S: Induction of pluripotent stem cells from mouse embryonic and adult fibroblast cultures by defined factors, *Cell* 126(4):663–676, 2006.
16. Jones PA, Baylin SB: The epigenomics of cancer, *Cell* 128(4):683–692, 2007.
17. Baylin SB, Ohm JE: Epigenetic gene silencing in cancer—a mechanism for early oncogenic pathway addiction? *Nat Rev Cancer* 6(2):107–116, 2006.
18. Lane AA, Chabner BA: Histone deacetylase inhibitors in cancer therapy, *J Clin Oncol* 27:5459–5468, 2009.
19. Voorhoeve PM: MicroRNAs: oncogenes, tumor suppressors or master regulators of cancer heterogeneity? *Biochim Biophys Acta* 1805:72–86, 2010.
20. Calin GA, Croce CM: Chronic lymphocytic leukemia: interplay between noncoding RNAs and protein-coding genes, *Blood* 114:4761–4770, 2009.
21. D'Andrea AD: Susceptibility pathways in Fanconi's anemia and breast cancer, *N Engl J Med* 362:1909–1919, 2010.
22. Weaver BA, Cleveland DW: Aneuploidy: instigator and inhibitor of tumorigenesis, *Cancer Res* 67:10103–10105, 2007.
23. Jorde LB, Carey JC, Bamshad MJ: *Medical genetics*, ed 4, St Louis, 2009, Mosby.
24. Shulman LP: Hereditary breast and ovarian cancer (HBOC): clinical features and counseling for BRCA1 and BRCA2, Lynch syndrome, Cowden syndrome, and Li-Fraumeni syndrome, *Obstet Gynecol Clin North Am* 37(1):109–133, 2010.
25. Vogelstein B, Kinzler KW: Cancer genes and the pathways they control, *Nat Med* 10:789–799, 2004.
26. Young A, et al: Ras signaling and therapies, *Adv Cancer Res* 102:1–17, 2009.
27. Folkman J: Angiogenesis: an organizing principle for drug discovery? *Nat Rev Drug Discov* 6(4):273–286, 2007.
28. Artandi SE, DePinho RA: Telomeres and telomerase in cancer, *Carcinogenesis* 31:9–18, 2010.
29. Van der Heiden MG, Cantley LC, Thompson CB: Understanding the Warburg effect: the metabolic requirements of cell proliferation, *Science* 324:1029–1033, 2009.
30. Dang CV: Cell metabolism and cancer: MYC micromanaging cancer cell metabolism and the Warburg effect. In *Cell metabolism and cancer*, pp 59–63, American Assocciation of Cancer Research.
31. Weinstein IB, Joe A: Oncogene addiction, *Cancer Res* 68:3077–3080, 2008:discussion 3080.

32. O'Brien CA, Kreso A, Jamieson CHM: Cancer stem cells and self-renewal, *Clin Cancer Res* 16:3113–3120, 2010.

33. Shackleton M, et al: Heterogeneity in cancer: cancer stem cells versus clonal evolution, *Cell* 138:822–829, 2009.

34. Joyce JA, Pollard JW: Microenvironmental regulation of metastasis, *Nat Rev Cancer* 9:239–252, 2009.

35. McAllister SS, Weinberg RA: Tumor-host interactions: a far-reaching relationship, *J Clin Oncol*, 2010 July 19:[Epub ahead of print].

36. Fitzpatrick FA: Inflammation, carcinogenesis and cancer, *Int Immunopharmacol* 1(9–10):1651–1667, 2001.

37. Mantovani A, et al: Tumor immunity: effector response to tumor and role of the microenvironment, *Lancet* 371:771–783, 2008.

38. Dubé C, et al: The use of aspirin for primary prevention of colorectal cancer: a systematic review prepared for the U.S. Preventive Services Task Force, *Ann Int Med* 146(5):365–375, 2007.

39. de Visser KE, Eichten A, Coussens LM: Paradoxical roles of the immune system during cancer development, *Nat Rev Cancer* 6:24–37, 2006.

40. Vajdic CM, et al: Cancer incidence before and after kidney transplantation, *J Am Med Assoc* 296:2823–2831, 2006.

41. Villeneuve PJ, et al: Cancer incidence among Canadian kidney transplant recipients, *Am J Transplant* 7:941–948, 2007.

42. Howley PM, Ganem D, Kieff E: Etiology of cancer: DNA viruses. In DeVita VT, et al: *Cancer: principles and practice of oncology*, ed 8, Philadelphia, 2008, Lippincott Williams & Wilkins.

43. Poeschla EM, et al: Etiology of cancer: RNA viruses. In DeVita VT, et al: *Cancer: principles and practice of oncology*, ed 8, Philadelphia, 2008, Lippincott Williams & Wilkins.

44. Paavonen J, Lehtinen M: Introducing human papillomavirus vaccines—questions remain, *Ann Med* 40(3):162–166, 2008.

45. Zafar S, Howell D, Gockerman J: Malignancy after solid organ transplantation: an overview, *Oncologist* 13:769, 2008.

46. Yang XR, et al: Evaluation of risk factors for nasopharyngeal carcinoma in high-risk nasopharyngeal carcinoma families in Taiwan, *Cancer Epidemiol Biomarkers Prev* 14(4):900–905, 2005.

47. Matsumoto Y, et al: *Helicobacter pylori* infection triggers aberrant expression of activation-induced cytidine deaminase in gastric epithelium, *Nat Med* 13:470–476, 2007.

48. Niwa T, et al: Inflammatory processes triggered by *Helicobacter pylori* infection cause aberrant DNA methylation in gastric epithelial cells, *Cancer Res* 70:1430–1440, 2010.

49. Wong BC, et al: *Helicobacter pylori* eradication to prevent gastric cancer in a high-risk region of China: a randomized controlled trial, *J Am Med Assoc* 291(2):187–194, 2004.

50. Gupta GP, Massagué J: Cancer metastasis: building a framework, *Cell* 127(4):697–708, 2006.

51. Talmadge JE, Fidler IJ: AACR centennial series: the biology of cancer metastasis: historical perspective, *Cancer Res* 70:5649–5669, 2010.

52. Tarin D, et al: Clinicopathological observations on metastasis in man studied in patients treated with peritoneovenous shunts, *Br Med J* 288(6419):749–751, 1984.

53. Maverakis E, et al: The etiology of paraneoplastic autoimmunity, *Clin Immunol*, 2011 Jan 19:[Epub ahead of print.].

54. Darnell RB, Posner JB: Paraneoplastic syndromes involving the nervous system, *N Engl J Med* 349:1543–1554, 2003.

55. Dy SM, et al: Evidence-based standards for cancer pain management, *J Clin Oncol* 26(23):3879–3885, 2008.

56. Shoemaker LK, et al: Symptom management: an important part of cancer care, *Clev Clin J Med* 78(1):25–34, 2011.

57. Miller AH, et al: Neuroendocrine-immune mechanisms of behavioral comorbidities in patients with cancer, *J Clin Oncol* 26(6):971–982, 2008.

58. Hess LM, Insel KC: Chemotherapy-related change in cognitive function: a conceptual model, *Oncol Nurs Forum* 34(5):981–994, 2007.

59. Blum D, et al: Cancer cachexia: a systematic literature review of items and domains associated with involuntary weight loss, *Crit Rev Oncol Hematol*, 2011 Jan 7:[Epub ahead of print.] (doi 10.1016/jcritrevonc.2010.10.004).

60. Porter D, et al: A neural survival factor is a candidate oncogene in breast cancer, *Proc Natl Acad Sci U S A* 100(10):10931–10936, 2003.

61. Adamson JW: *The anemia of inflammation/malignancy: mechanism and management, Hematology Am Soc Hematol Educ Program* 159–165, 2008.

62. Bohlius J, et al: Erythropoietin or Darbepoetin for patients with cancer—meta-analysis based on individual patient data, *Cochrane Database Syst Rev* (3), 2009:CD007303.

63. Kelly AM, Khuri FR: Unraveling the mystery of erythropoietin-stimulating agents in cancer promotion, *Cancer Res* 68:4013–4017, 2008.

64. Bhana N: Granulocyte colony-stimulating factors in the management of chemotherapy-induced neutropenia: evidence based review, *Curr Opin Oncol* 19(4):328–335, 2007.

65. DeVita VT Jr, Chu E: Principles of medical oncology. In DeVita VT, Lawrence TS, Rosenberg SA, editors: *Cancer: principles and practice of oncology*, ed 8, Philadelphia, 2008, Lippincott Williams & Wilkins, p 337.

66. Rebbeck TR, Kauff ND, Domchek SD: Meta-analysis of risk reduction estimates associated with risk-reducing salpingo-oophorectomy in *BRCA1* or *BRCA2* mutation carriers, *J Natl Cancer Inst* 101(2):80–87, 2009.

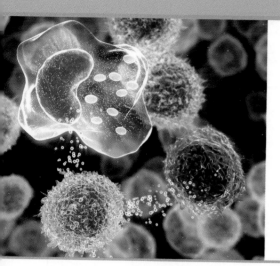

Cancer Epidemiology

Kathryn L. McCance

CHAPTER OUTLINE

Although cancer arises from a complicated and interacting web of multiple causes, avoiding exposure to individual carcinogens, or cancer-causing substances, may prevent many cancers. Research has shown that environmental-lifestyle factors and occupational exposure are responsible for the majority of cancer cases and deaths.[1-7] Widespread general exposure to pollutants from water, air, and the work environment; personal lifestyle choices (such as smoking, excessive alcohol use, and poor diet); and involuntary or unknown exposures to carcinogens in the air, water, and occupational environments are major contributors to cancer development. The National Cancer Institute (NCI) and the National Institute for Environmental Health Sciences (NIEHS) note in the document titled *Cancer and the Environment* that two thirds of all cancers are caused by environmental-lifestyle factors.[2]

GENES, ENVIRONMENTAL-LIFESTYLE FACTORS, AND RISK FACTORS

Cancers are caused by environmental-lifestyle and genetic factors. At the cellular level, cancer is a genetic process. Because relationships are unclear investigators are challenged to connect the complex web between genotype, phenotype, and the environment to understand a person's chances of developing cancer. Environmental-lifestyle factors include cigarette smoking, excessive alcohol consumption, poor diet, lack of exercise, excessive sunlight exposure, and sexual behavior that increases exposure to certain viruses. Additional factors include exposure to radiation, hormones, medical drugs, viruses, bacteria, pesticides, and other environmental chemicals present in air, water, food, soil, and the workplace. Investigations of occupational groups with high exposure to chemicals have identified numerous chemicals as carcinogens (Table 10-1).

Studies of gene-environmental interactions, whereby individuals with particular genetic predispositions may be more susceptible to the biologic effects of environmental exposures, do not explain the increased cancer risk found in most individuals exposed to carcinogens. Thus it appears that the majority of cancers are caused by carcinogen exposure rather than by rare genetic conditions.[2] For example, for women who have mutated cancer susceptibility genes, *BRCA1* or *BRCA2*, the risk of having breast cancer at age 50 is 24% for those born before 1940 but 67% for those born later.[8] The implication here is related to lifestyle factors that have changed since 1940 (e.g., hormone therapy, later age at first pregnancy, increased nulliparity). Investigations of more complex gene-gene environment interactions and proteins expressed by the genome (proteomics) may or may not alter these conclusions.

TABLE 10-1   SUMMARY OF ENVIRONMENTAL AND OCCUPATIONAL LINKS WITH CANCER

CATEGORY	CARCINOGENIC AGENT	SOURCE/USES	STRONG*	SUSPECTED†
Aromatic amines	Benzidine, 1-naphthylamine, 4,4'-methylenebis (2-chloroaniline) (MOCA), chloronaphthalene, heterocyclic aromatic amines	Antioxidants in production of rubber and cutting oils, intermediates in azo dye manufacturing, and as pesticides. Contaminant in chemical and mechanic industries and aluminum transformation and air contaminant from tobacco smoking. Used widely in textile industry and as hair dyes.	Bladder: benzidine, 2-naphthylamine, 4,4'-methylenebis (2-choloraniline) (MOCA), and chloronaphthalene	Prostate (heterocyclic aromatic amines)
Chlorination byproducts	Trihalomethanes	Chloroform, bromodichloromethane, chlorodibromomethane, and bromoform. Result from interaction of chlorine with organic chemicals. Several halogenated compounds may form from these reactions although trihalomethanes are most common. Brominated byproducts are also formed from reaction of chlorinated byproducts with low levels of bromide in drinking water.		Bladder, rectal
Environmental tobacco smoke	Contains more than 50 known carcinogens	Environmental tobacco smoke (ETS, also known as passive smoke) is combination of smoke emitted from burning end of cigarette, cigar, or pipe and smoke exhaled by smoker.	Lung, breast	
Metals	Arsenic	Byproduct of nonferrous metal production, mostly from copper production, comprising >10% of dust content in some smelter operations. Inorganic arsenic is commonly used to preserve wood but also as pesticide on cotton plants.	Bladder, lung, skin, soft tissue sarcoma (angiosarcoma of liver)	Brain/CNS, kidney, liver and biliary, prostate, soft tissue sarcoma
	Beryllium	Nuclear, aircraft, and medical devices industry. Alloy or in specialty ceramics for electric and electronic applications. Found as contaminant in combustion of coal and fuel oil.	Lung	
	Cadmium	Occurs naturally in ores together with zinc, lead, and copper. Used as stabilizers in PVC products, color pigment, several alloys, and now most commonly in rechargeable nickel-cadmium batteries. Also present as pollutant in phosphate fertilizers.	Lung	Pancreatic, kidney, prostate
	Chromium	Chromium is used in steel and other alloy production. Chromium III and chromium VI are used in chrome plating, manufacture of dyes and pigments, leather tanning, and wood preserving.	Lung, nasal and nasopharynx	
	Lead	Used primarily in production of batteries, ammunition, metal products such as solder and pipes, and devices to shield x-rays. Lead is also found in gasoline, paints, ceramic products, caulking, and pipe solder, but has been reduced dramatically in United States.		Brain/CNS, kidney, stomach
	Nickel	Used primarily as alloy in stainless steel. Also used in nickel plating and battery production.	Lung, nasal and nasopharynx	Laryngeal, pancreatic, stomach
Metal-working fluids and/or mineral oils	Straight oils, soluble oils, synthetic and semisynthetic fluids	Used in variety of industries including metal machining, print press operating, and cotton and jute spinning.	Bladder, laryngeal, lung, nasal and nasopharynx (mineral oils), rectal, skin, stomach	Esophageal, pancreatic, prostate
Natural fibers/dust	Asbestos	Inorganic naturally occurring fibrous silicate particle used primarily in acoustical and thermal insulation. Asbestos fibers can be divided into two groups: chrysolite (most widely used) and amphibole, which includes amosite, crocidolite, anthophyllite, actinolite, and tremolite fibers.	Laryngeal, lung, mesothelioma	
	Silica	Inorganic particle used in foundries, brick-making, and sand-blasting.	Lung	
	Talc containing asbestiform fibers	Mineral used in manufacture of pottery, paper, paint, and cosmetics.	Lung	
	Wood dust	Used primarily in carpentry, joinery, and furniture and cabinetry making.	Lung, nasal and nasopharynx	Laryngeal

TABLE 10-1 SUMMARY OF ENVIRONMENTAL AND OCCUPATIONAL LINKS WITH CANCER—cont'd

CATEGORY	CARCINOGENIC AGENT	SOURCE/USES	STRONG*	SUSPECTED†
Pesticides	Herbicides, fungicides, and insecticides	Used for preventing, destroying, repelling, or mitigating any pest or in use as plant regulator, defoliant, or desiccant. Majority of pesticides as registered with U.S. EPA are used in agricultural applications, although residential application is also important source.		Brain/CNS, breast, colon, Hodgkin lymphoma, leukemia, lung, multiple myeloma, non-Hodgkin lymphoma, ovarian, pancreatic, kidney, soft tissue sarcoma, stomach, testicular
Petrochemicals and combustion byproducts	Petroleum products, motor vehicle exhaust (including diesel), polycyclic aromatic hydrocarbons (PAHs), soot, and dioxins	Petrochemicals are derived from natural gas or petroleum and used to produce variety of other chemicals and materials including pesticides, plastics, medicines, and dyes. Substances can be produced as building blocks for other products, but mainly result from incomplete combustion of burning coal, oil, gas (diesel exhaust), household waste, tobacco, and other organic substances. Dioxins are a class of chemicals that are byproducts of combustion processes containing chlorine and chemicals such as PVC plastics. Dioxins are also created during chlorine-bleaching processes for whitening paper and wood pulp.	Lung (PAHs, air pollution including diesel exhaust, soot, dioxin), NHL (dioxin), soft tissue sarcoma (dioxin), skin (PAHs)	Bladder (PAHs), breast (dioxin), esophageal (soot), laryngeal (PAHs), multiple myeloma (dioxin), prostate (dioxin and PAHs)
Radiation	Ionizing radiation	Any of several types of particles and rays emitted by radioactive material, high-voltage equipment, nuclear reactions, and stars. Alpha and beta particles, x-rays, and γ-rays are radiation particles of concern to human health.	Bone, brain and CNS, breast, leukemia, liver and biliary, lung, multiple myelomas, soft tissue sarcoma, skin, thyroid	Bladder, colon, nasal and nasopharynx, ovarian, stomach
	Nonionizing radiation	Composed of microwaves and electromagnetic frequencies including radio waves and extremely low-frequency electromagnetic fields.		Brain, breast, leukemia
	Ultraviolet radiation	Ultraviolet radiation is part of solar radiation emitted by sun.	Skin	
Reactive chemicals	Butadiene	Used in production of polymers for manufacture of styrene-butadiene rubber for tires; nitrile rubber for hoses, gaskets, adhesives, and footwear; acrylonitrile-butadiene-styrene polymers for parts, pipes, and various appliances; and styrene-butadiene latexes for paints and carpet backing.		Leukemia
	Ethylene oxide	Used as sterilant, disinfectant, and pesticide. Also used as raw ingredient in making resins, films, and antifreeze.	Leukemia	Breast
	Formaldehyde	Primary use is in production of urea, phenol, or melamine resins for molded products such as appliances, electric controls, and telephones; in particle-board, plywood, and surface coatings.		Nasal and nasopharynx
	Mustard gas	Produced and used primarily in World War I as chemical warfare agent.	Lung	Laryngeal
	Vinyl chloride	Vinyl chloride is used in polyvinyl resins for production of plastic pipes and floor coverings and in electric and transportation applications.	Liver and biliary, soft tissue sarcoma (angiosarcoma of liver)	
	Sulfuric acid	Used widely in industry for production of isopropyl alcohol, ethanol; treatment of metals; and manufacture of soaps, detergents, and batteries.	Laryngeal	Lung
Solvents	Benzene	Used as intermediate in production of plastics, resins, and some synthetic and nylon fibers. Also used to make some types of rubbers, lubricants, dyes, detergents, drugs, and pesticides. Also found in crude oil, gasoline, and cigarette smoke.	Leukemia, NHL	Brain/CNS, lung, nasal and nasopharynx, multiple myeloma

Continued

TABLE 10-1   SUMMARY OF ENVIRONMENTAL AND OCCUPATIONAL LINKS WITH CANCER—cont'd

CATEGORY	CARCINOGENIC AGENT	SOURCE/USES	STRONG*	SUSPECTED†
	Carbon tetrachloride	Used primarily in various industrial applications. Before being banned, it also was used in production of refrigeration fluid and propellants for aerosol cans, as pesticide, as cleaning fluid and degreasing agent, in fire extinguishers, and in spot removers.		Leukemia
	Methylene chloride	Used primarily as solvent in industrial applications and as paint stripper. May also be found in some aerosol and pesticide products and in production of photographic film.		Brain/CNS, liver and biliary
	Styrene	Used in production of rubber, plastic, insulation, fiberglass, pipes, automobile parts, food containers, and carpet backing.		NHL
	Toluene	Used in production of paints, paint thinners, fingernail polish, lacquers, adhesives, and rubber. Also used in some printing and leather-tanning processes.		Brain/CNS, lung, rectal
	Trichloroethylene (TCE)	Mainly used for degreasing metal parts. Precious use as dry cleaning agent. TCE may be found in printing inks, varnishes, adhesives, paints, and lacquers. Important contaminant in general environment as a result of emissions and leakage from industrial settings.	Liver and biliary, kidney	Cervical, Hodgkin lymphoma, leukemia, NHL, kidney
	Tetrachloroethylene (PCE)	Used to degrease metal parts and as solvent in variety of industrial applications. Since the 1930s it was used by an increasingly large percentage of U.S. dry-cleaning operations.		Bladder, cervical, esophageal, NHL, kidney
	Xylene(s)	Used as cleaning agent, thinner for paint, and in paint and varnishes; in printing, rubber, and leather industries; found in small amounts in gasoline and airplane fuel.		Brain/CNS, rectal
Other	Creosotes	Includes coal tar and coal-tar pitch formed by high-temperature treatment of wood or coal or from resin of the creosote bush. Wood creosote was historically used as disinfectant, laxative, and cough treatment. Coal-tar products are used in medicine, animal and bird repellants, and pesticides. Coal-tar, coal-tar pitch, and coal-tar pitch volatiles are used in roofing, road paving, aluminum smelting, and coking.	Bladder (coal tars), lung, skin	
	Endocrine disruptors	A number of chemicals capable of mimicking body's natural hormones. See www.ourstolenfuture.org/Basics/chemlist.htm.	Breast (DES), cervical (DES)	Breast, prostate, testicular
	Hair dyes	Coloring products used on hair. Hair dyes usually fall into one of four categories: temporary, semipermanent, demi, and permanent. Chemical agents used in dyes are specific to color and degree of permanency.		Bladder, brain (SCNS), leukemia, multiple myeloma, NHL
	Nitrosamines and N-nitroso compounds	Class of chemicals that forms as result of chemical reaction of amines and nitrosating agents. Found in rubber, metal, and agricultural industries, in cosmetics, and in foods such as fried bacon and cured meats.		Brain/CNS
	Polychlorinated biphenyls (PCBs)	Used as coolants and lubricants in transformers, capacitors, and other electric equipment. PCBs have been banned in United States since 1997.	Liver and biliary	Breast, NHL

From Clapp RW, Jacobs MM, Loechler EL: Environmental and occupational causes of cancer: new evidence, 2005–2007, *Rev Environ Health* 23(1):1–37, review, 2008.

*Strong evidence of a causal link is based primarily on a Group 1 designation by the International Agency for Research on Cancer.
†Suspected evidence of a causal link is based on the assessment that results of epidemiologic studies are mixed, yet positive findings from well-designed and conducted studies warrant precautionary action and additional scientific investigation.
CNS, Central nervous system; *DES,* diethylstilbestrol; *EPA,* Environmental Protection Agency; *NHL,* non-Hodgkin lymphoma; *PVC,* polyvinyl chloride; *SCNS,* subcutaneous nerve stimulation.

Strong evidence suggests that certain environmental-lifestyle and occupational exposures are associated with cancers of the bladder, bone, brain, central nervous system (CNS), breast, liver, larynx, scrotum, kidney, skin, and thyroid as well as Ewing sarcoma, melanoma, mesothelioma, non-Hodgkin lymphoma (NHL), and soft tissue sarcoma (see Table 10-1).

Although tobacco smoke remains the single most preventable cause of cancer, it is not linked to the majority of cancers that have increased substantially in the United States. These cancers include melanoma, non-Hodgkin lymphoma, testicular, brain, and thyroid.[2] For example, testicular cancer, which affects men mostly in their 20s and 30s, increased about 75% from the 1970s to the 1980s; incidence rates remain about 11 to 12/100,000 in the United States. This increase is *not* attributed to improved diagnostic methods and cancer registration rates.[9] Among all population groups, brain and nervous system cancers increased from 10/100,000 in 1973 to 20.9/100,000 in 1992—an astounding 109% increase.[3,7,10]

Lung cancer rates have risen and fallen, paralleling the prevalence of smoking. Meanwhile, the prevalence of stomach cancer in the United States dropped dramatically over the past century.[2] The decrease may be caused by the adoption of healthier lifestyles or by the reduction of bacterial infection from *Helicobacter pylori*, or both.

Studies comparing the relationship between environmental-lifestyle factors and cancer risk for different populations around the world are compelling. Breast cancer, for example, is prevalent among northern Europeans and Americans but is relatively rare among women in developing countries. If ethnicity played a major role, then immigrants should retain the cancer incidence rates of their country of origin. Instead, within one or two generations immigrants acquire the cancer rates of their geographic relocation.[11,12] A particularly instructive group of studies has been the Multiethnic Cohort (MEC) study. These studies are focused on ethnic and migrant populations in Hawaii. The large populations of ethnic groups in Hawaii assist with establishing interethnic comparisons and disentangling the effects of genes, environment, and lifestyle on cancer rates. These results and others support the claim that cancer risk is substantially influenced by environmental factors (Box 10-1).

Elevated cancer rates are more common in cities, in farming locations, near hazardous waste sites, downwind of industrial and radiation activities, and near contaminated water wells. In addition, cancers are associated with areas of high pesticide use, toxic work exposures, waste incinerators, and other sources of pollution.[13,14]

Farmers have increased death rates from brain, multiple myeloma, prostate, Hodgkin lymphoma, leukemia, non-Hodgkin lymphoma, and lip and stomach cancers.[15] Migrant farmers also experience elevated rates of some of these cancers.[2] Public health advocates have argued that the manufacturers of environmental hazards (e.g., chemicals, tobacco, drugs, radiologic products) should be required to assess the health, safety, and environmental effects of their products before they are introduced to the marketplace; in addition, information regarding these products should be publicly available.

A new paradigm shift suggests that susceptibility to disease is established in utero or neonatally as the result of nutrition and exposures to environmental toxins or stressors, or both.[16] Children also may be affected by prenatal exposures, by parental exposures before conception, and by contaminated breast milk. Some epidemiologic studies have linked higher risks of childhood leukemia and brain and CNS cancers with parental and childhood exposure to particular solvents, pesticides, petrochemicals, dioxins, and polycyclic aromatic hydrocarbons.[17]

Environmental-lifestyle factors play important roles in cancer development, but there are major gaps in our knowledge of how

---

> **BOX 10-1   ESTABLISHED ENVIRONMENTAL-LIFESTYLE FACTORS AND RISK OF CANCER**
>
> Tobacco use
> Dietary choices (inadequate fruits, vegetables, and fiber; consumption of fat and alcohol)
> Obesity
> Reproductive/menstrual traits (age at menarche, age at menopause, parity, age at first birth, lactation)
> Sun exposure
> Ionizing radiation
> Viruses (hepatitis B and viruses, human papillomaviruses, Epstein-Barr virus)
> Bacteria *(Helicobacter pylori)*
> Occupational exposures (asbestos, rubber, others [see Table 10-1])
> Population-wide screening activities (prostate-specific antigen [PSA]), mammography, Pap smears*
>
> Data from Kolonel LN, Altshuler D, Henderson BE: *Nat Rev Cancer* 4(7):519–527, 2004.
> *Not a risk factor per se but increases the rates of cancer in the short term and in the long term can actually increase the number of cancer cases diagnosed by detecting latent, potentially noninvasive, but histopathologically apparent cancer.

these factors affect our individual resistance to cancer-causing agents. Research needed for shaping public policy concerning environmental exposures should focus on (1) the relationship between the timing of exposures (periods of vulnerability), multiple exposures, and chronic exposures; (2) risks among racial groups and gender; (3) human contamination (biomonitoring); and (4) scrutinization of unexplained patterns of risk. Table 10-2 summarizes the estimated new cases and deaths caused by cancer, by gender, for specified sites.

> **✔ QUICK CHECK 10-1**
> 1. Discuss what is meant by "environment is the main cause of cancer."
> 2. What are the types of cancers that have increased in the United States substantially?
> 3. What is the single most preventable cause of cancer?
> 4. For cancer prevalence, why is it important to study immigrant populations?

Epigenetics and Genetics

The idea that increased risk of disease originates from interactions among genes and environmental-lifestyle factors *may* not be directed by the genetic code. A source of heated debate has been the relative importance of genetic versus epigenetic processes. As discussed in Chapter 9, epigenetics is a change in the *expression* of the gene or phenotype that is heritable but does not involve deoxyribonucleic acid (DNA) mutation. The *epigenome* is sometimes called the code over the DNA code. Although it is clear that inherited variation in DNA sequence influences individual risk of cancer, this occurs in only a small percentage of the population.[18] In addition, the mechanism by which structural variation of the genome increases cancer risk is unknown. An explosion of recent data now indicates the importance of epigenetic processes, especially those with resultant gene silencing (not broken, but mute) of *key* regulatory genes (see Chapter 9). Epigenetic changes collaborate with genetic changes and environmental-lifestyle factors to *cause* the development of cancer (Figure 10-1). These changes are mitotically and meiotically

TABLE 10-2   ESTIMATED NEW U.S. CANCER CASES AND DEATHS BY GENDER, 2010*

	ESTIMATED NEW CASES			ESTIMATED DEATHS		
	BOTH GENDERS	MALE	FEMALE	BOTH GENDERS	MALE	FEMALE
All sites	1,529,560	789,620	739,940	569,490	299,200	270,290
Oral cavity and pharynx	36,540	25,420	11,120	7,880	5,430	2,450
Tongue	10,990	7,690	3,300	1,990	1,300	690
Mouth	10,840	6,430	4,410	1,830	1,140	690
Pharynx	12,660	9,880	2,780	2,410	1,730	680
Other oral cavity	2,050	1,420	630	1,650	1,260	390
Digestive system	274,330	148,540	125,790	139,580	79,010	60,570
Esophagus	16,640	13,130	3,510	14,500	11,650	2,850
Stomach	21,000	12,730	8,270	10,570	6,350	4,220
Small intestine	6,960	3,680	3,280	1,100	610	490
Colon†	102,900	49,470	53,430	51,370	26,580	24,790
Rectum	39,670	22,620	17,050			
Anus, anal canal, and anorectum	5,260	2,000	3,260	720	280	440
Liver and intrahepatic bile duct	24,120	17,430	6,690	18,910	12,720	6,190
Gallbladder and other biliary	9,760	4,560	5,310	3,320	1,240	2,080
Pancreas	43,140	21,370	21,770	36,800	18,770	18,030
Other digestive organs	4,880	1,660	3,220	2,290	810	1,480
Respiratory system	240,610	130,600	110,010	161,670	89,550	72,120
Larynx	12,720	10,110	2,610	3,600	2,870	730
Lung and bronchus	222,520	116,750	105,770	157,300	86,220	71,080
Other respiratory organs	5,370	3,740	1,630	770	460	310
Bones and joints	2,650	1,530	1,120	1,460	830	630
Soft tissue (including heart)	10,520	5,680	4,840	3,920	2,020	1,900
Skin (excluding basal and squamous)	74,010	42,610	31,400	11,790	7,910	3,880
Melanoma-skin	68,130	38,870	29,260	8,700	5,670	3,030
Other nonepithelial skin	5,880	3,740	2,140	3,090	2,240	850
Breast	209,060	1,970	207,090	40,230	390-	39,840
Genital system	311,210	227,460	83,750	60,420	32,710	27,710
Uterine cervix	12,200		12,200	4,210		4,210
Uterine corpus	43,470		43,470	7,950		7,950
Ovary	21,880		21,880	13,850		13,850
Vulva	3,900		3,900	920		912
Vagina and other genitalia, female	2,300		2,300	780		780
Prostate	217,730	217,730		32,050	32,050	
Testis	8,480	8,480		350	350	
Penis and other genitalia, male	1,250	1,250		310	310	
Urinary system	131,260	89,620	41,640	28,550	19,110	9,440
Urinary bladder	70,530	52,760	17,770	14,680	10,410	4,270
Kidney and renal pelvis	58,240	35,370	22,870	13,040	8,210	4,830
Ureter and other urinary organs	2,490	1,490	1,000	830	490	340
Eye and orbit	2,480	1,240	1,240	230	120	110
Brain and other nervous system	22,020	11,980	10,040	13,140	7,420	5,720
Endocrine system	46,930	11,890	35,040	2,570	1,140	1,430
Thyroid	44,670	10,740	33,930	1,690	730	960
Other endocrine	2,260	1,150	1,110	880	410	470
Lymphoma	74,030	40,050	33,980	21,530	11,450	10,080
Hodgkin lymphoma	8,490	4,670	3,820	1,320	740	580
Non-Hodgkin lymphoma	65,540	35,380	30,160	20,210	10,710	9,500
Myeloma	20,180	11,170	9,010	10,650	5,760	4,890
Leukemia	43,050	24,690	18,360	21,840	12,660	9,180
Acute lymphocytic leukemia	5,330	3,150	2,180	1,420	790	630
Chronic lymphocytic leukemia	14,990	8,870	6,120	4,390	2,650	1,740
Acute myeloid leukemia	12,330	6,590	5,740	8,950	5,280	3,670
Chronic myeloid leukemia	4,870	2,800	2,070	440	190	250
Other leukemias‡	5,530	3,280	2,250	6,640	3,750	2,890
Other and unspecified primary sites‡	30,580	15,170	15,510	44,030	23,690	20,340

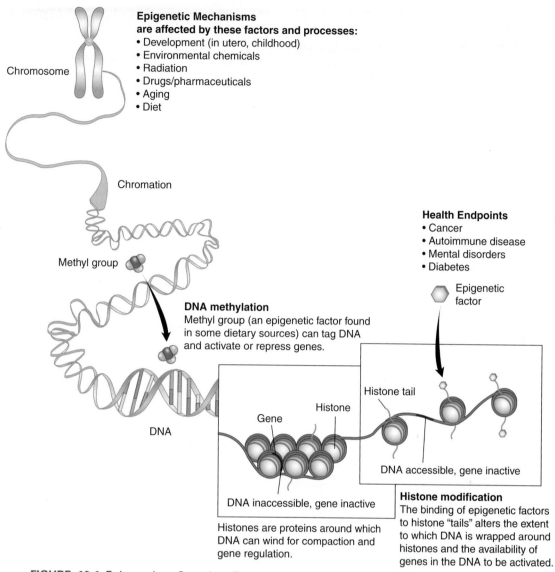

**Epigenetic Mechanisms
are affected by these factors and processes:**
• Development (in utero, childhood)
• Environmental chemicals
• Radiation
• Drugs/pharmaceuticals
• Aging
• Diet

Chromosome

Chromation

Methyl group

DNA methylation
Methyl group (an epigenetic factor found
in some dietary sources) can tag DNA
and activate or repress genes.

Health Endpoints
• Cancer
• Autoimmune disease
• Mental disorders
• Diabetes

Epigenetic
factor

DNA

Gene

Histone

Histone tail

DNA accessible, gene inactive

DNA inaccessible, gene inactive

Histones are proteins around which
DNA can wind for compaction and
gene regulation.

Histone modification
The binding of epigenetic factors
to histone "tails" alters the extent
to which DNA is wrapped around
histones and the availability of
genes in the DNA to be activated.

FIGURE 10-1 Epigenetics, Genetics, Environment, and Cancer. Epigenetic mechanisms are affected by many factors and processes including development in utero and during childhood, diet, environmental chemicals, radiation, drugs/pharmaceuticals, and aging. DNA methylation occurs when methyl groups, an epigenetic factor found in some dietary sources, for example, can tag DNA and activate or repress genes. Histones are proteins around which DNA can wind for compaction and gene regulation. Histone modification occurs when the binding of epigenetic factors to histone "tails" alters the extent to which DNA is wrapped around histones and the availability of genes in the DNA to be activated. All of these factors and processes can have an effect on and influence people's health, possibly resulting in cancer, autoimmune disease, mental disorders, diabetes, and other diseases. (Division of Program Coordination, Planning, and Strategic Initiatives. From National Institutes of Health Common Fund, National Institutes of Health, Washington, DC, U.S. Department of Health and Human Services.)

TABLE 10-2

Estimated new cases are based on 1995-2006 incidence rates from 44 states and the District of Columbia as reported by the North American Association of Central Cancer Registries (NAACCR), representing about 89% of the U.S. population. Estimated deaths are based on data from U.S. Mortality Data, 1969-2007, National Center for Health Statistics, Centers for Disease Control and Prevention, 2010. © 2010, American Cancer Society. Cancer Facts and Figures 2010. Atlanta: American Cancer Society, Inc.
*Rounded to the nearest 10; estimated new cases exclude basal and squamous cell skin cancers and in situ carcinomas except urinary bladder. About 54,010 cases of female carcinoma in situ of the breast and 46,770 cases of melanoma in situ will be newly diagnosed in 2010.
†Estimated deaths for colon and rectal cancers are combined.
‡More deaths than cases may reflect lack of specificity in recording underlying causes of death on death certificates of an undercount in the base estimate.

TABLE 10-3	**DIFFERENCES BETWEEN MULTIGENERATIONAL AND TRANSGENERATIONAL PHENOTYPES**	
PHENOTYPE	**EXPOSURE**	**DEFINITION**
Multigenerational	Direct	Simutaneous exposure of multiple generations to an environmental factor
Transgenerational	Initial germline exposure (ancestral)	Transgenerational phenotype is transmitted to future generations via germline inheritance

TABLE 10-4	**SOMATIC VERSUS GERM CELL INHERITANCE**
CELL TYPE	**BIOLOGIC RESPONSE**
Somatic cells	Critical for adult-onset disease in exposed individual; not transmitted to future generations as transgenerational effect
Germ cells	Allows transmission between generations; promotes transgenerational phenotype

heritable.[19,20] The following are the three major types of epigenetic processes:

1. Methylation (the addition of a methyl group [CH_3] to the cytosine ring) (see Figure 9-10); aberrant methylation can lead to silencing of tumor-suppressor genes.
2. Histone modifications (e.g., histone acetylation, alterations in chromatin) can result in gene silencing (see Figure 10-1).
3. Micro–ribonucleic acids (miRNAs) are small RNA molecules that can target gene expression post-transcriptionally. MicroRNAs act like a volume control lever to modulate the production of defined proteins in cells. The expression of miRNAs has been linked to carcinogenesis because they can act as either oncogenes or tumor-suppressor genes.[21]

An important feature of epigenetic mechanisms and their role in development and disease is that epigenetic processes can be modified by lifestyle, particularly diet and the environment, pharmacologic interventions, or both.[22] Data have also shown that aging affects DNA methylation in many cell types in various organisms.[23-25] The majority of environmental factors apparently do not promote genetic mutations or alterations in DNA sequence; however, environmental factors can alter the epigenome.[26] Significant evidence for environment-lifestyle as the major contributor to age-related effects on the "epigenome" was demonstrated in a recent study of monozygotic (MZ) twins. Cell types and patterns of DNA methylation across the genome were similar in young MZ twins, but diverged in older twins.[27] These data suggest that environmental-lifestyle factors act on individuals throughout life, changing gene expression through epigenetic mechanisms with subsequent implications for health. The heritable transmission to future generations of environmentally-caused phenotypes is called **transgenerational inheritance.** Most epigenetic changes from environmental causes involve somatic cells and will *not* promote transgenerational phenotypes. These somatic effects, however, are critical for the individual exposed because it can lead to adult-onset disease or other phenotype alterations.[26] An epigenetic alteration in germline cells (sex gametes) can lead to **transgenerational effects** independent of continued environmental exposure. Tables 10-3 and 10-4 include important explanations of these new findings.[26]

Nutrition has become a major focus because it influences DNA methylation in several ways (see p. 262). Biologically active food components modify DNA methylation directly. Nutrition influences metabolic effects associated with energy balance. Because adipose tissue is endocrine tissue, obese individuals accumulate macrophages that secrete various proinflammatory signaling molecules and cytokines (see p. 264). Inflammation is strongly associated with cancer development, and inflammatory bowel disease is related to methylation in the colon.[28,29] The role of nutrition and diet is discussed on p. 261.

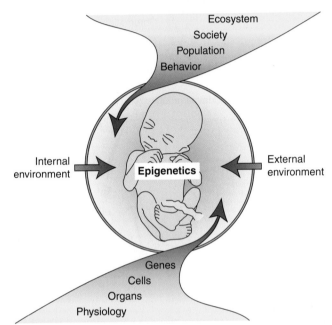

FIGURE 10-2 Fetal Vulnerability to External and Internal Environments. The fetus is particularly vulnerable to changes in the external and internal environments, which can have immediate and lifelong consequences. Such environmentally induced changes can occur at multiple levels, including molecular and behavioral. Ultimately these alterations may be epigenetic, inducing mitotically heritable alterations in gene expression without changing the DNA. (Adapted from Crews E, McLachlan JA: *Endocrinology* 147 [6 suppl]:S4–S10, 2006.)

In Utero and Early Life Conditions

From studies of the etiology of certain cancers, it is widely accepted that a long latency period precedes the onset of adult cancers. Accumulating data suggest early life events influence later susceptibility to certain chronic diseases (Figure 10-2).[30] **Developmental plasticity** is the degree to which an organism's development is contingent on its environment. It requires stable gene expression that in part appears to be modulated by epigenetic processes such as DNA methylation and histone modification.[30] Sensitivity to environmental-lifestyle factors influences the mature phenotype and is dependent on the interactions of both the genome and the epigenome.

Perhaps one of the best examples of early life events and future cancer is the chemical exposure to diethylstilbestrol (DES), a synthetic estrogen. This medication was prescribed between 1938 and 1971 in an attempt to prevent multiple pregnancy-related problems, such as miscarriage, premature birth, and abnormal bleeding.[31] In 1953 a clinical study found that DES did not reduce the risk of miscarriage, and by the 1950s it became clear that DES interfered with the *development* of the reproductive system in the fetus. Recent data suggest that a DES-associated increase in cancer of the female genital tract is elevated throughout a woman's reproductive years.[32] More recent studies have revealed that daughters of women who took DES during pregnancy may have a slight increased risk of breast cancer before age 40 (i.e., 1.9 times the risk compared with unexposed women at age 40).[33] For every 1000 DES-exposed women ages 45 to 49 it is estimated that 4 will be diagnosed with breast cancer.

Research from animal studies has demonstrated a relationship between DES exposure and an increased rate of a rare type of testicular cancer (rete testis) and prostate cancer.[34,35] In terms of in utero exposures, testicular cancer has been linked to exposure to abnormal levels of estrogen,[36] and testicular cancer is a risk factor for men with undescended testicles, a factor in some studies correlated with DES exposure. However, studies comparing the risk of testicular or prostate cancer in men and DES exposure are unclear and continuing.[37]

In summary, epidemiologic and animal studies reveal that small changes in the developmental environment can alter phenotypic changes, resulting in individual responses in adulthood. Continuing evidence indicates that epigenetic mechanisms are responsible for tissue-specific gene expression during cellular differentiation and that these mechanisms modulate developmental phenotypic changes.[30] The phenotypic effects of epigenetic modifications during development may need long latency periods, such as in cancer, thus manifesting later in life. In addition, epigenetic effects may help explain transgeneration effects (see Tables 10-3 and 10-4). For example, Newbold and colleagues[35] demonstrated that DES-related reproductive cancers in mice also occurred in the grandsons and granddaughters of mothers treated with DES.

In addition to altering some cancer risks, investigators are studying diet during pregnancy. Recently, a striking experiment in mice demonstrated how extra vitamin doses during pregnancy in the mother's diet changed the fur color of pups.[38] This was the first study to show maternal nutrition and subsequent phenotype changes. The nutrients (B_{12}, folic acid, choline, and betaine) silenced the gene that rendered mice fat and yellow but did not alter its DNA sequence. Silencing, or switching the gene off, linked prenatal diet to such diseases as diabetes, obesity, and cancer. These concepts, called the *developmental basis of health and disease,* are defining the hypothesis of disease onset. Subsequently, the focus of disease prevention and intervention needs to include the decades before onset—that is, in utero and neonatal periods.

> ✔ **QUICK CHECK 10-2**
> 1. Define epigenetics.
> 2. Discuss how epigenetic processes can be modified by environmental factors.
> 3. Define developmental plasticity.
> 4. Define the developmental basis of health and disease.

Tobacco Use

Cigarette smoking is carcinogenic and remains the most important cause of cancer. The risk is greatest in those who begin to smoke when young and continue throughout life.[39] Globally, tobacco use is greatest in developing countries, where 84% of 1.3 billion current smokers live.[40] The World Health Organization (WHO) reports tobacco use causes more than 5 million deaths per year from cancer, chronic lung disease, cardiovascular disease, and stroke.[41] Approximately 50% of regular smokers are killed by this habit. On average, smokers die 13 to 14 years earlier than nonsmokers;[42] about 25% will die prematurely during middle age (35 to 69 years).[43]

Cigarette smoking accounts for 1 of every 5 deaths each year in the United States.[44] About 21% of all U.S. adults smoke cigarettes. Estimates of cigarette smoking by age are as follows: 23.6% ages 18 to 24; 23.8% ages 25 to 44; 22.4% ages 45 to 64; and 8.8% ages 65 and older.[45] Cigarette smoking is more common among men (23.9%) than women (18.5%), and the prevalence of cigarette smoking is higher among Native Americans/Native Alaskans (36.4%) than whites (21.4%), blacks (19.8%), Hispanics (13.3%), and Asians (9.6%).[45] It is more common among adults living below the poverty level (30.6%) than those at or above the poverty level (20.4%).[45,46]

Overall, cigarette smoking in developed countries is responsible for 30% of all cancer deaths, and an epidemic of cancer deaths is expected in developing countries.[42] Tobacco use is associated primarily with squamous and small cell adenocarcinomas. In addition, smoking causes even more deaths from vascular, respiratory, and other diseases than from cancer. Smoking tobacco is linked to cancers of the lower urinary tract (renal, penis, and bladder), upper aerodigestive tract (oral cavity, pharynx, larynx, nasal cavity, paranasal sinuses, esophagus, and stomach), liver, kidney, pancreas, cervix, and uterus, as well as myeloid leukemia.[47] Evidence is lacking that smoking causes breast, prostate, or endometrial cancer of the uterus.[43] However, tobacco smoke is known to cause mammary tumors in animals. Smoking during the prepartum period of pregnancy, when breast tissue is less differentiated, appears to be relevant for breast cancer risk.[48-51] Japanese researchers reported that both active and passive smoking (secondhand smoke) increased the risk of breast cancer in premenopausal women.[52]

Secondhand smoke, also called environmental tobacco smoke (ETS), is the combination of sidestream smoke (burning end of a cigarette, cigar, or pipe) and mainstream smoke (exhaled by the smoker). More than 4000 chemicals have been identified in mainstream tobacco smoke (250 chemicals as toxic) of which 60 are considered carcinogenic.[53] Measuring secondhand smoke is difficult. Nonsmokers who live with smokers are at greatest risk for lung cancer as well as numerous noncancerous conditions.[53]

Cigar or pipe smoking, or both, is strongly and causally related to cancers of the oral cavity, oropharynx, hypopharynx, larynx, esophagus, and lung. Cigar smokers who inhale deeply may be at increased risk for developing coronary heart disease and chronic obstructive pulmonary disease.[54] Pipe smokers have a lower risk of dying from tobacco than cigarette smokers, but it is as harmful as and perhaps more harmful than cigar smoking.[55] Bidi smoking, a small amount of tobacco wrapped in the leaf of another plant (used in South Asia), delivers higher amounts of nicotine per gram of tobacco and comparable or greater amounts of tar compared with cigarettes.[47] Case-controlled studies indicate bidi smoking can cause cancers of the respiratory and digestive sites. Epidemiologic data from the United States and Asia show an increased risk of oral cancer with smokeless tobacco products.[56] These data, however, are not confirmed in northern European studies.[56]

Measures that prevent young adults from starting smoking would substantially avoid future disease burden. A public health approach is therefore needed that *prevents* young people from *starting* smoking and helps others *stop* smoking.

Diet

Understanding dietary factors that increase the risk for cancer can be difficult. The ways in which diet affects one's likelihood of developing cancer are complicated by the variety of foods consumed, the many constituents of foods, the metabolic consequences of eating, and the temporal changes in the patterns of food use. Cancer risks in older adults may depend as much on diet in early life as on current eating practices.[39,57] In addition, studies in humans targeting diet and disease associations face a variety of challenges including measurements of specific nutrients, food types, and dietary patterns.

Humans are constantly exposed to a variety of compounds termed **xenobiotics** (the Greek word *xenos* means "foreign;" *bios* means "life") that include toxic, mutagenic, and carcinogenic chemicals. Many of these chemicals are found in the human diet. Most xenobiotics are transported in the blood by lipoproteins and penetrate lipid membranes (see Chapter 3).

Dietary sources of carcinogenic substances include compounds produced in the cooking of fat, meat, or protein, and naturally occurring carcinogens associated with plant food substances, such as alkaloids or mold byproducts.[58] The most studied and most relevant carcinogens produced by cooking are the polycyclic aromatic hydrocarbon benzo[*a*]pyrene and the heterocyclic aromatic amines generated by meat protein. The greatest levels are found in well-done charbroiled beef. People, likewise, ingest xenobiotics that are found in environmental or industrial contaminants (e.g., particulate matter of diesel exhaust, contaminating pesticides in food and water supplies) and in certain prescribed and over-the-counter medicines. Dietary components can act directly as mutagens or interfere with mutagen elimination. Nutritional factors may alter cellular environments by modulating hormonal axes or influencing cellular proliferation, or both.[59]

Nutrition may directly influence epigenetic factors that silence genes that should be active or activate genes that should be silent.[59] Importantly, specific nutrients may directly affect the phenotype or expression of key genes, for example, epigenetically through abnormalities of methylation of the promoter regions of genes or histones. Epigenetic signals appear to act through remodeling of chromatin structure.[60] These alterations can affect DNA structure and mRNA for transcription.[59] Clearly, epigenetic events are susceptible to change, thus offering potential explanations of *how* environmental factors (e.g., diet) may modify cancer risk and tumor behavior. *DNA methylation*—the attachment of a methyl group to the 5-position of cytosine within cytosine guanine dinucleotides (CpGs)—is one of several epigenetic changes important in gene regulation and expression (Figure 10-3). DNA is also susceptible to hypomethylation, which can cause overexpression of transcription of proto-oncogenes, increased recombination and mutation (i.e., oncogenes), and failure to imprint. These alterations can all promote cancer.[61] Aberrant DNA methylation patterns occur in several cancers (colon, lung, prostate, and breast).

Specific nutritional factors seem to influence susceptibility to cancer (see *Nutrition & Disease:* Components of a Cancer Risk Reduction Diet). Continuing studies are determining whether certain deficiencies, such as vitamin D and compounds found in fruits and vegetables, can increase cancer incidence (Table 10-5).[61,62] Excess intake of alcohol can promote cancer (see p. 266). Aflatoxin (produced by mold), which can contaminate corn, peanuts, and rice stored in hot, humid environments, and Chinese-style salted fish are known to cause cancer. With emphasis on epigenetic and aberrant methylation (Figure 10-4) the role of folic acid in cancer is prominent and it is also complicated.[63] For example, low intake of folic acid is correlated with an increased risk of colorectal cancer. However, it is important to note that once a cancerous lesion is present folate intake may *increase* tumor growth.[64]

Selective dietary agents that inhibit histone deacetylase (HDAC), and thereby abnormal patterns of histone modification, include

Bioactive Food Substances in Epigenetics

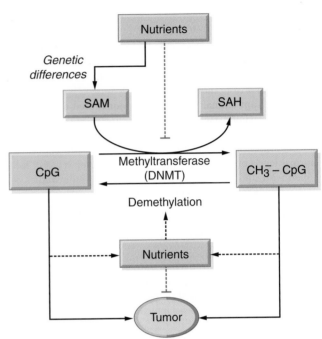

FIGURE 10-3 Dietary Factors, DNA Methylation, and Cancer. Certain dietary factors (see Table 10-5) may supply methyl groups (+CH$_3$) that can be donated through *S*-adenosylmethonine *(SAM)* to many acceptors in the cell (DNA, proteins, lipids, and metabolites). Donation and removal (demethylation) are affected by numerous enzymes, including DNA methyltransferase *(DNMT)*. Increased DNMT activity occurs in many tumor cells. Hypermethylation can inhibit or silence tumor-suppressor genes (see Chapter 9) and DNA methylation inhibitors as anticancer agents and can block DNMT, thus reactivating tumor-suppressor genes. DNA hypomethylation can reactivate and mutate genes, including cancer-causing oncogenes. *SAH, S*-Adenosylhomocysteine.

sulforaphane (SFN). SFN is an isothiocyanate found in cruciferous vegetables, such as broccoli and broccoli sprouts. A growing body of evidence suggests that SFN acts through epigenetic mechanisms to inhibit HDAC activity in human colon and prostate cancer lines.[65] In human subjects, a single ingestion of 68 g (1 cup) of broccoli sprouts inhibited HDAC activity in circulating white blood cells 3 to 6 hours after eating.[66]

In summary, epidemiologic and laboratory evidence suggests that diet is a significant factor in the cause, progression, and prevention of cancer (Box 10-2 and *Health Alert:* Snapshot of Foods as Therapeutic Nutrients). Diet affects many pathways to cancer including cell cycle control, differentiation, DNA repair, gene silencing, inflammation, apoptosis, and carcinogen metabolism. Many of these processes are likely influenced, if not regulated, by DNA methylation, an epigenetic mechanism that affects gene function. Imbalances of nutrients can lead to global hypomethylation, and there is reason to believe that diet can affect gene-specific hypomethylation or hypermethylation, or both.[67] Much more research is needed to identify how specific nutrients can alter DNA methylation and restore gene function as well as other pathways (e.g., apoptosis) that can prevent tumor development. Studies on diet and cancer need testing in a variety of settings and among different population groups.

TABLE 10-5   RELATIONSHIP OF DIETARY FACTORS TO RISK OF MAJOR CANCERS*

DIET	COLO-RECTAL	BREAST	PROSTATE	LUNG	STOMACH	ESOPHA-GEAL	ORAL	PANCREATIC	BLADDER	KIDNEY	ENDOMETRIAL	CERVICAL
Micronutrients/Energy Balance												
Obesity	↑↑	↑↑			↑†	↑†		↑		↑	↑↑	
GI/GL,‡ IGF, height, or metabolic syndrome	↑↑	↑	↑		↑			↑		↑	↑	
Animal fat			↑		↑						↑	↑
Nutrients												
Folic acid	↓↓ᵃ	↓‖		→	↑			↑				
Defects methionine pathway (folic acid, vitamin B12 deficiency)	↑	↑		↑	↑			↑				
Alcohol	↑↑	↑↑¶				↑↑	↑					
Calcium	↓		↑									
β-Carotene supplements				↑↑‖								
Lycopene-containing foods			→	→	→							
Vitamin C			↓?	↓??								
Vitamin E			↓?	→								
Selenium			↓?	→								
Foods												
Red or processed meat	↑	↑	↑	→	→	→	→					
Fruits§	→	→	↓	→	→	→	→				→	
Vegetables§	→		→	→	→	→	→		→		→	
Other												
Grilled meat	↑				↑							
Western diet pattern	↑											
High-fiber diet	↓											
Salt, preserved foods					↑	→	→					
Hot beverages						↑						

From Koushik A et al: *J Natl Cancer Inst* 99(19):1471–1483, 2007; McCullough ML, Giovannucci EL: *Oncogene* 23(38):6349–6364, 2004; Zhang SM et al: *Cancer Epidemiol Biomarkers Prev* 14(8):2004–2008, 2005.

*Two arrows indicate more consistent evidence.

†Cancers of the gastric cardia.

‡GI/GL signifies glycemic index/glycemic load.

§Evidence for a potential benefit from some components of fruits and vegetables (not necessarily blanket effect).

‖Increased risk limited to smokers.

¶Data support hypothesis that higher folate intake reduces estrogen receptor–breast cancer, particularly important with alcohol consumption.

IGF, Insulin-like growth factor; *?*, select trial; *??*, vital trial.

ᵃOnce colon cancer is present, folic acid may increase tumor growth.

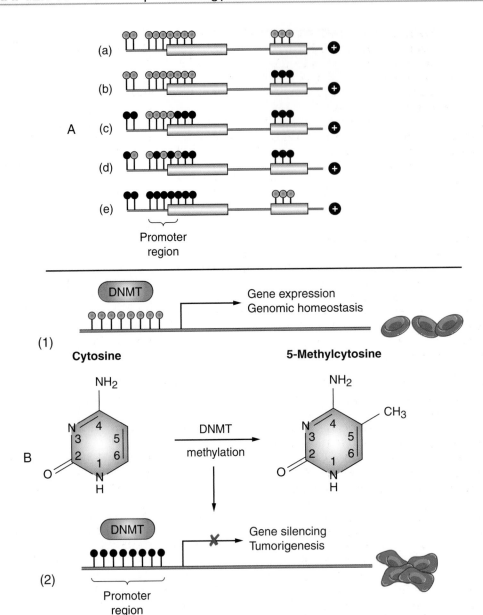

FIGURE 10-4 Methylation of a Gene Region and Its Effect on Gene Transcription. **(A)** (Green circles) Unmethylated cytosine guanine dinuceotide (CpG) sites *(a)* and (black circles) methylated CpG sites. Methylation of exons *(b, c)* does not block gene transcription. Mosaic methylation of promoter CpG island also does not block transcription *(d)*. However, dense methylation of promoter CpG islands completely blocks transcription, and is often associated with hypomethylation of downstream regions *(e)*. **(B)** DNA methylation in normal and cancer cells. DNA methylation in normal cells *(1)*. A *hypo*methylated promoter is related to gene expression. DNA methylation in cancer cells *(2)*. Aberrant DNA *hyper*methylation in the promoter leads to gene silencing (muting) and tumor development. The DNA methylation process is catalyzed by the enymes DNA methyltransferases (DNMTs) by adding a methyl group (CH_3) to the 5-position of the cytosine ring of CpG dinucleotides. (Green circles) Unmethylated cytosine guanine dinucleotide (CpG) sites; (black circles) hypermethylated CpG sites. **(A** from Ushijima T: *J Biochem Mol Biol* 40[2]:143, 2007; **B** adapted from Li Y, Tollefsbol TO: Impact on DNA methylation in cancer prevention and therapy by bioactive dietary components, *Curr Medicin Chem* 17[1]:2, 2010. [Epub ahead of print.])

Obesity

Obesity in most developed countries (and in urban areas of many developing countries) has been increasing rapidly over the past 20 years (Figure 10-5). The only globally accepted criteria for overweightness and obesity are based on the body mass index (BMI). Widely accepted standards based on BMI criteria for overweightness and obesity are recommended by the WHO[64] (Table 10-6) and supported by other panels and federal agencies.

Excess body weight, expressed in studies as increased BMI, is associated with the increased risk of some common cancers in men and women.[68-70] A recent hypothesis states that the observed increased incidence of such cancers as breast, endometrium, colon, liver, kidney,

NUTRITION & DISEASE
Components of a Cancer Risk Reduction Diet

Some foods increase the risk of cancer, whereas other foods decrease the risk. Observing the following dietary guidelines might reduce the risk of cancer.

Increase

Fruits and vegetables (especially broccoli, cauliflower, cabbage, spinach, onions, garlic, bok choy, brussels sprouts, kale, chard, collard greens, chicory, romaine, blueberries, and grapes)

Fiber (limiting glycemic index)

Foods containing vitamins A, C, D, and E; mineral selenium (not to exceed 200 mcg/day)

Vitamin B_6 (grains, beans, liver, avocados)

Vitamin D (see Chapter 2)

Vitamin C?

Foods containing folate (fruits, vegetables [asparagus, broccoli], legumes, grains*)

Epigallocatechin gallate (found in green tea)

Spices (curcumin [turmeric], garlic, cloves, capsaicin, ginger, coriander, fennel, fenugreek)

Whole grains instead of refined grains (wheat, rice, maize)

Lycopene (tomatoes, tomato paste, watermelon)[†]

Legumes (lentils, peas)

Nuts

Decrease

Fat (especially large amounts of omega-6 fatty acids)

High-glycemic-index carbohydrates, sugar

Foods with high amounts of preservatives

Alcohol

Grilled, blackened foods

Fried foods

High levels of calcium (≥2000 mg)

Refined grain products

Data from Ingraham BA et al: *Curr Med Res Opin* 24:139–149, 2008; Lee KW et al: *Am J Clin Nutr* 78:1074–1078, 2003.
*Whole grains.
[†]Recent data of inhibition of AK-signaling pathway.

BOX 10-2 DIET AND CANCER KEY POINTS

Cancer is not evenly distributed throughout the world.

Study of migrant populations shows extreme variations in incidence of cancers are linked to lifestyle differences.

Eating habits by some estimates account for 30% of the overall risk factors for cancer.

Adoption of the Western diet and habits has increased the rate of certain cancers.

Major research is needed on the effects of industrialization on food quality.

Nutrition is an important and a complementary approach in the treatment of cancer.

Continuing research is needed to refine the dietary origins of promoters and inhibitors of cancer in macronutrients and micronutrients.

Eat a balanced diet rich in fruits and vegetables; avoid obesity/weight gain.

Important areas of study are geographic latitude, ultraviolet/vitamin D related cancer research, and micronutrients/macronutrients.

Diet Composition: Macro and Micronutrients

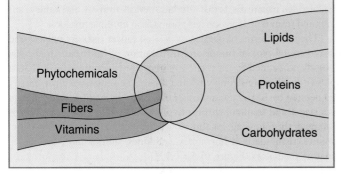

HEALTH ALERT
Snapshot of Foods as Therapeutic Nutrients

Investigators are studying food as a source of anticancer agents. Important is the understanding that some molecules in food have the ability to interfere with certain processes that occur in the development of cancer. Cancer development can be partially conceptualized as a malfunction in certain specialized proteins or enzymes. Molecules that block enzyme activity can be obtained both from pharmaceutical drugs and from foods that are eaten daily. A well-known example is genistein, a molecule that is abundant in soy. Genistein structurally resembles the estrogen hormone estradiol and is therefore known as a phytoestrogen. The genistein molecule can occupy the estrogen receptor, preventing or reducing estradiol's attachment to the receptor. Thus genistein reduces the biologic effects caused by estradiol. Molecules of dietary origin can interact with receptors, illustrating that molecules in food can affect selective downstream metabolic processes. Examples of particular foods that seem to provide phytochemicals important for risk reduction of cancer include tumeric (curcumin), blueberries (delpinidin), strawberries (ellagic acid), green tea (epigallocatechin 3-gallate), soybeans (genistein), grapes (reservatrol), citrus (limonene), garlic (diallyl sulfide), cabbage (especially Chinese, indole-3-carbinol), broccoli (sprouts; sulforaphane), and tomatoes (lycopene).

and esophagus (adenocarcinoma) may be associated with obesity.[71-73] Newer studies have added leukemia, multiple myeloma, pancreatic cancer, non-Hodgkin lymphoma, ovarian cancer,[69] gallbladder cancer, and thyroid cancer[70] to the list. Statistical associations were generally similar in studies from North America, Europe, Australia, and the Asia-Pacific region.[70]

A large prospective study of 900,000 American adults (mean age 57) showed obesity is linked to cancer. Individuals were followed for 16 years and cancer mortality data were collected during that interval.[74] Compared with individuals whose BMI was in the normal range (18.5 to 24.9), men and women with substantial obesity (BMI ≥40) showed significant increases in cancer mortality. Although significant, people with lesser

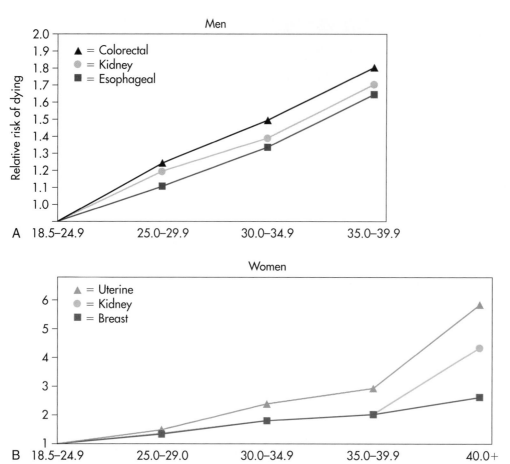

FIGURE 10-5 Weight and Risk of Dying from Cancer. **A,** As a man's body mass index (BMI) rises above the normal range (18.5 to 24.9), his risk of dying of colorectal, esophageal, kidney, and other cancers also rises. For example, the risk of dying from colorectal cancer is 10% higher for men who are overweight (BMI 25 to 29.9) than for men of normal or lower BMI. For the most obese men (BMI 35 or higher) the risk is almost double (84%). **B,** As a woman's BMI rises above the normal range (18.5 to 24.9), her risk of dying of breast, kidney, uterine, and other cancers rises. For example, the risk of dying of breast cancer is 34% higher for women who are overweight. For the most obese women (BMI >40), the risk of dying from breast cancer is double. The risk of kidney cancer is almost five times higher, and the risk of uterine cancer is six times higher. (Data from Calle EE et al: *N Engl J Med* 348:1625–1638, 2003.)

TABLE 10-6	WHO CLASSIFICATION OF BODY MASS INDEX (BMI)	
BMI (kg/m²)*	**WHO CLASSIFICATION**	**OTHER DESCRIPTIONS**
<18.5	Underweight	Thin
18.5-24.9	Normal range	"Healthy," "normal," or "acceptable" weight
25-29.9	Preobese	Overweight
30-34.9	Obese class I	Obesity
35-39.9	Obese class II	—*
>40	Obese class III	Morbidly overweight

Data available at http://apps.who.int/bmi/index.jsp?introPage=intro_3.html.
*The cutoffs are somewhat arbitrary, although they are derived from epidemiologic studies of BMI and overall mortality. It is important to understand that within each category of BMI there can be substantial individual variation in total and visceral adiposity and in related metabolic factors. These variations are also true for the normal range BMI. *WHO,* World Health Organization.

degrees of obesity had lower increases in cancer mortality. In men with higher BMI, there were higher rates of death from esophageal, stomach, colorectal, liver, gallbladder, pancreatic, prostate, and kidney cancers and non-Hodgkin lymphoma, multiple myeloma, and leukemia.[74] Among women, high BMI correlated to greater morbidity from colorectal, liver, gallbladder, pancreatic, breast, uterine, cervical, ovarian, and kidney cancers and from non-Hodgkin lymphoma, and multiple myeloma.

The mechanisms of obesity-associated cancer risks are unclear and may vary by type of tumor and distribution of body fat. Abdominal obesity, as defined by waist circumference or waist/hip ratio, has been shown to be more strongly related to some tumor types than obesity as defined by BMI.[72] Possible associated mechanisms include insulin resistance and resultant chronic hyperinsulinemia and increased levels of any of the following: insulin-like growth factors (IGFs), steroid hormones, tissue-derived hormones, cytokines (adipokines), or inflammatory mediators (Figure 10-6).[72,75-77]

Alcohol Consumption

Chronic alcohol consumption is a strong risk factor for cancer of the oral cavity, pharynx, hypopharynx, larynx, esophagus, and liver.[78] Although evidence is inconsistent, alcohol consumption is less strongly

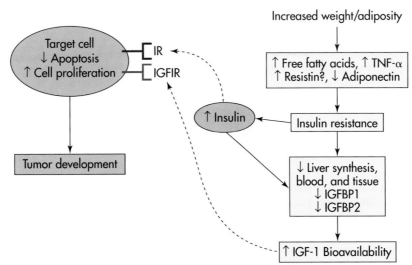

FIGURE 10-6 Energy Balance, Lipid Metabolism, and Insulin Sensitivity and Tumor Development. In obesity, increased release from adipose tissue of free fatty acids (FFAs), tumor necrosis factor-alpha *(TNF-α)*, and resistin and decreased release of adiponectin lead to insulin resistance and compensatory chronic hyperinsulinemia. Increased insulin levels ultimately lead to decreased liver synthesis and blood levels of insulin-like growth factor binding protein-1 *(IGFBP1)* and, theoretically, also decreased IGFBP1 synthesis locally in other tissues. Increased fasting levels of insulin in plasma are also correlated with decreased levels of IGFBP2 in the blood, leading to increased levels of bioavailable IGF-1. Insulin and IGF-1 signal through the insulin receptor *(IR)* and IGF-1 receptor *(IGF1R)* to stimulate cellular proliferation and inhibit apoptosis in many tissue types. These effects could promote tumor development. (Adapted from Calle EE, Kaaks R: *Nat Rev Cancer* 4[8]:579–591, 2004.)

related to breast cancer and colorectal cancer; however, it is known to increase cell growth of human breast cancer cells in vitro.[79] In addition, although the risk is lower, breast carcinogenesis can be enhanced with relatively low daily amounts of alcohol.[78] A meta-analysis showed no consistent relationship between alcohol and cancers of the pancreas, lung, prostate, or bladder.[80] However, alcohol and pancreatic cancer studies have produced conflicting findings. Alcohol interacts with smoke, increasing the risk of malignant tumors, possibly by acting as a solvent for the carcinogenic chemicals in smoke products. In individuals who have never smoked, substantial alcohol consumption (i.e., three or more drinks per day) has been associated with head and neck cancers.[81] Inherited factors also put some individuals at increased risk in DNA repair ability, carcinogen metabolism, and cell cycle control.[82] Individuals having the genes encoding *32-ADH* or the dominant negative allele for *ALDH2* are at reduced risk of alcoholism, despite being at much higher risk for oropharyngeal cancer.[83]

Mechanisms involved in alcohol-related carcinogenesis include the effect of acetaldehyde, the first metabolite of ethanol oxidation; the induction of cytochrome P-450 2E1 (genetic variant CYP2E1), leading to the generation of reactive oxygen species (ROS); increased procarcinogen activation (e.g., nitrosamines) and modulation of cellular regeneration (cell cycle); and nutritional deficiencies (retinol, retinyl esters, folic acid, other vitamins). Nutritional deficiencies may predispose to altered mucosal integrity, enzyme and metabolic dysfunction, and other structural abnormalities. The median age for diagnosis is the early 60s, with a male predominance, especially in laryngeal cancer.[81]

Ionizing Radiation

Much of the knowledge of the effects of ionizing radiation on human cancer has stemmed from observations of the Hiroshima and Nagasaki atomic bomb exposures, particularly the Life Span Study. These data provide the best estimate of human cancer risk over the dose range

from 20 to 250 cGy for low linear energy transfer (LET) radiation, such as x-rays or γ-rays. Other data are derived from groups exposed for medical reasons, underground miners exposed to radon gas, and workers exposed to high doses while in the nuclear weapons program of the former USSR. The atomic bomb exposures in Japan caused acute leukemias in adults and children and increased frequencies of thyroid and breast carcinomas. Lung, stomach, colon, esophageal, and urinary tract cancers and multiple myeloma have been added to the list. At Nagasaki and Hiroshima, leukemia incidence in individuals 15 years or younger reached its peak 6 to 7 years after the explosions and has steadily declined since 1952. People 45 years and older at the time of exposure had a latent period of 20 years before developing acute leukemia.

Recently, standard models and evaluations of age of exposure to radiation and radiation-induced cancer risks have been questioned.[84-87] Epidemiologic data from Japanese atomic bomb survivors and from children exposed to radiation for medical intervention suggest that excess relative risks (ERRs) for radiation-induced cancers at a given age are exceptionally higher for individuals exposed during childhood than for those exposed at older ages.[88] These data also are published by the International Commission on Radiological Protection (ICRP) and the National Academy of Sciences Committee on the Biological Effects of Ionizing Radiation (BEIR Committee).[89] What is at question is the ERRs of radiation exposure in *adulthood* and radiation-induced cancer risk. Recent analyses of Japanese bomb survivors suggest that the ERR for cancer induction decreases with increasing age at exposure only until exposure ages of 30 to 40 years; with radiation exposure at older ages, the ERR does not decrease further and for many individual cancer sites (liver, colon, lung, stomach, and bladder) the EER may actually increase in all solid cancers combined.[85,87,88,90] These new data present a challenge to our conceptual understanding of the mechanisms of cancer induction.[87] Biologic models of cancer development

All Categories *S* and *E*US

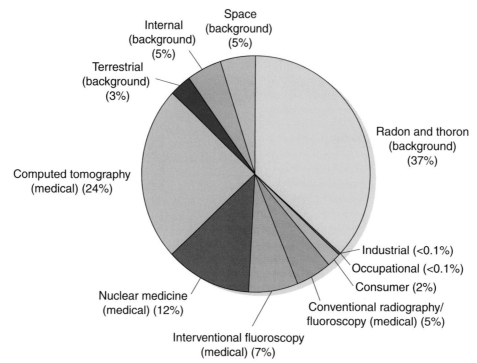

FIGURE 10-7 Pie Chart Showing Sources of Exposure to Ionizing Radiation. Percent contribution of various sources of exposure to the total collective effective dose (1,870,000 person-Sv) and the total effective dose per individual in the U.S. population (6.2 mSv) for 2006. Percent values have been rounded to the nearest 1%, except those <1%. *Sv,* Sievert. (From NCRP: *2009 Ionizing radiation exposure of the population of the United States,* NCRP Report no. 160. Bethesda, Maryland.)

all predict that ERRs should decrease continuously with increasing age of radiation exposure. Recent models, however, of radiation carcinogenesis show ionizing radiation acts not only as an *initiator* of premalignant cell clones but also as a *promoter* of preexisting premalignant cell alterations.[85,87,90] Promotion is used here to mean the process by which an initiated cell clonally expands. Therefore promotional processes from radiation can result in increasing excess lifetime cancer risks with increasing age at exposure. From these new data investigators propose that radiation-induced cancer risks after exposure in middle age may be almost twice as high as previously estimated.[87]

Human exposure to ionizing radiation includes emissions from the environment (e.g., radon), x-rays, radioisotopes, and other radioactive sources (Figure 10-7). Health risks involve not only neoplastic diseases but also cardiovascular disease and stroke following high doses in therapeutic medicine and lower doses in A-bomb survivors (BEIR VII).[89,91] Late effects of radiation in A-bomb survivors show persistent elevations of inflammatory markers (e.g., interleukin-6 [IL-6], C-reactive protein [CRP], tumor necrosis factor-alpha [TNF-α]), implying immunologic damage may be the cause of later cardiovascular effects.[92] Other risks include somatic mutations that may contribute to other diseases (e.g., birth defects and eye maladies) and, from animal studies, inherited mutations that may affect the incidence of diseases in future generations (see *Health Alert:* Radiation and Vulnerable Populations). Heritable mutations are of particular concern for women because the number of oocytes is presumably fixed at birth and mutations, if not repaired, are cumulative (see p. 272).[93] An important summary point in BEIR VII[89] is the concern from high-dose medical exposure, for example, computed tomography (CT) scans (see *Health Alert:* Increasing Use of Computed Tomography Scans and Risks). In

2009 the National Council on Radiation Protection and Measurements (NCRP)[94] reported Americans were exposed to more than seven times as much ionizing radiation from medical procedures as compared to the 1980s (Figure 10-8). The increased exposure is mostly because of the rapid increase in the use of CT imaging.[95]

The risks of low-dose radiation are being debated among radiobiologists, geneticists, physicists, and others because of the potential effect on the health of current and future generations.[96] Limiting is that general findings on the health risks of low-dose radiation are made by analyses of data on the risk of cancer alone.[93] The expression of radiation-induced damage depends not only on dose, fractionation, and protraction but also on repair mechanisms, bystander effects, radioprotective substances such as antioxidants, and the mechanism of radiation delivery.[93]

Radiation-Induced Cancer

Ionizing radiation (IR) is a mutagen and carcinogen and can penetrate cells and tissues and deposit energy in tissues at random in the form of ionizations (e.g., excitation or removal of an electron from the target atom). These ionizations can lead to irreversible or indirect damage from formation and attack by water-based free radicals (radiolysis).[96] IR affects many cell processes, including gene expression, disruption of mitochondrial function, cell cycle arrest, and cell death. IR is a potent DNA damaging agent causing cross-linking, nucleotide base damage, and single- and double-strand breaks (Figure 10-9).[97] Damage to DNA and disrupted cellular regulation processes can lead to carcinogenesis.[97-99] The double-strand break (DSB) (see Figure 10-9) is considered the characteristic lesion observed for the effects of IR. In certain experimental systems, a single DSB may lead to cell cycle

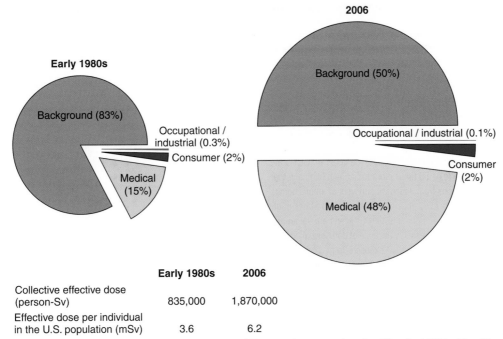

	Early 1980s	2006
Collective effective dose (person-Sv)	835,000	1,870,000
Effective dose per individual in the U.S. population (mSv)	3.6	6.2

FIGURE 10-8 NCRP estimates that 67 million CT scans (compared to 3 million in 1980), 18 million nuclear medicine procedures, and 17 million interventional fluoroscopy procedures, and 18 million nuclear medicine procedures were performed in the U.S. in 2006. (From NCRP: 2009 Ionizing radiation exposure of the population of the United States, NCRP Report no. 160. Bethesda, Md.)

HEALTH ALERT

Radiation and Vulnerable Populations: Pregnant Women, Embryos, Fetus, and Children

Protection of pregnant females against ionizing radiation is unique because of the high fetal radiosensitivity during various gestational stages. The main adverse effects to the embryo and fetus include malformations, mental retardation, induced cancer, hereditary effects, and death. These effects differ by absorbed dose, gestational period and exposure, and type of radiation. All of these concerns have demanded better radiation dosimetry (e.g., standards) for pregnant women. Although setting standards is extremely complex, models of pregnant women have, until very recently, been based on the same methodology developed 40 years ago. These models were developed by the Oak Ridge National Laboratory (ORNL) for the Medical Internal Radiation Dose (MIRD) Committee of the Society of Nuclear Medicine. Today published data on fetal doses for external neutron exposure are those by Chen and by Taranenko and Xu. The 2008 report by Taranenko and Xu noted that comparison with previously published data showed large deviations for the fetal doses at 50 keV. Previous data available of coefficients for photons were based on stylized models of simplified anatomy. To improve these earlier models, a new set of models, called RPI-P series, represent a pregnant female with the fetus at 3, 6, and 9 months' gestation. The deviations in data points are attributed to the differences in anatomic models.

In 2003 the American Academic of Pediatrics Committee on Environmental Health brought attention to the issue of radiation and children with the policy statement *Radiation Disasters and Children*. The following statements summarize the risks of radiation to children:

Children have a number of vulnerabilities that place them at greater risk of harm after radiation exposure. Because they have a relatively greater minute ventilation compared with adults, children are likely to have greater exposure to radioactive gases (e.g., those emitted from a nuclear power plant disaster). Nuclear fallout quickly settles to the ground, resulting in a higher concentration of radioactive material in the space where children most commonly live and breathe. Studies of airborne pollutants are needed to test the long-held belief that the short stature of children brings them into greater contact than adults with fallout as it settles to earth. Radioactive iodine is transmitted to human breast milk, contaminating this valuable source of nutrition to infants. Cow milk, a staple in the diet of most children, can also be quickly contaminated if radioactive material settles onto grazing areas.

In utero exposure to radiation also has important clinical effects, depending on the dose and form of the radiation; transmission of radionuclides across the placenta may occur, depending on the agent.

Radiation-induced cancers occur more often in children than in adults exposed to the same dose. Finally, children also have mental health vulnerabilities after any type of disaster, with a greater risk of long-term behavioral disturbances.

Radiation risks to infants and children per unit of exposure are far greater than they are to adults. In addition, a higher cancer risk is noted in females for most cancers.

Data from American Academic of Pediatrics Committee on Environmental Health: Radiation disasters and children, *Pediatrics* 111(6 Pt 1): 1455–1466, 2003; Chen J: *Health Phys* 86:285–295, 2004; Chen J: *Health Phys* 90:223–231, 2006; Chen J: *Radiat Prot Dosimetry* 126(1–4): 567–671, 2007; International Commission on Radiological Protection: *Ann ICRP* 30(1):iii–viii, 1–43, 2000; International Commission on Radiological Protection: *Ann ICRP* 31(1–3):19–515, 2001; International Commission on Radiological Protection: *Ann ICRP* 33(1–2):5–206, 2003; Suárez RC et al: *Radiat Prot Dosimetry* 127(1–4):19–22, 2007; Taranenko V, Xu XG: *Phys Med Biol* 53:1425–1445, 2008.

HEALTH ALERT

Increasing Use of Computed Tomography Scans and Risks

A review article in the *New England Journal of Medicine* on computed tomography (CT) and radiation exposure has received much media attention. The article was written by radiology researchers at Columbia University. In short, the numbers of CT scans have greatly increased in the United States. This increase has occurred both as a diagnostic treatment for individuals with symptoms and as a diagnostic modality for individuals without symptoms (heart, lung, colon, and whole-body screening). Faster scanning times are partly responsible for increased CT use in pediatric populations. Typical doses are larger from CT scans than a conventional examination (e.g., 50 times more radiation to stomach than an x-ray). Based on data correlations from Japanese survivors of atomic bombs, the authors estimated that 1.5% to 2.0% of cancers in the United States might be attributable to CT radiation. The authors note that CT scans are sometimes ordered excessively and repeated unnecessarily because of defensive medicine. They also include three ways to reduce radiation exposure from CT: (1) reduce radiation doses in individual studies (i.e., use modern scanners), (2) substitute ultrasonography with magnetic resonance imaging (MRI) for CT when possible, and (3) order CT scans only when absolutely necessary.

MEDIAN EFFECTIVE RADIATION DOSE FOR EACH TYPE OF CT STUDY

ANATOMIC AREA, STUDY TYPE	MEDIAN (mSv)	RANGE (mSv)	DOSE EQUIVALENT (NO. OF CHEST X-RAYS)
Head and Neck			
Routine head	2	0.3-6	30
Routine neck	4	0.7-9	55
Suspected stroke	14	4-56	199
Chest			
Chest, no contrast	8	2-24	117
Chest, with contrast	8	2-19	119
Suspected pulmonary embolus	10	2-30	137
Coronary angiogram	22	7-39	309
Abdomen-Pelvis			
Routine abdomen-pelvis, no contrast	15	3-43	220
Routine abdomen-pelvis, with contrast	16	4-45	234
Multiphase abdomen-pelvis	31	6-90	442
Suspected aneurysm or dissection	24	4-68	347

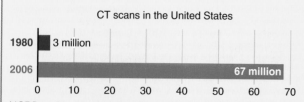

CT scans in the United States

1980 3 million
2006 67 million

NCRP estimates that 67 million CT scans (compared to 3 million in 1980), 18 million nuclear medicine procedures, and 17 million interventional fluoroscopy procedures, and 18 million nuclear medicine procedures were performed in the U.S. in 2006.

Data from Brenner DJ, Hall EJ: *N Engl J Med* 357:2277, 2007; Brett AS: *J Watch* 28(1):3, 2008.
Food and Drug Administration Public Health Notification: *Reducing radiation risk from computed tomography for pediatric and small adult patients.*

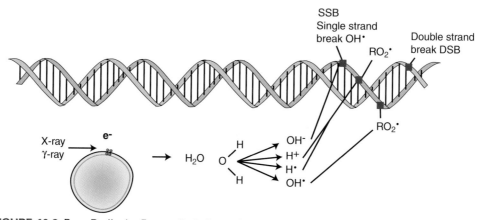

FIGURE 10-9 Free Radicals. Free radicals formed by water nearby and around DNA cause indirect effects. These effects have a short life of single free radicals. Oxygen can modify the reaction, enabling longer lifetimes of oxidative free radicals.

arrest and possible further repair. Yet many DSBs appear to result from clustered damage, a consequence of the pattern of distribution of ionizations with DNA. These patterns of clustered damage may be more difficult to accurately repair.[96] Importantly, DSBs are mostly repaired by the nonhomologous end joining (NHEJ) pathway. This pathway is efficient for joining the DNA broken ends; however, errors can occur. Irradiated human cells unable to execute the NHEJ pathway are supersensitive to the introduction of large-scale mutations and chromosomal aberrations.[96]

A long-held assumption is that cellular alterations—mutations and malignant transformation—occur only in cells directly radiated. It is now known that radiation may induce a type of genomic

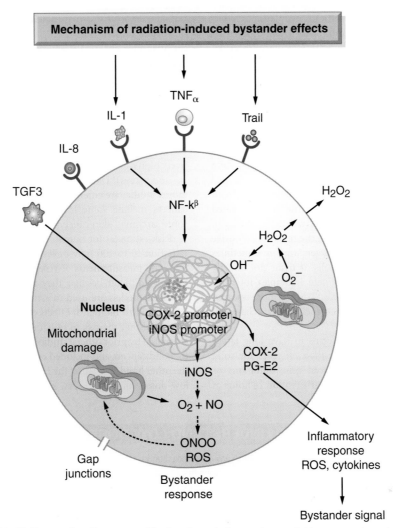

FIGURE 10-10 Bystander Response Mechanism. Inflammatory cytokines are strongly increased after exposure to ionizing radiation or oxidants. Membrane-associated cytokines, such as tumor necrosis factor-alpha *(TNF$_\alpha$)*, activate intracellular kinases (messengers), which release nuclear factor κβ *(NF-κ$^\beta$)*. NF-κ$^\beta$ enters the nucleus and promotes transcription of cyclooxygenase-2 *(COX-2)* and induces nitric oxide synthase *(iNOS)* genes, which stimulate production of nitric oxide *(NO)*. Mitochondrial damage promotes the production of hydrogen peroxide that easily crosses plasma membranes and is subjected to antioxidant removal. Activation of COX-2 provides a continuous supply of reactive radicals and cytokines propagating bystander signals through gap junctions or medium. *H$_2$O$_2$,* Hydrogen peroxide; *IL,* interleukin; *OH,* hydroxyl radical; *ONOO,* peroxynitrite anion; *PG-E2,* prostaglandin E2; *ROS,* reactive oxygen species; *TGF,* transforming growth factor; *TNF,* tumor necrosis factor; *Trail,* TNF-related apoptosis-inducing ligand. (Adapted from Hei-TK et al: Mechanism of radiation-induced bystander effects: a unifying model, *J Pharmacy Pharmacol* 60:943–950, 2008.)

instability to the progeny of the directly irradiated cells over many generations of cell radiation, leading to an increased rate at which the genetic effects (i.e., mutations/chromosomal aberrations) arise in these distant progeny called *transgeneration inheritance* or effects (see p. 260). The directly irradiated cells also can lead to genetic effects in so-called bystander cells or innocent cells (called bystander effects) even though they themselves received no direct radiation exposure.[96] For example, using an in vivo mouse model, investigators found that localized radiation to the head led to induced bystander effects in the lead-shielded distant spleen tissue.[100] These radiosensitive mice showed unexpected enhancement of medulloblastoma in their cerebellum. Both double-strand DNA breaks and apoptotic cell death were induced by bystander effects, supporting the role of signaling between the irradiated cells (the targeted cells) and unirradiated cells (the nontargeted or bystander cells). Such communication is thought to occur from direct physical connection between cells or gap junctions, called gap junctional intercellular communication (GJIC, see p. 274). Other mechanisms, however, may be involved. The bystander and genomic instability effects also have been termed "nontargeted" effects (see pp. 271-274). Numerous intercellular and intracellular signaling pathways are implicated in the bystander response and these effects have been shown to be transmitted to their descendants (Figure 10-10).

Although most of the reports on the bystander effect have been detrimental in nature, protective effects also have been reported (e.g., induction of terminal differentiation, apoptosis of potentially damaged cells).[101,102] Overall, bystander effects include mutations, sister chromatid exchanges, chromosomal aberrations, neoplastic transformation, genomic instability, cell death, proliferation, and differentiation. Although bystander and transgeneration IR effects are associated with induced genomic instability leading to chromosome aberrations, gene mutations, late cell death, and aneuploidy (an abnormal chromosome number), all of these effects may be epigenetically mediated (see p. 257). The epigenetic changes include DNA methylation, histone modification, and RNA-associated silencing (see Figure 10-1 and Chapter 9).[100]

Overall, the bystander effect raises questions about the validity of the linear no-threshold (LNT) model for estimating low-dose radiation risk because nonirradiated neighbor cells (not traversed by a charged particle) are still affected by the transfer of biologic "stress" factors. In addition, previous findings that mutations in the nuclei of irradiated hit cells can be induced by targeted cytoplasmic irradiation, which can further result in a bystander effect, suggest that the radiation-sensitive target is more than just the nucleus. This larger target is sometimes called abscopal, or effects found in other cells or tissue not directly radiated. Therefore bystander effects coordinate a complex interplay of radiation effects of organs, tissues, and cells.[103] Much more research needs to be done with the bystander effect, including mechanistic-based studies and clinical studies.

Radiation-induced cancer in humans seems to have long latent periods—10 years for leukemia and more than 30 years for solid tumors.[104] This implies that radiation-induced gene mutations or chromosomal alterations that can be detected early (within 24 hours of

radiation exposure) are not solely responsible for tumor development in normal human cells. Such mutations, however, provide a critical hit or induce genetic instability that makes cells more susceptible to accumulation of genetic alterations caused by other spontaneous or induced mutations. The accumulation of mutations leads to full transformation and cancer).[96]

The majority of evidence on radiation-induced human cancer risk is from epidemiologic studies of exposed populations. For example, an increase of total cancers after the Chernobyl radioactive fallout was reported in Sweden.[105] Most direct data are available only at relatively high doses (greater than 0.1 Gy) from mainly low-LET radiation (x- and γ-rays). Data, however, from cell-culture systems and in vivo mouse studies are emerging for low-dose radiation. Radiation-induced cancers include some leukemias and lymphomas, thyroid cancers, some sarcomas, skin cancers, and some lung and breast carcinomas.

Risk estimates for human exposure at low-dose, low-LET ionizing radiation (0 to 100 mSv or less than 0.1 Gy) are constantly debated. Accurate measurements of risks from low doses of radiation are statistically difficult because they require such large populations; thus theoretic models are used to estimate response curves (Box 10-3). In 1990 the Fifth Biological Effects of Ionizing Radiation Panel (BEIR V) estimated that the risk of radiation was considerably higher than that estimated by prior official studies.[104] It supported the LNT relationship for solid cancers and included estimates of cancer risk. Recent data, on the other hand, show that the LNT model underestimates the risk from low-dose radiation.[106] Yet, some laboratory studies in experimental

---

BOX 10-3   THEORETIC MODELS TO UNDERSTAND LOW-DOSE RADIATION

Several models include the linear no-threshold (LNT) relationship, in which any dose, including very low doses, has the potential to cause mutations (see **A**). Another model, the linear-quadratic relationship, proposes there is a risk mathematical term that is directly proportional to the dose (linear term) and another term proportional to the square of the dose (quadratic term) (see **B**). The threshold model proposes a threshold dose below which radiation may not cause cancer in humans (see **C**). Proponents of this model argue that such thresholds are derived, for example, from the ability to repair damage caused by lower doses of radiation. There is some evidence that low doses may actually produce a higher level of risk per unit of dose, which is called the supralinear hypothesis (see **D**). Currently, the shape of the response curve for the low-dose region is really unknown.

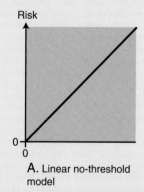

A. Linear no-threshold model

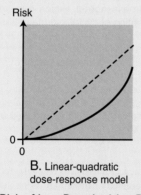

B. Linear-quadratic dose-response model

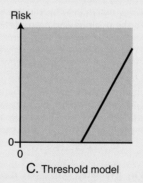

C. Threshold model

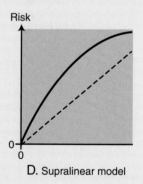

D. Supralinear model

Theoretic Models for Estimating Risk of Low-Dose Ionizing Radiation. Collective population dose is expressed as a person-rem (roentgen equivalent, man). Estimating a collective dose then enables an application of a "constant risk factor" to obtain a statistical estimate of the number of additional cancers (above background radiation) resulting from that exposure. These computations apply to low doses—low-dose rates only (**A**). Many propose the best fit is the linear no-threshold (LNT) model (**B**). The most common alternative to the LNT model is the linear-quadratic model. The quadratic term is the square of the dose. The linear term is equal to zero (**C**). The threshold model is a threshold below which there is *no* increase in cancer risk. Proponents of this model argue that because some toxic chemicals/materials exhibit such thresholds, radiation must also have a threshold. Their arguments are related to repair of the radiation damage caused by lower doses of radiation (**D**). Some evidence exists that low levels of radiation produce a higher level of risk per unit dose, which is called the supralinear model. (From Makhijani A, Smith B, Thorne MC: *Science for the vulnerable: setting radiation and multiple exposure environmental health standards to protect those at most risk,* Takoma Park, Md, 2006, IEER.)

Data from Hoel DG: Ionizing radiation and cardiovascular disease, *Ann N Y Acad Sci* 1076:309–317, 2006; Preston DL et al: Studies of mortality of atomic bomb survivors. Report 13: solid cancer and noncancer disease mortality: 1950–1997, *Radiat Res* 160:381–407, 2003.

TABLE 10-7	CANCER INCIDENCE AND FATALITY (BEIR VII) ESTIMATES OF LOW-LEVEL RADIATION PER GENDER*					
	SOLID CANCERS		**LEUKEMIA**		**ALL CANCERS**	
	MALES	**FEMALES**	**MALES**	**FEMALES**	**MALES**	**FEMALES**
Incidence	800 (400-1600)†	1300 (690-2500)	100 (30-300)	70 (20-250)	900	1370
Fatal cancers only	410 (200-830)	610 (300-1200)	70 (20-220)	50 (10-90)	480	660

*Estimated number of cancer cases and deaths expected to occur in 100,000 persons.
†Estimates correspond to 95% confidence interval in parentheses.

systems, not epidemiological data, indicate that extrapolation from high dose or dose rate down to very low doses and dose-rates may overestimate the cancer risks at low doses.[106a]

BEIR VII estimates of cancer risk from low-level radiation are different from those of BEIR V and are included in Table 10-7. The risk to women is now estimated to be considerably higher.[107] BEIR VII also provides estimates of risk of cancer incidence and fatal cancer risk as well as estimates of cancer risk by age.

Carcinogenesis: Genomic Instability

Genomic instability is an increased tendency of the genome to acquire mutations when various processes involved in maintaining and replicating the genome are dysfunctional. Chromosome instability (CIN) is the inability to maintain a correct chromosome complement after cell division.[108] Biologic consequences of exposure to ionizing radiation include cell death, gene mutations, and chromosome aberrations. Conventional dogma attributes these effects to alterations resulting from the deposition of energy to the DNA of an irradiated cell. Eventually the cell is presumed repaired by DNA enzymatic mechanisms that also can occur during DNA replication. It was widely accepted that most of these changes took place immediately after exposure. Thus if the damage was faithfully repaired, the descendants of an irradiated cell would be normal (Figure 10-11, *A*). If misrepaired, however, the descendants would be expected to pass on radiation-induced genetic change and all cells derived from such a cell would have the identical genetic alteration; in other words, the effect would be clonal (Figure 10-11, *B*). Yet many in vitro studies have demonstrated nonclonal chromosome aberrations and mutations in the clonal progeny of irradiated cells.[109] Furthermore, it has been known for many years that radiation-induced cellular alterations (cytotoxicity), identified as a loss of reproductive potential, might be delayed for several generations of cell replication, with death occurring randomly among the progeny cells.[109]

Now it is known that the progeny of irradiated cells can exhibit an increased death rate and a loss of reproductive potential that continue for several generations—perhaps indefinitely. This delayed cell death phenotype is known as "lethal mutation" and "delayed reproductive death." As introduced earlier, various genetic alterations are demonstrated in cells that are not themselves irradiated, but in so-called innocent cells (i.e., bystander effects; (see p. 271) and are considered manifestations of a radiation-induced genomic instability (see following and Figure 10-11, *C*). This instability is similar to inherited chromosome instability syndromes with spontaneously high levels of chromosomal alterations and mutations.[110] Why is radiation-induced genomic instability relevant to low-dose exposure? Little and Lauriston[111] provide a hypothetical model for multistep carcinogenesis incorporating radiation-induced genomic instability (RIGI). As part of this model, it is proposed that a number of mutations in individual genes must accumulate in a given group of cells to develop into an

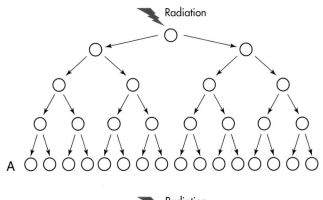

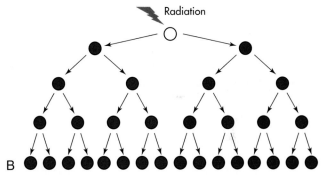

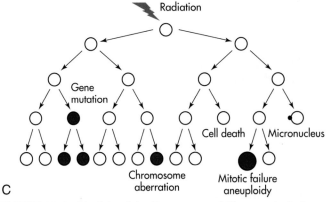

FIGURE 10-11 Models of the Responses of Clonogenic Cells to Ionizing Radiation. Mutations and/or chromosomal aberrations are shown as filled circles and apparently normal cells as open circles. *A,* If a cell faithfully repairs DNA damage, then its clonal descendants will appear normal. *B,* If a cell is directly mutated by radiation, then all of its descendants will express the same mutation. *C,* Radiation-induced genomic instability is characterized by nonclonal effects in descendant cells. (From Lorimore SA, Coates PJ, Wright EG: *Oncogene* 22[45]:7058–7069, 2003.)

invasive tumor. Thus hypothetically, radiation might act at an initial stage of carcinogenesis but could act at any time in later stages after one or more initiating mutations have occurred.[111] (A discussion of new models incorporating initiation and promotion can be found on p. 267.) Radiation may induce or increase genomic instability by facilitating new mutations in later generations. This effect may also be mediated by a nontargeted bystander mechanism.

Induction of genetic changes in bystander cells, as well as those directly radiated, could lead to a "hyperlinearity" response; that is, a disproportionately higher level of risk per unit dose, also called the supralinear model of the dose-response curve, for low doses (see Box 10-3) occurs when only a small number of the cells are irradiated.[111] Direct evidence of the dose-response relationship of a supralinear model was found with an increase in double-strand breaks (DSBs) (see Figure 10-9) in the dose range of 1.2 to 5 mGy and was largely from bystander effects.[112] In addition, Little and Lauriston[111] speculate that individuals with a decreased ability to repair their DNA might be more susceptible to bystander effects.

The genome is constantly challenged by destabilizing factors, including normal DNA replication and cell division; intracellular and extracellular environmental stresses, such as oxidative metabolism; exposure to genotoxic chemical agents; and background radiation. Cells have complex mechanisms for trying to maintain genomic stability. These processes include proofreading of DNA replication, enzymatic repair of DNA damage, and implementation of checkpoints to monitor progression through the cell cycle. Failure of any of these processes can result in destabilization of the genome, deleterious mutations, and alterations in cell proliferation.

Although similar to alterations to the chromosome instability syndromes, the radiation-induced genomic instability seems to reflect epigenetic phenomena rather than mutation of genome genes.[97] Experiments have shown that irradiation can induce growth factors and extracellular matrix (microenvironment) remodeling. A major function of the microenvironment is to control cell differentiation and proliferation, and its disruption is required for the establishment of cancer.[113]

Gap junction intercellular communication. Confluent cell cultures respond as an integrated whole rather than as separate individual cells that have been irradiated, indicating a critical role for cell-to-cell communication in mediating the bystander effect. This mediation could be controlled by gap junctions (see Figure 1-9). Gap junctions consist of a cell-to-cell channel spanning two plasma membranes; they result from the bridging of two half channels, or connexons, contributed separately by each of the two participating cells.[114] Exposure of cells to low levels of radiation (≤0.16 cGy) has been shown to induce the expression of connexin 43, suggesting that oxidizing mediators increase the expression of proteins involved in gap junction intercellular communication (GJIC).[115]

In conclusion, some data support a role for oxidative stress and GJIC in the radiation-induced bystander effects, and studies of the molecular mechanisms underlying bystander cells should increase our understanding of the overall risk of ionizing radiation.

Ultraviolet Radiation

Ultraviolet sunlight *causes* basal cell carcinoma and squamous cell carcinoma (i.e., photocarcinogenesis), two common skin cancers found in white individuals. Exposure to ultraviolet radiation (UVR) can emanate from natural and artificial sources; however, the principal source of exposure for most people is sunlight. With further depletion of the stratospheric ozone layer, people and the environment will be exposed to higher intensities of UVR. The degree of damage in skin depends on the intensity and wavelength content (i.e., ultraviolet A [UVA] or

ultraviolet B [UVB]) and the depth of penetration. UV radiation is known to cause specific gene mutations; for example, squamous cell carcinoma involves mutation in the *TP53* gene, basal cell carcinoma in the *patched* gene, and melanoma in the *p16* gene.[116] In addition, UV light induces the release of TNF-α in the epidermis, which may reduce immune surveillance against skin cancer.[117]

Skin exposure to UVR and ionizing radiation, as well as chemical (xenobiotic) agents/drugs, produces ROS in large quantities that can overwhelm tissue antioxidants and other oxygen-degrading pathways.[118] Uncontrolled release of ROS is an important contributor to skin carcinogenesis.[118] Imbalances in ROS and antioxidants can lead to oxidative stress, tissue injury, and direct DNA damage (Figure 10-12). ROS can induce a number of transcription factors (e.g., activator protein-1 [AP-1] and NF-κβ)[119] and increase regulating genes that induce inflammation.[118,120] Inflammation is a critical component of tumor progression.

Healthy genes are needed to coordinate the levels of antioxidants and decrease harmful ROS. Antioxidants decrease ROS and oxidative stress and other protective mechanisms including DNA repair and apoptosis (see Figure 10-12). The genetic alterations in proto-oncogenes and tumor-suppressor genes may make epidermal cells resistant to signals for terminal differentiation.[120] With oxidative stress, DNA damage occurs and calcium-dependent enzymes (endonucleases) are activated that produce DNA strand breaks.[120] In addition, ROS are involved in the activation of procarcinogens, such as polycyclic aromatic hydrocarbons including 7,12-dimethylbenzene[*a*]anthracene (DMBA). The pathophysiology of skin carcinogenesis is discussed further in Chapter 39.

Basal cell carcinoma commonly occurs on the head and neck. Individuals with these tumors generally have light complexions, light eyes, and fair hair. They tend to sunburn rather than tan and live in areas of high sunlight exposure. Usually these cancers arise on areas of the body that receive the greatest sun exposure, although they are not necessarily restricted to these skin sites. Squamous cell carcinoma is found more commonly in men who work outdoors. These tumors are distributed over the head, neck, and exposed areas of the upper extremities (see Chapter 39).

The incidence of melanoma has been increasing annually at rates of 2% to 7% for white populations;[121] because mortality rates have not risen as rapidly, however, controversy exists as to whether the incidence increase is a true increase in clinically significant melanoma or is a result of overdiagnosis.[122] Sun exposure and the risk of melanoma, a malignant pigmented mole, remain complex. Melanomas can appear suddenly without warning and can arise from or near a mole (melanocytic nevus). When detected in the early stages, melanoma is highly curable.[123] About 20% of melanomas, however, are diagnosed at nonlocalized and advanced stages.[123] According to Sekulic and colleagues,[124] the failure of current diagnostic methods to accurately predict individual risk of disease progression and outcome challenges the ability to diagnose melanoma in early stages. Recent progress in understanding the molecular alterations in melanoma will likely advance its diagnosis, prognosis, and treatment.

The pathogenesis of melanoma is very complex, involving genetic and environmental factors. The genetic factors can be inherited, for example, in high-susceptibility genes (i.e., *cyclin-dependent kinase inhibitor 2A [CDKN2A]*) or in low-susceptibility genes (i.e., *melanocortin-1*). The emerging molecular changes associated with melanoma emphasize that melanoma, like many other cancers, is not a single disease but a diverse group of disorders. Thus, understanding aberrant molecular alterations involved in important cellular processes, such as signaling networks, cell cycle regulation, and cell death (e.g., apoptosis,

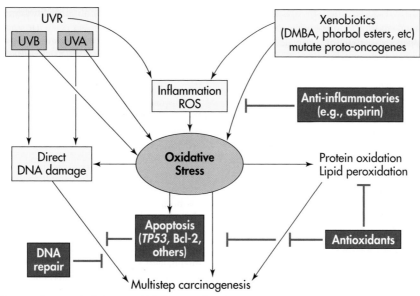

FIGURE 10-12 Theoretic Scheme of Multistep Skin Carcinogenesis. Ultraviolet radiation *(UVR)*, inflammation, and xenobiotics (see p. 262) lead to oxidative stress, resulting in direct DNA damage, protein oxidation, lipid peroxidation, and apoptosis. The protective mechanisms shown in *red* include apoptosis, DNA repair, and antioxidants. *DMBA,* Dimethylbenz[*a*]anthracene; *ROS,* reactive oxygen species; *UVA,* ultraviolet A; *UVB,* ultraviolet B. (Adapted from Sander CD et al: *Intl J Dermatol* 43[5]:326–340, 2004.)

autophagy), is essential for diagnosis and treatment. Epidemiologic and case-control studies suggest that UVR exposure is the most significant factor for the development of melanoma. Other evidence, however, reports rates of melanoma are uncommon in persons with outdoor occupations. An extensive review from the Nordic countries on occupation and cancer showed melanoma steadily increasing until the early 1990s in both men and women. After that, there was a plateau in Norway and Finland but a rapid increase in Iceland.[7] The highest rates of melanoma in men were observed among dentists, physicians, administrators, journalists, religious workers, and teachers. The highest rates among women were dentists followed by public safety workers, teachers, physicians, and other non-nurse healthcare workers. These occupations are all primarily indoor jobs. Dentists are exposed to lamps that emit no UVB but do emit low levels of UVA.[7] A recent analysis in Iceland suggests sunbed use as the reason for increased melanoma, especially in women.[125] Indoor tanning (sunbed use) is a risk factor for melanoma[126] (i.e., frequent indoor tanning increases melanoma risk). Certain skin conditions also are treated with UVA and UVB light therapy.

Although nonmelanoma skin cancers are related to cumulative exposure to UV radiation, melanoma is related to episodes of intense, intermittent exposure (measured as history of sunburn).[127] Melanomas more commonly occur in body areas less continually exposed to sunlight, such as the trunks in men and the backs of the legs in women. Family history (i.e., genetic factors), skin type, and the density of moles are important in determining the risk of developing melanoma. For example, the incidence of melanoma in white populations is 10 times greater than that in black, Asian, or Hispanic populations residing in the same area.[128] Most importantly, the risk of melanoma from sunlight is certainly modified by risk factors.[128] Traits associated with a high risk of melanoma are light-colored hair, eyes, and skin; an inability to tan; and a tendency to freckle, sunburn, and develop nevi.[129]

Until 1998 a direct causal relationship between UVB light and melanoma in humans had not been established. In the first experiment to show that UVB light and an exogenous carcinogen could result in a new malignant melanoma, newborn human foreskin (xenograft) was grafted onto immunodeficient mice.[130] Melanocytic hyperplasia occurred in 73% of UVB-treated xenografts. One graft treated with DMBA (chemical carcinogen) and UVB light developed a human malignant melanoma.

A similar study using UVB light and overexpression of an endogenous growth factor, basic fibroblast growth factor (bFGF), also induced human melanoma.[131] Numerous local factors may result in increased cytokine production, including trauma, infection, diet, obesity, hormones, and other causes of inflammation. Sunburn reflects an overdose of UV light, triggering inflammation with an increase in cytokine production.

In 2002 Davies and colleagues[132] stunned the field of melanoma research when they detected an activating point mutation in the *B-raf (BRAF)* proto-oncogene (i.e., somatic, not germline, mutation) in 60% to 70% of malignant melanomas. This mutation results in a marked increase in *BRAF* kinase activity, leading to activation of the mitogen-activated protein kinase (MAPK) pathway. This *BRAF* mutation and others have been linked to sun exposure.[133] The development of melanoma is associated with the loss of E-cadherin and the appearance of N-cadherin adhesion molecules. Cadherins are cell-surface glycoproteins that promote calcium-dependent cell-to-cell adhesion. The major adhesion molecule between keratinocytes and normal melanocytes is E-cadherin, which disappears during melanoma progression,[134] and thus allows the melanoma cells to survive as they migrate through the dermis.[135] (For further discussion, see Chapter 39.) Alterations in apoptotic signaling may be important in melanoma cell survival.

Sunscreens protect against sunburn but individuals use sunscreen to stay in the sun for longer periods. Consequently, individuals can be exposed to high doses of sunlight that are intermittent or sporadic.[136] Intermittent exposure is the strongest solar risk factor for the development of melanoma. More data are needed to understand if sunscreen prevents melanoma.

Increased knowledge of the intricate cellular interactions in melanoma will increase our understanding of melanoma etiology and pathogenesis. This knowledge is essential for early detection and treatment.

Electromagnetic Radiation

Health risks associated with electromagnetic radiation (EMR) are very controversial. Exposure to electric and magnetic fields is widespread. EMRs are a type of nonionizing, low-frequency radiation without enough energy to pull electrons from their orbits around atoms and ionize (charge) the atoms. Microwaves, radar, mobile and cell phones, mobile phone base stations, power frequency radiation associated with electricity and radio waves, fluorescent lights, computers, and other electric equipment create EMRs of varying strength. Despite the breadth of literature on microwaves (MW) the impact of EMR on human health has not been fully assessed. Scientific evidence is accumulating although hampered by the scarcity of methods to accurately measure exposure, the lack of a clear dose-response relationship, and the difficulty in reproducing effects. In addition, with competing priorities such as convenience, financial interest, and health necessity, a consensus of the risk/benefit ratio of EMR exposure may be difficult to achieve and safety standards significantly vary, up to a 1000 times among countries.[137,137a] In 1998 the National Institute of Environmental Health Sciences Electric and Magnetic Fields Working Group[138] recommended that low-frequency electromagnetic fields (EMFs) be classified as possible carcinogens.

A United Kingdom Childhood Cancer Study published in 1999 and updated in 2000[139,140] did not support a link between EMR exposure and childhood cancer. A pooled analysis from Europe showed no risk of childhood cancers with *average* exposures (less than 0.1 microtesla) and no increased risk at *intermediate* exposures; however, the *highest* average exposures (>0.3 microtesla in American studies or >0.4 microtesla in European studies) showed increased risk affecting a few children (1.4%) with a significant relative risk of 2.[141] In response to public concern, the WHO requested further studies in high-exposure areas such as Japan. A case-control study from Japan (N = 312 children) found acute lymphocytic leukemia (ALL) cases in the *highest* exposure category (>0.4 microtesla).[142,143] Another case-control study reported a link between childhood leukemia and prenatal proximity to high-voltage power lines.[144]

Sweden has officially categorized electrohypersensitivity as a functional impairment.[145] Their data show adverse EMR has the potential to induce certain skin abnormalities and is a positive factor in the development of melanoma.[146,147] Yet another recent study denied an association between EMR exposure and female breast cancer.[148] A recent population-based study (N = 5400 women), however, linked residential EMR exposure from high-voltage power lines to a 60% increased risk of breast cancer in Norwegian women of all ages.[149]

The controversy about potential health hazards associated with the exposure to EMFs has been stimulated by the increased use of mobile telecommunication devices and the increased emissions from cell towers. Cell phones emit electromagnetic radiation in the range of 800 to 2000 MHz, which is in the microwave range (300 MHz to 300 GHz). The output power of the phone is usually set to the highest level between network base stations as a user moves from one location to another or when signal interference is greatest. In rural areas, base station power output is much higher because of the great distances requiring coverage between sparsely distributed base stations. Cell phones in rural areas are often kept at their maximal power output during use to maintain better communication.[150]

EMR from a cell phone can penetrate the skull and deposit energy 4 to 6 cm into the brain (Figure 10-13).[151] This energy can result in thermal heating of the tissue. The debate therefore has been whether these thermal effects could induce carcinogenesis. One thermal mechanism proposed is a change in protein phosphorylation.[152,153] A linear increase in chromosome 17 aneuploidy was demonstrated from exposure of human peripheral blood lymphocytes to EMR associated with cell phones.[154] Control experiments (without EMR) involving temperature changes from 24.5° to 38.5° C (76° to 101.3° F) showed that elevated temperature is not associated with genetic or epigenetic alterations. Thus these findings indicated a genotoxic effect of the EMRs is not elicited by a thermal pathway.[154] There are four lines of evidence for the non-thermal MW effects: (1) altered cellular responses in laboratory in vitro studies and results of chronic exposures in vivo studies; (2) results of medical application of non-thermal MW in the former Soviet Union countries; (3) hypersensitivity to electromagnetic fields (EMF); (4) epidemiological studies suggesting increased cancer risks for mobile phone users.[137a] Increasing evidence indicates that the mechanism of harm from EMR is induction of cell stress and damage of intracellular components (e.g., free radical formation and altered protein conformation).[155] Adverse EMR has been reported to affect DNA synthesis, alter cell division, and change the electric charge of ions and the structures of molecules within cells.[156,157] Interference

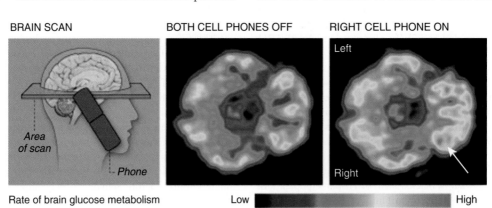

BRAIN SCAN   BOTH CELL PHONES OFF   RIGHT CELL PHONE ON

Area of scan   *Phone*   Left   Right

Rate of brain glucose metabolism   Low   High

Source: JAMA   *Note: Images are from a single participant*   THE NEW YORK TIMES; IMAGES BY JAMA

FIGURE 10-13 **Electromagnetic radiation from a cell phone can penetrate the skull.** EMR from a cell phone can penetrate the skull and deposit energy 4 to 6 cm into the brain.[132] 50-minute cell phone exposure was associated with increased brain glucose metabolism in the region closest to the antenna. This finding is of unknown clinical significance. (From Volkow ND et al: Effects of cell phone radiofrequency signal exposure on brain glucose metabolism, *JAMA* 305(8):808–813, 2011.)

with cellular electric charges may modify ionic structures, disturbing movement of ions across the membrane, including calcium ions.[134,158]

Some case-control studies[159] suggest a harmful association between the use of mobile phones and the risk of tumors (risk is highest on the same side of the head that the phone is used). Some meta-analyses of mobile phone use and malignant brain tumors showed no association or a slight increased risk.[160-162] The recent meta-analysis[159] of low-biased case-control studies included both malignant and benign conditions. Based on evidence from this study, the investigators report an increased risk of tumors for mobile phone use of 10 years or longer (i.e., gliomas and acoustic neuromas). These investigators also assessed the methodologic rigor and bias of previous studies. Unfortunately, they found poor quality and bias to have been prevalent in some (not all) previous studies. Relevant epidemiologic studies relating long-term cell phone use (>10 years) to central nervous system tumors are appearing.[163-166] These data show an increased risk of acoustic neuroma, glioma, and parotid gland tumors. Other studies have reported decreased human sperm motility and changes in sperm structure after exposure to cell phone radiation,[167] changes in sperm motility in rats exposed to cell phone radiation,[168] and a relationship between cell phone use and semen quality and fertility in men.[169-171]

There are no studies of adults who have used cell phones as children or adolescents. Concern is for children in whom the effects may be compounded because of increased vulnerability to radiation and their longer use of cell phones into adulthood. A recent review of 10 epidemiologic studies showed that 8 studies reported an increased prevalence of adverse neurobehavioral symptoms or cancer in populations living at distances <500 meters from base stations.[172] None of these studies reported exposure above accepted international guidelines. Ongoing unbiased research is desperately needed. A prospective cohort study is needed to reduce recall and selection biases. Absolute proof of causation may be hindered because of the ethical questions of exposing individuals to potentially harmful interventions.[135]

> **✔ QUICK CHECK 10-3**
> 1. What are the cancers associated with cigarette smoking?
> 2. How are dietary components related to cancer?
> 3. What are the possible pathophysiologic mechanisms of obesity-associated cancer risk?
> 4. How does ionizing radiation contribute to carcinogenesis?
> 5. Discuss the difficulty in determining cancer risks with electromagnetic radiation.

Sexual and Reproductive Behavior: Human Papillomaviruses

The past decade has demonstrated that sexually transmitted infection with carcinogenic types of human papillomavirus (HPV), referred to as *high-risk types of HPV*, is required for the development of most cervical cancers. HPV can cause other cancers, including vagina, vulva, penis, and anus, and is a newly identified causal factor for squamous cell carcinoma of the head and neck (SCCHN).[81,173] HPV infections, however, are very common in sexually active women, and the majority of these infections will resolve or only cause transient, minor problems.[174] There are more than 100 subtypes of HPV and the virus is found in 99.7% of women with cervical cancer.[175] Of the 100 subtypes of HPV, 30 infect the female and male genital tracts and two thirds of these are classified as high-risk types. HPV-16, in most countries, accounts for 50% to 60% of cervical cancer cases, followed by HPV-18 (10% to 12%) and HPV-31 and HPV-45 (4%

to 5% each).[176,177] HPV types correlated with genital warts, HPV-6 and HPV-11, are called *low risk* because they are rarely associated with cancer.[177] HPV-16 is directly mutagenic by inducing the viral genes *E6* and *E7* (sometimes called oncoproteins). Persistence of infection with high-risk HPV is a prerequisite for the development of cervical intraepithelial neoplasia (CIN) (see Figure 32-13) lesions and invasive cervical cancers.[176] Biologic factors that determine persistence are not understood; controversial risk factors include long-term use of oral contraceptives and smoking.[178] Newer risk factors being studied include drug addiction and reproductive factors (i.e., age at menarche and menopause). In fact, it has been shown that a second peak of high-risk HPV prevalence occurs in postmenopausal women.[178] Smoking has been implicated in acquiring high-risk HPV (HR-HPV) but not as an independent risk factor for high-grade CIN.[179] Earlier reported risk factors, for example, number of sexual partners, are probably indicators of HPV exposure rather than independent risk factors. HPV can be transmitted by genital contact (oral, touching, or sexual intercourse); therefore, condoms are not necessarily protective (see Chapter 32). The *Health Alert* contains information on the rising incidence of HPV-associated oropharyngeal cancers.

HEALTH ALERT

Rising Incidence of HPV-Associated Oropharyngeal Cancers

The incidence of head and neck cancers has fallen with a decrease in smoking in the United States; however, the incidence of HPV-associated oropharyngeal cancers (tonsil and tongue base) appears to be rising—especially in young white men. The two classes of oropharyngeal squamous cell carcinoma seem to have different causes: HPV-positive oral cancers are possibly associated with sex-related risk factors whereas HPV-negative cancers are associated with tobacco and alcohol consumption. Epidemiologic studies support little interaction between the two sets of risk factors, suggesting that HPV-positive cancer and HPV-negative cancer have *distinct* pathogenesis. Tobacco use and alcohol use are known etiologic factors in head and neck cancers; it is surprising that most cases of oropharyngeal cancers in non-smokers are HPV-related. Not yet known is whether this increase is attributed to changes in sexual norms (from past generations), with more oral sex partners or oral sex at an earlier age. Smoking, however, has an adverse effect on both HPV-positive and HPV-negative oral cancers. In Sweden the incidence of oropharyngeal cancers caused by HPV increased from 23% in the 1970s to 57% in the 1990s to 93% in 2007. Emerging data indicate that HPV is now the primary cause of tonsillar cancer in North America and Europe. The mechanism of HPV-oropharyngeal cancer is different than that related to tobacco use: *P53* degradation occurs (i.e., *P53* helps direct genetic repair and cell death [see Chapter 9]), the retinoblastoma *RB* pathway is inactivated (cell signaling pathway), and the risk of HPV-16 (i.e., *P16*) is increased. Tobacco-related oropharyngeal cancers are characterized by *TP53* mutation and a decrease in the *CDKN2A* mutation (cell cycle gene), and thus a decrease in *P16*. Individuals with *P16*-positive tumors have a better prognosis than those with *P16*-negative tumors.

Data from Lowy DR, Munger K: Prognostic implications of HPV in oropharyngeal cancer, *N Engl J Med* 363(1):82–84, 2010; Marur S et al: HPV-associated head and neck cancer: a virus-related cancer epidemic, *Lancet Oncol*, 2010 May 6 [Epub ahead of print]; Nasman A et al: Incidence of human papillomavirus (HPV) positive tonsillar carcinoma in Stockholm Sweden: an epidemic of viral-induced carcinoma? *Int J Cancer* 125:362–366, 2009.

Head and neck cancers are the sixth most common cancer worldwide with an annual incidence of about 563,826 and 310,408 deaths.[173] About 500,000 new cases of cervical cancer are diagnosed each year worldwide—the majority in developing countries, mainly Latin America, the Caribbean, sub-Saharan Africa, and Southeast Asia. About 80% of these cases affect women between the ages of 15 and 45 years.[175] Although HPV is the most prevalent sexually transmitted infection in the United States, less than one third of women and men in the general population have heard of it, and awareness is low among women in high school and college settings.[180] Cervical cancer mortality has decreased over the past five decades in the United States by more than 70%, probably attributable to screening with the Papanicolaou (Pap) test. HPV vaccination programs have made it possible to eliminate most invasive cervical cancers worldwide (see Chapter 32).[180] The World Health Organization (WHO) recommends the vaccine be given to girls between the ages of 9 and 13 years before their first coitus. U.S. Food and Drug Administration (FDA) did approve the use of the first HPV vaccine (marketed as Gardasil®) for boys or men age 9 through 26 for the prevention of genital warts caused by human papillomavirus (HPV) types 6 and 11. HPV may be transmitted by genital contact (oral, touching, or sexual intercourse); therefore condoms are not necessarily protective. The incidence of oropharyngeal cancers caused by HPV is increasing worldwide. Human immunodeficiency virus (HIV)–infected individuals have demonstrated an increase in oral and anogenital pathologic conditions because of HPV infection.[181] Consensus is that newborn babies can be exposed to cervical HPV infection of the mother. The possible modes of transmission in children, however, are controversial.[182]

Other Viruses and Microorganisms

A discussion of the relationship between viruses, bacteria, and cancer is contained in Chapter 9. Other microorganisms involved in carcinogenesis include parasites such as *Opisthorchis viverrini* and *Schistosoma haematobium*. Their specific roles in carcinogenesis are thought to be related to cofactors or carcinogens, or both.

Physical Activity

Physical activity reduces the risk of breast and colon cancers and may reduce the risk of other cancers. Several biologic mechanisms causing this effect have been proposed and include decreasing insulin and IGF levels; decreasing obesity; increasing free radical scavenger systems; altering inflammatory mediators; decreasing levels of circulating sex hormones and metabolic hormones; improving immune function; enhancing cytochrome P-450, thus modifying carcinogen activation; and increasing gut motility.[182-186] For colon cancer, physical activity increases gut motility, which reduces the length of time (transit time) that the bowel lining is exposed to potential mutagens.[187] For breast cancer, vigorous physical activity may decrease exposure of breast tissue to ovarian hormones, insulin, and IGF. A randomized trial found that after 12 months of moderate-intensity exercise, postmenopausal women had significantly decreased levels of serum estrogens.[188] Physical activity also helps prevent type 2 diabetes, which has been associated with risk of cancer of the colon and pancreas.[187,189]

Many questions are unanswered regarding frequency, intensity, and duration of exercise. Much of the literature suggests that between 3.5 and 4 hours of vigorous activity per week are necessary to optimize protection for colon cancer.[186] There is likely a dose-response relationship for colon cancer and breast cancer, and 30 to 60 minutes per day of moderate to vigorous intensity is proposed to decrease breast cancer risk.[190] A randomized controlled trial (12 months) recently supported the Institute of Medicine and Department of Agriculture guidelines

of 60 minutes per day of moderate to vigorous physical activity for decreasing weight, BMI, and percent of body fat and intra-abdominal fat.[191]

Chemicals and Occupational Hazards as Carcinogens

An estimated 80,000 synthetic chemicals are used in the United States. Of those, only about 7% have been tested for their health effects.[192] It is disturbing that another 1000 chemicals are added each year. Exposure to chemicals occurs every day—they are present in air, soil, food, water, household products, toys, personal care products, workplaces, and homes. Table 10-1 (pp. 254-256) provides a summary of chemicals according to strong and suspected links to various types of cancer. Box 10-4 identifies known occupational carcinogenic agents classified by the International Agency for Research on Cancer (IARC), and Box 10-5 identifies probable occupational carcinogenic agents classified by the IARC. A substantial percentage of cancers of the upper respiratory passages, lung, bladder, and peritoneum are attributed to occupational factors; however, fewer studies of nonsmokers exist.[193] One notable occupational factor is asbestos, which increases the risk of mesothelioma and lung cancer and possibly others. Asbestos was used in homes and buildings built before the 1970s to insulate ceiling tiles, flooring, and pipe covers. In Western Europe, the epidemic of mesothelioma in building workers and other workers born after 1940 did not become apparent until the 1990s because of long latency. No exposure to asbestos is without risk and a large number of countries still use, export, and import asbestos-containing products (see Table 10-1).

The central hypothesis, based on rat studies, for the mechanisms related to particle-induced lung carcinogenesis is that insoluble particles cause pulmonary inflammation (e.g., cytokine release, ROS), which leads to genotoxic stress, proliferative response, and tissue remodeling progressing toward fibrosis and tumor development. Additional research is needed to understand the surface chemistry and lung tissue remodeling in relation to insoluble particles, lung carcinogenesis, and other respiratory problems.[194]

Carcinoma of the bladder has been linked with the manufacture of dyes, rubber, paint, and aromatic amines, especially β-naphthylamine and benzidine. Benzol inhalation is linked to leukemia in shoemakers and in workers in the rubber cement, explosives, and dyeing industries. Other notable occupational hazards include heavy metals (e.g., high-nickel alloy, chromium VI compounds, inorganic arsenic), silica, polycyclic aromatic hydrocarbons, sulfuric acid, and chloromethyl ether. Studies of occupational exposure to diesel exhaust indicate an increased risk of lung cancer.[195] Other important exposures are included in Table 10-1. Disentangling data related to lung cancer, air pollution, and occupational risks is complex, especially in combination with active and passive smoking and the interplay of environmental factors and genetic polymorphisms at multiple loci.

Air Pollution

A person inhales about 20,000 L of air every day; thus even modest contamination of the atmosphere can result in inhalation of appreciable doses of pollutants. Airborne substances contaminate food, soil, and water. Contaminants include outdoor and indoor air pollutants. Concerns include industrial emissions, including arsenicals, benzene, chloroform, formaldehyde, sulfuric acid, mustard gas, vinyl chloride, and acrylonitrile.[196] Notable outdoor pollutants include ozone, carbon dioxide, particulates, and sulfur dioxide (Box 10-6) (see Chapter 3 for a discussion of the mechanism of action and side effects of carbon monoxide poisoning).

Living close to certain industries is a recognized cancer risk factor, although it is difficult to determine cancer risk from outdoor pollution

BOX 10-4   KNOWN CARCINOGENIC AGENTS CLASSIFIED BY THE INTERNATIONAL AGENCY FOR RESEARCH ON CANCER (IARC)

Agents or Group of Agents

4-Aminobiphenyl
Arsenic and arsenic compounds
Asbestos
Azathioprine
Benzene
Benzidine
Benzo[*a*]pyrene
Beryllium and beryllium compounds
N,N-Bis (2-chloromethyl)-2-naphthylamine ether and chloromethyl methyl ether*
1,3-Butadiene
1,4-Butanediol dimethanesulfonate (busulfan; Myleran)
Cadmium and cadmium compounds
Chlorambucil
1-(2-Chloroethyl)-3-(4-methylcyclohexyl)-1-nitrosourea (methyl-CCNU; semustine)
Chromium IV compounds
Cyclosporine
Cyclophosphamide
Diethylstilbestrol
Dyes metabolized to benzidine
Epstein-Barr virus
Eronite
Estrogen-progestogen menopausal therapy (combined)
Estrogen-progestogen oral contraceptives (combined)
Estrogens, nonsteroidal
Estrogens, steroidal
Estrogen therapy, postmenopausal
Ethanol
Ethylene oxide
Etoposide
Formaldehyde
Gallium arsenide
Gamma radiation: see x-ray and gamma (γ) radiation
Helicobacter pylori (infection with)
Hepatitis B virus (chronic infection with)
Hepatitis C virus (chronic infection with)
Human immunodeficiency virus type 1 (infection with)
Human papillomavirus types 16, 18, 31, 33, 35, 39, 45, 51, 52, 56, 58, 59, and 66
Human T cell lymphotropic virus type I
Melphalan
8-Methoxypsoralen (methoxsalen)
4,4′-Methylenebis(chloroaniline) (MBOCA)
MOPP and other combined chemotherapy including alkylating agents
Mustard gas (sulfur gas)
2-Naphthylamine
Nickel compounds
N′-Nitrosonornicotine (NNN)
Oestrogen: see Estrogen
Opisthorchis viverrini (infection with)
Oral contraceptives, combined estrogen-progestogen: see estrogen-progestogen oral contraceptives (combined)
Oral contraceptives, sequential
Ortho-toluidine
Phosphorus-32, as phosphate
Plutonium-239 and its decay products (may contain plutonium-240 and other isotopes) as aerosols
Radioiodines, short-lived isotopes, including iodine-131, from atomic reactor accidents and nuclear weapons detonation (exposure during childhood)

Radionuclides, α-particle-emitting, internally deposited
Radionuclides, β-particle-emitting, internally deposited
Radium-224 and its decay products
Radium-226 and its decay products
Radium-228 and its decay products
Radon-222 and its decay products
Schistosoma haematobium (infection with)
Silica, crystalline (inhaled in the form of quartz or cristobalite from occupational sources)
Solar radiation
Talc containing asbestiform fibers
Tamoxifen
2,3,7,8-Tetrachlorodibenzo-*para*-dioxin
Thiotepa
Thorium-232 and its decay products, administered intravenously as a colloidal dispersion of thorium-232 dioxide
Treosulfan
Vinyl chloride
x-ray and gamma (γ) radiation

Mixtures

Aflatoxins (naturally occurring mixtures of)
Alcoholic beverages
Areca nut
Betel quid with tobacco
Betel quid without tobacco
Coal-tar pitches
Coal tars
Herbal remedies containing plant species of the genus *Aristolochia*
Household combustion of coal, indoor emissions from
Mineral oils, untreated or mildly treated
Phenacetin, analgesic mixtures containing
Salted fish (Chinese-style)
Shale-oils
Soots
Tobacco, smokeless
Wood dust

Exposure Circumstances

Aluminum production
Arsenic in drinking water
Auramine production
Boot and shoe manufacture and repair
Chimney sweeping
Coal gasification
Coal-tar distillation
Coke production
Furniture and cabinet making
Hematite mining (underground) with exposure to radon
Involuntary smoking (exposure to secondhand or "environmental" tobacco smoke)
Iron and steel founding
Isopropyl alcohol manufacture (strong-acid process)
Magenta production
Painter (as occupational exposure)
Paving and roofing with coal-tar pitch
Rubber industry
Strong inorganic acid mists containing sulfuric acid (occupational exposure to)
Tobacco smoking and tobacco smoke

BOX 10-5 PROBABLE CARCINOGENIC AGENTS CLASSIFIED BY THE IARC

Agents and Group of Agents

Acrylamide
Adriamycin
Androgenic (anabolic) steroids
Aristolochic acids (naturally occurring mixtures of)
Azacitidine
Bis(chloroethyl)nitrosourea (BCNU)
Captafol
Chloramphenicol
α-Chlorinated toluenes (benzal chloride, benzotrichloride, benzyl chloride, and benzoyl chloride) (combined exposures)
1-(2-Chloroethyl)-3-cyclohexyl-1-nitrosourea (CCNU)
4-Chloro-*ortho*-toluidine
Chlorozotocin
Cisplatin
Clonorchis sinensis (infection with)
Cyclopeneta[*c,d*]pyrene
Dibenz[*a,i*]anthracene
Dibenz[*a,l*]pyrene
Diethyl sulfate
Dimethylcarbamoyl chloride
1,2-Dimethylhydrazine
Dimethyl sulfate
Epichlorohydrin
Ethyl carbamate (urethane)
Ethylene dibromide
N-Ethyl-*N*-nitrosourea
Etoposide
Glycidol
Indium phosphide
IQ (2-amino-3-methylimidazo[4,5-*f*]quinoline)
Kaposi sarcoma herpesvirus/human herpesvirus B
Lead compounds, inorganic
5-Methoxypsoralen
Methyl methanesulfonate
N-Methyl-*N'*-nitro-*N*-nitrosoguanidine (MNNG)
N-Methyl-*N*-nitrosourea

Nitrate or nitrite (ingested) under conditions that result in endogenous nitrosation
Nitrogen mustard
N-Nitrosodiethylamine
N-Nitrosodimethylamine
Phenacetin
Procarbazine hydrochloride
Styrene-7,8-oxide
Teniposide
Tetrachloroethylene
Trichloropropane
1,2,3-Trichloropropane
Tris(2,3-dibromoprophyl) phosphate
Ultraviolet radiation A
Ultraviolet radiation B
Ultraviolet radiation C
(Urethane: see Ethyl carbamate)
Vinyl bromide
Vinyl fluoride

Mixtures

Creosotes
Diesel engine exhaust
High-temperature frying, emissions from
Hot mate
Household combustion of biomass fuel (primarily wood), indoor emissions from
Nonarsenical insecticides (occupational exposures to spraying and application of)
Polychlorinated biphenyls

Exposure Circumstances

Art glass, glass container, and pressed ware (manufacture of)
Carbon electrode manufacture
Cobalt metal with tungsten carbide
Hairdresser and barber (occupational exposure as)
Petroleum refining (occupational exposure as)
Shiftwork that involves circadian disruption
Sunlamps and sunbeds

IARC, International Agency for Research on Cancer.

BOX 10-6 NOTABLE OUTDOOR POLLUTANTS

Ozone is created from the interaction of ultraviolet (UV) radiation and oxygen (O_2) in the stratosphere, leading to the formation of the ozone (O_3) layer *(good ozone)* that accumulates miles above the earth's surface. This layer protects life on earth by absorbing UV radiation emitted from the sun. The heavy use of propellants, such as aerosols, has decreased the good ozone layer, leading to the banning of chlorofluorocarbons. The accumulating ozone at the lower atmospheric level or ground level *(bad ozone)* is a toxic air pollutant. This ground-level ozone is a gas formed by reactions with nitrogen oxides, volatile organic compounds, and sunlight. This gas mixture is emitted from motor vehicle exhausts and industrial emissions. Nasty combinations of mixtures cause damage (i.e., ROS and inflammation) to lung tissue, especially in people with preexisting lung diseases. These mixtures can also affect healthy people when combined with other air

pollutants, such as sulfur dioxide. *Sulfur dioxide* is produced by power plants burning oil and coal, copper smelting, and paper mills.

Particulate matter, often called soot, is released by coal-fired and oil-fired power plants, by industries burning these compounds, and by diesel exhaust. Fine or ultrafine particles less than 10 micrometers in diameter are considered the most harmful. Fine or ultrafine particles are easily absorbed by the lungs and phagocytosed by macrophages and neutrophils that consequently release tissue-damaging inflammatory mediators. Acute exposure to diesel exhaust that contains fine particles can cause lung, throat, and eye irritation; asthma attacks; and myocardial ischemia. The nose and the epithelium of the airways trap particles greater than 10 micrometers in diameter, decreasing their toxic reactions.

Data from Puett RC et al: Chronic fine and course particulate exposure, mortality, and coronary heart disease in the Nurses' Health Study, *Environ Health Perspect*, 117(11):1697–1701, 2009. [Epub, June 15, 2009.]

alone because investigators must accurately control for smoking and radon. Studies that controlled or stratified for smoking demonstrated associations between excess lung cancer rates and heavy metal and aromatic hydrocarbon emissions in polluted air. Evidence for cancers, other than lung cancer and childhood cancer, is inconsistent.[197]

Indoor pollution generally is considered worse than outdoor pollution, partly because of cigarette smoke. Environmental tobacco smoke (ETS; passive smoking) can cause the formation of reactive oxygen free radicals and thus DNA damage. The IARC has classified ETS as a human carcinogen. Another significant indoor air pollutant is radon gas. Radon is a natural radioactive gas derived from the radioactive decay of uranium that is ubiquitous in rock and soil; it can become trapped in houses and form radioactive decay products known to be carcinogenic to humans. The most hazardous houses can be identified by testing and then by being modified to prevent further radon contamination. Exposure levels are greater from underground mines than from houses. Most of the lung cancers associated with radon are bronchogenic; however, small cell carcinoma does occur with greater frequency in underground miners. Radon increases the risk of lung cancer in underground miners whether they smoke or not.

In China, some regions report very high levels of lung cancer in women who spend much of their time indoors. Exposures from heating and cooking combustion sources (e.g., oil vapors) and asbestos are identified as risk factors for lung cancer.[198] In addition, domestic coal use and ETS increase the risk of lung cancer in women and men.[199]

Inorganic arsenic (known as a carcinogen since the late 1960s), found principally in underground water (at levels ranging from 1000 to 4000 mcg/L), is found in many regions of the world. According to the IARC, strong evidence indicates an increased risk of bladder, skin, and lung cancers following consumption of water with high levels of arsenic (generally greater than 200 mcg/L).[200] Evidence for cancers of the liver, colon, and kidney is weaker. Other sources of inorganic arsenic are related to occupational exposures (see Box 10-4).

✔ **QUICK CHECK 10-4**
1. Identify the high-risk types of HPV that are carcinogenic.
2. Chemicals present a notable challenge to the environment and cancer-why?
3. What components of air pollution are considered most important for carcinogenesis?

DID YOU UNDERSTAND?

Genes, Environmental-Lifestyle Factors, and Risk Factors

1. Environmental-lifestyle factors and occupational exposures are increasing the number of cancer cases and deaths.
2. Cancers are caused by environmental-lifestyle and genetic factors. Investigators are connecting the complex web between genotype, phenotype, and the environment and carcinogenesis.
3. Studies of individuals with particular genetic predispositions who may be more susceptible to the biologic effects of environmental exposures cannot explain the increased cancer risk in exposed groups.
4. It appears that the majority of cancers are caused by carcinogen exposure rather than by rare genetic conditions.
5. The cancers increasing substantially in the United States include melanoma, non-Hodgkin lymphoma, testicular, brain, and thyroid. These cancers are *not* linked to cigarette smoking.
6. Statistics have shown that immigrants acquire the cancer incidence rates of the country where they relocate within one or two generations; thus ethnicity or country of origin may not be as important as immediate environment.
7. A new paradigm shift suggests that susceptibility to disease may be established in utero or neonatally.

Epigenetics and Genetics

1. An explosion of new data indicate the relative importance of genetic versus epigenetic processes.
2. The importance of epigenetic processes includes gene silencing of key regulatory genes.
3. Epigenetic changes collaborate with the genetic changes and environmental-lifestyle factors to cause the development of cancer.
4. Developmental plasticity is the degree to which an organism's development is contingent on its environment. It requires stable gene expression that in part appears to be modulated by epigenetic processes such as DNA methylation, histone modification, and micro-RNAs.
5. Epidemiologic and animal studies reveal that small changes in the developmental environment can alter phenotypic changes, resulting in individual responses in adulthood.

Tobacco Use

1. Cigarette smoking is carcinogenic and the most important cause of cancer. The risk is greatest in those who begin to smoke when young and continue throughout life.
2. Cigarette smoking causes more than 5 million deaths per year from cancer, chronic lung disease, cardiovascular disease, and stroke.
3. Smoking tobacco is linked to cancers of the lung, lower urinary tract, upper aerodigestive tract, liver, kidney, pancreas, cervix, uterus, and myeloid leukemia.
4. Environmental tobacco smoke (ETS) is the combination of sidestream and mainstream smoke.
5. More than 60 chemicals in tobacco smoke are considered carcinogenic. Nonsmokers who live with smokers are at greatest risk for lung cancer as well as other noncancerous conditions.
6. Cigar or pipe smoking is strongly and causally related to cancers of the oral cavity, esophagus, and lung. Cigar smokers who inhale deeply may have other disease risks. Bidi smoking can cause cancers of the respiratory and digestive sites.

Diet

1. Diet can expose individuals to xenobiotics.
2. Carcinogenic substances from diet can develop from the cooking of fat, meat, or protein (e.g., heterocyclic aromatic amines), and from naturally occurring compounds associated with plant foods.
3. Nutrition may directly influence epigenetic factors that silence genes that should be active or activate genes that should be silent.
4. Dietary components can act directly as mutagens or interfere with their elimination.
5. Dietary factors may alter hormonal axes, influence cellular proliferation, and affect phenotype or expression of key genes, for example, epigenetically.
6. Diet affects pathways to cancer including cell cycle control, differentiation, DNA repair, gene silencing, inflammation, apoptosis, and carcinogenic metabolism.

DID YOU UNDERSTAND?—cont'd

Obesity

1. Obesity has been increasing in developed countries and in urban areas of developing countries. Studies in the United States have suggested obesity is associated with some cancers, though it may not be a causal factor in cancer mortality.
2. A recent hypothesis is obesity may be associated with the incidence of cancers of the breast, endometrium, colon, liver, kidney, and esophagus.
3. Biologic mechanisms of the association of obesity with cancer include insulin resistance, hyperinsulinemia, increased IGFs, increased steroid hormones, and increased tissue-derived hormones, cytokines, and/or inflammatory mediators.
4. Adipose tissue is active endocrine and metabolic tissue. Increased release of free fatty acids, resistin, and TNF-α and reduced release of adiponectin lead to insulin resistance. Adipose tissue cells produce steroid hormone—metabolizing enzymes and are an important source of estrogens in postmenopausal women. IGF-1 regulates cell proliferation and inhibits apoptosis and the synthesis and biologic availability of female and male sex hormones.
5. Numerous dietary factors are associated with cancer risk.

Alcohol Consumption

1. Chronic alcohol consumption is a *strong* risk factor for cancer of the oral cavity, pharynx, hypopharynx, larynx, esophagus, and liver.
2. Alcohol consumption is *less strongly* but consistently related to breast cancer and colorectal cancer. Also, it is known to increase cell growth of human breast cancer cells in vitro.

Ionizing Radiation (IR)

1. Human exposures to ionizing radiation include background radiation from soil or rocks, radon gas seeping into homes and other buildings, energy or matter moving through space, and sources within the human body.
2. Other sources of exposure to ionizing radiation include emissions from x-rays, radioisotopes, and other radioactive sources. The NCRP is concerned about the increased IR exposure from medical procedures, particularly CT scans and nuclear medicine procedures.
3. The risks from low-dose radiation are being debated among radiobiologists, geneticists, physicists, and others because of the potential effect on the health of current and future generations.
4. IR is a mutagen and carcinogen; it can penetrate cells and tissues and deposit energy in tissues at random in the form of ionizations.
5. IR affects many cellular processes, including gene expression, mitochondrial function, nucleotide base damage, and single- and double-strand DNA breaks. These changes can lead to carcinogenesis.
6. It is now known that radiation may induce a type of genomic instability to the progeny of the directly irradiated cells over many generations of cell radiation and can affect so-called innocent bystander cells.
7. New models of carcinogenesis identify ionizing radiation not only as an initiator of premalignant cell clones but also as a promoter of preexisting-premalignant damage.
8. Epigenetic events after radiation include alterations in pathways affecting cell adhesion, extracellular matrix interactions, and cell-to-cell communication.

Ultraviolet Radiation (UVR)

1. UVR causes basal cell carcinoma and squamous cell carcinoma. The principal source of UVR is sunlight.
2. The degree of damage in skin depends on the intensity and wavelength content—ultraviolet A (UVA) or ultraviolet B (UVB).
3. UVR is known to cause specific gene mutations: for example, squamous cell carcinoma involves mutation in the *TP53* gene, basal cell carcinoma in the *patched* gene, and melanoma in the *p16 gene*.

4. Skin exposure to UVR produces ROS in large quantities that can overwhelm tissue antioxidants and other oxygen-degrading pathways. Imbalances in ROS can lead to oxidative stress, tissue injury, and direct DNA damage.
5. UVR can activate the transcription factor NF-$\kappa\beta$ and other free radicals important in regulating genes that induce inflammation. Inflammation is a critical component of tumor progression.
6. Melanoma has been increasing annually at rates of 2% to 7% for white populations but mortality rates have not risen as rapidly. The pathogenesis of melanoma is complex, including genetic and environmental factors.

Electromagnetic Radiation (EMR)

1. EMRs are a type of nonionizing and low-frequency radiation. Health risks associated with EMRs are controversial. Exposure to electric and magnetic fields is widespread.
2. EMRs of varying strength include microwaves, radar, power frequency radiation associated with electricity and radio waves, fluorescent lights, computers, electric equipment, cell and cordless phones, and others.
3. Data regarding the effects of EMR have been slow because of methods to accurately measure exposure, the lack of clear dose-response relationships, reproducing effects, financial interests, and other priorities such as convenience.
4. Studies differ on findings, however, a pooled analysis with low and high exposures showed at the highest average exposures increased risks affecting few children with childhood cancer. The WHO requested studies in high-exposure areas like Japan and found (case-control study) acute lymphocytic leukemia in children in the highest exposure category.
5. Epidemiologic studies and a recent meta-analysis of low-bias studies found a consistent pattern of an increased risk for acoustic neuroma and glioma in those using cell phones for more than 10 years. The concern is more for children.

Sexual and Reproductive Behavior

1. High-risk types of HPV are required for the development of most cervical cancers. High-risk types include HPV-16 (50% to 60% of cervical cancer cases), HPV-18 (10% to 12%), and HPV-31 and HPV-45 (4% to 5% each). HPV can cause other cancers including vaginal, vulva, penis, anus, and oropharyngeal.
2. Biologic factors that may interact with HPV to promote persistent infection include oral contraceptives and smoking. Newer risk factors include drug addiction and reproductive factors such as age at menarche and menopause. A second peak of high-risk HPV prevalence occurs in postmenopausal women.
3. HPV may be transmitted by genital contact (oral, touching, or sexual intercourse); therefore condoms are not necessarily protective. The incidence of oropharyngeal cancers caused by HPV is increasing worldwide.
4. HPV vaccination programs have made it possible to eliminate the majority of all invasive cervical cancer worldwide.

Physical Activity

1. Physical activity reduces the risk for breast and colon cancers and may reduce the risk for other cancers.
2. Biologic mechanisms for the protective effects of physical activity include decreasing insulin and IGF levels, decreasing obesity, increasing free radical scavenger systems, altering inflammatory mediators, decreasing levels of circulating sex hormones and metabolic hormones, improving immune function, enhancing cytochrome P-450 activity (thus modifying carcinogen activation), and increasing gut motility.
3. Physical activity may prevent type 2 diabetes, which has been associated with cancer of the pancreas and colon.
4. Many unanswered questions remain regarding frequency of exercise, intensity, and duration.
5. Recent data encourage 60 minutes of vigorous activity daily for decreasing BMI, body fat, and intra-abdominal fat.

DID YOU UNDERSTAND?—cont'd

Chemicals and Occupational Hazards

1. The International Agency for Research on Cancer (IARC) has classified carcinogenic agents as known and probable.

2. An estimated 80,000 synthetic chemicals are used in the United States. Only 7% have been fully tested for their impact on health and another 1000 are added each year.

3. Chemicals are present in air, soil, food, water, personal care products, toys, household products, medications, workplaces, and homes. Table 10-1 is a summary of environmental and occupational links to cancer.

4. Chemicals can persist in the environment and accumulate in body fat and remain there indefinitely. Mechanisms of carcinogenesis for chemicals include direct carcinogenic action, hormonal disruptors, interference with cell signaling pathways, and other unknown effects.

5. A substantial percentage of cancers of the upper respiratory passages, lung, bladder, and peritoneum are attributed to occupational factors.

6. Disentangling data related to lung cancer, air pollution, and occupational factors is complex especially in combination with active and passive smoking, environmental factors, and multiple interacting genes.

7. Air pollution is a concern in regard to cancer because of inhalation of ozone, particulate matter, carbon dioxide, and other emissions, including arsenicals, benzene, chloroform, vinyl chloride, and acrylonitrile. Indoor pollution is considered worse than outdoor pollution because of cigarette smoke and possibly radon gas.

KEY TERMS

- Abscopal   272
- Bystander effect   271
- Cadherin   275
- Chromosome instability (CIN)   273
- Connexon   274
- Developmental plasticity   260
- Environmental tobacco smoke (ETS)   261
- Genomic instability   273
- Individual carcinogen   253
- "Nontargeted" effect   271
- Radon   281
- Transgenerational inheritance   260
- Transgeneration inheritance (effect)   260
- Xenobiotics   262

REFERENCES

1. Clapp RW, et al: Environmental and occupational causes of cancer; new evidence 2005–2007, *Rev Environ Health* 23(1):1–37, 2008.

2. Clapp RW, Howe GK, Jacobs MM: Environmental and occupational causes of cancer: a call to act on what we know, *Biomed Pharmacother* 61(10):631–639, 2007.

3. National Cancer Institute: *Cancer and the environment: what you need to know, what you can do,* Washington, DC, 2004, U.S. Department of Health and Human Services, Available at www.nci.nih.gov/newscenter/benchmarks-vol4-issue3.

4. National Toxicology Program: Final report on carcinogens background document for styrene, *Rep Carcinog Backgr Doc* (8–5978):1–398, 2008.

5. National Toxicology Program: Final report on carcinogens background document for formaldehyde, *Rep Carcinog Backgr Doc* (10–5981):1–512, 2010.

6. President's Cancer Panel: *Reducing environmental cancer risk: what we can do now,* Washington, DC, 2008–2009, U.S. Department of Health and Human Services, National Institutes of Health, National Cancer Institute.

7. Pukkala E, et al: Occupational and cancer—follow-up of 15 million people in five Nordic countries, *Acta Oncol* 48(5):646–790, 2009.

8. King MC, Marks JH, Mandell JB: *New York breast cancer study group: breast and ovarian cancer risks due to inherited mutations in BRCA1 and BRCA2, Science* 302:643–646, 2002.

9. Chia VM, et al: International trends in the incidence of testicular cancer, 1973–2002, *Cancer Epidemiol Biomarkers Prev* 19(5):1151–1159, 2010.

10. National Cancer Institute-DCCPS-Surveillance Research Program-Cancer Statistics Branch: Surveillance, epidemiology, and end results (SEER) program. Available at http://.seer.cancer.gov SEER* Stat Database: Incidence-SEER 9 Regs Public-Use, Nov 2005 Sub (1973-2003), SEER Cancer Query Systems, released April 2006. http://seer.cancer.gov/canques. Accessed July 2008.

11. Miller BA, et al: Cancer incidence and mortality patterns among specific Asian and Pacific Islander populations in the U.S., *Cancer Causes Control* 19(3):227–256, 2008.

12. Liao CK, et al: Endometrial cancer in Asian migrants to the United States and their descendants, *Cancer Causes Control* 11(5):357, 2003.

13. Knox EG: Childhood cancers, birthplaces, incinerators, and landfill sites, *Int J Epidemiol* 29:391, 2000.

14. Litt JS, Tran NL, Burke TA: Examining urban brownfields through the public health "macroscope," *Environ Health Perspect* 110(Suppl 2):183, 2002.

15. Blair A, Freeman LB: Epidemiologic studies in agricultural populations: observations and figure directions, *J Agromedicine* 14(2):125–131, 2009.

16. Skinner MK, Manikkam M, Guerro-Bosagna C: Epigenetic transgenerational actions of environmental factors in disease etiology, *Trends Endocrinol Metab* 21(4):214–222, 2010.

17. Gouveia-Vigeant T, Tickner J: *Lowell Center for Sustainable Production, Toxic chemicals and childhood cancer: a review of the evidence,* 2003, University of Massachusetts at Lowell. Available at www.sustainableproduction.org.

18. Kolonel LN, Altshuler D, Henderson BE: The multiethnic cohort study: exploring genes, lifestyle and cancer risk, *Nat Rev Cancer* 4(7):519–527, 2004.

19. Hajkova P, et al: Genome-wide reprogramming in the mouse germ line entails the base excision repair pathway, *Science* 329(5987):78–82, 2010.

20. Sasaki H, Matsui Y: Epigenetic events in mammalian germ-cell development: reprogramming and beyond, *Nat Rev Genet* 9(2):129–140, 2008.

21. Olson P, et al: Micro RNA dynamics in the stages of tumorigenesis correlate with hallmark capabilities of cancer, *Genes Dev* 23(18):2152–2165, 2009.

22. Boland CR, Shin SK, Goel A: Promoter methylation in the genesis of gastrointestinal cancer, *Yonsei Med J* 50(3):309–321, 2009.

23. Christensen BC, et al: Aging and environmental exposures after tissue-specific DNA methylation dependent upon CpG island context, *PLoS Genet* 5(8), 2009:e1000602.

24. Foley DL, et al: Prospects for epigenetic epidemiology, *Am J Epidemiol* 169(4):389–400, 2009.

25. Thompson RF, Fazzari MJ, Greally JM: Experimental approaches to the study of epidenomic dysregulation in ageing, *Exp Gerontol* 45(4): 255–268, 2003.

26. Skinner MK, Guerrero-Bosagna C: Environmental signals and transgender epigenetics, *Epigenomics* 1(1):111–117, 2009.

27. Poulsen P, et al: The epigenetic basis of twin discordance in age-related diseases, *Pediatr Res* 61(5 pt 2):38R–42R, 2007:review.

28. Kondo Y, Issa JP: DNA methylation profiling in cancer, *Exp Rev Mol Med* 12:e23, 2010.

29. Kim MS, Lee J, Sidransky D: DNA methylation markers in colorectal cancer, *Cancer Metastasis Rev* 29(1):181–206, 2010.

30. Gluckman PD, Hanson MA, Mitchell MD: Developmental origins of health and disease: reducing the burden of chronic disease in the next generation, *Genome Med* 2(2):14, 2010.

31. Rubin MM: Antenatal exposure to DES: lesions learned…future concerns, *Obstet Gynecol Surv* 62(8):548–555, 2007.

32. Park SK, et al: Intrauterine environments and breast cancer risk: meta-analysis and systematic review, *Breast Cancer Res* 10(1):R8, 2008. doi: 10.1186/ber 1850.

33. Palmer JR, et al: Prenatal diethylstilbestrol exposure and risk of breast cancer, *Cancer Epidemiol Biomarkers Prev* 15(8):1509–1514, 2006.

34. Newbold RR: Prenatal exposure to diethylstilbestrol (DES), *Fertil Steril* 89(2 suppl):e55–e56, 2008.

35. Newbold RR, Padilla-Banks E, Jefferson WN: Adverse effects of the model environmental estrogen diethylstilbestrol are transmitted to subsequent generations, *Endocrinology* 147(6 suppl):S11–S17, 2006.

36. Petridou E, et al: Baldness and other correlates of sex hormones in relation to testicular cancer, *Int J Cancer* 71(6):982–985, 1997.

37. Palmer JR, et al: Urogenital abnormalities in men exposed to diethylstilbestrol in utero: a cohort study, *Environ Health* 8:37, 2009.

38. Waterland RA: Early environmental effects on epigenetic regulation in humans, *Epigenet* 4(8):523–525, 2009.

39. Chen YC, Hunter DJ: Molecular epidemiology of cancer, *CA Cancer J Clin* 55(1):45–54, 2005:quiz 57.

40. Centers for Disease Control and Prevention: Global youth tobacco surveillance, 2000–2007, *MMWR Morb Mortal Wkly Rep* 57(5501):1–21, 2008.

41. World Health Organization: *WHO report on the global tobacco epidemic*, Geneva, 2008, Author.

42. Centers for Disease Control and Prevention: Annual smoking-attributable mortality, years of potential life lost, and productivity losses—United States, 1995–1999, *MMWR Morb Mortal Wkly Rep* 51(14):300–303, 2002:[serial online].

43. WHO World Cancer Report: Global cancer rates could increase by 50% to 15 million by 2020. Available at www.WHO.int/mediacentre/news/release/2003/pr27/en/. Accessed July 2008.

44. Centers for Disease Control and Prevention: Cigarette smoking among adults—United States, 2004, *MMWR Morb Mortal Wkly Rep* 54(44):1121–1124, 2005.

45. Centers for Disease Control and Prevention: Cigarette smoking among adults—United States, 2006, *MMWR Morb Mortal Wkly Rep* 56(44):1157–1161, 2007.

46. Centers for Disease Control and Prevention: Cigarette smoking among adults and trends in smoking cessation—United States, 2008, *MMWR Morb Mortal Wkly Rep* 58(44):1227–1232, 2008:[serial online]. Accessed April 30, 2010.

47. Taioli E: Gene-environment interaction in tobacco-related cancers, *Carcinogenesis* 29(8):1467–1474, 2008.

48. Egan KM, et al: Active and passive smoking in breast cancer: prospective results from the Nurses' Health Study, *Epidemiology* 13(2):138–145, 2002. Available at doi:10.1097/00001648-200203000-00007.

49. Gram IT, et al: Breast cancer risk among women who start smoking as teenagers, *Cancer Epidemiol Biomarkers Prev* 14(1):61–66, 2005.

50. Ha M, et al: Smoking cigarettes before first childbirth and risk of breast cancer, *Am J Epidemiol* 166(1):55–61, 2007. doi:10.1093/aje/kwm045.

51. Reynolds P, et al: Active smoking, household passive smoking, and breast cancer: evidence from the California Teachers Study, *J Natl Cancer Inst* 96(1):29–37, 2004.

52. Hanaoka T, et al: Active and passive smoking and breast cancer risk in middle-aged Japanese women, *Int J Cancer* 114:317–322, 2005.

53. Centers for Disease Control and Prevention: Smoking and secondhand smoke. Accessed July 2010. Available at www.cdc.gov/cancer/lung.

54. Centers for Disease Control and Prevention: Cigar smoking and cancer. Accessed July 2010. Available at www.cancer.gov/cancertopics/factsheet/Tobacco/cigars.

55. Henley SJ, et al: Association between exclusive pipe smoking and mortality from cancer and other diseases, *J Natl Cancer Inst* 96(11):853–861, 2004.

56. Boffetta P, et al: Smokeless tobacco and cancer, *Lancet Oncol* 9(7): 667–675, 2008.

57. Working Group on Diet and Cancer of the Committee on Medical Aspects of Food and Nutrition Policy: *Nutritional aspects of the development of cancer, Department of Health Rep Health Social Subjects 48,* London, 1998, The Stationery Office.

58. Jones DP, Delong MJ: Detoxification and protective functions of nutrients. In Stipanuk M, editor: *Biochemical and physiological aspects of nutrition,* Philadelphia, 2000, Saunders.

59. Wiseman M: The second World Cancer Research Fund/American Institute for Cancer Research expert report. Food, nutrition, physical activity, and the prevention of cancer: a global perspective, *Proc Nutr Soc* 67(3):253–256. [Epub May 1, 2008.]

60. Racki LR, et al: The chromatin remodeller ACF acts as a dimeric motor to space nucleosomes, *Nature* 462(7276):1016–1021, 2009.

61. Agrawal A, Murphy RF, Agrawal DK: DNA methylation in breast and colorectal cancers, *Mod Pathol* 20(7):711–721, 2007:review.

62. Gandini S, et al: Meta-analysis of observational studies of serum 25-hydroxvitamin D levels and colorectal, breast, and prostate cancer and colorectal adenoma, *Int J Cancer* 128(6):1414–1424, 2011.

63. Shames DS, et al: DNA methylation in health, disease, cancer, *Curr Mol Med* 7:85–102, 2007.

64. World Health Organization (WHO): *Global strategy on diet, physical activity, and health (online),* 2004:Available at www.who.int/dietphysical activity/strategy/eb11344/en/.

65. Dashwood RH, Ho E: Dietary histone deacetylase inhibitors: from cells to mice to man, *Semin Cancer Biol* 17:363–369, 2007.

66. Myzak MC, et al: Sulforaphane retards the growth of human PC-3 xenografts and inhibits HDAC activity in human subjects, *Exp Biol Med* 232:227–234, 2007.

67. Ross SA: Diet and DNA methylation interactions in cancer prevention, *Ann N Y Acad Sci* 983:197–207, 2003:review.

68. Calle EE, Kaaks R: Overweight, obesity and cancer: epidemiological evidence and proposed mechanisms, *Nat Rev Cancer* 4:579–591, 2004.

69. Reeves GK, et al: Cancer incidence and mortality in relation to body mass index in the Million Women Study: cohort study, *Br Med J* 335(7630):1134, 2007.

70. Renehan AG, et al: Body-mass index and incidence of cancer: a systematic review and meta-analysis of prospective observational studies, *Lancet* 371(9612):569–578, 2008.

71. Donohoe CL, et al: Obesity and gastrointestinal cancer, *Br J Surg* 97(5):628–642, 2010.

72. Pischon T, Nöthlings U, Boeing H: Obesity and cancer, *Proc Nutr Soc* 67(2):128–145, 2008.

73. World Cancer Research Fund: *Food, nutrition, and the prevention of cancer: a global perspective,* Washington, DC, 1997, American Institute for Cancer Research, 371–373.

74. Calle EE, et al: Overweight, obesity, and mortality from cancer in a prospectively studied cohort of U.S. adults, *N Engl J Med* 348(17): 1625–1638, 2003.

75. Palmqvist R, et al: Plasma insulin-like growth factor 1, insulin-like growth factor binding protein 3, and risk of colorectal cancer: a prospective study in northern Sweden, *Gut* 50(5):642–646, 2002.

76. Schumacher FR, et al: A comprehensive analysis of common IGF1, IGFBP1, and IGFBP3 genetic variation with prospective IGF-1 and IGFBP-3 blood levels and prostate cancer risk among Caucasians, *Hum Mol Genet* 19(15):3089–3101, 2010.

77. Stattin P, et al: Plasma insulin-like growth factor-I, insulin-like growth factor-binding proteins, and prostate cancer risk: a prospective study, *J Natl Cancer Inst* 92(2):1910–1917, 2000.

78. Poschl G, Seitz HK: Alcohol and cancer, *Alcohol Alcohol* 39(3):155–165, 2004.

79. Izevbigie EB, et al: Ethanol modulates the growth of human breast cancer cells in vitro, *Exp Biol Med* 227(4):260–265, 2002.

80. Bagnardi V, et al: A meta-analysis of alcohol drinking and cancer risk, *Br J Cancer* 85(11):1700–1705, 2001.

81. Argiris A, et al: Head and neck cancer, *Lancet* 9625(371):1695–1709, 2008.

82. Sturgis EM, Wei Q: Genetic susceptibility—molecular epidemiology of head and neck cancer, *Curr Opin Oncol* 14(3):310–317, 2002.

83. Crabb DW, et al: Overview of the role of alcohol dehydrogenese and aldehyde dehydrogenase and their variants in the genesis of alcohol-related pathology, *Proc Nutr Soc* 63(1):49–63, 2004.

84. Heidenreich WF, et al: Promoting action of radiation in the atomic bomb survivor carcinogenesis data?, *Radiat Res* 168(6):750–756, 2007.

85. Little MP: Heterogeneity of variation of relative risk by age at exposure in the Japanese atomic bomb survivors, *Radiat Environ Biophys* 48(3):253–262, 2009.

86. Shuryak I, et al: A new view of radiation-induced cancer: integrating short- and long-processes. Part l: Approach, *Radiat Environ Biophys* 48(3):263–274, 2009.

87. Shuryak I, Sachs RK, Brenner DJ: Cancer risks after radiation exposure in middle age, *J Natl Cancer Inst* 102(21):1606–1609, 2010.

88. Preston DL, et al: Solid cancer incidence in atomic bomb survivors: 1958–1998, *Radiat Res* 168(1):1–64, 2007.

89. Committee on the Biological Effects of Ionizing Radiation: *Health risks from exposure to low levels of ionizing radiation, BEIR VII Phase 2*, Washington, DC, 2006, National Academies Press.

90. Walsh L: Heterogeneity of variation of relative risk by age at exposure in Japanese atomic bomb survivors, *Radiat Environ Biophys* 48(3):345–347, 2009.

91. Preston DL, et al: Studies of mortality of atomic bomb survivors. Report 13: solid cancer and noncancer disease mortality: 1950–1997, *Radiat Res* 160:381–407, 2003.

92. Hoel DG: Ionizing radiation and cardiovascular disease, *Ann N Y Acad Sci* 1076:309–317, 2006.

93. Prasad KN, Cole WC, Hasse GM: Health risks of low dose ionizing radiation in humans: a review, *Exp Biol Med* 229(5):378–382, 2004.

94. NCRP: *1929–2009 medical radiation exposure of the U.S. population greatly increased since the early 1980s*, http://NCRPonline%2CorgMarch 2009:Available at.

95. Brenner DJ, Hall EJ: Computed tomography—an increasing source of radiation exposure, *N Engl J Med* 357(22):2277–2284, 2007.

96. Little JB: Cellular radiation effects and the bystander response, *Mutat Res* 597:113–118, 2006.

97. Kovalchuk O, Baulch JE: Epigenetic changes and nontargeted radiation effects—is there a link? *Environ Mol Mutagen* 49(1):16–25, 2008.

98. Barcellos-Hoff MH: Integrative radiation carcinogenesis: interactions between cell and tissue responses to DNA damage, *Semin Cancer Biol* 15:138–148, 2005.

99. Sowa M, et al: Effects of ionizing radiation on cellular structures, induced instability and carcinogenesis, *EXS* 96:293–301, 2006.

100. Koturbash I, et al: in vivo bystander effects: cranial x-irradiation leads to elevated DNA damage, altered cellular proliferation and apoptosis, and increased p53 levels in shielded spleen, *Int J Radiat Oncol Biol Phys* 70(2):554–562, 2008.

101. Coates PJ, Lorimore SA, Wright EG: Damaging and protective cell signaling in the untargeted effects of ionizing radiation, *Mutat Res* 568:5–20, 2004.

102. Belyakov OV, et al: Bystander induced differentiation: a major response to targeted irradiation of a urothelial explant model, *Mutat Res* 597:43–49, 2006.

103. Hei TK, et al: Mechanism of radiation-induced bystander effects: a unifying model, *J Pharm Pharmacol* 60:943–950, 2008.

104. Committee on the Biological Effects of Ionizing Radiation: *Biological effects of ionizing radiation BEIR V*, Washington, DC, 1990, National Academy Press.

105. Tondel M, et al: Increased incidence of malignancies in Sweden after the Chernobyl accident—a promoting effect?, *Am J Ind Med* 49(3):159–168, 2006.

106. Zhou H, et al: Induction of a bystander mutagenic effect of alpha particles in mammalian cells, *Proc Natl Acad Sci U S A* 97(5):2099–2104, 2000.

106a. Feinendegen LE, Brooks AL, Morgan WF: Final discussions, summary and recommendations, *Health Phys* 100(3):342–343, 2011.

107. Makhijani A, Smith B, Thorne MC: Science for the vulnerable setting radiation and multiple exposure environmental health standards to protect those at most risk, *Takoma Park, Md*, 2006:IEER.

108. Schvartzman JM, Sotillo R, Benezra R: Mitotic chromosomal instability and cancer: mouse modeling of the human disease, *Nat Rev Cancer* 10:102–115, 2010.

109. Lorimore SA, Coates PJ, Wright EG: Radiation-induced genomic instability and bystander effects: inter-related nontargeted effects of exposure to ionizing radiation, *Oncogene* 22(45):7058–7069, 2003.

110. Futaki M, Liu JM: Chromosomal breakage syndromes and the BRCA1 genome surveillance complex, *Trends Mol Med* 7(12):560–565, 2001.

111. Little JB, Lauriston S: Taylor lecture: nontargeted effects of radiation: implications for low dose exposures, *Health Phys* 91(5):416–426, 2006.

112. Ojima M, Ban N, Kai M: DNA double-strand breaks induced by very low x-ray doses are largely due to bystander effects, *Radiat Res* 170(3):365–371, 2008.

113. Park CC, et al: Ionizing radiation induces heritable disruption of epithelial cell interactions, *Proc Natl Acad Sci U S A* 100(19):10728–10733, 2003.

114. Spitz DR, et al: Metabolic oxidation/reduction reactions and cellular responses to ionizing radiation: a unifying concept in stress response biology, *Cancer Metastasis Rev* 23(3–4):311–322, 2004.

115. Azzam EI, de Toldeo SM, Little JB: Oxidative metabolism, gap junctions, and the ionizing radiation-induced bystander effect, *Oncogene* 22(45):7050–7057, 2003.

116. Cleaver JE, Crowley E: UV damage, DNA repair, and skin carcinogenesis, *Front Biosci* 7:d1024–d1043, 2002.

117. Streilein JW, et al: Immune surveillance and sunlight-induced skin cancer, *Immunol Today* 15(4):174–179, 1994.

118. Bickers DR, Ather M: Oxidative stress in the pathogenesis of skin disease, *J Invest Dermatol* 126:2562–2575, 2006.

119. Dhar A, Young MR, Colburn NH: The role of AP-1, NF-kappaB, and ROS/NOS in skin carcinogenesis: the JB6 model is predictive, *Mol Cell Biochem* 234(1–2):185–193, 2002.

120. Sander CD, et al: Role of oxidative stress and the antioxidant network in cutaneous carcinogenesis, *Intl J Dermatol* 43(5):326–335, 2004.

121. Lin J, et al: Genetics of melanoma, *Br J Dermatol* 159(2):286–291, 2008.

122. Welch HG, Black WC: Overdiagnosis in cancer, *J Natl Cancer Inst* 102:605–613, 2010.

123. Heymann WR: Screening for melanoma, *J Am Acad Dermatol* 56(1):144–145, 2007.

124. Sekulic A, et al: Malignant melanoma in the 21st century: the emerging molecular landscape, *Mayo Clin Proc* 83(7):825–846, 2008:review.

125. Héry C, et al: A melanoma epidemic in Iceland: possible influence of sunbed use, *Am J Epidemiol* 172(7):762–767, 2010.

126. Lazovich D, et al: Indoor tanning and risk of melanoma: A case-control study in a highly exposed population, *Cancer Epidemiol Biomarkers Prev* 19(60):1557–1568, 2010.

127. Perlis C, Herlyn M: Recent advances in melanoma biology, *Oncologist* 9(2):182–187, 2004.

128. Polsky D, et al: Molecular biology of melanoma. In Mendelsohn J, et al: *The molecular basis of cancer, ed 2,* Philadelphia, 2001, Saunders.

129. Rees JL: The melanocortin 1 receptor (MC1R): more than just red hair, *Pigment Cell Res* 13(3):135–140, 2000.

130. Berking C, et al: Basic fibroblast growth factor and ultraviolet B transform melanocytes in human skin, *Am J Pathol* 158(3):943–953, 1998.

131. Berking C, et al: Basic fibroblast growth factor and ultraviolet B transform melanocytes in human skin, *Am J Pathol* 158:943–954, 2002.

132. Davies H, et al: Mutations of the BRAF gene in human cancer, *Nature* 417(6892):949–954, 2002.

133. Besaratinia A, Pfeifer GP: Sunlight ultraviolet irradiation and BRAF V600 mutagenesis in human melanoma, *Hum Mutat* 29(8):983–1991, 2008.

134. Tang A, et al: E-cadherin is the major mediator of human melanocyte adhesion to keratinocytes in vitro, *J Cell Sci* 107(pt 4):983–992, 1994.

135. Li G, Satayamoorthy K, Herlyn M: *N*-cadherin-mediated intercellular interactions promote survival and migration of melanoma cells, *Cancer Res* 61(9):3819–3825, 2001.

136. Berwick M: The good, the bad, and the ugly of sunscreens, *Clin Pharmacol Ther* 89(1):31–33, 2011.

137. Genuis SJ: Fielding a current idea: exploring the public health impact of electromagnetic radiation, *Public Health* 122(2):113–124, 2008.

137a. Belyaev IY: Dependence of non-thermal biological effects of microwaves on physical and biological variables: implications for reproducibility and safety standards, *Eur J Oncol Library* 5:187–219, 2010.

138. National Institute of Environmental Health Sciences (NIEHS) Working Group Report: *Assessment of health effects from exposure to power-line frequency electric and magnetic fields,* Washington, DC, 1998, U.S. Government Printing Office.

139. UK Childhood Cancer Study Investigators: Exposure to power-frequency magnetic fields and the risk of childhood cancer, *Lancet* 354(9194):1925–1931, 1999.

140. UK Childhood Cancer Study Investigators: Childhood cancer and residential proximity to power lines, *Br J Cancer* 83(11):1573–1580, 2000.

141. Ahlbom A, et al: A pooled analysis of magnetic fields and childhood leukaemia, *Br J Cancer* 83(5):692–698, 2000.

142. Kabuto M, et al: Childhood leukemia and magnetic fields in Japan: a case-control study of childhood leukemia and residential power-frequency magnetic fields in Japan, *Int J Cancer* 119:643–650, 2006.

143. Hardell L, et al: Meta-analysis of long-term phone use and the association with brain tumours, *Int J Oncol* 32(5):1097–1103, 2008.

144. Draper G, et al: Childhood cancer in relation to distance from high voltage power lines in England and Wales: a case-control study, *Br Med J* 330:1290, 2005.

145. Johansson O: Electrohypersensitivity: state-of-art of a functional impairment, *Electromagn Biol Med* 25(4):245–258, 2006:review.

146. Hallberg O, Johansson O: Melanoma incidence and frequency modulation (FM) broadcasting, *Arch Environ Health* 57:32–40, 2002.

147. Hallberg O, Johansson O: Maligant melanomas of the skin—not a sunshine story! *Med Sci Monit* 10:CR336–CR340, 2004.

148. Feychting M, Forssén U: Electromagnetic fields and female breast cancer, *Cancer Causes Control* 17(4):553–558, 2006:review.

149. Kliukiene J, Tynes T, Andersen A: Residential and occupational exposure to 50-Hz magnetic fields and breast cancer in women: a population-based study, *Am J Epidemiol* 159(9):852–861, 2004.

150. Khurana VG, et al: Cell phones and brain tumors: a review including the long-term epidemiologic data, *Surg Neurol* 72(3):205–214, 2009.

151. Christensen HC, et al: Cellular telephone use and risk of acoustic neuroma, *Am J Epidemiol* 159(3):277–283, 2004.

152. Independent Expert Group on Mobile Phones: *Mobile phones and health (the Stewart report),* Didcot, Oxon, United Kingdom, 2000, National Radiological Protection Board. Available at www.iegmp.org.uk/report/text.htm.

153. Repacholi MH: Radiofrequency field exposure and cancer: what do the laboratory studies suggest? *Environ Health Perspect* 105(Suppl 6):1565–1568, 1997.

154. Mashevich M, et al: Exposure of human peripheral blood lymphocytes to electromagnetic fields associated with cellular phones leads to chromosomal instability, *Bioelectromagnetics* 24(2):82–90, 2003.

155. World Health Organization (WHO): Sensitivity of children to EMF exposure. Proceedings of a symposium sponsored by the WHO International EMF Project, June 9–10, 2004, Istanbul, Turkey, *Bioelectromagnetics* (Suppl 7)S1–S160, 2006:erratum 27(5):430.

156. Cherry N: *World conference on breast cancer—Ottawa, Canada, July 26–31, 1999,* Lincoln NZ, 2002, New Zealand Lincoln University, Available at: www.neilcherry.com/cart/specific+health+effect+review?mode=show_category.

157. Havas M: Biological effects of non-ionizing electromagnetic energy: a critical review of the reports by the US National Research Council and the US National Institute of Environment Health Sciences as they relate to the broad realm of EMF bioeffects, *Environ Rev* 89:173–253, 2000.

158. Blackman CF, Benane SG, House DE: The influence of temperature during electric- and magnetic-field-induced alteration of calcium-ion release from in vitro brain tissue, *Bioelectromagnetics* 12(3):173–182, 1991.

159. Myung S, et al: Mobile phone use and risk of tumors: a meta analysis, *J Clin Oncol* 27(33):5565–5572, 2009.

160. Hardell L, et al: Meta-analysis of long-term mobile phone use and the association with brain tumors, *Int J Oncol* 32:1097–1103, 2008.

161. Kan P, et al: Cellular phone use and brain tumor: a meta-analysis, *J Neurooncol* 86:71–78, 2008.

162. Lahkola A, Tokola K, Auvinen A: Meta-analysis of mobile phone use and intracranial tumors, *Scand J Work Environ Health* 32:171–177, 2006.

163. Hardell L, Mild KH, Carlberg M: Pooled analysis of two case-control studies on the use of cellular and cordless telephones and the risk for malignant brain tumors diagnosed in 1997–2003, *Int Arch Occup Environ Health* 79:630–639, 2006.

164. Lahkhola A, et al: Mobile phone use and risk of glioma in 5 North European Countries, *Int J Cancer* 120:1769–1775, 2007.

165. Sadetzki S, et al: Cellular phone use and risk of benign and malignant parotid gland tumors—a nationwide case-control study, *Am J Epidemiol* 167:457–467, 2008.

166. Schoemaker MJ, et al: Mobile phone use and risk of acoustic neuroma: results of the Interphone Case-control Study in five north European countries, *Br J Cancer* 93:842–848, 2005.

167. Erogul O, et al: Effects of electromagnetic radiation from a cellular phone on human sperm motility: an in vitro study, *Arch Med Res* 37:840–843, 2006.

168. Yan JG, et al: Effects of cellular phone emissions on sperm motility in rats, *Fert Steril* 88:957–964, 2007.

169. Agarwal A, et al: Effect of cell phone usage on semen analysis in men attending infertility clinic: an observational study, *Fert Steril* 89:124–128, 2008.

170. Fejes I, et al: Is there a relationship between cell phone use and semen quality? *Arch Androl* 51:385–393, 2005.

171. Wdowiak A, Wdowiak L, Wiktor H: Evaluation of the effect of using mobile phones on male fertility, *Ann Agric Environ Med* 14(1):169–172, 2007.

172. Kurhana VG, et al: Epidemiological evidence for a health risk from mobile phone base stations, *Int J Occup Environ Health* 16:263–267, 2010.

173. Marur S, et al: HPV-associated head and neck cancer: a virus-related cancer epidemic, *Lancet Oncol* 11(8):781–789, 2010.

174. Anhang R, Goodman A, Goldie SJ: HPV communication: review of existing research and recommendation for patient education, *CA Cancer J Clin* 54(5):248–259, 2004.

175. Nour NM: Cervical cancer: a preventable death, *Rev Obstet Gynecol* 2(4):240–244, 2009.

176. Bosch FX, de Sanjose S: Human papillomavirus and cervical cancer—burden and assessment of causality, *J Natl Cancer Inst Monogr* 31:3–13, 2003.

177. Stanley M: Immunobiology of HPV and HPV vaccines, *Gynecol Oncol* 109(Suppl 2):S15–S21, 2008:review.

178. Syrjänen K, et al: New concepts on risk factors of HPV and novel screening strategies for cervical cancer precursors, *Eur J Gynaecol Oncol* 29(3):205–221, 2008.

179. Syrjänen K, et al: Smoking is an independent risk factor for oncogenic human papillomavirus (HPV) infections but not for high-grade CIN, *Eur J Epidemiol* 22(10):723–735, 2007.

180. Herzog TJ, et al: Initial lessons learned in HPV vaccination, *Gynecol Oncol* 109(Suppl 2):S4–S11, 2008.

181. Hagensee ME, et al: Human papillomavirus infection and disease in HIV-infected individuals, *Am J Med Sci* 328(1):57–63, 2004.

182. Syrjänen S, Puranen M: Human papillomavirus infections in children: the potential role of maternal transmission, *Crit Rev Oral Biol Med* 11(2):259–274, 2000.

183. Eyre H, et al: Preventing cancer, cardiovascular disease, and diabetes: a common agenda for the American Cancer Society, the American Diabetes Association, and the American Heart Association, *Stroke* 35(8):1999–2010, 2004.

184. McTiernan A: Mechanisms linking physical activity with cancer, *Nat Rev Cancer* 8(3):205–211, 2008.

185. Rogers CJ, et al: Physical activity and cancer prevention: pathways and targets for intervention, *Sports Med* 38(4):271–296, 2008.

186. Slattery ML: Physical activity and colorectal cancer, *Sports Med* 34(4):239–252, 2004.

187. McTiernan A, et al: Physical activity and cancer etiology: associations and mechanisms, *Cancer Causes Control* 9(5):487–509, 1998:review.

188. McTiernan A, et al: Effect of exercise on serum estrogens in postmenopausal women: a 12-month randomized clinical trial, *Cancer Res* 64(8):2923–2928, 2004.

189. Calle EE, et al: Diabetes mellitus and pancreatic cancer mortality in a prospective cohort of United States adults, *Cancer Causes Control* 9(4):403–410, 1998.

190. Lee IM: Physical activity and cancer prevention…data from epidemiologic studies, *Med Sci Sports Exerc* 35(11):1823–1827, 2003.

191. McTiernan A, et al: Exercise effect on weight and body fat in men and women, *Obesity* 15(6):1496–1512, 2007.

192. Gray J: *State of the evidence 2008: the connection between breast cancer and the environment*, San Francisco, 2008, Breast Cancer Fund.

193. Neuberger JS, Field RW: Occupation and lung cancer in nonsmokers, *Rev Environ Health* 18(4):251–267, 2003:review.

194. Holguin F: Traffic, outdoor air pollution, and asthma, *Immunol Allergy Clin North Am* 28:577–588, 2008.

195. Vineis P, et al: Outdoor air pollution and lung cancer: recent epidemiologic evidence, *Int J Cancer* 111(5):647–652, 2004.

196. Blair A, Kazerouni N: Reactive chemicals and cancer, *Cancer Causes Control* 8(3):473–490, 1997.

197. Boffetta P, et al: Mortality among workers employed in the titanium dioxide production industry in Europe, *Cancer Causes Control* 15(7):697–706, 2004.

198. Boffetta P: Involuntary smoking and lung cancer, *Scand J Work Environ Health* 28(Suppl 2):30–40, 2002.

199. Zhao Y, et al: Air pollution and lung cancer risks in China—meta-analysis, *Sci Total Environ* 366(2–3):500–513, 2006.

200. Borm PJ, Schins RP, Albrecht C: Inhaled particles and lung cancer, part B: paradigms and risk assessment, *Int J Cancer* 110(1):3–14, 2004.

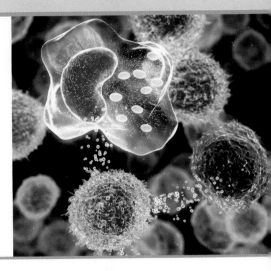

Cancer in children is rare; however, it is still the leading cause of death in children that is attributable to disease. Survival rates in children with cancer have dramatically improved in the past 30 years. Some of the factors leading to improved cure rates in children with cancer include the use of combination chemotherapy, the incorporation of research data obtained from clinical trials, and the utilization of multimodal treatment for childhood solid tumors.

INCIDENCE AND TYPES OF CHILDHOOD CANCER

In 2007 the mortality rates of children with cancer were 2.1 per 100,000 in children ages 1 to 4 years and 2.5 per 100,000 in children ages 5 to 14 years. In comparison, cancer is the second leading cause of death from disease in adults (second to heart disease), with an overall mortality rate of 185.2 per 100,000 individuals.[1]

The types of malignancies in children are vastly different from those that affect adults. The most common types of cancer among adults include prostate, breast, lung, and colon. Children tend to develop leukemias, brain tumors, and sarcomas. Although many adult cancers have associated lifestyle factors that could theoretically be avoided, such as smoking and exposure to sun, very few environmental factors have been linked to pediatric malignancies. Yet more data are emerging that the developing child may be affected by parental exposures before conception, exposures in utero, and the contents of breast milk.[2,3]

Most childhood cancers originate from the mesodermal germ layer, which develops into connective tissue, bone, cartilage, muscle, blood, blood vessels, gonads, kidney, and the lymphatic system. Thus the more common childhood cancers are leukemias, sarcomas, and embryonic tumors. Embryonic tumors originate during intrauterine life and contain abnormal cells that appear to be immature embryonic tissue unable to mature or differentiate into fully developed functional cells. Embryonic tumors (e.g., neuroblastoma, Wilms tumor) are diagnosed early in life (usually by 5 years of age) and therefore are rare in adults.

Sarcomas and lymphoreticular cancers seen in childhood also occur in adults, but most adult cancers involve epithelial tissue (and are therefore carcinomas). Carcinomas rarely occur in children because these cancers most commonly result from environmental carcinogens and require a long period from exposure to the appearance of the carcinoma. Carcinomas begin to increase in incidence between the ages of 15 and 19 years, becoming the most common cancer tissue type seen after adolescence.

By far the most common malignancy in children is leukemia, which accounts for more than one third of childhood cancers. The second most common group of cancers is tumors of the nervous system, primarily brain tumors. All other pediatric malignancies occur much less often. Neuroblastoma is a tumor of the sympathetic nervous system. Wilms tumor is a malignancy of the kidney (named after Max Wilms, who identified the tumor); the histologic name is *nephroblastoma*. Rhabdomyosarcoma is a soft tissue sarcoma of striated muscle. Two major bone tumors also occur in children. These are osteosarcoma and Ewing sarcoma.

Childhood cancers are usually diagnosed during peak times of physical growth and maturation. In general, they are extremely fast-growing cancers. Many childhood cancers have a peak incidence before the child is 5 years of age. Among these are the leukemias, neuroblastoma, Wilms tumor, and retinoblastoma. Bone tumors, soft tissue sarcomas, and lymphomas are more likely to occur in children ages 15 to 19 years (Table 11-1). Cancer is more common in white children than in other races (Table 11-2). In the United States childhood cancer also is slightly more common in boys than in girls. The male/female ratio for childhood cancers is 1.2:1.0.[1]

ETIOLOGY

The causes of cancer in children are largely unknown. A few environmental factors are known to predispose a child to cancer, but causal factors have not been established for most childhood cancers. A number of host factors, many of which are genetic risk factors or congenital conditions, have been implicated in the development of childhood cancer (Table 11-3).

Most childhood cancers, however, do not lend themselves to early cancer warning signs. Certainly the American Cancer Society's seven warning signs of cancer do not apply because they describe adult, environmentally caused carcinomas. Although host factors are important in identifying populations of children at risk for cancer, most children who are diagnosed with cancer do not demonstrate any predisposing environmental or host factors.

The multiple causation concept is useful when the results of epidemiologic studies are interpreted. For example, laboratory and epidemiologic studies may indicate that exposure to a certain chemical can cause leukemia, but not all children exposed to that chemical will develop leukemia. Additional studies will be needed to determine what other factors must interact with chemical exposure to cause the disease.

Genetic Factors

Genetic factors may involve chromosome aberrations or single-gene defects. These chromosome abnormalities include aneuploidy, deletions, amplifications, translocations, and fragility (see Chapter 2). Some congenital malformations herald the onset of pediatric malignancies. Several syndromes with diagnosed abnormalities are known to be related to a higher incidence of cancer development. Children identified with certain congenital syndromes can then be carefully followed and screened for tumor development. One of the more recognized syndromes is the association of trisomy 21 (Down syndrome)

TABLE 11-1	CHILDHOOD AGE-ADJUSTED INVASIVE CANCER INCIDENCE RATES BY PRIMARY SITE AND AGE, UNITED STATES*	
SITE	**BIRTH TO 14 YEARS**	**BIRTH TO 19 YEARS**
All sites	15.3	16.9
Leukemia	4.7	4.2
Acute lymphocytic	3.7	3.1
Acute myeloid	0.7	0.7
Brain and other nervous system	3.3	3.1
Soft tissue	1.0	1.0
Kidney and renal	0.8	0.7
Bones and joints	0.7	0.9
Non-Hodgkin lymphoma	0.9	1.1
Hodgkin lymphoma	0.6	1.2
Other	3.3	4.7

Data modified from U.S. Cancer Statistics Working Group: *United States cancer statistics: 1999–2006 incidence and mortality web-based report*, Atlanta, 2010, U.S. Department of Health and Human Services, Centers for Disease Control and Prevention, and National Cancer Institute; available at www.cdc.gov/uscs.
*Rates are per 100,000 persons and are age-adjusted to the 2000 U.S. standard population (19 age groups–Census P25-1130).

TABLE 11-2	CHILDHOOD AGE-ADJUSTED CANCER INCIDENCE RATES FOR CHILDREN UP TO 19 YEARS OF AGE BY PRIMARY SITE AND RACE AND ETHNICITY, UNITED STATES*				
CANCER SITE	**WHITE**	**BLACK**	**ASIAN/PACIFIC ISLANDER**	**AMERICAN INDIAN/ ALASKA NATIVE**	**HISPANIC[†]**
All cancer sites combined	18.7	12.9	13.9	10.7	18.0
Bones and joints	1.0	0.9	0.9	0.7	1.1
Brain and other nervous systems	3.4	2.3	2.1	1.6	2.8
Hodgkin lymphoma	1.3	1.0	1.0	—[‡]	1.2
Kidney and renal pelvis	0.6	0.3	0.3	—[‡]	0.5
Leukemia	5.0	4.5	4.5	3.7	5.9
Acute lymphocytic	3.8	3.3	3.3	2.5	4.6
Acute myeloid	0.7	0.8	0.8	—[‡]	0.9
Non-Hodgkin lymphoma	1.5	1.2	1.2	0.7	1.4
Soft tissue	1.1	0.9	0.9	—[‡]	0.9
Other	4.7	3.1	3.1	2.7	4.2

Data modified from U.S. Cancer Statistics Working Group: *United States cancer statistics: 1999–2006 incidence and mortality web-based report*, Atlanta, 2010, U.S. Department of Health and Human Services, Centers for Disease Control and Prevention, and National Cancer Institute; available at www.cdc.gov/uscs.
*Rates are per 100,000 persons and are age-adjusted to the 2000 U.S. standard population (19 age groups–Census P25-1130).
[†]Hispanic origin is not mutually exclusive from race categories (white, black, Asian/Pacific Islander, American Indian/Alaska Native).
[‡]Rates are suppressed if fewer than 16 cases were reported in a specific category (area, race, ethnicity).

TABLE 11-3 CONGENITAL FACTORS ASSOCIATED WITH CHILDHOOD CANCER

SYNDROME	ASSOCIATED CHILDHOOD CANCER
Chromosome Alterations	
Down syndrome	Acute leukemia
13q syndrome	Retinoblastoma
Chromosome Instability	
Ataxia-telangiectasia	Lymphoma
Bloom syndrome	Acute leukemia, lymphoma, Wilms tumor
Fanconi anemia	Nonlymphocytic leukemia, myelodysplastic syndrome, hepatic tumors
Hereditary Syndromes	
Beckwith-Wiedemann syndrome	Wilms tumor, sarcoma, brain tumors, neuroblastoma, hepatoblastoma
Neurofibromatosis type I	Brain tumor, sarcomas, neuroblastomas, Wilms tumor, nonlymphocytic leukemia
Neurofibromatosis type II	Meningioma (malignant or benign), acoustic neuroma/schwannoma, gliomas, ependymomas
Tuberous sclerosis	Glial tumors
Li-Fraumeni syndrome	Sarcoma, adrenocortical carcinoma
Von Hippel-Lindau disease	Cerebellar hemangioblastoma, retinal angioma, renal cell carcinoma, pheochromocytomas
Ataxia-telangiectasia	Leukemia, lymphoma, brain tumors
Gorlin syndrome	Medulloblastoma, skin tumors
Immunodeficiency Disorders	
Congenital	
Agammaglobulinemia	Lymphoma, leukemia, brain tumors
Immunoglobulin A (IgA) deficiency	Lymphoma, leukemia, brain tumors
Wiskott-Aldrich syndrome	Leukemia, lymphoma
Acquired	
Aplastic anemia	Leukemia
Organ transplantation	Leukemia, lymphoma
Congenital Malformation Syndromes	
Aniridia, hemihypertrophy, hamartoma, genitourinary anomalies	Wilms tumor
Cryptorchidism	Testicular tumor
Gonadal dysgenesis	Gonadoblastoma
Family Susceptibility	
Twin or sibling with leukemia	Leukemia

TABLE 11-4 SELECTED ONCOGENES AND TUMOR-SUPPRESSOR GENES ASSOCIATED WITH CHILDHOOD CANCER

GENE	ASSOCIATED PEDIATRIC TUMOR
Oncogenes	
bcr-abl	Acute lymphoblastic leukemia
N-myc	Neuroblastoma
c-myb	Neural tumors, leukemia, lymphoma, rhabdomyosarcoma, Wilms tumor, neuroblastoma
erb B	Glioblastomas
N-ras	Neuroblastoma, leukemia
H/K-ras	Neuroblastoma, rhabdomyosarcoma, leukemia
ATM	Lymphoma, leukemia
Tumor-Suppressor Genes	
Rb1	Retinoblastoma, sarcoma
WT1, WT2	Wilms tumor, leukemia
WTC	Wilms tumor
NF-1	Sarcoma, primitive neuroectodermal tumor, juvenile chronic myelocytic leukemia
NF-2	Brain tumors, melanoma, meningiomas
p16	Brain tumors, leukemia
TP53	Sarcoma, leukemia, brain tumors, lymphoma
DCC	Ewing sarcoma, rhabdomyosarcoma
*p16*INK4a	Glioma, leukemia
*p15*ARF	Glioblastoma, T cell ALL
CDC2L1	Non-Hodgkin lymphoma, neuroblastoma

Data from Dome JS, Coppes MS: *Curr Opin Pediatr* 14(1):5–11, 2002; Linblom A, Nordenskjold M: *Semin Cancer Biol* 10(4):251–254, 2000; Tischkowitz M, Rosser E: *Eur J Cancer* 40:2459–2470, 2004; Look A, Kirsch IR: Molecular basis of childhood cancer. In Pizzo PA, Poplack DG, editors: *Principles and practices of pediatric oncology*, ed 4, Philadelphia, 2002, Lippincott Williams & Wilkins. *ALL*, Acute lymphocytic leukemia.

(muscular overgrowth of half of the body or face), and mental retardation. Approximately 10% of children diagnosed with Wilms tumor demonstrate one of these congenital abnormalities.[5] Retinoblastoma, a malignant embryonic tumor of the eye, occurs either as an inherited defect or as an acquired mutation (see Chapter 16).

More than 150 single-gene defects, oncogenes and tumor-suppressor genes, have been associated with the subsequent development of both childhood and adult cancers (Table 11-4). Fanconi anemia and Bloom syndrome, two autosomal recessive conditions, are risk factors for the development of acute lymphocytic leukemia (ALL).

Although not determined to be genetically transmitted, a child who has a sibling with leukemia has a risk for the development of leukemia that is two to four times greater than that for children with healthy siblings. The occurrence of leukemia in monozygous twins is estimated as being as high as 25%.

In families with Li-Fraumeni syndrome (LFS) (an autosomal dominant disorder involving the *TP53* tumor-suppressor gene), the risk of developing cancer as a child or adult is significantly higher than the risk in the unaffected population. Children and adults in Li-Fraumeni families are at risk for soft tissue sarcoma, breast cancer, leukemia, osteosarcoma, melanoma, and cancer of the colon, pancreas, adrenal cortex, and brain. Individuals with LFS are at increased risk for developing multiple primary cancers.[6]

with an increased susceptibility to acute leukemia. For children with Down syndrome, the risk of developing leukemia is 10 to 20 times greater than the risk in healthy children. The risk is greatest between 1 and 4 years of age.[4]

Wilms tumor is particularly recognized for its association with a number of other abnormalities, including genitourinary anomalies, aniridia (congenital absence of the iris), hemihypertrophy

TABLE 11-5	DRUGS THAT MAY INCREASE RISK OF CHILDHOOD CANCER	
DRUG CLASS	**USES**	**CANCER RISK**
Anabolic androgenic steroids	Stimulate bone growth and appetite Induce puberty Increase muscle mass and physical strength	Hepatocellular carcinoma
Cytotoxic chemotherapy	Cancer treatment	Leukemia
Immunosuppressive agents	Prevent organ rejection following transplantation surgery	Lymphoma

Environmental Factors

Finding the cause of any disease is typically a long, slow process. It may take years for an epidemiologic study to determine whether a risk factor is possibly related to the development of a disease. No one factor determines whether an individual will develop cancer, even if a specific environmental exposure explains a high proportion of the occurrence of a specific cancer. Childhood cancer is no different. No single study, or even multiple epidemiologic studies, will tell a parent why his or her child developed cancer. The many factors that may play a role in the development of cancer include genetics, nutrition and diet, immune function, occupational exposure, hormonal variations, viral illnesses, and other individual characteristics such as biologic, social, or physical environments.

Prenatal Exposure

Prenatal exposure to some drugs and to ionizing radiation has been linked to childhood cancers. The most well-described drug is diethylstilbestrol (DES), which was prescribed by physicians to prevent spontaneous miscarriage (in women with previous miscarriage). In 1971 DES was identified as a transplacental chemical carcinogen because a small percentage of the daughters of women who took DES developed adenocarcinomas of the vagina. Since then, other studies have attempted to identify other drugs taken by pregnant women that may cause cancer in their offspring, but no other drugs have been found. Prior research suggested an association between antenatal x-ray exposure and childhood cancer but this has not been replicated or supported in recent literature.

Childhood Exposure

Childhood exposure to ionizing radiation, drugs, electromagnetic fields, or viruses has been associated with the risk of developing cancer. Retrospective research has shown a significant correlation between radiation-induced malignancies and either radiotherapy (cancer treatment) or radiation exposure from diagnostic imaging.[7] In addition to the drug and environmental agents that are known to cause cancer in adults and therefore also are risks for exposure during childhood, a few drugs may particularly increase cancer risk during childhood (Table 11-5).

The relationship between childhood cancer and other environmental factors (for example, electromagnetic fields, small appliances, radon) has been the focus of many epidemiologic studies, yet no conclusive evidence has been reported[7] (see *Health Alert:* Magnetic Fields and Development of Pediatric Cancer).

The strongest association between viruses and the development of cancer in children has been the Epstein-Barr virus (EBV), which is

Magnetic Fields and Development of Pediatric Cancer

Several recent reports have suggested that there is a possible association between environmental sources and the development of cancer in children. The presence of low-frequency and magnetic fields has been a concern for many years as causing leukemia in children, and although hundreds of epidemiologic studies have been published few have suggested a positive correlation. Recently, a research study reported pooled results from seven of the latest studies on magnetic fields and development of childhood leukemia. Although the samples of individual studies were small, the results support previous findings that magnetic fields are possibly carcinogenic to children. The World Health Organization (WHO) research agenda identified the importance of such an analysis as a high research priority in 2007. Ongoing research needs to be done in this area because it may take many years for exposure to environmental factors to cause disease. In addition, collection of the necessary epidemiologic data to examine the relationship between environmental exposure and childhood malignancies will be a time-consuming process.

Data from Khefits L et al: Pooled analysis of recent studies on magnetic fields and childhood leukemia, *Br J Cancer* 103:1128–1135, 2010 World Health Organization (WHO): *WHO research agenda for extremely low frequency fields,* 2007. Available at http://www.who.int/peh-emf/research/elf_research_agenda_2007.pdf. Accessed October 25, 2010.

linked to Burkitt lymphoma, nasopharyngeal carcinoma, and Hodgkin disease.[8] Children with acquired immunodeficiency syndrome (AIDS), caused by human immunodeficiency virus (HIV), have an increased risk of developing non-Hodgkin lymphoma and Kaposi sarcoma. However, with the use of highly active antiretroviral therapy in the developed world, the incidence of AIDS-related malignancies has declined dramatically.[9]

PROGNOSIS

More than 70% of children diagnosed with cancer are cured. Survival rates for children younger than 15 years of age have increased at a rate of 1.5% per year. Similar improvements have been noted in the survival rates of adults older than 50 years of age. However, adolescents and young adults between 15 and 24 years of age have experienced increases in survival of less than 0.5% per year.[10] A partial explanation for the relative lack of progress in curing the adolescent population at the same rate as that realized in the younger pediatric population is the lack of participation in clinical trials. Between 1997 and 2003, the percentage of 15- to 19-year-olds with cancer participating in clinical trials was estimated at 10% to 15%. This value is approximately one fourth the clinical trial participation rate of children younger than 15 years and is likely due to the fact that fewer trials are available for young adolescents. The National Cancer Institute (NCI) and pediatric and adult cooperative groups sponsored by the NCI have launched a national initiative to increase the numbers of adolescents and young adults in clinical trials.

Survivors of childhood cancer are at increased risk of developing a second malignancy later in life. This risk may be associated with a variety of factors, including previous chemotherapy or radiotherapy, genetic factors, and type of primary cancer (e.g., soft tissue sarcoma, neuroblastoma).

Because childhood cancer should be viewed as a chronic disease instead of a fatal illness, the focus of treatment is on the quality of life and symptom management. Even those cancers that cannot be cured generally can be treated, resulting in significantly improved quality of life. Although they may be cured, these children still face residual and late effects of their treatment. These late effects are more significant in children than in adults because treatment given during childhood occurs in a physically immature, growing individual. Late effects that need further study include physical impairments, reproductive dysfunction, soft tissue and bone atrophy, learning disabilities, secondary cancers, and psychologic sequelae. More must be learned about the genetic factors associated with childhood malignancies and about the genetic consequences of treatment. Genetic counseling is appropriate for children cured of cancers known to be transmitted genetically (e.g., retinoblastoma).

Some of the factors leading to improved cure rates in pediatric oncology include the use of combination chemotherapy or multimodal treatment for childhood solid tumors, improvements in nursing and supportive care, development of research centers for comprehensive childhood cancer treatment, cooperation among treatment institutions, development of cooperative study groups, recognition of the psychologic effects of cancer treatment, and continued follow-up to track trends in the late effects of cancer treatment. Young children are particularly prone to long-term sequelae of cancer therapy. It is imperative that more effective, targeted therapies with fewer side effects be found.

✔ **QUICK CHECK 11-1**
1. What are the most common childhood cancers?
2. Why are children less likely to develop carcinomas?
3. How are different etiologic factors associated with the development of childhood cancer?

DID YOU UNDERSTAND?

Incidence and Types of Childhood Cancers
1. Childhood cancer is a rare disease, but it remains the second leading cause of death in children.
2. The most common type of childhood cancer is leukemia, and the second most common type of pediatric malignancy is a tumor involving the brain or central nervous system.

Etiology
1. Because most carcinomas are caused by environmental exposure, these cancers are extremely rare in children because they have not lived long enough to be exposed to carcinogens.
2. Children with immunodeficiencies are at increased risk for developing cancer because of an ineffective immune system.

3. Children with Down syndrome are at increased risk for developing leukemia.
4. Risk factors that may be associated with the development of childhood cancer include genetics, nutrition and diet, immune function, occupational exposure, hormonal variations, and viral illnesses, as well as other individual characteristics such as biologic, social, or physical environments.

Prognosis
1. Survivors of childhood cancer are at increased risk for developing a second cancer during their lifetime, compared with the general population.
2. Improved survival for children with cancer is because of research aimed at identifying less toxic treatments that will minimize residual effects.

▋ KEY TERMS

- Embryonic tumor 288
- Mesodermal germ layer 288
- Multiple causation 289

REFERENCES

1. Kochanek KD, et al: Deaths: final data for 2004, *Natl Vital Stat Rep* 59(4), 2011. Available at www.cdc.gov/nchs/data/nvsr/nvsr55/nvsr55_19.pdf. Accessed May 20, 2011.
2. Clapp RW, Howe GK, Jacobs MM: Environmental and occupational causes of cancer: a call to act on what we know, *Biomed Pharmacother* 61(10):631–639, 2007.
3. Wigle DT, et al: Epidemiologic evidence of relationships between reproductive and child health outcomes and environmental chemical contaminants, *J Toxicol Environ Health B Crit Rev* 11(5–6):373–517, 2008.
4. Look AT, Aplan PD: Molecular and genetic basis of childhood cancer. In Pizzo PA, Poplack DG, editors: *Principles and practice of pediatric oncology*, ed 5, Philadelphia, 2006, Lippincott Williams & Wilkins, pp 38–85.
5. Dome JS, et al: Childhood cancer and heredity. In Pizzo PA, Poplack DG, editors: *Principles and practice of pediatric oncology*, ed 5, Philadelphia, 2006, Lippincott Williams & Wilkins, pp 905–932.
6. Tabori U, Malkin D: Risk stratification in cancer predisposition syndromes: lessons learned from novel molecular developments in Li-Fraumeni syndrome, *Cancer Res* 68(7):2053–2057, 2008.
7. Buka I, Koranteng S, Osomio Vargas AR: Trends in childhood cancer incidence: review of environmental linkages, *Pediatr Clin North Am* 54(1):177–203, 2007.
8. Powles T, et al: Head and neck cancer in patients with human immunodeficiency virus-1 infection: incidence, outcome and association with Epstein-Barr virus, *J Laryngol Otol* 118(3):207–212, 2004.
9. Mbulaiteye SM, et al: Spectrum of cancer among HIV-infected persons in Africa: the Uganda AIDS-Cancer Registry Match Study, *Int J Cancer* 118(4):985–990, 2006.
10. Bleyer A, et al: Relative lack of conditional survival improvement in young adults with cancer, *Semin Oncol* 36(5):460–467, 2009.

Structure and Function of the Neurologic System

Richard A. Sugerman and Sue E. Huether

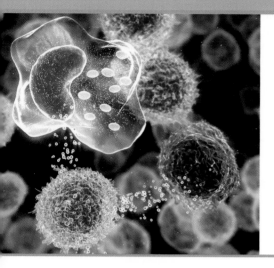

evolve WEBSITE

CHAPTER OUTLINE

The human nervous system is a remarkable structure responsible for conscious and unconscious muscle synergy and for the regulation of activities involving internal organs. The nervous system literally drives the other systems of the body. It is a network composed of complex structures that transmit electrical and chemical signals between the brain and the body's many organs and tissues.

OVERVIEW AND ORGANIZATION OF THE NERVOUS SYSTEM

Although the nervous system functions as a unified whole, structures and functions have been divided here to facilitate understanding. Structurally, the nervous system is divided into the central nervous system and the peripheral nervous system. The central nervous system (CNS) consists of the brain and spinal cord, enclosed within the protective cranial vault and vertebrae, respectively. The peripheral nervous system (PNS) is composed of the cranial nerves and the spinal nerves. Peripheral nerve pathways are differentiated into afferent pathways (ascending pathways), which carry sensory impulses toward the CNS, and efferent pathways (descending pathways), which innervate skeletal muscle or effector organs by transmitting motor impulses away from the CNS.

Functionally, the PNS can be divided into the somatic nervous system and the autonomic nervous system. The somatic nervous system consists of pathways that regulate voluntary motor control (e.g., skeletal muscle). The autonomic nervous system (ANS) is involved with regulation of the body's internal environment (viscera) through involuntary control of organ systems. The ANS is further divided into sympathetic and parasympathetic divisions. Organs innervated by specific components of the nervous system are called effector organs.

CELLS OF THE NERVOUS SYSTEM

Two basic types of cells constitute nervous tissue: neurons and supporting cells. The neuron is the primary cell of the nervous system, whereas cells such as neuroglial cells (in the CNS) and Schwann cells (in the PNS) provide structural support and nutrition for the neurons.[1]

The Neuron

Working alone or in units, neurons detect environmental changes and initiate body responses to maintain a dynamic steady state. Neuronal structure varies markedly, so that each neuron is adapted to perform specialized functions.

The fuel source for the neuron is predominantly glucose; insulin, however, is not required for cellular glucose uptake in the CNS. Among the cellular constituents of neurons are microtubules (transport substances within the cell), neurofibrils, microfilaments (thought to be involved in transport of cellular products), and Nissl substances (involved in protein synthesis).

A neuron (Figure 12-1) has three components: a cell body (soma), the dendrites (thin branching fibers of the cell), and the axons. Most cell bodies are located within the CNS; those in the PNS usually are

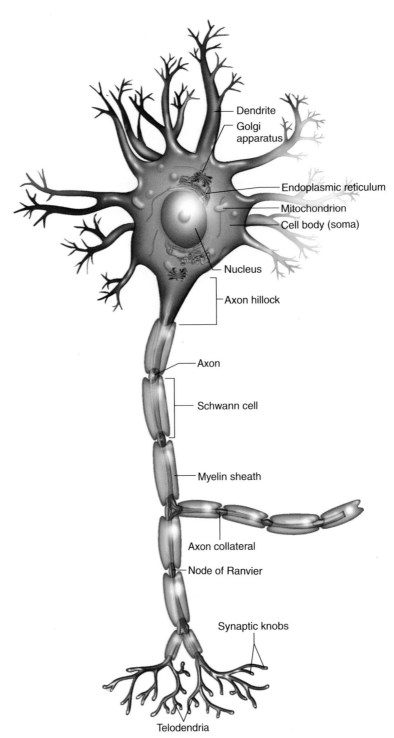

FIGURE 12-1 Neuron With Composite Parts. Multipolar neuron: neuron with multiple extensions from the cell body. (Modified from Patton KT, Thibodeau GA: *Anatomy & physiology,* ed 7, St Louis, 2010, Mosby.)

found in groups called ganglia (or plexuses). The dendrites are extensions that carry nerve impulses toward the cell body. Axons are long, conductive projections from the cell body that carry nerve impulses away from the cell body. The axon hillock is the cone-shaped process where the axon leaves the cell body. The first part of the axon hillock has the lowest threshold for stimulation, so action potentials begin there. A typical neuron has only one axon, which may be covered with a segmented layer of lipid material called myelin, an insulating substance that speeds impulse propagation. This entire membrane is referred to as the myelin sheath (see Figures 12-2 and 12-24, *B*) and is the cell membrane portion of a Schwann cell. The myelin sheaths are interrupted at regular intervals by the nodes of Ranvier. Axons can branch at the nodes of Ranvier.

The principle of *divergence* refers to the ability of axonal branches to influence many different neurons. *Convergence* applies when branches of various numbers of neurons "converge" on and influence a single neuron. Nutrient exchange is not possible through the myelin sheath, although it can occur at the nodes of Ranvier. Where there is myelin, the velocity of nerve impulses increases. Myelin acts as an insulator that allows ions to flow between segments

rather than along the entire length of the membrane, yielding the increased velocity. This mechanism is referred to as saltatory conduction. Disorders of the myelin sheath (demyelinating diseases), such as multiple sclerosis and Guillain-Barré syndrome, demonstrate the important role myelin plays in nerve function (see Chapter 15). Conduction velocities depend not only on the myelin coating but also on the diameter of the axon. Larger axons transmit impulses at a faster rate.

Neurons are structurally classified on the basis of the number of processes (projections) extending from the cell body. There are four basic types of cell configuration: (1) unipolar, (2) pseudounipolar, (3) bipolar, and (4) multipolar. Unipolar neurons have one process that branches shortly after leaving the cell body. One example is found in the retina. Pseudounipolar neurons (some authors call them *unipolar*) also have one process; the dendritic portion of each of these neurons extends away from the CNS and the axon portion projects into the CNS (Figure 12-2). This configuration is typical of sensory neurons in both cranial and spinal nerves. Bipolar neurons have two distinct processes arising from the cell body. This type of neuron connects the rod and cone cells of the retina. Multipolar neurons are the most

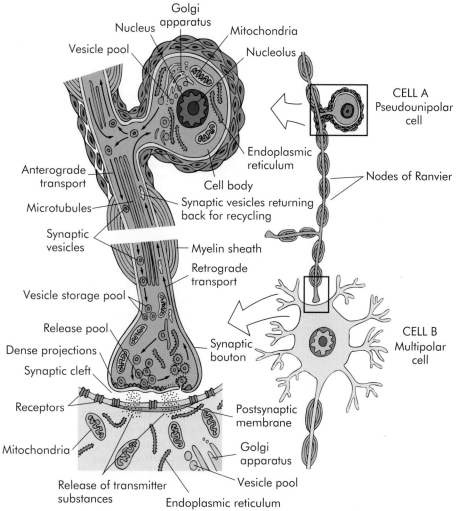

FIGURE 12-2 Neuronal Transmission and Synaptic Cleft. Electrical impulse travels along axon of first neuron to synapse. Chemical transmitter is secreted into synaptic space to depolarize membrane (dendrite or cell body) of next neuron in pathway. *Cell A* represents pseudounipolar cell; *cell B* represents multipolar cell.

CENTRAL NERVOUS SYSTEM NEUROGLIA

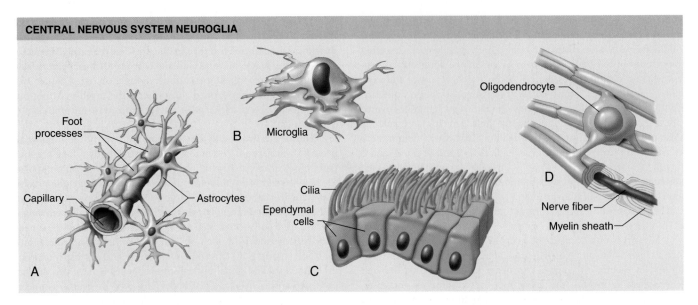

PERIPHERAL NERVOUS SYSTEM NEUROGLIA

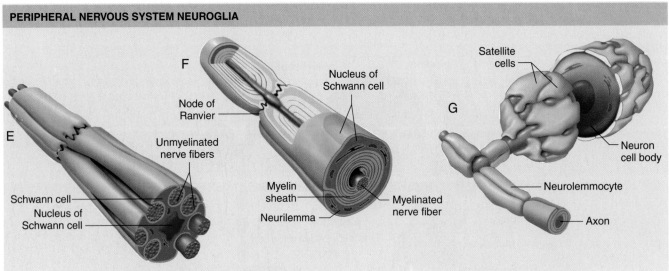

FIGURE 12-3 Types of Neuroglial Cells. Neuroglia of the CNS: **A,** Astrocytes attached to the outside of a capillary blood vessel in the brain. **B,** A phagocytic microglial cell. **C,** Ciliated ependymal cells forming a sheet that usually lines fluid cavities in the brain. **D,** An oligodendrocyte with processes that wrap around nerve fibers in the CNS to form myelin sheaths. Neuroglia of the peripheral nervous system (PNS): **E,** A Schwann cell supporting a bundle of nerve fibers in the PNS. **F,** Another type of Schwann cell encircling a peripheral nerve fiber to form a thick myelin sheath. **G,** Satellite cells, another type of Schwann cell, surround and support cell bodies of neurons in the PNS. (From Thibodeau GA, Patton KT: *Anatomy & physiology,* ed 7, St Louis, 2010, Mosby.)

common and have multiple processes capable of extensive branching. A motor neuron is typically multipolar (see Figure 12-2).

Functionally, there are three types of neurons (their direction of transmission and typical configuration are noted in parentheses): (1) sensory (afferent, mostly pseudounipolar), (2) associational (interneurons, multipolar), and (3) motor (efferent, multipolar). Sensory neurons carry impulses from peripheral sensory receptors to the CNS. Associational neurons (interneurons) transmit impulses from neuron to neuron—that is, sensory to motor neurons. They are located solely within the CNS. Motor neurons transmit impulses away from the CNS to an effector (i.e., skeletal muscle or organs). In skeletal muscle the end processes form a neuromuscular (myoneural) junction (see Figure 12-14).

Neuroglia and Schwann Cells

Neuroglia ("nerve glue") are the general classification of cells that support the neurons of the CNS. They comprise approximately half of the total brain and spinal cord volume and are 5 to 10 times more numerous than neurons. Different types of neuroglia serve different functions. Astrocytes, for example, fill the spaces between neurons and surround blood vessels in the CNS; oligodendroglia (oligodendrocytes) deposit myelin sheaths within the CNS. Oligodendroglia are the CNS counterpart of the Schwann cells. Ependymal cells line the cerebrospinal fluid (CSF)-filled cavities of the CNS. Microglia remove debris (phagocytosis) in the CNS. (Characteristics of neuroglia and Schwann cells are summarized in Figure 12-3 and Table 12-1.)

TABLE 12-1	SUPPORT CELLS OF THE NERVOUS SYSTEM
CELL TYPE	**PRIMARY FUNCTIONS**
Astrocytes	Form specialized contacts between neuronal surfaces and blood vessels
	Provide rapid transport for nutrients and metabolites
	Believed to form an essential component of blood-brain barrier
	Appear to be scar-forming cells of CNS, which may be foci for seizures
	Appear to work with neurons in processing information and memory storage
Oligodendroglia (oligodendrocytes)	Formation of myelin sheath in CNS
Schwann cells	Formation of myelin sheath in PNS
Microglia	Responsible for clearing cellular debris (phagocytic properties)
Ependymal cells	Serve as a lining for ventricles and choroid plexuses involved in production of cerebrospinal fluid

Some data from Martinez Banaclocha MA: Magnetic storage of information in the human cerebral cortex: a hypothesis for memory, *Int J Neurosci* 115(3):329–337, 2005; Sofroniew MV, Vinters HV: Astrocytes: biology and pathology, *Acta Neuropathol* 119(1):7–35, 2010. *CNS,* Central nervous system; *PNS,* peripheral nervous system.

Nerve Injury and Regeneration

Mature nerve cells do not divide, and injury can cause permanent loss of function. When an axon is severed, wallerian degeneration occurs in the distal axon: (1) a characteristic swelling appears within the portion of the axon distal to the cut; (2) the neurofilaments hypertrophy; (3) the myelin sheath shrinks and disintegrates; and (4) the axon degenerates and disappears. The myelin sheaths re-form into Schwann cells that align in a column between the severed part of the axon and the effector organ.

At the proximal end of the injured axon, similar changes occur but only back to the next node of Ranvier. The cell body responds to trauma by swelling and by dispersing the Nissl substance (chromatolysis). During the repair process, the cell increases all of the following: metabolic activity, protein synthesis, and mitochondrial activity. Approximately 7 to 14 days after the injury, new terminal sprouts project from the proximal segment and may enter the remaining Schwann cell pathway. (Figure 12-4 contains a more detailed representation of these events.) This process, however, is limited to myelinated fibers and generally occurs only in the PNS. The regeneration of axonal constituents in the CNS is limited by an increased incidence of scar formation and the different nature of myelin formed by the oligodendrocyte.

Nerve regeneration depends on many factors, such as location of the injury, the type of injury, the presence of inflammatory responses, and the process of scarring. The closer to the cell body of the nerve, the greater the chances that the nerve cell will die and not regenerate. A crushing injury allows recovery more fully than does a cut injury. Crushed nerves sometimes recover fully, whereas cut nerves form connective tissue scars that block or slow regenerating axonal branches.

THE NERVE IMPULSE

Neurons generate and conduct electrical and chemical impulses by selectively changing the electrical potential of the plasma membrane and influencing other nearby neurons by releasing chemicals (neurotransmitters). An unexcited neuron maintains a resting membrane

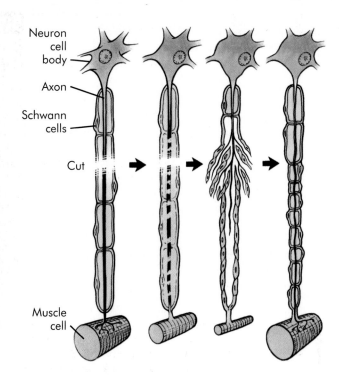

FIGURE 12-4 Repair of a Peripheral Nerve Fiber. When cut, a damaged motor axon can regrow to its distal connection only if the Schwann cells remain intact (to form a guiding tunnel) and if scar tissue does not block its way.

> ✓ **QUICK CHECK 12-1**
> 1. How do the functions of the somatic and autonomic nervous systems differ?
> 2. What are the three components of a neuron?
> 3. How does myelin affect nerve impulses?
> 4. Name the process through which injured axons are repaired, and describe the process.

potential (see Chapter 1). When the membrane potential is sufficiently raised, an action potential is generated and the nerve impulse then flows to all parts of the neuron. The action potential response occurs only when the stimulus is strong enough; if it is too weak, the membrane remains unexcited. This property is termed the *all-or-none response* (see Chapter 1 for a discussion of electrical impulse conduction).

Synapses

Neurons are not physically continuous with one another. The region between adjacent neurons is called a synapse (see Figure 12-2). Impulses are transmitted across the synapse by chemical and electrical conduction (see Figure 12-2); only chemical conduction is discussed here. Chapter 1 contains information on electrical conduction. The neurons that conduct a nerve impulse are named according to whether they relay impulses toward (presynaptic neurons) or away from (postsynaptic neurons) the synapse.

Impulses are transmitted across the synapse by chemical conduction. When an impulse originates in a presynaptic neuron, the impulse reaches the vesicles, where chemicals (neurotransmitters) are stored in the synaptic bouton. Once released from the vesicles, the

TABLE 12-2	SUBSTANCES THAT ARE NEUROTRANSMITTERS OR NEUROMODULATORS		
SUBSTANCE	**LOCATION**	**EFFECT**	**CLINICAL EXAMPLE**
Acetylcholine	Many parts of brain, spinal cord, neuromuscular junction of skeletal muscle, and many ANS synapses	Excitatory or inhibitory	Alzheimer disease (a type of dementia) is associated with a decrease in acetylcholine-secreting neurons. Myasthenia gravis (weakness of skeletal muscles) results from a reduction in acetylcholine receptors.
Monoamines			
Norepinephrine	Many areas of brain and spinal cord; also in some ANS synapses	Excitatory or inhibitory	Cocaine and amphetamines,* resulting in overstimulation of postsynaptic neurons.
Serotonin	Many areas of brain and spinal cord	Generally inhibitory	Involved with mood, anxiety, and sleep induction. Levels of serotonin are elevated in schizophrenia (delusions, hallucinations, withdrawal).
Dopamine	Some areas of brain and ANS synapses	Generally excitatory	Parkinson disease (depression of voluntary motor control) results from destruction of dopamine-secreting neurons. Drugs used to increase dopamine production induce vomiting and schizophrenia.
Histamine	Posterior hypothalamus	Excitatory (H1 and H2 receptors) and inhibitory (H3 receptors)	No clear indication of histamine-associated pathologic conditions. Histamine is involved with arousal and attention and links to other brain transmitter systems.
Amino Acids			
γ-Aminobutyric acid (GABA)	Most neurons of CNS have GABA receptors	Majority of postsynaptic inhibition in brain	Drugs that increase GABA function have been used to treat epilepsy by inhibiting excessive discharge of neurons.
Glycine	Spinal cord	Most postsynaptic inhibition in spinal cord	Glycine receptors are inhibited by strychnine.
Glutamate and aspartate	Widespread in brain and spinal cord	Excitatory	Drugs that block glutamate or aspartate, such as riluzole, used to treat amyotrophic lateral sclerosis. These drugs might prevent overexcitation from seizures and neural degeneration.
Neuropeptides			
Endorphins and enkephalins	Widely distributed in CNS and PNS	Generally inhibitory	Morphine and heroin bind to endorphin and enkephalin receptors on presynaptic neurons and reduce pain by blocking release of neurotransmitter.
Substance P	Spinal cord, brain, and sensory neurons associated with pain, GI tract	Generally excitatory	Substance P is a neurotransmitter in pain transmission pathways. Blocking release of substance P by morphine reduces pain.

From Seeley R, Stephens TD, Tate P: *Anatomy and physiology,* ed 7, New York, 2006, McGraw-Hill.
ANS, Autonomic nervous system; *CNS,* central nervous system; *GI,* gastrointestinal; *PNS,* peripheral nervous system.
*Increase the release and block the reuptake of norepinephrine.

neurotransmitters diffuse across the synaptic cleft (the space between the neurons) and bind to receptor sites on the plasma membrane of the postsynaptic neuron,[2] relaying the impulse (see Figure 12-2). Synapses can change in strength and number throughout life and this is known as synaptic plasticity or neuroplasticity (see *Health Alert:* Neuroplasticity).

Neurotransmitters

More than 30 substances are thought to be neurotransmitters, including norepinephrine, acetylcholine, dopamine, histamine, and serotonin. Many of these transmitters have more than one function.[3] For example, norepinephrine in the brain probably helps regulate mood, functions in dreaming sleep, and maintains arousal. Some neurotransmitters are amino acids, including gamma-aminobutyric acid (GABA), glutamic acid, and aspartic acid. Small chains of amino acids (neuropeptides), such as enkephalins and endorphins, also function as neurotransmitters. Neurotransmitter and neuromodulator substances are summarized in Table 12-2.

Because the neurotransmitter is normally stored on one side of the synaptic cleft and the receptor sites are on the other side, chemical synapses operate in one direction. Therefore action potentials are transmitted along a multineuronal pathway in one direction. The binding of the neurotransmitter at the receptor site changes the permeability of the postsynaptic neuron and, consequently, its membrane

potential. Two possible scenarios can then follow: (1) the postsynaptic neuron may be excited (depolarized; excitatory postsynaptic potentials [EPSPs]) or (2) the postsynaptic neuron's plasma membrane may be inhibited (hyperpolarized; inhibitory postsynaptic potentials [IPSPs]). Cannabinoid transmitters have been discovered that are released from postsynaptic neurons and modulate neurotransmitter release from the presynaptic neurons.[3,4] (Chapter 1 reviews electrical impulses and membrane potentials.)

Usually a single EPSP cannot induce a neuron's action potential and the propagation of the nerve impulse. Whether this occurs depends on the number and frequency of potentials the postsynaptic neuron receives—a concept known as summation. Temporal summation (time relationship) refers to the effects of successive, rapid impulses received from a single neuron at the same synapse. Spatial summation (spacing effect) is the combined effects of impulses from a number of neurons onto a single neuron at the same time. Facilitation refers to the effect of EPSP on the plasma membrane potential. The plasma membrane is facilitated when summation brings the membrane closer to the threshold potential and decreases the stimulus required to induce an action potential. The effect that a chemical neurotransmitter has on the plasma membrane potential depends on the balance of these effects.

HEALTH ALERT

Neuroplasticity

Neuroplasticity is the lifelong ability of the brain to adapt to new conditions by reorganizing neural pathways and forming new synapses, resulting in development, learning, and memory. The process is complex and the underlying mechanisms include environmental influences, genetics, neurochemical alterations, functional changes in excitatory and inhibitory synapses, and axonal and dendritic sprouting and turnover. Research is currently in progress to identify ways of delivering agents and therapies to promote neurorestoration and enhance brain or spinal cord reorganization of motor and sensory function following injury or disease. The new clinical area of neuro-optometry provides an example of neuroplasticity within the brain. The utilization of external prisms and computerized vision programs for visual rehabilitation can modify the visual processing system in children and adults to significantly improve visual performance.

Data from Alvarez TL et al: Vision therapy in adults with convergence insufficiency: clinical and functional magnetic resonance imaging measures, *Optom Vis Sci* 87(12):1–17, 2010; Barker AJ, Ullian EM: Astrocytes and synaptic plasticity, *Neuroscientist* 16(1):40–50, 2010; Galván A: Neural plasticity of development and learning, *Hum Brain Mapp* 31(6):879–890, 2010; Kujala T, Näätänen R: The adaptive brain: a neurophysiological perspective, *Prog Neurobiol* 91(1):55–67, 2010; Saver JL: Target brain: neuroprotection and neurorestoration in ischemic stroke, *Rev Neurol Dis* 7(suppl 1):S14–S21, 2010.

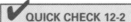

QUICK CHECK 12-2
1. Explain the process of the chemical conduction of impulses.
2. What are neurotransmitters? Give several examples.
3. Compare summation and facilitation.

THE CENTRAL NERVOUS SYSTEM

The Brain

The human brain enables a person to reason, function intellectually, express personality and mood, and interact with the environment. This pinkish gray organ weighs approximately 3 pounds and receives 15% to 20% of the total cardiac output. The three major divisions of the brain are (1) the forebrain, formed by the two cerebral hemispheres; (2) the midbrain, which includes the corpora quadrigemina and cerebral peduncles; and (3) the hindbrain, which includes the cerebellum, pons, and medulla (Table 12-3). The midbrain, medulla, and pons comprise the **brain stem,** which connects the hemispheres of the brain, cerebellum, and spinal cord. A collection of nerve cell bodies (nuclei) within the brain stem makes up the **reticular formation** (Figure 12-5). The reticular formation is a large network of diffuse nuclei that control vital reflexes, such as those controlling cardiovascular function and respiration. It is essential for maintaining wakefulness and therefore is referred to as the **reticular activating system** (see Figure 12-5). Some nuclei within the reticular formation cause specific motor movements.[3]

Divisions of the brain are associated with different functions, but attributing specific functions to definite regions of the brain is not entirely accurate. However, for clinical considerations functional specificity is very useful for localizing pathologic conditions in various nervous system regions. A neuropsychiatrist (Brodmann) is credited with postulating that various activities are correlated to many regions of the cerebral cortex. (Figure 12-6 illustrates these regions and describes some of the areas.)[5]

TABLE 12-3 DIVISIONS OF THE CENTRAL NERVOUS SYSTEM

PRIMARY BRAIN VESICLES	SECONDARY VESICLES	STRUCTURES IN SECONDARY VESICLES
Forebrain (prosencephalon)	Telencephalon	Cerebral hemispheres
		Cerebral cortex
		Limbic system
		Basal ganglia
	Diencephalon	Epithalamus
		Thalamus
		Hypothalamus
		Subthalamus
Midbrain (mesencephalon)	Mesencephalon	Corpora quadrigemina
		Cerebral peduncles
Hindbrain (rhombencephalon)	Metencephalon	Cerebellum
		Pons
	Myelencephalon	Medulla oblongata
Spinal cord	Spinal cord	Spinal cord

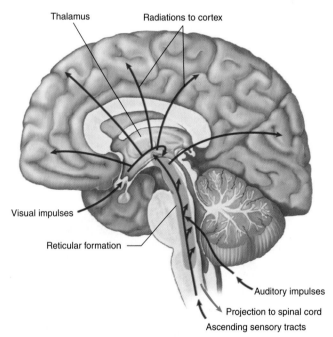

FIGURE 12-5 Reticular Activating System. System consists of nuclei in the brain stem reticular formation plus fibers that conduct to the nuclei from below and fibers that conduct from the nuclei to widespread areas of the cerebral cortex. Functioning of the reticular activating system is essential for consciousness.

Forebrain

Telencephalon. The **telencephalon** consists of the cerebrum (the largest portion of the brain), the limbic system, and some basal ganglia (composed of several *nuclei*). The surface of the cerebrum (cerebral cortex) is covered with convolutions called *gyri* (see Figure 12-6), which greatly increases the cortical surface area and the number of neurons. Grooves between adjacent gyri are termed **sulci;** deeper

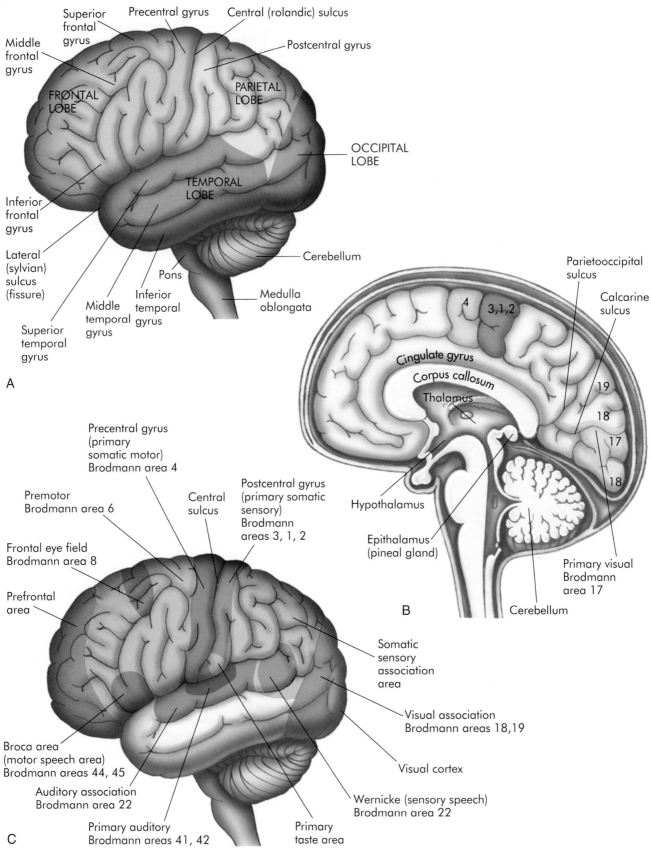

FIGURE 12-6 **The Cerebral Hemispheres. A,** Left hemisphere of cerebrum, lateral view. **B,** Functional areas of the cerebral cortex, midsagittal view. **C,** Functional areas of the cerebral cortex, lateral view.

grooves are fissures. The cerebral cortex contains the cell bodies of neurons (gray matter). White matter lies beneath the cerebral cortex and is composed of myelinated nerve fibers.

The two cerebral hemispheres are separated by a deep groove known as the longitudinal fissure. The surface of each hemisphere is divided into lobes named after the region of the skull under which each lobe lies. The frontal lobe's posterior margin is on the central sulcus (fissure of Rolando), and it borders inferiorly on the lateral sulcus (sylvian fissure, lateral fissure) (see Figure 12-6). The prefrontal area is responsible for goal-oriented behavior (e.g., ability to concentrate), short-term or recall memory, the elaboration of thought, and inhibition of the limbic areas of the CNS. The premotor area (Brodmann area 6) (see Figure 12-6, C) is involved in programming motor movements. This area contains the cell bodies that form part of the basal ganglia system (extrapyramidal system—efferent pathways outside the pyramids of the medulla oblongata). The frontal eye fields (the lower portion of Brodmann area 8), which are involved in controlling eye movements, are located on the middle frontal gyrus.

The primary motor area (Brodmann area 4) is located along the precentral gyrus forming the primary voluntary motor area, which has a somatotropic organization that is often referred to as a *homunculus* (little man) (Figure 12-7). Electrical stimulation of specific areas of this cortex causes specific muscles of the body to move. For example, stimulation of Brodmann area 4 in the medial longitudinal fissure affects the lower limb and foot, whereas stimulation of the superior lateral surface of the precentral gyrus affects the torso and arm, the middle third of the hand, and the lower third of the face and mouth/throat. The axons traveling from the cell bodies in and on either side of this gyrus project fibers (axons) that form the corticospinal tracts (pyramidal system) that descend into the spinal cord. Cerebral impulses control function on the opposite side of the body, a phenomenon called contralateral control (Figure 12-8, A). The Broca speech area (Brodmann areas 44, 45) is rostral on the inferior frontal gyrus. It is usually on the left hemisphere and is responsible for the motor aspects of speech. Damage to this area, commonly as a result of a cerebrovascular accident (stroke), results in the inability to form words or at least some difficulty in forming words (expressive aphasia or dysphasia) (see Chapter 14).

The parietal lobe lies within the borders of the central, parietooccipital, and lateral sulci. This lobe contains the major area for somatic sensory input, located primarily along the postcentral gyrus (Brodmann areas 3, 1, 2), which is adjacent to the primary motor area. Communication between the motor and sensory areas (and among other regions in the cortex) is provided by association fibers. Much of this region is involved in sensory association (storage, analysis, and interpretation of stimuli). (Figure 12-7 shows the distribution of functions associated with both the primary motor area and the primary sensory area of the cerebral cortex.)

The occipital lobe lies caudal to the parietooccipital sulcus and is superior to the cerebellum. The primary visual cortex (Brodmann area 17) is located in this region and receives input from the retinas. Much of the remainder of this lobe is involved in visual association (Brodmann areas 18, 19). The temporal lobe lies inferior to the lateral fissure and is composed of the superior, middle, and inferior temporal gyri. The primary auditory cortex (Brodmann area 41) and its related association area (Brodmann area 42) lie deep within the lateral sulcus on the superior temporal gyrus. The Wernicke area, along with adjacent portions of the parietal lobe, constitutes a *sensory speech area*. This area is responsible for reception and interpretation of speech, and dysfunction may result in receptive aphasia or dysphasia. The temporal lobe also is involved in memory consolidation and smell.

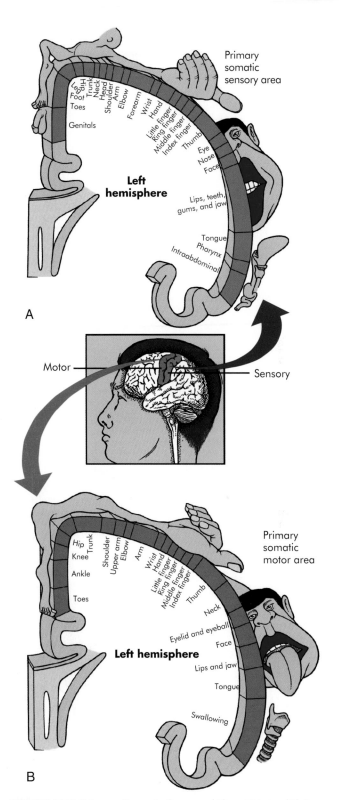

FIGURE 12-7 Primary Somatic Sensory (A) and Motor (B) Areas of the Cortex. This illustration shows which parts of the body are "mapped" to specific cortical areas. The exaggerated face indicates that more cortical area is devoted to processing information to and from the many receptors and motor units of the face than for the leg or arm, for example. (From Patton KT, Thibodeau GA: *Anatomy & physiology,* ed 7, St Louis, 2010, Mosby.)

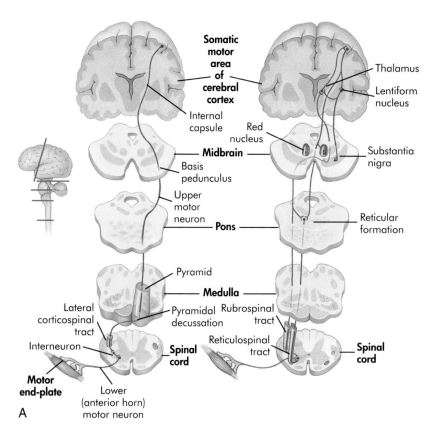

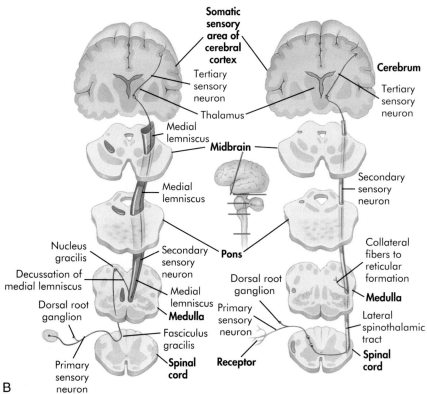

FIGURE 12-8 Examples of Somatic Motor and Sensory Pathways. A, Motor: pyramidal pathway illustrated by the lateral corticospinal tract and extrapyramidal pathways illustrated by the rubrospinal and reticulospinal tracts. **B,** Sensory: pathways of the medial lemniscal system that conducts information about discriminating touch and kinesthesis and the spinothalamic pathway that conducts information about pain and temperature. (Modified from Patton KT, Thibodeau GA: *Anatomy & physiology,* ed 7, St Louis, 2010, Mosby.)

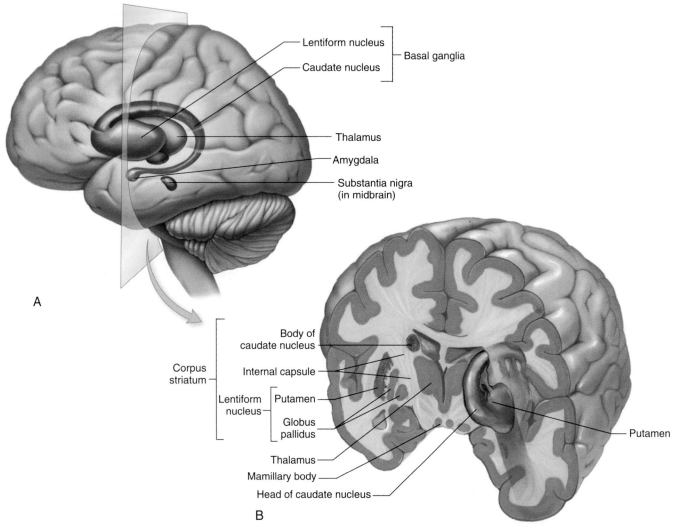

FIGURE 12-9 Basal Nuclei. **A,** The basal nuclei seen through the cortex of the left cerebral hemisphere. **B,** The basal nuclei seen in a frontal (coronal) section of the brain. (From Patton KT, Thibodeau GA: *Anatomy & physiology,* ed 7, p 432, St Louis, 2010, Mosby.)

Another lobe, the insula (insular lobe), lies hidden from view in the lateral sulci between the temporal and frontal lobe of each hemisphere. The insula processes sensory and emotional information and routes the information to other areas of the brain. Lying directly beneath the longitudinal fissure is a mass of white matter pathways called the corpus callosum (transverse or commissural fibers). This structure connects the two cerebral hemispheres and is essential in coordinating activities between hemispheres (see Figure 12-6).

Inside the cerebrum are numerous tracts (white matter) and nuclei (gray matter). The major cerebral nuclei are called basal ganglia and include the corpus striatum and amygdala. The corpus striatum consists of the lentiform nucleus (lens-shaped) (Figure 12-9), the putamen and globus pallidus, and the ram's horn–shaped caudate nucleus. The internal capsule (see Figure 12-9) is a thick white matter region in which afferent and efferent pathways, to and from the cerebral cortex, pass through the center of the cerebral hemispheres between the caudate and lentiform nuclei (see Figure 12-9).

Functionally, basal ganglia include, in addition to the corpus striatum, the subthalamic nucleus of the diencephalon and the substantia nigra of the mesencephalon. The basal ganglia plus their direct and indirect interconnections with the thalamus, premotor cortex, red nucleus, reticular formation, and spinal cord have been considered part of the basal ganglia system (extrapyramidal system). The basal ganglia system is believed to exert a stabilizing effect on motor movements. Parkinson disease and Huntington disease are conditions associated with defects of the basal ganglia. They are characterized by various involuntary or exaggerated motor movements (see Chapter 14).

The limbic system is a group of structures surrounding the corpus callosum that mediate emotion through connections in the prefrontal cortex. It is composed of the Papez circuit (amygdala, parahippocampal gyrus, hippocampus, fornix, mamillary body of the hypothalamus, thalamus, and cingulate gyrus), septal area, habenula, other portions of the hypothalamus, and related autonomic nuclei. It is an extension or modification of the olfactory system. Its principal effects are believed to be involved in primitive behavioral responses, visceral reaction to emotion, feeding behaviors, biologic rhythms, and the sense of smell.

Diencephalon. The diencephalon (interbrain), surrounded by the cerebrum, has four divisions: epithalamus, thalamus, hypothalamus, and subthalamus (see Table 12-3 and Figure 12-6).

BOX 12-1 FUNCTIONS OF THE HYPOTHALAMUS

- Visceral and somatic responses
- Affectual responses
- Hormone synthesis
- Sympathetic and parasympathetic activity
- Temperature regulation
- Feeding responses
- Physical expression of emotions
- Sexual behavior
- Pleasure-punishment centers
- Level of arousal or wakefulness

Data from Purves D et al: *Neuroscience,* ed 3, Sunderland, Mass, 2004, Sinauer Associates; Kiernan JA: *Barr's the human nervous system: an anatomical viewpoint,* ed 9, Philadelphia, 2009, Lippincott Williams & Wilkins.

The epithalamus forms the roof of the third ventricle (a brain cavity) and composes the most superior portion of the diencephalon. Its connections and functions are closely associated with those of the limbic system.

The thalamus borders and surrounds the third ventricle. It is a major integrating center for afferent impulses to the cerebral cortex. Various sensations are perceived at this level, but cortical processing is required for interpretation. The thalamus serves also as a relay center for information from the basal ganglia and cerebellum to the appropriate motor area.

The hypothalamus forms the base of the diencephalon. The hypothalamus functions to (1) maintain a constant internal environment and (2) implement behavioral patterns. Integrative centers control autonomic nervous system (ANS) function, regulate body temperature and endocrine function, and adjust emotional expression. The hypothalamus exerts its influence through the endocrine system, as well as through neural pathways (Box 12-1).

The subthalamus flanks the hypothalamus laterally. It serves as an important basal ganglia center for motor activities.

Midbrain

Mesencephalon. The midbrain (mesencephalon) is composed of three structures: the corpora quadrigemina (tectum) (composed of the superior and inferior colliculi), the tegmentum (containing the red nucleus and substantia nigra), and the basis pedunculi. (The tegmentum and basis pedunculi are collectively called the cerebral peduncles.)

The superior colliculi are involved with voluntary and involuntary visual motor movements (e.g., the ability of the eyes to track moving objects in the visual field). The inferior colliculi accomplish similar motor activities but involve movements affecting the auditory system (e.g., positioning the head to improve hearing). The red nucleus receives ascending sensory information from the cerebellum and projects a minor motor pathway, the rubrospinal tract, to the cervical spinal cord. The last portion of the basal ganglia is the substantia nigra, which synthesizes dopamine, a neurotransmitter and precursor of norepinephrine. Its dysfunction is associated with Parkinson disease and schizophrenia. The basis pedunculi are made up of efferent fibers of the corticospinal, corticobulbar, and corticopontocerebellar tracts.

Other notable structures of this region are the nuclei of the third and fourth cranial nerves. The cerebral aqueduct (aqueduct of Sylvius), which carries cerebrospinal fluid, also traverses this structure. Obstruction of this aqueduct is often the cause of hydrocephalus.

Hindbrain

Metencephalon. The major structures of the metencephalon are the cerebellum and the pons. The cerebellum (see Figure 12-6) is composed of gray and white matter, and its cortical surface is convoluted like the surface of the cerebrum. It also is divided by a central fissure into two lobes connected by the vermis.

The cerebellum is responsible for reflexive, involuntary fine-tuning of motor control and for maintaining balance and posture through extensive neural connections with the medulla (through the inferior cerebellar peduncle) and with the midbrain (through the superior cerebellar peduncle). The two hemispheres are connected to the pons by the middle cerebellar peduncles. These connections allow extensive sampling of visual, vestibular, and proprioceptive data from other regions of the CNS and periphery.

The pons (bridge) is easily recognized by its bulging appearance below the midbrain and above the medulla. Primarily it transmits information from the cerebellum to the brain stem and between the two cerebellar hemispheres. The nuclei of the fifth through eighth cranial nerves are located in this structure.

Myelencephalon. The myelencephalon usually is called the medulla oblongata and forms the lowest portion of the brain stem. Reflex activities, such as heart rate, respiration, blood pressure, coughing, sneezing, swallowing, and vomiting, are controlled in this area. The nuclei of cranial nerves IX through XII also are located in this region.

A major portion of the descending motor pathways (i.e., corticospinal tracts) cross to the other side, or decussate, at the medulla (see Figure 12-8). These pathways, together with other areas of decussation in the CNS, are the basis for the phenomenon of contralateral control. Sleep-wake rhythms also are processed by neural influences from lower brain centers and are associated with a complex group of diffuse structures and functions (see Chapter 13), including the reticular activating system (cells that receive collateral signals from the afferent sensory pathways and project the signals to the higher brain centers, thus controlling CNS activity) (see Figure 12-5).

 QUICK CHECK 12-3
1. Name the three major divisions of the brain and their component parts.
2. Describe the limbic system's functions.
3. What are the two major functions of the hypothalamus?

The Spinal Cord

The spinal cord is the portion of the CNS that lies within the vertebral canal and is surrounded and protected by the vertebral column. The spinal cord has many functions, which include a long nerve cable that connects the brain and body, somatic and autonomic reflexes, motor pattern control centers, and sensory and motor modulation. It originates in the medulla oblongata and ends at the level of the first or second lumbar vertebra in adults (Figure 12-10). The end of the spinal cord, the conus medullaris, is cone shaped. Spinal nerves continue from the end of the spinal cord and form a nerve bundle called the cauda equina. The filament anchor from the conus medullaris to the coccyx is the filum terminale (see Figure 12-10).

Grossly, the spinal cord is divided into vertebral sections (8 cervical, 12 thoracic, 5 lumbar, 5 sacral, and 1 coccygeal) that correspond to paired nerves (see Figure 12-10). A cross section of the spinal cord (Figure 12-11) is characterized by a butterfly-shaped inner core of gray matter (containing nerve cell bodies). The central canal lies in the

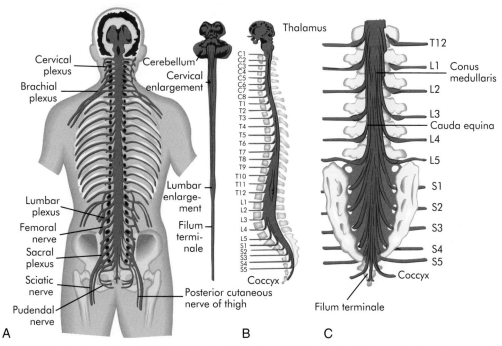

FIGURE 12-10 Spinal Cord Within Vertebral Canal and Exiting Spinal Nerves. **A**, Posterior view of brain stem and spinal cord in situ with spinal nerves and plexus. **B**, Lateral view of brain stem and spinal cord. **C**, Enlargement of caudal area showing termination of spinal cord (conus medullaris) and group of nerve fibers constituting the cauda equina. (Redrawn from Rudy EB, editor: *Advanced neurological and neurosurgical nursing,* St Louis, 1984, Mosby.)

center of this region and extends through the spinal cord from its origin in the fourth ventricle. The gray matter of the spinal cord is divided into three regions and displays specific functional characteristics. These regions include the posterior horn, or dorsal horn (composed primarily of interneurons and axons from sensory neurons whose cell bodies lie in the dorsal root ganglion). At the tip of the posterior horn is the substantia gelatinosa, a structure involved in pain transmission (see Chapter 13). The lateral horn contains cell bodies involved with the ANS. The anterior horn, or ventral horn, contains the nerve cell bodies for efferent pathways that leave the spinal cord by way of spinal nerves.

Surrounding the gray matter is white matter that forms ascending and descending pathways called spinal tracts. Spinal tracts are named to denote their beginning and ending points. For example, the spinothalamic tract (see Figure 12-8, *B*) carries nerve impulses from the spinal cord to the thalamus in the diencephalon. Numerous spinal tracts are grouped into columns according to their location within the white matter. These include the anterior columns, lateral columns, and posterior (dorsal) columns (Figure 12-12).

Neural circuits in the spinal cord, when activated, display specific sets of motor responses. Reflex arcs form basic units that respond to stimuli and provide protective circuitry for motor output. Structures needed for a reflex arc are a receptor, an afferent (sensory) neuron, an efferent (motor) neuron, and an effector muscle or gland. A simple reflex arc may contain only two neurons (Figure 12-13). Interneurons are usually present and provide a link between sensory and motor neurons.

The motor effects of reflex arcs generally occur before the event is perceived in the brain's higher centers. Much internal environmental regulation is mediated by reflex activity involving the ANS.

Afferent pathways transmit information from peripheral receptors and eventually terminate in the cerebral or cerebellar cortex, or

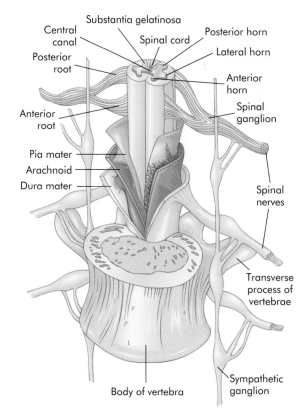

FIGURE 12-11 Coverings of the Spinal Cord. The dura mater is shown in natural color. Note how it extends to cover the spinal nerve roots and nerves. The arachnoid is highlighted in blue and the pia mater in pink. (Modified from Thibodeau GA, Patton KT: *Structure and function of the human body,* ed 3, St Louis, 2008, Mosby.)

both. Efferent pathways primarily relay information from the cerebrum to the brain stem or spinal cord. **Upper motor neurons** are completely contained within the CNS. Their primary roles are controlling fine motor movement and influencing/modifying spinal reflex arcs and circuits. Generally, upper motor neurons form synapses with interneurons, which then form synapses with lower motor neurons that project into the periphery. **Lower motor neurons** directly influence muscles. Their cell bodies lie in the gray matter of the brain stem and spinal cord, but their processes extend out of the CNS and into the PNS. Destruction of upper motor neurons usually results in initial

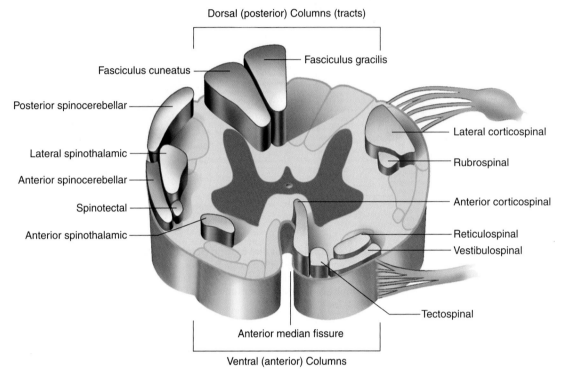

FIGURE 12-12 Major Tracts of the Spinal Cord. The major ascending (sensory) tracts, shown only on the left here, are highlighted in blue. The major descending (motor) tracts, shown only on the right, are highlighted in red. (From Patton KT, Thibodeau GA: *Anatomy & physiology*, ed 7, St Louis, 2010, Mosby.)

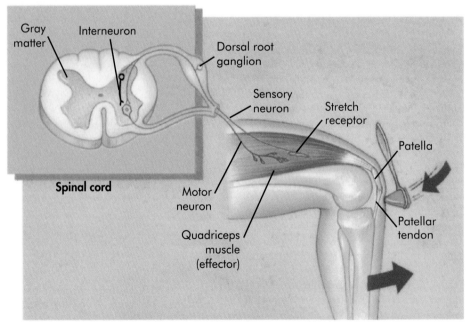

FIGURE 12-13 Cross Section of Spinal Cord Showing Simple Reflex Arc. (From Patton KT, Thibodeau GA: *Anatomy & physiology*, ed 7, St Louis, 2010, Mosby.)

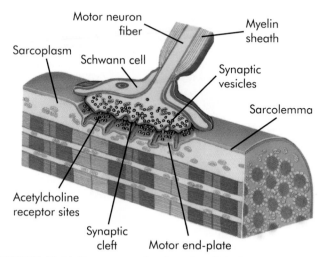

FIGURE 12-14 Neuromuscular Junction. This figure shows how the distal end of a motor neuron fiber forms a synapse, or "chemical junction," with an adjacent muscle fiber. Neurotransmitters (specifically, acetylcholine) are released from the neuron's synaptic vesicles and diffuse across the synaptic cleft. There they stimulate receptors in the motor end-plate region of the sarcolemma. (From Patton KT, Thibodeau GA: *Anatomy & physiology*, ed 7, St Louis, 2010, Mosby.)

paralysis followed within days or weeks by partial recovery, whereas destruction of the *lower motor neurons* leads to paralysis. Peripheral nerve damage may be followed by nerve regeneration and recovery (see Figure 12-4).

Muscle activity (i.e., stimulation and contraction) is regulated by nerve impulses. Motor neurons innervate one or more muscle cells, forming motor units, which consist of a neuron and the skeletal muscles it stimulates. The junction between the axon of the motor neuron and the plasma membrane of the muscle cell is called the neuromuscular (myoneural) junction (Figure 12-14). (Injury to motor neurons is discussed in Chapter 15.)

Motor Pathways

The four clinically relevant motor pathways are the lateral corticospinal, corticobulbar, reticulospinal, and vestibulospinal tracts.[5] The corticospinal (see Figure 12-8, *A*) and corticobulbar pathways are essentially the same tract and consist of a two-neuron chain. The cell bodies originate in and around the precentral gyrus; pass through the corona radiata of the cerebrum, the internal capsule, middle three fifths of the cerebral pedunculus, pons, and pyramid; and decussate (cross contralaterally) in the medulla oblongata and form the lateral corticospinal tract of the spinal cord (see Figure 12-12). The corticobulbar tract synapses on motor cranial nuclei within the brain stem. The lateral corticospinal tract axons (upper motor neurons) leave the tract to go to specific interneurons or motor neurons in the anterior horn. The lateral corticospinal tract has the same somatropic organization as the body (see Figures 12-7 and 12-8, *A*). These lower motor neurons project through nerves to specific muscles. These tracts are involved in precise motor movements. The reticulospinal tract (see Figure 12-12) modulates motor movement by inhibiting and exciting spinal activity. The vestibulospinal tract arises from a vestibular nucleus in the pons and causes the extensor muscles of the body to rapidly contract, most dramatically witnessed when a person starts to fall backward.

Sensory Pathways

The three clinically important spinal afferent pathways are the posterior column, anterior spinothalamic tract, and lateral spinothalamic tract (see Figures 12-7 and 12-8, *B*, and 12-12). The posterior (dorsal) column (fasciculus gracilis and fasciculus cuneatus) carries fine-touch sensation, two-point discrimination, and proprioceptive information (i.e., epicritic information). The posterior column is formed by a three-neuron chain. The primary afferent neuron is the sensory neuron (of the reflex arc), but it sends its axon ipsilaterally up the spinal cord to a specific part of the posterior funiculus and synapses in the posterior column nuclei in the medulla oblongata. A basketball playing center has primary afferent neurons that could be more than 6 feet long, running from the great toe up to the medulla oblongata. The second-order neuron crosses contralaterally at the medial lemniscus and ascends and synapses with a specific nucleus of the thalamus. The third-order neuron, originating in the thalamus, continues the tract into the internal capsule, corona radiata, and postcentral gyrus (Brodmann areas 3, 1, 2) (see Figures 12-6, 12-7, *A*, and 12-8, *B*). The anterior and lateral spinothalamic tracts are responsible for vague touch sensation and for pain and temperature perception, respectively (see Figure 12-8, *B*). These modalities are referred to as protopathic. These tracts also form a three-neuron chain. However, their primary afferent neurons synapse in the posterior horn of the spinal cord, not just at the level they enter the intervertebral foramen but in a number of spinal segments above and below their point of entry. This is an example of divergence. The second-order neurons in the posterior horn cross to the contralateral side in the spinal cord, ascend to the same thalamic nucleus as the posterior column pathway, and continue with the posterior column pathway to the postcentral gyrus.

Protective Structures of the Central Nervous System
Cranium

The cranium is composed of eight bones. The cranial vault encloses and protects the brain and its associated structures.

The galea aponeurotica, which is a thick, fibrous band of tissue overlying the cranium between the frontal and occipital muscles, affords added protection to the skull. The subgaleal space has venous connections with the dural sinuses, and with increased intracranial pressure, blood can be shunted to the space, thus reducing pressure in the intracranial cavity. The subgaleal space is also a common site for wound drains after intracranial surgery.

The floor of the cranial vault is irregular and contains many foramina (openings) for cranial nerves, blood vessels, and the spinal cord to exit. The cranial floor is divided into three fossae (depressions). The frontal lobes lie in the anterior fossa, the temporal lobes and base of the diencephalon lie in the middle fossa (temporal fossa), and the cerebellum lies in the posterior fossa. These terms are commonly used anatomic landmarks to describe the location of intracranial lesions.

Meninges

Surrounding the brain and spinal cord are three protective membranes: the dura mater, the arachnoid, and the pia mater. Collectively they are called the meninges (Figure 12-15, *B*). The dura mater (meaning literally "hard mother") is composed of two layers, with the venous sinuses formed between them. The outermost layer forms the periosteum (endosteal layer) of the skull. The inner dura (meningeal layer) is responsible for forming rigid membranes that support and separate various brain structures.

One of these membranes, the falx cerebri, dips between the two cerebral hemispheres along the longitudinal fissure. The falx cerebri

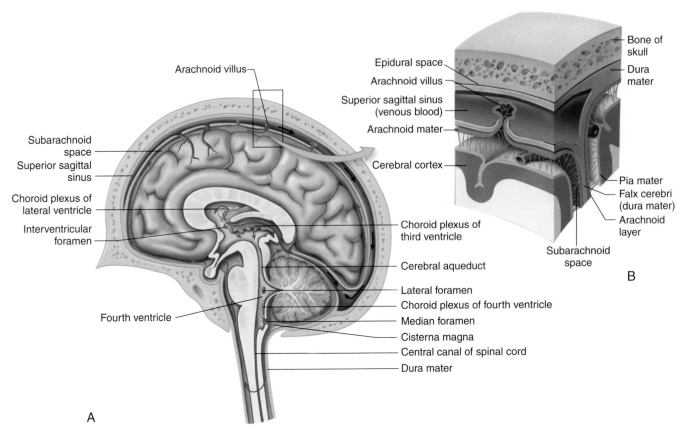

FIGURE 12-15 Flow of Cerebrospinal Fluid and Meninges of the Brain. **A,** The fluid produced by filtration of blood by the choroid plexus of each ventricle flows inferiorly through the lateral ventricles, interventricular foramen, third ventricle, cerebral aqueduct, fourth ventricle, and subarachnoid space to the blood. **B,** Meninges of the brain in relation to CSF and venous blood flow. (From Patton KT, Thibodeau GA: *Anatomy & physiology,* ed 7, St Louis, 2010, Mosby.)

is anchored anteriorly to the base of the brain at the crista galli of the ethmoid bone. The tentorium cerebelli, a common landmark, is a membrane that separates the cerebellum below from the cerebral structures above. Internal to the dura mater lies the arachnoid, a spongy, weblike structure that loosely follows the contours of the cerebral structures.

The subdural space lies between the dura and arachnoid. Many small bridging veins that have little support traverse the subdural space. Their disruption results in a subdural hematoma (see Chapter 15). The subarachnoid space lies between the arachnoid and the pia mater and contains cerebrospinal fluid (CSF) (see Figure 12-15, *A* and *B*). Unlike the dura mater and arachnoid, the delicate pia mater adheres to the contours of the brain and spinal cord. It provides support for blood vessels serving brain tissue. The choroid plexuses, structures that produce CSF, arise from the pial membrane (see Figure 12-15, *B*). The spinal cord is anchored to the vertebrae by extension of the meninges. The meninges continue beyond the end of the spinal cord (at vertebrae levels L1 and L2) to the lower portion of the sacrum. CSF contained within the subarachnoid space also circulates inferiorly to about the second sacral vertebra.

The meninges form potential and real spaces important to understanding functional and pathologic mechanisms. For example, between the dura mater and skull lies a potential space termed the epidural space (see Figure 12-15, *B*). The arterial supply to the meninges consists of blood vessels that lie within grooves in the skull. A skull fracture can sever one of these vessels and produce an epidural hematoma.

TABLE 12-4	**COMPOSITION OF CEREBROSPINAL FLUID**
CONSTITUENT	**NORMAL VALUE**
Na^+	148 mM
K^+	2.9 mM
Cl^-	125 mM
HCO_3^-	22.9 mM
Glucose (fasting)	50-75 mg/dl (60% of serum glucose)
pH	7.3
Protein	15-45 mg/dl
Albumin	80%
Globulin	6-10%
Cells	
White (lymphocyte)	0-6/mm³
Red	0

Cerebrospinal Fluid and the Ventricular System

Cerebrospinal fluid (CSF) is a clear, colorless fluid similar to blood plasma and interstitial fluid. The intracranial and spinal cord structures float in CSF and are thereby protected from jolts and blows. The buoyant properties of the CSF also prevent the brain from tugging on meninges, nerve roots, and blood vessels. (Constituents of CSF are listed in Table 12-4.) Between 125 and 150 ml of CSF is circulating

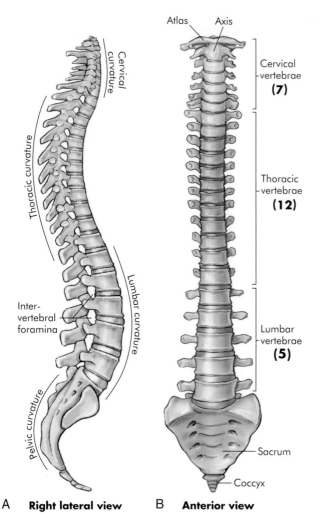

A **Right lateral view** B **Anterior view**

FIGURE 12-16 Vertebral Column. A, Right lateral view. B, Anterior view. (From Patton KT, Thibodeau GA: *Anatomy & physiology*, ed 7, St Louis, 2010, Mosby.)

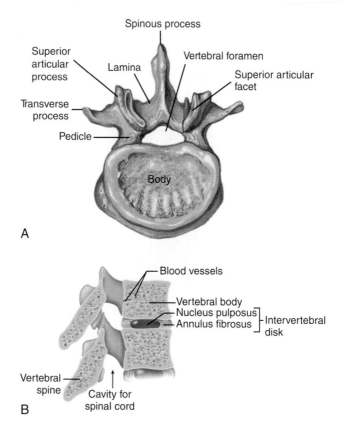

FIGURE 12-17 A, Lumbar Vertebra, Superior View; B, Intervertebral Disk. (A from Thibodeau GA, Patton KT: *Anatomy & physiology*, ed 6, St Louis, 2007, Mosby; B from Patton KT, Thibodeau GA: *Anatomy & physiology*, ed 7, St Louis, 2010, Mosby.)

within the **ventricles** (small cavities) and subarachnoid space at any given time. Approximately 600 ml of CSF is produced daily.

The choroid plexuses in the lateral, third, and fourth ventricles produce the major portion of CSF. (Ventricles are illustrated in Figure 12-15.) These plexuses are characterized by a rich network of blood vessels, supplied by the pia mater, that lie close to the ependymal cells of the ventricles.

The CSF exerts pressure within the brain and spinal cord. When a person is supine, CSF pressure is about 80 to 180 mm of water pressure, or approximately 5 to 14 mm of mercury pressure, but doubles when the person moves to an upright position. CSF flow results from the pressure gradient between the arterial system and the CSF-filled cavities. Beginning in the lateral ventricles, the CSF flows through the **interventricular foramen (foramen of Monro)** into the third ventricle and then passes through the cerebral aqueduct (aqueduct of Sylvius) into the fourth ventricle. From the fourth ventricle the CSF may pass through either the paired **lateral apertures (foramen of Luschka)** or the **median aperture (foramen of Magendie)** before communicating with the subarachnoid spaces of the brain and spinal cord. The CSF does not, however, accumulate. Instead, it is reabsorbed into the venous circulation through the arachnoid villi. The **arachnoid villi** protrude from the arachnoid space, through the dura mater, and lie

within the blood flow of the venous sinuses. CSF is reabsorbed through a pressure gradient between the arachnoid villi and the cerebral venous sinuses. The villi function as one-way valves directing CSF outflow into the blood but preventing blood flow into the subarachnoid space. Thus CSF is formed from the blood, and after circulating throughout the CNS, it returns to the blood.

Vertebral Column

The vertebral column (Figure 12-16) is composed of 33 vertebrae: 7 cervical, 12 thoracic, 5 lumbar, 5 fused sacral, and 4 fused coccygeal. Between each interspace (except for the fused sacral and coccygeal vertebrae) is an **intervertebral disk** (Figure 12-17). At the center of the intervertebral disk is the **nucleus pulposus,** a pulpy mass of elastic fibers. The intervertebral disk absorbs shocks, preventing damage to the vertebrae. The intervertebral disk is also a common source of back problems. If too much stress is applied to the vertebral column, the disk contents may rupture and protrude into the spinal canal, causing compression of the spinal cord or nerve roots.

✔ **QUICK CHECK 12-4**
1. What information is conveyed in the ascending and descending spinal tracts?
2. Contrast the functions of upper and lower motor neurons.
3. Name the protective structures of the central nervous system, and briefly describe each one.

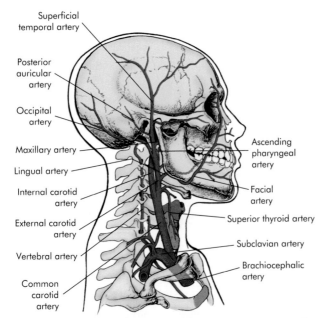

FIGURE 12-18 Major Arteries of the Head and Neck. (From Patton KT, Thibodeau GA: *Anatomy & physiology*, ed 7, St Louis, 2010, Mosby.)

Blood Supply of the Central Nervous System
Blood Supply to the Brain

The brain receives approximately 20% of the cardiac output, or 800 to 1000 ml of blood flow per minute. Carbon dioxide is a primary regulator for blood flow within the CNS. It is a potent vasodilator, and its effects ensure an adequate blood supply.

The brain derives its arterial supply from two systems: the internal carotid arteries and the vertebral arteries (Figure 12-18). The internal carotid arteries supply a proportionately greater amount of blood flow. They originate at the common carotid arteries, enter the cranium through the base of the skull, and pass through the cavernous sinus. After forming some small branches, these arteries divide into the anterior and middle cerebral arteries. The vertebral arteries originate at the subclavian arteries and pass through the transverse foramina of the cervical vertebrae, entering the cranium through the foramen magnum. They join at the junction of the pons and medulla to form the basilar artery (Figure 12-19). The basilar artery divides at the level of the midbrain to form paired posterior cerebral arteries.

The circle of Willis (see Figure 12-19) provides an alternative route for blood flow when one of the contributing arteries is obstructed (collateral blood flow). The circle of Willis is formed by the posterior cerebral arteries, posterior communicating arteries, internal carotid arteries, anterior cerebral arteries, and anterior communicating artery. The anterior cerebral, middle cerebral, and posterior cerebral arteries leave the

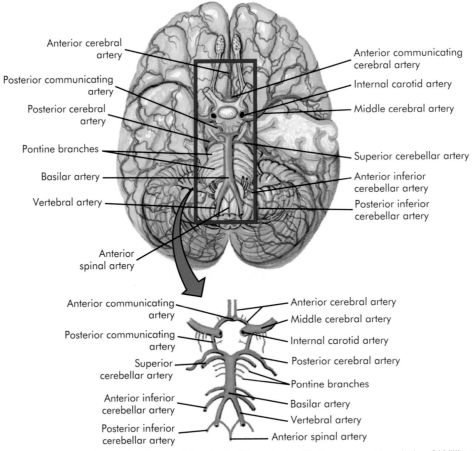

FIGURE 12-19 Arteries at the Base of the Brain. The arteries that compose the circle of Willis are the two anterior cerebral arteries, joined to each other by the anterior communicating artery and two short segments of the internal carotids, off of which the posterior communicating arteries connect to the posterior cerebral arteries. (From Patton KT, Thibodeau GA: *Anatomy & physiology*, ed 7, St Louis, 2010, Mosby.)

TABLE 12-5	ARTERIAL SYSTEMS SUPPLYING THE BRAIN	
ARTERIAL ORIGIN	**STRUCTURES SERVED**	**CONDITIONS CAUSED BY OCCLUSION**
Anterior cerebral artery	Basal ganglia; corpus callosum; medial surface of cerebral hemispheres; superior surface of frontal and parietal lobes	Hemiplegia on contralateral side of body, greater in lower than in upper extremities
Middle cerebral artery	Frontal lobe; parietal lobe; temporal lobe (primarily cortical surfaces)	Aphasia in dominant hemisphere and contralateral hemiplegia (see Chapter 14)
Posterior cerebral artery	Part of diencephalon and temporal lobe; occipital lobe	Visual loss; sensory loss; contralateral hemiplegia if cerebral peduncle affected

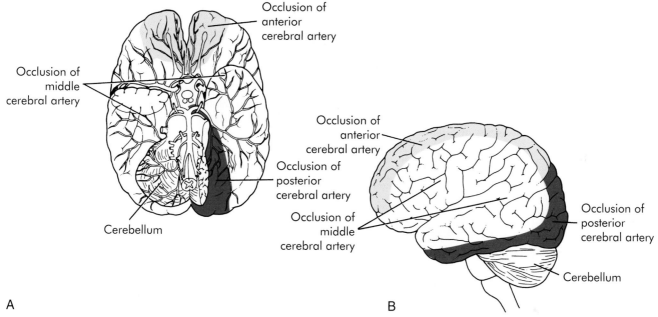

FIGURE 12-20 Areas of the Brain Affected by Occlusion of the Anterior, Middle, and Posterior Cerebral Artery Branches. **A,** Inferior view. **B,** Lateral view.

circle of Willis and extend to various brain structures. (Table 12-5 and Figure 12-20 illustrate structures served, functional relationships, and pathologic considerations related to occlusion of cerebral arteries.)

Cerebral venous drainage does not parallel its arterial supply, whereas the venous drainage of the brain stem and cerebellum does parallel the arterial supply of these structures. The cerebral veins are classified as superficial and deep veins. The veins drain into venous plexuses and dural sinuses (formed between the dural layers) and eventually join the internal jugular veins at the base of the skull (Figure 12-21). Adequacy of venous outflow can significantly affect intracranial pressure. For example, head-injured individuals who turn or let their heads fall to the side partially occlude venous return, and the intracranial pressure can increase then because of decreased flow through the jugular veins.

Blood-Brain Barrier

The blood-brain barrier describes cellular structures that selectively inhibit certain potentially harmful substances in the blood from entering the interstitial spaces of the brain or CSF. Supporting cells (neuroglia), particularly the astrocytes, and tight junctions between endothelial cells of brain cell capillaries (see Chapter 1) are likely involved in forming this barrier (Figure 12-22). The exact nature of this mechanism is controversial, but it appears that certain metabolites, electrolytes, and chemicals can cross into the brain to varying degrees. This has substantial implications for drug therapy because

certain types of antibiotics and chemotherapeutic drugs show a greater propensity than others for crossing this barrier.

Blood Supply to the Spinal Cord

The spinal cord derives its blood supply from branches off the vertebral arteries and from branches from various regions of the aorta (Figure 12-23). The anterior spinal artery and the paired posterior spinal arteries branch from the vertebral artery at the base of the cranium and descend alongside the spinal cord. Arterial branches from vessels exterior to the spinal cord follow the spinal nerve through the intervertebral foramina, pass through the dura, and divide into the anterior and posterior radicular arteries.

The radicular arteries eventually connect to the spinal arteries. Branches from the radicular and spinal arteries form plexuses whose branches penetrate the spinal cord, supplying the deeper tissues. Venous drainage parallels the arterial supply closely and drains into venous sinuses located between the dura and periosteum of the vertebrae.

THE PERIPHERAL NERVOUS SYSTEM

The cranial and spinal nerves, including their branches and ganglia, constitute the peripheral nervous system (PNS). A peripheral nerve (cranial or spinal) is composed of individual axons wrapped in a

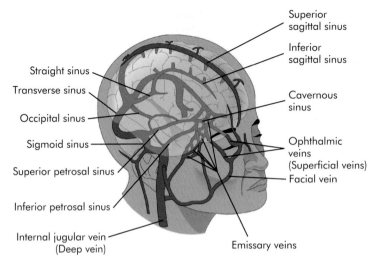

FIGURE 12-21 Large Veins of the Head. Deep veins and dural sinuses are projected on the skull. Note two superficial veins in the face are tributaries that send blood through emissary veins in the skull foramen into deep veins inside the skull terminating in the internal jugular vein. (From Patton KT, Thibodeau GA: *Anatomy & physiology,* ed 7, St Louis, 2010, Mosby.)

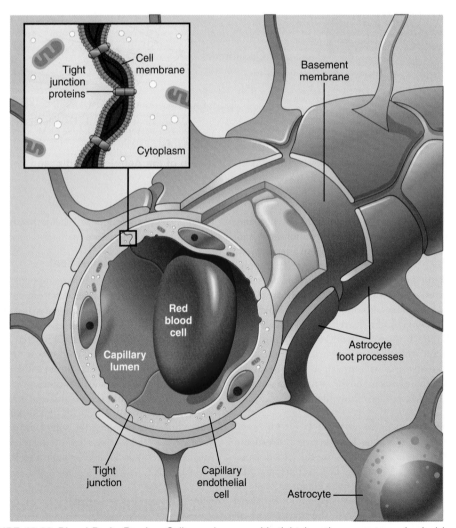

FIGURE 12-22 Blood-Brain Barrier. Cell membranes with tight junctions create a physical barrier between capillary blood and the cytoplasm of astrocytes. (From Bradley WG, editor: *Neurology in clinical practice,* ed 5, London, 2007, Butterworth-Heinemann.)

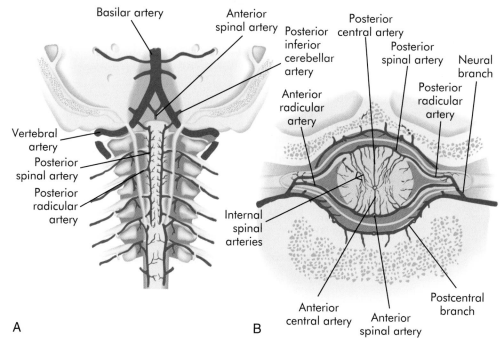

FIGURE 12-23 Arteries of the Spinal Cord. A, Arteries of cervical cord exposed from the rear. **B,** Arteries of spinal cord diagrammatically shown in horizontal section. (Redrawn from Rudy EB, editor: *Advanced neurological and neurosurgical nursing,* St Louis, 1984, Mosby.)

myelin sheath. These individual fibers are arranged in bundles called **fascicles** (Figure 12-24, *B*).

The 31 pairs of spinal nerves derive their names from the vertebral level from which they exit. There are 8 cervical, 12 thoracic, 5 lumbar, 5 sacral pair of spinal nerves, and 1 coccygeal. The first cervical nerve exits above the first cervical vertebra, and the rest of the spinal nerves exit below their corresponding vertebrae. From the thoracic region (and inferiorly), nerves correspond to the vertebral level above their exit.

Spinal nerves contain both sensory and motor neurons and are called **mixed nerves.** They arise as rootlets lateral to anterior and posterior horns of the spinal cord. These two spinal nerve roots converge in the region of the intervertebral foramen to form the spinal nerve trunk. Shortly after converging, the spinal nerve divides into anterior and posterior rami (branches). The anterior rami (except the thoracic) initially form **plexuses** (networks of nerve fibers), which then branch into the peripheral nerves. Instead of forming plexuses, the thoracic nerves pass through the intercostal spaces and innervate regions of the thorax.

The main spinal nerve plexuses innervate the skin and the underlying muscles of the limbs. The **brachial plexus,** for example, is formed by the last four cervical nerves (C5 to C8) and the first thoracic nerve (T1). The brachial plexus innervates the nerves of the arm, wrist, and hand. The **lumbar plexus** (L1 to L4) and **sacral plexus** (L5 to S5) contain nerves that innervate the anterior and posterior portions of the lower body, respectively.

The posterior rami of each spinal nerve, with their many processes, are distributed to a specific area in the body. Sensory signals thus arise from specific sites associated with a specific spinal cord segment. Specific areas of cutaneous innervation at these spinal cord segments are called **dermatomes.**

Like spinal nerves, cranial nerves are categorized as peripheral nerves. Most of these are mixed nerves (like the spinal nerves), although some are purely sensory or purely motor. Cranial nerves (see Figure 12-24, *A*) connect to nuclei in the brain and brain stem. (Figure 12-24 illustrates their structure, and Table 12-6 describes structural and functional characteristics.)

> ✔ **QUICK CHECK 12-5**
> 1. Describe the circle of Willis and explain its role in supplying blood to the brain.
> 2. What is the source of the spinal cord's blood supply?
> 3. What are the plexuses? Give two examples in the PNS.
> 4. What are the cranial nerves? Give three examples.
> 5. Describe the anatomy and function of the PNS.

THE AUTONOMIC NERVOUS SYSTEM

Components of the autonomic nervous system (ANS) are located in both the CNS and the PNS; however, the ANS is considered to be part of the efferent division of the PNS, even though visceral afferent neurons are certainly an important part of this system. Many neurons of the ANS travel in the spinal nerves and certain cranial nerves. The widespread activity of this system indicates that its components are distributed all over the body. The peripheral autonomic nerves carry mainly efferent fibers. The motor component of the ANS is a two-neuron system consisting of **preganglionic neurons** (myelinated) and **postganglionic neurons** (unmyelinated) (Figure 12-25). This arrangement contrasts with the somatic nervous system, where a single motor neuron travels from the CNS to the innervated structure. Visceral afferent neurons have their cell bodies in some sensory and cranial ganglia and their fiber processes traveling in peripheral nerves. The CNS has autonomic areas in the intermediolateral horns of the spinal cord, cardiovascular and respiratory centers in the reticular formation,

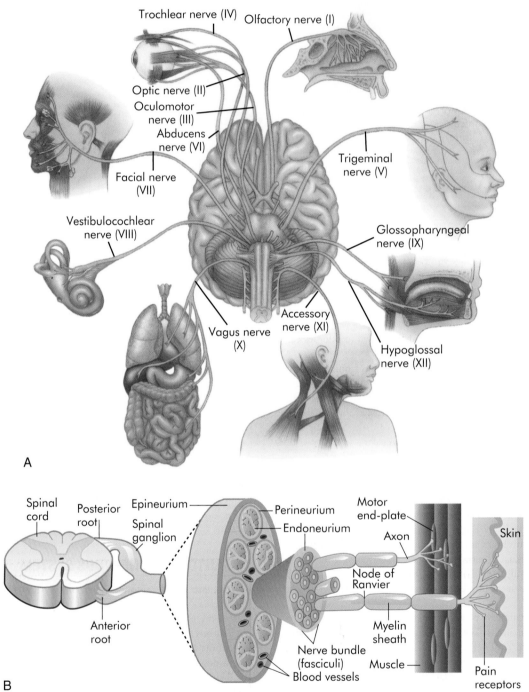

FIGURE 12-24 Cranial and Peripheral Nerves. A, Ventral surface of the brain showing attachment of the cranial nerves. **B,** Peripheral nerve trunk and coverings. (**A** from Patton KT, Thibodeau GA: *Anatomy & physiology,* ed 7, St Louis, 2010, Mosby.)

TABLE 12-6   THE CRANIAL NERVES

NUMBER AND NAME	ORIGIN AND COURSE	FUNCTION	HOW TESTED
I. Olfactory	Fibers arise from nasal olfactory epithelium and form synapses with olfactory bulbs, which transmit impulses to temporal lobe	Purely sensory; carries impulses for sense of smell	Person is asked to sniff aromatic substances, such as oil of cloves and vanilla, and to identify them
II. Optic	Fibers arise from retina of eye to form optic nerve, which passes through sphenoid bone; two optic nerves then form optic chiasma (with partial crossover of fibers) and eventually end in occipital cortex	Purely sensory; carries impulses for vision	Vision and visual field tested with an eye chart and by testing point at which person first sees an object (finger) moving into visual field; inside of eye is viewed with ophthalmoscope to observe blood vessels of eye interior
III. Oculomotor	Fibers emerge from midbrain and exit from skull to run to eye	Contains motor fibers to inferior oblique and to superior, inferior, and medial rectus extraocular muscles that direct eyeball; levator muscles of eyelid; smooth muscles of iris and ciliary body; and proprioception (sensory) to brain from extraocular muscles	Pupils examined for size, shape, and equality; pupillary reflex tested with a penlight (pupils should constrict when illuminated); ability to follow moving objects
IV. Trochlear	Fibers emerge from posterior midbrain and exit from skull to run to eye	Proprioceptor and motor fibers for superior oblique muscle of eye (extraocular muscle)	Tested in common with cranial nerve III relative to ability to follow moving objects
V. Trigeminal	Fibers emerge from pons and form three divisions that exit from skull and run to face and cranial dura mater	Both motor and sensory for face; conducts sensory impulses from mouth, nose, surface of eye, and dura mater; also contains motor fibers that stimulate chewing muscles	Sensations of pain, touch, and temperature tested with safety pin and hot and cold objects; corneal reflex tested with a wisp of cotton; motor branch tested by asking subject to clench teeth, open mouth against resistance, and move jaw from side to side
VI. Abducens	Fibers leave inferior pons and exit from skull to run to eye	Contains motor fibers to lateral rectus muscle and proprioceptor fibers from same muscle to brain	Tested in common with cranial nerve III relative to ability to move each eye laterally
VII. Facial	Fibers leave pons and travel through temporal bone to reach face	Mixed: (1) supplies motor fibers to muscles of facial expression and to lacrimal and salivary glands and (2) carries sensory fibers from taste buds of anterior part of tongue	Anterior two thirds of tongue tested for ability to taste sweet (sugar), salty, sour (vinegar), and bitter (quinine) substances; symmetry of face checked; subject asked to close eyes, smile, whistle, and so on; tearing tested with ammonia fumes
VIII. Vestibulocochlear (acoustic)	Fibers run from inner ear (hearing and equilibrium receptors in temporal bone) to enter brain stem just below pons	Purely sensory; vestibular branch transmits impulses for sense of equilibrium; cochlear branch transmits impulses for sense of hearing	Hearing checked by air and bone conduction by use of a tuning fork; vestibular tests: Bárány and caloric tests
IX. Glossopharyngeal	Fibers emerge from medulla and leave skull to run to throat	Mixed: (1) motor fibers serve pharynx (throat) and salivary glands, and (2) sensory fibers carry impulses from pharynx, posterior tongue (taste buds), and pressure receptors of carotid artery	Gag and swallow reflexes checked; subject asked to speak and cough; posterior one third of tongue may be tested for taste
X. Vagus	Fibers emerge from medulla, pass through skull, and descend through neck region into thorax and abdominal region	Fibers carry sensory and motor impulses for pharynx; a large part of this nerve is parasympathetic motor fibers, which supply smooth muscles of abdominal organs; receives sensory impulses from viscera	Same as for cranial nerve IX (IX and X are tested in common) because they both serve muscles of throat
XI. Spinal accessory	Fibers arise from medulla and superior spinal cord and travel to muscles of neck and back	Provides sensory and motor fibers for sternocleidomastoid and trapezius muscles and muscles of soft palate, pharynx, and larynx	Sternocleidomastoid and trapezius muscles checked for strength by asking subject to rotate head and shrug shoulders against resistance
XII. Hypoglossal	Fibers arise from medulla and exit from skull to travel to tongue	Carries motor fibers to muscles of tongue and sensory impulses from tongue to brain	Subject asked to stick out tongue, and any position abnormalities are noted

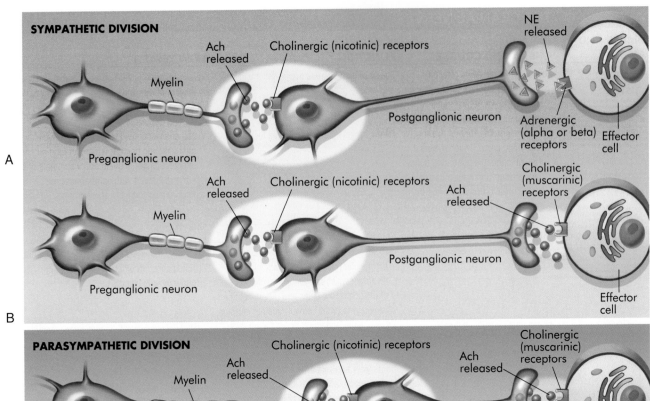

FIGURE 12-25 Locations of Neurotransmitters and Receptors of the Autonomic Nervous System. In all pathways, preganglionic fibers are cholinergic, secreting acetylcholine *(Ach)*, which stimulates nicotinic receptors in the postganglionic neuron. Most sympathetic postganglionic fibers are adrenergic, **A**, secreting norepinephrine *(NE)*, thus stimulating α- or β-adrenergic receptors. A few sympathetic postganglionic fibers are cholinergic, stimulating muscarinic receptors in effector cells, **B**, all parasympathetic postganglionic fibers are cholinergic, **C**, stimulating muscarinic receptors in effector cells. (From Patton KT, Thibodeau GA: *Anatomy & physiology*, ed 7, St Louis, 2010, Mosby.)

and both sympathetic and parasympathetic areas in the hypothalamus. CNS pathways interconnect all these areas.

The ANS coordinates and maintains a steady state among visceral (internal) organs, such as regulation of cardiac muscle, smooth muscle, and the glands of the body. This system is considered an involuntary system because one generally cannot *will* these functions to happen. The ANS is separated both structurally and functionally into two divisions: (1) the sympathetic nervous system (Figure 12-26) and (2) the parasympathetic nervous system (Figure 12-27).

Anatomy of the Sympathetic Nervous System

The sympathetic nervous system mobilizes energy stores in times of need (e.g., in the "fight or flight" response) (see Figure 8-1; see also Chapter 8). The sympathetic division is innervated by cell bodies located from the first thoracic (T1) through the second lumbar (L2) regions of the spinal cord and therefore is called the thoracolumbar division. The preganglionic axons of the sympathetic division form synapses shortly after leaving the cord in the sympathetic (paravertebral) ganglia. At this point the impulse may travel several ways: (1) directly across

the same ganglion level to form a synapse with the cell bodies of the postganglionic neuron, (2) up or down the sympathetic chain before forming synapses with a higher or lower postganglionic neuron, or (3) through the chain ganglion without synapsing (see Figure 12-26). Some preganglionic axons form pathways called splanchnic nerves, which lead to collateral ganglia on the front of the aorta. The collateral ganglia are named according to the branches of the aorta nearest them, namely, the celiac, superior mesenteric, and inferior mesenteric. The preganglionic neurons synapse with postganglionic neurons within the collateral ganglia. These postganglionic neurons leave the collateral ganglia and innervate the viscera below the diaphragm.

Preganglionic sympathetic neurons that innervate the adrenal medulla also travel in the splanchnic nerves and *do not* synapse before reaching the gland. The secretory cells in the adrenal medulla are considered modified postganglionic neurons. Because preganglionic sympathetic fibers are all myelinated, travel to the adrenal medulla is quick, and innervation causes the rapid release of epinephrine and norepinephrine. Epinephrine and norepinephrine are mediators of the fight or flight response (see Chapter 8).

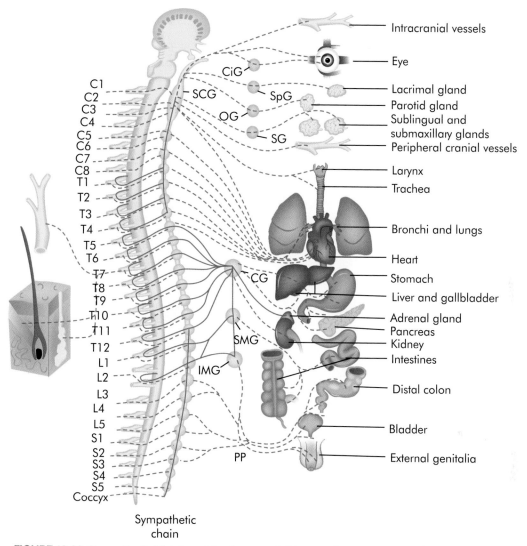

—— Preganglionic neuron
------ Postganglionic neuron

FIGURE 12-26 Sympathetic Division of the Autonomic Nervous System. *CG,* Celiac ganglion; *CiG,* ciliary ganglion; *IMG,* inferior mesenteric ganglion; *OG,* otic ganglion; *PP,* pelvic plexus; *SCG,* superior cervical ganglion; *SG,* submandibular ganglion; *SMG,* superior mesenteric ganglion; *SpG,* sphenopalatine ganglion. (Redrawn from Rudy EB, editor: *Advanced neurological and neurosurgical nursing,* St Louis, 1984, Mosby.)

Anatomy of the Parasympathetic Nervous System

The parasympathetic nervous system conserves and restores energy. The nerve cell bodies of this division are located in the cranial nerve nuclei and in the sacral region of the spinal cord and therefore constitute the craniosacral division. Unlike the sympathetic branch, the preganglionic fibers in the parasympathetic division travel close to the organs they innervate before forming synapses with the relatively short postganglionic neurons (see Figure 12-27). Parasympathetic nerves arising from nuclei in the brain stem travel to the viscera of the head, thorax, and abdomen within cranial nerves—including the oculomotor (III), facial (VII), glossopharyngeal (IX), and vagus (X) nerves.

Preganglionic parasympathetic nerves that originate from the sacral region of the spinal cord run either separately or together with some spinal nerves. The preganglionic axons unite to form the pelvic nerve, which innervates the viscera of the pelvic cavity. These preganglionic axons synapse with postganglionic neurons in terminal ganglia located close to the organs they innervate.

Neurotransmitters and Neuroreceptors

Sympathetic preganglionic fibers and parasympathetic preganglionic and postganglionic fibers release acetylcholine—the same neurotransmitter released by somatic efferent neurons (see Figures 12-26 and 12-28). These fibers are characterized by cholinergic transmission. Most postganglionic sympathetic fibers release norepinephrine (adrenaline) and thus are considered to function by adrenergic transmission. A few postganglionic sympathetic fibers, such as those that innervate the sweat glands, release acetylcholine.

The action of catecholamines varies with the type of neuroreceptor stimulated. It should be remembered that catecholamines also are

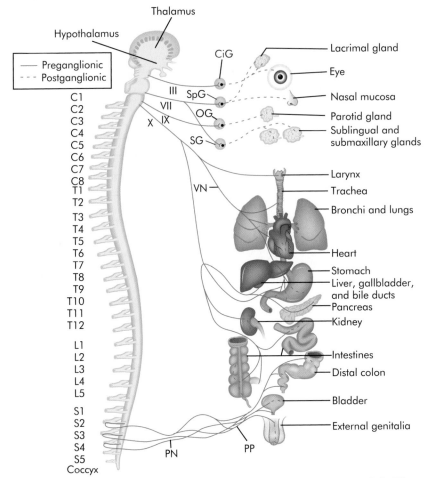

FIGURE 12-27 Parasympathetic Division of the Autonomic Nervous System. *CiG,* Ciliary ganglion; *OG,* otic ganglion; *PN,* pelvic nerve; *PP,* pelvic plexus; *SG,* submandibular ganglion; *SpG,* sphenopalatine ganglion; *VN,* vagus nerve. (Redrawn from Rudy EB, editor: *Advanced neurological and neurosurgical nursing,* St Louis, 1984, Mosby.)

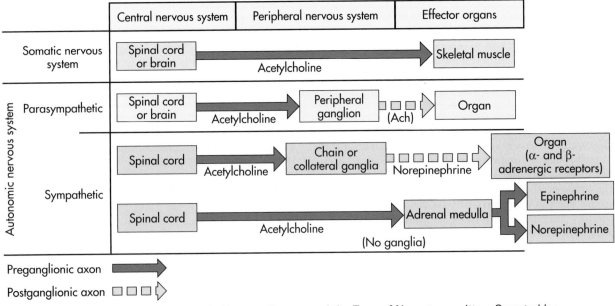

FIGURE 12-28 The Autonomic Nervous System and the Type of Neurotransmitters Secreted by Preganglionic and Postganglionic Fibers. Note that all preganglionic fibers are cholinergic (Ach). A somatic nerve is used for comparison.

TABLE 12-7   ACTIONS OF AUTONOMIC NERVOUS SYSTEM NEURORECEPTORS

EFFECTOR ORGAN OR TISSUE	ADRENERGIC RECEPTORS	ADRENERGIC EFFECTS	CHOLINERGIC EFFECTS (NICOTINE AND MUSCARINIC* RECEPTORS)
Eye, iris			
Radial muscle	α_1	Contraction (mydriasis)	—
Sphincter muscle	—	—	Contraction (miosis)
Eye, ciliary muscle	β_2	Relaxation for far vision	Contraction for near vision
Lacrimal glands	α	Secretion	Secretion
Nasopharyngeal glands	—	—	Secretion
Salivary glands	α_1	Secretion of potassium and water	Secretion of potassium and water
	β	Secretion of amylase	—
Heart			
SA node	β_1, β_2	Increase heart rate	Decrease heart rate; vagus arrest
Atrial	β_1, β_2	Increase contractility and conduction velocity	Decrease contractility; shorten action potential duration
AV junction	β_1, β_2	Increase automaticity and propagation velocity	Decrease automaticity and propagation velocity
Purkinje system	β_1, β_2	Increase automaticity and propagation velocity	—
Ventricles	β_1, β_2	Increase contractility	Slight decrease in contraction
Arterioles			
Coronary	$\alpha_1, \alpha_2, \beta_2$	Constriction, dilation	Dilation 1
Skin and mucosa	α_1, α_2	Constriction	Dilation 1
Skeletal muscle	α, β_2	Dilation, constriction	Dilation 1
Cerebral	α_1	Constriction (slight)	Dilation 1
Pulmonary	α_1, β_2	Constriction, dilation	Dilation 1
Mesenteric	α_1	Constriction	Dilation 1
Renal	$\alpha_1, \beta_1, \beta_2, D_2$	Constriction, dilation	Dilation 1
Salivary glands	α_1, α_2	Constriction	Dilation
Veins, systemic	$\alpha_1, \alpha_2, \beta_2$	Constriction, dilation	—
Lung			
Bronchial muscle	α_2	Relaxation	Contraction
Bronchial glands	α_1, β_2	Decrease secretion; increase secretion	Stimulation
Stomach			
Motility	$\alpha_1, \alpha_2, \beta_1, \beta_2$	Decrease (usually)	Increase
Sphincters	α_1	Contraction (usually)	Relaxation (usually)
Secretion	α_2	Inhibition	Stimulation
Liver	α_1, β_2	Glycogenolysis and gluconeogenesis	—
Gallbladder and ducts	β_2	Relaxation	Contraction
Pancreas			
Acini	α	Decrease secretion	Secretion
Islet cells	α_2, β_2	Decrease secretion; increase secretion	—
Intestine			
Motility and tone	$\alpha_1, \alpha_2, \beta_1, \beta_2$	Decrease	Increase
Sphincters	α_1	Contraction	Relaxation (usually)
Secretion	α_2	Inhibition	Stimulation
Adrenal medulla	—	Secretion of epinephrine and norepinephrine (nicotinic effect)	
Kidney			
Renin secretion	α_1, β_1	Decrease; increase	—
Ureter			
Motility and tone	β_1	Increase	Increase (?)
Urinary bladder			
Detrusor	β_2	Relaxation	Contraction
Trigone and sphincter	α_1	Contraction	Relaxation
Sex organs, male	α_1	Ejaculation	Erection
Skin			
Pilomotor muscles	α_1	Contraction	—
Sweat glands	α_1	Localized secretion	—
Fat cells	$\alpha_2, \beta_1, \beta_2, \beta_3$	Inhibition of lipolysis; stimulation of lipolysis	—
Pineal gland	β	Melatonin synthesis	—

Modified from Brunton LL, Lazo JS, Parker KL, editors: *Goodman & Gilman's: the pharmacological basis of therapeutics,* ed 11, New York, 2006, McGraw-Hill.

*Muscarinic receptors respond to circulating muscarinic antagonists.

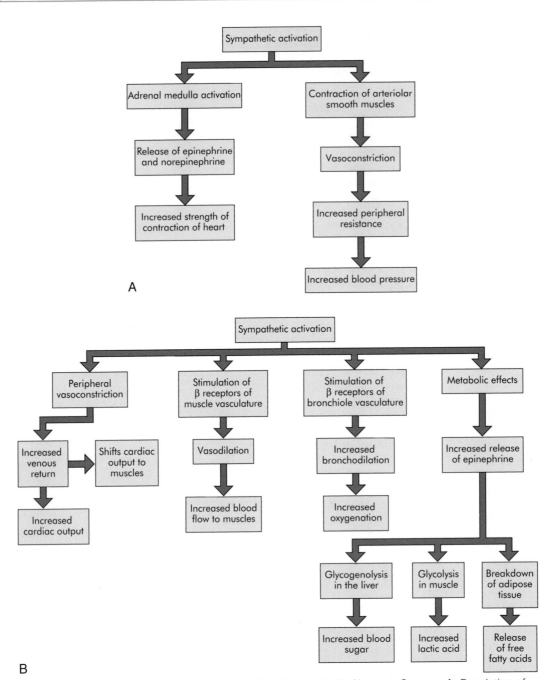

FIGURE 12-29 Some Important Functions of the Sympathetic Nervous System. **A,** Regulation of vasomotor tone. **B,** Regulation of strenuous muscular exercise ("fight or flight" response). (See also Chapter 8 and Figure 8-3 for more detail on the stress response.)

released by the adrenal medulla gland that physiologically and biochemically resembles the sympathetic nervous system. Two types of adrenergic receptors exist, α and β. Cells of the effector organs may have only one or both types of adrenergic receptors. The **α-adrenergic receptors** have been further subdivided according to the action produced. α_1-Adrenergic activity is associated mostly with excitation or stimulation; α_2-adrenergic activity is associated with relaxation or inhibition. Most of the α-adrenergic receptors on effector organs belong to the α_1 class. The **β-adrenergic receptors** are classified as β_1-adrenergic receptors (which facilitate increased heart rate and contractility and cause the release of renin from the kidney) and β_2-adrenergic receptors (which facilitate all remaining effects attributed to β receptors).[6]

Norepinephrine stimulates all α_1 and β_1 receptors and only certain β_2 receptors. The primary response from norepinephrine, however, is stimulation of the α_1-adrenergic receptors that cause vasoconstriction. Epinephrine strongly stimulates all four types of receptors and induces general vasodilation because of the predominance of β receptors in muscle vasculatures. (Table 12-7 summarizes the effects of neuroreceptors on their effector organs.)

Functions of the Autonomic Nervous System

Many body organs are innervated by both the sympathetic and parasympathetic nervous systems. The two divisions often cause opposite responses; for example, sympathetic stimulation of the stomach causes decreased peristalsis, whereas parasympathetic stimulation of the intestine increases peristalsis. In general, sympathetic stimulation promotes responses for the protection of the individual. For example, sympathetic activity increases blood glucose levels and temperature and raises the blood pressure. In emergency situations, a generalized and widespread discharge of the sympathetic system occurs. This is accomplished by an increased firing frequency of sympathetic fibers and by activation of sympathetic fibers normally silent and at rest (fibers to the sweat glands, pilomotor muscles, and the adrenal medulla, as well as vasodilator fibers to muscle). Regulation of vasomotor tone is considered the single most important function of the sympathetic nervous system. (Figure 12-29 illustrates some of the most important functions of the sympathetic nervous system.)

Increased parasympathetic activity promotes rest and tranquility and is characterized by reduced heart rate and enhanced visceral functions concerned with digestion. Stimulation of the vagus nerve (cranial nerve X) in the gastrointestinal tract increases peristalsis and secretion, as well as the relaxation of sphincters. Activation of parasympathetic fibers in the head, provided by cranial nerves III, VII, and IX, causes constriction of the pupil, tear secretion, and increased salivary

secretion. Stimulation of the sacral division of the parasympathetic system contracts the urinary bladder and facilitates the process of genital erection.

The parasympathetic system lacks the generalized and widespread response of the sympathetic system. Specific parasympathetic fibers are activated to regulate particular functions. Although the actions of the parasympathetic and sympathetic systems are usually antagonistic, there are exceptions. Peripheral vascular resistance, for example, is increased dramatically by sympathetic activation but is not altered appreciably by activity of the parasympathetic system. Most blood vessels involved in the control of blood pressure are innervated by sympathetic nerves. To decrease blood pressure, therefore, it is more important to block or paralyze the continuous (tonic) discharge of the sympathetic system than to promote parasympathetic activity.

QUICK CHECK 12-6
1. What are the structural and functional divisions of the ANS?
2. Compare cholinergic and adrenergic transmission.
3. What are the functions of the ANS?

GERIATRIC CONSIDERATIONS
Aging & the Nervous System

Structural Changes With Aging
Decreased brain weight and size, particularly frontal regions
Fibrosis and thickening of the meninges
Narrowing of gyri and widening of sulci
Increase in size of ventricles

Cellular Changes With Aging
Decrease in number of neurons not consistently related to changes in mental function
Decreased myelin
Lipofuscin deposition (a pigment resulting from cellular autodigestion)
Decreased number of dendritic processes and synaptic connections
Intracellular neurofibrillary tangles; significant accumulation in cortex associated with Alzheimer dementia
Imbalance in amount and distribution of neurotransmitters

Cerebrovascular Changes With Aging
Arterial atherosclerosis (may cause infarcts and scars)
Increased permeability of blood-brain barrier
Decreased vascular density

Functional Changes With Aging
Decreased tendon reflexes
Progressive deficit in taste and smell
Decreased vibratory sense
Decrease in accommodation and color vision
Decrease in neuromuscular control with change in gait and posture
Sleep disturbances
Memory impairments
Cognitive alterations associated with chronic disease
Functional changes and nervous system aging have significant individual variation

Data from Kumar A, Foster TC: Neurophysiology of old neurons and synapses. In Riddle DR, ed: *Brain aging: models, methods, and mechanisms,* Boca Raton, FL, 2007, CRC Press; Glorioso C, Sibille E: Between destiny and disease: genetics and molecular pathways of human central nervous system aging, *Prog Neurobiol* 93(2):165–181, 2011; Jang YC, Van Remmen H: Age-associated alterations of the neuromuscular junction, *Exp Gerontol* 46(2-3):193–198, 2011; Crowley K: Sleep and sleep disorders in older adults, *Neuropsychol Rev* 21(1):41–53, 2011; Brown WR, Thore CR: Review: cerebral microvascular pathology in ageing and neurodegeneration, *Neuropathol Appl Neurobiol* 37(1):56–74, 2011; Hof P, Mobbs C: *Neuroscience of aging,* Oxford, 2009, Academic Press.

DID YOU UNDERSTAND?

Overview and Organization of the Nervous System
1. The divisions of the nervous system have been categorized as either structural (central nervous system [CNS] and peripheral nervous system [PNS]) or functional (somatic nervous system and autonomic nervous system [ANS]).
2. The CNS is contained within the brain and spinal cord.
3. The PNS is composed of cranial and spinal nerves, which carry impulses toward the CNS (afferent) and away from the CNS (efferent) to target organs or skeletal muscle.

Cells of the Nervous System
1. The neuron and neuroglial cells constitute nervous tissue. The neuron is specialized to transmit and receive electrical and chemical impulses, whereas the neuroglial cell provides supportive functions. The neuron is further divided into unipolar, pseudounipolar, bipolar, and multipolar categories, according to its structure and particular mechanics of impulse transmission.
2. The neuron is composed of a cell body, dendrite(s), and an axon. A myelin sheath around selected axons forms insulation that allows quicker nerve impulse conduction.

Continued

DID YOU UNDERSTAND?—cont'd

The Nerve Impulse

1. The region between the neurons is the synapse, and the region between the neuron and muscle is the myoneural junction.
2. Neurotransmitters are responsible for chemical conduction across the synapse, and myoneural junction nerve impulse is regulated predominantly by a balance of inhibitory postsynaptic potentials (IPSPs) and excitatory postsynaptic potentials (EPSPs), temporal and spatial summation, and convergence and divergence.

The Central Nervous System

1. The brain is contained within the cranial vault and is divided into three distinct regions: (a) forebrain, (b) hindbrain, and (c) midbrain.
2. The forebrain comprises the two cerebral hemispheres and allows conscious perception of internal and external stimuli, thought and memory processes, and voluntary control of skeletal muscles. The deep portion of the forebrain is termed the *diencephalon* and processes incoming sensory data. The center for voluntary control of skeletal muscle movements is located along the precentral gyrus in the frontal lobe, whereas the center for perception is along the postcentral gyrus in the parietal lobe. The Broca area (inferior frontal gyrus) and the Wernicke area (superior temporal gyrus) are major speech centers.
3. The hindbrain allows sampling and comparison of sensory data, which are received from the periphery and motor impulses of the cerebral hemispheres, for the purpose of coordination and refinement of skeletal muscle movement.
4. The midbrain is primarily a relay center for motor and sensory tracts, as well as a center for auditory and visual reflexes.
5. The spinal cord contains most of the nerve fibers that connect the brain with the periphery. Reflex arcs are completed in the spinal cord and influenced by the higher centers in the brain.
6. The CNS is protected by the scalp, bony cranium, meninges, vertebral column, and cerebrospinal fluid (CSF). CSF is formed from blood components in the choroid plexuses of the ventricles and is reabsorbed in the arachnoid villi (located in the dural venous sinuses) after circulating through the brain and subarachnoid space.
7. The paired carotid and vertebral arteries supply blood to the brain and connect to form the circle of Willis. The major branches projecting from the circle of Willis are the anterior, middle, and posterior cerebral arteries. Drainage of blood from the brain is accomplished through the venous sinuses and jugular veins.
8. The blood-brain barrier is provided by tight junctions between the cells of brain capillaries and surrounding supporting cells.
9. Blood supply to the spinal cord originates from the vertebral arteries and branches arising from the aorta.

The Peripheral Nervous System

1. The PNS relays information from the CNS to muscle and effector organs through cranial and spinal nerve tracts arranged in fascicles (multiple fascicles bound together form the peripheral nerve).

The Autonomic Nervous System

1. The ANS is responsible for maintaining a steady state in the internal environment. Two opposing systems make up the ANS: (a) the sympathetic nervous system responds to stress by mobilizing energy stores and prepares the body to defend itself, and (b) the parasympathetic nervous system conserves energy and the body's resources. Both systems function, more or less, at the same time.

GERIATRIC CONSIDERATIONS: Aging & the Nervous System

1. Major structural changes with aging include a decrease in the number of neurons and a decrease in brain weight and size.
2. Deposition of lipofuscin and the presence of multiple neurofibrillary tangles are common cellular changes with aging.
3. A progressive slowing of neurologic function occurs with advancing age.

KEY TERMS

- Acetylcholine   317
- α-Adrenergic receptor   320
- β-Adrenergic receptor   320
- Adrenergic transmission   317
- Afferent (sensory) neuron   305
- Afferent pathway (ascending pathway)   293
- Amygdala   303
- Anterior column   305
- Anterior fossa   307
- Anterior horn (ventral horn)   305
- Anterior spinal artery   311
- Anterior spinothalamic tract   307
- Arachnoid   308
- Arachnoid villi   309
- Association fiber   301
- Associational neuron (interneuron)   296
- Astrocyte   296
- Autonomic nervous system (ANS)   293
- Axon   295
- Axon hillock   295
- Basal ganglia   303

- Basal ganglia system (extrapyramidal system)   301
- Basilar artery   310
- Basis pedunculi   304
- Bipolar neuron   295
- Blood-brain barrier   311
- Brachial plexus   313
- Brain stem   299
- Broca speech area (Brodmann areas 44, 45)   301
- Cauda equina   304
- Caudate nucleus   303
- Cavernous sinus   310
- Celiac   316
- Central canal   304
- Central nervous system (CNS)   293
- Central sulcus (fissure of Rolando)   301
- Cerebellum   304
- Cerebral aqueduct (aqueduct of Sylvius)   304
- Cerebral cortex   301
- Cerebral nuclei   303

- Cerebral peduncle   304
- Cerebrospinal fluid (CSF)   308
- Cholinergic transmission   311
- Choroid plexus   308
- Circle of Willis   310
- Collateral ganglia   316
- Contralateral control   301
- Conus medullaris   304
- Corpora quadrigemina (tectum)   304
- Corpus callosum (transverse fibers or commissural fibers)   303
- Corpus striatum   303
- Corticobulbar tract   307
- Corticospinal tract (pyramidal system)   301
- Cranial nerve   313
- Craniosacral division   317
- Dendrite   295
- Dermatome   313
- Diencephalon (interbrain)   303
- Dopamine   304
- Dorsal root ganglion   305

KEY TERMS—cont'd

- Dura mater   307
- Efferent (motor) neuron   305
- Effector organ   293
- Efferent pathway (descending pathway)   293
- Ependymal cell   296
- Epicritic information   307
- Epidural space   308
- Epithalamus   303
- Excitatory postsynaptic potential (EPSP)   298
- Facilitation   298
- Falx cerebri   307
- Fascicle   313
- Filum terminale   304
- Fissure   301
- Frontal lobe   301
- Galea aponeurotica   307
- Ganglia (plexus)   295
- Gray matter   301
- Hippocampus   303
- Hypothalamus   303
- Inferior colliculi   304
- Inferior mesenteric   316
- Inhibitory postsynaptic potential (IPSP)   298
- Inner dura (meningeal layer)   307
- Insula (insular lobe)   303
- Internal capsule   303
- Internal carotid artery   310
- Interventricular foramen (foramen of Monro)   309
- Intervertebral disk   309
- Lateral aperture (foramen of Luschka)   309
- Lateral column   305
- Lateral corticospinal tract   307
- Lateral horn   305
- Lateral spinothalamic tract   307
- Lateral sulcus (sylvian fissure, lateral fissure)   301
- Lentiform nucleus   303
- Limbic system   303
- Longitudinal fissure   301
- Lower motor neuron   306
- Lumbar plexus   313
- Median aperture (foramen of Magendie)   309
- Meninges   307
- Metencephalon   304
- Microfilament   294
- Microglia   296
- Microtubule   294
- Midbrain (mesencephalon)   304
- Middle fossa (temporal fossa)   307
- Mixed nerve   313
- Motor neuron   305
- Motor unit   307
- Multipolar neuron   295
- Myelencephalon (medulla oblongata)   304
- Myelin   295
- Myelin sheath   295
- Neurofibril   294
- Neuroglia   296
- Neuroglial cell   293
- Neuromuscular (myoneural) junction   296
- Neuron   293
- Neurotransmitter   297
- Nissl substance   294
- Node of Ranvier   295
- Norepinephrine   317
- Nucleus pulposus   309
- Occipital lobe   301
- Oligodendroglia (oligodendrocyte)   296
- Papez circuit   303
- Parasympathetic nervous system   316
- Parietal lobe   301
- Pelvic nerve   317
- Periosteum (endosteal layer)   307
- Peripheral nervous system (PNS)   311
- Pia mater   308
- Plexus   313
- Pons   304
- Postcentral gyrus   301
- Posterior (dorsal) column (fasciculus gracilis, fasciculus cuneatus)   307
- Posterior fossa   307
- Posterior horn (dorsal horn)   305
- Posterior spinal artery   311
- Postganglionic neuron   313
- Postsynaptic neuron   297
- Precentral gyrus   301
- Prefrontal area   301
- Preganglionic neuron   313
- Premotor area (Brodmann area 6)   301
- Presynaptic neuron   297
- Primary motor area (Brodmann area 4)   301
- Primary voluntary motor area   301
- Protopathic   307
- Pseudounipolar neuron   295
- Red nucleus   304
- Reflex arc   305
- Reticular activating system   299
- Reticular formation   299
- Reticulospinal tract   307
- Sacral plexus   313
- Saltatory conduction   295
- Schwann cell   293
- Sensory neuron   296
- Somatic nervous system   293
- Spatial summation   298
- Spinal cord   304
- Spinal nerve   313
- Spinal tract   305
- Spinothalamic tract   305
- Splanchnic nerve   316
- Subarachnoid space   308
- Subdural space   308
- Substantia gelatinosa   305
- Substantia nigra   304
- Subthalamus   303
- Sulci   299
- Summation   298
- Superior colliculi   304
- Superior mesenteric   316
- Sympathetic (paravertebral) ganglia   316
- Sympathetic nervous system   316
- Synapse   297
- Synaptic bouton   297
- Synaptic cleft   298
- Tegmentum   304
- Telencephalon   299
- Temporal lobe   301
- Temporal summation   298
- Tentorium cerebelli   308
- Thalamus   303
- Thoracolumbar division   316
- Unipolar neuron   295
- Upper motor neuron   306
- Ventricle   309
- Vermis   304
- Vertebral artery   310
- Vertebral column   304
- Vestibulospinal tract   307
- Wallerian degeneration   297
- Wernicke area   301
- White matter   301

REFERENCES

1. Martin JH: *Neuroanatomy: text and atlas*, ed 4, New York, 2012, McGraw-Hill.
2. Purves D, et al: *Neuroscience*, ed 3, Sunderland, Mass, 2008, Sinauer Associates.
3. Kolb B, Whishaw IQ: *An introduction to brain and behavior*, ed 3, New York, 2011, Worth.
4. Szabo B, Schlicker E: Effects of cannabinoids on neurotransmission, *Handb Exp Pharmacol* (168):327–365, 2005.
5. Kiernan JA: *Barr's the human nervous system: an anatomical viewpoint*, ed 9, Philadelphia, 2009, Lippincott Williams & Wilkins.
6. Siegel R, et al: *Basic neurochemistry: molecular, cellular, and medical aspects*, ed 8, Philadelphia, 2012, Academic Press.

13

Pain, Temperature, Sleep, and Sensory Function

Jan Belden, Curtis DeFriez, and Sue E. Huether

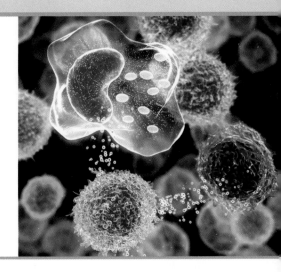

evolve WEBSITE

CHAPTER OUTLINE

Alterations in sensory function may involve dysfunctions of the general or the special senses. Dysfunctions of the general senses include chronic pain, abnormal temperature regulation, and tactile or proprioceptive dysfunction. Pain is an unpleasant but protective phenomenon that is uniquely experienced by each individual and it cannot be adequately defined, identified, or measured by an observer. Like pain, variations in temperature can signal disease. Fever is a common manifestation of dysfunction and is often the first symptom observed in an infectious or inflammatory condition.

Sleep is a normal cyclic process that restores the body's energy and maintains normal functioning. Sleep is so essential to both physiologic and psychologic function that sleep deprivation causes a wide range of clinical manifestations. The special senses of vision, hearing, touch, smell, and taste are the means by which individuals perceive stimuli that are essential in interacting with the environment. Dysfunctions of the special senses include visual, auditory, vestibular, olfactory, and gustatory (taste) disorders.

PAIN

The Experience of Pain

Pain is a complex experience. It is comprised of dynamic interactions between physical, cognitive, spiritual, emotional, and environmental factors and cannot be characterized as only a response to injury. McCaffery defined pain as "whatever the experiencing person says it is, existing whenever he says it does."[1] The International Association for the Study of Pain and the American Pain Society defined pain as "an unpleasant sensory and emotional experience associated with actual or potential tissue damage or described in terms of such damage."[2]

Evolution of Pain Theories

The **specificity theory of pain** was described by Descartes in the seventeenth century and proposes that there are specific pain receptors in the body that project to the brain[3] and that the intensity of pain is directly related to the amount of associated tissue injury. This theory is useful for pain associated with specific injury and acute pain but does not account for chronic pain or cognitive and emotional elements that contribute to more complex types of pain.[4] The **pattern theory**, initially proposed in the late nineteenth century, describes the role of impulse intensity and the repatterning of the central nervous system (CNS). Although the theory evolved to provide an explanation for neuropathic pain, the pattern theory does not account for all types of pain experiences.[5,6]

The **gate control theory (GCT)** proposed in 1965 by Melzack and Wall[4] integrates and builds upon features of other theories to explain the complex multidimensional aspects of pain perception. According to this theory, pain transmission is modulated by a balance of impulses conducted to the spinal cord, where cells in the substantia gelatinosa function as a "gate" that regulates the nociceptive (pain) transmission to higher centers in the CNS. Large myelinated A-delta fibers and small unmyelinated C fibers respond to a broad range of painful stimuli, including mechanical, thermal, and chemical (Figure 13-1). Nociceptive transmissions on these fibers "open" the spinal gate and increase the perception of pain. Partial closure of the spinal gates can occur from stimulating touch sensors in the skin, with impulses carried on non-nociceptive larger A-beta fibers. Non-nociceptive transmissions that serves to "close the gate," decrease pain perception. This is why rubbing a sore area may alleviate some of the discomfort. Other efferent pathways in the CNS descending to the spinal cord also may close, partially close, or open the gate. The gate control theory, bolstered by progresses in understanding neuronal pathways in the peripheral and central nervous system, have greatly advanced our understanding of pain.

As good as the GCT has been, however, there are observations on pain in paraplegics that "do not fit the theory." In 1999 Melzack and Wall outlined the concept of a "neuromatrix" to address these issues. The **neuromatrix theory** proposes that the brain produces patterns of nerve impulses drawn from various inputs, including genetic, psychologic, and cognitive experiences.[7] The qualities we normally feel from the body, including pain, also can be felt in the absence of inputs from the body (as noted with phantom limb pain). In other words, stimuli may trigger the patterns but do not produce them—neuromatrix patterns are normally activated by sensory inputs from the periphery but may originate independently in the brain with no external input.[8]

The neuromatrix theory illustrates the plasticity of the brain, but it does not supplant our understanding of the gate theory, and what we have learned about peripheral inflammation, spinal modulation, and midbrain descending control over the past 50 years. Gate control theory is an established part of our current conceptual model, and the proposition of the neuromatrix expounds upon that foundation by explicating a body-self that provides a holistic, integrated, dynamic consideration of pain.

Neuroanatomy of Pain

Three portions of the nervous system are responsible for the sensation and perception of pain:

1. The *afferent pathways*, which begin in the peripheral nervous system (PNS), travel to the spinal gate in the dorsal horn and then ascend to higher centers in the central nervous system (CNS).
2. The *interpretive centers* located in the brain stem, midbrain, diencephalon, and cerebral cortex.
3. The *efferent pathways* that descend from the CNS back to the dorsal horn of the spinal cord.

The processing of potentially harmful (noxious) stimuli through a normally functioning nervous system is called **nociception.**[2] Nociception involves four phases: transduction, transmission, perception, and modulation.[5,9]

Pain transduction begins when tissue is damaged by exposure to chemical, mechanical, or thermal noxious stimuli. This causes activation of **nociceptors**, which are free nerve endings in the afferent peripheral nervous system that selectively respond to different types of stimuli. Nociceptors are located throughout the body (Table 13-1) but are not evenly distributed so the relative sensitivity to pain differs according to their location.

Activation of nociceptors causes ion channels (sodium, calcium) to open, creating electrical impulses that travel through two primary types of nociceptors: **A-delta (Aδ) fibers** and **C fibers.** The medium sized thinly myelinated Aδ fibers rapidly transmit sharp, well-localized "fast" pain sensations. These fibers are responsible for causing reflex withdrawal of the affected body part from the stimulus before a pain sensation is perceived.[6] The smaller, unmyelinated C fibers slowly transmit dull, aching, or burning sensations that are poorly localized and often constant.[5,6,10] **A-beta (Aβ) fibers** are large myelinated fibers that transmit touch and vibration sensations. They normally do not transmit pain, but play a role in pain modulation.[10]

Pain transmission is the conduction of pain impulses along the Aδ and C fibers into the dorsal horn of the spinal cord (Figure 13-2). They

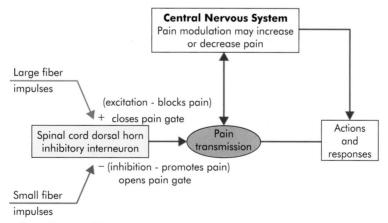

FIGURE 13-1 Gate Control Theory of Pain. Schematic diagram of the gate control theory of pain mechanism. Large A-beta (Aβ) fiber non-nociceptor impulses (i.e., mechanical and thermal) activate inhibitory interneuron in spinal cord dorsal horn and decrease pain transmission (close pain gate). Small fiber impulses block the inhibitory interneuron and promote pain transmission (open pain gate).

form synapses with interneurons in the substantia gelatinosa and cross the midline of the spinal cord, and then ascend to the thalamus (the major relay station of sensory information), brain stem, and cerebral cortex through multiple pathways, including the lateral spinothalamic tract, for further processing and interpretation[9] (see Figure 12-8, p. 302).

Pain perception is the conscious awareness of pain, which occurs primarily in the reticular and limbic systems and the cerebral cortex. Interpretation of pain is influenced by many factors including cultural preferences, male and female roles, and life experience, including past pain experiences and current expectations.[11] Three systems interact to produce the perception of pain.[12] The **sensory-discriminative system** is mediated by the somatosensory cortex and is responsible for identifying the presence, character, location, and intensity of pain. The **affective-motivational system** determines an individual's conditioned avoidance behaviors and emotional responses to pain. It is mediated through the reticular formation, limbic system, and brain stem. The **cognitive-evaluative system** overlies the individual's learned behavior concerning the experience of pain and therefore can modulate perception of pain. It is mediated through the cerebral cortex.

Pain modulation involves many different mechanisms that increase or decrease the transmission of pain signals throughout the nervous system. Depending on the mechanism, modulation can occur before, during, or after pain is perceived.[10] Pain modulation is discussed in the next section.

Neuromodulation of Pain

Neuromodulators of pain are found in the pathways that mediate information about painful stimuli throughout the nervous system.[13,14] Triggering mechanisms that initiate release of neuromodulators include tissue injury (prostaglandins, bradykinin) and chronic inflammatory lesions (lymphokines). Other **excitatory neuromodulators** include such substances as substance P, histamine, glutamate, and calcitonin gene–related peptide. These substances sensitize nociceptors in the peripheral nervous system (**peripheral sensitization**) or CNS (**central sensitization**), leading to an increased responsiveness and reduced threshold of nociceptors that cause them to fire with increased frequency, resulting in hyperalgesia (increased sensitivity to painful stimuli) and allodynia, (the perception of innocuous stimuli. A progressive buildup of repeated stimulation of neurons in the

TABLE 13-1	STIMULI THAT ACTIVATE NOCICEPTORS (PAIN RECEPTORS)
LOCATION OF RECEPTOR	**PROVOKING STIMULI**
Skin	Pricking, cutting, crushing, burning, freezing
Gastrointestinal tract	Engorged or inflamed mucosa, distention or spasm of smooth muscle, traction on mesenteric attachment
Skeletal muscle	Ischemia, injuries of connective tissue sheaths, necrosis, hemorrhage, prolonged contraction, injection of irritating solutions
Joints	Synovial membrane inflammation
Arteries	Piercing, inflammation
Head	Traction, inflammation, or displacement of arteries, meningeal structures, and sinuses; prolonged muscle contraction
Heart	Ischemia and inflammation
Bone	Periosteal injury: fractures, tumor, inflammation

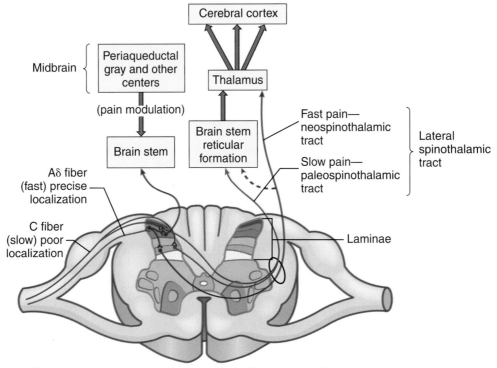

FIGURE 13-2 Transmission of Pain Sensations. The Aδ and C fibers synapse in the laminae of the dorsal horn, crossover to the contralateral spinothalamic tract, and then ascend to synapse in the midbrain through the neospinothalamic and paleospinothalamic tracts. Impulses are then conducted to the sensory cortex.

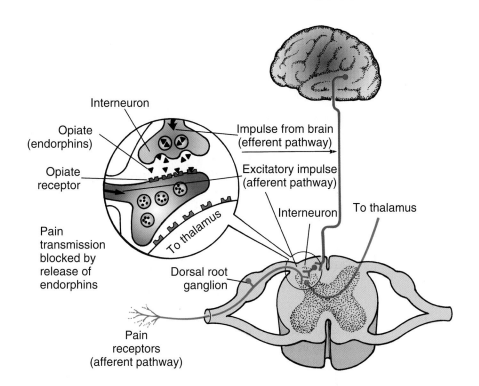

FIGURE 13-3 Descending Pathway and Endorphin Response. Endorphin receptors are located close to known pain receptors in the periphery and ascending and descending pain pathways.

dorsal horn by peripheral nerves leads to *wind-up,* which can result in pathologic changes in the CNS (central pain sensitization), prolonged pain, and increased sensitivity to future pain in the same location.[5,9,15] **Inhibitory neuromodulators** include gamma-aminobutyric acid (GABA), glycine, 5-hydroxytryptamine (serotonin), norepinephrine, and endogenous opioids (see below). Some neuromodulators, such as 5-hydroxytryptamine (serotonin) and norepinephrine, excite peripheral nerves but inhibit central nerves.[9]

Endogenous opioids are a family of morphine-like neuropeptides that block transmission of pain impulses in the spinal cord, brain, and periphery by binding with specific opioid receptors (mu [μ], kappa [κ], and delta [δ]). They inhibit the release of excitatory neurotransmitters, such as substance P in the dorsal horn or in other areas of the brain (Figure 13-3), and may also be responsible for general sensations of well-being.[16,17] **Enkephalins** are the most prevalent of the natural opioids. The best studied **endorphin** is β-endorphin, which is purported to produce the greatest sense of exhilaration as well as substantial natural pain relief. It is a strong μ receptor agonist. **Dynorphins** are the most potent of the endogenous opioids, binding strongly with κ receptors to impede pain signals. They can also incite pain by activating bradykinin receptors and may play a role in neuropathic pain.[18,19] Dynorphins are found in the hypothalamus, medulla, periaqueductal gray, and spinal dorsal horn. **Endomorphins** bind with μ receptors and have potent analgesic effects.[20]

Opiate drugs (exogenous opioids) relieve pain by attaching to the opiate receptors and enhancing the natural endogenous opioid response. Stress, excessive physical exertion, acupuncture, sexual intercourse, and other factors increase the levels of circulating neuromodulators, thereby raising the pain threshold.

Descending inhibitory pathways and nuclei also inhibit pain. Afferent stimulation of particularly the ventromedial medulla and periaqueductal gray (PAG) (gray matter surrounding the cerebral aqueduct) in the midbrain stimulates efferent pathways, which modulate or inhibit afferent pain signals at the dorsal horn.[21]

Diffuse noxious inhibitory control (DNIC) is an inhibitory pain system that involves a spinal-medullary-spinal pathway. Pain is relieved when two noxious stimuli occur at the same time in different sites (pain inhibiting pain). This is the basis for pain relief with acupuncture, deep massage, or intense cold or heat.[21a]

Clinical Descriptions of Pain

Pain can be described in a variety of ways, including temporal aspects (e.g., duration), inferred neurophysiologic mechanisms, etiology, and region affected (Box 13-1). Pain is commonly classified on the basis of duration (acute versus chronic) and inferred neurophysiologic mechanisms (nociceptive versus non-nociceptive). Because of the complex nature of pain, however, many terms overlap and more than one approach is often used.

Acute pain is a protective mechanism that alerts the individual to a condition or experience that is immediately harmful to the body and mobilizes the individual to take prompt action to relieve it.[11] Acute pain is transient, usually lasting seconds to days, sometimes up to 3 months.[22] It begins suddenly and is relieved after the chemical mediators that stimulate pain receptors are removed.[23] Stimulation of the autonomic nervous system results in physical manifestations including increased heart rate, hypertension, diaphoresis, and dilated pupils. Anxiety related to the pain experience, including its cause, treatment, and prognosis, is common as is the hope of recovery.[11]

Acute pain arises from cutaneous, deep somatic, or visceral structures and can be classified as (1) somatic, (2) visceral, or (3) referred. **Somatic pain** is superficial, arising from the skin. It is typically well localized and described as sharp, dull, aching, or throbbing. **Visceral pain** refers to pain in internal organs and lining of body cavities and tends to be poorly localized with an aching, gnawing, throbbing, or intermittent cramping quality. It is carried by sympathetic fibers and is associated with nausea and vomiting, hypotension, and, in some cases, shock. Visceral pain often radiates (spreads away from the actual site

BOX 13-1   CATEGORIES OF PAIN

I. Neurophysiologic pain
   A. Nociceptive pain
      1. Somatic (e.g., skin, muscle, bone)
      2. Visceral (e.g., intestine, liver, stomach)
   B. Neuropathic (non-nociceptive)
      1. Central pain (lesion in brain or spinal cord)
      2. Peripheral pain (lesion in PNS)
II. Neurogenic pain
   A. Neuralgia (pain in the distribution of a nerve)
   B. Constant
      1. Sympathetically independent
      2. Sympathetically dependent
III. Temporal pain (time related, duration)
   A. Acute pain
      1. Somatic
      2. Visceral
   B. Chronic
IV. Regional pain
   A. Abdominal pain
   B. Chest pain
   C. Headache
   D. Low back pain
   E. Orofacial pain
   F. Pelvic pain
V. Etiologic pain
   A. Cancer pain
   B. Dental pain
   C. Inflammatory pain
   D. Ischemic pain
   E. Vascular pain

Adapted from Derasari MD: Taxonomy of pain syndromes: classification of chronic pain syndromes. In Raj PP, editor: *Practical management of pain*, ed 3, St Louis, 2000, Mosby.

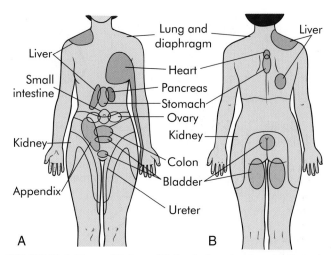

FIGURE 13-4 Sites of Referred Pain. **A,** Anterior view. **B,** Posterior view.

of the pain) or is referred. Referred pain is felt in an area removed or distant from its point of origin—the area of referred pain is supplied by the same spinal segment as the actual site of pain. Referred pain can be acute or chronic. Impulses from many cutaneous and visceral neurons converge on the same ascending neuron, and the brain cannot distinguish between the different sources of pain. Because the skin has more receptors, the painful sensation is experienced at the referred site instead of at the site of origin.[24] Figure 13-4 illustrates common areas of referred pain and their associated sites of origin.

Chronic or persistent pain has been defined as lasting for more than 3 to 6 months; however, a more accurate definition is pain lasting well beyond the expected normal healing time following the initial onset of tissue damage or injury. "Normal healing time" varies depending on the type of injury.[25]

Chronic or persistent pain serves no purpose and is poorly understood. It often appears to be out of proportion to any observable tissue injury. It may be ongoing (e.g., low back pain) or intermittent (e.g., migraine headaches). Changes in the peripheral and central nervous systems that cause dysregulation of nociception and pain modulation processes are thought to lead to chronic pain.[11,26] Additionally, neuroimaging studies have demonstrated brain atrophy in individuals with chronic pain, which may lead to cognitive deficits and decreased ability to cope with pain. These negative manifestations of chronic pain are

thought to be due, in part, to the stress of coping with continuous pain and may be reversible when pain is controlled.[27-29] Chronic pain often does not respond to usual therapy. Because it is not yet possible to predict when acute pain will develop into chronic pain, early treatment of acute pain is encouraged.[10]

Physiologic responses to intermittent chronic pain are similar to those for acute pain, whereas persistent pain allows for physiologic adaptation, producing normal heart rate and blood pressure. This leads many to mistakenly conclude that people with chronic pain are malingering because they do not appear to be in pain. As chronic pain progresses, certain behavioral and psychologic changes often emerge, including depression, difficulty eating and sleeping, preoccupation with the pain, and avoidance of pain-provoking stimuli.[30,31] The desire to relieve pain and the need to hide it become conflicting drives for those with chronic pain, who fear being labeled complainers.[32] Chronic pain is perceived as meaningless and is often associated with a sense of hopelessness as more time elapses and no cure seems possible. Common chronic pain conditions are listed in Table 13-2. Comparison of acute and chronic pain is summarized in Table 13-3.

Neuropathic pain is initiated or caused by a primary lesion or dysfunction in the nervous system and leads to long-term changes in pain pathway structure (neuroplasticity) and abnormal processing of sensory function.[2,33] It is often described as burning, shooting, shock-like, or tingling and is characterized by increased sensitivity to painful stimuli hyperalgesia, allodynia, and the development of spontaneous pain.[34] Neuropathic pain is primarily chronic so individuals present with some or all of the physiologic and behavioral changes described for chronic pain.

Neuropathic pain is classified as either peripheral or central.[35,36] Peripheral neuropathic pain is due to trauma or disease to one or more peripheral nerves. Examples include nerve entrapment and diabetic neuropathy. Central neuropathic pain is caused by a lesion or dysfunction in the brain or spinal cord. Examples include phantom pain or complex regional pain syndrome.

Pain Threshold and Pain Tolerance

Pain threshold and tolerance are subjective phenomena that influence an individual's perception of pain. They can be influenced by genetics, gender,[31,37] cultural perceptions, expectations, role socialization, and physical and mental health.

TABLE 13-2   COMPARISON OF ACUTE AND CHRONIC PAIN

CHARACTERISTIC	ACUTE PAIN	CHRONIC PAIN
Experience	An event	A situation; state of existence
Source	External agent or internal disease, injury, or inflammation	Unknown; if known, treatment is prolonged or ineffective
Onset	Usually sudden	May be sudden or develop insidiously
Duration	Transient (up to 3 months); usually of short duration Resolves with treatment and healing	Prolonged (months to years); lasts beyond expected normal healing time
Pain identification	Painful and nonpainful areas generally well identified	Painful and nonpainful areas less easily differentiated; change in sensations becomes more difficult to evaluate
Clinical signs	Typical response pattern with more visible signs Anxiety and emotional distress common	Response patterns vary; fewer overt signs (adaptation) Can interfere with sleep, productivity, and quality of life
Significance	Significant (informs person something is wrong); protective	Person looks for significance and meaning; serves no useful purpose
Pattern	Self-limiting or readily corrected	Continuous or intermittent; intensity may vary or remain constant
Course	Suffering usually decreases over time	Suffering usually increases over time
Actions	Leads to actions to relieve pain	Leads to actions to modify pain experience
Prognosis	Likelihood of eventual complete relief	Complete relief usually not possible

Data from Black RG: *Surg Clin North Am* 55(4):999, 1975.

TABLE 13-3   COMMON CHRONIC PAIN CONDITIONS

CONDITION	DESCRIPTION
Persistent low back pain	Most common chronic pain condition Results from poor muscle tone, inactivity, muscle strain, or sudden, vigorous exercise
Myofascial pain syndromes	Pain results from muscle spasm, tenderness, stiffness, or injury to muscle and fascia Examples include myositis, fibrositis, myalgia, fibromyalgia, and muscle strain Trigger points—small hypersensitive regions in muscle or connective tissues that, when stimulated, produce pain in a specific area As disorder progresses, pain becomes increasingly generalized
Chronic postoperative pain	Persistent pain that can occur with disruption or cutting of sensory nerves; examples include post-thoracotomy, post-mastectomy; risk factors may include preexisting pain and genetic susceptibility
Cancer pain	Attributed to advance of disease, treatment, or coexisting disease entities
Deafferentation pain	Pain due to loss of sensory input into CNS caused by lesion in peripheral nerves (e.g., brachial plexus injury) or pathology of CNS (e.g., complex regional pain syndrome); described as constant, vicelike ache with paroxysms of burning or shocklike sensations Common types include severe burning pain triggered by various stimuli, such as cold, light touch, or sound, and complex regional pain syndromes (occur after peripheral nerve injury and are characterized by continuous, severe, burning pain associated with vasomotor changes and muscle wasting)
Hyperesthesias	Increased sensitivity and decreased pain threshold to tactile and painful stimuli Pain is diffuse, modified by fatigue and emotion, and mixed with other sensations May result from chronic irritation of CNS areas
Hemiagnosia	Loss of ability to identify source of pain on one side of body Painful stimuli on that side produce discomfort, anxiety, moaning, agitation, and distress but no attempt to withdraw from stimulus Associated with stroke
Phantom limb pain	Pain experience in amputated limb after stump has completely healed; may be immediate or occur months later; associated with preamputation pain, acute postoperative pain Exact cause is unknown, thought to originate in brain; can be influenced by emotions/sympathetic stimulation

The **pain threshold** is defined as the lowest intensity of pain that a person can recognize.[2] Intense pain at one location may increase the threshold in another location. For example, a person with severe pain in one knee is more likely to experience less intense chronic back pain (this is called **perceptual dominance**). This means an individual with many painful sites may report only the most painful one. When the dominant pain is diminished, other painful areas are identified.

Pain tolerance is the duration of time or the intensity of pain that an individual will endure before initiating overt pain responses. It varies greatly among people and in the same person over time because of the body's ability to respond differently to noxious stimuli (Table 13-4). Pain tolerance generally *decreases* with repeated exposure to pain, fatigue, anger, boredom, apprehension, and sleep deprivation, and may *increase* with alcohol consumption, persistent use of opioid medications, hypnosis, distracting activities, and strong beliefs or faith.

> ✔ **QUICK CHECK 13-1**
> 1. Define the major categories of pain.
> 2. What portions of the nervous system are responsible for the sensation and perception of pain?
> 3. What physiologic responses are seen in acute pain?
> 4. List three common chronic pain conditions.

TABLE 13-4	PAIN PERCEPTION IN INFANTS, CHILDREN, AND ELDERLY PERSONS		
	INFANTS	**CHILDREN**	**ELDERLY PERSONS**
Pain threshold	Painful neonatal experiences increase pain sensitivity (lower threshold); pain may be increased with future procedures	Lower or same as adults	Individual responses may vary but pain threshold may be lower
Physiologic symptoms	Increased heart rate, blood pressure, and respiratory rate; flushing or pallor, sweating, and decreased oxygen saturation	Same as infants; nausea and vomiting	Same as infants and children; nausea and vomiting; may be decreased in individuals with cognitive impairment
Behavioral responses	Changes in facial expression, crying, and body movements, with lowered brows drawn together; vertical bulge and furrows in forehead between brows; broadened nasal root; tightly closed eyes; angular, square-shaped mouth, chin quiver; withdrawal of affected limbs, rigidity, flailing	Individual responses vary	Individual responses vary and may be influenced by presence of painful chronic diseases; individuals with cognitive impairment may demonstrate changes in behavior (e.g., combative or withdrawn, increased confusion)

Data from American Geriatric Society Panel in Persistent Pain in Older Adults: The management of persistent pain in older adults, *J Am Geriatr Soc* 50:S211, 2002; Fine PG: Chronic pain management in older adults: special considerations, *J Pain Symptom Manage* 38(2 suppl):S4–S14, 2009; Kunz M et al: Effects of age and mild cognitive impairment on the pain response system, *Gerontology* 55(6):674–682, 2009; Slover R, Coy J, Davids H: Advances in the management of pain in children: acute pain, *Adv Pediatr* 56:341–358, 2009; Weber F: Evidence for the need for anaesthesia in the neonate, *Best Pract Res Clin Anaesthesiol* 24(3):475-484, 2010.

TEMPERATURE REGULATION

Human thermoregulation is achieved through precise balancing of heat production, heat conservation, and heat loss. Body temperature is maintained in a range around 37° C (98.6° F). The normal range is considered to be 36.2° to 37.7° C (96.2° to 99.4° F) overall, but a person's individual body parts will vary in temperature. Body temperature rarely exceeds 41° C. The extremities are generally cooler than the trunk and the temperature at the core of the body (as measured by rectal temperature) is generally 0.5° C higher than the surface temperature (as measured by oral temperature). Internal temperature varies in response to activity, environmental temperature, and daily fluctuation (circadian rhythm). Oral temperatures fluctuate within 0.2° to 0.5° C during a 24-hour period. Women tend to have wider fluctuations that follow the menstrual cycle with a sharp rise in temperature just before ovulation. The daily fluctuating temperature in both genders peaks around 6 PM and is at its lowest during sleep. Maintenance of body temperature within the normal range is necessary for life.

Control of Body Temperature

Temperature regulation (thermoregulation) is mediated primarily by the hypothalamus. Peripheral thermoreceptors in the skin and central thermoreceptors in the hypothalamus, spinal cord, abdominal organs, and other central locations provide the hypothalamus with information about skin and core temperatures. If these temperatures are low or high, the hypothalamus triggers heat production and heat conservation or heat loss mechanisms. The endocrine system also operates to control body temperature.

Body heat is produced by the chemical reactions of metabolism and skeletal muscle tone and contraction. The heat-producing mechanism (chemical thermogenesis) begins with hypothalamic thyrotropin-stimulating hormone-releasing hormone (TSH-RH); it stimulates the anterior pituitary to release thyroid-stimulating hormone (TSH), which acts on the thyroid gland and stimulates the release of thyroxine. Thyroxine then acts on the adrenal medulla, causing the release of epinephrine into the bloodstream. Epinephrine causes vasoconstriction, stimulates glycolysis, and increases metabolic rate, thus increasing heat production.[38] Heat is distributed by the circulatory system.

The hypothalamus also triggers heat conservation by stimulating the sympathetic nervous system, which stimulates the adrenal cortex and results in increased skeletal muscle tone, initiating the shivering response and producing vasoconstriction. By constricting peripheral blood vessels, centrally warmed blood is shunted away from the periphery to the core of the body where heat can be retained. This involuntary mechanism takes advantage of the insulating layers of the skin and subcutaneous fat to protect core temperature. The hypothalamus relays information to the cerebral cortex about cold and voluntary responses result. Individuals typically bundle up, keep moving, or curl up in a ball. These types of voluntary physical activities respectively provide insulation, increase skeletal muscle activity, and decrease the amount of skin surface available for heat loss through radiation, convection, and conduction.[39]

The hypothalamus responds to warmer core and peripheral temperatures by reversing the same mechanisms resulting in heat loss. Heat loss is achieved through (1) radiation, (2) conduction, (3) convection, (4) vasodilation, (5) evaporation, (6) decreased muscle tone, (7) increased respiration, (8) voluntary measures, and (9) adaptation to warmer climates. Table 13-5 contains further information about heat production and loss.

Temperature Regulation in Infants and Elderly Persons

Infants (particularly low-birthweight infants) and elderly persons require special attention to maintenance of body temperature. Term infants produce sufficient body heat, primarily through metabolism of brown fat, but cannot conserve heat produced because of their small body size, greater ratio of body surface to body weight, and inability to shiver. Infants also have little subcutaneous fat and thus are not as well insulated as adults.[40] Elderly persons respond poorly to environmental temperature extremes because of their slowed blood circulation, structural and functional skin changes, and overall decreased heat-producing activities.[41] In addition, they have a decreased shivering response (delayed onset and decreased effectiveness), slowed metabolic rate, decreased vasoconstrictor response, diminished or absent ability to sweat, decreased peripheral sensation, desynchronized circadian rhythm, decreased perception of heat and cold, decreased thirst, decreased nutritional reserves, and decreased brown adipose tissue.[42]

Pathogenesis of Fever

Fever (febrile response) is a temporary "resetting of the hypothalamic thermostat" to a higher level in response to endogenous or exogenous pyrogens. The thermoregulatory mechanisms adjust heat

TABLE 13-5	MECHANISMS OF HEAT PRODUCTION AND HEAT LOSS
CONDITION	**DESCRIPTION**
Heat Production	
Chemical reactions of metabolism	Occur during ingestion and metabolism of food and while maintaining body at rest (basal metabolism); occur in body core (e.g., liver)
Skeletal muscle contraction	Gradual increase in muscle tone or rapid muscle oscillations (shivering)
Chemical thermogenesis	Epinephrine is released and produces rapid, transient increase in heat production by raising basal metabolic rate; quick, brief effect that counters heat lost through conduction and convection; involves brown adipose tissue, which decreases markedly in older adults; thyroid hormone increases metabolism
Heat Loss	
Radiation	Heat loss through electromagnetic waves emanating from surfaces with temperature higher than surrounding air
Conduction	Heat loss by direct molecule-to-molecule transfer from one surface to another, so that warmer surface loses heat to cooler surface
Convection	Transfer of heat through currents of gases or liquids; exchanges warmer air at body's surface with cooler air in surrounding space
Vasodilation	Diverts core-warmed blood to surface of body, with heat transferred by conduction to skin surface and from there to surrounding environment; occurs in response to autonomic stimulation under control of hypothalamus
Evaporation	Body water evaporates from surface of skin and linings of mucous membranes; major source of heat reduction connected with increased sweating in warmer surroundings
Decreased muscle tone	Exhausted feeling caused by moderately reduced muscle tone and curtailed voluntary muscle activity
Increased respiration	Air is exchanged with environment through normal process; minimal effect
Voluntary mechanisms	"Stretching out" and "slowing down" in response to high body temperatures; increasing body surface area available for heat loss; dressing in light-colored, loose-fitting garments
Adaptation to warmer climates	Gradual process beginning with lassitude, weakness, and faintness; proceeding through increased sweating, lowered sodium content, decreased heart rate, and increased stroke volume and extracellular fluid volume; and terminating in improved warm weather functioning and decreased symptoms of heat intolerance (work output, endurance, and coordination increase; subjective feelings of discomfort decrease)

production, conservation, and loss to maintain body core temperature at a normal level. During fever, this level is raised so that the thermoregulatory center now adjusts heat production, conservation, and loss to maintain the core temperature at the new, higher temperature, which functions as a new set point. This response is mediated in part by cytokines associated with the inflammatory response.[43] Exogenous pyrogens, or endotoxins produced by pathogens (see Chapter 7), stimulate the release of endogenous pyrogens from phagocytic cells, including tumor necrosis factor-alpha (TNF-α), interleukin-1 (IL-1), interleukin-6 (IL-6), and interferon (IFN), which raise the set point by inducing the hypothalamic synthesis of prostaglandin E_2 (PGE_2). In response, there is an increase in heat production and conservation to raise body temperature to the new set point (Figure 13-5). The individual feels colder, dresses more warmly, decreases body surface area by curling up, and may go to bed in an effort to get warm. Body temperature is maintained at the new level until the fever "breaks," when the set point begins to return to normal with decreased heat production and increased heat reduction mechanisms. The individual feels very warm, dons cooler clothes, throws off the covers, and stretches out. Once the body has returned to a normal temperature the individual feels more comfortable and the hypothalamus adjusts thermoregulatory mechanisms to maintain the new temperature.

Fever of unknown origin (FUO) is a body temperature of greater than 38.3° C (101° F) that remains undiagnosed after 3 days of hospital investigation or two or more outpatient visits. The clinical categories of FUO include infectious, rheumatic/inflammatory, neoplastic, and miscellaneous disorders.[44]

Benefits of Fever

Fever helps the body respond to infectious processes through several mechanisms[45,46]:

1. Raising of body temperature kills many microorganisms and adversely affects their growth and replication.
2. Higher body temperatures decrease serum levels of iron, zinc, and copper—minerals needed for bacterial replication.
3. Increased temperature causes lysosomal breakdown and autodestruction of cells, preventing viral replication in infected cells.
4. Heat increases lymphocytic transformation and motility of polymorphonuclear neutrophils, facilitating the immune response.
5. Phagocytosis is enhanced, and production of antiviral interferon is augmented.

Suppression of fever by treatment with antipyrogenic medications should be used when a fever produces serious side effects, such as cardiovascular stress, nerve damage, brain damage, or convulsion.[47,48]

Infection and fever responses in elderly persons and children may vary from those in normal adults. Box 13-2 lists the principal features associated with fever at these extremes of age.[49]

Disorders of Temperature Regulation
Hyperthermia

Hyperthermia is elevation of the body temperature without an increase in the hypothalamic set point. Hyperthermia can produce nerve damage, coagulation of cell proteins, and death. At 41° C (105.8° F), nerve damage produces convulsions in the adult. Death results at 43° C (109.4° F). Hyperthermia may be therapeutic, accidental, or associated with stroke or head trauma. Prevention of hyperthermia in stroke and head trauma assists in limiting brain injury.[50]

Therapeutic hyperthermia is a form of local or general body-induced hyperthermia used to destroy pathologic microorganisms or tumor cells by facilitating the host's natural immune process or tumor

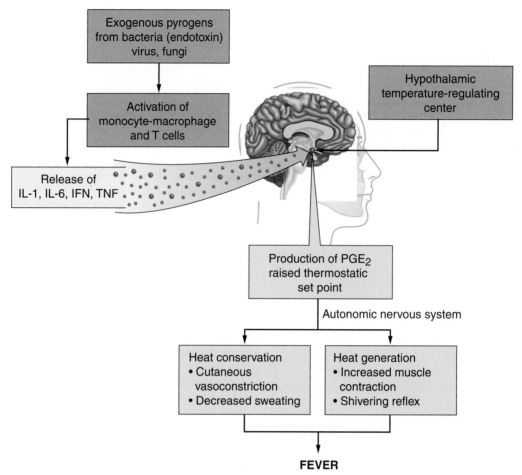

FIGURE 13-5 **Production of Fever.** Pathogens release exogenous pyrogens and activate monocytes/macrophages and other inflammatory cells that secrete endogenous pyrogenic cytokines, such as interleukin-1 (IL-1), interleukin-6 (IL-6), tumor necrosis factor (TNF), and interferon (IFN), which promote the synthesis and secretion of prostaglandin E_2 (PGE$_2$) in the anterior hypothalamus. PGE$_2$ increases the thermostatic set point, and the autonomic nervous system is stimulated, resulting in shivering, muscle contraction, peripheral vasoconstriction, and the production of fever. (From Lewis SM et al: *Medical-surgical nursing: assessment and management of clinical problems,* ed 7, St Louis, 2007, Mosby.)

BOX 13-2 **EFFECTS OF FEVER AT THE EXTREMES OF AGE**

Elderly Persons
Show decreased or no fever response to infection; therefore benefits of fever are reduced.
High morbidity and mortality result from lack of beneficial aspects.

Children
Develop higher temperatures than adults for relatively minor infections.
Febrile seizures before age 5 years are not uncommon.

---

blood flow.[51] The four forms of accidental hyperthermia are summarized as follows[52]:

1. **Heat cramps**—severe, spasmodic cramps in the abdomen and extremities that follow prolonged sweating and associated sodium loss. Usually occur in those not accustomed to heat or those performing strenuous work in very warm climates. Signs include fever, rapid pulse rate, and increased blood pressure.

2. **Heat exhaustion**—results from prolonged high core or environmental temperatures, which cause profound vasodilation and profuse sweating, leading to dehydration, decreased plasma volumes, hypotension, decreased cardiac output, and tachycardia. Symptoms include weakness, dizziness, confusion, nausea, and fainting.

3. **Heat stroke**—a potentially lethal result of an overstressed thermoregulatory center. With very high core temperatures (>40° C; 104° F), the regulatory center ceases to function and the body's heat loss mechanisms fail. Symptoms include high core temperature, absence of sweating, rapid pulse rate, confusion, agitation, and coma. Complications include cerebral edema, degeneration of the CNS, swollen dendrites, renal tubular necrosis, and hepatic failure with delirium, coma, and eventually death if treatment is not undertaken.

4. **Malignant hyperthermia**—a potentially lethal complication of a rare inherited muscle disorder that may be triggered by inhaled anesthetics and depolarizing muscle relaxants.[53,54] The syndrome involves altered calcium function in muscle cells with hypermetabolism, uncoordinated muscle contractions, increased muscle work, increased oxygen consumption, and a raised level of lactic

acid production. Acidosis develops, and body temperature rises, with resulting tachycardia and cardiac dysrhythmias, hypotension, decreased cardiac output, and cardiac arrest. Signs resemble those of coma—unconsciousness, absent reflexes, fixed pupils, apnea, and occasionally a flat electroencephalogram. Oliguria and anuria are common. It is most common in children and adolescents.

Hypothermia

Hypothermia (marked cooling of core temperature) produces depression of the central nervous and respiratory systems, vasoconstriction, alterations in microcirculation and coagulation, and ischemic tissue damage. Hypothermia may be accidental or therapeutic (Box 13-3). Most tissues can tolerate low temperatures in controlled situations, such as surgery. However, in severe hypothermia, ice crystals form on the inside of the cell, causing cells to rupture and die. Tissue hypothermia slows cell metabolism, increases the blood viscosity, slows microcirculatory blood flow, facilitates blood coagulation, and stimulates profound vasoconstriction (also see Frostbite, Chapter 39).

Trauma and Temperature

Major body trauma can affect temperature regulation through various mechanisms. Damage to the CNS, inflammation, increased intracranial pressure, or intracranial bleeding typically produces a body temperature of greater than 39° C (102.2° F). This sustained noninfectious fever, often referred to as a "central fever," appears with or without bradycardia. A central fever does not induce sweating and is very resistant to antipyretic therapy.

Other traumatic mechanisms that produce temperature alterations include accidental injuries, hemorrhagic shock, major surgery, and thermal burns. The severity and type of alteration (hyperthermia or hypothermia) vary with the severity of the cause and the body system affected.

✔ **QUICK CHECK 13-2**
1. Why is temperature regulation important?
2. What are the principal heat production methods? Heat loss methods?
3. How does the hypothalamus alter its set point to change body temperature?
4. Compare and contrast hyperthermia and hypothermia and their effects on the body.

SLEEP

Sleep is an active brain process that provides restorative functions and promotes memory consolidation. The suprachiasmatic nucleus (SCN) in the hypothalamus controls the timing of the sleep-wake cycle and coordinates this cycle with circadian rhythms (24-hour rhythm cycles) in other areas of the brain and other tissues.[55] Normal sleep has two phases that can be documented by electroencephalogram (EEG): rapid eye movement (REM) sleep (20% to 25% of sleep time) and slow-wave (non-REM) sleep. Non-REM sleep is further divided into four stages (I to IV) from light to deep sleep. There are four to six cycles of REM and non-REM sleep each night.[56]

REM (rapid eye movement) sleep is initiated by REM-on and REM-off neurons in the pons and mesencephalon. REM sleep occurs about every 90 minutes beginning 1 to 2 hours after non-REM sleep begins. This sleep is known as paradoxical sleep because the EEG pattern is similar to the normal awake pattern and the brain is very active with dreaming. REM and non-REM sleep alternate throughout the night, with lengthening intervals of REM sleep and fewer intervals of deeper stages of non-REM sleep toward morning. The changes

---

BOX 13-3 DEFINING CHARACTERISTICS OF HYPOTHERMIA

Accidental Hypothermia

The unintentional decrease in core temperature to less than 35° C (95° F) results from sudden immersion in cold water, prolonged exposure to cold environments, or altered thermoregulatory mechanisms. It is most common among young and elderly persons.

Factors that increase risk:
1. Hypothyroidism
2. Hypopituitarism
3. Malnutrition
4. Parkinson disease
5. Rheumatoid arthritis
6. Chronic increased vasodilation
7. Failure of thermoregulatory control resulting from cerebral injury, ketoacidosis, uremia, sepsis, and drug overdose

Response mechanisms:
1. Peripheral vasoconstriction—shunts blood away from cooler skin to core to decrease heat loss and produces peripheral tissue ischemia
2. Intermittent reperfusion of extremities (Lewis phenomenon) helps preserve peripheral oxygenation until core temperature drops dramatically
3. Hypothalamic center induces shivering; thinking becomes sluggish, and coordination is depressed
4. Stupor; heart rate and respiratory rate decline; cardiac output diminishes; metabolic rate falls; acidosis; eventual ventricular fibrillation and asystole occur at 30° C (86° F) and lower

Treatment:
1. Most changes are reversible with rewarming
2. Core temperature greater than 30° C (86° F)—active rewarming (external)
3. Core temperature less than 30° C (86° F) or with severe cardiovascular problems—active core rewarming (internal)

Therapeutic Hypothermia

Used to slow metabolism and preserve ischemic tissue during surgery (e.g., limb reimplantation), after cardiac arrest, or following neurologic injury

Effects and cautions:
1. Stresses the heart, leading to ventricular fibrillation and cardiac arrest (may be desired outcome in open heart surgery when heart must be stopped)
2. Exhausts liver glycogen stores by prolonged shivering
3. Surface cooling may cause burns, frostbite, and fat necrosis
4. Immunosuppression with increased infection risk
5. Slows drug metabolism

From Arrich J et al: Cochrane corner: hypothermia for neuroprotection in adults after cardiopulmonary resuscitation, *Anesth Analg* 110(4):1239, 2010; Mallet ML: Pathophysiology of accidental hypothermia, *QJM* 95(12):775–785, 2002; Lampe JW, Becker LB; State of the art in therapeutic hypothermia, *Annu Rev Med* 62:79–93, 2011; Varon J: Therapeutic hypothermia: implications for acute care practitioners, *Postgrad Med* 122(1):19–27, 2010.

---

associated with REM sleep include increased parasympathetic activity and variable sympathetic activity associated with rapid eye movement; muscle relaxation; loss of temperature regulation; altered heart rate, blood pressure, and respiration; penile erection in men and clitoral engorgement in women; release of steroids; and many memorable dreams. Respiratory control appears largely independent of metabolic requirements and oxygen variation. Loss of normal voluntary muscle control in the tongue and upper pharynx may produce some respiratory obstruction. Cerebral blood flow increases.

Non-REM sleep (NREM) accounts for 75% to 80% of sleep time in adults and is initiated when inhibitory signals are released from the hypothalamus. Sympathetic tone is decreased and parasympathetic activity is increased during NREM sleep, creating a state of reduced activity. The basal metabolic rate falls by 10% to 15%; temperature decreases 0.5° to 1.0° C (0.9° to 1.8° F); heart rate, respiration, blood pressure, and muscle tone decrease; and knee jerk reflexes are absent. Pupils are constricted. During the various stages, cerebral blood flow to the brain decreases and growth hormone is released, with corticosteroid and catecholamine levels depressed. Box 13-4 summarizes sleep characteristics in infants and elderly persons.

Sleep is an active multiphase process with complex neural circuits, interacting hormones, and neurotransmitters involving the hypothalamus, thalamus, brain stem, and cortex. The hypothalamus is a major sleep center and the hypocretins (orexins), acetylcholine, and glutamate are neuropeptides secreted by the hypothalamus that promote wakefulness. Prostaglandin D$_2$, adenosine, melatonin, serotonin, L-tryptophan, gamma-aminobutyric acid (GABA), and growth factors promote sleep. The pontine reticular formation is primarily responsible for generating REM sleep, and projections from the thalamocortical network produce non-REM sleep.[57,58]

Sleep Disorders

Because classification of sleep disorders is complex, a system has been established by the American Academy of Sleep Medicine and includes four classifications: (1) dyssomnias (disorders of initiating and maintaining sleep and disorders of excessive sleepiness), (2) parasomnias (disorders that primarily do not cause a complaint of insomnia or excessive sleepiness), (3) sleep disorders associated with medical/psychiatric disorders, and (4) proposed sleep disorders.[59] The most common dyssomnias and parasomnias are summarized here.

Common Dyssomnias

Insomnia. Insomnia is the inability to fall or stay asleep and may be mild, moderate, or severe. It may be transient, lasting a few days, and related to travel across time zones or caused by acute stress. Long-term insomnia can be idiopathic, start at an early age, and be associated with drug or alcohol abuse, chronic pain disorders, chronic depression, the use of certain drugs, obesity, and aging.[60]

Sleep disordered breathing and hypersomnia. Obstructive sleep apnea syndrome (OSAS) generally results from upper airway obstruction recurring during sleep with excessive snoring and multiple apneic episodes that last 10 seconds or longer. The periodic breathing eventually produces arousal, which interrupts the sleep cycle, reducing total sleep time and producing sleep and REM deprivation. Associated conditions include obesity, decreased sensitivity to carbon dioxide and oxygen tensions, and upper airway obstruction. Sleep apnea produces hypercapnia and low oxygen saturation and eventually leads to polycythemia, pulmonary hypertension, systemic hypertension, stroke, right-sided congestive heart failure, dysrhythmias, liver congestion, cyanosis, and peripheral edema.[61] Hypersomnia (excessive daytime sleepiness) is associated with OSAS. Individuals may fall asleep while driving a car, working, or even while conversing, with significant concerns for safety.[62]

Treatments for OSAS include use of nasal continuous positive airway pressure and dental devices, surgery of the upper airway and jaw in selected individuals, and management of obesity.[63] Adenotonsillar hypertrophy is the major cause of obstructive sleep apnea in children and obesity increases risk. Tonsillectomy and adenoidectomy are the treatments of choice.[64]

Narcolepsy is a primary hypersomnia of central origin characterized by hallucinations, sleep paralysis, and, rarely, cataplexy (brief spells of muscle weakness). The disorder is associated with hypothalamic hypocretin (orexin) deficiency and may be related to immune-mediated destruction of hypocretin-secreting cells. There is a genetic component to the disorder.[65]

Disorders of the sleep-wake schedule. Common disorders of the sleep-wake schedule (circadian rhythm sleep disorders) can result from rapid time-zone change (or jet-lag syndrome), alternating the sleep schedule (rotating work shifts) involving 3 hours or more in sleep time, or changing the total sleep time from day to day. These changes desynchronize circadian rhythm, which can depress the degree of vigilance, performance of psychomotor tasks, and arousal.[66]

Common Parasomnias

Parasomnias are unusual behaviors occurring during sleep.[67] These behaviors include sleepwalking, night terrors, rearranging furniture, eating food, violent behavior, and restless leg syndrome.

Two dysfunctions of sleep (somnambulism and night terrors) are common in children and may be related to central nervous system immaturity. Somnambulism (sleepwalking) is a disorder primarily of childhood and appears to resolve within a few years. Sleepwalking is therefore not associated with dreaming, and the child has no memory of the event on awakening. Sleepwalking in adults is often associated with sleep disordered breathing.[68] Night terrors are characterized by sudden apparent arousals in which the child expresses intense fear or emotion. However, the child is not awake and can be difficult to arouse. Once awakened, the child has no memory of the night terror event. Night terrors are not associated with dreams. Although this problem occurs most often in children, adults also may experience it with corresponding daytime anxiety.

Restless leg syndrome (RLS) is a common sensorimotor disorder associated with unpleasant sensations (prickling, tingling, crawling) that occurs at rest and is worse in the evening or at night. There is a

---

BOX 13-4   SLEEP CHARACTERISTICS OF INFANTS AND ELDERLY PERSONS

Infants

- Sleep 16 to 17 hours per day: 50% REM (active) sleep, 25% non-REM (inactive) sleep.
- Infant sleep cycles are 50 to 60 minutes in length; 10 to 45 minutes of REM sleep accompanied by movement of the arms, legs, and facial muscles followed by about 20 minutes of non-REM sleep.
- At 1 year, REM and non-REM sleep cycles are about equal in length and infants sleep through the night with about two naps per day.

Elderly Persons

- Total sleep time is decreased with a longer time to fall asleep and poorer quality sleep.
- Total time in slow-wave and final phase of non-REM sleep decreases by 15% to 30%.
- Alterations in sleep patterns occur about 10 years later in women than men.
- Sleep disorders more likely in elderly and increase risk of morbidity and mortality.

From Espiritu JR: Aging-related sleep changes, *Clin Geriatr Med* 24(1):1–14, v, 2008; McLaughlin Crabtree V, Williams NA: Normal sleep in children and adolescents, *Child Adolesc Psychiatr Clin N Am* 18(4):799–811, 2009; Neikrug AB, Ancoli-Israel S: Sleep disorders in the older adult—a mini-review, *Gerontology* 56(2):181–189, 2010.

compelling urge to move the legs for relief with a significant effect on sleep and quality of life. The disorder is more common in women, the elderly, and individuals with iron deficiency. RLS has a familial tendency and is associated with a circadian fluctuation of dopamine in the substantia nigra. Iron is a cofactor in dopamine production and some individuals respond to iron administration as well as dopamine agonists.[69]

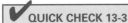

> **QUICK CHECK 13-3**
> 1. Describe REM and non-REM sleep.
> 2. What is the major difference between the dyssomnias and parasomnias?

THE SPECIAL SENSES

Vision

The eyes are complex sense organs responsible for vision. Within a protective casing, each eye has receptors, a lens system for focusing light on the receptors, and a system of nerves for conducting impulses from the receptors to the brain. Visual dysfunction may be caused by abnormal ocular movements or alterations in visual acuity, refraction, color vision, or accommodation. Visual dysfunction also may be the secondary effect of another neurologic disorder.

The Eye and Its External Structures

The wall of the eye consists of three layers: (1) sclera, (2) choroid, and (3) retina (Figure 13-6). The sclera is the thick, white, outermost layer. It becomes transparent at the cornea—the portion of the sclera in the central anterior region that allows light to enter the eye. The choroid is the deeply pigmented middle layer that prevents light from scattering inside the eye. The iris, part of the choroid, has a round opening, the pupil, through which light passes. Smooth muscle fibers control the size of the pupil so that it adjusts to bright light or dim light and to close or distant vision.

The retina is the innermost layer of the eye, and contains millions of rods and cones—special photoreceptors that convert light energy into nerve impulses. Rods mediate peripheral and dim light vision and are densest at the periphery. Cones, densest in the center of the retina, are color and detail receptors. There are no photoreceptors where the optic nerve leaves the eyeball; this creates the optic disc, or blind spot.

Lateral to each optic disc is the macula lutea, the area of most distinct vision, and in the center is the fovea centralis that contains only cones and provides the greatest visual acuity (see Figure 13-6).

As shown in Figure 13-10 (p. 330), nerve impulses pass through the optic nerves to the optic chiasm. The nerves from the inner (nasal) halves of the retinas cross to the opposite side and join fibers from the outer (temporal) halves of the retinas to form the optic tracts. The fibers of the optic tracts synapse in the dorsal lateral geniculate nucleus and pass by way of the optic radiation (or geniculocalcarine tract) to the primary visual cortex in the occipital lobe of the brain.[70] Light entering the eye is focused on the retina by the lens—a flexible, biconvex, crystal-like structure. The lens divides the anterior chamber into (1) the aqueous chamber and (2) the vitreous chamber. Aqueous humor fills the aqueous chamber and helps maintain pressure inside the eye, as well as provide nutrients to the lens and cornea. Aqueous humor is secreted by the ciliary processes and reabsorbed into the canal of Schlemm. If drainage is blocked, intraocular pressure increases (causing glaucoma). The vitreous chamber is filled with a gel-like substance called vitreous humor. Vitreous humor helps to prevent the eyeball from collapsing inward.

The central retinal artery provides blood to the inner retinal surface, and the choroid supplies nutrients to the outer surface of the retina. Six extrinsic eye muscles allow gross eye movements and permit eyes to follow a moving object (Figure 13-7).

The external structures protecting the eye include the eyelids (palpebrae), conjunctiva, and lacrimal apparatus (Figure 13-8). The eyelids are used to control the amount of light reaching the eyes, and the conjunctiva lines the eyelids. Tears released from the lacrimal apparatus bathe the surface of the eye and prevent friction, maintain hydration, and wash out foreign bodies and other irritants.

Visual Dysfunction

Alterations in ocular movements. Abnormal ocular movements result from oculomotor, trochlear, or abducens cranial nerve dysfunction (see Table 12-6). The three types of eye movement disorders are (1) strabismus, (2) nystagmus, and (3) paralysis of individual extraocular muscles.

In strabismus, one eye deviates from the other when the person is looking at an object. This is caused by a weak or hypertonic muscle in

FIGURE 13-6 Internal Anatomy of the Eye. (From Thibodeau GA, Patton KT: *Anatomy & physiology*, ed 6, St Louis, 2007, Mosby.)

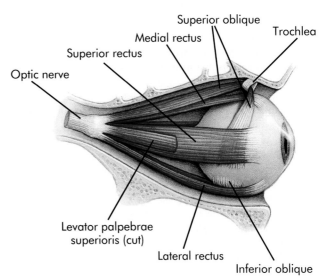

FIGURE 13-7 Extrinsic Muscles of the Right Eye. (From Thibodeau GA, Patton KT: *Anatomy & physiology*, ed 6, St Louis, 2007, Mosby.)

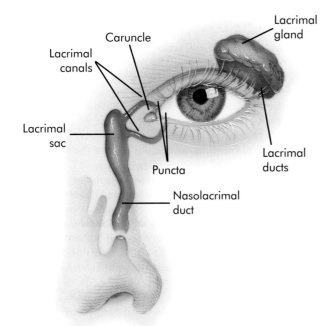

FIGURE 13-8 Lacrimal Apparatus. Fluid produced by lacrimal glands (tears) streams across the eye surface, enters the canals, and then passes through the nasolacrimal duct to enter the nose. (From Thibodeau GA, Patton KT: *Anatomy & physiology*, ed 6, St Louis, 2007, Mosby.)

TABLE 13-6	**CHANGES IN THE EYE CAUSED BY AGING**	
STRUCTURE	**CHANGE**	**CONSEQUENCE**
Cornea	Thicker and less curved	Increase in astigmatism
Formation of gray ring at edge of cornea (arcus senilis)	Not detrimental to vision	
Anterior chamber	Decrease in size and volume caused by thickening of lens	Occasionally exerts pressure on Schlemm canal and may lead to increased intraocular pressure and glaucoma
Lens	Increase in opacity	Decrease in refraction with increased light scattering (blurring) and decreased color vision (green and blue); can lead to cataracts
Ciliary muscles	Reduction in pupil diameter, atrophy of radial dilation muscles	Persistent constriction (senile miosis); decrease in critical flicker frequency*
Retina	Reduction in number of rods at periphery, loss of rods and associated nerve cells	Increase in minimum amount of light necessary to see an object

*The rate at which consecutive visual stimuli can be presented and still be perceived as separate.

one eye. The deviation may be upward, downward, inward (entropia), or outward (extropia). Strabismus in children requires early intervention to prevent **amblyopia** (reduced vision in the affected eye caused by cerebral blockage of the visual stimuli). The primary symptom of strabismus is **diplopia** (double vision). Causes of strabismus include neuromuscular disorder of the eye muscle, diseases involving the cerebral hemispheres, or thyroid disease.

Nystagmus is an involuntary unilateral or bilateral rhythmic movement of the eyes. It may be present at rest or when the eye moves. **Pendular nystagmus** is characterized by a regular back and forth movement of the eyes. In **jerk nystagmus,** one phase of the eye movement is faster than the other. Nystagmus may be caused by an imbalanced reflex activity of the inner ear, vestibular nuclei, cerebellum, medial longitudinal fascicle, or nuclei of the oculomotor, trochlear, and abducens cranial nerves (see Table 12-6 and Figure 12-24). Drugs, retinal disease, and diseases involving the cervical cord also may produce nystagmus.

Paralysis of specific extraocular muscles may cause limited abduction, abnormal closure of the eyelid, ptosis (drooping of the eyelid), or diplopia (double vision) as a result of unopposed muscle activity. Trauma or pressure in the area of the cranial nerves or diseases such as diabetes mellitus and myasthenia gravis also paralyze specific extraocular muscles.

Alterations in visual acuity. Visual acuity is the ability to see objects in sharp detail. With advancing age, the lens of the eye becomes less flexible and adjusts slowly, and there is altered refraction of light by the cornea and lens. Thus, visual acuity declines with age. Table 13-6 contains a summary of changes in the eye caused by aging. Specific causes of visual acuity changes are (1) amblyopia, (2) scotoma, (3) cataracts, (4) papilledema, (5) dark adaptation, (6) glaucoma, (7) retinal detachment, and (8) macular degeneration (Table 13-7). **Glaucoma** is the second leading cause of blindness and is characterized

by intraocular pressures greater than 12 to 20 mm Hg with death of retinal ganglion cells and their axons.[71] There are three primary types of glaucoma[71]:

1. *Open angle.* This type of glaucoma is characterized by outflow obstruction of aqueous humor at the trabecular meshwork or canal of Schlemm even though there is adequate space for drainage; often this is an inherited disease and is a leading cause of blindness with few preliminary symptoms.
2. *Angle closure.* In this type of glaucoma there is displacement of the iris toward the cornea with obstruction of the trabecular meshwork and obstruction of outflow of aqueous humor from the anterior chamber; it may occur acutely with a sudden rise in intraocular pressure, causing pain and visual disturbances.
3. *Congenital closure.* This is a rare disease associated with congenital malformations and other genetic anomalies.

Both medical and surgical therapies are available.[72]

Age-related macular degeneration (AMD) is a severe and irreversible loss of vision and a major cause of blindness in older individuals. Hypertension, cigarette smoking, diabetes mellitus and family history of AMD are risk factors. The degeneration usually occurs after the age of 60 years. There are two forms: atrophic (dry, nonexudative) and neovascular (wet, exudative). The atrophic form is slowly progressive with accumulation of drusen (waste products from photoreceptors) in the retina and may include limited night vision and difficulty reading. The neovascular form includes accumulation of drusen, abnormal choroidal blood vessel growth, leakage of blood or serum, retinal detachment, fibrovascular scarring, loss of photoreceptors, and more severe loss of central vision. Both medical and surgical therapies are available.[73]

TABLE 13-7	CAUSES OF VISUAL ACUITY CHANGES
DISORDER	**DESCRIPTION**
Amblyopia	Reduced or dimmed vision, cause unknown
	Associated with strabismus
	Accompanies such diseases as diabetes mellitus, renal failure, and malaria and use of drugs such as alcohol and tobacco
Scotoma	Circumscribed defect of central field of vision
	Often associated with retrobulbar neuritis and multiple sclerosis, compression of optic nerve by tumor, inflammation of optic nerve, pernicious anemia, methyl alcohol poisoning, and use of tobacco
Cataract	Cloudy or opaque area in ocular lens
	Incidence increases with age because most commonly a result of degeneration; other causes are congenital
Papilledema	Edema and inflammation of optic nerve where it enters eyeball
	Caused by obstruction of venous return from retina from one of three main sources: increased intracranial pressure, retrobulbar neuritis, or changes in retinal blood vessels
Dark adaptation	With age, eye does not adapt as readily to dark
	Also, changes in quantity and quality of rhodopsin are causative; vitamin A deficiencies can produce this at any age
Glaucoma	Increased intraocular pressures (>12-20 mm Hg)
	Loss of acuity results from pressure on optic nerve, which blocks flow of nutrients to optic nerve fibers, leading to their death; sixth leading cause of blindness
Retinal detachment	Tear or break in retina with accumulation of fluid and separation from underlying tissue; seen as floaters, flashes of light, or a curtain over visual field; risks include extreme myopia, diabetic retinopathy, sickle cell disease

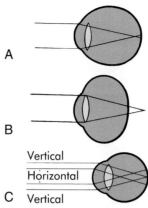

FIGURE 13-9 Alterations in Refraction. **A,** Myopic eye. Parallel rays of light are brought to a focus in front of the retina. **B,** Hyperopic eye. Parallel rays of light come to a focus behind the retina in the unaccommodative eye. **C,** Simple myopic astigmatism. The vertical bundle of rays is focused on the retina; the horizontal rays are focused in front of the retina. (From Stein HA, Slatt BJ, Stein RM: *The ophthalmic assistant: fundamentals and clinical practice,* ed 5, St Louis, 1998, Mosby.)

Alterations in color vision. Normal sensitivity to color diminishes with age because of the progressive yellowing of the lens that occurs with aging. All colors become less intense, although color discrimination for blue and green is greatly affected. Color vision deteriorates more rapidly for individuals with diabetes mellitus than for the general population.

Abnormal color vision also may be caused by color blindness, an inherited trait. Color blindness affects 8% of the male population and 0.5% of the female population. Although many forms of color blindness exist, most commonly the affected individual cannot distinguish red from green.[76] In the most severe form individuals see only shades of gray, black, and white.

Neurologic disorders causing visual dysfunction. Vision may be disrupted at many points along the visual pathway, causing various defects in the visual field. Visual changes may cause defects or blindness in the entire visual field or in half of a visual field (hemianopia). (Figure 13-10 illustrates the many areas along the visual pathway that may be damaged and the associated visual changes.)

Injury to the optic nerve causes same-side blindness. Injury to the optic chiasm (the X-shaped crossing of the optic nerves) can cause various defects, depending on the location of the injury.

External Eye Structure Disorders

Infection and inflammatory responses are the most common conditions affecting the supporting structures of the eyes. Blepharitis is an inflammation of the eyelids caused by *Staphylococcus* or seborrheic dermatitis. A hordeolum (stye) is an infection (usually staphylococcal) of the sebaceous glands of the eyelids usually centered near an eyelash. A chalazion is a noninfectious lipogranuloma of the meibomian (oil-secreting) gland that often occurs in association with a hordeolum and appears as a deep nodule within the eyelid. These conditions present with redness, swelling, and tenderness and are treated symptomatically.

Conjunctivitis is an inflammation of the conjunctiva caused by bacteria, viruses, allergies, or chemical irritants.[77] Acute bacterial conjunctivitis (pinkeye) is highly contagious and often caused by *Staphylococcus, Haemophilus, Streptococcus pneumoniae,* and *Moraxella catarrhalis,* although other bacteria may be involved. In children younger than 6 years, *Haemophilus* infection often leads to otitis media

Alterations in accommodation. Accommodation refers to changes in the thickness of the lens. Accommodation is needed for clear vision and is mediated through the oculomotor nerve. Pressure, inflammation, age, and disease of the oculomotor nerve may alter accommodation, causing diplopia, blurred vision, and headache.

Loss of accommodation with advancing age is termed presbyopia, a condition in which the ocular lens becomes larger, firmer, and less elastic. The major symptom is reduced near vision, causing the individual to hold reading material at arm's length. Treatment includes corrective forward, contact, and intraocular lenses or laser refractive surgery for monovision.[74,75]

Alterations in refraction. Alterations in refraction are the most common visual problem. Causes include irregularities of the corneal curvature, the focusing power of the lens, and the length of the eye. The major symptoms of refraction alterations are blurred vision and headache. Three types of refraction are as follows (Figure 13-9):

Myopia—nearsightedness: Light rays are focused in front of the retina when the person is looking at a distant object.

Hyperopia—farsightedness: Light rays are focused behind the retina when a person is looking at a near object.

Astigmatism—unequal curvature of the cornea: Light rays are bent unevenly and do not come to a single focus on the retina. Astigmatism may coexist with myopia, hyperopia, or presbyopia.

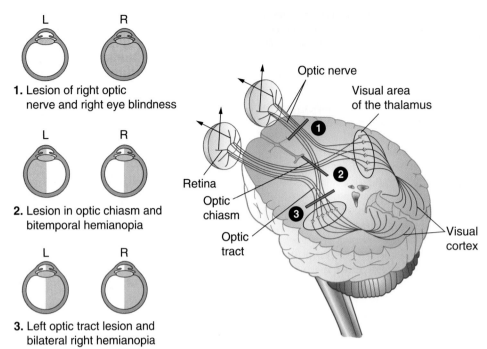

1. Lesion of right optic
   nerve and right eye blindness

2. Lesion in optic chiasm and
   bitemporal hemianopia

3. Left optic tract lesion and
   bilateral right hemianopia

FIGURE 13-10 Visual Pathways and Defects. (Modified from Thompson JM et al: *Mosby's clinical nursing,* ed 5, St Louis, 2002, Mosby.)

(conjunctivitis-otitis syndrome). Preventing spread of the microorganism with meticulous handwashing and use of separate towels is important. The disease also is treated with antibiotics.

Viral conjunctivitis is caused by an adenovirus. Again, it is contagious, with symptoms of watering, redness, and photophobia. Allergic conjunctivitis is associated with a variety of antigens, including pollens. Chronic conjunctivitis results from any persistent conjunctivitis. Trachoma (chlamydial conjunctivitis) is caused by *Chlamydia trachomatis* and often is associated with poor hygiene. It is the leading cause of preventable blindness in the world.

Keratitis is an infection of the cornea caused by bacteria or viruses. Bacterial infections cause corneal ulceration, and type 1 herpes simplex virus can involve both the cornea and the conjunctiva. Severe ulcerations with residual scarring require corneal transplantation.

Hearing

The external auditory canal is surrounded by the bones of the cranium. The opening (meatus) of the canal is just above the mastoid process. The air-filled sinuses, called mastoid air cells, of the mastoid process promote conductivity of sound between the external and the middle ear.

The Normal Ear

The ear is divided into three areas: (1) the external ear, involved only with hearing; (2) the middle ear, involved only with hearing; and (3) the inner ear, involved with both hearing and equilibrium.

The external ear is composed of the pinna (auricle), which is the visible portion of the ear, and the external auditory canal, a tube that leads to the middle ear (Figure 13-11). Sound waves entering the external auditory canal hit the tympanic membrane (eardrum) and cause it to vibrate. The tympanic membrane separates the external ear from the middle ear.

The middle ear is composed of the tympanic cavity, a small chamber in the temporal bone. Three ossicles (small bones known as the malleus [hammer], incus [anvil], and stapes [stirrup]) transmit the vibration of the tympanic membrane to the inner ear. When the tympanic membrane moves, the malleus moves with it and transfers the vibration to the incus, which passes it on to the stapes. The stapes presses against the oval window, a small membrane of the inner ear. The movement of the oval window sets the fluids of the inner ear in motion (Figure 13-12).

The eustachian (pharyngotympanic) tube connects the middle ear with the thorax. Normally flat and closed, the eustachian tube opens briefly when a person swallows or yawns, and it equalizes the pressure in the middle ear with atmospheric pressure. Equalized pressure permits the tympanic membrane to vibrate freely. Through the eustachian tube the mucosa of the middle ear is continuous with the mucosal lining of the throat.

The inner ear is a system of osseous labyrinths (bony, mazelike chambers) filled with perilymph. The bony labyrinth is divided into the cochlea, the vestibule, and the semicircular canals (see Figure 13-11). Suspended in the perilymph is the endolymph-filled membranous labyrinth that basically follows the shape of the bony labyrinth.

Within the cochlea is the organ of Corti, which contains hair cells (hearing receptors). Sound waves that reach the cochlea through vibrations of the tympanic membrane, ossicles, and oval window set the cochlear fluids into motion. Receptor cells on the basilar membrane are stimulated when their hairs are bent or pulled by fluid movement. Once stimulated, hair cells transmit impulses along the cochlear nerve (a division of the vestibulocochlear nerve) to the auditory cortex of the temporal lobe in the brain (see Figure 13-12). This is where interpretation of the sound occurs.

The semicircular canals and vestibule of the inner ear contain equilibrium receptors. In the semicircular canals the dynamic equilibrium receptors respond to changes in direction of movement. Within each semicircular canal is the crista ampullaris, a receptor region composed of a tuft of hair cells covered by a gelatinous cupula. When the head is rotated, the endolymph in the canal lags behind and moves in the direction opposite to the head's movement. The hair cells are stimulated, and impulses are transmitted through the vestibular nerve (a division of the vestibulocochlear nerve) to the cerebellum.

The vestibule in the inner ear contains maculae—receptors essential to the body's sense of static equilibrium. As the head moves, otoliths (small pieces of calcium salts) move in a gel-like material in response to changes in the pull of gravity. The otoliths pull on the gel, which in turn pulls on the hair cells in the maculae. Nerve impulses in the hair cells are triggered and transmitted to the brain (see Figure 13-12). Thus the ear not only permits the hearing of a large range of

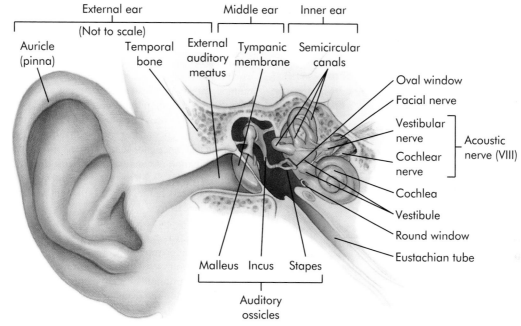

FIGURE 13-11 The Ear. External, middle, and inner ears. (Anatomic structures are not drawn to scale.) (From Thibodeau GA, Patton KT: *Anatomy & physiology,* ed 6, St Louis, 2007, Mosby.)

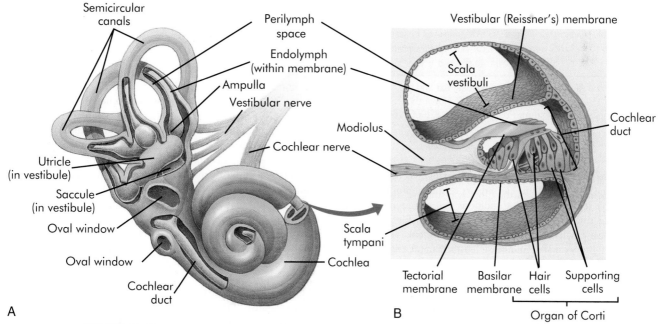

FIGURE 13-12 The Inner Ear. A, The bony labyrinth *(orange)* is the hard outer wall of the entire inner ear and includes the semicircular canals, vestibule, and cochlea. Within the bony labyrinth is the membranous labyrinth *(purple),* which is surrounded by perilymph and filled with endolymph. Each ampulla in the vestibule contains a crista ampullaris that detects changes in head position and sends sensory impulses through the vestibular nerve to the brain. **B,** The inset shows a section of the membranous cochlea. Hair cells in the organ of Corti detect sound and send the information through the cochlear nerve. The vestibular and cochlear nerves join to form the eighth cranial nerve. (From Thibodeau GA, Patton KT: *Anatomy & physiology,* ed 6, St Louis, 2007, Mosby.)

sounds but also assists with maintaining balance through the sensitive equilibrium receptors.

Auditory Dysfunction

Between 5% and 10% of the general population have impaired hearing, and it is the most common sensory defect. The major categories of auditory dysfunction are conductive hearing loss, sensorineural hearing loss, mixed hearing loss, and functional hearing loss.[78] Hearing loss may range from mild to profound. Auditory changes caused by aging are common and incremental (see the *Aging & Changes in Hearing* box).

GERIATRIC CONSIDERATIONS

Aging & Changes in Hearing

Hearing loss affects about 33% of older people.

CHANGES IN STRUCTURE	CHANGES IN FUNCTION
Cochlear hair cell degeneration	Inability to hear high-frequency sounds (presbycusis, sensorineural loss); interferes with understanding speech; hearing may be lost in both ears at different times
Loss of auditory neurons in spiral ganglia of organ of Corti	Inability to hear high-frequency sounds (presbycusis, sensorineural loss); interferes with understanding speech; hearing may be lost in both ears at different times
Degeneration of basilar (cochlear) conductive membrane of cochlea	Inability to hear at all frequencies but more pronounced at higher frequencies (cochlear conductive loss)
Decreased vascularity of cochlea	Equal loss of hearing at all frequencies (strial loss); inability to disseminate localization of sound
Loss of cortical auditory neurons	Equal loss of hearing at all frequencies (strial loss); inability to disseminate localization of sound

Data from Frisina RD: Age-related hearing loss: ear and brain mechanisms, *Ann N Y Acad Sci* 1170:708–717, 2009; Howarth A, Shone GR: Ageing and the auditory system, *Postgrad Med J* 82(965):166–171, 2009.

Conductive hearing loss. A conductive hearing loss occurs when a change in the outer or middle ear impairs conduction of the sound from the outer to the inner ear. Conditions that commonly cause a conductive hearing loss include impacted cerumen, foreign bodies lodged in the ear canal, benign tumors of the middle ear, carcinoma of the external auditory canal or middle ear, eustachian tube dysfunction, otitis media, acute viral otitis media, chronic suppurative otitis media, cholesteatoma, and otosclerosis.

Symptoms of conductive hearing loss include diminished hearing and soft speaking voice. The voice is soft because often the individual hears his or her voice, conducted by bone, as loud.

Sensorineural hearing loss. A sensorineural hearing loss is caused by impairment of the organ of Corti or its central connections. The loss may occur gradually or suddenly. Conditions causing sensorineural loss include congenital and hereditary factors, noise exposure, aging, Ménière disease, ototoxicity, systemic disease (syphilis, Paget disease, collagen diseases, diabetes mellitus), neoplasms, and autoimmune processes.[79] Congenital and neonatal sensorineural hearing loss may be caused by maternal rubella, ototoxic drugs, prematurity, traumatic delivery, erythroblastosis fetalis, and congenital hereditary malfunction. Diagnosis often is made when delayed speech development is noted.[80]

Presbycusis is the most common form of sensorineural hearing loss in elderly people. Its cause may be atrophy of the basal end of the organ of Corti, loss of auditory receptors, changes in vascularity, or stiffening of the basilar membranes. Drug ototoxicities (drugs that cause destruction of auditory function) have been observed after exposure to various chemicals; for example, antibiotics such as streptomycin, neomycin, gentamicin, and vancomycin; diuretics such as ethacrynic acid and furosemide; and chemicals such as salicylate, quinine, carbon monoxide, nitrogen mustard, arsenic, mercury, gold, tobacco, and alcohol. In most instances, the drugs and chemicals listed initially cause tinnitus (ringing in the ear), followed by a progressive high-tone sensorineural hearing loss that is permanent.

Mixed and functional hearing loss. A mixed hearing loss is caused by a combination of conductive and sensorineural losses. With functional hearing loss, which is rare, the individual does not respond to voice and appears not to hear. It is thought to be caused by emotional or psychologic factors.

Ménière disease. Ménière disease is a disorder of the middle ear with an unknown etiology that can be unilateral or bilateral. There is excessive endolymph and pressure in the membranous labyrinth that disrupts both vestibular and hearing functions. Recurring symptoms include profound vertigo, nausea and vomiting associated with deafness, and tinnitus (ringing in the ears). Treatment is symptomatic with either medical management or minimally invasive surgical management.[81]

Ear Infections

Otitis externa. Otitis externa is the most common inflammation of the outer ear and may be acute or chronic, infectious or noninfectious. The most common origins of acute infections are bacterial microorganisms including *Pseudomonas*, *Escherichia coli*, and *Staphylococcus aureus*. Fungal infections are less common. Infection usually follows prolonged exposure to moisture (swimmer's ear). The earliest symptoms are inflammation with pruritus, swelling, and clear drainage progressing to purulent drainage with obstruction of the canal. Tenderness and pain with earlobe retraction accompany inflammation. Acidifying solutions are used for early treatment and topical antimicrobials usually provide effective treatment for later stages of disease.[82] Chronic infections are more often related to allergy or skin disorders.

Otitis media. Otitis media is a common infection of infants and children. Most children have one episode by 3 years of age. The most common pathogens are *Streptococcus pneumoniae*, *Haemophilus influenzae*, and *Moraxella catarrhalis*. Predisposing factors include allergy, sinusitis, submucosal cleft palate, adenoidal hypertrophy, eustachian tube dysfunction, and immune deficiency. Breast-feeding is a protective factor. Recurrent acute otitis media may be genetically determined.[83]

Acute otitis media (AOM) is associated with ear pain, fever, irritability, inflamed tympanic membrane, and fluid in the middle ear. The appearance of the tympanic membrane progresses from erythema to opaqueness with bulging as fluid accumulates. There is an increasing prevalence of AOM caused by penicillin-resistant microorganisms. Otitis media with effusion (OME) is the presence of fluid in the middle ear without symptoms of acute infection.

Treatment includes symptom management, particularly of pain, with watchful waiting, antimicrobial therapy for severe illness, and placement of tympanotomy tubes when there is persistent bilateral effusion and significant hearing loss.[83] Complications include

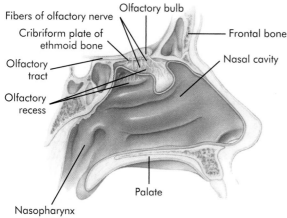

Fibers of olfactory nerve
Olfactory bulb
Cribriform plate of ethmoid bone
Olfactory tract
Olfactory recess
Frontal bone
Nasal cavity
Palate
Nasopharynx

FIGURE 13-13 Olfaction. Midsagittal section of the nasal area shows the location of major olfactory sensory structures. (From Thibodeau GA, Patton KT: *Anatomy & physiology*, ed 6, St Louis, 2007, Mosby.)

mastoiditis, brain abscess, meningitis, and chronic otitis media with hearing loss. Persistent middle ear effusions may affect speech, language, and cognitive abilities. Multivalent vaccines for prevention of otitis media are effective for reducing disease incidence.[84]

Olfaction and Taste

Olfaction (smell) is a function of cranial nerve I. Taste (gustation) is a function of multiple nerves in the tongue, soft palate, uvula, pharynx, and upper esophagus innervated by cranial nerves VII and IX. Both of these cranial nerves are influenced by hormones within the sensory cells. Dysfunctions of smell and taste may occur separately or jointly. The strong relationship between smell and taste creates the sensation of flavor. If either sensation is impaired, the perception of flavor is altered. Olfactory structures are illustrated in Figure 13-13.

Olfactory cells, located in the olfactory epithelium, are the receptor cells for smell. Seven different primary classes of olfactory stimulants have been identified: (1) camphoraceous, (2) musky, (3) floral, (4) peppermint, (5) ethereal, (6) pungent, and (7) putrid. The primary sensations of taste are (1) sour, (2) salty, (3) sweet, (4) bitter, and (5) umami (savoriness). Taste buds sensitive to each of the primary sensations are located in specific areas of the tongue.[85]

Sensitivity to odors declines steadily with aging. See the *Aging & Changes in Olfaction and Taste* box for a summary of changes in olfaction and taste with aging.

GERIATRIC CONSIDERATIONS

Aging & Changes in Olfaction and Taste

Decline in sensitivity to odors, usually after age 80, occurs.
Loss of olfaction may diminish appetite, taste, and food selection and may affect nutrition.
Inability to smell toxic fumes or gases can pose a safety hazard.
Decline in taste sensitivity is more gradual than decline in sense of smell.
Higher concentrations of flavors required to stimulate taste.
Taste may be influenced by decreased salivary secretion.

Olfactory and Taste Dysfunctions

Olfactory dysfunctions include the following:
1. Hyposmia—impaired sense of smell
2. Anosmia—complete loss of sense of smell

3. Olfactory hallucinations—smelling odors that are not really present
4. Parosmia—abnormal or perverted sense of smell

The sense of taste can be impaired by injury. Altered taste may be attributed to impaired smell associated with injury near the hippocampus.

Hypogeusia is a decrease in taste sensation, whereas ageusia is an absence of the sense of taste. These disorders result from cranial nerve injuries and can be specific to the area of the tongue innervated. Dysgeusia is a perversion of taste in which substances possess an unpleasant flavor (i.e., metallic). Alterations in taste may compromise adequate nutrition or cause anorexia.[86]

> ✔ **QUICK CHECK 13-4**
> 1. List the major structures of the eye.
> 2. Visual disorders fall into several categories; name them.
> 3. How does fluid accumulate in the middle ear during otitis media?
> 4. What factors are involved in the sensation of flavor?

SOMATOSENSORY FUNCTION

Touch

The sensation of touch involves four afferent fiber types that mediate tactile sensation and there may be an additional sensory nerve that transmits pleasurable touch.[87] Receptors sensitive to touch are present in the skin with high densities in the fingers and lips. Meissner and pacinian corpuscles are fast adapting receptors and sense movement across the skin and vibration, respectively. The slowly adapting Merkel disks sense sustained light touch, and Ruffini endings respond to deep sustained pressure, stretch, and joint position. Specific sensory input is carried to the higher levels of the CNS by the dorsal column of the spinal cord and the anterior spinothalamic tract.

The cutaneous senses develop before birth, but structural growth continues into early adulthood. Then a gradual decline occurs, with loss in tactile sensitivity with advancing age.[88]

Abnormal tactile perception may be caused by alterations at any level of the nervous system, from the receptor to the cerebral cortex. Factors that interrupt or impair reception, transmission, perception, or interpretation of touch—including trauma, tumor, infection, metabolic changes, vascular changes, and degenerative diseases—may cause tactile dysfunction. In addition, most tactile sensations evoke affective responses that determine whether the sensation is unpleasant, pleasant, or neutral.

Proprioception

Awareness of the position of the body and its parts depends on impulses from the inner ear and from receptors in joints and ligaments. Sensory data are transmitted to higher centers, primarily through the dorsal columns and the spinocerebellar tracts, with some data passing through the medial lemnisci and thalamic radiations to the cortex. These stimuli are necessary for the coordination of movements, the grading of muscular contraction, and the maintenance of equilibrium.

A progressive loss of proprioception has been reported in elderly persons.[89] As with tactile dysfunction, any factor that interrupts or impairs the reception, transmission, perception, or interpretation of proprioceptive stimuli also alters proprioception and increases risk for falls and injury. Two common causes are vestibular dysfunction and neuropathy.

Specific vestibular dysfunctions are vestibular nystagmus and vertigo. **Vestibular nystagmus** is the constant, involuntary movement of the eyeball and develops when the semicircular canal system is overstimulated. **Vertigo** is the sensation of spinning that occurs with inflammation of the semicircular canals in the ear. The individual may feel either that he or she is moving in space or that the world is revolving. Vertigo often causes loss of balance, and nystagmus may occur. Ménière disease can cause loss of proprioception during an acute attack, so that standing or walking is impossible.

Peripheral neuropathies also can cause proprioceptive dysfunction. They may be caused by several conditions and commonly are associated with renal disease and diabetes mellitus. Although the exact sequence of events is unknown, neuropathies cause a diminished or absent sense of body position or position of body parts. Gait changes often occur. (Neuropathies are discussed further in Chapter 14.)

✔ **QUICK CHECK 13-5**

1. How are different touch receptors distributed over the body?
2. What are two causes of alterations in proprioception?

DID YOU UNDERSTAND?

Pain

1. Pain is a complex phenomenon composed of sensory experiences (time, space, intensity) and emotion, cognition, and motivation.
2. The specificity theory of pain proposes that the intensity of pain is directly related to the degree of associated tissue injury. According to the gate control theory, specialized cells within the substantia gelatinosa act as a gate, opening and closing the afferent pathways to transmission of painful stimuli. The neuromatrix theory of pain proposes that chronic pain is related to multidimensional inputs triggered from the periphery or originating independently within the brain.
3. The portions of the nervous system responsible for the sensation and perception of pain may be divided into three areas: (a) the afferent fibers, (b) the central nervous system, and (c) the efferent pathways.
4. The afferent system is composed of nociceptors (Aδ and C fibers), the dorsal horn of the spinal column, and afferent neurons in the spinothalamic tract.
5. The thalamus, cortex, and postcentral gyrus perceive, describe, and localize pain. The reticular formation and limbic system control the emotional and affective response to pain.
6. Efferent pathways from the ventromedial thalamus and periaqueductal gray are responsible for modulation or inhibition of afferent pain signals.
7. Nociception is the processing of pain and includes four phases: transduction, transmission, perception, and modulation.
8. Neuromodulators of pain include substances that (a) stimulate pain nociceptors (e.g., prostaglandins, bradykinins, lymphokines, substance P, glutamate) and (b) suppress pain (e.g., GABA, endorphins). Some substances excite peripheral nerves but inhibit central nerves (e.g., serotonin, norepinephrine).
9. Endogenous opioids include enkephalins, endorphins, dynorphins, and endodorphins that inhibit pain transmission and are present in varying concentrations in the neurons of the brain, spinal cord, and gastrointestinal tract.
10. Classifications of pain include nociceptive pain (with a known physiologic cause), non-nociceptive pain (neurologic pain), acute pain (signal to the person of a harmful stimulus), and chronic pain (persistence of pain of unknown cause or unusual response to therapy).
11. Acute pain may be (a) somatic (superficial), (b) visceral (internal), or (c) referred (present in an area distant from its origin). The area of referred pain is supplied by the same spinal segment as the actual site of pain.
12. Chronic pain is pain lasting well beyond the expected normal healing time and may be intermittent (e.g., low back pain) or persistent (e.g., migraine headaches).
13. Psychologic, behavioral, and physiologic responses to chronic pain include depression, sleep disorders, preoccupation with pain, lifestyle changes, and physiologic adaptation.
14. Neuropathic pain is increased sensitivity to painful stimuli and results from abnormal processing of pain information in the peripheral or central nervous system.
15. *Pain threshold* is the least experience of pain that a person can recognize. *Pain tolerance* is the greatest level of pain that an individual is prepared to tolerate. Both are subjective and influenced by many factors.
16. Pain threshold in older individuals varies.
17. Newborns and young children have the anatomic and functional ability to perceive pain.
18. Older individuals tend to have a slightly higher pain threshold, probably because of changes in the thickness of the skin and peripheral neuropathies.
19. Women appear to be more sensitive to pain than are men in all age groups.

Temperature Regulation

1. Temperature regulation is achieved through precise balancing of heat production, heat conservation, and heat loss. Body temperature is maintained in a range around 37° C (98.6° F).
2. Temperature regulation is mediated by the hypothalamus through thermoreceptors in the skin, hypothalamus, spinal cord, and abdominal organs.
3. Heat is produced through chemical reactions of metabolism, skeletal muscle contraction, and vasoconstriction.
4. Heat is lost through radiation, conduction, convection, vasodilation, decreased muscle tone, evaporation of sweat, increased respiration, and voluntary mechanisms.
5. Heat conservation is accomplished through vasoconstriction and voluntary mechanisms.
6. Infants do not conserve heat well because of their greater body surface/mass ratio and decreased amounts of subcutaneous fat. Elderly persons have poor responses to environmental temperature extremes as a result of slowed blood circulation, structural and functional changes in the skin, and overall decrease in heat-producing activities.
7. Fever is triggered by the release of exogenous pyrogens from bacteria or the release of endogenous pyrogens (cytokines) from phagocytic cells. Fever is both a normal immunologic mechanism and a symptom of disease.
8. Fever involves the "resetting of the hypothalamic thermostat" to a higher level. When the fever breaks, the set point returns to normal.
9. Fever production aids responses to infectious processes. Higher temperatures kill many microorganisms and decrease serum levels of iron, zinc, and copper that are needed for bacterial replication.
10. Fever of unknown origin is a body temperature greater than 38.3° C (101° F) that remains undiagnosed.
11. Hyperthermia (marked warming of core temperature) can produce nerve damage, coagulation of cell proteins, and death. Forms of accidental hyperthermia include heat cramps, heat exhaustion, heat stroke, and malignant hyperthermia. Heat stroke and malignant hyperthermia are potentially lethal.

DID YOU UNDERSTAND?—cont'd

12. Hypothermia (marked cooling of core temperature) slows the rate of chemical reaction (tissue metabolism), increases the viscosity of the blood, slows blood flow through the microcirculation, facilitates blood coagulation, and stimulates profound vasoconstriction. Hypothermia may be accidental or therapeutic.

Sleep

1. Sleep is an active process and is divided into REM and non-REM stages, each of which has its own series of stages. While asleep, an individual progresses through REM and non-REM (slow wave) sleep in a predictable cycle.
2. REM sleep is controlled by mechanisms in the pons and mesencephalon. Non-REM sleep is controlled by release of inhibitory signals from the hypothalamus and accounts for 75% to 80% of sleep time.
3. The sleep patterns of the newborn and young child vary from those of the adult in total sleep time, cycle length, and percentage of time spent in each sleep cycle. Elderly persons experience a total decrease in sleep time.
4. The restorative, reparative, and growth processes occur during slow-wave (non-REM) sleep. Sleep deprivation can cause profound changes in personality and functioning.
5. Sleep disorders include (a) dyssomnias (disorders of initiating sleep [i.e., insomnia, sleep disordered breathing, hypersomnia, or disorders of the sleep-wake schedule]) and (b) parasomnias (i.e., sleepwalking or night terrors).
6. Restless leg syndrome is associated with unpleasant sensations and a compelling urge to move the legs that disrupts sleep.

The Special Senses

1. The wall of the eye has three layers: sclera, choroid, and retina. The retina contains millions of baroreceptors known as rods and cones that receive light through the lens and then convey signals to the optic nerve and subsequently to the visual cortex of the brain.
2. The eye is filled with vitreous and aqueous humor, which prevent it from collapsing.
3. The eyelids, conjunctiva, and lacrimal apparatus protect the eye. Infections are the most common disorders; they include blepharitis, conjunctivitis, chalazion, and hordeolum.
4. Structural eye changes caused by aging result in decreased visual acuity.
5. The major alterations in ocular movement include strabismus, nystagmus, and paralysis of the extraocular muscles.
6. Alterations in visual acuity can be caused by amblyopia, scotoma, cataracts, papilledema, glaucoma, and macular degeneration.
7. Alterations in accommodation develop with increased intraocular pressure, inflammation, and disease of the oculomotor nerve. Presbyopia is loss of accommodation caused by loss of elasticity of the lens with aging.
8. Alterations in refraction, including myopia, hyperopia, and astigmatism, are the most common visual disorders.
9. Alterations in color vision can be related to yellowing of the lens with aging and color blindness, an inherited trait.
10. Trauma or disease of the optic nerve pathways, or optic radiations, can cause blindness in the visual fields. Homonymous hemianopsia is caused by damage of one optic tract.
11. Blepharitis is an inflammation of the eyelid; a hordeolum (stye) is an infection of the eyelid's sebaceous gland; and chalazion is an infection of the eyelid's meibomian gland.

12. Conjunctivitis can be acute or chronic, bacterial, viral, or allergic. Redness, edema, pain, and lacrimation are common symptoms. Chlamydial conjunctivitis is the leading cause of blindness in the world and is associated with poor sanitary conditions.
13. Keratitis is a bacterial or viral infection of the cornea that can lead to corneal ulceration. Photophobia, pain, and tearing are common symptoms.
14. The ear is composed of external, middle, and inner structures. The external structures are the pinna, auditory canal, and tympanic membrane. The tympanic cavity (containing three bones: the malleus, the incus, and the stapes), oval window, eustachian tube, and fluid compose the middle ear and transmit sound vibrations to the inner ear.
15. The inner ear includes the bony and membranous labyrinths that transmit sound waves through the cochlea to the acoustic division of the eighth cranial nerve. The semicircular canals and vestibule help maintain balance through the equilibrium receptors.
16. Approximately one third of all people older than 65 years have hearing loss.
17. Hearing loss can be classified as conductive, sensorineural, mixed, or functional.
18. Conductive hearing loss occurs when sound waves cannot be conducted through the middle ear.
19. Sensorineural hearing loss develops with impairment of the organ of Corti or its central connections. Presbycusis is the most common form of sensorineural hearing loss in elderly people.
20. A combination of conductive and sensorineural loss is a mixed hearing loss.
21. Loss of hearing with no known organic cause is a functional hearing loss.
22. Ménière disease is a disorder of the middle ear that affects hearing and balance.
23. Otitis externa is an infection of the outer ear associated with prolonged exposure to moisture.
24. Otitis media is an infection of the middle ear that is common in children. Accumulation of fluid (effusion) behind the tympanic membrane is a common finding.
25. The perception of flavor is altered if olfaction or taste dysfunctions occur. Sensitivity to odor and taste decreases with aging.
26. Hyposmia is a decrease in the sense of smell, and anosmia is the complete loss of the sense of smell. Inflammation of the nasal mucosa and trauma or tumors of the olfactory nerve lead to a diminished sense of smell.
27. Hypogeusia is a decrease in taste sensation, and ageusia is the absence of the sense of taste. Loss of taste buds or trauma to the facial or glossopharyngeal nerves decreases taste sensation.

Somatosensory Function

1. Tactile sensation is a function of receptors present in the skin (pacinian corpuscles), and the sensory response is conducted to the brain through the dorsal column and anterior spinothalamic tract.
2. Alterations in touch can result from disruption of skin receptors, sensory transmission, or central nervous system perception.
3. Proprioception is the position and location of the body and its parts. Proprioceptors are located in the inner ear, joints, and ligaments. Proprioceptive stimuli are necessary for balance, coordinated movement, and grading of muscular contraction.
4. Disorders of proprioception can occur at any level of the nervous system and result in impaired balance and lack of coordinated movement.

KEY TERMS

- A-beta (Aβ) fiber 325
- Accidental hyperthermia 332
- Acute bacterial conjunctivitis (pinkeye) 337
- Acute otitis media (AOM) 340
- Acute pain 327
- A-delta (Aδ) fiber 325
- Affective-motivational system 326
- Age-related macular degeneration (AMD) 336
- Ageusia 341
- Allergic conjunctivitis 338
- Amblyopia 336
- Anosmia 341
- Aqueous humor 335
- Astigmatism 337
- Blepharitis 337
- Central neuropathic pain 328
- Central sensitization 326
- C fiber 325
- Chalazion 337
- Choroid 335
- Chronic conjunctivitis 338
- Chronic pain 328
- Circadian rhythm 330
- Cochlea 338
- Cognitive-evaluative system 326
- Color blindness 337
- Conductive hearing loss 340
- Cone 335
- Conjunctivitis 337
- Cornea 335
- Crista ampullaris 338
- Descending inhibitory pathway 327
- Diffuse noxious inhibitory control (DNIC) 327
- Diplopia 336
- Dynorphin 327
- Dysgeusia 341
- Dyssomnia 334
- Endogenous opioid 327
- Endogenous pyrogen 331
- Endomorphin 327
- Endorphin 327
- Enkephalin 327
- Equilibrium receptor 338
- Eustachian (pharyngotympanic) tube 338
- Excitatory neuromodulator 326
- Exogenous pyrogen 331
- External auditory canal 338
- Fever 331
- Fever of unknown origin (FUO) 331

- Fovea centralis 335
- Functional hearing loss 340
- Gate control theory (GCT) 325
- Glaucoma 336
- Hair cell 338
- Heat cramp 332
- Heat exhaustion 332
- Heat stroke 332
- Hordeolum (stye) 337
- Hyperopia 337
- Hypersomnia 334
- Hyperthermia 331
- Hypogeusia 341
- Hyposmia 341
- Hypothermia 333
- Incus (anvil) 338
- Inhibitory neuromodulator 327
- Insomnia 334
- Iris 335
- Jerk nystagmus 336
- Keratitis 338
- Lens 335
- Macula lutea 335
- Maculae 339
- Malignant hyperthermia 332
- Malleus (hammer) 338
- Mastoid air cell 338
- Mastoid process 338
- Meissner corpuscle 341
- Ménière disease 340
- Merkel disk 341
- Mixed hearing loss 340
- Myopia 337
- Narcolepsy 334
- Neuromatrix theory 325
- Neuropathic pain 328
- Night terrors 334
- Nociception 325
- Nociceptor 325
- Non-REM sleep (NREM) 334
- Nystagmus 336
- Obstructive sleep apnea syndrome (OSAS) 334
- Olfactory hallucination 341
- Optic chiasm 337
- Optic disc 335
- Organ of Corti 338
- Otitis externa 340
- Otitis media 340
- Otitis media with effusion (OME) 340
- Otolith 339
- Oval window 338

- Pacinian corpuscle 341
- Pain modulation 326
- Pain perception 326
- Pain threshold 329
- Pain tolerance 329
- Pain transduction 325
- Pain transmission 325
- Parasomnia 334
- Parosmia 341
- Pattern theory 325
- Pendular nystagmus 336
- Perceptual dominance 329
- Perilymph 338
- Peripheral neuropathic pain 328
- Peripheral sensitization 326
- Persistent pain 328
- Pinna 338
- Presbycusis 340
- Presbyopia 337
- Pupil 335
- Referred pain 328
- REM (rapid eye movement) sleep 333
- Restless leg syndrome (RLS) 334
- Retina 335
- Rod 335
- Ruffini ending 341
- Sclera 335
- Semicircular canal 338
- Sensorineural hearing loss 340
- Sensory-discriminative system 326
- Sleep 333
- Somatic pain 327
- Somnambulism (sleepwalking) 334
- Specificity theory of pain 324
- Stapes (stirrup) 338
- Strabismus 335
- Suprachiasmatic nucleus (SCN) 333
- Temperature regulation (thermoregulation) 330
- Therapeutic hyperthermia 331
- Tinnitus 340
- Trachoma 338
- Tympanic cavity 338
- Tympanic membrane 338
- Vertigo 342
- Vestibular nystagmus 342
- Vestibule 338
- Viral conjunctivitis 338
- Visceral pain 327
- Vitreous humor 335

REFERENCES

1. McCaffery M: *Nursing practice theories related to cognition, bodily pain and nonenvironment interactions*, Los Angeles Calif, 1968, University of California at Los Angeles Students' Store.
2. International Association for the Study of Pain (IASP): *IASP pain terminology*. Available at www.iasp-pain.org/AM/Template.cfm?Section=pain_Definitions&;Template=/CM/HTMLDisplay.cfm&ContentIK=1728#Pain. Accessed April, 2011.
3. American Society for Pain Management Nursing. In St. Marie B, editor: *Core curriculum for pain management nursing*, ed 2, Dubuque, Iowa, 2010, Kendall Hunt Publishing.
4. Melzack R, Wall PD: Pain mechanisms: a new theory, *Science* 150:971–979, 1965.
5. Arnstein P: *Clinical coach for effective pain management*, Philadelphia, 2010, FA Davis.
6. Helms JE, Barone CP: Physiology and treatment of pain, *Crit Care Nurs* 28:38–49, 2008.
7. Melzack R: Toward a new concept of pain for the new millenium. In Waldman SD, editor: *Interventional pain management*, ed 2, Philadelphia, 2001, Saunders.
8. Melzack R: Evolution of the neuromatrix theory of pain, *Pain Pract* 5(2):85–94, 2005.
9. Pasero C, McCaffery M: *Pain assessment and pharmacologic management*, St Louis, 2011, Mosby.
10. Marchand S: The physiology of pain mechanisms: from the periphery to the brain, *Rheum Dis Clin N Am* 34:285–309, 2008.
11. Argoff CE, et al: Multimodal analgesia for chronic pain: rationale and future directions, *Pain Med* 10(S2):S53–S66, 2009.
12. Casey KL: Forebrain mechanisms of nociception and pain: analysis through imaging, *Proc Natl Acad Sci U S A* 96(14):7668–7674, 1999.
13. Michael Ossipov H, Gregory Dussor O, Frank Porreca: Central modulation of pain, *J Clin Invest* 120(11):3779–3787, 2010.
14. Fields HL, Basbaum AL, Heinricher MM: Central nervous system mechanism of pain modulation. In McMahon S, Koltzenburg M, editors: *Wall and Melzack's textbook of pain*, ed 5, Edinburgh, Scotland, 2005, Churchill Livingstone.
15. Basbaum AI, et al: Cellular and molecular mechanisms of pain, *Cell* 139:267–284, 2009.
16. Bodnar RJ: Endogenous opiates and behavior: 2009, *Peptides* 31(12):2325–2359, 2010.
17. Busch-Dienstfertig M, Stein C: Opioid receptors and opioid peptide-producing leukocytes in inflammatory pain–basic and therapeutic aspects, *Brain Behav Immun* 24(5):683–694, 2010.
18. Lai J, et al: Pronociceptive actions of dynorphin via bradykinin receptors, *Neurosci Lett* 437(3):175–179, 2008.
19. Wolleman M, Benyhe S: Non-opioid actions of opioid peptides, *Life Sci* 75(30):257–270, 2004.
20. Fichna J, et al: The endomorphin system and its evolving neurophysiological role, *Pharmacol Rev* 59(1):88–123, 2007.
21. Mason P: Deconstructing endogenous pain modulations, *J Neurophysiol* 94(3):1659–1663, 2005.
21a. avanWijk G, Veldhuijzen DS: Perspective on diffuse noxious inhibitory controls as a model of endogenous pain modulation in clinical pain syndromes, *J Pain* 11(5):408–419, 2010.
22. American Pain Society: *Principles of analgesic use in the treatment of acute pain and cancer pain*, ed 6, Glenview, Ill, 2008, Author.
23. Costigan M, Scholz J, Woolf CJ: Neuropathic pain: a maladaptive response of the nervous system to damage, *Annu Rev Neurosci* 32:1–32, 2009.
24. Thibodeau GA, Patton KT: *Anatomy & physiology*, ed 5, St Louis, 2003, Mosby.
25. Apkarian AV, Baliki MN, Geha PY: Towards a theory of chronic pain, *Prog Neurobiol* 87(2):81–97, 2009.
26. Voscopoulos C, Lema M: When does acute pain become chronic? *Br J Anaesth* 105(Suppl 1):i69–i85, 2010.
27. May A: Chronic pain may change the structure of the brain, *Pain* 137:7–15, 2008.
28. Rodriquez-Raecke R, et al: Brain gray matter decrease in chronic pain is the consequence and not the cause of pain, *J Neurosci* 29(44):12746–12750, 2009.
29. Tracey I, Bushnell MC: How neuroimaging studies have challenged us to rethink: is chronic pain a disease? *J Pain* 10(11):1113–1120, 2009.
30. Gatchel RJ, et al: The biopsychosocial approach to chronic pain: scientific advances and future directions, *Psychol Bull* 133(4):581–624, 2007:review.
31. Morley S: Psychology of pain, *Br J Anaesth* 101(1):25–31, 2008.
32. Miles A, et al: Managing constraint: the experience of people with chronic pain, *Soc Sci Med* 61(2):431–441, 2005.
33. Zhou M: Neuronal mechanism for neuropathic pain, *Mol Pain* 3:14, 2007.
34. Vallejo R, et al: The role of glia and the immune system in the development and maintenance of neuropathic pain, *Pain Pract* 19(3):167–184, 2010.
35. Haanpaa ML, et al: Assessment of neuropathic pain in primary care, *Am J Med* 122(10A):S13–S21, 2009.
36. Schaible HG: Peripheral and central mechanisms of pain generation, *Handb Exp Pharmacol* 177:3–28, 2007.
37. Turk DC, Okifuji A: Psychological factors in chronic pain: evolution and resolution, *J Consult Clin Psychol* 70(3):678–690, 2002.
38. Sessler DI: Thermoregulatory defense mechanisms, *Crit Care Med* 37(7 suppl):S203–S210, 2009.
39. Rothwell NJ: CNS regulation of thermogenesis, *Crit Rev Neurobiol* 8(1–2):1–10, 1994.
40. Baumgart S: Iatrogenic hyperthermia and hypothermia in the neonate, *Clin Perinatol* 35(1):183–197, 2008:ix–x.
41. Holowatz LA, Thompson-Torgerson C, Kenney WL: Aging and the control of human skin blood flow, *Front Biosci* 15:718–739, 2010.
42. Degroot DW, et al: Compromised respiratory adaptation and thermoregulation in aging and age-related diseases, *Ageing Res Rev* 9(1):20–40, 2010.
43. Romanovsky AA, et al: Fever and hypothermia in systemic inflammation: recent discoveries and revisions, *Front Biosci* 10:2193–2216, 2005.
44. Tolan RW Jr: Fever of unknown origin: a diagnostic approach to this vexing problem, *Clin Pediatr (Phila)* 49(3):207–213, 2010.
45. Barone JE: Fever: fact and fiction, *J Trauma* 67(2):406–409, 2009.
46. Laupland KB: Fever in the critically ill medical patient, *Crit Care Med* 37(suppl 7):S273–S278, 2009.
47. BMJ Group: When the child has a fever, *Drug Ther Bull* 46(3):17–21, 2008.
48. Laupland KB: Fever in the critically ill medical patient, *Crit Care Med* 37(suppl 7):S273–S278, 2009.
49. Roghmann MC, Warner J, Mackowiak PA: The relationship between age and fever magnitude, *Am J Med Sci* 322(2):68–70, 2001.
50. Badjatia N: Hyperthermia and fever control in brain injury, *Crit Care Med* 37(suppl 7):S250–S257, 2009.
51. Palazzi M, et al: The role of hyperthermia in the battle against cancer, *Tumori* 96(6):902–910, 2010.
52. Glazer JL: Management of heatstroke and heat exhaustion, *Am Fam Physician* 71(11):2133–2140, 2005.
53. Litman RS, RosenbergH: Malignant hyperthermia: update on susceptibility testing, *J Am Med Assoc* 293(23):2918–2924, 2005.
54. Wappler F: Anesthesia for patients with a history of malignant hyperthermia, *Curr Opin Anaesthesiol* 23(3):417–422, 2010.
55. Moore RY: Suprachiasmatic nucleus in sleep-wake regulation, *Sleep Med* 8(suppl 3):27–33, 2007.
56. Datta S: Cellular and chemical neuroscience of mammalian sleep, *Sleep Med* 11(5):431–440, 2010.
57. McCarley RW: Neurobiology of REM and NREM sleep, *Sleep Med* 8(4):302–330, 2007.
58. Lu BS, Zee PC: Neurobiology of sleep, *Clin Chest Med* 31(2):309–318, 2010.
59. American Academy of Sleep Medicine, Diagnostic Classification Steering Committee: *International classification of sleep disorders, revised: diagnostic and coding manual*, 2005, Author, Westchester, Ill.
60. Mai E: Insomnia: prevalence, impact, pathogenesis, differential diagnosis, and evaluation, *Sleep Med Clin* 3(2):167–174, 2008.
61. Butt M, et al: Obstructive sleep apnea and cardiovascular disease, *Int J Cardiol* 139(1):7–16, 2010.

62. Lieberman JA III: Obstructive sleep apnea (OSA) and excessive sleepiness associated with OSA: recognition in the primary care setting, *Postgrad Med* 121(4):33–41, 2009.

63. Epstein LJ, et al: Adult Obstructive Sleep Apnea Task Force of the American Academy of Sleep Medicine: Clinical guideline for the evaluation, management and long-term care of obstructive sleep apnea in adults, *J Clin Sleep Med* 5(3):263–276, 2009.

64. Vlastos IM, Hajiioannou JK: Clinical practice: diagnosis and treatment of childhood snoring, *Eur J Pediatr* 169(3):261–267, 2010.

65. Mohsenin V: Narcolepsy—master of disguise: evidence-based recommendations for management, *Postgrad Med* 121(3):99–104, 2009.

66. Drake CL: The characterization and pathology of circadian rhythm sleep disorders, *J Fam Pract* 59(suppl 1):S12–S17, 2010.

67. Matwiyoff G, Lee-Chiong T: Parasomnias: an overview, *Indian J Med Res* 131:333–337, 2010.

68. Guilleminault C, et al: Adult chronic sleepwalking and its treatment based on polysomnography, *Brain* 128(Pt 5):1062–1069, 2005.

69. Salas RE, Gamaldo CE, Allen RP: Update in restless legs syndrome, *Curr Opin Neurol* 23(4):401–406, 2010.

70. Crossman AR, Neary D: *Neuroanatomy: an illustrated color text*, ed 4, London, 2010, Churchill Livingstone.

71. Agarwal R, et al: Current concepts in the pathophysiology of glaucoma, *Indian J Ophthalmol* 57(4):257–266, 2009.

72. Dietlein TS, Hermann MM, Jordan JF: The medical and surgical treatment of glaucoma, *Dtsch Arztebl Int* 106(37):597–605, 2009.

73. Prasad PS, Schwartz SD, Hubschman JP: Age-related macular degeneration, current and novel therapies, *Maturitas* 66(1):46–50, 2010.

74. Farid M, Steinert RF: Patient selection for monovision laser refractive surgery, *Curr Opin Ophthalmol* 20(4):251–254, 2009.

75. Gupta N, Wolffsohn JS, Naroo SA: Comparison of near visual acuity and reading metrics in presbyopia correction, *J Cataract Refract Surg* 35(8):1401–1409, 2009.

76. Deeb SS: The molecular basis of variation in human color vision, *Clin Genet* 67(5):369–377, 2005.

77. Cronau H, Kankanala RR, Mauger T: Diagnosis and management of red eye in primary care, *Am Fam Physician* 81(2):137–144, 2010.

78. Isaacson B: Hearing loss, *Med Clin North Am* 94(5):973–988, 2010.

79. Kozak AT, Grundfast KM: Hearing loss, *Otolaryngol Clin North Am* 42(1):79–85, 2009.

80. Katbamna B, Crumpton T, Patel DR: Hearing impairment in children, *Pediatr Clin North Am* 55(5):1175–1188, 2008.

81. Sajjadi H, Paparella MM: Ménière's disease, *Lancet* 372(9636):406–414, 2008.

82. Kaushik V, Malik T, Saeed SR: Interventions for acute otitis externa, *Cochrane Database Syst Rev* (1) CD004740, 2010.

83. Morris PS, Leach AJ: Acute and chronic otitis media, *Pediatr Clin North Am* 56(6):1383–1399, 2009.

84. Schuerman L, et al: Prevention of otitis media: now a reality? *Vaccine* 27(42):5748–5754, 2009.

85. Martin B, et al: Hormones in the naso-oropharynx: endocrine modulation of taste and smell, *Trends Endocrinol Metab* 20(4):163–170, 2009.

86. Visvanathan R, Chapman IM: Undernutrition and anorexia in the older person, *Gastroenterol Clin North Am* 38(3):393–409, 2009.

87. McGlone F, Reilly D: The cutaneous sensory system, *Neurosci Biobehav Rev* 34(2):148–159, 2010.

88. Humes LE, et al: The effects of age on sensory thresholds and temporal gap detection in hearing, vision, and touch, *Atten Percept Psychophys* 71(4):860–871, 2009.

89. Goble DJ, et al: Proprioceptive sensibility in the elderly: degeneration, functional consequences and plastic-adaptive processes, *Neurosci Biobehav Rev* 33(3):271–278, 2009.

Alterations in Cognitive Systems, Cerebral Hemodynamics, and Motor Function

Barbara J. Boss and Sue E. Huether

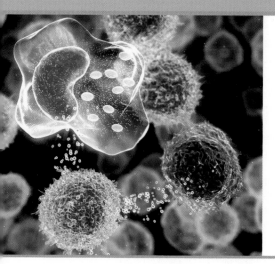

CHAPTER OUTLINE

A person achieves functional adequacy (competence) through complex integrated processes. Three major neural systems account for this functional adequacy: cognitive systems, sensory systems, and motor systems. Alterations in any or all of these affect functional adequacy. The neural systems that are essential to cognitive function are (1) attentional systems that provide arousal and maintenance of attention over time; (2) memory and language systems by which information is communicated; and (3) affective or emotive systems that mediate mood, emotion, and intention. These core systems are fundamental to the processes of abstract thinking and reasoning. The products of abstraction and reasoning are organized and made operational through the executive attentional networks. The normal functioning of these networks manifests through the motor network in a behavioral array viewed by others as appropriate to human activity and successful living.

ALTERATIONS IN COGNITIVE SYSTEMS

Full **consciousness** is a state of awareness both of oneself and the environment and a set of responses to that environment. The fully conscious individual responds to external stimuli with a wide array of responses. Any decrease in this state of awareness and varied responses is a decrease in consciousness.

Consciousness involves arousal and awareness (content of thought). **Arousal** is an individual's state of awakeness. Arousal is mediated by the reticular activating system, which regulates aspects of attention and information processing and maintains consciousness. When a person loses cerebral function, the reticular activating system and brain stem can maintain a crude waking state known as a **vegetative state (VS)**. Cognitive cerebral functions, however, cannot occur without a functioning reticular activating system.

Alterations in Arousal

The cause of an altered level of arousal may be organic or functional. Further distinction is then made between structural, metabolic, or psychogenic arousal alterations.

Pathophysiology. Structural alterations in arousal are divided according to whether the original location of the pathologic condition is above or below the tentorial plate. Structural causes include infectious, vascular, neoplastic, traumatic, congenital (developmental), degenerative, polygenic, and metabolic causes.

TABLE 14-1   CLINICAL MANIFESTATIONS OF METABOLIC AND STRUCTURAL CAUSES OF ALTERED AROUSAL

MANIFESTATIONS	METABOLICALLY INDUCED	STRUCTURALLY INDUCED
Blink to threat (cranial nerves II, VII)	Equal	Asymmetric
Optic discs (cranial nerve II)	Flat, good pulsation	Papilledema
Extraocular movement (cranial nerves III, IV, VI)	Roving eye movements; normal doll's eyes and calorics	Gaze paresis, nerve palsy
Pupils (cranial nerves II, III)	Equal and reactive; may be dilated (e.g., atropine), pinpoint (e.g., opiates), or midposition and fixed (e.g., glutethimide [Doriden])	Asymmetric or nonreactive; may be midposition (midbrain injury), pinpoint (pons injury), large (tectal injury)
Corneal reflex (cranial nerves V, VII)	Symmetric response	Asymmetric response
Grimace to pain (cranial nerve VII)	Symmetric response	Asymmetric response
Motor function movement	Symmetric	Asymmetric
Muscle tone	Symmetric	Paratonic (rigid), spastic, flaccid, especially if asymmetric
Posture	Symmetric	Decorticate, especially if symmetric; decerebrate, especially if asymmetric (see Figure 14-6)
Deep tendon reflexes	Symmetric	Asymmetric
Babinski sign	Absent or symmetric response	Present
Sensation	Symmetric	Asymmetric

Disorders above the tentorial plate (supratentorial) produce changes in arousal by either diffuse or localized dysfunction. Diffuse dysfunction may be caused by disease processes (e.g., encephalitis) and may affect the cerebral cortex or the underlying subcortical white matter. Disorders outside the brain but within the cranial vault can produce diffuse dysfunction. Examples include neoplasms, closed-head trauma with subsequent subdural bleeding, and accumulation of pus in the subdural space. Localized dysfunction generally is caused by masses that directly impinge on deep diencephalic structures (i.e., thalamus and hypothalamus) or that secondarily compress these structures in the process of herniation. Disorders within the brain substance—bleeding, infarcts, emboli, and tumors—function primarily as masses. Such localized destructive processes directly impair function of the thalamic or hypothalamic activating systems.

Disorders below the tentorial plate (infratentorial) produce a decline in arousal by direct destruction of the reticular activating system and its pathways or of the entire brain stem either by direct invasion or by indirect impairment of its blood supply. In addition, decreased arousal may result from compression of the reticular activating system by a disease process. This compression may result from direct pressure or compression as structures either expand or herniate. Causes include accumulations of blood or pus, neoplasms, and demyelinating disorders.

Metabolic alterations in arousal include hypoxia, electrolyte disturbances, hypoglycemia, drugs, and toxins (both endogenous and exogenous). All the systemic diseases that eventually produce nervous system dysfunction are part of this metabolic category. Alterations in arousal range from slight drowsiness to coma.

Psychogenic alterations in arousal (unresponsiveness), although uncommon, may signal general psychiatric disorders. Despite apparent unconsciousness, the person actually is physiologically awake.

Clinical manifestations and evaluation. Patterns of clinical manifestations help in determining the extent of brain dysfunction and serve as indexes for identifying increasing or decreasing central nervous system (CNS) function. Distinctions are made between metabolic and structurally induced manifestations (Table 14-1). The types of manifestations suggest the cause of the altered arousal state (Table 14-2). Five categories of neurologic function are critical to the evaluation process: (1) level of consciousness, (2) pattern of breathing, (3) pupillary reaction, (4) oculomotor responses, and (5) motor responses.

TABLE 14-2   DIFFERENTIAL CHARACTERISTICS OF STATES CAUSING ALTERED AROUSAL

MECHANISM	MANIFESTATIONS
Supratentorial mass lesions compressing or displacing diencephalon or brain stem	Initiating signs usually of focal cerebral dysfunction: vomiting, headache, hemiparesis, ocular signs, seizures, coma
	Signs of dysfunction progress rostral to caudal
	Neurologic signs at any given time point to one anatomic area (e.g., diencephalon, mesencephalon, medulla)
	Motor signs often asymmetric
Infratentorial mass of destruction causing coma	History of preceding brain stem dysfunction or sudden onset of coma
	Localizing brain stem signs precede or accompany onset of coma and always include oculovestibular abnormality
	Cranial nerve palsies usually manifest
Metabolic coma	"bizarre" respiratory patterns that appear at onset
	Confusion and stupor commonly precede motor signs
Psychiatric unresponsiveness	Motor signs usually are symmetric
	Pupillary reactions usually are preserved
	Asterixis, myoclonus, tremor, and seizures are common
	Acid-base imbalance with hyperventilation or hypoventilation is common
	Lids close actively
	Pupils reactive or dilated (cycloplegics)
	Oculocephalic reflexes are unpredictable; oculovestibular reflexes are physiologic (nystagmus is present)
	Motor tone is inconsistent or normal
	Eupnea or hyperventilation is usual
	No pathologic reflexes are present
	Electroencephalogram (EEG) is normal

Level of consciousness is the most critical clinical index of nervous system function, with changes indicating either improvement or deterioration of the individual's condition. A person who is alert and oriented to self, others, place, and time is considered to be functioning at the highest level of consciousness, which implies full use of all the person's cognitive capacities. From this normal alert state, levels of consciousness diminish in stages from confusion to coma, each of which is clinically defined (Table 14-3).

Patterns of breathing help evaluate the level of brain dysfunction and coma (Figure 14-1). Rate, rhythm, and pattern should be evaluated. Breathing patterns can be categorized as hemispheric or brain stem patterns (Table 14-4).

With normal breathing, a neural center in the forebrain (cerebrum) produces a rhythmic pattern. When consciousness decreases, lower brain stem centers regulate the breathing pattern by responding only to changes in $Paco_2$ levels; this is called *posthyperventilation apnea*. *Cheyne-Stokes respirations* are an abnormal pattern of ventilation with alternating periods of tachypnea and apnea (crescendo-decrescendo pattern). Increases in $Paco_2$ levels lead to tachypnea. The $Paco_2$ level then decreases to below normal and breathing stops (apnea) until the carbon dioxide reaccumulates and again stimulates tachypnea (see Figure 14-1). With opiate or sedative drug overdose, the respiratory center is depressed so the rate of breathing gradually decreases until respiratory failure occurs.

Pupillary changes indicate the presence and level of brain stem dysfunction because brain stem areas that control arousal are adjacent to areas that control the pupils (Figure 14-2). For example, severe ischemia and hypoxia usually produce dilated, fixed pupils. Hypothermia may cause fixed pupils.

Some drugs affect pupils and must be considered in evaluating individuals in comatose states. Large concentrations of atropine and scopolamine fully dilate and fix pupils. Doses of sedatives (e.g., glutethimide) may be sufficient to produce a coma, causing the pupils to become midposition or moderately dilated, unequal, and commonly fixed to light. Opiates cause pinpoint pupils. Severe barbiturate intoxication may produce fixed pupils.

Oculomotor responses (resting, spontaneous, and reflexive eye movements) change at various levels of brain dysfunction in comatose individuals. Persons with metabolically induced coma, except with barbiturate-hypnotic and phenytoin poisoning, generally retain ocular reflexes even when other signs of brain stem damage are present. Destructive or compressive injury to the brain stem causes specific abnormalities of the oculocephalic and oculovestibular reflexes

TABLE 14-3	LEVELS OF ALTERED CONSCIOUSNESS
STATE	**DEFINITION**
Confusion	Loss of ability to think rapidly and clearly; impaired judgment and decision making
Disorientation	Beginning loss of consciousness; disorientation to time followed by disorientation to place and impaired memory; lost last is recognition of self
Lethargy	Limited spontaneous movement or speech; easy arousal with normal speech or touch; may or may not be oriented to time, place, or person
Obtundation	Mild to moderate reduction in arousal (awakeness) with limited response to environment; falls asleep unless stimulated verbally or tactilely; answers questions with minimal response
Stupor	Condition of deep sleep or unresponsiveness from which person may be aroused or caused to open eyes only by vigorous and repeated stimulation; response is often withdrawal or grabbing at stimulus
Coma	No verbal response to external environment or to any stimuli; noxious stimuli such as deep pain or suctioning do not yield motor movement
Light coma	Associated with purposeful movement on stimulation
Coma	Associated with nonpurposeful movement only on stimulation
Deep coma	Associated with unresponsiveness or no response to any stimulus

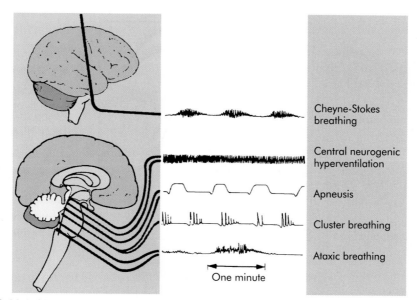

FIGURE 14-1 Abnormal Respiratory Patterns With Corresponding Level of Central Nervous System Activity. (From Urden LD, Davie JK, Lough ME: *Thelan's critical care nursing: diagnosis and management,* ed 5, St Louis, 2006, Mosby.)

TABLE 14-4 PATTERNS OF BREATHING

BREATHING PATTERN	DESCRIPTION	LOCATION OF INJURY
Hemispheric Breathing Patterns		
Normal	After a period of hyperventilation that lowers arterial carbon dioxide pressure ($Paco_2$), individual continues to breathe regularly but with reduced depth.	Response of nervous system to an external stressor—not associated with injury to CNS
Posthyperventilation apnea	Respirations stop after hyperventilation has lowered Pco_2 level below normal. Rhythmic breathing returns when Pco_2 level returns to normal.	Associated with diffuse bilateral metabolic or structural disease of cerebrum
Cheyne-Stokes respirations	Breathing pattern has a smooth increase (crescendo) in rate and depth of breathing (hyperpnea), which peaks and is followed by a gradual smooth decrease (decrescendo) in rate and depth of breathing to point of apnea, when cycle repeats itself. Hyperpneic phase lasts longer than apneic phase.	Bilateral dysfunction of deep cerebral or diencephalic structures; seen with supratentorial injury and metabolically induced coma states
Brain Stem Breathing Patterns		
Central neurogenic hyperventilation	A sustained, deep, rapid, but regular pattern (hyperpnea) occurs, with a decreased $Paco_2$ and a corresponding increase in pH and Po_2.	May result from CNS damage or disease that involves midbrain and upper pons; seen after increased intracranial pressure and blunt head trauma
Apneusis	A prolonged inspiratory cramp (a pause at full inspiration) occurs; a common variant of this is a brief end-inspiratory pause of 2 or 3 sec, often alternating with an end-expiratory pause.	Indicates damage to respiratory control mechanism located at pontine level; most commonly associated with pontine infarction but documented with hypoglycemia, anoxia, and meningitis
Cluster breathing	A cluster of breaths has a disordered sequence with irregular pauses between breaths.	Dysfunction in lower pontine and high medullary areas
Ataxic breathing	Completely irregular breathing occurs, with random shallow and deep breaths and irregular pauses. Rate is often slow.	Originates from a primary dysfunction of medullary neurons controlling breathing
Gasping breathing pattern (agonal gasps)	A pattern of deep "all-or-none" breaths is accompanied by a slow respiratory rate.	Indicative of a failing medullary respiratory center

CNS, Central nervous system.

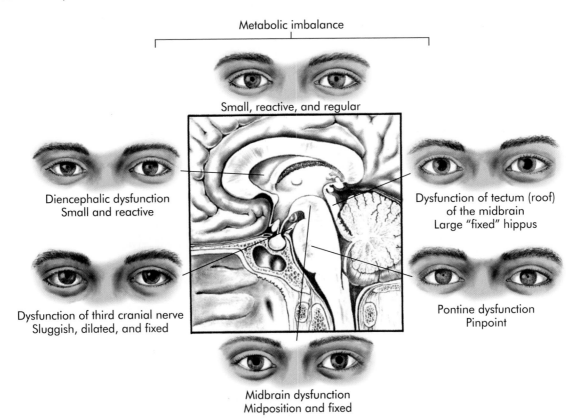

FIGURE 14-2 Pupils at Different Levels of Consciousness.

(Figures 14-3 and 14-4). Those that involve an oculomotor nucleus or nerve cause the involved eye to deviate outward, producing a resting dysconjugate lateral position of the eye.

Motor responses help evaluate the level of brain dysfunction and determine the most severely damaged side of the brain. The pattern of

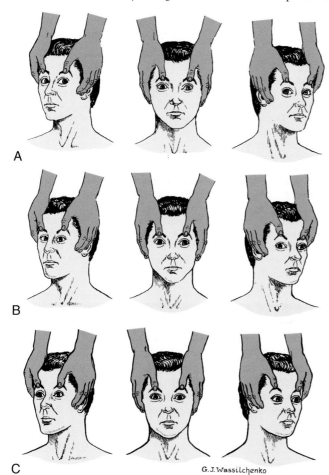

FIGURE 14-3 Test for Oculocephalic Reflex Response (Doll's Eyes Phenomenon). **A,** Normal response—eyes turn together to side opposite from turn of head. **B,** Abnormal response—eyes do not turn in conjugate manner. **C,** Absent response—eyes move in direction of head movement (brain stem injury). (From Rudy EB: *Advanced neurological and neurosurgical nursing,* St Louis, 1984, Mosby.)

response noted may be (1) purposeful; (2) inappropriate, generalized motor movement; or (3) not present. Motor signs indicating loss of cortical inhibition that are commonly associated with decreased consciousness include reflex grasping, reflex sucking, snout reflex, palmomental reflex, and rigidity (paratonia) (Figure 14-5). Abnormal flexor and extensor responses in the upper and lower extremities are defined in Table 14-5 and illustrated in Figure 14-6 (also see p. 372).

Vomiting, yawning, and **hiccups** are complex reflex-like motor responses that are integrated by neural mechanisms in the lower brain stem. These responses may be produced by compression or diseases involving tissues of the medulla oblongata (e.g., infection, neoplasm, infarct) but also occur relative to other more benign stimuli to the vagal nerve. Most CNS disorders produce nausea and vomiting. Vomiting without nausea indicates direct involvement of the central neural mechanism (or pyloric obstruction; see Chapters 33 and 34. Vomiting often accompanies CNS injuries that (1) involve the vestibular nuclei or its immediate projections, particularly when double vision (diplopia) also is present; (2) impinge directly on the floor of the fourth ventricle; or (3) produce brain stem compression secondary to increased intracranial pressure.

> ✔ **QUICK CHECK 14-1**
> 1. Why are structural as well as metabolic factors capable of producing coma?
> 2. Why is level of consciousness the most critical index of central nervous system function?
> 3. Why do Cheyne-Stokes respirations appear in coma?
> 4. Why are oculomotor changes associated with levels of brain injury?

Outcomes of Alterations in Arousal

Outcomes of alterations in arousal fall into two categories: *extent of disability (morbidity)* and *mortality.* Outcomes depend on the cause and extent of brain damage and the duration of coma. Some individuals may recover consciousness and an original level of function, some may have permanent disability, and some may never regain consciousness and experience neurologic death. Two forms of neurologic death—brain death and cerebral death—result from severe pathologic conditions and are associated with irreversible coma. Other possible outcomes are a vegetative state, a minimally conscious state, or locked-in syndrome. The extent of disability has four subcategories: recovery of consciousness, residual cognitive function, psychologic function, and vocational function.

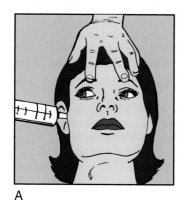
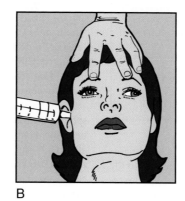
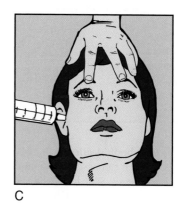

FIGURE 14-4 Test for Oculovestibular Reflex (Caloric Ice Water Test). **A,** Ice water is injected into the ear canal. Normal response—conjugate eye movements. **B,** Abnormal response—dysconjugate or asymmetric eye movements. **C,** Absent response—no eye movements.

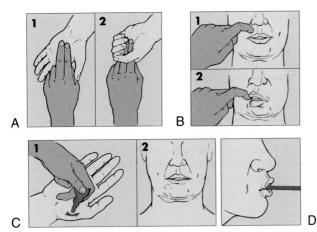

FIGURE 14-5 Pathologic Reflexes. **A,** Grasp reflex. **B,** Snout reflex. **C,** Palmomental reflex. **D,** Suck reflex.

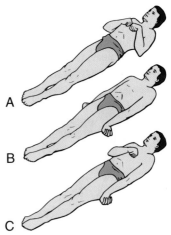

FIGURE 14-6 Decorticate and Decerebrate Responses. **A,** Decorticate response. Flexion of arms, wrists, and fingers with adduction in upper extremities. Extension, internal rotation, and plantar flexion in lower extremities. Both sides. **B,** Decerebrate response. All four extremities in rigid extension, with hyperpronation of forearms and plantar extension of feet. **C,** Decorticate response on right side of body and decerebrate response on left side of body. (From Rudy EB: *Advanced neurological and neurosurgical nursing,* St Louis, 1984, Mosby.)

TABLE 14-5	ABNORMAL MOTOR RESPONSES WITH DECREASED RESPONSIVENESS	
MOTOR RESPONSE	**DESCRIPTION**	**LOCATION OF INJURY**
Abnormal motor responses, upper extremity flexion with or without extensor responses in lower extremities (decorticate rigidity)	Slowly developing flexion of arm, wrist, and fingers with adduction in the upper extremity and extension, internal rotation, and plantar flexion of lower extremity	Suggest hemispheric damage above midbrain
Extensor responses in upper and lower extremities (decerebrate posturing, decerebrate rigidity)	Opisthotonos (hyperextension of vertebral column) with clenching of teeth; extension, abduction, and hyperpronation of arms; and extension of lower extremities	Associated with severe damage involving caudal diencephalon or midbrain
	In acute brain injury, shivering and hyperpnea may accompany unelicited recurrent decerebrate spasms	Acute injury often causes limb extension regardless of location
Extensor responses in upper extremities accompanied by flexion in lower extremities		Indicates pontine level dysfunction
Flaccid state with little or no motor response to stimuli		Damage to lower pons and upper myelencephalon

BOX 14-1 CRITERIA FOR BRAIN DEATH

1. Completion of all appropriate diagnostic and therapeutic procedures with no possibility of brain function recovery
2. Unresponsive coma (no motor or reflex movements)
3. No spontaneous respiration (apnea)
4. No brain stem functions (ocular responses to head turning or caloric stimulation; dilated, fixed pupils; no gag or corneal reflex)
5. Isoelectric (flat) EEG (electrocerebral silence)
6. Persistence of these signs for an appropriate observation period

Summarized from Wijdicks EF, Varelas PN, Gronseth GS et al: American Academy of Neurology. Evidence-based guideline update: determining brain death in adults: report of the Quality Standards Subcommittee of the American Academy of Neurology, *Neurology* 74(23):1911–1918, 2010.

abnormality of brain function must result from structural or known metabolic disease and must *not* be caused by a depressant drug, alcohol poisoning, or hypothermia. An isoelectric, or flat, electroencephalogram (EEG) (electrocerebral silence) for 6 to 12 hours in a person who is not hypothermic and has not ingested depressant drugs indicates brain death. The clinical criteria used to determine brain death are noted in Box 14-1. A task force for determination of brain death in children recommended the same criteria as for adults, but with a longer observation period.[2]

Cerebral death, or irreversible coma, is death of the cerebral hemispheres exclusive of the brain stem and cerebellum. Brain damage is permanent, and the individual is forever unable to respond behaviorally in any significant way to the environment. The brain stem may continue to maintain internal homeostasis (i.e., body temperature, cardiovascular functions, respirations, and metabolic functions). The survivor of cerebral death may remain in a coma or emerge into a persistent vegetative state (VS) or a minimally conscious state (MCS). In coma, the eyes are usually closed with no eye opening. The person does not follow commands, speak, or have voluntary movement.[3]

Brain death (total brain death) occurs when the brain is damaged so completely that it can never recover and cannot maintain the body's internal homeostasis. State laws define brain death as irreversible cessation of function of the entire brain including the brain stem and cerebellum. On postmortem examination, the brain is autolyzing (self-digesting) or already autolyzed. Brain death has occurred when there is no evidence of brain function for an extended period.[1] The

In a persistent vegetative state there is complete unawareness of the self or surrounding environment and complete loss of cognitive function. The individual does not speak any comprehensible words or follow commands. Sleep-wake cycles are present, eyes open spontaneously, and blood pressure and breathing are maintained without support. Brain stem reflexes (pupillary, oculocephalic, chewing, swallowing) are intact but cerebral function is lost. There is bowel and bladder incontinence. Recovery is unlikely if the state persists for 12 months. In a minimally conscious state (MCS) individuals may follow simple commands, manipulate objects, gesture or give yes/no responses, have intelligible speech, and have movements such as blinking or smiling.[3] In locked-in syndrome there is complete paralysis of voluntary muscles with the exception of eye movement. Content of thought and level of arousal are intact, but the efferent pathways are disrupted (injury at the base of the pons with the reticular formation intact, often caused by basilar artery occlusion). Thus, the individual cannot communicate through speech or body movement but is fully conscious, with intact cognitive function. Vertical eye movement and blinking are a means of communication.[4]

Alterations in Awareness

Awareness (content of thought) encompasses all cognitive functions, including awareness of self, environment, and affective states (i.e., moods). Awareness is mediated by all of the core networks (selective attention and memory) under the guidance of executive attention networks (i.e., the networks that involve abstract reasoning, planning, decision making, judgment, error correction, and self-control). Each attentional function is localized not in a single brain area, but as a network of interconnected brain areas.

Selective attention (orienting) refers to the ability to select specific information to be processed from available environmental and internal stimuli. Certain midbrain and thalamic structures contribute to selective attention, so the etiologic factors for coma potentially can alter selective attention. Selective attention also is mediated by the right parietal lobe. An isolated (pure) selective attention deficit rarely occurs clinically. Causes of temporary, permanent, or progressive attention deficits include seizure activity, parietal lobe contusions, subdural hematomas, stroke, gliomas or metastatic tumor, and late Alzheimer and frontotemporal dementia (see pp. 357-359).

Memory is the ability of the brain to store and retrieve information. Amnesia is the loss of memory and can be mild or severe. Two types of memory disorders are retrograde amnesia (loss of past personal history memories or past factual memories) and anterograde amnesia (retention of memory of events in the distant past but unable to form new personal or factual memories). Image processing is a higher level of memory function and includes the ability to use sensory data and language to form concepts, assign meaning, and make abstractions. Alterations in image processing include an inability to form concepts and generalizations or to reason. Thinking is very concrete. These memory disorders may be temporary (e.g., after a seizure) or permanent (e.g., after severe head injury or in Alzheimer disease). There may be only the memory disorder, or the memory disorder may be associated with other cognitive disorders.

Executive attention deficits include the inability to maintain sustained attention (an inability to set goals and recognize when an object meets a goal), and a working memory deficit (an inability to remember instructions and information needed to guide behavior). Executive attention deficits may be temporary, progressive, or permanent. Attention-deficit/hyperactivity disorder (ADHD) is a common disorder of childhood that can continue through adulthood (see *Health Alert*). Table 14-6 summarizes alterations in memory and attention.

HEALTH ALERT

Attention-Deficit/Hyperactivity Disorder (ADHD): Not Just a Childhood Disorder

Initially ADHD was viewed as a developmental disorder of childhood. It is now recognized that 50% to 75% of persons diagnosed in childhood have continuing symptoms into adulthood. Often the diagnosis is first made in adolescence or young adulthood when behavioral control and self-organization are expected of the person. The ability to function at work, at home, and in social situations is often impaired because of inattentiveness, hyperactivity, and impulsivity. Continued treatment including medications for symptomatic adults is supported; substance abuse, which is more common in persons with ADHD, is reduced with continued treatment. The multifactorial patterns of inheritance and gene-environment interactions are under investigation as are the pathogenesis and pathophysiology of this disorder. Hopefully new findings will lead to improved prevention, diagnosis, and treatment options.

Data from Cubillo A, Rubia K: Structural and functional brain imaging in adult attention-deficit/hyperactivity disorder, *Expert Rev Neurother* 10(4):603–620, 2010; Ficks CA, Waldman ID: Gene-environment interactions in attention-deficit/hyperactivity disorder, *Curr Psychiatr Rep* 11(5):387–392, 2009; Schmidt S, Petermann F: Developmental psychopathology: attention deficit hyperactivity disorder (ADHD), *BMC Psychiatr* 9:58, 2009.

Pathophysiology. Very generally, the primary pathophysiologic mechanisms that operate in disorders of awareness are (1) direct destruction caused by ischemia and hypoxia or indirect destruction resulting from compression and (2) the effects of toxins and chemicals. Disorders of selective attention, at least as they relate to visual orienting behavior, are produced by disease that involves portions of the midbrain. Disease affecting the superior colliculi manifests as a slowness in orienting attention. Parietal lobe disease may produce disengagement from a stimulus or unilateral neglect syndrome. Sensory inattentiveness is a form of neglect. The person is able to recognize individual sensory input from the dysfunctional side when asked but ignores the sensory input from the dysfunctional side when stimulated from both sides (extinction). The entire complex of denial of dysfunction, loss of recognition of one's own body parts, and extinction sometimes is referred to as the neglect syndrome. A disorder in vigilance may be produced by disease in the prefrontal areas. Right dysfunction in the anterior cingulate gyrus and basal ganglia may cause detection problems, whereas problems with working memory may be produced with left lateral frontal injury. Anterograde amnesia originates from pathologic conditions in the hippocampus and related temporal lobe structures; the diencephalic region including the thalamus; and the basal forebrain. Retrograde amnesia and higher level memory deficits originate from pathologic conditions in the widely distributed association areas of the cerebral cortex (see Figure 12-6, *C*). Executive attention deficits are associated with alterations in the frontal and prefrontal cortex including the anterior cingulate gyrus, supplementary motor area, and portions of the basal ganglia.

Clinical manifestations. Clinical manifestations of selective attention deficits, memory deficits, and executive attention function deficits are presented in Table 14-6.

Evaluation and treatment. Immediate medical management is directed at diagnosing the cause and treating reversible factors. Rehabilitative measures generally focus on compensatory or restorative activities and recently have been greatly facilitated by computer technology and other electronic devices.

TABLE 14-6	CLINICAL MANIFESTATIONS OF ALTERATIONS IN ATTENTION AND MEMORY	
DEFICIT	**CLINICAL SIGNS**	**SYMPTOMS**
Attention		
Selective attention (orienting)	Inability to focus attention; decreased eye, head, and body movements associated with focusing on stimuli; decreased search and scanning; faulty orientation to stimuli, causing safety problems	Person reports inability to focus attention, failure to perceive objects and other stimuli (history of injuries, falls, safety problems)
Memory		
Antegrade amnesia (inability to form new memories)	*Left hemisphere:* disorientation to time, situation, place, name, person (verbal identification); impaired language memory (e.g., names of objects); impaired semantic memory	Person reports disorientation, confusion, "not listening," "not remembering;" reports by others of person being disoriented, not able to remember, not able to learn new information
	Right hemisphere: disorientation to self, person (visual), place (visual); impaired episodic memory (personal history); impaired emotional memory	
	Either or both hemispheres: confusion; behavioral change	
Retrograde amnesia (loss of past memories)	*Left hemisphere:* inability to retrieve personal history, past medical history; unaware of recent current events	Person reports remote memory problems; others report that person cannot recall formerly known information
	Right hemisphere: inability to recognize persons, places, objects, music, and so on from past	
Image processing	Inability to categorize (identify similarities and differences) or sort; inability to form concepts; inability to analyze relationships; misinterpretations; inability to interpret proverbs	Reports by others of frequent misinterpretation of data, failure to conceptualize or generalize information
	Inability to perform deductive reasoning (convergent reasoning); inability to perform inductive reasoning (divergent reasoning); inability to abstract; concrete reasoning demonstrated; delusions	Reports by others of predominantly concrete thinking; lack of understanding of everyday situations, healthcare regimens, and such; delusional thinking
Executive Attention Deficits		
Vigilance	Failure to stay alert and orient to stimuli	Person reports decreased alertness or ability to orient
Detection	Lack of initiative (anergy); lack of ambition; lack of motivation; flat affect; no awareness of feelings; appears depressed, apathetic, and emotionless; fails to appreciate deficit; disinterested in appearance; lacks concern about childish or crude behavior	Reports by others of laziness or apathy, flat affect or lack of emotional expression; failing to exhibit or be aware of feelings
Mild	Responds to immediate environment but no new ideas; grooming and social graces are lacking	Reports by others of lack of ambition, motivation, or initiative; failure to carry out adult tasks; lack of social graces and new ideas
Severe	Motionless; lack of response to even internal cues; does not respond to physical needs; does not interact with surroundings	Reports by others of failure to groom or toilet self, unawareness of surroundings and own physical needs
	Inability to use feedback regarding behavior; failure to recognize omissions and errors in self-care, speech, writing, and arithmetic; impaired cue utilization; overestimation of performance	Reports by others of not changing behavior when requested; unawareness of limitations; does not recognize and correct errors in dressing, grooming, toileting, eating, and such; fails to recognize speech and arithmetic errors; careless speech
	Failure to shift response set; failure to change behavior when conditions change; cue utilization may be impaired	Reports by others of failure to use feedback; inability to incorporate feedback (does not correct when feedback is given)
Working memory	Inability to set goals or form goals; indecisiveness	Reports by others of failure to set goals, indecisiveness
	Failure to make plans; inability to produce a complete line of reasoning; inability to make up a story; appears impulsive	Reports by others of failure to plan, impulsiveness, "does not think things through"
	Failure to initiate behavior; failure to maintain behavior; failure to discontinue behavior; slowness to alternate response for the next step; motor perseveration	Reports by others of not knowing where to begin, inability to carry out sequential acts (maintain a behavior), inability to cease a behavior

Selective attention deficits and executive attention deficits can be confused with symptoms of other cognitive deficits. Differential diagnosis is difficult but essential for effective treatment.

Seizure Disorders

Seizure disorders represent a syndrome and not a specific disease entity. A **seizure** results from a sudden, explosive, disorderly discharge of cerebral neurons and is characterized by a sudden, transient alteration in brain function, usually involving motor, sensory, autonomic, or psychic clinical manifestations and a temporary altered level of arousal. A seizure produces a brief disruption in the brain's electrical functions.[5] **Convulsion,** a term sometimes applied to seizures, refers to the jerky, contract-relax (tonic-clonic) movement associated with some seizures. **Epilepsy** is seizure activity for which no underlying correctable cause for the seizure can be found; therefore seizure activity recurs without treatment. In the United

States 2.5 million people have epilepsy with about 200,000 new cases diagnosed per year.[6]

Conditions Associated With Seizure Disorders

Any disorder that alters the neuronal environment may cause seizure activity; therefore, theoretically, anyone may experience a seizure. The seizure threshold of some persons, however, is genetically lower.

Diseases or other processes that involve the nervous system can produce a seizure disorder. The onset may indicate the presence of an ongoing primary neurologic disease. Etiologic factors in seizures generally include (1) cerebral lesions, (2) biochemical disorders, (3) cerebral trauma, and (4) epilepsy, which can result from the following conditions:

- Metabolic defects
- Congenital malformation
- Genetic predisposition
- Perinatal injury
- Postnatal trauma
- Myoclonic syndromes
- Infection
- Brain tumor
- Vascular disease
- Fever
- Drug or alcohol abuse

Causes of recurrent seizures are age-related (Table 14-7). The cause of seizures is often unknown.

Seizures may be precipitated by hypoglycemia, fatigue or lack of sleep, emotional or physical stress, febrile illness, large amounts of water ingestion, constipation, use of stimulant drugs, withdrawal from depressant drugs (including alcohol), hyperventilation (respiratory alkalosis), and some environmental stimuli, such as blinking lights, a poorly adjusted television screen, loud noises, certain music, certain odors, or merely being startled. Women may have increased seizure activity immediately before or during menses.

Types of seizure disorders. Seizures are classified in different ways: by clinical manifestations, site of origin, EEG correlates, or response to therapy. A simplified version of the International Classification of Epileptic Seizures is presented in Table 14-8. Terms used to describe seizure activity are defined in Table 14-9.

Epilepsy now is considered to be the result of the interaction of complex genetic mutations with environmental effects that cause abnormalities in brain wiring, an imbalance in the brain's neurotransmitters, or the development of abnormal nerve connections after injury.[7] A group of neurons may exhibit a paroxysmal depolarization shift and function as an **epileptogenic focus.** These neurons are hypersensitive and are more easily activated by hyperthermia, hypoxia, hypoglycemia, hyponatremia, repeated sensory stimulation, and certain sleep phases. Epileptogenic neurons fire more frequently and with greater amplitude. When the intensity reaches a threshold point, cortical excitation spreads. Excitation of the subcortical, thalamic, and brain stem areas corresponds to the **tonic phase** (muscle contraction with increased muscle tone) and is associated with loss of consciousness.

The **clonic phase** (alternating contraction and relaxation of muscles) begins when inhibitory neurons in the cortex, anterior thalamus, and basal ganglia react to the cortical excitation. The seizure discharge is interrupted, producing intermittent muscle contractions that gradually decrease and finally cease. The epileptogenic neurons are exhausted.

During seizure activity, oxygen is consumed at a high rate—about 60% greater than normal. Although cerebral blood flow also increases, oxygen is rapidly depleted, along with glucose, and lactate accumulates

TABLE 14-7	CAUSES OF RECURRENT SEIZURES IN DIFFERENT AGE GROUPS
AGE AT ONSET	**PROBABLE CAUSE**
Neonates (<1 month)	Acute CNS infection (sepsis, meningitis, encephalitis)
	Cortical malformation
	Drug withdrawal or toxicity
	Genetic disorders
	Intracranial hemorrhage and trauma
	Kernicterus
	Metabolic disturbances (hypoglycemia, hypocalcemia, hypomagnesemia, pyridoxine deficiency)
	Perinatal hypoxic and ischemic encephalopathy
Infants and children (1 month to 12 yr)	Degenerative disorders (i.e., tuberous sclerosis, neurofibromatosis, Tay-Sachs disease)
	Febrile seizures
	Genetic disorders (metabolic, degenerative, primary epilepsy syndromes)
	Idiopathic
	Infantile spasms
	Trauma
Adolescents (12 to 18 yr)	Acute CNS infection (sepsis, meningitis, encephalitis)
	Brain tumor
	Genetic disorders
	Idiopathic
	Illicit drug use (i.e., cocaine, amphetamine)
	Trauma
Young adults (18 to 35 yr)	Alcohol or drug withdrawal (i.e., barbiturates, benzodiazepines)
	Brain tumor
	Idiopathic
	Illicit drug use (i.e., cocaine, amphetamine)
	Trauma
Older adults (>35 yr)	Alcohol or drug withdrawal (i.e., barbiturates, benzodiazepines)
	Brain tumor
	Cerebrovascular disease (i.e., stroke, aneurysm, arteriovenous malformations)
	CNS degenerative diseases (i.e., Alzheimer disease, multiple sclerosis)
	Idiopathic
	Metabolic disorders (i.e., uremia, hepatic failure, electrolyte abnormalities, hypoglycemia)

Data from Goetz CG, editor: *Textbook of clinical neurology,* ed 3, Philadelphia, 2007, Saunders; Nabbout R, Dulac O: *Curr Opin Neurol* 21(2):161–166, 2008; Waterhouse E, Towne A: *Cleve Clin J Med* 72(suppl 3):S26–S37, 2005.
CNS, Central nervous system.

in brain tissue. Continued, severe seizure activity has the potential for progressive brain injury and irreversible damage. In addition, if a seizure focus in the brain is active for a prolonged period, a **mirror focus** may develop in contralateral normal tissue.

Clinical manifestations. The clinical manifestations associated with seizure depend on its type (see Table 14-8). Two types of symptoms signal a generalized tonic-clonic seizure: an **aura,** a partial seizure that immediately precedes the onset of a generalized tonic-clonic

TABLE 14-8 INTERNATIONAL CLASSIFICATION OF EPILEPTIC SEIZURES

TRADITIONAL TERMINOLOGY	NEW NOMENCLATURE

Focal motor; jacksonian seizures (occasionally become secondarily generalized)	I. Partial seizures (seizures beginning locally)
	  A. Simple (without impairment of consciousness)
	    1. With motor signs
	    2. With special sensory or somatosensory symptoms
	    3. With autonomic symptoms or signs
	    4. With psychic symptoms

Temporal lobe or psychomotor seizures	B. Complex (with impairment of consciousness)
	    1. Simple partial onset followed by impaired consciousness
	    2. Impaired consciousness at onset—with or without automatisms
	  C. Secondarily generalized (partial onset evolving to generalized tonic-clonic seizures)

	II. Generalized seizures (bilaterally symmetric and without local onset)

Petit mal	A. Absence
	    1. Typical
	    2. Atypical
	  B. Myoclonic
	  C. Clonic
	  D. Tonic

Grand mal	E. Tonic-clonic
Drop attack	F. Atonic (astatic, akinetic)
	III. Unclassified epileptic seizures

TABLE 14-9 TERMINOLOGY APPLIED TO A SEIZURE DISORDER

TERM	DEFINITION
Aura	A partial seizure experienced as a peculiar sensation preceding onset of generalized seizure that may take the form of gustatory, visual, or auditory experience or a feeling of dizziness, numbness, or just "a funny feeling"
Prodroma	Early clinical manifestations, such as malaise, headache, or sense of depression, that may occur hours to a few days before onset of a seizure
Tonic phase	A state of muscle contraction in which there is excessive muscle tone
Clonic phase	A state of alternating contraction and relaxation of muscles
Postictal phase	Time period immediately following cessation of seizure activity

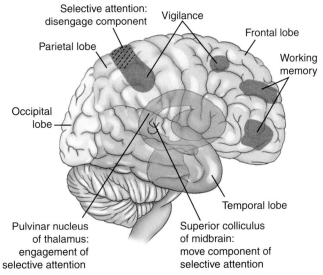

FIGURE 14-7 Right Cortical, Subcortical, and Brain Stem Areas of the Brain Mediating Cognitive Function. (From Boss GJ, Wilkerson R: Communication: language and pragmatics. In Hoeman SP, editor: *Rehabilitation nursing; prevention, intervention & outcomes,* ed 4, p 508, St Louis, 2008, Mosby.)

seizure; and a **prodroma**, early manifestations occurring hours to days before a seizure. Both may become familiar to the person experiencing recurrent generalized seizures and may enable the person to prevent injuries during the seizure.

Evaluation and treatment. The health history, physical examination, and laboratory tests of blood and urine (concentrations of blood glucose, serum calcium, blood urea nitrogen, and urine sodium; and creatinine clearance time) can identify systemic diseases known to promote seizures. Radiographic studies and cerebrospinal fluid (CSF) examination help identify neurologic diseases associated with seizures. The EEG is used to assess the type of seizure and determine its focus.

Treatment involves correcting or controlling the cause and, if none is identified, administering antiseizure medications to suppress seizure activity. Counseling also may be of value. Preventing and predicting epilepsy is a major area of research.[8]

> **✔ QUICK CHECK 14-2**
> 1. Why is irreversible coma different from brain death?
> 2. Why is a seizure different from epilepsy?
> 3. Why can so many conditions precipitate seizures?
> 4. Why is continued seizing dangerous? How does an epileptogenic focus differ from a mirror focus?

Data Processing Deficits

Data processing deficits are problems associated with recognizing and processing sensory information and include agnosia, dysphasia, and acute confusional states.

Agnosia

Agnosia is a defect of pattern recognition—a failure to recognize the form and nature of objects. Agnosia can be tactile, visual, or auditory, but generally only one sense is affected. For example, an individual may be unable to identify a safety pin by touching it with a hand but is able to name it when looking at it. Agnosia may be as minimal as a finger agnosia (failure to identify by name the fingers of one's hand) or more extensive, such as a color agnosia. Although agnosia is associated most commonly with cerebrovascular accidents, it may arise from any pathologic process that injures specific areas of the brain.

Dysphasia

Dysphasia is impairment of comprehension or production of language with impaired communication. Comprehension or use of symbols, in either written or verbal language, is disturbed or lost. Aphasia is a more severe form of dysphasia and an inability to communicate. Often the terms dysphasia and aphasia are used interchangeably. The term dysphasia is used here. Dysphasias usually are associated with cerebrovascular accident involving the middle cerebral artery or one of its many branches. Language disorders, however, may arise from a variety of injuries and diseases—vascular, neoplastic, traumatic, degenerative, metabolic, or infectious causes. Dysphasia results from dysfunction in the left cerebral hemisphere, usually the frontotemporal region (see Figures 14-7 and 12-6). Most language disorders result from acute processes or a chronic residual deficit of the acute process. Some progressive language disorders are the result of degenerative disorders.

Dysphasias have been classified both anatomically and functionally. Other classifications describe fluency, volume, or quantity of speech, although pure forms of any language dysfunction are rare. Expressive dysphasias involve primarily expression deficits, but verbal comprehension deficit also may be present. Receptive dysphasias may have expressive deficits. (Table 14-10 compares types of dysphasias; Table 14-11 illustrates some of the language disturbances.)

Some dysphasias are referred to as transcortical dysphasias and involve the ability to repeat (echolalia) and to recite. Speech is fluent but the words make no sense. The individual cannot read or write and has impaired comprehension. These dysphasias are caused by hypoxia or other mechanisms that destroy the border zone between the cerebral arteries (see Figure 12-19). The sensory and motor speech areas are functional, but connections with other sensory or motor areas are impaired. Information cannot be transmitted to Wernicke area and transformed into language.

Acute Confusional States

Acute confusional states (ACS) are transient disorders of awareness that result from cerebral dysfunction secondary to drug intoxication, metabolic disorders, nervous system disease, trauma, or surgery. Withdrawal from alcohol, barbiturate, or other sedative drug ingestion is a common cause. Acute confusional states may begin either suddenly or gradually, depending on the amount of exposure to the toxin. These states often occur with febrile illnesses, systemic diseases (e.g., heart failure), head injury, anesthesia use, or certain focal cerebral lesions and are seen postnatally.

Pathophysiology. Acute confusional states arise from disruption of a widely distributed neural network involving the reticular activating system of the upper brain stem and its projections into the thalamus, basal ganglion, and specific association areas of the cortex and limbic areas. Delirium (hyperkinetic confusional state) is an acute state of brain dysfunction associated with right-upper middle-temporal gyrus or left temporal-occipital junction disruption and several neurotransmitters are involved.[9]

Hypokinetic confusional states (hypoactive delirium) are more likely to be associated with right-sided frontal-basal ganglion disruption.

Most metabolic disturbances that produce an acute confusional state interfere with neuronal metabolism or synaptic transmission. Many drugs and toxins also interfere with neurotransmission function at the synapse.

Clinical manifestations. The predominant feature of an acute confusional state is impaired or lost detection. The person is highly distractible and unable to concentrate on incoming sensory information or on any one particular mental or motor task.

The onset of an ACS usually is abrupt. The first clinical manifestations are difficulty in concentration, restlessness, irritability, tremulousness, insomnia, and poor appetite. Later there are misperceptions, illusions, hallucinations, and delirium. Obsessions, compulsive behavior, and rituals may be evident.

Delirium is associated with autonomic nervous system overactivity; it typically develops over 2 to 3 days and most commonly occurs in critical care units, following surgery, or during withdrawal from central nervous system depressants (i.e., alcohol or narcotic agents). Delirium initially manifests as difficulty in concentrating, restlessness, irritability, insomnia, tremulousness, and poor appetite. Some persons experience seizures. Unpleasant, even terrifying, dreams or hallucinations may occur. In a fully developed delirium state, the individual is completely inattentive and perceptions are grossly altered, with extensive misperception and misinterpretation. The person appears distressed and often perplexed; conversation is incoherent. Frank tremor and high levels of restless movement are common. Violent behavior may be present. The individual cannot sleep, is flushed, and has dilated pupils, a rapid pulse rate (tachycardia), elevated temperature, and profuse sweating (diaphoresis). Delirium typically abates suddenly or gradually in 2 to 3 days, although occasionally delirium states persist for weeks.

Hypokinetic acute confusional states are associated with underactivity and may occur in individuals who have fevers or metabolic disorders (i.e., chronic liver or kidney failure), or who are under the influence of central nervous system depressants. The individual exhibits decreases in mental function, specifically alertness, attention span, accurate perception, interpretation of the environment, and reaction to the environment. Forgetfulness is prominent, and the individual dozes frequently.

Evaluation and treatment. The initial goals are to (1) establish that the individual is confused and (2) determine the cause of the confusion (organic or functional) (Table 14-12). The next step is to differentiate whether the confusion is delirium, a hypokinetic confusional state, or an underlying dementia. A complete history and physical examination as well as laboratory tests (electrocardiogram and blood, urine, cerebrospinal fluid, and radiologic studies) are needed. Once the cause is established, treatment is directed at controlling the primary disorder, with supportive measures used as appropriate. Delirium is preventable in some individuals.[10,10a] Table 14-13 contains a comparison of the features differentiating delirium and dementia.

> ✔ **QUICK CHECK 14-3**
> 1. Why are there so many cognitive disorders?
> 2. Why can so many disorders cause dysphasia?
> 3. Why is impaired detection the most common feature of acute confusional states (ACS)?
> 4. How is an ACS different from dementia?

Dementia

Dementia is a progressive failure of many cerebral functions that often includes a decrease in orienting, memory, language, judgment, and decision making. Because of declining intellectual ability, the individual exhibits alterations in behavior.

Pathophysiology. Mechanisms leading to dementia include neuron degeneration, compression, atherosclerosis, and trauma. Genetic predisposition is associated with the neurodegenerative diseases, including Alzheimer and Huntington diseases. CNS infections, including the human immunodeficiency virus (HIV) and slow-growing viruses associated with

TABLE 14-10	MAJOR TYPES OF DYSPHASIA			
TYPE	**EXPRESSION**	**VERBAL COMPREHENSION**	**REPETITION**	
Expressive Broca dysphasia, motor	Nonfluent; cannot find words, difficulty writing	Relatively intact	Impaired	
Receptive Wernicke dysphasia, sensory	Fluent; can produce verbal language but it is meaningless, with inappropriate words, similar sounds or meaning substituted for correct words, and neologisms that may be so extensive that speech is incomprehensible; unable to monitor language for correctness, so errors are not recognized Intonation, accent, cadence, rhythm, and articulation normal	Impaired (disturbance in understanding all language)	Impaired	
Others Global, conductive, anomia, transcortical motor, or transcortical sensory	Ranges from nonfluent and producing little speech to fluent with paraphrasia or impaired ability for naming	Can be relatively intact, impaired, or completely lost	Can be intact or impaired with an inability to repeat	

Creutzfeldt-Jakob disease, are associated with dementia in addition to changes in motor function (i.e., ataxia, rigidity, and shuffling gait). Progressive dementias produce nerve cell degeneration and brain atrophy.

Clinical manifestations. Clinical manifestations of the major dementias are presented in Table 14-14.

Evaluation and treatment. Establishing the cause for dementia may be complicated, but individuals with clinical manifestations of dementia should be evaluated with laboratory and neuropsychologic testing to identify underlying conditions that may be treatable. Unfortunately, no specific cure exists for most progressive dementias. Therapy is directed at maintaining and maximizing use of the remaining capacities, restoring functions if possible, and accommodating to lost abilities. Helping the family to understand the process and to learn ways to assist the individual is essential.

TABLE 14-11	EXAMPLES OF LANGUAGE DISTURBANCES
DISORDER	**EXAMPLE**
Verbal paraphrasia	Question: What did the car do? Patient: The car would spit sweetly down the road. (The car sped swiftly down the road.)
Literal paraphrasia	Request: Say "persistence is essential to success." Patient: Mesastence is instans to success.
Neologism	Question: What do you call this? (Pointing to a plant.) Patient: It's a logper.
Circumlocution	Question: What do you call this? (Pointing to a plant.) Patient: Something that grows.
Anomia	Patient: It's... *Or* Question: What did you do this morning? Patient: Reading. Question: Were you reading a book or newspaper? Patient: One of those.
Telegraphic style	Question: Where is your daughter? Patient: New Orleans...home...Monday.

From Boss BJ: Dysphasia, dyspraxia, and dysarthria: distinguishing features (part I), *J Neurosurg Nurs* 16(3):151–160, 1984.

TABLE 14-12	DIFFERENCES BETWEEN ORGANIC AND FUNCTIONAL CONFUSION	
FACTOR	**ORGANIC CONFUSION**	**FUNCTIONAL CONFUSION**
Memory impairment	Recent more impaired than remote	No consistent difference between recent and remote
Disorientation		
Time	Within own lifetime or reasonably near future	May not be related to person's lifetime
Place	Familiar place or one where person might easily be found	Bizarre or unfamiliar places
Person	Sense of identity usually preserved	Sense of identity diminished
	Misidentification of others as familiar	Misidentification of others based on delusion system
Hallucinations	Visual, vivid	Auditory more frequent
	Animals and insects common	Bizarre and symbolic
Illusions	Common	Not prominent
Delusions	Concern everyday occurrences and people	Bizarre and symbolic
Confused	Spotty confusion	More consistent
	Clear intervals mixed with confused episodes	No tendency to become worse at night
	Worse at night	

From Morris M, Rhodes M: Guidelines for the care of confused patients, *Am J Nurs* 72(9):1632, 1972.

READING COMPREHENSION	WRITING	LOCATION OF LESION	CAUSE OF LESION
Variable	Impaired	Left posteroinferior frontal lobe (Broca area)	Occlusion of one or several branches of left middle cerebral artery supplying inferior frontal gyrus
Impaired	Impaired	Left posterosuperior temporal lobe (Wernicke area)	Occlusion of inferior division of left middle cerebral artery
Variable; may be impaired or completely lost	Variable or impaired	Various areas including frontotemporal lobe; arcuate fasciculus, supramarginal gyrus, bundle of fibers from temporal lobe that project anteriorly to premotor area; angular gyrus and anterior or posterior presylvian fissures	Occlusion of left middle cerebral artery of left internal carotid artery, tumors, other mass lesions, hemorrhage, embolic occlusion of ascending parietal or posterior temporal branch of middle cerebral artery

Alzheimer Disease

Alzheimer disease (AD) (dementia of Alzheimer type [DAT], senile disease complex) is one of the most common causes of severe cognitive dysfunction in older persons and the leading cause of dementia.[10b]

TABLE 14-13   COMPARISON OF DELIRIUM AND DEMENTIA

FEATURE	DELIRIUM	DEMENTIA
Age	Usually older	Usually older
Onset	Acute—common during hospitalization	Usually insidious; acute in some cases of strokes/trauma
Associated conditions	Urinary tract infection, thyroid disorders, hypoxia, hypoglycemia, toxicity, fluid-electrolyte imbalance, renal insufficiency, trauma	May have no other conditions Brain trauma
Course	Fluctuating	Chronic slow decline
Duration	Hours to weeks	Months to years
Attention	Impaired	Intact early; often impaired late
Sleep-wake cycle	Disrupted	Usually normal
Alertness	Impaired	Normal
Orientation	Impaired	Intact early; impaired late
Behavior	Agitated, withdrawn/depressed	Intact early
Speech	Incoherent, rapid/slowed	Word-finding problems
Thoughts	Disorganized, delusions	Impoverished
Perceptions	Hallucinations/illusions	Usually intact early

Adapted from Caplan JP, Rabinowitz T: An approach to the patient with cognitive impairment: delirium and dementia, *Med Clin North Am* 94(6):1103–1116, ix, 2010.

The three forms of AD are early-onset AD (very rare), early-onset familial AD (FAD), and the most common (90%) form—late-onset AD.

Pathophysiology. The exact cause of Alzheimer disease is unknown. Early-onset FAD has been linked to three genes with mutations on chromosome 21 (abnormal amyloid precursor protein 14 *[APP14]*, abnormal presenilin 1 *[PSEN1]*, and abnormal presenilin 2 *[PSEN2]*). Late-onset AD may be related to the involvement of chromosome 19 with the apolipoprotein E gene-allele 4 (*APOE4*).[11] Pathologic alterations in the brain include formation of neuritic plaques containing a core of amyloid-beta protein, creation of neurofibrillary tangles, and degeneration of basal forebrain cholinergic neurons with loss of acetylcholine. Failure to process and clear amyloid precursor protein results in the accumulation of toxic fragments of amyloid-beta protein that leads to formation of diffuse neuritic plaques, disruption of nerve impulse transmission, and death of neurons. The tau protein, a microtubule-binding protein, in neurons detaches and forms an insoluble filament called a neurofibrillary tangle, contributing to neuronal death (Figure 14-8). Senile plaques and neurofibrillary tangles are more concentrated in the cerebral cortex and hippocampus. The loss of neurons results in brain atrophy with widening of sulci and shrinkage of gyri (see Figure 14-8). Loss of acetylcholine and other neurotransmitters contributes to the decline of memory and attention and the loss of other cognitive functions associated with AD.[11a]

Clinical manifestations. Initial clinical manifestations are insidious and often attributed to forgetfulness, emotional upset, or other illness. The individual becomes progressively more forgetful over time, particularly in relation to recent events. Memory loss increases as the disorder advances, and the person becomes disoriented and confused and loses the ability to concentrate. Abstraction, problem solving, and judgment gradually deteriorate, with failure in mathematic calculation ability, language, and visuospatial orientation. Dyspraxia may appear. The mental status changes induce behavioral changes, including irritability, agitation, and restlessness. Mood changes also result from the deterioration in cognition. The person may become anxious, depressed, hostile, emotionally labile, and prone to mood swings. Motor changes may occur if the posterior frontal lobes are involved,

TABLE 14-14 CLINICAL MANIFESTATIONS OF THE MAJOR DEGENERATIVE DEMENTIAS

DISEASE	FIRST SYMPTOM	MENTAL STATUS	NEUROBEHAVIOR	NEUROLOGIC EXAMINATION
Alzheimer disease	Memory loss; impaired learning	Episodic memory loss	Initially normal, progressive cognitive impairment	Initially normal
Creutzfeldt-Jakob disease	Dementia, mood, anxiety, movement disorders	Variable, frontal/executive, focal cortical, memory	Depression, anxiety	Myoclonus, rigidity, parkinsonism
Dementia with Lewy body	Visual hallucinations, REM sleep disorder, delirium; Capgras syndrome, parkinsonism	Drawing and frontal/executive; spares memory; delirium prone	Visual hallucinations, depression, sleep disorder, delusions	Parkinsonism
Frontotemporal dementia	Apathy; poor judgment/reasoning, speech/language; hyperorality	Frontal/executive, language; spares drawing	Apathy, decline in person or social conduct, hyperorality, euphoria, depression	Due to PSP/CBD overlap; vertical gaze palsy, axial rigidity, dystonia, alien hand
Vascular dementia	Often but not always sudden, usually within 3 months of a stroke; variable; apathy, falls, focal weakness	Frontal/executive, cognitive slowing; memory can be intact	Apathy, delusions, anxiety	Usually motor slowing, spasticity; can be normal

Adapted from Bird TD, Miller BL: Dementia. In Fauci AS et al, editors: *Harrison's principles of internal medicine,* ed 15, p 2538, New York, 2008, McGraw-Hill.
CBD, cortical basal degeneration; *PSP,* progressive supranuclear palsy; *REM,* rapid eye movement.

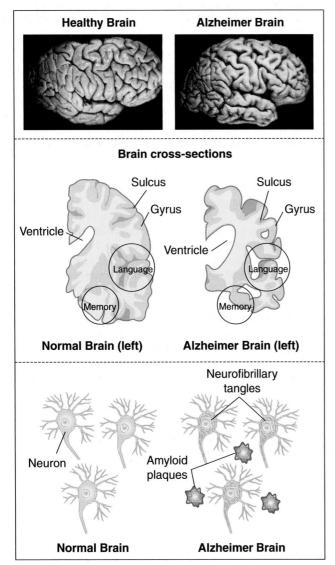

FIGURE 14-8 Common Pathologic Findings in Alzheimer Disease. The middle panel represents coronal slices through the left brain.

causing rigidity (paratonia, gegenhalten), with flexion posturing, propulsion, and retropulsion. Great variability in age of onset, intensity and sequence of symptoms, and location and extent of brain abnormalities is common. Stages for the progression of Alzheimer disease are summarized in Table 14-15.

Evaluation and treatment. The diagnosis of Alzheimer disease is made by ruling out other causes; clinical criteria have been developed to assist diagnosis.[12] The history, including mental status examinations (mini–mental status examination, clock drawing, and geriatric depression scale) and the course of the illness (which may span 5 years or more), is used to assess progression of the disease. Efforts are in progress to identify imaging and biochemical markers for early diagnosis and progression of Alzheimer type and other neurodegenerative causes of dementia (see *Health Alert*).[13,14]

HEALTH ALERT

Biomarkers and Neurodegenerative Dementia

Neurodegenerative disease processes that lead to dementia begin many years before clinical manifestations are evident for Alzheimer disease, Huntington disease, and Parkinson disease. Efforts are underway to identify neuroimaging techniques and predictive biomarkers in the brain, spinal fluid, and blood that will guide a more comprehensive understanding of the etiology and biologic pathways that mediate neurodegeneration. Identification and profiling of such molecules will promote early identification of risk factors, enhance preventive and protective measures, provide alerts for progression from mild to advanced stages, and accelerate development of presymptomatic treatment for these diseases.

Data from Seelaar H et al: Clinical, genetic, and pathological heterogeneity of frontotemporal dementia: a review, *J Neurol Neurosurg Psychiatr* 82(5):476–486, 2011; Patel B, Markus HS: Magnetic resonance imaging in cerebral small vessel disease and its use as a surrogate disease marker, *Int J Stroke* 6(1):47–59, 2011; Humpel C: Identifying and validating biomarkers for Alzheimer's disease, *Trends Biotechnol* 29(1):26–32, 2011; Forlenza OV, Diniz BS, Gattaz WF: Diagnosis and biomarkers of predementia in Alzheimer's disease, *BMC Med* 8:89, 2010.

TABLE 14-15	PROGRESSION OF ALZHEIMER DISEASE				
STAGE	**MILD COGNITIVE IMPAIRMENT**	**EARLY STAGE**	**MIDDLE STAGE**	**LATE STAGE**	**END-STAGE**
Cognitive	Mild memory loss	Measurable short-term memory loss; other cognition problems	Moderate to severe cognitive problems	Little cognitive ability; language not clear	No significant cognitive function
Functional	Possibly depression (vs. apathy); mild anxiety	Mild IADL problems	IADL-dependent; some ADL problems	ADL-dependent; incontinent	Nonambulatory/ bed-bound; unable to eat

Adapted from National Conference of Gerontological Nurse Practitioners and the National Gerontological Nursing Association: *Counseling Points* 1(1):6, 2008.
ADL, (Basic) activities of daily living; *IADL,* instrumental activities of daily living.

Treatment is directed at using devices to compensate for the impaired cognitive function, such as memory aids; maintaining unimpaired cognitive functions; and maintaining or improving the general state of hygiene, nutrition, and health. Cholinesterase inhibitors have shown a modest effect on cognitive function in mild to moderate Alzheimer disease. An *N*-methyl-D-aspartate (NMDA) receptor antagonist blocks glutamate activity and may slow progression of disease in moderate to severe AD.[15,16]

Frontotemporal Dementia

Frontotemporal dementia (FTD), previously known as Pick disease, is a rare, severe degenerative disease of the frontal and anterior frontal lobes that produces death of tissue and dementia. There is a familial association and an age of onset less than 60 years. The majority of cases involve mutations of genes encoding tau protein. The disease is difficult to distinguish clinically and pathologically from Alzheimer disease.[17]

ALTERATIONS IN CEREBRAL HEMODYNAMICS

An injured brain reacts with structural, chemical, and pathophysiologic changes that are called secondary brain injuries. Critical features of these changes include alterations in cerebral blood flow, intracranial pressure, and oxygen delivery (also see Chapter 15).

Cerebral blood flow (CBF) to the brain is normally maintained at a rate that matches local metabolic needs of the brain. Cerebral perfusion pressure (CPP) (70-90 mm Hg) is the pressure required to perfuse the cells of the brain, whereas cerebral blood volume (CBV) is the amount of blood in the intracranial vault at a given time. Cerebral oxygenation is the critical factor and is measured by oxygen saturation in the internal jugular vein.

Alterations in cerebral blood flow may be related to three injury states: inadequate cerebral perfusion (cerebral oligemia), normal cerebral perfusion with an elevated intracranial pressure, and excessive cerebral blood volume (cerebral hyperemia). Treatments for these injury states are directed at improving or maintaining CPP, as well as controlling intracranial pressure. An injured brain requires a CPP of greater than 70 mm Hg. Intracranial pressure (ICP) normally is 1 to 15 mm Hg, or 60 to 180 cm H_2O.

Increased Intracranial Pressure

Increased intracranial pressure (IICP) may result from an increase in intracranial content (as occurs with tumor growth), edema, excess CSF, or hemorrhage. It necessitates an equal reduction in volume of the other cranial contents. The most readily displaced content is CSF. If intracranial pressure remains high after CSF displacement out of the cranial vault, cerebral blood volume and blood flow are altered.

In *stage 1 of intracranial hypertension,* vasoconstriction and external compression of the venous system occur in an attempt to further decrease the intracranial pressure. Thus, during the first stage of intracranial hypertension, ICP may not change because of the effective compensatory mechanisms, and there may be few symptoms (Figure 14-9). Small increases in volume, however, cause an increase in pressure, and the pressure may take longer to return to baseline. This can be detected with ICP monitoring.

In *stage 2 of intracranial hypertension,* there is continued expansion of intracranial content. The resulting increase in ICP may exceed the brain's compensatory capacity to adjust. The pressure begins to compromise neuronal oxygenation, and systemic arterial vasoconstriction occurs in an attempt to elevate the systemic blood pressure sufficiently to overcome the IICP. Clinical manifestations at this stage usually are subtle and transient, including episodes of confusion, restlessness, drowsiness, and slight pupillary and breathing changes (see Figure 14-9).

In *stage 3 of intracranial hypertension,* ICP begins to approach arterial pressure, the brain tissues begin to experience hypoxia and hypercapnia, and the individual's condition rapidly deteriorates. Clinical manifestations include decreasing levels of arousal or central neurogenic hyperventilation, widened pulse pressure, bradycardia, and small, sluggish pupils (see Figure 14-9).

Dramatic sustained rises in ICP are not seen until all compensatory mechanisms have been exhausted. Then dramatic rises in ICP occur over a very short period. Autoregulation, the compensatory alteration in the diameter of the intracranial blood vessels designed to maintain a constant blood flow during changes in cerebral perfusion pressure, is lost with progressively increased ICP. Accumulating carbon dioxide may still cause vasodilation locally, but without autoregulation this vasodilation causes the hydrostatic (blood) pressure in the vessels to drop and the blood volume to increase. The brain volume is thus further enhanced, and ICP continues to rise. Small increases in volume cause dramatic increases in ICP, and the pressure takes much longer to return to baseline. As the ICP begins to approach systemic blood pressure, cerebral perfusion pressure falls and cerebral perfusion slows dramatically. The brain tissues experience severe hypoxia, hypercapnea, and acidosis.

In *stage 4 of intracranial hypertension,* brain tissue shifts (herniates) from the compartment of greater pressure to a compartment of lesser pressure and IICP in one compartment of the cranial vault is not evenly distributed throughout the other vault compartments (see Figures 14-9 and 14-10). With this shift in brain tissue, the herniating brain tissue's blood supply is compromised, causing further ischemia and hypoxia in the herniating tissues. The volume of content within the lower pressure compartment increases, exerting pressure on the brain tissue that normally occupies that compartment and impairing its blood supply.

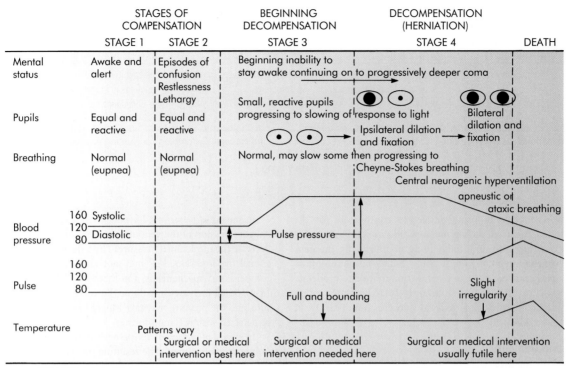

	STAGES OF COMPENSATION		BEGINNING DECOMPENSATION	DECOMPENSATION (HERNIATION)	
	STAGE 1	STAGE 2	STAGE 3	STAGE 4	DEATH
Mental status	Awake and alert	Episodes of confusion Restlessness Lethargy	Beginning inability to stay awake continuing on to progressively deeper coma		
Pupils	Equal and reactive	Equal and reactive	Small, reactive pupils progressing to slowing of response to light Ipsilateral dilation and fixation	Bilateral dilation and fixation	
Breathing	Normal (eupnea)	Normal (eupnea)	Normal, may slow some then progressing to Cheyne-Stokes breathing Central neurogenic hyperventilation apneustic or ataxic breathing		
Blood pressure	160 Systolic 120 80 Diastolic		Pulse pressure		
Pulse	160 120 80		Full and bounding	Slight irregularity	
Temperature		Patterns vary Surgical or medical intervention best here	Surgical or medical intervention needed here	Surgical or medical intervention usually futile here	

FIGURE 14-9 Clinical Correlates of Compensated and Uncompensated Phases of Intracranial Hypertension. (From Beare PG, Myers JL: *Principles and practice of adult health nursing,* ed 3, St Louis, 1998, Mosby.)

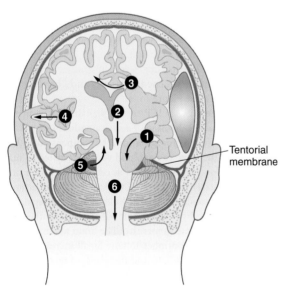

— Tentorial membrane

FIGURE 14-10 Herniation. Herniations can occur both above and below the tentorial membrane. **Suprateneorial:** *1,* uncal (transtentorial); *2,* central *3,* cinculate *4,* transcalvarial; **infratentorial:** *5,* upward, *6,* cerebellar tonsillar.

Small hemorrhages often develop in the involved brain tissue. Obstructive hydrocephalus may develop. The herniation process markedly and rapidly increases intracranial pressure. Mean systolic arterial pressure soon equals ICP, and cerebral blood flow ceases at this point. The types of herniation syndromes are outlined in Box 14-2.

Cerebral Edema

Cerebral edema is an increase in the fluid content of brain tissue (Figure 14-11). The result is increased extracellular or intracellular tissue volume. It occurs after brain insult from trauma, infection, hemorrhage, tumor, ischemia, infarct, or hypoxia. The harmful effects of cerebral edema are caused by distortion of blood vessels, displacement of brain tissues, and eventual herniation of brain tissue to a different brain compartment.

Three types of cerebral edema are (1) vasogenic edema, (2) cytotoxic (metabolic) edema, and (3) interstitial edema. Vasogenic edema is clinically the most important type and is caused by the increased permeability of the capillary endothelium of the brain after injury to the vascular structure. The blood-brain barrier (selective permeability of brain capillaries) is disrupted, and plasma proteins leak into the extracellular spaces, drawing water to them and increasing the water content of the brain parenchyma. Vasogenic edema starts in the area of injury and spreads, with fluid accumulating in the white matter of the ipsilateral side because the parallel myelinated fibers separate more easily. Edema promotes more edema because of ischemia from the increasing pressure.

Clinical manifestations of vasogenic edema include focal neurologic deficits, disturbances of consciousness, and a severe increase in ICP. Vasogenic edema resolves by slow diffusion.

In cytotoxic (metabolic) edema, toxic factors directly affect the cellular elements of the brain parenchyma (neuronal, glial, and endothelial cells), causing failure of the active transport systems. The cells lose their potassium and gain larger amounts of sodium. Water follows by osmosis into the cells, so that the cells swell. Cytotoxic edema occurs principally in the gray matter and may increase vasogenic edema.

BOX 14-2   HERNIATION SYNDROME

Supratentorial Herniation

1. *Uncal herniation.* Occurs when the uncus or hippocampal gyrus, or both, shifts from the middle fossa through the tentorial notch into the posterior fossa, compressing the ipsilateral third cranial nerve, the contralateral third cranial nerve, and the mesencephalon. Uncal herniation generally is caused by an expanding mass in the lateral region of the middle fossa. The classic manifestations of uncal herniation are a decreasing level of consciousness, pupils that become sluggish before fixing and dilating (first the ipsilateral, then the contralateral pupil), Cheyne-Stokes respirations (which later shift to central neurogenic hyperventilation), and the appearance of decorticate and then decerebrate posturing.

2. *Central herniation.* The straight downward shift of the diencephalon through the tentorial notch. It may be caused by injuries or masses located around the outer perimeter of the frontal, parietal, or occipital lobes; extracerebral injuries around the central apex (top) of the cranium; bilaterally positioned injuries or masses; and unilateral cingulate gyrus herniation. The individual rapidly becomes unconscious; moves from Cheyne-Stokes respirations to apnea; develops small, reactive pupils and then dilated, fixed pupils; and passes from decortication to decerebration.

3. *Cingulate gyrus herniation.* Occurs when the cingulate gyrus shifts under the falx cerebri. Little is known about its clinical manifestations.

Infratentorial Herniation

In the most common syndrome the cerebellar tonsil shifts through the foramen magnum because of increased pressure within the posterior fossa. The clinical manifestations are an arched stiff neck, paresthesias in the shoulder area, decreased consciousness, respiratory abnormalities, and pulse rate variations. Occasionally the force produces an upward transtentorial herniation of a cerebellar tonsil or the lower brain stem. No specific set of clinical manifestations is associated with infratentorial herniation (see Figure 14-10).

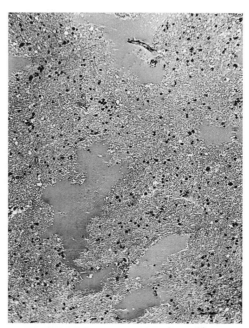

FIGURE 14-11 Brain Edema. Intercellular lakes of high protein content fluid. (Hematoxylin-eosin stain; ×90.) (From Kissane JM, editor: *Anderson's pathology*, ed 9, St Louis, 1993, Mosby.)

TABLE 14-16   TYPES OF HYDROCEPHALUS

TYPE	MECHANISM	CAUSE
Noncommunicating	Obstruction of CSF flow between ventricles	Congenital abnormality
	Aqueduct stenosis	
	Arnold-Chiari malformation (brain extension through foramen magnum)	
	Compression by tumor	
Communicating	Impaired absorption of CSF within subarachnoid space	Infection with inflammatory adhesions
	Compression of subarachnoid space by a tumor	
	High venous pressure in sagittal sinus	
	Head injury	
	Congenital malformation	
	Increased CSF secretion by choroid plexus	Secreting tumor

CSF, Cerebrospinal fluid.

Interstitial edema is seen most often with noncommunicating hydrocephalus. The edema is caused by transependymal movement of CSF from the ventricles into the extracellular spaces of the brain tissues. The brain fluid volume increases predominantly around the ventricles, with increased hydrostatic pressure within the white matter. The size of the white matter is reduced because of the rapid disappearance of myelin lipids.

Hydrocephalus

The term **hydrocephalus** refers to various conditions characterized by excess fluid in the cerebral ventricles, subarachnoid space, or both. Hydrocephalus occurs because of interference with CSF flow caused by increased fluid production, obstruction within the ventricular system, or defective reabsorption of the fluid. A tumor of the choroid plexus may, in rare instances, cause overproduction of CSF. The types of hydrocephalus are reviewed in Table 14-16.

Hydrocephalus may develop from infancy through adulthood. Congenital hydrocephalus (i.e., ventricular enlargement before birth) is rare. **Noncommunicating hydrocephalus (internal hydrocephalus, intraventricular hydrocephalus)**—obstruction within the ventricular system—is seen more often in children, and **communicating hydrocephalus**—defective resorption of CSF from the cerebral subarachnoid space—is found more often in adults.

Most cases of hydrocephalus develop gradually and insidiously over time. **Acute hydrocephalus,** however, may develop in a couple of hours in persons who have sustained head injuries. Acute hydrocephalus contributes significantly to IICP.

Pathophysiology. The obstruction of CSF flow associated with hydrocephalus produces increased pressure and dilation of the ventricles proximal to the obstruction. The increased pressure and dilation cause atrophy of the cerebral cortex and degeneration of the white matter tracts. Selective preservation of gray matter occurs. When excess CSF fills a defect caused by atrophy, a degenerative disorder, or a surgical excision, this fluid is not under pressure; therefore atrophy and degenerative changes are not induced.

Clinical manifestations. Acute hydrocephalus presents with signs of rapidly developing IICP. The person quickly deteriorates into a deep coma if not promptly treated. Normal-pressure hydrocephalus (dilation of the ventricles without increased pressure) develops slowly, with the individual or family noting declining memory and cognitive function. The triad symptoms of an unsteady, broad-based gait with a history of falling; incontinence; and dementia is common.[17a]

Evaluation and treatment. The diagnosis is based on physical examination, computed tomography (CT) scan, and magnetic resonance imaging (MRI). A radioisotopic cisternogram may be performed to diagnose normal-pressure hydrocephalus. Hydrocephalus can be treated by surgery to resect cysts, neoplasms, or hematomas or by ventricular bypass into the normal intracranial channel or into an extracranial compartment using a shunting procedure, one of the three most common neurosurgical procedures. Excision or coagulation of the choroid plexus occasionally is needed when a papilloma is present. In normal-pressure hydrocephalus, reduction in CSF is achieved through diuresis or placement of a ventriculoperitoneal shunt.

✔ **QUICK CHECK 14-4**
1. What are the four stages of intracranial hypertension (increased intracranial pressure)?
2. How does supratentorial herniation differ from infratentorial herniation?
3. What are the four different types of cerebral edema?
4. How is communicating hydrocephalus different from noncommunicating hydrocephalus?

ALTERATIONS IN NEUROMOTOR FUNCTION

Movements are complex patterns of activity controlled by the CNS. They are influenced by the cerebral cortex, the pyramidal system, the extrapyramidal system, and the motor units. Dysfunction in any of these areas can cause motor dysfunction. General neuromotor dysfunctions may produce changes in muscle tone, movement, and complex motor performance.

Alterations in Muscle Tone

Normal muscle tone involves a slight resistance to passive movement. Throughout the range of motion, the resistance is smooth, constant, and even. The alterations of muscle tone and their characteristics and causes are presented in Table 14-17.

Hypotonia

In hypotonia (decreased muscle tone), passive movement of a muscle occurs with little or no resistance. Causes include pure pyramidal tract damage (a rare occurrence) and cerebellar damage. A pure pyramidal tract injury produces hypotonia and weakness. The hypotonia contributes to the ataxia and intention tremor in cerebellar damage and manifests with minimal weakness and normal or slightly exaggerated reflexes. Hypotonia or flaccidity (a state in which the muscle may be moved rapidly without resistance) occurs when the nerve impulses needed for muscle tone are lost, such as in spinal cord injury or cerebrovascular accident.

Individuals with hypotonia tire easily (asthenia) or are weak. They may have difficulty rising from a sitting position, sitting down without using arm support, and walking up and down stairs, as well as an

---

TABLE 14-17 ALTERATIONS IN MUSCLE TONE

ALTERATIONS	CHARACTERISTICS	CAUSE
Hypotonia	Passive movement of a muscle mass with little or no resistance	Thought to be caused by decreased muscle spindle activity as a result of decreased excitability of neurons
	Muscles may be moved rapidly without resistance	
Flaccidity	Associated with limp, atrophied muscles, and paralysis	Occurs typically when nerve impulses necessary for muscle tone are lost
Hypertonia	Increased muscle resistance to passive movement	Results when lower motor unit reflex arc continues to function but is not mediated or regulated by higher centers
	May be associated with paralysis	
	May be accompanied by muscle hypertrophy	
Spasticity	A gradual increase in tone causing increased resistance until tone suddenly diminishes, which results in clasp-knife phenomenon; increased deep tendon reflexes (hyperreflexia); clonus (spread of reflexes)	Exact mechanism unclear; appears to arise from an increased excitability of alpha motor neurons to any input because of absence of descending inhibition of pyramidal systems
Gegenhalten (paratonia)	Resistance to passive movement, which varies in direct proportion to force applied	Exact mechanism unclear; associated with frontal lobe injury
Dystonia	Sustained involuntary twisting movement	Produced by slow muscular contraction; lack of reciprocal inhibition of muscle
Rigidity	Muscle resistance to passive movement of a rigid limb that is uniform in both flexion and extension throughout the motion	Occurs as a result of constant, involuntary contraction of muscle
Plastic, or lead pipe	Increased muscular tone relatively independent of degree of force used in passive movement; does not vary throughout the passive movement	Associated with basal ganglion damage
Cogwheel	Uniform resistance may be interrupted by a series of brief jerks, resulting in movements much like a ratchet, "cogwheel" phenomenon	Associated with basal ganglion damage
Gamma	Characterized by extensor posturing (decerebrate rigidity)	Loss of excitation of extensor inhibitory areas by cerebral cortex decreasing inhibition of alpha and gamma motor neurons
Alpha	Impaired relaxation characterized by extensor rigidity of skeletal muscle after contraction	Loss of cerebellum input to lateral vestibular nuclei

inability to stand on their toes. Because of their weakness, accidents during ambulatory and self-care activities are common. The joints become hyperflexible, so persons with hypotonia may be able to assume positions that require extreme joint mobility. The joints may appear loose, and the knee jerks are pendulous.

The muscle mass atrophies because of decreased input entering the motor unit, and muscles appear flabby and flat. Muscle cells are gradually replaced by connective tissue and fat. Fasciculations may be present in some cases.

Hypertonia

In hypertonia (increased muscle tone), passive movement of a muscle occurs with resistance. The four types of hypertonia are spasticity (Figure 14-12), gegenhalten (paratonia), dystonia (Figures 14-13 and 14-14), and rigidity. Four types of rigidity are described: plastic or lead-pipe, cogwheel, gamma, and alpha (see Table 14-17).

Individuals with hypertonia tire easily (asthenia) or are weak. Passive and active movement is affected equally, except in paratonia, in which more active than passive movement is possible. As a result of hypertonia and weakness, accidents occur during ambulatory and self-care activities.

The muscles may atrophy because of decreased use. However, hypertrophy occasionally occurs as a result of the overstimulation of muscle fibers. Overstimulation occurs when the motor unit reflex arc remains intact and functioning but is not inhibited by higher centers. This causes continual muscle contraction, resulting in enlargement of the muscle mass and the development of firm muscles.

Alterations in Movement

Movement requires a change in the contractile state of muscles. Abnormal movements occur when CNS dysfunctions alter muscle innervation. Currently, neuropharmacology and experimental therapeutics provide the knowledge base for movement disorders. Researchers have found that dopamine functions in several movement disorders. Some (e.g., the akinesias) result from too little dopaminergic activity, whereas others (e.g., chorea, ballism, tardive dyskinesia) result from too much dopaminergic activity. Still others are not primarily related to dopamine function. Movement disorders are not necessarily associated with mass, strength, or tone but are neurologic dysfunctions with either insufficient or excessive movement. Muscle strength is quantitatively evaluated on a scale of 0 to 4+ or 5+, in which 4+ or 5+ is normal and 0 indicates an inability to move against gravity.

Paresis/Paralysis

Paresis (weakness) is partial paralysis with incomplete loss of muscle power. Paralysis is loss of motor function so that a muscle group is unable to overcome gravity. Two subtypes of paresis/paralysis are described: upper motor neuron paresis/paralysis and lower motor neuron paresis/paralysis (Table 14-18).

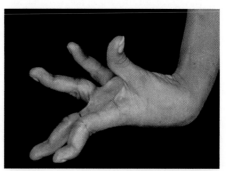

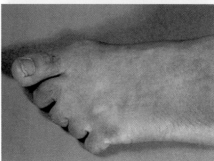

FIGURE 14-13 Dystonic Posturing of the Hand and Foot. (From Perkin GD: *Mosby's color atlas and text of neurology*, ed 2, London, 2002, Mosby.)

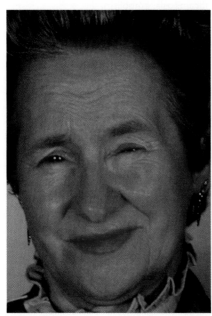

FIGURE 14-12 Paroxysm of Left-Sided Hemifacial Spasm. (From Perkin GD: *Mosby's color atlas and text of neurology*, ed 2, London, 2002, Mosby.)

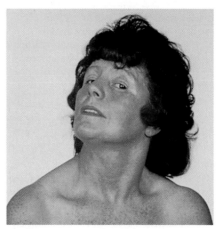

FIGURE 14-14 Spasmodic Torticollis. A characteristic head posture. (From Perkin GD: *Mosby's color atlas and text of neurology*, ed 2, London, 2002, Mosby.)

TABLE 14-18	UPPER AND LOWER MOTOR NEURON SIGNS AND SYMPTOMS
UPPER MOTOR NEURON (PYRAMIDAL CELLS [MOTOR CORTEX])	**LOWER MOTOR NEURON (VENTRAL HORN [SPINAL CORD], MOTOR NUCLEI [BRAIN STEM])**
Muscle groups are affected	Individual muscles may be affected
Mild weakness	Mild weakness
Minimal disuse muscle atrophy	Marked muscle atrophy
No fasciculations	Fasciculations
Increased muscle stretch reflexes (clasp-knife spasticity; resistance to passive flexion that releases abruptly to allow easy flexion)	Decreased muscle stretch reflexes
Clonus may be present	Clonus not present
Hypertonia, spasticity	Hypotonia, flaccidity
	Hyporeflexia
Pathologic reflexes (Babinski and Hoffmann signs, loss of abdominal reflexes)	No Babinski sign
Often initial impairment of only skilled movements	Asymmetric and may involve one limb only in beginning to become generalized as disease progresses

Upper Motor Neuron Syndromes

Upper motor neuron paresis/paralysis is known also as *spastic paresis/paralysis,* and different terms are used to describe the specific disorders. **Hemiparesis/hemiplegia** is paresis/paralysis of the upper and lower extremities on one side. **Diplegia** is paralysis of corresponding parts of both sides of the body as a result of cerebral hemisphere injuries. **Paraparesis/paraplegia** refers to weakness/paralysis of the lower extremities. **Quadriparesis/quadriplegia** refers to paresis/paralysis of all four extremities. Both paraparesis/paraplegia and quadriparesis/quadriplegia may be caused by dysfunction of the spinal cord. Upper cord damage results in quadriparesis/quadriplegia, and lower cord damage preserves upper extremity function and causes paraparesis/paraplegia. (Spinal cord injury is discussed in Chapter 15.)

Upper motor neuron paresis/paralysis is associated with a **pyramidal motor syndrome,** which involves a series of motor dysfunctions resulting from interruption of the pyramidal system (Figures 14-15 and 14-16). The injury may be in the cerebral cortex, the subcortical white matter, the internal capsule, the brain stem, or the spinal cord. The clinical manifestations reflect muscle overactivity and include excessive movements, such as clonus and spasms, occurring regularly as a result of loss of higher motor center control. There is great variation depending on the suddenness of onset and the age of the individual.

Spinal shock is the complete cessation of spinal cord functions below the lesion (below the level of the pons). It is characterized by complete flaccid paralysis, absence of reflexes, and marked

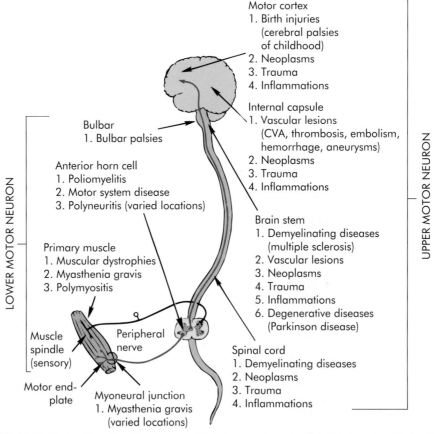

FIGURE 14-15 Motor Function Syndromes. Disturbances in motor function are classified pathologically along upper and lower motor neuron structures. It should be noted that the same pathologic condition occurs at more than one site in an upper motor neuron (above right). A few pathologic conditions involve both upper and lower motor neuron structures, as in amyotrophic lateral sclerosis, for example. Other lesion sites include myoneural junction and primary muscle, making it possible to classify conditions as neuromuscular and muscular, respectively.

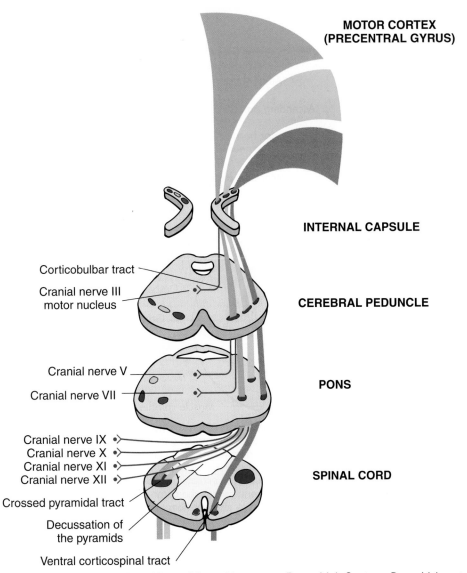

MOTOR CORTEX (PRECENTRAL GYRUS)

INTERNAL CAPSULE

Corticobulbar tract

Cranial nerve III motor nucleus

CEREBRAL PEDUNCLE

Cranial nerve V

Cranial nerve VII

PONS

Cranial nerve IX
Cranial nerve X
Cranial nerve XI
Cranial nerve XII

SPINAL CORD

Crossed pyramidal tract

Decussation of the pyramids

Ventral corticospinal tract

FIGURE 14-16 Structures of the Upper Motor Neuron, or Pyramidal, System. Pyramidal system fibers are shown to originate primarily in cells in precentral gyrus of motor cortex; to converge at internal capsule; to descend to form central third of cerebral peduncle; to descend further through pons, where small fibers supply cranial nerve motor nuclei along the way; to form pyramids at medulla, where most of the fibers decussate; and then to continue to descend in lateral column of white matter of spinal cord. A few fibers descend without crossing at medulla level (see Figure 12-8).

disturbances of bowel and bladder function. A major factor in spinal shock is the sudden destruction of the efferent pathways. If destruction occurs more slowly, spinal shock may not develop (see Chapter 15).

If the pyramidal system is interrupted above the level of the pons, the hand and arm muscles are greatly affected. Paralysis rarely involves all the muscles on one side of the body, even when the hemiplegia results from complete damage to the internal capsule. Bilateral movements, such as those of the eye, jaw, and larynx, as well as those of the trunk, are affected only slightly if at all. Predominantly the limbs are influenced.

Paralysis associated with a pyramidal motor syndrome rarely remains flaccid for a prolonged time. After a few days or weeks, a gradual return of spinal reflexes marks the end of spinal shock. Reflexes then become hyperactive, and muscle tone increases significantly, particularly in antigravity muscles. Spasticity is common, although

rigidity occasionally occurs. Most often, passive range-of-motion movements cause the "clasp-knife" phenomenon, probably by activating the stretch receptors in the muscle spindles and the Golgi tendon organ. (Muscle function is discussed in Chapter 36.) With pyramidal motor syndrome, predominantly the flexors of the arms and extensors of the legs are affected.

Lower Motor Neuron Syndromes

Lower (primary, alpha) motor neurons are the large motor neurons in the anterior (or ventral) horn of the spinal cord, the motor nuclei of the brain stem, and the axons that originate from these nerve cell bodies (to course in the anterior spinal roots or in the cranial nerves to reach skeletal muscles) (Figure 14-17). Dysfunction in this motor system impairs both voluntary hand involuntary movement. The degree of paralysis or paresis is proportional to the number of lower motor

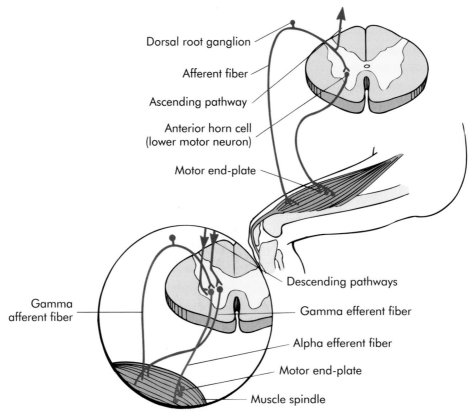

FIGURE 14-17 Structures Composing Lower Motor Neuron, Including Motor (Efferent) and Sensory (Afferent) Elements. *(Top)* Anterior horn cell (in anterior gray column of spinal cord and its axon), terminating in motor end-plate as it innervates extrafusal muscle fibers in quadriceps muscle. *(Detailed enlargement)* Sensory and motor elements of gamma loop system. Gamma efferent fibers shown innervating the muscle spindle (sensory receptor of skeletal muscle). Contraction of muscle spindle fibers stretches central portion of the spindle and causes the gamma afferent spindle fiber to transmit impulse centrally to cord. Muscle spindle gamma afferent fibers in turn synapse on the anterior horn cell and impulses are transmitted by way of alpha efferent fibers to skeletal (extrafusal) muscle, causing it to contract. Muscle spindle discharge is interrupted by active contraction of skeletal muscle fibers.

neurons affected. If only some of the motor units that supply a muscle are affected, only partial paralysis (or paresis) results. If all motor units are affected, a complete paralysis results. Other clinical manifestations also are proportional to the degree of dysfunction, but the precise manifestations depend on the location of the dysfunction in the motor unit and in the CNS.

Small motor (gamma) neurons, which maintain muscle tone and protect the muscle from injury, are needed for normal motor movement. They depend on input from the muscle spindle (arriving through an afferent limb rising to the cord). Dysfunction in this motor system (the gamma loop) impairs tone and reduces tendon reflexes, causing hyporeflexia. The muscles become susceptible to damage from hyperextensibility.

Generally, the large and small motor neuron systems are equally affected. Therefore the muscle has reduced or absent tone and is accompanied by hyporeflexia or areflexia (loss of tendon reflexes) and flaccid paresis/paralysis.

Denervated muscles (i.e., muscles that have lost their nervous system input) atrophy over weeks to months, mostly from disuse, and demonstrate fasciculations (muscle rippling or quivering under the skin). Occasionally, denervated muscles cramp. Fibrillation (isolated contraction of a single muscle fiber due to metabolic changes in denervated muscle not visible clinically).

Amyotrophies. Lower motor neuron syndromes originating in the anterior horn cells or the motor nuclei of the cranial nerves are called amyotrophies. Paralytic poliomyelitis is a contagious viral disease that involves a severe inflammatory reaction in motor neurons, some of which do not survive, leaving an irreversible paralysis (1 in 200 infections).[18] It has been eradicated in most of the world by vaccines.

A virally induced or postinfectious/postvaccination inflammatory process may injure or destroy anterior horn cells or cranial nerve cell bodies. Most of these inflammatory processes are mild and are followed by rapid cellular recovery.

In the amyotrophies, muscle strength, muscle tone, and muscle bulk are affected in the muscles innervated by the involved motor neurons. The paresis and paralysis associated with anterior horn cell injury are segmental, but because each muscle is supplied by two or more roots, the segmental character may be difficult to see. When cranial nerve motor nuclei are affected (these lack nerve roots and have only small rootlets near the point of exit from the brain stem), the distribution of the motor weakness follows that of the cranial nerve. The weakness may involve distal muscles, proximal muscles, or the muscles of midline structures. Hypotonia and hyporeflexia/areflexia are present.

The atrophy associated with amyotrophy is segmental when the anterior horn cells of the spinal cord are involved and follows the distribution of the cranial nerve when the motor nuclei of the cranial nerves are affected. It may be in distal, proximal, or midline muscles. Fasciculations are associated particularly with primary motor neuron injury, and muscle cramps and mild fatigue are common. If the pathologic process is limited to the primary motor neuron, no sensory changes are evident.

Several brain stem syndromes, called nuclear palsies, involve damage to one or more of the cranial nerve nuclei. Causes include vascular occlusion, tumor, aneurysm, tuberculosis, and hemorrhage.

The anterior horn cells and the motor nuclei of the cranial nerves may be secondarily affected in many severe pathologic processes involving primarily the cranial nerves. The condition may extend proximally to affect the nerve roots or rootlets and the motor neurons themselves, a process commonly seen, for example, in Guillain-Barré syndrome. If enough motor neurons are destroyed, permanent loss of motor function results because regeneration of the damaged axons requires a living neuronal cell body.

In progressive spinal muscular atrophy, the anterior horn cells of the spinal cord are affected. This disorder occurs in adults and closely resembles the familial progressive muscular atrophies that occur in infants and children and are considered inherited metabolic disorders (see Chapter 38). If the motor nuclei of the cranial nerves are affected instead of the anterior horn cells, the disorder is called a progressive bulbar palsy, so named because the myelencephalon originally was called the *bulb* and a degenerative process causes a progressively more serious condition. When any lower motor neuron syndrome involves the cranial nerves that arise from the bulb (i.e., cranial nerves IX, X, XII), the dysfunction is called a bulbar palsy.

The clinical manifestations of bulbar palsy include paresis or paralysis of the jaw, face, pharynx, and tongue musculature. Articulation is affected, especially articulation of the lingual *(r, n, l)*, labial *(b, m, p, f)*, dental *(d, t)*, and palatal *(k, g)* consonants. Modulation is impaired, making the voice rasping or nasal. Pharyngeal reflexes are diminished or lost, palate and vocal cord movement during phonation is impaired, and chewing and swallowing are affected. The facial muscles are weak, and the face appears to droop, with decreased jaw jerk. Atrophy and fasciculations eventually occur. All these manifestations become progressively worse, leading to aspiration, malnutrition, possible dehydration, and an inability to communicate verbally.

Hyperkinesia

Hyperkinesia (excessive movements) represents the second broad category of abnormal movements. Within this category are a number of specific dysfunctions including tremors (Table 14-19). Also included under the general category of hyperkinesias are dyskinesias—abnormal involuntary movements.

Paroxysmal dyskinesias are abnormal, involuntary movements that occur as spasms. The type of dyskinesia varies depending on the specific disorder.

Tardive dyskinesia is the involuntary movement of the face, trunk, and extremities. Although the condition occurs occasionally in individuals with Parkinson disease, it usually occurs as a side effect of prolonged phenothiazine drug therapy. The most common symptom of tardive dyskinesia is rapid, repetitive, stereotypic movements. Most characteristic is continual chewing with intermittent protrusions of the tongue, lip smacking, and facial grimacing.

Other movement disorders in this category are (1) complex repetitive movements, including automatism, stereotype, complex tics, e.g., Tourette syndrome (see *Health Alert*), compulsions, perseverations, and mannerisms; (2) positivism (excessive reactions to certain stimuli); and (3) paroxysmal excessive activity, including cataplexy and excessive startle reaction.

Huntington Disease

Huntington disease (HD), also known as *chorea,* is a relatively rare, hereditary, degenerative hyperkinetic movement disorder diffusely involving the basal ganglia and cerebral cortex. The onset of Huntington disease is usually between 25 and 45 years of age, when the trait may already have been passed to the person's children. The disorder has a prevalence rate of approximately 3 to 7 per 100,000 persons and occurs in all races.[19]

HEALTH ALERT

Tourette Syndrome

There is growing evidence that Tourette syndrome (TS) occurs worldwide and has common features across all races and cultures. The hallmark of TS is the presence of multiple motor and vocal tics. The tics may be either simple, involving only an individual muscle group (e.g., eye blinking or grunting), or complex, requiring coordinated movement of muscle groups (e.g., head banging or repeating of another person's words). Sensory tics involve unpleasant sensations in the face, head, and neck areas. Probably underdiagnosed, the onset of TS is typically between the ages of 2 and 15 years, with the tics lessening in adulthood. The syndrome has a complex multifactorial etiology with undetermined genetic, environmental, immune, and hormonal factors. The pathophysiology of TS is unclear and currently under study. There is evidence of frontal-striatal-thalamic dysfunction and, in some cases, altered dopaminergic neurotransmission. TS is often diagnosed in association with anxiety, depression, attention-deficit/hyperactivity disorder (ADHD), and obsessive-compulsive disorder.

Data from Robertson MM: Gilles de la Tourette syndrome: the complexities of phenotype and treatment, *Br J Hosp Med (Lond)* 72(2):100–117, 2011; Worbe Y et al: Distinct structural changes underpin clinical phenotypes in patients with Gilles de la Tourette syndrome, *Brain* 133(Pt 12):3649–3660, 2010; Worbe Y et al: Repetitive behaviours in patients with Gilles de la Tourette syndrome: tics, compulsions, or both? *PLoS One* 5(9):e12959, 2010; Jankovic J, Gelineau-Kattner R, Davidson A: Tourette's syndrome in adults, *Mov Disord* 25(13):2171–2175, 2010.

Pathophysiology. Huntington disease (HD) is inherited from both mothers and/or fathers who have the autosomal dominant trait with high penetrance. The Huntingtin gene (*HTT*) is located on the short arm of chromosome 4. Mutated forms of the HD gene contain abnormally repeated segments of deoxyribonucleic acid (DNA), called CAG trinucleotide repeats. These repeated segments result in the synthesis of huntingtin proteins. CAG repeat allele lengths are defined as fully penetrant at ≥40, reduced penetrance at 36 to 39, high normal at 27 to 35, and normal at ≤26. Fathers, but not mothers, with high normal alleles do not develop HD but are at risk of transmitting potentially penetrant HD alleles (≥36) to their offspring, who can develop HD.[20]

The principal pathologic feature of Huntington disease is severe degeneration of the basal ganglia, particularly the caudate nucleus. Tangles of protein (huntingtin protein) collect in the brain cells and chains of glutamine on the abnormal molecules stick to each other and contribute to neuronal loss.[21] Basal ganglia and nigral depletion of gamma-aminobutyric acid (GABA), an inhibitory neurotransmitter, is the principal biochemical alteration in Huntington disease. It alters the integration of motor and mental function.[22] Frontal cerebral atrophy occurs late in the disease. The triggers and timing of pathogenesis are not clearly understood.

TABLE 14-19   TYPES OF HYPERKINESIA AND TREMOR

TYPE	CHARACTERISTICS	CAUSES
Hyperkinesia		
Chorea*	Nonrepetitive muscular contractions, usually of extremities of face; random pattern of irregular, involuntary rapid contractions of groups of muscles; disappears with sleep, decreases with resting; increases with emotional stress and attempted voluntary movement	Associated with excess concentration of or supersensitivity to dopamine within basal ganglia
Athetosis*	Disorder of distal muscle postural fixation; slow, sinuous, irregular movements most obvious in distal extremities, more rhythmic than choreiform movements and always much slower; movements accompany characteristic hand posture; slowly fluctuating grimaces	Occurs most commonly as result of injury to putamen of basal ganglion; exact pathophysiologic mechanism is not known
Ballism	Disorder of proximal muscle postural fixation with wild flinging movement of limbs; movement is severe and stereotyped, usually lateral; does not lessen with sleep; ballism is most common on one side of body, a condition termed *hemiballism*	Results from injury to subthalamic nucleus (one of nuclei that comprise basal ganglia); thought to be caused by reduced inhibitory influence in nucleus, a release phenomenon; hemiballism results from injury to contralateral subthalamic nucleus
Hyperactivity	State of prolonged, generalized, increased activity that is largely involuntary but may be subject to some voluntary control; not highly stereotyped but rather manifests as continuous changes in total body posture or in excessive performance of some simple activity, such as pacing under inappropriate circumstances	May be caused by frontal and reticular activating system injury
Wandering	Tendency to wander without regard for environment	"Release phenomenon" associated with bilateral injury to globus pallidus or putamen
Akathisia	Special type of hyperactivity; mild compulsion to move (usually more localized to legs); severe, frenzied motion possible; movements are partly voluntary and may be transiently suppressed; carrying out movement brings sense of relief; frequent complication of antipsychotic drugs	Dopaminergic transmission may be involved
Tremor at Rest		
Parkinsonian tremor	Rhythmic, oscillating movement affecting one or more body parts	Caused by regular contraction of opposing groups of muscles
	Regular, rhythmic, slower flexion-extension contraction; involves principally metacarpophalangeal and wrist joints; alternating movements between thumb and index finger described as "pill rolling;" disappears during voluntary movement	Loss of inhibitory influence of dopamine in the basal ganglia, causing instability of basal ganglial feedback circuit within cerebral cortex
Postural Tremor		
Asterixis (tremor of hepatic encephalopathy)	Irregular flapping movement of hands accentuated by outstretching arms	Exact mechanisms responsible unknown; thought to be related to accumulation of products normally detoxified by liver, i.e., ammonia
Metabolic	Rapid, rhythmic tremor affecting fingers, lips, and tongue; accentuated by extending body part; enhanced physiologic tremor	Occurs in conditions associated with disturbed metabolism or toxicity, as in thyrotoxicosis (hyperthyroidism), alcoholism, and chronic use of barbiturates, amphetamines, lithium, or amitriptyline [Elavil]; exact mechanism responsible unknown
Essential (familial)	Tremor of fingers, hands, and feet; absent at rest but accentuated by extension of body part, prolonged muscular activity, and stress	Not associated with any other neurologic abnormalities; cause unknown
Intention Tremor		
Cerebellar	Tremor initiated by movement, maximal toward end of movement	Occurs in disease of dentate nucleus (one of deep cerebellar nuclei responsible for efferent output) and superior cerebellar peduncle (stalklike structure connected to pons); caused by errors in feedback from periphery and errors in preprogramming goal-directed movement
Rubral	Rhythmic tremor of limbs that originates proximally by movement	Results from lesions involving dentatorubrothalamic tract (a spinothalamic tract connecting red nucleus in reticular formation and dentate nucleus in cerebellum)
Myoclonus	Series of shocklike nonpatterned contractions of portion of a muscle, entire muscle, or group of muscles that cause throwing movements of a limb; usually appear at random but frequently triggered by sudden startle; do not disappear during sleep	Associated with an irritable nervous system and spontaneous discharge of neurons; structures associated with myoclonus include cerebral cortex, cerebellum, reticular formation, and spinal cord

*Choreoathetosis involves both chorea and athetosis; precise pathophysiology unknown.

Clinical manifestations. Symptoms of Huntington disease progress slowly and include involuntary fragmentary movements, such as chorea (irregular, uncontrolled, excessive movement), athetosis (writhing movements), and ballism (flinging movements). Chorea, the most common type of abnormal movement, begins in the face and arms, eventually affecting the entire body. There is progressive dysfunction of intellectual and thought processes (dementia). Any one of these features may mark the onset of the disease. Cognitive deficits include loss of working memory and reduced capacity to plan, organize, and sequence. Thinking is slow, and apathy is present. Restlessness, disinhibition, and irritability are common. Euphoria or depression may be present.

Evaluation and treatment. The diagnosis of Huntington disease is based on family history and clinical presentation of the disorder. No known treatment is effective in halting the degeneration or progression of symptoms. Drug therapies are being explored.[23]

Hypokinesia

Hypokinesia (decreased movement) is loss of voluntary movement despite preserved consciousness and normal peripheral nerve and muscle function. Types of hypokinesia include akinesia, bradykinesia, and loss of associated movement.

Akinesia and bradykinesia. Akinesia is a decrease in voluntary and associated movements. It is related to dysfunction of the extrapyramidal system and caused by either a deficiency of dopamine or a defect of the postsynaptic dopamine receptors, which occurs in parkinsonism. Bradykinesia is slowness of voluntary movements. All voluntary movements become slow, labored, and deliberate, with difficulty in (1) initiating movements, (2) continuing movements smoothly, and (3) performing synchronous (at the same time) and consecutive tasks. Both akinesia and bradykinesia involve a delay in the time it takes to start to perform a movement.

Loss of associated movement. In hypokinesia, the normal, habitually associated movements that provide skill, grace, and balance to voluntary movements are lost. Decreased associated movements accompanying emotional expression cause an expressionless face, a statue-like posture, absence of speech inflection, and absence of spontaneous gestures. Decreased associated movements accompanying locomotion cause reduction in arm and shoulder movements, in hip swinging, and in rotary motion of the cervical spine.

Parkinson Disease

Parkinson disease (PD) is a commonly occurring disorder of movement. Either primary Parkinson disease or secondary parkinsonism may occur. Secondary parkinsonism is parkinsonism caused by disorders other than Parkinson disease (i.e., head trauma, infection, neoplasm, atherosclerosis, toxins, drug intoxication). Drug-induced parkinsonism, caused by neuroleptics, antiemetics, and antihypertensives, is the most common secondary form and usually is reversible.

Parkinson (primary) disease begins after the age of 40 years, with the incidence increasing after 60 years. It is more prevalent in males and a leading cause of neurologic disability in individuals older than 60 years. The prevalence is about 1 in 272 persons, with approximately 60,000 new cases diagnosed in the United States each year.[24]

Pathophysiology. The pathogenesis of primary Parkinson disease is unknown. Several genes have been identified. Epidemiologic data also suggest viral and environmental toxins as possible causes. There is degeneration of the basal ganglia (see Figure 12-9) with dysfunctional or misfolded α-synuclein protein and loss of dopamine-producing neurons in the substantia nigra and dorsal striatum. The resulting depletion of dopamine, an inhibitory neurotransmitter, and relative excess of cholinergic (excitatory) activity in the feedback circuit are manifested by hypertonia (tremor and rigidity) and akinesia, producing a syndrome of abnormal movement called parkinsonism (Parkinson syndrome, parkinsonian syndrome, paralysis agitans) (Figure 14-18). Dementia may develop over decades with infiltration of Lewy bodies (accumulation of abnormal protein in nerve cells) and plaque formation similar to Alzheimer disease.[25]

Clinical manifestations. The classic manifestations of Parkinson disease are tremor at rest (resting tremor), rigidity (muscle stiffness), bradykinesia/akinesia (poverty of movement), postural disturbance, dysarthria, and dysphagia. They may develop alone or in combination, but as the disease progresses, all are usually present. There is no true paralysis. The symptoms are always bilateral but usually involve one side early in the illness. Because the onset is insidious, the beginning of symptoms is difficult to document. Early in the disease, reflex status, sensory status, and mental status usually are normal. Postural abnormalities (flexed, forward leaning), difficulty walking, and weakness develop. Speech may be slurred. Autonomic-neuroendocrine symptoms include inappropriate diaphoresis, orthostatic hypotension, drooling, gastric retention, constipation, and urinary retention. Depression is also prevalent.

Disorders of equilibrium result from postural abnormalities (Figure 14-19). The person with Parkinson disease cannot make the appropriate postural adjustment to tilting or falling and falls like a post when starting to tilt. The festinating gait (short, accelerating steps) of the individual with Parkinson disease is an attempt to maintain an upright position while walking. Individuals are also unable to right themselves when changing from a reclining or crouching position to a standing position and when rolling over from a supine to a lateral or prone position. Sleep disorders and excessive daytime sleepiness are commonly experienced.[26] Sensory disturbances (pain and impaired smell and vision), difficulty concentrating, and hallucinations are some of the nonmotor symptoms of Parkinson disease.[27]

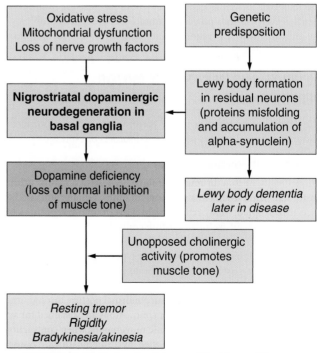

FIGURE 14-18 Pathophysiology of Parkinson Disease.

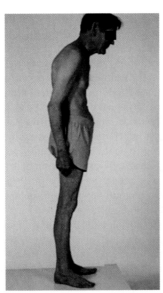

FIGURE 14-19 Stooped Posture of Parkinson Disease. (From Perkin DG: *Mosby's color atlas and text of neurology*, ed 2, London, 2002, Mosby.)

Progressive dementia is more common in persons older than 70 years. Mental status may be further compromised by the side effects of the medication taken to control symptoms.

Evaluation and treatment. The diagnosis of Parkinson disease is based on the history and physical examination. Causes of secondary parkinsonism are first excluded. No specific diagnostic tests are available, except positron emission tomography (PET). Treatment of Parkinson disease is symptomatic with drug therapy to decrease akinesia. Because of troublesome side effects and loss of effectiveness, however, drug therapy may not be started until the symptoms become incapacitating. Deep brain stimulation is replacing surgery to treat persons unresponsive to drug therapy. Implants of stem cells and fetal cells as well as gene therapy hold promise for future treatments.[28,29] Dysphagia and general immobility are special problems of the individual with PD requiring interdisciplinary efforts to improve functional status.[30]

ALTERATIONS IN COMPLEX MOTOR PERFORMANCE

The alterations in complex motor performance include disorders of posture (stance), disorders of gait, and disorders of expression.

Disorders of Posture (Stance)

An inequality of tone in muscle groups, because of a loss of normal postural reflexes, results in a posturing of limbs. Equilibrium and balance are disrupted. Many reflex systems govern tone and posture, but the most important factor in posture control is the stretch reflex, in which extensor (antigravity) muscle stretching causes increased extensor tone and inhibited flexor tone. Four types of disorders of postures are (1) dystonic posture, (2) decerebrate posture, (3) basal ganglion posture, and (4) senile posture.

Dystonia is the maintenance of an abnormal posture through muscular contractions. When muscular contractions are sustained for several seconds, they are called dystonic movements; when contractions last for longer periods, they are called dystonic postures. Dystonic postures may last for weeks, causing permanent, fixed contractures.

Dystonia has been associated with basal ganglia abnormality, but the exact pathophysiologic mechanisms are unknown. One dystonic posture already discussed in this chapter is decorticate posture (striatal posture or upper motor neuron dysfunction posture), which may be unilateral or bilateral. Decorticate posture (also referred to as antigravity posture or hemiplegic posture) is characterized by upper extremities flexed at the elbows and held close to the body and by lower extremities that are externally rotated and extended (see Figure 14-6). Decorticate posture is thought to occur when the brain stem is not inhibited by the cerebral cortex motor area. Upper motor neuron posture is more commonly described as the arm flexed at the elbow with a wrist drop, the leg inadequately bent at the knee, the hip excessively circumabducted, and the presence of footdrop.

Decerebrate posture refers to increased tone in extensor muscles and trunk muscles, with active tonic neck reflexes. When the head is in a neutral position, all four limbs are rigidly extended. The decerebrate posture is caused by severe injury to the brain and brain stem, resulting in overstimulation of the postural righting and vestibular reflexes.

Basal ganglion posture refers to a stooped, hyperflexed posture with a narrow-based, short-stepped gait. This posture abnormality results from the loss of normal postural reflexes and not from defects in proprioceptive, labyrinthine, or visual function. Dysfunctional equilibrium results when the individual loses stability and cannot make the appropriate postural adjustment to tilting or loss of balance, falling instead. Dysfunctional righting is the inability to right oneself when changing from a lying or crouching to a standing position or when rolling from the supine to the lateral or prone position. Dysfunctional postural fixation is the involuntary flexion of the head and neck, causing the person difficulty in maintaining an upright trunk position while standing or walking. Basal ganglion dysfunction accounts for this posture.

Senile posture is characterized by an increasingly flexed posture similar to that caused by basal ganglion dysfunction. The posture is associated with frontal lobe dysfunction, but the primary pathophysiology is not known.

Disorders of Gait

Four predominant types of gait are (1) upper motor neuron dysfunction gait, (2) cerebellar (ataxic) gait, (3) basal ganglion gait, and (4) senile gait (pseudoparkinsonian gait). As with posture, equilibrium and balance are affected with gait disturbances.

Several upper motor neuron gaits exist. With mild forms, the individual may have footdrop with fatigue and hip and leg pain. A spastic gait, which is associated with unilateral injury, manifests by a shuffling gait with the leg extended and held stiff, causing a scraping over the floor surface. The leg swings improperly around the body rather than being appropriately lifted and placed. The foot may drag on the ground, and the person tends to fall to the affected side. A scissors gait is associated with bilateral injury and spasticity. The legs are adducted so they touch each other. As the person walks, the legs are swung around the body but then cross in front of each other because of adduction. Injury to the pyramidal system accounts for these gaits.

A cerebellar gait is wide-based with the feet apart and often turned outward or inward for greater stability. The pelvis is held stiff, and the individual staggers when walking. Cerebellar dysfunction accounts for this particular gait.

A basal ganglion gait and a senile gait are both broad-based gaits in which the person walks with small steps and a decreased arm swing. The head and body are flexed and the arms semiflexed and abducted, whereas the legs are flexed and rigid in more advanced states. Basal ganglion and frontal lobe dysfunction, respectively, account for these two gaits.

Disorders of Expression

Disorders of expression involve the motor aspects of communication and include (1) hypermimesis, (2) hypomimesis, and (3) dyspraxias/apraxias. **Hypermimesis** commonly manifests as pathologic laughter or crying. Pathologic laughter is associated with right hemisphere injury, and pathologic crying is associated with left hemisphere injury. The exact pathophysiology is not known. **Hypomimesis** manifests as *aprosody*—the loss of emotional language. *Receptive aprosody* involves an inability to understand emotion in speech and facial expression. *Expressive aprosody* involves the inability to express emotion in speech and facial expression. Aprosody is associated with right hemisphere damage.

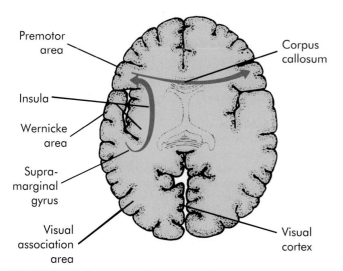

FIGURE 14-20 Pathways Disrupted in Dyspraxias. Formulation of the idea of the motor act is thought to originate in the region of the supramarginal gyrus in the inferior left parietal lobe. This area is connected via associational pathways to the left premotor cortex. The left premotor cortex is connected through the corpus callosum to the right premotor and motor areas. An injury that interrupts the pathways between the left supramarginal gyrus and the premotor region produces a dyspraxia that involves the entire body. An injury that disrupts the callosal pathways produces a dyspraxia of the left side of the body only.

Dyspraxia/apraxia is a disorder of learned motor skills with difficulty planning and executing coordinated motor movements. It can be developmental, beginning at birth (developmental dyspraxia), or associated with vascular disorders (common in stroke), trauma, tumors, degenerative disorders, infections, or metabolic disorders. People with dyspraxia have difficulty performing tasks requiring motor skills including speaking, writing, using tools or utensils, playing sports, following instructions, and focusing.[31]

True dyspraxias occur when the connecting pathways between the left and right cortical areas are interrupted (Figure 14-20). Dyspraxias may result from any pathologic process that disrupts the cortical areas necessary for the conceptualization and execution of a complex motor act or the communication pathways within the left hemisphere or between the hemispheres.

EXTRAPYRAMIDAL MOTOR SYNDROMES

Because the extrapyramidal system encompasses all the motor pathways except the pyramidal system, two types of motor dysfunction make up the **extrapyramidal motor syndromes:** (1) the basal ganglia motor syndromes and (2) the cerebellar motor syndromes. Unlike pyramidal motor syndromes, both extrapyramidal motor syndromes result in movement or posture disturbance without significant paralysis, along with other distinctive symptoms (Table 14-20).

Basal ganglia motor syndromes are caused by an imbalance of dopaminergic and cholinergic activity in the corpus striatum. A relative excess of cholinergic activity produces akinesia and hypertonia. A relative excess of dopaminergic activity produces hyperkinesia and hypotonia. Symptoms associated with Parkinson and Huntington diseases are exemplary of disorders of the basal ganglia. **Cerebellar motor syndromes** are associated with ataxia and other symptoms affecting coordinated movement. Cerebellar disorders primarily influence the same side of the body, so that damage to the right cerebellum generally causes symptoms on the right side of the body.

> **QUICK CHECK 14-5**
> 1. Why are there so many causes of hypertonia?
> 2. How is chorea different from athetosis?
> 3. Why is paresis/paralysis a type of hypokinesia?
> 4. What structures are involved in alterations of complex motor performance?

TABLE 14-20 PYRAMIDAL VS. EXTRAPYRAMIDAL MOTOR SYNDROME

MANIFESTATIONS	PYRAMIDAL MOTOR SYNDROME	EXTRAPYRAMIDAL MOTOR SYNDROME
Unilateral movement	Paralysis of voluntary movement	Little or no paralysis of voluntary movement
Tendon reflexes	Increased tendon reflexes	Normal or slightly increased tendon reflexes
Babinski sign	Present	Absent
Involuntary movements	Absence of involuntary movements	Presence of tremor, chorea, athetosis, or dystonia
Muscle tone	Spasticity in muscles (e.g., clasp-knife phenomenon)	Plastic (equal throughout movement) rigidity or intermittent (generalized but predominantly in flexors of limbs and trunk) rigidity (cogwheel rigidity)
	Hypertonia present in flexors of arms and extensors of legs	Hypotonia, weakness and gait disturbances in cerebellar disease

DID YOU UNDERSTAND?

Alterations in Cognitive Systems

1. Full consciousness is an awareness of oneself and the environment with an ability to respond to external stimuli with a wide variety of responses.
2. Consciousness has two components: arousal and awareness.
3. An altered level of arousal occurs by diffuse bilateral cortical dysfunction, bilateral subcortical (reticular formation, brain stem) dysfunction, and localized hemispheric dysfunction.
4. An alteration in breathing pattern and level of consciousness reflect the level of brain dysfunction.
5. Pupillary changes reflect changes in level of brain stem function, drug action, and response to hypoxia and ischemia.
6. Abnormal eye movements, including nystagmus and divergent gaze, reflect alterations in brain stem function.
7. Level of brain function manifests by changes in generalized motor responses or no responses.
8. Loss of cortical inhibition associated with decreased consciousness produces abnormal flexor and extensor movements.
9. Cerebral death or irreversible coma represents permanent brain damage, with an ability to maintain cardiac, respiratory, and other vital functions.
10. Brain death results from irreversible brain damage, with an inability to maintain internal homeostasis.
11. Arousal returns in vegetative states, but awareness is absent.
12. With a deficit in selective attention, mediated by midbrain, thalamus, and parietal lobe structures, the individual cannot focus on selective stimuli and thus neglects those stimuli.
13. In amnesia, some past memories are lost and new memories cannot be stored.
14. Frontal areas mediate vigilance, detection, and working memory.
15. With vigilance deficits, the person cannot maintain sustained concentration.
16. With detection deficits, the person is unmotivated and unable to set goals and plan.
17. Seizures represent a sudden, chaotic discharge of cerebral neurons, with transient alterations in brain function. Seizures may be generalized or focal and can result from cerebral lesions, biochemical disorders, trauma, or epilepsy.
18. Data processing deficits include agnosias, dysphasias, acute confusional states, and dementias.
19. Agnosias are defects of recognition and may be tactile, visual, or auditory. They are caused by dysfunction in the primary sensory area or the interpretive areas of the cerebral cortex.
20. Dysphasia (aphasia) is an impairment of comprehension or production of language. Dysphasia may be expressive or receptive.
21. Acute confusional states are characterized chiefly by a loss of detection and, in the case of delirium, an intense autonomic nervous system hyperactivity.
22. Alzheimer disease is a chronic irreversible dementia that is related to altered production or failure to clear amyloid from the brain.
23. Frontotemporal dementias are rare early-onset degenerative diseases similar to Alzheimer disease.

Alterations in Cerebral Hemodynamics

1. Increased intracranial pressure may result from edema, excess cerebrospinal fluid, hemorrhage, or tumor growth. When intracranial pressure approaches arterial pressure, hypoxia and hypercapnia produce brain damage.
2. Cerebral edema is an increase in the fluid content of the brain resulting from infection, hemorrhage, tumor, ischemia, infarct, or hypoxia.
3. The shifting or herniation of brain tissue from one compartment to another disrupts the blood flow of both compartments and damages brain tissue.

4. Supratentorial herniation involves temporal lobe and hippocampal gyrus shifting from the middle fossa to posterior fossa; transtentorial herniation involves a downward shift of the diencephalon through the tentorial notch; and shifting of the cingulate gyrus can occur under the falx cerebri.
5. The most common infratentorial herniation is a shift of the cerebellar tonsils through the foramen magnum.
6. Hydrocephalus comprises a variety of disorders characterized by an excess of fluid within the ventricles, subarachnoid space, or both. Hydrocephalus occurs because of interference with cerebrospinal fluid flow caused by increased fluid production or obstruction within the ventricular system or by defective reabsorption of the fluid.

Alterations in Neuromotor Function

1. Motor dysfunction may be characterized as alterations of motor tone, movement, and complex motor performance.

Alterations in Tone

1. Hypotonia and hypertonia are the main categories of altered tone.
2. The four types of hypertonia are spasticity, gegenhalten, dystonia, and rigidity.

Alterations in Movement

1. Paresis, paraplegia, hyperkinesias, and hypokinesia are the main categories of altered movement.
2. Two subtypes of paresis/paralysis are described: upper motor neuron spastic paresis/paralysis and lower motor neuron flaccid paresis/paralysis.
3. An upper motor neuron syndrome is characterized by paresis/paralysis, hypertonia, and hyperreflexia.
4. Interruption of the pyramidal tract below the pons results in spinal shock.
5. Lower motor neuron syndromes manifest by impaired voluntary and involuntary movements and flaccid paralysis.
6. Partial paralysis occurs with only partial loss of alpha motor neurons, and total paralysis is complete loss of alpha motor neurons. Loss of gamma motor neurons impairs muscle tone and decreases tendon reflexes.
7. Amyotrophy (e.g., poliomyelitis) is a lower motor neuron syndrome involving the anterior horn cells, with loss of muscle tone and strength resulting in segmental paresis and hyporeflexia.
8. Nuclear palsies involve damage to the cranial nerve nuclei.
9. Bulbar palsies involve cranial nerves IX, X, and XII.
10. Included in the category of hyperkinesias are chorea, athetosis, ballism, akathisia, tremor, and myoclonus.
11. Huntington disease (chorea) is a rare hereditary disease involving the basal ganglia and cerebral cortex. It is inherited as an autosomal dominant trait and commonly manifests between 25 and 45 years of age with involuntary fragmentary movements.
12. The major pathologic feature of Huntington disease is severe degeneration of the basal ganglia and the frontal cerebral cortex. The basal ganglia and the substantia nigra exhibit a depletion of gamma-aminobutyric acid (an inhibitory neurotransmitter) secreting neurons. This depletion leads to an excess of dopaminergic activity that causes involuntary, fragmentary movements.
13. Types of hypokinesia include akinesia, bradykinesia, and loss of associated movements.
14. Parkinson disease is a commonly occurring degenerative disorder of the basal ganglia (corpus striatum) involving degeneration of the dopamine-secreting nigrostriatal pathway. The pathogenesis of Parkinson disease is unknown, but researchers suggest genetic, viral, and environmental toxins as possible causes.

DID YOU UNDERSTAND?—cont'd

15. Degeneration of the dopaminergic nigrostriatal pathway causes dopamine depletion in the basal ganglia and excess of cholinergic activity in the cortex, basal ganglia, and thalamus. Tremor and rigidity are caused by the excess cholinergic activity. Progressive dementia may be associated with an advanced stage of the disease.

16. Treatment of Parkinson disease is symptomatic, involving levodopa (L-dopa), a precursor of dopamine.

Alterations in Complex Motor Performance

1. Alterations in complex motor performance include disorders of posture (stance), disorders of gait, and disorders of expression.

2. Disorders of posture include dystonic posture, decerebrate posture, basal ganglion posture, and senile posture.

3. Disorders of gait include upper motor neuron gait, cerebellar gait, basal ganglion gait, and senile gait.

4. Disorders of expression include hypermimesis, hypomimesis, and dyspraxia/apraxia.

5. Dyspraxia is an impairment of the conceptualization or execution of a complex motor act.

Extrapyramidal Motor Syndromes

1. Extrapyramidal motor syndromes include basal ganglia and cerebellar motor syndromes.

2. Basal ganglia disorders manifest by alterations in muscle tone and posture, including rigidity, involuntary movements, and loss of postural reflexes.

3. Cerebellar motor syndromes result in loss of muscle tone, difficulty with coordination, and disorders of equilibrium and gait.

KEY TERMS

- Acute confusional state (ACS)   357
- Acute hydrocephalus   363
- Agnosia   356
- Akinesia   371
- Alzheimer disease (AD) (dementia of Alzheimer type [DAT], senile disease complex)   359
- Amnesia   353
- Amyotrophy   368
- Anterograde amnesia   353
- Aphasia   357
- Apraxia   373
- Areflexia   368
- Arousal   347
- Aura   355
- Autoregulation   361
- Awareness (content of thought)   353
- Basal ganglia motor syndrome   373
- Basal ganglion gait   372
- Basal ganglion posture   372
- Bradykinesia   371
- Brain death (total brain death)   352
- Bulbar palsy   369
- Cerebellar gait   372
- Cerebellar motor syndrome   373
- Cerebral blood flow (CBF)   361
- Cerebral blood volume (CBV)   361
- Cerebral death (irreversible coma)   352
- Cerebral edema   362
- Cerebral oxygenation   361
- Cerebral perfusion pressure (CPP)   361
- Clonic phase   355
- Communicating hydrocephalus   363
- Consciousness   347
- Convulsion   354
- Cytotoxic (metabolic) edema   362
- Decerebrate posture   372
- Decorticate posture (antigravity posture, hemiplegic posture)   372

- Delirium (hyperkinetic confusional state)   357
- Dementia   357
- Diplegia   366
- Dysphasia   357
- Dyspraxia   373
- Dystonia   365
- Dystonic movement   372
- Dystonic posture   372
- Echolalia   357
- Epilepsy   354
- Epileptogenic focus   355
- Executive attention deficit   353
- Expressive dysphasia   357
- Extinction   353
- Extrapyramidal motor syndrome   373
- Fibrillation   368
- Flaccid paresis/paralysis   368
- Frontotemporal dementia (FTD) (Pick disease)   361
- Gegenhalten (paratonia)   365
- Guillain-Barré syndrome   369
- Hemiparesis   366
- Hemiplegia   366
- Hiccup   351
- Huntington disease (HD)   369
- Hydrocephalus   363
- Hyperkinesia   369
- Hypermimesis   373
- Hypertonia   365
- Hypokinesia   371
- Hypokinetic confusional state (hyperactive delirium)   357
- Hypomimesis   373
- Hypotonia   364
- Image processing   353
- Increased intracranial pressure (IICP)   361
- Interstitial edema   363
- Level of consciousness   349

- Locked-in syndrome   353
- Memory   353
- Memory disorder   353
- Metabolic alteration in arousal   348
- Minimally conscious state (MCS)   353
- Mirror focus   355
- Motor response   351
- Neglect syndrome   353
- Neurofibrillary tangle   359
- Noncommunicating hydrocephalus (internal hydrocephalus, intraventricular hydrocephalus)   363
- Normal-pressure hydrocephalus   364
- Nuclear palsy   369
- Oculomotor response   349
- Paralysis   365
- Paraparesis   366
- Paraplegia   366
- Paresis   365
- Parkinson disease   371
- Parkinsonism (Parkinson syndrome, parkinsonian syndrome, paralysis agitans)   371
- Paroxysmal dyskinesia   368
- Pattern of breathing   349
- Persistent vegetative state   353
- Poliomyelitis   368
- Prodroma   356
- Progressive bulbar palsy   369
- Progressive spinal muscular atrophy   369
- Psychogenic alteration in arousal (unresponsiveness)   348
- Pupillary change   349
- Pyramidal motor syndrome   366
- Quadriparesis   366
- Quadriplegia   366
- Receptive dysphasia   357
- Retrograde amnesia   353
- Rigidity   365
- Scissors gait   372

▎ KEY TERMS—cont'd

- Secondary parkinsonism 371
- Seizure 354
- Selective attention 353
- Selective attention deficit 353
- Senile gait 372
- Senile posture 372
- Sensory inattentiveness 353

- Spastic gait 372
- Spasticity 365
- Spinal shock 366
- Structural alteration in arousal 347
- Tardive dyskinesia 369
- Tonic phase 355
- Transcortical dysphasia 357

- Upper motor neuron gait 372
- Upper motor neuron paresis/paralysis 366
- Vasogenic edema 362
- Vegetative state (VS) 347
- Vomiting 351
- Yawning 351

REFERENCES

1. Wijdicks EF, et al: American Academy of Neurology. Evidence-based guideline update: determining brain death in adults: report of the Quality Standards Subcommittee of the American Academy of Neurology, *Neurology* 74(23):1911–1918, 2010.
2. American Academy of Pediatrics: Task Force on Brain Death in Children: Report of special task force: guidelines for the determination of brain death in children, *Pediatrics* 80(2):298–300, 1987.
3. Overgaard M: How can we know if patients in coma, vegetative state or minimally conscious state are conscious? *Prog Brain Res* 177:11–19, 2009.
4. Lulé D, et al: Life can be worth living in locked-in syndrome, *Prog Brain Res* 177:339–351, 2009.
5. Placantonakis DG, Schwartz TH: Localization in epilepsy, *Neurol Clin* 27(4):1015–1030, 2009.
6. Centers for Disease Control and Prevention: Targeting epilepsy: improving the lives of people with one of the nation's most common neurological conditions: at a glance, accessed Jan 29, 2010, available at www.cdc.gov/chronicdisease/resources/publications/AAG/epilepsy.htm.
7. Baulac S, Baulac M: Advances on the genetics of mendelian idiopathic epilepsies, *Neurol Clin* 27(4):1041–1061, 2009.
8. Dichter MA: Emerging concepts in the pathogenesis of epilepsy and epileptogenesis, *Arch Neurol* 66(4):443–447, 2009.
8a. Berg AT: Epilepsy, cognition, and behavior: the clinical picture, *Epilepsia* 52(Suppl 1):7–12, 2011.
9. Smith DA: Delirium as an emerging frontier in the management of critically ill children, *Crit Care Clin* 25(3):593–614, 2009:x.
10. Caplan JP, Rabinowitz T: An approach to the patient with cognitive impairment: delirium and dementia, *Med Clin North Am* 94(6):1103–1116, 2010:ix.
10a. Vasilevskis EE, et al: Reducing iatrogenic risks: ICU-acquired delirium and weakness–crossing the quality chasm, *Chest* 138(5):1224–1233, 2010.
10b. Reitz C, Brayne C, Mayeux R: Epidemiology of Alzheimer disease, *Nat Rev Neurol* 7(3):137–152, 2011.
11. Bekris LM, et al: Genetics of Alzheimer disease, *J Geriatr Psychiatry Neurol* 23(4):213–227, 2010.
11a. Mondragón-Rodríguez S, et al: Causes versus effects: the increasing complexities of Alzheimer's disease pathogenesis, *Expert Rev Neurother* 10(5):683–691, 2010.
12. McKhann GM, et al: The diagnosis of dementia due to Alzheimer's disease: recommendations from the National Institute on Aging and the Alzheimer's Association workgroup, Alzheimer's & Dementia, *The Journal of the Alzheimer's Association* 7(3):1–7, 2011.
13. Ballard C, et al: Alzheimer's disease, *Lancet* 377(9770):1019–1031, 2011.
14. Humpel C: Identifying and validating biomarkers for Alzheimer's disease, *Trends Biotechnol* 29(1):26–32, 2011.
15. Galimberti D, Scarpini E: Treatment of Alzheimer's disease: symptomatic and disease-modifying approaches, *Curr Aging Sci* 3(1):46–56, 2010.
16. Riordan KC, et al: Effectiveness of adding memantine to an Alzheimer dementia treatment regimen which already includes stable donepezil therapy: a critically appraised topic, *Neurologist* 17(2):121–123, 2011.
17. Rabinovici GD, Miller BL: Frontotemporal lobar degeneration: epidemiology, pathophysiology, diagnosis and management, *CNS Drugs* 24(5):375–398, 2010.
17a. Siraj S: An overview of normal pressure hydrocephalus and its importance: how much do we really know? *J Am Med Dir Assoc* 12(1):19–21, 2011.
18. World Health Organization: Poliomyelitis fact sheet No 114, updated November 2010. Accessed April 11, 2011. Available at www.who.int/mediacentre/factsheets/fs114/en/.
19. Cardoso F: Huntington disease and other choreas, *Neurol Clin* 27(3):719–736, 2009:vi.
20. Ross CA, Tabrizi SJ: Huntington's disease: from molecular pathogenesis to clinical treatment, *Lancet Neurol* 10(1):83–98, 2011.
21. Ross CA, Tabrizi SJ: Huntington's disease: from molecular pathogenesis to clinical treatment, *Lancet Neurol* 10(1):83–98, 2011.
22. Kumar P, Kalonia H, Kumar A: Huntington's disease: pathogenesis to animal models, *Pharmacol Rep* 62(1):1–14, 2010.
23. Mason SL, Barker RA: Emerging drug therapies in Huntington's disease, *Expert Opin Emerg Drugs* 14(2):273–297, 2009.
24. 2011 Parkinson Disease Foundation, Inc.: Statistics on Parkinson's available at www.pdf.org/en/parkinson_statistics.
25. Halliday GM, McCann H: The progression of pathology in Parkinson's disease, *Ann N Y Acad Sci* 1184:188–195, 2010.
26. Stavitsky K, et al: Sleep in Parkinson's disease: a comparison of actigraphy and subjective measures, *Parkinsonism Relat Disord* 16(4):280–283, 2010.
27. Löhle M, Storch A, Reichmann H: Beyond tremor and rigidity: non-motor features of Parkinson's disease, *J Neural Transm* 116(11):1483–1492, 2009.
28. Chan DK, Cordato DJ, O'Rourke F: Management for motor and nonmotor complications in late Parkinson's disease, *Geriatrics* 63(5):22–27, 2008.
29. Yuan H, et al: Treatment strategies for Parkinson's disease, *Neurosci Bull* 26(1):66–76, 2010.
30. Hayes MW, et al: Current concepts in the management of Parkinson disease, *Med J Aust* 192(3):144–149, 2010.
31. Gross RG, Grossman M: Update on apraxia, *Curr Neurol Neurosci Rep* 8(6):490–496, 2008.

Disorders of the Central and Peripheral Nervous Systems and Neuromuscular Junction

Barbara J. Boss and Sue E. Huether

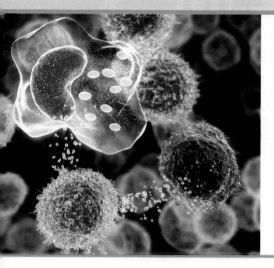

CHAPTER OUTLINE

Alterations in central nervous system (CNS) function are caused by traumatic injury, vascular disorders, tumor growth, infectious and inflammatory processes, metabolic derangements (including those arising from nutritional deficiencies and drugs or chemicals), and degenerative processes. Alterations in peripheral nervous system function involve the nerve roots, a nerve plexus or the nerves themselves, or the neuromuscular junction.

CENTRAL NERVOUS SYSTEM DISORDERS

Traumatic Brain and Spinal Cord Injury
Brain Trauma

Major head injury is traumatic insult to the brain capable of producing physical, intellectual, emotional, social, and vocational changes. Those at highest risk for traumatic brain injury (TBI) are children 4 years and younger, adolescents 15 to 19 years, and adults 65 years and older. Males have the highest incidence in every age group. Traumatic brain injury is highest among blacks and in lower- and median-income families. Most traumatic brain injuries are caused by transportation-related events, falls, sports-related events, and violence.[1] The causative mechanisms are summarized in Table 15-1.

In recent years, individuals with traumatic brain injury have improved survival outcomes mostly because of advancements in safety measures (e.g., passive seat restraints, air bags, protective head gear), reduced transport time to hospitals or trauma centers, and improved on-scene medical management. Prevention and management of secondary and tertiary brain injuries also have improved outcomes.

The damage from brain trauma can be focal, affecting one area of the brain, or diffuse (diffuse axonal injury), involving more than one area of the brain. Usually both types of injuries are associated with an event of primary brain injury.

Head injuries can be caused by closed (blunt) trauma and open (penetrating) trauma. **Closed (blunt) trauma** is more common and involves either the head striking a hard surface or a rapidly moving object striking the head. The dura remains intact, and brain tissues are not exposed to the environment. Blunt trauma may result in both focal brain injuries and diffuse axonal injuries (Table 15-2). **Open trauma** occurs when a break in (penetration of) the dura results in exposure of the cranial contents to the environment. The most common type of blunt trauma is mild (75% to 90%) and causes mild concussion and classical cerebral concussion (Table 15-3). Focal brain injury and

TABLE 15-1 CAUSES OF BRAIN INJURIES

TYPE OF INJURY	MECHANISM
Focal Brain Injury	Localized injury from direct impact
Blunt trauma	Closed injury
Coup	Injury is directly below site of forceful impact
Contrecoup	Injury is on opposite side of brain from site of forceful impact
Extradural (epidural) hematoma	Vehicular accidents, minor falls, sporting accidents
Subdural hematoma	Vehicular accidents or falls, especially in elderly persons or persons with chronic alcohol abuse
Intracerebral hemorrhage; subarachnoid hemorrhage	Contusions caused by forceful impact, usually vehicular accidents or long distance falls
Compound fracture	Objects strike head with great force or head strikes object forcefully; temporal blows, occipital blows, upward impact of cervical vertebrae (basilar skull fracture)
Penetrating trauma	Open injury
	Missiles (bullets) or sharp projectiles (knives, ice picks, axes, screwdrivers)
Diffuse Brain Injury (diffuse axonal injury)	Traumatic shearing forces; tearing of axons from twisting and rotational forces with injury over widespread area
	Moving head strikes hard, unyielding surface or moving object strikes stationary head; vehicular accidents (occupant or pedestrian); torsional head motion

TABLE 15-2 SEVERITY OF TRAUMA RELATED TO TRAUMA STATE INDUCED AND ONSET AND PERSISTENCE OF CLINICAL MANIFESTATIONS

SEVERITY OF TRAUMA	TRAUMA STATE INDUCED		ONSET OF CLINICAL MANIFESTATIONS	PERSISTENCE OF DAI CLINICAL MANIFESTATIONS
	FOCAL INJURY	**DIFFUSE AXONAL INJURY (DAI)**		
Mild blunt trauma		Mild concussion	Immediate	Hours to days
Moderate blunt trauma		Classic cerebral concussion	Immediate	Up to 6 months or longer
	Paraplegia (associated with injury to top of head)		Immediate	
	Blindness (associated with occipital injury)		Immediate	
	Delayed development of unresponsiveness (vasomotor or vasovagal syncopal episode)		Delayed	
Severe blunt trauma		Mild DAI	Immediate	Recovery in days to weeks
		Moderate DAI	Immediate	Residual manifestation
		Severe DAI	Immediate	Permanent severe disability
	Acute epidural hemorrhage		Immediate to delayed (2-3 hr)	
	Acute contusional swelling		Delayed onset (few hours after injury)	
	Acute subdural hematoma		Delayed onset (few hours to 1 week after injury)	
	Subacute subdural hematoma*		Delayed onset (1 to few weeks)	
	Subdural hygroma (fluid accumulation)		Delayed onset	
	Traumatic cerebral hemorrhage*		Delayed onset (as late as 1 week after injury)	

*May be seen after moderate head injury, especially in elderly people.

diffuse axonal injury (DAI) each account for half of all injuries. Focal brain injury accounts for more than two thirds of head injury deaths; DAI accounts for fewer than one third. However, more severely disabled survivors, including those in an unresponsive state or reduced level of consciousness, have DAI.

Three mechanisms produce brain damage: primary, secondary, and tertiary injury. Primary injury is caused by the impact and involves neural injury, primary glial injury, and vascular responses. Secondary injury is an indirect consequence of the primary injury and includes a cascade of cellular and molecular events (i.e., altered cerebral blood flow, hypoxia, ischemia, inflammation, cerebral edema, increased intracranial pressure, and herniation) that cause further neural injury or death. Tertiary injury develops days or months later as a consequence of primary and secondary injury and can result from systemic

TABLE 15-3	CATEGORIES OF DIFFUSE BRAIN INJURY
TYPE OF INJURY	**MECHANISM**
Mild concussion	Temporary axonal disturbance affecting attentional and memory systems; consciousness not lost
Grade I	Confusion and disorientation with amnesia (momentary)
Grade II	Momentary confusion and retrograde amnesia after 5-10 min
Grade III	Confusion and retrograde amnesia from impact; also anterograde amnesia
Classic cerebral concussion	Same as grade IV mild concussion—diffuse cerebral disconnection from brain stem reticular activating system; physiologic neurologic dysfunction without substantial anatomic disruption; immediate loss of consciousness lasting less than 6 hr; retrograde and anterograde amnesia (post-traumatic); may be uncomplicated or complicated
Diffuse axonal injury (DAI)	Prolonged traumatic coma (longer than 6 hr)
Mild	Post-traumatic coma lasts 6-24 hr; persistent residual cognitive, psychologic, and sensorimotor deficits; rare—only 8% of severe head injuries; reversible memory loss, confusion, disorientation
Moderate	Widespread physiologic impairment throughout cerebral cortex and diencephalon; coma longer than 24 hr; tearing of axons in both hemispheres; prolonged incomplete recovery among survivors with headaches, nausea, and memory difficulty; common—20% of severe head injuries
Severe	Formerly called *primary brain stem injury* or *brain stem contusion;* prolonged coma—days to months; irreversible coma or death; severe mechanical disruption of axons in both hemispheres, diencephalon, and brain stem; 16% of severe head injuries

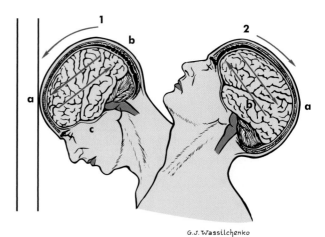

G.J. Wassilchenko

FIGURE 15-1 Coup and Contrecoup Head Injury After Blunt Trauma. *1, Coup injury:* impact against object; *a,* site of impact and direct trauma to brain; *b,* shearing of subdural veins; *c,* trauma to base of brain. *2, Contrecoup injury:* impact within skull; *a,* site of impact from brain hitting opposite side of skull; *b,* shearing forces through brain. These injuries occur in one continuous motion—the head strikes the wall (coup) and then rebounds (contrecoup). (Modified from Rudy EB: *Advanced neurological and neurosurgical nursing,* St Louis, 1984, Mosby.)

complications, such as pneumonia, fever, infections, and immobility, that contribute to further brain injury.

Primary brain injury

Focal brain injury. Focal brain injuries are specific, grossly observable brain lesions that occur in a precise location (e.g., cortical contusions, epidural hemorrhage, subdural hematoma, intracerebral hematoma, and open brain trauma). The force of impact typically produces **contusions** (blood leaking from injured blood vessels) from injury to the vault, vessels, and supporting structures that, in turn, produce epidural hemorrhage and subdural and intracerebral hematomas. The mechanisms of injury are depicted in Figure 15-1.

Focal brain injury results from compression of the skull at the point of impact and rebound effects. The injury may be coup or contrecoup (see Figure 15-1 and Table 15-1) and produces contusions (brain bruising). The severity of contusion varies with the amount of energy transmitted by the skull to underlying brain tissue. The smaller the area of impact, the greater the severity of injury because the force

is concentrated into a smaller area. Brain edema forms around and in damaged neural tissues, contributing to the increasing intracranial pressure (see Chapter 14). Within the contused areas, infarction, necrosis, multiple hemorrhages, and edema occur. The tissue has a pulpy quality. The maximal effects of these injuries peak 18 to 36 hours after severe head injury.

Contusions are found most commonly in the frontal lobes, particularly at the poles and along the inferior orbital surfaces; in the temporal lobes, especially at the anterior poles and along the inferior surface; and at the frontotemporal junction. They cause changes in attention, memory, executive attention functions (see Chapter 14), affect, emotion, and behavior. Less commonly, contusions occur in the parietal and occipital lobes. Focal cerebral contusions are usually superficial, involving just the gyri. Hemorrhagic contusions may coalesce into a large confluent intracranial hematoma.

A contusion may be evidenced by immediate loss of consciousness (generally accepted to last no longer than 5 minutes), loss of reflexes (individual falls to the ground), transient cessation of respiration, brief period of bradycardia, and decrease in blood pressure (lasting 30 seconds to a few minutes). Increased cerebrospinal fluid (CSF) pressure and electrocardiogram (ECG) and electroencephalogram (EEG) changes occur on impact. Vital signs may stabilize to normal values in a few seconds; reflexes then return and the person regains consciousness over minutes to days. Residual deficits may persist and some persons never regain a full level of consciousness.

Evaluation includes a complete history and physical examination. Skull and spinal x-ray films are often taken and a computed tomography (CT) scan or magnetic resonance imaging (MRI) may be performed. Large contusions and lacerations with hemorrhage may be surgically excised. Treatment is otherwise directed at controlling intracranial pressure and managing symptoms.

Extradural hematomas (bleeding between the dura mater and the skull [i.e., epidural hematomas, epidural hemorrhages]) represent 1% to 2% of major head injuries and occur in all age groups, but most commonly in those 20 to 40 years old. An artery is the source of

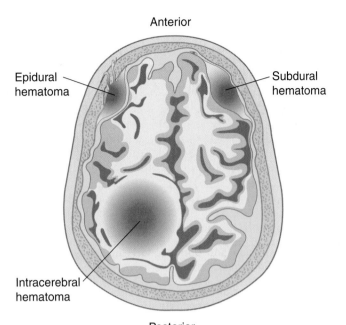

FIGURE 15-2 Brain Hematomas.

bleeding in 85% of extradural hematomas; 15% result from injury to the meningeal vein or dural sinus (Figure 15-2). The temporal fossa is the most common site of extradural hematoma caused by injury to the middle meningeal artery or vein. The temporal lobe shifts medially, precipitating uncal (see Figure 14-10) and hippocampal gyrus herniation through the tentorial notch. Extradural hemorrhages are found occasionally in the subfrontal area, especially in the young and elderly populations, caused by injury to the anterior meningeal artery or a venous sinus, and in the occipital-suboccipital area, resulting in herniation of the posterior fossa contents through the foramen magnum.

Individuals with classic temporal extradural hematomas lose consciousness at injury; one third of those affected then become lucid for a few minutes to a few days (if a vein is bleeding). As the hematoma accumulates, a headache of increasing severity, vomiting, drowsiness, confusion, seizure, and hemiparesis may develop. Because temporal lobe herniation occurs, the level of consciousness is rapidly lost, with ipsilateral pupillary dilation and contralateral hemiparesis.

A CT scan or MRI usually is needed to diagnose extradural hematoma. The prognosis is good if intervention is initiated before bilateral dilation of the pupils occurs. Extradural hematomas are almost always medical emergencies requiring surgical ligation of bleeding vessels.

Subdural hematomas (bleeding between the dura mater and the brain) arise in 10% to 20% of persons with traumatic brain injury. *Acute subdural hematomas* develop rapidly, commonly within hours, and usually are located at the top of the skull (the cerebral convexities). Bilateral hematomas occur in 15% to 20% of persons. Subacute subdural hematomas develop more slowly, often over 48 hours to 2 weeks. *Chronic subdural hematomas* (commonly found in elderly persons and persons who abuse alcohol and have some degree of brain atrophy with a subsequent increase in extradural space) develop over weeks to months. Bridging veins tear, causing both rapidly and subacutely developing subdural hematomas, although torn cortical veins or venous sinuses and contused tissue also may be the source. These subdural hematomas act like expanding masses, increasing intracranial pressure that eventually compresses the bleeding vessels (see Figure 15-2). Brain herniation can result. With a chronic subdural

hematoma, the existing subdural space gradually fills with blood. A vascular membrane forms around the hematoma in approximately 2 weeks. Further enlargement may take place.

In acute, rapidly developing subdural hematomas, the expanding clots directly compress the brain. As intracranial pressure rises, bleeding veins are compressed. Thus, bleeding is self-limiting, although cerebral compression and displacement of brain tissue can cause temporal lobe herniation.

An acute subdural hematoma classically begins with headache, drowsiness, restlessness or agitation, slowed cognition, and confusion. These symptoms worsen over time and progress to loss of consciousness, respiratory pattern changes, and pupillary dilation (i.e., the symptoms of temporal lobe herniation). Homonymous hemianopia (defective vision in either the right or the left field [see Figure 13-10]), disconjugate gaze, and gaze palsies also may occur.

Of those individuals affected by chronic subdural hematomas, 80% have chronic headaches and tenderness over the hematoma on palpation. Most persons appear to have a progressive dementia with generalized rigidity (paratonia). Chronic subdural hematomas require a craniotomy to evacuate the gelatinous blood. Percutaneous drainage for chronic subdural hematomas has proven successful. However, reaccumulation often occurs unless the surrounding membrane is removed.

Intracerebral hematomas (bleeding within the brain) occur in 2% to 3% of persons with head injuries, may be single or multiple, and are associated with contusions. Although most commonly located in the frontal and temporal lobes, they may occur in the hemispheric deep white matter. Penetrating injury or shearing forces traumatize small blood vessels. The intracerebral hematoma then acts as an expanding mass, increasing intracranial pressure, compressing brain tissues, and causing edema (see Figure 15-2). Delayed intracerebral hematomas may appear 3 to 10 days after the head injury.

Intracerebral hematomas cause a decreasing level of consciousness. Coma or a confusional state from other injuries, however, can make the cause of this increasing unresponsiveness difficult to detect. Contralateral hemiplegia also may occur and, as intracranial pressure rises, temporal lobe herniation may appear. In delayed intracerebral hematoma, the presentation is similar to that of a hypertensive brain hemorrhage—sudden, rapidly progressive decreased level of consciousness with pupillary dilation, breathing pattern changes, hemiplegia, and bilateral positive Babinski reflexes.

History and physical examination help to establish the diagnosis and CT scan, MRI, and cerebral angiography confirm it. Evacuation of a singular intracerebral hematoma has only occasionally been helpful, mostly for subcortical white matter hematomas. Otherwise, treatment is directed at reducing the intracranial pressure and allowing the hematoma to reabsorb slowly.

Open (penetrating) brain trauma (trauma that penetrates the dura mater) produces discrete (focal) injuries and includes compound skull fractures and missile injuries. A **compound skull fracture** opens a communication between the cranial contents and the environment and should be investigated whenever lacerations of the scalp, tympanic membrane, sinuses, eye, or mucous membranes are present. Such fractures may involve the cranial vault or the base of the skull (basilar skull fracture). Bone fragments cause tangential injury (injury caused by direct contact) and, occasionally, penetrating injuries. Cranial nerves may be damaged with a basilar skull fracture.

Missiles include bullets, rocks, shell fragments, knives, and blunt instruments. The mechanisms of injury are crush injury (laceration and crushing of whatever the missile touches) and stretch injury (blood vessels and nerves damaged without direct contact as a result of stretching). The tangential injury is to the coverings and the brain (scalp and brain lacerations) and may also include skull fractures and meningeal or cerebral lacerations. When driven into the brain substance, projectiles and debris from scalp and skull injury produce a penetrating brain injury.

Most persons lose consciousness with open-head injury. The depth and duration of the coma are related to the location of injury, extent of damage, and amount of bleeding. Open-head injury often requires débridement of the traumatized tissues to prevent infection and to remove blood clots, thereby reducing intracranial pressure. Intracranial pressure also is managed with steroids, dehydrating agents, osmotic diuretics, or a combination of these drugs. Broad-spectrum antibiotics are administered.

A compound fracture may be diagnosed through physical examination, skull x-ray films, or both. Basilar skull fracture is determined on the basis of clinical findings. Skull x-rays often do not demonstrate the fracture, although intracranial air or air in the sinuses on x-ray film, CT scan, or MRI is indirect evidence of a basilar skull fracture.

Bed rest and close observation for meningitis and other complications are prescribed for a basilar skull fracture. Prophylactic antibiotics are controversial and may or may not be given.

Diffuse brain injury. Diffuse brain injury (diffuse axonal injury [DAI]) involves widespread areas of the brain. Damage to delicate axonal fibers and white matter tracts that project to the cerebral cortex cause concussion. Mechanical effects from shaking (high levels of acceleration and deceleration [whiplash]) and rotational and twisting movements are the primary mechanisms of injury, producing strains and distortions within the brain. The freely moving head is attached to the neck, allowing rotational forces to trigger shearing forces on brain tissues. The most severe axonal injuries are located more peripheral to the brain stem, causing extensive cognitive and affective impairments, as seen in survivors of traumatic brain injury from vehicular crashes. Axonal damage reduces the speed of informational processing and responding and disrupts the individual's attention span.

Pathophysiologically, axonal damage can be seen only with an electron microscope and involves numerous axons, either alone or in conjunction with actual tissue tears. Areas where axons and small blood vessels are torn appear as small hemorrhages, particularly in the corpus callosum and dorsolateral quadrant of the rostral brain stem at the superior cerebellar peduncle. More and more damaged axons are visible 12 hours to several days after the injury (secondary brain injury). The severity of diffuse injury correlates with how much shearing force was applied to the brain stem. DAI is not associated with intracranial hypertension immediately after injury; however, acute brain swelling caused by increased intravascular blood flow within the brain, vasodilation, and increased cerebral blood volume is seen often and can result in death.

Several categories of diffuse brain injury exist: mild concussion, classic concussion, mild DAI, moderate DAI, and severe DAI (see Table 15-2). DAI has the following consequences:

1. *Physical consequences:* spastic paralysis, peripheral nerve injury, swallowing disorders, dysarthria, visual and hearing impairments, taste and smell deficits
2. *Cognitive deficits:* disorientation and confusion, short attention span, memory deficits, learning difficulties, dysphasia, poor judgment, perceptual deficits
3. *Behavioral manifestations:* agitation, impulsiveness, blunted affect, social withdrawal, depression

Mild concussion is characterized by immediate but transitory clinical manifestations. CSF pressure rises, and ECG and EEG changes occur without loss of consciousness. The initial confusional state lasts for 1 to

several minutes, possibly with amnesia for events preceding the trauma (retrograde amnesia). Anterograde amnesia (lack of memories) may also exist transiently. Persons may experience head pain and complain of nervousness and "not being themselves" for up to a few days.

In classic cerebral concussion, consciousness is lost for up to 6 hours and reflexes fail, causing falls. Reflexes are regained as responsiveness returns. Transiently, breathing stops, bradycardia occurs, and blood pressure falls. Vital signs quickly stabilize to within normal limits. Retrograde and anterograde amnesia exist (see Chapter 14), along with a confusional state lasting for hours to days. Head pain, nausea, fatigue, attentional and memory system impairments (inability to concentrate and forgetfulness), and mood and affect changes (nervousness, anxiety reactions, depression, irritability, fatigability, insomnia) occur. A postconcussive syndrome, including headache, nervousness or anxiety, irritability, insomnia, depression, inability to concentrate, forgetfulness, and fatigability, may exist. Treatment entails reassurance and symptomatic relief in addition to 24 hours of close observation.

In mild diffuse axonal injury, 30% of persons display decerebrate or decorticate posturing and may experience prolonged periods of stupor or restlessness (see Figure 14-6).

In moderate diffuse axonal injury, the score on the Glasgow Coma Scale (GCS) is 4 to 8 initially and 6 to 8 by 24 hours. Thirty-five percent of victims have transitory decerebration or decortication, with unconsciousness lasting days or weeks. On awakening, the person is confused and suffers a long period of post-traumatic anterograde and retrograde amnesia. There is often permanent deficit in memory, attention, abstraction, reasoning, problem solving, executive functions, vision or perception, and language. Mood and affect changes range from mild to severe.

In severe diffuse axonal injury, the person experiences immediate autonomic dysfunction that disappears in a few weeks. Increased intracranial pressure appears 4 to 6 days after injury. Pulmonary complications occur often. Profound sensorimotor and cognitive system deficits are present. Severely compromised coordinated movements and verbal and written communication skills, inability to learn and reason, and failure to modulate behavior are found also.

High-resolution CT scan and MRI assist in the diagnosis of focal and diffuse injuries. Medical management must address endocrine and metabolic derangements. Early and late seizures must be prevented and controlled. Mortality associated with acute head injury is significantly higher in persons treated with corticosteroids within 8 hours of the injury.[2,3]

Secondary brain trauma. Secondary brain trauma is the result of both systemic and intracranial processes and is an indirect result of primary brain trauma. Systemic hypotension, hypoxia, anemia, and hypercapnia and hypocapnia contribute to secondary brain insults. Mechanisms of secondary injury include cerebral edema, increased intracranial pressure (IICP), decreased cerebral perfusion pressure, ischemia, and brain herniation. Cellular and molecular brain damage from the effects of primary injury develops hours to days later. Astrocyte swelling and proliferation alter the blood-brain barrier and cause IICP. Release of excitatory neurotransmitters, such as glutamate and aspartate, cause neuronal depolarization and alter postsynaptic receptor function. A hypermetabolic state, mitochondrial influx of calcium, fluctuations in sodium and potassium levels, poor perfusion, influx of inflammatory mediators, and mitochondrial failure all contribute to cytotoxic edema, axonal swelling, and neuronal death.[4,5]

The management of secondary brain trauma is related to prevention and includes removal of hematomas and management of hypotension, hypoxemia, anemia, intracranial pressure, replacement fluids, body temperature, and ventilation. Research is in progress to find specific pharmacologic interventions and neuroprotective agents that limit the progression of secondary injury.[6,7]

Spinal Cord Trauma

Each year 12,000 persons experience serious spinal cord injury. Male gender and ages 16 to 30 years are strong risk factors. Motor vehicle accidents are the leading cause of injury (41%); falls are the next most common cause (27%) followed by violence and sports activities.[8] Elderly people are particularly at risk for minor trauma that results in serious spinal cord injury because of preexisting degenerative vertebral disorders.

PATHOPHYSIOLOGY Spinal cord injuries most commonly occur because of vertebral injuries that result from acceleration, deceleration, or deformation forces usually applied at a distance. These forces compress the tissues, pull or exert traction (tension) on the tissues, or shear tissues so that they slide into one another (Figures 15-3 to 15-6). The bones,

ligaments, and joints of the vertebral column may be damaged through fracture and compression of one or more elements, dislocation of elements, or both fracture and dislocation. Vertebral injuries can be classified as (1) simple fracture—a single break usually affecting transverse or spinous processes; (2) compressed (wedged) vertebral fracture—vertebral body compressed anteriorly; (3) comminuted (burst) fracture—vertebral body shattered into several fragments; and (4) dislocation.

The vertebrae fracture readily with both direct and indirect trauma. When the supporting ligaments are torn, the vertebrae move out of alignment and dislocations occur. A horizontal force moves the vertebrae straight forward; if the individual is in a flexed position at the time of injury, the vertebrae are then angulated. Flexion and extension injuries may result in dislocations. (Bone, ligament, and joint injuries are presented in Table 15-4.)

Vertebral injuries in adults occur most often at vertebrae C1 to C2 (cervical), C4 to C7, and T10 (thoracic) to L2 (lumbar) (see Figure 12-10), the most mobile portions of the vertebral column. The cord occupies most of the vertebral canal in the cervical and lumbar regions, so it is easily injured. (Injuries to the cord are summarized in Table 15-5.)

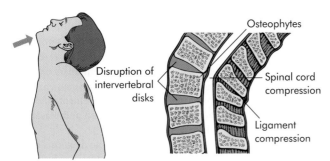

FIGURE 15-3 Hyperextension Injuries of the Spine. Hyperextension injuries of the spine can result in fracture or nonfracture injuries with spinal cord damage.

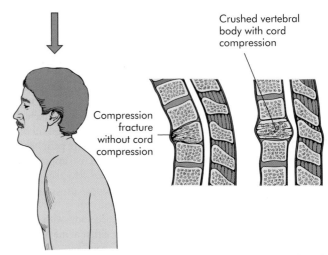

FIGURE 15-5 Axial Compression Injuries of the Spine. In axial compression injuries of the spine, the spinal cord is contused directly by retropulsion of bone or disk material into the spinal canal.

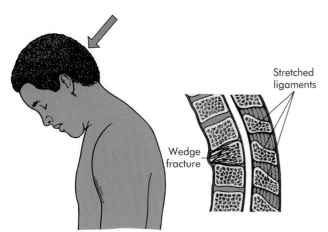

FIGURE 15-4 Flexion Injury of the Spine. Hyperflexion produces translation (subluxation) of vertebrae that compromises the central canal and compresses spinal cord parenchyma or vascular structures.

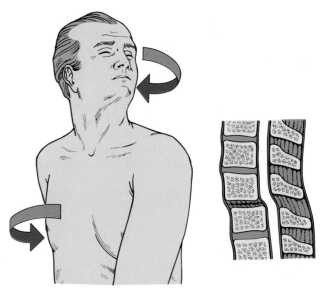

FIGURE 15-6 Flexion-Rotation Injuries of the Spine.

TABLE 15-4   MECHANISMS OF VERTEBRAL INJURY INVOLVING BONE, LIGAMENTS, AND JOINTS

MECHANISM OF INJURY	LOCATION OF VERTEBRAL INJURY	FORCES OF INJURY	LOCATION OF INJURY
Hyperextension	Fracture and dislocation of posterior elements, such as spinous processes, transverse processes, laminae, pedicles, or posterior ligaments	Results from forces of acceleration-deceleration and sudden reduction in anteroposterior diameter of spinal cord	Cervical area
Hyperflexion	Fracture or dislocation of vertebral bodies, disks, or ligaments	Results from sudden and excessive force that propels neck forward or causes an exaggerated lateral movement of neck to one side	Cervical area
Vertical compression (axial loading)	Shattering fractures	Results from a force applied along an axis from top of cranium through vertebral bodies	T12 to L2
Rotational forces (flexion-rotation)	Rupture support ligaments in addition to producing fractures	Adds shearing force to acceleration forces	Cervical area

TABLE 15-5   SPINAL CORD INJURIES

INJURY	DESCRIPTION
Cord concussion	Results in temporary disruption of cord-mediated functions
Cord contusion	Bruising of neural tissue causes swelling and temporary loss of cord-mediated functions
Cord compression	Pressure on cord causes ischemia to tissues; must be relieved (decompressed) to prevent permanent damage to spinal cord
Laceration	Tearing of neural tissues of spinal cord; may be reversible if only slight damage sustained by neural tissues; may result in permanent loss of cord-mediated functions if spinal tracts are disrupted
Transection	Severing of spinal cord causes permanent loss of function
Complete	All tracts in spinal cord are completely disrupted; all cord-mediated functions below transection are completely and permanently lost
Incomplete	Some tracts in spinal cord remain intact, together with functions mediated by these tracts; has potential for recovery although function is temporarily lost
Preserved sensation only	Some demonstrable sensation below level of injury
Preserved motor nonfunctional	Preserved motor function without useful purpose; sensory function may or may not be preserved
Preserved motor functional	Preserved voluntary motor function that is functionally useful
Hemorrhage	Bleeding into neural tissue as a result of blood vessel damage; usually no major loss of function
Damage or obstruction of spinal blood supply	Causes local ischemia

With injury, microscopic hemorrhages appear in the central gray matter and pia-arachnoid, increasing in size until the entire gray matter is hemorrhagic and necrotic. Edema in the white matter occurs, impairing the microcirculation of the cord. Localized hemorrhaging and edema are followed by reduced vascular perfusion and development of ischemic areas. Oxygen tension in the tissue at the injury site is decreased. The microscopic hemorrhages and edema are maximal at the level of injury and two cord segments above and below it.

Cellular and subcellular alterations and tissue necrosis occur. Cord swelling increases the individual's degree of dysfunction, making it hard to distinguish functions permanently lost from those temporarily impaired. In the cervical region, cord swelling may be life-threatening because it may impair the diaphragm function (phrenic nerves exit at C3 to C5) and vegetative functions (mediated by the medulla oblongata).

Circulation in the white matter tracts of the spinal cord returns to normal in about 24 hours, but gray matter circulation remains altered. Phagocytes appear 36 to 48 hours after injury, and microglia proliferate with altered astrocytes. Red blood cells then begin to disintegrate, and resorption of hemorrhages begins. Degenerating axons are engulfed by macrophages in the first 10 days after injury. The traumatized cord is replaced by acellular collagenous tissue, usually in 3 to 4 weeks. Meninges thicken as part of the scarring process.

CLINICAL MANIFESTATIONS   Normal activity of the spinal cord cells at and below the level of injury ceases because of loss of the continuous tonic discharge from the brain or brain stem and inhibition of suprasegmental impulses immediately after cord injury, thus causing spinal shock. In spinal shock, reflex function is completely lost in all segments below the lesion. This condition involves all skeletal muscles; bladder, bowel, and sexual function; and autonomic control. Severe impairment below the level of the lesion is obvious; it includes paralysis and flaccidity in muscles, absence of sensation, loss of bladder and rectal control, transient drop in blood pressure, and poor venous circulation. The condition also results in disturbed thermal control because the sympathetic nervous system is damaged. The hypothalamus cannot regulate body heat through vasoconstriction and increased metabolism; therefore the individual assumes the temperature of the air (poikilothermia).

Spinal shock generally lasts 7 to 20 days, with a range of a few days to 3 months. It terminates with the reappearance of reflex activity, hyperreflexia, spasticity, and reflex emptying of the bladder.

Loss of motor and sensory function depends on the level of injury. All motor, sensory, reflex, and autonomic functions cease below any transected area and also may cease below concussive, contused, compressed, or ischemic areas. Table 15-6 summarizes the clinical manifestations of spinal cord injury.

TABLE 15-6 CLINICAL MANIFESTATIONS OF SPINAL CORD INJURY

STAGE	MANIFESTATIONS

Spinal Shock Stage
Complete spinal cord transection
	Loss of motor function
	    1. Quadriplegia with injuries of cervical spinal cord
	    2. Paraplegia with injuries of thoracic spinal cord
	Muscle flaccidity
	    Loss of all reflexes below level of injury
	    Loss of pain, temperature, touch, pressure, and proprioception below level of injury
	    Pain at site of injury caused by zone of hyperesthesia above injury
	    Atonic bladder and bowel
	    Paralytic ileus with distention
	    Loss of vasomotor tone in lower body parts; low and unstable blood pressure
	    Loss of perspiration below level of injury
	    Loss or extreme depression of genital reflexes such as penile erection and bulbocavernous reflex
	    Dry and pale skin; possible ulceration over bony prominences
	    Respiratory impairment

Partial spinal cord transection	Asymmetric flaccid motor paralysis below level of injury
	Asymmetric reflex loss
	Preservation of some sensation below level of injury
	Vasomotor instability less severe than that seen with complete cord transection
	Bowel and bladder impairment less severe than that seen with complete cord transection
	Preservation of ability to perspire in some portions of body below level of injury
	Brown-Séquard syndrome (associated with penetrating injuries, hyperextension and flexion, locked facets, and compression fractures)
	    1. Ipsilateral paralysis or paresis below level of injury
	    2. Ipsilateral loss of touch, pressure, vibration, and position sense below level of injury
	    3. Contralateral loss of pain and temperature sensations below level of injury
	Central cervical cord syndrome (acute cord compression between bony bars or spurs anteriorly and thickened ligamentum flavum posteriorly associated with hyperextension)
	    1. Motor deficits in upper extremities, especially hands, more dense than in lower extremities
	    2. Varying degrees of bladder dysfunction
	Burning hand syndrome (variant of central cord syndrome; in 50% of cases an underlying spine fracture/dislocation is present)
	    1. Severe burning paresthesias and dysesthesias in the hands or feet
	Anterior cord syndrome (compromise of anterior spinal artery by occlusion or pressure effect of disk)
	    1. Loss of motor function below level of injury
	    2. Loss of pain and temperature sensations below level of injury
	    3. Touch, pressure, position, and vibration senses intact
	Posterior cord syndrome (associated with hyperextension injuries with fractures of vertebral arch)
	    1. Impaired light touch and proprioception
	Conus medullaris syndrome (compression injury at T12 from disk herniation or burst fracture of body of T12)
	    1. Flaccid paralysis of legs
	    2. Flaccid paralysis of anal sphincter
	    3. Variable sensory deficits
	Cauda equina syndrome (compression of nerve roots below L1 caused by fracture and dislocation of spine or large posterocentral intervertebral disk herniation)
	    1. Lower extremity motor deficits
	    2. Variable sensorimotor dysfunction
	    3. Variable reflex dysfunction
	    4. Variable bladder, bowel, and sexual dysfunction
	Syndrome of neuropraxia (postathletic injury, associated with congenital spinal stenosis)
	    1. Dramatic but transient neurologic deficits including quadriplegia
	Horner syndrome (injury to preganglionic sympathetic trunk or postganglionic sympathetic neurons of superior cervical ganglion)
	    1. Ipsilateral pupil smaller than contralateral pupil
	    2. Sunken ipsilateral eyeball
	    3. Ptosis of affected eyeball
	    4. Lack of perspiration on ipsilateral side of face

TABLE 15-6	**CLINICAL MANIFESTATIONS OF SPINAL CORD INJURY—cont'd**
STAGE	**MANIFESTATIONS**
Heightened Reflex Activity Stage	Emergence of Babinski reflexes, possibly progressing to a triple reflex; possible development of still later flexor spasms Reappearance of ankle and knee reflexes, which become hyperactive Contraction of reflex detrusor muscle leading to urinary incontinence Appearance of reflex defecation Mass reflex with flexion spasms, profuse sweating, piloerection, and bladder and occasional bowel emptying may be evoked by autonomic stimulation of skin or from full bladder Episodes of hypertension Defective heat-induced sweating Eventual development of extensor reflexes, first in muscles of hip and thigh, later in leg Possible paresthesias below level of transection: dull, burning pain in lower back, abdomen, buttocks, and perineum

Autonomic hyperreflexia (dysreflexia) may occur after spinal shock resolves. The syndrome is associated with a massive, uncompensated cardiovascular response to stimulation of the sympathetic nervous system (Figure 15-7). The condition is life-threatening and requires immediate treatment. Individuals most likely to be affected have lesions at the T6 level or above. Characteristics include paroxysmal hypertension (up to 300 mm Hg, systolic), a pounding headache, blurred vision, sweating above the level of the lesion with flushing of the skin, nasal congestion, nausea, piloerection caused by pilomotor spasm, and bradycardia (30 to 40 beats/min). The symptoms may develop singly or in combination (syndrome) and often are associated with a distended bladder or rectum.

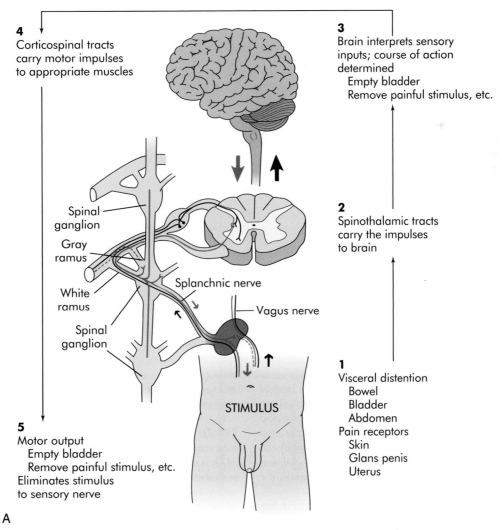

FIGURE 15-7 Autonomic Hyperreflexia. **A,** Normal response pathway.

Continued

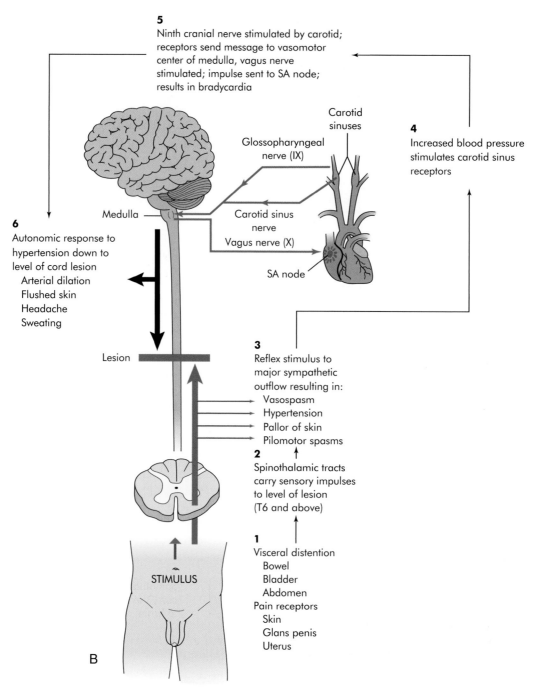

5
Ninth cranial nerve stimulated by carotid; receptors send message to vasomotor center of medulla, vagus nerve stimulated; impulse sent to SA node; results in bradycardia

Carotid sinuses

Glossopharyngeal nerve (IX)

4
Increased blood pressure stimulates carotid sinus receptors

Medulla

Carotid sinus nerve

Vagus nerve (X)

SA node

6
Autonomic response to hypertension down to level of cord lesion
Arterial dilation
Flushed skin
Headache
Sweating

Lesion

3
Reflex stimulus to major sympathetic outflow resulting in:
Vasospasm
Hypertension
Pallor of skin
Pilomotor spasms

2
Spinothalamic tracts carry sensory impulses to level of lesion (T6 and above)

1
Visceral distention
Bowel
Bladder
Abdomen
Pain receptors
Skin
Glans penis
Uterus

STIMULUS

B

FIGURE 15-7, cont'd B, Autonomic dysreflexia pathway. *SA,* Sinoatrial. (Modified from Rudy EB: *Advanced neurological and neurosurgical nursing,* St Louis, 1984, Mosby.)

In autonomic hyperreflexia, sensory receptors below the level of the cord lesion are stimulated. The intact autonomic nervous system reflexively responds with an arteriolar spasm that increases blood pressure. Baroreceptors in the cerebral vessels, the carotid sinus, and the aorta sense the hypertension and stimulate the parasympathetic system. The heart rate decreases, but the visceral and peripheral vessels do not dilate because efferent impulses cannot pass through the cord.

The most common cause is a distended bladder or rectum, but any sensory stimulation can elicit autonomic hyperreflexia. Stimulation of the skin or pain receptors may cause autonomic hyperreflexia. Bladder or bowel emptying usually relieves the syndrome, and drugs such as phenoxybenzamine may facilitate this result.

EVALUATION AND TREATMENT Diagnosis of spinal cord injury is based on physical examination, radiologic examination, CT scan, MRI, and myelography. For a suspected or confirmed vertebral fracture or dislocation, regardless of the presence or absence of spinal cord injury, the immediate intervention is immobilization of the spine to prevent further injury. Decompression and surgical fixation may be necessary. Corticosteroids are given at the time of injury to decrease secondary cord injury from inflammation and thereafter for several days. Nutrition, lung function, skin integrity, and bladder and bowel management must be addressed. Plans for rehabilitation need early consideration.

In cases of autonomic hyperreflexia, intervention must be prompt because cerebrovascular accident is possible. The head of the bed should be elevated, and the stimulus should be found and removed. Antihypertensive medications may be used if blood pressure remains elevated.

Degenerative Disorders of the Spine
Degenerative Joint Disease (DJD)

Degenerative disk disease. Degenerative disk disease (DDD) is common in individuals 30 years of age and older. It is, in part, a process of normal aging and includes a genetic component, involving genes that code the cartilage intermediate layer protein (CILP), as well as environmental interactions that may increase susceptibility to lumbar disk disease by disrupting normal building and maintenance of cartilage.[9] Causes include biochemical (e.g., inflammatory mediators) and biomechanical alterations (e.g., mechanical loading and compression) of the intervertebral disk tissue. Diminished blood supply and loss of disk proteoglycans cause subsequent disk dehydration, alterations in disk structure, and impaired disk function. The disk can herniate, pinching nerves or placing strain on the spine. The pathologic findings in DDD include disk protrusion, spondylolysis and/or subluxation (spondylolisthesis), degeneration of vertebrae, and spinal stenosis. Lumbar disk disease causes one third of all back pain that affects 70% to 90% of adults at some point in their lives. However, only a small percentage of people with degenerative disk disease have any functional incapacity because of pain.

Spondylolysis. Spondylolysis is a structural defect (degeneration or developmental defect) of the spine involving the lamina or neural arch of the vertebra. The lumbar spine is affected most often. Mechanical pressure may cause a forward displacement of the deficient vertebra (spondylolisthesis). Heredity plays a significant role, and spondylolysis is associated with an increased incidence of other congenital spinal defects. Symptoms include lower back and lower limb pain.

Spondylolisthesis. Spondylolisthesis occurs when a vertebra slides forward and onto the vertebra below it, and may include a fracture of the pars interarticularis, commonly occurring at L5-S1. Spondylolisthesis is graded from 1 to 4 based on the percentage of slip that occurs. Grades 1 and 2 usually are managed symptomatically and nonsurgically. Individuals with grade 3 or 4 usually require operative decompression, stabilization, or both.

Spinal stenosis. Spinal stenosis is a narrowing of the spinal canal that causes pressure on the spinal nerves or cord and can be congenital or acquired (more common) and associated with trauma or arthritis. The lumbar and cervical areas of the spine are most often involved. Acquired conditions include a bulging disk, facet hypertrophy, or a thick ossified posterior longitudinal ligament. Symptoms can produce pain, numbness, and tingling in the legs. Surgical decompression is recommended for those with chronic symptoms and those who do not respond to medical management.

Low Back Pain

Low back pain affects the area between the lower rib cage and gluteal muscles and often radiates into the thighs. About 1% of individuals with acute low back pain have pain along the distribution of a lumbar nerve root (radicular pain), most commonly involving the sciatic nerve (sciatica). Sciatica often is accompanied by neurosensory and

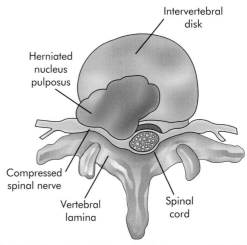

FIGURE 15-8 Herniated Nucleus Pulposus. (Modified from Thompson JM et al: *Mosby's clinical nursing,* ed 5, St Louis, 2002, Mosby.)

motor deficits, such as tingling, numbness, and weakness in various parts of the leg and foot. The percentage of the population affected with low back pain at some point in their lives is 60% to 80%, and the annual prevalence is 5%. Men and women are equally affected. Women report low back symptoms more often after 60 years of age.

PATHOGENESIS Most cases of low back pain are idiopathic, and no precise diagnosis is possible. The local processes include tension caused by tumors or disk prolapse, bursitis, synovitis, rising venous and tissue pressures (found in degenerative joint disease), abnormal bone pressures, spinal immobility, inflammation caused by infection (as in osteomyelitis), bony fractures, or ligamentous sprains to pain referred from viscera or the posterior peritoneum. General processes resulting in low back pain include bone diseases, such as osteoporosis or osteomalacia, and hyperparathyroidism.

Risk factors include occupations that require repetitious lifting in the forward bent-and-twisted position; exposure to vibrations caused by vehicles or industrial machinery; obesity; and cigarette smoking. Osteoporosis increases the risk of spinal compression fractures and may be why elderly women report more symptoms than men. Genetic predispositions for low back pain include isthmic spondylolisthesis (vertebra slides forward or slips in relation to a vertebra below), spinal osteochondrosis, and spinal stenosis associated with achondroplasia.

The most commonly encountered causes of low back pain include lumbar disk herniation, degenerative disk disease, spondylolysis, spondylolisthesis, and spinal stenosis. Anatomically, low back pain must originate from innervated structures, but deep pain is widely referred and varies. The nucleus pulposus has no intrinsic innervation, but when extruded or herniated through a prolapsed disk, it irritates the dural membranes and causes pain referred to the segmental area (Figure 15-8). The interspinous bursae can be a source of pain between L3, L4, L5, and S1 but also may affect L1, L2, and L3 spinous processes. The anterior and posterior longitudinal ligaments of the spine and the interspinous and supraspinous ligaments are abundantly supplied with pain receptors, as is the ligamentum flavum. All of these ligaments are vulnerable to traumatic tears (sprains) and fracture. Muscle injury may contribute to low back pain, with sprains and strains the most common diagnoses.

EVALUATION AND TREATMENT Diagnosis of low back injury is based on physical examination, electromyelography, CT with or without myelography, MRI, nerve conduction studies, diskography, and epidurography. Most individuals with acute low back pain benefit from a nonspecific short-term treatment regimen of bed rest, analgesic medications, exercises, physical therapy, and education. Surgical treatments, specifically diskectomy and spinal fusions, are used for individuals not responding to medical management. Individuals with chronic low back pain also are prescribed anti-inflammatory and muscle relaxant medications; exercise programs; massage, topical heat, spinal manipulation, and cognitive-behavioral therapies; and interdisciplinary care.[10]

Herniated Intervertebral Disk

Herniation of an intervertebral disk is a displacement of disk material (nucleus pulposus or annulus fibrosus [the fibrous capsule enclosing the gelatinous center of the disk]) beyond the intervertebral disk space (see Figure 15-8). Rupture of an intervertebral disk usually is caused by trauma, degenerative disk disease, or both. Risk factors are weight-bearing sports, light weight lifting, and certain work activities, such as repeated lifting. Men are affected more often than women, with the highest incidence in the 30- to 50-year age group. Most commonly affected are the lumbosacral disks—that is, L5-S1 and L4-L5. Herniation is typically at a higher vertebrae in older persons. Disk herniation occasionally occurs in the cervical area, usually at C5-C6 and C6-C7. Herniations at the thoracic level are extremely rare. The injury may occur immediately, within a few hours, or months to years after injury.

PATHOPHYSIOLOGY In a herniated disk, the ligament and posterior capsule of the disk are usually torn, allowing the gelatinous material (the nucleus pulposus) to extrude and compress the nerve root. Occasionally the injury tears the entire disk loose, and it protrudes onto the nerve root or compresses the spinal cord. Multiple nerve root compression may be found at the L5-S1 level, where the cauda equina may be compressed. Large amounts of extruded nucleus pulposus or complete disk herniation (i.e., of both the capsule and the nucleus pulposus) may compress the spinal cord.

CLINICAL MANIFESTATIONS The location and size of the herniation into the spinal canal, together with the amount of space in the canal, determine the clinical manifestations associated with the injury (Figure 15-9). A herniated disk in the lumbosacral area is associated with pain that radiates along the sciatic nerve course over the buttock and into the calf or ankle. The pain occurs with straining, including coughing and sneezing, and usually on straight leg raising. Other clinical manifestations include limited range of motion of the lumbar spine; tenderness on palpation in the sciatic notch and along the sciatic nerve; impaired pain, temperature, and touch sensations in the L5-S1 or L4-L5 dermatomes of the leg and foot; decreased or absent ankle jerk reflex; and mild weakness of the foot.

With the herniation of a lower cervical disk, paresthesias and pain are present in the upper arm, forearm, and hand along the affected nerve root distribution. Neck motion and straining, including coughing and sneezing, may increase neck and nerve root pain. Neck range of motion is diminished. Slight weakness and atrophy of biceps or triceps muscles may occur; the biceps or triceps reflex may decrease. Occasionally, signs of corticospinal and sensory tract impairments appear, including motor weakness of the lower extremities, sensory disturbances in the lower extremities, and presence of a Babinski reflex.

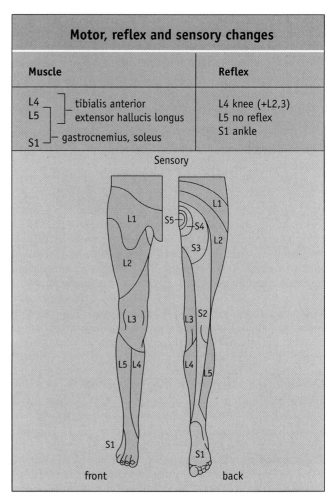

FIGURE 15-9 Clinical Features of a Herniated Nucleus Pulposus.

EVALUATION AND TREATMENT Diagnosis of a herniated intervertebral disk is made through the history and physical examination, spinal x-ray films, electromyelography, CT scan, MRI, myelography, diskography, and nerve conduction studies. Multiple avenues of therapy are available, although there is little evidence to support use of analgesics, muscle relaxants, systemic corticosteroids, or antidepressants. Nonsteroidal anti-inflammatory drugs, bed rest, or traction does not improve sciatica related to disk herniation.[11] Most herniated disks heal spontaneously over time and do not require surgery. A surgical approach is indicated if there is evidence of severe compression (weakness or decreased deep tendon, bladder, or bowel reflexes) or if a conservative approach is unsuccessful.[12]

Cerebrovascular Disorders

Cerebrovascular disease is the most frequently occurring neurologic disorder, accounting for more than 50% of the persons admitted to general hospitals with neurologic problems. Any abnormality of the brain caused by a pathologic process in the blood vessels is referred to as a *cerebrovascular disease*. Included in this category are lesions of the vessel wall, occlusion of the vessel lumen by thrombus or embolus, rupture of the vessel, and alteration in blood quality such as increased blood viscosity.

The brain abnormalities induced by cerebrovascular disease are either (1) ischemia with or without infarction (death of brain tissues) or (2) hemorrhage. The common clinical manifestation of cerebrovascular disease is a cerebrovascular accident (CVA, stroke): a sudden, nonconvulsive focal neurologic deficit.

Cerebrovascular Accidents (Stroke Syndromes)

Cerebrovascular accidents are the leading cause of disability and the third cause of death in the United States. About 75% of CVAs occur among those older than 65 years. Stroke tends to run in families and is more common in men at younger ages. The incidence is about 2 times greater in blacks than whites.[13] Blacks between the ages of 55 and 64 who live in the Southern states are about 50% more likely to die of stroke than blacks of the same age who live in the North.[14] In addition, persons with both hypertension and type 2 diabetes mellitus have a fourfold increase in stroke incidence and an eightfold increase in stroke mortality.[15] In its mildest form, a cerebrovascular accident is so minimal that it is almost unnoticed. In its most severe state, hemiplegia, coma, and death result.

Cerebrovascular accidents (stroke syndromes) are classified pathophysiologically as global hypoperfusion (as in shock), ischemic (thrombotic, embolic), or hemorrhagic. Risk factors for stroke include the following:

- Arterial hypertension (both elevated systolic and diastolic blood pressures) increases the risk for stroke.
- Smoking increases the risk of stroke by 50%.
- Compared to a nondiabetic person, a person with diabetes is 2½ to 3½ times more likely to have an ischemic stroke.
- Insulin resistance increases the risk for ischemic stroke.
- Polycythemia and thrombocythemia place the person at risk for ischemic stroke.
- The presence of lipoprotein-A is a risk factor for ischemic stroke.
- Impaired cardiac function increases the risk for ischemic stroke.
- Hyperhomocysteinemia increases the risk for ischemic stroke.
- Nonrheumatic atrial fibrillation is associated with a fivefold increase in the incidence of ischemic stroke.
- *Chlamydia pneumoniae* can increase the risk of stroke by infiltrating and inflaming the vascular endothelium.

Thrombotic stroke. Thrombotic strokes (cerebral thromboses) arise from arterial occlusions caused by thrombi formation in arteries supplying the brain or intracranial vessels. Cerebral thrombosis develops most often from atherosclerosis and inflammatory disease processes (arteritis) that damage arterial walls. Increased coagulation can lead to thrombus formation. Conditions causing inadequate cerebral perfusion (e.g., dehydration, hypotension, prolonged vasoconstriction from malignant hypertension) increase the risk of thrombosis. It may take as long as 20 to 30 years for atheromatous plaques (stenotic lesions) to develop at the branches and curvature found in the cerebral circulation. The smooth stenotic area can degenerate, forming an ulcerated area of the vessel wall. Platelets and fibrin adhere to the damaged wall, and a clot forms, gradually occluding the artery. The clot may enlarge both distally and proximally. Thrombotic strokes occur when parts of the clot detach, travel upstream, and obstruct blood flow, causing acute ischemia.

The distinction between transient ischemic attacks (TIAs) and thrombotic stroke is losing importance. With increasing use of brain imaging modalities, many persons with symptoms lasting less than 24 hours are diagnosed as having a brain infarction. The new definition for transient ischemic attack (TIA) is a brief episode of neurologic dysfunction caused by a focal disturbance of brain or retinal ischemia with clinical symptoms typically lasting no more than 1 hour; no evidence of infarction; and complete clinical recovery.[16]

TIAs likely represent platelet clumps or vessel narrowing with spasm causing an intermittent blockage of circulation. Without definitive diagnosis and treatment, 80% of persons have a recurrence of symptoms by 1 year and are at higher risk for subsequent stroke.

Embolic stroke. An embolic stroke involves fragments that break from a thrombus formed outside the brain or in the heart, aorta, or common carotid artery. The embolus usually involves small brain vessels and obstructs at a bifurcation or other point of narrowing, thus causing ischemia. An embolus may plug the lumen entirely and remain in place or shatter into fragments and become part of the vessel's blood flow. Risk factors for an embolic stroke include atrial fibrillation, left ventricular aneurysm or thrombus, left atrial thrombus, recent myocardial infarction, endocarditis, rheumatic valve disease, mechanical valvular prostheses, atrioseptal defects, patent foramen ovale, and primary cardiac tumors. In persons who experience an embolic stroke, a second stroke usually follows because the source of emboli continues to exist. Embolization is usually in the distribution of the middle cerebral artery (the largest cerebral artery).

Hemorrhagic stroke. Hemorrhagic stroke (intracranial hemorrhage) is the third most common cause of cerebrovascular accident. Hypertension, ruptured aneurysms or vascular malformation, bleeding into a tumor, or hemorrhage associated with anticoagulants or clotting disorders, head trauma, or illicit drug use are common causes.

A hypertensive hemorrhage is associated with significantly increased systolic and diastolic blood pressure measurements over several years and usually occurs in the brain tissue. A mass of blood is formed and grows, displacing and compressing adjacent brain tissue. Rupture or seepage into the ventricular system occurs in many cases. Hemorrhages are described as massive, small, slit, or petechial. Massive hemorrhages are several centimeters in diameter; small hemorrhages are 1 to 2 cm in diameter; a slit hemorrhage lies in the subcortical area; and a petechial hemorrhage is the size of a pinhead bleed. The most common sites for hypertensive hemorrhages are in the putamen of the basal ganglia (a portion of the lentiform nucleus) (40%), the thalamus (15%), the cortex and subcortex (22%), the pons (7%), the caudate nucleus (7%), and the cerebellar hemispheres (8%).

Lacunar stroke. Lacunar strokes (lacunar infarcts or small vessel disease) are caused by occlusion of a single deep perforating artery that supplies small penetrating subcortical vessels, causing ischemic lesions (0.5 to 15 mm or lacunes) predominantly in the basal ganglia, internal capsules, and pons. Because of the location and small area of infarction, these strokes may have pure motor or sensory deficits.[17]

PATHOPHYSIOLOGY

Cerebral infarction. Cerebral infarction results when an area of the brain loses its blood supply because of vascular occlusion. Causes include (1) abrupt vascular occlusion (e.g., embolus), (2) gradual vessel occlusion (e.g., atheroma), and (3) partial occlusion of stenotic vessels. Cerebral thrombi and cerebral emboli most commonly produce occlusion, but atherosclerosis and hypotension are the dominant underlying processes.

Cerebral infarctions are ischemic or hemorrhagic. In ischemic infarcts, the affected area becomes slightly discolored and softens 6 to 12 hours after the occlusion. Necrosis, swelling around the insult, and mushy disintegration appear by 48 to 72 hours after infarction. The necrosis resolves by about the second week, leaving a cavity.

In hemorrhagic infarcts, bleeding occurs into the infarcted area when blood flow is restored. The embolic fragments may be moved or lysed, or compressive forces may lessen, allowing blood flow to be reestablished.

Cerebral hemorrhage. The primary cause of cerebral hemorrhage is hypertension. Other causes include ruptured aneurysms or arteriovenous malformations, tumors, coagulation disorders, and trauma.

Hypertension involves primarily smaller arteries and arterioles, resulting in thickening of the vessel walls and increased cellularity of the vessels and hyalinization. Necrosis may be present. Microaneurysms in these smaller vessels or arteriolar necrosis may precipitate the bleeding.

A mass of blood is formed as bleeding continues into the brain tissue. Adjacent brain tissue is deformed, compressed, and displaced, producing ischemia, edema, and increased intracranial pressure. Rupture or seepage of blood into the ventricular system often occurs.

The cerebral hemorrhage resolves through reabsorption. Macrophages and astrocytes clear blood from the area. A cavity forms, surrounded by a dense gliosis (glial scar) after removal of the blood.

Because neurons surrounding the ischemic or infarcted areas undergo changes that disrupt plasma membranes, cellular edema results, causing further compression of capillaries. Maximal cerebral edema develops in approximately 72 hours and takes about 2 weeks to subside. Most persons survive an initial hemispheric ischemic stroke unless there is massive cerebral edema, which is nearly always fatal.

CLINICAL MANIFESTATIONS Clinical manifestations of thrombotic stroke vary, depending on the artery obstructed. Different sites of obstruction create different occlusion syndromes (e.g., carotid artery syndromes, middle cerebral artery syndromes, or vertebrobasilar system syndromes).

With hemorrhagic stroke, clinical manifestations vary, depending on the location and size of the bleed. Once a deep unresponsive state occurs, the person rarely survives. The immediate prognosis is grave. If the person survives, however, recovery of function often is possible.

Individuals experiencing intracranial hemorrhage from a ruptured or leaking aneurysm have one of three sets of symptoms: (1) onset of an excruciating generalized headache with an almost immediate lapse into an unresponsive state, (2) headache but with consciousness maintained, and (3) sudden lapse into unconsciousness. If the hemorrhage is confined to the subarachnoid space, there may be no local signs. If bleeding spreads into the brain tissue, hemiparesis/paralysis, dysphasia, or homonymous hemianopia may be present. Warning signs of an impending aneurysm rupture include headache, transient unilateral weakness, transient numbness and tingling, and transient speech disturbance. However, such warning signs often are absent.

EVALUATION AND TREATMENT MRI and magnetic resonance angiography (MRA) are used to diagnose stroke. In thrombotic stroke, thrombolytic therapy for acute ischemic stroke is within 3 hours of onset of symptoms. The American Heart Association/American Stroke Association (AHA/ASA) guidelines for the administration of recombinant tissue plasminogen activator (rtPA) following acute stroke were revised to expand the window of treatment from 3 hours to 4.5 hours; however, this has not been approved by the Food and Drug Administration.[18] Treatment is directed at prevention of ischemic injury and supportive management to control cerebral edema and increased intracranial pressure. Arresting the disease process by control of risk factors is critical and antiplatelet therapy may be instituted.[19]

In embolic strokes treatment is directed at preventing further embolization by instituting anticoagulation therapy and correcting the primary problem. Rehabilitation is indicated in both thrombotic and embolic strokes. Treatment of an intracranial bleed, regardless of cause, focuses on stopping or reducing the bleeding, controlling the increased intracranial pressure, preventing a rebleed, and preventing vasospasm. Occasionally an attempt is made to evacuate or aspirate the blood. Some surgeons drain the blood in a cerebral bleed but the benefit is not documented in studies.

Intracranial Aneurysm

Intracranial aneurysms may result from arteriosclerosis, congenital abnormality, trauma, inflammation, and cocaine abuse. The size may vary from 2 mm to 2 or 3 cm. Most aneurysms are located at bifurcations in or near the circle of Willis, in the vertebrobasilar arteries, or within the carotid system (see Figures 12-18 and 12-19). Aneurysms may be single, but in 20% to 25% of the cases, more than one is present. In these instances, the aneurysms may be unilateral or bilateral. Peak incidence of rupture occurs in persons 50 to 59 years of age, with the incidence in women slightly higher than that in men.

PATHOPHYSIOLOGY No single pathologic mechanism exists. Aneurysms may be classified on the basis of shape and form. Saccular aneurysms (berry aneurysms) occur frequently (in approximately 2% of the population) and likely result from congenital abnormalities in the tunica media of the arterial wall and degenerative changes.[20] The sac gradually grows over time. A saccular aneurysm may be (1) round with a narrow stalk connecting it to the parent artery, (2) broad-based without a stalk, or (3) cylindrical (Figure 15-10). Saccular aneurysms are rare in childhood; their highest incidence of rupturing or bleeding (subarachnoid hemorrhage) is among persons 20 to 50 years of age (Figure 15-11).

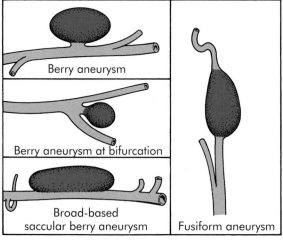

FIGURE 15-10 Types of Aneurysms.

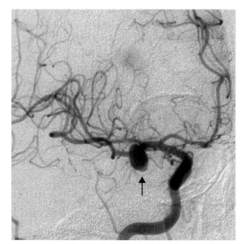

FIGURE 15-11 Berry Aneurysm, Angiogram. In this lateral view with contrast filling a portion of the cerebral arterial circulation can be seen a berry aneurysm *(arrow)* involving the middle cerebral artery of the circle of Willis at the base of the brain. (From Klatt EC: *Robbins and Cotran atlas of pathology,* Philadelphia, 2006, Saunders.)

Fusiform aneurysms (giant aneurysms) occur as a result of diffuse arteriosclerotic changes and are found most commonly in the basilar arteries or terminal portions of the internal carotid arteries (see Figure 15-10). They act as space-occupying lesions.

Aneurysms rupture through thin areas, causing hemorrhage into the subarachnoid space that spreads rapidly, producing localized changes in the cerebral cortex and focal irritation of nerves and arteries (see the discussion of the Laplace law in Chapter 22). Bleeding ceases when a fibrin-platelet plug forms at the point of rupture and as a result of compression. Blood undergoes reabsorption through arachnoid villi within 3 weeks.

CLINICAL MANIFESTATIONS Aneurysms often are asymptomatic. Of all persons undergoing routine autopsy, 5% are found to have one or more intracranial aneurysms. Clinical manifestations may arise from cranial nerve compression, but the signs vary, depending on the location and size of the aneurysm. Cranial nerves III, IV, V, and VI are affected most often (see Table 12-6). Unfortunately, the most common first indication of the presence of an aneurysm is an acute subarachnoid hemorrhage, intracerebral hemorrhage, or combined subarachnoid-intracerebral hemorrhage (see Subarachnoid Hemorrhage).

EVALUATION AND TREATMENT Diagnosis before a bleeding episode is made through arteriography. After a subarachnoid or intracerebral hemorrhage, a tentative diagnosis of an aneurysm is based on clinical manifestations, history, CT scan, and MRI. Treatments for intracranial aneurysm include surgical management and endovascular coil embolization for selected individuals.[21,22] The location and size of the aneurysm and the person's clinical status determine whether invasive therapy is feasible.

Vascular Malformation

An arteriovenous malformation (AVM) is a tangled mass of dilated blood vessels creating abnormal channels between the arterial and venous systems (arteriovenous fistula). AVMs may occur in any part of the brain and vary in size from a few millimeters to large malformations extending from the cortex to the ventricle. AVMs occur equally in males and females and occasionally occur in families. Although AVMs are usually present at birth, symptoms exhibit a delayed age of onset and commonly occur before 30 years of age.

PATHOPHYSIOLOGY AVMs have abnormal blood vessel structure, are abnormally thin, and have complex growth and remodeling patterns.[23] One or several arteries may feed the AVM and become tortuous and dilated over time. With moderate to large AVMs, sufficient blood is shunted into the malformation to deprive surrounding tissue of adequate blood perfusion.

CLINICAL MANIFESTATIONS Twenty percent of persons with an AVM have a characteristic chronic, nondescript headache, although some experience migraine. Fifty percent of persons experience seizures caused by compression. The other 50% experience an intracerebral, subarachnoid, or subdural hemorrhage. Bleeding from an AVM into the subarachnoid space causes symptoms identical to those associated with a ruptured aneurysm. If bleeding is into the brain tissue, focal signs that develop resemble a stroke-in-evolution. Ten percent of persons experience hemiparesis or other focal signs. At times, noncommunicating hydrocephalus (see Chapter 14) develops with a large AVM that extends into the ventricular lining.

EVALUATION AND TREATMENT A systolic bruit over the carotid artery in the neck, the mastoid process, or the eyeball in a young person is almost diagnostic of an AVM. Confirming diagnosis is made by CT and MRI followed by MRA. Treatment options are direct surgical intervention, embolization, or radiotherapy.

Subarachnoid Hemorrhage

With a subarachnoid hemorrhage, blood escapes from a defective or injured vessel into the subarachnoid space. Individuals at risk for a subarachnoid hemorrhage are those with intracranial aneurysm, intracranial arteriovenous malformation, or hypertension and those who have sustained head injuries. Subarachnoid hemorrhages often recur, especially from a ruptured intracranial aneurysm.

PATHOPHYSIOLOGY When a vessel is leaking, blood oozes into the subarachnoid space. When a vessel tears, blood under pressure is pumped into the subarachnoid space. The blood increases intracranial volume, and it is also extremely irritating to the neural tissues and produces an inflammatory reaction. In addition, the blood coats nerve roots, clogs arachnoid granulations (impairing CSF reabsorption), and obstructs foramina within the ventricular system (impairing CSF circulation). Intracranial pressure immediately increases to almost diastolic levels but returns to near baseline in about 10 minutes. Cerebral blood flow and cerebral perfusion pressure decrease. Autoregulation of blood flow is impaired, and there is a compensatory increase in systolic blood pressure.[24] The expanding hematoma acts like a space-occupying lesion, compressing and displacing brain tissue. Granulation tissue is formed, and meningeal scarring with impairment of CSF reabsorption and secondary hydrocephalus often results. Mortality in subarachnoid hemorrhage is 50% at 1 month.

Delayed cerebral ischemia, a syndrome of progressive neurologic deterioration, is associated with cerebral artery vasospasm. From 40% to 60% of persons with a subarachnoid hemorrhage experience vasospasms in adjacent and, occasionally, in nonadjacent vessels. Vasospasm may occur because of leukocyte-endothelial cell interactions or the effects of vasoactive substances (e.g., calcium, prostaglandins, serotonin, catecholamines) on the arteries of the subarachnoid space. Edema, medial necrosis, and proliferation of the tunica intima have been found. Vasospasm causes decreased cerebral blood flow, ischemia, and possibly infarct and can lead to delayed ischemic injury and death 3 to 14 days after the initial hemorrhage.[25]

CLINICAL MANIFESTATIONS Early manifestations associated with leaking vessels are episodic and include headache, changes in mental status or level of consciousness, nausea or vomiting, and focal neurologic defects. A ruptured vessel causes a sudden, throbbing, "explosive" headache, accompanied by nausea and vomiting, visual disturbances, motor deficits, and loss of consciousness related to a dramatic rise in intracranial pressure. Meningeal irritation and inflammation often occur, causing neck stiffness (nuchal rigidity), photophobia, blurred vision, irritability, restlessness, and low-grade fever. A positive Kernig sign (straightening the knee with the hip and knee in a flexed position produces pain in the back and neck regions) and a positive Brudzinski sign (passive flexion of the neck produces neck pain and increased rigidity) may appear. No localizing signs are present if the bleed is confined completely to the subarachnoid space.

The Hunt and Hess subarachnoid hemorrhage (SAH) grading system is based on description of the clinical manifestations (Table 15-7).[26] Rebleeding is a significant risk with a high mortality (up to 70%). The period of greatest risk is the first month, with the peak incidence of rebleeding during the first 2 weeks after the initial bleed.

Rebleeding is manifested by a sudden increase in blood pressure and intracranial pressure, along with a deteriorating neurologic status.

Seizures occur in 25% of persons with an SAH, and hydrocephalus after a bleed occurs in 20% of cases. Hypothalamic dysfunction, manifested by salt wasting, hyponatremia, and ECG changes, is common.

EVALUATION AND TREATMENT The diagnosis of an SAH is based on the clinical presentation as well as the results of a noncontrast CT scan and a lumbar puncture. Arteriography is the definitive diagnostic measure for identifying an aneurysm or arteriovenous malformation. Treatment is directed at controlling intracranial pressure, improving cerebral perfusion pressure, preventing ischemia and hypoxia of neural tissues, and avoiding rebleeding episodes.[27] The primary problem must be diagnosed and corrected as well.

> ✔ **QUICK CHECK 15-2**
> 1. Why is atherosclerosis a risk factor for thrombotic stroke?
> 2. Why do TIA's signs and symptoms resolve completely?
> 3. Why do lacunar strokes involve small infarcts?
> 4. How is an AVM different from an aneurysm?

TABLE 15-7 SUBARACHNOID HEMORRHAGE CLASSIFICATION SCALE

CATEGORY	DESCRIPTION
Grade I	Neurologic status intact; mild headache, slight nuchal rigidity
Grade II	Neurologic deficit evidenced by cranial nerve involvement; moderate to severe headache with more pronounced meningeal signs (e.g., photophobia, nuchal rigidity)
Grade III	Drowsiness and confusion with or without focal neurologic deficits; pronounced meningeal signs
Grade IV	Stuporous with pronounced neurologic deficits (e.g., hemiparesis, dysphasia); nuchal rigidity
Grade V	Deep coma state with decerebrate posturing and other brain stem functioning

From Cook HS: Aneurysmal subarachnoid hemorrhage: neuroscience frontiers and nursing challenges. In Winkelman C, editor: *AACN clinical issues in critical nursing*, Philadelphia, 1991, Lippincott.

Headache

Headache is a common neurologic disorder and is usually a benign symptom. However, it can be associated with serious disease such as brain tumor, meningitis, or cerebral vascular disease (e.g., giant cell arteritis, cerebral aneurysm, or cerebral bleeds). The headache syndromes discussed here are the chronic, recurring type not associated with structural abnormalities or systemic disease and include migraine, cluster, and tension headaches. Characteristics of the major types of headache syndromes are summarized in Table 15-8.

Migraine

Migraine is a familial, episodic neurological disorder whose marker is headache[28] and is defined as repeated, episodic headache lasting 4 to 72 hours. It is diagnosed when any two of the following features occur: unilateral head pain, throbbing pain, pain worsens with activity, moderate or severe pain intensity; *and* at least one of the following: nausea and/or vomiting, or photophobia and phonophobia.[29] Migraine can occur in children and is more common in women and those 25 to 55 years of age. In susceptible women, migraine occurs most frequently before and during menstruation and is decreased during pregnancy and menopause. The cyclic withdrawal of estrogen and progesterone may trigger attacks of migraine.[30]

Migraine is caused by a combination of multiple genetic and environmental factors. Persons with migraine have an increased risk for epilepsy, depression, anxiety disorders, cardiovascular disease, and stroke. Triggers believed to precipitate migraine attacks include altered sleep patterns (becoming tired or oversleeping), missed meals, overexertion, weather change, stress or relaxation from stress, hormonal changes (menstrual periods), excess afferent stimulation (bright lights, strong smells), and chemicals (alcohol or nitrates).

The pathophysiologic basis for migraine is not clearly established and includes neurologic, vascular, hormonal, and neurotransmitter components.[28] Migraine is broadly classified as (1) *migraine with aura* with visual, sensory, or motor symptoms and, more commonly, (2) migraine without aura. The clinical phase of a migraine attack and the associated pathophysiologic manifestations follow:

1. *Premonitory phase:* Up to one third of persons have premonitory symptoms (tiredness, irritability, loss of concentration, food craving) hours to days before onset of aura or headache; the pathogenesis is unknown.
2. *Migraine aura:* Up to one third of persons have aura symptoms at least some of the time that may last 1 hour or sometimes much longer; the pathophysiologic basis appears to involve a cortical

TABLE 15-8 CHARACTERISTICS OF COMMON HEADACHES

	MIGRAINE		CLUSTER HEADACHE/ PROXIMAL HEMICRANIA	TENSION TYPE OF HEADACHE
	WITHOUT AURA	**WITH AURA**		
Age of onset	Childhood, adolescence, or young adulthood	Childhood, adolescence, or young adulthood	Young adulthood, middle age	Young adulthood, middle age
Gender	Female	Female	Male	Not gender specific
Family history of headaches	Yes	Yes	No	Yes
Onset and evolution	Slow to rapid	Slow to rapid	Rapid	Slow to rapid
Time course	Episodic	Episodic	Clusters in time	Episodic, may become constant
Quality	Usually throbbing	Usually throbbing	Steady	Steady
Location	Variable, often unilateral	Variable, often unilateral	Orbit, temple, cheek	Variable
Associated features	Prodrome, vomiting	Prodrome, vomiting	Lacrimation, rhinorrhea, Horner syndrome	None

spreading depression (CSD) (a spreading wave of depolarization accompanied by transient increased cerebral perfusion followed by reduction in electrical activity, and a decrease in blood flow that slowly spreads across the cerebral cortex from the occipital region).

3. *Headache phase:* Includes associated symptoms and may last from 4 to 72 hours (usually about a day); pain mechanisms are initiated in the brain with disturbances in serotonin and other neurotransmitters, resulting in compensatory overactivity in the trigeminovascular system of the brain because afferents from dural-vascular structures are innervated by branches of the trigeminal nerve. Triggers can include strong odors, lack of sleep, sun glare, high altitude, and foods containing vasoactive amines.

Differentiation of types of migraine headache is summarized in Table 15-8. The diagnosis of migraine is made from medical history and physical examination. Differential diagnosis is confirmed with CT and MRI scans and EEG. The management of migraine includes avoidance of triggers and education that migraine is a chronic physiologic disorder and not psychosomatic. Darkening the room, applying ice, and sleeping can provide some relief with the onset of acute migraine. Pharmacologic management varies and is related to the severity of attack. Drug prophylaxis for migraine is considered when attacks cannot be treated effectively.[31,32]

Cluster Headache

Cluster headaches are one of a group of disorders referred to as trigeminal autonomic cephalagias.[33] They occur in one side of the head primarily in men between 20 and 50 years of age. These uncommon headaches occur in clusters for a period of days followed by a long period of spontaneous remission. Cluster headache has an episodic and a chronic form with extreme pain intensity and short duration. If the cluster of attacks occurs more frequently without sustained spontaneous remission, they are classified as *chronic cluster headaches* (20% of cases) (see Table 15-8). Triggers are similar to those that cause migraine headache.

Trigeminal activation occurs but the mechanism is unclear. There is unilateral trigeminal distribution of severe pain with ipsilateral autonomic manifestations including tearing on affected side, ptosis of the ipsilateral eye, and congestion of the nasal mucosa. The pathogenic mechanism for pain is related to the release of vasoactive peptides and the formation of neurogenic inflammation. Autonomic dysfunction is characterized by sympathetic underactivity and parasympathetic activation. The rhythmicity of attacks is associated with changes in the inferior posterior hypothalamus. There may be altered serotonergic nerve transmission, but at different loci than in migraine headache.[33] Prophylactic drugs are used to treat cluster headache, as well as avoidance of triggers. Acute attacks are managed with oxygen inhalation, sumatriptan or inhaled ergotamine administration, and nerve stimulation.[34]

Tension-type headache. Tension-type headache is the most common type of headache. The average age of onset is during the second decade of life. It is a mild to moderate bilateral headache with a sensation of a tight band or pressure around the head with gradual onset of pain. The headache occurs in episodes and may last for several hours or several days. It is not aggravated by physical activity. Chronic tension-type headache (CTTH) evolves from episodic tension-type headache and represents headache that occurs at least 15 days per month for at least 3 months. A central pain mechanism is associated with chronic tension headache and a peripheral mechanism with episodic tension headache. The mechanism involves hypersensitivity of pain fibers from the trigeminal nerve and contraction of jaw and neck muscles, but the exact mechanisms are

unknown. Headache sufferers have more localized pain and tenderness of craniocervical muscles. Many individuals have both tension-type and migraine headaches.

Mild headaches are treated with ice, and more severe forms are treated with aspirin or nonsteroidal anti-inflammatory drugs. Chronic tension-type headaches are best managed with a tricyclic antidepressant and behavioral therapy. Long-term use of analgesics or other drugs, such as muscle relaxants, antihistamines, tranquilizers, caffeine, and ergot alkaloids, should be avoided.[35]

Infection and Inflammation of the Central Nervous System

The CNS may be infected by bacteria, viruses, fungi, parasites, and mycobacteria. The invading organisms enter the nervous system either by spreading through arterial blood vessels (Figure 15-12) or by directly invading the nervous tissue from another site of infection. Neurologic infections produce disease by several mechanisms: direct neuronal or glial infection, mass lesion formation, inflammation with subsequent edema, interruption of cerebrospinal fluid pathways, neuronal or vascular damage, and secretion of neurotoxins. An immune process may initiate an inflammatory reaction.

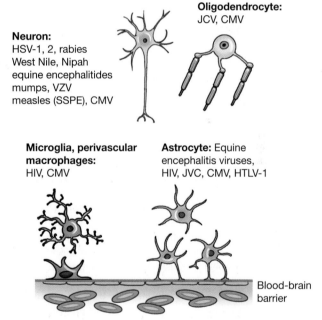

Oligodendrocyte: JCV, CMV

Neuron: HSV-1, 2, rabies West Nile, Nipah equine encephalitides mumps, VZV measles (SSPE), CMV

Microglia, perivascular macrophages: HIV, CMV

Astrocyte: Equine encephalitis viruses, HIV, JVC, CMV, HTLV-1

Blood-brain barrier

Endothelia: Nipah virus, CMV

FIGURE 15-12 Viral Infection in the Central Nervous System (CNS). Viruses infect specific cell types within the CNS depending on the particular properties of the virus together with individual cell membrane proteins expressed on permissive cell types. Normally the brain is protected from circulating pathogens and toxins by the blood-brain barrier. *CMV,* Cytomegalovirus; *HIV,* human immunodeficiency virus; *HSV,* herpes simplex virus; *HTLV-1,* human T cell lymphotropic virus (causes T cell leukemia); *JCV,* John Cunningham virus (a polyomavirus causing progressive multifocal leukoencephalopathy); *SSPE,* subacute sclerosing panencephalitis; *VZV,* varicella-zoster virus. (Adapted from Power C, Noorbakhsh G: Central nervous system viral infections: clinical aspects and pathogenic mechanisms. In Gilman S, editor, Neurobiology of disease, p 488, Burlington, Mass, 2007, Elsevier.)

Meningitis

Meningitis is inflammation of the brain or spinal cord. The causes of meningitis (infection of the meninges) include bacteria, viruses, fungi, parasites, or toxins. The infection may be acute, subacute, or chronic with the pathophysiology, clinical manifestations, and treatment differing for each type of microorganism.

Bacterial meningitis is primarily an infection of the pia mater and arachnoid, the subarachnoid space, the ventricular system, and the CSF. Meningococcus (*Neisseria meningitidis*) and pneumococcus (*Streptococcus pneumoniae*) are the most common causes of bacterial meningitis. About 1.3 in 100,000 persons are affected annually.[36] Meningococcus has been identified worldwide. Meningococcal meningitis occurs predominantly in men and boys and in the fall, winter, and spring of the year. Epidemics of meningococcal meningitis occur in approximately 10-year cycles, predominantly affecting children and adolescents. With pneumococcal meningitis, young persons and those over 40 years of age are mostly affected. Predisposing conditions are otitis or sinusitis (25%), immunocompromise (16%), and pneumonia (12%).[37,38]

Aseptic meningitis (viral meningitis, nonpurulent meningitis) is believed to be limited to the meninges. It produces various symptoms and is caused by several infectious agents, primarily viruses. Bacterial infections not adequately treated also cause aseptic meningitis.

Fungal meningitis is a chronic, much less common condition than bacterial or viral meningitis. The infection occurs most often in persons with impaired immune responses or alterations in normal body flora. It develops insidiously, usually over days or weeks.

PATHOPHYSIOLOGY A systemic or bloodstream infection or a direct extension from an infected area, usually respiratory, is the access route to the subarachnoid space. With bacterial infection, large numbers of neutrophils are recruited to the subarachnoid space. Release of cytotoxic inflammatory agents and bacterial toxins alter the blood-brain barrier and damage brain tissue. Prognosis depends on the type of pathogen.[39] The meningeal vessels become hyperemic and increasingly permeable. The inflammatory exudate thickens the CSF and interferes with normal CSF flow around the brain and spinal cord, possibly obstructing arachnoid villi and producing hydrocephalus. Meningeal cells become edematous, and the combined exudate and edematous cells increase intracranial pressure. Engorged blood vessels and thrombi can disrupt blood flow, causing further injury.

Fungi in the nervous system usually produce a granulomatous reaction, forming granulomata or gelatinous masses in the meninges at the base of the brain. Fungi also may extend along the perivascular sites in the subarachnoid space and into the brain tissue, producing arteritis with thrombosis, infarction, and communicating hydrocephalus. Meningeal fibrosis develops later in the inflammatory process. Cranial nerve dysfunction, caused by compression, often results from the granulomata and fibrosis.

CLINICAL MANIFESTATIONS The clinical manifestations of bacterial meningitis can be grouped into infectious signs, meningeal signs, and neurologic signs. The clinical manifestations of systemic infection include fever, tachycardia, chills, and a petechial rash. The clinical manifestations of meningeal irritation are a severe throbbing headache, severe photophobia, nuchal rigidity, and positive Kernig and Brudzinski signs. The neurologic signs include a decrease in consciousness, cranial nerve palsies, focal neurologic deficits (such as hemiparesis/hemiplegia and ataxia), and seizures. Often there is projectile vomiting. With meningococcal meningitis, a petechial or purpuric rash covers the skin and mucous membranes. As intracranial

pressure increases, papilledema develops and delirium may progress to unconsciousness and death.

The clinical manifestations of aseptic meningitis are similar to those of bacterial meningitis but milder. Fungal meningitis develops slowly and insidiously. The first manifestations are often those of dementia (see Chapter 14) or communicating hydrocephalus (see Chapter 14). The individual is characteristically afebrile.

EVALUATION AND TREATMENT Diagnosis of bacterial meningitis is based on physical examination and the results of nasopharyngeal smear and antigen tests. CSF cultures are required for differential diagnosis. Bacterial meningitis and fungal meningitis are treated with appropriate antibiotic therapy and other supportive measures. Aseptic meningitis is managed pharmacologically with antiviral drugs and steroids. There are vaccinations to prevent meningococcal, pneumococcal, and *Haemophilus influenzae* meningitis.[40]

Brain or Spinal Cord Abscess

Abscesses are localized collections of pus within the parenchyma of the brain or spinal cord. They develop in about 1 of every 100,000 hospital admissions and are more common in middle-aged men. They occur (1) after open trauma and during neurosurgery; (2) from contiguous spread of infection from the middle ear, mastoid cells, nasal cavity, and nasal sinuses; (3) through metastatic or hematogenous distribution from distant foci, such as the heart, lungs, pelvic organs, skin, tonsils, abscessed teeth, osteomyelitis (with the exception of cranial bones), and dirty needles (especially in compromised hosts); and (4) from cryptogenic factors, arising without other associated areas of infection. Streptococci, staphylococci, and *Bacteroides*, often combined with anaerobes, are the most common bacteria that cause abscesses; however, yeast and fungi may also be involved. *Toxoplasma gondii* is producing an ever-increasing number of CNS abscesses in persons with acquired immunodeficiency syndrome (AIDS). Most CNS abscesses are located in the cerebrum and immunosuppressed persons are particularly at risk.

Brain abscesses are classified as extradural or intracerebral. **Extradural brain abscesses** are associated with osteomyelitis in a cranial bone. **Intracerebral brain abscesses** arise from a vascular source. **Spinal cord abscesses** are classified as epidural or intramedullary. Epidural spinal abscesses usually originate as osteomyelitis in a vertebra; the infection then spreads into the epidural space. (Osteomyelitis is discussed in Chapter 37.)

PATHOPHYSIOLOGY Microorganisms gain entrance to the CNS by direct extension or distribution along the wall of a vein. Infective emboli carry organisms from distant sites. Brain abscesses evolve through four stages:

1. In *early cerebritis* (days 1 to 3) localized inflammation and the presence of inflammatory cells surrounding a core of necrosis are seen; marked cerebral edema is evident (Figure 15-13).
2. During *late cerebritis* (days 4 to 9) a necrotic center surrounded by macrophages and fibroblasts is present; new blood vessels form rapidly around the abscess, a thin capsule develops, and edema still persists.
3. During *early capsule formation* (days 10 to 13) the necrotic center decreases in size, more fibroblasts and macrophages are present, and mature collagen evolves, forming a capsule.
4. In the *late capsule formation* stage (days 14 and longer), a well-formed necrotic center surrounded by a dense collagen capsule develops.

Existing abscesses also tend to spread and form daughter abscesses.

CLINICAL MANIFESTATIONS Clinical manifestations of brain abscesses are associated with (1) an intracranial infection or (2) an expanding intracranial mass. Early manifestations include low-grade fever, headache (most common symptom), neck pain and stiffness with mild nuchal rigidity, confusion, drowsiness, sensory deficits, and communication deficits. Later clinical manifestations include inattentiveness (distractibility), memory deficits, decreased visual acuity and narrowed visual fields, papilledema, ocular palsy, ataxia, and dementia. The development of symptoms may be very insidious, often making an abscess difficult to diagnose.

Extradural brain abscesses are associated with localized pain, purulent drainage from the nasal passages or auditory canal, fever, localized tenderness, and neck stiffness. Occasionally the individual experiences a focal seizure.

Clinical manifestations of spinal cord abscesses have four stages: (1) spinal aching; (2) severe root pain, accompanied by spasms of the back muscles and limited vertebral movement; (3) weakness caused by progressive cord compression; and (4) paralysis.

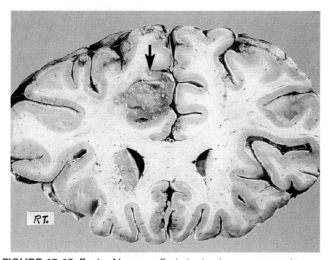

FIGURE 15-13 Brain Abscess. Early brain abscess appearing as a poorly demarcated area *(arrow)* of cerebritis at the gray-white junction. (From Damjanov I, Linder J, editors: *Anderson's pathology*, ed 10, St Louis, 1996, Mosby.)

EVALUATION AND TREATMENT The diagnosis is suggested by clinical features and confirmed by imaging studies. Aspiration through a burr hole and excision through craniotomy accompanied by antibiotic therapy are treatment options. In addition, intracranial pressure may have to be managed.

Because decompression is necessary, spinal cord abscesses are treated with surgical excision or aspiration. Antibiotic therapy and support therapy also are instituted.

Encephalitis

Encephalitis is an acute febrile illness, usually of viral origin, with nervous system involvement. The most common forms are caused by arthropod-borne (mosquito-borne) viruses and herpes simplex type 1. Viruses infect specific cell types in the CNS as shown in Figure 15-12, p. 393. Referred to as infectious viral encephalitides, encephalitis may occur as a complication of systemic viral diseases such as poliomyelitis, rabies, or mononucleosis, or it may arise after recovery from viral infections such as rubella or rubeola. Encephalitis also may follow vaccination with a live attenuated virus vaccine if the vaccine has an encephalitis component, for example, measles, mumps, and rubella. Typhus, trichinosis, malaria, and schistosomiasis also are associated with encephalitis. Toxoplasmosis may acutely reactivate in immunosuppressed persons when the once-dormant parasite in cyst form disseminates in brain tissues.

With the exception of the California viral encephalitis, which is endemic, the arthropod-borne (mosquito-borne) encephalitides occur in epidemics, varying in geographic and seasonal incidence (Table 15-9 and *Health Alert:* West Nile Virus). Eastern equine encephalitis is the most serious but least common of the encephalitides.

PATHOPHYSIOLOGY Meningeal involvement is present in all encephalitides. The various encephalitides may cause widespread nerve cell degeneration. Edema, necrosis with or without hemorrhage, and increased intracranial pressure develop. Infectious encephalitis may result from a postinfectious autoimmune response to the virus or from direct invasion of the CNS.

CLINICAL MANIFESTATIONS Encephalitis ranges from a mild infectious disease to a life-threatening disorder. Dramatic clinical manifestations include fever, delirium, or confusion progressing to

| | PERIOD | | | |
INCUBATION VIRUSES	(DAYS)	LOCATION	SEASON	AFFECTED POPULATION
Eastern equine encephalitis	5-15	Atlantic, Gulf Coast, and Great Lakes regions	Midsummer to early fall	Infants, children, and adults >50 yr
Western equine encephalitis	5-10	All parts of United States, especially western two thirds of country	Summer to early fall	Infants and young children
Venezuelan equine encephalitis	2-5	Texas, Florida, Mexico, Central and South America	All seasons	Infants and young children
St Louis encephalitis	4-21	United States and Canada, especially Mississippi River, Pacific Coast, Texas, and Florida	Summer and fall	Adults >40 yr; elderly more often affected than younger ages
California encephalitis	5-15	Midwestern United States, Eastern seaboard, and Canada	Late summer and early fall	Children <15 yr
West Nile encephalitis	3-14	Lower 48 states of United States	Summer and fall	Elderly most seriously
Dengue encephalitis	5-10	Florida, Texas, Mexico, Asia, Central and South America, and the Caribbean	All seasons	Adults and children

TABLE 15-9 CLASSIFICATION AND CHARACTERISTICS OF ARBOVIRUSES CAUSING ENCEPHALITIS

Modified from Barker E: *Neuroscience nursing,* ed 2, St Louis, 2002, Mosby.

West Nile Virus

West Nile virus (WNV) is the most common cause of epidemic meningoencephalitis in North America and the leading cause of arboviral encephalitis in the United States. It is spread by infected mosquitoes. The illness is seasonal in the summer and continues into the fall.

Symptoms: There may be no symptoms or there may be illness of varying severity with central nervous system involvement including fever, headache, stiff neck, vision loss, and altered mental status ranging from confusion to coma with or without additional signs of brain dysfunction (e.g., paresis or paralysis, cranial nerve palsies, sensory deficits, abnormal reflexes, generalized convulsions, and abnormal movements). When the central nervous system is affected, clinical syndromes ranging from febrile headache to aseptic meningitis to encephalitis may occur, and these are usually indistinguishable from similar syndromes caused by other viruses. Symptoms usually develop between 3 and 14 days after a bite by an infected mosquito and may last for a few days to several weeks. The diagnosis is made by serologic examination.

Transmission: WNV is generally distributed by the bite of an infected mosquito. Mosquitoes are WNV carriers that become infected when they feed on infected birds. The bite of infected mosquitoes can then spread WNV to humans and other animals. In a very small number of cases, WNV also has been transferred through blood transfusions, organ transplants, breast-feeding, and even maternal-fetal contact, but the risk is low. WNV is not distributed through casual contact such as touching or kissing a person with the virus.

Risk: Less than 20% of people who are bitten by mosquitoes develop any symptoms of the disease, and relatively few mosquitoes actually carry WNV. People older than age 50 and immunocompromised persons are more likely to develop serious symptoms.

Prevention: Prevent mosquito bites. Avoid outdoor activities dusk to dawn or wear protective clothing—long sleeves, long pants, and socks. Treat clothes with insect repellents containing DEET. Higher concentrations of active ingredients provide longer protection. Maintain fully functioning screens on windows and doors. Eradicate mosquito breeding sites by eliminating or treating standing water. Do not handle dead birds with bare hands. No West Nile vaccine has been developed for humans. Since 2003 all blood banks use blood-screening tests for West Nile virus. In addition, blood banks will not take donations from people who had a fever and headache in the week before they volunteered to donate blood.

Treatment: There is no specific treatment for WNV infection. Severe symptoms require hospital care. A subset of persons remain profoundly weak and limited in daily functioning 1 year following acute illness. Work is in progress to develop a vaccine and antiviral therapy.

Data from Avalos-Bock SA: West Nile virus and the US blood supply: new tests substantially reduce the risk of transmission via donated blood products, *Am J Nurs* 105(12):34–37, 2005; Centers for Disease Control and Prevention: Surveillance for human West Nile disease-United States 1999–2008, *MMWR* 59(SS2), 2010; Centers for Disease Control and Prevention, Division of Vector Borne Infectious Diseases: *West Nile virus*. Available at: http://www.cdc.gov/mmwr/preview/mmwrhtml/ss5902a1.htm; Davis LE et al: West Nile virus neuroinvasive disease, *Ann Neurol* 60(3):286–300, 2006; Beasley DW: Vaccines and immunotherapeutics for the prevention and treatment of infections with West Nile virus, *Immunotherapy* 3(2):269–285, 2011.

unconsciousness, seizure activity, cranial nerve palsies, paresis and paralysis, involuntary movement, and abnormal reflexes. Signs of marked intracranial pressure may be present.

EVALUATION AND TREATMENT Diagnosis is made by history and clinical presentation aided by CSF examination and culture, serologic studies, white blood cell count, CT scan, or MRI. Most cases of viral meningitis are self-limiting, and until recently no definitive treatment was available. However, herpes encephalitis in immunocompromised persons is now being treated with antiviral agents, such as acyclovir and steroids. Measures to control intracranial pressure are paramount.

Neurologic Complications of AIDS

From 40% to 60% of all persons with AIDS have neurologic complications. The most common neurologic disorder is HIV-associated dementia (HIV encephalopathy). Others are peripheral neuropathies, vacuolar (spongy softening) myelopathy, opportunistic infections of the CNS, and neoplasms.

Human immunodeficiency virus–associated dementia (HIV encephalopathy). HIV-associated dementia (HIV-associated cognitive dysfunction, HIV encephalopathy, subacute encephalitis, HIV-associated dementia complex, HIV cognitive motor complex, AIDS encephalopathy, AIDS dementia complex, AIDS-related dementia) may affect adults or children and is characterized by progressive cognitive dysfunction with motor and behavioral alterations. The syndrome typically develops later in the disease but may be an early or singular manifestation in some persons.

In HIV–associated dementia, HIV-infected macrophages and monocytes from blood accumulate in the brain by up-regulation of proinflammatory mediators that enable activated macrophages and monocytes to penetrate the blood-brain barrier, promoting chronic neuroinflammation and neurodegeneration. The virus can be isolated in the CSF at approximately the time of seroconversion. Chronic drug abuse (cocaine, opiates, methamphetamine) potentiates neurotoxicity.[41]

HIV-associated dementia is insidious in onset and unpredictable in its course. Most persons experience a steady progression with abrupt accelerations of signs over several months to more than 1 year. Impaired concentration and memory deficits are common, and apathy, lack of motivation, social withdrawal, irritability, and emotional lability appear. Later, difficulties with language, spatial or temporal disorientation, and visual construction are present. Some persons manifest an organic psychosis with agitation, inappropriate behavior, and hallucinosis. Motor signs include difficulty speaking, progressive loss of balance, gait ataxia, spastic paraparesis or paralysis, and generalized hyperreflexia sometimes accompanied by decreased writing ability, tremor, myoclonus, and seizure.

Diagnosis is difficult, especially in early stages, and CSF analysis, CT scan, and MRI data help establish the diagnosis. Treatment consists of controlling the disease with antiretroviral agents, protease inhibitors, and reverse transcriptase inhibitors.[42]

HIV myelopathy. Myelopathy involving diffuse degeneration of the spinal cord may occur in persons with AIDS (HIV myelopathy). **Vacuolar myelopathy** is believed to be a direct consequence of HIV. The lateral and posterior columns of the lumbar spinal cord are affected. Progressive spastic paraparesis with ataxia is the predominant clinical manifestation. Leg weakness, upper motor neuron signs, incontinence, and posterior column sensory loss may be present. Diagnosis is made on the basis of history, physical findings, and supporting data from diagnostic procedures. Treatment is supportive.

HIV peripheral neuropathy. HIV has been isolated from peripheral nerves; consequently, the virus may directly infect nerves and cause neuropathy (HIV distal symmetric polyneuropathy), most commonly sensory. Persons experience neuropathic pain including painful, burning dysesthesias and paresthesias, typically in the extremities. Weakness and decreased or absent distal reflexes may be present. Diagnosis is established through history and physical findings, laboratory data, and nerve conduction and electromyogram (EMG) studies.

Aseptic viral meningitis. Some persons develop acute aseptic meningitis at approximately the time of seroconversion. This may represent the initial infection of the nervous system by the virus. Symptoms include headache, fever, and meningismus (headache, photophobia, nuchal rigidity). Cranial nerve involvement, especially V and VII, may appear, but the disease is self-limiting and requires only symptomatic treatment.

Opportunistic infections. Opportunistic infections may be bacterial, fungal, or viral in origin and may produce disease. Typically, bacterial infections are caused by unusual microorganisms. Cryptococcal infection is the most common fungal disorder and the third leading cause of neurologic disease in persons with AIDS. The symptoms are vague, such as fever, headache, malaise, and meningismus. Herpes encephalitis and herpes varicella-zoster radiculitis may develop. Papovavirus may produce a demyelinating disorder. Cytomegalovirus encephalitis and toxoplasmosis (a protozoal infection) are common in persons with AIDS. Tuberculosis has a high incidence, particularly in African countries.

CNS neoplasms. CNS neoplasms associated with AIDS include CNS lymphoma, systemic non-Hodgkin lymphoma, and metastatic Kaposi sarcoma. Primary CNS lymphoma is a large-cell tumor that presents as rapidly developing and expanding multicentric intracranial mass lesions. The meninges and, possibly, the cranial nerves and spinal cord are invaded in systemic non-Hodgkin lymphoma. Metastasis of a Kaposi sarcoma to the CNS is uncommon.

Other CNS complications. Persons with AIDS may develop multifocal ischemic infarctions, hemorrhagic infarctions, hemorrhage into tumors, subdural hematomas, and epidural hemorrhage. Reported neurologic symptoms produced by AIDS therapeutics include extrapyramidal movements, myoclonus, dysphasia, delirium, and acute myelopathy.

Demyelinating Degenerative Disorders

Demyelinating disorders result from damage to the myelin nerve sheath and affect neural transmission. Either the central or the peripheral nervous system can be affected. CNS demyelinating disorders are subclassified as primary or secondary. Multiple sclerosis is a major demyelinating syndrome. A disorder is classified as degenerative when the cause of the degeneration is unclear, which is the case with amyotrophic lateral sclerosis.

Multiple Sclerosis

Multiple sclerosis (MS) is a relatively common acquired autoimmune inflammatory disorder involving destruction of axonal myelin in the brain and spinal cord. The onset of MS is usually between 20 and 40 years of age and is more common in women. Men may have a more severe progressive course. The prevalence rate is affected by gene-environment interactions in susceptible individuals.[43]

PATHOPHYSIOLOGY   MS involves an autoimmune process that develops when a previous viral insult to the nervous system has occurred in a genetically susceptible individual. B lymphocytes, plasma cells, and activated T cells, along with proinflammatory cytokines, cause inflammation, oligodendrocyte injury, and demyelination. Early

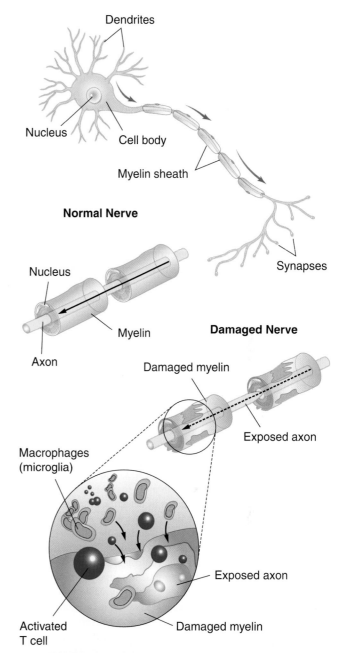

FIGURE 15-14 Pathogenesis of Multiple Sclerosis.

inflammation and demyelination lead to irreversible axonal degeneration and scarring (sclerosis). Activated microglia and macrophages release nitric acid and oxygen free radicals, and activated immune cells also produce glutamate, a neurotoxin (Figure 15-14).[43a]

MS not only has focal inflammatory changes but also manifests diffuse injury throughout the CNS called MS lesions (see Figure 15-14). MS lesions can occur anywhere in gray or white matter with localized areas of demyelination (plaques), changes in the constituents of myelin, damage to oligodendrocytes, substantial loss of neurons over time, and atrophy of the brain. Even normal appearing white matter is microscopically very abnormal. The multifocal, multistaged features of MS lesions in established disease produce symptoms that are multiple and variable.

CLINICAL MANIFESTATIONS   Various events occur immediately before the onset or exacerbation of symptoms and are regarded as precipitating factors, including infection, trauma, and pregnancy. The most common initial symptoms are paresthesias of the face, trunk, or limbs; weakness; visual disturbances; or urinary incontinence, indicating diffuse CNS involvement.

The subtypes of MS are based on the clinical course: remitting-relapsing (RR), primary-progressive (PP), secondary-progressive (SP), and progressive-relapsing (PR). Initially, 90% of persons present with a remitting-relapsing course and without treatment transition to the progressive types with insidious neurologic decline. Early cognitive changes are common and may include poor judgment, apathy, emotional lability, and depression. Short-lived attacks of neurologic deficits (paresthesias, dysarthria, and ataxia) are the temporary appearance or worsening of symptoms. The mechanism of these attacks is complete, reversible conduction block in partially demyelinated axons. Conditions that cause short-lived attacks include (1) minor increases in body temperature or serum calcium (Ca^{++}) concentration and (2) functional demands exceeding conduction capacity. An increase in body temperature or serum Ca^{++} level increases current leakage through demyelinated neurons. Other triggering events include hypercalcemia and physical and emotional stress. Paroxysmal attacks may persist for weeks or months and may be followed by progressive symptoms of MS.

Individuals with advanced MS have cerebellar symptoms including ataxia, slurred speech, and intention tremor. Painful sensory events, spastic paralysis, and bowel and bladder incontinence are common and disabling with progressive disease.[44]

EVALUATION AND TREATMENT There is no single test available to diagnose or rule out MS and the diagnosis is based on the history and physical examination in combination with MRI and CSF findings. Persistently elevated levels of CSF immunoglobulin G (IgG) are found in about two thirds of individuals with MS, and oligoclonal (IgG) bands on electrophoresis are found in more than 90% of MS patients. Evoked potential studies aid diagnosis by detecting decreased conduction velocity in visual, auditory, and somatosensory pathways. MRI is the most sensitive available method of detecting the disease.

The treatment goal in MS is prevention of exacerbations and permanent neurologic damage and control of symptoms. Disease-modifying drugs include corticosteroids, immunosuppressants, and immune system modulators. Drugs are also available for symptom control.[45] Supportive care includes participation in a regular exercise program, cessation of smoking, and avoidance of overwork, extreme fatigue, and heat exposure. Vitamin D may prevent disease progression.[46] Stem cell therapy is under investigation (see *Health Alert:* Stem Cells: Neuroprotection and Restoration).

HEALTH ALERT

Stem Cells: Neuroprotection and Restoration

Transplantation of adult neural stem cells can protect and restore brain functions in animal models of ischemic and inflammatory brain injury. Some subsets of stem cells replace damaged tissue and also have modulated immune responses, providing neuroprotection and potential benefit in diseases such as multiple sclerosis. Progress toward the use of stem cells for neuroprotective and regenerative interventions holds much promise for the future.

Data from Martino G et al: Stem Cells in Multiple Sclerosis (STEMS) Consensus Group. Stem cell transplantation in multiple sclerosis: current status and future prospects, *Nat Rev Neurol* 6(5):247–255, 2010; Ucelli A, Mancardi G: Stem cell transplantation in multiple sclerosis, *Curr Opin Neurol* 23(3):218–225, 2010.

Amyotrophic Lateral Sclerosis

Amyotrophic lateral sclerosis (ALS, sporadic motor neuron disease, sporadic motor system disease, motor neuron disease [MND]) is a worldwide neurodegenerative disorder that diffusely involves lower and upper motor neurons, resulting in progressive muscle weakness. *Amyotrophic* (without muscle nutrition or progressive muscle wasting) refers to the predominant lower motor neuron component of the syndrome. *Lateral sclerosis,* scarring of the corticospinal tract in the lateral column of the spinal cord, refers to the upper motor neuron component of the syndrome.

Classic ALS (Lou Gehrig disease) may begin at any time from the fourth decade of life; its peak occurrence is in the early fifties. The male/female ratio is about 1.5:1, equalizing after menopause. Ten percent of persons with ALS have a familial form and specific genes have been identified.[47]

PATHOPHYSIOLOGY The cause of motor neuron death in ALS is unknown. A subset of persons with familial ALS have a genetic mutation in copper-zinc superoxide dismutase (SODI) on the glial cells surrounding the motor neuron that contributes to neurotoxicity through oxidative stress, mitochondrial dysfunction, and impaired axonal transport.[48,49] The reuptake of glutamate by glial cells also is diminished, and glutamate-induced neurotoxicity contributes to neuron degeneration.

The principal pathologic feature of ALS is lower and upper motor neuron degeneration, although without inflammation. There are fewer large motor neurons in the spinal cord, brain stem, and cerebral cortex (premotor and motor areas), with ongoing degeneration in the remaining motor neurons. Death of the motor neuron results in axonal degeneration and secondary demyelination with glial proliferation and sclerosis (scarring). Widespread neural degeneration of nonmotor neurons in the spinal cord and motor cortices, as well as in the premotor, sensory, and temporal cortices, has been found.

Lower motor neuron degeneration denervates motor units. Adjacent, still viable lower motor neurons attempt to compensate by distal intramuscular sprouting, reinnervation, and enlargement of motor units. The initial symptoms of the disease may be related to lower or upper motor neuron dysfunction or to both.

CLINICAL MANIFESTATIONS About 60% of individuals have a spinal form of the disease with focal muscle weakness beginning in the arms and legs and progressing to muscle atrophy, spasticity, and loss of manual dexterity and gait. No associated mental, sensory, or autonomic symptoms are present. ALS with progressive bulbar palsy presents with difficulty speaking and swallowing, and peripheral muscle weakness and atrophy usually occur within 1 to 2 years. Progressive muscle atrophy and paralysis lead to respiratory failure and death within 2 to 5 years although a small percentage of individuals may live 10 years or longer.[50]

EVALUATION AND TREATMENT Diagnosis of the syndrome is based predominantly on the history and physical examination with no evidence of other neuromuscular disorders. Electromyography and muscle biopsy results verify lower motor neuron degeneration and denervation. Imaging studies and cerebrospinal fluid biomarkers can assist in making the diagnosis. Little treatment is available to alter the overall course of the ALS syndrome. The drug riluzole (Rilutek) has extended time not requiring ventilatory assistance. Supportive management and rehabilitative management are directed toward preventing complications of immobility. Psychologic support of the affected individual and the family is extremely important.[51]

TABLE 15-10 PERIPHERAL NERVOUS SYSTEM DISORDERS

DISORDER	PATHOLOGY	CLINICAL MANIFESTATIONS
Radiculopathies	Injury to spinal roots as they exit or enter vertebral canal; caused by compression, inflammation, direct trauma	Affects strength, tone, and bulk of muscles innervated by involved roots; pattern similar to that seen in amyotrophies, with tone and deep tendon reflexes decreased, rarely absent; fasciculations; mild fatigue; sensory alterations, pain
Plexus injuries	Involve nerve plexus distal to spinal roots but proximal to formation of peripheral nerves; caused by trauma, compression, infiltration, or iatrogenic (positioning or intramuscular injection)	Motor weakness, muscle atrophy, sensory loss in affected areas; paralysis common
Neuropathies	Called sensorimotor if sensory, motor, and reflex effects; pure sensory caused by leprosy, industrial solvents, chloramphenicol, and hereditary mechanisms; motor caused by Guillain-Barré syndrome, infectious mononucleosis, viral hepatitis, acute porphyria, or lead, mercury, and triorthocresylphosphate (TCP) poisoning	Affects muscle strength, tone, and bulk; whole muscles or groups may be paretic or paralyzed; muscles of feet and legs first, then hands and arms; tone and deep tendon reflexes generally decreased with atrophy and fasciculation; mild fatigue; some specific symptoms of paresthesia and dysesthesia; altered reflexes; autonomic disturbances; deformities; metabolic changes
Guillain-Barré syndrome (several antibody subtypes have been identified)	Acute onset of motor, sensory, or autonomic symptoms caused by autoimmune inflammatory response, resulting in axonal demyelination; most commonly manifests as ascending motor paralysis; often preceded by respiratory or gastrointestinal viral infection	Clinical manifestations are related to antibody subtypes; manifestations can include paresis of legs to complete quadriplegia, paralysis of eye muscles, respiratory insufficiency, autonomic nervous system instability; sensory symptoms (pain, numbness, paresthesias); may progress to respiratory arrest or cardiovascular collapse

From Vucic S, Kiernan MC, Cornblath DR: Guillain-Barré syndrome: an update, *J Clin Neurosci* 16(6):733–741, 2009.

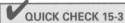

QUICK CHECK 15-3
1. Why is multiple sclerosis an autoimmune disease?
2. Why is amyotrophic lateral sclerosis a motor neuron disease?

PERIPHERAL NERVOUS SYSTEM AND NEUROMUSCULAR JUNCTION DISORDERS

Peripheral Nervous System Disorders

Disease processes may injure the axons traveling to and from the brain stem and spinal cord neuronal cell bodies. The injury may affect a distinct anatomic area on the axon, or the spinal nerves may be injured at the roots, at the plexus before peripheral nerve formation, or at the nerves themselves. The cranial nerves do not have roots or plexuses and are affected only within themselves. Autonomic nerve fibers may be injured as they travel in certain cranial nerves and emerge through the ventral root and plexuses to pass through the peripheral nerves of the body. Peripheral nervous system disorders are summarized in Table 15-10.

Neuromuscular Junction Disorders

Transmission of the nerve impulse at the neuromuscular junction requires the release of adequate amounts of neurotransmitter from the presynaptic terminals of the axon and effective binding of the released transmitter to the receptors on the membranes of muscle cells (see Figure 12-14). Four neuromuscular junction disorders have been identified: acetylcholine receptor (AChR) myasthenia gravis, muscle-specific-kinase protein (MuSK) antibody-associated myasthenia gravis, Lambert-Eaton myasthenic syndrome (*presynaptic* antibodies to voltage-dependent calcium channels), and acquired neuromyotonia. Nutritional deficits, certain drugs (e.g., reserpine, methyldopa [Aldomet]), certain toxins (e.g., botulism), some venoms, and certain disorders that interfere with the synthesis or packaging of the neurotransmitter or its release into the synaptic cleft may result in weakness.

Myasthenia Gravis

Myasthenia gravis is an acquired chronic autoimmune disease mediated by antibodies against the acetylcholine receptor (AChR) at the neuromuscular junction, and is characterized by muscle weakness and fatigability. The incidence is about 9 to 21 per million population[52] and it is more common in women. Thymic tumors, pathologic changes in the thymus, and other autoimmune diseases are associated with the disorder. (Autoimmune mechanisms are discussed in Chapter 7.) Ocular myasthenia, more common in males, involves weakness of the eye muscles and eyelids, and may include swallowing difficulties and slurred speech.

PATHOPHYSIOLOGY Myasthenia gravis results from a defect in nerve impulse transmission at the neuromuscular junction. The postsynaptic AChRs on the muscle cell's plasma membrane are no longer recognized as "self" and elicit the generation of autoantibodies. IgG antibody is produced against the AChR and fixes onto the receptor sites, blocking the binding of acetylcholine. Eventually the antibody action destroys receptor sites. This causes diminished transmission of the nerve impulse across the neuromuscular junction and lack of muscle depolarization. Symptomatic individuals without anti-AChR antibodies may have antibodies against muscle-specific-kinase (MuSK) with similar symptoms. Why this autosensitization occurs is unknown.

CLINICAL MANIFESTATIONS Myasthenia gravis has an insidious onset with the foremost complaint of muscle fatigue and progressive weakness. Clinical manifestations may first appear during pregnancy, during the postpartum period, or in conjunction with the administration of certain anesthetic agents. The person often complains of fatigue after exercise and the muscles of the eyes, face, mouth, throat, and neck usually are affected first. The muscles of the neck, shoulder girdle, and hip flexors are less frequently affected. The respiratory muscles of the diaphragm and chest wall can become weak with impaired ventilation. Myasthenic crisis occurs when severe muscle weakness causes extreme quadriparesis or quadriplegia, respiratory insufficiency with shortness of breath, and extreme difficulty in swallowing. The individual in myasthenic crisis is in danger of respiratory arrest.

Cholinergic crisis may arise from anticholinesterase drug toxicity with increased intestinal motility, episodes of diarrhea and complaints of intestinal cramping, bradycardia, pupillary constriction, increased salivation, and diaphoresis. These are caused by the smooth muscle hyperactivity secondary to excessive accumulation of acetylcholine at the neuromuscular junctions and excessive parasympathetic-like activity. As in myasthenic crisis, the individual is in danger of respiratory arrest.

EVALUATION AND TREATMENT   The diagnosis of myasthenia gravis is made on the basis of a response to edrophonium chloride (Tensilon), results of EMG studies, and detection of anti-AChR or MuSK antibodies. With the intravenous administration of the drug, immediate demonstrable improvement in muscle strength usually persists for several minutes. Mediastinal tomography and MRI help determine whether a thymoma is present. The progression of myasthenia gravis varies, appearing first as a mild case that spontaneously remits, with a series of relapses and symptom-free intervals ranging from weeks to months. Over time the disease can progress, leading to death. Ocular myasthenia has a very good prognosis.

Anticholinesterase drugs, steroids, and immunosuppressant drugs (e.g., azathioprine and cyclosporine) are used to treat myasthenia gravis and myasthenic crisis. For individuals with cholinergic crisis, anticholinergic drugs are withheld until blood levels are nontoxic; in addition, ventilatory support is provided and respiratory complications are prevented. Thymectomy is the treatment of choice in individuals with a thymoma and those with anti-AChR antibodies because this terminates the produciton self-reactive T cells and B cells that produce the antibodies.[53,54]

> 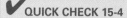 **QUICK CHECK 15-4**
> 1. Where in the peripheral nervous system can disease occur?
> 2. Why do antibodies contribute to the symptoms of myasthenia gravis?

TUMORS OF THE CENTRAL NERVOUS SYSTEM

CNS tumors include both brain and spinal cord tumors. No proven causative agents for CNS tumors have been established. Carcinogenesis is discussed in Chapter 9.

Cranial Tumors

Tumors within the cranium can be either primary or metastatic as follows:
- *Primary*—Intracerebral tumors originate from brain substance, including neuroglia, neurons, cells of blood vessels, and connective tissue. Extracerebral tumors originate outside substances of brain and include meningiomas, acoustic nerve tumors, and tumors of pituitary and pineal glands.
- *Metastatic*—These tumors are found inside or outside brain substance.
- Sites of intracranial tumors are illustrated in Figure 15-15.

Primary brain tumors (both malignant and nonmalignant) have an estimated incidence rate of 20,020 with 13,140 deaths in the United States for 2010.[55] The incidence of CNS tumors increases to age 70 years and then decreases. CNS tumors are the second most common group of tumors occurring in children. Approximately 70% to 75% of all intracranial tumors in children are located infratentorially, and in adults 70% are located supratentorially. Peripheral nerve tumors are rare in children and common in adults.

Local effects of cranial tumors are caused by the destructive action of the tumor itself on a particular site in the brain and by compression causing decreased cerebral blood flow. Effects include seizures, visual disturbances, unstable gait, and cranial nerve dysfunction. Generalized effects result from increased intracranial pressure caused by obstruction of the ventricular system, hemorrhages in and around the tumor, or cerebral edema (Figure 15-16).

Intracranial brain tumors do not metastasize as readily as tumors in other organs because there are no lymphatic channels within the brain substance. If metastasis does occur, it is usually through seeding of cerebral blood or CSF during cranial surgery or through artificial shunts.

Primary Brain (Intracerebral) Tumors

Primary brain (intracerebral) tumors, also called **gliomas**, include astrocytomas, oligodendrogliomas, and ependymomas. They comprise 50% to 60% of all adult brain tumors and make up about 2% of all cancers in the United States (Table 15-11). The World Health Organization (WHO) divides gliomas into four grades based on histopathologic

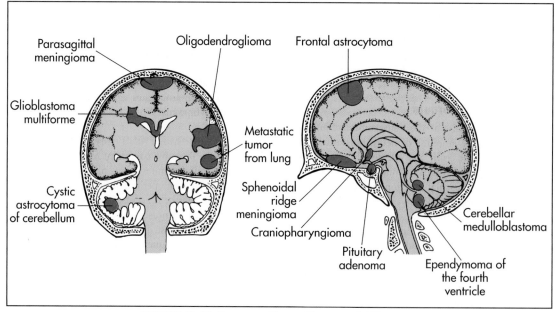

FIGURE 15-15 Common Sites of Intracranial Tumors.

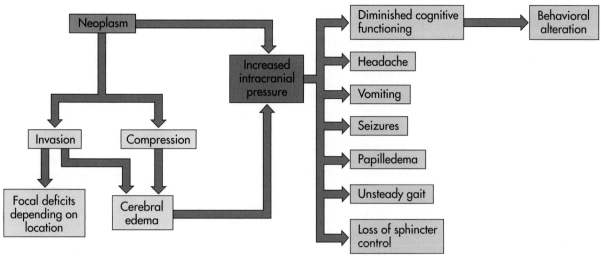

FIGURE 15-16 Origin of Clinical Manifestations Associated With an Intracranial Neoplasm.

TABLE 15-11 BRAIN AND SPINAL CORD TUMORS

NEOPLASM	LOCATION	CHARACTERISTICS	CELL OF ORIGIN
Gliomas			
Astrocytoma	Anywhere in brain or spinal cord	Slow growing, invasive	Astrocytes
Glioblastoma multiforme	Predominantly in cerebral hemispheres	Highly invasive and malignant	Thought to arise from mature astrocytes
Oligodendrocytoma	Most commonly in frontal lobes deep in white matter; may arise in brain stem, cerebellum, and spinal cord	Relatively avascular; tends to be encapsulated; more malignant form called *oligodendroblastoma*	Oligodendrites
Ependymoma	Intramedullary: wall of ventricles; may arise in caudal tail of spinal cord	More common in children, variable growth rates; more malignant, invasive form is called *ependymoblastoma;* may extend into ventricle or invade brain tissue	Ependymal cells
Neuronal Cell			
Medulloblastoma	Posterior cerebellar vermis, roof of fourth ventricle	Well-demarcated but infiltrating, rapid growing; fills fourth ventricle	Embryonic cells
Mesodermal Tissue			
Meningioma	Intradural, extramedullary: sylvian fissure region, superior parasagittal surface of frontal and parietal lobes, olfactory groove, wing of sphenoid bone, superior surface of cerebellum, cerebellopontine angle, spinal cord	Slow growing, circumscribed, encapsulated, sharply demarcated from normal tissues, compressive in nature	Arachnoid cells; may be from fibroblasts
Choroid Plexus			
Papillomas	Choroid plexus of ventricular system, lateral ventricle in children, fourth ventricle in adults	Usually benign; slow expansion inducing hemorrhage and hydrocephalus; malignant tumor is rare	Epithelial cells
Cranial Nerves and Spinal Nerve Roots			
Neurilemmoma	Cranial nerves (most commonly vestibular division of cranial nerve VIII)	Slow growing	Schwann cells
Neurofibroma	Extramedullary—spinal cord	Slow growing	Neurilemma, Schwann cells

Continued

TABLE 15-11	BRAIN AND SPINAL CORD TUMORS—cont'd		
NEOPLASM	**LOCATION**	**CHARACTERISTICS**	**CELL OF ORIGIN**
Pituitary Tumors	Pituitary gland; may extend to or invade floor of third ventricle	Age linked, several types, slow growing, macroadenomas and microadenomas	Pituitary cells, pituitary chromophobes, basophils, eosinophils
Germ Cell Tumors	Neurohypophysis, hypothalamus, pineal region Primarily in adolescents Male > female Variable prognosis	Rare, 0.5% of all primary brain tumors	Several types—germinoma, embryonal carcinoma, yolk sac tumor, choriocarcinoma, teratoma, mixed germ cell tumor—with different cell origins
Pineal region	Pineal region; pineal parenchyma	Several types (germinoma, pineocytoma, teratoma)	Several types with different cell origins
Blood Vessel Tumors			
Angioma	Predominantly in posterior cerebral hemispheres	Slow growing	Arising from congenitally malformed arteriovenous connections
Hemangioblastomas	Predominantly in cerebellum	Slow growing	Embryonic vascular tissue

TABLE 15-12	CLASSIFICATION SYSTEMS FOR ASTROCYTOMAS		
GRADE*	**TYPE**	**DESCRIPTION**	**CHARACTERISTICS**
I	Pilocytic astrocytoma	Common in children and young adults and people with neurofibromatosis type 1; common cerebellum	Least malignant, well differentiated, grow slowly, near normal microscopic appearance, non-infiltrating
II	Diffuse, low grade astrocytoma (fibrillary, gemistocytic protoplasmic)	Common in young adults, more common in cerebrum but can occur in any part of brain	Abnormal microscopic appearance, grows slowly, infiltrates to adjacent tissue, may recur at higher grade
III	Anaplastic (malignant) astrocytoma	Common in young adults	Malignant, many cells undergoing mitosis, infiltrates adjacent tissue, frequently recur at higher grade
IV	Glioblastoma (glioblastoma multiforme)	Common in older adults particularly men	Poorly differentiated, increased number of cells undergoing cell division, bizarre microscopic appearance, widely infiltrates, neovascularization, central necrosis

*World Health Organization grading of central nervous system tumors.
Data from: Louis DN et al: The 2007 WHO classification of tumours of the central nervous system, *Acta Neuropathol* 114(2):97-109, 2007.
American Brain Tumor Association: *A Primer of Brain Tumors*, Updated January, 2009. Available at http://www.abta.org/Tumor_&_Treatment_Info/A_Primer_of_Brain_Tumors/170.

features, cellular density, atypia, mitotic activity, microvascular proliferation, and necrosis (Table 15-12). Etiology for primary brain tumors is unknown.

Surgical or radiosurgical excision, surgical decompression, chemotherapy, radiotherapy, and hyperthermia are treatment options for these tumors. Supportive treatment is directed at reducing edema. (Cancer treatment is discussed in Chapters 10 and 11.)

Astrocytoma. Astrocytomas are the most common glioma (about 50% of all tumors of the brain and spinal cord)[56] and are graded by two classification systems (see Table 15-12). These tumor cells are believed to have lost normal growth restraint and thus proliferate uncontrollably. Astrocytomas are graded I through IV with grades I and II being slow-growing tumors that may form cavities.

They may occur anywhere in the brain or spinal cord; they generally are located in the cerebrum, hypothalamus, or pons. Low-grade astrocytomas tend to be located laterally or supratentorially in adults and in a midline or near-midline position in children.

Headache and subtle neurobehavioral changes may be early signs with other neurologic symptoms evolving slowly and increased intracranial pressure occurring late in the tumor's course. Onset of a focal seizure disorder between the second and sixth decade of life suggests an astrocytoma. Low-grade astrocytomas are treated with surgery or by external radiation. Fifty percent of persons survive 5 years when surgery is followed by radiation therapy (RT).[55] Grade I and II astrocytomas commonly progress to a higher grade tumor.

Grades III and IV astrocytomas are found predominantly in the frontal lobes and cerebral hemispheres, although they may occur in the brain stem, cerebellum, and spinal cord. Men are twice as likely to have astrocytomas as women; in the 15- to 34-year-old age group they are the third most common brain cancer, whereas in the 35- to 54-year-old age group they are the fourth most common.

Grade IV astrocytoma, **glioblastoma multiforme,** is the most lethal and common type of primary brain tumor. They are highly vascular and extensively infiltrative. Fifty percent of glioblastomas are bilateral or at least occupy more than one lobe at the time of death. The typical clinical presentation for a glioblastoma multiforme is that of diffuse, nonspecific clinical signs, such as headache, irritability, and "personality changes" that progress to more clearcut manifestations of increased intracranial pressure, headache on position change, papilledema, vomiting, or seizure activity. Symptoms may progress to include definite focal signs, such as hemiparesis, dysphasia, dyspraxia, cranial nerve palsies, and visual field deficits.

Higher grade astrocytomas are treated surgically and with radiotherapy and chemotherapy. Recurrence is common and survival time is about 1 to 5 years.[57] (See *Health Alert:* Stereotactic Radioneurosurgery.)

HEALTH ALERT

Stereotactic Radioneurosurgery

Stereotactic radiosurgery is a treatment modality in which a minimally invasive series of radiation beams converge on a specific target from various angles; no incision is needed. A high dose of radiation can be directed to a specific target with minimal radiation to adjacent normal tissue. Applications in the brain include benign and malignant brain tumors, vascular lesions such as arteriovenous malformations, pain syndromes such as trigeminal neuralgia, movement disorders, and epilepsy. The techniques can be used with exceptional geometric and dosimetric accuracy for primary treatment or as an adjuvant to surgical resection or whole-brain radiation therapy. Radiographs and CT and/or MRI scans are required for precise localization of the target in three dimensions. The skull is secured in position by either a headframe or a plastic mask. Frameless and maskless positioning systems will soon be available.

From Suh JH: Stereotactic radiosurgery for the management of brain metastases, *N Engl J Med* 362(12):1119–1127, 2010; Rahman M et al: Stereotactic radiosurgery and the linear accelerator: accelerating electrons in neurosurgery, *Neurosurg Focus* 27(3):E13, 2009; Hoeffelt CS: Gamma Knife vs CyberKnife, *Oncology Issues* September, October 18–29, 2006. Available at http://www.swmedicalcenter.com/documents/Cyberknife/OncologyIssuesVol21No5.pdf; Kilby W et al: The CyberKnife Robotic Radiosurgery System in 2010, *Technol Cancer Res Treat* 9(5):433–452, 2010; Cerviño LI et al: Frame-less and maskless cranial stereotactic radiosurgery: a feasibility study, *Phys Med Biol* 55(7):1863–1873, 2010.

Oligodendroglioma. Oligodendrogliomas constitute about 2% of all brain tumors and 10% to 15% of all gliomas. They are typically slow-growing tumors, and most oligodendrogliomas are macroscopically indistinguishable from other gliomas and may be a mixed type of oligodendroglioma and astrocytoma. The majority are found in the frontal and temporal lobes, often in the deep white matter, but they are found also in other parts of the brain and spinal cord. Many are found in young adults with a history of temporal lobe epilepsy.

Malignant degeneration occurs in approximately one third of persons with oligodendrogliomas, and the tumors are then referred to as **oligodendroblastomas.**

More than 50% of individuals experience a focal or generalized seizure as the first clinical manifestation. Only half of those with an oligodendroglioma have increased intracranial pressure at the time of diagnosis and surgery, and only one third develop focal manifestations. Treatment includes surgery, radiotherapy, and chemotherapy and these tumors may be more sensitive to treatment than other gliomas.[58]

Ependymoma. Ependymomas are nonencapsulated gliomas that arise from ependymal cells; they are rare in adults, usually occurring in the spinal cord.[59] However, in children ependymomas are typically located in the brain. They constitute about 6% of all primary brain tumors in adults and 10% in children and adolescents. Approximately 70% of these tumors occur in the fourth ventricle, with others found in the third and lateral ventricles and caudal portion of the spinal cord. Approximately 40% of infratentorial ependymomas occur in children younger than 10 years. Cerebral (supratentorial) ependymomas occur at all ages.

Fourth ventricle ependymomas present with difficulty in balance, unsteady gait, uncoordinated muscle movement, and difficulty with fine motor movement. The clinical manifestations of a lateral and third ventricle ependymoma that involves the cerebral hemispheres are seizures, visual changes, and hemiparesis. Blockage of the CSF pathway produces hydrocephalus and presents with headache, nausea, and vomiting.

The interval between first manifestations and surgery may be as short as 4 weeks or as long as 7 or 8 years. Ependymomas are treated with radiotherapy, radiosurgery, and chemotherapy. About 20% to 50% of persons survive 5 years. Some persons benefit from a shunting procedure when the ependymoma has caused a noncommunicating hydrocephalus.

Primary Extracerebral Tumors

Meningioma. Meningiomas constitute about 30% of all intracranial tumors. These tumors usually originate from the arachnoidal (meningeal) cap cells in the dura mater and rarely from arachnoid cells of the choroid plexus of the ventricles. Meningiomas are located most commonly in the olfactory grooves, on the wings of the sphenoid bone (at the base of the skull), in the tuberculum sellae (a structure next to the sella turcica), on the superior surface of the cerebellum, and in the cerebellopontine angle and spinal cord. The cause of meningiomas is unknown.

A meningioma is sharply circumscribed and adapts to the shape it occupies. It may extend to the dural surface and erode the cranial bones or produce an osteoblastic reaction. A few meningiomas exhibit malignant, invasive qualities.

Meningiomas are slow growing and clinical manifestations occur when they reach a certain size and begin to indent the brain parenchyma. Focal seizures are often the first manifestation and increased intracranial pressure is less common than with gliomas.

There is a 20% recurrence rate even with complete surgical excision. If only partial resection is possible, the tumor recurs. Radiation therapies also are used to slow growth.

Nerve sheath tumors. Neurofibromas (benign nerve sheath tumors) are a group of autosomal dominant disorders of the nervous system. They include neurofibromatosis type 1 (NF1, previously known as von Recklinghausen disease) and neurofibromatosis type 2 (NF2), also known as peripheral and central neurofibromatosis, respectively.

Neurofibromatosis type 1 is the most prevalent with an incidence of about 1 in 3500 people and causes multiple cutaneous neurofibromas, cutaneous macular lesions (café-au-lait spots and freckles), and less commonly bone and soft tissue tumors.[60] Inactivation of the *NF1* gene results in loss of function of neurofibromin in Schwann cells and promotes tumorigenesis (neurofibromas). Learning disabilities are present in about 50% of affected individuals.[61]

Neurofibromatosis type 2 is rare and occurs in about 1 in 60,000 people. The *NF2* gene product is neurofibromin 2 (merlin), a tumor-suppressor protein, and mutations promote development of central nervous system tumors, particularly schwannomas, although other tumor types can occur (meningiomas, ependymomas, astrocytomas, and neurofibromas). Schwannomas of the vestibular nerves present with hearing loss and deafness. Other symptoms may include loss of balance and dizziness. Schwannomas also may develop in other cranial, spinal, and peripheral nerves and cutaneous signs are less prominent. Intracranial meningiomas can involve the optic nerve with loss of visual acuity and cataracts, or be intraspinal with formation of ependymomas.[62]

Genetic testing is available for the management of NF families and prenatal diagnosis is possible. Diagnosis is based on clinical manifestations and neuroimaging studies, and diagnostic criteria have been established for NF1.[63] Surgery is the major treatment. Individuals with NF2 have extensive morbidity and reduced life expectancy, particularly with early age of onset. Genetically tailored drugs are likely to provide huge improvements for both of these devastating conditions.

Pituitary tumors are discussed in Chapter 18 and cerebral tumors in children are discussed in Chapter 16.

Metastatic carcinoma. Metastatic brain tumors from systemic cancers are 10 times more common than primary brain tumors and 20% to 40% of persons with cancer have metastasis to the brain.[64] Common primary sites include lung, breast, skin (e.g., melanomas), kidney, and colorectal.[65] Other types of cancer can also metastasize to the brain.

Metastatic brain tumors produce signs resembling those of glioblastomas, although several unusual syndromes do exist. Carcinomatous encephalopathy causes headache, nervousness, depression, trembling, confusion, and forgetfulness. In carcinomatosis of the cerebellum, headache, dizziness, and ataxia are found. Carcinomatosis of the craniospinal meninges (carcinomatous meningitis) manifests with headache, confusion, and symptoms of cranial or spinal nerve root dysfunction.

Metastatic brain tumors carry a poor prognosis. If one to three tumors are present, surgical excision is indicated. Radiotherapy is used frequently. With the development of new drugs that cross the blood-brain barrier, chemotherapy is increasingly recommended.[66] Survival is about 1 year.

Spinal Cord Tumors

Spinal cord tumors are rare and represent about 2% of CNS tumors. They may be **intramedullary tumors** (originating within the neural tissues) or **extramedullary tumors** (originating from tissues outside the spinal cord). Intramedullary tumors are primarily gliomas (astrocytomas and ependymomas). Gliomas are difficult to resect completely and radiotherapy is required. Spinal ependymomas may be completely resected and are more common in adults. Extramedullary tumors are either peripheral nerve sheath tumors (neurofibromas or schwannomas) or meningiomas. Neurofibromas are generally found in the thoracic and lumbar region, whereas meningiomas are more evenly distributed through the spine. Complete resection of these tumors can be curative. Other extramedullary tumors are sarcomas, vascular tumors, chordomas, and epidermoid tumors.

Metastatic spinal cord tumors are usually carcinomas, lymphomas, or myelomas. Their location is often extradural, having proliferated to the spine through direct extension from tumors of the vertebral structures or from extraspinal sources extending through the interventricular foramen or bloodstream.

PATHOPHYSIOLOGY Extramedullary spinal cord tumors produce dysfunction by compressing adjacent tissue, not by direct invasion. Intramedullary spinal cord tumors produce dysfunction by both invasion and compression. Metastases from spinal cord tumors occur from direct extension or seeding through the CSF or bloodstream.

CLINICAL MANIFESTATIONS The acute onset of clinical manifestations suggests a vascular occlusion of vessels supplying the spinal cord whereas gradual and progressive symptoms suggest compression. The **compressive syndrome (sensorimotor syndrome)** involves both the anterior and the posterior spinal tracts, and motor function and sensory function are affected as the tumor grows. Pain is usually present.

The **irritative syndrome (radicular syndrome)** combines the clinical manifestations of a cord compression with radicular pain (occurs in the sensory root distribution and indicates root irritation). The segmental manifestations include segmental sensory changes (paresthesias and impaired pain and touch perception); motor disturbances, including cramps, atrophy, fasciculations, and decreased or absent deep tendon reflexes; and continuous spinal pain.

EVALUATION AND TREATMENT The diagnosis of a spinal cord tumor is made through bone scan, PET, CT-guided needle biopsy, or open biopsy. Involvement of specific cord segments is established. Any metastases also are identified. Treatment varies depending on the nature of the tumor and the person's clinical status, but surgery is essential for all spinal cord tumors.[67]

> ✔ **QUICK CHECK 15-5**
> 1. How is an encapsulated CNS tumor different from a nonencapsulated CNS tumor?
> 2. What are three types of spinal cord tumors?
> 3. What are some common signs and symptoms of compressive and irritative spinal cord tumor syndromes?

DID YOU UNDERSTAND?

Central Nervous System Disorders

1. Motor vehicle crashes are the major cause of traumatic CNS injury. Traumatic injuries to the head are classified as closed-head trauma (blunt) or open-head trauma (penetrating). Closed-head trauma is the more common type of trauma.

2. Different types of focal brain injury include contusion (bruising of the brain), laceration (tearing of brain tissue), extradural hematoma (accumulation of blood between the bony skull and the dura mater), subdural hematoma (blood between the dura mater and arachnoid membrane), intracerebral hematoma (bleeding into the brain), and open-head trauma.

3. Open-head trauma involves a skull fracture with exposure of the cranial vault to the environment. The types of open-head trauma (compound fracture, perforated fracture are linear, comminuted, compound, and basilar skull fractures) of the cranial vault or at the base of the skull.

4. Diffuse brain injury (diffuse axonal injury [DAI]) results from the effects of head rotation. The brain experiences shearing stresses that result in axonal damage ranging from concussion to a severe DAI state.

5. Secondary brain trauma develops from systemic and intracranial responses to primary brain trauma that result in further brain injury and neuronal death.

6. Spinal cord injury involves damage to vertebral or neural tissues by compressing tissue, pulling or exerting tension on tissue, or shearing tissues so that they slide into one another.

7. Spinal cord injury may cause spinal shock with cessation of all motor, sensory, reflex, and autonomic functions below the transected area. Loss of motor and sensory function depends on the level of injury.

8. Paralysis of the lower half of the body with both legs involved is called *paraplegia*. Paralysis involving all four extremities is called *quadriplegia*.

9. Return of spinal neuron excitability occurs slowly. Reflex activity can return in 1 to 2 weeks in most persons with acute spinal cord injury. A pattern of flexion reflexes emerges, involving first the toes, then the feet and the legs. Eventually, reflex voiding and bowel elimination appear and mass reflex (flexor spasms accompanied by profuse sweating, piloerection, and automatic bladder emptying) may develop.

10. Degenerative disk disease is an alteration in intervertebral disk tissue and can be related to normal aging.

11. Spondylolysis is a structural defect of the spine with displacement of the vertebra.

12. Spondylolisthesis involves forward slippage of the vertebra and can include a crack or fracture of the pars interarticularis, usually at the L5-S1 vertebrae.

13. Low back pain is pain between the lower rib cage and gluteal muscles and often radiates into the thigh.

14. Most causes of low back pain are unknown; however, some secondary causes are disk prolapse, tumors, bursitis, synovitis, degenerative joint disease, osteoporosis, fracture, inflammation, and sprain.

15. Herniation of an intervertebral disk is a protrusion of part of the nucleus pulposus. Herniation most commonly affects the lumbosacral disks (L5-S1 and L4-5). The extruded pulposus compresses the nerve root, causing pain that radiates along the sciatic nerve course.

16. Cerebrovascular disease is the most frequently occurring neurologic disorder. Any abnormality of the blood vessels of the brain is referred to as a cerebrovascular disease.

17. Cerebrovascular disease is associated with two types of brain abnormalities: (a) ischemia with or without infarction and (b) hemorrhage.

18. Cerebrovascular accidents (stroke syndromes) are classified according to pathophysiologic mechanisms and include global hypoperfusion, ischemic (thrombotic or embolic), and hemorrhagic (intracranial hemorrhage).

19. Transient ischemic attacks (TIAs) are temporary decreases in brain blood flow.

20. Intracranial aneurysms result from defects in the vascular wall and are classified on the basis of form and shape. They are often asymptomatic, but the signs vary depending on the location and size of the aneurysm.

21. An arteriovenous malformation (AVM) is a tangled mass of dilated blood vessels. Although sometimes present at birth, AVM exhibits a delayed age of onset.

22. A subarachnoid hemorrhage occurs when blood escapes from defective or injured vasculature into the subarachnoid space. When a vessel tears, blood under pressure is pumped into the subarachnoid space. The blood produces an inflammatory reaction in these tissues.

23. Migraine headache is an episodic headache that can be associated with triggers, and may have an aura associated with a cortical spreading depression that alters cortical blood flow. Pain is related to overactivity in the trigeminovascular system.

24. Cluster headaches are a group of disorders known as trigeminal autonomic cephalalgias and occur primarily in men. They occur in clusters over a period of days with extreme pain intensity and short duration, and are associated with trigeminal activation.

25. Tension-type headache is the most common headache. Episodic-type headaches involve a peripheral pain mechanism and the chronic type involves a central pain mechanism and may be related to hypersensitivity to pain in craniocervical muscles.

26. Infection and inflammation of the CNS can be caused by bacteria, viruses, fungi, protozoa, and rickettsiae. Bacterial infections are pyogenic or pus producing.

27. Meningitis (infection of the meninges) is classified as bacterial, aseptic (nonpurulent), or fungal. Bacterial meningitis primarily is an infection of the pia mater, the arachnoid, and the fluid of the subarachnoid space. Aseptic meningitis is believed to be limited to the meninges. Fungal meningitis is a chronic, less common type of meningitis.

28. The meningeal vessels become hyperemic, and neutrophils migrate into the subarachnoid space with bacterial meningitis. An inflammatory reaction occurs, and exudate is formed and increases rapidly.

29. Brain abscesses often originate from infections outside the CNS. Organisms gain access to the CNS from adjacent sites or spread along the wall of a vein. A localized inflammatory process develops with formation of exudate, thrombosis of vessels, and degeneration of leukocytes. After a few days, the infection becomes delimited with a center of pus and a wall of granular tissue.

30. Clinical manifestations of brain abscesses include headache, nuchal rigidity, confusion, drowsiness, and sensory and communication deficits. Treatment includes antibiotic therapy and surgical excision or aspiration.

31. Encephalitis is an acute, febrile illness of viral origin with nervous system involvement. The most common encephalitides are caused by arthropod-borne (mosquito-borne) viruses and herpes simplex type 1. Meningeal involvement appears in all encephalitides.

32. Clinical manifestations of encephalitis include fever, delirium, confusion, seizures, abnormal and involuntary movement, and increased intracranial pressure.

33. Herpes encephalitis is treated with antiviral agents. No definitive treatment exists for the other encephalitides.

34. The common neurologic complications of AIDS are HIV-associated dementia, HIV myelopathy, opportunistic infections, cytomegalovirus, parasitic infection, and neoplasms. Pathologically, there may be diffuse CNS involvement, focal pathologic changes, and obstructive hydrocephalus.

DID YOU UNDERSTAND?—cont'd

Demyelinating Degenerative Disorders

1. Multiple sclerosis (MS) is a relatively common demyelinating disorder involving CNS myelin. Although the pathogenesis is unknown, the demyelination is thought to result from an immunogenetic-viral cause. A previous viral insult to the nervous system in a genetically susceptible individual yields a subsequent abnormal immune response in the CNS.
2. Amyotrophic lateral sclerosis (ALS) is a degenerative disorder diffusely involving lower and upper motor neurons. The pathogenesis of ALS is not fully known; however, there is lower and upper motor neuron degeneration.

Peripheral Nervous System and Neuromuscular Junction Disorders

1. With disorders of the roots of spinal cord nerves, the roots may be compressed, inflamed, or torn. Clinical manifestations include local pain or paresthesias in the sensory root distribution. Treatment may involve surgery, antibiotics, steroids, radiation therapy, and chemotherapy
2. **Plexus injuries** involve the plexus distal to the spinal roots. Paralysis can occur with complete plexus involvement.
3. When peripheral nerves are affected, axon and myelin degeneration may be present. These syndromes are classified as sensorimotor, sensory, or motor and are characterized by varying degrees of sensory disturbance, paresis, and paralysis. Secondary atrophy may be present.
4. **Guillain-Barré syndrome** is a demyelinating disorder caused by a humoral and cell-mediated immunologic reaction directed at the peripheral nerves. The clinical manifestations may vary from paresis of the legs to complete quadriplegia, respiratory insufficiency, and autonomic nervous system instability. Plasmapheresis is used during the acute phase and followed by aggressive rehabilitation.

5. Myasthenia gravis is a disorder of voluntary muscles characterized by muscle weakness and fatigability. It is considered an autoimmune disease and is associated with an increased incidence of other autoimmune diseases.
6. Myasthenia gravis results from a defect in nerve impulse transmission at the neuromuscular junction. IgG antibody is secreted against the "self" AChR receptors and blocks the binding of acetylcholine. The antibody action destroys the receptor sites, causing decreased transmission of the nerve impulse across the neuromuscular junction.

Tumors of the Central Nervous System

1. Two main types of tumors occur within the cranium: primary and metastatic. Primary tumors are classified as intracerebral tumors (astrocytomas, oligodendrogliomas, and ependymomas) or extracerebral tumors (meningioma or nerve sheath tumors). Metastatic tumors can be found inside or outside the brain substance.
2. CNS tumors cause local and generalized manifestations. The effects are varied, and local manifestations include seizures, visual disturbances, loss of equilibrium, and cranial nerve dysfunction.
3. Spinal cord tumors are classified as intramedullary tumors (within the neural tissues) or extramedullary tumors (outside the spinal cord). Metastatic spinal cord tumors are usually carcinomas, lymphomas, or myelomas.
4. Extramedullary spinal cord tumors produce dysfunction by compression of adjacent tissue, not by direct invasion. Intramedullary spinal cord tumors produce dysfunction by both invasion and compression.
5. The onset of clinical manifestations of spinal cord tumors is gradual and progressive, suggesting compression. Specific manifestations depend on the location of the tumor; for example, there may be paresis and spasticity of one leg with thoracic tumors, followed by involvement of the opposite leg.

KEY TERMS

- Amyotrophic lateral sclerosis (ALS, sporadic motor neuron disease, sporadic motor system disease, motor neuron disease [MND]) 398
- Arteriovenous malformation (AVM) 391
- Aseptic meningitis (viral meningitis, non-purulent meningitis) 394
- Autonomic hyperreflexia (dysreflexia) 385
- Bacterial meningitis 394
- Brain abscess 394
- Brudzinski sign 391
- Cerebrovascular accident (CVA, stroke) 389
- Cholinergic crisis 400
- Classic ALS (Lou Gehrig disease) 398
- Classic cerebral concussion 381
- Closed (blunt) trauma 377
- Cluster headache 393
- Compound skull fracture 380
- Compressive syndrome (sensorimotor syndrome) 404
- Contrecoup injury 379
- Contusion 379
- Coup injury 379
- Degenerative disk disease (DDD) 387
- Diffuse brain injury (diffuse axonal injury [DAI]) 381

- Embolic stroke 389
- Encephalitis 395
- Ependymoma 403
- Extradural brain abscess 394
- Extradural hematoma 379
- Extramedullary tumor 404
- Focal brain injury 379
- Fungal meningitis 394
- Fusiform aneurysm (giant aneurysm) 391
- Glioblastoma multiforme 403
- Glioma 400
- Guillain-Barré syndrome 406
- Headache 392
- Hemorrhagic stroke (intracranial hemorrhage) 389
- HIV distal symmetric polyneuropathy 397
- HIV myelopathy 396
- HIV-associated dementia (HIV-associated cognitive dysfunction, HIV encephalopathy, subacute encephalitis, HIV-associated dementia complex, HIV cognitive motor complex, AIDS encephalopathy, AIDS dementia complex, AIDS-related dementia) 396
- Intracerebral brain abscess 394
- Intracerebral hematoma 380

- Intramedullary tumor 404
- Irritative syndrome (radicular syndrome) 404
- Kernig sign 391
- Lacunar stroke (lacunar infarct) 389
- Meningioma 403
- Meningitis 394
- Migraine headache 392
- Mild concussion 381
- Mild diffuse axonal injury 381
- Moderate diffuse axonal injury 381
- Multiple sclerosis (MS) 397
- Myasthenia gravis 399
- Myasthenic crisis 399
- Neurofibroma (benign nerve sheath tumor) 403
- Neurofibromatosis type 1 404
- Neurofibromatosis type 2 404
- Ocular myasthenia 399
- Oligodendroblastoma 403
- Oligodendroglioma 403
- Open (penetrating) brain tumor 380
- Open trauma 377
- Plexus injuries 406
- Postconcussive syndrome 381
- Primary brain (intracerebral) tumor (glioma) 400

KEY TERMS—cont'd

- Saccular aneurysm (berry aneurysm)   390
- Secondary brain trauma   381
- Severe diffuse axonal injury   381
- Spinal cord abscess   391
- Spinal shock   383
- Spinal stenosis   387
- Spondylolisthesis   387
- Spondylolysis   387
- Subarachnoid hemorrhage   391
- Subdural hematoma   380
- Tension-type headache   393
- Thrombotic stroke (cerebral thrombosis)   389
- Toxoplasmosis   395
- Transient ischemic attack (TIA)   389
- Vacuolar myelopathy   396
- West Nile virus (WNV)   396

REFERENCES

1. Centers for Disease Control and Prevention: Traumatic brain injury statistic. Available at www.cdc.gov/TraumaticBrainInjury/statistics.html. Accessed March 17, 2010.
2. Edwards P, et al: Final results of MRC CRASH, a randomised placebo-controlled trial of intravenous corticosteroid in adults with head injury—outcomes at 6 months, *Lancet* 365(9475):1957–1959, 2005.
3. Sauerlaud S, Maegele MA: CRASH landing in severe head injury, *Lancet* 364:729–782, 2004.
4. Maas AIR, Stocchetti N, Bullock R: Moderate and severe traumatic brain injury in adults, *Lancet Neurol* 7(8):728–741, 2008.
5. Park E, et al: Traumatic brain injury: can the consequences be stopped?, *CMAJ* 178(9):1163–1170, 2008. Available at www.cmaj.ca/cgi/content/full/178/9/11632008.
6. Beauchamp K, et al: Pharmacology of traumatic brain injury: where is the "golden bullet"? *Mol Med* 14(11–12):731–740, 2008.
7. Maas AI, Roozenbeek B, Manley GT: Clinical trials in traumatic brain injury: past experience and current developments, *Neurotherapeutics* 7(1):115–126, 2010.
8. National Spinal Cord Injury Statistical Center: Spinal cord injury facts and figures at a glance. Available at www.nscisc.uab.edu. Accessed June 2011.
9. Battié MC: The twin spine study: contributions to a changing view of disc degeneration, *Spine J* 9(1):47–59, 2009.
10. Chou R, Huffman LH: Nonpharmacologic therapies for acute and chronic low back pain; a review of the evidence from an American Pain Society/American College of Physicians clinical practice guideline, *Ann Intern Med* 147(7):492–504, 2007.
11. Legrand E, et al: Sciatica from disk herniation: medical treatment or surgery? *Joint Bone Spine* 74(6):530–535, 2007.
12. Benson RT, et al: Conservatively treated massive prolapsed discs: a 7-year follow-up, *Ann R Coll Surg Engl* 92(2):147–153, 2010.
13. Lloyd-Jones D, et al: American Heart Association Statistics Committee and Stroke Statistics Subcommittee: heart disease and stroke statistics—2010 update: a report from the American Heart Association, *Circulation* 121(7):e46–e215, 2010.
14. Seppa N: Southern blacks face excess risk of stroke, *Sci News* 167:126, 2005.
15. Bradley WG, et al: *Neurology in clinical practice*, ed 5, Philadelphia, 2008, Butterworth-Heinemann, pp 1165–1169.
16. Easton JD, et al: Definition and evaluation of transient ischemic attack: a scientific statement for healthcare professionals from the American Heart Association/American Stroke Association Stroke Council, Council on Cardiovascular Surgery and Anesthesia, Council on Cardiovascular Radiology and Intervention, Council on Cardiovascular Nursing and the Interdisciplinary Council on Peripheral Vascular Disease. The American Academy of Neurology affirms the value of this statement as an educational tool for neurologists, *Stroke* 40(6):2276–2293, 2009.
17. Wardlaw JM, et al: Lacunar stroke is associated with diffuse blood-brain barrier dysfunction, *Ann Neurol* 65(2):194–202, 2009.
18. Del Zoppo GJ, et al: Expansion of the time window for treatment of acute ischemic stroke with intravenous tissue plasminogen activator. A science advisory from the American Heart Association/American Stroke Association, *Stroke* 40(8):2945–2948, 2009.
19. Simmons BB, Yeo A, Fung K: American Heart Association, American Stroke Association current guidelines on antiplatelet agents for secondary prevention of noncardiogenic stroke: an evidence-based review, *Postgrad Med* 122(2):49–53, 2010.
20. Selman WR, et al: Vascular diseases of the nervous system: intracranial aneurysm and subarachnoid hemorrhage. In Bradley WB et al: *Neurology in clinical practice*, ed 5, Philadelphia, 2008, Butterworth-Heinemann.
21. Colby GP, Coon AL, Tamargo RJ: Surgical management of aneurysmal subarachnoid hemorrhage, *Neurosurg Clin N Am* 21(2):247–261, 2010.
22. Jabbour PM, Tjoumakaris SI, Rosenwasser RH: Endovascular management of intracranial aneurysms, *Neurosurg Clin N Am* 20(4):383–398, 2010.
23. Moftakhar P, et al: Cerebral arteriovenous malformations. Part 2: physiology, *Neurosurg Focus* 26(5):E11, 2009.
24. Blissit PA, et al: Cerebrovascular dynamics with head-of-bed elevation in patients with mild or moderate vasospasm after aneurysmal subarachnoid hemorrhage, *Am J Crit Care* 15(2):206–216, 2006.
25. Jordan JD, Nyquist P: Biomarkers and vasospasm after aneurysmal subarachnoid hemorrhage, *Neurosurg Clin N Am* 21(2):381–391, 2010.
26. Cavanaugh SJ: GordonVL: Grading scales used in the management of aneurismal subarachnoid hemorrhage: a critical review, *J Neurosci Nurs* 34:288–295, 2002.
27. Lazaridis C, Naval N: Risk factors and medical management of vasospasm after subarachnoid hemorrhage, *Neurosurg Clin N Am* 21(2):353–364, 2010.
28. Goadsby PJ: Pathophysiology of migraine, *Neurol Clin* 27(2):335–360, 2009.
29. Headache Classification Committee of The International Headache Society: The International Classification of Headache Disorders, ed 2, *Cephalalgia*, 24(suppl 1):9–160, 2004.
30. Lay CL, Broner SW: Migraine in women, *Neurol Clin* 27(2):503–511, 2009.
31. Kostic MA, et al: A prospective, randomized trial of intravenous prochlorperazine versus subcutaneous sumatriptan in acute migraine therapy in the emergency department, *Ann Emerg Med* 56(1):1–6, 2010.
32. Silberstein SD: Preventive migraine treatment, *Neurol Clin* 27(2):429–443, 2009.
33. Massimo L, Gennaro B: Pathophysiology of trigeminal autonomic cephalalgias, *Lancet Neurol* 8(8):755–764, 2009.
34. Halker R, Vargas B, Dodick DW: Cluster headache: diagnosis and treatment, *Semin Neurol* 30(2):175–185, 2010.
35. Ailani J: Chronic tension-type headache, *Curr Pain Headache Rep* 13(6):479–483, 2009.
36. Thigpen MC, et al: Emerging Infections Programs Network. Bacterial meningitis in the United States, 1998-2007, *N Engl J Med* 364(21):2016–2025, 2011.
37. van de Beek D, et al: Clinical features and prognostic factors in adults with bacterial meningitis, *N Engl J Med* 351(18):1849–1859, 2004.
38. Swartz MN: Bacterial meningitis—a view of the past 90 years, *N Engl J Med* 351:1826–1828, 2004.
39. Koedel U, Klein M, Pfister HW: New understandings on the pathophysiology of bacterial meningitis, *Curr Opin Infect Dis* 23(3):217–223, 2010.
40. Poland GA: Prevention of meningococcal disease: current use of polysaccharide and conjugate vaccines, *Clin Infect Dis* 50(suppl 2):S45–S53, 2010.
41. Nath A: Human immunodeficiency virus-associated neurocognitive disorder: pathophysiology in relation to drug addiction, *Ann N Y Acad Sci* 1187:122–128, 2010.

42. Liner KJ II, Ro MJ, Robertson KR: HIV, antiretroviral therapies, and the brain, *Curr HIV/AIDS Rep* 7(2):85–91, 2010.

43. Koch-Henriksen N, Sørensen PS: The changing demographic pattern of multiple sclerosis epidemiology, *Lancet Neurol* 9(5):520–532, 2010.

43a. Kakalacheva K, Münz C, Lünemann JD: Viral triggers of multiple sclerosis, *Biochim Biophys Acta* 1812(2):132–140, 2011.

44. Courtney AM: Multiple sclerosis, *Med Clin North Am* 93(2):451–476, 2009:ix–x.

45. Milo R, Panitch H: Combination therapy in multiple sclerosis, *J Neuroimmunol* 231(1-2):23–31, 2011.

46. Hanwell HE, Banwell B: Assessment of evidence for a protective role of vitamin D in multiple sclerosis, *Biochim Biophys Acta* 1812(2):202–212, 2011.

47. Deng HX, et al: FUS-immunoreactive inclusions are a common feature in sporadic and non-SOD1 familial amyotrophic lateral sclerosis, *Ann Neurol* 67(6):739–748, 2010.

48. Gordon PH: Amyotrophic lateral sclerosis: pathophysiology, diagnosis, and management, *CNS Drugs* 25(1):1–15, 2011.

49. Chattopadhyay M, Valentine JS: Aggregation of copper-zinc superoxide dismutase in familial and sporadic ALS, *Antioxid Redox Signal* 11(7):1603–1614, 2009.

50. Wijesekera LC, Leigh PN: Amyotrophic lateral sclerosis, *Orphanet J Rare Dis* 4:3, 2009.

51. Miller RG, et al: Practice parameter update: the care of the patient with amyotrophic lateral sclerosis: drug, nutritional, and respiratory therapies (an evidence-based review): report of the Quality Standards Subcommittee of the American Academy of Neurology, *Neurology* 73(15):1218–1226, 2009.

52. Meyer A, Levy Y: Chapter 33: geoepidemiology of myasthenia gravis, *Autoimmun Rev* 9(5):A383–A386, 2010.

53. Mehndiratta MM, Pandey S, Kuntzer T: Acetylcholinesterase inhibitor treatment for myasthenia gravis, *Cochrane Database Syst Rev* 2:CD006986, 2011.

54. Zieliński M: Management of myasthenic patients with thymoma, *Thorac Surg Clin* 21(1):47–57, vi, 2011.

55. American Cancer Society: Cancer facts and figures, estimated new cancer cases and deaths by sex for all sites, US. Available at www.cancer.org/docroot/stt/stt_0.asp. Accessed June, 2011.

56. Brain Tumor Society: Brain tumor facts & statistics. Available at www.tbts.org/itemDetail.asp?categoryID=384&itemID=16535. Accessed June, 2011.

57. Tran B, Rosenthal MA: Survival comparison between glioblastoma multiforme and other incurable cancers, *J Clin Neurosci* 17(4):417–421, 2010.

58. Ney DE, Lassman AB: Molecular profiling of oligodendrogliomas: impact on prognosis, treatment, and future directions, *Curr Oncol Rep* 11(1):62–67, 2009.

59. Gilbert MR, Ruda R, Soffietti R: Ependymomas in adults, *Curr Neurol Neurosci Rep* 10(3):240–247, 2010.

60. Boyd KP, Korf BR, Theos A: Neurofibromatosis type 1, *J Am Acad Dermatol* 61(1):1–14, 2009.

61. Jett K, Friedman JM: Clinical and genetic aspects of neurofibromatosis 1, *Genet Med* 12(1):1–11, 2010.

62. Evans D: Neurofibromatosis type 2 (NF2): a clinical and molecular review, *Orphanet J Rare Dis* 4:16, 2009.

63. DeBella K, Szudek J, Friedman JM: Use of the National Institutes of Health criteria for diagnosis of neurofibromatosis 1 in children, *Pediatrics* 105(3 Pt 1):608–614, 2000.

64. Walbert T, Gilbert MR: The role of chemotherapy in the treatment of patients with brain metastases from solid tumors, *Int J Clin Oncol* 14(4):299–306, 2009.

65. Nguyen TD: Brain metastases, *Neurol Clin* 25(4):1173–1192, 2007.

66. Chamberlain MC: Brain metastases: a medical neuro-oncology perspective, *Expert Rev Neurother* 10(4):563–573, 2010.

67. Grimm S, Chamberlain MC: Adult primary spinal cord tumors, *Expert Rev Neurother* 9(10):1487–1495, 2009.

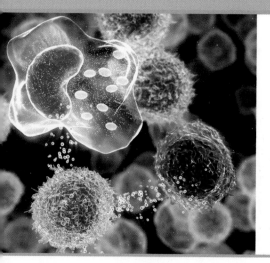

Alterations of Neurologic Function in Children

Vinodh Narayanan

CHAPTER OUTLINE

Neurologic disorders in children can occur from infancy through adolescence and include congenital malformations, genetic defects in metabolism, brain injuries, infection, tumors, and other disorders that affect neurologic function. Compared to adults, the symptoms, diagnosis, and management of neurologic disorders in children are often different.

NORMAL GROWTH AND DEVELOPMENT OF THE NERVOUS SYSTEM

The nervous system develops from the embryonic ectoderm through a complex, sequential process that can be arbitrarily divided into stages. These include (1) formation of the neural tube (3 to 4 weeks' gestation), (2) development of the forebrain from the neural tube (2 to 3 months' gestation), (3) neuronal proliferation and migration (3 to 5 months' gestation), (4) formation of network connections and synapses (5 months' gestation to many years postnatally), and (5) myelination (birth to many years postnatally). Environmental factors (e.g., nutrition, hormones, oxygen levels, toxins, alcohol, drugs, maternal infections, maternal disease) can have a significant effect on neural development. The effect of an environmental factor depends on the developmental stage at which it acts. Nutritional deficiency (in particular, folic acid deficiency) during formation of the neural tube (3 to 4 weeks' gestation) can result in failure of neural tube closure, whereas a fetal viral infection during the proliferative stage (3 to 5 months' gestation) can cause the development of a small brain. Micronutrients, including iron, are also important for the development of the nervous system[1,2] (see *Health Alert:* Iron and Cognitive Function).

The growth and development of the brain occur rapidly during the third and fourth months of gestation and again from the fifth month of gestation through the first year of life, reflecting the proliferation of neurons and glial cells. The head is the fastest growing body part during infancy. One half of postnatal brain growth is achieved by the first year and is 90% complete by age 6 years. The cortex thickens with maturation, and the sulci deepen as a result of rapid expansion of the surface area of the brain. Cerebral blood flow and oxygen consumption during these years are about twice those of the adult brain.

The bones of the infant's skull are separated at the suture lines, forming two **fontanelles** or "soft spots": one diamond-shaped anterior fontanelle and one triangular-shaped posterior fontanelle. The sutures allow for expansion of the rapidly growing brain. The posterior fontanelle may be open until 2 to 3 months of age; the anterior fontanelle normally does not fully close until 18 months of age (Figure 16-1). Head growth almost always reflects brain growth. Monitoring the fontanelles and careful measurement and plotting of the head circumference on standardized growth charts are essential elements of the pediatric examination.[3] A common cause of accelerating head growth and macrocephaly is hydrocephalus, a condition in which the cerebral spinal fluid (CSF) compartment (ventricles) is enlarged. Increased intracranial pressure, with distention or bulging of the fontanelles, and separation of the sutures are key signs of hydrocephalus. Microcephaly (head circumference below the 2nd percentile for age) can be the result of prenatal infection, toxin exposure, or malnutrition, or have a primary genetic etiology.

Because of the immaturity of much of the human forebrain at birth, neurologic examination of the infant detects mostly reflex responses that require an intact spinal cord and brain stem. Some of these reflex patterns are inhibited as cerebral cortical function matures, and these patterns disappear at predictable times during infancy (Table 16-1).

Absence of expected reflex responses at the appropriate age indicates general depression of central or peripheral motor functions. Asymmetric responses may indicate lesions in the motor cortex or peripheral nerves, or may occur with fractures of bones after traumatic delivery or postnatal injury. As the infant matures, the neonatal reflexes disappear in a predictable order as voluntary motor functions supersede them. Abnormal persistence of these reflexes is seen in infants with developmental delays or with central motor lesions.

STRUCTURAL MALFORMATIONS

Central nervous system (CNS) malformations are responsible for 75% of fetal deaths and 40% of deaths during the first year of life. CNS malformations account for 33% of all apparent congenital malformations, and 90% of CNS malformations are defects of neural tube closure.

Defects of Neural Tube Closure

The incidence of neural tube defects ranges from 1.0 to 10 per 1000 live births in the United States each year.[4] Fetal death often occurs in the more severe forms, thereby reducing the actual prevalence of neural defects at birth.[5] These defects are divided into two categories: (1) posterior defects (dorsal induction) and (2) anterior midline defects (ventral induction). Posterior defects are more common and include anencephaly (*an* = without; *enkephalos* = brain) and a group

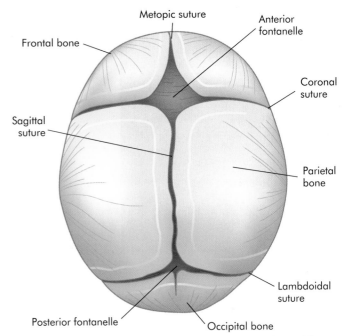

FIGURE 16-1 Cranial Sutures and Fontanelles in Infancy. Fibrous union of suture lines and interlocking of serrated edges (occurs by 6 months; solid union requires approximately 12 years). (Head growth charts are available from the Centers for Disease Control and Prevention at www.cdc.gov/nchs/data/series/sr_11/sr11_246.pdf.)

TABLE 16-1	REFLEXES OF INFANCY	
REFLEX	**AGE OF APPEARANCE OF REFLEX**	**AGE AT WHICH REFLEX SHOULD NO LONGER BE OBTAINABLE**
Moro	Birth	3 months
Stepping	Birth	6 weeks
Sucking	Birth	4 months awake
		7 months asleep
Rooting	Birth	4 months awake
		7 months asleep
Palmar grasp	Birth	6 months
Plantar grasp	Birth	10 months
Tonic neck	2 months	5 months
Neck righting	4-6 months	24 months
Landau	3 months	24 months
Parachute reaction	9 months	Persists indefinitely

Also see demonstration of primitive or postural reflexes at http://library.med.utah.edu/pedineurologicexam/html/home_exam.html.

of disorders collectively referred to as the **myelodysplasias** (*dys* = bad; *plassein* = to form). Anterior midline defects may cause brain and face abnormalities, with the most extreme form being **cyclopia**, in which the child has a single midline orbit and eye with a protruding nose-like proboscis above the orbit. Disorders of embryonic development are summarized in Figure 16-2. The cause of neural tube defects is believed to be multifactorial (a combination of genes and environment). No single gene has been found to cause neural tube defects.[6] Folic acid deficiency during early stages of pregnancy increases the risk for neural tube defects,[7] but preconceptional supplementation ensures adequate

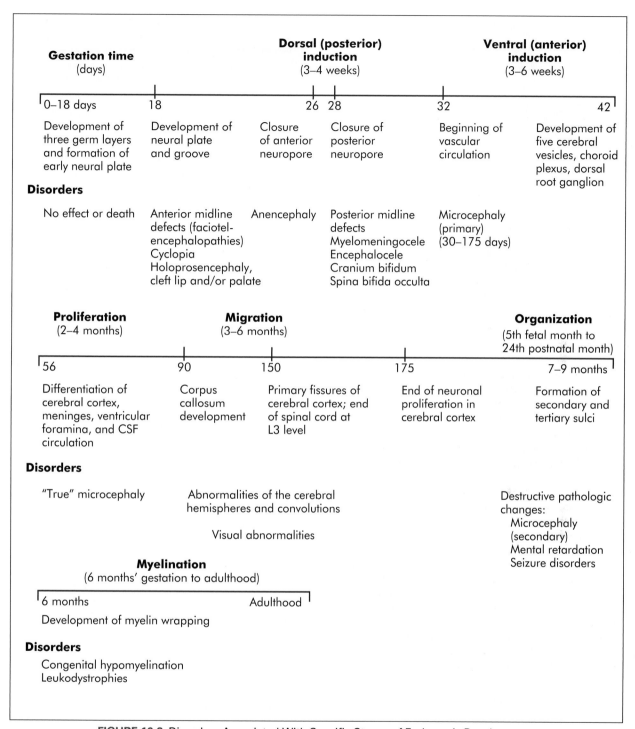

FIGURE 16-2 Disorders Associated With Specific Stages of Embryonic Development.

folate status. Other risk factors include heredity, maternal blood glucose concentrations, use of anticonvulsant drugs (particularly valproic acid), and maternal hyperthermia.[4,5]

The most severe malformation that results from complete failure of posterior neural tube closure is craniorachischisis totalis. A platelike structure is present on the back without overlying skeleton or skin. In anencephaly, the soft, bony component of the skull and part of the brain are missing. This is a relatively common disorder, with an incidence of approximately 1 per 8000 total live births in the United States each year.[8] The infant's head has a froglike appearance when viewed face-on at birth. Both of these malformations result in spontaneous abortion or early neonatal death.

Encephalocele refers to a herniation or protrusion of brain and meninges through a defect in the skull, resulting in a saclike structure. The incidence is approximately 1.4 per 10,000 live births in the United States each year.[9,10] In Europe and the United States, most encephaloceles occur in the occipital region, whereas in Russia and Southeast Asia, encephaloceles are most often in the frontonasal region.[10]

Meningocele, which is a saclike cyst of meninges filled with spinal fluid, is a mild form of posterior neural tube closure defect

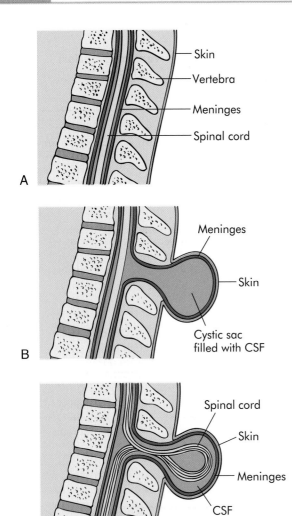

A

B

C

FIGURE 16-3 Normal Spine, Meningocele, and Myelomeningocele. Diagram showing section through normal spine (**A**), meningocele (**B**), and myelomeningocele (**C**).

TABLE 16-2	FUNCTIONAL ALTERATIONS IN MYELODYSPLASIA RELATED TO LEVEL OF LESION
LEVEL OF LESION	**FUNCTIONAL IMPLICATIONS**
Thoracic	Flaccid paralysis of lower extremities; variable weakness in abdominal trunk musculature; high thoracic level may mean respiratory compromise; absence of bowel and bladder control
High lumbar	Voluntary hip flexion and adduction; flaccid paralysis of knees, ankles, and feet; may walk with extensive braces and crutches; absence of bowel and bladder control
Mid lumbar	Strong hip flexion and adduction; fair knee extension; flaccid paralysis of ankles and feet; absence of bowel and bladder control
Low lumbar	Strong hip flexion, extension, and adduction and knee extension; weak ankle and toe mobility; may have limited bowel and bladder function
Sacral	Normal function of lower extremities; normal bowel and bladder function

Modified from Farley JA, Dunleavy MJ: Myelodysplasia. In Allen PJ, Vessey JA, editors: *Primary care of the child with a chronic condition,* ed 4, St Louis, 2004, Mosby.

(Figure 16-3). This cystic dilation of meninges protrudes through the vertebral defect but does not involve the spinal cord or nerve roots and may produce no neurologic deficit. Meningoceles occur with equal frequency in the cervical, thoracic, and lumbar spine areas. *Spina bifida occulta* is a term used to describe a purely vertebral defect and is the mildest form of posterior neural tube closure defect (see p. 413).

Myelomeningocele (meningomyelocele; spina bifida cystica) is a hernial protrusion of a saclike cyst (containing meninges, spinal fluid, and a portion of the spinal cord with its nerves) through a defect in the posterior arch of a vertebra. Eighty percent of myelomeningoceles are located in the lumbar and lumbosacral regions, the last regions of the neural tube to close. Myelomeningocele is one of the most common developmental anomalies of the nervous system, with an incidence rate ranging from 0.2 to 0.4 per 1000 live births.[11]

CLINICAL MANIFESTATIONS Most cases of myelomeningocele are diagnosed prenatally by a combination of maternal serologic testing (alpha-fetoprotein) and prenatal ultrasound. In these cases, the fetus is usually delivered by elective cesarean section to minimize trauma during labor. Myelomeningoceles are evident at birth as a pronounced skin defect on the infant's back (see Figure 16-3). The bony prominences of the unfused neural arches can be palpated at the lateral border of the defect. The defect usually is covered by a transparent membrane that may have neural tissue attached to its inner surface. This membrane may be intact at birth or may leak cerebrospinal fluid (CSF), thereby increasing the risks of infection and neuronal damage. Surgical repair is critical and is usually performed during the first 24 to 48 hours of life.

The spinal cord and nerve roots are malformed at the level of the myelomeningocele, resulting in loss of motor, sensory, reflex, and autonomic functions below the level of the lesion. A brief neurologic examination concentrating on motor function in the legs, reflexes, and sphincter tone is usually sufficient to determine the level above which spinal cord and nerve root function is preserved (Table 16-2). This is useful to predict if the child will ambulate, require bladder catheterization, or be at high risk for developing scoliosis.

Hydrocephalus occurs in 85% of infants with myelomeningocele.[12] Seizures also occur in 30% of those with myelodysplasia. Visual and perceptual problems, including ocular palsies, astigmatism, and visuoperceptual deficits, are common. Motor and sensory functions below the level of the lesions are altered. Often these problems worsen as the child grows and the cord ascends within the vertebral canal, pulling primary scar tissue and tethering the cord.[13] Several musculoskeletal deformities are related to this diagnosis, as are spinal deformities.

Myelomeningoceles are almost always associated with the type II Chiari malformation (also known as the Arnold-Chiari malformation).[14] This is a complex malformation of the brain stem and cerebellum in which the cerebellar tonsils are displaced downward into the cervical spinal canal; the upper medulla and lower pons are elongated and thin; and the medulla is also displaced downward and sometimes has a "kink" (Figure 16-4). The Chiari II malformation also is associated with hydrocephalus and syringomyelia, an abnormality causing cysts at multiple levels within the spinal cord. Other forms of Chiari malformation include type I, which is a milder form of type II and

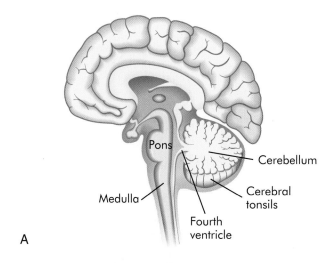

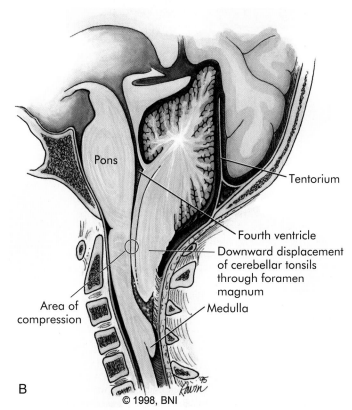

FIGURE 16-4 Normal Brain and Arnold-Chiari II Malformation. **A,** Diagram of normal brain. **B,** Diagram of Arnold-Chiari II malformation with downward displacement of cerebellar tonsils and medulla through foramen magnum causing compression and obstruction to flow of CSF. (**B** modified from Barrow Neurological Institute of St Joseph's Hospital and Medical Center. Reprinted with permission.)

may be asymptomatic; type III, in which the brain stem or cerebellum extend into a high cervical myelomeningocele; and type IV, which is characterized by lack of cerebellar development.

Malformations of the Axial Skeleton
Spina Bifida
When defects of neural tube closure, such as meningocele and myelomeningocele, occur, an accompanying vertebral defect allows the protrusion of the neural tube contents. Such a defect is called spina bifida.

Periconceptual maternal folate deficiency and genetic alterations are commonly associated with the defect.[7] Approximately 80% of these vertebral defects are located in the lumbosacral region, most commonly in the fifth lumbar vertebra and the first sacral vertebra. Certain cutaneous or subcutaneous abnormalities suggest underlying spina bifida, including the following:

1. Abnormal growth of hair along the spine, which often is either very coarse or very silky
2. A midline dimple with or without a sinus tract
3. A cutaneous angioma, usually of the "port wine" variety
4. A subcutaneous mass, usually representing a lipoma or dermoid cyst

When the defect occurs without any visible exposure of meninges or neural tissue, the term spina bifida occulta is used. In spina bifida occulta, the posterior vertebral laminae have failed to fuse. Extremely common, the defect occurs to some degree in 10% to 25% of infants. About 3% of normal adults have spina bifida occulta of the atlas (C1). Spina bifida occulta usually causes no serious neurologic dysfunctions. Symptoms become evident during periods of rapid growth and are a result of tethering of the spinal cord (attachment of the spinal cord to adjacent tissue that results in abnormal stretching of the cord). Neurologic signs of spina bifida occulta include gait abnormality (toe walking), foot deformity (equinovarus), and sphincter disturbance of the bladder. Surgical treatment is usually directed at associated intraspinal abnormalities (tethered cord, sacral lipoma, or dermoid cyst).

Cranial Deformities
Skull malformations range from minor, insignificant defects to major defects that are incompatible with life. In acrania, the cranial vault is almost completely absent, and an extensive defect of the vertebral column often is present. Acrania associated with anencephaly (absence of brain) occurs in approximately 1 per 1000 live births and is incompatible with life.

Craniosynostosis (craniostenosis) is the premature closure of one or more of the cranial sutures (sagittal, coronal, lambdoid, metopic) during the first 18 to 20 months of the infant's life. The incidence of craniosynostosis is 1 per 2100 live births.[15] Males are affected twice as often as females. Fusion of a cranial suture prevents growth of the skull perpendicular to the suture line, resulting in an asymmetric shape of the skull. The general term *plagiocephaly,* meaning "misshapen skull," is used to describe deformities that result from craniosynostosis or from asymmetric head posture (positional). When a single coronal suture fuses prematurely, the head is flattened on that side in front. When the sagittal suture fuses prematurely, the head is elongated in the anteroposterior direction (scaphocephaly).[16] Single suture craniosynostosis is usually only a cosmetic issue. Rarely, when multiple sutures fuse prematurely, brain growth may be restricted, and surgical repair may prevent neurologic dysfunction (Figure 16-5).

Microcephaly is a defect in brain growth as a whole (see Figure 16-5). Cranial size is significantly below average for the infant's age, gender, race, and gestation. True (primary) microcephaly is usually caused by an autosomal recessive genetic or chromosomal defect. Secondary (acquired) microcephaly is associated with various causes. Infection, toxin or radiation exposure, trauma, metabolic disorders, and anoxia experienced during the third trimester of pregnancy, the perinatal period, or early infancy may be responsible. Table 16-3 summarizes the causes of microcephaly. Microcephaly may develop later in life in certain genetic disorders (e.g., Rett syndrome) or in degenerative brain disorders.

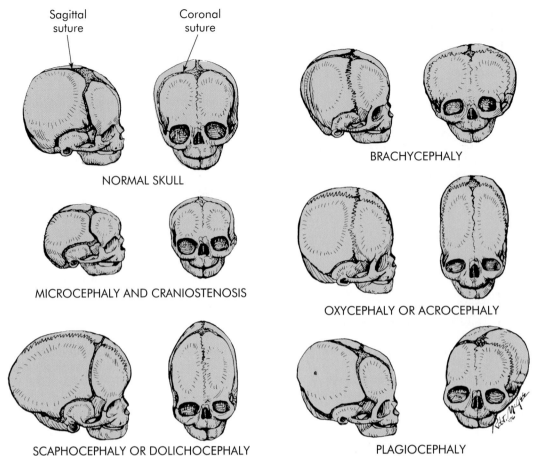

Sagittal suture

Coronal suture

NORMAL SKULL

BRACHYCEPHALY

MICROCEPHALY AND CRANIOSTENOSIS

OXYCEPHALY OR ACROCEPHALY

SCAPHOCEPHALY OR DOLICHOCEPHALY

PLAGIOCEPHALY

FIGURE 16-5 Normal and Abnormal Head Configurations. *Normal skull:* Bones separated by membranous seams until sutures gradually close. *Microcephaly and craniostenosis:* Microcephaly is head circumference more than 2 standard deviations below the mean for age, gender, race, and gestation and reflects a small brain; craniosynostosis is premature closure of sutures. *Scaphocephaly or dolichocephaly* (frequency 56%): Premature closure of sagittal suture, resulting in restricted lateral growth. *Brachycephaly:* Premature closure of coronal suture, resulting in excessive lateral growth. *Oxycephaly or acrocephaly* (frequency 5.8% to 12%): Premature closure of all coronal and sagittal sutures, resulting in accelerated upward growth and small head circumference. *Plagiocephaly* (frequency 13%): Unilateral premature closure of coronal suture, resulting in asymmetric growth. (From Hockenberry MJ: *Wong's nursing care of infants and children,* ed 7, St Louis, 2003, Mosby.)

TABLE 16-3	**CAUSES OF MICROCEPHALY**	
DEFECTS IN BRAIN DEVELOPMENT	**INTRAUTERINE INFECTIONS**	**PERINATAL AND POSTNATAL DISORDERS**
Hereditary (recessive) microcephaly	Congenital rubella	Intrauterine or neonatal anoxia
Down syndrome and other trisomy syndromes	Cytomegalovirus infection	Severe malnutrition in early infancy
Fetal ionizing radiation exposure	Congenital toxoplasmosis	Neonatal herpesvirus infection
Maternal phenylketonuria		
Cornelia de Lange syndrome		
Rubinstein-Taybi syndrome		
Smith-Lemli-Opitz syndrome		
Fetal alcohol syndrome		
Angelman syndrome		
Seckel syndrome		

Congenital hydrocephalus is characterized by enlargement of the cerebral ventricles. It may be caused by blockage within the ventricular system where the CSF flows, an imbalance in the production of CSF, or a reduced reabsorption of CSF.[17] The pressure within the ventricular system pushes and compresses the brain tissue against the skull cavity. When hydrocephalus develops before fusion of the cranial sutures, the skull can expand to accommodate this additional space-occupying volume and preserve neuronal function. The overall incidence of hydrocephalus is approximately 3 per 1000 live births. The incidence of hydrocephalus that is not associated with myelomeningocele is approximately 0.5 to 1 per 1000 live births.[18] (Types of hydrocephalus are discussed in Chapter 14.)

The **Dandy-Walker malformation (DWM)** is a congenital defect of the cerebellum characterized by a large posterior fossa cyst that communicates with the fourth ventricle and an atrophic, upwardly rotated cerebellar vermis.[19] DWM is commonly associated with hydrocephalus caused by compression of the aqueduct of Sylvius. Other causes of obstructions within the ventricular system that can result in hydrocephalus include brain tumors, cysts, trauma, arteriovenous malformations, blood clots, and infections.

Congenital hydrocephalus may cause fetal death in utero, or the increased head circumference may require cesarean delivery of the infant. Symptoms depend directly on the cause and rate of hydrocephalus development. When there is separation of the cranial sutures, a resonant note sounds when the skull is tapped, a manifestation termed Macewen sign or "cracked pot" sign. The eyes may assume a staring expression, with sclera visible above the cornea, called *sunsetting*. Cognitive impairment in children with hydrocephalus is often related to associated brain malformations, or episodes of shunt failure or infection. Approximately two thirds of children with uncomplicated congenital hydrocephalus who have been treated successfully with shunting may have normal to borderline normal intelligence.[20]

> ✔ **QUICK CHECK 16-1**
> 1. List two defects of neural tube closure.
> 2. Why do motor and sensory functions worsen with growth in a child with a neural tube defect?

ENCEPHALOPATHIES

Encephalopathy, meaning brain dysfunction, is a general category that includes a number of syndromes and diseases (see Chapter 15). These disorders may be acute or chronic, as well as static or progressive.

Static Encephalopathies

Static or nonprogressive encephalopathy describes a neurologic condition caused by a fixed lesion without active and ongoing disease. Causes include brain malformations (disorders of neuronal migration) or brain injury that may occur during the fetal period, around birth, or later during childhood. The degree of neurologic impairment is directly related to the extent of the injury or malformation. Anoxia, trauma, and infections are the most common factors that cause injury to the nervous system in the perinatal period. Infections, metabolic disturbances (acquired or genetic), trauma, toxins, and vascular disease may injure the nervous system in the postnatal period.

Cerebral palsy is a term used to describe a group of nonprogressive syndromes that affect the brain and cause motor dysfunction beginning in early infancy. The causes include prenatal or perinatal cerebral hypoxia, hemorrhage, or infection. It can be classified on the basis of neurologic signs and motor symptoms, with the major types involving spasticity, ataxia, or dystonia, or a combination of these symptoms. Diplegia, hemiplegia, or tetraplegia may be present.[21] Cerebral palsy is one of the most common crippling disorders of childhood, affecting approximately 764,000 children and adults in the United States alone. The incidence of cerebral palsy is about 2 to 2.5 cases per 1000 live births.[22]

Spastic cerebral palsy is associated with increased muscle tone, persistent primitive reflexes, hyperactive deep tendon reflexes, clonus, rigidity of the extremities, scoliosis, and contractures. This accounts for approximately 70% to 80% of cerebral palsy cases. Dystonic cerebral palsy is associated with extreme difficulty in fine motor coordination and purposeful movements. Movements are stiff, uncontrolled, and abrupt, resulting from injury to the basal ganglia or extrapyramidal tracts. This form of cerebral palsy accounts for approximately 10% to 20% of cases. Ataxic cerebral palsy manifests with gait disturbances and instability. The infant with this form of cerebral palsy may have hypotonia at birth, but stiffness of the trunk muscles develops by late infancy. Persistence of this increased tone in truncal muscles affects the child's gait and ability to maintain equilibrium. This form of cerebral palsy accounts for approximately 5% to 10% of cases. A child may have

symptoms of each of these cerebral palsy types, which leads to a mixed disorder accounting for approximately 13% of cases.[23]

Children with cerebral palsy often have associated neurologic disorders, such as seizures (about 50%), and intellectual impairment ranging from mild to severe (about 67%). Other complications include visual impairment, communication disorders, respiratory problems, bowel and bladder problems, and orthopedic disabilities.[24]

Although often caused by a fixed lesion (remote injury), the clinical picture of cerebral palsy may change with growth and development. Therefore an effective treatment regimen includes ongoing assessment, evaluation, and revision of the child's overall management plan. The use of oral baclofen, intrathecal baclofen infusion, and botulinum toxin injections, has positively impacted many children with cerebral palsy. Family-focused interdisciplinary team management provides the best treatment outcomes.[25,26]

Inherited Metabolic Disorders of the Central Nervous System

A large number of inherited metabolic disorders have been identified, typically leading to diffuse brain dysfunction. Early diagnosis and treatment is vital if these infants are to survive without severe neurologic problems. Table 16-4 lists some of these inherited metabolic disorders.

TABLE 16-4	INHERITED METABOLIC DISORDERS OF THE CENTRAL NERVOUS SYSTEM
AGE OF ONSET	**DISORDER**
Neonatal period	Pyridoxine dependency, galactosemia, urea cycle defects, maple syrup urine disease and its variant, phenylketonuria (PKU), Menkes kinky hair syndrome
Early infancy	Tay-Sachs disease and its variants, infantile Gaucher disease, infantile Niemann-Pick disease, Krabbe disease (leukodystrophy), Farber lipogranulomatosis, Pelizaeus-Merzbacher disease and other sudanophilic leukodystrophies, spongy degeneration of CNS (Canavan disease), Alexander disease, Alpers disease, Leigh disease (subacute necrotizing encephalomyelopathy), congenital lactic acidosis, Zellweger encephalopathy, Lowe disease (oculocerebrorenal disease)
Late infancy and early childhood	Disorders of amino acid metabolism, metachromatic leukodystrophy, adrenoleukodystrophy, late infantile GM₁ gangliosidosis, late infantile Gaucher and Niemann-Pick diseases, neuroaxonal dystrophy, mucopolysaccharidosis, mucolipidosis, fucosidosis, mannosidosis, aspartylglycosaminuria, neuronal ceroid lipofuscinoses (Jansky-Bielschowsky disease, Batten disease, Vogt-Spielmeyer disease, neuronal ceroid lipofuscinosis), Cockayne syndrome, ataxia telangiectasia (AT)
Later childhood and adolescence	Progressive cerebellar ataxias of childhood and adolescence, hepatolenticular degeneration (Wilson disease), Hallervorden-Spatz disease, Lesch-Nyhan syndrome, Aicardi-Goutieres syndrome, progressive myoclonus epilepsies, homocystinuria, Fabry disease

Data from Lyon G, Kolodny E, Pastores GM, editors: *Neurology of hereditary metabolic diseases of children*, ed 3, New York, 2006, McGraw Hill.

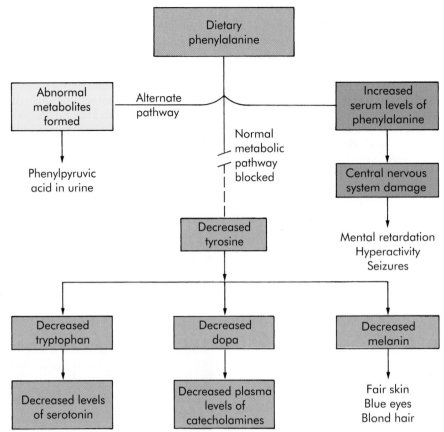

FIGURE 16-6 Metabolic Error and Consequences in Phenylketonuria. (From Hockenberry MJ: *Wong's nursing care of infants and children*, ed 8, St Louis, 2007, Mosby.)

Defects in amino acid and lipid metabolism are among the most common. Some of these disorders (e.g., urea cycle defects, organic acidurias) present in the newborn period with hyperammonemia and coma.

Defects in Amino Acid Metabolism

Biochemical defects in amino acid metabolism include (1) those in which the transport of an amino acid is impaired, (2) those involving an enzyme or cofactor deficiency, and (3) those encompassing certain chemical components, such as branched-chain or sulfur-containing amino acids. Most of these disorders are caused by genetic defects resulting in lack of a normal protein and absence of enzymatic activity.

Phenylketonuria. Phenylketonuria (PKU) is an inborn error of metabolism characterized by the inability of the body to convert the essential amino acid phenylalanine to tyrosine (Figure 16-6). PKU is caused by phenylalanine hydroxylase deficiency and has an incidence of 1:15,000 in the United States.[27,27a] Most natural food proteins contain about 15% phenylalanine, an essential amino acid. Phenylalanine hydroxylase controls the conversion of this essential amino acid to tyrosine in the liver. The body uses tyrosine in the biosynthesis of proteins, melanin, thyroxine, and the catecholamines in the brain and adrenal medulla. Phenylalanine hydroxylase deficiency causes an accumulation of phenylalanine in the serum. Other types of PKU involve impaired synthesis of cofactors (e.g., tetrahydrobiopterin [BH$_4$]), which contributes to elevated levels of phenylalanine. Elevated phenylalanine levels result in developmental abnormalities of the cerebral cortical layers, defective myelination, and cystic degeneration of the gray and white matter. Unfortunately, brain damage occurs before the metabolites can be detected in the urine, and damage continues as long as phenylalanine

levels remain high. Nonselective newborn screening is used to detect PKU in the United States and in more than 30 other countries. Treatment, consisting of reduction of dietary phenylalanine (PKU diet), is effective and allows for normal development of most of these children. Some individuals have a positive response when sapropterin, a synthetic form of tetrahydrobiopterin, is included in their treatment.[28]

Defects in Lipid Metabolism

Disorders of lipid metabolism are termed lysosomal storage diseases because each disorder in this group can be traced to a missing lysosomal enzyme. Lysosomal storage disorders include more than 50 known genetic disorders caused by an inborn error of metabolism. The incidence of lysosomal storage disorders is approximately 1 in 7500 live births.[29] These disorders cause an excessive accumulation of a particular cell product, occurring in the brain, liver, spleen, bone, and lung, and thus involving several organ systems. Some of these disorders may be treated with enzyme replacement therapy.[29a]

Perhaps the best known of the lysosomal storage disorders is Tay-Sachs disease (GM$_2$ gangliosidosis), an autosomal recessive disorder related to a deficiency of the enzyme hexosaminidase A (HEXA). Approximately 80% of individuals diagnosed are of Jewish ancestry, although sporadic cases appear in the non-Jewish population. In Tay-Sachs disease, GM$_2$ ganglioside accumulates in neurons throughout the body, although the pathologic progressive changes prevail in the CNS. Onset of this disease usually occurs when the infant is 4 to 6 months old. Symptoms of Tay-Sachs include an exaggerated startle response to loud noise, seizures, developmental regression, dementia, and blindness. Death from this disease is almost universal and occurs

TABLE 16-5 MAJOR TYPES OF SEIZURE DISORDERS FOUND IN CHILDREN

DISORDER	PATHOLOGY
Generalized Seizure	First clinical manifestations indicate that seizure activity starts in or involves both cerebral hemispheres; consciousness may be impaired
Convulsive Activity	
Tonic-clonic	Musculature stiffens, then intense jerking as trunk and extremities undergo rhythmic contraction and relaxation
Atonic	Sudden, momentary loss of muscle tone; drop attacks
Myoclonic	Sudden, brief contractures of a muscle or group of muscles
Nonconvulsive Activity	
Absence	Brief loss of consciousness with minimal or no loss of muscle tone; may experience 20 or more episodes a day lasting approximately 5-10 sec each; may have minor movement, such as lip smacking, twitching of eyelids
Epilepsy Syndromes	Seizure disorders that display a group of signs and symptoms that occur collectively and characterize or indicate a particular condition
Infantile spasms (West syndrome)	Form of epilepsy with episodes of sudden flexion or extension involving neck, trunk, and extremities; clinical manifestations range from subtle head nods to violent body contractions (jackknife seizures); onset between 3 and 12 months of age; may be idiopathic, genetic, result of metabolic disease, or in response to CNS insult; spasms occur in clusters of 5-150 times per day; EEG shows large-amplitude, chaotic, and disorganized pattern called "hypsarrhythmia"
Lennox-Gastaut syndrome	Epileptic syndrome with onset in early childhood, 1-5 yr of age; includes various generalized seizures—tonic-clonic, atonic (drop attacks), akinetic, absence, and myoclonic; EEG has characteristic "slow spike and wave" pattern; results in mental retardation and delayed psychomotor developments
Juvenile myoclonic epilepsy	Onset in adolescence; multifocal myoclonus; seizures often occur early in morning, aggravated by lack of sleep or after excessive alcohol intake; occasional generalized convulsions; require long-term medication treatment
Partial Seizure Types	Seizure activity that begins and usually is limited to one part of left or right hemisphere
Simple	Seizure activity that occurs without loss of consciousness
Complex	Seizure activity that occurs with impairment of consciousness
Benign rolandic epilepsy	Epileptic syndrome typically occurring in the pre-adolescent age (6-12 yr); strong association with sleep (seizures typically occur few hours after sleep onset or just before waking in morning); complex partial seizures with orofacial signs (drooling, distortion of facial muscles); characteristic EEG with centrotemporal (Rolandic fissure) spikes
Unclassified Epileptic Seizures	
Neonatal seizures	Wide variety of abnormal clinical activity, including rhythmic eye movements, chewing, and swimming movements; common in neonatal seizures
Simple febrile seizures	Common in children younger than 5-6 yr of age; brief (less than a few minutes) generalized convulsions associated with high fever; important to exclude meningitis as cause of seizures; usually do not develop epilepsy
Pseudoseizures	Non-epileptic phenomena that look like epileptic seizures; diagnosis often requires video-EEG monitoring to capture spells, and determine that EEG is normal during clinical events; frequently occurs in setting of child abuse
Status Epilepticus	
Nonconvulsive	Continuing or recurring seizure activity in which recovery from seizure activity is incomplete; unrelenting seizure activity can
Convulsive	last 30 min or more; other forms can evolve into status epilepticus; medical emergency that requires immediate intervention

by 5 years of age. Screening for carriers of the gene defect concomitant with counseling to prevent disease transmission is possible.[30]

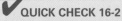

QUICK CHECK 16-2
1. List three types of cerebral palsy.
2. Why does failure to metabolize phenylalanine produce such widespread and devastating consequences?

Seizure Disorders

Epilepsy

Seizures are the abnormal discharge of electrical activity within the brain. **Epilepsy** is a neurologic condition characterized by a predisposition to recurrent seizures. Seizures may result from diseases that are primarily neurologic (CNS) or are systemic and affect CNS function secondarily (such as diabetes). Seizures can be caused by structural abnormalities of the brain, hypoxia, intracranial hemorrhage, CNS infection, traumatic injury, electrolyte imbalance, or inborn metabolic disturbances. Febrile seizures occur in up to 5% of children between ages 6 months and 5 years and are usually benign. Seizures are sometimes clearly familial. Often the cause of epilepsy is unknown and presumed to have a genetic basis.

The incidence of epilepsy varies greatly with age and is estimated to occur in 0.5% to 1% of children, with onset developing during infancy or childhood.[31] It decreases with age; 75% to 80% of epilepsy cases initially occur before 20 years of age, with 30% of the cases initially occurring within the first 4 years of life. Approximately 200,000 individuals in the United States are newly affected each year; 45,000 are under age 15 years.[32] Table 16-5 summarizes the major types of seizures.

Acute Encephalopathies

Reye Syndrome

Reye syndrome is characterized by encephalopathy, hyperammonemia, and fatty changes in the liver. The incidence of Reye syndrome has declined sharply since the 1980s, coinciding with increased public awareness of the association between ingestion of aspirin or aspirin-containing products during illness and subsequent development of Reye syndrome.[33]

An overview of Reye syndrome is important for the following reasons: (1) it may be considered a prototype for acute hepatic encephalopathies, (2) the potential for recurrence is a factor, and (3) the use of acetaminophen rather than aspirin during childhood febrile illnesses should be discussed with the parents.

Typically, Reye syndrome develops in a previously healthy child who is recovering from varicella, influenza B, upper respiratory tract infection, or gastroenteritis. The manifestations of the various clinical states are as follows:

Stage I: vomiting, lethargy, drowsiness

Stage II: disorientation, delirium, aggressiveness and combativeness, central neurologic hyperventilation, shallow breathing, hyperactive reflexes, stupor

Stage III: obtundation, coma, hyperventilation, decorticate rigidity

Stage IV: deepening coma, decerebrate rigidity, loss of ocular reflexes, large fixed pupils, divergent eye movements

Stage V: seizures, loss of deep tendon reflexes, flaccidity, respiratory arrest

Reye syndrome is a result of a toxin interfering with normal mitochondrial function. Treatment and outcome depend on the stage of development at diagnosis and the individual child's symptoms.

Intoxications of the Central Nervous System

Drug-induced encephalopathies must always be considered a possibility in the child with unexplained neurologic changes. Such encephalopathies may result from accidental ingestion, therapeutic overdose, intentional overdose, or ingestion of environmental toxins (the most commonly ingested poisons are listed in Table 16-6). Approximately 1.6 million children were exposed to poisons and approximately 650 children died in the United States in 2007 as a result of poisoning.[34,34a]

High blood levels of lead occur in lead poisoning. If lead poisoning is untreated, lead encephalopathy results and is responsible for serious and irreversible neurologic damage. Those at greatest risk are children ages 2 to 3 years and children prone to the practice of pica—the habitual, purposeful, and compulsive ingestion of non–food substances, such as clay, soil, and paint chips. Lead intoxication also may occur from chronic exposure to lead in cosmetics, inhalation of gasoline vapors, and ingestion of airborne lead.[35]

An estimated 250,000 children ages 1 to 5 years in the United States (2.2% of children 1 month to 5 years of age) have excessive amounts of lead in their blood.[36] The incidence in black children is five times greater than that in white children. Most lead exposures are preventable.[37]

Meningitis

Meningitis refers to the inflammation of the meningeal coverings of the brain. In most cases, meningitis is a result of viral or bacterial infection. It also can develop secondary to a chemical irritant (e.g., drugs, contrast agents) or result from diffuse infiltration with malignant cells (cancer).

Bacterial meningitis. Bacterial meningitis is one of the most serious infections to which infants and children are susceptible. In general,

TABLE 16-6	COMMONLY INGESTED POISONS		
PHARMACOLOGIC AGENTS	**HEAVY METALS**	**MISCELLANEOUS AGENTS**
Acetaminophen	Arsenic	Alcohols
Amphetamines	Lead	Ethyl
Anticonvulsants	Acute	Isopropyl
Antidepressants	Chronic	Methyl
Antihistamines	Mercury	Botulism toxin
Atropine	Thallium	Chlorinated hydrocarbons
Barbiturates		Ethylene glycol
Methadone		Mushrooms
Phencyclidine		Organophosphates
Salicylates		Pesticides
Tranquilizers		Snakebite
		Tick bites
		Venoms

Data from Swaiman KF, Ashwal S, Ferriero DM: *Pediatric neurology: principles and practice,* ed 4, St Louis, 2006, Mosby.

bacterial meningitis affects males more often than females and is most prevalent during infancy.[38] Conditions associated with increased incidence of respiratory tract infection heighten the occurrence of bacterial meningitis. The introduction of the protein conjugate vaccines against *Haemophilus influenzae* type B, *Streptococcus pneumoniae,* and *Neisseria meningitidis* has decreased the incidence of bacterial meningitis.[39] *Haemophilus influenzae* type B was once the most common pathogen of bacterial meningitis in children younger than 5 years, but *H. influenzae* meningitis has declined dramatically since the introduction of the Hib vaccine.[40-41]

Now the most common microorganism to cause bacterial meningitis is *Neisseria meningitidis* (meningococcus)—60% of all pediatric cases of meningitis.[42] Approximately 4% to 5% of infants and 23% to 27% of 19 year olds are carriers of *N. meningitidis.*[43] The risk of developing meningitis from day-care center contact of children with meningococcal disease is 1 per 1000.[44]

The second most common microorganism that causes meningitis is *Streptococcus pneumoniae,* which is likely to be found in children older than 4 years. Staphylococcal or streptococcal meningitis shows a predilection for children who have undergone neurosurgical procedures or fractured their skull; it also can develop as a complication of systemic bacterial infection. Infections that originate in the middle ear, sinuses, or mastoid cells also may lead to *S. pneumoniae* meningitis in children. In addition, 1 in every 24 children with sickle cell disease develops pneumococcal meningitis by the age of 4 years. *Escherichia coli* and group B β-hemolytic streptococci are the most common causes of meningitis in the newborn.

Viral meningitis. The hallmark of viral meningitis, or aseptic meningitis, is a mononuclear response in the CSF and the presence of normal glucose levels as well. Viral meningitis may result from a direct infection of a virus, or it may be secondary to disease, such as measles, mumps, herpes, or leukemia.

Onset of symptoms may be sudden or gradual. Malaise, fever, headache and stiff neck, abdominal pain, and nausea and vomiting are common. Sore throat, chest pain, photophobia, and maculopapular rash can develop also. The child usually recovers spontaneously within 3 to 10 days. Treatment is usually symptomatic.

CEREBROVASCULAR DISEASE IN CHILDREN

Cerebrovascular disease in children differs from that in adults in three ways:

1. An absence of predisposing factors, such as high blood pressure and arteriosclerosis
2. Significant differences in the clinical response related to the developing nervous system, and thus greater capacity for the pediatric brain to recovery from vascular insult
3. The anatomic site of the pathologic condition

Occlusive cerebrovascular disease is rare in children and may result from embolism, sinovenous thrombosis, or congenital or iatrogenic narrowing of vessels, which leads to a decreased flow of blood and oxygen to areas of the brain. Stroke is among the top 10 causes of death in children. Risk factors include cardiac diseases, hematologic and vascular disorders, and infection. Half of acute ischemic strokes occur with no known risk factors.[45] *Sickle cell disease* is the most common hematologic risk factor for ischemic stroke and is more common at 2 to 5 years of age, with hemorrhagic stroke more frequent at 20 to 30 years of age. A combination of chronic hemolytic anemia and vaso-occlusion contributes to brain ischemia and infarction. Congenital cerebral arteriovenous malformations are the most common cause of intracranial bleeding and hemorrhagic stroke in children.[46]

Moyamoya disease is a rare, chronic, progressive vascular stenosis of the circle of Willis with obstruction of arterial flow to the brain and the development of basal arterial collateral vessels that vascularize hypoperfused brain distal to the occluded vessels.[47] Moyamoya means a "puff of smoke" in Japanese. The disease is idiopathic or associated with other disorders (moyamoya syndrome).

Clinical presentation varies according to the vessels involved, the cause of the disease, and the age of the individual. Symptoms include hemiplegia, weakness, seizures, headaches, high fever, nuchal rigidity, hemianopia, sensory changes, facial palsy, and temporary aphasia. Obtaining a thorough history of evolving symptoms and risk factors is important for diagnosis. Laboratory studies may be indicated. Neuroimaging studies assist in determining the cause of the disease.[48] Surgery is an option for treatment and anticoagulants and antithrombotics may be used in selected cases.

TUMORS

Brain Tumors

Brain tumors are the most common solid tumor and most prevalent primary neoplasm in children. Overall, brain tumors account for nearly 20% of all childhood cancers, with an annual incidence of 2.4 to 4 per 100,000 in the United States; approximately 4150 brain tumors are diagnosed each year.[49,50] Five year survival for childhood brain tumors is about 72%.[51] Astrocytomas are the most frequent type of brain tumor in children.[52]

The cause of brain tumors is largely unknown, although genetic, environmental, and immune factors have been implicated in some tumor development. Factors that have been investigated as the cause of brain tumors include familial tendencies as well as exposure to radiation, oncologic viruses, and chemical carcinogens.[53] Alterations in embryologic development may play a part in the occurrence of childhood brain tumors.

Two thirds of all pediatric brain tumors are found in the posterior fossa (infratentorial) region of the brain, and approximately one third of childhood brain tumors are located in the supratentorial space. Brain tumors can arise from any CNS cell, and tumors are classified by cell type. The types and characteristics of childhood brain tumors are summarized in Table 16-7.

Medulloblastoma, ependymoma, astrocytoma, brain stem glioma, craniopharyngioma, and optic nerve glioma constitute approximately 75% to 80% of all pediatric brain tumors. Most brain tumors in children are located in the posterior fossa (Figure 16-7); treatment strategies and prognosis are listed in Table 16-8.

Signs and symptoms of brain tumors in children vary from generalized and vague to localized and related specifically to an anatomic area. Signs of increased intracranial pressure may occur, including headache, vomiting, lethargy, and irritability. If a young child complains of repeated and worsening headache, a thorough investigation should take place because headache is an uncommon complaint in young children. Headache caused by increased intracranial pressure usually is worse in the morning and gradually improves during the day when the child is upright and venous drainage is enhanced. The frequency of headache and other symptoms increases as the tumor grows. Irritability or possible apathy and increased somnolence also may result. Like headache, vomiting occurs more commonly in the morning. Often it is *not* preceded by nausea and may become projectile, differing from a gastrointestinal disturbance in that the child may be ready to eat immediately after vomiting. Other signs and symptoms include increased head circumference with bulging fontanelle in the child younger than 2 years, cranial nerve palsies, and papilledema (Box 16-1).

Localized findings relate to the degree of disturbance in physiologic functioning in the area where the tumor is located. Children with infratentorial tumors exhibit localized signs of impaired coordination and balance, including ataxia, gait difficulties, truncal ataxia, and loss of balance. Medulloblastoma occurs as an invasive malignant tumor that develops in the vermis of the cerebellum and may extend into the fourth ventricle. Ependymoma develops in the fourth ventricle and arises from the ependymal cells that line the ventricular system. Because both tumors are located in the posterior fossa region along the midline, presenting signs and symptoms are similar and are usually related to hydrocephalus and increased intracranial pressure. In contrast, cerebellar astrocytomas are located on the surface of the right or left cerebellar hemisphere and cause unilateral symptoms (occurring

TABLE 16-7	**BRAIN TUMORS IN CHILDREN**
TYPE	**CHARACTERISTICS**
Astrocytoma	Arises from astrocytes, often in cerebellum or lateral hemisphere
	Slow growing, solid or cystic
	Often very large before diagnosed
	Varies in degree of malignancy
Optic nerve glioma	Arises from optic chiasm or optic nerve (association with neurofibromatosis type 1)
	Slow-growing, low-grade astrocytoma
Medulloblastoma (infiltrating glioma)	Often located in cerebellum, extending into fourth ventricle and spinal fluid pathway
	Rapidly growing malignant tumor
	Can extend outside CNS
Brain stem glioma	Arises from pons
	Numerous cell types
	Compresses cranial nerves V through X
Ependymoma	Arises from ependymal cells lining ventricles
	Circumscribed, solid, nodular tumors
Craniopharyngioma	Arises near pituitary gland, optic chiasm, and hypothalamus
	Cystic and solid tumors that affect vision, pituitary, and hypothalamic functions

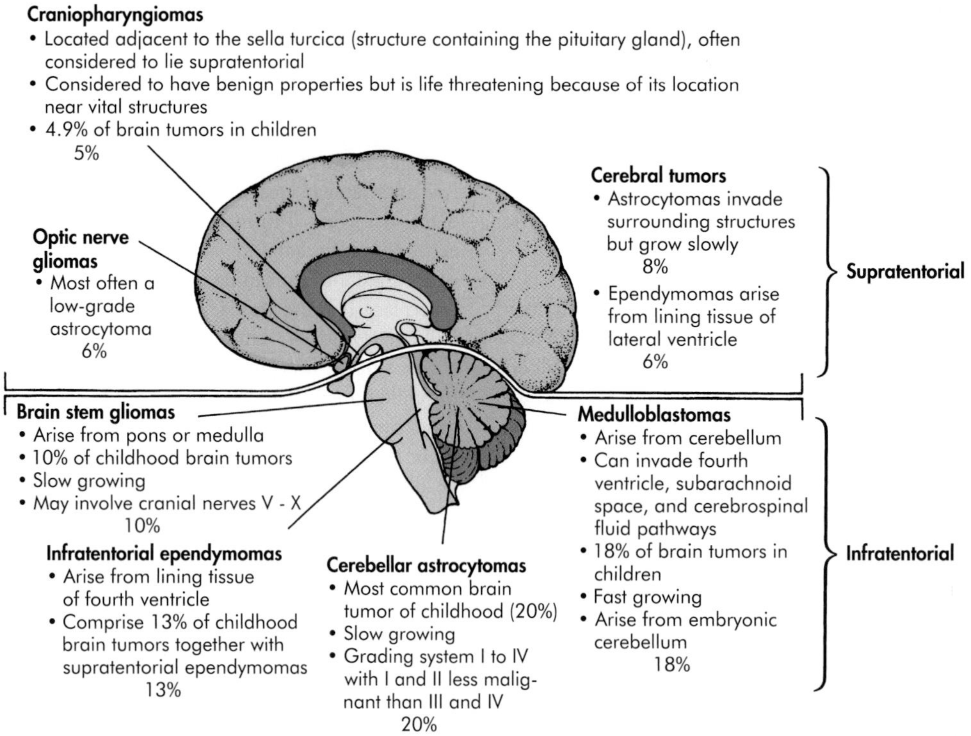

Craniopharyngiomas
- Located adjacent to the sella turcica (structure containing the pituitary gland), often considered to lie supratentorial
- Considered to have benign properties but is life threatening because of its location near vital structures
- 4.9% of brain tumors in children
  5%

Optic nerve gliomas
- Most often a low-grade astrocytoma
  6%

Cerebral tumors
- Astrocytomas invade surrounding structures but grow slowly
  8%
- Ependymomas arise from lining tissue of lateral ventricle
  6%

} **Supratentorial**

Brain stem gliomas
- Arise from pons or medulla
- 10% of childhood brain tumors
- Slow growing
- May involve cranial nerves V - X
  10%

Infratentorial ependymomas
- Arise from lining tissue of fourth ventricle
- Comprise 13% of childhood brain tumors together with supratentorial ependymomas
  13%

Cerebellar astrocytomas
- Most common brain tumor of childhood (20%)
- Slow growing
- Grading system I to IV with I and II less malignant than III and IV
  20%

Medulloblastomas
- Arise from cerebellum
- Can invade fourth ventricle, subarachnoid space, and cerebrospinal fluid pathways
- 18% of brain tumors in children
- Fast growing
- Arise from embryonic cerebellum
  18%

} **Infratentorial**

FIGURE 16-7 Location of Brain Tumors in Children.

TABLE 16-8 TREATMENT STRATEGIES FOR CHILDHOOD BRAIN TUMORS

TUMOR TYPE	TREATMENT AND PROGNOSIS
Cerebellar astrocytoma	Surgery; possibly curative
	Radiation and chemotherapy not proved successful but may delay recurrence
	90%-100% 5-yr survival rate if pilocytic type; if tumor recurs, it does so very slowly
Medulloblastoma	Surgery, primarily as partial resection to relieve increased intracranial pressure and "debulk" tumor
	Type of treatment is age and tumor type dependent
	Radiation as primary treatment; may include spinal radiation
	Chemotherapy showing some promise in conjunction with craniospinal radiation
	65%-85% 5-yr survival rate depending on stage/type
Brain stem glioma	Surgery, resection occasionally possible
	Radiation, primarily palliative treatment
	Chemotherapy not yet proven beneficial, but new protocols being studied
	20%-40% 5-yr survival rate
Ependymoma	Tumor possibly indolent for many years
	Surgery rarely curative; risk of resecting an infratentorial tumor too great
	Radiation for palliation (current controversy over whether local or craniospinal radiation is best)
	Chemotherapy used for recurrent disease but with disappointing results
	20%-80% 5-yr survival rate dependent on total resection
Craniopharyngioma	Surgery possibly successful when complete resection is performed (partial resection usually requires further treatment)
	Radiation after partial surgical resection
	Chemotherapy not commonly used
	80%-95% 5-yr survival rate
Optic nerve glioma	In setting of visual impairment, or progression (increase in size), chemotherapy is usual initial treatment
	Surgery for hydrocephalus or other complications; rarely for diagnosis
	Radiation therapy for those tumors that progress or recur in spite of chemotherapy
Cerebral astrocytoma	Surgery used if resection is possible
	Radiation useful for all grades of astrocytoma
	Chemotherapy beneficial in higher grade tumors but further study required
	75% 5-yr survival rate with lower grade tumors

Data from Packer RJ, Macdonald T, Vezina G: Central nervous system tumors, *Hematol-Oncol Clin North Am* 24(1):87–108, 2010; Merchant TE, Pollack IF, Loeffler JS: Brain tumors across the age spectrum: biology, therapy, and late effects, *Semin Radiat Oncol* 20(1):58–66, 2010; Gurney JG, Smith, MA, Bunin GR: CNS and miscellaneous intracranial and intraspinal neoplasms, ICCC III, *Cancer incidence and survival among children and adolescents: United States SEER Program 1975–1995*, National Cancer Institute, pp 51–63. Available at http://seer.cancer.gov/publications/childhood/cns.pdf.

BOX 16-1   CLINICAL MANIFESTATIONS OF BRAIN TUMORS

Headache
Recurrent and progressive
In frontal or occipital area
Worse on arising, pain lessens during the day
Intensified by lowering head and straining, such as when defecating, coughing, sneezing

Vomiting
With or without nausea or feeding
Progressively more projectile
More severe in morning
Relieved by moving and changing position

Neuromuscular Changes
Uncoordination or clumsiness
Loss of balance (use of wide-based stance, falling, tripping, banging into object)
Poor fine motor control
Weakness
Hyporeflexia or hyperreflexia
Positive Babinski sign
Spasticity
Paralysis

Behavioral Changes
Irritability
Decreased appetite
Failure to thrive
Fatigue (frequent naps)
Lethargy
Coma
Bizarre behavior (staring, automatic movements)

Cranial Nerve Neuropathy
Cranial nerve involvement varies according to tumor location
Most common signs
  Head tilt
  Visual defects (nystagmus, diplopia, strabismus, episodic "graying out" of vision, and visual field defects)

Vital Sign Disturbances
Decreased pulse and respiratory rates
Increased blood pressure
Decreased pulse pressure
Hypothermia or hyperthermia

Other Signs
Seizures
Cranial enlargement*
Tense, bulging fontanelle at rest*
Nuchal rigidity
Papilledema (edema of optic nerve)

From Hockenberry MN: *Wong's essentials of pediatric nursing,* ed 7, St Louis, 2005, Mosby.
*Present only in infants and young children.

on the same side as the tumor), such as head tilt, limb ataxia, and nystagmus.

Brain stem gliomas often cause a combination of cranial nerve involvement (facial weakness, limitation of horizontal eye movement), cerebellar signs of ataxia, and corticospinal tract dysfunction. Increased intracranial pressure generally does not occur.

The area of the sella turcica, the structure containing the pituitary gland, is the site of several childhood brain tumors; most common of this group is the craniopharyngioma. This tumor originates from the pituitary gland or hypothalamus. Usually slow growing, it may be quite large by the time of diagnosis. Symptoms include headache, seizures, diabetes insipidus, early onset of puberty, and growth delay. Other tumors located in this region of the brain include optic gliomas. Optic nerve gliomas are associated with neurofibromatosis type 1, a neurocutaneous condition characterized by café-au-lait macules on the skin and benign tumors of the skin. Tumors that involve the optic tract may cause complete unilateral blindness and hemianopia of the other eye. Optic atrophy is another common finding. Supratentorial tumors of the cerebral hemispheres in children are uncommon.

Embryonal Tumors
Neuroblastoma

Neuroblastoma is an embryonal tumor originating in neural crest cells that normally develop into sympathetic ganglia and the adrenal medulla. Because neuroblastoma involves a defect of embryonic tissue, it most commonly is diagnosed during the first 2 years of life, and 75% of neuroblastomas are found before the child is 5 years old.

Occasionally, these tumors have been diagnosed at birth with metastasis apparent in the placenta. It is seen more commonly in white children (9.6 per million) than in black children (7 per million). Although it accounts for only 8% to 10% of pediatric malignancies,[54] neuroblastoma causes 15% of cancer deaths in children.

Neuroblastoma is the most common and immature form of the sympathetic nervous system tumors. Areas of necrosis and calcification often are present in the tumor. More than with any other cancer, neuroblastoma has been associated with spontaneous remission, commonly in infants. Prognosis is worse for children older than 2 years of age with disseminated disease.[55]

Although familial tendency has been noted in individual cases, a nonfamilial or sporadic pattern is found in most children with neuroblastoma. Familial cases of neuroblastoma are considered to have an autosomal dominant pattern of inheritance (mechanisms of inheritance are discussed in Chapter 2).

The most common location of neuroblastoma is in the retroperitoneal region (65% of cases), most often the adrenal medulla. The tumor is evident as an abdominal mass and may cause anorexia, bowel and bladder alteration, and sometimes spinal cord compression. The second most common location of neuroblastoma is the mediastinum (15% of cases), where the tumor may cause dyspnea or infection related to airway obstruction. Less commonly, neuroblastoma may arise from the cervical sympathetic ganglion (3% to 4% of cases). Cervical neuroblastoma often causes Horner syndrome, which consists of miosis (pupil contraction), ptosis (drooping eyelid), enophthalmos (backward displacement of the eyeball), and anhidrosis (sweat deficiency). Neuroblastoma rarely presents with a neurologic syndrome

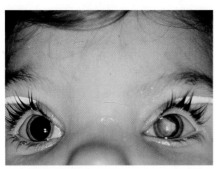

FIGURE 16-8 Retinoblastoma. The tumor occupies a large portion of the inside of the eye bulbus. (From Damjanov I: *Pathology for the health professions,* ed 3, St Louis, 2006, Saunders. Courtesy Dr. Walter Richardson and Dr. Jamsheed Khan, Kansas City, Kan.)

called opsoclonus-myoclonus syndrome.[56] Children develop conjugate chaotic eye movements, jerky movements of the limbs, and ataxia.

A number of systemic signs and symptoms are characteristic of neuroblastoma, including weight loss, irritability, fatigue, and fever. Intractable diarrhea occurs in 7% to 9% of children and is caused by tumor secretion of a hormone called *vasoactive intestinal polypeptide (VIP).*

More than 90% of children with neuroblastoma have increased amounts of catecholamines and associated metabolites in their urine. High levels of urinary catecholamines and serum ferritin are associated with a poor prognosis.

Retinoblastoma

Retinoblastoma is a rare congenital eye tumor of young children that originates in the retina of one or both eyes (Figure 16-8). Two forms of retinoblastoma are exhibited: inherited and acquired. The inherited

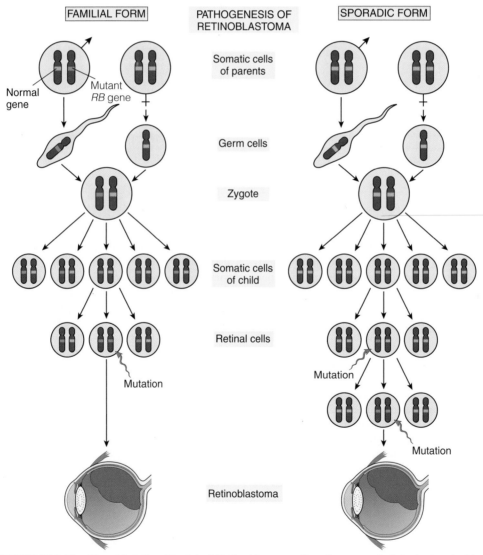

FIGURE 16-9 The Two-Mutation Model of Retinoblastoma Development. In inherited retinoblastoma, the first mutation is transmitted through the germline of an affected parent. The second mutation occurs somatically in a retinal cell, leading to development of the tumor. In sporadic retinoblastoma, development of a tumor requires two somatic mutations.

form of the disease generally is diagnosed during the first year of life. The acquired disease most commonly is diagnosed in children 2 to 3 years of age and involves unilateral disease.

Approximately 40% of retinoblastomas are inherited as an autosomal dominant trait with incomplete penetrance (see Figure 2-2). The remaining 60% are acquired. In the early 1970s, Knudson proposed the "two-hit" hypothesis to explain the occurrence of both hereditary and acquired forms of the disease.[57] This hypothesis predicts that two separate transforming events or "hits" must occur in a normal retinoblast cell to cause the cancer. Further, it proposes that in the inherited form, the first hit or mutation occurs in the germ cell (inherited from either parent), and the mutation is contained in every cell of the child's body. Only a second, random mutation in a retinoblast cell is needed to transform that cell into cancer. Multiple tumors are observed in the inherited form because these second mutations are likely to occur in several of the approximately 1 to 2 million retinoblast cells. In contrast, the acquired form of retinoblastoma requires two independent hits or mutations to occur in the same somatic cell (after the egg is fertilized) for the transformation to cancer. This is much less likely to happen. Figure 16-9 illustrates the two-mutation model for these two patterns of mutation.

The primary sign of retinoblastoma is leukocoria, a white pupillary reflex also called *cat's eye reflex*, which is caused by the mass behind the lens (see Figure 16-8). Other signs and symptoms include strabismus; a red, painful eye; and limited vision.

Because retinoblastoma is a treatable tumor, dual priorities are saving the child's life and restoring useful vision. The prognosis for most children with retinoblastoma is excellent, with a greater than 90% long-term survival.

QUICK CHECK 16-3
1. Why are the principal symptoms of brain tumors in children related to brain stem function?

DID YOU UNDERSTAND?

Normal Growth and Development of the Nervous System
1. Growth and development of the brain occur most rapidly during fetal development and during the first year of life.
2. The bones of the skull are joined by sutures, and the wide, membranous junctions of the sutures (known as *fontanelles*) allow for brain growth and close by 18 months of age.
3. At birth neurologic function is primarily at the subcortical level with transition in reflexes as motor development progresses during the first year.

Structural Malformations
1. Defects of neural tube closure include anencephaly (absence of part of the skull and brain), encephalocele (herniation of the meninges and brain through a skull defect), meningocele (a saclike meningeal cyst that protrudes through a vertebral defect), and myelomeningocele that occurs with spina bifida (failure of the vertebrae to close and the resulting protrusion of neural tube contents).
2. Spina bifida occulta is a vertebral defect without visible exposure of meninges or neural tissue.
3. Acrania is nearly complete absence of the cranial vault.
4. Premature closure of the cranial sutures causes craniosynostosis and prevents normal skull expansion, resulting in compression of growing brain tissue.
5. Microcephaly is lack of brain growth with retarded mental and motor development.
6. Congenital hydrocephalus results from overproduction, impaired absorption, or blockage of circulation of cerebrospinal fluid. Dandy-Walker deformity is caused by cystic dilation of the fourth ventricle and aqueductal compression.

Encephalopathies
1. Static encephalopathies are nonprogressive disorders of the brain that can occur during gestation, birth, or childhood and can be caused by endogenous or exogenous factors.
2. Cerebral palsy can be caused by prenatal cerebral hypoxia or perinatal trauma, with symptoms of motor dysfunction (including increased muscle tone, increased reflexes, and loss of fine motor coordination), mental retardation, seizure disorders, or developmental disabilities.

3. Inherited metabolic disorders that damage the nervous system include defects in amino acid metabolism (phenylketonuria) and lipid metabolism (Tay-Sachs disease) and result in abnormal behavior, seizures, and deficient psychomotor development.
4. Seizure disorders are abnormal discharges of electrical activity within the brain. They are associated with numerous nervous system disorders and more often are a generalized rather than a partial type of seizure.
5. Generalized forms of seizures include tonic-clonic, myoclonic, atonic, akinetic, and infantile spasms.
6. Partial seizures suggest more localized brain dysfunction.
7. Febrile seizures usually are limited to children ages 6 months to 6 years, with a pattern of one seizure per febrile illness.
8. Reye syndrome is an encephalopathy with fatty changes in the liver and hyperammonemia associated with influenza B, varicella viruses, and aspirin ingestion. Progressive manifestations include lethargy, stupor, rigidity, seizures, and respiratory arrest.
9. Accidental poisonings from a variety of toxins can cause serious neurologic damage.
10. Bacterial meningitis is commonly caused by *Neisseria meningitidis* or *Streptococcus pneumoniae* and may result from respiratory or gastrointestinal infections; symptoms include fever, headaches, photophobia, seizures, rigidity, and stupor.
11. Viral meningitis may result from direct infection or be secondary to a systemic viral infection (e.g., measles, mumps, herpes, or leukemia).

Cerebrovascular Disease in Children
1. Occlusive cerebrovascular disease is rare in children but can occur from embolism, sinovenous thrombosis, or congenital narrowing of vessels.
2. Stroke can occur in association with cardiac disease, hematologic disorders (e.g., sickle cell disease), vascular disorders, and infection.
3. Moyamoya is a rare, progressive vascular stenosis of the circle of Willis that obstructs arterial blood flow to the brain.

Continued

DID YOU UNDERSTAND?—cont'd

Tumors

1. Brain tumors are the most common tumors of the nervous system and the second most common type of childhood cancer.
2. Tumors in children most often are located below the tentorial plate.
3. Fast-growing tumors produce symptoms early in the disease, whereas slow-growing tumors may become very large before symptoms appear.
4. Symptoms of brain tumors may be generalized or localized. The most common general symptoms are the result of increased intracranial pressure and include headache, irritability, vomiting, somnolence, and bulging of fontanelles.
5. Localized signs of infratentorial tumors in the cerebellum include impaired coordination and balance. Cranial nerve signs occur with tumors in or near the brain stem.
6. Supratentorial tumors may be located near the cortex or deep in the brain. Symptoms depend on the specific location of the tumor.
7. Neuroblastoma is an embryonal tumor of the sympathetic nervous system and can be located anywhere there is sympathetic nervous tissue. Symptoms are related to tumor location and size of metastasis.
8. Retinoblastoma is a congenital eye tumor that has two forms: inherited and acquired.

KEY TERMS

- Acrania 413
- Anencephaly 411
- Ataxic cerebral palsy 415
- Bacterial meningitis 418
- Brain stem glioma 421
- Cerebellar astrocytoma 419
- Cerebral palsy 415
- Congenital hydrocephalus 414
- Craniopharyngioma 421
- Craniorachischisis totalis 411
- Craniosynostosis 413
- Cyclopia 410
- Dandy-Walker malformation (DWM) 414
- Dystonic cerebral palsy 415
- Encephalocele 411
- Encephalopathy 415
- Ependymoma 419
- Epilepsy 417
- Fontanelle 409
- Lysosomal storage disease 416
- Macewen sign ("cracked pot" sign) 415
- Medulloblastoma 419
- Meningitis 418
- Meningocele 411
- Microcephaly 413
- Moyamoya disease 419
- Myelodysplasia 410
- Myelomeningocele 412
- Neuroblastoma 421
- Occlusive cerebrovascular disease 419
- Optic glioma 421
- Phenylketonuria (PKU) 416
- Pica 418
- Retinoblastoma 422
- Reye syndrome 418
- Spastic cerebral palsy 415
- Spina bifida 413
- Spina bifida occulta 413
- Stroke 419
- Tay-Sachs disease (GM$_2$ gangliosidosis) 416
- Type II Chiari malformation (Arnold-Chiari malformation) 412
- Viral meningitis 418

REFERENCES

1. Beard JL: Why iron deficiency is important in infant development, *J Nutr* 138(12):2534–2536, 2008.
2. Todorich B, et al: Oligodendrocytes and myelination: the role of iron, *Glia* 57(5):467–478, 2009.
3. Rollins JD, Collins JS, Holden KR: United States head circumference growth reference charts: birth to 21 years, *J Pediatr* 156(6):907–913, 2010.
4. Mitchell LE: Epidemiology of neural tube defects, *Am J Med Genet Part C: Sem Med Genet* 135C(1):88–94, 2005.
5. Kaufman B: Neural tube defects, *Pediatr Clin North Am* 51(2):389–419, 2004.
6. Copp AJ, Greene ND: Genetics and development of neural tube defects, *J Pathol* 220(2):217–230, 2010.
7. Blencowe H, et al: Folic acid to reduce neonatal mortality from neural tube disorders, *Int J Epidemiol* 39(suppl 1):i110–i121, 2010.
8. Quinn L, Thompson S, Ott MK: Application of the social ecological model; in folic acid public health initiatives, *J Obstet Gynecol Neonat Nurs* 34(6):672–681, 2005.
9. Rowland CA, et al: Are encephaloceles neural tube defects? *Pediatrics* 118(3):916–923, 2006.
10. Wen S, et al: Prevalence of encephalocele in Texas, 1999–2002, *Am J Med Genet Part A* 143A:2150–2155, 2007.
11. Behrman R, Kleigman R, Jenson H: *Nelson's textbook of pediatrics*, ed 17, Philadelphia, 2004, Saunders.
12. Adzick N, Walsh D: Myelomeningocele: prenatal diagnosis, pathophysiology, and management, *Semin Pediatr Surg* 12(2):168–174, 2003.
13. Adzick NS: Fetal myelomeningocele: natural history, pathophysiology, and in-utero intervention, *Semin Fetal Neonatal Med* 15(1):9–14, 2009.
14. Juranek J, Salman MS: Anomalous development of brain structure and function in spina bifida myelomenigocele, *Dev Disabil Res Rev* 16(1):23–30, 2010.
15. Cartwright C: Assessing asymmetrical infant head shapes, *Nurse Pract* 27(8):33–36, 2002:39.
16. Raj S, et al: *Craniosynostosis emedicine from WebMD*, updated July 23, 2010. Available at http://emedicine.medscape.com/article/1175957-overview. Accessed June, 2011.
17. Rekate HL: The definition and classification of hydrocephalus: a personal recommendation to stimulate debate, *Cerebrospinal Fluid Res* 5:2, 2008.
18. Garton HJ, Piatt JH Jr: Hydrocephalus, *Pediatr Clin North Am* 51:305–325, 2004.
19. Hu CF, et al: Successful treatment of Dandy-Walker syndrome by endoscopic third ventriculostomy in a 6-month-old girl with progressive hydrocephalus: a case report and literature review, *Pediatr Neonatol* 52(1):42–45, 2011.
20. Del Bigio MR: Neuropathology and structural changes in hydrocephalus, *Dev Disabil Res Rev* 16(1):16–22, 2010.
21. Kuban KC, et al: ELGAN Study Cerebral Palsy-Algorithm Group. An algorithm for identifying and classifying cerebral palsy in young children, *J Pediatr* 153(4):466–472, 2008.
22. Longo M, Hankins GD: Defining cerebral palsy: pathogenesis, pathophysiology and new intervention, *Minerva Ginecol* 61(5):421–429, 2009.
23. Krigger KW: Cerebral palsy: an overview, *Am Fam Physician* 73(1):91–100, 2006.
24. Pruitt DW, Tsai T: Common medical comorbidities associated with cerebral palsy, *Phys Med Rehabil Clin North Am* 20(3):453–467, 2009.

25. Blair: Epidemiology of the cerebral palsies, *Orthop Clin North Am* 41(4):441–455, 2010.

26. Delgado MR, Hirtz D, Aisen M, et al: Quality Standards Subcommittee of the American Academy of Neurology and the Practice Committee of the Child Neurology Society, Practice parameter: pharmacologic treatment of spasticity in children and adolescents with cerebral palsy (an evidence-based review): report of the Quality Standards Subcommittee of the American Academy of Neurology and the Practice Committee of the Child Neurology Society, *Neurology* 74(4):336–343, 2010.

27. Mijuskovic Z, Karadaglic D, Stojanov L: Phenylketonuria, Emedicine. Accessed June, 2011 from http://emedicine.medscape.com/article/1115450-overview.

27a. Blau N, van Spronsen FJ, Levy HL: Phenylketonuria, *Lancet* 376(9750):1417–1427, 2010

28. Vernon HJ, et al: Introduction of sapropterin dihydrochloride as standard of care in patients with phenylketonuria, *Mol Genet Metab* 100(3):229–233, 2010.

29. Hodges BL, Cheng SH: Cell and gene-based therapies for the lysosomal storage diseases, *Curr Gene Ther* 6(2):227–241, 2006

29a. Urbanelli L, et al: Developments in therapeutic approaches for lysosomal storage diseases, *Recent Pat CNS Drug Discov* 6(1):1–19, 2011.

30. Schneider A, et al: Population-based Tay-Sachs screening among Ashkenazi Jewish young adults in the 21st century: hexosaminidase A enzyme assay is essential for accurate testing, *Am J Med Genet A* 149A(11):2444–2447, 2009.

31. Schmidt K: Phenylketonuria. In Jackson PL, Vessey JA, editors: *Primary care of the child with chronic conditions*, ed 4, St Louis, 2003, Mosby.

32. Epilepsy Foundation of American: *Epilepsy and seizure statistics*, Accessed June, 2011. Available at www.epilepsyfoundation.org/about/statistics.cfm.

33. Pugliese A, Beltramo T, Torre D: Reye's and Reye's-like syndromes, *Cell Biochem Funct* 26(7):741–746, 2008.

34. Bronstein AC, et al: 2009 Annual Report of the American Association of Poison Control Centers' National Poison Data System (NPDS): 27th Annual Report, *Clinical Toxicology* 48:979–1178, 2010. Available at http://www.aapcc.org/dnn/Portals/0/correctedannualreport.pdf:page 991.

34a. National Center for Injury Prevention and Control: WISQARS Injury Mortaliity Reports, *Centers for Disease Control*, 1999-2007. Available at http://webappa.cdc.gov/sasweb/ncipc/mortrate10_sy.html. http://webappa.cdc.gov/cgi-bin/broker.exe.

35. Advisory Committee on Childhood Lead Poisoning Prevention: Interpreting and managing blood lead levels <10 μg/dL in children and reducing childhood exposures to lead: recommendations of CDC's Advisory Committee on Childhood Lead Poisoning Prevention, *MMWR Recommend Rep* 56(RR-8):1–14, 16, 2007. Available at www.cdc.gov/mmwr/preview/mmwrhtml/rr5608a1.htm.

36. Centers for Disease Control and Prevention: *Lead*. Last updated July 27, 2010. Available from www.cdc.gov/nceh/lead/Last updated July 27, 2010.

37. Centers for Disease Control and Prevention: *Lead: prevention tips*, Updated June 1, 2009. Available at www.cdc.gov/nceh/lead/tips.htm.

38. Chang CJ, et al: Bacterial meningitis in infants: the epidemiology, clinical features, and prognostic factors, *Brain Dev* 26(3):168–175, 2004.

39. Kim KS: Acute bacterial meningitis in infants and children, *Lancet Infect Dis* 10(1):32–42, 2010.

40. Trück J, Pollard AJ: Challenges in immunisation against bacterial infection in children, *Early Hum Dev* 86(11):695–701, 2010.

41. Thigpen MC, et al: Emerging Infections Programs Network. Bacterial meningitis in the United States, 1998-2007, *N Engl J Med* 364(21):2016–2025, 2011.

42. Harrison LH: Epidemiological profile of meningococcal disease in the United States, *Clin Infect Dis* 50(suppl 2):S37–S44, 2010.

43. Christensen H, May M, Bowen L, Hickman M, Trotter CL: Meningococcal carriage by age: a systematic review and meta-analysis, *Lancet Infect Dis* 10(12):853–861, 2010.

44. Nigrovic LE, Kuppermann N, Malley R: Development and validation of a multivariable predictive model to distinguish bacterial from aseptic meningitis in children in post-*Haemophilus influenzae* era, *Pediatrics* 110(4):712–719, 2002.

45. Lopez-Vicente M, et al: Diagnosis and management of pediatric arterial ischemic stroke, *J Stroke Cerebrovasc Dis* 19(3):175–183, 2010.

46. Breslow LA, et al: Predictors of outcome in childhood intracerebral hemorrhage: a prospective consecutive cohort study, *Stroke* 41(2):313–318, 2009.

47. Smith JL: Understanding and treating moyamoya disease in children, *Neurosurg Focus* 26(4):E4, 2009.

48. Diamini N, Kirkham FJ: Stroke and cerebrovascular disorders, *Curr Opin Pediatr* 21(6):751–761, 2009.

49. Packer RJ, Macdonald T, Vezina G: Central nervous system tumors, *Hematol-Oncol Clin North Am* 24(1):87–108, 2010.

50. Children's Brain Tumor Foundation: *Pediatric brain tumors*. Updated March 24, 2011. Available at http://www.pbtfus.org/medcomm/research/Pediatric-brain-tumor-facts-updated.html.

51. American Cancer Society. *Cancer Facts and Figures 2010*. Atlanta Georgia available at http://www.cancer.org/acs/groups/content/@epidemiologysurveilance/documents/document/acspc-026238.pdf.

52. Kaatsch P: Epidemiology of childhood cancer, *Cancer Treat Rev* 36(4):277–285, 2010.

53. Pediatric Brain Tumor Foundation: *Facts about pediatric brain tumors*, Asheville, NC, 2006, Author. Available at www.pbtfus.org/medcomm/research/facts.html.

54. Esiashvili N, Anderson C, Katzenstein HM: Neuroblastoma, *Curr Probl Cancer* 33(6):333–360, 2009.

55. Maris JM: Recent advances in neuroblastoma, *N Engl J Med* 362(23):2202–2211, 2010.

56. De Grandis E, et al: Long-term follow-up of neuroblastoma-associated opsoclonus-myoclonus-ataxia syndrome, *Neuropediatrics* 40(3):103–111, 2009.

57. Knudson AG Jr: Mutation and cancer: a statistical study of retinoblastoma, *Proc Natl Acad Sci U S A* 68(4):820–823, 1971.

Mechanisms of Hormonal Regulation

Valentina L. Brashers and Sue E. Huether

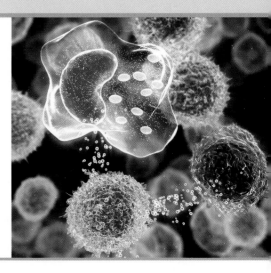

℮volve WEBSITE

CHAPTER OUTLINE

The endocrine system is composed of various glands located throughout the body (Figure 17-1). These glands can synthesize and release special chemical messengers called hormones. The endocrine system has five general functions: (1) differentiation of the reproductive and central nervous systems in the developing fetus; (2) stimulation of sequential growth and development during childhood and adolescence; (3) coordination of the male and female reproductive systems, which makes sexual reproduction possible; (4) maintenance of an optimal internal environment throughout life; and (5) initiation of corrective and adaptive responses when emergency demands occur. Hormones convey specific regulatory information among cells and organs and are integrated with the nervous system to maintain communication and control. The mechanisms of communication include *autocrine* (within the cell), *paracrine* (between local cells), and *endocrine* (between remote cells).

MECHANISMS OF HORMONAL REGULATION

The endocrine glands respond to specific signals by synthesizing and releasing hormones into the circulation, which then trigger intracellular responses. All hormones share certain general characteristics:
1. Have specific rates and rhythms of secretion. Three basic secretion patterns are (a) diurnal patterns, (b) pulsatile and cyclic patterns,

and (c) patterns that depend on levels of circulating substrates (e.g., calcium, sodium, potassium, or the hormones themselves). Diurnal, pulsatile, and cyclic patterns of hormone release involve consistent patterns of secretion.
2. Operate within feedback systems, either positive or negative, to maintain an optimal internal environment.
3. Affect only target cells with specific receptors for the hormone and then act on these cells to initiate specific cell functions or activities.
4. Are excreted by the kidneys or are deactivated by the liver or cellular mechanisms.

Hormones may be classified according to structure, gland of origin, effects, or chemical composition. (Table 17-1 categorizes known hormones based on structure.) The secretion and mechanisms of action of hormones represent an extremely complex system of integrated responses. The endocrine and nervous systems work together to regulate responses to the internal and external environments.

Regulation of Hormone Release

Hormones are released either in response to an altered cellular environment or in the maintenance of a regulated level of another hormone or substance. One or more of the following mechanisms regulates hormone release: (1) chemical factors (such as blood glucose or calcium

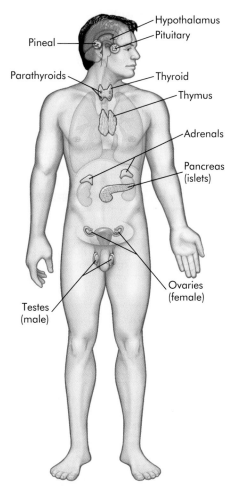

FIGURE 17-1 Principal Endocrine Glands. (From Patton KT, Thibodeau GA: *Anatomy & physiology,* ed 7, St Louis, 2010, Mosby.)

TABLE 17-1	STRUCTURAL CATEGORIES OF HORMONES
STRUCTURAL CATEGORY	**EXAMPLES**
Water Soluble	
Peptides	Growth hormone
	Insulin
	Leptin
	Parathyroid hormone
	Prolactin
Glycoproteins	Follicle-stimulating hormone
	Luteinizing hormone
	Thyroid-stimulating hormone
Polypeptides	Adrenocorticotropic hormone
	Antidiuretic hormone
	Calcitonin
	Endorphins
	Glucagon
	Hypothalamic hormones
	Lipotropins
	Melanocyte-stimulating hormone
	Oxytocin
	Somatostatin
	Thymosin
	Thyrotropin-releasing hormone
Amines	Epinephrine
	Norepinephrine
Lipid Soluble	
Thyroxine (an amine but lipid soluble)	Both thyroxine (T_4) and triiodothyronine (T_3)
Steroids (cholesterol is a precursor for all steroids)	Estrogens
	Glucocorticoids (cortisol)
	Mineralocorticoids (aldosterone)
	Progestins (progesterone)
	Testosterone
Derivatives of arachidonic acid (autocrine or paracrine action)	Leukotrienes
	Prostacyclins
	Prostaglandins
	Thromboxanes

levels), (2) endocrine factors (a hormone from one endocrine gland controlling another endocrine gland), and (3) neural control. For example, insulin is secreted by the chemical stimulation of increased plasma glucose levels, cortisol from the adrenal cortex is an endocrine factor that regulates and stimulates insulin secretion, and direct stimulation of the insulin-secreting cells of the pancreas by the autonomic nervous system is a form of neural control.

Feedback systems provide precise monitoring and control of the cellular environment. The most common feedback system, **negative feedback,** occurs because the changing chemical, neural, or endocrine response to a stimulus negates the initiating change that triggered the release of the hormone. An example of hormone negative feedback is shown in Figure 17-2, *A.* Thyroid-stimulating hormone (TSH) secretion from the anterior pituitary is stimulated by **thyrotropin-releasing hormone (TRH)** from the hypothalamus and by decreased serum levels of the thyroid hormones thyroxine (T_4) and triiodothyronine (T_3). Secretion of TSH stimulates the synthesis and secretion of thyroid hormones. Increasing levels of T_4 and T_3 then generate negative feedback on the pituitary and hypothalamus to inhibit TRH and TSH synthesis. Negative feedback systems are important for maintaining hormone levels within physiologic ranges. These negative feedback regulatory systems are diagrammed in Figure 17-2, *B.*

The lack of negative feedback inhibition on hormonal release often results in pathologic excessive hormone production (see Chapter 18).

Hormone Transport

Once hormones are released into the circulatory system, they are distributed throughout the body. The protein (peptide) hormones (see Table 17-1) are water soluble and generally circulate in free (unbound) forms. This process immediately exposes these water-soluble hormones to circulating catabolizing enzymes, giving them an expected half-life of seconds to minutes. Lipid-soluble hormones (see Table 17-1) are transported bound to a carrier or transport protein. Lipid-soluble hormones can remain in the blood for hours to days. Water-soluble hormones mediate short-acting responses, and lipid-soluble hormones mediate both rapid-acting and long-acting responses. Water-soluble hormones bind to cell-surface receptors, and lipid-soluble hormones may bind to plasma membrane receptors or diffuse through the cellular plasma membrane and bind to cytosolic or nuclear receptors.[1]

Because an equilibrium exists between the concentrations of free hormones and hormones bound to plasma proteins, a significant change in the concentration of binding proteins can affect the concentration of free hormones in the plasma (Table 17-2). Only free hormones can signal a target cell. (Mechanisms of hormone binding are discussed in Chapter 1.)

Mechanisms of Hormone Action

Although a hormone is distributed throughout the body, only those cells with appropriate receptors for that hormone are affected. *Hormone receptors* of the **target cell** have two main functions: (1) to recognize

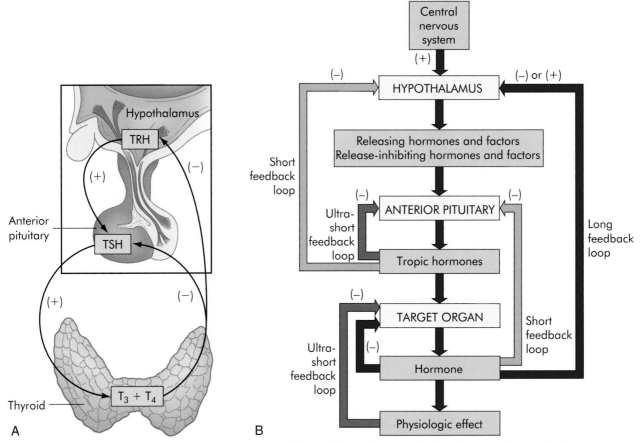

FIGURE 17-2 Feedback Loops. A, Endocrine feedback loops involving the hypothalamus-pituitary gland and end organs; in this example, the thyroid gland is illustrated (endocrine regulation). **B,** General model for control and negative feedback to hypothalamic-pituitary target organ systems. Negative feedback regulation is possible at three levels: target organ (ultra-short feedback), anterior pituitary (short feedback), and hypothalamus (long feedback). *TRH,* Thyroid-releasing hormone; *TSH,* thyroid-stimulating hormone; T_3, triiodothyronine; T_4, tetraiodothyronine (thyroxine).

TABLE 17-2	BINDING PROTEINS, THEIR HORMONES, AND VARIABLES THAT AFFECT THEIR CIRCULATING LEVELS		
BINDING PROTEIN	**HORMONE**	**FACTORS THAT INCREASE BINDING PROTEIN LEVELS**	**FACTORS THAT DECREASE BINDING PROTEIN LEVELS**
Corticosteroid-binding globulin	Cortisol	Estrogen	Liver disease
	Progesterone		
Sex hormone–binding globulin	Dihydrotestosterone	—	Androgens
	Testosterone	Hypothyroidism	
	Estradiol	Liver disease	
Thyroid-binding globulin	Thyroxine (T_4)	Estrogen	Testosterone
	Triiodothyronine (T_3)	Hyperthyroidism	Glucocorticoids
			Liver disease
Albumin	All lipid-soluble hormones	Estrogen	Liver disease
			Malnutrition
			Renal disease

and bind specifically and with high affinity to their particular hormones and (2) to initiate a signal to appropriate intracellular effectors.

The sensitivity of the target cell to a particular hormone is related to the total number of receptors per cell: the more receptors, the more sensitive the cell. Low concentrations of hormone increase the number of receptors per cell; this is called **up-regulation**. High concentrations of hormone decrease the number of receptors; this is called **down-regulation** (Figure 17-3). Thus the cell can adjust its sensitivity to the concentration of the signaling hormone. The receptors on the plasma membrane are continuously synthesized and degraded, so that changes in receptor concentration may occur within hours. Various physiochemical conditions can affect both the receptor number and the affinity of the hormone for its receptor. Some of these physiochemical conditions are the fluidity and structure of the plasma membrane, pH, temperature, ion concentration, diet, and the presence of other chemicals (e.g., drugs).

Hormones affect target cells directly or permissively. **Direct effects** are the obvious changes in cell function that result specifically from stimulation by a particular hormone. **Permissive effects** are less obvious hormone-induced changes that facilitate the maximal response or functioning of a cell. For example, insulin via insulin receptors has a direct effect on skeletal muscle cells, causing increased glucose transport into these cells. Insulin also has a permissive effect on mammary cells, facilitating the response of these cells to the direct effects of prolactin.

Some hormones have biphasic effects that are dependent on the concentration of the hormone. For example, physiologic levels of antidiuretic hormone (ADH) released in response to dehydration stimulate renal tubular reabsorption of sodium and water. However, at very high levels (i.e., achieved with exogenous administration), ADH acts as a vasoconstrictor.

Hormone Receptors

Hormone receptors may be located in the plasma membrane or in the intracellular compartment of the target cell. Water-soluble (peptide) hormones, which include the protein hormones and the catecholamines, have a high molecular weight and cannot diffuse across the cell membrane. They interact or bind with receptors located in or on the cell membrane. Fat-soluble steroid, vitamin D, retinoic acid, and thyroid hormones diffuse freely across the plasma and nuclear membranes and bind with cytosolic or nuclear receptors (Figure 17-4). The hormone-receptor complex binds to a specific region in the deoxyribonucleic acid (DNA) and stimulates the expression of a specific gene. Some fat-soluble hormones (i.e., estrogen [see Chapter 31] may also bind with plasma membrane receptors and can have rapid cellular effects.[1-3]

First and Second Messengers

Receptors for most water-soluble hormones and some steroid hormones are located in the plasma membranes of cells. The hormone is the **first messenger** and is secreted into the bloodstream and carries a message to the target cell. At the target cell it interacts with the receptor on the plasma membrane. The interaction initiates a signal that generates a **second messenger** inside the cell. Second messengers are small molecules, such as cyclic adenosine monophosphate (cAMP), cyclic guanosine monophosphate (cGMP), calcium, and inositol triphosphate (IP_3), and the tyrosine kinase system (Table 17-3). The second messenger transduces the signal from the receptor to the cytoplasm and nucleus of the cell and mediates the effect of the hormone on the target cell (e.g., membrane transport, contractile protein control, enzyme activation, protein synthesis, or cellular growth).

When hormones, such as adrenocorticotropic hormone and thyroid-stimulating hormone, bind to a cell membrane receptor, intracellular levels of cAMP increase. cAMP activates protein kinases, leading to phosphorylation of cellular proteins. This either activates

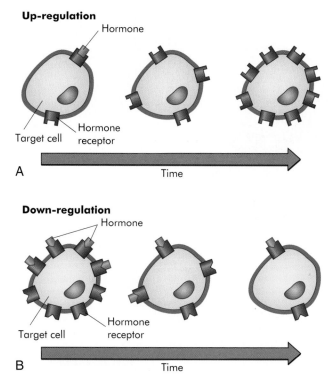

FIGURE 17-3 Regulation of Target Cell Sensitivity. A, Low hormone level and up-regulation, or an increase in the number of receptors. **B,** High hormone level and down-regulation, or a decrease in the number of receptors. (From Patton KT, Thibodeau GA: *Anatomy & physiology,* ed 7, St Louis, 2010, Mosby.)

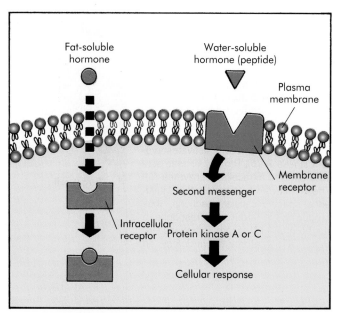

FIGURE 17-4 Hormone Binding at Target Cell.

TABLE 17-3 SECOND MESSENGERS IDENTIFIED FOR SPECIFIC HORMONES

SECOND MESSENGER	ASSOCIATED HORMONES
Cyclic AMP	Adrenocorticotropic hormone (ACTH)
	Luteinizing hormone (LH)
	Human chorionic gonadotropin (hCG)
	Follicle-stimulating hormone (FSH)
	Thyroid-stimulating hormone (TSH)
	Antidiuretic hormone (ADH)
	Thyrotropin-releasing hormone (TRH)
	Parathyroid hormone (PTH)
	Glucagon
Cyclic GMP	Atrial natriuretic peptide
Calcium and IP$_3$	Angiotensin II
	Gonadotropin-releasing hormone (GnRN)
	Antidiuretic hormone (ADH)
	Luteinizing hormone–releasing hormone (LHRH)
Tyrosine kinases	Insulin
	Growth hormone
	Leptin
	Prolactin

AMP, Adenosine monophosphate; *GMP,* guanosine monophosphate; *IP$_3$,* inositol triphosphate.

or deactivates intracellular enzymes, thus directing the actions or products of specific cells (Figure 17-5).

cGMP functions as a second messenger for receptor binding by atrial natriuretic peptide and nitric oxide. These hormones play crucial roles in cardiovascular and pulmonary health and disease; thus drugs such as phosphodiesterase inhibitors that target cGMP are being explored.[4,5]

Calcium and inositol triphosphate function as second messengers for non–steroid hormones, such as angiotensin II and antidiuretic hormone. Hormone receptor binds through a plasma membrane G protein and results in generation of inositol triphosphate. Inositol triphosphate triggers a release of intracellular calcium stores. Increased intracellular calcium levels can lead to the formation of the calcium-calmodulin complex, which mediates the effects of calcium on intracellular activities that are crucial for cell metabolism and growth. For example, calmodulin-dependent protein kinases control intracellular contractile components (myosin and actin, which cause contraction), alter plasma membrane permeability to calcium, and regulate the intracellular enzyme activity that promotes hormone secretion.

Some hormones, such as insulin, growth hormone, and prolactin, bind to surface receptors that directly activate tyrosine kinases. These tyrosine kinases include the Janus family of tyrosine kinases (JAK) and signal transducers and activators of transcription (STAT). They regulate a wide range of intracellular processes that contribute to cellular metabolism and growth, and are being targeted in emerging treatments for diabetes and cancer.[1,6,7]

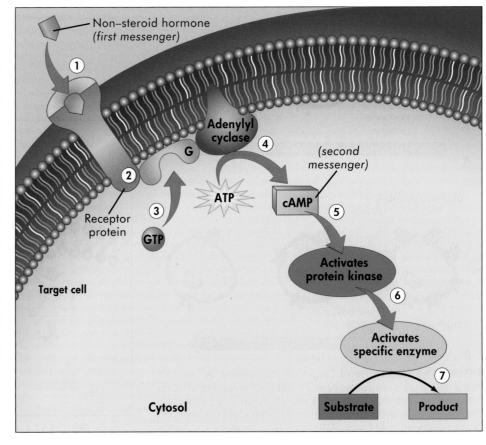

FIGURE 17-5 Example of First- and Second-Messenger Mechanisms. A non–steroid hormone (first messenger) binds to a fixed receptor in the plasma membrane of the target cell *(1).* The hormone-receptor complex activates the G protein *(2).* The activated G protein *(G)* reacts with guanosine triphosphate *(GTP),* which in turn activates the membrane-bound enzyme adenylyl cyclase *(3).* Adenylyl cyclase catalyzes the conversion of adenosine triphosphate *(ATP)* to cyclic adenosine monophosphate *(cAMP)* (second messenger) *(4).* cAMP activates protein kinase A *(5).* Protein kinases activate specific intracellular enzymes *(6).* These activated enzymes then influence specific cellular reactions, thus producing the target cell's response to the hormone *(7).* (From Thibodeau GA, Patton KT: *Anatomy & physiology,* ed 6, St Louis, 2007, Mosby.)

Steroid (Lipid-Soluble) Hormone Receptors

The lipid-soluble hormones are steroid hormones and are synthesized from cholesterol. They include androgens, estrogens, progestins, glucocorticoids, mineralocorticoids, thyroid hormones, vitamin D, and retinoid. Because these are relatively small, lipophilic, hydrophobic molecules, they can cross the lipid plasma membrane by simple diffusion (see Chapter 1). Receptors for steroid hormones are in the cytosol and nucleus and direct gene expression (Figure 17-6). Modulation of gene expression can take hours to days. Studies also reveal that steroid hormone receptors are in the plasma membrane and are associated with rapid responses that may have genomic and nongenomic effects.[8,9]

> **✔ QUICK CHECK 17-1**
> 1. What are hormones? By what mechanisms do they function?
> 2. What is meant by a negative feedback regulation of hormone release?
> 3. How do first messengers differ from second messengers?
> 4. Where are the receptors for steroid (lipid-soluble) hormones located?

STRUCTURE AND FUNCTION OF THE ENDOCRINE GLANDS

Hypothalamic-Pituitary System

The hypothalamic-pituitary axis (HPA) forms the structural and functional basis for central integration of the neurologic and endocrine systems, creating what is called the neuroendocrine system. The HPA produces several hormones that affect a number of diverse body functions (Figure 17-7), including thyroid, adrenal, and reproductive functions.

The **hypothalamus** contains special neurosecretory cells and is located at the base of the brain. It is connected to the pituitary gland by the pituitary stalk (Figure 17-8). The hypothalamus is connected to the anterior pituitary through hypophysial portal blood vessels (Figure 17-9) and to the posterior pituitary via a nerve tract referred to as the *hypothalamohypophysial tract* (Figure 17-10). These connections are vital to the functioning of the hypothalamus-pituitary system. The special cells of the hypothalamus are like other neurons in that they have similar electrical properties, organelles, membranes, and synapses. Neurosecretory cells, however, can synthesize and secrete the hypothalamic-releasing hormones that regulate the release of hormones from the anterior pituitary; in addition, these cells synthesize the hormones antidiuretic hormone (ADH) and oxytocin that are released from the posterior pituitary gland. These hormones are summarized in Table 17-4.

The **pituitary gland** is located in the sella turcica (a saddle-shaped depression of the sphenoid bone at the base of the skull). It weighs approximately 0.5 g, except during pregnancy when its weight approaches 1 g. It is composed of two distinctly different lobes: (1) the anterior pituitary, or adenohypophysis, and (2) the posterior pituitary, or neurohypophysis (see Figure 17-7). These two lobes differ in their embryonic origins, cell types, and functional relationship to the hypothalamus.

The Anterior Pituitary

The **anterior pituitary** (adenohypophysis) accounts for 75% of the total weight of the pituitary gland. It is composed of three regions: (1) the pars distalis, (2) the pars tuberalis, and (3) the pars intermedia. The **pars distalis** is the major component of the anterior pituitary and is the source of the anterior pituitary hormones. The **pars tuberalis** is a thin layer of cells on the anterior and lateral portions of the pituitary stalk. The **pars intermedia** lies between the two. In the adult, the distinct pars intermedia disappears and the individual cells are distributed diffusely throughout the pars distalis and pars nervosa (neural lobe) of the posterior pituitary.

The anterior pituitary is composed of two main cell types: (1) the **chromophobes,** which appear to be nonsecretory, and (2) the

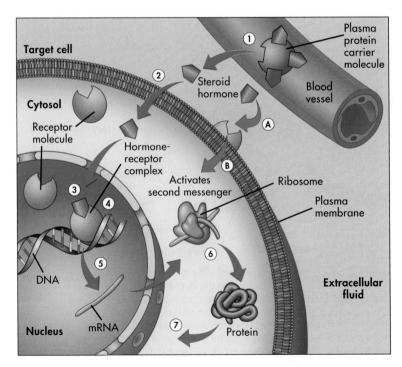

FIGURE 17-6 Steroid Hormone Mechanism. Lipid-soluble steroid hormone molecules detach from the carrier protein *(1)* and pass through the plasma membrane *(2)*. Hormone molecules then diffuse into the nucleus, where they bind to a receptor to form a hormone-receptor complex *(3)*. This complex then binds to a specific site on a deoxyribonucleic acid *(DNA)* molecule *(4)*, triggering transcription of the genetic information encoded there *(5)*. The resulting messenger ribonucleic acid *(mRNA)* molecule moves to the cytosol, where it associates with a ribosome, initiating synthesis of a new protein *(6)*. This new protein—usually an enzyme or channel protein—produces specific effects on the target cell *(7)*. The classic genomic action is typically slow *(red arrows)*. Steroids also may exact rapid effects *(green arrows)* by binding to receptors on the plasma membrane *(A)* and activating an intercellular second messenger *(B)*. (Modified from Patton KT, Thibodeau GA: *Anatomy & physiology,* ed 7, St Louis, 2010, Mosby.)

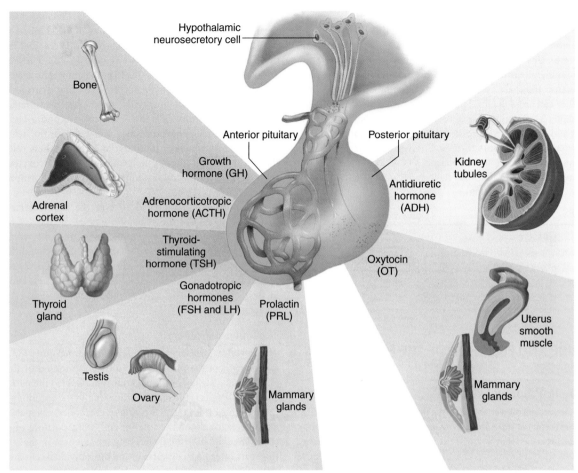

FIGURE 17-7 Pituitary Hormones and Their Target Organs. *FSH,* Follicle-stimulating hormone; *ICSH,* male analog of LH (interstitial cell–stimulating hormone); *LH,* luteinizing hormone. (Modified from Patton KT, Thibodeau GA: *Anatomy & physiology,* ed 7, St Louis, 2010, Mosby.)

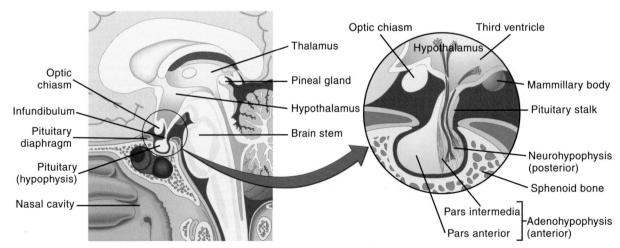

FIGURE 17-8 Location and Structure of the Pituitary Gland (Hypophysis). The pituitary gland is located within the sella turcica of the skull's sphenoid bone and is connected to the hypothalamus by a stalklike infundibulum. The infundibulum passes through a gap in the portion of the dura mater that covers the pituitary (the pituitary diaphragm). The inset shows that the pituitary is divided into an anterior portion, the adenohypophysis, and a posterior portion, the neurohypophysis. The adenohypophysis is further subdivided into the pars anterior and pars intermedia. The pars intermedia is almost absent in the adult pituitary. (Modified from Patton KT, Thibodeau GA: *Anatomy & physiology,* ed 7, St Louis, 2010, Mosby.)

chromophils, which are considered the secretory cells of the adeno-hypophysis. The chromophils are subdivided into seven secretory cell types, and each cell type secretes a specific hormone or hormones. In general, the anterior pituitary hormones are regulated by (1) secretion of hypothalamic peptide hormones or releasing factors, (2) feedback effects of the hormones secreted by target glands, and (3) direct effects of other mediating neurotransmitters. (These are summarized in Figure 17-2.)

The anterior pituitary secretes tropic hormones that affect the physiologic function of specific target organs (see Figure 17-7 and Table 17-5). Melanocyte-stimulating hormone (MSH) promotes the pituitary secretion of melanin, which darkens skin color. The glycoprotein hormones follicle-stimulating hormone (FSH) and luteinizing hormone (LH) influence reproductive function and are discussed in Chapter 31. Adrenocorticotropic hormone (ACTH) regulates the release of cortisol from the adrenal cortex. Thyroid-stimulating hormone (TSH) regulates the activity of the thyroid gland. The roles of ACTH and TSH are discussed later in this chapter. Growth hormone (GH)

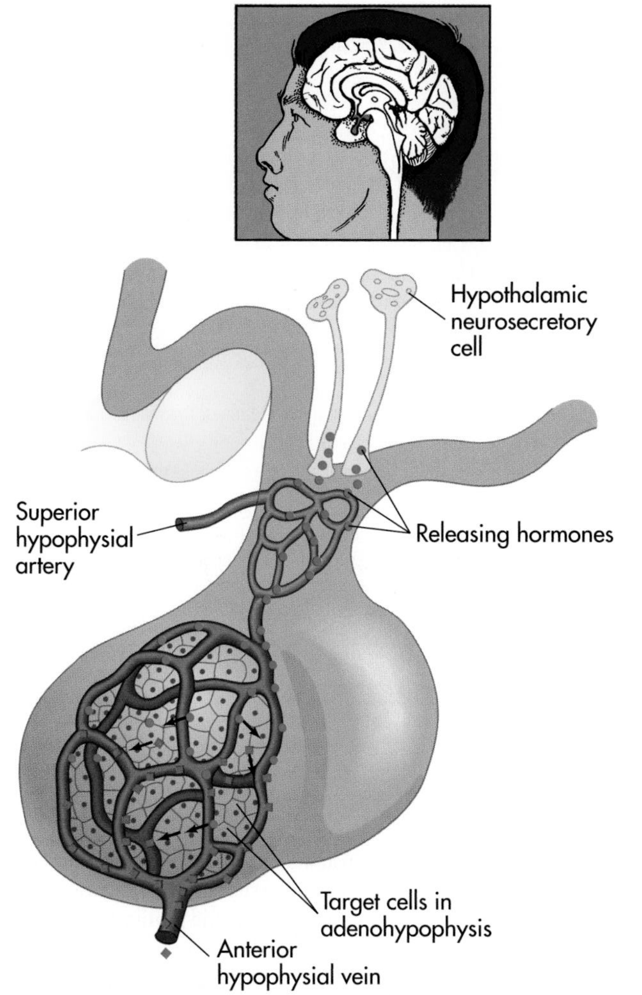

FIGURE 17-9 Hypophysial Portal System. Neurons in the hypothalamus secrete releasing hormones into veins that carry the releasing hormones directly to the vessels of the adenohypophysis, thus bypassing the normal circulatory route. (From Patton KT, Thibodeau GA: *Anatomy & physiology,* ed 7, St Louis, 2010, Mosby.)

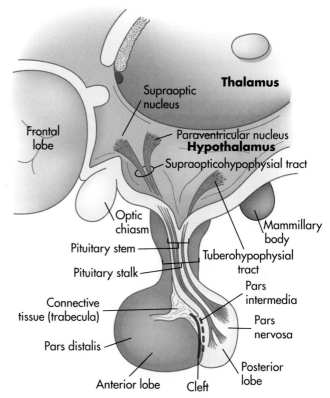

FIGURE 17-10 Nerve Tracts From Hypothalamus to Posterior Lobe of Pituitary Gland. Nerve tracts from hypothalamus to posterior lobe of pituitary gland.

TABLE 17-4 HYPOTHALAMIC HORMONES (HYPOPHYSIOTROPIC HORMONES)

HORMONE	TARGET TISSUE	ACTION
Thyrotropin-releasing hormone (TRH)	Anterior pituitary	Stimulates release of thyroid-stimulating hormone (TSH)
		Modulates prolactin secretion
Gonadotropin-releasing hormone (GnRH)	Anterior pituitary	Stimulates release of follicle-stimulating hormone (FSH) and luteinizing hormone (LH)
Somatostatin	Anterior pituitary	Inhibits release of growth hormone (GH) and TSH
Growth hormone–releasing hormone (GHRH)	Anterior pituitary	Stimulates release of GH
Corticotropin-releasing hormone (CRH)	Anterior pituitary	Stimulates release of adrenocorticotropic hormone (ACTH) and β-endorphin
Substance P	Anterior pituitary	Inhibits synthesis and release of ACTH
		Stimulates secretion of GH, FSH, LH, and prolactin
Prolactin-inhibiting factor (PIF, dopamine)	Anterior pituitary	Inhibits synthesis and secretion of prolactin
Prolactin-releasing factor (PRF)	Anterior pituitary	Stimulates secretion of prolactin

TABLE 17-5 TROPIC HORMONES OF THE ANTERIOR PITUITARY AND THEIR FUNCTIONS

HORMONE	SECRETORY CELL TYPE	TARGET ORGANS	FUNCTIONS
Adrenocorticotropic hormone (ACTH)	Corticotropic	Adrenal gland (cortex)	Increased steroidogenesis (cortisol and androgenic hormones)
			Synthesis of adrenal proteins contributing to maintenance of adrenal gland
Melanocyte-stimulating hormone (MSH)	Melanotropic	Anterior pituitary	Promotes secretion of melanin and lipotropin by anterior pituitary; makes skin darker
Somatotropic Hormones			
Growth hormone (GH)	Somatotropic	Muscle, bone, liver	Regulates metabolic processes related to growth and adaptation to physical and emotional stressors, muscle growth, increased protein synthesis, increased liver glycogenolysis, increased fat mobilization
		Liver	Induces formation of somatomedins, or insulin-like growth factors (IGFs) that have actions similar to insulin
Prolactin	Lactotropic	Breast	Milk production
Glycoprotein Hormones			
Thyroid-stimulating hormone (TSH)	Thyrotropic	Thyroid gland	Increased production and secretion of thyroid hormone
			Increased iodide uptake
			Promotes hypertrophy and hyperplasia of thymocytes
Luteinizing hormone (LH)	Gonadotropic	In women: granulosa cells	Ovulation, progesterone production
		In men: Leydig cells	Testicular growth, testosterone production
Follicle-stimulating hormone (FSH)	Gonadotropic	In women: granulosa cells	Follicle maturation, estrogen production
		In men: Sertoli cells	Spermatogenesis
β-Lipotropin	Corticotropic	Adipose cells	Fat breakdown and release of fatty acids
β-Endorphins	Corticotropic	Adipose cells	Analgesia; may regulate body temperature, food and water intake
		Brain opioid receptors	

and prolactin are called the somatotropic hormones and have diverse effects on body tissues. GH secretion is controlled by two hormones from the hypothalamus: growth hormone–releasing hormone (GHRH), which increases GH secretion; and somatostatin, which inhibits GH secretion. GH is essential to normal tissue growth and maturation and also impacts aging, sleep, nutritional status, stress, and reproductive hormones. Many of the anabolic functions of GH are mediated, at least in part, by the insulin-like growth factors (IGFs), which are also known as the somatomedins.[10] There are two primary forms of IGF: IGF-1 and IGF-2, of which IGF-1 is the most biologically active. They both circulate bound to a group of IGF binding proteins (IGFBP). IGF-1 binds to both insulin receptors, providing an insulin-like effect on skeletal muscle, and to IGF-1 receptor, which mediates the anabolic effects of GH. The IGF-2 receptor causes a negative effect on tissue growth, thus balancing the activity of the IGF-1 receptor. Because of the anabolic effects of GH and IGF, they can be used to treat growth disorders and increase muscle mass but their use has also been linked to increased rates of cancer.[11-13]

Prolactin primarily functions to induce milk production during pregnancy and lactation and also has effects on ovulation and immune function. Synthesis is stimulated by vasoactive intestinal polypeptide, serotonin, and growth factors with release inhibited by dopamine.

The Posterior Pituitary

The embryonic posterior pituitary (neurohypophysis) is derived from the hypothalamus and is comprised of three parts: (1) the median eminence, located at the base of the hypothalamus; (2) the pituitary stalk; and (3) the pars nervosa or neural lobe. The median eminence is composed largely of the nerve endings of axons from the ventral hypothalamus. It often is designated as part of the posterior pituitary but contains at least 10 biologically active hypothalamic-releasing hormones, as well as the neurotransmitters dopamine, norepinephrine, serotonin, acetylcholine, and histamine. The pituitary stalk contains the axons of neurons that originate in the supraoptic and paraventricular nuclei of the hypothalamus and connects the pituitary gland to the brain. Axons originating in the hypothalamus terminate in the pars nervosa, which secretes the hormones of the posterior pituitary (see Figure 17-10).

The posterior pituitary secretes two polypeptide hormones: (1) antidiuretic hormone (ADH), also called arginine vasopressin, and (2) oxytocin. These hormones differ by only two amino acids. They are synthesized—along with their binding proteins, the neurophysins—in the supraoptic and paraventricular nuclei of the hypothalamus (see Figure 17-10). They are packaged in secretory vesicles and are moved down the axons of the pituitary stalk to the pars nervosa for storage. The posterior pituitary thus can be seen as a storage and releasing site for hormones synthesized in the hypothalamus. The release of ADH and oxytocin is mediated by cholinergic and adrenergic neurotransmitters. The major stimulus to both ADH and oxytocin release is glutamate, whereas the major inhibitory input is through gamma-aminobutyric acid (GABA).[14] Before release into the circulatory system, ADH and oxytocin are split from the neurophysins and are secreted in unbound form.

Antidiuretic hormone. The major homeostatic function of the posterior pituitary is the control of plasma osmolality as regulated by ADH, or arginine vasopressin (see Chapter 4). At physiologic levels, ADH increases the permeability of the distal renal tubules and collecting ducts (see Chapter 28. This increased permeability leads to increased water reabsorption into the blood, thus reducing serum osmolality and concentrating the urine. Hypercalcemia, prostaglandin E, and hypokalemia can inhibit this water reabsorption.

The secretion of ADH is regulated primarily by the osmoreceptors of the hypothalamus, located near or in the supraoptic nuclei. As plasma osmolality increases these osmoreceptors are stimulated, the rate of ADH secretion increases, more water is reabsorbed from the kidney, and the plasma is diluted back to its set-point osmolality. ADH has no direct effect on electrolyte levels, but by increasing water reabsorption, serum electrolyte concentrations may decrease because of a dilutional effect.

ADH secretion also is increased by changes in intravascular volume, which are monitored by baroreceptors in the left atrium, in the carotid arteries, and in the aortic arches. A volume loss of 7% to 25% stimulates ADH secretion. Stress, trauma, pain, exercise, nausea, nicotine, exposure to heat, and drugs such as morphine also increase ADH secretion. ADH secretion decreases with decreased plasma osmolality, increased intravascular volume, hypertension, and alcohol ingestion.

ADH was originally named *vasopressin* because in extremely high levels it causes vasoconstriction and a resulting increase in arterial blood pressure. This baroreceptor-mediated response is much less sensitive than the ADH response to changes in osmolality. Therefore physiologic levels of ADH do not significantly impact vessel tone. However, significant vasoconstriction may be achieved pharmacologically. For example, high doses of ADH (given as the drug vasopressin) may be administered to achieve hemostasis during hemorrhage and to raise blood pressure in shock states.[15,16]

Oxytocin. Oxytocin is responsible for contraction of the uterus and milk ejection in lactating women and may affect sperm motility in men. In both genders, oxytocin has an antidiuretic effect similar to that of ADH.

In women, oxytocin is secreted in response to suckling and mechanical distention of the female reproductive tract. Oxytocin binds to its receptors on myoepithelial cells in the mammary tissues and causes contraction of those cells, which increases intramammary pressure and milk expression ("let-down" reflex).

Oxytocin also acts on the uterus to stimulate contractions. Oxytocin functions near the end of labor to enhance effectiveness of contractions, promote delivery of the placenta, and stimulate postpartum uterine contractions, thereby preventing excessive bleeding. The function of this hormone is discussed in detail in Chapter 31.

> ✔ **QUICK CHECK 17-2**
> 1. What is the relationship between the hypothalamus and the pituitary?
> 2. What is the action of antidiuretic hormone (ADH)?

Pineal Gland

The pineal gland is located near the center of the brain and is composed of photoreceptive cells that secrete melatonin. It is innervated by noradrenergic sympathetic nerve terminals controlled by pathways within the hypothalamus. Melatonin release is stimulated by exposure to dark and inhibited by light exposure. It is synthesized from tryptophan, which is first converted to serotonin and then to melatonin. Melatonin regulates circadian rhythms and reproductive systems, including the secretion of the gonadotropin-releasing hormones and the onset of puberty. It also plays an important role in immune regulation and is postulated to impact the aging process. Further effects of melatonin include increasing nitric oxide release from blood

vessels, removing toxic oxygen free radicals, and decreasing insulin secretion.[17]

Thyroid and Parathyroid Glands

The thyroid gland, located in the neck just below the larynx, produces hormones that control the rates of metabolic processes throughout the body. The four parathyroid glands are near the posterior side of the thyroid and function to control serum calcium levels (Figure 17-11).

Thyroid Gland

The two lobes of the thyroid gland lie on either side of the trachea, inferior to the thyroid cartilage and joined by the isthmus (see Figure 17-11). The normal thyroid gland is not visible on inspection, but it may be palpated on swallowing, which causes it to be displaced upward.

The thyroid gland consists of follicles that contain follicular cells surrounding a viscous substance called *colloid* (Figure 17-12). The follicular cells synthesize and secrete the thyroid hormones. Neurons terminate on blood vessels within the thyroid gland and on the follicular cells themselves, so neurotransmitters (acetylcholine, catecholamines) may directly affect the secretory activity of follicular cells.

Also found in the thyroid are parafollicular cells, or C cells (see Figure 17-12). C cells secrete calcitonin and somatostatin. Calcitonin, also called *thyrocalcitonin*, lowers serum calcium levels by inhibition of bone-resorbing osteoclasts (Table 17-6). High levels of calcitonin are required for these effects; however, deficiencies of calcitonin do not lead to hypocalcemia. Consequently, the metabolic consequences of calcitonin deficiency or excess do not appear to be significant in humans. (Bone resorption is explained in Chapter 36.) Calcitonin and parathyroid hormone together regulate calcium balance.

Regulation of thyroid hormone secretion. Thyroid hormone (TH) is regulated through a negative feedback loop involving the hypothalamus, the anterior pituitary, and the thyroid gland (see Figure 17-2). Thyrotropin-releasing hormone (TRH), which is synthesized and stored within the hypothalamus, initiates this loop. TRH is released into the hypothalamic-pituitary portal system and circulates to the anterior pituitary, where it stimulates the release of TSH. TRH levels increase with exposure to cold or stress and from decreased levels of T_4.

Thyroid-stimulating hormone (TSH) is a glycoprotein synthesized and stored within the anterior pituitary. When TSH is secreted by the

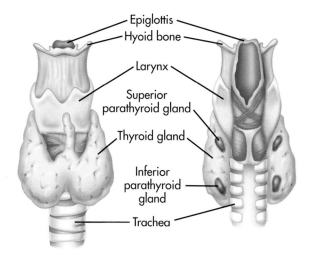

FIGURE 17-11 Thyroid and Parathyroid Glands. Note the relationship of the thyroid and parathyroid glands to each other, to the larynx (voice box), and to the trachea. (From Patton KT, Thibodeau GA: *Anatomy & physiology,* ed 7, St Louis, 2010, Mosby.)

anterior pituitary, it circulates to bind with receptors on the plasma membrane of the thyroid follicular cells. The primary effect of TSH on the thyroid gland is to cause an immediate release of stored TH and an increase in TH synthesis. Another effect of TSH is to affect growth of the thyroid gland by stimulating thymocyte hyperplasia and hypertrophy. As TH levels rise, there is a negative feedback effect on the HPA to inhibit TRH and TSH release, which then results in decreased TH synthesis and secretion. TH synthesis is also controlled by serum iodide levels and by circulating selenium-dependent enzymes, called deiodinases, which inactivate the precursor molecule thyroxine. Thyroid gland hormones and their regulation and function are summarized in Table 17-6.[18,19]

Synthesis of thyroid hormone. The first step in the synthesis of TH is the concentration of iodide by the thyroid gland. Iodide is the inorganic or ionic form of iodine and is the form in which iodine enters the thyroid gland. Because there is an iodide concentration gradient of about 30:1 to 40:1 between the thyroid gland and the blood, iodide is moved by active transport from the extracellular fluid to the thyroid follicular cells (called the iodide trap). The iodide must then be oxidized to iodine by the enzyme thyroidal peroxidase inside the follicular cells.

Thyroglobulin (TG), a large glycoprotein synthesized within the follicular cell, is the precursor of TH. Uniodinated TG is released into the colloid, and iodine combines with tyrosine in the TG to form iodotyrosines. Coupling of iodotyrosines by the enzyme thyroperoxidase

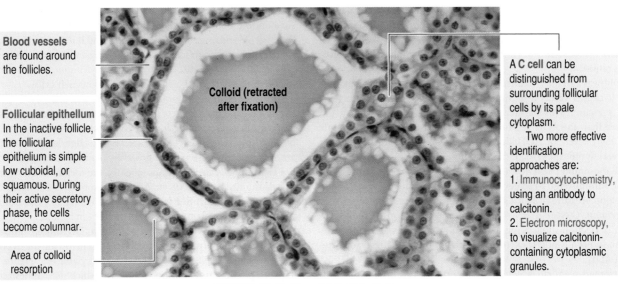

Blood vessels are found around the follicles.

Follicular epithelium In the inactive follicle, the follicular epithelium is simple low cuboidal, or squamous. During their active secretory phase, the cells become columnar.

Area of colloid resorption

Colloid (retracted after fixation)

A **C cell** can be distinguished from surrounding follicular cells by its pale cytoplasm.
   Two more effective identification approaches are:
1. Immunocytochemistry, using an antibody to calcitonin.
2. Electron microscopy, to visualize calcitonin-containing cytoplasmic granules.

FIGURE 17-12 Thyroid Follicle Cells.

TABLE 17-6	THYROID GLAND HORMONES AND THEIR REGULATION AND FUNCTIONS	
HORMONE	**REGULATION**	**FUNCTIONS**

Thyroxine (T$_4$) and triiodothyronine (T$_3$)	T$_4$ and T$_3$ levels are controlled by TSH
	Released in response to metabolic demand
	Influences on amount secreted:
	  Gender
	  Pregnancy
	  Gonadal- and adrenocortical-increased steroids = ↑ levels
	  Exposure to extreme cold = ↑ levels
	  Nutritional state
	  Chemicals
	  GHIH = ↓ levels
	  Dopamine = ↓ levels
	  Catecholamines = ↑ levels
		Regulates protein, fat, and carbohydrate catabolism in all cells
		Regulates metabolic rate of all cells
		Regulates body heat production
		Insulin antagonist
		Maintains growth hormone secretion, skeletal maturation
		Affects CNS development
		Necessary for muscle tone and vigor
		Maintains cardiac rate, force, and output
		Maintains secretion of GI tract
		Affects respiratory rate and oxygen utilization
		Maintains calcium mobilization
		Affects RBC production
		Stimulates lipid turnover, free fatty acid release, and cholesterol synthesis

Calcitonin	Elevated serum calcium level—major stimulant for calcitonin
	Other stimulants:
	  Gastrin
	  Calcium-rich foods (regardless of serum Ca^{++} levels)
	  Pregnancy
	Lowered serum calcium level—suppresses calcitonin release
		Lowers serum calcium level by opposing bone-resorbing effects of PTH, prostaglandins, and calciferols by inhibiting osteoclastic activity
		Lowers serum phosphate levels
		Decreases calcium and phosphorus absorption in GI tract

From Monohan FD et al: Phipps' medical-surgical nursing: health and illness perspective, ed 8, St Louis, 2007, Mosby.
CNS, Central nervous system; *GHIH,* growth hormone–inhibiting hormone; *GI,* gastrointestinal; *PTH,* parathyroid hormone; *RBC,* red blood cell; *TSH,* thyroid-stimulating hormone.

forms TH. Triiodothyronine (T_3) is formed from the coupling of monoiodotyrosine (one iodine atom and tyrosine) and diiodotyrosine (two iodine atoms and tyrosine). Thyroxine is tetraiodothyronine (T_4) and is formed from the coupling of two diiodotyrosines. Nearly 90% of TH is synthesized as T_4; however, most of the T_4 is then converted to T_3, which acts on the target cell.

TH is transported in the blood in bound and free forms. Most of the TH is transported bound to **thyroxine-binding globulin (TBG)** and to a lesser extent by thyroxine-binding prealbumin or albumin. The free form is generally considered to be biologically active, and the bound form serves as a reservoir.[20]

Actions of thyroid hormone. TH affects many body tissues and has a significant effect on the growth and maturation of tissues. TH is essential for normal growth and neurologic development in the fetus and infant and affects neurologic functioning in adults. Similar to some steroid hormones, TH binds to intracellular receptor complexes that then influence the genetic expression of specific proteins. TH also affects cell metabolism by altering protein, fat, and glucose metabolism and, as a result, heat production and oxygen consumption are increased. Thus these hormones are essential for maintaining healthy metabolic processes, and their use is being explored for the therapy of many metabolic disorders.[21]

Parathyroid Glands

Normally two pairs of small parathyroid glands are present behind the upper and lower poles of the thyroid gland (see Figure 17-11). However, their number may range from two to six.

The parathyroid glands produce **parathyroid hormone (PTH)**, which is the single most important factor in the regulation of serum calcium concentration. The overall effect of PTH secretion is to increase serum calcium concentration and decrease serum phosphate level. A decrease in serum-ionized calcium level stimulates PTH secretion. PTH acts directly on the bone to release calcium by stimulating osteoclast activity. PTH also acts on the kidney to increase calcium reabsorption and to decrease phosphate reabsorption. The resultant increase in serum calcium concentration inhibits PTH secretion. **1,25-Dihydroxy-vitamin D_3** (the active form of vitamin D) works as a cofactor with PTH to promote calcium and phosphate absorption in the gut and enhance bone mineralization. Vitamin D also plays an important role in metabolic processes and controlling inflammation. It has been found to be deficient in the majority of individuals in the United States (see *Health Alert:* Vitamin D).

Phosphate and magnesium concentrations also affect PTH secretion. An increase in serum phosphate level decreases serum calcium level by causing calcium-phosphate precipitation into soft tissue and bone, which indirectly stimulates PTH secretion. Hypomagnesemia in persons with normal calcium levels acts as a mild stimulant to PTH secretion; however, in persons with hypocalcemia, hypomagnesemia decreases PTH secretion.[22]

> ✔ **QUICK CHECK 17-3**
> 1. How does the anterior pituitary regulate the thyroid gland?
> 2. What form of thyroid hormone is biologically active?
> 3. What two organs are the sites of action of parathyroid hormone (PTH)?

Endocrine Pancreas

The **pancreas** is both an endocrine gland that produces hormones and an exocrine gland that produces digestive enzymes. (The exocrine function of the pancreas is discussed in Chapter 33.) The pancreas is located behind the stomach, between the spleen and the duodenum.

HEALTH ALERT

Vitamin D

Vitamin D is essential for bone health and is widely used for the prevention and treatment of postmenopausal osteoporosis and renal osteodystrophy. More recently, vitamin D deficiency has been found to affect more than 75% of all Americans, and more than 90% of Americans with pigmented skin. Inadequate serum levels of vitamin D have been linked to infections, cancer, heart disease, dementia, diabetes, chronic pain syndromes, and autoimmune disorders. Recommendations for vitamin D supplementation include increased intake of vitamin D–containing foods (seafood, vitamin D–fortified juices, and milk products), increased exposure to sunlight, and vitamin D supplementation with a goal of achieving a serum level of 35 to 50 ng/mL.

Data from Holick MF et al: Evaluation, treatment, and prevention of vitamin D deficiency: an Endocrine Society clinical practice guideline, *J Clin Endocrinol Metab* 96(7):1911–1930, 2011. Bruner RL et al: Calcium, vitamin D supplementation and physical function in the Women's Health Initiative, *J Am Dietetic Assoc* 108:1472–1479, 2008; Dimeglio LA: Pediatric endocrinology: vitamin D and cardiovascular disease risk in children, *Nat Rev Endocrinol* 6(1):12–13, 2010; Pearce SH, Cheetham TD: Diagnosis and management of vitamin D deficiency, *BMJ* 340:b5664, 2010; Institute of Medicine: *Dietary reference intakes for vitamin D and calcium*, National Acadamies of Science, November 30, 2010. Available at http://www.iom.edu/Reports/2010/Dietary-Reference-Intakes-for-Calcium-and-Vitamin-D.aspx.

It houses the **islets of Langerhans.** The islets of Langerhans have four types of hormone-secreting cells: **alpha cells,** which secrete glucagon; **beta cells,** which secrete insulin and amylin; **delta cells,** which secrete gastrin and somatostatin; and **F (or PP) cells,** which secrete pancreatic polypeptide. These hormones regulate carbohydrate, fat, and protein metabolism. (The pancreas is illustrated in Figure 17-13.) Nerves from both the sympathetic and parasympathetic divisions of the autonomic nervous system innervate the pancreatic islets.

Insulin

The beta cells of the pancreas synthesize **insulin** from the precursor proinsulin, which is formed from a larger precursor molecule, preproinsulin. Proinsulin is composed of A peptide and B peptide connected by a C peptide and two disulfide bonds. C peptide is cleaved by proteolytic enzymes, leaving the bonded A and B peptides as the insulin molecule. C peptide level can be measured in the blood and used as an indirect measurement of serum insulin synthesis.[23] Secretion of insulin is regulated by chemical, hormonal, and neural control. Insulin secretion is promoted when blood levels of glucose, amino acids (arginine and lysine), and gastrointestinal hormones (glucagon, gastrin, cholecystokinin, secretin) increase, and when the beta cells are stimulated parasympathetically. Insulin secretion diminishes in response to low blood levels of glucose (hypoglycemia), high levels of insulin (through negative feedback to the beta cells), and sympathetic stimulation of the alpha cells in the islets. Prostaglandins also inhibit insulin secretion.

At the target cell, insulin combines with an enzyme-linked plasma membrane receptor that contains tyrosine kinase on the cytosolic surface. Insulin receptor binding activates tyrosine kinase autophosphorylation and sends a cascade of signals to activate glucose transporters (GLUT) for entry of glucose into the cell, and to phosphorylate protein kinase.[24] Protein kinase then activates or deactivates target enzymes for glucose metabolism (Figure 17-14).

The sensitivity of the insulin receptor is a key component in maintaining normal cellular function; insulin resistance has been implicated

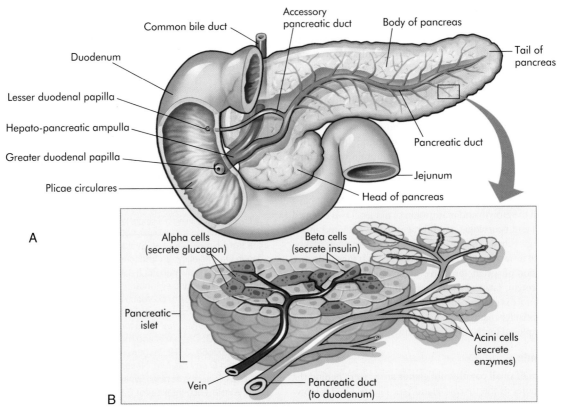

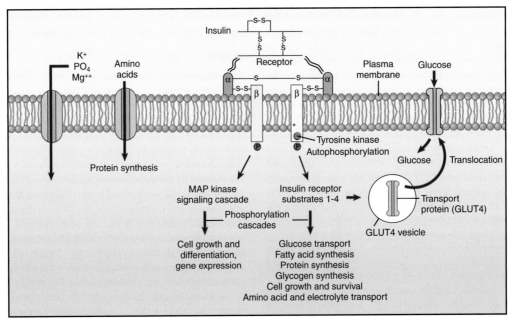

FIGURE 17-13 The Pancreas. **A,** Pancreas dissected to show main and accessory ducts. The main duct may join the common bile duct, as shown here, to enter the duodenum by a single opening at the major duodenal papilla, or the two ducts may have separate openings. The accessory pancreatic duct is usually present and has a separate opening into the duodenum. **B,** Exocrine glandular cells (around small pancreatic ducts) and endocrine glandular cells of the pancreatic islets (adjacent to blood capillaries). Exocrine pancreatic cells secrete pancreatic juice, alpha endocrine cells secrete glucagon, and beta cells secrete insulin. (From Thibodeau GA, Patton KT: *Anatomy & physiology,* ed 6, St Louis, 2007, Mosby.)

FIGURE 17-14 Insulin Action on Cells. Binding of insulin to its receptor causes autophosphorylation of the receptor, which then itself acts as a tyrosine kinase that phosphorylates insulin receptor substrate 1 *(IRS-1).* Numerous target enzymes, such as protein kinase B and MAP kinase, are activated and these enzymes have a multitude of effects on cell function. The glucose transporter *(GLUT4)* is recruited to the plasma membrane, where it facilitates glucose entry into the cell. The transport of amino acids, potassium, magnesium, and phosphate into the cell is also facilitated. The synthesis of various enzymes is induced or suppressed, and cell growth is regulated by signal molecules that modulate gene expression. *IREs,* Insulin responsive elements; *mRNA,* messenger ribonucleic acid. (Redrawn from Berne RM, Levy MN: *Principles of physiology,* ed 3, St Louis, 2000, Mosby.)

in numerous cardiovascular diseases, including hypertension and diabetes. Adipocytes release a number of hormones that are altered in obesity and have an important impact on insulin sensitivity (see *Health Alert:* Hormones from Adipose Tissue—The Adipokines).

HEALTH ALERT

Hormones from Adipose Tissue—The Adipokines

Several hormones are released from adipose cells that affect many other tissues. The best known of these substances are leptin and adiponectin. *Leptin* decreases appetite but in obese individuals levels of leptin are chronically elevated and lead to resistance to its appetite-suppressive functions. Chronically elevated levels of leptin also can result in many adverse effects on tissues and contribute to vascular diseases, such as atherosclerosis and hypertension. In contrast, *adiponectin* is a protective hormone that is decreased in obesity. It normally helps maintain insulin sensitivity and protect vascular function. Finally, *resistin* is another less well-known adipokine that is increased in obesity and that decreases insulin sensitivity. These hormones also have been implicated in bone diseases and cancer. The roles of these hormones in health and disease are being intensively studied in the search for new therapeutic modalities to treat obesity-related disorders.

Data from Kelesidis T et al: Narrative review: the role of leptin in human physiology: emerging clinical applications, *Ann Intern Med* 152(2):93–100, 2010; Maury E, Brichard SM: Adipokine dysregulation, adipose tissue inflammation and metabolic syndrome, *Mol Cell Endocrinol* 314(1):1–16, 2010; Oswal A, Yeo G: Leptin and the control of body weight: a review of its diverse central targets, signaling mechanisms, and role in the pathogenesis of obesity, *Obesity* 18(2):221–229, 2010; Ouchi N, et al: Adipokines in inflammation and metabolic disease, *Nat Rev Immunol* 11(2):85–97, 2011; Cui J, Panse S, Falkner B: The role of adiponectin in metabolic and vascular disease: a review, *Clin Nephrol* 75(1):26–33, 2011.

Insulin is an anabolic hormone that promotes glucose uptake and the synthesis of proteins, carbohydrates, lipids, and nucleic acids and functions mainly in the liver, muscle, and adipose tissue. Table 17-7 summarizes the actions of insulin. The net effect of insulin in these tissues is to stimulate protein and fat synthesis and decrease blood glucose level. The brain, red blood cells, kidney, and lens of the eye do not require insulin for glucose transport. Insulin also facilitates the intracellular transport of potassium (K^+), phosphate, and magnesium.

Amylin

Amylin (or islet amyloid polypeptide) is a hormone co-secreted with insulin in response to nutrient stimuli. It regulates blood glucose concentration by delaying nutrient uptake and suppressing glucagon secretion after meals. Amylin also has a satiety effect. Through these mechanisms, amylin has an antihyperglycemic effect.[25]

Glucagon

Glucagon is produced by the alpha cells of the pancreas and by cells lining the gastrointestinal tract. Glucagon acts primarily in the liver and increases blood glucose concentration by stimulating glycogenolysis and gluconeogenesis in muscle and lipolysis in adipose tissue. Amino acids, such as alanine, glycine, and asparagine, stimulate glucagon secretion. Glucagon release is inhibited by high glucose levels and stimulated by low glucose levels and sympathetic stimulation; thus it is antagonistic to insulin.[26]

Pancreatic Somatostatin

The somatostatin produced by delta cells of the pancreas is essential in carbohydrate, fat, and protein metabolism (homeostasis of ingested nutrients). It is different from hypothalamic somatostatin, which inhibits the release of growth hormone and TSH. Pancreatic somatostatin is involved in regulating alpha-cell and beta-cell function within the islets by inhibiting secretion of insulin, glucagon, and pancreatic polypeptide.[26]

Gastrin, Grehlin, and Pancreatic Polypeptide

The function of pancreatic gastrin has not been established. It is postulated that fetal pancreatic gastrin secretion is necessary for adequate islet cell development. Grehlin stimulates GH secretion, controls appetite, and plays a role in the regulation of insulin sensitivity. Pancreatic polypeptide is released by F cells in response to hypoglycemia and protein-rich meals. It inhibits gallbladder contraction and exocrine pancreas secretion and is frequently increased in individuals with pancreatic tumors or diabetes.[25]

Adrenal Glands

The adrenal glands are paired, pyramid-shaped organs behind the peritoneum and close to the upper pole of each kidney. Each gland is surrounded by a capsule, embedded in fat, and well supplied with blood from the phrenic and renal arteries and the aorta. Venous return from the left adrenal gland is to the renal vein and from the right adrenal gland is to the inferior vena cava.

Each adrenal gland consists of two separate portions—an inner medulla and an outer cortex. These two portions have different embryonic origins, structures, and hormonal functions. In effect, each adrenal gland functions like two separate glands, although there are interrelationships (Figure 17-15).

The adrenal cortex, or outer region of the gland, accounts for 80% of the weight of the adult gland. The cortex is histologically subdivided into the following three zones[27]:

1. The zona glomerulosa, the outer layer, constitutes about 15% of the cortex and primarily produces the mineralocorticoid aldosterone.
2. The zona fasciculata, the middle layer, constitutes 78% of the cortex and secretes the glucocorticoids cortisol, cortisone, and corticosterone.
3. The zona reticularis, the inner layer, constitutes 7% of the cortex and secretes mineralocorticoids (aldosterone), adrenal androgens and estrogens, and glucocorticoids.

TABLE 17-7   INSULIN ACTIONS

ACTIONS	SITES OF INSULIN ACTION		
	LIVER CELLS	MUSCLE CELLS	ADIPOSE CELLS
Glucose uptake	Increased	Increased	Increased
Glucose use	—	—	Increased glycerol phosphate
Glycogenesis	Increased	Increased	—
Glycogenolysis	Decreased	Decreased	—
Glycolysis	Increased	Increased	Increased
Gluconeogenesis	Increased	—	—
Other	Increased fatty acid synthesis	Increased amino acid uptake	Increased fat esterification
	Decreased ketogenesis	Increased protein synthesis	Decreased lipolysis
	Decreased urea cycle activity	Decreased proteolysis	Increased fat storage

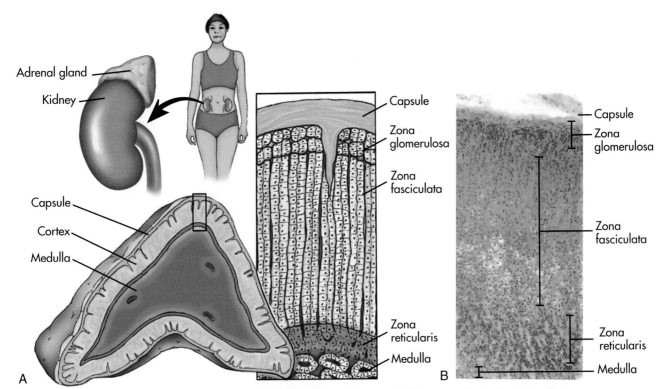

FIGURE 17-15 Structure of the Adrenal Gland Showing Cell Layers (Zonae) of the Cortex. **A,** Zona glomerulosa secretes aldosterone. Zona fasciculata secretes abundant amounts of glucocorticoids, chiefly cortisol. Zona reticularis secretes minute amounts of sex hormones and glucocorticoids. **B,** A portion of the medulla is visible at the lower right in the photomicrograph (×35) and at the bottom of the drawing. (**A** from Patton KT, Thibodeau GA: *Anatomy & physiology,* ed 7, St Louis, 2010, Mosby; **B** from Kierszenbaum A: *Histology and cell biology,* St Louis, 2002, Mosby.)

The adrenal medulla, which accounts for 20% of the gland's total weight, secretes the catecholamines epinephrine (adrenaline) and norepinephrine (noradrenaline). Both sympathetic and parasympathetic cholinergic fibers innervate the adrenal medulla.

Adrenal Cortex

The adrenal cortex secretes several steroid hormones, including the glucocorticoids, the mineralocorticoids, and the adrenal androgens and estrogens. These hormones are all synthesized from cholesterol. The cells of the adrenal cortex are stimulated by adrenocorticotropic hormone (ACTH) from the pituitary gland.[27] The best known pathway of steroidogenesis involves the conversion of cholesterol to pregnenolone, which is then converted to the major corticosteroids. The adrenal cortex also contains a high concentration of ascorbic acid (vitamin C) and vitamin A.

Glucocorticoids

Functions of the glucocorticoids. The glucocorticoids are steroid hormones that have metabolic, anti-inflammatory, and growth-suppressing effects and influence levels of awareness and sleep patterns. (These functions are summarized in Box 17-1). Glucocorticoids have direct effects on carbohydrate metabolism. These hormones increase blood glucose concentration by promoting gluconeogenesis in the liver and by decreasing uptake of glucose into muscle cells, adipose cells, and lymphatic cells. In extrahepatic tissues, they stimulate protein catabolism and inhibit amino acid uptake and protein synthesis.

The glucocorticoids act at several sites to influence immune and inflammatory reactions. One major immune suppressant effect is the glucocorticoid-mediated decrease in the proliferation of T lymphocytes, primarily T-helper lymphocytes. There is a greater effect on T-helper 1 (Th1) cytokine production (including antiviral interferons) than there is T-helper 2 (Th2) cytokine production and therefore greater depression of cellular immunity than humoral immunity (see Chapter 7). Glucocorticoids affect innate immunity through several pathways, including decreasing the activity of pattern receptors on the surface of macrophages (see Chapter 5). Glucocorticoids also have anti-inflammatory effects related to decreased function of natural killer cells, suppression of inflammatory cytokines, and stabilization of lysosomal membranes, which decreases the release of proteolytic enzymes.[27] This suppression of innate and adaptive immunity by glucocorticoids means that infection and poor wound healing are some of the most problematic complications of the use of glucocorticoids in the treatment of disease. Similarly, psychologic and physiologic stress increases glucocorticoid production, which provides a pathway for the well-described decrease in immunity seen in both acute and chronic stress conditions (see Chapter 8).

Other effects of glucocorticoids include inhibition of bone formation, inhibition of ADH secretion, and stimulation of gastric acid secretion. Glucocorticoids appear to potentiate the effects of catecholamines, including sensitizing the arterioles to the vasoconstrictive effects of norepinephrine. Thyroid hormone and growth hormone effects on adipose tissue are also potentiated by glucocorticoids. A metabolite of cortisol may act like a barbiturate and depress nerve cell function in the brain, accounting for the noted effects on mood associated with steroid level fluctuation in disease or stress.

Pathologically high levels of glucocorticoids increase the number of circulating erythrocytes (leading to polycythemia), increase the

BOX 17-1 MAJOR FUNCTIONS OF GLUCOCORTICOIDS

Metabolic
Increase blood glucose concentration
  Increase hepatic gluconeogenesis
  Decease glucose use in muscle, adipose, and lymphatic tissue
  Antagonize insulin
Stimulate protein catabolism and decrease protein synthesis

Inflammatory and Immune
Decrease cellular immunity
  Decrease T lymphocyte proliferation
  Decrease natural killer cell activity
  Decrease macrophage activity
Anti-inflammatory
  Decrease number of eosinophils
  Decrease number of fibroblasts
  Decrease inflammatory cytokines (interleukins, bradykinin, serotonin, and histamine)
  Stimulate anti-inflammatory cytokines (interleukin-10, transforming growth factor-beta)
  Stabilize lysosomal membranes

Other
Inhibit bone formation
Inhibit ADH and ACTH secretion
Stimulate gastric acid secretion
Potentiate the effects of catecholamines, thyroid hormone, and growth hormone on adipose tissue
Affect nerve function in the brain (affects mood and sleep)

Data from Stewart PM, Krone NP: The adrenal cortex. In Melmed S, et al: *Williams textbook of endocrinology,* ed 12, Philadelphia, 2011, Saunders.

appetite, promote fat deposition in the face and cervical areas, increase uric acid excretion, decrease serum calcium levels (possibly by inhibiting gastrointestinal absorption of calcium), suppress the secretion and synthesis of ACTH, and interfere with the action of growth hormone so that somatic growth is inhibited.

Cortisol. The most potent naturally occurring glucocorticoid is cortisol. It is the main secretory product of the adrenal cortex and is needed to maintain life and protect the body from stress (see Figure 8-1). Cortisol has a biologic half-life of approximately 90 minutes, with the liver primarily responsible for its deactivation.

Cortisol secretion is regulated primarily by the hypothalamus and the anterior pituitary gland (Figure 17-16). **Corticotropin-releasing hormone (CRH)** is produced by several nuclei in the hypothalamus and stored in the median eminence. Once released, CRH travels through the portal vessels to stimulate the production of ACTH, β-lipotropin, γ-lipotropin, endorphins, and enkephalins by the anterior pituitary. ACTH is the main regulator of cortisol secretion and adrenocortical growth.

ACTH is synthesized as part of a precursor called pro-opiomelanocortin (POMC). Three factors appear to be primarily involved in regulating the secretion of ACTH: (1) high circulating levels of cortisol and synthetic glucocorticoids suppress both CRH and ACTH, whereas low cortisol levels stimulate their secretion; (2) diurnal rhythms affect ACTH and cortisol levels (in persons with regular sleep-wake patterns, ACTH peaks 3 to 5 hours after sleep begins and declines throughout the day, and cortisol

levels follow a similar pattern); and (3) psychologic and physiologic (e.g., hypoxia, hypoglycemia, hyperthermia, exercise) stress increases ACTH secretion, leading to increased cortisol levels. (Neurologic mechanisms regulating sleep are discussed in Chapter 13.) A form of immunoreactive ACTH (ir ACTH) is produced by the cells of the immune system and may account, in part, for integration of the immune and endocrine systems.

Once ACTH is secreted, it binds to specific plasma membrane receptors on the cells of the adrenal cortex and on other extraadrenal tissues. Because both adrenal and extraadrenal tissues have ACTH receptors, a number of effects result from stimulation by ACTH. In addition to increasing adrenocortical secretion of cortisol, ACTH maintains the size and synthetic functions of the adrenal cortex through activation of crucial enzymes and storage of cholesterol for metabolism into steroid hormones. Extraadrenal effects of ACTH include stimulation of melanocytes and activation of tissue lipase.

Once ACTH stimulates the cells of the adrenal cortex, cortisol synthesis and secretion immediately occur. In the healthy person, the secretory patterns of ACTH and cortisol are nearly identical. After secretion, some cortisol circulates in bound form attached to albumin but primarily it is bound to the plasma protein transcortin. A smaller amount circulates in the free form and diffuses into cells with specific intracellular receptors for cortisol. ACTH is rapidly inactivated in the circulation, and the liver and kidneys remove the deactivated hormone.

Mineralocorticoids: aldosterone. Mineralocorticoid steroids directly affect ion transport by epithelial cells, causing sodium retention and potassium and hydrogen loss. Aldosterone is the most potent naturally occurring mineralocorticoid and conserves sodium by increasing the activity of the sodium pump of epithelial cells. (The sodium pump is described in Chapter 1.)

The initial stages of aldosterone synthesis occur in the zona fasciculata and zona reticularis. The final conversion of corticosterone to aldosterone is confined to the zona glomerulosa. Aldosterone synthesis and secretion are regulated primarily by the renin-angiotensin system (described in Chapter 28). The renin-angiotensin system is activated by sodium and water depletion, increased potassium levels, and a diminished effective blood volume (Figure 17-17). Angiotensin II is the primary stimulant of aldosterone synthesis and secretion; however, sodium and potassium levels also may directly affect aldosterone secretion. ACTH may transiently stimulate aldosterone synthesis but does not appear to be a major regulator of secretion.

When sodium and potassium levels are within normal limits, approximately 50 to 250 mg of aldosterone is secreted daily. Of the secreted aldosterone, 50% to 75% binds to plasma proteins. The large proportion of unbound aldosterone contributes to its rapid metabolic turnover in the liver, its low plasma concentration, and its short half-life (about 15 minutes). Aldosterone is degraded in the liver and is excreted by the kidney.

Aldosterone maintains extracellular volume by acting on distal nephron epithelial cells to increase sodium reabsorption and potassium and hydrogen excretion. This renal effect takes 90 minutes to 6 hours. Other effects of aldosterone include enhancement of cardiac muscle contraction, stimulation of ectopic ventricular activity through secondary cardiac pacemakers in the ventricles, stiffening of blood vessels with increased vascular resistance, and decreased fibrinolysis. Pathologically elevated levels of aldosterone have been implicated in the myocardial changes associated with heart failure, resistant hypertension, insulin resistance, and systemic inflammation.[28,29]

Adrenal estrogens and androgens. The healthy adrenal cortex secretes minimal amounts of estrogen and androgens. ACTH appears to be the major regulator. Some of the weakly androgenic substances secreted by the cortex (dehydroepiandrosterone [DHEA], androstenedione) are converted by peripheral tissues to stronger androgens, such as testosterone,

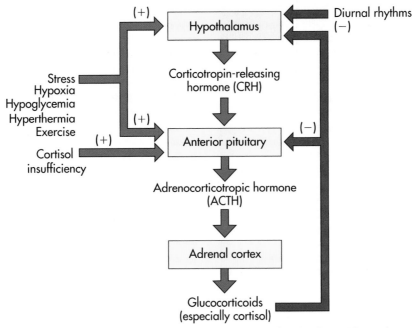

FIGURE 17-16 Feedback Control of Glucocorticoid Synthesis and Secretion.

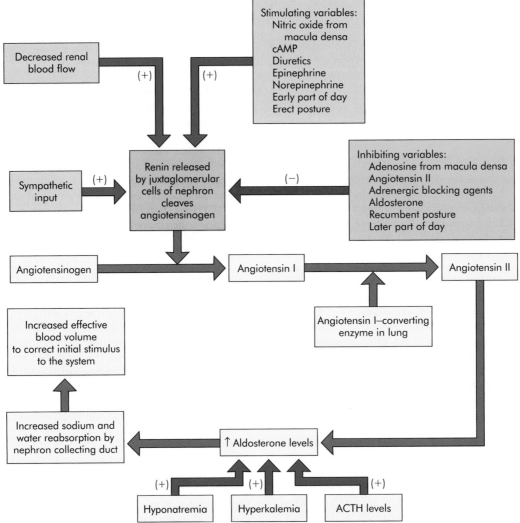

FIGURE 17-17 The Feedback Mechanisms Regulating Aldosterone Secretion. *ACTH,* Adrenocorticotropic hormone; *cAMP,* cyclic adenosine monophosphate.

thus accounting for some androgenic effects initiated by the adrenal cortex. Peripheral conversion of adrenal androgens to estrogens is enhanced in aging or obese persons as well as in those with liver disease or hyperthyroidism.[30] The biologic effects and metabolism of the adrenal sex steroids do not vary from those produced by the gonads (see Chapter 31).

Adrenal Medulla

The adrenal medulla, together with the sympathetic division of the autonomic nervous system, is embryonically derived from neural crest cells. Chromaffin cells (pheochromocytes) are the cells of the adrenal medulla. The major products stored and secreted by the chromaffin cells are the catecholamines epinephrine (adrenaline) and norepinephrine, which are synthesized from the amino acid phenylalanine (Figure 17-18). Only 30% of circulating epinephrine comes from the adrenal medulla; the other 70% is released from nerve terminals. The medulla is only a minor source of norepinephrine. The adrenal medulla functions as a sympathetic ganglion without postganglionic processes. Sympathetic cholinergic preganglion fibers terminate on the chromaffin cells and secrete catecholamines directly into the bloodstream. The catecholamines are therefore hormones and not neurotransmitters.

Physiologic stress to the body (e.g., traumatic injury, hypoxia, hypoglycemia, and many others) triggers release of adrenal catecholamines through acetylcholine (from the preganglionic sympathetic fibers), which depolarizes the chromaffin cells. Depolarization causes exocytosis of the storage granules from the chromaffin cells with release of epinephrine and norepinephrine into the bloodstream. Secretion of adrenal catecholamines also is increased by ACTH and the glucocorticoids.[31]

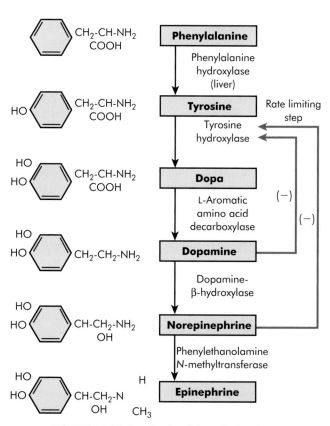

FIGURE 17-18 Synthesis of Catecholamines.

Once released, the catecholamines remain in the plasma for only seconds to minutes. The catecholamines exert their biologic effects after binding to plasma membrane receptors (α_1, α_2, β_1, β_2, and β_3) in target cells. This binding activates the adenylyl cyclase system. Catecholamines are rapidly removed from the plasma by being absorbed by neurons for storage in new cytoplasmic granules, or they may be metabolically inactivated and excreted in the urine. The catecholamines directly inhibit their own secretion by decreasing the formation of the enzyme tyrosine hydroxylase (the rate-limiting step).

Catecholamines have diverse effects on the entire body. Their release and the body's response have been characterized as the fight-or-flight response (stress response) (see Figure 8-2 and Figure 8-3 and Tables 8-3 and 8-4). Metabolic effects of catecholamines promote hyperglycemia through a variety of mechanisms including interference with the usual glucose regulatory feedback mechanisms.

> **✓ QUICK CHECK 17-4**
> 1. What are the islets of Langerhans? Where are they located?
> 2. Compare and contrast the actions of alpha, beta, delta, and F cells.
> 3. What is the most potent naturally occurring glucocorticoid, and how is its secretion related to that of adrenocorticotropic hormone (ACTH)?
> 4. How does aldosterone influence fluid and electrolyte balance?
> 5. What are catecholamines?

Neuroendocrine Response to Stressors

The endocrine system acts together with the nervous and immune systems to respond to stressors. Perception that an event is stressful may be essential to the emotional arousal and initiation of the stress response. Some events, such as bacterial invasion, can activate the stress response without emotional arousal. Details of the stress response are presented in Chapter 8. Methods of hormone measurement are given in Box 17-2.

BOX 17-2   METHODS OF HORMONE MEASUREMENT

Radioimmunoassay (RIA)
In this immunologic technique, known amounts of antibody and radiolabeled hormone are placed in an assay tube with the unlabeled hormone. The radiolabeled hormone competes chemically with the nonlabeled hormone molecules for binding sites on the antibodies. When increasing amounts of unlabeled hormones are added to the assay, the limited binding sites of the antibody can bind less of the radiolabeled hormone. Therefore, the higher the concentration of unlabeled hormone, the fewer the number of radioactive *counts,* or labeled hormone, that bind with the fixed concentration of antibody. A quantitative value is established by use of standard reference curves.

Enzyme-Linked Immunosorbent Assay (ELISA)
Used to determine circulating hormone levels. The method is similar to that of RIA but is less expensive and easier to conduct. Instead of radiolabeled hormones, an enzyme-labeled hormone is used. The enzyme activity in either the bound or the unbound fraction is determined and related to the concentration of the unlabeled hormone.

Bioassay
This assay uses graded doses of hormone in a reference preparation and then compares the results with an unknown sample. Bioassays are used more commonly in investigative endocrinology than in clinical laboratories.

GERIATRIC CONSIDERATIONS
Aging & Its Effects on Specific Endocrine Glands

General Endocrine Changes With Aging

Atrophy and weight loss with vascular changes; decreased secretion and clearance of hormones often occurs; variable change in receptor binding and intracellular responses.

Pituitary

Posterior: Decrease in size; reduced antidiuretic hormone (ADH) secretion.

Anterior: Increased fibrosis and moderate increase in size of gland; decline in growth hormone release.

Thyroid

Glandular atrophy, fibrosis, nodularity, and increased inflammatory infiltrates; possible changes in thyroid hormone (TH) are difficult to determine because of concurrent disease in elderly persons; may find decreased T_4 secretion and turnover, decline in T_3 (especially in men), diminished thyroid-stimulating hormone (TSH) secretion; reduced response of plasma TSH concentration to thyroid-releasing hormone (TRH) administration (especially in men).

Growth Hormone and Insulin-like Growth Factors

The amounts of GH and IGF decline with aging, which contributes to decreases in muscle size and function, reduced fat and bone mass, and changes in reproductive and cognitive function. Increased visceral fat, decreased lean body mass, and decreased bone density are common in older adults.

Pancreas

Nearly half of older individuals have glucose intolerance or diabetes, and these disorders frequently are undiagnosed in aging adults. Mechanisms include decreased insulin receptor activity and decreased beta-cell secretion of insulin.

Adrenal

Decreased DHEA levels lead to decreased synthesis of androgen-derived estrogen and testosterone; decreased metabolic clearance of glucocorticoids and cortisol causes decreased cortisol secretion; there also are decreased levels of aldosterone. Circadian patterns of ACTH and cortisol secretion may change with aging.

Gonads

Postmenopausal women have decreased estrogen and progesterone, increased follicle-stimulating hormone, and relative increases in androgen levels; these changes have numerous physiologic and pathophysiologic consequences (see Chapter 31); in men there is a gradual decrease in serum testosterone levels, leading to decreased sexual activity, decreased muscle strength, and decreased bone mineralization.

DID YOU UNDERSTAND?

Mechanisms of Hormonal Regulation

1. The endocrine system has diverse functions, including sexual differentiation, growth and development, and continuous maintenance of the body's internal environment.
2. Hormones are chemical messengers synthesized by endocrine glands and released into the circulation.
3. Hormones have specific negative and positive feedback mechanisms. Most hormone levels are regulated by negative feedback, in which hormone secretion raises the level of a specific hormone, ultimately causing secretion to subside.
4. Endocrine feedback is described in terms of short, long, and ultra-short feedback loops.
5. Water-soluble hormones circulate throughout the body in unbound form, whereas lipid-soluble hormones (e.g., steroid and thyroid hormones) circulate throughout the body bound to carrier proteins.
6. Hormones affect only target cells with appropriate receptors and then act on these cells to initiate specific cell functions or activities.
7. Hormones have two general types of effects on cells: (a) direct effects, or obvious changes in cell function, and (b) permissive effects, or less obvious changes that facilitate cell function.
8. Receptors for hormones may be located on the plasma membrane or in the intracellular compartment of a target cell.
9. Water-soluble hormones act as first messengers, binding to receptors on the cell's plasma membrane. The signals initiated by hormone-receptor binding are then transmitted into the cell by the action of second messengers.
10. Lipid-soluble hormones (including steroid and thyroid hormones) cross the plasma membrane by diffusion. These hormones diffuse directly into the cell nucleus and bind to nuclear receptors. Rapid responses of steroid hormones may be mediated by plasma membrane receptors.

Structure and Function of the Endocrine Glands

1. The pituitary gland, consisting of anterior and posterior portions, is connected to the central nervous system through the hypothalamus.
2. The hypothalamus regulates anterior pituitary function by secreting releasing or inhibiting hormones and factors into the portal circulation.
3. Hypothalamic hormones include prolactin-releasing factor (PRF), which stimulates secretion of prolactin; prolactin-inhibiting factor (PIF, dopamine), which inhibits prolactin secretion; thyrotropin-releasing hormone (TRH), which affects release of thyroid hormones; growth hormone–releasing hormone (GHRH), which stimulates the release of growth hormone (GH); somatostatin, which inhibits the release of GH; gonadotropin-releasing hormone (GnRH), which facilitates the release of follicle-stimulating hormone (FSH) and luteinizing hormone (LH); corticotropin-releasing hormone (CRH), which facilitates the release of adrenocorticotropic hormone (ACTH) and endorphins; and substance P, which inhibits ACTH release and stimulates the release of a variety of other hormones.
4. The posterior pituitary secretes antidiuretic hormone (ADH), which also is called vasopressin, and oxytocin.
5. Hormones of the anterior pituitary are regulated by (a) secretion of hypothalamic-releasing hormones or factors, (b) negative feedback from hormones secreted by target organs, and (c) mediating effects of neurotransmitters.
6. Hormones of the anterior pituitary include ACTH, melanocyte-stimulating hormone (MSH), somatotropic hormones (growth hormone [GH], prolactin), and glycoprotein hormones—follicle-stimulating hormone (FSH), luteinizing hormone (LH), and thyroid-stimulating hormone (TSH).
7. ADH controls serum osmolality, increases permeability of the renal tubules to water, and causes vasoconstriction when administered pharmacologically in high doses. ADH also may regulate some central nervous system functions.

DID YOU UNDERSTAND?—cont'd

8. Oxytocin causes uterine contraction and lactation in women and may have a role in sperm motility in men. In both men and women, oxytocin has an antidiuretic effect similar to that of ADH.

9. The two-lobed thyroid gland contains follicles, which secrete some of the thyroid hormones, and C cells, which secrete calcitonin and somatostatin.

10. Regulation of thyroid hormone (TH) levels is complex and involves the hypothalamus, anterior pituitary, thyroid gland, and numerous biochemical variables.

11. Thyroid hormone (TH) secretion is regulated by thyroid-releasing hormone (TRH) through a negative feedback loop that involves the anterior pituitary and hypothalamus.

12. Thyroid-stimulating hormone (TSH), which is synthesized and stored in the anterior pituitary, stimulates secretion of TH by activating intracellular processes, including uptake of iodine necessary for the synthesis of TH.

13. Once secreted, TH acts on the thyroid gland, the anterior pituitary, and the median eminence to regulate further TH production.

14. Synthesis of TH depends on the glycoprotein thyroglobulin (TG), which contains a precursor of TH, tyrosine. Tyrosine then combines with iodine to form precursor molecules of the thyroid hormones thyroxine (T_4) and triiodothyronine (T_3).

15. When released into the circulation, T_3 and T_4 are bound by carrier proteins in the plasma, which store these hormones and provide a buffer for rapid changes in hormone levels. The free form is the active form.

16. Thyroid hormones alter protein synthesis and have a wide range of metabolic effects on proteins, carbohydrates, lipids, and vitamins. TH also affects heat production and cardiac function.

17. The paired parathyroid glands normally are located behind the upper and lower poles of the thyroid. These glands secrete parathyroid hormone (PTH), an important regulator of serum calcium levels.

18. PTH secretion is regulated by levels of ionized calcium in the plasma and by cyclic adenosine monophosphate (cAMP) within the cell.

19. In bone, PTH causes bone breakdown and resorption. In the kidney, PTH increases reabsorption of calcium and decreases reabsorption of phosphorus and bicarbonate.

20. The endocrine pancreas contains the islets of Langerhans, which secrete hormones responsible for much of the carbohydrate metabolism in the body.

21. The islets of Langerhans consist of alpha cells, beta cells, delta cells, and F cells.

22. Alpha cells produce glucagon, which is secreted inversely to blood glucose concentrations.

23. Delta cells secrete somatostatin, which inhibits glucagon and insulin secretion.

24. Beta cells secrete preproinsulin, which is ultimately converted to insulin.

25. F cells secrete pancreatic polypeptide.

26. Insulin is a hormone that regulates blood glucose concentrations and overall body metabolism of fat, protein, and carbohydrates.

27. The paired adrenal glands are situated above the kidneys. Each gland consists of an adrenal medulla, which secretes catecholamines, and an adrenal cortex, which secretes steroid hormones.

28. The steroid hormones secreted by the adrenal cortex are synthesized from cholesterol. These hormones include glucocorticoids, mineralocorticoids, and adrenal androgens and estrogens.

29. Glucocorticoids directly affect carbohydrate metabolism by increasing blood glucose concentration through gluconeogenesis in the liver and by decreasing use of glucose. Glucocorticoids inhibit immune and inflammatory responses.

30. The most potent naturally occurring glucocorticoid is cortisol, which is necessary for the maintenance of life and for protection from stress. Secretion of cortisol is regulated by the hypothalamus and anterior pituitary.

31. Cortisol secretion is related to secretion of adrenocorticotropic hormone (ACTH), which is stimulated by corticotropin-releasing hormone (CRH). ACTH binds with receptors of the adrenal cortex, which activates intracellular mechanisms (specifically cyclic AMP) and leads to cortisol release.

32. Mineralocorticoids are steroid hormones that directly affect ion transport by renal tubular epithelial cells, causing sodium retention and potassium and hydrogen loss.

33. Aldosterone is the most potent of the naturally occurring mineralocorticoids. Its primary role is to conserve sodium.

34. Aldosterone secretion is regulated primarily by the renin-angiotensin system and by the serum sodium concentration.

35. Aldosterone acts by binding to a site on the cell nucleus and altering protein production within the cell. Its principal site of action is the kidney, where it causes sodium reabsorption and potassium and hydrogen excretion.

36. Androgens and estrogens secreted by the adrenal cortex act in the same way as those secreted by the gonads.

37. The adrenal medulla secretes the catecholamines epinephrine and norepinephrine. Epinephrine is 10 times more potent than norepinephrine in exerting metabolic effects. Their release is stimulated by sympathetic nervous system stimulation, ACTH, and glucocorticoids.

38. Catecholamines bind with various target cells and are taken up by neurons or excreted in the urine. They cause a range of metabolic effects characterized as the fight-or-flight response and include hyperglycemia and immune suppression.

39. The endocrine system acts together with the nervous system to respond to stressors.

40. The response to stressors involves (a) activation of the sympathetic division of the autonomic nervous system and (b) activation of the endocrine system.

41. Other hormones that are secreted in response to stress include growth hormone (GH), prolactin, testosterone, antidiuretic hormone (ADH), and insulin.

42. The adrenal glands and the sympathetic neurons that innervate these glands form the sympathoadrenal axis.

GERIATRIC CONSIDERATIONS: Aging & Its Effects on Specific Endocrine Glands

1. The general changes in the endocrine glands that occur with older age include atrophy and weight loss with vascular changes, decreased secretion and clearance of hormones, and variable change in receptor binding and intracellular responses

KEY TERMS

- Adrenal cortex   439
- Adrenal gland   439
- Adrenal medulla   440
- Adrenocorticotropic hormone (ACTH)   433
- Aldosterone   441

- Alpha cell   437
- Amylin   439
- Anterior pituitary   431
- Antidiuretic hormone (ADH)   434
- Beta cell   437
- C cell   435

- Calcitonin   435
- Chromophil   433
- Chromophobe   431
- Corticotropin-releasing hormone (CRH)   441
- Cortisol   441

Continued

KEY TERMS—cont'd

- Delta cell   437
- 1,25-Dihydroxy-vitamin D_3 437
- Direct effect   429
- Down-regulation   429
- F (or PP) cell   437
- First messenger   429
- Follicle   435
- Follicle-stimulating hormone (FSH)   433
- Gastrin   439
- Glucagon   439
- Glucocorticoid   440
- Grehlin   439
- Growth hormone   433
- Hormone   426
- Hormone receptor   429
- Hypothalamus   431
- Insulin   437
- Islet of Langerhans   437
- Isthmus   435
- Luteinizing hormone (LH)   433
- Median eminence   434
- Melanocyte-stimulating hormone (MSH)   433
- Melatonin   435
- Mineralocorticoid   441
- Negative feedback   427
- Oxytocin   435
- Pancreas   437
- Pancreatic polypeptide   439
- Parathyroid hormone (PTH)   437
- Pars distalis   431
- Pars intermedia   431
- Pars nervosa (neural tube)   434
- Pars tuberalis   431
- Permissive effect   429
- Pituitary gland   431
- Pituitary stalk   434
- Posterior pituitary   434
- Prolactin   434
- Second messenger   429
- Somatostatin   439
- Target cell   428
- Thyroglobulin (TG)   436
- Thyroid gland   435
- Thyroid hormone (TH)   435
- Thyroid-stimulating hormone (TSH)   433
- Thyrotropin-releasing hormone (TRH)   427
- Thyroxine-binding globulin (TBG)   437
- Tropic hormone   433
- Up-regulation   429
- Zona fasciculata   439
- Zona glomerulosa   439
- Zona reticularis   439

REFERENCES

1. Gardner DG, Nissenson RA: Mechanisms of hormone action. In Gardner DG, Shoback D, editors: *Greenspan's basic & clinical endocrinology*, ed 8, New York, 2007, McGraw-Hill.
2. Evanson NK, et al: Nongenomic actions of adrenal steroids in the central nervous system, *J Neuroendocrinol* 22(8):846–861, 2010.
3. Spiegel A, Carter-Su C, Taylor SI: Mechanisms of action of hormones that act at the cell surface. In Kronenberg HM, et al, editor: *Williams textbook of endocrinology*, ed 11, Philadelphia, 2008, Saunders.
4. Fellner SK, Arendshorst WJ: Complex interactions of NO/cGMP/PKG systems on Ca^{2+} signaling in afferent arteriolar vascular smooth muscle, *Am J Physiol Heart Circ Physiol* 298(1):H144–H151, 2010.
5. Reffelmann T, Kloner RA: Phosphodiesterase 5 inhibitors: are they cardioprotective? *Cardiovasc Res* 83(2):204–212, 2009.
6. Belfiore A, et al: Insulin receptor isoforms and insulin receptor/insulin-like growth factor receptor hybrids in physiology and disease, *Endocr Rev* 30(6):586–623, 2009.
7. Takeuchi K, Ito F: EGF receptor in relation to tumor development: molecular basis of responsiveness of cancer cells to EGFR-targeting tyrosine kinase inhibitors, *FEBS J* 277(2):316–326, 2010.
8. Haller J, Mikics E, Makara GB: The effects of non-genomic glucocorticoid mechanisms on bodily functions and the central neural system. A critical evaluation of findings, *Front Neuroendocr* 29(2):273–291, 2008.
9. Kronenberg HM, et al: Principles of endocrinology. In Kronenberg HM, et al, editor: *Williams textbook of endocrinology*, ed 11, Philadelphia, 2008, Saunders.
10. Annunziata M, Granata R, Ghigo E: The IGF system, *Acta Diabetol* 48(1):1–9, 2011.
11. Bright GM, Mendoza JR, Rosenfeld RG: Recombinant human insulin-like growth factor-1 treatment: ready for primetime, *Endocr Metab Clin North Am* 38(3):625–638, 2009.
12. Clemmons DR: Role of IGF-I in skeletal muscle mass maintenance, *Trends Endocr Metab* 20(7):349–356, 2009.
13. Yang SY, et al: Growth factors and their receptors in cancer metastases, *Front Biosci* 16:531–538, 2011.
14. Robinson AG, Verbalis J: Posterior pituitary. In Kronenberg HM, et al, editor: *Williams textbook of endocrinology*, ed 12, Philadelphia, 2011, Saunders.
15. Kampmeier TG, et al: Vasopressin in sepsis and septic shock, *Minerva Anestesiol* 76(10):844–850, 2010.
16. Bauer SR, Lam SW: Arginine vasopressin for the treatment of septic shock in adults, *Pharmacotherapy* 30(10):1057–1071, 2010.
17. Zawilska JB, Skene DJ, Arendt J: Physiology and pharmacology of melatonin in relation to biological rhythms, *Pharmacol Rep* 61(3):383–410, 2010.
18. St Germain DL, Galton VA, Hernandez A: Minireview: defining the roles of the iodothyronine deiodinases: current concepts and challenges, *Endocrinology* 150(3):1097–1107, 2009.
19. Triggiani V, et al: Role of iodine, selenium and other micronutrients in thyroid function and disorders, *Endocr Metab Immune Disorders Drug Targets* 9(3):277–294, 2009.
20. Salvatore D, et al: Thyroid physiology and diagnostic evaluation of patients with thyroid disorders. In Melmed S, et al: *Williams textbook of endocrinology*, ed 12, Philadelphia, 2011, Saunders.
21. Tancevski I, et al: A selective thyromimetic for the treatment of dyslipidemia, *Recent Pat Cardiovasc Drug Discov* 6(1):16–19, 2011.
22. Rude RK, Singer FR, Gruber HE: Skeletal and hormonal effects of magnesium deficiency, *J Am Coll Nutr* 28(2):131–141, 2009.
23. Buse JB, Polonsky KS, Burant CF: Disorders of carbohydrate and metabolism. In Kronenberg HM, et al, editor: *Williams textbook of endocrinology*, ed 12, Philadelphia, 2011, Saunders.
24. Foley K, Boguslavsky S, Klip A: Endocytosis, recycling, and regulated exocytosis of glucose transporter 4, *Biochemistry* 50(15):3048–3061, 2011.
25. Stores RD, Cone JK: Neuroendocrine control of energy stores. In Melmed S, et al: *Williams textbook of endocrinology*, ed 12, Philadelphia, 2011, Saunders.
26. Vella A, Drucker DJ, et al: Gastrointestinal hormones and gut endocrine tumors. In Melmed S, et al: *Williams textbook of endocrinology*, ed 12, Philadelphia, 2011, Saunders.
27. Stewart PM, Krone NP: The adrenal cortex. In Melmed S, et al: *Williams textbook of endocrinology*, ed 12, Philadelphia, 2011, Saunders.
28. Dooley R, Harvey BJ, Thomas W: The regulation of cell growth and survival by aldosterone, *Front Biosci* 16:440–457, 2011.
29. Whaley-Connell A, Johnson MS, Sowers JR: Aldosterone: role in the cardiometabolic syndrome and resistant hypertension, *Prog Cardiovasc Dis* 52(5):401–409, 2010.
30. Lambers SW: Endocrinology of aging. In Melmed S, et al: *Williams textbook of endocrinology*, ed 12, Philadelphia, 2011, Saunders.
31. Young WF: Endocrine hypertension. In Melmed S, et al: *Williams textbook of endocrinology*, ed 12, Philadelphia, 2011, Saunders.

Alterations of Hormonal Regulation

Robert E. Jones, Valentina L. Brashers, and Sue E. Huether

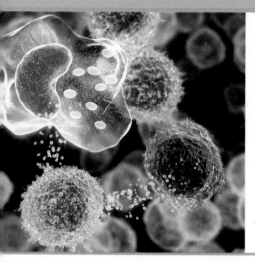

Functions of the endocrine system involve complex interrelationships and interactions that maintain dynamic steady states and provide growth and reproductive capabilities. Endocrine system dysfunction includes excessive or insufficient function of the endocrine gland with alterations in hormone levels. These alterations are caused by either hypersecretion or hyposecretion of the various hormones, leading to abnormal hormone concentrations in the blood. Dysfunction also may result from abnormal cell receptor function or from altered intracellular response to the hormone-receptor complex.

MECHANISMS OF HORMONAL ALTERATIONS

Significantly elevated or significantly depressed hormone levels may result from various causes (Table 18-1). Dysfunction of an endocrine gland may involve its failure to produce adequate amounts of biologically free or active hormone, or a gland may synthesize or release too much hormone. Feedback systems that recognize the need for a particular hormone may fail to function properly or may respond to inappropriate signals. Once hormones are released into the circulation, they may be degraded at an altered rate or be inactivated before reaching the target cell by antibodies that function as circulating hormone inhibitors. Other causes of decreased hormone delivery to the target cell include an inadequate blood supply to the gland or target tissues or an insufficient amount of the appropriate carrier proteins in the serum. Ectopic sources of hormones (hormones produced by nonendocrine tissues) may cause abnormally elevated hormone levels without the benefit of the normal feedback system for hormone control; in this case, the ectopic hormone production is said to be autonomous.

Target cells may not respond appropriately to hormonal stimulation for a number of reasons. The following are the two general types of target cell insensitivity to hormones:
1. *Cell surface receptor–associated disorders.* These disorders have been identified primarily in water-soluble hormones, such as insulin. They may involve a decrease in the number of receptors, leading to decreased or defective hormone-receptor binding; impaired receptor function, resulting in insensitivity to the hormone; presence of

TABLE 18-1   MECHANISMS OF HORMONE ALTERATIONS

INAPPROPRIATE AMOUNTS OF HORMONE DELIVERED TO TARGET CELL	INAPPROPRIATE RESPONSE BY TARGET CELL
Inadequate Hormone Synthesis 1. Inadequate quantity of hormone precursors 2. Secretory cell unable to convert precursors to active hormone	**Cell Surface Receptor–Associated Disorders** 1. Decrease in the number of receptors 2. Impaired receptor function (altered affinity for hormones) 3. Presence of antibodies against specific receptors 4. Unusual expression of receptor function
Failure of Feedback Systems 1. Do not recognize positive feedback, leading to inadequate hormone synthesis 2. Do not recognize negative feedback, leading to excessive hormone synthesis	
Inactive Hormones 1. Inadequate biologically free hormone 2. Hormone degraded at an altered rate 3. Circulating inhibitors	**Intracellular Disorders** 1. Acquired defects in postreceptor signaling cascades 2. Inadequate synthesis of a second messenger 3. Intracellular enzymes or proteins are altered 4. Alterations in nuclear co-regulators 5. Altered protein synthesis
Dysfunctional Delivery System 1. Inadequate blood supply 2. Inadequate carrier proteins 3. Ectopic production of hormones	

antibodies against specific receptors that either reduce available binding sites or mimic hormone action, suppressing or exaggerating, respectively, the target cell response; or unusual expression of receptor function, for example, tumor cells with abnormal receptor activity.

2. *Intracellular disorders.* These disorders involve acquired defects in postreceptor signaling cascades or inadequate synthesis of a second messenger, such as cyclic adenosine monophosphate (cAMP), needed to transduce the hormonal signal into intracellular events. The target cell for water-soluble hormones may have a faulty response to hormone-receptor binding and thus fail to generate the required second messenger, or the cell may respond abnormally to the second messenger if levels of intracellular enzymes or proteins are altered. (Second messengers for various hormones are listed in Table 17-3.) As a result, the target cell fails to express the usual hormonal effect.

Pathogenic mechanisms affecting target cell response for lipid-soluble hormones are recognized less often than those affecting water-soluble hormones. When they do occur, the mechanisms are similar to those for water-soluble hormones, including changes in the number and binding affinity of intracellular receptors or altered generation of new messenger ribonucleic acid (RNA) and substrates for new protein synthesis.

ALTERATIONS OF THE HYPOTHALAMIC-PITUITARY SYSTEM

Perhaps the most common cause of apparent hypothalamic dysfunction is interruption of the pituitary stalk caused by destructive lesions, rupture after head injury, surgical transection, or tumor. In these cases, interruption of the physical connections between the hypothalamus and the pituitary gland causes apparent pituitary disease. For example, without hypothalamic hormones (Figure 18-1), women cease to menstruate and men experience hypogonadism and impaired spermatogenesis. Adrenocorticotropic hormone (ACTH) response to low serum cortisol levels is decreased because of the absence of corticotropin-releasing hormone (CRH). Hypothalamic hypothyroidism is caused by the absence of thyrotropin-releasing hormone (TRH). Low levels

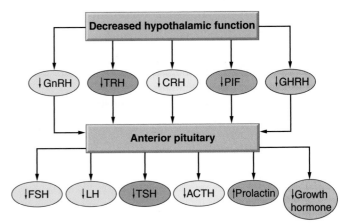

FIGURE 18-1 Loss of Hypothalamic Hormones. *GnRH,* Gonadotropin-releasing hormone; *TRH,* thyrotropin-releasing hormone; *CRH,* corticotropin-releasing hormone; *PIF,* prolactin inhibitory factor (probably dopamine); *GHRH,* growth hormone–releasing hormone; *FSH,* follicle-stimulating hormone; *LH,* luteinizing hormone; *TSH,* thyroid-stimulating hormone; *ACTH,* adrenocorticotropic hormone.

of growth hormone–releasing hormone (GHRH) result in growth hormone (GH) deficiency and growth failure in children. Hyperprolactinemia is caused by an absence of the usual inhibitory control of prolactin secretion (dopamine).

Diseases of the Posterior Pituitary

Diseases of the posterior pituitary that cause clinically significant alterations in hormone function usually are related to abnormal secretion of antidiuretic hormone (ADH, arginine vasopressin). An excess amount of this hormone results in water retention and a hypoosmolar state, whereas deficiencies in the amount or response to ADH result in serum hyperosmolarity. These complex pathophysiologic states not only have significant clinical effects on the modulation of body fluids and electrolytes but also affect cognitive and emotional responses to stress.

Syndrome of Inappropriate Antidiuretic Hormone Secretion

Syndrome of inappropriate ADH secretion (SIADH), also known as **vasopressin dysregulation**, is characterized by high levels of ADH without normal physiologic stimuli for its release.

The most common cause of SIADH is the ectopic production of ADH by tumors such as small cell carcinoma of the duodenum, stomach, and pancreas; cancers of the bladder, prostate, and endometrium; lymphomas; and sarcomas. Pulmonary disorders associated with SIADH include bronchogenic carcinoma, pneumonia (e.g., tuberculosis), asthma, cystic fibrosis, and respiratory failure requiring mechanical ventilation.[1,2] Central nervous system disorders that may cause SIADH include encephalitis, meningitis, intracranial hemorrhage, tumors, and trauma.[3]

Any surgery can result in increased ADH secretion for as long as 5 to 7 days after surgery. The precise mechanism is uncertain but is likely related to fluid and volume changes following surgery, the amount and type of intravenous fluids given, and the use of narcotic analgesics. Transient SIADH also may follow pituitary surgery because stored ADH is released in an unregulated fashion.

Medications are an important cause of SIADH, especially in the elderly. These include hypoglycemic medications (e.g., chlorpropamide), narcotics, general anesthetics, chemotherapeutic agents, nonsteroidal anti-inflammatory drugs, and synthetic ADH analogs. Finally, SIADH may be associated with psychiatric disease treated with antidepressants or antipsychotics.[4]

PATHOPHYSIOLOGY The cardinal features of SIADH are the result of enhanced renal water retention. ADH increases renal collecting duct permeability to water by inducing the insertion of aquaporin-2, a water channel protein, into the tubular luminal membrane, which increases water reabsorption by the kidneys. (Renal function is discussed in Chapter 28.) This results in an expansion of extracellular fluid volume that leads to dilutional hyponatremia (low serum sodium concentration), hypoosmolarity, and urine that is inappropriately concentrated with respect to serum osmolarity.[3]

CLINICAL MANIFESTATIONS The symptoms of SIADH result from hyponatremia and are determined by its severity and rapidity of onset. Thirst, impaired taste, anorexia, dyspnea on exertion, fatigue, and dulled sensorium occur when the serum sodium level decreases rapidly from 140 to 130 mEq/L. Peripheral edema is absent. Severe gastrointestinal symptoms, including vomiting and abdominal cramps, occur with a drop in sodium concentration from 130 to 120 mEq/L. Even if hyponatremia develops slowly, serum sodium levels below 110 to 115 mEq/L cause confusion, lethargy, muscle twitching, and convulsions; severe and sometimes irreversible neurologic damage may occur. Symptoms usually resolve with correction of hyponatremia.

EVALUATION AND TREATMENT A diagnosis of SIADH requires the following manifestations: (1) serum hypoosmolality and hyponatremia, (2) urine hyperosmolarity (i.e., urine osmolality is greater than expected for the concomitant serum osmolarity), (3) urine sodium excretion that matches sodium intake, (4) normal adrenal and thyroid function, and (5) absence of conditions that can alter volume status (e.g., congestive heart failure, hypovolemia from any cause, or renal insufficiency).[5]

The treatment of SIADH involves the correction of any underlying causal problems and fluid restriction with careful monitoring. In severe SIADH, emergency correction of severe hyponatremia by careful administration of hypertonic saline may be required. Resolution usually occurs within 3 days, with a 2- to 3-kg weight loss and correction of hyponatremia and salt wasting. Demeclocycline, which causes the renal tubules to develop resistance to ADH, may be used to treat resistant or chronic SIADH. ADH receptor antagonists have been used in selective instances of ADH excess.[6]

Diabetes Insipidus

Diabetes insipidus (DI) is a disorder of insufficient activity of ADH, leading to polyuria (frequent urination) and polydipsia (frequent drinking). The two forms of DI are as follows:

1. *Neurogenic or central DI.* Caused by the insufficient secretion of ADH, it occurs when any organic lesion of the hypothalamus, pituitary stalk, or posterior pituitary interferes with ADH synthesis, transport, or release. Causative lesions include primary brain tumors, hypophysectomy, aneurysms, thrombosis, infections, and immunologic disorders. Central DI is a well-recognized complication of closed-head injury. It can also be caused by hereditary disorders that affect ADH genes or result in structural changes in the pituitary gland.
2. *Nephrogenic DI.* Caused by inadequate response of the renal tubules to ADH, which is usually acquired or may be genetic. Acquired nephrogenic DI is generally related to disorders and drugs that damage the renal tubules or inhibit the generation of cAMP in the tubules. These disorders include pyelonephritis, amyloidosis, destructive uropathies, and polycystic kidney disease, all of which lead to irreversible diabetes insipidus. Drugs that may induce a reversible form of nephrogenic diabetes insipidus include lithium carbonate, colchicines, amphotericin B, loop diuretics, general anesthetics (such as methoxyflurane), and demeclocycline. Several genetic causes of nephrogenic DI have been identified.[7] One of the best described is a mutation in the gene that codes for aquaporin-2, which is one of the four water transport channels in the renal tubule.[8]

Psychogenic polydipsia may be confused with diabetes insipidus. It is caused by the chronic ingestion of extremely large quantities of fluid that wash out the renal medullary concentration gradient, which results in a partial resistance to ADH. This condition resolves with decreased fluid ingestion. Psychogenic polydipsia must be differentiated from true DI because administering an ADH analog to an individual with psychogenic DI will result in severe hypoosmolality.

PATHOPHYSIOLOGY Individuals with diabetes insipidus have a partial to total inability to concentrate urine. Insufficient ADH activity causes excretion of large volumes of dilute urine, leading to increased plasma osmolality. In conscious individuals, the thirst mechanism is stimulated and induces polydipsia—usually a craving for cold drinks. The urine output is varied but can increase from the normal output of 1 to 2 L/day to as much as 8 to 12 L/day and the urine specific gravity is low. Dehydration develops rapidly without ongoing fluid replacement. If the individual with DI cannot conserve as much water as is lost in the urine, serum hypernatremia and hyperosmolality occur. Other serum electrolytes generally are not affected.

CLINICAL MANIFESTATIONS The clinical manifestations of diabetes insipidus include polyuria, nocturia, continuous thirst, and polydipsia. Individuals with long-standing diabetes insipidus develop a large bladder capacity and hydronephrosis (see Chapter 28).[9] Neurogenic diabetes insipidus usually has an abrupt onset and many individuals can specifically recall the date of onset of their symptoms. Nephrogenic DI usually has a more gradual onset.

EVALUATION AND TREATMENT Diabetes insipidus must be distinguished from other polyuric states, including diabetes mellitus, osmotically induced diuresis, and psychogenic polydipsia. The criteria for the

TABLE 18-2   SIGNS AND SYMPTOMS OF DIABETES INSIPIDUS (DI) AND SYNDROME OF INAPPROPRIATE ANTIDIURETIC HORMONE (SIADH) SECRETION

SIGNS AND SYMPTOMS	DI	SIADH
Urine output	High	Low (no hypovolemia)
Urine osmolality	Low (<100-200 mOsm/L)	High (>800 mOsm/L)
Urine specific gravity	Low (<1.010)	High (>1.020)
Serum sodium	Hypernatremia (>145 mEq/L)	Hyponatremia (<135 mEq/L)
Serum osmolality	Hyperosmolar (>300 mOsm/L)	Hypoosmolar (<285 mOsm/L)
Symptoms	Polyuria, thirst	Nausea, vomiting, mental changes

diagnosis of DI include low urine specific gravity, low urine osmolality, hypernatremia, high serum osmolality, and continued diuresis despite a serum sodium concentration of 145 mEq/L or greater. The diagnosis of DI is generally confirmed through water deprivation testing. Psychogenic polydipsia can be differentiated from nephrogenic DI based on plasma ADH levels. ADH levels are low in psychogenic polydipsia and normal or high in nephrogenic DI.

Treatment of neurogenic DI is based on the extent of the ADH deficiency and on age, endocrine and cardiovascular status, and lifestyle. Some individuals require ADH replacement, but oral hydration often is adequate. ADH replacement therapy for symptomatic central or neurogenic diabetes insipidus includes intravascular or, more commonly, oral or intranasal administration of the synthetic vasopressin analog DDAVP (desmopressin).[10] Management of nephrogenic DI requires treatment of any reversible underlying disorders, discontinuation of etiologic medications, and correction of associated electrolyte disorders. Surprisingly, thiazide diuretics may improve renal tubular salt and water retention in individuals with moderate nephrogenic DI. Drugs that potentiate the action of otherwise insufficient amounts of endogenous ADH, such as chlorpropamide, carbamazepine, and clofibrate, may be used in individuals with incomplete ADH deficiency.[11] Table 18-2 compares the signs and symptoms of DI and SIADH.

Diseases of the Anterior Pituitary
Hypopituitarism

Hypopituitarism can be characterized by the absence of selective pituitary hormones or the complete failure of all pituitary hormone functions. Hypopituitarism results from either an inadequate supply of hypothalamic-releasing hormones, because of damage to the pituitary stalk, or an inability of the gland to produce hormones.[12] The most common causes of hypopituitarism lie within the pituitary gland itself and result from pituitary infarction or space-occupying lesions, such as pituitary adenomas or aneurysms. Other causes of hypopituitarism include removal or destruction of the gland, head trauma, infections (e.g., meningitis, syphilis, tuberculosis), autoimmune hypophysitis, certain drugs (e.g., bexarotene, carbamazepine), or mutation of the prophet of pituitary transcription factor *(PROP-1)* gene involved in early embryonic pituitary development.[13,14]

PATHOPHYSIOLOGY   The pituitary gland is highly vascular and relies heavily upon portal blood flow from the hypothalamus. It is, therefore, vulnerable to ischemia and infarction. Pituitary infarction may be seen with Sheehan syndrome (postpartum pituitary necrosis), pituitary apoplexy, traumatic brain injury, shock, sickle cell disease, and diabetes mellitus. Infarction results in tissue necrosis and edema with swelling of the gland. Expansion of the pituitary within the fixed compartment of the sella turcica further impedes blood supply to the pituitary. Over time the pituitary undergoes shrinkage and fibrosis of

pituitary tissue and the symptoms of hypopituitarism develop.[12,13] Adenomas and aneurysms may compress otherwise normal secreting pituitary cells and lead to compromised hormonal output.[15]

CLINICAL MANIFESTATIONS   The signs and symptoms of hypofunction of the anterior pituitary are variable and depend on which hormones are affected. In panhypopituitarism, all hormones are deficient and the individual suffers from multiple complications including cortisol deficiency from lack of ACTH, thyroid deficiency from lack of thyroid-stimulating hormone (TSH), and loss of secondary sex characteristics because of the lack of follicle-stimulating hormone (FSH) and luteinizing hormone (LH). Low levels of growth hormone (GH) and insulin-like growth factor 1 (IGF-1) affect growth in children and can cause physiologic and psychologic symptoms in adults. In addition, postpartum women cannot lactate because of decreased or absent prolactin.

ACTH deficiency with associated loss of cortisol is a potentially life-threatening disorder. ACTH deficiency usually is encountered with generalized pituitary hypofunction; it rarely occurs as an isolated event. Within 2 weeks of the complete absence of ACTH, symptoms of cortisol insufficiency develop, including nausea, vomiting, anorexia, fatigue, and weakness. Hypoglycemia results from increased insulin sensitivity, decreased glycogen reserves, and decreased gluconeogenesis associated with hypocortisolism. ACTH deficiency also limits maximal aldosterone secretion, although the renin-angiotensin system can stimulate some aldosterone secretion. The glomerular filtration rate decreases, causing decreased urine output. (Renal function is described in Chapter 28.)

TSH deficiency is rarely seen in isolation but often occurs with other pituitary hormone deficiencies. Symptoms develop 4 to 8 weeks after hypothyrotropinemia occurs and include cold intolerance, skin dryness, mild myxedema, lethargy, and decreased metabolic rate. The symptoms usually are less severe than those of primary hypothyroidism.

The onset of FSH and LH deficiencies in women of reproductive age is associated with amenorrhea and an atrophic vagina, uterus, and breasts. In postpubertal males, testicles atrophy and beard growth is stunted. Both men and women experience decreased body hair and diminished libido.

GH deficiency occurs in both children and adults. Several genetic defects have been identified in the growth hormone axis in children including a recessive mutation in the GH gene, resulting in a failure of growth hormone secretion.[16] Mutations also may involve the GH receptor, IGF-1 biosynthesis, IGF-1 receptors, or defects in GH signal transduction. In adults, GH deficiency is most often caused by structural or functional abnormalities of the pituitary. GH deficiency in children is manifested by growth failure and a condition known as hypopituitary dwarfism (Figure 18-2); however, not all children with short stature have growth hormone deficiency. Symptoms of adult GH deficiency syndrome are vague and include social withdrawal, fatigue,

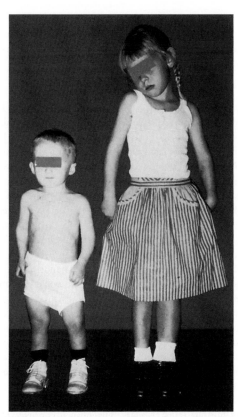

FIGURE 18-2 Hypopituitary Dwarfism. A 4-year-old boy whose height is 25 inches. Girl is also 4 years old and has a normal height of 39 inches. Boy (dwarf) has a normal face, as well as head, trunk, and limbs of approximately normal proportions. (From Brashear HR, Raney RB: *Handbook of orthopaedic surgery,* ed 10, St Louis, 1986, Mosby.)

loss of motivation, and a diminished feeling of well-being. Osteoporosis and alterations in body composition (i.e., reduced lean body mass) are typical concomitant symptoms of adult GH deficiency.[17]

EVALUATION AND TREATMENT The diagnostic evaluation of suspected pituitary disease is often challenging and must be carefully interpreted together with the individual's signs and symptoms. Simultaneous measurements of the tropic hormones from the pituitary and target endocrine glands are crucial and dynamic testing of the various axes may be indicated. Imaging of the pituitary (magnetic resonance imaging [MRI] or computed tomography [CT] scans) is critical to assess for anatomic lesions, such as tumors.

Management of hypopituitarism requires correction of the underlying disorder as quickly as possible. Replacement of target gland hormones that are deficient because of lack of tropic anterior pituitary hormones is essential (such as cortisol, thyroid hormone, growth hormone, and gender-specific steroid hormones). In cases of circulatory collapse, immediate therapy with glucocorticoids and intravenous fluids is critical.

Hyperpituitarism: Primary Adenoma

Pituitary adenomas usually are benign, slow-growing tumors that arise from cells of the anterior pituitary. The cause of pituitary adenomas is not known. Most are microscopic (microadenomas) and are found only on postmortem examinations or incidentally discovered on MRI examinations. The vast majority of pituitary microadenomas

are hormonally silent and do not pose significant hazards to the individual. More significant adenomas are associated with morbidity and mortality attributable to alterations in hormone secretion or to invasion or impingement of surrounding structures.

PATHOPHYSIOLOGY Local expansion of the adenoma may impinge on the optic chiasma and cause various visual disturbances, depending on the portion of the nerve compressed. If the tumor is locally aggressive, invasion of the cavernous sinuses may occur, resulting in compromise of the oculomotor, trochlear, abducens, and trigeminal nerves with attending symptoms. Extension to the hypothalamus disturbs control of wakefulness, thirst, appetite, and temperature.

Hormonal effects of adenomas include hypersecretion from the adenoma itself and hyposecretion from surrounding pituitary cells. The adenomatous tissue secretes the hormone of the cell type from which it arose, without regard to the needs of the body and without benefit of regulatory feedback mechanisms. Because of the pressure exerted by the tumor in the unexpandable bony sella turcica, hyposecretion from those cells that are most sensitive to pressure is common (GH-, FSH-, and LH-secreting cells).

CLINICAL MANIFESTATIONS The clinical manifestations of pituitary adenomas are related to tumor growth and hormone hypersecretion or hyposecretion. Increased tumor size causes headache, fatigue, neck pain or stiffness, and seizures. Visual changes include visual field impairments (often beginning in one eye and progressing to the other) and temporary blindness. If the tumor infiltrates other cranial nerves, neuromuscular function is affected.

Pituitary adenomas are most often associated with increased secretion of growth hormone and prolactin (see Hypersecretion of Growth Hormone: Acromegaly and Prolactinoma sections in this chapter).[18] Gonadotropic hyposecretion results in menstrual irregularity in women, decreased libido, and receding secondary sex characteristics in both men and women. If the tumor exerts sufficient pressure, thyroid and adrenal hypofunction may occur because of lack of TSH and ACTH, resulting in the symptoms of hypothyroidism and hypocortisolism, respectively.

EVALUATION AND TREATMENT Diagnosis of pituitary adenoma involves physical and laboratory evaluations, including pertinent hormone assays and radiographic examination of the skull (MRI [preferred] or contrast-enhanced CT). The goal of treatment is to protect the individual from the effects of tumor growth and to control hormone hypersecretion while minimizing damage to appropriately secreting portions of the pituitary. Depending on tumor size and type, individuals may be treated by administration of specific medications to suppress tumor growth, transsphenoidal tumor resection, or radiation therapy including stereotactic treatments.[19]

 QUICK CHECK 18-1

1. What is the mechanism of receptor-associated hormonal disorder?
2. Why do individuals with the syndrome of inappropriate antidiuretic hormone (SIADH) secrete concentrated urine?
3. Why may individuals with a pituitary adenoma develop visual disturbances?

Hypersecretion of Growth Hormone: Acromegaly

Acromegaly results from continuous exposure to high levels of growth hormone (GH) and insulin-like growth factor 1 (IGF-1); it almost always is caused by a GH-secreting pituitary adenoma (it rarely results from the ectopic production of GHRH).[20,21]

Acromegaly usually occurs in adults in the 40- to 59-year-old age group, although it is often present for years before diagnosis. It is a slowly progressive disease and, if untreated, is associated with a decreased life expectancy. Deaths from acromegaly are caused by heart disease secondary to hypertension and atherosclerosis, diabetes mellitus, or malignancy (colon or lung cancers).[21]

PATHOPHYSIOLOGY With a GH-secreting adenoma, the usual GH baseline secretion pattern and sleep-related GH peaks are lost, and a totally unpredictable secretory pattern ensues. However, GH levels in acromegalics are never completely suppressed. Only slight elevations of GH and IGF-1 stimulate growth. In children and adolescents whose epiphyseal plates have not yet closed, the effect of increased GH levels is termed **giantism** (Figure 18-3). Skeletal growth is excessive, with some individuals becoming 8 or 9 feet tall. In the adult, epiphyseal closure has occurred, and increased amounts of GH and IGF-1 cause connective tissue proliferation and increased cytoplasmic matrix, as well as bony proliferation that results in the characteristic appearance of acromegaly (Figure 18-4).[21]

GH also has significant effects on glucose, lipid, and protein metabolism.[22] Hyperglycemia results from GH's inhibition of peripheral glucose uptake and increased hepatic glucose production, followed by compensatory hyperinsulinism and, finally, insulin resistance. Diabetes mellitus occurs when the pancreas cannot secrete enough insulin to offset the effects of GH. Excessive levels of GH and IGF-1 also affect the cardiovascular system. Although the associated pathophysiologic mechanism is not clearly understood at present, hypertension and left ventricular heart failure are seen in one third to one half of individuals with acromegaly. Cardiomyopathy associated with progressive and unrestrained myocardial growth is a significant factor.[21] GH also acts on the renal tubules to increase phosphate reabsorption, leading to mild hyperphosphatemia. Because the adenoma becomes increasingly a space-occupying lesion, hypopituitarism may occur because of compression of surrounding hormone-secreting cells.

CLINICAL MANIFESTATIONS With connective tissue proliferation, individuals with acromegaly have an enlarged tongue, interstitial edema, enlarged and overactive sebaceous and sweat glands (leading to increased body odor), and coarse skin and body hair. Bony proliferation involves periosteal vertebral growth and enlargement of the bones of the face, hands, and feet (see Figure 18-4). The lower jaw and forehead also protrude.

Increased IGF-1 levels cause ribs to elongate at the bone-cartilage junction, leading to a barrel-chested appearance, and increased proliferation of cartilage in joints, which causes backache and arthralgias. With bony and soft tissue overgrowth, nerve entrapment occurs, leading to peripheral nerve damage manifested by weakness, muscular atrophy, footdrop, and sensory changes in the hands.

Symptoms of diabetes, such as polyuria and polydipsia, may occur. Acromegaly-associated hypertension is usually asymptomatic until heart failure symptoms develop. Increased tumor size results in central nervous system symptoms of headache, seizure activity, visual disturbances, and papilledema. If compression hypopituitarism occurs, gonadotropin secretion may be affected, causing amenorrhea in women and sexual dysfunction in men. Approximately 20% of growth hormone–secreting tumors also secrete prolactin, resulting in hypogonadism.

EVALUATION AND TREATMENT Diagnosis is confirmed by clinical features of the disease, MRI scans, and elevated levels of GH that are not suppressed by oral glucose intake. IGF-1 levels also are elevated. The goals of treatment are to normalize or reduce GH secretion and relieve or prevent complications related to tumor expansion. The treatment of choice in acromegaly is transsphenoidal surgical removal of the GH-secreting adenoma. Radiation therapy may be effective when rapid control of GH levels is not essential, when the individual is not a good surgical candidate, or when hyperfunction persists after subtotal

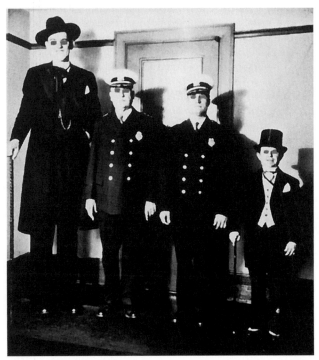

FIGURE 18-3 Giantism. A pituitary giant and dwarf contrasted with normal-size men. Excessive secretion of growth hormone by the anterior lobe of the pituitary gland during the early years of life produces giants of this type, whereas deficient secretion of this substance produces well-formed dwarfs. (From Thibodeau GA, Patton KT: *Anatomy & physiology,* ed 6, St Louis, 2007, Mosby.)

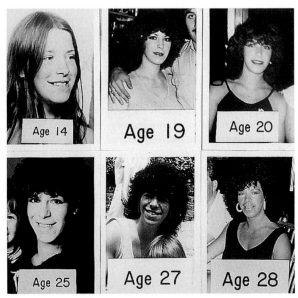

FIGURE 18-4 Acromegaly. Chronologic sequence of photographs showing slow development of acromegaly. (From Belchetz P, Hammond P: *Mosby's color atlas and text of diabetes and endocrinology,* Edinburgh, 2003, Mosby.)

resection. Somatostatin analogs, such as octreotide, octreotide LAR, and lanreotide, normalize IGF-1 levels and lower growth hormone levels. Dopaminergic agonists, such as cabergoline, also may be helpful, especially if the tumor also secretes prolactin. Pegvisomant is an effective drug that induces tissue insensitivity to GH by blocking the GH receptor.[23]

Prolactinoma

Pituitary tumors that secrete prolactin, prolactinomas, are the most common hormonally active pituitary tumors.[24] Other conditions or medications can elevate prolactin levels in the absence of pituitary pathologic condition. For example, renal failure, polycystic ovarian disease, primary hypothyroidism, breast stimulation, or even venipuncture can increase prolactin levels. Prolactin is under tonic inhibitory hypothalamic control through the secretion of dopamine. Thus medications that block the effects of dopamine can increase prolactin level and stimulate proliferation of prolactin-secreting cells (lactotrophs). These include antipsychotics (risperidone, chlorpromazine), metoclopramide, tricyclic antidepressants, and methyldopa. Estrogens increase prolactin concentration by stimulating hyperplasia of prolactin-secreting cells. Any process that interferes with the delivery of dopamine from the hypothalamus to the lactotrophs (pituitary stalk tumor, pituitary stalk transection, or compressive pituitary tumor) also results in hyperprolactinemia. Because thyrotropin-releasing hormone (TRH) stimulates prolactin secretion, in addition to enhancing TSH release, prolactin concentration may be elevated in individuals with primary hypothyroidism.

PATHOPHYSIOLOGY The hallmark of a prolactinoma is sustained increases in the levels of serum prolactin. The physiologic actions of prolactin include breast development during pregnancy, postpartum milk production, and suppression of ovarian function in nursing women. Pathologic elevation of prolactin levels in women results in amenorrhea, nonpuerperal milk production (galactorrhea), hirsutism, and osteopenia resulting from estrogen deficiency. Hyperprolactinemia in men causes hypogonadism and erectile dysfunction.

Because the adenoma becomes an increasingly space-occupying lesion, hypopituitarism may occur because of the compression of surrounding hormone secreting cells. Central nervous system symptoms may develop because of growth and pressure of the adenoma within the sella turcica.

CLINICAL MANIFESTATIONS Women with hyperprolactinemia generally present with galactorrhea (nonpuerperal milk production) and menstrual disturbances including amenorrhea. In susceptible women, hirsutism develops because of estrogen deficiency. If not detected until after many years, this estrogen deficiency also may result in osteoporosis. Men often present late with symptoms related to the increasing size of the adenoma (i.e., headache or visual impairment).[24]

EVALUATION AND TREATMENT The diagnostic evaluation of hyperprolactinemia includes a careful history to exclude medications that may cause elevations in prolactin concentration. Symptoms of hypothyroidism should be elicited, and screening with a serum TSH level is mandatory. MRI scanning of the pituitary is indicated to determine the size and location of an adenoma. If serum prolactin level is less than 50 ng/ml, a careful search for a nonpituitary cause should be pursued.

Dopaminergic agonists (bromocriptine and cabergoline) are the treatment of choice for prolactinomas.[24] Restoration of fertility in previously anovulatory women is common. In individuals resistant or intolerant to these medications, transsphenoidal surgery and radiotherapy are options.[25]

ALTERATIONS OF THYROID FUNCTION

Disorders of thyroid function develop as a result of primary dysfunction or disease of the thyroid gland or, secondarily, as a result of pituitary or hypothalamic alterations. Primary thyroid disorders result in alterations of thyroid hormone (TH) levels with secondary feedback effects on pituitary thyroid-stimulating hormone (TSH). For example, when there are primary elevations in TH level, TSH level will secondarily decrease because of negative feedback. When TH level is decreased because of a condition affecting the thyroid gland, TSH level will be elevated. Thyroid disease also can present with minimal or no symptoms but with abnormal laboratory values, known as subclinical thyroid disease (see Health Alert: Subclinical Thyroid Dysfunction). Central (secondary) thyroid disorders are related to disorders of pituitary gland TSH production. When there is excessive TSH production, TH level is elevated secondary to the primary elevation of TSH concentration. The reverse is true with inadequate TSH production.

HEALTH ALERT
Subclinical Thyroid Dysfunction

Subclinical hypothyroidism is defined as a condition in which thyroid hormone levels are within normal limits but serum TSH level is mildly elevated. This condition occurs in 3% to 8% of the population overall, and in 10% of individuals over the age of 60. Risk factors for the spontaneous form of this condition include female gender, aging, and the presence of thyroid antibodies. Subclinical hypothyroidism can also occur in neonates and children with certain genetic disorders and in individuals being inadequately treated for other hypothyroid conditions. Although the most common complication is the high likelihood of progression to clinical hypothyroidism, some studies suggest an associated increase in risk for dyslipidemia, atherosclerosis, and left ventricular dysfunction.

Subclinical hyperthyroidism is defined as a condition in which thyroid hormone levels are within normal limits but serum TSH level is mildly decreased. This condition affects between 2% and 6% of the population, women more commonly than men. The recognized complications of subclinical hyperthyroidism include osteoporosis, diminished arterial elasticity, reduced cognitive performance, diminished muscle strength, and increased risk of atrial fibrillation.

Monitoring and treatment of subclinical thyroid dysfunction is controversial although some studies link treatment with a reduced risk of complications.

Data from Biondi B: Cardiovascular mortality in subclinical hyperthyroidism: an ongoing dilemma, Eur J Endocrinol 162(3):587–589, 2010; Diez JJ, Iglesias P: An analysis of the natural course of subclinical hyperthyroidism, Am J Med Sci 337(4):225–232, 2009; Fatourechi V: Subclinical hypothyroidism: an update for primary care physicians, Mayo Clin Proc 84(1):65–71, 2009; Kim SK et al: Regression of the increased common carotid artery-intima media thickness in subclinical hypothyroidism after thyroid hormone replacement, Endocr J 56(6):753–758, 2009; O'Grady MJ, Cody D: Subclinical hypothyroidism in childhood, Arch Dis Child 96(3):280–284, 2011; Karmisholt J, et al: Variation in thyroid function in subclinical hypothyroidism: importance of clinical follow-up and therapy. Eur J Endocrinol 164(3):317–323, 2011.

Hyperthyroidism
Thyrotoxicosis

Thyrotoxicosis is a condition that results from increased levels of thyroid hormones (TH). Hyperthyroidism is a form of thyrotoxicosis in which excess amounts of TH are secreted from the thyroid gland. The terms *thyrotoxicosis* and *hyperthyroidism* are often used interchangeably. Common diseases that cause primary hyperthyroidism include

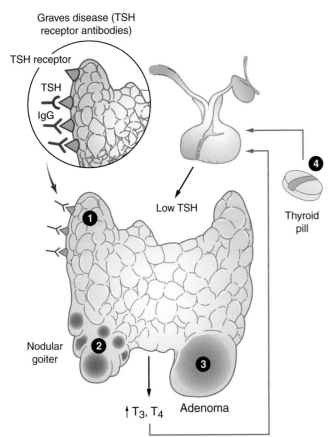

FIGURE 18-5 Common Causes of Hyperthyroidism. Hyperthyroidism may have several causes, among them: *1,* Graves disease; *2,* toxic multinodular goiter; *3,* follicular adenoma; *4,* thyroid medication. (From Damjanov I: *Pathology for the health professions,* ed 3, St Louis, 2006, Saunders.)

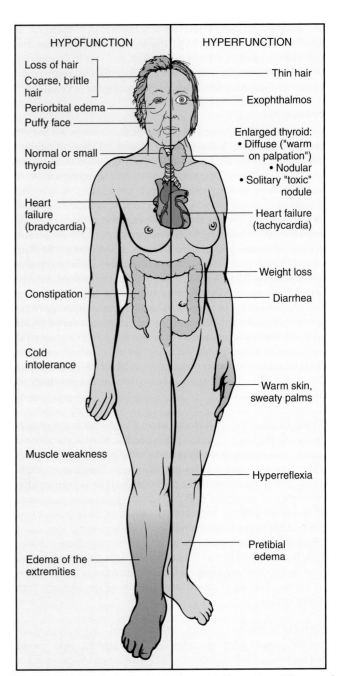

FIGURE 18-6 Clinical Manifestations of Hyperthyroidism and Hypothyroidism. (From Damjanov I: *Pathology for the health professions,* ed 4, St Louis, 2012, Saunders.)

Graves disease, toxic multinodular goiter, and solitary toxic adenoma (Figure 18-5). **Central (secondary) hyperthyroidism** is less common and is caused by TSH-secreting pituitary adenomas. Thyrotoxicosis not associated with hyperthyroidism includes subacute thyroiditis, ectopic thyroid tissue, and ingestion of excessive TH. Each condition is associated with a specific pathophysiology and manifestations; however, all forms of thyrotoxicosis share some common characteristics.

CLINICAL MANIFESTATIONS The clinical features of thyrotoxicosis are attributable to the metabolic effects of increased circulating levels of thyroid hormones. This usually results in an increased metabolic rate with heat intolerance and increased tissue sensitivity to stimulation by the sympathetic division of the autonomic nervous system. The major manifestations are summarized in Figure 18-6. Enlargement of the thyroid gland (goiter) is common in hyperthyroid conditions caused by stimulation of TSH receptors.

EVALUATION AND TREATMENT Elevated serum thyroxine (T_4) and triiodothyronine (T_3) and suppressed serum TSH levels are diagnostic for primary hyperthyroidism. By contrast, central (secondary) hyperthyroidism caused by TSH-secreting pituitary tumors is characterized by normal to increased TSH levels despite elevated thyroid hormone concentrations. Radioactive iodine is used to test for increased uptake in primary hyperthyroidism (Figure 18-7). Treatment is directed at controlling excessive TH production, secretion, or action and employs antithyroid drug therapy, radioactive iodine therapy, and surgery.[26] A major complication of all forms of treatment for hyperthyroidism is excessive ablation of the gland leading to hypothyroidism.

Hyperthyroid Conditions

Graves disease. Graves disease is the underlying cause of 50% to 80% of cases of hyperthyroidism with a prevalence of approximately 0.5% in the U.S. population. It occurs more commonly in women. Although the cause of Graves disease is not known, genetic factors interacting with environmental triggers play an important role in the pathogenesis of this autoimmune thyroid disease. Graves disease results from a form of type II hypersensitivity (see Chapter 7) in which

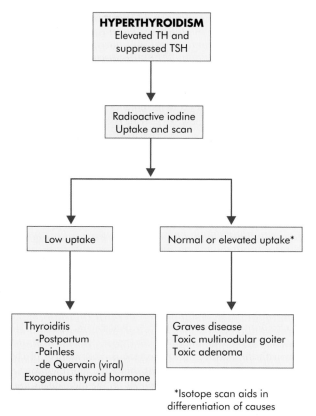

FIGURE 18-7 Evaluation of Hyperthyroidism. Radioactive iodine is used in the differential diagnosis of hyperthyroidism.

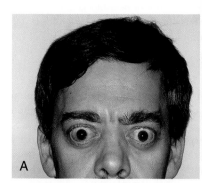
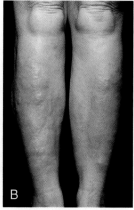

FIGURE 18-8 Thyrotoxicosis (Graves Disease). A, Exophthalmos (large and protruding eyeballs often in association with a large goiter); B, Pretibial myxedema associated with Graves disease; note lumpy and swollen appearance from accumulation of connective tissue and pinkish purple discoloration. (A from Belchetz P, Hammond P: *Mosby's color atlas and text of diabetes and endocrinology*, Edinburgh, 2003, Mosby; B from Habif T: *Clinical dermatology*, ed 5, 2009.)

there is stimulation of the thyroid by autoantibodies directed against the TSH receptor. These autoantibodies, called thyroid-stimulating immunoglobulins (TSIs), override the normal regulatory mechanisms. The TSI stimulation of TSH receptors in the gland results in hyperplasia of the gland (goiter) and increased synthesis of TH, especially of triiodo-L-thyronine (T_3). Increased levels of TH result in the classic signs and symptoms of hyperthyroidism illustrated in Figure 18-6. TSI stimulation of the gland also causes diffuse thyroid enlargement (goiter). TSH production by the pituitary is inhibited through the usual negative feedback loop.[27]

TSI also contributes to the two major distinguishing clinical manifestations of Graves disease (ophthalmopathy and, perhaps, dermopathy [pretibial myxedema]). Two categories of ophthalmopathy associated with Graves disease (Figure 18-8) are (1) functional abnormalities resulting from hyperactivity of the sympathetic division of the autonomic nervous system (lag of the globe on upward gaze and of the upper lid on downward gaze) and (2) infiltrative changes involving the orbital contents with enlargement of the ocular muscles. These changes affect more than half of individuals with Graves disease. Orbital fat accumulation, inflammation, and edema of the orbital contents result in exophthalmos (protrusion of the eyeball), periorbital edema, and extraocular muscle weakness, leading to diplopia (double vision).[28] The individual may experience irritation, pain, lacrimation, photophobia, blurred vision, decreased visual acuity, papilledema, visual field impairment, exposure keratosis, and corneal ulceration.

A small number of individuals with Graves disease and very high levels of TSI experience pretibial myxedema (Graves dermopathy), characterized by subcutaneous swelling on the anterior portions of the legs and by indurated and erythematous skin. Graves dermopathy is associated with thyrotropin receptor antigens on fibroblasts and recruited T lymphocytes.[29] These manifestations occasionally appear on the hands, giving the appearance of clubbing of the fingers (thyroid acropachy).

Hyperthyroidism resulting from nodular thyroid disease. The thyroid gland normally enlarges in response to the increased demand for TH that occurs in puberty, pregnancy, and iodine-deficient states as well as in individuals with immunologic, viral, or genetic disorders. When the condition requiring increased TH resolves, TSH secretion normally subsides and the thyroid gland returns to its original size.

Irreversible changes may have occurred in some follicular cells so these cells function autonomously and produce excessive amounts of TH. On the other hand, some follicular cells may cease to function. The balance between the amount of TH produced by hyperfunctioning nodules and that produced by the remainder of the gland determines whether an individual develops hyperthyroidism. Toxic multinodular goiter occurs when there are several hyperfunctioning nodules leading to hyperthyroidism. If only one nodule is hyperfunctioning, it is termed toxic adenoma. The classic clinical manifestations of hyperthyroidism (see Figure 18-6) usually develop slowly, and exophthalmos and pretibial myxedema do not occur. Nodules may be palpable on physical examination. The incidence of malignancy in toxic nodular goiter is estimated to be as high as 9%, so most individuals should undergo a fine needle aspiration biopsy of suspicious nodules before treatment. Treatment consists of a combination of radioactive iodine, surgery, and antithyroid medications.[30]

Thyrotoxic crisis. Thyrotoxic crisis (thyroid storm) is a rare but dangerous worsening of the thyrotoxic state in which death can occur within 48 hours without treatment. The condition may develop spontaneously, but it usually occurs in individuals who have undiagnosed or partially treated Graves disease and are subjected to excessive stress, such as infection, pulmonary or cardiovascular disorders, trauma, seizures, emotional distress, dialysis, plasmapheresis, or inadequate preparation for thyroid surgery.

The systemic symptoms of thyrotoxic crisis include hyperthermia; tachycardia, especially atrial tachydysrhythmias; high-output heart failure; agitation or delirium; and nausea, vomiting, or diarrhea contributing to fluid volume depletion. The symptoms may be attributed to increased β-adrenergic receptors and catecholamines. Treatment includes (1) the use of drugs that block TH synthesis (i.e., propylthiouracil or methimazole), (2) the use of beta-blockers for control of cardiovascular symptoms, the administration of (3) steroids or (4) iodine (e.g., saturated solution of potassium iodide [SSKI]), and (5) supportive care.

Hypothyroidism

Deficient production of TH by the thyroid gland results in the clinical state termed hypothyroidism. Hypothyroidism is the most common disorder of thyroid function, affects between 1% and 2% of the U.S. population, and occurs more commonly in women. It may be primary or central. Primary hypothyroidism accounts for 99% of all cases. Causes of central (secondary) hypothyroidism are less common and are related to either pituitary or hypothalamic failure.

PATHOPHYSIOLOGY In primary hypothyroidism, loss of thyroid function leads to decreased production of TH and increased secretion of TSH and TRH (Figure 18-9). The most common causes of primary hypothyroidism in adults include autoimmune thyroiditis (Hashimoto disease), iatrogenic loss of thyroid tissue after surgical or radioactive treatment for hyperthyroidism or after head and neck radiation therapy, medications, and endemic iodine deficiency.[31] Infants and children may present with hypothyroidism because of congenital defects. Central (secondary) hypothyroidism is caused by the pituitary's failure to synthesize adequate amounts of TSH or a lack of TRH. Pituitary tumors that compress surrounding pituitary cells or the consequences of their treatment are the most common causes of central hypothyroidism. Other causes include traumatic brain injury, subarachnoid hemorrhage, or pituitary infarction. Hypothalamic dysfunction results in low levels of TH, TSH, and TRH.[32]

CLINICAL MANIFESTATIONS Hypothyroidism generally affects all body systems and occurs insidiously over months or years. The decrease in TH level lowers energy metabolism and heat production. The individual develops a low basal metabolic rate, cold intolerance, lethargy, and slightly lowered basal body temperature (see Figure 18-6). The decrease in the level of TH can lead to excessive TSH production, which stimulates thyroid tissue and causes goiter.

The characteristic sign of severe or long-standing hypothyroidism is myxedema, which results from the altered composition of the dermis and other tissues. The connective tissue fibers are separated by large amounts of protein and mucopolysaccharide. This complex binds water, producing nonpitting, boggy edema, especially around the eyes, hands, and feet and in the supraclavicular fossae (Figure 18-10). The tongue and laryngeal and pharyngeal mucous membranes thicken, producing thick, slurred speech and hoarseness. Myxedema coma, a medical emergency, is a diminished level of consciousness associated with severe hypothyroidism. Signs and symptoms include hypothermia without shivering, hypoventilation, hypotension, hypoglycemia, and lactic acidosis. Older individuals with severe vascular disease and with moderate or untreated hypothyroidism are particularly at risk for developing myxedema coma. It also may occur after overuse of narcotics or sedatives or after an acute illness in hypothyroid individuals.[33] Symptoms of hypothyroidism in older adults should not be attributed to normal aging changes.

EVALUATION AND TREATMENT The diagnosis of primary hypothyroidism is made by documentation of the clinical symptoms of hypothyroidism, and measurement of increased levels of TSH and decreased levels of TH (total T_3 and both total and free T_4). When hypothyroidism is caused by pituitary deficiencies, serum TSH levels and basal metabolic rate (BMR) decrease. Hormone replacement therapy with the hormone levothyroxine is the treatment of choice. The restoration of normal TH levels should be timed appropriately; a regimen of hormonal therapy depends on the individual's age, the duration and severity of the hypothyroidism, and the presence of other disorders, particularly cardiovascular disorders.[34]

Hypothyroid Conditions

Primary hypothyroidism. The most common cause of hypothyroidism in the United States is autoimmune thyroiditis (Hashimoto disease, chronic lymphocytic thyroiditis), which results in gradual

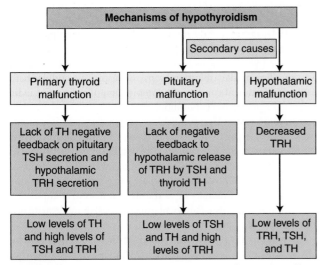

FIGURE 18-9 Mechanisms of Primary and Secondary Hypothyroidism.

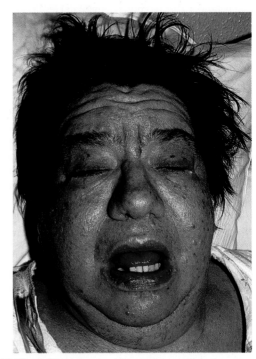

FIGURE 18-10 Myxedema. Note edema around eyes and facial puffiness. The hair is dry. (From Bolognia: *Dermatology*, ed 2, 2008, Mosby.)

inflammatory destruction of thyroid tissue by infiltration of lymphocytes and circulating thyroid autoantibodies (antithyroid peroxidase and antithyroglobulin antibodies).[35] This disorder is linked with several genetic risk factors and is commonly associated with other autoimmune conditions.[36] Infiltration of thyroid autoantibodies, autoreactive T lymphocytes, natural killer cells, and inflammatory cytokines and induction of apoptosis are involved in the tissue destruction seen in Hashimoto thyroiditis.[37]

Spontaneous recovery of thyroid function is seen in three conditions: subacute thyroiditis, painless thyroiditis, and postpartum thyroiditis. Subacute thyroiditis is a nonbacterial inflammation of the thyroid gland often preceded by a viral infection. It is accompanied by fever, tenderness, and enlargement of the thyroid gland. The inflammatory process initially results in elevated levels of thyroid hormone through the release of stored thyroglobulin, which then is associated with transient hypothyroidism before the gland recovers normal activity. Symptoms may last for 2 to 4 months, and nonsteroidal anti-inflammatory drugs or corticosteroids usually resolve symptoms. Painless thyroiditis has a course similar to that of subacute thyroiditis but is pathologically identical to Hashimoto disease. Postpartum thyroiditis is pathologically related to Hashimoto disease and generally occurs up to 6 months after delivery with a course similar to that seen in subacute thyroiditis. Thus a hyperthyroid phase (with a low thyroid radioiodine uptake) precedes the hypothyroid phase in typical cases of subacute, painless, or postpartum thyroiditis. Spontaneous recovery occurs in 95% of these conditions.

Congenital hypothyroidism. Hypothyroidism in infants occurs when thyroid tissue is absent (thyroid dysgenesis) or with hereditary defects in TH synthesis. Thyroid dysgenesis occurs more often in female infants, with permanent abnormalities in 1 of every 4000 live births. Because TH is essential for embryonic growth, particularly of brain tissue, the infant will be cognitively disabled if there is no thyroxine during fetal life.[38] Hypothyroidism at birth presents clinically with high birthweight, hypothermia, delay in passing meconium, and neonatal jaundice. Cord blood can be examined in the first days of life for T_4 and TSH levels. The probability of normal growth and intellectual function is high if treatment with levothyroxine is started before the child is 3 or 4 months old. The earlier thyroid hormone replacement is initiated, the better the child's outcome.[39]

Without early screening, hypothyroidism may not be evident until after 4 months of age. Symptoms include difficulty eating, hoarse cry, and protruding tongue caused by myxedema of oral tissues and vocal cords; hypotonic muscles of the abdomen with constipation, abdominal protrusion, and umbilical hernia; subnormal temperature; lethargy; excessive sleeping; slow pulse rate; and cold, mottled skin. Skeletal growth is stunted because of impaired protein synthesis, poor absorption of nutrients, and lack of bone mineralization. The child will be dwarfed with short limbs, if not treated. Dentition is often delayed. Cognitive disability varies with the severity of hypothyroidism and the length of delay before treatment is initiated.

Thyroid Carcinoma

Thyroid carcinoma is the most common endocrine malignancy and accounts for 4% of all cancer cases in women in the United States.[40] Exposure to ionizing radiation, especially during childhood, is the most consistent causal factor. Papillary and follicular thyroid carcinomas are the most frequent and medullary and anaplastic thyroid carcinomas are less common. Most tumors are well differentiated.

Most individuals with thyroid carcinoma have normal T_3 and T_4 levels and are therefore euthyroid. The cancer is typically discovered as a small thyroid nodule or metastatic tumor in the lungs, brain, or bone. Changes in voice and swallowing and difficulty breathing are related to tumor growth impinging on the trachea or esophagus. The diagnosis of thyroid cancer is generally made by fine needle aspiration of a thyroid nodule. Ultrasonographic characteristics may be suggestive of malignancy, but radioisotope scanning is rarely helpful in a euthyroid individual. Treatment may include partial or total thyroidectomy, TSH suppression therapy (levothyroxine), radioactive iodine therapy (in iodine-concentrating tumors), postoperative radiation therapy, and chemotherapy (especially in anaplastic carcinoma). New insights into the molecular pathogenesis of thyroid carcinoma are leading to new therapies.[41]

> ✔ **QUICK CHECK 18-2**
> 1. Compare the clinical manifestations of hyperthyroidism and hypothyroidism.
> 2. What is Graves disease?
> 3. What is myxedema?

ALTERATIONS OF PARATHYROID FUNCTION

Hyperparathyroidism

Hyperparathyroidism is characterized by greater than normal secretion of parathyroid hormone (PTH) and hypercalcemia. Hyperparathyroidism is classified as primary or secondary. Calcium levels are either low or normal in secondary hyperparathyroidism.

PATHOPHYSIOLOGY   Primary hyperparathyroidism is characterized by inappropriate excess secretion of PTH by one or more of the parathyroid glands. It is one of the most common endocrine disorders. Approximately 80% to 85% of cases are caused by parathyroid adenomas, another 10% to 15% result from parathyroid hyperplasia, and approximately 1% is caused by parathyroid carcinoma. In addition, primary hyperparathyroidism may be caused by a variety of genetic causes, especially the genes that cause multiple endocrine neoplasia.[42]

In primary hyperparathyroidism, PTH secretion is increased and is not under the usual feedback control mechanisms. The calcium level in the blood increases because of increased bone resorption and gastrointestinal absorption of calcium, but fails to inhibit PTH secretion by the parathyroid gland.

Secondary hyperparathyroidism is a compensatory response of the parathyroid glands to chronic hypocalcemia, which can be associated with decreased renal activation of vitamin D (renal failure) (see Chapter 29. Secretion of PTH is elevated, but PTH cannot achieve normal calcium levels because of insufficient levels of activated vitamin D. Other causes of secondary hyperparathyroidism include dietary deficiency in vitamin D or calcium; decreased intestinal absorption of vitamin D or calcium; and ingestion of drugs, such as phenytoin, phenobarbital, and laxatives, which either accelerates the metabolism of vitamin D or decreases intestinal absorption of calcium.

CLINICAL MANIFESTATIONS   Hypercalcemia and hypophosphatemia are the hallmarks of primary hyperparathyroidism. Hypercalcemia and hypophosphatemia may be asymptomatic or affected individuals may present with symptoms related to the muscular, nervous, and gastrointestinal systems, including fatigue, headache, depression, anorexia, and nausea and vomiting. Excessive osteoclastic and osteocytic activity resulting in bone resorption may cause pathologic fractures, kyphosis of the dorsal spine, and compression fractures of the vertebral bodies. (Bone resorption is discussed in Chapter 37.)

The increased renal filtration load of calcium leads to hypercalciuria. Hypercalcemia also affects proximal renal tubular function, causing metabolic acidosis and production of an abnormally alkaline urine.[43] PTH hypersecretion enhances renal phosphate excretion and results in hypophosphatemia and hyperphosphaturia (see Chapter 4). The combination of these three variables—hypercalciuria, alkaline urine, and hyperphosphaturia—predisposes the individual to the formation of calcium stones, particularly in the renal pelvis or renal collecting ducts. These may be associated with infections. Both kidney stones and renal infection can lead to impaired renal function. Hypercalcemia also impairs the concentrating ability of the renal tubule by decreasing its response to ADH. Chronic hypercalcemia of hyperparathyroidism is associated with mild insulin resistance, necessitating increased insulin secretion to maintain normal glucose levels.

Secondary hyperparathyroidism caused by renal disease presents clinically not only with bone resorption but also with the symptoms of hypocalcemia and hyperphosphatemia. Hypocalcemia can cause many significant clinical problems (see Chapter 4 and hyperphosphatemia can cause deleterious effects on the cardiovascular system.

EVALUATION AND TREATMENT The concurrent findings of increased ionized calcium concentration despite elevated PTH concentration are suggestive of primary hyperparathyroidism. Imaging procedures are used to localize adenomas before surgery. Observation of asymptomatic individuals with mild hypercalcemia is recommended; these individuals are advised to avoid dehydration and limit dietary calcium intake. Definitive treatment of severe primary hyperparathyroidism involves surgical removal of the solitary adenoma or, in the case of hyperplasia, complete removal of three and partial removal of the fourth hyperplastic parathyroid glands. In those individuals who fail surgery, other treatments such as bisphosphonates and calcimimetics (e.g., cinacalcet, a new class of calcium-lowering drugs) may be considered.

If serum calcium concentration is low but PTH level is elevated, secondary hyperparathyroidism is likely. Evaluation for renal function may indicate chronic renal disease. Treatment for secondary hyperparathyroidism in chronic renal disease requires calcium replacement, dietary phosphate restriction and phosphate binders, and vitamin D replacement. Treatment also may include calcimimetics, which work to increase parathyroid calcium receptor sensitivity, thus lowering PTH levels.[44]

Hypoparathyroidism

Hypoparathyroidism (abnormally low PTH levels) is most commonly caused by damage to the parathyroid glands during thyroid surgery. This occurs because of the anatomic proximity of the parathyroid glands to the thyroid. Hypoparathyroidism also is associated with genetic syndromes, including familial hypoparathyroidism and DiGeorge syndrome (velocardiofacial syndrome). Hypomagnesemia also can cause a decrease in both PTH secretion and PTH function. An idiopathic or autoimmune form of hypoparathyroidism also is recognized.[45] There is an inherited condition associated with hypocalcemia but with normal to elevated levels of PTH called pseudohypoparathyroidism; it is caused by a postreceptor defect in PTH action.

PATHOPHYSIOLOGY A lack of circulating PTH causes depressed serum calcium levels and increased serum phosphate levels. In the absence of PTH, resorption of calcium from bone and regulation of calcium reabsorption from the renal tubules are impaired. Phosphate reabsorption by the renal tubules is therefore increased, causing hyperphosphatemia (PTH causes a phosphaturia).

The effects of hypomagnesemia on the peripheral metabolism and clearance of PTH are not clearly understood. Once serum magnesium levels return to normal, however, PTH secretion returns to normal, as does the responsiveness of peripheral tissues to PTH. Hypomagnesemia may be related to chronic alcoholism, malnutrition, malabsorption, increased renal clearance of magnesium caused by the use of aminoglycoside antibiotics or certain chemotherapeutic agents, or prolonged magnesium-deficient parenteral nutritional therapy.

CLINICAL MANIFESTATIONS Symptoms associated with hypoparathyroidism are primarily those of hypocalcemia. Hypocalcemia causes a lowered threshold for nerve and muscle excitation so that a nerve impulse may be initiated by a slight stimulus anywhere along the length of a nerve or muscle fiber. This creates tetany, a condition characterized by muscle spasms, hyperreflexia, clonic-tonic convulsions, laryngeal spasms, and, in severe cases, death by asphyxiation. Chvostek and Trousseau signs may be used to evaluate for neuromuscular irritability. Chvostek sign is elicited by tapping the cheek, resulting in twitching of the upper lip. Trousseau sign is elicited by sustained inflation of a sphygmomanometer placed on the upper arm to a level above the systolic blood pressure with resultant painful carpal spasm. Other symptoms of hypocalcemia include dry skin, loss of body and scalp hair, hypoplasia of developing teeth, horizontal ridges on the nails, cataracts, basal ganglia calcifications (which may be associated with a parkinsonian syndrome), and bone deformities, including brachydactyly and bowing of the long bones.

Phosphate retention caused by increased renal reabsorption of phosphate is also associated with hypoparathyroidism. Hyperphosphatemia results from PTH deficiency and, in turn, hyperphosphatemia further lowers calcium concentration by inhibiting the activation of vitamin D, thereby lowering the gastrointestinal absorption of calcium.

EVALUATION AND TREATMENT A low serum calcium concentration and a high phosphorus level in the absence of renal failure, intestinal disorders, or nutritional deficiencies suggest hypoparathyroidism. PTH levels are low in hypoparathyroidism and measurement of serum magnesium level and urinary calcium excretion also can help in diagnosis. Treatment is directed toward alleviation of the hypocalcemia.[45] In acute states, this involves parenteral administration of calcium, which corrects serum calcium concentration within minutes. Maintenance of serum calcium level is achieved with pharmacologic doses of an active form of vitamin D and oral calcium. Hypoplastic dentition, cataracts, bone deformities, and basal ganglia calcifications do not respond to the correction of hypocalcemia, but the other symptoms of hypocalcemia are reversible.

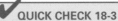

> **✓ QUICK CHECK 18-3**
> 1. How does excessive parathyroid hormone (PTH) affect bones?
> 2. What are the results of a lack of circulating PTH?

DYSFUNCTION OF THE ENDOCRINE PANCREAS: DIABETES MELLITUS

Diabetes mellitus is a group of metabolic diseases characterized by hyperglycemia resulting from defects in insulin secretion, insulin action, or both. 25.8 million people, or 8.3% of the U.S. population, have diabetes and another 7 million are estimated to be undiagnosed. It is the seventh cause of death and costs $174 billion dollars per year in

TABLE 18-3 CLASSIFICATION AND CHARACTERISTICS OF DIABETES MELLITUS

NAME	CHARACTERISTICS
Type 1 (beta-cell destruction leading to absolute insulin deficiency) Immune-mediated diabetes common form (≈90%)	Cellular-mediated autoimmune destruction of pancreatic beta cells Individual prone to ketoacidosis Little or no insulin secretion Insulin dependent 75% of individuals develop before 30 yr of age; can occur up to the tenth decade Usually not obese
Idiopathic (≈10%)	No defined etiologies; absolute requirement for insulin replacement therapy in affected individuals may vary
Type 2 diabetes (may range from pre-dominantly insulin resistance with rela-tive insulin deficiency to predominantly secretory defect with insulin resistance)	Usually not insulin dependent but may be insulin requiring Individual not ketosis prone (but may form ketones under stress) Obesity common in abdominal region Generally occurs in those older than 40 yr, but frequency is rapidly increasing in children Strong genetic predisposition Often associated with hypertension and dyslipidemia
Other Specific Types	
Genetic defects of beta-cell function	Genetic abnormalities that decrease ability of beta-cell to secrete insulin: 1. Maturity-onset of youth (MODY) includes six specific autosomal dominant mutations including genes for hepatocyte nuclear factor-1α (HNF-1α; *MODY 3*), glucokinase *(MODY 2)*, HNF-4α *(MODY 1)*, insulin promoter factor-1 (IPF-1; *MODY 4*), HNF-1β *(MODY 5)*, and NeuroD1 *(MODY 6)* 2. Defects in mitochondrial deoxyribonucleic acid (DNA) 3. Other (including inability to convert proinsulin to insulin)
Genetic defects in insulin action	Mutations in insulin receptor with hyperinsulinism or hyperglycemia or severe diabetes
Diseases of exocrine pancreas	Any process that diffusely injures the pancreas, including pancreatitis, neoplasia, and cystic fibrosis
Endocrinopathies	Endocrine disorders including acromegaly, Cushing syndrome, glucagonoma, pheochromocytoma, hyperthyroid-ism, somatostatinoma, and aldosteronoma
Drug- or chemical-induced beta-cell dysfunction	Commonly associated drugs include glucocorticoids and thiazide diuretics, although many others may be implicated
Infections	Beta-cell destruction by viruses including cytomegalovirus, congenital rubella
Uncommon forms of immune-mediated diabetes mellitus	Anti–insulin receptor antibodies Reported with "stiff man syndrome" and individuals receiving interferon-α
Other genetic syndromes sometimes as-sociated with diabetes mellitus	Down, Klinefelter, Turner, and Wolfram syndromes
Gestational Diabetes Mellitus (GDM)	
Any degree of glucose intolerance with onset of first recognition during pregnancy	Insulin resistance combined with inadequate insulin secretion in relation to hyperglycemia Women who are obese, older than 25 yr, have a family history of diabetes, have a history of previous GDM, or are of certain ethnic groups (Hispanic, Native Americans, Asians, or blacks) are at increased risk of developing GDM Metabolic stress of pregnancy may uncover a genetic tendency for type 2 diabetes mellitus

From American Diabetes Association: Diagnosis and classification of diabetes mellitus, *Diabetes Care* 33:S62–S69, 2010.

the United States.[45a] The American Diabetes Association (ADA) classi-fies four categories of diabetes mellitus[46] (Table 18-3):

1. Type 1 (beta-cell destruction, usually leading to absolute insulin deficiency)
2. Type 2 (ranging from predominantly insulin resistance with rela-tive insulin deficiency to predominantly an insulin secretory defect with insulin resistance)
3. Other specific types
4. Gestational diabetes

The diagnosis of diabetes mellitus is based on glycosylated hemo-globin (HbA_{1C}) levels; fasting plasma glucose (FPG) levels; 2-hour plasma glucose levels during oral glucose tolerance testing (OGTT) using a 75-g oral glucose load; or random glucose levels in an indi-vidual with symptoms (Box 18-1). **Glycosylated hemoglobin** refers to the permanent attachment of glucose to hemoglobin molecules and reflects the average plasma glucose exposure over the life of a red blood

cell (approximately 120 days). This test is critically dependent upon the method of measurement and must be related to established stan-dards. The ADA classification "categories at increased risk for diabetes" describes nondiabetic elevations of HbA_{1C}, FPG, or the 2-hour plasma glucose value during OGTT (see Box 18-1). This classification includes impaired glucose tolerance (IGT), which results from diminished insu-lin secretion, and impaired fasting glucose (IFG), which is caused by enhanced hepatic glucose output. Individuals with IGT and IFG are at increased risk of cardiovascular disease and premature death and carry a 3% to 7% yearly risk of developing diabetes.[46]

Types of Diabetes Mellitus
Type 1 Diabetes Mellitus

Type 1 diabetes mellitus is the most common pediatric chronic disease and affects 0.17% of U.S. children and the incidence is increasing.[47,47a] Between 10% and 13% of individuals with newly diagnosed type 1

BOX 18-1 DIAGNOSTIC CRITERIA FOR DIABETES MELLITUS

1. HbA$_{1C}$ (as measured in a DCCT-referenced assay) ≥6.5%*
OR
2. FPG ≥126 mg/dl (7.0 mmol/L); fasting is defined as no caloric intake for at least 8 hr*
OR
3. 2-hr plasma glucose ≥200 mg/dl (11.1 mmol/L) during OGTT*
OR

4. In an individual with classic symptoms of hyperglycemia or hyperglycemic crisis, a random plasma glucose ≥200 mg/dl (11.1 mmol/L)

Categories of Increased Risk for Diabetes
1. FPG 100 to 125 mg/dl
2. 2-hr PG 75 to 199 mg/dl during OGTT
3. HbA$_{1C}$ 5.7% to 6.4%

The Diabetes Control and Complications Trial Research Group: The effect of intensive treatment of diabetes on the development and progression of long-term complications in insulin-dependent diabetes mellitus, *N Engl J Med* 329(14):977–986, 1993.
*In the absence of unequivocal hyperglycemia, criteria 1 through 3 should be confirmed by repeat testing.
From American Diabetes Association: Diagnosis and classification of diabetes mellitus, *Diabetes Care* 33:S62–S69, 2010.
FPG, Fasting plasma glucose; *HbA$_{1C}$ (hemoglobin A$_{1C}$)*, glycosylated hemoglobin; *DCCT*, Diabetes Control and Complications Trial; *OGTT*, oral glucose tolerance testing; *PG*, plasma glucose.

TABLE 18-4 EPIDEMIOLOGY AND ETIOLOGY OF DIABETES MELLITUS IN THE UNITED STATES

	TYPE 1 DIABETES: PRIMARY BETA-CELL DEFECT OR FAILURE	TYPE 2 DIABETES: INSULIN RESISTANCE WITH INADEQUATE INSULIN SECRETION
Incidence		
Frequency	One of most common childhood diseases (5-10% of all cases of diabetes mellitus) Prevalence rate is 0.17%	Accounts for most cases (≈90%-95%) Prevalence rate for ages 45-64 yr is 10.5%, for ages 65-74 yr is 18.4%
Change in incidences	No documented increase in incidence in United States	Incidence in all age groups has doubled since 1980
Characteristics		
Age at onset	Peak onset at age 11-13 yr (slightly earlier for girls than for boys) Rare in children younger than 1 yr and adults older than 30 yr	Risk of developing diabetes increases after age 40 yr; in general, incidence increases with age into 70s; among Pima Indians, incidence peaks between ages 40 and 50 yr, then falls
Gender	Similar in males and females	Similar in males and females overall, although black females have highest incidence and prevalence of all groups
Racial distribution	Rates for whites 1.5-2 times higher than for nonwhites Higher rates for those of Scandinavian descent than for those of Central or Southern European descent	Risk is highest for blacks and Native Americans
Obesity	Generally normal or underweight	Frequent contributing factor to precipitate type 2 diabetes among those susceptible; a major factor in populations recently exposed to westernized environment Increased risk related to duration, degree, and distribution of obesity
Etiology		
Common theory	*Autoimmune:* genetic and environmental factors, resulting in gradual process of autoimmune destruction in genetically susceptible individuals *Nonautoimmune:* Unknown Strong association with *HLA-DQA* and *HLA-DQB* genes	Disease results from genetic susceptibility (polygenic) combined with environmental determinants and other risk factors; inherited defects in beta-cell mass and function combined with peripheral tissue insulin resistance Associated with long-duration obesity
Heredity	Risk to sibling: 5%-10%; risk to offspring: 2-5%	Risk to first-degree relative (child or sibling): 10%-15%
Presence of antibody	Islet cell autoantibodies (ICAs) and/or autoantibodies to insulin, and autoantibodies to glutamic acid decarboxylase (GAD$_{65}$) and tyrosine phosphatases IA-2 and IA-2β are present in 85%-90% of individuals when fasting hyperglycemia is initially detected	Islet cell antibodies not present
Insulin resistance	Insulin resistance at diagnosis is unusual, but insulin resistance may occur as individual ages and gains weight	Insulin resistance is generally caused by altered cellular metabolism and intracellular postreceptor defect
Insulin secretion	Severe insulin deficiency or no insulin secretion at all	Typically increased at time of diagnosis, but progressively declines over course of illness

Data from American Diabetes Association: *Diabetic Care* 30(suppl 1): S42–S47, 2007; National Diabetes Clearinghouse: National Diabetes Statistics, 2011, NIH Publication No. 11–3892, February 2011. Available at http://diabetes.niddk.nih.gov/dm/pubs/statistics/#fast.

diabetes have a first-degree relative (parent or sibling) with type 1 diabetes. There is a 50% concordance rate in twins.[48] Diagnosis is rare during the first 9 months of life and peaks at 12 years of age. Two distinct types of type 1 diabetes have been identified: autoimmune and nonimmune.[49] Autoimmune type 1 diabetes is called *type 1A.* Nonimmune type 1 diabetes is far less common than immune. It occurs secondary to other diseases, such as pancreatitis, or to a more fulminant disorder termed *idiopathic (type 1B) diabetes.* Type 1B diabetes occurs mostly in people of Asian or African descent and affected individuals have varying degrees of insulin deficiency. Table 18-4 summarizes the epidemiology of diabetes mellitus.

PATHOPHYSIOLOGY Type 1A diabetes mellitus is a slowly progressive autoimmune T cell–mediated disease that destroys beta cells of the pancreas. Destruction of beta cells is related to genetic susceptibility and environmental factors. The strongest genetic association is with histocompatibility leukocyte antigen (HLA) class II alleles *HLA-DQ* and *HLA-DR.* The *HLA-DR* marker is associated with other autoimmune disorders, such as celiac, Graves, Hashimoto, and Addison diseases.[50] Environmental factors that have been implicated include exposure to certain drugs, foods, and viruses. These gene-environment interactions result in the formation of autoantigens that are expressed on the surface of pancreatic beta cells and circulate in the bloodstream and lymphatics (Figure 18-11). Cellular immunity (T cytotoxic cells and macrophages) and humoral immunity (autoantibodies) are stimulated, resulting in beta-cell destruction and apoptosis.[51,52] Over time, insulin synthesis declines and hyperglycemia develops.

Insulin, amylin, and glucagon. For insulin synthesis to decline enough such that hyperglycemia occurs, 80% to 90% of the insulin-secreting beta cells of the islet of Langerhans must be destroyed. Insulin normally suppresses secretion of glucagon and, thus, hypoinsulinemia leads to a marked increase in glucagon secretion. Glucagon, a hormone produced by the alpha cells of the islets, acts in the liver to increase blood glucose level by stimulating glycogenolysis and gluconeogenesis. In addition to the decline in insulin secretion, there is decreased secretion of amylin, another beta-cell hormone. One of the critical actions of amylin is to suppress glucagon release from the alpha cells.[53] Thus both alpha-cell and beta-cell functions are abnormal and both a lack of insulin and a relative excess of glucagon contribute to hyperglycemia in type 1 diabetes.

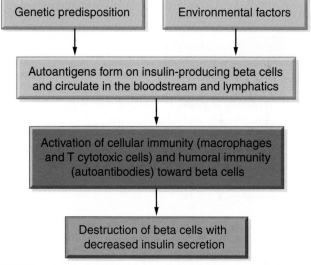

FIGURE 18-11 Pathophysiology of Type 1 Diabetes Mellitus.

CLINICAL MANIFESTATIONS Historically, type 1 diabetes mellitus was believed to have an abrupt onset. It is now known, however, that the natural history involves a long preclinical period with gradual destruction of beta cells, eventually leading to insulin deficiency and hyperglycemia. Generally, this latent period is longer in older individuals with type 1 diabetes and often results in misclassification of those affected as having type 2 diabetes.

Type 1 diabetes mellitus affects the metabolism of fat, protein, and carbohydrates. Glucose accumulates in the blood and appears in the urine as the renal threshold for glucose is exceeded, producing an osmotic diuresis and symptoms of polyuria and thirst (Table 18-5). Wide fluctuations in blood glucose levels occur. In addition, protein and fat breakdown occurs because of the lack of insulin, resulting in weight loss. Increased metabolism of fats and proteins leads to high levels of circulating ketones, causing a condition known as diabetic ketoacidosis (DKA) (see p. 465).

EVALUATION AND TREATMENT The criteria for diagnosis of type 1 diabetes are the same as those for type 2 diabetes (see Box 18-1). The diagnosis of diabetes is not difficult when the symptoms of polydipsia,

TABLE 18-5	CLINICAL MANIFESTATIONS AND MECHANISMS FOR TYPE 1 DIABETES MELLITUS
MANIFESTATION	**RATIONALE**
Polydipsia	Because of elevated blood glucose levels, water is osmotically attracted from body cells, resulting in intracellular dehydration and stimulation of thirst in hypothalamus
Polyuria	Hyperglycemia acts as an osmotic diuretic; amount of glucose filtered by glomeruli of kidney exceeds that which can be reabsorbed by renal tubules; glycosuria results, accompanied by large amounts of water lost in urine
Polyphagia	Depletion of cellular stores of carbohydrates, fats, and protein results in cellular starvation and a corresponding increase in hunger
Weight loss	Weight loss occurs because of fluid loss in osmotic diuresis and loss of body tissue as fats and proteins are used for energy
Fatigue	Metabolic changes result in poor use of food products, contributing to lethargy and fatigue
Recurrent infections (e.g., boils and carbuncles)	Growth of microorganisms is stimulated by increased glucose levels and diabetes is associated with some immunocompromise
Prolonged wound healing	Impaired blood supply hinders healing
Genital pruritus	Hyperglycemia and glycosuria favor fungal growth; candidal infections, resulting in pruritus, are a common presenting symptom in women
Visual changes	Blurred vision occurs as water balance in eye fluctuates because of elevated blood glucose levels; diabetic retinopathy may ensue
Paresthesias	Paresthesias are common manifestations of diabetic neuropathies
Cardiovascular symptoms (e.g., chest pain, extremity pain and neurologic deficits)	Diabetes contributes to formation of atherosclerotic plaques that involve coronary, peripheral, and cerebrovascular circulations

polyuria, polyphagia, weight loss, and hyperglycemia are present in fasting and postprandial states. C-peptide, a component of proinsulin released during insulin production, can be measured in the serum as a surrogate for insulin levels and is indicative of residual beta-cell mass and function. Other important aspects of evaluation include looking for evidence of the chronic complications of type 1 diabetes, including renal, nervous system, cardiac, peripheral vascular, retinal, and bony tissue damage.

Nearly 50% of children ages 4 years and younger and nearly 25% of those between the ages of 5 and 15 with type 1 diabetes are first diagnosed when they present with the signs and symptoms of DKA.[54] In DKA, acetone (a volatile form of ketones) is exhaled by hyperventilation and gives the breath a sweet or "fruity" odor. Occasionally, diabetic coma is the initial symptom of the disease.

Currently, treatment regimens are designed to achieve optimal glucose level control (as measured by the HbA_{1C} value) without causing episodes of significant hypoglycemia. Management requires individual planning according to type of disease, age, and activity level, but all individuals require some combination of insulin therapy, meal planning, and exercise regimen. There are several different types of insulin preparations available and there are new technologies for more physiologic insulin delivery systems.[55] Many different kinds of therapies are being tested to prevent the autoimmune destruction of beta cells,

including immunosuppression with antirejection drugs.[56] Finally, islet cell and whole pancreas transplantation has been successful in selected individuals.[57]

Type 2 Diabetes Mellitus

Type 2 diabetes mellitus (non–insulin-dependent diabetes mellitus) is much more common than type 1 and has been rising in incidence since 1940. In the United States, type 2 diabetes affects 10.5% of those ages 45 to 64 years and 18.4% of those ages 65 to 74 years and has doubled in all adult age groups in the past two decades.[58] Prevalence varies by ethnic group and gender and is highest in black women with an overall prevalence of 34% in those ages 65 to 74. There also is an increased prevalence of type 2 diabetes in children, especially in Native American and obese children (see Table 18-4).

A genetic-environmental interaction appears to be responsible for type 2 diabetes. The most well-recognized risk factors are age, obesity, hypertension, physical inactivity, and family history. The metabolic syndrome is a constellation of disorders (central obesity, dyslipidemia, prehypertension, and an elevated fasting blood glucose level) that together confer a high risk of developing type 2 diabetes and associated cardiovascular complications (Box 18-2). The metabolic syndrome develops during childhood and is highly prevalent among overweight children and adolescents, affecting approximately 55 million Americans. These individuals should be screened on a regular basis for diabetes mellitus. Early recognition and treatment, including vigorous lifestyle changes, are critical to reducing cardiovascular events and improving clinical outcomes.[59,60]

PATHOPHYSIOLOGY Many genes have been identified that are associated with type 2 diabetes, including those that code for beta-cell mass, beta-cell function (ability to sense blood glucose levels, insulin synthesis, and insulin secretion), proinsulin and insulin molecular structures, insulin receptors, hepatic synthesis of glucose, glucagon synthesis, and cellular responsiveness to insulin stimulation. These genetic abnormalities combined with environmental influences, such as obesity, result in the basic pathophysiologic mechanisms of type 2 diabetes: insulin resistance and decreased insulin secretion by beta cells (Figure 18-12).

Insulin resistance is defined as a suboptimal response of insulin-sensitive tissues (especially liver, muscle, and adipose tissue) to insulin and is associated with obesity. Cellular insulin resistance and obesity are present in 60% to 80% of those with type 2 diabetes. Obesity

---

BOX 18-2   CRITERIA FOR THE DIAGNOSIS OF METABOLIC SYNDROME

Three of the following five traits:
- Increased waist circumference (>40 inches in men; >35 inches in women)
- Plasma triglycerides ≥150 mg/dl
- Plasma high-density lipoprotein (HDL) cholesterol <40 mg/dl (men) or <50 mg/dl (women)
- Blood pressure ≥130/85 mm Hg
- Fasting plasma glucose ≥100 mg/dl*

From Third Report of the National Cholesterol Education Program (NCEP) expert panel on detection, evaluation, and treatment of high blood cholesterol in adults (Adult Treatment Panel III): final report, *Circulation* 106:3143–3421, 2002.
*Criterion decreased from 110 to 100 mg/dl based on 2010 diagnostic category for persons at risk for diabetes mellitus (see Box 18-1).

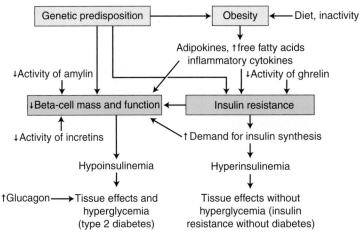

FIGURE 18-12 Pathophysiology of Type 2 Diabetes Mellitus.

contributes to the development of insulin resistance and diabetes through several important mechanisms:

1. Adipokines (leptin and adiponectin) are hormones produced in adipose tissue. Obesity results in increased serum levels of leptin and decreased levels of adiponectin. These changes are associated with inflammation and decreased insulin sensitivity.[61]
2. Elevated levels of serum free fatty acids (FFAs) and intracellular deposits of triglycerides and cholesterol are also found in obese individuals. These changes interfere with intracellular insulin signaling and thus decrease tissue responses to insulin and contribute to beta-cell apoptosis, a process known as lipotoxicity.[62]
3. Inflammatory cytokines (tumor necrosis factor-alpha [TNF-α], interleukin-1-beta [IL-1β], and interleukin-6 [IL-6]) are released from intra-abdominal adipocytes or adipocyte-associated mononuclear cells; they induce insulin resistance and are cytotoxic to beta cells.[63,64]
4. Obesity is correlated with hyperinsulinemia and decreased insulin receptor density.

Compensatory hyperinsulinemia prevents the clinical appearance of diabetes for many years. Eventually, however, beta-cell dysfunction develops and leads to a relative deficiency of insulin activity. The islet dysfunction is caused by a combination of a decrease in beta-cell mass and a reduction in normal beta-cell function. A progressive decrease in the weight and number of beta cells occurs and many of the remaining cells develop "exhaustion" from increased demand for insulin biosynthesis.[65]

Glucagon concentration is increased in type 2 diabetes because pancreatic alpha cells become less responsive to glucose inhibition, resulting in an increase in glucagon secretion. These abnormally high levels of glucagon increase blood glucose level by stimulating glycogenolysis and gluconeogenesis. As was discussed under type 1 diabetes, type 2 diabetes also is associated with a deficiency in amylin, further increasing glucagon levels. Drugs aimed at improving amylin function are being evaluated.[62]

Hormones released from the gastrointestinal (GI) tract play a role in insulin resistance, beta-cell function, and diabetes. Ghrelin is a peptide produced in the stomach and pancreatic islets that stimulates growth hormone release. Decreased levels of circulating ghrelin have been associated with insulin resistance and increased fasting insulin levels.[66] The incretins are a class of peptides that are released from the GI tract in response to food intake and function to increase the sensitivity of beta cells to circulating glucose levels, thus improving insulin responsiveness to meals. Incretins also suppress glucagon secretion, delay gastric emptying, suppress appetite, reduce beta-cell apoptosis, and induce pancreatic acinar cells to differentiate into new beta cells. Between meals they are inactivated by the enzyme dipeptidyl peptidase IV (DPP-IV). Incretin analogs and DPP-IV inhibitors are being used for the treatment of type 2 diabetes[67] (see *Health Alert:* Incretin Hormones for Type 2 Diabetes Mellitus Therapy).

CLINICAL MANIFESTATIONS The clinical manifestations of type 2 diabetes are nonspecific. Although many more children and adolescents are now developing type 2 diabetes, it generally affects those older than 30 years of age.[68] The affected individual is often overweight, dyslipidemic, hyperinsulinemic, and hypertensive. The individual with type 2 diabetes may show some classic symptoms of diabetes, such as polyuria and polydipsia, but more often will have nonspecific symptoms such as fatigue, pruritus, recurrent infections, visual changes, or symptoms of neuropathy (paresthesias or weakness). In those whose diabetes has progressed without treatment, symptoms related to coronary artery, peripheral artery, and cerebrovascular disease may develop.

HEALTH ALERT

Incretin Hormones for Type 2 Diabetes Mellitus Therapy

The incretin hormones are secreted from endocrine intestinal cells in the presence of carbohydrates, proteins, and fats. The major incretin hormone is glucagon-like peptide-1 (GLP-1) and it controls postprandial glucose levels by promoting glucose-dependent insulin secretion, inhibiting glucagon synthesis, and delaying gastric emptying. It may also enhance beta-cell mass and replenish intracellular stores of insulin. These many positive effects on glucose metabolism without hypoglycemia have led to the use of incretin hormones and incretin enhancers for the treatment of type 2 diabetes. In addition to improving glucose control, many people taking these medications experience weight loss and improvements in measurements of blood pressure, serum lipids, and myocardial function.

Data from Majumdar ID, Weber HC: Gastrointestinal regulatory peptides and their effects on fat tissue, *Curr Opin Endocrinol Diabetes Obes* 17(1):51–56, 2010; Mudaliar S, Henry RR: Effects of incretin hormones on beta-cell mass and function, body weight, and hepatic and myocardial function, *Am J Med* 123(3 Suppl):S19–S27, 2010; Peters A: Incretin-based therapies: review of current clinical trial data, *Am J Med* 123(3 Suppl):S28–S37, 2010; Jellinger PS: Focus on incretin-based therapies: targeting the core defects of type 2 diabetes, *Postgrad Med* 123(1):53–65, 2011; Nauck MA: Incretin-based therapies for type 2 diabetes mellitus: properties, functions, and clinical implications, *Am J Med* 124(1 Suppl):S3–S18, 2011.

EVALUATION AND TREATMENT The diagnostic criteria for type 2 diabetes are the same as those for type 1 (see Box 18-1). As with type 1 diabetes, the goal of treatment for individuals with type 2 diabetes is the restoration of near-euglycemia (a normal blood glucose level) and correction of related metabolic disorders. Dietary measures and exercise are of primary importance in both the prevention and the treatment of type 2 diabetes.[69] As the obese individual loses weight, the body's resistance to insulin often diminishes so that weight loss results in improved glucose tolerance. In those individuals with morbid obesity unresponsive to diet and exercise interventions, bariatric surgery may be indicated. Recent studies suggest that gastric bypass surgery is associated with a decrease in the incidence of type 2 diabetes and marked improvements in glycemic control in those with established diabetes.[70]

Although the first approach to treatment of the individual with type 2 diabetes is maintaining an appropriate diet and exercise program, medications are usually needed for optimal management. Oral hypoglycemic agents are useful in many individuals with type 2 diabetes (Table 18-6). Insulin therapy may be needed in the later stage of type 2 diabetes because of loss of beta-cell function, which is progressive over time.[69,71]

Other Specific Types of Diabetes Mellitus and Gestational Diabetes Mellitus

As listed in Table 18-3, the American Diabetes Association classification of diabetes mellitus not only includes the most common forms of diabetes (type 1 and type 2) but also encompasses "other specific types of diabetes mellitus" and "gestational diabetes mellitus." Other specific types of diabetes include genetic defects in beta-cell function, genetic defects in insulin action, diseases of the exocrine pancreas, endocrinopathies, drug- or chemical-induced beta-cell dysfunction, infections, and other uncommon autoimmune and inherited disorders that are associated with diabetes. The best-described of these other specific types of diabetes is termed maturity-onset diabetes of youth (MODY). MODY includes six specific autosomal dominant mutations that affect critical enzymes involved in beta-cell function or insulin action. It is

TABLE 18-6 TYPES OF ORAL HYPOGLYCEMIC DRUGS

DRUG TYPE	MECHANISM OF ACTION
α-Glucosidase inhibitor	Delays carbohydrate absorption in GI tract by inhibiting disaccharidases
Biguanide (metformin)	Decreases hepatic glucose production
Meglitinides	
Amino acid derivatives	Stimulate insulin release from pancreatic beta cells
Sulfonylureas	Stimulate insulin release from pancreatic beta cells
Thiazolidinediones	Increase insulin sensitivity, particularly in adipose tissue
DPP-IV inhibitors	Increase GLP-1 levels, increasing insulin secretion (see *Health Alert*, p. 463)
GLP-1 agonists	Mimic GLP-1, which increases insulin sensitivity and promotes weight loss (see *Health Alert*, p. 463)

estimated that only 2% to 5% of cases of diabetes are monogenic and, therefore, are classified as MODY. Diagnosis and management are similar to those used for type 2 diabetes.[72]

Gestational diabetes mellitus (GDM) has been defined as any degree of glucose intolerance with onset or first recognition during pregnancy. However, this definition meant that many women with previously undiagnosed type 1 or type 2 diabetes were diagnosed with GDM, and many of them had progressive disease after delivery. Therefore the ADA recently recommended that high-risk women found to have diabetes at their initial prenatal visit receive a diagnosis of type 1 or type 2 diabetes, not gestational diabetes.[73] GDM complicates approximately 7% of all pregnancies. Diagnosis of GDM is based on the presence of risk factors (older age, family history, history of glucose intolerance, membership in certain ethnic or racial group, and history of poor obstetric outcomes in the past), plus the measurement of an elevated fasting or casual FPG level. OGTT is often required to confirm the diagnosis. Careful glucose control prenatally, during pregnancy, and after delivery is essential to the short- and long-term health of both mother and baby.[69,74] Women who have GDM have a 35% to 60% chance of developing DM in the next 10-20 years. Making continued evaluation is important.[45a]

TABLE 18-7 COMMON ACUTE COMPLICATIONS OF DIABETES MELLITUS

HYPOGLYCEMIA IN PERSONS WITH DM	DIABETIC KETOACIDOSIS	HYPERGLYCEMIC NONKETOTIC SYNDROMES
Synonyms		
Insulin shock, insulin reaction	Diabetic coma syndrome	Hyperosmolar hyperglycemia nonketotic coma
Persons at Risk		
Individuals taking insulin	Individuals with type 1 diabetes	Older adults or very young individuals with type 2 diabetes, nondiabetics with predisposing factors, such as pancreatitis; individuals with undiagnosed diabetes
Individuals with rapidly fluctuating blood glucose levels	Individuals with nondiagnosed diabetes	
Individuals with type 2 diabetes taking sulfonylurea agents		
Predisposing Factors		
Excessive insulin or sulfonylurea agent intake, lack of sufficient food intake, excessive physical exercise, abrupt decline in insulin needs (e.g., renal failure, immediately postpartum), simultaneous use of insulin-potentiating agents or beta-blocking agents that mask symptoms	Stressful situation such as infection, accident, trauma, emotional stress; omission of insulin; medications that antagonize insulin	Infection, medications that antagonize insulin, comorbid condition
Typical Onset		
Rapid	Slow	Slowest
Presenting Symptoms		
Adrenergic reaction: pallor, sweating, tachycardia, palpitations, hunger, restlessness, anxiety, tremors	Malaise, dry mouth, headache, polyuria, polydipsia, weight loss, nausea, vomiting, pruritus, abdominal pain, lethargy, shortness of breath, Kussmaul respirations, fruity or acetone odor to breath	Polyuria, polydipsia, hypovolemia, dehydration (parched lips, poor skin turgor), hypotension, tachycardia, hypoperfusion, weight loss, weakness, nausea, vomiting, abdominal pain, hypothermia, stupor, coma, seizures
Neurogenic reaction: fatigue, irritability, headache, loss of concentration, visual disturbances, dizziness, hunger, confusion, transient sensory or motor defects, convulsions, coma, death		
Laboratory Analysis		
Serum glucose <30 mg/dl in newborn (first 2-3 days) and <55-60 mg/dl in adults	Glucose levels >250 mg/dl, reduction in bicarbonate concentration, increased anion gap, increased plasma levels of β-hydroxybutyrate, acetoacetate, and acetone	Glucose levels >600 mg/dl, lack of ketosis, serum osmolarity >320 mOsm/L, elevated blood urea nitrogen and creatinine levels

Acute Complications of Diabetes Mellitus

The major acute complications of diabetes mellitus are hypoglycemia, diabetic ketoacidosis, and hyperosmolar hyperglycemic nonketotic syndrome (see comparison in Table 18-7). Somogyi phenomenon and dawn phenomenon also may be seen.

Hypoglycemia in diabetes is sometimes called *insulin shock* or *insulin reaction.* Individuals with type 2 diabetes are at less risk for hypoglycemia than those with type 1 diabetes because they retain relatively intact glucose counterregulatory mechanisms. However, hypoglycemia does occur in type 2 diabetes when treatment involves insulin secretogogues (e.g., sulfonylureas) or exogenous insulin. Symptoms include pallor, tremor, anxiety, tachycardia, palpitations, diaphoresis, headache, dizziness, irritability, fatigue, poor judgment, confusion, visual disturbances, hunger, seizures, and coma. Treatment requires immediate replacement of glucose either orally or intravenously. Prevention is achieved with individualized management of medications and diet, blood glucose monitoring, and education.

Diabetic ketoacidosis (DKA) is a serious complication related to a deficiency of insulin and an increase in the levels of insulin counterregulatory hormones (catecholamines, cortisol, glucagon, growth hormone) (Figure 18-13). The American Diabetes Association criteria for the diagnosis of DKA are (1) a serum glucose level >250 mg/dl, (2) a serum bicarbonate level <18 mg/dl, (3) a serum pH <7.30, (4) the presence of an anion gap, and (5) the presence of urine and serum ketones.[75] DKA is much more common in type 1 diabetes because insulin is more deficient (see Table 18-7). Insulin normally stimulates lipogenesis and inhibits lipolysis, thus preventing fat catabolism. With insulin deficiency, lipolysis is enhanced and there is an increase in the amount of nonesterified fatty acids delivered to the liver. The consequence is increased glyconeogenesis contributing to hyperglycemia and production of ketone bodies (acetoacetate, hydroxybutyrate, and acetone) by the mitochondria of the liver at a rate that exceeds peripheral use. Accumulation of ketone bodies causes a drop in pH, resulting in metabolic acidosis. Symptoms of diabetic ketoacidosis include Kussmaul respirations (hyperventilation in an attempt to compensate for the acidosis), postural dizziness, central nervous system depression, ketonuria, anorexia, nausea, abdominal pain, thirst, and polyuria.

Hyperosmolar hyperglycemic nonketotic syndrome (HHNKS) is an uncommon but significant complication of type 2 diabetes mellitus with a high overall mortality. It occurs more often in elderly individuals who have other comorbidities, including infections or cardiovascular or renal disease. HHNKS differs from DKA in the degree of insulin deficiency (which is more profound in DKA) and the degree of fluid deficiency (which is more marked in HHNKS) (see Table 18-6). The clinical features of HHNKS include a serum glucose level >600 mg/dl, a serum pH >7.30, a serum bicarbonate level >15 mg/dl, a serum osmolarity >320 mOsm/L, and either absent or small numbers of ketones in the urine and serum.[75] Glucose levels are considerably higher in HHNKS than in DKA because of volume depletion. Because the amount of insulin required to inhibit fat breakdown is less than that needed for effective glucose transport, insulin levels are sufficient to prevent excessive lipolysis and ketosis (see Figure 18-13). Clinical manifestations include severe dehydration; loss of electrolytes, including potassium; and neurologic changes, such as stupor.

The Somogyi effect is a unique combination of hypoglycemia followed by rebound hyperglycemia. The rise in blood glucose concentration occurs because of counterregulatory hormones (epinephrine, GH, corticosteroids), which are stimulated by hypoglycemia. They produce gluconeogenesis. Excessive carbohydrate intake may contribute to the rebound hyperglycemia. The clinical occurrence of Somogyi effect is controversial.

The dawn phenomenon is an early morning rise in blood glucose concentration with no hypoglycemia during the night. It is related to nocturnal elevations of GH, which decrease metabolism of glucose by muscle and fat. Increased clearance of plasma insulin also may be involved. Altering the time and dose of insulin administration manages the problem.

Chronic Complications of Diabetes Mellitus

A number of serious complications are associated with any type of long-term diabetes mellitus, including microvascular (retinopathies, nephropathies, and neuropathies) and macrovascular (coronary artery, peripheral vascular, and cerebral vascular) disease (Table 18-8). Most complications are associated with chronic hyperglycemia (also

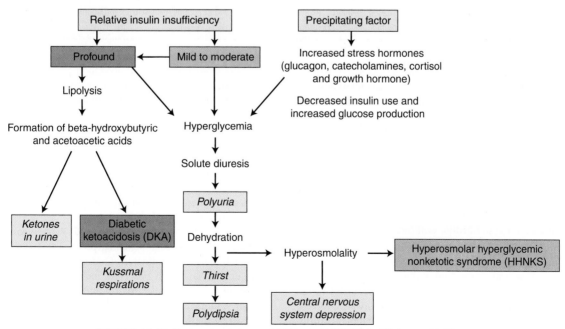

FIGURE 18-13 Pathophysiology of DKA and HHNKS in Diabetes Mellitus.

TABLE 18-8 CHRONIC COMPLICATIONS OF DIABETES MELLITUS

COMPLICATIONS	PATHOLOGIC MECHANISMS	ASSOCIATED SYMPTOMS
Microvascular		
Retinopathy		
Nonproliferative	Microaneurysms, capillary dilation, soft and hard exudates, dot and flame hemorrhages, arteriovenous shunts	May have no visual changes
Proliferative	Formation of new blood vessels, vitreal hemorrhage, scarring, retinal detachment	Loss of visual acuity
Maculopathy	Macular edema	Loss of central vision
Hyperglycemic lens edema	Shunting of glucose to polyol pathway: hyperosmolar fluid in lens	Blurring of vision
Cataract formation	Chronic hyperglycemia	Decreasing visual acuity
Nephropathy	Glomerular basement membrane thickening, mesangial expansion, glomerulosclerosis, focal tubular atrophy; hyperperfusion and hyperfiltration	Microalbuminuria and hypertension slowly progressing to end-stage kidney failure
Neuropathy	Oxidative stress, poor perfusion and ischemia, loss of nerve growth factor	Nerve dysfunction and degeneration
Peripheral neuropathy	Same as above	Distal symmetric sensorimotor polyneuropathy with glove and stocking loss of sensation (pain, vibration, temperature, proprioception); loss of motor nerve function with clawed toes and small muscle wasting in hands and flexor muscles; Charcot joints (loss of sensation results in joint and ligament degeneration, particularly of foot) Acute painful neuropathy with burning pain in legs and feet
Autonomic neuropathy	Same as above	Heart rate variability and postural hypotension Gastroparesis (delayed gastric emptying) and diarrhea Loss of bladder tone, urinary retention, and risk for bladder infection Erectile dysfunction and impotence in men
Skin and foot lesions	Loss of sensation, poor perfusion, suppressed immunity, and increased risk of infection	High risk for pressure ulcers and delayed wound healing; abscess formation; development of necrosis and gangrene, particularly of toes and foot; infection and osteomyelitis
Macrovascular		
Cardiovascular	Endothelial dysfunction, hyperlipidemia, accelerated atherosclerosis, coagulopathies	Hypertension, coronary artery disease, cardiomyopathy, and heart failure
Cerebrovascular	Same as above	Increased risk for ischemic and thrombotic stroke
Peripheral vascular	Same as above	Claudication, nonhealing ulcers, gangrene
Infection	Impaired immunity, decreased perfusion, recurrent trauma, delayed wound healing, urinary retention	Wound infections, urinary tract infections, increased risk for sepsis

known as glucose toxicity). Strict control of blood glucose level reduces some complications, particularly non-fatal myocardial infarction, but increases 5-year mortality. Strict control is not recommended for high-risk individuals with type 2 DM.[76] Several complex metabolic pathways have been associated with persistent hyperglycemia and the chronic complications of diabetes mellitus. They include shunting of glucose into the polyol pathway, activation of protein kinase C, production of advanced glycation end products, increased activation of the hexosamine pathway, and overproduction of reactive oxygen species (oxidative stress).

Metabolic Mechanisms of Chronic Complications

Hyperglycemia and the polyol pathway. Tissues that do not require insulin for glucose transport, such as kidney, red blood cells (RBCs), blood vessels, eye lens, and nerves, cannot down-regulate the cellular uptake of glucose; consequently, intracellular glucose is shunted into an alternate metabolic pathway, known as the polyol pathway. Overactivation of the polyol pathway results in two processes that may contribute to the complications of diabetes. One is the excessive accumulation

of sorbitol (a six-carbon sugar alcohol, or polyol) through the action of the enzyme aldose reductase. The accumulated sorbitol increases intracellular osmotic pressure and attracts water in tissue; for example, sorbitol buildup in the lens of the eye causes swelling and visual changes and predisposition to cataracts. In nerves sorbitol interferes with ion pumps, damages Schwann cells, and disrupts nerve conduction. RBCs become swollen and stiff, which interferes with perfusion. Activation of the polyol pathway also reduces the level of glutathione, an important antioxidant, and consequently there is oxidative injury in cells and tissues. Aldose reductase inhibitors are being evaluated for treatment of these complications.[77]

Hyperglycemia and protein kinase C. Protein kinase C (PKC) is a family of intracellular signaling proteins that can become inappropriately activated in different tissues by hyperglycemia.[78] Various consequences have been observed, including insulin resistance and production of extracellular matrix and proinflammatory cytokines; vascular endothelial proliferation and enhanced contractility and increased permeability. These effects contribute to the microvascular complications of diabetes.

Hyperglycemia and nonenzymatic glycation. Nonenzymatic glycation is a normal process that involves the *reversible* attachment of glucose to proteins, lipids, and nucleic acids without the action of enzymes. With recurrent or persistent hyperglycemia, glucose becomes *irreversibly* bound to proteins in blood vessel walls, interstitial tissue, and cells, forming advanced glycation end products (AGEs). When AGEs attach to their receptor (RAGE) or act independently they have a number of properties that may cause tissue injury or pathologic conditions associated with the chronic complications of diabetes.[79,79a] These include the following:

1. Cross-linking and trapping of proteins, including albumin, low-density lipoprotein (LDL), immunoglobulin, and complement, with thickening of the basement membrane or increased permeability in small blood vessels and nerves
2. Binding to cell receptors, such as macrophages, and inducing release of cytokines and growth factors that stimulate cellular proliferation in the glomeruli and smooth muscle of blood vessels
3. Induction of lipid oxidation, oxidative stress, and inflammation
4. Inactivation of nitric oxide with loss of vasodilation
5. Procoagulant changes on endothelial cells and promotion of platelet adhesion

Pharmacologic agents that inhibit AGE formation or block their receptor (RAGE) are being evaluated.[80]

Hyperglycemia and the hexosamine pathway. Chronic hyperglycemia causes shunting of excess intracellular glucose into the hexosamine pathway and leads to O-linked glycosylation (attachment of groups of oligosaccharides directly to proteins) of several enzymes and proteins with alteration in signal transduction pathways and oxidative stress. These reactions are associated with insulin resistance and cardiovascular complications of diabetes mellitus.[81]

Microvascular Disease

Diabetic microvascular complications (disease in capillaries) are a leading cause of blindness, end-stage kidney failure, and various neuropathies. Thickening of the capillary basement membrane, endothelial hyperplasia, thrombosis, and pericyte degeneration are characteristic of diabetic microangiopathy. The frequency and severity of lesions appear to be proportional to the duration of the disease (more or less than 10 years) and the status of glycemic control. Hypoxia and ischemia accompany microangiopathy, especially in the eye, kidney, and nerves. Many individuals with type 2 diabetes will present with microvascular complications because of the long duration of asymptomatic hyperglycemia that generally precedes diagnosis. This underscores the need to screen for diabetes.

Diabetic retinopathy. Diabetic retinopathy is a leading cause of blindness worldwide and in adults less than 60 years of age in the United States.[82] In comparison to type 1 diabetes, retinopathy seems to develop more rapidly in individuals with type 2 diabetes because of the likelihood of long-standing hyperglycemia before diagnosis. Most individuals with diabetes will eventually develop retinopathy and they are also more likely to develop cataracts and glaucoma (see Chapter 13).

Diabetic retinopathy results from relative hypoxemia, damage to retinal blood vessels, and RBC aggregation. The three stages of retinopathy that lead to loss of vision are *nonproliferative* (stage I), characterized by an increase in retinal capillary permeability, vein dilation, microaneurysm formation, and superficial (flame-shaped) and deep (blot) hemorrhages; *preproliferative* (stage II), a progression of retinal ischemia with areas of poor perfusion that culminate in infarcts; and *proliferative* (stage III), the result of neovascularization (angiogenesis) and fibrous tissue formation within the retina or optic disc. Traction of the new vessels on the vitreous humor may cause retinal detachment or hemorrhage into the vitreous humor. Macular edema is the leading cause of decreased vision among persons with diabetes. Blurring of vision also can be a consequence of hyperglycemia and sorbitol accumulation in the lens. Dehydration of the lens, aqueous humor, and vitreous humor also reduces visual acuity.

Diabetic nephropathy. Diabetes is the most common cause of end-stage kidney disease.[83] Hyperglycemia, AGEs, activation of the polyol pathway, protein kinase C all contribute to kidney tissue injury; yet the exact process responsible for destruction of kidneys in diabetes is unknown. The glomeruli are injured by protein denaturation from high glucose levels, by hyperglycemia with high renal blood flow (hyperfiltration), and by intraglomerular hypertension exacerbated by systemic hypertension. Renal glomerular changes occur early in diabetes mellitus, occasionally preceding the overt manifestation of the disease. Progressive changes include glomerular enlargement and glomerular basement membrane thickening with proliferation of mesangial cells and mesangial matrix. This results in diffuse and nodular glomerulosclerosis and progressively decreased glomerular blood flow and glomerular filtration. Alterations in glomerular membrane permeability occur with loss of negative charge and albuminuria. Ultimately, there also is tubular and interstitial fibrosis contributing to loss of function.[84]

Microalbuminuria is the first manifestation of kidney dysfunction. Continuous proteinuria generally heralds a life expectancy of less than 10 years. Before proteinuria, no clinical signs or symptoms of progressive glomerulosclerosis are likely to be evident. Later, hypoproteinemia, reduction in plasma oncotic pressure, fluid overload, anasarca (generalized body edema), and hypertension may occur. As renal function continues to deteriorate, individuals with type 1 diabetes may experience hypoglycemia (because of loss of renal insulin metabolism), which necessitates a decrease in insulin therapy. As the glomerular filtration rate drops below 10 ml/min, uremic signs, such as nausea, lethargy, acidosis, anemia, and uncontrolled hypertension, occur (see Chapter 29 for a discussion of renal failure). Death from kidney failure is much more common in individuals with type 1 diabetes mellitus than in those with type 2 diabetes because the appearance of proteinuria in these individuals is strongly correlated with death from cardiovascular disease.[85] Control of hypertension and hyperglycemia delays the onset of end-stage kidney disease.

Diabetic neuropathies. Diabetic neuropathy is the most common cause of neuropathy in the Western world and is the most common complication of diabetes. The underlying pathologic mechanism includes both metabolic and vascular factors related to chronic hyperglycemia with ischemia and demyelination contributing to neural changes. Oxidative stress from advanced glycosylation end products and increased formation of polyols contribute to nerve degeneration and delayed conduction.[86] Both somatic and peripheral nerve cells show diffuse or focal damage, resulting in polyneuropathy. Sensory deficits (loss of pain, temperature, and vibration sensation) are more common than motor involvement and often involve the extremities first in a "stocking and glove" pattern.

Some neuropathies are progressive, but many—such as painful peripheral neuropathy, mononeuropathy (wristdrop, footdrop), diabetic amyotrophy, diabetic neuropathic cachexia, and visceral manifestations associated with autonomic neuropathy (e.g., delayed gastric emptying, diabetic diarrhea, altered bladder function, impotence, orthostatic hypotension, and heart rate variability)—may spontaneously appear to improve. Neuropathy may occur during periods of "good" glucose control and may be the initial clinical manifestation of diabetes. Chronic hyperglycemia also can cause cognitive dysfunction, perhaps by promoting microvascular disease.[87]

Macrovascular Disease

Macrovascular disease (lesions in large- and medium-sized arteries) increases morbidity and mortality and increases risk for accelerated atherosclerosis and coronary artery disease, stroke, and peripheral vascular disease, particularly among individuals with type 2 diabetes mellitus. Unlike microangiopathy, atherosclerotic disease is unrelated to the severity of diabetes and is often present in those with insulin resistance and impaired glucose tolerance.[88] (Atherosclerosis is discussed in Chapter 23.) Children with poorly controlled type 2 diabetes have high risk for macrovascular complications within one to two decades.[89] Advanced glycosylated end products attach to proteins in the walls of blood vessels, promoting oxidative stress and endothelial and vascular smooth muscle dysfunction (Figure 18-14). The process tends to be more severe and accelerated in the presence of other risk factors, including hyperlipidemia, hypertension, and smoking.

Coronary artery disease. Cardiovascular disease is the ultimate cause of death in up to 75% of people with diabetes. Coronary artery disease (CAD) is the most common cause of morbidity and mortality in individuals with diabetes mellitus. Mechanisms of disease include hyperglycemia and insulin resistance, high levels of low-density lipoproteins (LDLs) and triglycerides, low levels of high-density lipoproteins (HDLs), platelet abnormalities, and endothelial cell dysfunction.[90] Mortality is high for both men and women. In general, the prevalence of CAD increases with the duration but not the severity of diabetes.

The incidence of congestive heart failure is higher in individuals with diabetes, even without myocardial infarction. This may be related to the presence of increased amounts of collagen in the ventricular wall, which reduces the mechanical compliance of the heart during filling. Increased platelet adhesion and decreased fibrinolysis promote thrombus formation in persons with diabetes.[91] (Heart disease is described in Chapter 23.) Guidelines have been developed to reduce the risk and improve treatment of cardiovascular and coronary artery disease in individuals with diabetes.[69,92]

Stroke. Stroke is twice as common in those with diabetes (particularly type 2 diabetes) as in the nondiabetic population.[93] The survival rate for individuals with diabetes after a massive stroke is typically shorter than that for nondiabetic individuals. Hypertension, hyperglycemia, hyperlipidemia, and thrombosis are definite risk factors (see Chapter 23).

Peripheral vascular disease. The increased incidence of peripheral vascular disease (PVD), with claudication, ulcers, gangrene, and amputation, in the individual with diabetes has been well documented.[94] Age, duration of diabetes, genetics, and additional risk factors influence the development and management of PVD. Peripheral vascular disease in those with diabetes is more diffuse and often involves arteries below the knee. Occlusions of the small arteries and arterioles cause most of the gangrenous changes of the lower extremities and occur in patchy areas of the feet and toes. The lesions begin as ulcers and progress to osteomyelitis or gangrene requiring amputation. Loss of sensation and increased risk for infection advance the disease. Significant morbidity and mortality are associated with major amputation.

Infection

The individual with diabetes is at an increased risk for infection throughout the body for several reasons[95]:
1. *The senses.* Impaired vision caused by retinal changes and impaired touch caused by neuropathy lead to loss of protection with injury and repeated trauma, open wounds, and soft tissue or osseous infection.
2. *Hypoxia.* Once skin integrity is compromised, tissues' susceptibility to infection increases as a result of hypoxia. In addition, the glycosylated hemoglobin in the RBCs impedes the release of oxygen to tissues.

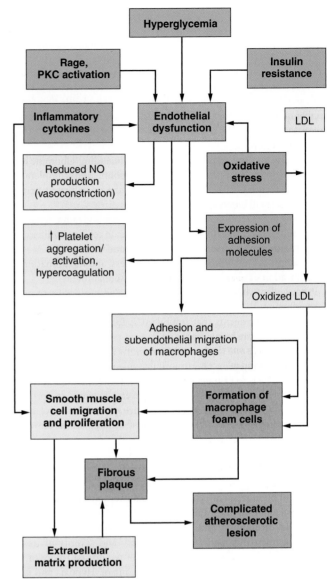

FIGURE 18-14 Diabetes Mellitus and Atherosclerosis. Diabetes with its associated hyperglycemia, relative hypoinsulinemia, oxidative stress, and proinflammatory state contributes to atherogenesis by causing arterial endothelial dysfunction (impaired vasodilation and adhesion of inflammatory cells), dyslipidemia, and smooth muscle proliferation. *LDL,* Low-density lipoprotein; *NO,* nitric oxide; *PKC,* protein kinase C; *Rage,* receptor advanced glycation end product. (Data from D'Souza A et al: Pathogenesis and pathophysiology of accelerated atherosclerosis in the diabetic heart, *Mol Cell Biochem* 331[1–2]:89–116, 2009; Stratmann B, Tschoepe D: Atherogenesis and atherothrombosis—focus on diabetes mellitus, *Best Pract Res Clin Endocrinol Metab* 23[3]:291–303, 2009.)

3. *Pathogens.* Some pathogens proliferate rapidly because of increased glucose in body fluids, which provides an excellent source of energy.
4. *Blood supply.* Decreased blood supply results from vascular changes and reduces the supply of white blood cells to the affected area.
5. *Suppressed immune response.* Chronic hyperglycemia impairs both the innate and adaptive immune responses, including abnormal chemotaxis and vasoactive responses, and defective phagocytosis. Clinical signs of infection may be absent.

ALTERATIONS OF ADRENAL FUNCTION

Disorders of the Adrenal Cortex

Disorders of the adrenal cortex are related either to hyperfunction or to hypofunction. Hyperfunction that causes hypercortisolism leads to Cushing disease or Cushing syndrome; that which causes increased secretion of adrenal androgens and estrogens leads to virilization or feminization; and that which causes increased levels of aldosterone leads to hyperaldosteronism, which may be primary or secondary. Hypofunction of the adrenal cortex leads to Addison disease.

Hypercortical Function (Cushing Syndrome, Cushing Disease)

Cushing syndrome refers to the clinical manifestations resulting from chronic exposure to excess cortisol (hypercortisolism). Cushing disease refers to excess endogenous secretion of ACTH. *ACTH-dependent hypercortisolism* results from overproduction of pituitary ACTH by a pituitary adenoma (which can occur at any age) or by an ectopic secreting nonpituitary tumor, such as a small cell carcinoma of the lung (more common in older adults). *ACTH-independent hypercortisolism* is caused by cortisol secretion from a rare benign or malignant tumor of one or both adrenal glands (more common in children).

A Cushing-like syndrome may develop as a result of the exogenous administration of glucocorticoids.[96]

PATHOPHYSIOLOGY Whatever the cause, two observations consistently apply to individuals with hypercortisolism: (1) the normal diurnal or circadian secretion patterns of ACTH and cortisol are lost, and (2) there is no increase in ACTH and cortisol secretion in response to a stressor.[97] With ACTH-dependent hypercortisolism, the excess ACTH stimulates excess production of cortisol and there is loss of feedback control of ACTH secretion. In individuals with ACTH-dependent hypercortisolism, secretion of both cortisol and adrenal androgens is increased, and cortisol-releasing hormone is inhibited. ACTH-independent secreting tumors of the adrenal cortex, however, generally secrete only cortisol. When the secretion of cortisol by the tumor exceeds normal cortisol levels, symptoms of hypercortisolism develop.

CLINICAL MANIFESTATIONS Weight gain is the most common feature and results from the accumulation of adipose tissue in the trunk, facial, and cervical areas. These characteristic patterns of fat deposition have been respectively described as "truncal obesity," "moon face," and "buffalo hump" (Figures 18-15 and 18-16).

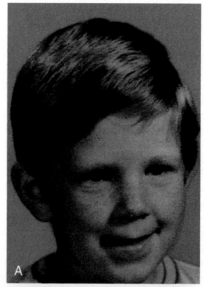
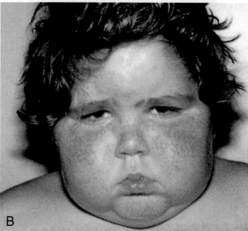

FIGURE 18-16 Cushing Syndrome. A, Patient before onset of Cushing syndrome. **B,** Patient 4 months later. Moon facies is clearly demonstrated. (From Zitelli BJ, Davis HW: *Atlas of pediatric physical diagnosis,* ed 3, London, 1997, Gower.)

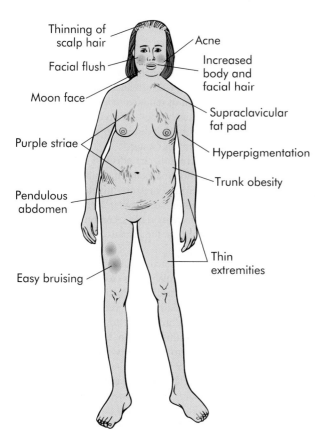

Thinning of scalp hair
Facial flush
Moon face
Purple striae
Pendulous abdomen
Easy bruising
Acne
Increased body and facial hair
Supraclavicular fat pad
Hyperpigmentation
Trunk obesity
Thin extremities

FIGURE 18-15 Symptoms of Cushing Disease.

Glucose intolerance occurs because of cortisol-induced insulin resistance and increased gluconeogenesis and glycogen storage by the liver. Overt diabetes mellitus develops in approximately 20% of individuals with hypercortisolism. Polyuria is a manifestation of hyperglycemia and resultant glycosuria.

Protein wasting is caused by the catabolic effects of cortisol on peripheral tissues. Muscle wasting leads to muscle weakness. In bone, loss of the protein matrix leads to osteoporosis, with pathologic fractures, vertebral compression fractures, bone and back pain, kyphosis, and reduced height. Cortisol interferes with the action of GH in long bones; thus children who present with short stature may be experiencing growth retardation related to Cushing syndrome rather than GH deficiency. Bone disease may contribute to hypercalciuria and resulting renal stones.

In the skin, loss of collagen leads to thin, weakened integumentary tissues through which capillaries are more visible and are easily stretched by adipose deposits. Together, these changes account for the characteristic purple striae seen in the trunk area. Loss of collagenous support around small vessels makes them susceptible to rupture, leading to easy bruising, even with minor trauma. Thin, atrophied skin is also easily damaged, leading to skin breaks and ulcerations. Bronze or brownish hyperpigmentation of the skin, mucous membranes, and hair occurs when there are very high levels of ACTH.

With elevated cortisol levels, vascular sensitivity to catecholamines increases significantly, leading to vasoconstriction and hypertension. Mineralocorticoid effects promote sodium and water retention and hypokalemia with transient weight gain. Suppression of the immune system and increased susceptibility to infections also occur. Approximately 50% of individuals with Cushing syndrome experience alterations in their mental status that range from irritability and depression to severe psychiatric disturbances, such as schizophrenia.[97] Females with ACTH-dependent hypercortisolism may experience symptoms of increased adrenal androgen levels, increased hair growth (especially facial hair), acne, and oligomenorrhea. Rarely, unless an adrenal carcinoma is involved, do androgen levels become high enough to cause changes of the voice, recession of the hairline, and hypertrophy of the clitoris.

EVALUATION AND TREATMENT Routine laboratory examinations may reveal hyperglycemia, glycosuria, hypokalemia, and metabolic alkalosis. A variety of laboratory tests are used to confirm the diagnosis of hypercortisolism and to determine the underlying disorder. These include urinary free cortisol level higher than 50 mcg in 24 hours, abnormal dexamethasone suppressibility of either urinary or serum cortisol, and simultaneous measurement of ACTH and cortisol levels. Late evening salivary cortisol levels are used as a screening test and to document alterations in the diurnal variation of cortisol level. Tumors are diagnosed using imaging procedures.[98]

Treatment is specific for the cause of hypercorticoadrenalism and includes medication, radiation, and surgery. Differentiation between pituitary ectopic and adrenal causes is essential for effective treatment. Without treatment, approximately 50% of individuals with Cushing syndrome die within 5 years of onset as a result of overwhelming infection, suicide, complications from generalized arteriosclerosis, and hypertensive disease.

Congenital Adrenal Hyperplasia

Congenital adrenal hyperplasia results from the deficiency of an enzyme that is critical in cortisol biosynthesis. Because cortisol production is low, the concentration of ACTH increases and causes adrenal hyperplasia, which results in the overproduction of either mineralocorticoids or androgens. The most common form is a 21-hydroxylase deficiency, which involves both mineralocorticoid and cortisol synthesis. Affected female infants are virilized, and infants of both genders exhibit salt wasting. Disease management requires life-long treatment with glucocorticoids and mineralocorticoids.[98a]

Hyperaldosteronism

Hyperaldosteronism is characterized by excessive aldosterone secretion by the adrenal glands. Both primary and secondary forms of hyperaldosteronism can occur in individuals.

Primary hyperaldosteronism (Conn syndrome, primary aldosteronism) is caused by excessive secretion of aldosterone from an abnormality of the adrenal cortex, usually a single benign aldosterone-producing adrenal adenoma. Bilateral adrenal nodular hyperplasia and adrenal carcinomas account for the remainder of cases. The incidence is estimated to be about 10% of all hypertensive individuals; however, approximately 33% of people with resistant hypertension will have evidence of primary hyperaldosteronism.[98b]

Secondary hyperaldosteronism results from an extra-adrenal stimulus of aldosterone secretion, most often angiotensin II through a renin-dependent mechanism. This occurs in various situations, including decreased circulating blood volume (e.g., in dehydration, shock, or hypoalbuminemia) and decreased delivery of blood to the kidneys (e.g., renal artery stenosis, heart failure, or hepatic cirrhosis). Here, the activation of the renin-angiotensin system and subsequent aldosterone secretion may be seen as compensatory, although in some instances (e.g., congestive heart failure) the increased circulating volume further worsens the condition. Other causes of secondary hyperaldosteronism are Bartter syndrome, in which the underlying disorder is a renal tubular defect leading to hypokalemia, and renin-secreting tumors of the kidney.

PATHOPHYSIOLOGY In *primary hyperaldosteronism,* pathophysiologic alterations are caused by excessive aldosterone secretion and the fluid and electrolyte imbalances that ensue. Hyperaldosteronism promotes (1) increased renal sodium and water reabsorption with corresponding hypervolemia (see Chapter 4) and hypertension and (2) renal excretion of potassium. The extracellular fluid volume overload, hypertension, and suppression of renin secretion are characteristic of primary disorders. Edema usually does not occur with primary aldosteronism because hypervolemia-induced atrial natriuretic factor release results in loss of sodium and water.[99]

In *secondary hyperaldosteronism,* the effect of increased extracellular volume on renin secretion may vary. If renin secretion is being stimulated by variables other than pressure-initiated cellular changes at the juxtaglomerular apparatus (see Chapter 28), increased circulating blood volume may not decrease renin secretion through feedback mechanisms. This process occurs, for instance, in states of increased estrogen levels.

Potassium secretion is promoted by aldosterone; therefore with excessive aldosterone, hypokalemia occurs (see Chapter 4). Hypokalemic alkalosis, changes in myocardial conduction, and skeletal muscle alterations may be seen, particularly with severe potassium depletion. The renal tubules may become insensitive to ADH, thus promoting excessive loss of free water. In this situation, hypernatremia also may occur because water is not able to follow the sodium that is reabsorbed.

CLINICAL MANIFESTATIONS Hypertension and hypokalemia are the hallmarks of primary hyperaldosteronism. With sustained hypertension, the chronic effects of elevated arterial pressure become evident, for example, left ventricular dilation and hypertrophy and progressive arteriosclerosis.[100] Aldosterone-stimulated potassium loss can be substantial, resulting in typical manifestations of hypokalemia. Hypokalemic alkalosis may develop (see Chapter 4).

EVALUATION AND TREATMENT Various clinical and laboratory measurements are useful in assessing hyperaldosteronism. Tests include the following:

1. Blood pressure is elevated.
2. Serum and urinary electrolyte levels: serum sodium level is normal or elevated and serum potassium level is depressed, but urinary potassium level is elevated.
3. Serum and urinary levels of aldosterone increase.
4. Aldosterone suppression testing: fludrocortisone acetate (Florinef) is used.
5. Plasma renin activity is suppressed.
6. Imaging techniques may be used to localize an aldosterone-secreting adenoma.

Treatment includes management of hypertension and hypokalemia, as well as correction of any underlying causal abnormalities. If an aldosterone-secreting adenoma is present, it must be surgically removed.[101]

Hypersecretion of Adrenal Androgens and Estrogens

Hypersecretion of adrenal androgens and estrogens may be caused by adrenal tumors, either adenomas or carcinomas, Cushing syndrome, or defects in steroid synthesis. The clinical syndrome that results depends on the hormone secreted, the gender of the individual, and the age at which the hypersecretion is initiated. Hypersecretion of estrogens causes feminization, the development of female secondary sex characteristics. Hypersecretion of androgens causes virilization, the development of male secondary sex characteristics (Figure 18-17).

The effects of an estrogen-secreting tumor are most evident in males and result in gynecomastia (98% of cases), testicular atrophy, and decreased libido. In female children, such tumors may lead to early development of secondary sex characteristics. The changes caused by an androgen-secreting tumor are more easily observed in females and include excessive face and body hair growth (hirsutism), clitoral enlargement, deepening of the voice, amenorrhea, acne, and breast atrophy. In children, virilizing tumors promote precocious sexual development and bone aging. Treatment of androgen-secreting tumors usually involves surgical excision.

Adrenocortical Hypofunction

Hypocortisolism (low levels of cortisol secretion) develops because of either inadequate stimulation of the adrenal glands by ACTH or a primary inability of the adrenals to produce and secrete the adrenocortical hormones. Sometimes there is partial dysfunction of the adrenal cortex, so only synthesis of cortisol and aldosterone or the adrenal androgens is affected. Hypofunction of the adrenal cortex may affect glucocorticoid or mineralocorticoid secretion, or both.

Addison disease. Primary adrenal insufficiency is termed Addison disease. It is relatively rare, occurring most often in adults ages 30 to 60 years, although it may appear at any time. Addison disease is caused by autoimmune mechanisms that destroy adrenal cortical cells and is more common in women. Chronic infections, such as tuberculosis, account for the majority of cases of primary adrenal insufficiency in underdeveloped countries.

PATHOPHYSIOLOGY Addison disease is characterized by inadequate corticosteroid and mineralocorticoid synthesis and elevated levels of serum ACTH (loss of negative feedback). Before clinical manifestations of hypocortisolism are evident, more than 90% of total adrenocortical tissue must be destroyed.

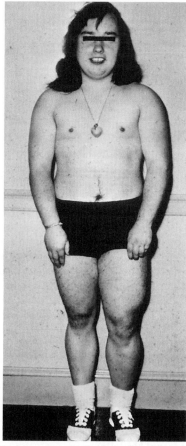

FIGURE 18-17 Virilization. Virilization of a young girl by an androgen-secreting tumor of the adrenal cortex. Masculine features include lack of breast development, increased muscle bulk, and hirsutism (excessive hair). (From Thibodeau GA, Patton KT: *Anatomy & physiology,* St Louis, 1987, Mosby.)

Idiopathic Addison disease (organ-specific autoimmune adrenalitis) causes adrenal atrophy and hypofunction and is an organ-specific autoimmune disease. It may occur in childhood (type 1) or adulthood (type 2). 21-Hydroxylase autoantibodies and autoreactive T cells specific to adrenal cortical cells are present in 50% to 70% of individuals with idiopathic Addison disease, and this percentage increases in younger persons and in those with other autoimmune diseases. This deficiency allows the proliferation of immunocytes directed against specific antigens within the adrenocortical cells.[102] The adrenal glands in idiopathic Addison disease are smaller than normal and may be misshapen.

Idiopathic Addison disease is often associated with other autoimmune diseases, especially Hashimoto thyroiditis, pernicious anemia, and idiopathic hypoparathyroidism. In these cases, Addison disease may be inherited as an autosomal recessive trait. (Mechanisms of inheritance are described in Chapter 2.)

CLINICAL MANIFESTATIONS The symptoms of Addison disease are primarily a result of hypocortisolism and hypoaldosteronism. With mild to moderate hypocortisolism, symptoms usually begin with weakness and easy fatigability. Skin changes, including hyperpigmentation and vitiligo, may occur. As the condition progresses, anorexia, nausea, vomiting, and diarrhea may develop. Of greatest concern is the development of hypotension that can progress to complete vascular collapse and shock.

EVALUATION AND TREATMENT Serum and urine levels of cortisol are depressed with primary hypocortisolism and ACTH levels are increased. Because of dehydration, blood urea nitrogen levels may increase. Serum glucose level is low. Eosinophil and lymphocyte counts often are elevated. Hyperkalemia is seen in Addison disease and may cause mild alkalosis (see Chapter 4). The ACTH stimulation test may be used to evaluate serum cortisol levels.

The treatment of Addison disease involves lifetime glucocorticoid and possibly mineralocorticoid replacement therapy, together with dietary modifications and correction of any underlying disorders.[103] With acute stressors, additional cortisol must be administered to approximate the amount of cortisol that might be expected if normal adrenal function were present (approximately 100 to 300 mg/day). The individual's diet should include at least 150 mEq of sodium per day, and sodium intake should be increased if the individual experiences excessive sweating or diarrhea.

Secondary hypocortisolism. Secondary hypocortisolism commonly results from prolonged administration of exogenous glucocorticoids; they suppress ACTH secretion and cause adrenal atrophy, resulting in inadequate corticosteroidogenesis once the exogenous glucocorticoids are withdrawn. Decreased ACTH secretion also can result from pituitary infarction, pituitary tumors that compress ACTH-secreting cells, or hypophysectomy. In all instances of low ACTH levels, adrenal atrophy occurs and endogenous adrenal steroidogenesis is depressed. Clinical manifestations of secondary hypocortisolism are similar to those of Addison disease, although hyperpigmentation usually does not occur. The renin-angiotensin system usually is normal, so aldosterone and potassium levels also tend to be normal.

Disorders of the Adrenal Medulla
Tumor of the Adrenal Medulla

Adrenomedullary hyperfunction is caused by pheochromocytomas (chromaffin cell tumors) or sympathetic paragangliomas of the adrenal medulla that secrete catecholamines on a continual basis. They are rare, and about 10% are malignant. Those that are malignant metastasize to the lungs, liver, bones, or para-aortic lymph nodes. These tumors are rare and usually sporadic although up to 30% of them can be inherited.[103a]

PATHOPHYSIOLOGY Pheochromocytomas and sympathetic paragangliomas cause excessive production of catecholamines because of autonomous secretion of the tumor. Approximately 5% of people with these tumors have no symptoms, apparently because the tumor is nonfunctioning. Such tumors can, however, release catecholamines, especially in response to a stressor, such as surgery.

CLINICAL MANIFESTATIONS The clinical manifestations of a pheochromocytoma and sympathetic paragangliomas are related to the chronic effects of catecholamine secretion and include persistent hypertension, headache, pallor, diaphoresis, tachycardia, and palpitations. Hypertension results from increased peripheral vascular resistance and may be sustained or paroxysmal. An acute episode of hypertension related to hypersecretion of catecholamines may follow specific events, such as exercise, excessive ingestion of tyrosine-containing foods (aged cheese, red wine, beer, yogurt), ingestion of caffeine-containing foods, external pressure on the tumor, and induction of anesthesia. Headaches appear because of sudden changes in catecholamine levels in the blood, affecting cerebral blood flow. Hypermetabolism and sweating are related to chronic activation of sympathetic receptors in adipocytes, hepatocytes, and other tissues. Glucose intolerance may occur because of catecholamine-induced inhibition of insulin release by the pancreas. These tumors tend to be extremely vascular and can rupture, causing massive and potentially fatal hemorrhage.

EVALUATION AND TREATMENT A diagnosis of pheochromocytoma is made when increased catecholamine production is demonstrated in the blood or urine. The site of the tumor is then determined using abdominal imaging techniques. Because of the possibility of metastasis, whole-body scanning may be done.

Management of catecholamine excess is essential to prevent hypertensive emergencies and requires the use of α- and β-adrenergic blockers. The usual treatment of pheochromocytoma is laparoscopic surgical excision of the tumor, although open resection is still completed for large tumors or when metastasis is suspected. Medical therapy is continued to stabilize blood pressure before, during, or after surgery.[104] Malignant pheochromocytoma is rarely curable and is usually managed by a combination of surgical debulking of the tumor combined with chemotherapy.[105]

> ✔ **QUICK CHECK 18-5**
> 1. What are the symptoms of hyperaldosteronism?
> 2. What major diseases are classified as hypocortisolism?
> 3. What are pheochromocytomas?

DID YOU UNDERSTAND?

Mechanisms of Hormonal Alterations
1. Abnormalities in endocrine function may be caused by elevated or depressed hormone levels that result from (a) faulty feedback systems, (b) dysfunction of the gland, (c) altered metabolism of hormones, or (d) production of hormones from nonendocrine tissues.
2. Target cells may fail to respond to hormones because of (a) cell surface receptor–associated disorders, (b) intracellular disorders, or (c) circulating inhibitors.

Alterations of the Hypothalamic-Pituitary System
1. Dysfunction in the action of hypothalamic hormones is most commonly related to interruption of the connection between the hypothalamus and pituitary—the pituitary stalk.
2. Disorders of the posterior pituitary include syndrome of inappropriate ADH secretion (SIADH) and diabetes insipidus. SIADH secretion is characterized by abnormally high ADH secretion; diabetes insipidus is characterized by abnormally low ADH secretion.

3. In SIADH, high ADH levels interfere with renal free water clearance, leading to hyponatremia and hypoosmolality, and are associated with brain injury and with certain forms of cancer, apparently because of ectopic secretion of ADH by tumor cells.
4. Diabetes insipidus may be neurogenic (caused by insufficient amounts of ADH) or nephrogenic (caused by an inadequate response to ADH). Its principal clinical features are polyuria and polydipsia.
5. Hypopituitarism can be primary (dysfunction of the pituitary) or secondary (dysfunction of the hypothalamus). Primary hypopituitarism can result from a pituitary tumor, trauma, infections, stroke, or surgical removal.
6. Hypopituitarism can affect any or all of the pituitary hormones and symptoms may range from mild to life-threatening.
7. Hyperpituitarism is caused by pituitary adenomas. These are usually benign, slow-growing tumors that arise from cells of the anterior pituitary.

DID YOU UNDERSTAND?—cont'd

8. Expansion of a pituitary adenoma causes both neurologic and secretory effects. Pressure from the expanding tumor causes hyposecretion of cells, dysfunction of the optic chiasma (leading to visual disturbances), and dysfunction of the hypothalamus and some cranial nerves.

9. Hypersecretion of growth hormone (GH) in adults causes acromegaly, in which GH secretion becomes high and unpredictable. Pituitary adenoma is the most common cause of acromegaly.

10. Prolonged, abnormally high levels of GH lead to proliferation of body and connective tissue and slowly developing renal, thyroid, and reproductive dysfunction.

11. Prolactinomas result in galactorrhea, hirsutism, amenorrhea, hypogonadism, and osteopenia.

Alterations of Thyroid Function

1. Thyrotoxicosis is a general condition in which elevated thyroid hormone (TH) levels cause greater than normal physiologic responses. The condition can be caused by a variety of specific diseases, each of which has its own pathophysiology and course of treatment.

2. In general, hyperthyroidism has a range of endocrine, reproductive, gastrointestinal, integumentary, and ocular manifestations. These are caused by increased circulating levels of TH and by stimulation of the sympathetic division of the autonomic nervous system.

3. Graves disease, the most common form of hyperthyroidism, is caused by an autoimmune mechanism that overrides normal mechanisms for control of TH secretion and is characterized by thyrotoxicosis, ophthalmopathy, and circulating thyroid-stimulating immunoglobulins.

4. Toxic nodular goiter and toxic multinodular goiter occur when TH-regulating mechanisms and abnormal hypertrophy of the thyroid gland cause hyperthyroidism. Toxic multinodular goiter is caused by independently functioning follicular cell adenomas.

5. Thyrotoxic crisis is a severe form of hyperthyroidism that is often associated with physiologic or psychologic stress. Without treatment, death occurs quickly.

6. Primary hypothyroidism is caused by deficient production of TH by the thyroid gland. Secondary hypothyroidism is caused by hypothalamic or pituitary dysfunction. Symptoms depend on the degree of TH deficiency. Common manifestations include decreased energy metabolism, decreased heat production, and myxedema.

7. Primary hypothyroidism is characterized by an increased level of TSH, which stimulates goiter formation.

8. Autoimmune thyroiditis (Hashimoto disease) is associated with humoral (antibodies) and cellular autoimmune destruction of the thyroid and gradual loss of thyroid function. Autoimmune thyroiditis occurs in those individuals with genetic susceptibility to an autoimmune mechanism that causes thyroid damage and eventual hypothyroidism.

9. Subacute thyroiditis is a self-limiting nonbacterial inflammation of the thyroid gland. The inflammatory process damages follicular cells, causing leakage of T_3 and T_4. Hyperthyroidism then is followed by transient hypothyroidism, which is corrected by cellular repair and a return to normal levels in the thyroid.

10. Myxedema is a sign of hypothyroidism caused by alterations in connective tissue with water-binding proteins that lead to edema and thickened mucous membranes.

11. Myxedema coma is a severe form of hypothyroidism that may be life-threatening without emergency medical treatment.

12. Congenital hypothyroidism is the absence of thyroid tissue during fetal development or defects in hormone synthesis.

13. Thyroid carcinoma is a relatively rare cancer. The most consistent causal risk factor associated with thyroid carcinoma is exposure to ionizing radiation, especially in childhood.

Alterations of Parathyroid Function

1. Hyperparathyroidism, which may be primary or secondary, is characterized by greater than normal secretion of parathyroid hormone (PTH).

2. Primary hyperparathyroidism is caused by an interruption of the normal mechanisms that regulate calcium and PTH levels. Manifestations include chronic hypercalcemia, increased bone resorption, and hypercalciuria.

3. Secondary hyperparathyroidism is a compensatory response to hypocalcemia and often occurs with chronic renal failure and vitamin D deficiency.

4. Hypoparathyroidism, defined by abnormally low PTH levels, is caused by thyroid surgery, autoimmunity, or genetic mechanisms.

5. The lack of circulating PTH in hypoparathyroidism causes depressed serum calcium levels, increased serum phosphate levels, decreased bone resorption, and hypocalciuria.

Dysfunction of the Endocrine Pancreas: Diabetes Mellitus

1. Diabetes mellitus is a group of disorders characterized by glucose intolerance, chronic hyperglycemia, and disturbances of carbohydrate, protein, and fat metabolism.

2. A diagnosis of diabetes mellitus is based on elevated plasma glucose concentrations and measurement of glycosylated hemoglobin. Classic signs and symptoms are often present as well.

3. The two most common types of diabetes mellitus are type 1 and type 2.

4. Type 1 diabetes mellitus is characterized by loss of beta cells, presence of islet cell antibody, lack of insulin, and excess of glucagon, which causes improper metabolism of fat, protein, and carbohydrates.

5. Type 1 diabetes mellitus seems to be caused by a gradual process of autoimmune destruction of beta cells in genetically susceptible individuals.

6. In type 1 diabetes mellitus, hyperglycemia causes polyuria and polydipsia resulting from osmotic diuresis.

7. Ketoacidosis is caused by increased levels of circulating ketones without the inhibiting effects of insulin. Increased levels of circulating fatty acids and weight loss are both manifestations of type 1 uncontrolled diabetes mellitus.

8. Type 2 diabetes mellitus is caused by genetic susceptibility that is triggered by environmental factors. The most compelling environmental risk factor is obesity.

9. In the obese, many factors, such as altered adipokines, increased fatty acids, inflammation, and hyperinsulinemia, contribute to the development of insulin resistance.

10. Some insulin production continues in type 2 diabetes mellitus, but the weight and number of beta cells decrease. There are dysfunctional levels of both insulin and glucagon.

11. Other specific types of diabetes mellitus include monogenetic forms of diabetes called maturity-onset diabetes mellitus (MODY).

12. Gestational diabetes is glucose intolerance during pregnancy.

13. Acute complications of diabetes mellitus include hypoglycemia, diabetic ketoacidosis, and hyperosmolar hyperglycemic nonketotic syndrome.

14. Hypoglycemia in diabetes is a complication related to insulin treatment.

15. Diabetic ketoacidosis develops when there is an absolute or relative deficiency of insulin and an increase in the insulin counterregulatory hormones of catecholamines—cortisol, glucagon, and growth hormone.

16. Hyperosmolar hyperglycemic nonketotic syndrome is pathophysiologically similar to diabetic ketoacidosis, although levels of free fatty acids are lower in hyperosmolar nonacidotic diabetes and lack of ketosis indicates that some level of insulin is present.

17. The Somogyi effect is a combination of hypoglycemia with rebound hyperglycemia.

18. The dawn phenomenon is an early morning rise in glucose levels caused by nocturnal elevations in growth hormone.

19. Chronic complications of diabetes mellitus include microvascular disease (e.g., neuropathy, retinopathy, nephropathy), macrovascular disease (e.g., coronary artery disease, stroke, peripheral vascular disease), and infection.

Continued

DID YOU UNDERSTAND?—cont'd

20. Microvascular disease is characterized by thickening of the capillary basement membrane and eventual decreased tissue perfusion affecting the microcirculation.
21. Macrovascular disease associated with diabetes mellitus is most often related to the proliferation of atherosclerotic plaques in the arterial wall.
22. The incidence of coronary heart disease, peripheral vascular disease, and stroke is greater in those with diabetes than in nondiabetic individuals.
23. Individuals with diabetes are at risk for a variety of infections. Infection may be related to sensory impairment and resulting injury, hypoxia, increased proliferation of pathogens in elevated concentrations of glucose, decreased blood supply associated with vascular damage, and impaired white cell function.

Alterations of Adrenal Function

1. Disorders of the adrenal cortex are related to hyperfunction or hypofunction. No known disorders are associated with hypofunction of the adrenal medulla, but medullary hyperfunction causes clinically defined syndromes.
2. Cortical hyperfunction, or hypercortisolism, causes Cushing syndrome, which does not involve the pituitary gland, and Cushing disease, which is hypercortisolism with pituitary involvement.
3. Hypercortisolism is usually caused by Cushing disease (pituitary-dependent) and very rarely can be caused by ectopic production of ACTH. Complications include obesity, diabetes, protein wasting, immune suppression, and mental status changes.
4. Excessive aldosterone secretion causes hyperaldosteronism, which may be primary or secondary. Primary hyperaldosteronism is caused by an abnormality of the adrenal cortex. Secondary hyperaldosteronism involves an extra-adrenal stimulus, often angiotensin.

5. Hyperaldosteronism promotes increased sodium reabsorption, corresponding hypervolemia, increased extracellular volume (which is variable), hypokalemia related to renal reabsorption of sodium, and excretion of potassium.
6. Hypersecretion of adrenal androgens and estrogens can be a result of adrenal tumors, either adenomas or carcinomas. Hypersecretion of estrogens causes feminization, the development of female secondary sexual characteristics. Hypersecretion of androgens causes virilization, the development of male secondary sexual characteristics.
7. Hypofunction of the adrenal cortex can affect glucocorticoid or mineralocorticoid secretion, or both. Hypofunction can be caused by a deficiency of ACTH or by a primary deficiency in the gland itself.
8. Hypocortisolism, or low levels of cortisol, is caused by inadequate adrenal stimulation by ACTH or by primary cortisol hyposecretion. Primary adrenal insufficiency is termed Addison disease.
9. Addison disease is characterized by elevated ACTH levels with inadequate corticosteroid synthesis and output.
10. Manifestations of Addison disease are related to hypocortisolism and hypoaldosteronism. Symptoms include weakness, fatigability, hypoglycemia and related metabolic problems, lowered response to stressors, hyperpigmentation, vitiligo, and manifestations of hypovolemia and hyperkalemia.
11. Hyperfunction of the adrenal medulla is usually caused by a pheochromocytoma, a catecholamine-producing tumor. Symptoms of catecholamine excess are related to their sympathetic nervous system effects and include hypertension, palpitations, tachycardia, glucose intolerance, excessive sweating, and constipation.

▮ KEY TERMS

- Acromegaly   451
- Addison disease (primary adrenal insufficiency)   471
- Advanced glycation end product (AGE)   467
- Aldose reductase   466
- Amylin   461
- Autoimmune thyroiditis (Hashimoto disease, chronic lymphocyte thyroiditis)   456
- Beta-cell dysfunction   463
- Central (secondary) hyperthyroidism   454
- Central (secondary) hypothyroidism   456
- Central (secondary) thyroid disorders   453
- Congenital adrenal hyperplasia   470
- Cushing disease   469
- Cushing-like syndrome   469
- Cushing syndrome   469
- Dawn phenomenon   465
- Diabetes insipidus (DI)   449
- Diabetes mellitus   458
- Diabetic ketoacidosis (DKA)   465
- Diabetic neuropathy   467
- Diabetic retinopathy   467
- Feminization   471
- Gestational diabetes mellitus (GDM)   464
- Ghrelin   463
- Giantism   452
- Glucagon   461

- Glycosylated hemoglobin   459
- Graves disease   454
- Hyperaldosteronism   470
- Hypercortisolism   469
- Hyperosmolar hyperglycemic nonketotic syndrome (HHNKS)   465
- Hyperparathyroidism   457
- Hypocortisolism   471
- Hypoglycemia   465
- Hypoparathyroidism   458
- Hypopituitarism   450
- Hypothyroidism   456
- Idiopathic Addison disease (organ-specific autoimmune adrenalitis)   471
- Incretin   463
- Insulin resistance   462
- Macular edema   467
- Maturity-onset diabetes of youth (MODY)   463
- Myxedema   456
- Myxedema coma   456
- Nonenzymatic glycation   467
- Painless thyroiditis   457
- Panhypopituitarism   450
- Pheochromocytoma (chromaffin cell tumor)   472
- Pituitary adenoma   451
- Polyol pathway   466

- Postpartum thyroiditis   457
- Pretibial myxedema (Graves dermopathy)   455
- Primary hyperaldosteronism (Conn syndrome, primary aldosteronism)   470
- Primary hyperparathyroidism   457
- Primary hyperthyroidism   453
- Primary hypothyroidism   456
- Primary thyroid disorder   453
- Prolactinoma   453
- Protein kinase C (PKC)   466
- Secondary hyperaldosteronism   470
- Secondary hyperparathyroidism   457
- Secondary hypocortisolism   472
- Somogyi effect   465
- Subacute thyroiditis   457
- Subclinical thyroid disease   453
- Syndrome of inappropriate ADH secretion (SIADH)   449
- Thyrotoxic crisis (thyroid storm)   455
- Thyrotoxicosis   453
- Toxic adenoma   455
- Toxic multinodular goiter   455
- Type 1 diabetes mellitus   459
- Type 2 diabetes mellitus (non–insulin-dependent diabetes mellitus)   462
- Vasopressin dysregulation   449
- Virilization   471

REFERENCES

1. Peri A, et al: Hyponatremia and the syndrome of inappropriate secretion of antidiuretic hormone (SIADH), *J Endocrinol Invest* 33(9):671–682, 2010.
2. Gustafsson BI, et al: Bronchopulmonary neuroendocrine tumors, *Cancer* 113(1):5–21, 2008.
3. Hannon MJ, Thompson CJ: The syndrome of inappropriate antidiuretic hormone: prevalence, causes and consequences, *Eur J Endocrinol* 162(Suppl 1):S5–S12, 2010.
4. Meulendijks D, et al: Antipsychotic-induced hyponatraemia: a systematic review of the published evidence, *Drug Safety* 33(2):101–114, 2010.
5. Decaux G, Musch W: Clinical laboratory evaluation of the syndrome of inappropriate secretion of antidiuretic hormone, *Clin J Am Soc Nephrol* 3(4):1175–1184, 2008.
6. Sherlock M, Thompson CJ: The syndrome of inappropriate antidiuretic hormone: current and future management options, *Eur J Endocrinol* 162(Supp 1):S13–S18, 2010.
7. Chadha V, Alon US: Hereditary renal tubular disorders, *Semin Nephrol* 29(4):399–411, 2009.
8. Bircan Z, Mutlu H, Cheong HI: Differential diagnosis of hereditary nephrogenic diabetes insipidus with desmopressin infusion test, *Indian J Pediatr* 77(11):1329–1331, 2010.
9. Yang H, et al: Severe hydronephrosis in nephrogenic diabetes insipidus, *Clin Med Res* 7(4):170–171, 2009.
10. Loh JA, Verbalis JG: Disorders of water and salt metabolism associated with pituitary disease, *Endocrinol Metab Clin North Am* 37(1):213–234, 2008.
11. Boussemart T, et al: Nephrogenic diabetes insipidus: treat with caution, *Pediatr Nephrol* 24(9):1761–1763, 2009.
12. Toogood AA, Stewart PM: Hypopituitarism: clinical features, diagnosis, and management, *Endocrinol Metab Clin North Am* 37(1):235–261, 2008:x.
13. Tessnow AH, Wilson JD: The changing face of Sheehan's syndrome, *Am J Med Sci* 340(5):402–406, 2010.
14. Romero CJ, Nesi-Franca S, Radovick S: The molecular basis of hypopituitarism, *Trends Endocrinol Metab* 20(10):506–516, 2009.
15. Schneider HJ, et al: Hypopituitarism, *Lancet* 369(9571):1461–1470, 2007.
16. Richmond EJ, Rogol AD: Growth hormone deficiency in children, *Pituitary* 11(2):115–120, 2008.
17. Thomas JD, Monson IP: Adult GH deficiency throughout lifetime, *Eur J Endocrinol* 161(Suppl 1):S97–S106, 2009.
18. Dworakowska D, Grossman AB: The pathophysiology of pituitary adenomas, *Best Pract Res Clin Endocrinol Metab* 23(5):525–541, 2009.
19. Buchfelder M, Schlaffer S: Surgical treatment of pituitary tumours, *Best Pract Res Clin Endocrinol Metab* 23(5):677–692, 2009.
20. Chanson P, et al: Pituitary tumours: acromegaly, *Best Pract Res Clin Endocrinol Metab* 23(5):555–574, 2009.
21. Melmed S: Acromegaly pathogenesis and treatment, *J Clin Invest* 119(11):3189–3202, 2009.
22. Moller N, Jorgensen JO: Effects of growth hormone on glucose, lipid, and protein metabolism in human subjects, *Endocr Rev* 30(2):152–177, 2009.
23. Bronstein MD: Optimizing acromegaly treatment, *Front Horm Res* 38:174–183, 2010.
24. Melmed S, et al: Endocrine Society. Diagnosis and treatment of hyperprolactinemia: an Endocrine Society clinical practice guideline, *J Clin Endocrinol Metab* 96(2):273–288, 2011.
25. Schaberg MR, et al: Microscopic versus endoscopic transnasal pituitary surgery, *Curr Opin Otolaryngol Head Neck Surg* 18(1):8–14, 2010.
26. Kharlip J, Cooper DS: Recent developments in hyperthyroidism, *Lancet* 373(9679):1930–1932, 2009.
27. Brent GA: Clinical practice. Graves' disease, *N Engl J Med* 358(24):2594–2605, 2008.
28. Bahn RS: Graves' ophthalmopathy, *N Engl J Med* 362(8):726–738, 2010.
29. Fatourechi V: Pretibial myxedema: pathophysiology and treatment options, *Am J Clin Dermatol* 6(5):295–309, 2005.
30. Porterfield JR Jr, et al: Evidence-based management of toxic multinodular goiter (Plummer's Disease), *World J Surg* 32(7):1278–1284, 2008.
31. McDermott MT: In the clinic. Hypothyroidism, *Ann Intern Med* 151(11):ITC61, 2009.
32. Yamada M, Masatomo M: Mechanisms related to the pathophysiology and management of central hypothyroidism, *Nat Clin Pract Endocrinol Metab* 4(12):683–694, 2008.
33. Mallipedhi A, Vali H, Okosieme O: Myxedema coma in a patient with subclinical hypothyroidism, *Thyroid* 21(1):87–99, 2011.
34. Vaidya B, Pearce SH: Management of hypothyroidism in adults, *Br Med J* 337:801, 2008.
35. Takami HE, Miyabe R, Kameyama K: Hashimoto's thyroiditis, *World J Surg* 32(5):688–692, 2008.
36. Boelaert K, et al: Prevalence and relative risk of other autoimmune diseases in subjects with autoimmune thyroid disease, *Am J Med* 123(2)183:e1–e9, 2010.
37. Figueroa-Vega N, et al: Increased circulating pro-inflammatory cytokines and Th17 lymphocytes in Hashimoto's thyroiditis, *J Clin Endocrinol Metab* 95(2):953–962, 2010.
38. Peter F, Muzsnai A: Congenital disorders of the thyroid: hypo/hyper, *Endocrinol Metab Clin North Am* 38(3):491–507, 2009.
39. Raymond J, LaFranchi SH: Fetal and neonatal thyroid function: review and summary of significant new findings, *Curr Opin Endocrinol Diabetes Obes* 17(1):1–7, 2010.
40. American Cancer Society: *Cancer Facts and Figures 2010.* Available at http://www.cancer.org/acs/groups/content/@epidemiologysurveilance/documents/document/acspc-026238.pdf.
41. Kouniavsky G, Zeiger MA: Thyroid tumorigenesis and molecular markers in thyroid cancer, *Curr Opin Oncol* 22(1):23–29, 2010.
42. Fraser WD: Hyperparathyroidism, *Lancet* 374(9684):145–158, 2009.
43. Riccardi D, Brown EM: Physiology and pathophysiology of the calcium-sensing receptor in the kidney, *Am J Physiol Renal Physiol* 298(3):F485–F499, 2010.
44. Komaba H, Shiizaki K, Fukagawa M: Pharmacotherapy and interventional treatments for secondary hyperparathyroidism: current therapy and future challenges, *Expert Opin Biol Ther* 10(12):1729–1742, 2010.
45. Shoback D: Clinical practice. Hypoparathyroidism, *N Engl J Med* 359(4):391–403, 2008.
45a. Centers for Disease Control and Prevention (2011). *National diabetes fact sheet.* Available at http://www.cdc.gov/diabetes/pubs/estimates11.htm#3. Accessed June, 2011.
46. American Diabetes Association: Diagnosis and classification of diabetes mellitus, *Diabetes Care* 33:S62–S69, 2010.
47. Centers for Disease Control and Prevention: *Diabetes data and trends,* 2007. Available at http://apps.nccd.cdc.gov/DDTSTRS/default.aspx.
47a. Vehik K, Dabelea D: The changing epidemiology of type 1 diabetes: why is it going through the roof? *Diabetes Metab Res Rev* 27(1):3–13, 2011.
48. Ferrannini E, et al: Progression to diabetes in relatives of type 1 diabetic patients: mechanisms and mode of onset. DPT-1 Study Group, *Diabetes* 59(3):679–685, 2010.
49. Daneman D: Type 1 diabetes, *Lancet* 367:847–858, 2006.
50. van Belle TL, Coppieters KT, von Herrath MG: Type 1 diabetes: etiology.
51. Faustman DL, Davis M: The primacy of CD8 T lymphocytes in type 1 diabetes and implications for therapies, *J Mol Med* 87(12):1173–1178, 2009.
52. Todd JA: Etiology of type 1 diabetes, *Immunity* 32(4):457–477, 2010.
53. Raman VS, Heptulla RA: New potential adjuncts to treatment of children with type 1 diabetes mellitus, *Pediatr Res* 65(4):370–374, 2009.
54. Bui H, et al: Is diabetic ketoacidosis at disease onset a result of missed diagnosis? *J Pediatr* 156(3):472–477, 2010.
55. Jacobsen IB, et al: Evidence-based insulin treatment in type 1 diabetes mellitus, *Diabetes Res Clin Pract* 86(1):1–10, 2009.
56. Wherrett DK, Daneman D: Prevention of type 1 diabetes, *Endocrinol Metab Clin North Am* 38(4):777–790, 2009.
57. Vardanyan M, et al: Pancreas vs. islet transplantation: a call on the future, *Curr Opin Organ Transplant* 15(1):1224–1230, 2010.
58. Centers for Disease Control and Prevention: *2007 national diabetes fact sheet,* May 25, 2010. Available at www.cdc.gov/diabetes/pubs/estimates07.htm#1. Accessed June, 2011.

59. Stolar M: Addressing cardiovascular risk in patients with type 2 diabetes: focus on primary care, *Am J Med Sci* 341(2):132–140, 2011.

60. Bruce KD, Hanson MA: The developmental origins, mechanisms, and implications of metabolic syndrome, *J Nutr* 140(3):648–652, 2010.

61. Maury E, Brichard SM: Adipokine dysregulation, adipose tissue inflammation and metabolic syndrome, *Mol Cell Endocrinol* 314(1):1–16, 2010.

62. Elsner M, Gehrmann W, Lenzen S: Peroxisome-generated hydrogen peroxide as important mediator of lipotoxicity in insulin-producing cells, *Diabetes* 60(1):200–208, 2011.

63. Donath MY, Shoelson SE: Type 2 diabetes as an inflammatory disease, *Nat Rev Immunol* 11(2):98–107, 2011.

64. Iyer A, et al: Inflammatory lipid mediators in adipocyte function and obesity, *Nat Rev Endocrinol* 6(2):71–82, 2010.

65. Grill V, Bjorklund A: Impact of metabolic abnormalities for beta cell function: clinical significance and underlying mechanisms, *Mol Cell Endocrinol* 297(1–2):86–92, 2009.

66. Castaneda TR, et al: Ghrelin in the regulation of body weight and metabolism, *Front Neuroendocrinol* 31(1):44–60, 2010.

67. Peters A: Incretin-based therapies: review of current clinical trial data, *Am J Med* 123(3 suppl):S28–S37, 2010.

68. Rosenbloom AL, et al: Type 2 diabetes in children and adolescents, *Peds Diabetes* 10(suppl 12):17–32, 2009.

69. American Diabetes Association: Standards of medical care in diabetes—2010, *Diabetes Care* 3:S11–S61, 2010.

70. Rubino F, et al: The Diabetes Surgery Summit consensus conference: recommendations for the evaluation and use of gastrointestinal surgery to treat type 2 diabetes mellitus, Diabetes Surgery Summit Delegates, *Ann Surg* 251(3):399–405, 2010.

71. Blonde L: Current antihyperglycemic treatment guidelines and algorithms for patients with type 2 diabetes mellitus, *Am J Med* 123(3A):S3–S11, 2010.

72. Hattersley A, et al: The diagnosis and management of monogenic diabetes in children and adolescents, *Peds Diabetes* 10(suppl 12):33–42, 2009.

73. American Diabetes Association: Diagnosis and classification of diabetes mellitus, *Diabetes Care* 33:S62–S69, 2010.

74. Nolan CJ: Controversies in gestational diabetes, *Best Pract Res Clin Obstet Gynaecol* 25(1):37–49, 2011.

75. Kitabchi AE, Nyenwe EA: Hyperglycemic crises in diabetes mellitus: diabetic ketoacidosis and hyperglycemic hyperosmolar state, *Endocrinol Metab Clin North Am* 35(4):725–751, 2006:viii.

76. ACCORD Study Group, Gerstein HC, et al: Long-term effects of intensive glucose lowering on cardiovascular outcomes, *N Engl J Med* 364(9):818–828, 2011.

77. Obrosova IG, Kador PF: Aldose reductase / polyol inhibitors for diabetic retinopathy, *Curr Pharm Biotechnol* 12(3):373–385, 2011.

78. Geraldes P, King GL: Activation of protein kinase C isoforms and its impact on diabetic complications, *Circ Res* 106(8):1319–1331, 2010.

79. Goh SY, Cooper ME: Clinical review: the role of advanced glycation end products in progression and complications of diabetes, *J Clin Endocrinol Metab* 93(4):1143–1152, 2008.

79a. Méndez JD, et al: Molecular susceptibility to glycation and its implication in diabetes mellitus and related diseases, *Mol Cell Biochem* 344(1-2):185–193, 2010.

80. Yan SF, Ramasamy R, Schmidt AM: The RAGE axis: a fundamental mechanism signaling danger to the vulnerable vasculature, *Circ Res* 106(5):842–853, 2010.

81. Yamagishi S: Advanced glycation and end products and receptor-oxidative stress system in diabetic vascular complications, *Ther Apher Dial* 13(6):534–539, 2009.

82. Fante RJ, Jurairaj VD, Oliver SC: Diabetic retinopathy: an update on treatment, *Am J Med* 123(3):213–216, 2010.

83. Kanwar YS, Sun L, Xie P, Liu FY, Chen S: A glimpse of various pathogenetic mechanisms of diabetic nephropathy, *Annu Rev Pathol* 6:395–423, 2011.

84. Magri CJ, Fava S: The role of tubular injury in diabetic nephropathy, *Eur J Intern Med* 20(6):551–555, 2009.

85. Olivero JJ, Nguyen PT: Chronic kidney disease: a marker of cardiovascular disease, *Methodist Debakey Cardiovasc J* 5(2):24–29, 2009.

86. Tomlinson DR, Gardiner NJ: Diabetic neuropathies: components of etiology, *J Peripher Nerv Syst* 13(2):112–121, 2008.

87. Strachan MW, et al: Cognitive function, dementia and type 2 diabetes mellitus in the elderly, *Nat Rev Endocrinol* 7(2):108–114, 2011.

88. Ford ES, Zhao G, Li C: Pre-diabetes and the risk for cardiovascular disease: a systematic review of the evidence, *J Am Coll Cardiol* 55(13):1310–1317, 2010.

89. Shah AS, et al: Influence of duration of diabetes, glycemic control, and traditional cardiovascular risk factors on early atherosclerotic vascular changes in adolescents and young adults with type 2 diabetes mellitus, *J Clin Endocrinol Metab* 94(10):3740–3745, 2009.

90. Mytas DZ, et al: Diabetic myocardial disease: pathophysiology, early diagnosis and therapeutic options, *J Diabetes Complications* 23(4):273–282, 2008.

91. Vinik A, Flemmer M: Diabetes and macrovascular disease, *J Diabetes Complications* 16(3):235–245, 2002.

92. Highlander P, Shaw GP: Current pharmacotherapeutic concepts for the treatment of cardiovascular disease in diabetics, *Ther Adv Cardiovas Dis* 4(1):43–54, 2010.

93. Sander D, Kearney MT: Reducing the risk of stroke in type 2 diabetes: pathophysiology and therapeutic perspectives, *J Neurol* 256(10):1603–1619, 2009.

94. Jude EB, Eleftheriadou I, Tentolouris N: Peripheral arterial disease in diabetes—a review, *Diabet Med* 27(1):4–14, 2010.

95. Gupta S, et al: Infections in diabetes mellitus and hyperglycemia, *Infect Dis Clin North Am* 21(3):617–638, 2007.

96. De Martin M, Pecori Giraldi F, Cavagnini F: Cushing's disease, *Best Pract Res Clin Endocrinol Metab* 23(5):607–623, 2009.

97. Findling JW, Raff H: Cushing's syndrome: important issues in diagnosis and management, *J Clin Endocrinol Metab* 91(10):3746–3753, 2006.

98. Reimondo G, et al: Laboratory differentiation of Cushing's syndrome, *Clin Chim Acta* 388(1–2):5–14, 2008.

98a. Dauber A, Kellogg M, Majzoub JA: Monitoring of therapy in congenital adrenal hyperplasia, *Clin Chem* 56(8):1245–1251, 2010.

98b. Quinkler M, Stewart PM: Treatment of primary aldosteronism, *Best Pract Res Clin Endocrinol Metab* 24(6):923–932, 2010.

99. Moneva MH, Gomez-Sanchez CE: Pathophysiology of adrenal hypertension, *Semin Nephrol* 22(1):44–53, 2002.

100. Tomaschitz A, et al: Aldosterone and arterial hypertension, *Nat Rev Endocrinol* 6(2):83–93, 2010.

101. Hennings J, et al: Long-term effects of surgical correction of adrenal hyperplasia and adenoma causing primary aldosteronism, *Langenbecks Arch Surg* 395(2):133–137, 2010.

102. Neary N, Nieman L: Adrenal insufficiency: etiology, diagnosis and treatment, *Curr Opin Endocrinol Diabetes Obes* 17(3):217–223, 2010.

103. Betterle C, Morlin L: Autoimmune Addison's disease, *Endocr Dev* 20:161–172, 2011.

103a. Karasek D, Frysak Z, Pacak K: Genetic testing for pheochromocytoma, *Curr Hypertens Rep* 12(6):456–464, 2010.

104. Zelinaka T, Elsenhofer G, Pacak K: Pheochromocytoma as a catecholamine producing tumor: implications for practice, *Stress* 10(2):195–203, 2007.

105. Adjalle R, et al: Treatment of malignant pheochromocytoma, *Horm Metabolic* 41(9):687–696, 2009.

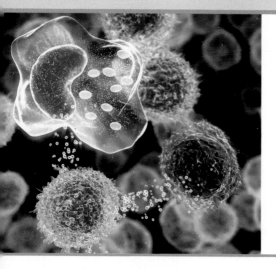

Structure and Function of the Hematologic System

Neal S. Rote and Kathryn L. McCance*

ℰvolve WEBSITE

CHAPTER OUTLINE

All the body's tissues and organs require oxygen and nutrients to survive. These essential needs are provided by the blood that flows through miles of vessels throughout the human body. The red blood cells provide the oxygen, and the fluid portion of the blood carries the nutrients. The blood also cleans discarded waste from the tissues and transports cells (white blood cells) and other ingredients that are necessary for protecting the entire body from injury and infection.

COMPONENTS OF THE HEMATOLOGIC SYSTEM

Composition of Blood

Blood consists of various cells that circulate suspended in a solution of protein and inorganic materials (plasma), which is approximately 92% water and 8% dissolved substances (solutes). The blood volume amounts to about 6 quarts (5.5 L) in adults. The continuous movement of blood guarantees that critical components are available to all parts

of the body to carry out their chief functions: (1) delivery of substances needed for cellular metabolism in the tissues, (2) removal of the wastes of cellular metabolism, (3) defense against invading microorganisms and injury, and (4) maintenance of acid-base balance.

Plasma and Plasma Proteins

In adults, plasma accounts for 50% to 55% of blood volume (Figure 19-1). Plasma is a complex aqueous liquid containing a variety of organic and inorganic elements (Table 19-1). The concentration of these elements varies depending on diet, metabolic demand, hormones, and vitamins. Plasma differs from serum in that serum is plasma that has been allowed to clot in the laboratory in order to remove fibrinogen and other clotting factors that may interfere with some diagnostic tests.

The plasma contains a large number of proteins (plasma proteins). These vary in structure and function and can be classified into two major groups, albumin and globulins. Most plasma proteins are produced by the liver. The major exception is antibody, which is produced by plasma cells in the lymph nodes and other lymphoid tissues (see Chapter 6).

---

*Thom J. Mansen, RN, PhD, contributed to this chapter in the previous edition.

TABLE 19-1 ORGANIC AND INORGANIC COMPONENTS OF ARTERIAL PLASMA

CONSTITUENT	AMOUNT/CONCENTRATION	MAJOR FUNCTIONS
Water	92% of plasma weight	Medium for carrying all other constituents
Electrolytes	Total >1% of plasma	Maintain H_2O in extracellular compartment; act as buffers; function in membrane excitability
Na^+	142 mEq/L (142 mM)	
K^+	4 mEq/L (4 mM)	
Ca^{++}	5 mEq/L (2.5 mM)	
Mg^{++}	3 mEq/L (1.5 mM)	
Cl^-	103 mEq/L (103 mM)	
HCO_3^-	27 mEq/L (27 mM)	
Phosphate (mostly HPO_4^-)	2 mEq/L (1 mM)	
S_4^{--}	1 mEq/L (0.5 mM)	
Proteins	7.3 g/dl (2.5 mM)	Provide colloid osmotic pressure of plasma; act as buffers; see text for other functions
Albumins	4.5 g/dl	
Globulins	2.5 g/dl	
Fibrinogen	0.3 g/dl	
Transferrin	250 mg/dl	
Ferritin	15-300 mg/L	
Gases		
CO_2 content	22-20 mmol/L plasma	By-product of oxygenation, most CO_2 content is from HCO_3^- and acts as buffer
O_2	Pa_{O_2} 80 torr or greater (arterial); Pv_{O_2} 30-40 torr (venous)	Oxygenation
N_2	0.9 ml/dl	By-product of protein catabolism
Nutrients		Provide nutrition and substances for tissue repair
Glucose and other carbohydrates	100 mg/dl (5.6 mM)	
Total amino acids	40 mg/dl (2 mM)	
Total lipids	500 mg/dl (7.5 mM)	
Cholesterol	150-250 mg/dl (4-7 mM)	
Individual vitamins	0.0001-2.5 mg/dl	
Individual trace elements	0.001-0.3 mg/dl	
Iron	50-150 mg/dl	
Waste Products		
Urea (BUN)	7-18 mg/dl (5.7 mM)	End product of protein catabolism
Creatinine (from creatine)	1 mg/dl (0.09 mM)	End product from energy metabolism
Uric acid (from nucleic acids)	5 mg/dl (0.3 mM)	End product from protein metabolism
Bilirubin (from heme)	0.2-1.2 mg/dl (0.003-0.018 mM)	End product of red blood cell destruction
Individual hormones	0.000001-0.5 mg/dl	Functions specific to target tissue

Data from Vander AJ, Sherman JH, Luchiano DS: *Human physiology: the mechanisms of body function*, New York, 2001, McGraw-Hill.

Albumin (about 60% of total plasma protein) serves as a carrier molecule for both normal components of blood and drugs. Its most essential role is regulation of the passage of water and solutes through the capillaries. Albumin molecules are large and do not diffuse freely through the vascular endothelium, and thus they maintain the critical colloidal osmotic pressure (or oncotic pressure) that regulates the passage of water and solutes into the surrounding tissues (see Chapters 1 and 3). Water and solute particles tend to diffuse out of the arterial portions of the capillaries because blood pressure is greater in arterial than in venous blood vessels. Water and solutes move from tissues into the venous portions of the capillaries where the pressures are reversed, oncotic pressure being greater than intravascular pressure or hydrostatic pressure. In the case of decreased production (e.g., cirrhosis, other diffuse liver diseases, protein malnutrition) or excessive loss of albumin (e.g., certain kidney diseases), the reduced oncotic pressure leads to excessive movement of fluid and solutes into the tissue and decreased blood volume.[1]

The remaining plasma proteins, or **globulins**, are often classified by their properties in an electric field (serum electrophoresis). Under the normal conditions used to perform serum electrophoresis, albumin is the most rapidly moving protein. The globulins are classified by their movement relative to albumin: alpha globulins (those moving most closely to albumin), beta globulins, and gamma globulins (those with the least movement). The alpha and beta globulins may be subdivided into subregions (alpha-1, alpha-2, beta-1, or beta-2 globulins).

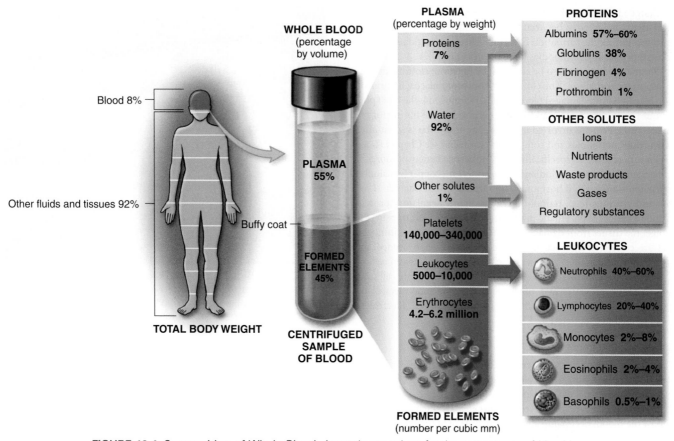

FIGURE 19-1 Composition of Whole Blood. Approximate values for the components of blood in a normal adult. (From Patton KT, Thibodeau GA: *Anatomy & Physiology,* ed 7, St Louis, 2010, Mosby.)

TABLE 19-2	CELLULAR COMPONENTS OF THE BLOOD			
CELL	**STRUCTURAL CHARACTERISTICS**	**NORMAL AMOUNTS OF CIRCULATING BLOOD**	**FUNCTION**	**LIFE SPAN**
Erythrocyte (red blood cell)	Nonnucleated cytoplasmic disk containing hemoglobin	4.2-6.2 million/mm³	Gas transport to and from tissue cells and lungs	80-120 days
Reticulocyte	60,000/mm³	Immature erythrocyte		
Absolute reticulocyte count	0.5-2.0% of erythrocytes			
Leukocyte (white blood cell)	Nucleated cell	5000-10,000/mm³	Body defense mechanisms	See below
Lymphocyte	Mononuclear immunocyte	25-36% of leukocyte count (leukocyte differential)	Humoral and cell-mediated immunity (see Chapter 6)	Days or years depending on type
Natural killer cell	Large granular lymphocyte	5-10% circulatory pool (some in spleen)	Defense against some tumors and viruses (see Chapters 5 and 6)	Unknown
Monocyte and macrophage	Large mononuclear phagocyte	3-8% of leukocyte differential	Phagocytosis; mononuclear phagocyte system	Months or years
Eosinophil	Segmented polymorphonuclear granulocyte	2-4% of leukocyte differential	Control of inflammation, phagocytosis, defense against parasites, allergic reactions	Unknown
Neutrophil	Segmented polymorphonuclear granulocyte	40-60% of leukocyte differential	Phagocytosis, particularly during early phase of inflammation	4 days
Basophil	Segmented polymorphonuclear granulocyte	0.5-1% of leukocyte differential	Mast cell–like functions, associated with allergic reactions and mechanical irritation	Unknown
Platelet	Irregularly shaped cytoplasmic fragment (not a cell)	150,000-400,000/mm³	Hemostasis after vascular injury; normal coagulation and clot formation/retraction	8-11 days

Fibrinogen is a major plasma protein (about 4% of total plasma protein) that would move between the beta and gamma regions but is removed during the formation of serum. The gamma-globulin region consists primarily of antibodies (see Chapter 6).

Plasma proteins can also be classified by function: clotting, defense, transport, or regulation. The clotting factors promote coagulation and stop bleeding from damaged blood vessels. Fibrinogen is the most plentiful of the clotting factors and is the precursor of the fibrin clot (see Figure 19-7). Proteins involved in defense, or protection, against infection include antibodies and complement proteins (see Chapters 5 and 6). Transport proteins specifically bind and carry a variety of inorganic and organic molecules, including iron (transferrin), copper (ceruloplasmin), lipids and steroid hormones (lipoproteins) (see Chapters 1 and 22), and vitamins (e.g., retinol-binding protein). Regulatory proteins include a variety of enzymatic inhibitors (e.g., alpha-1 antitrypsin) that protect the tissues from damage, precursor molecules (e.g., kininogen) that are converted into active biologic molecules when needed, and protein hormones (e.g., cytokines) that communicate between cells.

Plasma also contains several inorganic ions that regulate cell function, osmotic pressure, and blood pH. These include electrolytes, sodium, potassium, calcium, chloride, and phosphate. (Electrolytes are described in Chapters 1 and 3.)

Cellular Components of the Blood

The cellular elements of the blood are broadly classified as red blood cells (i.e., erythrocytes), white blood cells (i.e., leukocytes), and platelets. The components of the blood are listed in Table 19-2.

Erythrocytes. Erythrocytes (red blood cells) are the most abundant cells of the blood, occupying approximately 48% of the blood volume in men and about 42% in women. Erythrocytes are primarily responsible for tissue oxygenation. Hemoglobin (Hb) carries the gases, and electrolytes regulate gas diffusion through the cell's plasma membrane. The mature erythrocyte lacks a nucleus and cytoplasmic organelles (e.g., mitochondria), so it cannot synthesize protein or carry out oxidative reactions. Because it cannot undergo mitotic division, the erythrocyte has a limited life span (approximately 120 days).

The erythrocyte's size and shape are ideally suited to its function as a gas carrier. It is a small disk with two unique properties: (1) a *biconcave* shape and (2) the capacity to be *reversibly deformed*. The flattened, biconcave shape provides a surface area/volume ratio that is optimal for gas diffusion into and out of the cell. During its life span, the erythrocyte, which is 6 to 8 μm in diameter, repeatedly circulates through splenic sinusoids (see Figure 19-5) and capillaries that are only 2 μm in diameter. Reversible deformity enables the erythrocyte to assume a more compact torpedo-like shape, squeeze through the microcirculation, and return to normal.[2]

Leukocytes. Leukocytes (white blood cells) defend the body against organisms that cause infection and also remove debris, including dead or injured host cells of all kinds (Figure 19-2). The leukocytes act primarily in the tissues but are transported in the circulation. The average adult has approximately 5000 to 10,000 leukocytes/mm³ of blood.

Leukocytes are classified according to structure as either granulocytes or agranulocytes and according to function as either phagocytes or immunocytes. The granulocytes, which include neutrophils, basophils, and eosinophils, are all phagocytes. (Phagocytic action is described in Chapter 5.) Of the agranulocytes, the monocytes and macrophages are phagocytes, whereas the lymphocytes are immunocytes (cells that create immunity; see Chapter 6).

Granulocytes. The granulocytes have many membrane-bound granules in their cytoplasm. These granules contain enzymes capable

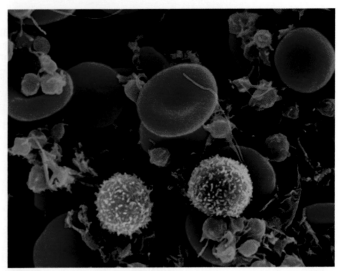

FIGURE 19-2 Blood Cells. Leukocytes are spherical and have irregular surfaces with numerous extending pili. Leukocytes are the cotton candy–like cells in yellow. Erythrocytes are flattened spheres with a depressed center (red). (Copyright Dennis Kunkel Microscopy, Inc.)

of killing microorganisms and catabolizing debris ingested during phagocytosis. The granules also contain powerful biochemical mediators with inflammatory and immune functions. These mediators, along with the digestive enzymes, are released from granulocytes in response to specific stimuli and affect other cells in the circulation. Granulocytes are capable of ameboid movement, by which they migrate through vessel walls (diapedesis) and then to sites where their action is needed.

The neutrophil (polymorphonuclear neutrophil [PMN]) is the most numerous and best understood of the granulocytes (Figure 19-3).[3] Neutrophils constitute about 55% of the total leukocyte count in adults.

Neutrophils are the chief phagocytes of early inflammation. Soon after bacterial invasion or tissue injury, neutrophils migrate out of the capillaries and into the damaged tissue, where they ingest and destroy contaminating microorganisms and debris. Neutrophils are sensitive to the environment in damaged tissue (e.g., low pH, enzymes released from damaged cells) and die in 1 or 2 days. The breakdown of dead neutrophils releases digestive enzymes from their cytoplasmic granules. These enzymes dissolve cellular debris and prepare the site for healing.

Eosinophils, which have large, coarse granules, constitute only 2% to 4% of the normal leukocyte count in adults.[4] Like neutrophils, eosinophils are capable of ameboid movement and phagocytosis. Unlike neutrophils, eosinophils ingest antigen-antibody complexes and are induced by immunoglobulin E (IgE)-mediated hypersensitivity reactions to attack parasites (see Chapters 5 and 6). The eosinophil granules contain a variety of enzymes (e.g., histaminase) that help to control inflammatory processes. During type I hypersensitivity, allergic reactions and asthma are characterized by high eosinophil counts, which may be involved in limiting the inflammatory response but may also contribute to the destructive inflammatory processes observed in the lungs of asthmatics.

Basophils, which make up less than 1% of the leukocytes, are structurally similar to the mast cells found throughout extravascular tissue (see Figure 19-3).[5] Like the mast cells, basophils have cytoplasmic granules that contain vasoactive amines (e.g., histamine) and an anticoagulant (heparin). Their function is similar to that of tissue mast cells (see Chapter 5).

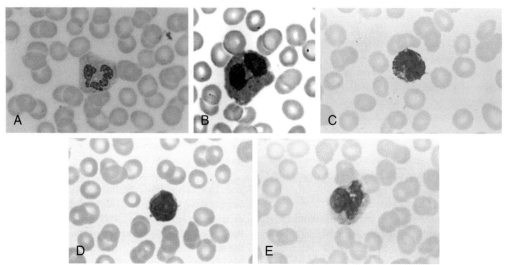

FIGURE 19-3 Leukocytes. An example of leukocytes in human blood smear. **A,** Neutrophil. **B,** Eosinophil. **C,** Basophil with obscured nucleus. **D,** Typical monocyte showing vacuolated cytoplasm and cerebriform nucleus. **E,** Lymphocyte. (**A, C, D,** and **E** from Rodak BF: *Hematology: clinical principles and applications,* ed 2, Philadelphia, 2002, Saunders; **B** from Carr JC, Rodak BF: *Clinical hematology atlas,* Philadelphia, 1999, Saunders.)

Agranulocytes. The agranulocytes—monocytes, macrophages, and lymphocytes—contain relatively fewer granules than granulocytes. Monocytes and macrophages make up the mononuclear phagocyte system (or MPS, described on p. 483). Both monocytes and macrophages participate in the immune and inflammatory response, being powerful phagocytes. They also ingest dead or defective host cells, particularly blood cells.

Monocytes are immature macrophages (see Figure 19-3). Monocytes are formed and released by the bone marrow into the bloodstream. As they mature, monocytes migrate into a variety of tissues (e.g., liver, spleen, lymph nodes, peritoneum, gastrointestinal tract) and fully mature into tissue **macrophages.** Other monocytes may mature into macrophages and migrate out of the vessels in response to infection or inflammation.

Lymphocytes constitute approximately 20-40% of the total leukocyte count and are the primary cells of the immune response (see Figure 19-3) (see Chapter 6). Most lymphocytes transiently circulate in the blood and eventually reside in lymphoid tissues as mature T cells, B cells, or plasma cells. (Lymphocyte function and dysfunction are described in detail in Unit 2.)

Natural killer (NK) cells, which resemble lymphocytes, kill some types of tumor cells (in vitro) and some virus-infected cells without prior exposure (see Chapter 6). They develop in the bone marrow and circulate in the blood.

Platelets. Platelets (thrombocytes) are not true cells but disk-shaped cytoplasmic fragments that are essential for blood coagulation and control of bleeding. They lack a nucleus, have no deoxyribonucleic acid (DNA), and are incapable of mitotic division. They do, however, contain cytoplasmic granules capable of releasing proinflammatory biochemical mediators when stimulated by injury to a blood vessel (Figure 19-4) (see Chapter 5).

The normal platelet concentration is 150,000 to 400,000 platelets/mm^3 of circulating blood, although the normal ranges may vary slightly from laboratory to laboratory. An additional one third of the body's available platelets are in a reserve pool in the spleen. A platelet circulates for approximately 10 days, ages, and is removed by macrophages of the MPS, mostly in the spleen. **Thrombopoietin (TPO),**

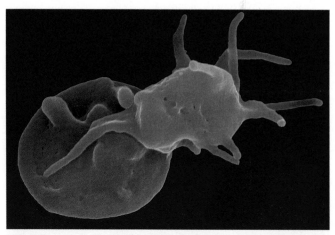

FIGURE 19-4 Colored Micrograph of Platelets. The platelet on the left is moderately activated, with a generally round shape and the beginning of formation of pseudopodia (foot-like extensions from the membrane). The platelet on the right is fully activated, with extensive pseudopodia. (Copyright Dennis Kunkle Microscopy, Inc.)

a hormone growth factor, is the main regulator of the circulating platelet mass. TPO is primarily produced by the liver and induces platelet production in the bone marrow.[6] Platelets express receptors for TPO, and when circulating platelet levels are normal, TPO is adsorbed onto the platelet surface and prevented from accessing the bone marrow and initiating further platelet production. When platelet levels are low, however, the amount of TPO exceeds the number of available platelet TPO receptors, and free TPO can enter the bone marrow.

> ✔ **QUICK CHECK 19-1**
> 1. Why are plasma proteins important to blood volume?
> 2. Which leukocytes are granulocytes?
> 3. Compare and contrast granulocytes, agranulocytes, phagocytes, and immunocytes.

Lymphoid Organs

The lymphoid system is closely integrated with the circulatory system. The role of lymphoid organs in the immune response was discussed in Chapter 6. Lymphoid organs are sites of residence, proliferation, differentiation, and function of lymphocytes and mononuclear phagocytes (monocytes, macrophages). (The liver, which also has hematologic functions, is primarily a digestive organ and is described in Chapter 33.)

Spleen

The spleen is the largest of the lymphoid organs. It is a site of fetal hematopoiesis, its mononuclear phagocytes filter and cleanse the blood, its lymphocytes mount immune responses to blood-borne microorganisms, and it serves as a blood reservoir.

The spleen is a concave, encapsulated organ that weighs about 150 g and is about the size of a fist (see Figure 6-2). It is located in the left upper abdominal cavity, curved around a portion of the stomach. Strands of connective tissue (trabeculae) extend throughout the spleen from the splenic capsule, dividing it into compartments that contain masses of lymphoid tissue called *splenic pulp*. The spleen is interlaced with many blood vessels, some of which can distend to store blood.

Blood that circulates through the spleen first encounters the white splenic pulp, which consists of masses of lymphoid tissue containing lymphocytes and macrophages. The white pulp forms clumps around the splenic arterioles and is the chief site of immune and phagocytic function within the spleen. Here blood-borne antigens encounter lymphocytes, initiating the immune response (see Chapter 6).[7]

Some of the blood continues through the microcirculation and enters highly distensible storage areas called *venous sinuses*. Most of the blood, however, oozes through the capillary walls into the principal site of splenic filtration, the red pulp (Figure 19-5). Here the resident macrophages of the MPS phagocytose damaged or old blood cells of all kinds (but chiefly erythrocytes), microorganisms, and particles of

debris. Hemoglobin from phagocytosed erythrocytes is catabolized, and heme (iron) is stored in the cytoplasm of the macrophages or released back into the blood plasma (see Figure 19-13). Blood that filters through the red pulp then moves through the venous sinuses and into the portal circulation.

The venous sinuses (and the red pulp) can store more than 300 ml of blood. Sudden reductions in blood pressure cause the sympathetic nervous system to stimulate constriction of the sinuses and expel as much as 200 ml of blood into the venous circulation, helping to restore blood volume or pressure in the circulation and increasing the hematocrit by as much as 4%.

The spleen is not necessary for life or for adequate hematologic function. Its absence, however, has several effects that indicate its function. For example, leukocytosis (high levels of circulating leukocytes) often occurs after splenectomy, so the spleen must exert some control over the rate of proliferation of leukocytes. After splenectomy iron levels in the circulation are decreased, immune function is diminished, and the blood contains more structurally defective blood cells than normal.

Lymph Nodes

Structurally, lymph nodes are part of the lymphatic system. Thousands are clustered around the lymphatic veins, which collect interstitial fluid from the tissues and transport it, as lymph, back into the circulatory system near the heart. Functionally, however, lymph nodes are part of the hematologic and immune systems because large numbers of lymphocytes, monocytes, and macrophages develop or function within the lymph nodes.[8] As the lymph filters through the bean-shaped lymph nodes clustered in the inguinal, axillary, and cervical regions of the body, it is cleansed of foreign particles and microorganisms by the monocytes and macrophages. The microorganisms in lymph stimulate the resident lymphocytes to develop into antibody-producing plasma cells. During an infection, the rate of proliferation of lymphocytes within the nodes is so great that the nodes enlarge and become tender.[9]

Each lymph node is enclosed in a fibrous capsule (Figure 19-6), with strands of connective tissue (trabeculae) extending inward,

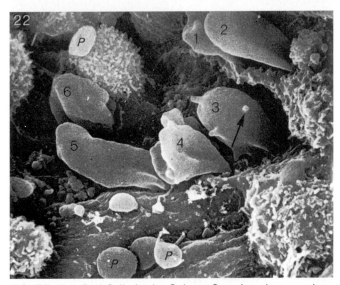

FIGURE 19-5 Red Cells in the Spleen. Scanning electron micrograph of spleen, demonstrating erythrocytes (numbered *1* through *6*) squeezing through the fenestrated wall in transit from the splenic cord to the sinus. The view shows the endothelial lining of the sinus wall, to which platelets (*P*) adhere, along with "hairy" white cells, probably macrophages. The arrow shows a protrusion on a red blood cell (×5000). (From Weiss L: A scanning electron microscope study of the spleen, *Blood* 43:665, 1974; reprinted with permission.)

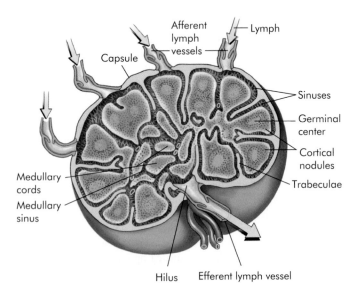

FIGURE 19-6 Cross Section of Lymph Node. Several afferent valved lymphatics bring lymph to node. A single efferent lymphatic leaves the node at the hilus. *Note that the artery and vein also enter and leave at the hilus. Arrows show direction of lymph flow.* (From Thibodeau GA, Patton KT: *Anatomy & physiology,* ed 6, St Louis, 2007, Mosby.)

dividing the node into several compartments. Reticular fibers divide the compartments into smaller sections and trap and store large numbers of lymphocytes, monocytes, and macrophages. The node has an outer cortex area and an inner medullary area. Within the cortex are germinal centers, or separate masses of lymphoid tissue (see Figure 19-6). Lymph enters the node, slowly filters through its sinuses, and leaves through efferent lymphatic vessels.[10]

The Mononuclear Phagocyte System

The mononuclear phagocyte system (MPS) consists of cells that originate in the bone marrow, are transported by the bloodstream, and, after differentiation to blood monocytes, finally settle in the tissues as mature macrophages. Table 19-3 lists the various names given to macrophages localized in specific tissues.

The cells of the MPS ingest and destroy (by phagocytosis) unwanted materials, such as foreign protein particles, microorganisms, debris from dead or injured cells, defective or injured erythrocytes, and dead neutrophils (see Figure 5-10). The MPS (mostly in the liver and spleen) is also the main line of defense against bacteria in the bloodstream. In addition, the MPS cleanses the blood of old, injured, or dead erythrocytes, leukocytes, platelets, coagulation products, antigen-antibody complexes, and macromolecules. Recently, the osteoclast was classified as a true member of the MPS. Osteoclasts are multinucleated cells specialized for the function of lacunar bone resorption; however, they are also known to have phagocytic abilities. The osteoclast originates from the monocyte cell lineage (Figure 19-7). Macrophages also play a role in blood coagulation, wound healing, tissue remodeling, and the control of blood production.

The origin and turnover time of all the tissue macrophages named in Table 19-3 are not precisely known. Once monocytes leave the circulation, they do not return. In the tissues, monocytes differentiate into macrophages without dividing and can survive for many months or perhaps even years.

✔ **QUICK CHECK 19-2**

1. Why is the spleen considered a hematologic organ? Why can humans live without it?
2. Why are lymph nodes considered part of the hematologic system?
3. What is the MPS?

TABLE 19-3	MONONUCLEAR PHAGOCYTE SYSTEM (FORMERLY CALLED THE RETICULOENDOTHELIAL SYSTEM)
NAME OF CELL	**LOCATION**
Monocytes/macrophages	Bone marrow and peripheral blood
Kupffer cells (inflammatory macrophages)	Liver
Alveolar macrophages	Lung
Histiocytes	Connective tissue
Macrophages	Bone marrow
Fixed and free macrophages	Spleen and lymph nodes
Pleural and peritoneal macrophages	Serous cavities
Microglial cells	Nervous system
Mesangial cells	Kidney
Osteoclasts	Bone
Langerhans cells	Skin
Dendritic cells	Lymphoid tissue

DEVELOPMENT OF BLOOD CELLS

Hematopoiesis

The typical human requires about 100 billion new blood cells per day. Blood cell production, termed hematopoiesis, is constantly ongoing, occurring in the liver and spleen of the fetus and only in bone marrow after birth, and is known as *medullary hematopoiesis*. This process involves the biochemical stimulation of populations of relatively undifferentiated cells to undergo mitotic division (i.e., proliferation) and maturation (i.e., differentiation) into mature hematologic cells. Certain blood cells proliferate and differentiate simultaneously. Proliferation usually ceases after a number of doubling divisions, but differentiation continues. Erythrocytes and neutrophils generally differentiate fully before entering the blood, but monocytes and lymphocytes do not.

Hematopoiesis continues throughout life, increasing in response to proliferative disease, hemorrhage, hemolytic anemia (in which erythrocytes are destroyed), chronic infection, thrombocytopenic purpura (bleeding caused by platelet insufficiency; see Chapter 20), and other disorders that deplete blood cells. In general, long-term stimuli, such as chronic diseases, cause a greater increase in hematopoiesis than acute conditions, such as hemorrhage. Abnormal proliferation of erythrocytes occurs in polycythemia vera, a myeloproliferative disease (discussed in Chapter 20). In adults, extramedullary hematopoiesis—blood cell production in tissues other than bone marrow—is usually a sign of disease, occurring in pernicious anemia, sickle cell anemia, thalassemia, hemolytic disease of the newborn (erythroblastosis fetalis), hereditary spherocytosis, and certain leukemias. Extramedullary hematopoiesis of apparently normal blood cells has been reported in the spleen, liver, and, less frequently, lymph nodes, adrenal glands, cartilage, adipose tissue, intrathoracic areas, and kidneys.

Bone Marrow

Bone marrow is confined to the cavities of bone. It consists of blood vessels, nerves, mononuclear phagocytes, stromal cells, blood cells in various stages of differentiation, and fatty tissue. Adults have two kinds of bone marrow: red, or active (hematopoietic), marrow (also called myeloid tissue); and yellow, or inactive, marrow. The large quantities of fat in inactive marrow make it yellow. Not all bones contain active marrow. In adults, active marrow is found primarily in the flat bones of the pelvis (34%), vertebrae (28%), cranium and mandible (13%), sternum and ribs (10%), and in the extreme proximal portions of the humerus and femur (4% to 8%). Inactive marrow predominates in cavities of other bones. (Bones are discussed further in Chapter 36.)

Hematopoietic marrow receives oxygen and nutrients needed for cellular differentiation from the primary arteries of the bones. Branches of these arteries terminate in a capillary network that coalesces into large venous sinuses, which eventually drain into a central vein. Hematopoietic marrow and fat fill the spaces surrounding the network of venous sinuses. Newly produced blood cells traverse narrow openings in the venous sinus walls and thus enter the circulation. Normally, cells do not enter the circulation until they have differentiated to a certain extent, but premature release occurs in certain diseases.

Cellular Differentiation

The hematologic system arises from the proliferation and differentiation of hematopoietic stem cells. All humans originate from a single cell (the fertilized egg) that has the capacity to proliferate and eventually differentiate into the huge diversity of cells of the human body. After fertilization, the egg divides over a 5-day period to form a hollow ball (blastocyst) that implants on the uterus. Until about 3 days after fertilization, each cell (blastomere) is undifferentiated and retains the capacity to differentiate into any cell type. In the 5-day blastocyst, the outer layer of cells has undergone differentiation and commitment to become the placenta. Cells of the inner cell mass, however, continue to have unlimited differentiation potential (currently referred to as being *pluripotent*) and can grow into different kinds of tissue—blood, nerves, heart, bone, and so forth. After implantation, cells of the inner cell mass begin differentiation into other cell types. Differentiation is a multistep process and results in intermediate groups of stem cells with more limited, but still impressive, abilities to differentiate into many different types of cells.[11]

The bone marrow contains a population of hematopoietic stem cells that have partially differentiated (see Figure 19-7).[12] They have the capacity to differentiate into any of the hematologic cell populations but can no longer differentiate into other cell types, like nerve or muscle cells. As with all stem cells, the hematopoietic stem cells are self-renewing (they have the ability to proliferate without further differentiation)

so that a relatively constant population of stem cells is available. Some hematopoietic stem cells will continue differentiation into hematopoietic progenitor cells. Progenitor cells retain proliferative capacity but are committed to possible further differentiation into particular types of hematologic cells: lymphoid (lymphocytes, NK cells), granulocyte/ monocyte (granulocytes, monocytes, macrophages), and megakaryocyte/erythroid (platelets, erythrocytes) progenitor cells.

As with all other forms of cellular differentiation, successful hematopoiesis requires that progenitor cells interact with neighboring cells (stromal cells of the bone marrow) through a variety of adhesion molecules and are exposed to particular signaling molecules (cytokines).[13] Populations of stromal stem cells differentiate into many different bone marrow cell types, including bone cells (chondrocytes that produce cartilage and osteoblasts that produce bone), fat cells (adipocytes), muscle (myocytes), and fibroblasts. Interactions between osteoclasts and hematopoietic stem cells appear to be the most important for hematopoiesis.

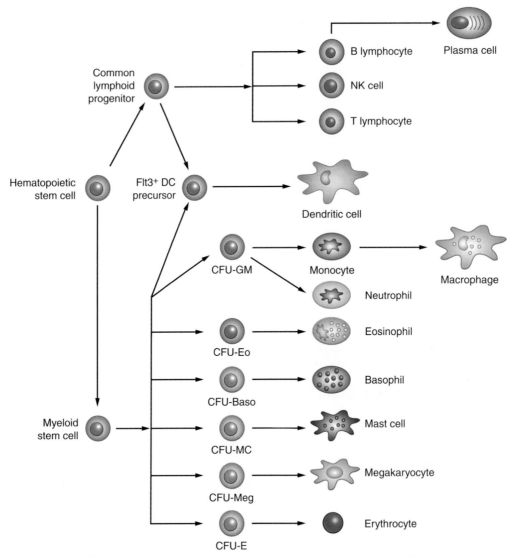

FIGURE 19-7 Differentiation of Hematopoietic Cells. Curved arrows indicate proliferation and expansion of pre-hematopoietic stem cell populations. *EPO,* Erythropoietin; *G-CSF,* granulocyte colony-stimulating factor; *GM-CSF,* granulocyte-macrophage colony-stimulating factor; *IL,* interleukin; *M-CSF,* macrophage colony-stimulating factor; *NK,* natural killer; *SCF,* stem cell factor; *TPO,* thrombopoietin. (Mast cells are discussed in Chapter 5.)

Several cytokines participate in hematopoiesis, particularly **colony-stimulating factors (CSFs or hematopoietic growth factors)**, which stimulate the proliferation of progenitor cells and their progeny and initiate the maturation events necessary to produce fully mature cells. Multiple cell types, including endothelial cells, fibroblasts, and lymphocytes, produce CSFs.

Hematopoiesis in the bone marrow occurs in two separate pools, the stem cell pool and the bone marrow pool, with eventual release of mature cells into the peripheral circulation (Figure 19-8). The stem cell pool contains pluripotent stem cells and partially committed progenitor cells. In addition, there is a bone marrow pool that contains cells that are proliferating and maturing and cells that are stored for later release into the peripheral blood. In the peripheral blood, two pools of cells are also categorized: those circulating and those stored around the walls of the blood vessels (often called the **marginating storage pool**). The marginating storage pool primarily consists of neutrophils that adhere to the endothelium in vessels where the blood flow is relatively slow. These cells can rapidly move into tissues and mucous membranes when needed. Cells from the circulating pool join the marginating pool to replace the cells that have migrated out of the capillaries.

Under certain conditions, the levels of circulating hematologic cells need to be rapidly replenished. Medullary hematopoiesis can be accelerated by any or all of three mechanisms: (1) conversion of yellow bone marrow, which does not produce blood cells, to red marrow, which does, by the actions of **erythropoietin** (a hormone that stimulates erythrocyte production); (2) faster differentiation of daughter cells; and presumably (3) faster proliferation of stem cells.

> ✔ **QUICK CHECK 19-3**
> 1. Why is the stem cell system important to hematopoiesis?
> 2. Why are some stem cells called pluripotent?
> 3. What role do stromal cells play in hematopoiesis?

Development of Erythrocytes

For almost 100 years it was believed that erythrocytes developed in the spleen. It was not until the 1950s that the bone marrow was identified as the site of **erythropoiesis**, or development of red blood cells (Figure 19-9).

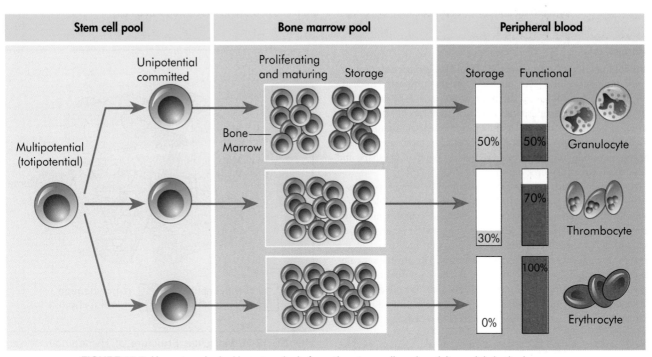

FIGURE 19-8 Hematopoiesis. Hematopoiesis from the stem cell pool; activity mainly in the bone marrow and in the peripheral blood.

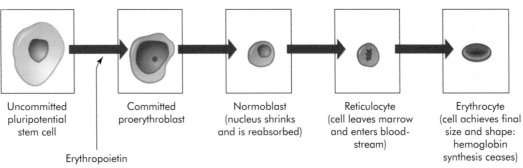

FIGURE 19-9 Erythrocyte Differentiation. Erythrocyte differentiation from large, nucleated stem cell to small, nonnucleated erythrocyte.

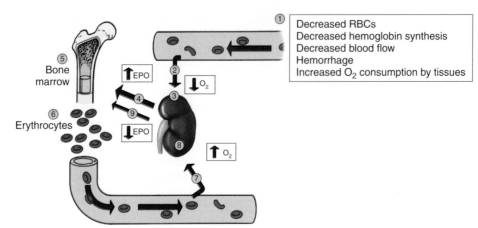

FIGURE 19-10 Role of Erythropoietin in Regulation of Erythropoiesis. *(1)* Decreased arterial oxygen levels result in *(2)* decreased tissue oxygen (hypoxia) that *(3)* stimulates the kidney to increase *(4)* production of erythropoietin. Erythropoietin is carried to the bone marrow *(5)* and binds to erythropoietin receptors on proerythroblasts, resulting in increased red cell production and maturation and expansion of the erythron *(6)*. The increased release of red cells into the circulation frequently corrects the hypoxia in the tissues *(7)*. *(8)* Perception of normal oxygen levels by the kidney causes *(9)* diminished production of erythropoietin (negative feedback) and return to normal levels of erythrocyte production. *EPO,* Erythropoietin; O_2, oxygen in the blood and tissue; *RBCs,* red blood cells.

Erythropoiesis

In the confines of the bone marrow erythroid progenitor cells proliferate and differentiate into large, nucleated **proerythroblasts,** which are committed into producing cells of the erythroid series. The proerythroblast differentiates through several intermediate forms of **erythroblast** (sometimes called **normoblast**) while progressively eliminating most intracellular structures, including the nucleus, synthesizing hemoglobin, and becoming more compact, eventually taking on the shape and characteristics of an erythrocyte.

The last immature form is the **reticulocyte,** which contains a mesh-like (reticular) network of ribosomal RNA that is visible microscopically after staining with certain dyes. Reticulocytes remain in the marrow approximately 1 day and are released into the venous sinuses. They continue to mature in the bloodstream and may travel to the spleen for several days of additional maturation. The normal reticulocyte count is 1% of the total red blood cell count. Approximately 1% of the body's circulating erythrocyte mass normally is generated every 24 hours. Therefore, the reticulocyte count is a useful clinical index of erythropoietic activity and indicates whether new red cells are being produced.

Most steps of this process are primarily under the control of erythropoietin.[14] In healthy humans, the total volume of circulating erythrocytes remains surprisingly constant. In conditions of tissue hypoxia, erythropoietin is secreted by the kidney (Figure 19-10). It causes a compensatory increase in erythrocyte production if the oxygen content of blood decreases because of anemia, high altitude, or pulmonary disease. The normal steady-state rate of production (2.5 million erythrocytes per second) can increase (to 17 million per second) under anemic or low-oxygen states. Thus, the body responds to reduced oxygenation of blood in two ways: (1) by increasing the intake of oxygen through increased respiration and (2) by increasing the oxygen-carrying capacity of the blood through increased erythropoiesis.

Hemoglobin Synthesis

Hemoglobin (Hb), the oxygen-carrying protein of the erythrocyte, constitutes approximately 90% of the cell's dry weight. Hemoglobin-packed blood cells take up oxygen in the lungs and exchange it for

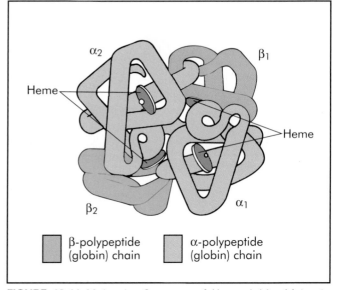

FIGURE 19-11 Molecular Structure of Hemoglobin. Molecule is a spherical tetramer weighing approximately 64,500 daltons. It contains a pair of α-polypeptide chains and a pair of β-polypeptide chains and several heme groups.

carbon dioxide in the tissues. A single erythrocyte can contain as many as 300 hemoglobin molecules. Hemoglobin increases the oxygen-carrying capacity of blood by 100-fold. Each hemoglobin molecule is composed of two pairs of polypeptide chains (the **globins**) and four colorful complexes of iron plus protoporphyrin (the hemes) (Figure 19-11). Hemoglobin is responsible for blood's ruby-red color.[15]

Several variants of hemoglobin exist, but they differ only slightly in primary structure based on the use of different polypeptide chains: alpha, beta, gamma, delta, epsilon, or zeta (α, β, γ, δ, ε, or ζ). Hemoglobin A, the most common type in adults, is composed of two α- and two β-polypeptide chains.

Heme is a large, flat, iron-protoporphyrin disk that can carry one molecule of oxygen (O_2). Thus, an individual hemoglobin molecule with its four hemes can carry four oxygen molecules.[16] If all four oxygen-binding sites are occupied by oxygen, the molecule is said to be saturated. Through a series of complex biochemical reactions, protoporphyrin, a complex four-ringed molecule, is produced and bound with ferrous iron. It is crucial that the iron be correctly charged; reduced ferrous iron (Fe^{2+}) can bind oxygen, whereas ferric iron (Fe^{3+}) cannot. Binding of oxygen to ferrous iron temporarily oxidizes Fe^{2+} to Fe^{3+} (oxyhemoglobin), but after the release of oxygen the body reduces the iron to Fe^{2+} and reactivates the hemoglobin (deoxyhemoglobin [reduced hemoglobin]). Without reactivation, the Fe^{3+}-containing hemoglobin (methemoglobin) cannot bind oxygen. An excess of ferric iron occurs with certain drugs and chemicals, such as nitrates and sulfonamides.

Several other molecules can competitively bind to deoxyhemoglobin. Carbon monoxide (CO) directly competes with oxygen for binding to ferrous ion with an affinity that is about 200-fold greater than that of oxygen. Thus, even a small amount of CO can dramatically decrease the ability of hemoglobin to bind and transport oxygen. Hemoglobin also binds carbon dioxide (CO_2), but at a binding site separate from where oxygen binds. In the lungs, CO_2 is released allowing hemoglobin to bind oxygen.

Erythrocytes may play a role in the maintenance of vascular relaxation. Nitric oxide (NO) produced by blood vessels is a major mediator of relaxation and dilation of the vessel walls.[16] In the lungs, hemoglobin can concurrently bind oxygen to the ferrous ion and NO to cysteine residues in the globins (Figure 19-12). As hemoglobin transfers its oxygen to tissue, it may also shed small amounts of nitric oxide contributing to dilation of the blood vessels and helping get the oxygen into tissues.

Nutritional Requirements for Erythropoiesis

Normal development of erythrocytes and synthesis of hemoglobin depend on an optimal biochemical state and adequate supplies of the necessary building blocks, including protein, vitamins, and minerals (Table 19-4). If these components are lacking for a prolonged time, erythrocyte production slows and anemia (insufficient numbers of functional erythrocytes) may result (see Chapter 20).

Iron cycle. Approximately 67% of total body iron is bound to heme in erythrocytes (hemoglobin) and muscle cells (myoglobin), and approximately 30% is stored in mononuclear phagocytes (i.e., macrophages) and hepatic parenchymal cells as either ferritin or hemosiderin. The remaining 3% (less than 1 mg) is lost daily in urine, sweat,

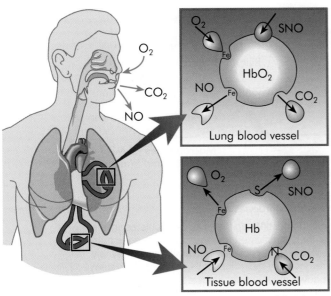

FIGURE 19-12 Hemoglobin (Hb) Binding to Nitric Oxide. In the lungs, hemoglobin (Hb) binds to nitric oxide (NO) as *S*-nitrosothiol (SNO). In tissue, this SNO is released, and free, circulating NO is bound to a different site for exhalation. *Fe,* Iron; *N,* nitrogen.

TABLE 19-4 NUTRITIONAL REQUIREMENTS FOR ERYTHROPOIESIS

NUTRIENT	ROLE IN ERYTHROPOIESIS	CONSEQUENCE OF DEFICIENCY (See Chapter 20)
Protein (amino acids)	Structural component of plasma membrane	Decreased strength, elasticity, and flexibility of membrane; hemolytic anemia
Synthesis of hemoglobin	Decreased erythropoiesis and life span of erythrocytes	
Intrinsic factor	Gastrointestinal absorption of vitamin B_{12}	Pernicious anemia
Cobalamin (vitamin B_{12})	Synthesis of DNA, maturation of erythrocytes, facilitator of folate metabolism	Macrocytic (megaloblastic) anemia
Folate (folic acid)	Synthesis of DNA and RNA, maturation of erythrocytes	Macrocytic (megaloblastic) anemia
Vitamin B_6 (pyridoxine)	Heme synthesis, possibly increases folate metabolism	Hypochromic-microcytic anemia
Vitamin B_2 (riboflavin)	Oxidative reactions	Normochromic-normocytic anemia
Vitamin C (ascorbic acid)	Iron metabolism, acts as reducing agent to maintain iron in its ferrous (Fe^{++}) form	Normochromic-normocytic anemia
Pantothenic acid	Heme synthesis	Unknown in humans*
Niacin	None, but needed for respiration in mature erythrocytes	Unknown in humans
Vitamin E	Synthesis of heme; possible protection against oxidative damage in mature erythrocytes	Hemolytic anemia with increased cell membrane fragility; shortens life span of erythrocytes in individual with cystic fibrosis
Iron	Hemoglobin synthesis	Iron deficiency anemia
Copper	Structural component of plasma membrane	Hypochromic-microcytic anemia

Data from Lee GR et al: *Wintrobe's clinical hematology,* ed 9, Philadelphia, 1993, Lee & Febiger; Harmening DM: *Clinical hematology and fundamentals of hemostasis,* ed 3, Philadelphia, 1997, FA Davis.

DNA, Deoxyribonucleic acid; *RNA,* ribonucleic acid.

*Although pantothenic acid is important for optimal synthesis of heme, experimentally induced deficiency failed to produce anemia or other hematopoietic disturbances.

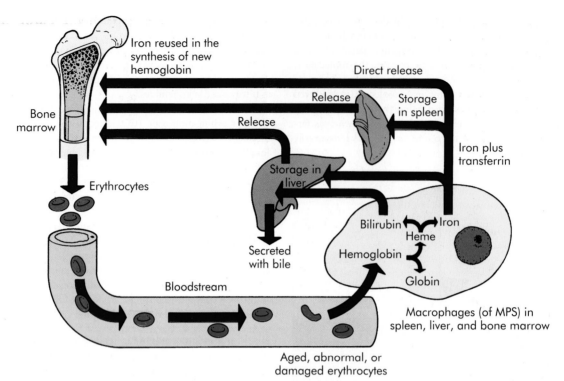

FIGURE 19-13 Iron Cycle. Iron (Fe) released from gastrointestinal epithelial cells circulates in the bloodstream associated with its plasma carrier, transferrin. It is delivered to erythroblasts in bone marrow, where most of it is incorporated into hemoglobin. Mature erythrocytes circulate for approximately 120 days, after which they become senescent and are removed by the mononuclear phagocyte system (MPS). Macrophages of MPS (mostly in spleen) break down ingested erythrocytes and return iron to the bloodstream directly or after storing it as ferritin or hemosiderin.

bile, and epithelial cells shed from the gut. Iron is transported in the blood bound to **transferrin,** a glycoprotein synthesized primarily by the liver but also by tissue macrophages, submaxillary and mammary glands, and ovaries or testes (Figure 19-13).

Iron for hemoglobin production is carried by transferrin to erythroblasts in the bone marrow, where it binds to transferrin receptors on erythroblasts. The iron is transported to the erythroblast's mitochondria (the site of hemoglobin production) and incorporated into protoporphyrin by the action of the enzyme heme synthetase.

Aged or damaged erythrocytes are removed from the bloodstream by macrophages of the MPS—chiefly in the spleen. Within the phagolysosomes (digestive vacuoles) of the macrophage, the erythrocyte is broken down, the hemoglobin molecule catabolized, and the iron stored as ferritin or hemosiderin. The stored iron is released into the bloodstream, where it binds to transferrin (see Figure 19-13).[17]

Iron balance is maintained through controlled absorption rather than excretion. Regulation of iron transport across the plasma membrane of gastrointestinal epithelial cells is related to the cell's iron content and the overall rate of erythropoiesis.[18] If the body's iron stores are low or the demand for erythropoiesis increases, iron is transported rapidly through the epithelial cell and into the plasma. If body stores are high and erythropoiesis is not increased, iron crosses the epithelial cell's plasma membrane passively and is stored as ferritin. Excretion of iron occurs when the epithelial cells of the intestinal mucosa slough off.

Normal Destruction of Senescent Erythrocytes

Although mature erythrocytes lack nuclei, mitochondria, and endoplasmic reticula, they do have cytoplasmic enzymes capable of glycolysis (anaerobic glucose metabolism) and production of small quantities

of adenosine triphosphate (ATP). ATP provides the energy needed to maintain cell function and its plasma membrane pliable (see Figure 1-1). Metabolic processes diminish as the erythrocyte ages, so less ATP is available to maintain plasma membrane function. The aged or senescent red cell becomes increasingly fragile and loses its reversible deformability, becoming susceptible to rupture while passing through narrowed regions of the microcirculation.[19]

Additionally, the plasma membrane of senescent red cells undergoes phospholipid rearrangement that is recognized by receptors on macrophages (primarily in the spleen), which selectively remove and sequester the red cells. If the spleen is dysfunctional or absent, macrophages in the liver (Kupffer cells) take over. During digestion of hemoglobin in the macrophage, porphyrin reduces to bilirubin, which is transported to the liver, conjugated, and finally excreted in the bile as glucuronide (Figure 19-14). Bacteria in the intestinal lumen transform conjugated bilirubin into urobilinogen. Although a small portion is reabsorbed, most urobilinogen is excreted in feces.

Conditions causing accelerated erythrocyte destruction increase the load of bilirubin for hepatic clearance, leading to increased serum levels of unconjugated bilirubin and increased urinary excretion of urobilinogen. Gallstones (cholelithiasis) can result from a chronically elevated rate of bilirubin excretion.

> ✔ **QUICK CHECK 19-4**
> 1. Why is the reticulocyte count important?
> 2. Why is iron important to erythropoiesis?
> 3. What happens to aging erythrocytes?

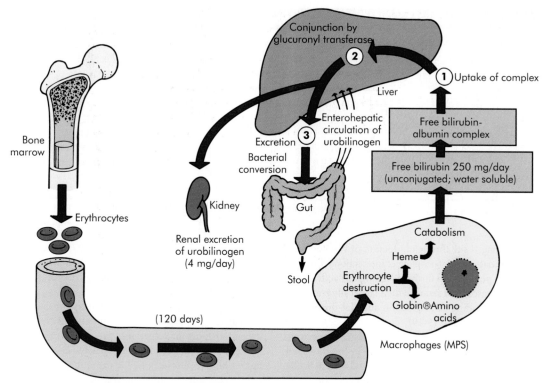

FIGURE 19-14 Metabolism of Bilirubin Released by Heme Breakdown. *MPS,* Mononuclear phagocyte system.

Development of Leukocytes

All leukocytes arise from stem cells in the bone marrow (their pathways of differentiation are shown in Figure 19-7). Lymphoid progenitor cells develop into lymphocytes, which are released into the bloodstream to undergo further maturation in the primary and secondary lymphoid organs (see Chapter 6). Monocyte progenitors develop into monocytic cells, which continue maturing into macrophages after release into the bloodstream and entrance into various tissues.[20] Progenitor cells for granulocytes normally fully mature in the marrow into neutrophils, eosinophils, and basophils and are released into the blood.

The bone marrow selectively retains immature granulocytes as a reserve pool that can be rapidly mobilized in response to the body's needs.[3] Further maturation is under the control of several hematopoietic growth factors, including interleukins, granulocyte-macrophage colony-stimulating factor (GM-CSF), and granulocyte colony-stimulating factor (G-CSF).

Leukocyte production increases in response to infection, to the presence of steroids, and to reduction or depletion of reserves in the marrow. It is also associated with strenuous exercise, convulsive seizures, heat, intense radiation, increased heart rates, pain, nausea and vomiting, and anxiety.

Development of Platelets

Platelets (thrombocytes) are derived from stem cells and progenitor cells that differentiate into megakaryocytes.[6] During thrombopoiesis, the megakaryocyte progenitor is programmed to undergo an endomitotic cell cycle (endomitosis) during which DNA replication occurs, but anaphase and cytokinesis are blocked (see Chapter 1) (see Figures 19-4 and 19-7). Thus, the megakaryocyte nucleus enlarges and becomes extremely polyploidy (up to 100-fold or more of the normal amount of DNA) without cellular division. Concurrently, the numbers of cytoplasmic organelles (e.g., internal membranes, granules) increase, and

the cell develops cellular surface elongations and branches that progressively fragment into platelets. Like erythrocytes, platelets released from the bone marrow lack nuclei.

An optimal number of platelets and committed platelet precursors (megakaryoblasts) in the bone marrow is maintained primarily by thrombopoietin, with other factors such as GM-CSF, produced by the liver and kidney. These factors affect the rate of differentiation into megakaryocytes and the rate of platelet release.[6] About two thirds of platelets enter the circulation, and the remainder resides in the splenic pool. Platelets circulate in the bloodstream for about 10 days before beginning to lose their ability to carry out biochemical reactions. Senescent platelets are sequestered and destroyed in the spleen by mononuclear cell phagocytosis.

MECHANISMS OF HEMOSTASIS

Hemostasis means arrest of bleeding. As a result of hemostasis, damaged blood vessels may maintain a relatively steady state of blood volume, pressure, and flow. Three equally important components of the control of hemostasis are platelets, blood proteins (clotting factors), and the vasculature (endothelial cells and subendothelial matrix) (Figure 19-15). The role of platelets is to (1) contribute to regulation

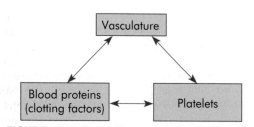

FIGURE 19-15 Three Hemostatic Compartments.

TABLE 19-5 TYPES OF BLEEDING: SOURCES, VESSEL SIZE, AND SEALING REQUIREMENTS			
TYPES AND SOURCES OF BLEEDING	**INVOLVED VESSEL**	**SIZE**	**SEALING REQUIREMENTS**
Pinpoint petechial hemorrhage (blood leakage from small vessels)	Capillary	Smallest	Generally direct-sealing
	Venule		Mostly fused platelets
	Arteriole		Mostly fused platelets
Ecchymosis (large, soft tissue bleeding)	Vein		Vascular contraction, fused platelets, perivascular and intravascular hemostatic factor activation (see Figure 19-16)
Rapidly expanding "blowout" hemorrhage	Artery		Greater vascular contraction, more fused platelets, greater perivascular, and intravascular hemostatic factor activation
		Largest	

Modified from Harmening DM, editor: *Clinical hematology and fundamentals of hemostasis,* ed 3, Philadelphia, 1997, FA Davis.

of blood flow into a damaged site through induction of vasoconstriction (vasospasm), (2) initiate platelet-to-platelet interactions resulting in formation of a platelet plug to stop further bleeding, (3) activate the coagulation (or clotting) cascade to stabilize the platelet plug, and (4) initiate repair processes including clot retraction and clot dissolution (fibrinolysis) (see Figures 19-18 and 19-19).

The relative importance of the hemostatic mechanisms clearly varies with vessel size. Damage to large vessels cannot easily be controlled by hemostasis but requires vascular contraction and dramatically decreased blood flow into the damaged vessels (Table 19-5).

Function of Platelets and Blood Vessels

The normal platelet count ranges from 150,000 to 400,000/mm^3, and a count below 150,000/mm^3 is defined as thrombocytopenia. However, the thrombocytopenia is usually asymptomatic unless the count drops below 100,000/mm^3, at which time abnormal bleeding may occur in response to trauma. Spontaneous major bleeding episodes do not generally occur unless the platelet count falls below 20,000/mm^3.

Platelets normally circulate freely, suspended in plasma, in an unactivated state. The state of platelet activation is primarily under the control of endothelial cells lining the vessels. Endothelial products, such as nitric oxide (NO) and the prostaglandin derivative prostacyclin I$_2$ (PGI$_2$), maintain platelets in an inactive state. When a vessel is damaged, platelet activation may be initiated. Activation proceeds through a process of increasing platelet adhesion, aggregation, and activation.[21] Initially, platelets adhere weakly to the vessel wall, followed by increased strength of adherence to the vessels, adherence between platelets (aggregation), and finally the development of an immobilizing meshwork of platelets and fibrin (Figure 19-16) (see *Health Alert:* Sticky Platelets, Genetic Variations, and Cardiovascular Complications).

This process can begin in several ways. If the vessel lining remains intact in an area of inflammation, the endothelial cells may become activated and begin expressing new proteins on their surface. Several of these, particularly P-selectin, bind specifically yet weakly with receptors on the surface of inactive platelets (e.g., GPIb) (Figure 19-17). As inflammation progresses, the platelets adhere more avidly through additional receptors that bind through a fibrinogen bridge with the endothelial cell surface.[22] The principal fibrinogen receptor is the integrin α$_{IIb}$β$_3$ (also known as GPIIb/IIIa).

During vessel damage, the endothelial layer is frequently compromised resulting in exposure of the underlying matrix that contains collagen and other components including fibronectin. The matrix also contains von Willebrand factor (vWF), and the exposed collagen can bind additional vWF from the circulation (see Figure 19-17). Platelets adhere strongly to collagen through the receptor GPVI and to vWF

through the receptor complex GPIb/IX/V. Progressively the platelets undergo further aggregation through platelet-to-platelet adhesion involving further fibrinogen bridging between receptors (particularly GPIIb/IIIa) on adjacent platelets.

As a result of interactions with the endothelium or the subendothelial matrix, as well as exposure to inflammatory mediators produced by the endothelium and other cells, the platelets are activated.[23] Activation results in dynamic changes in platelet shape from smooth spheres to those with spiny projections and degranulation (also called the platelet-release reaction) resulting in the release of various potent biochemicals.

HEALTH ALERT

Sticky Platelets, Genetic Variations, and Cardiovascular Complications

Investigators report that a genetic trait induces some people to make sticky platelets. People with platelets that tend to stick together have an increased risk of suffering complications from heart procedures. After individuals received angioplasty, in which a balloon-tipped catheter opens a blocked artery, investigators compared complications in the group with more sticky, or reactive, platelets with those with less reactive platelets. Of 112 participants, 3 months after the procedure, 15 individuals with sticky platelets experienced chest pain or a heart attack; 4 individuals with less reactive platelets experienced such complications. In addition, 10 people with sticky platelets needed another angioplasty, compared with only 2 from the less reactive platelet group.

In another study, investigators analyzed the receptor glycoprotein GP11b/111a for weaknesses that might direct attempts to prevent clotting, heart attack, and stroke. Blood samples from 1340 people revealed that 72% had inherited from both parents a gene for a version of GP11b/111a called *P1*[A1], whereas 28% had inherited 1 or 2 copies of a gene encoding a version called *P1*[A2]. The blood from the group with two copies of *P1*[A1] clotted less readily than did the blood of the other group. The degree of clotting also depended on fibrinogen levels in the blood. In individuals with unusually high fibrinogen levels, the presence of *P1*[A1] glycoprotein seemed to increase clotting more than did *P1*[A2]. Thus, testing for platelet stickiness and GP11b/111a status could determine which people need anticlotting drugs and for how long.

Data from Furlan M: Sticky and promiscuous plasma proteins maintain the equilibrium between bleeding and thrombosis, *Swiss Med Wkly* 132(15–16):181–189, 2002; Lohse J et al: Platelet function in obese children and adolescents, *Hamostaseologie* 30(suppl 1):S126–S132, 2010; Mammen EF: Sticky platelet syndrome, *Semin Thromb Hemost* 25(4):361–365, 1999.

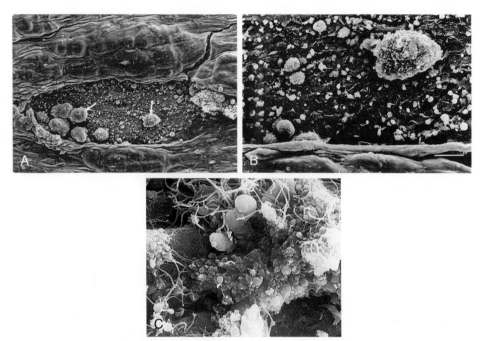

FIGURE 19-16 Platelet Activation. A, After endothelial denudation, platelets and leukocytes adhere to the subendothelium in a monolayer fashion. **B,** Higher-power view showing leukocytes and platelets adherent to the subendothelium. **C,** High magnification of a thrombus showing a mixture of red cells and platelets incorporated into the fibrin meshwork. (**A** and **B** from Libby P et al: *Braunwald's heart disease: a textbook of cardiovascular medicine,* ed 8, Philadelphia, 2007, Saunders; as reproduced from Faggiotto A, Ross R: Studies of hypercholesterolemia in the nonhuman primate. II. Fatty streak conversion to fibrous plaque, *Arteriosclerosis* 4(4):341–356, 1984; **C** from Damjanov I, Linder J, editors: *Anderson's pathology,* ed 10, St Louis, 1996, Mosby.)

Platelets contain three types of granules: lysosomes, dense bodies, and alpha granules. The contents of the dense bodies and alpha granules are particularly important in hemostasis. The dense bodies contain ADP, serotonin, and calcium. ADP reacts with specific receptors on platelets to induce further adherence and subsequent degranulation of nearby platelets and causing their plasma membranes to become ruffled and sticky. The activated platelets cause a platelet plug to seal the injured endothelium. Serotonin is a vasoactive amine that functions like histamine and has immediate effects on smooth muscle in the vascular endothelium, causing an immediate temporary constriction of the injured vessel (see Chapter 5). Vasoconstriction reduces blood flow and diminishes bleeding. Vasodilation soon follows, permitting the inflammatory response to proceed (see Figures 22-24 and 22-25). Calcium is necessary for many of the intracellular signaling mechanisms that control platelet activation.

Alpha granules contain a large number of clotting factors (e.g., fibrinogen, factor V), growth factors (e.g., platelet-derived growth factor), and heparin-binding proteins (e.g., platelet factor 4). Many of these mediators either promote or inhibit platelet activity and the eventual process of clot formation (see Figure 19-17). Platelet-derived growth factor stimulates smooth muscle cells and promotes tissue repair. Heparin-binding proteins enhance clot formation at the site of injury.

Platelets also begin producing the prostaglandin derivative **thromboxane A$_2$ (TXA$_2$)**, which counters the effects of prostacyclin I$_2$ (PGI$_2$), produced by endothelial cells (see Figure 19-17). TXA$_2$ causes vasoconstriction and promotes the degranulation of platelets, whereas PGI$_2$ promotes vasodilation and inhibiting platelet degranulation. In platelets, an isoform of **cyclooxygenase (COX-1)** converts arachidonic acid to TXA$_2$. Aspirin, particularly at low doses, specifically and irreversibly inhibits COX-1, decreasing production of TXA$_2$ and decreasing platelet activation.

If blood vessel injury is minor, hemostasis is achieved temporarily by formation of the platelet plug, which usually forms within 3 to 5 minutes of injury. Platelet plugs seal the many minute ruptures that occur daily in the microcirculation, particularly in capillaries. With too few platelets, numerous small hemorrhagic areas called *purpuras* develop under the skin and throughout the tissues (see Chapter 20).

Function of Clotting Factors

A **blood clot** is a meshwork of protein strands that stabilizes the platelet plug and traps other cells, such as erythrocytes, phagocytes, and microorganisms (Figure 19-18). The strands are made of fibrin, which is produced by the **clotting (coagulation) system.** The clotting system was described in Chapter 5 and consists of a family of proteins that circulate in the blood in inactive forms. Initiation of the system results in sequential activation (cascade) of multiple members of the system until a fibrin clot is created. As was described for the clotting, complement, and kinin systems (see Chapter 5), each is usually diagrammed with multiple pathways of activation that unite in a common pathway. This organization is purely for convenience, and many members of each pathway may be activated by several alternative means and members of one system frequently activate members of another (e.g., activated members of the complement system can activate members of the clotting system).

The clotting system is usually presented as two pathways of initiation (intrinsic and extrinsic pathways) that join in a common pathway.

I. Subendothelial exposure

- Occurs after endothelial sloughing
- Platelets begin to fill endothelial gaps
- Promoted by thromboxane A_2 (TXA_2)
- Inhibited by prostacyclin I_2 (PGI_2)
- Platelet function depends on many factors, especially calcium

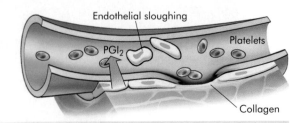

II. Adhesion

- Adhesion is initiated by loss of endothelial cells (or rupture or erosion of atherosclerotic plaque), which exposes adhesive glycoproteins such as collagen and von Willebrand factor (vWF) in the subendothelium. vWF and, perhaps, other adhesive glycoproteins in the plasma deposit on the damaged area. Platelets adhere to the subendothelium through receptors that bind to the adhesive glycoproteins (GPIb, GPIa/IIa, GPIIb/IIIa).

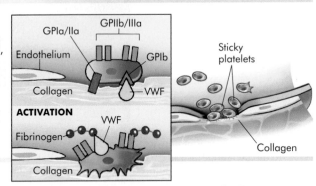

III. Activation

- After platelets adhere they undergo an activation process that leads to a conformational change in GPIIb/IIIa receptors, resulting in their ability to bind adhesive proteins, including fibrinogen and von Willebrand factor
- Changes in platelet shape
- Formation of pseudopods
- Activation of arachidonic pathway

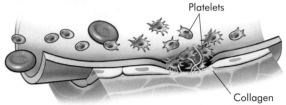

IV. Aggregation

- Induced by release of TXA_2
- Adhesive glycoproteins bind simultaneously to GPIIb/IIIa on two different platelets
- Stabilization of the platelet plug (blood clot) occurs by activation of coagulation factors, thrombin, and fibrin
- Heparin neutralizing factor enhances clot formation

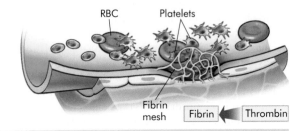

V. Platelet plug formation

- RBCs and platelets enmeshed in fibrin

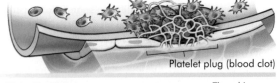

VI. Clot retraction and clot dissolution

- Clot retraction, using large number of platelets, joins the edges of the injured vessel
- Clot dissolution is regulated by thrombin and plasminogen activators

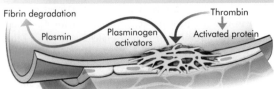

FIGURE 19-17 Blood Vessel Damage, Blood Clot, and Clot Dissolution.

The intrinsic pathway is activated when Hageman factor (factor XII) in plasma contacts negatively charged subendothelial substances exposed by vascular injury. The extrinsic pathway is activated when tissue thromboplastin, a substance released by damaged endothelial cells, reacts with clotting factors, particularly factor VII. Both pathways lead to the common pathway and activation of factor X (Stuart-Prower factor), which proceeds to clot formation. As with complement and kinin systems, the clotting system is complex with a large number of alternative activators and inhibitors. Also, there is interaction between the pathways so that an activated member of one pathway may activate a member of the other pathway.

Activated platelets are important participants in clotting. During activation, phospholipids in the platelet plasma membrane undergo redistribution so that a particular phospholipid, phosphatidyl serine (PS), is greatly enriched on the platelet surface. PS provides a matrix for formation of several important complexes of clotting factors, including the tenase complex (factor X and activated factors VIII and IX) that activates factor X and the prothrombinase complex (prothrombin and activated factors X and V) that activated prothrombin into thrombin. Thrombin then converts fibrinogen into fibrin, which polymerizes into a fibrin clot (e.g., factor VIIa of the extrinsic pathway can directly activate factor IX of the intrinsic pathway).

A variety of substances, some of which are products of the coagulation system itself, control coagulation. For example, excess thrombin is inactivated by antithrombin III. Other anticoagulants, most notably heparin, are produced and secreted locally by tissue mast cells and basophils activated by the injury (see Chapter 5).

Retraction and Lysis of Blood Clots

After a clot is formed, it retracts, or "solidifies." Fibrin strands shorten, becoming denser and stronger, which approximates the edges of the injured vessel wall and seals the site of injury. Retraction is facilitated by the large numbers of platelets trapped within the fibrin meshwork. The platelets contract and "pull" the fibrin threads closer together while releasing a factor that stabilizes the fibrin. Contraction expels protein-free serum from the fibrin meshwork (see Figure 19-18). This process usually begins within a few minutes after a clot has formed, and most of the serum is expelled within 20 to 60 minutes.

Lysis (breakdown) of blood clots is carried out by the fibrinolytic system (Figure 19-19). Another plasma protein, plasminogen, is converted to plasmin by several products of coagulation and inflammation (e.g., activated factor XII, thrombin, lysosomal enzymes). Plasmin is an enzyme that dissolves clots (fibrinolysis) by degrading fibrin and fibrinogen into fibrin degradation products (FDPs).[24] The fibrinolytic system removes clotted blood from tissues and dissolves small clots (thrombi) in blood vessels. A balance between the amounts of thrombin and plasmin in the circulation maintains normal coagulation and lysis.

Blood tests for evaluating the hematologic system are listed in Table 19-6.

✔ **QUICK CHECK 19-5**
1. Why are platelets necessary to stop bleeding?
2. Briefly describe the steps of platelet adhesion and aggregation.
3. How does plasminogen initiate fibrinolysis?

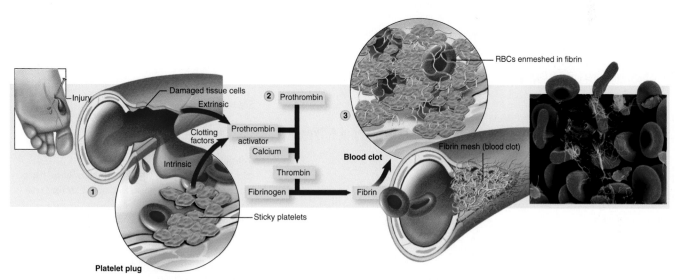

FIGURE 19-18 Blood Clotting Mechanism. A, The complex clotting mechanism can be distilled into three basic steps: *(1)* release of clotting factors from both injured tissue cells and sticky platelets at the injury site (which form temporary platelet plug), *(2)* series of chemical reactions that eventually result in the formation of thrombin, and *(3)* formation of fibrin and trapping of blood cells to form a clot. **B,** An electron micrograph showing entrapped RBCs in a fibrin clot. (**A** from Patton KT, Thibodeau GA: *Anatomy & physiology,* ed 7, St Louis, 2010, Mosby; **B** copyright Dennis Kunkel Microscopy, Inc.)

TABLE 19-6 COMMON BLOOD TESTS FOR HEMATOLOGIC DISORDERS

CELL TYPE AND TEST	PROPERTY EVALUATED BY TEST	POSSIBLE HEMATOLOGIC CAUSE OF ABNORMAL FINDINGS
Erythrocyte		
Red cell count	Number (in millions) of erythrocytes/μl of blood	Altered erythropoiesis, anemias, hemorrhage, Hodgkin disease, leukemia
Mean corpuscle volume (MCV)	Size of erythrocytes	Anemias, thalassemias
Mean corpuscle hemoglobin (MCH)	Amount of hemoglobin in each erythrocyte (by weight)	Anemias, hemoglobinopathy
Mean corpuscular hemoglobin concentration (MCHC)	Concentration of hemoglobin in each erythrocyte (percentage of erythrocyte occupied by hemoglobin)	Anemias, hereditary spherocytosis
Hemoglobin determination	Amount of hemoglobin (by weight)/dl of blood	Anemias
Hematocrit determination	Percentage of a given volume of blood that is occupied by erythrocytes	Hemorrhage, polycythemia, erythrocytosis, anemias, leukemia
Reticulocyte count	Number of reticulocytes/μl of blood (also expressed as percentage of reticulocytes in total red blood cell count)	Hyperactive or hypoactive bone marrow function
Erythrocyte osmotic fragility test	Cellular shape (biconcavity), structure of plasma membrane	Anemias, hemolytic disease caused by ABO or Rh incompatibility, Hodgkin disease, polycythemia vera, thalassemia major
Hemoglobin electrophoresis	Relative percentage of different types of hemoglobin in erythrocytes	Sickle cell disease, sickle cell trait, hemoglobin C disease, hemoglobin C trait, thalassemias
Sickle cell test	Presence of hemoglobin S in erythrocytes	Sickle cell trait, sickle cell anemia
Glucose-6-phosphate dehydrogenase (G6PD) deficiency test	Deficiency of G6PD in erythrocytes	Hemolytic anemia
Hemoglobin Metabolism		
Serum ferritin determination	Depletion of body iron (potential deficiency of heme synthesis)	Iron deficiency anemias
Total iron-building capacity (TIBC)	Amount of iron in serum plus amount of transferrin available in serum (μγ/δγ)	Hemorrhage, iron deficiency anemia, hemochromatosis, hemosiderosis, iron overload, anemias, thalassemia
Transferrin saturation	Percentage of transferrin that is saturated with iron	Acute hemorrhage, hemochromatosis, hemosiderosis, sideroblastic anemia, iron deficiency anemia, iron overload, thalassemia
Porphyrin analysis (protoporphyrin analysis)	Concentration of protoporphyrin in erythrocytes (mcg/dl), an indicator of iron-deficient erythropoiesis	Megaloblastic anemia, congenital erythropoietic porphyria
Direct antiglobulin test (DAT)	Antibody binding to erythrocytes	Hemolytic disease of newborn, autoimmune hemolytic anemia, drug-induced hemolytic anemia, transfusion reaction
Antibody screen test (indirect Coombs test)	Detection of antibodies to erythrocyte antigens (other than ABO antigens) See below	Same as for DAT See below
Leukocytes: Differential White Cell Count (Absolute Number of A Type of Leukocyte/μl of Blood		
Neutrophil count	Neutrophils/μl	Myeloproliferative disorders, hematopoietic disorders, hemolysis, infection
Lymphocyte count	Lymphocytes/μl	Infectious lymphocytosis, infectious mononucleosis, hematopoietic disorders, anemias, leukemia, lymphosarcoma, Hodgkin disease
Plasma cell count	Plasma cells/μl	Infectious mononucleosis, lymphocytosis, plasma cell leukemia
Monocyte count	Monocytes/μl	Hodgkin disease, infectious mononucleosis, monocytic leukemia, non-Hodgkin lymphoma, polycythemia vera
Eosinophil count	Eosinophils/μl	Hematopoietic disorders
Basophil count	Basophils/μl	Chronic myelogenous leukemia, hemolytic anemias, Hodgkin disease, polycythemia vera

TABLE 19-6   COMMON BLOOD TESTS FOR HEMATOLOGIC DISORDERS—cont'd

CELL TYPE AND TEST	PROPERTY EVALUATED BY TEST	POSSIBLE HEMATOLOGIC CAUSE OF ABNORMAL FINDINGS
Platelets and Clotting Factors		
Platelet count	Number of circulating platelets (in thousands)/μl of blood	Anemias, multiple myeloma, myelofibrosis, polycythemia vera, leukemia, disseminated intravascular coagulation (DIC), hemolytic disease of the newborn, transfusion reaction, lymphoproliferative disorders
Bleeding time	Duration of bleeding following a standardized superficial puncture wound of skin, integrity of platelet plug, measured in minutes following puncture	Leukemia, anemias, DIC, fibrinolytic activity, purpuras, hemorrhagic disease of the newborn, infectious mononucleosis, multiple myeloma, clotting factor deficiencies, thrombasthenia, thrombocytopenia, von Willebrand disease
Clot retraction test	Platelet number and function, fibrinogen quantity and use, measured in hours required for expression of serum from a clot incubated in a test tube	Acute leukemia, aplastic anemia, factor XIII deficiency, increased fibrinolytic activity, Hodgkin disease, hyperfibrinogenemia or hypofibrinogenemia, idiopathic thrombocytopenic purpura, multiple myeloma, polycythemia vera, secondary thrombocytopenia, thrombasthenia
Platelet adhesion studies	Ability of platelets to adhere to foreign surfaces	Anemia, macroglobulinemia, Bernard-Soulier syndrome, multiple myeloma, myeloid metaplasia, plasma cell dyscrasias, thrombasthenia, thrombocytopathy, von Willebrand disease
Platelet aggregation tests	Ability of platelets to adhere to one another	Afibrinogenemia, Bernard-Soulier syndrome, thrombasthenia, hemorrhagic thrombocythemia, myeloid metaplasia, plasma cell dyscrasias, platelet release defects, polycythemia vera, preleukemia, sideroblastic anemia, von Willebrand disease, Waldenström macroglobulinemia, hypercoagulability
Whole blood clotting time (Lee-White coagulation time)	Overall ability of blood to clot, as measured in minutes in a test tube	Afibrinogenemia, clotting factor deficiencies, excessive fibrinolysis, hemorrhagic disease of the newborn, hypofibrinogenemia, hypoprothrombinemia, leukemia
Circulating anticoagulants (immunoglobulin G [IgG] antibodies that inhibit coagulation)	Presence of antibodies that neutralize clotting factors and inhibit coagulation, as indicated by prolonged clotting time, prothrombin time, or partial thromboplastin time	Afibrinogenemia, presence of fibrin-fibrinogen degradation products, macroglobulinemia, multiple myeloma, DIC, plasma cell dyscrasias
Partial thromboplastin time (PTT)	Effectiveness of clotting factors (except factors VII and VIII), effectiveness of intrinsic pathway of coagulation cascade, as measured by a test tube (in seconds)	Presence of circulating anticoagulants, DIC, clotting factor deficiencies, excessive fibrinolysis, hemorrhagic disease of the newborn, hypofibrinogenemia and afibrinogenemia, prothrombin deficiency, von Willebrand disease, acute hemorrhage
Prothrombin time	Effectiveness of activity of prothrombin, fibrinogen, and factors V, VII, and X; effectiveness of vitamin K–dependent coagulation factors of extrinsic and common pathways of coagulation cascade as measured in a test tube (in seconds)	Hypofibrinogenemia, dysfibrinogenemia, and afibrinogenemia; presence of circulating anticoagulants; DIC; deficiency of factors V, VII, or X; presence of fibrin degradation products, increased fibrinolytic activity, hemolytic jaundice, hemorrhagic disease of the newborn; acute leukemia, polycythemia vera, prothrombin deficiency, multiple myeloma
Thrombin time	Quantity and activity of fibrinogen as measured in a test tube (in seconds)	Hypofibrinogenemia, dysfibrinogenemia, and afibrinogenemia; presence of circulating anticoagulants; hemorrhagic disease of the newborn, polycythemia vera; increase in fibrinogen-fibrin degradation products; increased fibrinolytic activity
Fibrinogen assay	Amount of fibrinogen available for fibrin formation	Acute leukemia, congenital hypofibrinogenemia or afibrinogenemia, DIC, increased fibrinolytic activity, severe hemorrhage
Fibrin-fibrinogen degradation products (fibrin-fibrinogen split products)	Fibrinogenic activity as measured by levels of fibrin-fibrinogen degradation products (in μl/ml of blood)	Transfusion reactions, DIC, internal hemorrhage in the newborn, deep vein thrombosis, pulmonary embolism

Data from Bick RL et al: *Hematology: clinical and laboratory practice*, St Louis, 1993, Mosby; Byrne CJ et al: *Laboratory tests: implications for nursing care*, Menlo Park, Calif, 1986, Addison-Wesley.

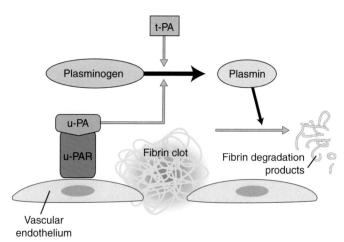

FIGURE 19-19 The Fibrinolytic System. Fibrinolysis is initiated by the binding of plasminogen to fibrin. Although tissue plasminogen activator *(t-PA)* initiates intravascular fibrinolysis, urokinase plasminogen activator *(u-PA)* is the major activator of fibrinolysis in tissue (extravascular). Plasmin digests the fibrin into smaller soluble pieces (fibrin degradation products). *u-PAR,* Urokinase-like plasminogen activator receptor.

PEDIATRICS & HEMATOLOGIC VALUE CHANGES

Blood cell counts tend to rise above adult levels at birth and then decline gradually throughout childhood. Table 19-7 lists normal ranges during infancy and childhood. The immediate rise in values is the result of accelerated hematopoiesis during fetal life and the increased numbers of cells that result from the trauma of birth and cutting of the umbilical cord.

Average blood volume in the full-term neonate is 85 ml/kg of body weight. The premature infant has a slightly larger blood volume of 90 ml/kg of body weight, with the mean increasing to 150 ml/kg during the first few days after birth. In both full-term and premature infants, blood volume decreases during the first few months. Thereafter the average blood volume is 75 to 77 ml/kg, which is similar to that of older children and adults.

The hypoxic intrauterine environment stimulates erythropoietin production in the fetus and accelerates fetal erythropoiesis, producing polycythemia (excessive proliferation of erythrocyte precursors) in the newborn. After birth, the oxygen from the lungs saturates arterial blood, and more oxygen is delivered to the tissues. In response to the change from a placental to a pulmonary oxygen supply during the first few days of life, levels of erythropoietin and the rate of blood cell formation decrease. The active rate of fetal erythropoiesis is reflected by the large numbers of immature erythrocytes (reticulocytes) in the peripheral blood of full-term neonates. After birth, the number of reticulocytes decreases about 50% every 12 hours, so it is rare to find an elevated reticulocyte count after the first week of life. During this period of rapid growth, the rate of erythrocyte destruction is greater than that in later childhood and adulthood. In full-term infants, the normal erythrocyte life span is 60 to 80 days; in premature infants, it may be as short as 20 to 30 days; and in children and adolescents, it is the same as that in adults—120 days.

The postnatal fall in hemoglobin and hematocrit values is more marked in premature infants than it is in full-term infants. In preschool and school-aged children, hemoglobin, hematocrit, and red blood cell counts gradually rise. Metabolic processes within the erythrocytes of neonates differ significantly from those found in erythrocytes of normal adults. The relatively young population of erythrocytes in newborns consumes greater quantities of glucose than do erythrocytes in adults.

The lymphocytes of children tend to have more cytoplasm and less compact nuclear chromatin than do the lymphocytes of adults. A possible explanation is that children tend to have more frequent viral infections, which are associated with atypical lymphocytes. Minor infections, in which the child fails to exhibit clinical manifestations of illness, and the administration of immunizations also may account for the lymphocyte changes.

At birth the lymphocyte count is high, and it continues to rise during the first year of life. Then it steadily declines until the lower value seen in adults is reached. It is unknown whether these developmental variations are physiologic or a pathologic response to frequent viral infection and immunizations in children.

The neutrophil count, like the lymphocyte count, is high at birth and rises during the first days of life. After 2 weeks, the neutrophil count falls to within or below the normal adult range. By approximately 4 years of age, the neutrophil count is the same as that of an adult.

The eosinophil count is high in the first year of life and higher in children than in teenagers or adults. Monocyte counts too are high in the first year of life but then decrease to adult levels. Platelet counts in full-term neonates are comparable with platelet counts in adults and remain so throughout infancy and childhood.

AGING & HEMATOLOGIC VALUE CHANGES

Blood composition changes little with age. The erythrocyte life span in elderly persons is normal, although the erythrocytes are replenished more slowly after bleeding, probably because of iron depletion. Total serum iron, total iron-binding capacity, and intestinal iron absorption are all decreased somewhat in elderly persons. Iron deficiency is often responsible for the low hemoglobin levels noted in elderly persons. The plasma membranes of erythrocytes become increasingly fragile, with portions being lost, presumably because of physical trauma inflicted during circulation.

Lymphocyte function decreases with age (see Chapters 6 and 7), causing changes in cellular immunity and some decline in T cell function. The humoral immune system is less able to respond to antigenic challenge.

No changes in platelet numbers or structure have been observed in elderly persons, yet evidence shows that platelet adhesiveness probably increases. Although fibrinogen levels and factors V, VII, and IX tend to be increased in elderly people, evidence concerning hypercoagulability is inconclusive.

TABLE 19-7   HEMATOLOGIC VALUES FROM BIRTH TO ADULTHOOD

AGE	HEMOGLOBIN (g/dl): MEAN	HEMATOCRIT (%): MEAN	RETICULOCYTES (%): MEAN	LEUKOCYTES (WBC/mm³): MEAN	DIFFERENTIAL COUNTS				
					NEUTROPHILS (%): MEAN	LYMPHOCYTES (%): MEAN	EOSINOPHILS (%): MEAN	MONOCYTES (%): MEAN	PLATELETS (10³/mm³): MEAN
Newborn (cord blood)	16.8	55	5.0	18,000	61	31	2	6	290
2 wk	16.5	50	1.0	12,000	40	48	3	9	252
3 months	12.0	36	1.0	12,000	30	63	2	5	140-340
6 months to 6 yr	12.0	37	1.0	10,000	45	48	2	5	140-340
7-12 yr	13.0	38	1.0	8,000	55	38	2	5	140-340
Adult	13.0	40	1.0	8,000	55	35	2	5	140-340
Female	14	41	0.8-4.1	7,400	54-62	25-33	1-4	3-7	140-340
Male	16	47	0.8-2.5	7,400	54-62	25-33	1-4	3-7	140-340

DID YOU UNDERSTAND?

Components of the Hematologic System

1. Blood consists of a variety of components: about 92% water and 8% solutes. In adults, the total blood volume is approximately 5.5 L.
2. Plasma, a complex aqueous liquid, contains two major groups of plasma proteins: (a) albumins and (b) globulins.
3. The cellular elements of blood are the red blood cells (erythrocytes), white blood cells (leukocytes), and platelets.
4. Erythrocytes are the most abundant cells of the blood, occupying approximately 48% of the blood volume in men and approximately 42% in women. Erythrocytes are responsible for tissue oxygenation.
5. Leukocytes are fewer in number than erythrocytes and constitute approximately 5000 to 10,000 cells/mm^3 of blood. Leukocytes defend the body against infection and remove dead or injured host cells.
6. Leukocytes are classified as either granulocytes (neutrophils, basophils, eosinophils) or agranulocytes (monocytes/macrophages, lymphocytes).
7. Platelets are not cells but disk-shaped cytoplasmic fragments. Platelets are essential for blood coagulation and control of bleeding.
8. The lymphoid organs are sites of residence, proliferation, differentiation, or function of lymphocytes and mononuclear phagocytes.
9. The spleen is the largest lymphoid organ and functions as the site of fetal hematopoiesis, filters and cleanses the blood, and acts as a reservoir for lymphocytes and other blood cells.
10. The lymph nodes are the site of development or activity of large numbers of lymphocytes, monocytes, and macrophages.
11. The mononuclear phagocyte system (MPS) is composed of monocytes in bone marrow and peripheral blood and macrophages in tissue.
12. The MPS is the main line of defense against bacteria in the bloodstream and cleanses the blood by removing old, injured, or dead blood cells; antigen-antibody complexes; and macromolecules.

Development of Blood Cells

1. Hematopoiesis, or blood cell production, occurs in the liver and spleen of the fetus and in the bone marrow after birth.
2. Hematopoiesis involves two stages: (a) proliferation and (b) differentiation, or maturation. Each type of blood cell has parent cells called *stem cells*.
3. Hematopoiesis continues throughout life to replace blood cells that grow old and die, are killed by disease, or are lost through bleeding.
4. Bone marrow consists of blood vessels, nerves, mononuclear phagocytes, stem cells, blood cells in various stages of differentiation, and fatty tissue.
5. Hemoglobin, the oxygen-carrying protein of the erythrocyte, enables the blood to transport 100 times more oxygen than could be transported dissolved in plasma alone.

6. Erythropoiesis depends on the presence of vitamins (especially vitamin B$_{12}$, folate vitamin, vitamin B$_6$, riboflavin, pantothenic acid, niacin, ascorbic acid, and vitamin E).
7. Regulation of erythropoiesis is mediated by erythropoietin. Erythropoietin is secreted by the kidneys in response to tissue hypoxia and causes a compensatory increase in erythrocyte production if the oxygen content of the blood decreases because of anemia, high altitude, or pulmonary disease.
8. Maintenance of optimal levels of granulocytes and monocytes in the blood depends on the availability of pluripotential stem cells in the marrow, induction of these into committed stem cells, and timely release of new cells from the marrow.
9. Specific humoral colony-stimulating factors (CSFs) are necessary for the adequate growth of myeloid, erythroid, lymphoid, and megakaryocytic lineages.
10. Platelets develop from megakaryocytes by a process called *endomitosis*. In endomitosis, the megakaryocytes undergo DNA replication but not cell division; thus, the cell does not divide into two daughter cells.

Mechanisms of Hemostasis

1. Hemostasis, or arrest of bleeding, involves (a) vasoconstriction (vasospasm), (b) formation of a platelet plug, (c) activation of the clotting cascade, (d) formation of a blood clot, and (e) clot retraction and clot dissolution.
2. The normal vascular endothelium prevents clotting by producing factors such as nitric oxide (NO) and prostacyclin I$_2$ (PGI$_2$) that relax the vessels and prevent platelet activation.
3. Lysis of blood clots is the function of the fibrinolytic system. Plasmin, a proteolytic enzyme, splits fibrin and fibrinogen into fibrin degradation products that dissolve the clot.

Pediatrics & Hematologic Value Changes

1. Blood cell counts tend to rise above adult levels at birth and then decline gradually throughout childhood.
2. The lymphocytes of children tend to have more cytoplasm and less compact nuclear chromatin than do the lymphocytes of adults.

Aging & Hematologic Value Changes

1. Blood composition changes little with age. Erythrocyte replenishment may be delayed after bleeding, presumably because of iron deficiency.
2. Lymphocyte function appears to decrease with age. Particularly affected is a decrease in cellular immunity.
3. Platelet adhesiveness probably increases with age.

KEY TERMS

- Agranulocyte 480
- Albumin 478
- Basophil 480
- Blood clot 491
- Bone marrow (myeloid tissue) 483
- Clotting (coagulation) system 491
- Clotting factor 480
- Collagen 490
- Colony-stimulating factor (CSF, hematopoietic growth factor) 485
- Cyclooxygenase (COX-1) 491
- Deoxyhemoglobin 487
- Endomitosis 489
- Eosinophil 480
- Erythroblast (normoblast) 486
- Erythrocyte (red blood cell) 480
- Erythropoiesis 485
- Erythropoietin 485
- Fibrin degradation product (FDP) 493
- Fibrinolysis 490
- Fibrinolytic system 493
- Globin 486
- Globulin 478
- Granulocyte 480
- Hematopoiesis 483
- Hematopoietic stem cell 483
- Heme 487
- Hemoglobin (Hb) 486
- Hemostasis 489
- Immunocyte 480
- Integrin $\alpha_{IIb}\beta_3$ (GPIIb/IIIa) 490
- Leukocyte (white blood cell) 480
- Lipoprotein 480
- Lymph node 482
- Lymphocyte 481
- Macrophage 481
- Marginating storage pool 485
- Methemoglobin 487
- Monocyte 481
- Mononuclear phagocyte system (MPS) 483
- Myoglobin 487
- Natural killer (NK) cells 481
- Neutrophil (polymorphonuclear neutrophil [PMN]) 480
- Nitric oxide (NO) 490
- Oxyhemoglobin 487
- Phagocyte 480
- Plasma 477
- Plasma protein 477
- Plasmin 493
- Platelet (thrombocyte) 481
- Platelet-release reaction 490
- Proerythroblast 486
- Prostacyclin I_2 (PGI$_2$) 490
- Protoporphyrin 487
- Reticulocyte 486
- Serum 477
- Spleen 482
- Stromal cell 484
- Stromal stem cell 484
- Thrombopoietin (TPO) 481
- Thromboxane A_2 (TXA$_2$) 491
- Tissue thromboplastin 493
- Transferrin 488
- von Willebrand factor (vWF) 490

REFERENCES

1. Chuang VT, Otagiri M: Recombinant human serum albumin, *Drugs Today (Barc)* 43(8):547–561, 2007.
2. Mohandas N, Gallagher PG: Red cell membrane: past, present, and future, *Blood* 112(10):3939–3948, 2008.
3. Borregaard N: Neutrophils, from marrow to microbes, *Immunity* 33(5):657–670, 2010.
4. Bochner BS, Gleich GJ: What targeting eosinophils has taught us about their role in diseases, *J Allergy Clin Immunol* 126(1):16–25, 2010.
5. Karasuyama H, et al: Role for basophils in systemic anaphylaxis, *Chem Immunol Allergy* 95:85–97, 2010.
6. Stasi R, et al: Thrombopoietic agents, *Blood Rev* 24(4–5):179–190, 2010.
7. Turley SJ, Fletcher AL, Elpek KG: The stromal and haematopoietic antigen-presenting cells that reside in secondary lymphoid organs, *Nat Rev Immunol* 10(12):813–825, 2010.
8. Gatto D, Brink R: The germinal center reaction, *J Allergy Clin Immunol* 126(5):898–907, 2010.
9. van de Pavert SA, Mebius RE: New insights into the development of lymphoid tissues, *Nat Rev Immunol* 10(9):664–674, 2010.
10. Hume DA: The mononuclear phagocyte system, *Curr Opin Immunol* 18(1):49–53, 2005.
11. National Institutes of Health: *Stem cell information*, Bethesda, Md, 2010, National Institutes of Health, U.S. Department of Health and Human Services [cited January 10, 2011]. Available at http://stemcells.nih.gov/info 2010.
12. Ratajczak MZ: Phenotypic and functional characterization of hematopoietic stem cells, *Curr Opin Hematol* 15(4):293–300, 2008.
13. Del Fattore A, Capannolo M, Rucci N: Bone and bone marrow: the same organ, *Arch Biochem Biophys* 503(1):28–34, 2010.
14. Lippi G, Franchini M, Favaloro EJ: Thrombotic complications of erythropoiesis-stimulating agents, *Semin Thromb Hemost* 36(5):537–549, 2010.
15. Schechter AN: Hemoglobin research and the origins of molecular medicine, *Blood* 112(10):3927–3938, 2008.
16. Mozzarelli A, et al: Haemoglobin-based oxygen carriers: research and reality towards an alternative to blood transfusions, *Blood Transfus* 8(suppl 3):s59–s68, 2010.
17. Edison ES, Bajel A, Chandy M: Iron homeostasis: new players, newer insights, *Eur J Haematol* 1(6):411–424, 2008.
18. West AR, Oates PS: Mechanisms of heme iron absorption: current questions and controversies, *World J Gastroenterol* 14(26):4101–4110, 2008.
19. Antonelou MH, Kriebardis AG, Papassideri IS: Aging and death signaling in mature red cells: from basic science to transfusion practice, *Blood Transfus* 8(suppl 3):s39–s47, 2010.
20. Geissmann F, et al: Development of monocytes, macrophages, and dendritic cells, *Science* 27(5966):656–661, 2010.
21. Kunicki TJ, Nugent DJ: The genetics of normal platelet reactivity, *Blood* 116(15):2627–2634, 2010.
22. Li Z, Delaney MK, O'Brien KA, et al: Signaling during platelet adhesion and activation, *Arterioscler Thromb Vasc Biol* 30(12):2341–2349, 2010.
23. Totani L, Evangelista V: Platelet-leukocyte interactions in cardiovascular disease and beyond, *Arterioscler Thromb Vasc Biol* 30(12):2357–2361, 2010.
24. Weisel JW, Litvinov RI: The biochemical and physical process of fibrinolysis and effects of clot structure and stability on the lysis rate, *Cardiovasc Hematol Agents Med Chem* 6(3):161–180, 2008.

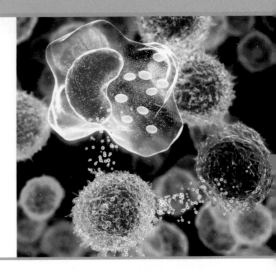

evolve WEBSITE

CHAPTER OUTLINE

Alterations of erythrocyte function involve either insufficient or excessive numbers of erythrocytes in the circulation or normal numbers of cells with abnormal components. Anemias are conditions in which there are too few erythrocytes or an insufficient volume of erythrocytes in the blood. Polycythemias are conditions in which erythrocyte numbers or volume is excessive. All of these conditions have many causes and are pathophysiologic manifestations of a variety of disease states.

Many disorders involving leukocytes range from increased numbers of leukocytes (i.e., leukocytosis) in response to infections to proliferative disorders (such as leukemia). Many hematologic disorders are malignancies, and many nonhematologic malignancies metastasize to bone marrow, affecting leukocyte production. Thus a large portion of this chapter is devoted to malignant disease.

The primary role of clotting (hemostasis) is to stop bleeding through an interaction of endothelium lining the vessels, platelets, and clotting factors. A large number of disease states may be associated with a clinically significant increase or decrease in clotting resulting from alterations in any of the three main components of the clotting process.

ALTERATIONS OF ERYTHROCYTE FUNCTION

Strictly speaking, anemia is a reduction in the total number of circulating erythrocytes or a decrease in the quality or quantity of hemoglobin. The causes of anemia are (1) altered production of erythrocytes, (2) blood loss, (3) increased erythrocyte destruction, or (4) a combination of all three.

Classification of Anemias

Anemias are classified by their causes (e.g., anemia of chronic disease) or by the changes that affect the size, shape, or substance of the erythrocyte. The most common classification of anemias is based on the changes that affect the cell's size and hemoglobin content (Table 20-1). Terms used to identify anemias reflect these characteristics. Terms that end with *cytic* refer to cell size, and those that end with *chromic* refer to

TABLE 20-1 MORPHOLOGIC CLASSIFICATION OF ANEMIAS

MORPHOLOGY OF REMAINING ERYTHROCYTES	NAME AND MECHANISM OF ANEMIA	PRIMARY CAUSE
Macrocytic-normochromic anemia: large, abnormally shaped erythrocytes, normal hemoglobin concentrations	Pernicious anemia: lack of vitamin B_{12}; abnormal DNA and RNA synthesis in erythroblast; premature cell death	Congenital or acquired deficiency of intrinsic factor (IF); genetic disorder of DNA synthesis
	Folate deficiency anemia: lack of folate; premature cell death	Dietary folate deficiency
Microcytic-hypochromic anemia: small, abnormally shaped erythrocytes and reduced hemoglobin concentration	Iron deficiency anemia: lack of iron for hemoglobin; insufficient hemoglobin	Chronic blood loss, dietary iron deficiency, disruption of iron metabolism or iron cycle
	Sideroblastic anemia: dysfunctional iron uptake by erythroblasts and defective porphyrin and heme synthesis	Congenital dysfunction of iron metabolism in erythroblasts, acquired dysfunction of iron metabolism as result of drugs or toxins
	Thalassemia: impaired synthesis of α- or β-chain of hemoglobin A; phagocytosis of abnormal erythroblasts in marrow	Congenital genetic defect of globin synthesis
Normocytic-normochromic anemia: normal size, normal hemoglobin concentration	Aplastic anemia: insufficient erythropoiesis	Depressed stem cell proliferation
Posthemorrhagic anemia: blood loss	Increased erythropoiesis; iron depletion	
	Hemolytic anemia: premature destruction (lysis) of mature erythrocytes in circulation	Increased fragility of erythrocytes
	Sickle cell anemia: abnormal hemoglobin synthesis, abnormal cell shape with susceptibility to damage, lysis, and phagocytosis	Congenital dysfunction of hemoglobin synthesis
	Anemia of chronic inflammation; abnormally increased demand for new erythrocytes	Chronic infection or inflammation; malignancy

DNA, Deoxyribonucleic acid; *RNA*, ribonucleic acid.

hemoglobin content. Additional terms describing erythrocytes found in some anemias are anisocytosis (assuming various sizes) and poikilocytosis (assuming various shapes).

CLINICAL MANIFESTATIONS The fundamental alteration of anemia is a reduced oxygen-carrying capacity of the blood resulting in tissue hypoxia. Symptoms of anemia vary, depending on the body's ability to compensate for the reduced oxygen-carrying capacity. Anemia that is mild and starts gradually is usually easier to compensate for and may cause problems for the individual only during physical exertion. As red cell reduction continues, symptoms become more pronounced and alterations in specific organs and compensation effects are more apparent. Compensation generally involves the cardiovascular, respiratory, and hematologic systems (Figure 20-1).

A reduction in the number of blood cells in the blood causes a reduction in the consistency and volume of blood. Initial compensation for cellular loss is movement of interstitial fluid into the blood causing an increase in plasma volume. This movement maintains an adequate blood volume, but the viscosity (thickness) of the blood decreases. The "thinner" blood flows faster and more turbulently than normal blood, causing a hyperdynamic circulatory state. This hyperdynamic state creates cardiovascular changes— increased stroke volume and heart rate. These changes may lead to cardiac dilation and heart valve insufficiency if the underlying anemic condition is not corrected.

Hypoxemia, reduced oxygen level in the blood, further contributes to cardiovascular dysfunction by causing dilation of arterioles, capillaries, and venules, thus increasing flow through them. Increased peripheral blood flow and venous return further contributes to an increase in heart rate and stroke volume in a continuing effort to meet normal oxygen demand and prevent cardiopulmonary congestion. These compensatory mechanisms may lead to heart failure.

Tissue hypoxia creates additional demands and effects on the pulmonary and hematologic systems. The rate and depth of breathing increases in an effort to increase oxygen availability accompanied by an increase in the release of oxygen from hemoglobin. All of these compensatory mechanisms may cause individuals to experience shortness of breath (dyspnea), a rapid and pounding heartbeat, dizziness, and fatigue. In mild chronic cases, these symptoms may be present only when there is an increased demand for oxygen (e.g., during physical exertion), but in severe cases, symptoms may be experienced even at rest.

Manifestations of anemia may be seen in other parts of the body. The skin, mucous membranes, lips, nail beds, and conjunctivae become either pale because of reduced hemoglobin concentration or yellowish (jaundiced) because of accumulation of end products of red cell destruction (hemolysis) if that is the cause of the anemia. Tissue hypoxia of the skin results in impaired healing and loss of elasticity, as well as thinning and early graying of the hair. Nervous system manifestations may occur where the cause of anemia is a deficiency of vitamin B_{12}. Myelin degeneration occurs, causing a loss of nerve fibers in the spinal cord, resulting in paresthesias (numbness), gait disturbances, extreme weakness, spasticity, and reflex abnormalities. Decreased oxygen supply to the gastrointestinal (GI) tract often produces abdominal pain, nausea, vomiting, and anorexia. Low-grade fever ($<101°$ F) occurs in some anemic individuals and may result from the release of leukocyte pyrogens from ischemic tissues.

When the anemia is severe or acute in onset (e.g., hemorrhage), the initial compensatory mechanism is peripheral blood vessel constriction, diverting blood flow to essential vital organs. Decreased blood flow detected by the kidneys activates the renin-angiotensin response, causing salt and water retention in an attempt to increase blood volume. These situations are considered to be emergencies and require immediate intervention to correct the underlying problem that caused

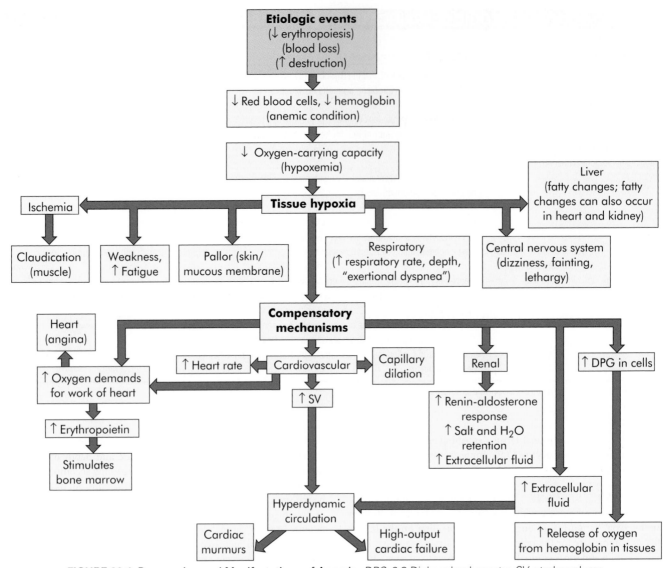

FIGURE 20-1 Progression and Manifestations of Anemia. *DPG*, 2,3-Diphosphoglycerate; *SV*, stroke volume.

the acute blood loss; therefore, long-term compensatory mechanisms do not develop.

Therapeutic interventions for slowly developing anemic conditions require treatment of the underlying condition and palliation of associated symptoms.[1] Therapies include transfusion, dietary correction, and administration of supplemental vitamins or iron.

Macrocytic-Normochromic Anemias

The **macrocytic (megaloblastic) anemias** are characterized by unusually large stem cells (megaloblasts) in the marrow that mature into erythrocytes that are unusually large in size (macrocytic), thickness, and volume.[2] The hemoglobin content is normal, thus allowing them to be classified as normochromic.

These anemias are the result of ineffective erythrocyte deoxyribonucleic acid (DNA) synthesis, commonly caused by deficiencies of vitamin B_{12} (cobalamin) or folate (folic acid). These defective erythrocytes die prematurely, which decreases their numbers in the circulation, causing anemia.

Defective DNA synthesis in megaloblastic anemias causes red cell growth and development to proceed at unequal rates. DNA synthesis

and cell division is blocked or delayed. However, ribonucleic acid (RNA) replication and protein (hemoglobin) synthesis proceed normally. Asynchronous development leads to an overproduction of hemoglobin during prolonged cellular division, creating a larger than normal erythrocyte with a disproportionately small nucleus. With each cell division, the disproportion between RNA and DNA becomes more apparent.

Pernicious Anemia

Pernicious anemia (PA), the most common type of macrocytic anemia, is caused by vitamin B_{12} deficiency, which often accompanies the end stage of type A chronic atrophic (autoimmune) gastritis (Figure 20-2, *C*).[3] *Pernicious* means highly injurious or destructive and reflects the fact that this condition was once fatal. It most commonly affects individuals over the age of 30 who are of Northern European descent, as well as blacks and Hispanics. Females are more prone to develop PA, with black females having an earlier onset.

PATHOPHYSIOLOGY The underlying alteration in PA is the absence of **intrinsic factor (IF),** an enzyme required for gastric absorption of

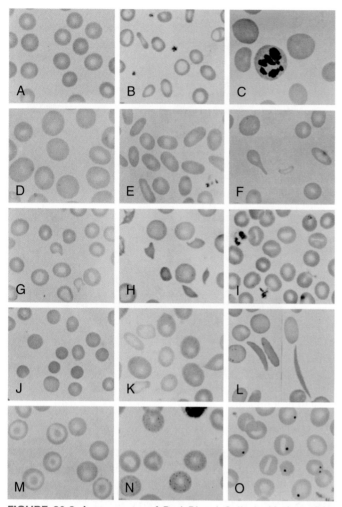

FIGURE 20-2 Appearance of Red Blood Cells in Various Disorders. **A,** Normal blood smear. **B,** Hypochromic-microcytic anemia (iron deficiency). **C,** Macrocytic anemia (pernicious anemia). **D,** Macrocytic anemia in pregnancy. **E,** Hereditary elliptocytosis. **F,** Myelofibrosis (teardrop). **G,** Hemolytic anemia associated with prosthetic heart valve. **H,** Microangiopathic anemia. **I,** Stomatocytes. **J,** Spherocytes (hereditary spherocytosis). **K,** Sideroblastic anemia; note the double population of red blood cells. **L,** Sickle cell anemia. **M,** Target cells (after splenectomy). **N,** Basophil stippling in case of unexplained anemia. **O,** Howell-Jolly bodies (after splenectomy). (From Wintrobe MM et al: *Clinical hematology,* ed 8, Philadelphia, 1981, Lea & Febiger.)

dietary vitamin B_{12}, a vitamin essential for nuclear maturation and DNA synthesis in red blood cells. Deficiency of IF may be congenital or may be the result of adult-onset gastric mucosal atrophy in which the parietal cells are destroyed. Subsequently, all secretions of the stomach—hydrochloric acid, pepsin, and IF—are deficient. PA is associated with autoimmune conditions that affect the endocrine system. Gastric atrophy may be caused by type A chronic gastritis, an autoimmune disorder that causes destruction of parietal and zymogenic cells. These destroyed cells are replaced with mucus-containing cells (intestinal metaplasia). In addition, PA may be caused by heavy alcohol ingestion, hot tea, and cigarette smoking. Complete or partial removal of the stomach (gastrectomy) causes IF deficiency and results in PA. Individuals with chronic gastritis are at risk for the development of gastric cancer and must be followed regularly to prevent this condition.

CLINICAL MANIFESTATIONS Pernicious anemia develops slowly (over 20 to 30 years), so by the time an individual seeks treatment, it is usually severe. Early symptoms are often ignored because they are nonspecific and vague and include infections, mood swings, and gastrointestinal, cardiac, or kidney ailments. When the hemoglobin level has decreased to 7 to 8 g/dl, the individual experiences the classic symptoms of anemia: weakness, fatigue, paresthesias of feet and fingers, difficulty walking, loss of appetite, abdominal pain, weight loss, and a sore tongue that is smooth and beefy red. The skin may become "lemon yellow" (sallow), caused by a combination of pallor and jaundice. Hepatomegaly, indicating right-sided heart failure, may be present in the elderly along with splenomegaly, which is nonpalpable.

EVALUATION AND TREATMENT Evaluation is based on blood tests, bone marrow aspiration, serologic studies, gastric biopsy, clinical manifestations, and the Schilling test. The Schilling test uses cobalt radioisotopes and labeled B_{12} to evaluate IF production. The test is performed by administering radioactive cobalamin and then measuring its excretion in the urine. Low urinary excretion is significant for PA. Serologic studies show the presence of antibodies against gastric cells and gastric biopsy reveals achlorhydria, a total absence of hydrochloric acid (HCl).

Untreated PA is fatal, usually because of heart failure. With replacement therapy of vitamin B_{12}, mortality has decreased significantly. Death from PA is now rare and relapses are often the result of noncompliance with therapy. Initial replacement of vitamin B_{12} is accomplished by weekly injections until the deficiency is corrected. Monthly injections are then required for the remainder of an individual's life. Conventional wisdom and practice determined that oral preparations were ineffective because there was no IF to facilitate absorption of B_{12}. However, recent practice has shown that oral administration of higher doses of B_{12} is beneficial. Apparently, an alternative mechanism for B_{12} absorption exists that is independent of IF. PA is not curable; therefore, treatment must be continued throughout the individual's lifetime.

Folate Deficiency Anemias

Folate (folic acid) is an essential vitamin required for RNA and DNA synthesis within the erythrocyte. Humans are totally dependent on dietary intake to meet the daily requirement of 50 to 200 mg/day. Increased amounts are required for lactating and pregnant females. Folate is absorbed from the upper small intestine and does not require any other element (i.e., IF) to facilitate absorption. After absorption, folate circulates through and is stored in the liver. Folate deficiency occurs more often than B_{12} deficiency, particularly in alcoholics and individuals who are malnourished because of fad diets or diets low in vegetables. It is estimated that at least 10% of North Americans are folate deficient.

Clinical manifestations are similar to the malnourished appearance of individuals with PA, except for the absence of neurologic symptoms. Specific manifestations include cheilosis (scales and fissures of the mouth), stomatitis (inflammation of the mouth), and painful ulcerations of the buccal mucosa and tongue. Dysphagia, flatulence, and watery diarrhea also may be present, as well as histologic changes in the GI tract suggestive of sprue (chronic absorption disorder). Neurologic manifestations, if present, may be caused by thiamine deficiency, which often accompanies folate deficiency.

Evaluation of folate deficiency is based on blood tests, measurement of serum folate levels, and clinical manifestations. Treatment requires administration of oral folate preparations until adequate blood levels are obtained and manifestations are reduced or eliminated. Long-term therapy is not necessary except for maintenance of an adequate daily intake of folate. Folate is essential for reducing blood levels of homocysteine, which has been recently recognized as a risk factor for the development of coronary artery disease.

Microcytic-Hypochromic Anemias

The microcytic-hypochromic anemias are characterized by abnormally small erythrocytes that contain abnormally reduced amounts of hemoglobin (see Figure 20-2, *B*). Hypochromia occurs even in cells of normal size.

Microcytic-hypochromic anemia can result from (1) disorders of iron metabolism, (2) disorders of porphyrin and heme synthesis, or (3) disorders of globin synthesis. Specific conditions include iron deficiency anemia, sideroblastic anemia, and thalassemia.

Iron Deficiency Anemia

Iron deficiency anemia (IDA) is the most common type of anemia throughout the world, occurring in both developing and developed countries.[2,4] The overall incidence of IDA is difficult to establish because of the lack of standardized methods and techniques to determine hypoferremia and IDA. Certain populations are at high risk for developing hypoferremia and IDA and include individuals living in poverty, women of childbearing age, and children. Females in the United States have a higher incidence than males for both hypoferremia and IDA, with the peak incidence occurring in the reproductive years and decreasing at menopause. Males have a higher incidence during childhood and adolescence. Children under 2 years of age are often affected because of their increased demand for iron during growth.

PATHOPHYSIOLOGY In developed countries, pregnancy and a continuous loss of blood are the most common causes of IDA. A blood loss of 2 to 4 ml/day (1 to 2 mg of iron) is enough to cause IDA. Males may experience bleeding as a result of ulcers, hiatal hernia, esophageal varices, cirrhosis, hemorrhoids, ulcerative colitis, or cancer. Menorrhagia (excessive menstrual bleeding) causes primary IDA in females. Other causes of blood loss for both genders include: (1) use of medications that cause GI bleeding; (2) surgical procedures that decrease stomach acidity, intestinal transit time, and absorption (e.g., gastric bypass); (3) insufficient dietary intake of iron; and (4) eating disorders such as pica—the craving and eating of nonnutritional substances, such as dirt, chalk, and paper.

Iron in the form of hemoglobin is in constant use in the body. An important attribute of iron is that it can be recycled; therefore, the body maintains a balance between iron that is in use as hemoglobin and iron that is stored and available for future hemoglobin synthesis (see Figure 19-13). Blood loss disrupts this balance by creating a need for more iron, thus depleting the iron stores more rapidly to replace the iron lost from bleeding.

IDA develops slowly through three overlapping stages. In stage I, the body's iron stores for red cell production and hemoglobin synthesis are depleted. Red cell production proceeds normally with the hemoglobin content of red cells also remaining normal. In stage II, insufficient amounts of iron are transported to the marrow, and iron-deficient red cell production begins. Stage III begins when the hemoglobin-deficient red cells enter the circulation to replace normal, aged erythrocytes that have been destroyed. The manifestations of IDA appear in stage III when there is an insufficient iron supply and diminished hemoglobin synthesis.

CLINICAL MANIFESTATIONS The onset of symptoms is gradual, and individuals usually do not seek medical attention until hemoglobin levels drop to 7 or 8 g/dl. Early symptoms are nonspecific and include fatigue, weakness, shortness of breath, and pale earlobes, palms, and conjunctiva (Figure 20-3).

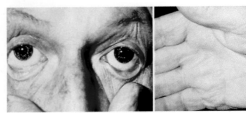

FIGURE 20-3 Pallor and Iron Deficiency. Pallor of the skin, mucous membranes, and palmar creases in an individual with hemoglobin level of 9 g/dl. Palmar creases become as pale as the surrounding skin when the hemoglobin level approaches 7 g/dl. (From Hoffbrand AV, Pettit JE: *Sandoz atlas of clinical hematology,* London, 1988, Gower Medical.)

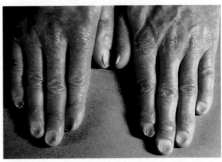

FIGURE 20-4 Koilonychia. The nails are concave, ridged, and brittle. (From Hoffbrand AV, Pettit JE: *Sandoz atlas of clinical hematology,* London, 1988, Gower Medical.)

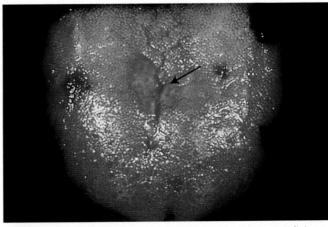

FIGURE 20-5 Glossitis. Tongue of individual with iron deficiency anemia has bald, fissured appearance *(arrow)* caused by loss of papillae and flattening. (From Hoffbrand AV, Pettit JE: *Sandoz atlas of clinical hematology,* London, 1988, Gower Medical.)

As the condition progresses and becomes more severe, structural and functional changes occur in epithelial tissue. The fingernails become brittle and "spoon shaped" or concave (koilonychia) (Figure 20-4). Tongue papillae atrophy and cause soreness along with redness and burning (Figure 20-5). These changes can be reversed within 1 to 2 weeks of iron replacement. The corners of the mouth become dry and sore (angular stomatitis), and an individual may experience difficulty with swallowing because of a "web" that develops from mucus and inflammatory cells at the opening of the esophagus. These lesions have the potential to become cancerous.

Iron is a component of many enzymes in the body, and lack of iron may alter other physiologic processes and contribute to the clinical manifestations. Individuals with IDA exhibit gastritis, neuromuscular changes, irritability, headache, numbness, tingling, and vasomotor disturbances. Gait disturbances are rare. In the elderly, mental confusion, memory loss, and disorientation may be wrongly perceived as normal events associated with aging.

EVALUATION AND TREATMENT Evaluation is based on clinical manifestations and laboratory tests. Iron stores are measured directly, by bone marrow biopsy, or indirectly, by tests that measure serum ferritin, transferrin saturation, or total iron-binding capacity. A sensitive indicator of heme synthesis is the amount of free erythrocyte protoporphyrin (FEP) within erythrocytes. A test that determines the concentration of soluble fragment transferrin receptor differentiates primary IDA from IDA that is associated with chronic disease.

The first step in treatment of IDA is to find and eliminate, or rule out, sources of blood loss. If this is not done, replacement therapy is ineffective. Iron replacement therapy is required and very effective. Initial doses are 150 to 200 mg/day and are continued until the serum ferritin level reaches 50 mg/L, indicating that adequate replacement has occurred. A rapid decrease in fatigue, lethargy, and other associated symptoms is generally seen within the first month of therapy. Replacement therapy usually continues for 6 to 12 months after the bleeding has stopped but may continue for as long as 24 months. Menstruating females may need daily oral iron replacement therapy (325 mg/day) until menopause.

Sideroblastic Anemia

Sideroblastic anemias (SAs) are a heterogeneous group of disorders characterized by anemia of varying severity because of inefficient iron uptake, resulting in abnormal hemoglobin synthesis. SA is characterized by the presence of ringed sideroblasts in the bone marrow. These are red cells that contain iron granules that have not been synthesized into hemoglobin but instead are arranged in a circle around the nucleus. Individuals with SA also have increased tissue levels of iron.

PATHOPHYSIOLOGY Sideroblastic anemias have various causes but all share the commonality of altered heme synthesis in the erythroid cells in bone marrow. SAs are either acquired or hereditary. Acquired sideroblastic anemias, which are the most common, occur as a primary disorder with no known cause (idiopathic) or are associated with other myeloproliferative or myeloplastic disorders. Another form is described as reversible SAs; these are secondary to various conditions such as alcoholism, drug reactions, copper deficiency, and hypothermia.

Hereditary sideroblastic anemias are rare and occur almost exclusively in males, supporting a recessive X-linked transmission; however, autosomal transmission affecting females has been reported. Other genetic, chromosomal, or enzyme dysfunctions also have been associated with hereditary SA. In all instances, SA anemia is present in infancy or childhood but may remain undetected until midlife, when other conditions, such as diabetes or cardiac failure from iron overload, cause it to be manifest.

Reversible sideroblastic anemia, associated with alcoholism, results from nutritional deficiencies of folate. Alcohol impairs heme synthesis by reducing the activity of specific enzymes along the biosynthetic pathway and also by direct effects of alcohol or acetaldehyde, or both, on the heme biosynthetic steps or mitochondrial metabolism. Some specific drugs also cause reversible SA and include antituberculous agents (isoniazid [INH], pyrazinamide, cycloserine, and chloramphenicol), which interfere with B_{12} metabolism or directly injure the mitochondria. Copper deficiency also causes reversible SA by interfering with conversion of ferric iron to ferrous iron. This is extremely rare and is associated with gastrectomy and prolonged parenteral nutrition without copper supplements. Hypothermia causes decreased heme synthesis and incorporation into hemoglobin.

CLINICAL MANIFESTATIONS Along with the cardiovascular and respiratory manifestations common to all anemias, individuals with SA may show signs of iron overload (hemosiderosis), including mild to moderate enlargement of the liver (hepatomegaly) and spleen (splenomegaly); however, liver function remains normal or only mildly affected. Occasionally the skin may become abnormally colored (bronze-tinted). Neurologic and skin alterations associated with other anemias are absent. Hemosiderosis of cardiac tissue may result in heart rhythm disturbances, which is a significant but uncommon complication and generally occurs late in the course of the disease. Growth and development impairment may occur in infants and young children who are severely affected.

EVALUATION AND TREATMENT Initially, SA may be mistaken for deficiency of stem cells in the marrow (hypoplastic anemia) or iron deficiency anemia. The diagnosis of SA is established by bone marrow biopsy, which documents the presence of sideroblasts and confirms the diagnosis.

Hereditary SA is initially treated with pyridoxine therapy (50 to 200 mg/day), which is effective in approximately one third of individuals treated; however, response is variable. An optimal response is reticulocytosis with normal levels of hemoglobin and FEP returning within 1 to 2 months; cellular morphologic abnormalities do not disappear. A less optimal response is an elevated hemoglobin level that stabilizes at less than normal levels. A therapeutic response to pyridoxine may be maintained with lifelong administration of a reduced dosage. Nonresponse to pyridoxine requires blood transfusions for symptom relief and to promote growth and development.

Evidence of iron overload requires iron depletion therapy to prevent or minimize organ damage. Phlebotomy, or removal of blood from the circulation, is used in individuals with mild to moderate anemia without other complications (i.e., heart disease). After iron removal, maintenance phlebotomies are continued. Severely anemic individuals who may require transfusions become extremely iron overloaded, which mandates use of deferoxamine, an iron-chelating agent, to reduce iron levels.

Individuals with acquired SA are less likely to respond to pyridoxine, but SA rarely incapacitates them. When SA is secondary to an identifiable cause, treatment or removal of the cause is essential. In the absence of blood cell abnormalities and iron overload, progression takes place over years. Transfusion and iron overload therapy is the same as for hereditary SA when indicated.

Death from SA is rare and often secondary to complications such as infection, bone marrow failure, liver failure, or cardiac failure, or arrhythmias. Idiopathic SA has the potential to convert to myelodysplastic syndrome, or abnormal marrow proliferation, which may then convert to acute myeloblastic leukemia.

Normocytic-Normochromic Anemias

Normocytic-normochromic anemias (NNAs) are characterized by erythrocytes that are relatively normal in size and hemoglobin content but insufficient in number.[5] These anemias do not share any common etiology, pathologic mechanism, or morphologic characteristics. They are less common than the macrocytic-normochromic and the microcytic-hypochromic anemias. Five distinct anemias—aplastic, posthemorrhagic, hemolytic, sickle cell, and anemia of chronic inflammation—exemplify the diversity of the NNA characteristics and are summarized in Table 20-2. (Sickle cell anemia is discussed in Chapter 21.)

✔ QUICK CHECK 20-1

1. How do cell size and content determine classification of anemia?
2. Why is iron important to hemoglobin synthesis, and why is iron deficiency related to anemia?
3. How is anemia diagnosed?

MYELOPROLIFERATIVE RED CELL DISORDERS

Hematologic dysfunction results from an overproduction of cells, as well as a deficiency. One or more marrow elements may be produced in excess, responding to exogenous (e.g., exposure to radiation, drugs) or endogenous (e.g., physiologic compensatory response, immune disorder) signals. Excessive red cell production is classified as **polycythemia**

(Table 20-3). Polycythemia exists in two forms: relative and absolute. Relative polycythemia results from hemoconcentration of the blood associated with dehydration. It is of minor consequence and resolves with fluid administration or treatment of underlying conditions.

Absolute polycythemia consists of two forms: primary and secondary. Secondary polycythemia, the most common of the two, is a physiologic response resulting from erythropoietin secretion caused by hypoxia. This hypoxia is noted in individuals living at higher altitudes (>10,000 ft), smokers with increased blood levels of CO, and individuals with chronic obstructive pulmonary disease or coronary heart failure, or both. Abnormal types of hemoglobin (e.g., San Diego, Chesapeake), which have a greater affinity for oxygen, also cause secondary polycythemia, as does inappropriate secretion of erythropoietin by certain tumors (e.g., renal cell carcinoma, hepatoma, and cerebellar hemangioblastomas). The absolute primary form of polycythemia is referred to as *polycythemia vera*.

Polycythemia Vera

Polycythemia vera (PV) is a chronic, clonal alteration characterized by overproduction of red cells (frequently with increased white cells and platelets) accompanied by splenomegaly.[6] Hypercellularity of bone

TABLE 20-2 NORMOCYTIC-NORMOCHROMIC ANEMIAS

ANEMIA	PATHOPHYSIOLOGY	CLINICAL MANIFESTATIONS	EVALUATION AND TREATMENT
Aplastic	Rare; may result from infiltrative disorders of bone marrow, autoimmune diseases, renal failure, splenic dysfunction, vitamin B_{12} or folate deficiency, parvovirus infection, or exposure to radiation, drugs, and toxins; also may be congenital Common stem cell population may be altered so it cannot proliferate or differentiate, or stem cell environment is altered to inhibit erythropoiesis Outcome ranges from death to minimal manifestations	Classic cardiovascular and respiratory manifestations with thrombocytopenia, hemorrhage into tissues, leukopenia, and infection	Bone marrow biopsy determines whether anemia is caused by pure red cell aplasia or hypoplasia Treat underlying disorder or prevent further exposure to causative agent Blood transfusions, marrow transplant, and pharmacologic stimulation of bone marrow function
Posthemorrhagic	Caused by sudden blood loss with normal iron stores	Often obscured by cardiovascular manifestations of acute hemorrhage Severe shock, lactic acidosis, and death can occur if blood loss exceeds 40-50% of plasma volume	Restoration of blood volume by intravenous administration of saline, dextran, albumin, or plasma Transfusion of whole blood also required occasionally
Hemolytic	Acquired: caused by infection, systemic disease, drugs or toxins, liver disease, kidney disease, abnormal immune responses Hereditary: caused by abnormalities of RBC membrane or cytoplasmic contents; present at birth Hemolysis: in blood vessels or lymphoid tissues that filter blood (e.g., spleen, liver) Erythrocytes: rigid, slowing their passage and making them vulnerable to phagocytosis Types: warm antibody disease (mediated by IgG antibody specific for erythrocyte antigens), cold antibody disease (mediated by IgM), and drug induced	Splenomegaly, jaundice, aplastic hemolytic, or megaloblastic crises can develop with viral infection With severe disease, bones become deformed and pathologic fractures occur Cardiovascular and respiratory manifestations correspond with severity of anemia	Blood and bone marrow studies Erythroid hyperplasia is found in marrow and blood smears Treatment of acquired disease involves removing cause or treating underlying disorder Other forms of treatment are transfusions, splenectomy, and steroids or folate
Anemia of chronic inflammation	Associated with chronic infections (e.g., AIDS), chronic inflammatory diseases (e.g., rheumatoid arthritis, SLE), and malignancies Causes are decreased erythrocyte life span, failure of mechanisms of compensatory erythropoiesis, or disturbance of iron cycle	Manifestations fewer and milder than most other anemias General disability caused by chronic disease limits physical activity so hemoglobin levels adequate; if they drop, signs of iron deficiency anemia develop	Blood tests show iron deficiency in marrow despite normal or increased iron stores elsewhere No treatment is needed unless anemia becomes symptomatic Erythropoietin may be used

AIDS, Acquired immunodeficiency syndrome; *RBC,* red blood cell; *SLE,* systemic lupus erythematosus.

TABLE 20-3   DISORDERS CLASSIFIED AS POLYCYTHEMIA

TYPE OF POLYCYTHEMIA	MECHANISM OF INCREASED ERYTHROPOIESIS	CAUSE OF ASSOCIATED DISORDER
Primary polycythemia (polycythemia vera)	Excessive proliferation of erythroid precursors in marrow; increased sensitivity of stem cell to erythropoietin	Possible mutation in erythropoietin receptor
Secondary polycythemia	Physiologic increase in erythropoietin secretion by kidneys in response to underlying systemic disorder	Tissue hypoxia caused by cardiopulmonary disorders (chronic obstructive pulmonary disease, congestive heart failure), decreased barometric pressure, cardiovascular malformations causing mixing of arterial and venous blood, methemoglobinemia, carboxyhemoglobinemia, smoking, obesity
	"Nonphysiologic"* increase in erythropoietin secretion	Renal disorders, cerebellar hemangioblastomas, hepatoma (liver tumor), ovarian carcinoma, uterine leiomyoma, pheochromocytoma, adrenocortical hypersecretion
Familial polycythemia	Genetically induced increase in erythroid precursors of marrow Abnormal Hb† with increased oxygen affinity Decreased 2,3-DPG Increased sensitivity of stem cells to erythropoietin Increased erythropoietin in secretion	Genetic defect

*Nonphysiologic means that there is no obvious physiologic explanation for hypersecretion of erythropoietin.
†*2,3-DPG*, 2,3-Diphosphoglycerate; *Hb*, hemoglobin.

marrow, along with hyperplasia of myeloid, erythroid, and megakaryocytes, is a distinguishing feature. PV is quite rare, occurring mostly in white males of Eastern European Jewish origin from 55 to 80 years of age, with a median age of 55 to 60 years, but it has been observed in females and individuals less than 40 years of age. It is rarely seen in children or in multiple members of a single family; however, an autosomal dominant form exists that causes increased secretion of erythropoietin.

PATHOPHYSIOLOGY   PV is a neoplastic, nonmalignant condition characterized by an abnormal proliferation of bone marrow stem cells with subsequent self-destructive expansion of red cells. This aberrant proliferation occurs despite normal to below normal erythropoietin levels. The underlying cause remains unknown, with the most likely etiology thought to be an acquired genetic stem cell alteration of the erythropoietin receptor that causes the abnormal proliferation. Laboratory studies have found red cell precursors that are capable of growth independent of erythropoietin. These red blood cell precursors also demonstrate sensitivity to other growth factors, such as interleukin-3 (IL-3), granulocyte-macrophage colony-stimulating factor (GM-CSF), or insulin-like growth factor.

CLINICAL MANIFESTATIONS   Clinical manifestations of PV are due to increased blood volume, which increases blood viscosity, creating a hypercoagulable state resulting in clogging and occlusion of blood vessels. Tissue injury (ischemia) and death (infarction) is the outcome of blood vessel blockage, and this occurs about 40% of the time. These outcomes are directly correlated with hematocrit levels. Increases in numbers of thrombocytes, as well as production of dysfunctional platelets, also contribute to this hypercoagulable condition.

Circulatory alterations caused by the thick, sticky blood give rise to other manifestations, such as plethora (ruddy, red color of the face, hands, feet, ears, and mucous membranes) and engorgement of retinal and cerebral veins. Other symptoms may include headache, drowsiness, delirium, mania, psychotic depression, chorea, and visual disturbances. Death from cerebral thrombosis is approximately five times greater in individuals with PV.[6,7]

Cardiovascular function, despite the vascular alterations, remains relatively normal. Cardiac workload and output remain constant; however, increased blood volume does increase blood pressure. Coronary blood flow may be affected, precipitating angina, although cardiovascular infarctions are uncommon. Other cardiovascular manifestations include Raynaud phenomenon and thromboangiitis obliterans.

A unique feature of PV, and helpful in diagnosis, is the development of intense, painful itching that appears to be intensified by heat or exposure to water (aquagenic pruritus) so that individuals avoid exposure to water, particularly warm water when bathing or showering. The intensity of itching is related to the concentration of mast cells in the skin and is generally not responsive to antihistamines or topical lotions.

EVALUATION AND TREATMENT   Blood and laboratory findings, characterized by an absolute increase in red blood cells and in total blood volume, confirm the diagnosis. Erythrocytes appear normal, but anisocytosis may be present. There also may be moderate increases in white blood cells and platelets. A bone marrow examination may be done; however, it cannot definitively confirm the diagnosis. Treatment of PV consists of reducing red cell proliferation and blood volume, controlling symptoms, and preventing clogging and clotting of the blood vessels. Phlebotomy (approximately 300 to 500 ml) is used to reduce red cell mass and blood volume. Initial phlebotomies are done two to three times a week until hematocrit levels drop sufficiently and then are repeated every 3 to 4 months to maintain appropriate hematocrit levels (<45%). Frequent phlebotomies also reduce iron levels, a condition that impedes erythropoiesis, but they also may contribute to the development of thrombosis; thus, use of phlebotomies needs to be individualized. Smokers are urged to quit smoking, and individuals with congestive heart failure and chronic obstructive pulmonary disease require appropriate drug intervention.

Hydroxyurea, a nonalkylating myelosuppressive, is the drug of choice for myelosuppression because of a reduced incidence to cause leukemia and thrombosis. Radioactive phosphorus (^{32}P) also is used as an effective and easily tolerated intervention to suppress erythropoiesis. Its effects may last up to 18 months. Side effects of ^{32}P include suppression of hematopoiesis resulting in anemia, leukopenia, and thrombocytopenia. Acute leukemia is also a side effect, although most often it occurs only after 7 or more years of treatment, making its use in elderly persons more common. Interferon is gaining popularity as an effective drug therapy because of its ability to inhibit growth of the abnormal clone, which diminishes the clinical and laboratory manifestations of myeloproliferation. Interferon use for this purpose is still new, and long-term effects are as yet unknown.

Survival for 10 to 15 years is common. However, without proper treatment, 50% of individuals with PV die within 18 months of the onset of initial symptoms because of thrombosis or hemorrhage. A significant potential outcome of PV is the conversion to acute myeloid leukemia (AML), occurring spontaneously in 10% of individuals and generally being resistant to conventional therapy. Conversion to AML is most likely related to treatment methods associated with cytotoxic myelosuppressive agents, chlorambucil, and busulfan. Although PV is a chronic disorder, appropriate therapy results in remissions and prevention of significant pathologic outcomes.

Iron Overload

Iron overload can be primary, as in hereditary hemochromatosis (HH), or secondary. The secondary causes of iron overload include anemias with inefficient erythropoiesis (e.g., sideroblastic anemia, aplastic anemia), dietary iron overload, or conditions that require repeated blood transfusions or iron dextran injections.

Hereditary Hemochromatosis

Hereditary hemochromatosis (HH) is a common inherited, autosomal recessive disorder of iron metabolism,[8] and is characterized by increased gastrointestinal iron absorption with subsequent tissue iron deposition. Excess iron is deposited in the liver, pancreas, heart, joints, and endocrine gland causing tissue damage that can lead to diseases such as cirrhosis, diabetes, heart failure, arthropathies, and impotence.

HH is caused by two genetic base-pair alterations, C282Y and H63D. These are mutations in the *HFE* gene on chromosome 6. Homozygosity of C282Y is the most common genotype and accounts for 82% to 90% of HH cases. The remaining cases appear to be caused by environmental factors or other genotypes. *HFE* mutations are common in the United States with 1 in 10 white persons heterozygous for *HFE* C282Y mutation and 4.4 in 1000 homozygous for the C282Y mutation. C282Y homozygosity is much lower among Hispanics (0.27 in 1000), Asian Americans (<0.001 per 1000), Pacific islanders (0.12 per 1000), and black persons (0.14 per 1000).

PATHOPHYSIOLOGY Mouse studies have confirmed that the *HFE* gene is responsible for HH. HFE protein, found in the crypt cells of the duodenum, facilitates transferring receptor-dependent iron uptake into crypt cells. Mutant HFE protein loses its functional ability and causes a relative iron deficiency in duodenal crypt cells. The deficiency results in an increase in the expression of an iron transport protein, divalent metal ion transporter 1 (DMT-1), which is responsible for dietary iron absorption in the villus cells of the small intestine. This inappropriate intestinal iron absorption leads to iron overload and, eventually, end-organ damage that can result in cirrhosis, diabetes mellitus, hypothyroidism, cardiomyopathies, and arthritis.

Although the natural history of HH is not well understood, there appears to be a long latent period with individual variation in biochemical expression modified by environmental factors, such as blood loss from menstruation or donation, alcohol intake, and diet. Cirrhosis is a late-stage development of HH that can shorten life expectancy. Cirrhosis also is a risk factor for hepatocellular carcinoma that occurs between 40 and 60 years old. Cirrhosis prevention is a major goal of HH screening and treatment.

CLINICAL MANIFESTATIONS Clinical manifestations of HH include symptoms such as fatigue, malaise, abdominal pain, arthralgias and impotence, and clinical findings of hepatomegaly, abnormal liver enzymes, bronzed skin, diabetes, and cardiomegaly. Many individuals are diagnosed as a result of serum iron studies as part of a health screening panel. Most (>75%) are asymptomatic and have a low frequency (<25%) of cirrhosis, diabetes, or skin pigmentation.

EVALUATION AND TREATMENT Laboratory findings in individuals with HH show elevations in serum iron levels, transferrin saturation, and ferritin levels. Documentation of iron overload relies on quantitative phlebotomy with calculation of the amount of iron removed or liver biopsy with determination of quantitative hepatic iron. With the advent of genetic testing, individuals who are C282Y homozygous or compound heterozygous, less than 40 years old, and have normal liver functions, no further workup is necessary.

Treatment of HH is simple and consists of phlebotomy of 550 ml of whole blood, which is equivalent to 200 to 250 mg of iron. Frequency of phlebotomy depends on ferritin levels and should continue until the ferritin level is between 20 and 50 ng/ml. Initially, phlebotomy may be needed weekly but once therapeutic ferritin levels are reached, phlebotomy may only be needed every 2 to 3 months. Blood banks now accept blood donations from persons with documented HH. Iron chelating agents are sometimes used in addition to phlebotomy, but this is not the mainstay of treatment. Individuals with HH should be instructed to refrain from taking iron and vitamin C supplements and consuming raw shellfish; in addition, alcohol should be used in moderation. Family screening is recommended and necessary for all first-degree relatives of a person with HH.

ALTERATIONS OF LEUKOCYTE FUNCTION

Leukocyte function is affected if too many or too few white cells are present in the blood or if the cells that are present are structurally or functionally defective. Phagocytic cells (granulocytes, monocytes, macrophages) may lose their ability to act as effective phagocytes, and the lymphocytes may lose their ability to respond to antigens. (Disruptions of inflammatory and immune processes caused by leukocyte disorders are described in Chapter 5.) Other leukocyte alterations include infectious mononucleosis and cancers of the blood—leukemia and multiple myeloma.

Quantitative Alterations of Leukocytes

Quantitative alterations are increases or decreases in numbers of leukocytes in the blood. Leukocytosis is present when the count is higher than normal; leukopenia is present when the count is lower than normal. Leukocytosis and leukopenia may affect a specific type of white blood cell and may result from a variety of physiologic conditions and alterations.

Leukocytosis occurs as a normal protective response to physiologic stressors, such as invading microorganisms, strenuous exercise, emotional changes, temperature changes, anesthesia, surgery, pregnancy, and some drugs, hormones, and toxins. It also is caused by pathologic conditions, such as malignancies and hematologic disorders. Unlike leukocytosis, leukopenia is never normal. When the leukocyte count falls to less than $1000/mm^3$, the risk of infection increases drastically. With counts below $500/mm^3$, the possibility for life-threatening infections is high. Leukopenia may be caused by radiation, anaphylactic shock, autoimmune disease (e.g., systemic lupus erythematosus), immune deficiencies (see Chapter 7), and certain chemotherapeutic agents.

Granulocyte and Monocyte Alterations

Increased levels of circulating granulocytes (neutrophils, eosinophils, basophils) and monocytes are chiefly a physiologic response to microbial invasion. Increased numbers also occur as a result of myeloproliferative disorders (polycythemia vera, chronic myelocytic leukemia [CML]) that increase stem cell proliferation in the bone marrow.[9]

Decreases occur when infectious processes deplete the supply of circulating granulocytes and monocytes, drawing them out of the circulation and into infected tissues faster than they can be replaced. Decreases also can be caused by disorders that suppress marrow function, such as Shwachman-Diamond syndrome, severe congenital neutropenia, or immune-related neutropenia.[10]

Granulocytosis—an increase in granulocytes (neutrophils, eosinophils, or basophils)—begins when stored blood cells are released. Neutrophilia is another term that may be used to describe *granulocytosis* because neutrophils are the most numerous of the granulocytes (Table 20-4). Neutrophilia is seen in the early stages of infection or inflammation and is established when the absolute count exceeds 7500/mm³. Release and depletion of stored neutrophils stimulates granulopoiesis to replenish neutrophil reserves. Specific conditions associated with neutrophilia are identified in Table 20-4.

When the demand for circulating mature neutrophils exceeds the supply, immature neutrophils (and other leukocytes) are released from the bone marrow. Premature release of the immature cells is responsible for the phenomenon known as a shift-to-the-left or leukemoid reaction. This refers to the microscopic detection of disproportionate numbers of immature leukocytes in peripheral blood smears. To understand this phenomenon, visualize cellular differentiation, maturation, and release (see Figure 19-7) as progressing from left to right instead of vertically. The early release of immature white cells prevents the completion of the sequence and shifts the distribution of leukocytes in the blood toward those on the left side of the diagram. This phenomenon is also seen in the blood smear of individuals with leukemia, hence the term *leukemoid reaction*. As infection or inflammation diminishes, and granulopoiesis replenishes circulating granulocytes, a shift-to-the-right, or return to normal, occurs.

Neutropenia is a condition associated with a reduction in circulating neutrophils and exists clinically when the neutrophil count is less than 2000/mm³. Reduction in neutrophils occurs in severe prolonged infections when production of granulocytes cannot keep up with demand.[9,10]

Other causes of neutropenia, in the absence of overwhelming infection, may be (1) decreased neutrophil production or ineffective granulopoiesis, (2) reduced neutrophil survival, and (3) abnormal neutrophil distribution and sequestration. Hematologic disorders that cause ineffective or decreased production include hypoplastic or aplastic anemia, megaloblastic anemias, leukemia, or drug-/toxin-induced neutropenia. Neutropenia also is seen in starvation and anorexia nervosa because of an inadequate supply of protein building blocks. Decreased neutrophil survival is seen in autoimmune disorders (e.g., systemic lupus erythematosus, rheumatoid arthritis). Abnormal neutrophil distribution and sequestration are associated with hypersplenism and a pseudoneutropenia, which in the presence of rheumatoid arthritis constitute Felty syndrome. Viral infections (human immunodeficiency virus [HIV], Epstein-Barr virus [EBV]) also may cause neutropenia, as does chemotherapy and other toxic drugs received for cancer treatment and transplantation.

If neutrophils are drastically reduced (<500/mm³) and the entire granulocyte count is extremely low, granulocytopenia or agranulocytosis results. Usually, when this occurs, hematopoiesis is arrested in the bone marrow or cell destruction increases in the circulation.

Chemotherapeutic agents used to treat hematologic and other malignancies cause bone marrow suppression. Several other drugs cause agranulocytosis, which occurs rarely but carries a high mortality rate of 10% to 48%. Clinical manifestations of agranulocytosis include infection (particularly of the respiratory system), general malaise, septicemia, fever, tachycardia, and ulcers in the mouth and colon. If untreated, sepsis results in death within 3 to 6 days. Other conditions associated with neutropenia are identified in Table 20-4.

Eosinophilia is an absolute increase (>450/mm³) in the total number of circulating eosinophils. Allergic disorders (type 1) associated with asthma, hay fever, and drug reactions often cause eosinophilia. Hypersensitivity reactions trigger the release of eosinophilic chemotaxic factor of anaphylaxis (ECF-A) and histamine from mast cells, attracting eosinophils to the area. Areas with abundant mast cells, such as the respiratory and GI tracts, are commonly affected. Eosinophilia also may occur in dermatologic disorders, eosinophilia-myalgia syndrome, and parasitic invasion. Other conditions that cause eosinophilia are detailed in Table 20-4.

Eosinopenia, a decrease in circulating eosinophils, generally is caused by migration of eosinophils into inflammatory sites. It may be seen in Cushing syndrome and as a result of stress caused by surgery, shock, trauma, burns, or mental distress. Other conditions that cause eosinopenia are detailed in Table 20-4.

Basophilia is a response to inflammation and immediate hypersensitivity reactions. Basophils contain histamine that is released during an allergic reaction. Increased basophils are seen in myeloproliferative disorders, such as chronic myeloid leukemia and myeloid metaplasia. Other conditions that are associated with basophilia are listed in Table 20-4.

Basopenia is seen in hyperthyroidism, acute infection, and long-term therapy with steroids. Other conditions associated with basopenia are listed in Table 20-4.

Monocytosis, an increase in monocytes, is often transient and correlates poorly with disease states. It is usually associated with neutropenia during bacterial infections, particularly in the late stages or recovery stage, when monocytes are needed to phagocytize surviving microorganisms and debris. Increased monocytes also may indicate marrow recovery from agranulocytosis. Monocytosis is often seen in chronic infections such as tuberculosis (TB) and subacute bacterial endocarditis (SBE), and it has been found to correlate with the extent of myocardial damage following myocardial infarctions. Other conditions associated with monocytosis are identified in Table 20-4. Monocytopenia, a decrease in monocytes, is rare but has been identified with hairy cell leukemia and prednisone therapy.

Lymphocyte Alterations

Quantitative alterations of lymphocytes occur when lymphocytes are activated by antigenic stimuli, usually microorganisms (see Chapter 6). Lymphocytosis is rare in acute bacterial infections and is seen most commonly in acute viral infections, particularly those caused by the Epstein-Barr virus (EBV)—a causative agent in infectious mononucleosis. Other specific disorders associated with lymphocytosis are listed in Table 20-4.

Lymphocytopenia may be attributed to (1) abnormalities of lymphocyte production associated with neoplasias and immune deficiencies and (2) destruction by drugs, viruses, or radiation. It is also known to occur without any detectable cause. Conditions associated with lymphocytopenia are identified in Table 20-4. The lymphocytopenia associated with heart failure and other acute illnesses may be caused by elevated levels of cortisol. Lymphocytopenia is a major problem in acquired immunodeficiency syndrome (AIDS). AIDS-related lymphocytopenia is caused by HIV, which destroys T-helper lymphocytes. (For a detailed discussion of AIDS, see Chapter 7.)

TABLE 20-4 OTHER CONDITIONS ASSOCIATED WITH NEUTROPHILS, EOSINOPHILS, BASOPHILS, MONOCYTES, AND LYMPHOCYTES

CONDITION	CAUSE	EXAMPLE
Neutrophil		
Neutrophilia (granulocytosis)	Inflammation or tissue necrosis	Surgery, burns, MI, pneumonitis, rheumatic fever, rheumatoid arthritis
	Infection	Bacterial: gram-positive (staphylococci, streptococci, pneumococci), gram-negative (*Escherichia coli, Pseudomonas* species)
	Physiologic	Exercise, extreme heat or cold, third-trimester pregnancy, emotional distress
	Hematologic	Acute hemorrhage, hemolysis, myeloproliferative disorder, chronic granulocytic leukemia
	Drugs or chemicals	Epinephrine, steroids, heparin, histamine, endotoxin
	Metabolic	Diabetes (acidosis), eclampsia, gout, thyroid storm
	Neoplasm	Liver, GI tract, bone marrow
Neutropenia	Decreased marrow production	Radiation, chemotherapy, leukemia, aplastic anemia, abnormal granulopoiesis
	Increased destruction	Splenomegaly, hemodialysis, autoimmune disease
	Infection	Gram-negative (typhoid), viral (influenza, hepatitis B, measles, mumps, rubella), severe infections, protozoal infections (malaria)
Eosinophil		
Eosinophilia	Allergy	Asthma, hay fever, drug sensitivity
	Infection	Parasites (trichinosis, hookworm), chronic (fungal, leprosy, TB)
	Malignancy	CML, lung, stomach, ovary, Hodgkin disease
	Dermatosis	Pemphigus, exfoliative dermatitis (drug-induced)
	Drugs	Digitalis, heparin, streptomycin, tryptophan (eosinophilia-myalgia syndrome), penicillins, propranolol
Eosinopenia	Stress response	Trauma, shock, burns, surgery, mental distress
	Drugs	Steroids (Cushing syndrome)
Basophil		
Basophilia	Inflammation	Infection (measles, chickenpox), hypersensitivity reaction (immediate)
	Hematologic	Myeloproliferative disorders (CML, polycythemia vera, Hodgkin lymphoma, hemolytic anemia)
	Endocrine	Myxedema, antithyroid therapy
Basopenia	Physiologic	Pregnancy, ovulation, stress
	Endocrine	Graves disease
Monocyte		
Monocytosis	Infection	Bacterial (subacute bacterial endocarditis, TB), recovery phase of infection
	Hematologic	Myeloproliferative disorders, Hodgkin disease, agranulocytosis
	Physiologic	Normal newborn
Monocytopenia	Rare	
Lymphocyte		
Lymphocytosis	Physiologic	4 months to 4 years
	Acute infection	Infectious mononucleosis, CMV infection, pertussis, hepatitis, mycoplasma pneumonia, typhoid
	Chronic infection	Congenital syphilis, tertiary syphilis
	Endocrine	Thyrotoxicosis, adrenal insufficiency
	Malignancy	ALL, CLL, lymphosarcoma cell leukemia
Lymphocytopenia	Immunodeficiency syndrome	AIDS, agammaglobulinemia
	Lymphocyte destruction	Steroids (Cushing syndrome), radiation, chemotherapy
	Hodgkin lymphoma	
	CHF, renal failure, TB, SLE, aplastic anemia	

AIDS, Acquired immunodeficiency syndrome; *ALL,* acute lymphocytic leukemia; *CHF,* congestive (left) heart failure; *CLL,* chronic lymphocytic leukemia; *CML,* chronic myelogenous leukemia; *CMV,* cytomegalovirus; *GI,* gastrointestinal; *MI,* myocardial infarction, *SLE,* systemic lupus erythematosus; *TB,* tuberculosis.

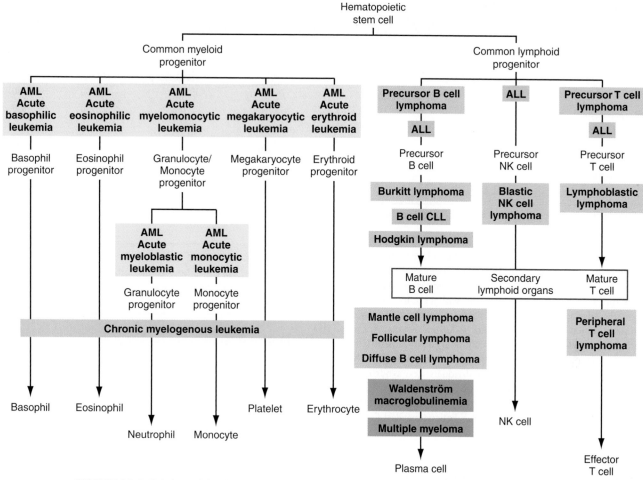

FIGURE 20-6 Origins of Leukemias and Lymphomas. Differentiation pathways of blood-forming cells and reported sites from which specific leukemias and lymphomas originate. Tumors of similar types are given the same background coloring. *ALL,* Acute lymphocytic leukemia; *AML,* acute myelogenous leukemia; *CLL,* chronic lymphocytic leukemia; *NK,* natural killer.

Infectious Mononucleosis

Infectious mononucleosis (IM) is an acute infection of B lymphocytes (B cells) with Epstein-Barr virus (EBV).[11] Infections with EBV are common in children, particularly those from low socioeconomic environments. Approximately 50% to 85% of these children are infected with EBV by age 4, and more than 90% of adults have indications of exposure to EBV. These early infections are usually asymptomatic and provide immunity to EBV; thus children with an early infection rarely develop IM. Mononucleosis may arise when the initial infection with EBV occurs during adolescence or later, but it results in mononucleosis in only 35% to 50% of these individuals.

The incidence of IM is approximately 45 in 10,000 individuals and is most commonly seen in young adults between 15 and 35 years of age, with the peak incidence between 15 and 19 years. It is rarely seen in individuals over 40 years, and when it does occur, is more commonly caused by cytomegalovirus (CMV).

Transmission of EBV is usually through saliva from close personal contact (e.g., kissing, hence the term *kissing disease*). The virus also may be secreted in other mucosal secretions of the genital, rectal, and respiratory tract, as well as blood. Transmission through sneezing or coughing has not been documented. The infection begins with widespread invasion of the B lymphocytes, which have receptors for EBV.

The virus initially infects the oropharynx, nasopharynx, and salivary epithelial cells with later extension into lymphoid tissues and B cells.

Unaffected B cells produce antibodies (IgG, IgA, IgM) against the virus. Cytotoxic T lymphocytes (Tc cells) are activated and multiply to assist the B cells in attacking the virus and virus-infected cells directly (see Chapter 6). The production of B and T cells and the process of removing dead and damaged leukocytes are largely responsible for lymphoid tissue swelling (lymph nodes, spleen, tonsils, and, occasionally, liver). Sore throat and fever, two initial manifestations of IM, are caused by inflammation and infection at the site of initial viral entry—the mouth and throat.

CLINICAL MANIFESTATIONS The incubation period for IM is approximately 30 to 50 days. Early flulike symptoms, such as headache, malaise, joint pain, and fatigue, may appear during the first 3 to 5 days, although some individuals are without symptoms. At the time of diagnosis, the individual commonly presents with the classic group of symptoms: fever, sore throat, cervical lymph node enlargement, and fatigue. As the condition progresses, generalized lymph node enlargement also may develop as well as enlargement of the spleen and liver (25% to 75% of individuals). Splenic rupture is rare and can occur spontaneously or as a result of mild trauma, occurring primarily in males (90%) between day 4 and day 21 after symptom onset. It is the most common cause of death related to IM. Other causes of the

TABLE 20-5	ESTIMATED NEW CASES AND DEATHS FROM LEUKEMIA IN THE UNITED STATES—2007					
	TOTAL NEW CASES	**NEW CASES BY GENDER**		**DEATHS BY GENDER**		
TYPES OF LEUKEMIA	**(PROPORTION OF NEW CASES)**	**MALE**	**FEMALE**	**MALE**	**FEMALE**
All types	43,050 (100%)	24,690	19,440	12,660	9,180
Acute lymphocytic leukemia	5,330 (12%)	3,150	2,180	790	630
Chronic lymphocytic leukemia	14,990 (35%)	8,870	6,120	2,650	1,740
Acute myelogenous leukemia	12,330 (29%)	6,590	5,740	5,280	3,670
Chronic myelogenous leukemia	4,870 (11%)	2,800	2,070	190	250
Other	5,530 (13%)	3,280	2,250	3,750	2,890

Data from American Cancer Society: *Cancer facts and figures—2010,* Atlanta, 2010, The Society.

rare fatalities associated with IM are hepatic failure, extensive bacterial infection, or viral myocarditis. Other organ systems are rarely involved, but such involvement may be present with characteristic manifestations, such as fulminant hepatitis with jaundice and anemia, encephalitis, meningitis, Guillain-Barré syndrome, and Bell palsy. Eye manifestations may include eyelid and periorbital edema, dry eyes, keratitis, uveitis, and conjunctivitis. Pulmonary involvement is rare, although incidences of pneumonia and respiratory failure have been documented in immunocompromised individuals. Reye syndrome has been known to develop in children with EBV infection.

IM is usually self-limiting, and recovery occurs in a few weeks; severe clinical complications are rare (5%). Fatigue may last for 1 to 2 months after resolution of other symptoms.

EVALUATION AND TREATMENT The blood of affected individuals contains an increased number of white blood cells with many atypical forms. Serologic tests to determine a heterophile antibody response are necessary to diagnose EBV infection.[12] Heterophilic antibodies are a heterogeneous group of IgM antibodies that are agglutinins against nonhuman red blood cells (e.g., horse, sheep) and are detected by qualitative (Monospot) or quantitative (heterophile antibody test) methods. Use of the Monospot test is limited because other infections (e.g., CMV, adenovirus) and toxoplasmosis also produce heterophilic antibodies. Thus 5% to 15% of Monospot tests yield false-positive results. Heterophilic antibodies in the blood increase as the condition progresses, although some individuals and children under 4 years of age do not produce them. Diagnosis of EBV infection specifically may be increased with newer viral-specific tests that identify EBV-specific antibodies. Because these tests are more expensive and labor intensive, they are reserved for instances when the Monospot is not appropriate.

Treatment is supportive and consists of rest and alleviation of symptoms with analgesics and antipyretics. Aspirin is avoided with children because of its association with Reye syndrome. Streptococcal pharyngitis, which occurs in 20% to 30% of cases, is treated with penicillin or erythromycin, not ampicillin—ampicillin is known to cause a rash. Bed rest with avoidance of strenuous activity and contact sports is indicated. Steroids are used when severe complications, such as impending airway obstruction, or other organ involvement (central nervous system [CNS] manifestations, thrombocytopenic purpura, myocarditis, pericarditis) is evident. Acyclovir has been used in immunocompromised individuals but is not considered standard therapy. IM and EBV infection were thought to be associated with chronic fatigue syndrome, but that is no longer the case.

> **✔ QUICK CHECK 20-2**
> 1. Explain the relationship between the early release of premature white blood cells and a "shift-to-the-left."
> 2. What is meant by "shift-to-the-right"?

Qualitative Alterations of Leukocytes
Leukemias

Leukemia is a clonal malignant disorder of the blood and blood-forming organs.[13] The common pathologic feature of all forms of leukemia is an uncontrolled proliferation of malignant leukocytes, causing an overcrowding of bone marrow and decreased production and function of normal hematopoietic cells.

The classification of leukemia is based on (1) the predominant cell of origin (either myeloid or lymphoid) and (2) the degree of differentiation that took place before the cell became malignant (acute, with a rapid growth of immature blood cells, or chronic, with a slow growth of more differentiated cells) (Figure 20-6). Thus there are four types of leukemia: acute lymphocytic (ALL) or myelogenous (AML) and chronic lymphocytic (CLL) or myelogenous (CML).[13-15] Further classification of acute leukemias is based on characteristics that may provide significant therapeutic prognostic information, such as structure, number of cells, genetics, identification of surface markers, and histochemical staining (see Figure 20-6).

Acute leukemia is characterized by undifferentiated or immature cells, usually a blast cell. The onset of disease is abrupt and rapid. Disease progression results in a short survival time. In chronic leukemia, the predominant cell is more mature but does not function normally. The onset of the disease is gradual, and the prolonged clinical course results in a relatively longer survival time.

Leukemia occurs with varying frequencies at different ages and is more common in adults than in children. It is estimated that more than 43,050 cases of leukemia will be newly diagnosed in 2010, with males having a slightly higher incidence than females (Table 20-5). ALL is the least common type (12% of all leukemias) overall, but it is the most common in children. Leukemia accounts for about 31% of all childhood cancers; ALL accounts for almost 74% of all new cases of leukemia in children. CLL and AML (35% and 29% of leukemias, respectively) are the most common types in adults. CML (11% of leukemias) is found mostly in adults. The sites of highest overall incidence are the United States, Canada, Sweden, and New Zealand.

Over the past 2 decades, remission induction rate and survival in most forms of leukemia have increased. Current survival rates range from 23% for AML to 74% for CLL. This progress is the result of more effective chemotherapeutic agents, improved blood product and

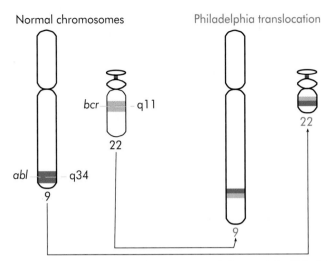

Normal chromosomes

Philadelphia translocation

bcr — q11

22

abl — q34

9

9

22

FIGURE 20-7 **Philadelphia Chromosome.** Schema of the Philadelphia (Ph) translocation (+) seen in chronic myelocytic leukemia. The Ph[1] chromosome results from an exchange of materials between chromosomes 9 and 22—that is, t(9;22)(q34;q11). Because chromosome 22 loses much more of its long arm than is translocated to it from chromosome 9, chromosome 22 becomes much abbreviated and is known as Ph[1]. (From Damjanov I, Linder J, editors: *Anderson's pathology,* ed 10, St Louis, 1996, Mosby.)

antimicrobial support, and specialized nursing care. Chemotherapy and bone marrow transplants have significantly increased the survival time for individuals with acute leukemia.

PATHOPHYSIOLOGY   Although the exact cause of leukemia is unknown, several risk factors and related genetic aberrations are associated with the onset of malignancy. There is a statistically significant tendency for leukemia to reappear in families. There is also an increased incidence of leukemia in association with other hereditary abnormalities such as Down syndrome, Fanconi aplastic anemia, Bloom syndrome, trisomy 13, Patau syndrome, and some immune deficiencies (ataxia-telangiectasia, Wiskott-Aldrich syndrome, congenital X-linked agammaglobulinemia; see Chapter 7).

Several genetic translocations (mitotic errors) are observed in leukemic cells. One of these translocations, the Philadelphia chromosome, is observed in 95% of those with CML and 30% of adults with ALL (Figure 20-7). The Philadelphia chromosome results from a reciprocal translocation between the long arms of chromosomes 9 and 22. A unique protein (*bcr-abl* protein) is encoded from two genes (*BCR* from chromosome 22 and *ABL* from chromosome 9) artificially linked at the junction of translocation. The *bcr-abl* protein affects a variety of cell cycle control genes leading to an increased rate of cellular division, inhibition of DNA repair, and other dysregulations of cell growth.

Risk factors for the onset of leukemia include environmental factors as well as other diseases. Increased risk has been linked to cigarette smoke, exposure to benzene, and ionizing radiation. Large doses of ionizing radiation particularly result in an increased incidence of myelogenous leukemia. Infections with HIV or hepatitis C virus increase the risk for leukemia, and it is now widely accepted that some types of leukemia are caused by infection with the human T cell leukemia/lymphoma virus-1 (HTLV-1). Drugs that cause bone marrow depression (e.g., chloramphenicol, phenylbutazone, and certain alkylating agents, such as Cytoxan) also can predispose an individual to leukemia. AML is the most frequently reported secondary cancer after high doses of

chemotherapy for Hodgkin lymphoma, non-Hodgkin lymphoma, multiple myeloma, ovarian cancer, and breast cancer. Acute leukemia also may develop secondary to certain acquired disorders, including CML, CLL, polycythemia vera, myelofibrosis, Hodgkin lymphoma, multiple myeloma, ovarian cancer, and sideroblastic anemia.

The leukemia blasts literally "crowd out" the marrow and cause cellular proliferation of the other cell lines to cease. Normal granulocytic-monocytic, lymphocytic, erythrocytic, and megakaryocytic progenitor cells cease to function, resulting in pancytopenia (a reduction in all cellular components of the blood).

Acute leukemias. About 85% of ALL arise from the B cell line, and about 15% arise from T cell lineage. A small percentage of ALL cases have neither B nor T cell origination and are called *null cell.* Acute leukemias are seen in both genders and in all ages, with the incidence increasing dramatically in individuals older than 50 years. Mortality for all acute leukemias in the United States is about 7 per 100,000. In children younger than 15 years, leukemia accounts for more deaths than any other cancer. However, leukemia deaths have declined 76% in children, ages newborn to 14 years, in the United States from 1969 to 2007. North American and Scandinavian countries have the highest mortality; Eastern European countries, Asia (except Japan), and Central America have the lowest mortality. In past years, Japan's mortality has been higher because of the atomic bombs dropped in World War II. Blacks have consistently shown a lower mortality than whites.

CLINICAL MANIFESTATIONS   The clinical manifestations of all varieties of acute leukemia are generally similar. Mechanisms associated with common manifestations are summarized in Table 20-6. Signs and symptoms related to bone marrow depression include fatigue caused by anemia, bleeding resulting from thrombocytopenia, and fever caused by infection. Bleeding may occur in the skin, gums, mucous membranes, and GI tracts. Visible signs include petechiae and ecchymosis, as well as discoloration of the skin, gingival bleeding, hematuria, and midcycle or heavy menstrual bleeding.

Infection sites include the mouth, throat, respiratory tract, lower colon, urinary tract, and skin and may be caused by gram-negative bacilli (*Escherichia coli*), *Pseudomonas*, and *Klebsiella*). Fever is an early sign often accompanied by chills.

Anorexia is accompanied by weight loss, diminished sensitivity to sour and sweet tastes, wasting of muscle, and difficulty swallowing. Liver, spleen, and lymph node enlargement occurs more commonly in ALL than in CML. Liver and spleen enlargement commonly occur together. The leukemic individual often experiences abdominal pain and tenderness and also breast tenderness.

Neurologic manifestations are common and may be caused by either leukemic infiltration or cerebral bleeding. Headache, vomiting, papilledema, facial palsy, blurred vision, auditory disturbances, and meningeal irritation can occur if leukemic cells infiltrate the cerebral or spinal meninges. Because most chemotherapeutic agents do not penetrate the blood-brain barrier, leukemia cells can grow easily in these locations.

EVALUATION AND TREATMENT   Because leukemia often is confused with other conditions, early detection is difficult. Persistent symptoms need intensive medical investigation. The diagnosis is made through blood tests and examination of bone marrow.

Chemotherapy, used in various combinations, is the treatment of choice for leukemia. Supportive measures include blood transfusions, antibiotics, antifungals, and antivirals. Allopurinol is used to prevent uric acid production and elevation that occurs because of cellular death caused by treatment. Bone marrow transplantation as a treatment has

TABLE 20-6 CLINICAL MANIFESTATIONS AND RELATED PATHOPHYSIOLOGY IN LEUKEMIA

CLINICAL MANIFESTATIONS	LABORATORY ABNORMALITIES	CAUSE	COMMENTS
Anemia	Relative *proportion* of erythroblasts to total count (decreased in anemia) is key	Decreased stem cell input or ineffective erythropoiesis or both	In acute leukemia, anemia is usually present from beginning, often first symptom noticed, and severe; mild form without symptoms is common in CML and CLL; hemorrhage common in acute forms, occasional in CML, but rare in CLL
Bleeding (purpura, petechiae, ecchymosis, hemorrhage)	Decreased and possibly abnormal platelets	Reduction in megakaryocytes leading to thrombocytopenia	Bleeding more common in acute than in chronic leukemia
Infection	Increased multisegmented neutrophils	Opportunistic organisms; decreased protection resulting from granulocytopenia or immune deficiency secondary to chemotherapy, corticosteroids, and disease process	Major sites of infection: oral cavity, throat, lower colon, urinary tract, lungs, and skin; prevention of infection focuses on restoration of host defenses, decreasing invasive procedures, and reducing colonization of organisms
Weight loss	Decreased 24-hr urinary creatinine excretion; hypoalbuminemia	Condition can be attributed to pain, depression, chemotherapy, radiation therapy, loss of appetite, and alterations in taste	Severe weight loss may be related to excess production of TNF-α
Bone pain	Often no radiographic evidence of bone problems	Result of bone infiltration by leukemic cells or intramedullary infection	If combination drug regimens are ineffective, radiation therapy is used
Liver, spleen, and lymph node enlargement	Biopsy abnormal for liver and spleen	Leukemic cell infiltration; lymph nodes also undergo leukemia proliferation in CLL	
Elevated uric acid level	Normal excretion of uric acid is 300-500 mg/day; leukemic individual can excrete 50 times more	Increased catabolism of protein and nucleic acid; urate precipitation increased from dehydration caused by anorexia or fever and drug therapy	Hyperuricemia is present in both acute leukemia and CML; increasing urine pH or decreasing acid production with drug allopurinol

CLL, Chronic lymphocytic leukemia; *CML,* chronic myelocytic leukemia; *RBC,* red blood cell.

increased since the 1980s. Survival rates have dramatically increased because of improvements in donor matching, transfusion support, conditioning regimens, and antibiotics.

The 5-year survival rate for those with leukemia is 38%, largely because of poor survival rates of individuals with certain types of leukemia (e.g., acute myelogenous). Since the 1970s, 5-year survival rates for those with ALL have increased from 38% to 66% for adults and from 53% to 91% for children. Factors influencing increased survival rate include the use of combined and multimodality treatment methods, improved supportive services such as blood banking and nutritional support, and antimicrobial treatment. The presence of the Philadelphia chromosome (observed in about 5% of children with ALL, in 30% of adults with ALL, and occasionally in AML) is a poor prognostic indicator.

Stimulation of blood cell growth and development with hematopoietic drugs has increased neutrophil recovery during chemotherapy and bone marrow transplant. Blood granulocyte numbers (e.g., eosinophils, neutrophils, basophils/mast cells) are normally in the range of 4000 to 6000 cells/μl, and susceptibility to infection develops below 1000 cells/μl. During a natural response to a bacterial infection, granulocytes usually rise in number to 10,000 to 20,000 cells/μl. Leukemia itself as well as the chemotherapeutic agents used to treat the disease can result in dramatic decreases in circulating granulocytes. The advent and administration of colony-stimulating factors (CSFs) (e.g., granulocytestimulating factors) can stimulate bone marrow production and raise white cell numbers and afford protection from infections (Table 20-7).

Chronic leukemias. The two main types of chronic leukemia are (1) myelogenous (CML) and (2) lymphocytic (CLL). Several forms of CML can occur, depending on the lineage of the malignant cells (e.g., chronic neutrophilic leukemia [CNL], chronic eosinophilic leukemia [CEL]). Unlike cells in acute leukemia, chronic leukemic cells are well differentiated and can be readily identified. Individuals with chronic leukemia have a longer life expectancy, usually extending several years from the time of diagnosis.

The chronic leukemias account for the majority of cases in adults (see Table 20-5). The incidences of CLL and CML increase significantly in individuals over 40 years of age, with prevalence in the sixth through eighth decades. CML is a group of diseases called **myeloproliferative disorders,** which also include polycythemia vera, primary thrombocytosis, and idiopathic myelofibrosis (invasion of bone marrow by fibrous tissue).

PATHOPHYSIOLOGY AND CLINICAL MANIFESTATIONS Chronic leukemia advances slowly and insidiously. Individuals are generally unaware of the condition until symptoms appear. When symptoms do appear, they present as splenomegaly, extreme fatigue, weight loss, night sweats, and low-grade fever. Individuals with CML may progress through three phases of the disease: a chronic phase lasting 2 to 5 years during which symptoms may not be apparent, an accelerated phase of 6 to 18 months during which the primary symptoms develop, and a terminal blast phase with a survival of only 3 to 6 months. The accelerated phase is characterized by excessive proliferation and accumulation of malignant cells. Splenomegaly is prominent and becomes painful, but lymphadenopathy generally is not present. Liver enlargement also occurs, but liver function is rarely altered. Hyperuricemia is common

TABLE 20-7 SOME EXAMPLES OF HUMAN COLONY-STIMULATING FACTORS

CSF	CELL ORIGIN	CELL STIMULATED
M-CSF	Macrophage, fibroblast	Macrophage
GM-CSF	T cell, macrophage, fibroblast	Neutrophil, monocyte, macrophage, eosinophils
G-CSF	Macrophage, fibroblast	Neutrophil, eosinophil, basophil
IL-3	T cell	Neutrophil, macrophage
Erythropoietin	Kupffer and peritubular kidney cells	Erythrocyte

Morphologic Effects of Growth Factor. Marrow aspirate from a patient receiving granulocyte colony-stimulating factor (G-CSF) showing an early neutrophil response. There is a marked shift toward immaturity in the neutrophils with the majority at the promyelocyte and early myelocyte stages of maturation. (Wright-Giemsa stain.) (Courtesy Laura Schmitz, MD, Hennepin County Medical Center, Minneapolis, Minn. From Damjanov I, Linder J, editors: Anderson's pathology, ed 10, St Louis, 1996, Mosby.)

and produces gouty arthritis. Infections, fever, and weight loss also are seen often. The terminal blast phase is characterized by rapid and progressive leukocytosis with an increase in basophils. In the later stages of the terminal phase, which then resembles AML, blast cells or promyelocytes predominate, and the individual experiences a "blast crisis."

The Philadelphia chromosome is a useful diagnostic marker for CML and is observed in 95% of individuals with CML. The median age for persons with Philadelphia chromosome-positive CML is 40 to 45 years. The Philadelphia chromosome, although present in red cells, white cells, and platelets, appears to affect only white cell function and production. Although it is difficult to identify alterations within the cell's structure, absent or low levels of the enzyme neutrophil alkaline phosphatase, along with decreased phagocytic capabilities, indicate that cells fail to differentiate normally. The only known cause of CML is exposure to ionizing radiation.

CLL involves predominantly malignant transformation of B cells; rarely (<5%) are T cells involved. The malignant transformation is thought to be caused by failure of the normal mechanisms of programmed cell destruction (apoptosis), allowing these cells to have an extended life, thus the chronic nature of the disease. These cells fail to develop into antibody-producing cells and fail to respond to stimulation by helper T cells.

Suppression of normal antibody production is the most significant effect in CLL. Individuals are thus at risk for recurrent bacterial and other infections that are commonly sensitive to antibodies. Anemia, thrombocytopenia, and neutropenia are typically present with overt CLL. Invasion of most organs by leukemic cells is uncommon, but infiltration of lymph nodes, liver, spleen, and salivary glands is observed. Central nervous system involvement and elevated blood levels of calcium are rare, whereas elevated levels of lactic dehydrogenase (LDH) and uric acid are common.

EVALUATION AND TREATMENT Therapeutic approaches include bone marrow transplantation, biologic response modifiers, and combination chemotherapy. Alone, state-of-the-art chemotherapy for CML does not cure the disease, prevent blastic transformation, or prolong the average survival time. New drugs, including imatinib mesylate, which is highly specific for CML, are being utilized. Bone marrow transplantation, when compared with biologic response modifiers

and combination chemotherapy, appears to increase the survival time more significantly. Allogeneic bone marrow transplant survival rates have increased from 20% to 30% in 1977 to approximately 55% in 2006 with the use of concurrent high-dose radiation, chemotherapy, and interferon therapy.

When to begin treatment for CLL is difficult to determine and is related to the degree of symptoms. Treatment consists of alkylating agent or purine analog chemotherapy. Steroids and, later, splenectomy also may be used to control leukocytosis and cytopenias. Radiation therapy may be used to alleviate lymphadenopathy. Late stages of the disease require combination chemotherapy. Regardless of the approach, cure rates for CLL are poor.

> ✔ **QUICK CHECK 20-3**
> 1. How are leukemias classified?
> 2. What is the pathogenesis of ALL?
> 3. What is the significance of the Philadelphia chromosome, and how is it related to leukemia?

ALTERATIONS OF LYMPHOID FUNCTION

Lymphadenopathy

Lymphadenopathy is characterized by enlarged lymph nodes (Figure 20-8). Lymph node enlargement occurs because of an increase in size and number of its germinal centers caused by proliferation of lymphocytes and monocytes (immature phagocytes) or invasion by malignant cells. Normally, lymph nodes are not palpable or are barely palpable. Enlarged lymph nodes are characterized by being palpable and often also may be tender or painful to touch, although not in all situations.

Localized lymphadenopathy (reactive lymph nodes) usually indicates drainage of an area associated with an inflammatory or infectious lesion. Generalized lymphadenopathy, associated with infection, occurs less often and is generally seen in the presence of malignant or nonmalignant disease. Lymphadenopathy is of more significance in adult disease than in children. The location and size of the enlarged nodes are important factors in diagnosing the cause of the lymphadenopathy, as are the individual's age, gender, and geographic location.

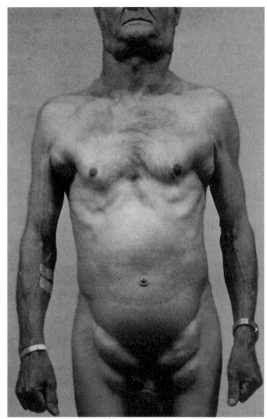

FIGURE 20-8 Lymphadenopathy. Individual with lymphocyte leukemia with extreme but symmetric lymphadenopathy. (Courtesy Dr. A.R. Kagan, Los Angeles. From del Regato JA, Spjut HJ, Cox JD: *Cancer: diagnosis, treatment, and prognosis*, ed 6, St Louis, 1985, Mosby.)

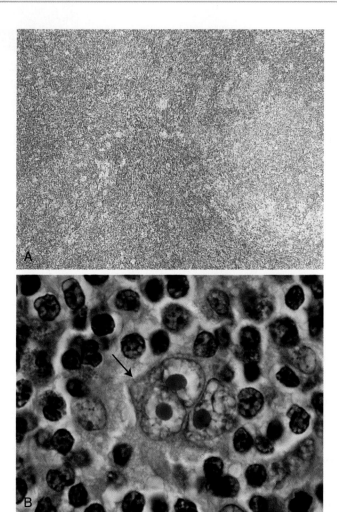

FIGURE 20-9 Lymph Nodes. **A,** Lymphocytes and histiocytes of Hodgkin lymphoma, nodular type. Large nodules with small, round lymphocytes, histiocytes, and scattered lymphocyte and histiocyte cells. **B,** Diagnostic Reed-Sternberg cell *(arrow)*. A large multinucleated or multilobed cell with inclusion body–like nucleoli surrounded by a halo of clear nucleoplasm. (From Damjanov I, Linder J, editors, *Anderson's pathology*, ed 10, St Louis, 1996, Mosby.)

Generalized lymphadenopathy occurs with non-Hodgkin lymphomas, chronic lymphocytic leukemia, histiocytosis, and disorders that produce lymphocytosis. In general, lymphadenopathy results from four types of conditions: (1) neoplastic disease, (2) immunologic or inflammatory conditions, (3) endocrine disorders, or (4) lipid storage diseases. Diseases of unknown cause, including autoimmune diseases and reactions to drugs, also may lead to generalized lymphadenopathy.

Malignant Lymphomas

Lymphomas consist of a diverse group of neoplasms that develop from the proliferation of malignant lymphocytes in the lymphatic system. The most recent classification of lymphomas was published by the World Health Organization (WHO) and is derived from the Revised European-American Lymphoma (REAL) Classification. This classification is based on the cell type from which the lymphoma probably originated. The groups include Hodgkin lymphoma and two that were previously classified as non-Hodgkin lymphoma (B cell neoplasms, T cell and NK cell neoplasms). With the new classification, multiple myeloma, which was previously classified independently, is included as a B cell lymphoma.

Incidence rates of lymphoma differ with respect to age, gender, geographic location, and socioeconomic class. The estimated new cases of lymphoma, including multiple myeloma, for 2010 are approximately 94,210 individuals. These consist of 8490 cases of Hodgkin lymphoma, 65,540 cases of non-Hodgkin lymphoma (except multiple myeloma), and 20,180 cases of multiple myeloma. It is estimated that 32,180 people will die from these diseases in 2010. Since the early 1970s, the

incidence of non-Hodgkin lymphoma has nearly doubled. The exact reason for this increase remains a mystery; however, a modest portion of the increase had been attributed to lymphomas developing in association with immune deficiencies, including AIDS and organ transplants. Conversely, the incidence of Hodgkin lymphoma has declined over the same time period, especially among elderly persons. In children under 15 years, Hodgkin lymphoma accounts for about 7.2% of childhood cancer and non-Hodgkin lymphoma for 6.6%. Currently the 5-year survival rates for children are 79% for all childhood cancers and 96% for Hodgkin lymphoma.

Hodgkin Lymphoma

PATHOPHYSIOLOGY Hodgkin lymphoma (HL) is characterized by its progression from one group of lymph nodes to another, the development of systemic symptoms, and the presence of Reed-Sternberg (RS) cells (Figure 20-9).[16] It is widely accepted that the RS cell represents the malignant transformation of lymph cells.[17] The RS cells are often large and binucleate, with occasional mononuclear variants. The RS cells

TABLE 20-8 SUBTYPES OF CLASSIC HODGKIN LYMPHOMA

SUBTYPE	INCIDENCE	PRESENTATION
Nodular sclerosis HL	Most common subtype in developing countries Found in all ages but most common in adolescents and young adults (median age of onset is about 28 yr) Incidence in females exceeds that in males	Large tumor nodules with RS cells surrounded by collagen and fibrous bands
Mixed cellularity HL	Second most common subtype Incidence in males exceeds that in females	RS cells with mixed inflammatory cell (lymphocytes, monocytes/macrophages, eosinophils, plasma cells) infiltrate
Lymphocyte-rich classic HL	Uncommon subtype Found in all ages but most common in adults Incidence in males exceeds that in females	Few RS cells and predominantly lymphocytic infiltration Usually localized at diagnosis Survival is long with or without treatment
Lymphocyte depletion HL	Uncommon subtype Most common type in elderly persons, HIV-positive individuals, and persons in nonindustrialized countries Incidence in males exceeds that in females	Large number of RS cells with less additional cellular infiltrate Usually widespread disease: abdominal lymphadenopathy; spleen, liver, and bone marrow involvement, without peripheral lymphadenopathy Stage is usually more advanced at diagnosis

are necessary for the diagnosis of HL; however, they are not specific to HL. In rare instances, cells resembling RS cells can be found in benign illnesses, as well as in other forms of cancer, including non-Hodgkin lymphomas and solid tissue cancers and in infectious mononucleosis.

The incidence of HL is approximately 3.0/100,000 males and 2.6/100,000 females and peaks at two different times—during the second and third decades of life and later during the sixth and seventh decades. The incidence is greater in whites than blacks, with Denmark, the Netherlands, and the United States having the highest incidence and Japan and Australia having the lowest. The overall incidence is lower in economically disadvantaged countries, although a greater proportion of HL is observed in the elderly in those countries.

The triggering mechanism for the malignant transformation of cells remains unknown. Classical HL appears to be derived from a B cell in the germinal center that has not undergone successful immunoglobulin gene rearrangement (see Chapter 6) and would normally be induced to undergo apoptosis. Survival of this cell may be linked to infection with Epstein-Barr virus (EBV). Laboratory and epidemiologic studies have linked HL with EBV infections and EBV DNA, RNA, and proteins are frequently observed in HL cells.[18] The RS cells secrete and release cytokines (e.g., IL-10, transforming growth factor-beta [TGF-β]) that result in the accumulation of inflammatory cells that produces the local and systemic effects. Classical HL is subclassified into four types (Table 20-8) based on the morphology of RS cells, and the characteristics of the inflammatory cell infiltrate in the tumor.

CLINICAL MANIFESTATIONS Many clinical features of HL can be explained by the complex action of cytokines and other growth factors that are secreted and released by the malignant cells. These substances induce infiltration and proliferation of inflammatory cells, resulting in an enlarged, painless lymph node in the neck (often the first sign of HL) (Figure 20-10). The discovery of an asymptomatic mediastinal mass on routine chest x-ray is not uncommon. The cervical, axillary, inguinal, and retroperitoneal lymph nodes are commonly affected in HL (Figure 20-11). Local symptoms caused by pressure and obstruction of the lymph nodes are the result of the lymphadenopathy.

About a third of individuals will have some degree of systemic symptoms. Intermittent fever, without other symptoms of infection, drenching night sweats, itchy skin (pruritus), and fatigue are relatively common. These constitutional symptoms accompanied by weight loss are associated with a poor prognosis. The Cotswold

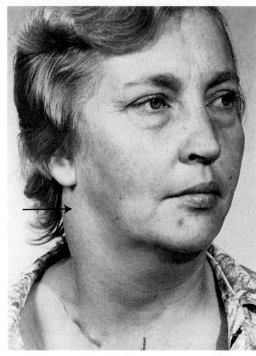

FIGURE 20-10 Hodgkin Lymphoma and Enlarged Cervical Lymph Node. Typical enlarged cervical lymph node in the neck *(arrow)* of a 35-year-old woman with Hodgkin lymphoma. (From del Regato JA, Spjut HJ, Cox JD: *Cancer: diagnosis, treatment, and prognosis,* ed 6, St Louis, 1985, Mosby.)

staging classification system used for HL is able to establish a correlation between the anatomic extent of the disease and the prognosis (Table 20-9). This classification system is based on the individual's medical history, examination (presence of symptoms and palpable lymph nodes), and other radiologic and hematologic results. Prognostic indicators include clinical stage, histologic type, tumor cell concentration and tumor burden, constitutional symptoms, and age.

Although HL rarely arises in the lung, mediastinal and hilar node adenopathy can cause secondary involvement of the trachea, bronchi, pleura, or lungs. Retroperitoneal nodes can involve vertebral bodies and nerves and also can cause displacement of ureters. Spinal cord

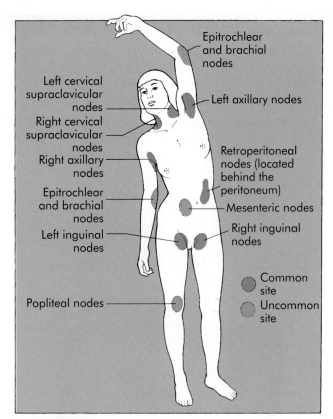

FIGURE 20-11 Common and Uncommon Involved Lymph Node Sites for Hodgkin Lymphoma.

TABLE 20-9	DEFINITIONS OF STAGES OF HODGKIN DISEASE
STAGE	**CRITERIA**
I	Involvement of a single lymph node region (I) or localized involvement of a single extralymphatic organ or site (I_E)*
II	Involvement of two or more lymph node regions on same side of diaphragm (II) or localized involvement of a single associated extralymphatic organ or site and its regional lymph node(s), with or without involvement of other lymph node regions on same side of diaphragm (II_E)
III	Involvement of lymph node regions on both sides of diaphragm (III), which may also be accompanied by localized involvement of an associated extralymphatic organ or site (III_E), by involvement of spleen (III_S), or by both (III_{E+S}).
IV	Disseminated (multifocal) involvement of one or more extralymphatic organs, with or without associated lymph node involvement, or isolated extralymphatic organ involvement with distant (nonregional) nodal involvement

A: No systemic symptoms present
B: Unexplained fevers >38° C, drenching night sweats, or weight loss >10% of body weight

From NCCN: Hodgkin lymphoma. In *NCCN practice guidelines in oncology Cold Spring Publishing Huntington New York,* vol 2, 2010. (Originally adapted from Carbono PP et al: Report of the Committee on Hodgkin's Disease Staging Classification, *Cancer Res* 31[11]: 1860–1861, 1971.)
*NOTE: The number of lymph node regions involved may be indicated by a subscript (e.g., II_3).

involvement is more common in the dorsal and lumbar regions than in the cervical region. Skin lesions, although uncommon, include psoriasis and eczematoid lesions, causing itching and scratching.

As a result of direct invasion from mediastinal lymph nodes, pericardial involvement can cause pericardial friction rub, pericardial effusion, and engorgement of neck veins. The GI tract and urinary tract are rarely involved. Anemia is often found in individuals with HL accompanied by a low serum iron level and reduced iron-binding capacity. Other laboratory findings include elevated sedimentation rate, leukocytosis, and eosinophilia. Leukopenia occurs in advanced stages of HL.

Splenic involvement in HL depends on histologic type. In mixed cellularity and lymphocytic deletion types of HL, the spleen is involved in 60% of cases. With lymphocyte and nodular sclerosis types, 34% of cases involve the spleen.

EVALUATION AND TREATMENT Because of the variability in symptoms, early definitive detection may be difficult. Asymptomatic lymphadenopathy can progress undetected for several years. Careful evaluation, including chest x-ray films, positron emission tomography (PET) scans, and biopsy, should be carried out for individuals with fever of unknown origin and peripheral lymphadenopathy. A lymph node biopsy with scattered RS cells and a cellular infiltrate is highly indicative of HL. The effectiveness of treatment is related to the age of the individual and the extent of the disease. Approximately 75% of individuals diagnosed with HL can be cured, largely because of successful treatment of HL with irradiation and chemotherapy. The 5-year survival rate is 83%.

Persons with stage III or IV disease, bulky disease (>10-cm mass or mediastinal disease with a transverse diameter exceeding 33% of the transthoracic diameter), or presence of B symptoms require combined chemotherapy with or without additional radiation treatment. Those with stage I or II disease are candidates for chemotherapy, combined chemotherapy, or radiation therapy alone. The survival rate depends on many factors, including the age and gender of the individual, the stage of the disease, and other variables. The 5-year survival rate in persons under age 20 is 96%; the survival rate for adults is 88%.

Non-Hodgkin Lymphomas

The previously used generic classification of **non-Hodgkin lymphoma** has been reclassified in the WHO/REAL scheme into (1) **B cell neoplasms,** a group that consists of a variety of lymphomas including myelomas that originate from B cells at various stages of differentiation, and (2) **T cell** and **NK cell neoplasms,** a group that includes lymphomas that originate from either T or NK cells. These cancers are differentiated from HL by lack of RS cells and other cellular changes not characteristic of HL.

Because malignant changes can occur at various stages of B cell, T cell, or NK cell development, these cancers present with a variety of clinical states. In the following section, the types of tumors previously classified as non-Hodgkin lymphoma are considered together, and myeloma is described separately.

PATHOPHYSIOLOGY As with all cancers, lymphomas most likely originate from mutations in cellular genes (many of which are environmentally induced) in a single cell that lead to loss of control of proliferation and other aspects of cell growth. The most common type of chromosomal alteration in non-Hodgkin lymphoma (NHL) is translocation, which disrupts the genes encoded at the breakpoints. Risk factors include a family history, exposure to a variety of mutagenic chemicals, irradiation, infection with certain cancer-related viruses

CHARACTERISTICS	NON-HODGKIN LYMPHOMA	HODGKIN LYMPHOMA
Nodal involvement	Multiple peripheral nodes	Localized to single axial group of nodes (i.e., cervical, mediastinal, paraaortic)
	Mesenteric nodes and Waldeyer ring commonly involved	Mesenteric nodes and Waldeyer ring rarely involved
Spread	Noncontiguous	Orderly spread by contiguity
B symptoms*	Uncommon	Common
Extranodal involvement	Common	Rare
Extent of disease	Rarely localized	Often localized

TABLE 20-10 CLINICAL DIFFERENCES BETWEEN NON-HODGKIN LYMPHOMA AND HODGKIN LYMPHOMA

*Fever, weight loss, night sweats.

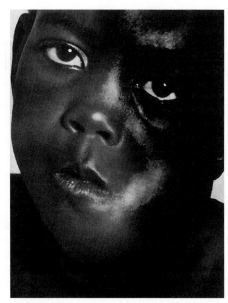

FIGURE 20-12 Burkitt Lymphoma. Burkitt lymphoma involving the jaw in a young African boy. (Courtesy Dr. J.N.P. Davies, Albany, NY. From del Regato JA, Spjut HJ, Cox JD: *Cancer: diagnosis, treatment, and prognosis,* ed 6, St Louis, 1985, Mosby.)

(e.g., Epstein-Barr virus, human herpesvirus-8, HIV, HTLV-1, hepatitis C), and immune suppression related to organ transplantation. Gastric infection with *Helicobacter pylori* increases the risk for gastric lymphomas. NHL is a disease of middle age, usually found in persons over 50 years old.

CLINICAL MANIFESTATIONS Clinical manifestations of NHL usually begin as localized or generalized lymphadenopathy, similar to HL. Differences in clinical features are noted in Table 20-10. The cervical, axillary, inguinal, and femoral chains are the most commonly affected sites. Generally, the swelling is painless and the nodes have enlarged and transformed over a period of months or years. Other sites of involvement are the nasopharynx, GI tract, bone, thyroid, testes, and soft tissue. Some individuals have retroperitoneal and abdominal masses with symptoms of abdominal fullness, back pain, ascites (fluid in the peritoneal cavity), and leg swelling.

EVALUATION AND TREATMENT Individuals with NHL can survive for extended periods. Survival with nodular lymphoma ranges up to 15 years. Individuals with diffuse disease generally do not survive as long. Overall, the survival rates for NHL are less than those for Hodgkin lymphoma. For NHL, the survival rates are 1 year, 80%; 5 years, 67%; and 10 years, 56%. Many investigators think that more aggressive treatment increases the cure rate. High-grade NHL is seen with increasing frequency in persons with AIDS and has an extremely poor prognosis.

Success of treatment is dependent on several parameters, including the type of lymphoma, stage of disease, cell type, involvement of organs outside the lymph nodes, age of the person, and the severity of the body's reaction to the disease (e.g., fever, night sweats, weight loss).[19] Treatment includes chemotherapy alone in many cases, although radiation therapy is frequently included. Low-dose chemotherapy has been followed by autologous stem cell transplantation in some individuals with NHL or for recurrent disease. Treatment of B cell lymphomas with rituximab has proven effective. Rituximab is a commercial monoclonal antibody against antigen CD20, which is expressed on the surface of all B cells, including malignant ones. Administration of rituximab depletes most B cells and allows the replenishment of normal B cells from the lymphoid stem cell pool. It has also proven useful

in a variety of autoimmune diseases, including immune thrombocytopenia purpura, autoimmune anemias, systemic lupus erythematosus, and rheumatoid arthritis.

Burkitt lymphoma. Burkitt lymphoma is a B cell tumor with unique clinical and epidemiologic features that accounts for 30% of childhood lymphomas worldwide. It occurs in children from east-central Africa and New Guinea and is characterized by a facial mass around the jaw (Figure 20-12). In the United States, Burkitt lymphoma is rare, usually involves the abdomen, and is characterized by extensive bone marrow invasion and replacement.

PATHOPHYSIOLOGY Epstein-Barr virus (EBV) is associated with almost all cases (>90%) of Burkitt lymphoma. It is suspected that suppression of the immune system by other illnesses (e.g., HIV infection, chronic malaria) increases the individual's susceptibility to EBV. B cells are particularly sensitive because of specific surface receptors for EBV. As a result, the B cell undergoes chromosomal translocations that result in overexpression of the *c-myc* proto-oncogene and loss of control of cell growth. The most common translocation (75% of individuals) is between chromosomes 8 (containing the *c-myc* gene) and 14 (containing the immunoglobulin heavy chain genes). Other translocations have been reported between chromosome 8 and chromosomes 2 or 22, which contain genes for immunoglobulin light chains.

CLINICAL MANIFESTATIONS In non-African Burkitt lymphoma the most common presentation is abdominal swelling. More advanced disease may involve other organs—eyes, ovaries, kidneys, glandular tissue (breast, thyroid, tonsil)—and presents with type B symptoms (night sweats, fever, weight loss).

EVALUATION AND TREATMENT The distribution of tumors and the results of biopsy of enlarged lymph nodes or the bone marrow containing malignant B cells are usually indicative of Burkitt lymphoma. It is one of the most aggressive and quickly growing malignancies. However, the African variety in children has been successfully treated with radiotherapy and cyclophosphamide (60% survival overall; 90%

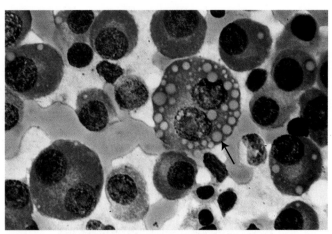

FIGURE 20-13 Multiple Myeloma, Bone Marrow Aspirate. Normal marrow cells are largely replaced by plasma cells, including atypical forms with multiple nuclei *(arrow),* and cytoplasmic droplets containing immunoglobulin. (From Kumar V, Abbas AK, Fausto N: *Robbins and Cotran pathologic basis of disease,* ed 7, Philadelphia, 2005, Saunders.)

survival with limited disease). The American type is more resistant to treatment.

Multiple myeloma. Multiple myeloma (MM) is a B cell cancer characterized by the proliferation of malignant plasma cells that infiltrate the bone marrow and aggregate into tumor masses throughout the skeletal system (Figure 20-13).[20] The reported incidence of MM has doubled in the past 2 decades, possibly as a result of more sensitive testing used for diagnosis. The annual incidence rate in the United States is 5/100,000, with 20,180 new cases estimated for 2010. Multiple myeloma occurs in all races, but the incidence in blacks is about twice that of whites. It rarely occurs before the age of 40 years—the peak age of incidence is about 70 years. It is slightly more common in men (11,170 estimated new cases) than women (9010 new cases). It is estimated that approximately 10,650 people in the United States will die of MM in 2010.

Neoplastic cells of multiple myeloma reside in the bone marrow and are usually not found in the peripheral blood. Occasionally, however, it may spread to other tissues, especially in very advanced disease. The basic defect is genetic, which may result from chronic stimulation of B cells with bacterial or viral antigens.

PATHOPHYSIOLOGY Most, if not all, multiple myelomas involve chromosomal translocations (breakpoints), which recur in many individuals. In about half of MM cases, one of the chromosomal partners is 14 (site of genes for the immunoglobulin heavy chain), which recombines with a number of other chromosomal sites of oncogenes, most commonly 11(q13), 4(p16), 16(q23), 20(q11), and 6(p25), resulting in probable dysregulation of the oncogenes. Breaks in 11q13 occur in about 25% of multiple myelomas and are associated with a more aggressive disease and a poorer prognosis. Deletions in chromosome 13 are observed in about 50% of cases. The molecular pathogenesis of multiple myeloma also involves proto-oncogene mutations and, more rarely, inactivation of tumor-suppressor genes. The precise timing and reason for the genetic alteration and accumulation are unknown.

Malignant plasma cells arise from one clone of B cells that produce abnormally large amounts of one class of immunoglobulin (usually IgG, occasionally IgA, and rarely IgM, IgD, or IgE). The malignant transformation may begin early in B cell development, possibly before encountering antigen in the secondary lymphoid organs. The myeloma

cells return to either the bone marrow or other soft tissue sites. Their return is aided by cell adhesion molecules that help them target favorable sites that promote continued expansion and maturation. Cytokines, particularly interleukin-6 (IL-6), have been identified as essential factors that promote the growth and survival of multiple myeloma cells. (Lymphocytes and cytokines are described in Chapter 6.)

Myeloma cells in the bone marrow produce several cytokines themselves (e.g., IL-6, IL-1, TNF-α). IL-6 in particular acts as an osteoclast-activating factor and stimulates osteoclasts to reabsorb bone. This process results in bone lesions and hypercalcemia (high calcium levels in the blood) attributable to the release of calcium from the breakdown of bone.

The antibody produced by the transformed plasma cell is frequently defective, containing truncations, deletions, and other abnormalities, and is often referred to as a paraprotein (abnormal protein in the blood). Because of the large number of malignant plasma cells, the abnormal antibody, called the **M protein,** becomes the most prominent protein in the blood (see Figure 20-15). Suppression of normal plasma cells by the myeloma results in diminished or absent normal antibodies. The excessive amount of M protein may also contribute to many of the clinical manifestations of the disease. If the myeloma produces IgM (Waldenström macroglobulinemia), the excessive amount of large molecule weight proteins (about 900,000 daltons) can lead to abnormally high blood viscosity (hyperviscosity syndrome). Frequently, the myeloma produces free immunoglobulin light chain (Bence Jones protein) that is present in the blood and urine and contributes to damage of renal tubular cells.

CLINICAL MANIFESTATIONS The common presentation of MM is characterized by elevated levels of calcium in the blood (hypercalcemia), renal failure, anemia, and bone lesions. The hypercalcemia and bone lesions result from infiltration of the bone by malignant plasma cells and stimulation of osteoclasts to reabsorb bone. This process results in the release of calcium (hypercalcemia) and development of "lytic lesions" (round, "punched out" regions of bone) (Figure 20-14). Destruction of bone tissue causes pain, the most common presenting symptom, and pathologic fractures. The bones most commonly involved, in decreasing order of frequency, are the vertebrae, ribs, skull, pelvis, femur, clavicle, and scapula. Spinal cord compression, because of the weakened vertebrae, occurs in about 10% of individuals.

Proteinuria is observed in 90% of individuals. Renal failure may be either acute or chronic and is usually secondary to the hypercalcemia. Bence Jones protein is present in about 80% of cases and may also lead to damage of the proximal tubules. Anemia is usually normocytic and normochromic and results from inhibited erythropoiesis caused by tumor cell infiltration of the bone marrow.

The high concentration of paraprotein in the blood, particularly associated with the large-molecular-weight IgM produced in Waldenström macroglobulinemia, may lead to hyperviscosity syndrome. The increased viscosity interferes with blood circulation to various sites (brain, kidneys, extremities). IgM paraprotein may also result in cryoglobulins (proteins that precipitate from the blood at lower than body temperature). Hyperviscosity syndrome is observed in up to 20% of persons. Additional neurologic symptoms (e.g., confusion, headaches, blurred vision) may occur secondary to hypercalcemia or hyperviscosity.

Suppression of the humoral (antibody-mediated) immune response results in repeated infections, primarily pneumonias and pyelonephritis. The most commonly involved organisms are encapsulated bacteria that are particularly sensitive to the effects of antibody; pneumonia caused by *Streptococcus pneumoniae, Staphylococcus aureus,* or *Klebsiella pneumoniae* or pyelonephritis caused by *Escherichia coli* or other

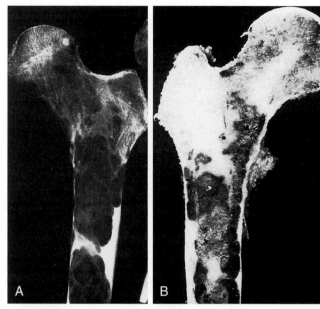

FIGURE 20-14 Multiple (Plasma Cell) Myeloma. A, Roentgeno-gram of femur showing extensive bone destruction caused by tumor. Note absence of reactive bone formation. B, Gross speci-men from same individual; myelomatous sections appear as dark granular sections. (From Kissane JM, editor: *Anderson's pathology*, ed 9, St Louis, 1990, Mosby.)

gram-negative organisms. Cell-mediated (T cell) function is relatively normal. Overwhelming infection is the leading cause of death from MM.

EVALUATION AND TREATMENT   Diagnosis of MM is made by symptoms, radiographic and laboratory studies, and a bone marrow biopsy. Quantitative measurements of immunoglobulins (IgG, IgM, IgA) are usually performed. Typically, one class of immunoglobulin (the M protein produced by the myeloma cell) is greatly increased, whereas the others are suppressed. Serum electrophoretic analysis shows increased levels of M protein (Figure 20-15). Because the M protein is monoclonal, each molecule has the same electric charge and migrates at about the same site on electrophoresis, resulting in a highly concentrated protein (M spike) (see Figure 20-15). Bence Jones protein is observed in the urine or serum by immunoelectrophoresis or in the serum using newly available enzyme-linked immunosorbent (ELISA) assays. Usually an intact antibody paraprotein coexists with Bence Jones protein. However, variants of MM include individuals in which free light chain only is produced and a rare variant that produces only free heavy chain. Measurement of another protein, free β_2-microglobulin, is used as an indicator of prognosis or effectiveness of therapy.

Although chemotherapy, radiation therapy, and marrow transplant have been used for treatment, the prognosis for persons with MM remains poor. A mainstay of all treatments is corticosteroids (prednisone and/or dexamethasone). Autologous peripheral blood stem cell transplantation is preferred to bone marrow transplantation. Controversial is whether tandem transplant offers the best outcome. Biphosphonate therapy is the primary treatment for bone lesions. However, individuals with multiple bone lesions, if untreated, rarely survive more than 6 to 12 months. Individuals with inactive (indolent) myeloma, however, can survive for many years. With chemotherapy and aggressive management of complications, the prognosis can improve significantly, with a median survival of 24 to 30 months and a 10-year survival rate of 3%. The 3-year survival for all stages of MM is 58%.

A recent addition to treatment of MM in individuals who have a relapse after conventional chemotherapy is the drug thalidomide. The use of thalidomide in treating MM is based on its suppression of TNF-α and its anti-angiogenesis ability.

> ✔ **QUICK CHECK 20-4**
> 1. Define multiple myeloma and discuss its pathogenesis.
> 2. Describe the features of a clonal disorder. Give an example.
> 3. How is lymphadenopathy related to infection?

Lymphoblastic lymphoma. Lymphoblastic lymphoma (LL) is a relatively rare variant of NHL overall (2% to 4%) but accounts for almost a third of cases of NHL in children and adolescents, with a male predominance. The vast majority of LL (90%) is of T cell origin, and the remainder arises from B cells. LL is similar to acute lymphoblastic leukemia and may be considered a variant of that disease.

PATHOPHYSIOLOGY   The disease arises from a clone of relatively immature T cells that becomes malignant in the thymus. As with most lymphoid tumors, LL is frequently associated with translocations, primarily of the chromosomes that encode for the T cell receptor (chromosomes 7 and 14). These aberrations result in increased expression of a variety of transcription factors and loss of growth control.

CLINICAL MANIFESTATIONS   The first sign of LL is usually a painless lymphadenopathy in the neck. Peripheral lymph nodes in the chest become involved in about 70% of individuals. Involved nodes are located mostly above the diaphragm. LL is a very aggressive tumor that presents as stage IV in most people. T cell LL is associated with a unique mediastinal mass (up to 75%) because of the apparent origin of the tumor in the thymus. The mass results in dyspnea and chest pain and may cause compression of bronchi or the superior vena cava. The tumor may infiltrate the bone marrow in about half of those affected, and suppression of bone marrow hematopoiesis leads to increased susceptibility to infections. Other organs, including the liver, kidney, spleen, and brain, may also be affected. Many individuals express type B symptoms: fever, night sweats, and significant weight loss.

EVALUATION AND TREATMENT   The most common therapeutic approach is combined chemotherapy. In early disease, the response rate is high with increased survival; the 5-year survival in children is 80% to 90%, and it is 45% to 55% in adults. Disease-free survival rates at 5 years range from 70% to 90% in children and from 45% to 55% in adults. Although LL is easily treated, there is a high relapse rate: 40% to 60% of adults.

ALTERATIONS OF SPLENIC FUNCTION

In the past, splenomegaly (enlargement of the spleen) has been associated with various disease states. It is now recognized that splenomegaly is not necessarily pathologic; an enlarged spleen may be present in certain individuals without any evidence of disease. Splenomegaly may be, however, one of the first physical signs of underlying conditions, and its presence should not be ignored. In conditions where splenomegaly is present, the normal functions of the spleen may become overactive, producing a condition known as hypersplenism.

Current diagnostic criteria for hypersplenism include: (1) anemia, leukopenia, thrombocytopenia, or combinations of these; (2) cellular bone marrow; (3) splenomegaly; and (4) improvement after

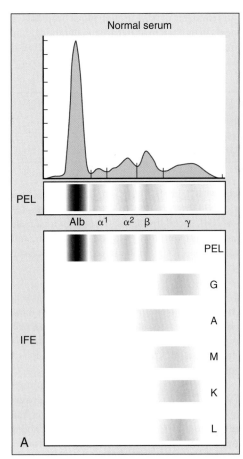

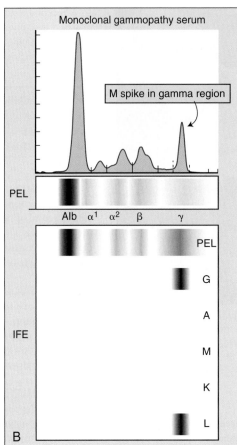

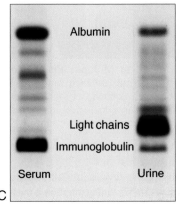

FIGURE 20-15 M Protein. Serum protein electrophoresis (PEL) is used to screen for M proteins in multiple myeloma. **A,** In normal serum the proteins separate into several regions between albumin (Alb) and a broad band in the gamma (γ) region, where most antibodies (gamma globulins) are found. Immunofixation (IFE) can identify the location of IgG (G), IgA (A), IgM (M), and kappa (K) and lambda (L) light chains. **B,** Serum from an individual with multiple myeloma contains a sharp M protein (M spike). The M protein is monoclonal and contains only one heavy chain and one light chain. In this instance the IFE identifies the M protein as an IgG containing a lambda light chain. **C,** Serum and urine protein electrophoretic patterns in an individual with multiple myeloma. Serum demonstrates an M protein (immunoglobulin) in the gamma region, and the urine has a large amount of the smaller-sized light chains with only a small amount of the intact immunoglobulin. (**A** and **B** from Abeloff M et al: *Abeloff's clinical oncology,* ed 4, Philadelphia, 2008, Churchill Livingstone. **C** from McPherson R, Pincus M: *Henry's clinical diagnosis and management by laboratory methods,* ed 21, Edinburgh, 2006, Saunders.)

splenectomy. Some individuals may seek treatment for problems even though they have not met all the above clinical criteria; therefore, the relevance and significance of hypersplenism are still uncertain. Primary hypersplenism is recognized when no etiologic factor has been identified; secondary hypersplenism occurs in the presence of another condition.

PATHOPHYSIOLOGY Overactivity of the spleen results in hematologic alterations that affect all three blood components. Splenic sequestering of red cells, white cells, and platelets results in a reduction of all circulating blood cells. Up to 50% of red cells may be sequestered; however, the rate of splenic pooling is directly related to spleen size and the degree of increased blood flow through it. Sequestering exposes the red cells to splenic activities, which accelerates their destruction, causing further reductions in red cell concentration. Anemia is the result of these combined actions. Anemia is further potentiated by an increased blood volume, producing a dilutional effect on the already reduced red cell concentration.

The white cells and platelets also are affected by sequestering, although not to the same degree as the red cell. The degree of red cell destruction and the diluting effect are determined by the degree of spleen enlargement.

CLINICAL MANIFESTATIONS Specific diseases or particular conditions related to the various classifications of splenomegaly are detailed in Box 20-1. Different pathologic processes that produce splenomegaly are briefly described here.

Acute inflammatory or infectious processes cause splenomegaly because of increased demand for defensive activities. An acutely enlarged spleen secondary to infection may become so filled with erythrocytes that its natural rubbery resilience is lost and it becomes fragile and vulnerable to blunt trauma. Splenic rupture is a complication associated with infectious mononucleosis.

Congestive splenomegaly is accompanied by ascites, portal hypertension, and esophageal varices and is most commonly seen in hepatic cirrhosis. Splenic hyperplasia develops in any disorder in which splenic workload is increased and is most commonly associated with various types of anemias (hemolytic) and chronic myeloproliferative disorders (i.e., polycythemia vera).

Infiltrative splenomegaly is caused by engorgement of the macrophages with indigestible materials associated with various "storage diseases." Tumors and cysts are neoplastic disorders that cause actual growth of the spleen. Metastatic tumors of the spleen are rare and may result from skin, lungs, breast, and cervical primary sites.

EVALUATION AND TREATMENT Treatment for hypersplenism is splenectomy; however, it may not always be indicated. A splenectomy is performed when its removal is considered necessary, eliminating its destructive effects on red cells. Clinical indicators should determine the needs for splenectomy, not necessarily specific conditions. Splenectomy for splenic rupture is no longer considered mandatory because of the possibility of overwhelming sepsis after removal. Repair and preservation should be considered before the decision to remove the spleen is made.

> ✔ **QUICK CHECK 20-5**
> 1. Contrast the principal features of Hodgkin lymphoma with those of non-Hodgkin lymphoma.
> 2. What is Burkitt lymphoma?
> 3. Identify the major causes of splenomegaly. How does it differ from hypersplenism?

ALTERATIONS OF PLATELETS AND COAGULATION

Disorders of Platelet Function

Quantitative or qualitative abnormalities of platelets can interrupt normal blood coagulation and prevent hemostasis. The quantitative abnormalities are thrombocytopenia, a decrease in the number of circulating platelets, and thrombocythemia, an increase in the number of platelets. Qualitative disorders affect the structure or function of individual platelets and can coexist with the quantitative disorders. Qualitative disorders usually prevent platelet adherence and aggregation, thereby preventing formation of a platelet plug.

Thrombocytopenia

Thrombocytopenia is defined as a platelet count below $150,000/mm^3$ of blood, although most individuals do not consider the decrease significant unless it falls below $100,000/mm^3$, and the risk for hemorrhage associated with minor trauma does not appreciably increase until the count falls below $50,000/mm^3$. Spontaneous bleeding without trauma can occur with counts ranging from $10,000/mm^3$ to $15,000/mm^3$. When this happens, skin manifestations (i.e., petechiae, ecchymoses, and larger purpuric spots) are observed or frank bleeding from mucous membranes occurs. Severe bleeding results if the count falls below $10,000/mm^3$ and can be fatal if it occurs in the gastrointestinal tract, respiratory tract, or central nervous system.

Before thrombocytopenia is diagnosed, the presence of a pseudothrombocytopenia must be ruled out. This phenomenon is seen in approximately 1 in 1000 to 10,000 samples and results from an error in platelet counting when a blood sample is analyzed by an automated cell counter. Platelets in the blood can become nonspecifically agglutinated by immunoglobulins in the presence of ethylenediaminetetraacetic acid (EDTA) and are not counted, thus giving an apparent, but false, thrombocytopenia. Thrombocytopenia also may be falsely diagnosed because of a dilutional effect observed after massive transfusion of platelet-poor packed cells to treat a hemorrhage. This is observed when more than 10 units of blood have been transfused within a 24-hour period. The precipitating hemorrhage also depletes platelets, contributing to the pseudothrombocytopenic state. Splenic sequestering of platelets in hypersplenism also stimulates thrombocytopenia. Hypothermia ($<25°$ C) also predisposes to a thrombocytopenic state, which is reversed when temperatures return to normal, suggesting sequestering and release.

PATHOPHYSIOLOGY Thrombocytopenia results from decreased platelet production, increased consumption, or both. The condition may also be either congenital or acquired and may be either primary or secondary to other conditions.[21,22] Thrombocytopenia secondary to congenital conditions occurs in a large number of different diseases, although each is relatively rare.[23] These include thrombocytopenia–absent radius (TAR) syndrome, Wiskott-Aldrich syndrome (see Chapter 7), various forms of *MYH9* gene mutation (e.g., May-Hegglin syndrome), X-linked thrombocytopenia, and many other examples.

Acquired thrombocytopenia is more common and may occur in relationship to acute viral infections (EBV, rubella, CMV, and HIV), drug reactions, autoimmune diseases, nutritional deficiencies, anemia (e.g., aplastic anemia), or cancer. Thrombocytopenia that results from decreased platelet production is usually the result of nutritional deficiencies (vitamin B_{12} or folic acid, in particular), some infections (e.g., HIV), drugs (e.g., thiazides, estrogens, quinine-containing medications, chemotherapeutic agents, ethanol), radiation therapy, bone marrow infiltration by some cancers, bone marrow hypoplasia (aplastic anemia), or chronic renal failure.

Most common forms of thrombocytopenia are the result of increased platelet consumption. Examples include heparin-induced thrombocytopenia, idiopathic (immune) thrombocytopenia purpura, thrombotic thrombocytopenia purpura, and disseminated intravascular coagulation (discussed later in this chapter).

Heparin-induced thrombocytopenia. Heparin is the most common cause of drug-induced thrombocytopenia.[24] Approximately 4%

of individuals treated with unfractionated heparin develop **heparin-induced thrombocytopenia (HIT).** The incidence is lower (about 0.1%) with the use of low-molecular-weight heparin. The onset of HIT is most common in people undergoing surgery. HIT is an immune-mediated, adverse drug reaction caused by IgG antibodies primarily against the heparin–platelet factor 4 complex. The IgG binds to platelet Fc receptors and activates platelet aggregation, release of additional platelet factor 4, and activation of thrombin, resulting in decreased platelet counts 5 to 10 days after heparin administration. If HIT is not recognized and treated, intravascular aggregation of platelets causes rapid development of arterial and venous thrombosis.

CLINICAL MANIFESTATIONS The hallmark of HIT is thrombocytopenia. However, 30% or more of those with thrombocytopenia are also at risk for thrombosis. Venous thrombosis is more common and results in deep venous thrombosis and pulmonary emboli. Arterial thrombosis affects the lower extremities, causing limb ischemia. Cardiovascular accidents and myocardial infarctions also may be experienced. Other major arteries (e.g., renal, mesenteric, upper limb) may be affected too.

EVALUATION AND TREATMENT Diagnosis is primarily based on clinical observations. The individual presents with dropping platelet counts after 5 days or longer of heparin treatment. On average, platelet counts may reach 60,000/mm^3. The onset of symptoms, including thrombosis, may be delayed until after release from the hospital. Most individuals are affected by HIT following surgery; therefore other possible causes of thrombocytopenia (e.g., infection, other drugs) must be considered. ELISAs and other tests are available to measure anti-heparin–platelet factor 4 antibodies. The sensitivity of this test is extremely high (>90%), but the specificity is less because of false-positive reactions (e.g., those receiving dialysis).

Treatment is the withdrawal of heparin and use of alternative anticoagulants. A switch to low-molecular-weight heparin is not indicated, and warfarin should not be used until the symptoms of HIT have resolved because of an increased risk of initiating skin necrosis. The thrombocytopenia should then progressively resolve. The chance of blood clots can be diminished using thrombin inhibitors (e.g., argatroban, lepirudin).

Idiopathic (immune) thrombocytopenia purpura. Most of the literature refers to thrombocytopenic purpura as **idiopathic** (no known cause) **thrombocytopenia purpura (ITP),** although the majority of cases are immune in nature.[25] ITP may be acute or chronic. The acute form is frequently observed in children and typically lasts 1 to 2 months with a complete remission. In some instances it may last for up to 6 months, and some children (7% to 28%) may progress to the chronic condition (see Chapter 19). Acute ITP is usually secondary to infections (particularly viral) or other conditions (such as systemic lupus erythematosus [SLE]) that lead to large amounts of antigen in the blood, such as exposure to some drugs. Under these conditions, the antigen usually forms immune complexes with circulating antibody, and it is thought that the immune complexes bind to Fc receptors on platelets, leading to their destruction in the spleen. The acute form of ITP usually resolves as the source of antigen is removed.

Chronic ITP is the primary form of the disease associated with the presence of autoantibodies against platelet-associated antigens. This form is more commonly observed in adults, being most prevalent in women between 20 and 40 years old, although it can be found in all age categories. The chronic form tends to get progressively worse. The autoantibodies are generally of the IgG class and are against one or more of several platelet glycoproteins (e.g., GPIIb/IIIa, GPIIb/IX,

GPIa/IIa). The antibodies bind directly to the platelet antigens, after which the antibody-coated platelets are recognized and removed from the circulation by macrophages in the spleen.

CLINICAL MANIFESTATIONS Initial manifestations range from minor bleeding problems (development of petechiae and purpura) over the course of several days to major hemorrhage from mucosal sites (epistaxis, hematuria, menorrhagia, bleeding gums). Rarely will an individual present with intracranial bleeding or other sites of internal bleeding.

EVALUATION AND TREATMENT Diagnosis is based on a history of bleeding and associated symptoms (weight loss, fever, headache). Physical examination includes notations on the types of bleeding, location, and severity of bleeding. In addition, evidence of infections (bacterial, HIV and other viral), medication history, family history, and evidence of thrombosis are assessed. Other diagnostic tests include complete blood count (CBC) and peripheral blood smear. Unlike some other forms of thrombocytopenia, there is usually no evidence of splenectomy. Testing for antiplatelet antibodies is usually not helpful. Although most cases of ITP are associated with elevated levels of IgG on platelets, other forms of thrombocytopenia also have a high incidence of platelet-associated IgG; thus, the sensitivity is low (50% to 65%). In addition, some cases of ITP will not present with elevated platelet-associated antibodies; the specificity is 75% to 94%, so that a negative test does not rule out ITP.

Treatment is palliative, not curative, focusing on prevention of platelet destruction by the spleen. Initial therapy for ITP is glucocorticoids (e.g., prednisone), which suppress the immune response and prevent sequestering and further destruction of platelets. If steroid therapy is ineffective, other reagents have been used. Treatment with intravenous immunoglobulin (IVIg) is used to prevent major bleeding. The response rate is 80%, but the effects are transient, lasting only days to a few weeks. Anti-Rh$_o$(D) (RhoGAM) has been used with limited success to treat individuals who are Rh positive.

If platelet counts do not increase appropriately, splenectomy is considered to remove the site of platelet destruction. However, splenectomy is not without risks, and approximately 10% to 20% of individuals who undergo a splenectomy suffer a relapse and require further treatment. In that situation, it is believed that the liver has become the site for platelet destruction. If splenectomy is unsuccessful, more aggressive immunosuppressive medications (e.g., azathioprine, cyclophosphamide) are usually recommended. Because of potential complications, these medications are reserved for individuals who are severely thrombocytopenic and refractive to other therapies.

Thrombotic thrombocytopenia purpura. **Thrombotic thrombocytopenia purpura (TTP)** is a life-threatening multisystem disorder that is characterized by thrombotic microangiopathy, which includes microangiopathic hemolytic anemia and occlusion of arterioles and capillaries by aggregated platelets within the microcirculation.[26,27] Aggregation may lead to increased platelet consumption and organ ischemia. TTP is relatively uncommon, occurring in about 5:1,000,000 individuals per year. The incidence of TTP is increasing and does appear to be an actual increase and not just the result of improved recognition.

There are two types of TTP: familial and acquired idiopathic. The familial type is the more rare type and is usually chronic, relapsing, and usually seen in children. When recognized and treated early, the child experiences predictable recurring episodes approximately every 3 weeks that are responsive to treatment. Acquired TTP is more common and more acute and severe. It occurs mostly in females in their thirties and is rarely observed in infants and the elderly.

Most cases of TTP are related to a dysfunction of the plasma metalloprotease ADAMTS13. This enzyme is responsible for cutting large precursor molecules of von Willebrand factor (vWF) produced by endothelial cells into smaller molecules. Defects in ADAMTS13 result in expression of large-molecular-weight vWF on the endothelial cell surface and the formation of large aggregates of platelets, which can break off and form occlusions in smaller vessels. People with TTP (about 80%) have <5% of normal plasma ADAMTS13 levels. Most individuals with familial TTP are homozygous for mutations in ADAMTS13. Acquired TTP of unexplained origin is associated in most (44% to 94%) people with an IgG autoantibody against ADAMTS13 that is able to neutralize the enzyme's activity and accelerate its clearance from the plasma.

CLINICAL MANIFESTATIONS TTP is clinically related to and must be distinguished from other thrombotic microangiopathic conditions, including hemolytic uremic syndrome, malignant hypertension, preeclampsia, and pregnancy-induced HELLP (*h*emolysis, *e*levated *l*iver enzymes, *l*ow *p*latelet count) syndrome. Early diagnosis and treatment is essential because TTP may prove fatal within 90 days of onset if untreated.

Acute idiopathic TTP is characterized by a pentad of symptoms, including extreme thrombocytopenia (<20,000/mm³), intravascular hemolytic anemia, ischemic signs and symptoms most often involving the central nervous system (about 65% present with memory disturbances, behavioral irregularities, headaches, or coma), kidney failure (65%), and fever (33%).

EVALUATION AND TREATMENT A routine blood smear usually shows fragmented red cells (*schizocytes*) produced by shear forces when red cells are in contact with the fibrin mesh in clots that form in the vessels. As a result of tissue injury, serum levels of lactate dehydrogenase (LDH) may be very high, and low-density lipoprotein (LDL) levels may be elevated. Tests for antibody on red cells are negative, excluding immune hemolytic anemia.

Plasma exchange with fresh frozen plasma, which replenishes functional ADAMTS13, is the treatment of choice, achieving a 70% to 80% response rate. Additionally, steroids (glucocorticoids) are administered. Nonresponse to conventional therapy may require a splenectomy; however, postoperative hemorrhage remains a dangerous complication. Immunosuppressive (azathioprine) therapy has been successful in some individuals. Agents that target ADAMTS13 autoantibody production by B cells (e.g., anti-CD20 monoclonal antibodies) are being studied and may potentially shorten the duration of plasma exchange treatment and reduce relapses.

Thrombocythemia

Thrombocythemia (also called thrombocytosis) is defined as a platelet count greater than 400,000/mm³ of blood.[28] Thrombocythemia may be primary or secondary (reactive) and is usually asymptomatic until the count exceeds 1 million/mm³. Then intravascular clot formation (thrombosis), hemorrhage, or other abnormalities can occur.

PATHOPHYSIOLOGY Essential (primary) thrombocythemia (ET) is a myeloproliferative disorder in which platelet production increases, resulting in platelet counts in excess of 600,000/mm³. It can occur in individuals at most any age. Manifestations include increased numbers of bone marrow megakaryocytes, splenomegaly, and periodic episodes of hemorrhage or thrombosis, or both. The thrombocythemia is secondary to increased plasma thrombopoietin levels resulting from defects in the thrombopoietin receptor. The defective receptor cannot adequately bind and remove thrombopoietin from the blood; thus circulating levels remain high. Along with increased platelets, there may be a concomitant increase in the number of red cells, indicating a myeloproliferative disorder; however, the increase in red cells is not to the extent seen in polycythemia vera.

Secondary thrombocythemia may occur after splenectomy because platelets that normally would be stored in the spleen remain in circulating blood. The increase in platelets may be gradual, with thrombocythemia not occurring for up to 3 weeks after splenectomy. Reactive thrombocythemia may occur during some inflammatory conditions, such as rheumatoid arthritis and cancers. In these conditions, excessive production of some cytokines (e.g., IL-6, IL-11) may induce increased production of thrombopoietin in the liver, resulting in increased megakaryocyte proliferation. Reactive thrombocythemia may also occur during a variety of physiologic conditions, such as after exercise.

CLINICAL MANIFESTATIONS Clinical manifestations vary among individuals. Those with ET are at risk for large-vessel arterial or venous thrombosis, and ischemia in the fingers, toes, or cerebrovascular regions is common. Digital ischemia is characterized by warm, congested red extremities with a burning sensation, particularly on the forefoot sole and toes. The lower extremities are affected more often, and only one side may be involved. Standing, exercising, or applying heat precipitates the pain, which is relieved by elevation and cooling of the affected extremity. In extreme situations, acrocyanosis and gangrene may result.

Thrombosis of arteries is more common than of veins, and myocardial and renal arteries may be involved. The carotid, mesenteric, and subclavian arteries also may be affected. Myocardial ischemia and infarction have occurred without clear evidence of coronary artery disease.

Involvement of the nervous system is manifested by headache and dizziness, with paresthesias, transient ischemic attacks, strokes, visual disturbances, and seizures also being reported. Major thrombotic events, not directly related to platelet count, occur in about 20% to 30% of individuals with ET. Other risk factors (prior thrombosis, age, and duration of ET) are better predictors of future thrombosis.

Although thrombosis is the more common symptom, hemorrhage can also occur. Sites for bleeding include the GI tract, skin, urinary tract, gums, joints, and brain. GI bleeding may be mistaken for a duodenal ulcer. Hemorrhage is not severe and generally occurs in the presence of very high platelet counts; transfusions are required only occasionally. Bleeding and clotting may occur simultaneously, and individuals are not necessarily prone to one or the other.

EVALUATION AND TREATMENT Initial diagnosis is not difficult; as many as two thirds of cases are diagnosed from a routine complete blood cell count (CBC). Secondary thrombocytosis also may occur as a moderate rise in the platelet count that resolves with treatment or resolution of the underlying condition.

Essential thrombocythemia is diagnosed by a platelet count that exceeds 600,000/mm³ and remains elevated, with no other indicated cause, such as arthritis, iron deficiency anemia, cancer, or splenectomy. Many individuals present with a mild anemia and a slightly elevated white blood cell count.

Hydroxyurea (HU), a nonalkylating myelosuppressive agent, is used to suppress platelet production and at one time was the drug of choice for treating ET; however, long-term therapy with this drug may cause progression to other myeloplastic disorders, particularly acute myeloid leukemia. Other drugs used to treat ET include aspirin and interferon-alpha (IFNα). IFNα may not be effective for everyone and aspirin, with its blood thinning properties, may cause hemorrhage. Anagrelide is now the drug of choice. Anagrelide interferes with platelet maturation rather than production, thus not interfering with red and white cell growth and development.

Alterations of Platelet Function

Qualitative alterations in platelet function are characterized by an increased bleeding time in the presence of a normal platelet count. Associated clinical manifestations include spontaneous petechiae and purpura and bleeding from the GI tract, genitourinary tract, pulmonary mucosa, and gums. Congenital alterations in platelet function (thrombocytopathies) are quite rare and may be categorized into several types of disorders: (1) platelet–vessel wall adhesion (e.g., defect in GPIb expression [Bernard-Soulier syndrome]), (2) platelet-platelet interactions (e.g., defect in GPIIb/IIIa expression [Glanzmann thrombasthenia]), (3) platelet granules and secretion (e.g., receptor defects [ADP, collagen]), (4) arachidonic acid pathways (e.g., thromboxane synthase deficiency), (5) cytoskeletal function (e.g., Wiskott-Aldrich syndrome [see Chapter 7]), and (6) membrane phospholipid regulation (coagulation protein-platelet interactions) (e.g., Scott syndrome).

Acquired disorders of platelet function are more common than the congenital disorders and may be categorized into three principal causes: (1) drugs, (2) systemic conditions, and (3) hematologic alterations.

Multiple drugs are known to affect platelet function by interfering with platelet function in three ways: (1) inhibition of platelet membrane receptors, (2) inhibition of prostaglandin pathways, and (3) inhibition of phosphodiesterase activity. Aspirin is the most commonly used drug that affects platelets. It irreversibly inhibits cyclooxygenase function for several days after administration. Nonsteroidal anti-inflammatory drugs also affect cyclooxygenase, although in a reversible fashion. Diet can affect platelet function (see *Health Alert:* Dark Chocolate, Wine, and Platelet-Inhibitory Functions).

Systemic disorders that affect platelet function are chronic renal disease, liver disease, cardiopulmonary bypass surgery, and severe deficiencies of iron or folate. Hematologic disorders associated with platelet dysfunction include chronic myeloproliferative disorders, multiple myeloma, leukemias, and myelodysplastic syndromes.

HEALTH ALERT

Dark Chocolate, Wine, and Platelet-Inhibitory Functions

An increasing number of foods have been reported to have platelet-inhibitory functions. Recent studies showed flavanol-rich cocoa inhibited several measures of platelet activity. Dark chocolate contains much more cocoa than does light chocolate. Additional cardioprotective effects may include antioxidant properties and activation of nitric oxide (NO). Low to moderate consumption of red wine reportedly has a greater benefit than other alcoholic beverages on cardioprotective mechanisms. Emerging are the effects of the polyphenol resveratrol known to be abundant in red wine. Investigators documented that the polyphenolic antioxidants, resveratrol, and proanthocyanidins provide cardioprotection by their function in vivo as antioxidants.

Data from Corti R et al: Cocoa and cardiovascular health, *Circulation* 119(10):1433–1441, 2009; Djousse L et al: Chocolate consumption is inversely associated with prevalent coronary heart disease: The National Health, Lung and Blood Institute Heart Study, *Clin Nutr* 2010 Sept 9 [Epub ahead of print]; Flammer AJ et al: Dark chocolate improves coronary vasomotion and reduces platelet reactivity, *Circulation* 116(21):2376–2382, 2007; Pearson DA et al: Flavanols and platelet reactivity, *Clin Dev Immunol* 12(1):1–9, 2005.

Disorders of Coagulation

Disorders of coagulation are usually caused by defects or deficiencies of one or more of the clotting factors. (Normal function of the clotting factors is described in Chapter 19.) Qualitative or quantitative abnormalities interfere with or prevent the enzymatic reactions that transform clotting factors, circulating as plasma proteins, into a stable fibrin clot (see Figure 19-17).

Some clotting factor defects are inherited and involve one single factor, such as the hemophilias and von Willebrand disease, caused by deficiencies of clotting factors. Other coagulation defects are acquired and tend to result from deficient synthesis of clotting factors by the liver. Causes include liver disease and dietary deficiency of vitamin K.

Other coagulation disorders are attributed to pathologic conditions that trigger coagulation inappropriately, engaging the clotting factors and causing detrimental clotting within blood vessels. For example, any cardiovascular abnormality that alters normal blood flow by acceleration, deceleration, or obstruction can create conditions in which coagulation proceeds within the vessels. An example of this is thromboembolic disease, in which blood clots obstruct blood vessels. Coagulation is also stimulated by the presence of tissue factor that is released by damaged or dead tissues. Vasculitis, or inflammation of the blood vessels, along with vessel damage activates platelets, which in turn activates the coagulation cascade. In extensive or prolonged vasculitis, blood clot formation can suppress mechanisms that normally control clot formation and dissolution, leading to clogging of the vessels. In each of these acquired conditions, normal hemostatic function proves detrimental to the body by consuming coagulation factors excessively or by overwhelming normal control of clot formation and breakdown (fibrinolysis) (see Figure 19-19).

Impaired Hemostasis

Impaired hemostasis, or the inability to promote coagulation and the development of a stable fibrin clot, is commonly associated with liver dysfunction, which may be caused by either specific liver disorders or lack of vitamin K.

Vitamin K deficiency. Vitamin K, a fat-soluble vitamin, is required for the synthesis of prothrombin; the procoagulant factors II, VII, IX, and X; and the anticoagulant factors (proteins C and S). Parenteral administration of vitamin K is the treatment of choice and usually results in correction of the deficiency. Fresh frozen plasma also may be administered but is usually reserved for individuals with life-threatening hemorrhages or those who require emergency surgery.

Liver disease. Individuals who have liver disease present with a broad range of hemostatic derangements that may be characterized by defects in the clotting or fibrinolytic system and by platelet dysfunction. The usual sequence of events is an initial reduction in clotting factors, which parallels the degree of liver cell damage or destruction. Factor VII is the first to decline because of its rapid turnover, followed by a decrease in the levels of factors II and X. Factor IX levels are less affected and do not decline until the liver destruction is well advanced. Protein C (an antithrombin) levels decline early, similar to levels of factor VII, and protein S (also an antithrombin) levels decline in the later stages of liver disease. Declines of factor V levels are of special importance because factor V plasma levels appear to be a direct reflection of liver cell damage.

Other alterations of hemostasis in liver disease include an increase in fibrinolytic activity that either is primary in origin or is a manifestation secondary to disseminated intravascular coagulation (DIC). This increased fibrinolysis results from excessive fibrinolytic activators and decreased levels of inhibitors, such as α_2-antiplasmin.

Thrombocytopenia and thrombocytopathies are manifestations of liver disease. Thrombocytopenia is caused by splenomegaly, which often accompanies liver disease. Splenic pooling of platelets is the major cause of thrombocytopenia. Thrombocytopathies are associated with elevated levels of fibrin split products, ethanol, or drugs.

Treatment of hemostasis alterations in liver disease must be comprehensive to cover all aspects of dysfunctions. Fresh frozen plasma (FFP) administration is the treatment of choice; however, not all individuals tolerate the volume needed to adequately replace all deficient factors. Alternative modalities include the addition of exchange transfusions and platelet concentration to FFP administration.

Consumptive Thrombohemorrhagic Disorders

Consumptive thrombohemorrhagic disorders are a heterogeneous group of conditions that demonstrate the entire spectrum of hemorrhagic and thrombotic pathologic findings. The symptoms of these disorders also range from the subtle to the devastating and are generally considered to be intermediary disease processes that complicate a vast number of primary disease states. These disorders are also characterized by confusion and controversy related to their diagnosis, treatment, and management. No one term is capable of covering all the possible varieties of these disorders; however, DIC is most commonly used in the clinical setting to describe a pathologic condition that is associated with hemorrhage and thrombosis.

Disseminated intravascular coagulation. **Disseminated intravascular coagulation (DIC)** is an acquired clinical syndrome characterized by widespread activation of coagulation, resulting in formation of fibrin clots in medium and small vessels throughout the body.[29] Widespread clotting may lead to blockage of blood flow to organs, resulting in multiple organ failure. The magnitude of clotting may cause consumption of platelets and clotting factors, leading to severe bleeding.

The clinical course of DIC is largely determined by the intensity of the stimulus, the response of the host, and the comorbidities, ranging from an acute, severe, life-threatening process that is characterized by massive hemorrhage and thrombosis to a chronic, low-grade condition. The chronic condition is characterized by subacute hemorrhage and diffuse microcirculatory thrombosis. DIC may be localized to one specific organ or generalized, involving multiple organs.

PATHOPHYSIOLOGY   Coagulation is designed to function at local areas of vascular damage, resulting in cessation of bleeding and activation of repair to the vessels. DIC results from abnormally widespread and ongoing activation of clotting.

A variety of conditions are associated with DIC (Box 20-2). Infectious disease, particularly involving sepsis, is the most common condition associated with DIC. Although all types of infections may cause DIC, bacterial infections (both gram-negative and gram-positive) are the most commonly observed underlying causes. DIC may occur in up to 50% of persons with gram-negative sepsis. Most solid tumors and hematologic cancers may trigger DIC. Approximately 15% of those with metastatic cancer or acute leukemia have symptoms of DIC. Severe trauma, especially to the brain, can induce DIC. DIC occurs in about two thirds of individuals with a systemic inflammatory response to the trauma. Some complications of pregnancy are also associated with DIC; incidences range from 50% for women with placental abruptions to less than 10% for severe preeclampsia.

Regardless of the underlying disease that initiates DIC, the common pathway appears to be excessive and widespread exposure of tissue factor (TF or tissue thromboplastin) (Figure 20-16). This may occur

---

BOX 20-2   CONDITIONS ASSOCIATED WITH DIC

Malignancy: acute leukemias, metastatic solid malignancies
Infections: bacterial (gram-negative endotoxin, gram-positive mucopolysaccharides), viral (hepatitis, varicella, cytomegalovirus), fungal, parasitic
Pregnancy complications: eclampsia/preeclampsia, placental abruption, amniotic fluid embolism
Severe trauma: head injury, burns, crush injuries, tissue necrosis
Liver disease: obstructive jaundice, acute liver failure
Intravascular hemolysis: transfusion reactions, drug-induced hemolysis
Medical devices: aortic balloon, prosthetic devices
Hypoxia and low blood flow states: arterial hypotension secondary to shock, cardiopulmonary arrest

Data from Bick RL et al: *Hematology: clinical and laboratory practice,* St Louis, 1993, Mosby.

---

by several mechanisms. Widespread damage to vascular endothelium results in exposure of subendothelial tissue factor. Several types of cells either alter induction by cytokines or constitutively express TF on their surface. Endothelial cells and monocytes do not normally express surface TF unless stimulated by inflammatory cytokines (particularly IL-6 and TNF-α). These cytokines are abundantly produced during many of the conditions listed in Box 20-2. Many tumors express surface TF or produce cytokines that can stimulate TF expression by endothelium, monocytes, or both.

TF binds clotting factor VII, which undergoes activation to factor VIIa (also see Figure 19-18). The TF-VIIa complex is a potent activator of clotting factors IX and X, which leads to conversion of prothrombin to thrombin and formation of fibrin clots. This pathway appears to be the primary route by which DIC is initiated; in animal models of DIC, inhibition of TF or factor VIIa completely prevents the generation of thrombi by gram-negative bacterial endotoxin.

Not only is the clotting system extensively activated in DIC, but also the predominant natural anticoagulants (tissue factor pathway inhibitor, antithrombin III, protein C) are greatly diminished. Tissue factor pathway inhibitor (TFPI) in association with factor Xa inactivates the TF-VIIa complex, preventing further activation of clotting. Antithrombin III (AT-III) is the principal inhibitor of thrombin, preventing further activation of fibrinogen to fibrin. Protein C is activated by thrombin to form activated protein C, which uses protein S as a cofactor to degrade factors Va and VIIIa. The rate of protein C activation increases dramatically if thrombin has first bound to the membrane protein thrombomodulin on the endothelial cell surface. During DIC, the activation of clotting is prolonged by the increased rate of consumption, as well as decreased synthesis, of these inhibitors and protein S and by cytokine-mediated decreased expression of thrombomodulin on the endothelial cell surface. Thus clotting is initiated concurrently with loss of regulation of the extent of thrombosis.

The rate of fibrinolysis is also diminished in DIC. The primary component of fibrinolysis is **plasmin,** which exists in the circulation as an inactive precursor, plasminogen. Plasminogen is activated to plasmin by a variety of substances, including thrombin, fibrin, tissue plasminogen activator (t-PA), and other molecules. Plasmin is an enzyme that digests fibrin clots, thus controlling the extent of fibrin deposition in the vessels. During DIC, the activity of plasmin is diminished by increased production of its natural inhibitor, plasminogen-activator inhibitor type I. Although some fibrinolytic activity remains, the level

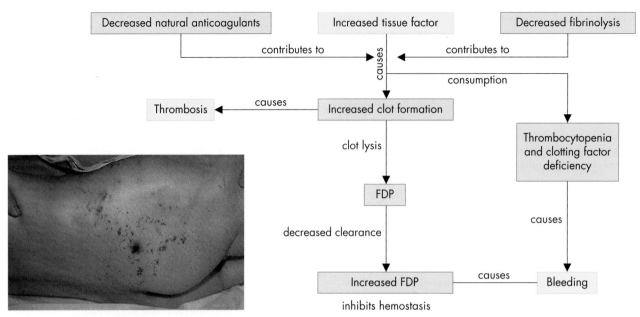

FIGURE 20-16 Pathophysiology of Disseminated Intravascular Coagulation (DIC). Tissue factor initiates clot formation and this effect is increased by a decrease in natural anticoagulants (tissue factor inhibitor, antithrombin-III, and protein C). There also is a reduction in clot breakdown or fibrinolysis by plasmin. The combined effect is to cause thrombosis. The thrombotic activity consumes (uses up) coagulation factors and platelets, which can increase bleeding. Slow degradation of the fibrin clot produces fibrin degradation products (FDPs). FDPs have inhibitory effects on thrombin and platelets. The inhibition of coagulation, combined with the depletion of factors and platelets, then creates a bleeding tendency. Uncontrolled DIC will eventually lead to multiple end-organ failure. For further details of these mechanisms see Chapters 5 and 23. Inset is an example of DIC resulting from staphylococcal septicemia. Note the characteristic skin hemorrhage ranging from small purpuric lesions to larger ecchymoses.

is inadequate to control the systemic deposition of fibrin. The slow breakdown of fibrin by plasmin produces fibrin degradation products that are released into the blood. These are potent anticoagulants that are normally removed from blood by fibronectin and macrophages. During DIC, the presence of fibrin degradation products is prolonged, probably because of diminished production of fibronectin. Low levels of fibronectin suggest a poor prognosis.

Although thrombosis is generalized and widespread, individuals with DIC are paradoxically at risk for hemorrhage. Hemorrhage is secondary to the abnormally high consumption of clotting factors and platelets, as well as the anticoagulant properties of fibrin degradation products. Thrombin causes platelet activation and aggregation—an event that occurs early in the development of DIC—which facilitates microcirculatory coagulation and obstruction in the initial phase. However, platelet consumption exceeds production, resulting in a thrombocytopenia that increases bleeding.

Activation of clotting also leads to activation of other inflammatory pathways, including the kallikrein-kinin and complement systems (see Chapter 5). Factor XIIa, generated in DIC, converts prekallikrein to kallikrein, ultimately resulting in conversion to circulating kinins. Activation of these systems contributes to increased vascular permeability, hypotension, and shock. Activated complement components also induce platelet destruction, which initially contributes to the thrombosis and later to the thrombocytopenia.

The deposition of fibrin clots in the circulation interferes with blood flow, causing widespread organ hypoperfusion. This condition may lead to ischemia, infarction, and necrosis, further potentiating and complicating the existing DIC process by causing further release of TF and eventually organ failure.

In addition to initiation of clotting by tissue factor, DIC may be precipitated by direct proteolytic activation of factor X. This has been described as thrombin mimicry and is the result of proteases directly converting fibrinogen to fibrin. These proteases may come from snake venom, some tumor cells, or the pancreas and liver, where they are respectively released during episodes of pancreatitis and various stages of liver disease. Direct proteolytic activity appears to be independent of any type of damage to the endothelium or tissue.

Whatever initiates the process of DIC, the cycle of thrombosis and hemorrhage persists until the underlying cause of the DIC is removed or appropriate therapeutic interventions are used.

CLINICAL MANIFESTATIONS Clinical signs and symptoms of DIC present a wide spectrum of possibilities, depending on the underlying disease process that initiates DIC and whether the DIC is acute or chronic in nature (Box 20-3). Most symptoms are the results of either bleeding or thrombosis. Acute DIC presents with rapid development of hemorrhaging (oozing) from venipuncture sites, arterial lines, or surgical wounds or development of ecchymotic lesions (purpura, petechiae) and hematomas. Other sites of bleeding include the eyes (sclera, conjunctiva), the nose, and the gums. Most individuals with DIC demonstrate bleeding at three or more unrelated sites, and any combination may be observed. Shock of variable intensity, out of proportion to the amount of blood loss, also may be observed. Hemorrhaging into closed compartments of the body also can occur and may precede the development of shock.

Manifestations of thrombosis are not always as evident, even though it is often the first pathologic alteration to occur. Several organ

BOX 20-3 CLINICAL MANIFESTATIONS ASSOCIATED WITH DIC*

Integumentary System
Widespread hemorrhage and vascular lesions
Oozing from puncture sites, incisions, mucous membranes
Acrocyanosis (irregular-shaped cyanotic patches)
Gangrene

Central Nervous System
Subarachnoid hemorrhage
Altered state of consciousness (slight confusion to convulsions and coma)

Gastrointestinal System
Occult bleeding to massive gastrointestinal bleeding
Abdominal distention
Malaise
Weakness

Pulmonary System
Pulmonary infarctions
ARDS
Cyanosis
Tachypnea
Hypoxemia

Renal System
Hematuria
Oliguria
Renal failure

Modified from Bailes BK: Disseminated intravascular coagulation. Principles, treatment, nursing management, *AORN J* 55(2):517–529, 1992. *ARDS,* Adult respiratory distress syndrome; *DIC,* disseminated intravascular coagulation.

systems are susceptible to microvascular thrombosis associated with dysfunction: cardiovascular, pulmonary, central nervous, renal, and hepatic systems. Acute and accurate clinical interpretations are critical to preventing progression of DIC that may lead to multisystem organ dysfunction and failure. (Multiple organ dysfunction and failure are discussed further in Chapter 23.) Indicators of multisystem dysfunction include changes in level of consciousness or behavior, confusion, seizure activity, oliguria, hematuria, hypoxia, hypotension, hemoptysis, chest pain, and tachycardia. Symmetric cyanosis of fingers and toes (blue finger/toe syndrome), nose, and breast may be observed and indicates macrovascular thrombosis. This may lead to infarction and gangrene that may require amputation. Jaundice also is observed and most likely results from red cell destruction rather than liver dysfunction.

Individuals with chronic or low-grade DIC do not present with the overt manifestations of hemorrhaging and thrombosis but instead have subacute bleeding and diffuse thrombosis and are described as having compensated DIC. The major characteristic of this state is an increased turnover and decreased survival time of the components of hemostasis: platelets and clotting factors. Occasionally, diffuse or localized thrombosis develops, but this is infrequent.

EVALUATION AND TREATMENT No single laboratory test can be used to effectively diagnose DIC. Diagnosis is based primarily on clinical symptoms and confirmed by a combination of laboratory tests. The person must present with a clinical condition that is known to be associated with DIC. The most commonly used combination of laboratory tests usually confirms thrombocytopenia or a rapidly decreasing platelet count on repeated testing, prolongation of clotting times, the presence of fibrin degradation products, and decreased levels of coagulation inhibitors.

Platelet counts below $100,000/mm^3$ or a progressive decrease in platelet counts is very sensitive for DIC, although not greatly specific. These changes usually indicate consumption of platelets.

The standard coagulation tests (e.g., prothrombin time [PT], activated partial thromboplastin time [aPTT]) also have a high degree of sensitivity, but they are not highly specific for DIC. As a result of consumption of circulating clotting factors, these tests are usually abnormal, ranging from shortened to prolonged times. However, conditions other than DIC may prolong clotting times.

Detection of fibrin degradation products is more specific for DIC. Detection of D-dimers is a widely used test for DIC. A D-dimer is a molecule produced by plasmin degradation of cross-linked fibrin in clots. D-dimers in the blood can be quantified using ELISA tests that include commercially available and highly specific monoclonal antibody against the D-dimer. Agglutination tests for other fibrin degradation products are available. Fibrin degradation products are elevated in the plasma in 95% to 100% of cases; however, they are less specific for DIC than D-dimers and only document the presence of plasmin and its action on fibrin. ELISAs for markers of thrombin activity are sometimes used. For instance, ELISAs for fibrinopeptide A, a breakdown product of fibrinogen produced during activation by thrombin, are available. However, these assays are also less specific for DIC.

Levels of coagulation inhibitors (e.g., antithrombin III [AT-III], protein C) can be measured by assays that rely on function or by ELISAs that quantify the amount of the specific inhibitor. AT-III levels can provide key information for diagnosing and monitoring therapy of DIC. Initial levels of functional AT-III are low in DIC because thrombin is irreversibly complexed with activated clotting factors and AT-III.

Treatment of DIC is directed toward (1) eliminating the underlying pathologic condition, (2) controlling ongoing thrombosis, and (3) maintaining organ function. Elimination of the underlying pathologic condition is the initial intervention in the treatment phase in order to eliminate the trigger for activation of clotting. Once the stimulus is gone, production of coagulation factors in the liver leads to restoration of normal plasma levels within 24 to 48 hours.

Control of thrombosis is more difficult to attain. Heparin has been used for this; however, its use is controversial because its mechanism of action is binding to and activating AT-III, which is deficient in many types of DIC. Currently, heparin is only indicated in certain types of situations related to DIC. For instance, heparin seems to be effective in DIC caused by a retained dead fetus or associated with acute promyelocytic leukemia. Organ function is compromised by microthrombi, and there is a risk of losing an extremity because of vascular occlusion; thus heparin is also indicated in these conditions. Heparin's usefulness, however, for DIC that is precipitated by septic shock has not been established and so is contraindicated in that instance; heparin is also contraindicated when there is evidence of postoperative bleeding, peptic ulcer, or central nervous system bleeding.

Replacement of deficient coagulation factors, platelets, and other coagulation elements is gaining recognition as an effective treatment modality. Their use is not without controversy, however, because a major concern with replacement therapy is the possible risk of adding components that will increase the rate of thrombosis. Clinical judgment is the key factor in determining whether replacement is to be used as a treatment modality.

Several clinical trials are evaluating replacement of anticoagulants (i.e., AT-III, protein C). Replacement of AT-III appears to be effective in DIC caused by sepsis. Low levels of AT-III correlate with sepsis-initiated DIC, which makes a case for its use. AT-III inactivates thrombin, factor Xa, factor IXa, and other activated components of the clotting system. Heparin augments AT-III, but the combination of heparin with AT-III replacement has not been established. Antifibrinolytic drugs also are used in treatment but are limited to instances of life-threatening bleeding that have not been controlled by blood component replacement therapy.

Maintenance of organ function is achieved by fluid replacement to sustain adequate circulating blood volume and maintain optimal tissue and organ perfusion. Fluids may be required to restore blood pressure, cardiac output, and urine output to normal parameters.

Thromboembolic Disorders

Certain conditions within the blood vessels predispose an individual to develop clots spontaneously. A clot attached to the vessel wall is called a thrombus (Figure 20-17). A thrombus is composed of fibrin and blood cells and can develop in either the arterial or the venous system. Arterial clots form under conditions of high blood flow and are composed mostly of platelet aggregates held together by fibrin strands. Venous clots form in conditions of low flow and are composed mostly of red cells with larger amounts of fibrin and few platelets.

A thrombus eventually reduces or obstructs blood flow to tissues or organs, such as the heart, brain, or lungs, depriving them of essential nutrients critical to survival. A thrombus also has the potential of detaching from the vessel wall and circulating within the bloodstream (referred to as an embolus). The embolus may become lodged in smaller blood vessels, blocking blood flow into the local tissue or organ and leading to ischemia. Whether episodes of thromboembolism are life-threatening depends on the site of vessel occlusion.

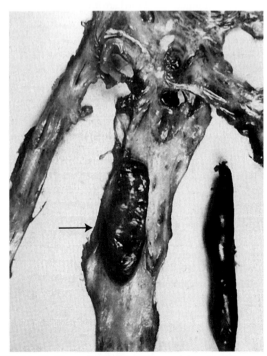

FIGURE 20-17 Thrombus. Thrombus arising in valve pocket at upper end of superficial femoral vein *(arrow)*. Postmortem clot on the right is shown for comparison. (From McLachlin J, Paterson JC: Some basic observations on venous thrombosis and pulmonary embolism, *Surg Gynecol Obstet* 93[1]:1–8, 1951.)

Therapy consists of removal or dissolution of the clot and supportive measures. Anticoagulant therapy is effective in treating or preventing venous thrombosis; it is not as useful in treating or preventing arterial thrombosis. Parenteral heparin is the major anticoagulant used to treat thromboembolism. Oral coumarin drugs also are widely used, particularly for individuals not hospitalized. More aggressive therapy may be indicated for such conditions as pulmonary embolism, coronary thrombosis, or thrombophlebitis. Streptokinase and urokinase activate the fibrinolytic system and are administered to accelerate the lysis of known thrombi. Thrombolytic therapy has limited uses and is prescribed with a high degree of caution because it can cause hemorrhagic complications.

The risk for developing spontaneous thrombi is related to several factors, referred to as the Virchow triad: (1) injury to the blood vessel endothelium, (2) abnormalities of blood flow, and (3) hypercoagulability of the blood.

Endothelial injury to blood vessels can result from atherosclerosis (plaque deposits on arterial walls) (see Chapter 23). Atherosclerosis initiates platelet adhesion and aggregation, promoting the development of atherosclerotic plaques that enlarge, causing further damage and occlusion. Other causes of vessel endothelial injury may be related to hemodynamic alterations associated with hypertension and turbulent blood flow. Injury also is caused by radiation injury, exogenous chemical agents (e.g., toxins from cigarette smoke), endogenous agents (e.g., cholesterol), bacterial toxins or endotoxins, or immunologic mechanisms. Whatever the precipitating cause of endothelial injury, it is a potent thrombogenic agent.

Sites of turbulent blood flow in the arteries and stasis of blood flow in the veins are at risk for thrombus formation. In areas of turbulence, platelets and endothelial cells may be activated, leading to thrombosis. In sites of stasis, platelets may remain in contact with the endothelium for prolonged lengths of time, and clotting factors that would normally be diluted with fresh flowing blood are not diluted and may become activated. The most common clinical conditions that predispose to venous stasis and subsequent thromboembolic phenomena are major surgery (e.g., orthopedic surgery), acute myocardial infarction, congestive heart failure, limb paralysis, spinal injury, malignancy, advanced age, the postpartum period, and bed rest longer than 1 week. Turbulence and stasis occur with ulcerated atherosclerotic plaques (myocardial infarction), hyperviscosity (polycythemia), and conditions with deformed red cells (sickle cell anemia).

Hypercoagulability is the condition in which an individual is at risk for thrombosis, but by itself it is a rare cause of thrombosis. Hypercoagulability is differentiated according to whether it results from primary (hereditary) or secondary (acquired) causes.

Hereditary hypercoagulability and thrombosis. Hereditary thrombophilias that increase the risk to develop thrombosis include factor V Leiden mutation; prothrombin mutation; methylenetetrahydrofolate reductase (MTHFR) mutation, leading to high homocysteine levels; and deficiencies in protein C, protein S, and antithrombin III (AT-III).[30] Most are autosomal dominant. Factor V Leiden results from a single nucleotide mutation that confers partial resistance to inactivation by activated protein C, resulting in prolonged high levels of activated factor V (factor Va) and overproduction of thrombin. It is the most common hereditary thrombophilia and is primarily observed in individuals of European ancestry. It is observed in about 5% of whites in the United States and in about 30% of individuals presenting with deep venous thrombosis (DVT) or pulmonary embolism.

Other hereditary thrombophilias are less common. Prothrombin mutation is observed in about 5% of individuals and leads to high levels of circulating prothrombin. More than 100 different known mutations lead to defects of protein C, protein S, and AT-III and increase the risk of venous thrombosis. Mutations may lead to either quantitative (low levels of protein) or qualitative (production of defective protein) changes. MTHFR mutation leads to alterations in the metabolism of the amino acid homocysteine into methionine and abnormally elevated levels of that amino acid in the blood (hyperhomocysteinemia). Acquired hyperhomocysteinemia may result from deficiencies in vitamins B_6 or B_{12}, endocrine diseases (e.g., diabetes mellitus, hypothyroidism), pernicious anemia, inflammatory bowel disease, renal failure, and therapy with some drugs. The mechanism of hypercoagulability conferred by hyperhomocysteinemia is unclear but may be related to direct injury of endothelial cells or platelets or to alteration of some components of the clotting system.

Tests to diagnosis inherited thrombophilias include prothrombin time, partial thromboplastin time, and levels of protein C, protein S, and AT-III. More elaborate tests to detect precise mutations in factor V, prothrombin, or MTHFR may be indicated.

Acquired hypercoagulability and thrombosis. Acquired hypercoagulable states include antiphospholipid syndrome (APS).[31] APS is an autoimmune syndrome characterized by autoantibodies against plasma membrane phospholipids and phospholipid-binding proteins. As with most autoimmune diseases, the predominate individual is

female and of reproductive age. Those with APS are at risk for both arterial and venous thrombosis and a variety of obstetric complications, including pregnancy loss and preeclampsia/eclampsia. The pathophysiology is related to autoantibodies directly reacting with platelets or endothelial cells (increasing the risk for thrombosis) or the placental surface (resulting in damage to the placenta). The predominant diagnostic tests measure prolongation of laboratory blood coagulation tests related to an antibody inhibitor (lupus anticoagulant) and specific ELISAs for antibodies against phospholipids (e.g., anticardiolipin antibody) or proteins that bind to phospholipids (e.g., β_2-glycoprotein I). Highly effective therapy (i.e., unfractionated or low-molecular-weight heparin with low-dose aspirin) is available to prevent the obstetric complications.

✔ **QUICK CHECK 20-6**

1. Identify three pathologic causes of DIC, and describe the manifestations associated with DIC.
2. Compare and contrast thrombocytopenia with thrombocytosis.
3. Why does vitamin K deficiency predispose an individual to a coagulation disorder?
4. Compare and contrast a thrombus with an embolus.

DID YOU UNDERSTAND?

Alterations of Erythrocyte Function

1. Anemia is generally defined as a reduction in the number or volume of circulating red cells or an alteration in hemoglobin.
2. The most common classification of anemias is based on changes in the cell size—represented by the suffix *cytic*—and changes in the cell's hemoglobin content—represented by the suffix *chromic.*
3. Clinical manifestations of anemia can be found in all organs and tissues throughout the body. Decreased oxygen delivery to tissues causes fatigue, dyspnea, syncope, angina, compensatory tachycardia, and organ dysfunction.
4. Macrocytic (megaloblastic) anemias are caused most commonly by deficiency of vitamin B_{12}. Pernicious anemia can be fatal unless vitamin B_{12} replacement is given.
5. Microcytic-hypochromic anemias are characterized by abnormally small red cells with insufficient hemoglobin content. The most common cause is iron deficiency.
6. Iron deficiency anemia usually develops slowly, with a gradual insidious onset of symptoms, including fatigue, weakness, dyspnea, alteration of various epithelial tissues, and vague neuromuscular complaints.
7. Iron deficiency anemia is usually a result of a chronic blood loss or decreased iron intake. Once the source of blood loss is identified and corrected, iron replacement therapy can be initiated.
8. Sideroblastic anemia results from impaired iron metabolism and abnormal sequestration of iron within the red cell. Treatment varies depending on the cause.
9. Normocytic-normochromic anemias are characterized by insufficient numbers of normal erythrocytes. Included in this category are aplastic, posthemorrhagic, and hemolytic anemia and anemia of chronic inflammation.
10. In aplastic anemia, erythrocyte stem cells are underdeveloped, defective, or absent. Unless the cause is determined, bone marrow aplasia results in death.
11. Posthemorrhagic anemia results from a sudden blood loss. Restoration of blood volume by plasma expanders or transfusions may diminish subjective symptoms of anemia. Hemoglobin restoration may take 6 to 8 weeks.
12. Hemolytic anemia results from premature destruction of red cells and may be acquired or hereditary. Of the acquired forms, autoimmune reaction and drug-induced hemolysis are the most common causes.
13. Anemia of chronic inflammation is associated with chronic infections, chronic inflammatory diseases, and malignancies.

Myeloproliferative Red Cell Disorders

1. Polycythemia vera is characterized by excessive proliferation of erythrocyte precursors in the bone marrow. Signs and symptoms result directly from increased blood volume and viscosity. Therapeutic phlebotomy to remove excessive blood volume and use of radioactive phosphorus have been helpful in decreasing the excessive red cell pool.
2. Polycythemia vera may spontaneously convert to acute myelogenous leukemia.

Alterations of Leukocyte Function

1. Quantitative alterations of leukocytes (too many or too few) can be caused by bone marrow dysfunction or premature destruction of cells in the circulation. Many quantitative changes in leukocytes occur in response to invasion by microorganisms.
2. Leukocytosis is a condition in which the leukocyte count is higher than normal and is usually a response to stress and invasion of microorganisms.
3. Leukopenia is a condition in which the leukocyte count is lower than normal and is caused by pathologic conditions, such as malignancies and hematologic disorders.
4. Granulocytosis (particularly as a result of an increase in neutrophils) occurs in response to infection. The marrow releases immature cells, causing a shift-to-the-left, when responding to an infection that has created a demand for neutrophils that exceeds the supply in the circulation.
5. Eosinophilia results most commonly from parasitic invasion and ingestion or inhalation of toxic foreign particles.
6. Basophilia is seen in hypersensitivity reactions because of the high content of histamine and subsequent release.

Continued

7. Monocytosis occurs during the late or recuperative phase of infection when macrophages (mature monocytes) phagocytose surviving microorganisms and debris.

8. Granulocytopenia, a significant decrease in neutrophils, can be a life-threatening condition if sepsis occurs; it is often caused by chemotherapeutic agents, severe infection, and radiation.

9. Infectious mononucleosis is an acute infection of B lymphocytes most commonly associated with the Epstein-Barr virus (EBV), a type of herpesvirus. Transmission of EBV is through close personal contact, commonly via saliva, thus its nickname, the *kissing disease*.

10. Two of the earliest manifestations of infectious mononucleosis are sore throat and fever caused by inflammation at the primary site of viral entry.

11. Most causes of EBV infectious mononucleosis include fever lasting 7 to 10 days, sore throat, and enlargement and tenderness of the cervical lymph nodes. It is self-limiting and treatment consists of rest and symptomatic treatment.

12. The common pathologic feature of all forms of leukemia is an uncontrolled proliferation of leukocytes, overcrowding the bone marrow and resulting in decreased production and function of the other blood cell lines.

13. All leukemias are classified by the cell type involved—lymphocytic or myelogenous—and are differentiated by onset—acute or chronic. Thus there are four major types of leukemia: acute lymphocytic leukemia (ALL), chronic lymphocytic leukemia (CLL), acute myelogenous leukemia (AML), and chronic myelogenous leukemia (CML).

14. Although the exact cause of leukemia is unknown, it is considered a clonal disorder. A high incidence of acute leukemias and CLL is reported in certain families, suggesting a genetic predisposition.

15. The major clinical manifestation of leukemia includes fatigue caused by anemia, bleeding caused by thrombocytopenia, fever secondary to infection, anorexia, and weight loss.

16. Chemotherapy is the treatment of choice for leukemia. Acute leukemias are associated with an increasing survival rate of 80% to 90%, with long-term survival of 30% to 40%. Chronic leukemias are associated with a longer life expectancy than are acute leukemias.

17. Chronic leukemias progress differently than acute leukemias, advancing slowly and without warning. The presence of the Philadelphia chromosome is a diagnostic marker for CML.

Alterations of Lymphoid Function

1. The number of lymphocytes is decreased (lymphocytopenia) in most acute infections and in some immunodeficiency syndromes.

2. Lymphocytosis occurs in viral infections (infectious mononucleosis and infectious hepatitis, in particular), leukemia, lymphomas, and some chronic infections.

3. Lymphomas are tumors of primary lymphoid tissue (thymus, bone marrow) or secondary lymphoid tissue (lymph nodes, spleen, tonsils, intestinal lymphoid tissue). The two major types of malignant lymphomas are Hodgkin lymphoma and non-Hodgkin lymphoma.

4. Distinctive abnormal chromosomes are present in multiple cells of the lymph nodes of an individual with Hodgkin lymphoma. The abnormal cell is called the Reed-Sternberg cell.

5. A virus might be involved in the pathogenesis of Hodgkin lymphoma. Some familial clustering suggests an unknown genetic mechanism.

6. An enlarged, painless mass or swelling, most commonly in the neck, is an initial sign of Hodgkin lymphoma. Local symptoms are produced by lymphadenopathy, usually caused by pressure or obstruction.

7. Treatment of Hodgkin lymphoma includes radiation therapy and chemotherapy. A cure is possible regardless of the stage of Hodgkin lymphoma; however, individuals treated with chemotherapy who relapse in less than 2 years have a poorer prognosis.

8. The cause of lymph node enlargement and cancerous transformation in non-Hodgkin lymphoma is unknown. Immunosuppressed persons have a higher incidence of non-Hodgkin lymphoma, suggesting an immune mechanism.

9. Generally, with non-Hodgkin lymphoma, the swelling of lymph nodes is painless, and the nodes enlarge and transform over a period of months or years.

10. Individuals with non-Hodgkin lymphoma can survive for long periods. The treatment used is chemotherapy.

11. Burkitt lymphoma involves the jaw and facial bones and occurs in children from east-central Africa and New Guinea.

12. Multiple myeloma is a neoplasm of B cells (immature plasma cells) and mature plasma cells. It is characterized by multiple malignant tumor masses of plasma cells scattered throughout the skeletal system and sometimes found in soft tissue.

13. The exact cause of multiple myeloma is unknown, but genetic factors and chronic stimulation of the mononuclear phagocyte system by bacteria, viral agents, and chemicals have been suggested.

14. The major clinical manifestations for multiple myeloma include recurrent infections caused by suppression of the humoral immune response and renal disease as a result of Bence Jones proteinuria.

15. Chemotherapy is the treatment of choice for multiple myeloma. Survival is still only 2 to 3 years with chemotherapy, however. Treatment with thalidomide combination therapies and blood cell transplantation are showing promise for producing long-term remissions.

Alterations of Splenic Function

1. Splenomegaly (enlargement of the spleen) may be considered normal in certain individuals, but its presence should not be ignored.

2. Splenomegaly results from (a) acute inflammatory or infectious processes, (b) congestive disorders, (c) infiltrative processes, and (d) tumors or cysts.

3. Hypersplenism (overactivity of the spleen) results from splenomegaly. Hypersplenism results in sequestering of the blood cells, causing increased destruction of red blood cells, which leads to the development of anemia.

Alterations of Platelets and Coagulation

1. Thrombocytopenia is characterized by a platelet count below $100,000/mm^3$ of blood; a count below $50,000/mm^3$ increases the potential for hemorrhage associated with minor trauma.

2. Thrombocytopenia exists in primary or secondary forms and is commonly associated with autoimmune diseases and viral infections; bacterial sepsis with DIC also results in thrombocytopenia.

3. Thrombocythemia is characterized by a platelet count more than 400,000 platelets/mm^3 of blood and is symptomatic when the count exceeds $1,000,000/mm^3$, at which time the risk for intravascular clotting (thrombosis) is high.

4. Thrombocythemia is caused by accelerated platelet production in the bone marrow.

5. Qualitative alterations in normal platelet adherence or aggregation prevent platelet plug formation and may result in prolonged bleeding times.

6. Platelet dysfunction results from changes in the cellular contents and integrity.

7. Disorders of coagulation are usually caused by defects or deficiencies of one or more clotting factors.

8. Coagulation is impaired when there is a deficiency of vitamin K because of insufficient production of prothrombin and synthesis of clotting factors II, VII, IX, and X, often associated with liver diseases.

9. Disseminated intravascular coagulation (DIC) is a complex syndrome resulting from a variety of clinical conditions that release tissue factor, causing an increase in fibrin and thrombin activity in the blood and producing augmented clot formation and accelerated fibrinolysis. Sepsis is a condition that is often associated with DIC.

DID YOU UNDERSTAND?—cont'd

10. DIC is characterized by a cycle of intravascular clotting followed by active bleeding caused by the initial consumption of coagulation factors and platelets and diffuse fibrinolysis.

11. Diagnosis of DIC is based on measurement in the blood of end products characteristic of dysfunctional coagulation activity. Treatment is complex and nonstandardized and focused on removing the primary cause, restoring hemostasis, and preventing further organ damage.

12. Thromboembolic disease results from a fixed (thrombus) or moving (embolus) clot that blocks flow within a vessel, denying nutrients to tissues distal to the occlusion; death can result when clots obstruct blood flow to the heart, brain, or lungs.

13. Hypercoagulability is the result of deficient anticoagulation proteins. Secondary causes are conditions that promote venous stasis.

14. The term *Virchow triad* refers to three factors that can cause thrombus formation: (a) loss of integrity of the vessel wall, (b) abnormalities of blood flow, and (c) alterations in the blood constituents.

KEY TERMS

- Absolute polycythemia 506
- Acquired sideroblastic anemia 505
- Agranulocytosis 509
- Anemia 500
- Anisocytosis 501
- Basopenia 509
- Basophilia 509
- B cell neoplasm 518
- Bence Jones protein 520
- Blast cell 512
- Burkitt lymphoma 519
- Consumptive thrombohemorrhagic disorder 527
- D-dimer 529
- Disseminated intravascular coagulation (DIC) 527
- Embolus 530
- Eosinopenia 509
- Eosinophilia 509
- Essential (primary) thrombocythemia (ET) 525
- Felty syndrome 509
- Folate 503
- Granulocytopenia 509
- Granulocytosis 509
- Hemolysis 501
- Hemosiderosis 505
- Heparin-induced thrombocytopenia (HIT) 524
- Hereditary hemochromatosis (HH) 508
- Hereditary sideroblastic anemia 505
- Heterophilic antibody 512
- Hodgkin lymphoma (HL) 516
- Hypercoagulability 530
- Hypersplenism 521
- Hypoplastic anemia 505
- Hypoxemia 501
- Idiopathic thrombocytopenia purpura (ITP) 524
- Impaired hemostasis 526
- Infectious mononucleosis (IM) 511
- Intrinsic factor (IF) 502
- Iron deficiency anemia (IDA) 504
- Koilonychia 504
- Leukemia 512
- Leukocytosis 508
- Leukopenia 508
- Lymphoblastic lymphoma (LL) 521
- Lymphocytopenia 509
- Lymphocytosis 509
- Macrocytic (megaloblastic) anemia 502
- Microcytic-hypochromic anemia 504
- Monocytopenia 509
- Monocytosis 509
- M protein 520
- Multiple myeloma (MM) 520
- Myelodysplastic syndrome 505
- Myeloproliferative disorder 514
- Neutropenia 509
- Neutrophilia 509
- NK cell neoplasm 518
- Non-Hodgkin lymphoma (NHL) 518
- Normocytic-normochromic anemia (NNA) 505
- Pancytopenia 513
- Pernicious anemia (PA) 502
- Phlebotomy 505
- Plasmin 527
- Poikilocytosis 501
- Polycythemia 506
- Polycythemia vera (PV) 506
- Reed-Sternberg (RS) cell 516
- Relative polycythemia 506
- Reversible sideroblastic anemia 505
- Secondary thrombocythemia 525
- Shift-to-the-left (leukemoid reaction) 509
- Shift-to-the-right 509
- Sideroblastic anemia (SA) 505
- Splenomegaly 521
- T cell neoplasm 518
- Thrombocythemia (thrombocytosis) 525
- Thrombocytopenia 523
- Thrombotic thrombocytopenia purpura (TTP) 524
- Thrombus 530
- Vasculitis 526
- Virchow triad 530

REFERENCES

1. Theurl I, et al: Regulation of iron homeostasis in anemia of chronic disease and iron deficiency anemia: diagnostic and therapeutic implications, *Blood* 113(21):5277–5286, 2009.

2. Muñoz M, García-Erce JA, Remacha AF: Disorders of iron metabolism. Part II: iron deficiency and iron overload, *J Clin Pathol* 2010 Dec 20:[Epub ahead of print.]

3. den Elzen WP, et al: Subnormal vitamin B_{12} concentrations and anaemia in older people: a systematic review, *BMC Geriatr* 10:42, 2010.

4. Guidi GC, Lechi Santonastaso C: Advancements in anemias related to chronic conditions, *Clin Chem Lab Med* 48(9):1217–1226, 2010.

5. Young NS, Calado RT, Scheinberg P: Current concepts in the pathophysiology and treatment of aplastic anemia, *Blood* 108(8):2509–2519, 2006.

6. Vannucchi AM, Guglielmelli P: Advances in understanding and management of polycythemia vera, *Curr Opin Oncol* 22(6):636–641, 2010.

7. Beer PA, et al: How we treat essential thrombocythemia, *Blood* 2010 Nov 24:[Epub ahead of print.]

8. Franchini M, Veneri D: Recent advances in hereditary hemochromatosis, *Ann Hematol* 84(6):347–352, 2005.

9. Greenberg PL: Myelodysplastic syndromes, *J Natl Compr Canc Netw* 9(1):30–56, 2011.

10. Leguit RJ, van den Tweel JG: The pathology of bone marrow failure, *Histopathology* 57(5):655–670, 2010.

11. Odumade OA, Hogquist KA, Balfour HH: Progress and problems in understanding and managing primary Epstein-Barr virus infections, *Clin Microbiol Rev* 24(1):193–209, 2011.

12. Bell AT, Fortune B, Sheeler R: Clinical inquiries: what test is the best for diagnosing infectious mononucleosis? *J Fam Pract* 55(9):799–802, 2006.

13. Konopleva MY, Jordan CT: Leukemia stem cells and microenvironment: biology and therapeutic targeting, *J Clin Oncol* 2011 Jan 10:[Epub ahead of print.]

14. Hodgson K, et al: Chronic lymphocytic leukemia and autoimmunity: a systematic review, *Haematologica* 2011 Jan 17:[Epub ahead of print.]

15. Roboz GJ, Guzman M: Acute myeloid leukemia stem cells: seek and destroy, *Exp Rev Hematol* 2(6):663–672, 2009.

16. Bomken S, et al: Understanding the cancer stem cell, *Br J Cancer* 103(4):439–445, 2010.

17. Monroy CM, et al: Hodgkin disease risk: role of genetic polymorphisms and gene-gene interactions in inflammation pathway genes, *Mol Carcinog* 50(1):36–46, 2011.

18. Vereide DT, Sugden B: Lymphomas differ in their dependence on Epstein-Barr virus, *Blood* 117(6):1977–1985, 2011.

19. Zelentz AD, et al: NCCN clinical practice guidelines in oncology; non-Hodgkin's lyphomas, *J Natl Compr Canc Netw* 8(3):288–334, 2010.

20. Surveillance Epidemiology and End Results (SEER): *SEER stat fact sheets: myeloma,* Bethesda, Md, 2009, National Cancer Institute. Accessed Jan 22, 2011. Available at http//seer.cancer.gov. (Based on Nov 2009 SEER data submission, posted to the SEER website, 2010.)

21. Anguilillo DJ, Ueno M, Goto S: Basic principles of platelet biology and clinical implications, *Circ J* 74(4):597–607, 2010.

22. Thijs T, et al: Review: platelet physiology and antiplatelet agents, *Clin Chem Lab Med* 2010 Nov 5:[Epub ahead of print.]

23. Handin RI: Inherited platelet disorders, *Hematology Amer Soc Hematol Educ Program* 396–402, 2005.

24. Butt A, Aronow WS, Chandy D: Heparin-induced thrombocytopenia and thrombosis, *Compr Ther* 36:23–27, 2010.

25. Bennett CN, de Jong JLO, Neufeld EJ: Targeted ITP strategies: do they elucidate the biology of ITP and related disorders? *Pediatr Blood Cancer* 47(Suppl 5):706–709, 2006.

26. Kiss JE: Thrombotic thrombocytopenic purpura: recognition and management, *Int J Hematol* 9(1):36–45, 2010.

27. Tsai HM: Pathophysiology of thrombotic thrombocytopenic purpura, *Int J Hematol* 91(1):1–19, 2010.

28. Harrison CN, et al: Guideline for investigation and management of adults and children presenting with a thrombocytosis, *Br J Haematol* 149(3):352–375, 2010.

29. Bick RL: Disseminated intravascular coagulation current concepts of etiology, pathology, diagnosis, and treatment, *Hematol Oncol Clin North Am* 17(1):149–176, 2003.

30. Bockenstedt PL: Management of hereditary hypercoagulable disorders, *Hematology Amer Soc Hematol Educ Program* 2006:444–449, 2006.

31. Tripodi A, de Groot PG, Pengo V: Antiphospholipid syndrome: Laboratory detection, mechanisms of action and treatment, *J Jntern Med* Feb 15. doi: 10.111/j. 1365–2796, 2011. 02362, 2011 [Epub ahead of print].

Alterations of Hematologic Function in Children

Nancy E. Kline

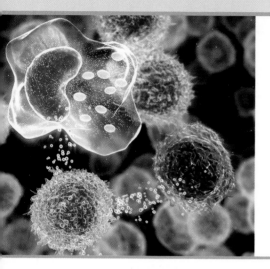

CHAPTER OUTLINE

Among the diseases that affect erythrocytes in children are acquired disorders, such as iron deficiency anemia and hemolytic disease of the newborn, and inherited disorders, such as glucose-6-phosphate dehydrogenase deficiency, sickle cell disease, and the thalassemias.

Childhood disorders that involve the coagulation process and platelets include inherited hemorrhagic diseases, such as the hemophilias, and antibody-mediated hemorrhagic diseases, including idiopathic thrombocytopenic purpura. Finally, leukocyte disorders, such as leukemia and the lymphomas (both Hodgkin lymphoma and non-Hodgkin lymphoma), are discussed in this chapter.

DISORDERS OF ERYTHROCYTES

Anemia is the most common blood disorder in children. Like the anemias of adulthood, the anemias of childhood are caused by ineffective erythropoiesis or premature destruction of erythrocytes. The most common cause of insufficient erythropoiesis is iron deficiency, which may result from insufficient dietary intake or chronic loss of iron caused by bleeding. The hemolytic anemias of childhood may be divided into (1) disorders that result from premature destruction caused by intrinsic abnormalities of the erythrocytes and (2) disorders that result from damaging extraerythrocytic factors. The hemolytic anemias are either inherited or acquired.

The most dramatic form of acquired congenital hemolytic anemia is hemolytic disease of the newborn (HDN), also termed erythroblastosis fetalis. HDN is an alloimmunity (isoimmunity) disease in which maternal blood and fetal blood are antigenically incompatible, causing the mother's immune system to produce antibodies against fetal erythrocytes. Fetal erythrocytes attacked by (i.e., bound to) maternal antibodies are recognized as foreign or defective by the fetal mononuclear phagocyte system and are removed from the circulation by phagocytosis, usually in the fetal spleen. (For a complete examination of HDN, see the discussion that follows.) Other acquired hemolytic anemias—some of which begin in utero—include those caused by infections or the presence of toxic chemicals.

The inherited forms of hemolytic anemia result from intrinsic defects of the child's erythrocytes, any of which can lead to erythrocyte removal by the mononuclear phagocyte system. Structural defects include abnormal cellular size or shape and abnormalities of plasma membrane structure (spherocytosis). Intracellular defects include enzyme deficiencies, the most common of which is glucose-6-phosphate dehydrogenase (G6PD) deficiency, and defects of hemoglobin synthesis, which manifest as sickle cell disease or thalassemia, depending on which component of hemoglobin is defective. These and other causes of childhood anemia are listed in Table 21-1.

TABLE 21-1	ANEMIAS OF CHILDHOOD	
CAUSE	**ANEMIC CONDITION**
Deficient Erythropoiesis or Hemoglobin Synthesis	
Decreased stem cell population in marrow (congenital or acquired pure red cell aplasia)	Normocytic-normochromic anemia
Decreased erythropoiesis despite normal stem cell population in marrow (infection, inflammation, cancer, chronic renal disease, congenital dyserythropoiesis)	Normocytic-normochromic anemia
Deficiency of a factor or nutrient needed for erythropoiesis	
Cobalamin (vitamin B_{12}), folate	Megaloblastic anemia
Iron	Microcytic-hypochromic anemia
Increased or Premature Hemolysis	
Alloimmune disease (maternal-fetal Rh, ABO, or minor blood group incompatibility)	Autoimmune hemolytic anemia
Autoimmune disease (idiopathic autoimmune hemolytic anemia, symptomatic systemic lupus erythematosus, lymphoma, drug-induced autoimmune processes)	Autoimmune hemolytic anemia
Inherited defects of plasma membrane structure (spherocytosis, elliptocytosis, stomatocytosis) or cellular size or both (pyknocytosis)	Hemolytic anemia
Infection (bacterial sepsis, congenital syphilis, malaria, cytomegalovirus infection, rubella, toxoplasmosis, disseminated herpes)	Hemolytic anemia
Intrinsic and inherited enzymatic defects (deficiencies) of glucose-6-phosphate dehydrogenase [G-6-PD], pyruvate kinase, 5'-nucleotidase, glucose phosphate isomerase	Hemolytic anemia
Inherited defects of hemoglobin synthesis	Sickle cell anemia
	Thalassemia
Disseminated intravascular coagulation (see Chapter 20)	Hemolytic anemia
Galactosemia	Hemolytic anemia
Prolonged or recurrent respiratory or metabolic acidosis	Hemolytic anemia
Blood vessel disorders (cavernous hemangiomas, large vessel thrombus, renal artery stenosis, severe coarctation of aorta)	Hemolytic anemia

Acquired Disorders

Iron Deficiency Anemia

Iron deficiency anemia is the most common blood disorder of infancy and childhood, with the highest incidence occurring between 6 months and 2 years of age. Incidence is not related to gender or race, but socioeconomic factors are important because they affect nutrition.[1] Iron deficiency anemia is common in children because they need an extremely high amount of iron for normal growth to occur.

Between 4 years of age and the onset of puberty, dietary iron deficiency is uncommon. During adolescence, however, it is relatively common, especially in menstruating females. Rapid growth, together with the average teenager's dietary habits, causes iron depletion.

PATHOPHYSIOLOGY Blood loss is a common cause of iron deficiency anemia in childhood. Chronic iron deficiency anemia from occult (hidden) blood loss may be caused by a gastrointestinal lesion, parasitic infestation, or hemorrhagic disease. As many as one third of infants with severe iron deficiency anemia have chronic intestinal blood loss induced by exposure to a heat-labile protein in cow's milk. Such exposure causes an inflammatory gastrointestinal reaction that damages the mucosa and results in diffuse hemorrhage.

CLINICAL MANIFESTATIONS The symptoms of mild anemia—listlessness and fatigue—usually are not present or are undetectable in infants and young children, who are unable to describe these symptoms. Therefore parents generally do not note any change in the child's behavior or appearance until moderate anemia has developed. General irritability, decreased activity tolerance, weakness, and lack of interest in play are nonspecific indications of anemia. When hemoglobin levels fall below 5 g/dl, pallor, anorexia, tachycardia, and systolic murmurs may occur.

Other symptoms and signs include splenomegaly, widened skull sutures, decreased physical growth and developmental delays, pica (a behavior in which nonfood substances are eaten), and altered neurologic and intellectual functions, especially those involving attention span, alertness, and learning ability.

EVALUATION AND TREATMENT The most definitive test for differentiating iron deficiency from other microcytic states is the absence of iron stores in the bone marrow. However, measurements of serum ferritin concentration, transferrin saturation, and free erythrocyte protoporphyrin level can help avoid a painful bone marrow evaluation to make a diagnosis. Evaluation and treatment of iron deficiency anemia in children are similar to those in adults. Dietary modification is required to prevent recurrences of iron deficiency anemia.

Hemolytic Disease of the Newborn

The most common cause of hemolytic anemia in newborns is alloimmune disease (HDN). HDN can occur only if antigens on fetal erythrocytes differ from antigens on maternal erythrocytes. Maternal-fetal incompatibility exists if mother and fetus differ in ABO blood type or if the fetus is Rh-positive and the mother is Rh-negative. Some minor blood antigens also may be involved. (The antigenic properties of erythrocytes are described in Chapter 7.)

ABO incompatibility occurs in about 20% to 25% of all pregnancies, but only 1 in 10 cases of ABO incompatibility results in HDN. Rh incompatibility occurs in fewer than 10% of pregnancies and rarely causes HDN in the first incompatible fetus. Even after five or more pregnancies, only 5% of women have babies with hemolytic disease. Usually erythrocytes from the first incompatible fetus cause the mother's immune system to produce antibodies that affect the fetuses of subsequent incompatible pregnancies. Only one in three cases of

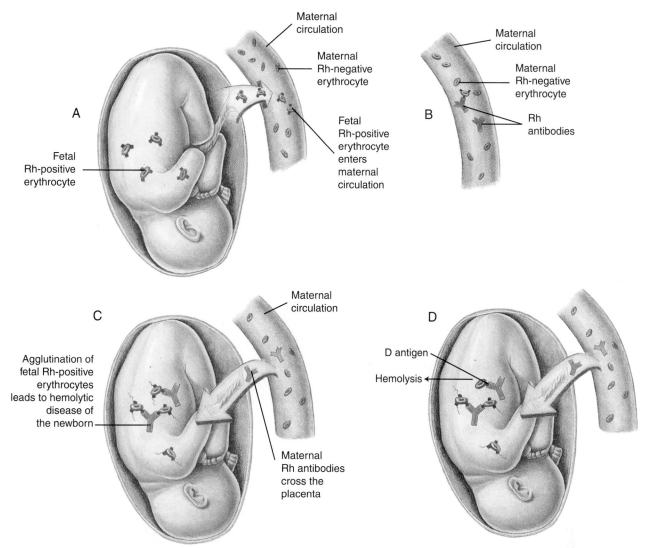

FIGURE 21-1 Hemolytic Disease of the Newborn (HDN). **A,** Before or during delivery, Rh-positive erythrocytes from the fetus enter the blood of an Rh-negative woman through a tear in the placenta. **B,** The mother is sensitized to the Rh antigen and produces Rh antibodies. Because this usually happens after delivery, there is no effect on the fetus in the first pregnancy. **C,** During a subsequent pregnancy with an Rh-positive fetus, Rh-positive erythrocytes cross the placenta, enter the maternal circulation, and (**D**) stimulate the mother to produce antibodies against the Rh antigen. (Modified from Seeley RR, Stephens TD, Tate P: *Anatomy and physiology,* ed 3, St Louis, 1995, Mosby.)

HDN is caused by Rh incompatibility; most cases are caused by ABO incompatibility.

PATHOPHYSIOLOGY   HDN will result (1) if the mother's blood contains preformed antibodies against fetal erythrocytes or produces them on exposure to fetal erythrocytes, (2) if sufficient amounts of antibody (usually immunoglobulin G [IgG]) cross the placenta and enter fetal blood, and (3) if IgG binds with sufficient numbers of fetal erythrocytes to cause widespread antibody-mediated hemolysis or splenic removal. (Antibody-mediated cellular destruction is described in Chapter 7.)

Maternal antibodies may be formed against type B erythrocytes if the mother is type A or against type A erythrocytes if the mother is type B. Usually, however, the mother is type O and the fetus is A or B. ABO incompatibility can cause HDN even if fetal erythrocytes do not escape into the maternal circulation during pregnancy. This occurs because the blood of most adults already contains anti-A or anti-B antibodies,

which are produced on exposure to certain foods or infection by gram-negative bacteria. (Anti-O antibodies do not exist because type O erythrocytes are not antigenic.) Therefore IgG against type A or B erythrocytes usually is preformed in maternal blood and can enter the fetal circulation throughout the first incompatible pregnancy.

Anti-Rh antibodies, on the other hand, are formed only in response to the presence of incompatible (Rh-positive) erythrocytes in the blood of an Rh-negative mother. Sources of exposure include fetal blood that is mixed with the mother's blood at the time of delivery, transfused blood, and, rarely, previous sensitization of the mother by her own mother's incompatible blood (Figure 21-1).

The first Rh-incompatible pregnancy generally presents no difficulties because few fetal erythrocytes cross the placental barrier during gestation. When the placenta detaches at birth, however, a large number of fetal erythrocytes usually enter the mother's bloodstream. If the mother is Rh-negative and the fetus is Rh-positive, the mother

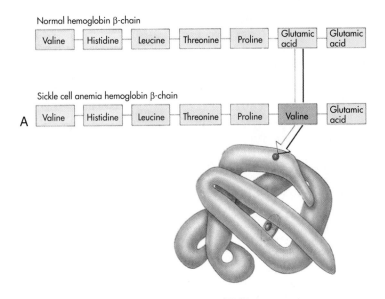

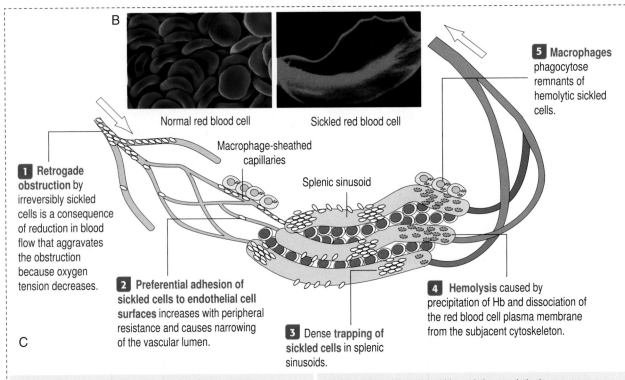

FIGURE 21-2 Sickle Cell Hemoglobin. A, Sickle cell hemoglobin is produced by a recessive allele of the gene encoding the beta-chain of the protein hemoglobin. It represents a single amino acid change—from glutamic acid to valine at the sixth position of the chain. In this model of a hemoglobin molecule, the position of the mutation can be seen near the end of the upper arm. **B,** Color-enhanced electron micrograph shows normal erythrocytes and sickled blood cell. **C,** Brief summary of sickle cell. (**A** from Raven PH, Johnson GB: *Biology,* ed 3, St Louis, 1992, Mosby; **B** copyright Dennis Kunkel Microscopy, Inc; **C** from Kierszenbaum A and Tres L: *Histology and cell biology: an introduction to pathology,* ed 3, St Louis, 2012, Mosby.)

produces anti-Rh antibodies. Anti-Rh antibodies persist in the bloodstream for a long time, and if the next offspring is Rh-positive, the mother's anti-Rh antibodies can enter the bloodstream of the fetus and destroy the erythrocytes. Antibodies against Rh antigen D are of the IgG class and easily cross the placenta.

IgG-coated fetal erythrocytes usually are destroyed in the spleen. As hemolysis proceeds, the fetus becomes anemic. Erythropoiesis accelerates, particularly in the liver and spleen, and immature nucleated cells (erythroblasts) are released into the bloodstream (hence the name *erythroblastosis fetalis*). The degree of anemia depends on the length of time the antibody has been in the fetal circulation, the concentration of the antibody, and the ability of the fetus to compensate for increased hemolysis. Unconjugated (indirect) bilirubin, which is formed during breakdown of hemoglobin, is transported across the placental barrier into the maternal circulation and is excreted by the mother. Hyperbilirubinemia occurs in the neonate after birth because excretion of lipid-soluble unconjugated bilirubin through the placenta no longer is possible.

The pathophysiologic effects of HDN are more severe in Rh incompatibility than in ABO incompatibility. ABO incompatibility may resolve after birth without life-threatening complications. Maternal-fetal incompatibility in which a mother with type O blood has a child with type A or B blood usually is so mild that it does not require treatment.

Rh incompatibility is more likely than ABO incompatibility to cause severe or even life-threatening anemia, death in utero, or damage to the central nervous system. Severe anemia alone can cause death as a result of cardiovascular complications. Extensive hemolysis also results in increased levels of unconjugated bilirubin in the neonate's circulation. If bilirubin levels exceed the liver's ability to conjugate and excrete bilirubin, some of it is deposited in the brain, causing cellular damage and eventually, if the neonate does not receive exchange transfusions, death.

Fetuses that do not survive anemia in utero usually are stillborn, with gross edema in the entire body, a condition called **hydrops fetalis.** Death can occur as early as 17 weeks' gestation and results in spontaneous abortion.

CLINICAL MANIFESTATIONS Neonates with mild HDN may appear healthy or slightly pale, with slight enlargement of the liver or spleen. Pronounced pallor, splenomegaly, and hepatomegaly indicate severe anemia, which predisposes the neonate to cardiovascular failure and shock. Life-threatening Rh incompatibility is rare today, largely because of the routine use of Rh immunoglobulin.

Because the maternal antibodies remain in the neonate's circulatory system after birth, erythrocyte destruction can continue. This causes **hyperbilirubinemia** and **icterus neonatorum (neonatal jaundice)** shortly after birth. Without replacement transfusions, in which the child receives Rh-negative erythrocytes, the bilirubin is deposited in the brain, a condition termed **kernicterus.** Kernicterus produces cerebral damage and usually causes death **(icterus gravis neonatorum).** Infants who do not die may have mental retardation, cerebral palsy, or high-frequency deafness.

EVALUATION AND TREATMENT Routine evaluation of fetuses at risk for HDN (i.e., fetuses resulting from Rh- or ABO-incompatible matings) includes the Coombs test. The indirect Coombs test measures antibody in the mother's circulation and indicates whether the fetus is at risk for HDN. The direct Coombs test measures antibody already bound to the surfaces of fetal erythrocytes and is used primarily to confirm the diagnosis of antibody-mediated HDN. With a prior history of fetal hemolytic disease, diagnostic tests are done to determine risk with the current pregnancy. These tests include maternal antibody titers,

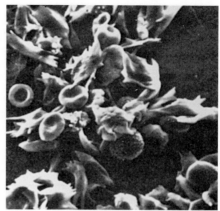

FIGURE 21-3 Normal and Sickle-Shaped Blood Cells. Scanning electron micrograph of normal and sickle-shaped red blood cells. The irregularly shaped cells are the sickle cells; the circular cells are the normal blood cells. (From Raven PH, Johnson GB: *Biology,* ed 3, St Louis, 1992, Mosby.)

fetal blood sampling, amniotic fluid spectrophotometry, and ultrasound fetal assessment.

The key to treatment of HDN resulting from Rh incompatibility lies in prevention (immunoprophylaxis). One of the success stories of immunology has been the result obtained with Rh immune globulin (RhoGAM), a preparation of antibody against Rh antigen D. If an Rh-negative woman is given Rh immune globulin within 72 hours of exposure to Rh-positive erythrocytes, she will not produce antibody against the D antigen, and the next Rh-positive baby she conceives will be protected.

If antigenic incompatibility of the mother's erythrocytes is not discovered in time to administer prophylactic immune globulin (RhoGAM) and a child is born with HDN, treatment consists of exchange transfusions in which the neonate's blood is replaced with new Rh-positive blood that is not contaminated with anti-Rh antibodies. Phototherapy also is used to reduce the toxic effects of unconjugated bilirubin.

Inherited Disorders
Sickle Cell Disease

Sickle cell disease is a group of disorders characterized by the production of abnormal **hemoglobin S (Hb S)** within the erythrocytes. Hb S is formed by a genetic mutation in which one amino acid (valine) replaces another (glutamic acid) (Figure 21-2). Hb S, the so-called sickle hemoglobin, reacts to deoxygenation and dehydration by solidifying and stretching the erythrocyte into an elongated sickle shape, producing hemolytic anemia (Figure 21-3).

Sickle cell disease is an inherited, autosomal recessive disorder expressed as sickle cell anemia, sickle cell–thalassemia disease, or sickle cell–hemoglobin C disease, depending on mode of inheritance (Table 21-2). (See Chapter 2 for a discussion of genetic inheritance of disease.) Sickle cell anemia, a homozygous form, is the most severe. Sickle cell–thalassemia and sickle cell–Hb C disease are heterozygous forms in which the child simultaneously inherits another type of abnormal hemoglobin from one parent. Sickle cell trait, in which the child inherits Hb S from one parent and normal hemoglobin (Hb A) from the other, is a heterozygous carrier state that rarely has clinical manifestations. All forms of sickle cell disease are lifelong conditions and have no known cure.

Sickle cell disease tends to occur in persons with origins in equatorial countries, particularly central Africa, the Near East, the

TABLE 21-2 INHERITANCE OF SICKLE CELL DISEASE

HEMOGLOBIN INHERITED FROM FIRST PARENT	HEMOGLOBIN INHERITED FROM SECOND PARENT	FORM OF SICKLE CELL DISEASE IN CHILD
Hb S (an abnormal hemoglobin)	Hb S	Sickle cell anemia: homozygous inheritance in which child's hemoglobin is mostly Hb S, with remainder Hb F (fetal hemoglobin)
Hb S	Defective or insufficient alpha or beta chains of Hb A (alpha- or beta-thalassemia)	Sickle cell–thalassemia disease (heterozygous inheritance of Hb S and alpha- or beta-thalassemia)
Hb S	Hb C or D (both abnormal hemoglobins)	Sickle cell–hemoglobin C (or D) disease (heterozygous inheritance of hemoglobin S and either C or D)
Hb S	Normal hemoglobins (mostly Hb A)	Sickle cell trait, carrier state (heterozygous inheritance of Hb S and normal hemoglobin)

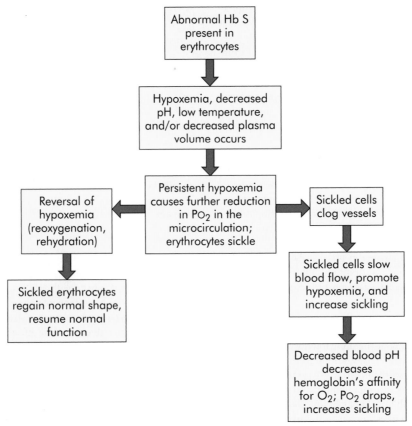

FIGURE 21-4 Sickling of Erythrocytes.

Mediterranean area, and parts of India. In the United States, sickle cell disease is most common in blacks, with a reported incidence ranging from 1:400 to 1:500 live births. In the general population, the risk of two black parents having a child with sickle cell anemia is 0.7%. Sickle cell–hemoglobin C disease is less common (1 in 800 births), and sickle cell–thalassemia occurs in 1 in 1700 births.

Sickle cell trait occurs in 7% to 13% of African Americans, whereas its incidence among East Africans may be as high as 45%. The sickle cell trait may provide protection against lethal forms of malaria, a genetic advantage to carriers who reside in endemic regions for malaria (Mediterranean and African zones) but no advantage to carriers living in the United States.

PATHOPHYSIOLOGY Hemoglobin S is soluble and usually causes no problem when properly oxygenated. When oxygen tension decreases, the single amino acid substitution in the beta-globin chain of Hb S

polymerizes, forming abnormal fluid polymers. As these polymers realign, they cause the red cell to deform into the sickle shape. Sickling depends on the degree of oxygenation, pH, and dehydration of the individual. A decrease in oxygenation (hypoxemia) and pH, as well as dehydration, increases sickling. Deoxygenation is probably the most important variable in determining the occurrence of sickling.[2] Sickle-trait cells sickle at oxygen tensions of about 15 mm Hg, whereas those from an individual with sickle cell disease begin to sickle at about 40 mm Hg. Sickled erythrocytes tend to plug the blood vessels, increasing the viscosity of the blood, which slows circulation and causes vascular occlusion, pain, and organ infarction. Viscosity increases the time of exposure to less oxygenation, promoting further sickling. Sickled cells undergo hemolysis in the spleen or become sequestered there, causing blood pooling and infarction of splenic vessels. The anemia that follows triggers erythropoiesis in the marrow and, in extreme cases, in the liver (Figure 21-4).

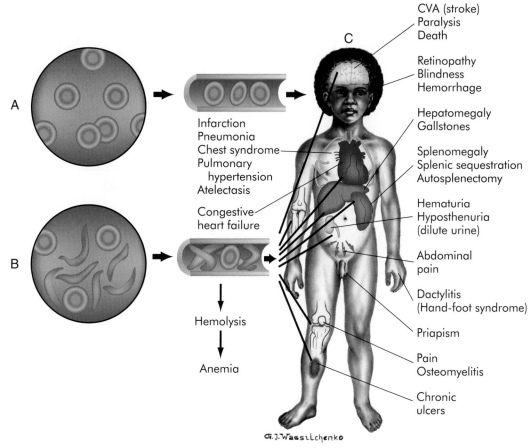

FIGURE 21-5 Differences Between Effects of (A) Normal and (B) Sickled RBCs on Blood Circulation and Selected Consequences in a Child. C, Tissue Effects of Sickle Cell Anemia. *CVA,* Cerebrovascular accident. (**A** and **B** adapted from Hockenberry MJ et al, editors: *Wong's nursing care of infants and children,* ed 8, St Louis, 2007, Mosby.)

Sickling usually is not permanent; most sickled erythrocytes regain a normal shape after reoxygenation and rehydration. Irreversible sickling is caused by irreversible plasma membrane damage caused by sickling. In persons with sickle cell anemia, in which the erythrocytes contain a high percentage of Hb S (75% to 95%), up to 30% of the erythrocytes can become irreversibly sickled. Occasionally, irreversible sickling occurs in sickle cell disease but not in the carrier state (sickle cell trait). Sickling also can be triggered by increased plasma osmolality, decreased plasma volume, and low environmental temperature.

CLINICAL MANIFESTATIONS   When sickling occurs, the general manifestations of hemolytic anemia—pallor, fatigue, jaundice, and irritability—sometimes are accompanied by acute manifestations called *crises.* Extensive sickling can precipitate the following four types of crises:

1. **Vaso-occlusive crisis (thrombotic crisis).** This begins with sickling in the microcirculation. As blood flow is obstructed by sickled cells, vasospasm occurs and a "logjam" effect blocks all blood flow through the vessel. Unless the process is reversed, thrombosis and infarction (death caused by lack of oxygen) of local tissue follow. Vasoocclusive crisis is extremely painful and may last for days or even weeks, with an average duration of 4 to 6 days. The frequency of this type of crisis is variable and unpredictable.
2. **Sequestration crisis.** Large amounts of blood become acutely pooled in the liver and spleen. This type of crisis is seen only in the young child. Because the spleen can hold as much as one fifth of the body's blood supply at one time, up to 50% mortality has been reported, with death being caused by cardiovascular collapse.
3. **Aplastic crisis.** Profound anemia is caused by diminished erythropoiesis despite an increased need for new erythrocytes. In sickle cell anemia, erythrocyte survival is only 10 to 20 days. Normally a compensatory increase in erythropoiesis (five to eight times normal) replaces the cells lost through premature hemolysis. If this compensatory response is compromised, aplastic crisis develops in a very short time.
4. **Hyperhemolytic crisis.** Although unusual, this may occur in association with certain drugs or infections.

The clinical manifestations of sickle cell disease usually do not appear until the infant is at least 6 months old, at which time the postnatal decrease in concentrations of Hb F causes concentrations of Hb S to rise (Figure 21-5). Infection is the most common cause of death related to sickle cell disease. Sepsis and meningitis develop in as many as 10% of children with sickle cell anemia during the first 5 years of life, with a death rate of 25%. Survival time is unpredictable, but many individuals die in their twenties.

Sickle cell–Hb C disease is usually milder than sickle cell anemia. The main clinical problems are related to vaso-occlusive crises and are believed to result from higher hematocrit values and viscosity. In older children, sickle cell retinopathy, renal necrosis, and aseptic necrosis of the femoral heads occur along with obstructive crises.

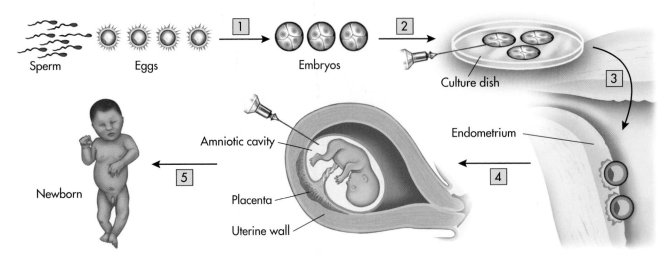

FIGURE 21-6 Prepregnancy Sickle Cell Test. This technique has potential for detection of other inherited diseases. *1,* Fertilization produces several embryos. *2,* The embryos are tested for the presence of the gene. *3,* The embryos without the gene are implanted. *4,* Amniocentesis confirms whether the fetus (or fetuses) has the sickle cell gene. *5,* Woman has a normal child.

Sickle cell–thalassemia has the mildest clinical manifestations of all the sickle cell diseases. The normal hemoglobins, particularly Hb F, inhibit sickling. In addition, the erythrocytes tend to be small (microcytic) and to contain relatively little hemoglobin (hypochromic), making them less likely to occlude the microcirculation, even when in a sickled state.

EVALUATION AND TREATMENT The sickle cell trait does not affect life expectancy or interfere with daily activities. However, on rare occasions, severe hypoxia caused by shock, vigorous exercising at high altitudes, flying at high altitudes in unpressurized aircraft, or undergoing anesthesia is associated with vaso-occlusive episodes in persons with sickle cell trait. These cells form an ivy shape instead of a sickle shape.

The parents' hematologic history and clinical manifestations may suggest that a child has sickle cell disease, but hematologic tests are necessary for diagnosis. If the sickle solubility test confirms the presence of Hb S in peripheral blood, hemoglobin electrophoresis provides information about the amount of Hb S in erythrocytes. Prenatal diagnosis can be made after chorionic villus sampling as early as 8 to 10 weeks' gestation or by amniotic fluid analysis at 15 weeks' gestation (Figure 21-6). Newborn screening for sickle cell disease should be performed according to state law.

Treatment of sickle cell disease consists of supportive care aimed at preventing consequences of anemia and avoiding crises. Genetic counseling and psychologic support are important for the child and family.

Hydroxyurea is an antimetabolite that inhibits deoxyribonucleic acid (DNA) synthesis and causes an increase in the synthesis of hemoglobin F. It is used in the treatment of children with severe sickle cell disease to increase hemoglobin level and reduce the incidence of vaso-occlusive crises and hospitalization. It is well tolerated, with the most common side effect being myelosuppression.[3]

Thalassemias

The alpha- and beta-thalassemias are inherited autosomal recessive disorders that cause an impaired rate of synthesis of one of the two chains—alpha or beta—of adult hemoglobin (Hb A). The disorder was named thalassemia, which is derived from the Greek word for sea, because it was discovered initially in persons with origins near the Mediterranean Sea. Beta-thalassemia, in which synthesis of the beta-globin chain is slowed or defective, is prevalent among Greeks, Italians, and some Arabs and Sephardic Jews. Alpha-thalassemia, in which the alpha chain is affected, is most common among Chinese, Vietnamese, Cambodians, and Laotians. Both alpha- and beta-thalassemias are common among blacks.

Both alpha- and beta-thalassemias are referred to as major or minor, depending on how many of the genes that control alpha- or beta-chain synthesis are defective and whether the defects are inherited homozygously (thalassemia major) or heterozygously (thalassemia minor). Pathophysiologic effects range from mild microcytosis to death in utero, depending on the number of defective genes and mode of inheritance. The anemic manifestation of thalassemia is microcytic-hypochromic hemolytic anemia.

PATHOPHYSIOLOGY The fundamental defect in beta-thalassemia is the uncoupling of alpha- and beta-chain synthesis. Beta-chain production is depressed—moderately in the heterozygous form, beta-thalassemia minor, and severely in the homozygous form, beta-thalassemia major (also called Cooley anemia). This results in erythrocytes having a reduced amount of hemoglobin and accumulations of free alpha chains. The free alpha chains are unstable and easily precipitate in the cell. Most erythroblasts that contain precipitates are destroyed by mononuclear phagocytes in the marrow, resulting in ineffective erythropoiesis and anemia. Some of the precipitate-carrying cells do mature and enter the bloodstream, but they are destroyed prematurely in the spleen, resulting in mild hemolytic anemia.

There are four forms of alpha-thalassemia: (1) alpha trait (the carrier state), in which a single alpha-chain–forming gene is defective; (2) alpha-thalassemia minor, in which two genes are defective; (3) hemoglobin H disease, in which three genes are defective; and (4) alpha-thalassemia major, a fatal condition in which all four alpha-forming genes are defective. Death is inevitable because alpha chains are absent and oxygen cannot be released to the tissues.

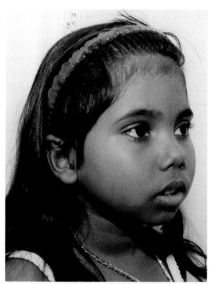

FIGURE 21-7 Young Girl with Beta-Thalassemia Demonstrating Mild Frontal Bossing (Prominence) of the Right Forehead and Mild Maxillary Prominence. (From Hockenberry MJ et al, editors: *Wong's nursing care of infants and children*, ed 8, St Louis, 2007, Mosby.)

CLINICAL MANIFESTATIONS   Beta-thalassemia occurs more commonly than does alpha-thalassemia. Occasionally, synthesis of gamma or delta polypeptide chains is defective, resulting in gamma- or delta-thalassemia. (Hemoglobin chains are described in Chapter 19.)

Beta-thalassemia minor causes mild to moderate microcytic-hypochromic anemia, mild splenomegaly, bronze coloring of the skin, and hyperplasia of the bone marrow. The degree of reticulocytosis depends on the severity of the anemia and results in skeletal changes (Figure 21-7). Hemolysis of immature (and therefore fragile) erythrocytes may cause a slight elevation in serum iron and indirect bilirubin levels. Persons with beta-thalassemia minor are usually asymptomatic.

Persons with beta-thalassemia major may become quite ill. Anemia is severe and results in a significant cardiovascular burden with high-output congestive heart failure. In the past, death resulted from cardiac failure. Today, blood transfusions can increase life span by 1 to 2 decades, and death usually is caused by hemochromatosis (from transfusions). Liver enlargement occurs as a result of progressive hemosiderosis, whereas enlargement of the spleen is caused by extramedullary hemopoiesis and increased destruction of red blood cells (Figure 21-8). Growth and maturation are retarded, and a characteristic chipmunk deformity develops on the face, caused by expansion of bones to accommodate hyperplastic marrow (see Figure 21-7).

Persons who inherit the mildest form of alpha-thalassemia (the alpha trait) usually are symptom free or have mild microcytosis. Alpha-thalassemia minor has clinical manifestations that are virtually identical to those of beta-thalassemia minor: mild microcytic-hypochromic reticulocytosis, bone marrow hyperplasia, increased serum iron concentrations, and moderate splenomegaly.

Signs and symptoms of alpha-thalassemia major are similar to those of beta-thalassemia major, but milder. Moderate microcytic-hypochromic anemia, enlargement of the liver and spleen, and bone marrow hyperplasia are evident.

Alpha-thalassemia major causes hydrops fetalis and fulminant intrauterine congestive heart failure. In addition to edema and massive ascites, the fetus has a grossly enlarged heart and liver. Diagnosis usually is made postmortem. Prenatal screening for this disorder can be performed by use of chorionic villus sampling. These cells can be

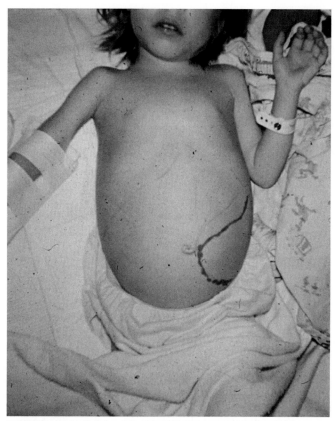

FIGURE 21-8 Child with Beta-Thalassemia Major Who Has Severe Splenomegaly. (From Jorde LB et al: *Medical genetics*, ed 3, updated, St Louis, 2006, Mosby.)

analyzed, and a DNA genetic map can be constructed and evaluated for the abnormalities characteristic of hydrops fetalis.

Both alpha- and beta-thalassemia major are life-threatening. Children with thalassemia major generally are weak, fail to thrive, show poor development, and experience cardiovascular compromise with high-output failure secondary to anemia. Untreated, they will die by 5 to 6 years of age.

EVALUATION AND TREATMENT   Evaluation of thalassemia is based on familial disease history, clinical manifestations, and blood tests. Peripheral blood smears that show microcytosis and hemoglobin electrophoresis that demonstrates diminished amounts of alpha or beta chains are used to make the diagnosis. Analysis of fetal DNA from withdrawn amniotic fluid is used as a screening test to detect hydrops fetalis (alpha-thalassemia major). Newborn screening for thalassemia should be done according to state law.

Persons who are silent carriers or have thalassemia minor generally have few if any symptoms and require no specific treatment. Therapies to support and prolong life are necessary, however, for thalassemia major. There is no cure for either condition. For both symptom-free carriers and those with the disease, prenatal diagnosis and genetic counseling may be the most important therapeutic measures that can be offered.

✔ **QUICK CHECK 21-1**

1. Why do clinical manifestations of sickle cell disease not appear until the infant is at least 6 months old?
2. Why is Rh incompatibility rare today?
3. Why do children with thalassemia major develop cardiovascular complications?

DISORDERS OF COAGULATION AND PLATELETS

Inherited Hemorrhagic Disease

Hemophilias

Awareness of a serious bleeding disorder in males was documented nearly 2000 years ago in the Babylonian Talmud, which exempted from the rite of circumcision those boys having male relatives prone to excessive bleeding. In 1803 the first description of this disorder appeared in the medical literature, where it was noted to be X-linked in nature and associated with joint bleeding and crippling.

Table 21-3 lists the coagulation factors that are associated with clinical bleeding. Until 1952 the term *hemophilia* was reserved for deficiency of factor VIII (antihemophilic factor). Since that time, two additional coagulation proteins, factor IX (plasma thromboplastin component [PTC]) and factor XI (plasma thromboplastin antecedent [PTA]), have been identified and their deficiency has been associated with similar clinical manifestations. Congenital deficiencies of these three plasma clotting factors—VIII, IX, and XI—account for 90% to 95% of the hemorrhagic bleeding disorders collectively called *hemophilia*. Table 21-3 lists coagulation factors and associated disorders, and the major types of hemophilia are summarized in Table 21-4.

PATHOPHYSIOLOGY Two types of defects dominate the hereditary defects of hemophilia to date: gene deletions and point mutations (base pair substitutions). Both types of genetic defects are associated with severe hemophilia A, in which no factor VIII circulates in the blood. Numerous gene mutations and deletions have been identified at the molecular level in factor VII and IX deficiency. The molecular defect that leads to hemophilia is identical among members of a given family; however, the deletion mutation has been unique in each family studied.[4]

Point mutations, in which a single base in the DNA is mutated to another base, represent a second type of mutation that causes hemophilia. When a point mutation becomes a de novo stop codon (nonsense mutation), translation of the protein ceases and a shortened version of the protein is synthesized. Usually the protein is destroyed intracellularly and never reaches the plasma. This type of defect is associated with severe hemophilia—that is, with coagulant activity levels below 1%. Point mutations in which one amino acid is substituted for another can cause phenotypes of varying severity. The mutation of an important amino acid can destroy protein function, activation, or folding; inhibit intracellular processing; or cause protein clearance. Unlike deletion mutations, point mutations at the same site have been recorded in different families with hemophilia.

Not all coagulation disorders are discussed in this chapter because some are extremely rare (e.g., congenital dysfibrinogenemias), whereas others have no clinical significance (e.g., Hageman factor deficiency, a condition in which profound laboratory deficiency of factor XII has absolutely no clinical effects on the child).

CLINICAL MANIFESTATIONS Children with severe hemophilia start to bleed at different ages. There is no transfer of maternal clotting factor to the fetus, yet many boys with hemophilia are circumcised without excessive bleeding. Normal hemostasis is achieved in these infants because clotting is activated through the extrinsic coagulation cascade.

During the first year, spontaneous bleeding often is minimal, but hematoma formation may result from injections and from firm holding (e.g., under the arms). Easy bruising, hemarthrosis (bleeding into joints), or both occur with ambulation. By age 3 to 4 years, 90% of children with hemophilia have shown episodes of persistent bleeding from relatively minor traumatic lacerations (e.g., to the lip or tongue). This usually is the first clinical manifestation of hemophilia. Hemorrhage into the elbows, knees, and ankles causes pain, limits joint movement,

TABLE 21-3	THE COAGULATION FACTORS AND ASSOCIATED DISORDERS	
CLOTTING FACTORS	**SYNONYM**	**DISORDER**
I	Fibrinogen	Congenital deficiency (afibrinogenemia) and dysfunction (dysfibrinogenemia)
II	Prothrombin	Congenital deficiency or dysfunction
V	Labile factor, proaccelerin	Congenital deficiency (parahemophilia)
VII	Stable factor or proconvertin	Congenital deficiency
VIII	Antihemophilic factor (AHF)	Congenital deficiency is hemophilia A (classic hemophilia)
IX	Christmas factor	Congenital deficiency is hemophilia B
X	Stuart-Prower factor	Congenital deficiency
XI	Plasma thromboplastin antecedent	Congenital deficiency, sometimes referred to as hemophilia C
XII	Hageman factor	Congenital deficiency is *not* associated with clinical symptoms
XIII	Fibrin-stabilizing factor	Congenital deficiency

TABLE 21-4	THE HEMOPHILIAS
TYPE	**DESCRIPTION**
Hemophilia A (classic hemophilia)	Caused by factor VIII deficiency; most common of hemophilias; inherited as X-linked recessive disorder; factor VIII gene has been mapped to distal arm of X chromosome and clones; affects males and is transmitted by females; 1:5000–10,000 male births; occurs with varying degrees of severity
Hemophilia B (Christmas disease)	Caused by factor IX deficiency; transmitted as X-linked recessive trait; clinically indistinguishable from factor VIII deficiency, however, less severe than hemophilia A (IX gene also has been cloned); 1:30,000 male births; occurs with varying degrees of severity
Hemophilia C	Caused by factor XI deficiency; inherited as autosomal recessive disease; occurs equally in males and females; bleeding is usually less severe than with A or B
von Willebrand disease	Also caused by factor VIII deficiency; results from inherited autosomal dominant trait encoded by a gene on chromosome 12; has variable clinical manifestations and hematologic findings; infusion of plasma causes factor VIII activity to increase

TABLE 21-5 LABORATORY TESTS OF COAGULATION

TEST	SIGNIFICANCE
Thrombin time	Measures fibrinogen level; usually elevated first because without fibrinogen, blood cannot clot
Prothrombin time (PT)	Decrease indicates a deficiency of factors II, V, VII, or X; also used to monitor warfarin sodium (Coumadin) therapy
Activated partial thromboplastin time (PTT or APTT)	Assesses for factors XII, XI, IX, and VIII; also used to monitor heparin therapy
PT or APTT mixing study	Differentiates between factor deficiency and factor antibody activity
Specific factor assay	Measures specific factors; XIII, XII, XI, X, IX, VIII, VII, V, II, fibrinogen (factor I)

and predisposes the child to degenerative joint changes. Spontaneous hematuria and epistaxis are troublesome but minor complications.

Recurrent bleeding, both spontaneous and after minor trauma, is a lifelong problem. Many affected persons experience phases or cycles of spontaneous bleeding episodes. Mechanisms that cause this phenomenon are unknown. Intracranial hemorrhage and bleeding into the tissues of the neck or abdomen constitute life-threatening emergencies.

EVALUATION AND TREATMENT Although laboratory tests are of primary value in the evaluation of hemorrhagic disorders, the history and physical assessment also are important. The phases of coagulation can be individually assessed by simple, reliable tests (Table 21-5).

The majority of children with hemophilia A (factor VIII deficiency) are treated with recombinant factor VIII, and children with hemophilia B (factor IX deficiency) are treated with recombinant factor IX. Plasma-derived factor is available and less expensive but carries with it the risk of viral infection (e.g., human immunodeficiency virus [HIV], hepatitis).[5]

The prognosis for children with hemophilia is promising. Programs of comprehensive care and home treatment have improved the quality of life for those with hemophilia and enhanced their general physical capabilities.

Antibody-Mediated Hemorrhagic Disease

The antibody-mediated hemorrhagic diseases are a group of disorders caused by the immune response. Antibody-mediated destruction of platelets or antibody-mediated inflammatory reactions to allergens damage blood vessels and cause seepage into tissues. The thrombocytopenic purpuras may be intrinsic or idiopathic, or they may be transient phenomena transmitted from mother to fetus. The inflammatory, or "allergic," purpuras, although rare, occur in response to allergens in the blood. All of these disorders first appear during infancy or childhood.

Idiopathic Thrombocytopenic Purpura

Acute **idiopathic thrombocytopenic purpura (ITP; autoimmune [primary] thrombocytopenic purpura)** is the most common disorder of platelet consumption. Antiplatelet antibodies bind to the plasma membranes of platelets, causing platelet sequestration and destruction by mononuclear phagocytes in the spleen and other lymphoid tissues at a rate that exceeds the ability of the bone marrow to produce them.

PATHOPHYSIOLOGY In approximately 70% of cases of ITP, there is an antecedent viral disease (e.g., cytomegalovirus [CMV], Epstein-Barr virus [EBV], parvovirus, or respiratory tract infection) that precedes the eruption of petechiae or purpura by 1 to 3 weeks. High levels of IgG have been found bound to platelets and may represent immune complexes on the platelet surface (see *Health Alert:* Vaccine-Associated ITP in Early Childhood).

HEALTH ALERT
Vaccine-Associated ITP in Early Childhood

Over the last several years, there has been growing concern that childhood vaccinations are associated with an increased incidence of ITP. A retrospective study in 2010 was performed to examine the relationship between vaccination and ITP in 20 children younger than age 3 years. Of these 20 children, 12 developed ITP following vaccination: 5 after hepatitis B virus vaccine at 1 month of age, 4 after the first dose of diphtheria-tetanus-acellular pertussis (DTaP) vaccine at 2 to 3 months of age, 2 after the first dose of measles-mumps-rubella (MMR) vaccine at 16 months of age, and 1 after the first dose of varicella vaccine at 14 months of age. Although this is a small sample, vaccination may be a risk factor for ITP in infancy and early childhood.

Data from Hsieh Y, Lin L: Thrombocytopenic purpura following vaccination in early childhood: experience of a medical center in the past 2 decades, *J Chin Med Assoc* 73(12):634–637, 2010.

CLINICAL MANIFESTATIONS Bruising and a generalized petechial rash often occur with acute onset. Asymmetric bruising is typical and is found most often on the legs and trunk. Hemorrhagic bullae of the gums, lips, and other mucous membranes may be prominent, and epistaxis (nose bleeding) may be severe and difficult to control. Otherwise, the child appears well. The acute phase lasts 1 to 2 weeks, but thrombocytopenia often persists. Although the incidence is less than 1%, intracranial hemorrhage is the most serious complication of ITP. In some cases, the onset is more gradual, and clinical manifestations consist of moderate bruising and a few petechiae.

EVALUATION AND TREATMENT Laboratory examination reveals a low platelet count, and the few platelets observed on a smear are large, reflecting increased bone marrow production. The Ivy bleeding time is prolonged. Bone marrow aspiration shows normal or increased numbers of megakaryocytes and normal levels of erythrocytes and granulocytes.

Even without treatment, the prognosis for children with ITP is excellent: 75% recover completely within 3 months. After the initial acute phase, spontaneous clinical manifestations subside. By 6 months after onset, 80% of affected children have regained normal platelet counts.[6]

✔ QUICK CHECK 21-2
1. List the major disorders of coagulation and platelets found in children.
2. How do gene deletions differ from point mutations?
3. Why are persons with hemophilia at risk for developing degenerative joint changes?
4. What is the major abnormality in idiopathic thrombocytopenic purpura (ITP)?

TABLE 21-6	MAJOR CLASSIFICATIONS OF LEUKEMIA
MAJOR TYPES	**ORIGINS**
Lympho	Leukemia involving lymphoid tissue and lymphatic system (e.g., lymphatic vessels, lymph nodes, spleen, thymus)
Myelo	Leukemias of bone marrow (myeloid) origin
Blastic and acute	Leukemias involving immature cells
Cytic and chronic	Leukemias involving mature cells

NEOPLASTIC DISORDERS

Leukemia and Lymphoma

Leukemia, cancer of the blood-forming tissues, is the most common malignancy of childhood, representing approximately 33% of all childhood cancers. Childhood lymphoma, or cancer of the lymphoid system (primarily lymph nodes), is the third most common malignant neoplasm of children in the United States, representing approximately 11% of all childhood cancers. (See Chapter 20 for a discussion of leukemia in adults.) Table 21-6 defines the major classifications of leukemia.

Leukemia

Approximately 80% to 85% of leukemias in children are acute lymphoblastic leukemia (ALL). The remaining 15% to 20% are acute nonlymphocytic leukemias (ANLLs) (which include myeloblastic, promyelocytic, monocytic, and myelomonoblastic) and erythroleukemia, the rare red blood cell leukemia. Because the vast majority of ANLL cases involve the myeloblastic cell, many experts refer to the disease as acute myelogenous leukemia (AML). Both a juvenile form and an adult form of chronic myelocytic leukemia (CML) develop in children but are uncommon and account for only 2% of all leukemias in childhood. Chronic lymphocytic leukemia (CLL) is virtually nonexistent in children.

ALL is the most common malignancy in children, representing nearly one third of all pediatric cancers. The annual incidence of ALL is about 30 cases per million people, with a peak incidence in children 2 to 5 years of age, and affects almost twice as many white children as nonwhite children (4.2:100,000 versus 2.4:100,000, respectively). Childhood ALL also is more common in boys than in girls (1.3:1.0).

PATHOGENESIS Investigations into the causes of childhood leukemia have focused on genetic susceptibility, environmental factors, and viral infections. Observations of a familial tendency and links with a number of inherited disorders have implicated genetic factors in the origin of leukemia.

Inherited diseases that predispose a child to leukemia (both ALL and AML) include Down syndrome, Fanconi anemia, Bloom syndrome, and ataxia-telangiectasia. Leukemia also has been associated with known genetic diseases, such as congenital agammaglobulinemia. AML is attributable to prior chemotherapy, especially alkylating agents. AML can develop from preexisting myeloproliferative disorders that also are preleukemia syndromes. When these disorders progress to ANLL, an insidious pattern of leukemic dysfunction usually is revealed.

Many environmental factors (e.g., exposure to ionizing radiation and electromagnetic fields, parental use of alcohol and tobacco) have been investigated as potential risk factors, but none has been definitively shown to cause lymphoblastic leukemia in children.

There is no evidence that radon gas exposure causes cancer in children. Likewise, electromagnetic field (EMF) exposure has not been demonstrated to be a causative factor in acute leukemias.[7] In addition, no evidence suggests a chemical or drug association.[8]

The multiple causation concept is useful when results of epidemiologic studies are interpreted. For example, laboratory and epidemiologic studies may indicate that exposure to a certain chemical can cause leukemia, but not all children exposed to that chemical will develop leukemia. Additional studies are needed to determine what other factors must interact with chemical exposure to cause the disease.

Leukemic clusters that represent a greater number of leukemia cases occurring in a particular geographic location have raised speculation about environmental factors and infectious patterns of transmission. Careful follow-up, however, has failed to document the abnormal clustering. Explanations for this phenomenon therefore are statistical artifact and coincidence.

Viruses clearly have been known to cause leukemia in a number of animals, including cats, fowl, and mice. Scientists have linked retroviruses with other types of cancer, but retroviruses have not been linked with childhood leukemia.

CLINICAL MANIFESTATIONS The onset of leukemia may be abrupt or insidious, but the most common symptoms reflect the consequence of bone marrow failure: decreased levels of both red blood cells and platelets and changes in white blood cells. Pallor, fatigue, petechiae, purpura, bleeding, and fever generally are present. Approximately 45% of children have a hemoglobin level below 7 g/dl. If acute blood loss occurs, characteristic symptoms of tachycardia, air hunger, restlessness, and thirst may be present. Epistaxis often occurs in children with severe thrombocytopenia.

Fever is usually present as a result of (1) infection associated with the decrease in functional neutrophils and (2) hypermetabolism associated with the ongoing rapid growth and destruction of leukemic cells. White blood cell counts greater than 200,000/mm³ can cause leukostasis, an intravascular clumping of cells that results in infarction and hemorrhage, usually in the brain and lung.

Renal failure as a result of hyperuremia (high uric acid levels) can be associated with ALL, particularly at diagnosis or during active treatment. Extramedullary invasion with leukemic cells can occur in nearly all body tissue. The central nervous system (CNS) is a common site of infiltration of extramedullary leukemias, although fewer than 10% of children with ALL have CNS involvement at diagnosis. CNS infiltration manifests later in the course of the disease. The most common symptoms of CNS involvement relate to increased intracranial pressure, causing early morning headaches, nausea, vomiting, irritability, and lethargy.

Gonadal involvement can occur and leukemic infiltration into bones and joints is common. Reports of bone or joint pain actually lead to the diagnosis of leukemia in some children. In most children, bone pain is characterized as migratory, vague, and without areas of swelling or inflammation. If joint pain is the primary symptom and some swelling is associated with the pain, however, misdiagnoses of rheumatoid arthritis and rheumatic fever have occurred.

Other organs reported to be sites of leukemic invasion include the kidneys, heart, lungs, thymus, eyes, skin, and gastrointestinal tract. Children with leukemia usually have shown symptoms for only 1 week before diagnosis.

EVALUATION AND TREATMENT Although blood test results can raise the clinician's suspicion of leukemia, a bone marrow aspiration is required to establish the diagnosis. The blast cell is the hallmark of

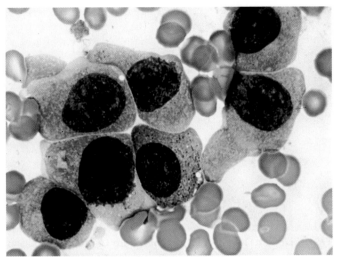

FIGURE 21-9 Monoblasts From Acute Monoblastic Leukemia. Monoblasts in a marrow smear from an individual with acute monoblastic leukemia. The monoblasts are larger than myeloblasts and usually have abundant cytoplasm, often with delicate scattered azurophilic granules (an element that stains well with blue aniline dyes). (From Damjanov I, Linder J, editors: *Anderson's pathology,* ed 10, St Louis, 1996, Mosby.)

acute leukemia (Figure 21-9). This relatively undifferentiated cell is characterized by diffusely distributed nuclear chromatin, with one or more nucleoli and basophilic cytoplasm. Healthy children have fewer than 5% blast cells in the bone marrow and none in the peripheral blood. In ALL, the bone marrow often is replaced by 80% to 100% blast cells, with a reduction in normal developing red blood cells and granulocytes. Occasionally, the marrow appears hypocellular, making the diagnosis difficult to differentiate from aplastic anemia. When this occurs, bone marrow biopsy or biopsy of extramedullary sites is necessary to confirm the diagnosis.

Combination chemotherapy, with or without radiation therapy to localized sites, such as the CNS, is the treatment of choice for acute leukemia. In ALL, identification of various risk groups has led to the development of different intensities of drug protocols. Thus treatment is tailored specifically for a particular risk group. The 5-year relative survival rate for ALL is about 80% (see *Health Alert:* Dasatinib: A Promising Agent to Treat Refractory Chronic Myeloid Leukemia).

HEALTH ALERT

Dasatinib: A Promising Agent to Treat Refractory Chronic Myeloid Leukemia

Dasatinib is in a class of medications called protein-tyrosine kinase inhibitors; these medications block the action of an abnormal protein that signals cancer cells to multiply. Dasatinib has been demonstrated to treat chronic myeloid leukemia (CML) in adults whose disease has not responded to other medications, including imatinib (Gleevec), or in those who cannot take these medications because of severe side effects. A phase I study recently conducted in children with refractory CML demonstrated that this drug is well tolerated in children. Further phase II studies are needed to determine the efficacy of this oral medication that may hold promise as an additional line of therapy for children.

Data from Aplenc R et al: Pediatric phase I trial and pharmacokinetic study of dasatinib: a report from the Children's Oncology Group Phase I Consortium, *J Clin Oncol*, 2011 Jan 24. (Epub ahead of print.)

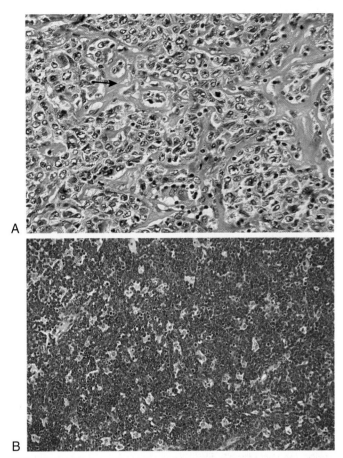

FIGURE 21-10 Lymphomas. A, Large cell lymphoma. The tumor contains prominent areas of sclerosis *(arrow).* **B,** Burkitt lymphoma. A starry sky pattern is seen at low magnification. (From Damjanov I, Linder J: *Pathology: a color atlas,* St Louis, 2000, Mosby.)

Lymphomas

Non-Hodgkin lymphoma (NHL) and Hodgkin lymphoma constitute approximately 11% of all cases of childhood cancer. Approximately 750 cases of lymphoma occur in children between birth and 14 years of age in the United States each year.[9] NHL occurs more often than Hodgkin lymphoma (4.5% versus 3.5% of all pediatric malignancies). Either group of diseases is rare before the age of 5 years, and the relative incidence increases throughout childhood. Boys are more likely to be diagnosed with a malignant lymphoma than are girls. At particular risk are children with inherited or acquired immunodeficiency syndromes, who have increased rates of lymphoreticular cancers that range between 100 and 10,000 times the rate of normal children.

Non-Hodgkin lymphoma. Generally, most classification systems divide NHL into two categories—nodular or diffuse—on the basis of cellular pattern. Whereas half of all adults with NHL have a nodular form of the disease, children rarely demonstrate this pattern. Nodular disease represents a less aggressive form of lymphoma. Almost without exception, childhood NHL becomes evident as a diffuse disease and can be further subdivided into three groups: (1) large cell (histiocytic), (2) lymphoblastic, and (3) small noncleaved cell (Burkitt or non-Burkitt lymphoma) (Figure 21-10). Large cell NHL often involves chromosomal translocations. Disease sites commonly involve extranodal sites, such as brain, lung, bone, and skin. Lymphoblastic NHL also shows chromosomal translocations, particularly chromosomes 7 and 14. Disease sites commonly include the mediastinum and peripheral lymph nodes. Small noncleaved cell NHL involves translocations of chromosomes 8 and 14. Children with small noncleaved cell NHL commonly have intra-abdominal disease at diagnosis.

As in ALL, immunophenotyping is an important part of the classification of childhood NHL. Almost 45% of cases of the disease in children originate from T cells; an equal number originate from B cells. The remaining group, which represents less than 10% of childhood NHLs, is classified as non-T, non-B.

PATHOGENESIS Viral etiology is suggested, with the strongest correlation between the Epstein-Barr virus and African Burkitt lymphoma. The relationship outside Africa is weak, however, even though the tumor is histopathologically and clinically indistinguishable. Chronic immunostimulation also has been suggested as a factor in the development of lymphomas, because these diseases are seen more often when chronic persistent antigenic stimulation occurs from infection, such as that caused by malaria or intestinal parasites. Genetic susceptibility also may play a role in the process of malignant transformation. There is increased evidence of NHL in children with congenital immunodeficiency syndromes, such as Wiskott-Aldrich syndrome, ataxia-telangiectasia, and Bloom syndrome. Children with acquired immunodeficiency syndrome (AIDS) have an increased risk of developing NHL. However, the incidence of AIDS-related malignancies has declined dramatically with the use of highly active antiretroviral therapy in the developed world.[10]

CLINICAL MANIFESTATIONS NHL has been found to arise from any lymphoid tissue. Signs and symptoms therefore are specific for the site involved. Because childhood NHL is a rapidly progressive disease, symptoms generally are present only a few weeks before diagnosis is made. Rapidly enlarging lymphoid tissue and painless lymphadenopathy are common with abdominal sites of involvement, usually representing a gastrointestinal origin for the disease. Symptoms often include abdominal pain and vomiting, but a palpable mass is not always present. Most children with abdominal symptoms have diffuse, small noncleaved cell NHL (Burkitt or non-Burkitt) of B cell origin. If the tumor recurs, it appears again in the abdomen before distant metastasis.

The other common site of childhood NHL is the chest region. An anterior mediastinal mass, with or without pleural effusion, often is present. If the mass is large enough, respiratory compromise, tracheal compression, and superior vena cava syndrome may arise, which constitute a medical emergency. Children with anterior mediastinal involvement often are male adolescents and usually have diffuse lymphoblastic lymphoma of T cell origin. This often evolves into extensive bone marrow involvement and is considered to be an overt leukemic phase, therefore referred to as *leukemic transformation*. CNS involvement and testicular infiltration often occur.

CNS involvement is common. A relatively small number (10% to 20%) of children with NHL have lymphoid tissue involvement of the head and neck (Waldeyer ring, nasopharynx, sinuses). Signs and symptoms include tonsillitis, sinusitis, and a painless nasopharynx mass. In African Burkitt lymphoma, involvement of facial bones, particularly the jaw, is common.

EVALUATION AND TREATMENT Diagnosis is made by biopsy of disease sites, usually the involved lymph nodes, tonsils, bone marrow, spleen, liver, bowel, or skin. Most children with NHL are cured of the disease. Optimal treatment is still being developed, but combination chemotherapy, with or without radiation therapy for prevention of CNS involvement, is being used successfully.

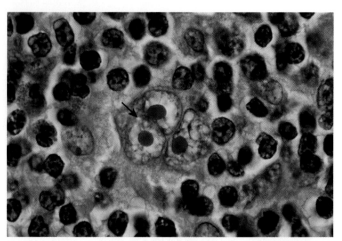

FIGURE 21-11 Diagnostic Reed-Sternberg Cell. A large multinucleated or multilobated cell with *(arrow)* inclusion body–like nucleoli surrounded by a halo of clear nucleoplasm. (From Damjanov I, Linder J: *Pathology: a color atlas,* St Louis, 2000, Mosby.)

Children with advanced small noncleaved cell lymphoma of the abdomen have the poorest prognosis. Although remission occurs in more than 90% of these children, most experience subsequent relapses. Even in the presence of advanced lymphoblastic lymphoma, however, 60% to 80% of children can be cured. Overall, children with localized disease have a 90% survival rate and those with advanced disease have a 60% to 70% survival rate.[9]

Hodgkin Lymphoma

Although the etiologic agent for Hodgkin lymphoma, a lymphoma, has not been identified in children, an infectious mode of transmission, particularly focused on viruses, has been implicated. Many persons with Hodgkin lymphoma have high Epstein-Barr virus titers. At this time, however, the evidence is not sufficient to link an Epstein-Barr virus infection to Hodgkin lymphoma.

Genetic susceptibility has been suggested, because observations show that siblings have a sevenfold increase in risk, particularly siblings of the same gender. In general, Hodgkin lymphoma is more common in males—in childhood, 60% of all cases occur in males.

Hodgkin lymphoma is rare in childhood. It occurs only infrequently in children younger than 2 years, and few cases are observed before the age of 5 years. A gradual rise in incidence occurs through the age of 11 years, with a marked increase through adolescence that continues into the 30 to 39 year age group. The annual incidence of Hodgkin lymphoma in the United States is 4:1,000,000 in children younger than 15 years. Histologically, the tumor consists of neoplastic Reed-Sternberg cells that are typically found surrounded by small lymphocytes, macrophages, neutrophils, and plasma cells (Figure 21-11).

Painless adenopathy in the lower cervical chain, with or without fever, is the most common symptom in children. Other lymph nodes and organs also may be involved (Figure 21-12). Mediastinal involvement can cause pressure on the trachea or bronchi, leading to airway obstruction. Extranodal primary sites in Hodgkin lymphoma are rare. Initial symptoms consist of anorexia, malaise, and lassitude. Intermittent fever is present in 30% of children, and weight loss also may accompany these symptoms. Hodgkin lymphoma has a well-defined staging system that considers the extent and location of disease and the presence of fever, weight loss, or night sweats at diagnosis.

Treatment for Hodgkin lymphoma includes chemotherapy and radiation therapy. For many years, the standard chemotherapy was a

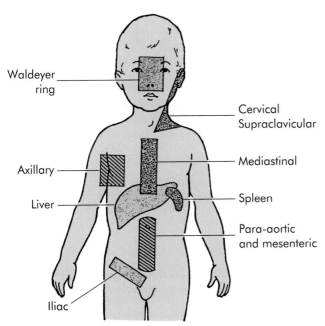

Waldeyer ring

Cervical Supraclavicular

Axillary

Mediastinal

Liver

Spleen

Para-aortic and mesenteric

Iliac

FIGURE 21-12 Main Areas of Lymphadenopathy and Organ Involvement in Hodgkin Lymphoma. (From Hockenberry MJ et al, editors: *Wong's nursing care of infants and children,* ed 8, St Louis, 2007, Mosby.)

regimen of *m*echlorethamine, Oncovin (*v*incristine), *p*rocarbazine, and *p*rednisone (MOPP) given for 6 to 12 cycles. Although hematologic toxicities and associated infections were minimal with MOPP therapy, sterility was reported in male children. Currently, chemotherapy-only trials have been based on alternative regimens of MOPP/ABVD (*A*driamycin [doxorubicin], *b*leomycin, *v*inblastine, *d*acarbazine) or COPP (cyclophosphamide, *v*incristine [Oncovin], procarbazine, prednisone). Although long-term follow-up data are not available, it is hoped that gonadal toxicity will be minimized.[11]

The survival rate for children with Hodgkin lymphoma is high. Most children are seen initially with limited disease and have a 90% survival rate. Even children who are first seen with advanced disease have a 70% to 90% survival rate.

> **QUICK CHECK 21-3**
> 1. List the childhood leukemias in order of rate of incidence.
> 2. Why do children with leukemia experience bone or joint pain?
> 3. What are the common types of non-Hodgkin lymphoma (NHL) in children?

DID YOU UNDERSTAND?

Disorders of Erythrocytes

1. Iron deficiency anemia is the most common blood disorder of infancy and childhood; the highest incidence occurs between 6 months and 2 years of age.
2. Hemolytic disease of the newborn (HDN) results from incompatibility between the maternal and the fetal blood, which may involve differences in Rh factors or blood type (ABO). Maternal antibodies enter the fetal circulation and cause hemolysis of fetal erythrocytes. Because the immature liver is unable to conjugate and excrete the excess bilirubin that results from the hemolysis, icterus neonatorum, kernicterus, or both can develop. Kernicterus, which also may develop from other causes, results in increased breakdown of red blood cells or decreased liver output of enzymes.
3. Infections of the newborn, often acquired by the mother and transmitted to the infant, may result in hemolytic anemia.
4. Sickle cell disease is a genetically determined defect of hemoglobin synthesis inherited by an autosomal recessive transmission; it causes a change in the shape of a red blood cell that results in decreased oxygen or hydration. It is most common among Africans and those of Mediterranean descent.
5. The thalassemias are a heterogeneous group of hereditary hypochromic anemias of varying severity. Basic genetic defects include abnormalities of messenger-RNA processing or deletion of genetic materials, resulting in a decrease in the chains for hemoglobin.

Disorders of Coagulation and Platelets

1. Hemophilia is a condition characterized by impairment of the coagulation of blood and a subsequent tendency to bleed. The classic disease is hereditary and limited to males, being transmitted through the female to the second generation. Many similar conditions attributable to the absence of various clotting factors are now recognized.

2. The antibody-mediated hemorrhagic diseases are a group of disorders caused by the immune response. Antibody-mediated destruction of platelets or antibody-mediated inflammatory reactions to allergens damage blood vessels and cause seepage into tissues.
3. ITP, the most common of the childhood thrombocytopenic purpuras, is a disorder of platelet consumption in which antiplatelet antibodies bind to the plasma membranes of platelets. This results in platelet sequestration and destruction by mononuclear phagocytes at a rate that exceeds the ability of the bone marrow to produce them.

Neoplastic Disorders

1. The childhood leukemias include, in order of their rate of incidence, acute lymphoblastic, acute myeloblastic, and the very rare chronic myelocytic leukemia.
2. Although the cause of childhood leukemia is not known for certain, it is probably the result of multiple interactions between hereditary or genetic predisposition and environmental influences.
3. Acute lymphoblastic leukemia is a potentially curable disease, with about 80% of cases cured.
4. The lymphomas of childhood are Hodgkin lymphoma and non-Hodgkin lymphoma.
5. The origin of non-Hodgkin lymphoma is unknown. Factors that have been implicated include defective host immunity, exposure to a viral agent, chronic immunostimulation, and genetic predisposition.
6. Non-Hodgkin lymphoma has a favorable prognosis, with a 60% to 80% rate of cure.
7. Hodgkin lymphoma is thought to be caused by a still unidentified etiologic agent.
8. Hodgkin lymphoma in children is a readily curable disease with a 90% survival rate in children with limited disease and a 70% to 90% survival rate in those with advanced disease.

REFERENCES

1. Schneider JM, et al: Anemia, iron deficiency, and iron deficiency anemia in 12-36-mo-old children from low-income families, *Am J Clin Nutr* 82(6):1269–1275, 2005.
2. Kyung P: Sickle cell disease and other hemoglobinopathies, *Int Anesthesiol Clin* 42(3):77–93, 2004.
3. Stallworth J, Jerrell J, Tripathi A: Cost-effectiveness of hydroxyurea in reducing the frequency of pain episodes and hospitalization in pediatric sickle cell disease, *Am J Hematol* 85(10):795–797, 2010.
4. Mariani G, Bernardi F: Factor II deficiency, *Semin Thromb Hemost* 35(4):400–406, 2009.
5. Bergman G: Progress in the treatment of bleeding disorders, *Thromb Res* 127(suppl 1):S3–S5, 2011.
6. Gupta V, Tilak V, Bhatia BD: Immune thrombocytopenic purpura, *Indian J Pediatr* 75(7):723–728, 2008.
7. Buka I, Kotsntrng S, Osomio Vargas AR: Trends in childhood cancer incidence: review of environmental linkages, *Pediatr Clin North Am* 54(1):177–203, 2007.
8. Davies SM, Ross JA: Childhood cancer etiology: recent reports, *Med Pediatr Oncol* 40:35–38, 2003.
9. U.S. Cancer Statistics Working Group: *United States cancer statistics: 1999–2005, incidence and mortality web-based report*, Atlanta, 2010, U.S. Department of Health and Human Services, Centers for Disease Control and Prevention, and National Cancer Institute. Available at www.cdc.gov/uscs.
10. Mbulaiteye SM, et al: Spectrum of cancer among HIV-infected persons in Africa: the Uganda AIDS-Cancer Registry Match Study, *Int J Cancer* 118(4):985–990, 2006.
11. Metzger M, et al: Hodgkin lymphoma. In Pizzo PA, Poplack DG, editors: *Principles and practice of pediatric oncology*, ed 6, Philadelphia, 2011, Lippincott, pp 638–662.

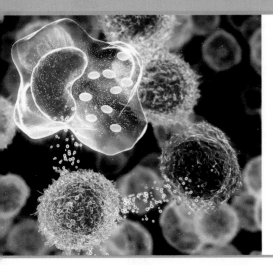

Structure and Function of the Cardiovascular and Lymphatic Systems

Valentina L. Brashers and Kathryn L. McCance

℮volve WEBSITE

CHAPTER OUTLINE

The function of the circulatory system is to deliver oxygen, nutrients, and other substances to all the body's cells and to remove the waste products of cellular metabolism. Delivery and removal are achieved by a complex array of tubing (the blood vessels) connected to a pump (the heart). The heart pumps blood continuously through the blood vessels with cooperation from other systems, particularly the nervous and endocrine systems, which are intrinsic regulators of the heart and blood vessels. Nutrients and oxygen are supplied by the digestive and respiratory systems. Gaseous wastes of cellular metabolism are exhaled by the lungs and other wastes are removed by the kidneys. Of critical importance to cardiovascular function is the vascular endothelium. As a multifunctional organ, its health is essential to normal vascular physiology, and its dysfunction is a critical factor in the development of vascular disease.

THE CIRCULATORY SYSTEM

The heart pumps blood through two separate circulatory systems: one to the lungs and one to all other parts of the body. Structures on the right side of the heart, or **right heart**, pump blood through the lungs. This system is termed the **pulmonary circulation**. The left side of the heart, or **left heart**, sends blood throughout the **systemic circulation**, which supplies all of the body except the lungs (Figure 22-1). These two systems are serially connected; thus the output of one becomes the input of the other.

Arteries carry blood flow from the heart to all parts of the body, where they branch into increasingly smaller vessels and ultimately become a fine meshwork of capillaries. Capillaries allow the closest contact and exchange between the blood and the interstitial space, or interstitium—the environment in which the cells live. Veins channel blood flow from capillaries in all parts of the body back to the heart. The plasma passes through the walls of the capillaries into the interstitial space. This fluid is eventually returned to the cardiovascular system by vessels of the lymphatic system.

THE HEART

The adult heart weighs less than 1 pound (2.2 kg) and is about the size of a fist. It lies obliquely (diagonally) in the **mediastinum,** an area above the diaphragm and between the lungs. Heart structures can be described with respect to three general categories of function:

1. *Structural support of heart tissues and circulation of pulmonary and systemic blood through the heart.* This includes the heart wall and fibrous skeleton, which enclose and support the heart and divide it into four chambers; the valves that direct flow through the chambers; and the great vessels that conduct blood to and from the heart.

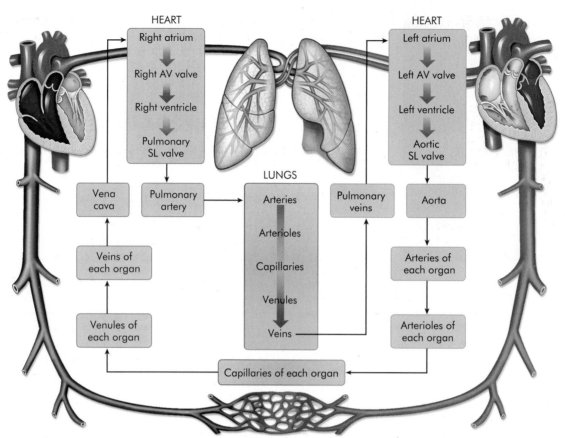

FIGURE 22-1 Diagram Showing Serially Connected Pulmonary and Systemic Circulatory Systems and How to Trace the Flow of Blood. Right heart chambers propel unoxygenated blood through the pulmonary circulation, and the left heart propels oxygenated blood through the systemic circulation. (From Patton KT, Thibodeau GA: *Anatomy & physiology*, ed 7, St Louis, 2010, Mosby.)

2. *Maintenance of heart cells.* This comprises vessels of the coronary circulation—the arteries and veins that serve the metabolic needs of all the heart cells—and the lymphatic vessels of the heart.

3. *Stimulation and control of heart action.* Among these structures are the nerves and specialized muscle cells that direct the rhythmic contraction and relaxation of the heart muscles, propelling blood throughout the pulmonary and systemic circulatory systems.

Structures That Direct Circulation Through the Heart
The Heart Wall

The heart wall has three layers: the pericardium, myocardium, and endocardium (Figure 22-2). The **pericardium** is a double-walled membranous sac that encloses the heart and (1) prevents displacement of the heart during gravitational acceleration or deceleration, (2) serves as a physical barrier that protects the heart against infection and inflammation from the lungs and pleural space, and (3) contains pain receptors and mechanoreceptors to elicit reflex changes in blood pressure and heart rate. The two layers of the pericardium are the parietal and the visceral pericardia (see Figure 22-2). These are separated by a fluid-containing space called the **pericardial cavity.** The **pericardial fluid** (10 to 30 ml) is secreted by cells of the mesothelium and lubricates the membranes that line the pericardial cavity, enabling them to slide over one another with a minimum amount of friction as the heart beats. The amount and character of the pericardial fluid are altered if the pericardium is inflamed (see Chapter 23).

The thickest layer of the heart wall, the **myocardium,** is composed of cardiac muscle and is anchored to the heart's fibrous skeleton. The

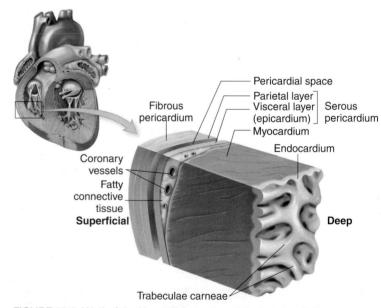

FIGURE 22-2 Wall of the Heart. This section of the heart wall shows the fibrous pericardium, the parietal and visceral layers of the serous pericardium (with the pericardial space between them), the myocardium, and the endocardium. Note the fatty connective tissue between the visceral layer of the serous pericardium (epicardium) and the myocardium. Note also that the endocardium covers beamlike projections of myocardial muscle tissue called *trabeculae*. (From Patton KT, Thibodeau GA: *Anatomy & physiology*, ed 7, St Louis, 2010, Mosby.)

myocardial cells provide the contractile force needed for blood to flow through the heart and into the pulmonary and systemic circulations.

The internal lining of the myocardium, the endocardium, comprises connective tissue and squamous cells (see Figure 22-2). This lining is continuous with the endothelium that lines all the arteries, veins, and capillaries of the body, creating a continuous, closed circulatory system.

Chambers of the Heart

The heart has four chambers: the left atrium, the right atrium, the right ventricle, and the left ventricle. (Blood flow through these chambers is illustrated in Figure 22-3.) The atria are smaller than the ventricles and have thinner walls. The ventricles have a thicker myocardial

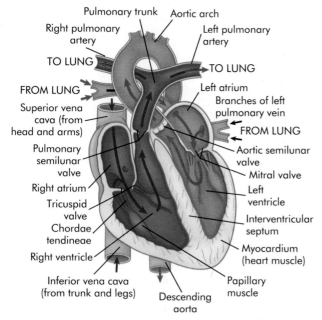

Pulmonary trunk
Aortic arch
Right pulmonary artery
Left pulmonary artery
TO LUNG
TO LUNG
FROM LUNG
Left atrium
Branches of left pulmonary vein
Superior vena cava (from head and arms)
FROM LUNG
Aortic semilunar valve
Pulmonary semilunar valve
Mitral valve
Right atrium
Left ventricle
Tricuspid valve
Interventricular septum
Chordae tendineae
Myocardium (heart muscle)
Right ventricle
Inferior vena cava (from trunk and legs)
Papillary muscle
Descending aorta

FIGURE 22-3 Structures That Direct Blood Flow Through the Heart. Arrows indicate path of blood flow through chambers, valves, and major vessels.

layer and constitute much of the bulk of the heart. The ventricles are formed by a continuum of muscle fibers originating from the fibrous skeleton at the base of the heart.

The myocardial thickness of each cardiac chamber depends on the amount of pressure or resistance it must overcome to eject blood. The two atria have the thinnest walls because they are low-pressure chambers that serve as storage units and conduits for blood that is emptied into the ventricles. Normally, there is little resistance to flow from the atria to the ventricles. The ventricular myocardium, on the other hand, must be strong enough to pump against pressures in the pulmonary or systemic vessels. The mean pulmonary artery pressure is only 15 mm Hg, whereas the mean systemic arterial pressure is about 92 mm Hg. For this reason, the left ventricle's myocardium is several times thicker than that of the right ventricle.

The right ventricle is shaped like a crescent, or triangle, enabling a bellows-like action that efficiently ejects large volumes of blood through a very small valve into the low-pressure pulmonary system. The left ventricle is larger than the right ventricle and is bullet shaped, helping it to eject blood through a relatively large valve opening into the high-pressure systemic circulation.

The septal membrane separates the right and left sides of the heart and prevents blood from crossing over. The atria are separated by the interatrial septum, and the ventricles by the interventricular septum. Indentations of the endocardium form valves that separate the atria from the ventricles and the ventricles from the aorta and pulmonary arteries.

Fibrous Skeleton of the Heart

Four rings of dense fibrous connective tissue provide a firm anchorage for the attachments of the atrial and ventricular musculature, as well as the valvular tissue (Figure 22-4). The fibrous rings are adjacent and form a central, fibrous supporting structure collectively termed the *annuli fibrosi cordis.*

Valves of the Heart

One-way blood flow through the heart is ensured by the four heart valves. During ventricular relaxation, the two atrioventricular valves open and blood flows from the atria to the relaxed ventricles. As the

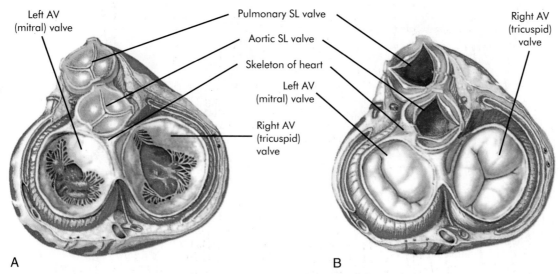

Left AV (mitral) valve
Pulmonary SL valve
Right AV (tricuspid) valve
Aortic SL valve
Skeleton of heart
Left AV (mitral) valve
Right AV (tricuspid) valve

A
B

FIGURE 22-4 Structure of the Heart Valves. A, The heart valves in this drawing are depicted as viewed from above (looking down into the heart). Note that the semilunar *(SL)* valves are closed and the atrioventricular *(AV)* valves are open, as when the atria are contracting. View **B** is similar to view **A** except that the semilunar valves are open and the atrioventricular valves are closed, as when the ventricles are contracting. (From Patton KT, Thibodeau GA: *Anatomy & physiology,* ed 7, St Louis, 2010, Mosby.)

ventricles contract, increasing ventricular pressure causes these valves to close and prevent backflow into the atria. The semilunar valves of the heart open when intraventricular pressure exceeds aortic and pulmonary pressures, and blood flows out of the ventricles and into the pulmonary and systemic circulations. After ventricular contraction and ejection, intraventricular pressure falls and the pulmonic and aortic semilunar valves close, preventing backflow into the right and left ventricles, respectively. The coordinated actions of the heart valves are shown in Figures 22-3 and 22-4.

The atrioventricular (tricuspid and mitral) valve openings are guarded by flaps of tissue called *leaflets* or *cusps,* which are attached to the papillary muscles by the chordae tendineae cordis (see Figure 22-3). The papillary muscles are extensions of the myocardium that pull the cusps together and downward at the onset of ventricular contraction, thus preventing their backward expulsion into the atria.

The right atrioventricular valve is called the tricuspid valve because it has three cusps. The left atrioventricular valve is a bicuspid (two-cusp) valve called the mitral valve. The tricuspid and mitral valves function as a unit because the atrium, fibrous rings, valvular tissue, chordae tendineae, papillary muscles, and ventricular walls are connected. Collectively, these six structures are known as the mitral and tricuspid complex. Damage to any one of the six components of this complex can alter function significantly.

Blood leaves the right ventricle through the pulmonic semilunar valve, and it leaves the left ventricle through the aortic semilunar valve (see Figures 22-3 and 22-4). Both the pulmonic and aortic semilunar valves have three cup-shaped cusps that arise from the fibrous skeleton.

The Great Vessels

Blood moves in and out of the heart through several large vessels (see Figure 22-3). The right heart receives venous blood from the systemic circulation through the superior and inferior venae cavae, which enter the right atrium. Blood leaves the right ventricle and enters the pulmonary circulation through the pulmonary artery. This artery divides into right and left branches to transport unoxygenated blood from the right heart to the right and left lungs. The pulmonary arteries branch further into the pulmonary capillary bed, where oxygen and carbon dioxide exchange occurs.

The four pulmonary veins, two from the right lung and two from the left lung, carry oxygenated blood from the lungs to the left side of the heart. The oxygenated blood moves through the left atrium and ventricle and out into the aorta, which delivers it to systemic vessels that supply the body.

Blood Flow During the Cardiac Cycle

The pumping action of the heart consists of contraction and relaxation of the myocardial layer of the heart wall. Each ventricular contraction and the relaxation that follows it constitute one cardiac cycle. (Blood flow through the heart during a single cardiac cycle is illustrated in Figure 22-5.) During relaxation, termed diastole, blood fills the ventricles. The ventricle fills rapidly in early diastole and again in late diastole when the atrium contracts. The ventricular contraction that follows, termed systole, propels the blood out of the ventricles and into the circulation. Contraction of the left ventricle is slightly earlier than contraction of the right ventricle.

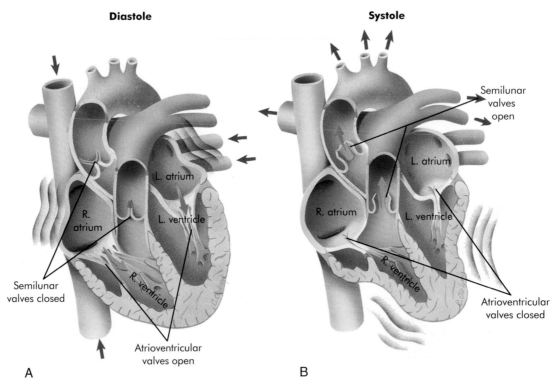

Diastole

Systole

Semilunar valves open

L. atrium

L. ventricle

R. atrium

R. ventricle

Atrioventricular valves closed

L. atrium

L. ventricle

R. atrium

R. ventricle

Semilunar valves closed

Atrioventricular valves open

A

B

FIGURE 22-5 Blood Flow Through the Heart During a Single Cardiac Cycle. A, During diastole, blood flows into atria, atrioventricular valves are pushed open, and blood begins to fill ventricles. Atrial systole squeezes any blood remaining in atria out into ventricles. **B,** During ventricular systole, ventricles contract, pushing blood out through semilunar valves into pulmonary artery (right ventricle) and aorta (left ventricle). (Modified from Patton KT, Thibodeau GA: *Anatomy & physiology,* ed 7, St Louis, 2010, Mosby.)

The phases of the cardiac cycle can be identified on initiation of ventricular myocardial contraction (Figures 22-6 and 22-7). Expulsion of blood from the ventricles marks the end of one cardiac cycle.

Normal Intracardiac Pressures

Normal intracardiac pressures are shown in Table 22-1.

TABLE 22-1	NORMAL INTRACARDIAC PRESSURES	
	MEAN (MM HG)	**RANGE (MM HG)**
Right atrium	4	0-8
Right ventricle		
Systolic	24	15-28
End-diastolic	4	0-8
Left atrium	7	4-12
Left ventricle		
Systolic	130	90-140
End-diastolic	7	4-12

> ✔ **QUICK CHECK 22-1**
> 1. Why are the two separate circulatory systems said to be "serially connected"?
> 2. Why does the thickness of the myocardium vary dramatically in the different heart chambers?
> 3. Trace blood flow through the heart during a single cardiac cycle.

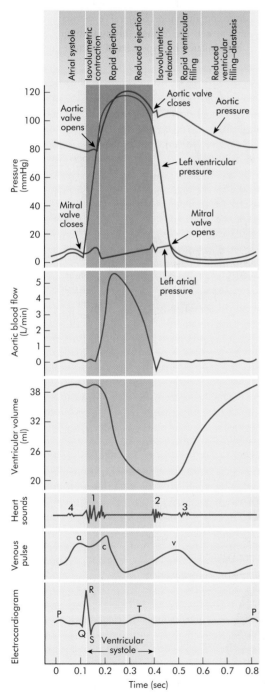

FIGURE 22-6 Composite Chart of Heart Function. This chart is a composite of several diagrams of heart function (cardiac pumping cycle, blood pressure, blood flow, volume, heart sounds, venous pulse, and electrocardiogram [ECG]), all adjusted to the same timescale.

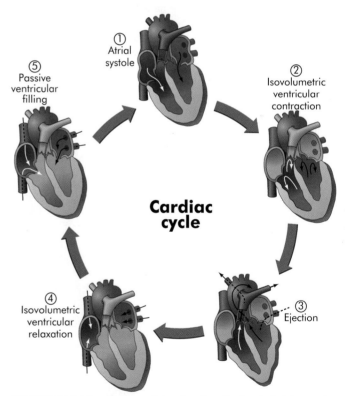

FIGURE 22-7 The Phases of the Cardiac Cycle. *1,* Atrial systole. *2,* Isovolumetric ventricular contraction. Ventricular volume remains constant as pressure increases rapidly. *3,* Ejection. *4,* Isovolumetric ventricular relaxation. Both sets of valves are closed, and the ventricles are relaxing. *5,* Passive ventricular filling. The atrioventricular (AV) valves are forced open, and the blood rushes into the relaxing ventricles. (From Patton KT, Thibodeau GA: *Anatomy & physiology,* ed 7, St Louis, 2010, Mosby.)

Structures That Support Cardiac Metabolism: The Coronary Vessels

The blood within the heart chambers does not supply oxygen and other nutrients to the cells of the heart. Like all other organs, including the lungs, heart structures are nourished by vessels of the systemic circulation. The branch of the systemic circulation that supplies the heart is termed the coronary circulation and consists of coronary arteries, which receive blood through openings in the aorta called the coronary ostia, and the cardiac veins, which empty into the right atrium through the opening of a large vein called the coronary sinus (Figure 22-8). (Regulation of the coronary circulation, which is similar to regulation of flow through systemic and pulmonary vessels, is described elsewhere.)

Coronary Arteries

The right coronary artery and the left coronary artery (see Figure 22-8) traverse the epicardium, myocardium, and endocardium and branch to become arterioles and then capillaries. Their main branches are outlined in Box 22-1.

Collateral Arteries

The collateral arteries are actually connections, or anastomoses, between two branches of the same or the opposite coronary artery.[1] The epicardium contains more collateral vessels than the endocardium. New collateral vessels are formed through the process of angiogenesis, which is stimulated by hypoxia and vascular endothelial growth

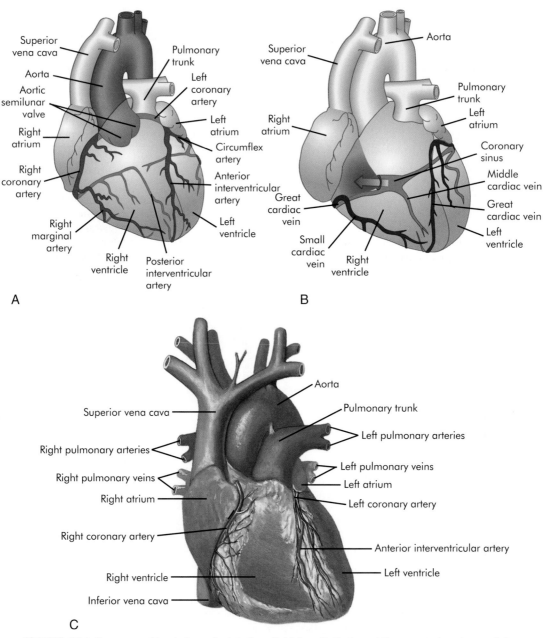

FIGURE 22-8 Coronary Circulation. A, Arteries. **B,** Veins. Both **A** and **B** are anterior views of the heart. Vessels near the anterior surface are more darkly colored than vessels of the posterior surface seen through the heart. **C,** View of the anterior (sternocostal) surface. (**A** and **B** modified from Patton KT, Thibodeau GA: *Anatomy & physiology,* ed 7, St Louis, 2010, Mosby; **C** from Seeley RR, Stephens TD, Tate P: *Anatomy and physiology,* ed 3, St Louis, 1995, Mosby.)

BOX 22-1   **MAIN BRANCHES OF THE CORONARY ARTERIES**

Left coronary artery. Arises from single ostium behind left cusp of aortic semilunar valve; ranges from a few millimeters to a few centimeters long; passes between left arterial appendage and pulmonary artery and generally divides into two branches: the left anterior descending artery and the circumflex artery; other branches are distributed diagonally across the free wall of the left ventricle.

Left anterior descending artery (or anterior interventricular artery). Delivers blood to portions of left and right ventricles and much of interventricular septum; travels down the anterior surface of the interventricular septum toward apex of the heart.

Circumflex artery. Travels in a groove *(coronary sulcus)* that separates left atrium from left ventricle and extends to left border of heart; supplies blood to left atrium and lateral wall of left ventricle; often branches to posterior surfaces of left atrium and left ventricle.

Right coronary artery. Originates from an ostium behind the right aortic cusp, travels from behind the pulmonary artery, and extends around the right heart to the heart's posterior surface, where it branches to atrium and ventricle; three major branches are conus (supplies blood to upper right ventricle), right marginal branch (supplies right ventricle to the apex), and posterior descending branch (lies in posterior interventricular sulcus and supplies smaller branches to both ventricles).

factors. The collateral circulation is responsible for supplying blood and oxygen to the myocardium that has become ischemic following gradual narrowing of one or more major coronary arteries (coronary artery disease). Unfortunately, diabetes, which predisposes to coronary artery disease, also impedes collateral formation because of increased production of antiangiogenic factors, such as endostatin and angiostatin. An increased understanding of the process of angiogenesis has led to the use of angiogenic factors in the treatment of coronary artery disease that is not responsive to more conventional therapies.[2]

Coronary Capillaries

The heart has an extensive capillary network. Blood travels from the arteries to the arterioles and then into the capillaries, where exchange of oxygen and other nutrients takes place. At rest, the heart extracts 70% to 80% of the oxygen delivered to it and coronary blood flow is directly correlated with myocardial oxygen consumption.[3] Any alteration of the cardiac muscles dramatically affects blood flow in the capillaries.

Coronary Veins and Lymphatic Vessels

After passing through the extensive capillary network, blood from the coronary arteries drains into the cardiac veins, which travel alongside the arteries. Most of the venous drainage of the heart occurs through veins in the visceral pericardium. The veins then feed into the great cardiac vein (see Figure 22-8) and coronary sinus on the posterior surface of the heart, between the atria and ventricles, in the coronary sulcus.

The myocardium has an extensive system of lymphatic vessels. With cardiac contraction, the lymphatic vessels drain fluid to lymph nodes in the anterior mediastinum that eventually empty into the superior vena cava. The lymphatics are important for protecting the myocardium against infection and injury.

Structures That Control Heart Action

The continuous, rhythmic repetition of the cardiac cycle (systole and diastole) depends on the transmission of electrical impulses, termed cardiac action potentials, through the myocardium. (Action potentials are described in Chapters 1 and 4.) The muscle fibers of the myocardium are uniquely joined so that action potentials pass from cell to cell rapidly and efficiently.

The myocardium also contains its own conduction system—specialized cells that enable it to generate and transmit action potentials without stimulation from the nervous system (Figure 22-9). These cells are concentrated at certain sites in the myocardium called nodes. The cardiac cycle is stimulated by these nodes of specialized cells. Although the heart is innervated by the autonomic nervous system (both sympathetic and parasympathetic fibers), neural impulses are not needed to maintain the cardiac cycle. Thus the heart will beat in the absence of any innervation.

Heart action is also influenced by substances delivered to the myocardium in coronary blood. Nutrients and oxygen are needed for cellular survival and normal function, whereas hormones and biochemicals affect the strength and duration of myocardial contraction and the degree and duration of myocardial relaxation. Normal or appropriate function depends on the availability of these substances, which is why coronary artery disease can seriously disrupt heart function.

The Conduction System

Normally, electrical impulses arise in the sinoatrial node (SA node, sinus node), which is often called the pacemaker of the heart. The SA node is located at the junction of the right atrium and superior vena cava, just superior to the tricuspid valve. The SA node is heavily innervated by both sympathetic and parasympathetic nerve fibers.[4] In the resting adult the SA node generates about 75 action potentials per minute. Each one travels rapidly from cell to cell and through special pathways in the atrial myocardium, causing both atria to contract. There are three pathways in the atria called the anterior, middle, and posterior internodal pathways. These pathways consist of ordinary myocardial cells and specialized conducting fibers. The anterior interatrial myocardial band, or Bachmann bundle, conducts the impulse from the SA node to the left atrium. The posterior internodal pathway connects the right and left atria and the SA node and AV node for conduction from the SA node to the atrioventricular node (AV node).[4,5]

The AV node is well situated for mediating conduction between the atria and ventricles. It is located in the right atrial wall superior to the tricuspid valve and anterior to the ostium of the coronary sinus. Behind it are numerous autonomic parasympathetic ganglia. These ganglia serve as receptors for the vagus nerve and cause slowing of impulse conduction through the AV node.

Conducting fibers from the AV node converge to form the bundle of His (atrioventricular bundle), within the posterior border of the interventricular septum. The bundle of His then gives rise to the right and left bundle branches. The right bundle branch (RBB) is thin and travels without much branching to the right ventricular apex. Because of its thinness and relative lack of branches, the RBB is susceptible to interruption by damage to the endocardium. The left bundle branch (LBB) arises perpendicularly from the bundle of His and, in some hearts, divides into two branches, or fascicles. The left anterior bundle branch (LABB) passes the left anterior papillary muscle and the base of the left ventricle and crosses the aortic outflow tract. Damage to the aortic valve or the left ventricle can interrupt this branch. The left posterior bundle branch (LPBB) travels posteriorly, crossing the left ventricular inflow tract to the base of the left posterior papillary muscle. This branch spreads diffusely through the posterior inferior left ventricular wall. Blood flow through this portion of the left ventricle is relatively nonturbulent, so the LBB is somewhat protected from injury caused by wear and tear.

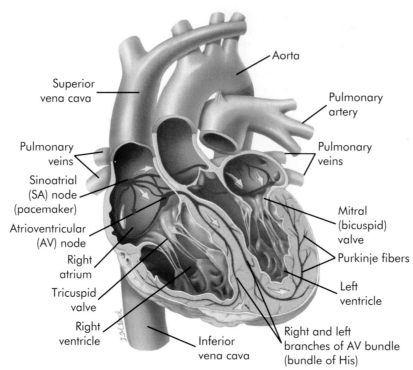

FIGURE 22-9 Conduction System of Heart. Specialized cardiac muscle cells in the wall of the heart rapidly conduct an electrical impulse throughout the myocardium. The signal is initiated by the sinoatrial (SA) node (pacemaker) and spreads to the rest of the atrial myocardium and to the atrioventricular (AV) node. The AV node then initiates a signal that is conducted through the ventricular myocardium by way of the atrioventricular bundle (of His) and Purkinje fibers. (Modified from Patton KT, Thibodeau GA: *Anatomy & physiology*, ed 7, St Louis, 2010, Mosby.)

The Purkinje fibers are the terminal branches of the RBB and LBB. They extend from the ventricular apexes to the fibrous rings and penetrate the heart wall to the outer myocardium. The first areas of the ventricles to be excited are portions of the interventricular septum. The septum is activated from both the RBB and the LBB. The extensive network of Purkinje fibers promotes the rapid spread of the impulse to the ventricular apices. The basal and posterior portions of the ventricles are the last to be activated.

✔ **QUICK CHECK 22-2**
1. Outline the conduction system of the heart.
2. What happens ionically during depolarization and during repolarization?
3. Why are the left and right coronary vessels considered the major coronary vessels?

TABLE 22-2	INTERCELLULAR AND EXTRACELLULAR ION CONCENTRATIONS IN THE MYOCARDIUM	
	INTRACELLULAR CONCENTRATION (mM)	**EXTRACELLULAR CONCENTRATION (mM)**
Sodium (Na+)	15	145
Potassium (K+)	150	4
Chloride (Cl-)	5	120
Calcium (Ca++)	10^{-7}	2

mM, Micromolar (millimoles per kilogram).

Propagation of cardiac action potentials. Electrical activation of the muscle cells, termed depolarization, is caused by the movement of electrically charged solutes (ions) across cardiac cell membranes. Deactivation, called repolarization, occurs the same way. (Movement of ions across cell membranes is described in Chapter 1; electrical activation of muscle cells is described in Chapter 36.)

When ions move into and out of the cell, an electrical (voltage) difference across the cell membrane, called the *membrane potential,* is created. The resting membrane potential of myocardial cells is between −80 and −90 millivolts (mV), whereas that of the SA node is between −50 and −60 mV and that of the AV node is between −60 and −70 mV.[4] During depolarization, the inside of the cell becomes less negatively charged. In cardiac cells, the difference between resting membrane potential (in millivolts) and the decreased negative charge caused by depolarization is the cardiac action potential. Table 22-2 summarizes the intracellular and extracellular ionic concentrations of cardiac muscle. Hence, drugs that alter ion movement (e.g., calcium) have profound effects on the action potential and can alter heart rate. The various phases of the cardiac action potential are related to changes in the permeability of the cell membrane, primarily to sodium and potassium changes. Threshold is the point at which the cell membrane's selective permeability to sodium and potassium is temporarily disrupted, leading to depolarization. If the resting membrane potential becomes more negative because of a decrease in extracellular potassium concentration (hypokalemia), it is termed *hyperpolarization.*

A refractory period, during which no new cardiac action potential can be initiated by a stimulus, follows depolarization. This effective or absolute refractory period corresponds to the time needed for the reopening of channels that permit sodium and calcium influx. A relative refractory period occurs near the end of repolarization, following the effective refractory period. During this time, the membrane can be depolarized again but only by a greater-than-normal stimulus. Abnormal refractory periods as a result of disease can cause abnormal heart rhythms or dysrhythmias (see Chapter 23).

The normal electrocardiogram. The normal electrocardiogram is recorded from electrical activity transmitted by skin electrodes and reflects the sum of all the cardiac action potentials (Figure 22-10). The P wave represents atrial depolarization. The PR interval is a measure of time from the onset of atrial activation to the onset of ventricular activation (normally 0.12 to 0.20 second). The PR interval represents the time necessary for electrical activity to travel from the sinus node through the atrium, AV node, and His-Purkinje system to activate ventricular myocardial cells. The QRS complex represents the sum of all ventricular muscle cell depolarizations. The configuration and amplitude of the QRS complex vary considerably among individuals. The duration is normally between 0.06 and 0.10 second. During the ST interval, the entire ventricular myocardium is depolarized. The QT interval is sometimes called the "electrical systole" of the ventricles. It lasts about 0.4 second but varies inversely with the heart rate. The T wave represents ventricular repolarization.

Automaticity. Automaticity, or the property of generating spontaneous depolarization to threshold, enables the SA and AV nodes to generate cardiac action potentials without any stimulus. Cells capable of spontaneous depolarization are called automatic cells. Those of the cardiac conduction system can stimulate the heart to beat even when it is removed from the body. Spontaneous depolarization is possible in automatic cells because the membrane potential does not "rest" during return to the resting membrane potential. Instead, it slowly creeps toward threshold during the diastolic phase of the cardiac cycle.

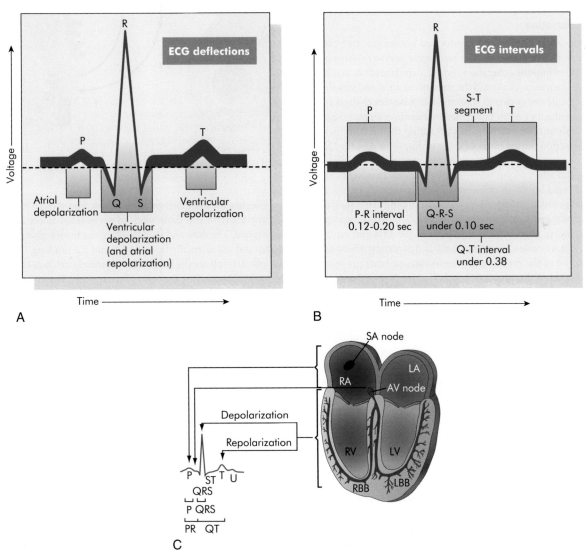

FIGURE 22-10 Electrocardiogram (ECG) and Cardiac Electrical Activity. A, Normal ECG. Depolarization and repolarization. **B,** ECG intervals among P, QRS, and T waves. **C,** Schematic representation of ECG and its relationship to cardiac electrical activity. *AV,* Atrioventricular; *LA,* left atrium; *LBB,* left bundle branch; *LV,* left ventricle; *RA,* right atrium; *RBB,* right bundle branch; *RV,* right ventricle. (**A** and **B** from Patton KT, Thibodeau GA: *Anatomy & physiology,* ed 7, St Louis, 2010, Mosby.)

Because threshold is approached during diastole, return to the resting membrane potential in automatic cells is called diastolic depolarization. The electrical impulse normally begins in the SA node because its cells depolarize more rapidly than other automatic cells.

Rhythmicity. Rhythmicity is the regular generation of an action potential by the heart's conduction system. The SA node sets the pace because normally it has the fastest rate. The SA node depolarizes spontaneously 60 to 100 times per minute. If the SA node is damaged, the AV node will become the heart's pacemaker at a rate of about 40 to 60 spontaneous depolarizations per minute. Eventually, however, conduction cells in the atria usually take over from the AV node. Purkinje fibers are capable of spontaneous depolarization but at a rate of only 30 to 40 beats/min.[4]

> ✔ **QUICK CHECK 22-3**
> 1. What are the pathways of conduction through the heart?
> 2. What does each of the electrocardiogram waves (P, Q, R, S, T) represent?
> 3. Define automaticity and rhythmicity.

Cardiac Innervation

Although the heart's nodes and conduction system generate cardiac action potentials independently, the autonomic nervous system influences the rate of impulse generation (firing), depolarization, and repolarization of the myocardium and the strength of atrial and ventricular contraction. Autonomic neural transmission produces changes in the heart and circulatory system faster than metabolic or humoral agents. Speed is important, for example, in stimulating the heart to increase its pumping action during times of stress or fear—the so-called fight-or-flight response. Although increased delivery of oxygen, glucose, hormones, and other blood-borne factors sustains increased cardiac activity, the rapid initiation of increased activity depends on the sympathetic and parasympathetic fibers of the autonomic nervous system.

Sympathetic and parasympathetic nerves. Sympathetic and parasympathetic nerve fibers innervate all parts of the atria and ventricles and the SA and AV nodes. The sympathetic and parasympathetic nerves affect the speed of the cardiac cycle (heart rate, or beats per minute) and the diameter of the coronary vessels (Figure 22-11). Sympathetic nervous activity enhances myocardial performance. Stimulation of the SA node by the sympathetic nervous system rapidly increases heart rate. Furthermore, neurally released norepinephrine or circulating catecholamines interact with β-adrenergic receptors on the cardiac cell membranes. The overall effect is an increased influx of Ca^{++}, which increases the contractile strength of the heart and increases the speed of electrical impulses through the heart muscle and the nodes. Finally, increased sympathetic discharge dilates the coronary vessels.[4]

The parasympathetic nervous system affects the heart through the vagus nerve, which releases acetylcholine. Acetylcholine causes decreased heart rate and slows conduction through the AV node. Acetylcholine also causes coronary vasodilation.[4]

Myocardial Cells

The cells of cardiac muscle (the myocardium) are composed of long, narrow fibers that contain bundles of longitudinally arranged myofibrils; a nucleus (cardiac muscle) or many nuclei (skeletal muscle); mitochondria; an internal membrane system (the sarcoplasmic reticulum); cytoplasm (sarcoplasm); and a plasma membrane (the sarcolemma), which encloses the cell. Cardiac and skeletal muscle cells also have an "external" membrane system made up of transverse tubules (T tubules) formed by invaginations of the sarcolemma. The sarcoplasmic reticulum forms a network of channels that surrounds the muscle fiber.

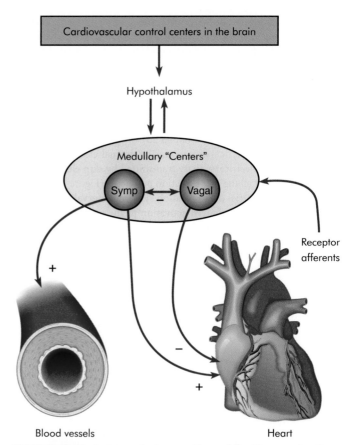

FIGURE 22-11 Autonomic Innervation of Cardiovascular System. Inhibition (−); activation (+).

Because the myofibrils in both cardiac and skeletal fibers consist of alternating light and dark bands of protein, the fibers appear striped, or striated. The dark and light bands of the myofibrils are called *sarcomeres* and are normally between 1.6 and 2.2 μm long (Figure 22-12). Length determines the limits of myocardial stretch at the end of diastole and subsequently the force of contraction during systole.

Differences between cardiac and skeletal muscle reflect heart function. Cardiac cells are arranged in branching networks throughout the myocardium, whereas skeletal muscle cells tend to be arranged in parallel units throughout the length of the muscle. Cardiac fibers have only one nucleus, whereas skeletal muscle cells have many nuclei. Other differences enable cardiac fibers to:

1. *Transmit action potentials quickly from cell to cell.* Electrical impulses are transmitted rapidly from cardiac fiber to cardiac fiber because the network of fibers is connected at intercalated disks, which are thickened portions of the sarcolemma. The intercalated disks contain two junctions: desmosomes, which attach one cell to another; and gap junctions, which allow the electrical impulse to spread from cell to cell (see Chapter 1). Together, these junctions provide a low-resistance pathway for impulse propagation.

2. *Maintain high levels of energy synthesis.* Unlike skeletal muscle, the heart cannot rest and is in constant need of energy compounds such as adenosine triphosphate (ATP). Therefore the cytoplasm surrounding the bundles of myofibrils in each cardiac muscle cell contains a superabundance of mitochondria (25% of the cellular volume). Cardiac muscle cells have more mitochondria than do skeletal muscle cells to provide the necessary respiratory enzymes for aerobic metabolism and supply quantities of ATP sufficient for the constant action of the myocardium.

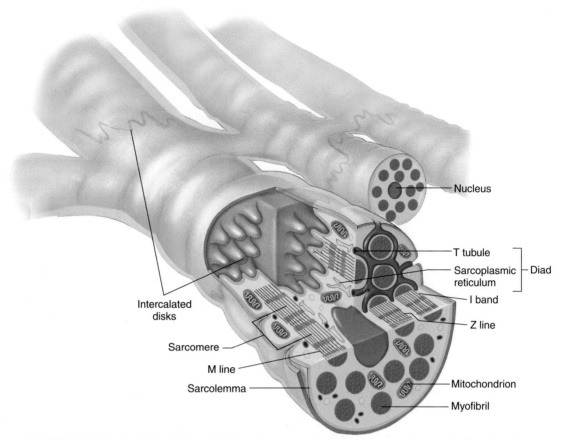

FIGURE 22-12 Cardiac Muscle Fiber. Unlike other types of muscle fibers, cardiac muscle fiber is typically branched and forms junctions, called *intercalated disks,* with adjacent cardiac muscle fibers. Like skeletal muscle fibers, cardiac muscle fibers contain sarcoplasmic reticula and T tubules—although these structures are not as highly organized as in skeletal muscle fibers. (From Patton KT, Thibodeau GA: *Anatomy & physiology,* ed 7, St Louis, 2010, Mosby.)

3. *Gain access to more ions, particularly sodium and potassium, in the extracellular environment.* Cardiac fibers contain more T tubules than do skeletal muscle fibers. This gives each myofibril in the myocardium ready access to molecules needed for the continuous transmission of action potentials, which involves transport of sodium and potassium through the walls of the T tubules. Because the T tubule system is continuous with the extracellular space and the interstitial fluid, it facilitates the rapid transmission of the electrical impulses from the surface of the sarcolemma to the myofibrils inside the fiber. This activates all the myofibrils of one fiber simultaneously. The sarcoplasmic reticulum is located around the myofibrils. When an action potential is transmitted through the T tubules, it induces the sarcoplasmic reticulum to release its stored calcium, which activates the contractile proteins actin and myosin.

Actin, myosin, and the troponin-tropomyosin complex. The thick filaments of **myosin** constitute the central dark band called the **anisotropic,** or **A, band** (see Figure 22-12). The myosin molecule resembles a golf club with two large bulbous heads protruding from one end of a straight shaft (Figure 22-13, *A*). The bilobed heads contain an actin-binding site and a site of ATPase activity. A thick filament contains about 200 myosin molecules bundled together with the heads of the molecules (called *cross-bridges*) facing outward (Figure 22-14, *C*). The **actin** molecules are part of the thin filaments (Figure 22-14, *A*). The light bands are called **isotropic,** or **I, bands** (see Figure 22-12). The thin filaments of actin appear light and extend from the **Z line,** a dense fibrous line that crosses

the center of each I band. The area from one dark Z line to an adjacent Z line is the sarcomere. In the center of the sarcomere is the H zone, a somewhat less dense region. A thin, dark **M line** travels through the center of the H zone. A single **tropomyosin** molecule (a relaxing protein) lies alongside seven actin molecules. Troponin, another relaxing protein, associates with the tropomyosin molecule, forming the **troponin-tropomyosin complex** (see Figure 22-14). The troponin complex itself has three components. **Troponin T** aids in the binding of the troponin complex to actin and tropomyosin; **troponin I** inhibits the ATPase of actomyosin; and **troponin C** contains binding sites for the calcium ions involved in contraction. These troponin molecules are released into the bloodstream during myocardial infarction or injury, where they can be measured.

Myocardial metabolism. Cardiac muscle, like other muscle tissue, depends on the constant production of ATP for energy. ATP is produced within the mitochondria mainly from glucose, fatty acids, and lactate. If the myocardium is inadequately perfused because of coronary artery disease, anaerobic metabolism becomes an essential source of energy (see Chapter 1). The energy produced by metabolic processes is used for muscle contraction and relaxation, electrical excitation, membrane transport, and synthesis of large molecules. Normally, the amount of ATP produced supplies sufficient energy to pump blood throughout the system.

Cardiac work is often expressed in terms of **myocardial oxygen consumption** ($M\dot{V}O_2$), which correlates closely with total cardiac

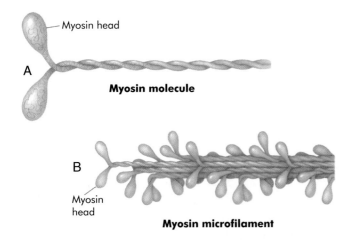

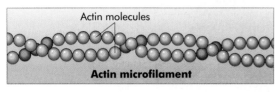

C

FIGURE 22-13 Structure of Myosin. A, Each myosin molecule is a coil of two chains wrapped around one another. At the end of each chain is a globular region, much like a golf club, called the *head.* **B,** Myosin molecules usually are combined into filaments, which are stalks of myosin from which the heads protrude. **C,** Actin microfilament. (From Raven PH, Johnson GB: *Understanding biology,* ed 3, Dubuque, Iowa, 1995, Brown.)

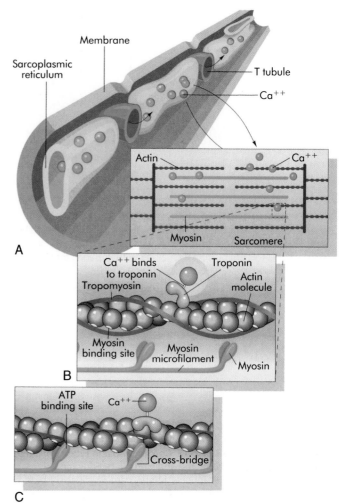

FIGURE 22-14 Myofilaments and Mechanisms of Muscle Contraction. A, Thin and thick myofilaments. In resting muscle, calcium ions are stored in the sarcoplasmic reticulum. When an action potential reaches the muscle cell, the T tubules carry the action potential deep into the sarcoplasm. The action potential causes the sarcoplasmic reticulum to release the store of calcium ions. **B,** In resting muscle the myosin binding sites are covered by troponin and tropomyosin. The calcium ions released into the sarcoplasm as a result of action potential bind to the troponin. **C,** This binding causes the tropomyosin and troponin to move out of the way of the myosin binding sites, leaving the myosin heads free to bind to the actin microfilament. *ATP,* Adenosine triphosphate. (From Raven PH, Johnson GB: *Understanding biology,* ed 3, Dubuque, Iowa, 1995, Brown.)

energy requirements. $M\dot{V}O_2$ is determined by the following three major factors: (1) amount of wall stress during systole, which can be estimated by measuring the systolic blood pressure; (2) duration of systolic wall tension, which is measured indirectly by the heart rate; and (3) contractile state of the myocardium, for which no clinical measurement exists. $M\dot{V}O_2$ can increase several-fold with exercise and decrease moderately under conditions such as hypotension and hypothermia.

The oxygen supply to the myocardium is delivered exclusively by the coronary arteries. Approximately 70% to 75% of the oxygen from the coronary arteries is used immediately by cardiac muscle, leaving little oxygen in reserve. The oxygen content of the blood cannot be increased under normal atmospheric conditions nor can the amount of O_2 extracted from the blood be appreciably increased from the resting level. Any increased energy needs can be met only by increasing coronary blood flow. When oxygen content decreases, the local concentration of metabolic factors increases. One of these, adenosine, dilates coronary arterioles, increasing coronary blood flow.

Myocardial Contraction and Relaxation

Myocardial contractility is a change in developed tension at a given resting fiber length. In functional terms, contractility is the ability of the heart muscle to shorten. On a molecular basis, thin filaments of actin slide over thick filaments of myosin, according to the cross-bridge theory of muscle contraction.[4] Anatomically, contraction occurs when the sarcomere shortens, so adjacent Z lines move closer together (see Figures 22-12 and 22-15). The A band width, including thick myosin filaments, is unchanged, with the movement coming from the long sets of filaments. The degree of shortening depends on how much the thin filaments overlap the thick filaments.

Calcium and excitation-contraction coupling. Excitation-contraction coupling is the process by which an action potential in the plasma membrane of the muscle fiber triggers the cycle, leading to cross-bridge activity and contraction. Activation of this cycle depends on the availability of calcium.

Calcium is stored in the tubule system and the sarcoplasmic reticulum. It enters the myocardial cell from the interstitial fluid after electrical excitation, which increases membrane permeability to calcium. Two types of calcium channels (L-type, T-type) are identified in cardiac tissues.[4,6] The L-type, or long-lasting, channels predominate and are the channels blocked by calcium channel–blocking drugs (verapamil, nifedipine, diltiazem).[6] The T-type, or transient, channels are much less abundant in

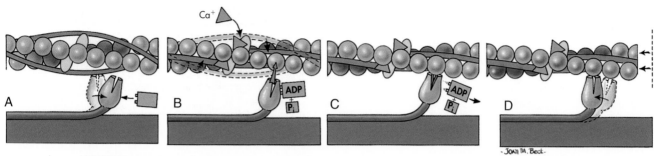

FIGURE 22-15 Cross-Bridge Theory of Muscle Contraction. A, Each myosin cross-bridge in the thick filament moves into a resting position after an adenosine triphosphate (ATP) molecule binds and transfers its energy. **B,** Calcium ions released from the sarcoplasmic reticulum bind to troponin in the thin filament, allowing tropomyosin to shift from its position blocking the active sites of actin molecules. **C,** Each myosin cross-bridge then binds to an active site on a thin filament, displacing the remnants of ATP hydrolysis—adenosine diphosphate (ADP) and inorganic phosphate (P_i). **D,** The release of stored energy from step **A** provides the force needed for each cross-bridge to move back to its original position, pulling actin along with it. Each cross-bridge will remain bound to actin until another ATP molecule binds to it and pulls it back into its resting position, **A.** (From Patton KT, Thibodeau GA: *Anatomy & physiology,* ed 7, St Louis, 2010, Mosby.)

the heart. T-type channels are not blocked by currently available calcium channel–blocking drugs; therefore T-type channel blockers are being developed.[7] Calcium entering the cell triggers the release of calcium from the storage sites, particularly the sarcoplasmic reticulum. Calcium then diffuses toward the myofibrils and binds with troponin.

The calcium-troponin complex interaction facilitates the contraction process. In the resting state, troponin I is bound to actin and the tropomyosin molecule covers the sites where the myosin heads bind to actin. Therefore interaction between actin and myosin is prevented. Calcium binding to troponin inhibits troponin C (which enhances troponin I–actin binding) and causes tropomyosin to be displaced, consequently uncovering the binding sites on the myosin heads. Myosin and actin can now form cross-bridges, and ATP can be dephosphorylated to adenosine diphosphate (ADP). Under these circumstances, sliding of the thick and thin filaments can occur, and the muscle contracts.

Myocardial relaxation. Adequate relaxation is just as vital to optimal cardiac function as contraction; and calcium, troponin, and tropomyosin also facilitate relaxation. After contraction, free calcium ions are actively pumped out of the cell back into the interstitial fluid or reaccumulated in the sarcoplasmic reticulum and stored. Troponin releases its bound calcium. The tropomyosin complex blocks the active sites on the actin molecule, preventing cross-bridges with the myosin heads. A decreased ability by the myocardium to relax leads to increased diastolic filling pressures and eventually heart failure.[8]

> ✔ **QUICK CHECK 22-4**
> 1. What features distinguish myocardial cells from skeletal cells?
> 2. Describe the interactions of actin, myosin, and the troponin-tropomyosin complex in controlling heart function.
> 3. Define excitation-contraction coupling.

Factors Affecting Cardiac Output

Cardiac performance can be quantified by measuring the **cardiac output.** Cardiac output is the volume of blood flowing through either the systemic or the pulmonary circuit per minute and is expressed in liters per minute (L/min). To determine cardiac output, heart rate (beats per minute) is multiplied by stroke volume (liters per beat). Normal cardiac output is about 5 L/min for a resting adult.

The ventricle does not eject all the blood it contains, and the amount ejected per beat is called the **ejection fraction.** The ejection fraction can be estimated by echocardiography and is the stroke volume divided by the end-diastolic volume. The end-diastolic volume of the normal ventricle is about 70 to 80 ml/m^2, and the stroke volume is about 40 to 60 ml/beat; thus the normal ejection fraction of the resting heart is about 60% to 75%. The ejection fraction is increased by factors that increase contractility (e.g., sympathetic nervous system activity). A decrease in ejection fraction is a hallmark of ventricular failure. The effects of aging on cardiovascular function are summarized in Table 22-3.

The factors that determine cardiac output are (1) preload, (2) afterload, (3) myocardial contractility, and (4) heart rate. Preload, afterload, and contractility affect stroke volume.

Preload

Preload is the volume and associated pressure generated in the ventricle at the end of diastole (**ventricular end-diastolic volume [VEDV]** and **pressure [VEDP]**). Preload is determined by two primary factors: (1) the amount of venous return entering the ventricle during diastole, and (2) the blood left in the ventricle after systole (end-systolic volume). Venous return is dependent on blood volume and flow through the venous system and the atrioventricular valves. End-systolic volume is dependent on the strength of ventricular contraction and the resistance to ventricular emptying.

The **Laplace law** describes the relationship by which the amount of tension generated in the wall of the ventricle (or any chamber or vessel) to produce a given intraventricular pressure depends on the size (radius and wall thickness) of the ventricle. Ventricular end-diastolic volume, which determines the size of the ventricle and the stretch of the cardiac muscle fibers, therefore affects the tension (or force) for contraction. The **Frank-Starling law of the heart** describes the length-tension relationship of VEDV (preload) to myocardial contractility (as measured by stroke volume). Muscle fibers have an optimal resting length from which to generate the maximum amount of contractile strength. Within a physiologic range of muscle stretching, increased preload increases stroke volume (and therefore cardiac output and stroke work) (Figure 22-16, curve *B*). Excessive ventricular filling and preload (increased VEDV) stretches the heart muscle beyond optimal length and stroke volume begins to fall. Factors that increase

TABLE 22-3 CARDIOVASCULAR FUNCTION IN ELDERLY PERSONS

DETERMINANT	RESTING CARDIAC PERFORMANCE	EXERCISE CARDIAC PERFORMANCE
Cardiac output	Unchanged or slightly decreased in women only	Declines because of a decrease in heart rate and stroke volume
Heart rate	Slight decrease	Increases less than in younger people, possibly because of decreased cardiovascular response to catecholamines; overall slight decrease
Stroke volume	Slight increase	Slight increase
Ejection fraction	Unchanged	Increases less from rest to exercise in younger people
Afterload	Increased	Uncertain
End-diastolic volume	Unchanged	Smaller for women
End-systolic volume	Unchanged	Lesser increase
Contraction	Increased because of prolonged relaxation	Decreases with vigorous exercise*
Cardiac dilation	No change	Increases at end-diastole and end-systole
$\dot{V}O_2$ max	Not applicable	Declines because of a decline in skeletal muscle mass

Data from Gerstenblith G, Lakatta EG: Aging and the cardiovascular system. In Willerson JT, Cohn JN, editors: *Cardiovascular medicine*, New York, 1995, Churchill Livingstone; Kaye D, Esler M: Sympathetic neuronal regulation of the heart in aging and heart failure, *Cardiovasc Res* 66(2):256–264, 2005; Kenny RA, Ceifer CM: Aging and geriatric heart disease. In Crawford MH, DiMarco JP, editors: *Cardiology*, London, 2001, Mosby.
*As measured by end-systolic volume/systolic blood pressure (ESV/SBP), an index of contractility.

contractility cause the heart to operate on a higher length-tension curve (Figure 22-16, curve *A*). Factors that decrease contractility (Figure 22-16, curve *C*) cause the heart to operate at a lower length-tension curve. Figure 22-17 illustrates the relationship between VEDV and stroke volume, cardiac output, and stroke work.

Increases in preload (VEDV) not only cause a decline in stroke volume, but also result in increases in VEDP. These changes can lead to heart failure (see Chapter 23). Increased VEDP causes pressures to "back up" into the pulmonary or systemic venous circulation, where they force plasma out through vessel walls, causing fluid to accumulate in lung tissues (pulmonary edema; see Chapter 26) or in the peripheral tissues (peripheral edema).

Afterload

Left ventricular **afterload** is the resistance to ejection of blood from the left ventricle. It is the load the muscle must move after it starts to contract. Aortic systolic pressure is a good index of afterload. Pressure in the ventricle must exceed aortic pressure before blood can be pumped out during systole. Low aortic pressures (decreased afterload) enable the heart

to contract more effectively, whereas high aortic pressures (increased afterload) slow contraction and cause higher workloads against which the heart must function so it can eject less blood. Increased aortic pressure is usually the result of increased **peripheral vascular resistance (PVR)**, also called **total peripheral resistance (TPR)**. In individuals with hypertension, increased PVR means that afterload is chronically elevated, resulting in increased ventricular workload and hypertrophy of the myocardium. In some individuals, changes in afterload are the result of aortic valvular disease (see Figure 22-17).

Myocardial Contractility

Stroke volume, or the volume of blood ejected per beat during systole, also depends on the *force* of contraction, which depends on myocardial contractility or the degree of myocardial fiber shortening. Three major factors determine the force of contraction (see Figure 22-17):

1. *Changes in the stretching of the ventricular myocardium caused by changes in VEDV (preload).* As discussed previously, increased blood flow from the veins into the heart distends the ventricle by increasing preload, which increases the stroke volume and, subsequently, cardiac output, up to a certain point. However, an excessive increase in preload leads to decreased stroke volume.

2. *Alterations in the inotropic stimuli of the ventricles.* Chemicals affecting contractility are called **inotropic agents**. The most important positive inotropic agents are epinephrine and norepinephrine released from the sympathetic nervous system. Other positive inotropes include thyroid hormone and dopamine. The most important negative inotropic agent is acetylcholine released from the vagus nerve. Many drugs have positive or negative inotropic properties that can have profound effects on cardiac function.

3. *Adequacy of myocardial oxygen supply.* Myocardial contractility also is affected by oxygen and carbon dioxide levels (tensions) in the coronary blood. With severe hypoxemia (arterial oxygen saturation less than 50%), contractility is decreased. With less severe hypoxemia (saturation more than 50%), contractility is stimulated. Moderate degrees of hypoxemia may increase contractility by enhancing the myocardial response to circulating catecholamines.[1]

Preload, afterload, and contractility all interact with one another to determine stroke volume and cardiac output. Changes in any one of these factors can result in deleterious effects on the others, resulting in heart failure (see Chapter 23).

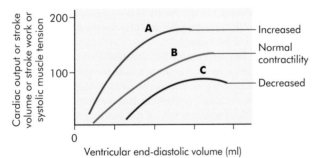

FIGURE 22-16 Frank-Starling Law of the Heart. Relationship between length and tension in heart. End-diastolic volume determines end-diastolic length of ventricular muscle fibers and is proportional to tension generated during systole, as well as to cardiac output, stroke volume, and stroke work. A change in myocardial contractility causes the heart to perform on a different length-tension curve. *A,* Increased contractility; *B,* normal contractility; *C,* heart failure or decreased contractility. (See text for further explanation.)

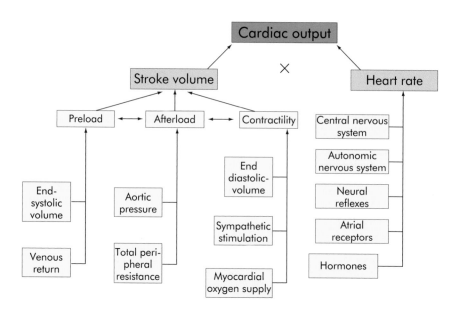

FIGURE 22-17 Factors Affecting Cardiac Performance. Cardiac output, which is the amount of blood (in liters) ejected by the heart per minute, depends on heart rate (beats per minute) and stroke volume (milliliters of blood ejected during ventricular systole).

Heart Rate

As described previously, the activity of the SA node is the primary determinant of the heart rate. The average heart rate in healthy adults is about 70 beats/min. This diminishes by 10 to 20 beats/min during sleep and can accelerate to more than 100 beats/min during muscular activity or emotional excitement. In well-conditioned athletes at rest, the heart rate is normally about 50 to 60 beats/min. In highly trained or elite athletes, the resting heart rate can be below 50 beats/min; these athletes also have a greater stroke volume and lower peripheral resistance in active muscles than they had before training. The control of heart rate includes activity of the central nervous system, autonomic nervous system, neural reflexes, atrial receptors, and hormones (see Figure 22-17).

Cardiovascular control centers in the brain. The cardiovascular control center is in the brain stem in the medulla, with secondary areas in the hypothalamus, cerebral cortex, and thalamus along with complex networks of excitatory or inhibitory interneurons (connecting neurons) throughout the brain. The hypothalamic centers regulate cardiovascular responses to changes in temperature; the cerebral cortex centers adjust cardiac reaction to a variety of emotional states; and the medullary control center regulates heart rate and blood pressure (see Figure 22-11).

The nerve fibers from the cardiovascular control center synapse with autonomic neurons that influence the rate of firing of the SA node. As previously discussed, increased heart rate occurs with sympathetic (adrenergic) stimulation. Thus the interneurons that cause sympathetic neuronal excitation are collectively called the cardioexcitatory center.[9] When the parasympathetic nerves to the heart are stimulated (primarily via the vagus nerve), heart rate slows and the sympathetic nerves to the heart, arterioles, and veins are inhibited. Because parasympathetic excitation and simultaneous sympathetic inhibition generally depress cardiac function, these interneurons are often referred to as the cardioinhibitory center. At rest, the heart rate in healthy individuals is primarily under the control of parasympathetic stimulation. Administration of drugs that block parasympathetic function (anticholinergic) or physical interruption of the vagus nerve causes significant tachycardia (abnormally fast heart rate) because this inhibitory parasympathetic influence is lost.

Neural reflexes. The baroreceptor reflex facilitates both blood pressure changes and heart rate changes. It is mediated by tissue pressure receptors (pressoreceptors) in the aortic arch and carotid arteries.

If blood pressure is decreased, the baroreceptor reflex accelerates heart rate and causes vessels to constrict. These responses raise blood pressure back toward normal. This reflex is critical to maintaining adequate tissue perfusion. When blood pressure is increased, the pressoreceptors increase their rate of discharge, sending neural impulses over the glossopharyngeal nerve (ninth cranial nerve) and through the vagus nerve to the cardiovascular control centers in the medulla. These reflexes increase parasympathetic activity and decrease sympathetic activity, causing blood vessels to dilate and heart rate to decrease (see Figure 22-18). The role of baroreceptors in influencing blood pressure is discussed in more detail later in this chapter.

Atrial receptors. Receptors that influence heart rate exist in both atria (Figure 22-18).[1,4] They are located in the right atrium at its junctions with the venae cava and in the left atrium at its junctions with the pulmonary veins. Distention of the atria causes stimulation of these atrial receptors (for example, when intravascular volume is increased by intravenous infusions). This causes activation of the Bainbridge reflex, which increases heart rate (see Figure 22-18). The magnitude of the change in heart rate depends on the relative contributions of this reflex with baroreceptor activity.[10]

Stimulation of these atrial receptors also increases urine volume, presumably because of a neurally mediated reduction in antidiuretic hormone. In addition, atrial natriuretic peptide (ANP) and brain natriuretic peptide (BNP) are released from atrial tissue in response to the increases in blood volume. ANP and BNP have powerful diuretic and natriuretic (salt excretion) properties, resulting in decreased blood volume and pressure.[4,11]

Hormones and biochemicals. Hormones and biochemicals affect the arteries, arterioles, venules, capillaries, and contractility of the myocardium. Norepinephrine increases heart rate, enhances myocardial contractility, and constricts blood vessels. Epinephrine dilates vessels of the liver and skeletal muscle and also causes an increase in myocardial contractility. Some adrenocortical hormones, such as hydrocortisone, potentiate the effects of these catecholamines.

Thyroid hormones enhance sympathetic activity, promoting increased cardiac output. A decrease in growth hormone, as well as in thyroid and adrenal hormones, results in bradycardia (heart rate below 60 beats/min), reduced cardiac output, and low blood pressure. (See other hormones in the Regulation of Blood Pressure section.)

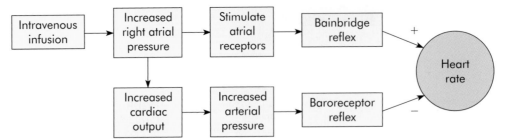

FIGURE 22-18 Heart Rate and Intravenous Infusions. Intravenous infusions of blood or electrolyte solutions tend to increase heart rate through the Bainbridge reflex and to decrease heart rate through the baroreceptor reflex. The actual change in heart rate induced by such infusions is the result of these two opposing effects. (From Berne RM, Levy MN: *Cardiovascular physiology*, ed 8, St Louis, 2001, Mosby.)

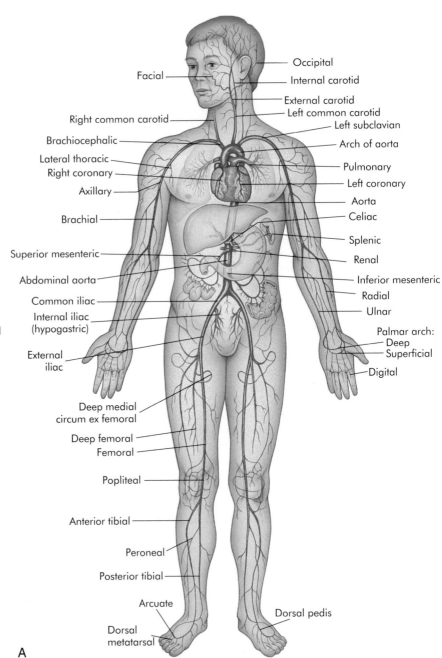

FIGURE 22-19 Circulatory System. A, Principal arteries of body.

THE SYSTEMIC CIRCULATION

The arteries and veins of the systemic circulation are illustrated in Figure 22-19. Blood from the left side of the heart flows through the aorta and into the systemic arteries. The arteries branch into small arterioles, which branch further into the smallest vessels, the capillaries, where nutrient exchange between the blood and tissues occurs. Blood from the capillaries then enters tiny venules that join to form the larger veins, which return venous blood to the right heart. Peripheral vascular system is an imprecise term used to describe the part of the systemic circulation that supplies the skin and the extremities, particularly the legs and feet.

Structure of Blood Vessels

Blood vessel walls are composed of three layers: (1) the tunica intima (innermost, or intimal, layer), (2) the tunica media (middle, or medial, layer), and (3) the tunica externa or adventitia (outermost, or external, layer). These structures are illustrated in Figure 22-20. Blood vessel

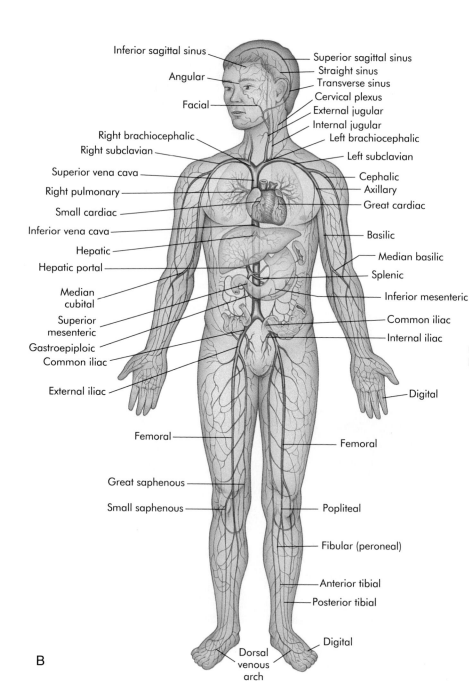

FIGURE 22-19, cont'd B, Principal veins of body. (From Patton KT, Thibodeau GA: *Anatomy & physiology,* ed 7, St Louis, 2010, Mosby.)

B

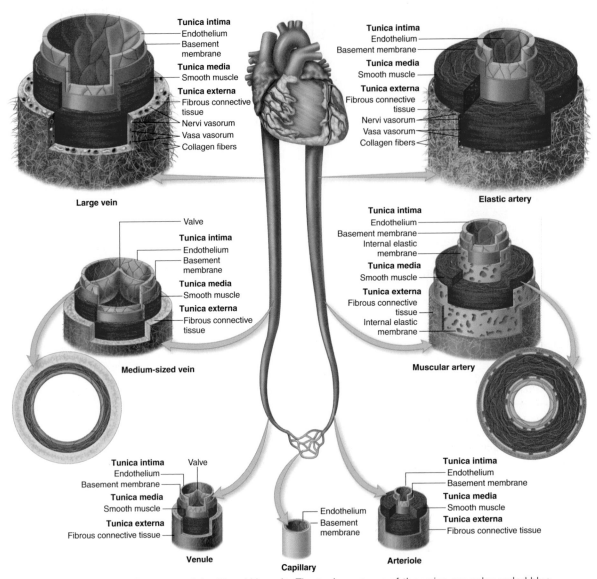

FIGURE 22-20 Structure of the Blood Vessels. The tunica externa of the veins are color-coded blue and the arteries red. (From Patton KT, Thibodeau GA: *Anatomy & physiology*, ed 7, St Louis, 2010, Mosby.)

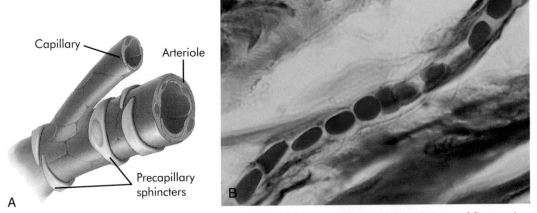

FIGURE 22-21 Capillary Wall. A, Capillaries have a wall composed of only a single layer of flattened cells, whereas the walls of the larger vessels also have smooth muscle. **B,** Capillary with red blood cells in single file (× 500). (**A** from Patton KT, Thibodeau GA: *Anatomy & physiology*, ed 7, St Louis, 2010, Mosby; **B,** Copyright Ed Reschke.)

walls vary in thickness depending on the thickness or absence of one or more of these three layers. Cells of the larger vessels are nourished by the vasa vasorum, small vessels located in the tunica externa.

Arterial Vessels

Arterial walls are composed of elastic connective tissue, fibrous connective tissue, and smooth muscle. Elastic arteries have a thick tunica media with more elastic fibers than smooth muscle fibers. Examples include the aorta and its major branches and the pulmonary trunk. Elasticity allows the vessel to stretch as blood is ejected from the heart during systole. During diastole, elasticity promotes recoil of the arteries, maintaining blood pressure within the vessels.

Muscular arteries are medium- and small-sized arteries and are farther from the heart than the elastic arteries. They contain more muscle fibers than the elastic arteries because they need less stretch and recoil. The muscular arteries distribute blood to arterioles throughout the body and help control blood flow because their smooth muscle can be stimulated to contract or relax. Contraction narrows the vessel lumen (the internal cavity of the vessel), which diminishes flow through the vessel (vasoconstriction). When the smooth muscle layer relaxes, more blood flows through the vessel lumen (vasodilation).

An artery becomes an arteriole where the diameter of its lumen narrows to less than 0.5 mm. The arterioles are composed almost exclusively of smooth muscle and regulate the flow of blood into the capillaries by vasoconstriction, which retards the flow of blood into the capillaries, and vasodilation, which permits blood to enter the capillaries freely (Figure 22-21). The thick smooth muscle layer of the arterioles is a major determinant of the resistance blood encounters as it flows through the systemic circulation.

The capillary network is composed of connective channels, or thoroughfares, called metarterioles, and "true" capillaries (Figure 22-22).

The capillaries branch from the metarterioles, meeting at a ring of smooth muscle called the precapillary sphincter. As the sphincters contract and relax, they regulate blood flow through the capillaries. Appropriately stimulated, the precapillary sphincters help to maintain arterial pressure and regulate selective flow to vascular beds.

The capillary walls are very thin, making possible the rapid exchange of substrates, metabolites, and special products (e.g., hormones) between the blood and the interstitial fluid, from which they are taken up by the cells. A single endothelial cell may form the entire vessel wall if the capillary has no tunica media or tunica externa. In some capillaries, the endothelial cells contain oval windows or pores termed fenestrations, which are generally covered by a thin diaphragm.

Substances pass between the capillary lumen and the interstitial fluid (1) through junctions between endothelial cells, (2) through fenestrations in endothelial cells, (3) in vesicles moved by active transport across the endothelial cell membrane, or (4) by diffusion through the endothelial cell membrane. A single capillary may be only 0.5 to 1 mm in length and 0.01 mm in diameter, but the capillaries are so numerous that their total surface area may be more than 600 m², or larger than 100 football fields.

Endothelium

All tissues depend on a blood supply and the blood supply depends on endothelial cells, which form the lining, or endothelium, of the blood vessel (Figure 22-23). Endothelial cells are really quite remarkable in that they can adjust their number and arrangement to accommodate local requirements. They are a life-support tissue extending and remodeling the network of blood vessels to enable tissue growth, motion, and repair. Vascular endothelial cells produce a number of essential chemicals including vasodilators, vasoconstrictors, anticoagulants, and growth factors. The endothelium performs these vital functions through synthesis and release of vasoactive chemicals.

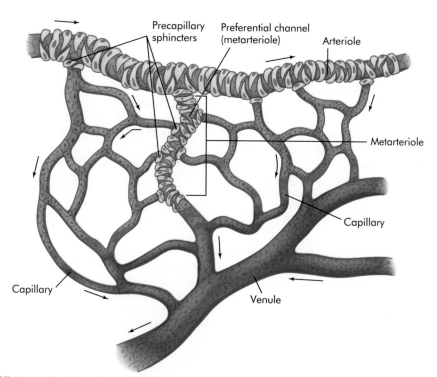

FIGURE 22-22 Capillary Network. Blood enters network as arterial blood and exits as venous blood.

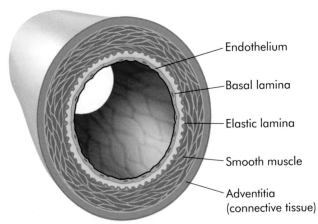

- Endothelium
- Basal lamina
- Elastic lamina
- Smooth muscle
- Adventitia (connective tissue)

FIGURE 22-23 Endothelium. Practically imperceptible, the endothelial cells arrange themselves as a fine lining that has numerous life-support functions (see Table 22-4).

Table 22-4 and Figures 22-24 and 22-25 summarize some of the more important endothelial functions. Dysfunction of the endothelium has been implicated in virtually every type of vascular disorder, including atherosclerosis and hypertension (see Chapter 23).[4,12]

Veins

Compared with arteries, veins are thin walled and fibrous and have a larger diameter (see Figure 22-20). Veins also are more numerous than arteries. The smallest venules closest to the capillaries have an inner lining composed of the endothelium of the tunica intima and surrounded by fibrous tissue. The largest venules are surrounded by a few smooth muscle fibers constituting a thin tunica media. In veins, the tunica externa has less elastic tissue than in arteries, so veins do not recoil after distention as quickly as do arteries. Like arteries, veins receive nourishment from the tiny vasa vasorum.

Some veins, most commonly in the lower limbs, contain valves to regulate the one-way flow of blood toward the heart (Figure 22-26). These valves are folds of the tunica intima and resemble the semilunar valves of the heart. When a person stands up, contraction of the skeletal muscles of the legs compresses the deep veins of the legs and assists the flow of blood toward the heart. This important mechanism of venous return is called the muscle pump (Figure 22-27).

Factors Affecting Blood Flow

Blood flow is the amount of fluid moved per unit of time and is usually expressed as liters per minute (L/min) or milliliters per minute (ml/min), or as cubic centimeters per second (cm³/sec). Flow is regulated by the same physical properties that govern the movement of simple fluids in a closed, rigid system—that is, pressure, resistance, velocity, turbulent versus laminar flow, and compliance.

Pressure and Resistance

Pressure in a liquid system is the force exerted on the liquid per unit area and is expressed as dynes per square centimeter (dynes/cm²), millimeters of mercury (mm Hg), or units of pressure (torr). Blood flow depends partly on the difference between pressures in the arterial and venous vessels supplying the organ. Fluid moves from the arterial "side" of the capillaries, a region of greater pressure, to the venous side, a region of lesser pressure.

Resistance is the opposition to force. In the cardiovascular system, most opposition to blood flow is provided by the diameter and length of the blood vessels themselves. Therefore changes in blood flow

TABLE 22-4	**FUNCTIONS OF THE ENDOTHELIUM**
FUNCTION	**ACTIONS INVOLVED**
Filtration and permeability	Facilitates transport of large molecules via vesicular transport movement through intercellular junctions
	Facilitates transport of small molecules via movement of vesicles, through opening of tight junctions, and across cytoplasm
Vasomotion	Stimulates vascular relaxation through production of nitric oxide, prostacyclin, and other vasodilators
	Stimulates vascular constriction through production of endothelin and angiotensin II
Clotting	Stimulates clotting by inducing platelet adhesion via production of von Willebrand factor, platelet-activating factor, and others
	Prevents clotting through production of endogenous anticoagulants such as heparin sulfate
	Promotes fibrinolysis via production of tissue plasminogen activating factor (t-PH) and plasminogen activator inhibitor (PAI-A)
Inflammation	Expresses adhesion molecules that allow for monocyte and polymorphonucleocyte margination and diapedesis
	Expresses receptors for oxidized lipoproteins, allowing them to enter vascular intima

From Hansson GK, Nilsson J: Pathogenesis of atherosclerosis. In Crawford MH, DiMarco JP, editors: *Cardiology,* ed 2, London, 2004, Mosby.

through an organ result from changes in the vascular resistance within the organ. Resistance in a vessel is inversely related to blood flow—that is, increased resistance leads to decreased blood flow. Poiseuille law shows the relationship among blood flow, pressure, and resistance:

$$Q = \frac{\delta P}{R}$$

where Q = blood flow, P = pressure difference ($P_1 - P_2$), and R = resistance. Resistance to flow cannot be measured directly, but it can be calculated if the pressure difference and flow volumes are known. Resistance to blood flow in a single vessel is determined by the radius and length of the blood vessel and by the blood viscosity.

The most important factor determining resistance *in a single vessel* is the radius or diameter of the vessel's lumen (Figure 22-28, *A*). Small changes in the lumen's radius or diameter lead to large changes in vascular resistance. Another important factor is the length of the vessel. Resistance to flow is generally greater in longer tubes because resistance increases with length. Blood flow varies inversely with the viscosity of the fluid. Thick fluids move more slowly and experience greater resistance to flow than thin fluids. For example, blood that contains a high percentage of red cells is more viscous. This relationship is expressed as the hematocrit—the ratio of the volume of red blood cells to the volume of whole blood. A high hematocrit level reduces flow through the blood vessels, particularly the microcirculation (arterioles, capillaries, venules).

Resistance to flow through a *system of vessels,* or total resistance, depends not only on characteristics of individual vessels but also on

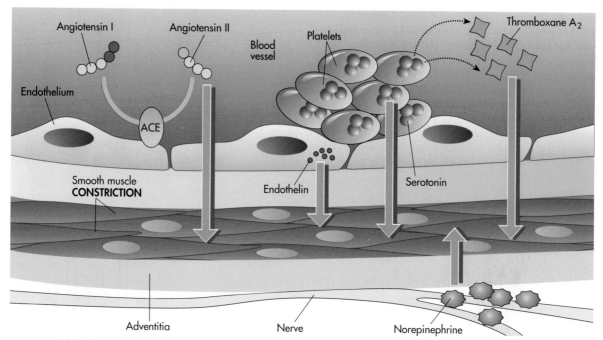

FIGURE 22-24 Endothelium Regulation of Vasomotion (Constriction and Dilation) and Platelet Aggregation by Release of a Variety of Constricting and Dilating Substances. Constricting factors include arachidonic acid and metabolites, such as thromboxane A_2 (which aspirin inhibits), and a potent amino acid peptide called *endothelin.* The endothelium also converts angiotensin I into angiotensin II by the membrane-bound angiotensin-converting enzyme that also metabolizes the endogenous endothelium-dependent vasodilator, bradykinin. (Modified from Stern S: *Silent myocardial ischemia,* St Louis, 1998, Mosby.)

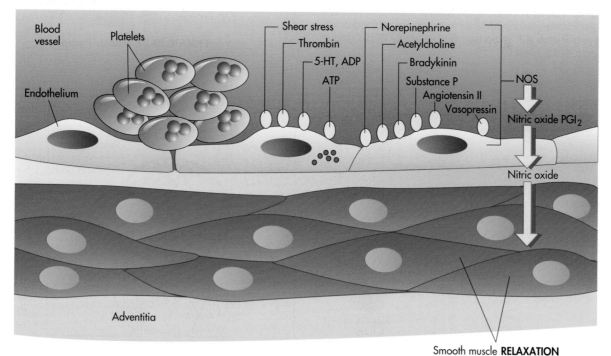

FIGURE 22-25 Factors Causing Endothelium-Dependent Vasodilation. A variety of exogenous pharmacologic substances, platelet-derived factors, and shear stress can promote release of nitric oxide by stimulating nitric oxide synthase *(NOS).* Prostacyclin *(PGI2)* causes relaxation of vascular smooth muscle cells by a cyclic adenosine monophosphate (cAMP)-dependent mechanism, and both nitric oxide and PGI_2 inhibit platelet aggregation. *ADP,* Adenosine diphosphate; *ATP,* adenosine triphosphate; *5-HT,* serotonin. (Modified from Stern S: *Silent myocardial ischemia,* St Louis, 1998, Mosby.)

whether the vessels are arranged in series or in parallel and on the total cross-sectional area of the system. Vessels arranged in series will generally provide less resistance than vessels arranged in parallel. Blood flowing through the distributing arteries, beginning with branches off the aorta and ending at arterioles in the capillary bed, encounters more resistance than blood flowing through the capillary bed itself, where flow is distributed among many short, tiny branches arranged in parallel (see Figure 22-28, *B*). The total cross-sectional area of the arteriolar system is greater than that of the arterial system, yet the greater number of arterioles arranged in parallel leads to great resistance to flow

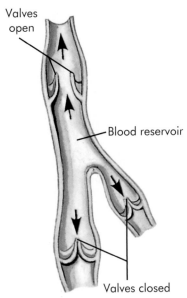

FIGURE 22-26 Valves of Vein. Pooled blood is moved toward heart as valves are forced open by pressure from volume of blood downstream. (From Patton KT, Thibodeau GA: *Anatomy & physiology,* ed 7, St Louis, 2010, Mosby.)

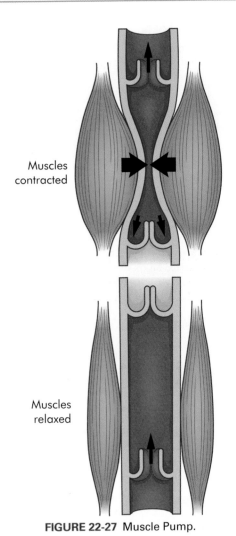

FIGURE 22-27 Muscle Pump.

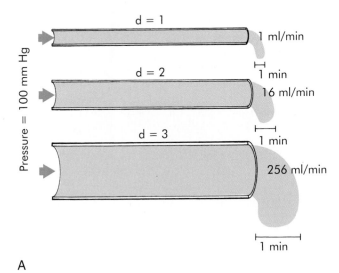

A

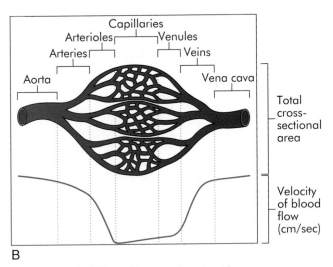

B

FIGURE 22-28 Lumen Diameter, Blood Flow, and Resistance. A, Effect of lumen *diameter (d)* on flow through vessel. **B,** Blood flows with great speed in the large arteries. However, branching of arterial vessels increases the total cross-sectional area of the arterioles and capillaries, reducing the flow rate. When capillaries merge into venules and venules merge into veins, the total cross-sectional area decreases, causing the flow rate to increase. (**B** from Patton KT, Thibodeau GA: *Anatomy & physiology,* ed 7, St Louis, 2010, Mosby.)

in the arteriolar system. In contrast, the capillary system has a larger number of vessels arranged in parallel than the arteriolar system, and the total cross-sectional area is much greater; thus there is lower resistance overall through the capillary system. This, plus the slow velocity of flow in each capillary, promotes optimal capillary-tissue exchange.

Velocity

Blood velocity is the *distance* blood travels in a unit of time, usually centimeters per second (cm/sec). It is directly related to blood flow (*amount* of blood moved per unit of time) and inversely related to the cross-sectional area of the vessel in which the blood is flowing. As blood moves from the aorta to the capillaries, the total cross-sectional area of the vessels increases and the velocity of flow decreases.

Laminar Versus Turbulent Flow

Normally, blood flow through the vessels is *laminar* (**laminar flow**), meaning that concentric layers of molecules move "straight ahead." Each concentric layer flows at a different velocity (Figure 22-29). The cohesive attraction between the fluid and the vessel wall prevents the molecules of blood that are in contact with the wall from moving. The next thin layer of blood is able to slide slowly past the stationary layer and so on until, at the center, the blood velocity is greatest. Large vessels have room for a large center layer; therefore they have less resistance to flow and greater flow and velocity than smaller vessels.

Where flow is obstructed, the vessel turns, or blood flows over rough surfaces, the flow becomes *turbulent* (**turbulent flow**), with whorls or eddy currents that produce noise, causing a murmur to be heard on auscultation. Resistance increases with turbulence.

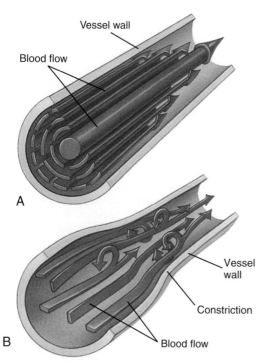

FIGURE 22-29 Laminar and Turbulent Blood Flow. A, Laminar flow. Fluid flows in long, smooth-walled tubes as if it is composed of a large number of concentric layers. **B,** Turbulent flow. Turbulent flow is caused by numerous small currents flowing crosswise or oblique to the long axis of the vessel, resulting in flowing whorls and eddy currents. (From Seeley RR, Stephens TD, Tate P: *Anatomy and physiology*, ed 3, St Louis, 1995, Mosby.)

Vascular Compliance

Vascular compliance is the increase in volume a vessel can accommodate for a given increase in pressure. Compliance depends on the ratio of elastic fibers to muscle fibers in the vessel wall. The elastic arteries are more compliant than the muscular arteries. The veins are more compliant than either type of artery, and they can serve as storage areas for the circulatory system.

Compliance determines a vessel's response to pressure changes. For example, a large volume of blood can be accommodated by the venous system with only a small increase in pressure. In the less compliant arterial system, where smaller volumes and higher pressures are normal, even small changes in the volume of blood can cause significant changes in pressure within the arterial vessels.

Stiffness is the opposite of compliance. Several conditions and disorders can cause stiffness, with the most common being arteriosclerosis (see Chapter 23).

> **QUICK CHECK 22-6**
> 1. What is the function of the arterioles?
> 2. Identify the functions of the endothelium.
> 3. Why does the total cross-sectional area in the capillary system lower the resistance to flow?

Regulation of Blood Pressure
Arterial Pressure

Arterial blood pressure is determined by the cardiac output times the peripheral resistance (see Figure 22-30). The **systolic blood pressure** is the arterial blood pressure during ventricular contraction or systole. The **diastolic blood pressure** is the arterial blood pressure during ventricular filling or diastole. The **mean arterial pressure (MAP)**, which is the average pressure in the arteries throughout the cardiac cycle, depends on the elastic properties of the arterial walls and the mean volume of blood in the arterial system. MAP can be approximated from the measured values of the systolic (P_s) and diastolic (P_d) pressures as follows:

$$MAP = P_d + \frac{1}{3}(P_s - P_d)$$

where $P_s - P_d$ is the pulse pressure.

Arterial pressure is constantly regulated to maintain tissue **perfusion,** or blood supply to the capillary beds, during a wide range of physiologic conditions, such as changes in body position, muscular activity, and circulating blood volume. The major factors and relationships that regulate arterial blood pressure are summarized in Figure 22-30.

Effects of Cardiac Output

The cardiac output (minute volume) of the heart can be changed by alterations in heart rate, stroke volume (volume of blood ejected during each ventricular contraction), or both. An increase in cardiac output without a decrease in peripheral resistance will cause both arterial volume and arterial pressure to increase. The higher arterial pressure increases blood flow through the arterioles. On the other hand, a decrease in the cardiac output causes an immediate drop in the mean arterial blood pressure and arteriolar flow.

Effects of Total Peripheral Resistance

Total resistance in the systemic circulation, sometimes called *total peripheral resistance,* is determined by changes in the diameter of the arterioles. Arteriolar constriction increases mean arterial pressure by

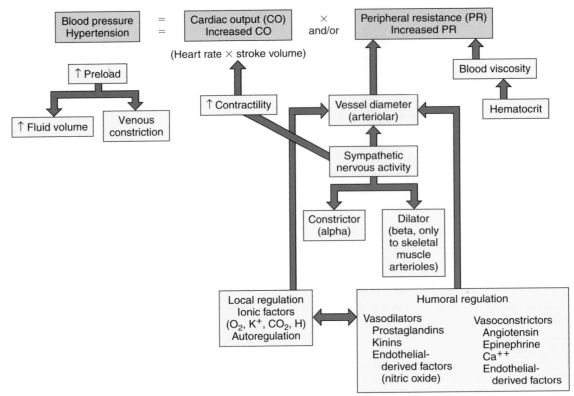

FIGURE 22-30 Factors Regulating Blood Pressure.

preventing the free flow of blood into the capillaries. Dilation has the opposite effect. Reflex control of total cardiac output and peripheral resistance includes (1) sympathetic stimulation of heart, arterioles, and veins; and (2) parasympathetic stimulation of the heart (Figure 22-31). The autonomic nervous system is monitored by the cardiovascular control center in the brain. Vasoconstriction is regulated by an area of the brain stem that maintains a constant (tonic) output of norepinephrine from sympathetic fibers in the peripheral arterioles. This tonic activity is essential for maintenance of blood pressure. Information about pressure and resistance is sensed by neural receptors (baroreceptors, chemoreceptors) in arterial walls and delivered to the medullary centers.

Baroreceptors. As discussed previously, baroreceptors are stretch receptors located in the aorta and in the carotid sinus (see Figure 22-31, *A*). They respond to changes in smooth muscle fiber length by altering their rate of discharge and supply sensory information to the cardioinhibitory center in the brain stem. When activated, these baroreceptors decrease cardiac output (heart rate and stroke volume) and peripheral resistance, and thus lower blood pressure. (Postural changes and the baroreceptor reflex are discussed in Chapter 23.)

Arterial chemoreceptors. Specialized areas within the aortic and carotid arteries are sensitive to concentrations of oxygen, carbon dioxide, and hydrogen ions (pH) in the blood (see Figure 22-31, *B*). These chemoreceptors are most important for the control of respiration but also transmit impulses to the medullary cardiovascular centers that regulate blood pressure. If arterial oxygen concentration or pH falls, a reflexive increase in blood pressure occurs, whereas an increase in carbon dioxide concentration causes a slight increase in blood pressure. The major chemoreceptive reflex is the result of alterations in arterial oxygen concentration, with only minor effects resulting from altered pH or carbon dioxide levels.

Effect of Hormones

Antidiuretic hormone. Antidiuretic hormone (ADH) is released by the posterior pituitary and causes reabsorption of water by the kidney. With reabsorption, the blood plasma volume will increase, increasing blood pressure. Antidiuretic hormone, also known as arginine vasopressin, is also a potent vasoconstrictor, thus increasing peripheral resistance (Figure 22-32, and see Chapters 4 and 17).

Renin-angiotensin system. Renin is an enzyme synthesized and secreted by the juxtaglomerular cells of the kidney. It also has been found in the adrenal cortex, salivary gland, brain, pituitary gland, arterial smooth muscle cells in the vascular endothelium, and myocardium. Renin is an essential factor that interacts with many other systems to control vascular tone and renal sodium excretion.[13] The primary factor that stimulates renin release is a drop in renal perfusion as detected by the juxtaglomerular cells. Other factors that stimulate renin release include a decrease in the amount of sodium chloride delivered to the kidney, β-adrenergic stimuli, and low potassium concentrations in plasma. Once in the circulation, renin splits off a polypeptide from angiotensinogen to generate angiotensin I (Ang I). This is converted by an enzyme, angiotensin-converting enzyme (ACE), to angiotensin II (Ang II), a powerful vasoconstrictor that stimulates the secretion of aldosterone from the adrenal gland (see Figures 22-33, *A*, and 17-18). This kidney-based renin-angiotensin system serves as an important regulatory loop. For example, decreases in blood pressure or renal blood flow (as might occur after hemorrhage or dehydration) stimulate secretion of renin. This causes the formation of Ang I, which is then converted to Ang II. Ang II causes vasoconstriction and aldosterone secretion. The resultant increase in TPR and sodium retention restores blood pressure. Overall, the renin-angiotensin system is activated after volume depletion or hypotension, and is suppressed after volume repletion.

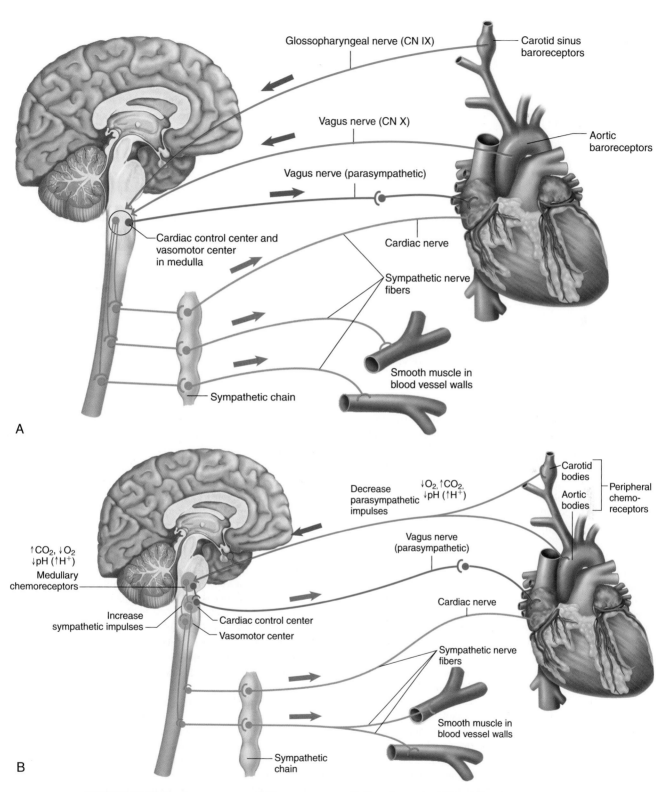

FIGURE 22-31 Baroreceptors and Chemoreceptor Reflex Control of Blood Pressure. A, Baroreceptor reflexes. **B,** Vasomotor chemoreflexes. (Modified from Patton KT, Thibodeau GA: *Anatomy & physiology,* ed 7, St Louis, 2010, Mosby.)

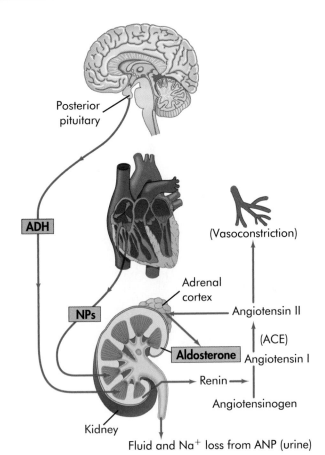

FIGURE 22-32 Three Mechanisms That Influence Total Plasma Volume. The antidiuretic hormone *(ADH)* mechanism and renin-angiotensin and aldosterone mechanisms tend to increase water retention and thus increase total plasma volume. The natriuretic peptides antagonize these mechanisms by promoting water loss and sodium loss, thus promoting a decrease in total plasma volume. *ACE,* Angiotensin-converting enzyme; *ANP,* atrial natriuretic peptide; *NPs,* natriuretic peptides. (Modified from Patton KT, Thibodeau GA: *Anatomy & physiology,* ed 7, St Louis, 2010, Mosby.)

Ang II has two primary receptors, AT_1 and AT_2 (Figure 22-34). Both subtypes, AT_1 and AT_2, are expressed in human hearts. AT_1 also is found on vascular smooth muscle and endothelial cells, nerve endings, conduction tissues, adrenal cortex, liver, kidney, and brain. AT_2 has been found in fetal mesenchymal tissue, adrenal medulla, uterus and ovarian follicles, renal tubules, and vasculature. A third type of Ang II receptor, AT_4, has been described although its effects are still being evaluated.[14] The majority of Ang II actions occur through the AT_1 receptor, including vasoconstriction, stimulation of aldosterone release, myocyte hypertrophy, fibroblast proliferation, collagen synthesis, smooth muscle cell growth, endothelial adhesion molecule expression, and catecholamine synthesis.[15] There also exists a tissue-based renin-angiotensin system that can be independently regulated from the circulation. The tissue renin-angiotensin system is activated in response to tissue injury.[16] Through stimulation of the AT_1 receptor and through the tissue renin-angiotensin system, Ang II is involved in maladaptive alterations, such as ventricular and vascular remodeling, atherosclerosis, alterations in renal function, and heart failure[17-19] (see Figure 22-33, *B*, and Chapter 23). Therefore treatments such as angiotensin-converting enzyme (ACE) inhibitors and angiotensin receptor blockers (ARBs) that inhibit mostly AT_1

receptors are a main target in preventive and reparative strategies in cardiovascular diseases. Aldosterone also has direct deleterious effects on cardiovascular tissues.[20]

The role of AT_2 receptors remains controversial. AT_2 stimulation results in NO-mediated vasodilation in many vascular beds and it is suggested that this receptor plays a modulating and protective role when AT_1 is activated.[21] However, other investigators suggest that AT_2 receptor stimulation may actually contribute to cardiovascular remodeling.[22] Numerous studies are under way to further elucidate the role of these important vascular receptors. In addition, a second form of ACE, called ACE_2, helps to degrade Ang II into Ang 1-7, which balances the effects of Ang II on the vasculature[23] (see *Health Alert:* Multiple Effects of the Renin-Angiotensin-Aldosterone System).

Natriuretic peptides. Another mechanism that can change blood plasma volume and, therefore, blood pressure involves the natriuretic peptides (NPs) (see Figure 22-32). The natriuretic peptides include atrial natriuretic peptide (ANP), brain natriuretic peptide (BNP), C-type natriuretic peptide (CNP), and urodilatin. These peptides help regulate sodium excretion (natriuresis), diuresis, vasodilation, and antagonism of the renin-angiotensin system. Atrial natriuretic peptide (ANP) is a hormone secreted from cells in the right atrium when right atrial blood pressure increases. ANP increases urine sodium loss, leading to the formation of a large volume of dilute urine that decreases blood volume and blood pressure.[24] Brain natriuretic peptide (BNP) is secreted from cardiac cells and also increases sodium loss from the kidney. It is used both as a marker and as a treatment for acute heart failure.[25,26] C-type natriuretic peptide (CNP) is found throughout the vascular endothelium and in cardiac, renal, skeletal, and reproductive tissues. It has been found to promote vasodilation, increase cardiac contractility, and inhibit smooth muscle proliferation and vascular remodeling.[27] Urodilatin is made in the kidneys and promotes natriuresis and is being explored for the treatment of heart failure.[28]

Adrenomedullin. Adrenomedullin (ADM) is present in cardiovascular, pulmonary, renal, gastrointestinal, cerebral, and endocrine tissues. ADM is secreted by the adrenal medulla and from endothelial and smooth muscle cells and mediates vasodilation and sodium excretion. Thus ADM plays an important role in fluid and electrolyte balance and cardiorenal regulation. ADM also plays an important role in vascular protection by decreasing oxidative stress, limiting endothelial injury, causing vasodilation, and promoting angiogenesis.[29,30] Other functions of ADM include neurotransmission, vascular growth, hormone secretion regulation, down-regulation of the proinflammatory cytokines, and modulation of anticoagulant properties.[31] Therefore changes in ADM levels have been correlated with several diseases including cardiovascular and renal sepsis, cancer, and diabetes[31] (see *Health Alert:* Adrenomedullin).

Insulin. Insulin has direct vascular actions that contribute to both vascular protection and vascular injury.[32,33] The vascular protection and injury properties are summarized in Box 22-2. Insulin resistance and diabetes have a profound effect on cardiovascular disorders, including hypertension and atherosclerotic disease (see Chapter 23).

Adipokines. Adipocytes synthesize and release several hormones that influence blood pressure, including adiponectin, leptin, and resistin.[34,35] Leptin and resistin levels are increased in obesity and are associated with increased blood pressure and hypertension. Adiponectin is a protective factor for the cardiovascular system that is found in reduced levels in patients with obesity-related hypertension. Increasing evidence suggests that aberrant production and release of these factors from adipocytes may contribute not only to hypertension but also to atherosclerosis and heart failure (see Chapter 23).

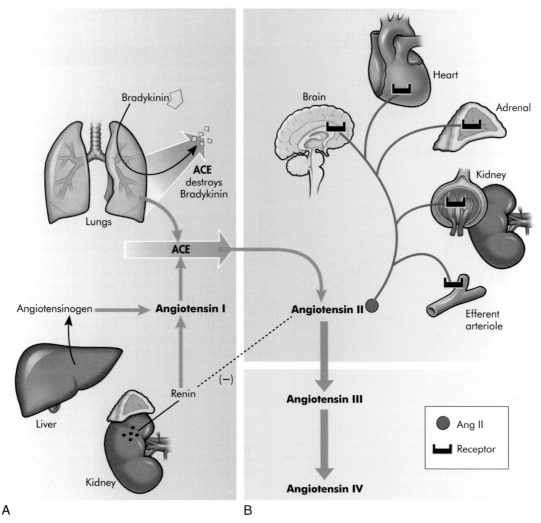

A   B

FIGURE 22-33 Angiotensins and the Organs Affected. **A,** The shaded blue area is the classic pathway of biosynthesis that generates the renin and angiotensin I. Angiotensinogen is synthesized in the liver and is released into the blood where it is cleaved to form angiotensin I by renin secreted by cells in the kidneys. Angiotensin-converting enzyme (ACE) in the lungs catalyzes the formation of angiotensin II from angiotensin I and destroys the potent vasodilator bradykinin. Further cleavage generates the angiotensins III and IV. The reddish shading shows the organs affected by angiotensin II, including brain, heart, adrenals, kidney, and the kidney's efferent arterioles. The *dashed arrow (left)* shows the inhibition of renin by angiotensin II. **B,** Summary of angiotensin II effects on blood vessel structure and function leading to atherosclerosis. (Adapted from Goodfriend TL et al: *N Engl J Med* 334:2649–2654, 1996.)

HEALTH ALERT

Multiple Effects of the Renin-Angiotensin-Aldosterone System

Exciting research is uncovering additional roles of the renin-angiotensin-aldosterone system (RAA) in cardiovascular and systemic conditions:

1. The RAA has profound effects on glucose metabolism, endothelial cell function, and renal disease, which has led to new uses for drugs that block angiotensin receptors, especially in individuals with diabetes and kidney disease.
2. Activation of angiotensin 1 receptor (AT_1) promotes systemic inflammation and mediates inflammatory myocyte hypertrophy, fibroblast proliferation, collagen synthesis, smooth muscle cell growth, endothelial adhesion molecule expression, and catecholamine synthesis. Thus there is likely an important role for the RAA in many diseases including atherosclerosis, heart failure, and shock.

3. A new angiotensin receptor (AT_4) has been described that is concentrated in the brain and may be involved in cerebral processing, cerebroprotection, local blood flow, stress, anxiety, and depression.
4. A new type of angiotensin-converting enzyme (ACE_2) has been identified that decreases Ang II levels and may offer an entirely new approach to combating hypertension.
5. Vaccines for Ang II and its receptors are being developed that might provide a more targeted and potent blockade of the RAA.
6. Aldosterone has a number of deleterious effects, including myocardial necrosis and fibrosis, vascular stiffening and injury, reduced fibrinolysis, endothelial dysfunction, catecholamine release, and promotion of dysrhythmias.

Data from Bader M: Tissue renin-angiotensin-aldosterone systems: targets for pharmacological therapy, *Annu Rev Pharmacol Toxicol* 50:439–465, 2010; Benigni A, Cassis P, Remuzzi G: Angiotensin II revisited: new roles in inflammation, immunology and aging, *EMBO Mol Med* 2(7):247–257, 2010; Briet M, Schiffrin EL: Aldosterone: effects on the kidney and cardiovascular system, *Nat Rev Nephrol* 6(5):261–273, 2010; Vanderheyden PM: From angiotensin IV binding site to AT4 receptor, *Mol Cell Endocrinol* 302(2):159–166, 2009; Zhong J et al: Angiotensin-converting enzyme 2 suppresses pathological hypertrophy, myocardial fibrosis, and cardiac dysfunction, *Circulation* 122(7):717–728, 18 p following 728, 2010.

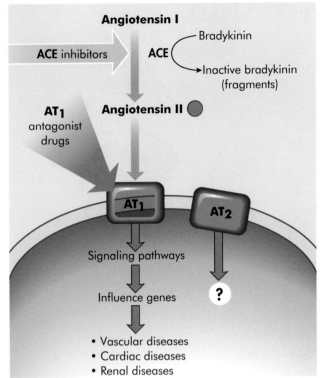

FIGURE 22-34 Angiotensins and Their Receptors, AT₁ and AT₂. Blocking the angiotensin-converting enzyme (ACE) with ACE inhibitors decreases the amount of angiotensin II. Blocking the receptor AT₁ with drugs (AT₁ antagonists) blocks the attachment of angiotensin II to the cell, preventing the cellular effects and decreasing the vascular, cardiac, and renal effects.

HEALTH ALERT

Adrenomedullin

ADM is a vasodilator secreted by the adrenal medulla and by endothelial cells. It also increases sodium excretion and antagonizes the effects of aldosterone and angiotensin II on tissues. Thus ADM agonists are being evaluated as potential treatments for hypertension, kidney disease, and heart failure. More recently, the role of adrenomedullin in improving ion channel function and angiogenesis (growth of new blood vessels) has been explored as a potential mechanism to reduce ischemic and reperfusion injury to the myocardium. Other areas for which adrenomedullin may present new therapeutic options include pulmonary hypertension, postmenopausal hot flashes, pregnancy-induced hypertension, hepatic cirrhosis, and bone disorders.

Data from Alonso-Martínez JL et al: Hemodynamic effects of chronic smoking in liver cirrhosis: a role for adrenomedullin, *Eur J Gastroenterol Hepatol* 22(5):513–518, 2010; Kim S et al: Adrenomedullin protects against hypoxia/reoxygenation-induced cell death by suppression of reactive oxygen species via thiol redox systems, *FEBS Lett* 584(1):213–218, 2010; Kita T, Tokashiki M, Kitamura K: Aldosterone antisecretagogue and antihypertensive actions of adrenomedullin in patients with primary aldosteronism, *Hypertens Res* 33(4):374–379, 2010; Nishida H et al: New aspects for the treatment of cardiac diseases based on the diversity of functional controls on cardiac muscles: mitochondrial ion channels and cardioprotection, *J Pharmacol Sci* 109(3):341–347, 2009; Shah K et al: Attenuation of renal ischemia and reperfusion injury by human adrenomedullin and its binding protein, *J Surg Res* 163(1):110–117, 2010; Takahashi K et al: The renin-angiotensin system, adrenomedullins and urotensin II in the kidney: possible renoprotection via the kidney peptide systems, *Peptides* 30(8):1575–1585, 2009.

Venous Pressure

The main determinants of venous blood pressure are (1) the volume of fluid within the veins and (2) the compliance (distensibility) of the vessel walls. The venous system accommodates approximately 60% of the total blood volume at any given moment, with venous pressure averaging less than 10 mm Hg. The arteries accommodate about 15% of the total blood volume, with an average arterial pressure (blood pressure) of about 100 mm Hg.

The sympathetic nervous system controls venous compliance. The walls of the veins are highly innervated by sympathetic fibers that, when stimulated, cause venous smooth muscle to contract and increase muscle tone. This stiffens the wall of the vein, which reduces distensibility and increases venous blood pressure, forcing more blood through the veins and into the right heart.

Two other mechanisms that increase venous pressure and venous return to the heart are (1) the skeletal muscle pump and (2) the respiratory pump. During skeletal muscle contraction, the veins within the muscles are partially compressed, causing decreased venous capacity and increased return to the heart (see Figure 22-27). The respiratory pump acts during inspiration, when the veins of the abdomen are partially compressed by the downward movement of the diaphragm. Increased abdominal pressure moves blood toward the heart.

Regulation of the Coronary Circulation

Flow of blood in the coronary circulation is directly proportional to the perfusion pressure and inversely proportional to the vascular resistance of the bed. Coronary perfusion pressure is the difference between pressure in the aorta and pressure in the coronary vessels of the right atrium. Aortic pressure is the driving pressure that perfuses vessels of the myocardium. Vasodilation and vasoconstriction normally maintain coronary blood flow despite stresses imposed by the constant contraction and relaxation of the heart muscle and despite shifts (within a physiologic range) of coronary perfusion pressure.

Several anatomic factors influence coronary blood flow. The aortic valve cusps obstruct coronary blood flow by pushing against the openings of the coronary arteries during systole. Also during systole, the coronary arteries are compressed by ventricular contraction. The resulting systolic compressive effect is particularly evident in the subendocardial layers of the left ventricular wall and can greatly increase resistance to coronary blood flow. Therefore most coronary blood flow in the left ventricle occurs during diastole. During the period of systolic compression, when flow is slowed or stopped, oxygen is supplied by myoglobin, a protein present in heart muscle that binds oxygen during diastole and then releases it when blood levels of oxygen drop during systole.

Autoregulation

Autoregulation (automatic self-regulation) enables individual vessels to regulate blood flow by altering their own arteriolar resistances. Autoregulation in the coronary circulation maintains constant blood flow at perfusion pressures (mean arterial pressure) between 60 and 180 mm Hg, provided that other influencing factors are held constant. Thus autoregulation ensures constant coronary blood flow despite shifts in the perfusion pressure within the stated range.

BOX 22-2   VASCULAR PROTECTION AND INJURY PROPERTIES OF INSULIN

Protection

Insulin has numerous protective actions on blood vessels:

1. Increases endothelial cell production of nitric oxide
   a Nitric oxide (NO) (in vitro) inhibits growth of vascular smooth muscle cells
   b NO decreases the inflammatory reaction by inhibiting the expression of adhesion molecules, inhibiting the activity of proinflammatory cytokines (e.g., tumor necrosis factor-alpha [TNF-α], monocyte chemoattractant protein-1 [MCP-1]). Thus NO decreases the binding of monocytes/macrophages to the vessel wall
2. Enhances acetylcholine-mediated vasodilation
3. Reduces platelet adherence and thus decreases thrombus formation
   a Increased NO also inhibits the thrombotic process by preventing platelet adhesion and enhancing the effect of prostacyclin to inhibit platelet aggregation
   b Insulin increases the endogenous anticoagulant plasminogen activator inhibitor
4. Is anti-inflammatory
   a Reduces toxic oxygen free radical production
   b Decreases levels of C-reactive protein

Injury

Hyperinsulinemia has some deleterious effects on blood vessels:

1. Increases growth of vascular smooth muscle cells (VSMCs)
   a Increases activity of insulin-like growth factor-1
   b Increases angiotensin II–mediated vascular remodeling
2. Increases the effect of platelet-derived growth factor
3. Increases sympathetic nervous system activity and thus contributes to increased blood pressure

Insulin resistance is likely more important to the development of hypertension and the atherogenesis process than hyperinsulinemia:

1. Reduces NO production and increases vasoconstrictors such as angiotensin II and catecholamines
2. Promotes inflammation with increased production of toxic oxygen free radicals and other inflammatory mediators
3. Increases clot formation
4. Contributes to endothelial damage
5. Contributes to deleterious lipid changes

Data from Bloomgarden ZT: Inflammation, atherosclerosis, and aspects of insulin action, *Diabetes Care* 28(9):2312–2319, 2005; Duckles SP, Miller VM: Hormonal modulation of endothelial NO production, *Pflugers Arch* 459(6):841–851, 2010; Kuritzky L, Nelson SE: Beneficial effects of insulin on endothelial function, inflammation, and atherogenesis and their implications, *J Fam Pract* 54(6):S7–S9, 2005; Richards OC, Raines SM, Attie AD: The role of blood vessels, endothelial cells, and vascular pericytes in insulin secretion and peripheral insulin action, *Endocr Rev* 31(3):343–363, 2010; Sowers JR, Frohlich ED: Insulin and insulin resistance: impact on blood pressure and cardiovascular disease, *Med Clin North Am* 88(1): 63–82, 2004.

The mechanism of autoregulation is not known, but two explanations have been proposed. The myogenic hypothesis proposes that autoregulation originates in vascular smooth muscle, presumably that of the arterioles, as a response to changes in arterial perfusion pressure. Increased coronary perfusion pressure increases the pressure against the vessel wall and the stretch increases the vessel's radius, resulting in an increase in wall tension. Initially, coronary blood flow increases with the abrupt distention of the blood vessels. The stretching eventually stimulates contraction of the smooth muscles, which increases vascular resistance. The return of more normal flow follows constriction of the arterioles. Because stretching of vascular smooth muscle increases intracellular Ca^{++} concentration, it is proposed that an increase in transmural pressure activates membrane calcium channels.[1] This mechanism also works in the opposite direction—that is, vasodilation is stimulated by decreased arterial pressure.

The metabolic hypothesis of autoregulation proposes that autoregulation of coronary vessels originates in the myocardium. The stimulus is an increase in the metabolic needs of the myocardium (e.g., because of strenuous exercise). With an increased myocardial oxygen requirement, myocardial cells release substances that promote vasodilation. The best known of these substances is adenosine, a potent vasodilator released in response to a decrease in myocardial oxygenation. Low coronary blood flow, hypoxemia, or increased metabolic activity of the heart can all increase the heart muscle's need for oxygen.[1,35] An increased concentration of adenosine in the interstitial fluid decreases the resistance of the coronary arterioles and increases blood flow. Perfusion strongly correlates with the amount of adenosine released.[35] When coronary perfusion pressure is increased, the increased flow washes out the vasodilatory substances. As the dilators are removed, vasoconstriction occurs and returns flow toward normal.

Autonomic Regulation

Although the coronary vessels themselves contain sympathetic (α- and β-adrenergic) and parasympathetic neural receptors, coronary blood flow is regulated locally through metabolic autoregulation. Metabolic autoregulation overrides neurogenic influences.[4]

✔ **QUICK CHECK 22-7**
1. Why is capillary flow increased with increased mean arterial pressure?
2. Why is angiotensin significant in blood flow?
3. Identify the factors regulating blood pressure.
4. Define natriuretic peptides and adrenomedullin.

THE LYMPHATIC SYSTEM

The lymphatic system is a special vascular system that picks up excess tissue fluid and returns it to the bloodstream (Figure 22-35). Normally, fluid is forced out of the blood at the arterial end of the capillary bed and is reabsorbed into the bloodstream at the venous end. However, capillary outflow exceeds venous reabsorption by about 3 L/day, so some fluid lags behind in the interstitium. To maintain sufficient blood volume in the cardiovascular system, this fluid must eventually rejoin the bloodstream; this is the function of the lymphatic system.

The components of the lymphatic system are the lymphatic vessels and the lymph nodes (Figure 22-36). (Lymph nodes and lymphoid tissues are described in Chapters 5 and 7.) In this pumpless system, a series of valves ensures one-way flow of the excess interstitial fluid (now called lymph) toward the heart. The lymphatic capillaries are closed at the ends, as shown in Figure 22-37.

Lymph consists primarily of water and small amounts of dissolved proteins, mostly albumin that are too large to be reabsorbed into the

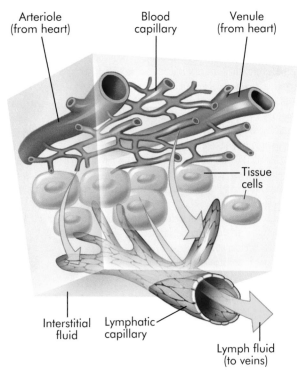

FIGURE 22-35 Role of the Lymphatic System in Fluid Balance.
Fluid from plasma flowing through the capillaries moves into interstitial spaces. Although much of this interstitial fluid is either absorbed
by tissue cells or reabsorbed by capillaries, some of the fluid tends
to accumulate in the interstitial spaces. As this fluid builds up, it
tends to drain into lymphatic vessels that eventually return the fluid
to the venous blood. (From Patton KT, Thibodeau GA: *Anatomy &
physiology,* ed 7, St Louis, 2010, Mosby.)

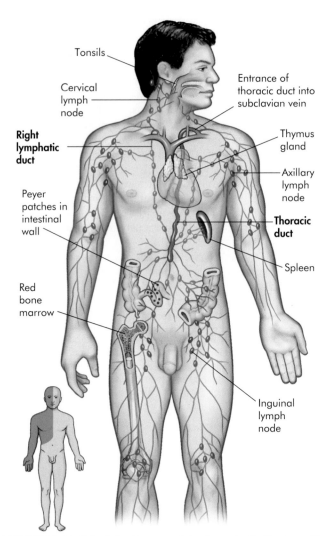

FIGURE 22-36 Principle Organs of the Lymphatic System. The
inset shows the areas drained by the right lymphatic duct *(green)*
and the thoracic duct *(blue).* (From Patton KT, Thibodeau GA: *Anatomy & physiology,* ed 7, St Louis, 2010, Mosby.)

less permeable blood capillaries. Once within the lymphatic system,
lymph travels through larger vessels called lymphatic venules and
lymphatic veins. The lymphatic vessels run alongside the arteries and
veins and eventually drain into one of two large ducts in the thorax—
the right lymphatic duct and the thoracic duct. The right lymphatic
duct drains lymph from the right arm and the right side of the head
and thorax, whereas the larger thoracic duct receives lymph from the
rest of the body (see Figure 22-36). The right lymphatic duct and the
thoracic duct drain lymph into the right and left subclavian veins,
respectively.

The lymphatic veins are thin walled like the veins of the cardiovascular system. In the larger lymphatic veins, endothelial flaps form
valves similar to those in the circulatory veins (see Figure 22-26).
The valves permit lymph to flow in only one direction because
lymphatic vessels are compressed intermittently by contraction of
skeletal muscles, pulsatile expansion of an artery in the same sheath,
and contraction of the smooth muscles in the walls of the lymphatic
vessel.

As lymph is transported toward the heart, it is filtered through
thousands of bean-shaped lymph nodes clustered along the lymphatic

vessels (see Figure 22-36). Lymph enters the node through several
afferent lymphatic vessels, filters through the sinuses in the node,
and leaves by way of efferent lymphatic vessels. Lymph flows slowly
through the node, which facilitates the phagocytosis of foreign substances within the node and prevents them from reentering the bloodstream. (Phagocytosis is described in Chapter 6.)

> ✓ **QUICK CHECK 22-8**
> 1. Why is the lymphatic system considered a circulatory system?
> 2. What happens to lymph in lymph nodes?

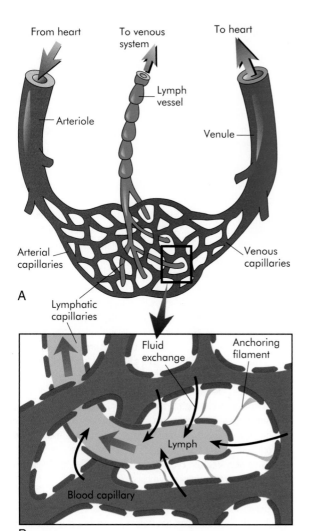

From heart

To venous system

To heart

Lymph vessel

Arteriole

Venule

Arterial capillaries

Venous capillaries

A

Lymphatic capillaries

Fluid exchange

Anchoring filament

Lymph

Blood capillary

B

FIGURE 22-37 Lymphatic Capillaries. A, Schematic representation of lymphatic capillaries. **B,** Anatomic components of microcirculation.

DID YOU UNDERSTAND?

The Circulatory System

1. The circulatory system is the body's transport system. It delivers oxygen, nutrients, metabolites, hormones, neurochemicals, proteins, and blood cells through the body and carries metabolic wastes to the kidneys and lungs for excretion.

2. The circulatory system consists of the heart and blood vessels and is made up of two separate, serially connected systems: the pulmonary circulation and the systemic circulation.

3. The pulmonary circulation is driven by the right side of the heart; its function is to deliver blood to the lungs for oxygenation.

4. The systemic circulation is driven by the left side of the heart, and its function is to move oxygenated blood throughout the body.

5. The lymphatic vessels collect fluids from the interstitium and return the fluids to the circulatory system.

The Heart

1. The heart consists of four chambers (two atria and two ventricles), four valves (two atrioventricular valves and two semilunar valves), a muscular wall, a fibrous skeleton, a conduction system, nerve fibers, systemic vessels (the coronary circulation), and openings where the great vessels enter the atria and ventricles.

2. The heart wall, which encloses the heart and divides it into chambers, is made up of three layers: the pericardium (outer layer), the myocardium (muscular layer), and the endocardium (inner lining).

3. The myocardial layer of the two atria, which receive blood entering the heart, is thinner than the myocardial layer of the ventricles, which have to be stronger to squeeze blood out of the heart.

4. The right and left sides of the heart are separated by portions of the heart wall called the *interatrial septum* and the *interventricular septum*.

5. Deoxygenated (venous) blood from the systemic circulation enters the right atrium through the superior and inferior venae cavae. From the atrium, the blood passes through the right atrioventricular (tricuspid) valve into the right ventricle. In the ventricle, the blood flows from the inflow tract to the outflow tract and then through the pulmonary semilunar valve (pulmonary valve) into the pulmonary artery, which delivers it to the lungs for oxygenation.

6. Oxygenated blood from the lungs enters the left atrium through the four pulmonary veins (two from the left lung and two from the right lung). From the left atrium, the blood passes through the left atrioventricular valve (mitral valve) into the left ventricle. In the ventricle, the blood flows from the inflow tract to the outflow tract and then through the aortic semilunar

Continued

valve (aortic valve) into the aorta, which delivers it to systemic arteries of the entire body.

7. The heart valves ensure the one-way flow of blood from atrium to ventricle and from ventricle to artery.

8. Oxygenated blood enters the coronary arteries through an opening in the aorta, and unoxygenated blood from the coronary veins enters the right atrium through the coronary sinus.

9. The pumping action of the heart consists of two phases: diastole, during which the myocardium relaxes and the ventricles fill with blood; and systole, during which the myocardium contracts, forcing blood out of the ventricles. A cardiac cycle consists of one systolic contraction and the diastolic relaxation that follows it. Each cardiac cycle constitutes one "heartbeat."

10. The conduction system of the heart generates and transmits electrical impulses (cardiac action potentials) that stimulate systolic contractions. The autonomic nerves (sympathetic and parasympathetic fibers) can adjust heart rate and systolic force, but they do not stimulate the heart to beat.

11. The normal electrocardiogram is the sum of all action potentials. The P wave represents atrial depolarization; the QRS complex is the sum of all ventricular cell depolarizations. The ST interval occurs when the entire ventricular myocardium is depolarized.

12. Cardiac action potentials are generated by the sinoatrial node at the rate of about 75 impulses per minute. The impulses can travel through the conduction system of the heart, stimulating myocardial contraction as they go.

13. Cells of the cardiac conduction system possess the properties of automaticity and rhythmicity. Automatic cells return to threshold and depolarize rhythmically without an outside stimulus. The cells of the sinoatrial node depolarize faster than other automatic cells, making it the natural pacemaker of the heart. If the sinoatrial node is disabled, the next fastest pacemaker, the atrioventricular node, takes over.

14. Each cardiac action potential travels from the sinoatrial node to the atrioventricular node to the bundle of His (atrioventricular bundle), through the bundle branches, and finally to the Purkinje fibers. There the impulse is stopped. It is prevented from reversing its path by the refractory period of cells that have just been polarized. The refractory period ensures that diastole (relaxation) will occur, thereby completing the cardiac cycle.

15. Adrenergic receptor number, type, and function govern autonomic (sympathetic) regulation of heart rate, contractile force, and the dilation or constriction of coronary arteries. The presence of specific receptors (α_1, α_2, β_1, β_2) on the myocardium and coronary vessels determines the effects of the neurotransmitters norepinephrine and epinephrine.

16. Unique features that distinguish myocardial cells from skeletal cells enable myocardial cells to transmit action potentials faster (through intercalated disks), synthesize more ATP (because of a large number of mitochondria), and have readier access to ions in the interstitium (because of an abundance of transverse tubules). These combined differences enable the myocardium to work constantly, which is not required by skeletal muscle.

17. Cross-bridges between actin and myosin enable contraction. Calcium and its interaction with the troponin complex facilitate the contraction process. With troponin release of calcium, myocardial relaxation begins.

18. Cardiac performance is affected by preload, afterload, myocardial contractility, and heart rate.

19. Preload, or pressure generated in the ventricles at the end of diastole, depends on the amount of blood in the ventricle. Afterload is the resistance to ejection of the blood from the ventricle. Afterload depends on pressure in the aorta.

20. The Frank-Starling law of the heart states that the myocardial stretch determines the force of myocardial contraction (the greater the stretch, the stronger the contraction).

21. Contractility is the potential for myocardial fiber shortening during systole. It is determined by the amount of stretch during diastole (i.e., preload) and by sympathetic stimulation of the ventricles.

22. Heart rate is determined by the sinoatrial node and by components of the autonomic nervous system, including cardiovascular control centers in the brain, neuroreceptors in the atria and aorta, hormones, and catecholamines (epinephrine, norepinephrine).

The Systemic Circulation

1. Blood flows from the left ventricle into the aorta and from the aorta into arteries that eventually branch into arterioles and capillaries, the smallest of the arterial vessels. Oxygen, nutrients, and other substances needed for cellular metabolism pass from the capillaries into the interstitium, where they are available for uptake by the cells. Capillaries also absorb products of cellular metabolism from the interstitium.

2. Venules, the smallest veins, receive capillary blood. From the venules, the venous blood flows into larger and larger veins until it reaches the venae cavae, through which it enters the right atrium.

3. Vessel walls consist of three layers: the tunica intima (inner layer), the tunica media (middle layer), and the tunica externa (the outer layer).

4. Layers of the vessel wall differ in thickness and composition from vessel to vessel, depending on the vessel's size and location within the circulatory system. In general, the tunica media of arteries close to the heart contains a greater proportion of elastic fibers because these arteries must be able to distend during systole and recoil during diastole. Distributing arteries farther from the heart contain a greater proportion of smooth muscle fibers because these arteries must be able to constrict and dilate to control blood pressure and volume within specific capillary beds.

5. Blood flow into the capillary beds is controlled by the contraction and relaxation of smooth muscle bands (precapillary sphincters) at junctions between metarterioles and capillaries.

6. Endothelial cells form the lining or endothelium of blood vessels. The endothelium is a life-support tissue; it functions as a filter (altering permeability), changes in vasomotion (constriction and dilation), and is involved in clotting and inflammation.

7. Blood flow through the veins is assisted by the contraction of skeletal muscles (the muscle pump), and one-way valves prevent backflow in the lower body, particularly in the deep veins of the legs.

8. Blood flow is affected by blood pressure, resistance to flow within the vessels, blood consistency (which affects velocity), anatomic features that may cause turbulent or laminar flow, and compliance (distensibility) of the vessels.

9. Poiseuille law describes the relationship of blood flow, pressure, and resistance as the difference between pressure at the inflow end of the vessel and pressure at the outflow end divided by resistance within the vessel.

10. The greater the vessel's length and the blood's viscosity and the narrower the radius of the vessel's lumen, the greater the resistance within the vessel.

11. Total peripheral resistance, or the resistance to flow within the entire systemic circulatory system, depends on the combined lengths and radii of all the vessels within the system and on whether the vessels are arranged in series (greater resistance) or in parallel (lesser resistance).

12. Peripheral resistance is based on physical laws governing the behavior of fluids in a straight tube. In the body, blood flow is also influenced by neural stimulation (vasoconstriction or vasodilation) and by autonomic features that cause turbulence within the vascular lumen (e.g., protrusions from the vessel wall, twists and turns, bifurcations).

DID YOU UNDERSTAND?—cont'd

13. Arterial blood pressure is influenced and regulated by factors that affect cardiac output (heart rate, stroke volume), total resistance within the system, and blood volume.

14. Antidiuretic hormone, renin-angiotensin system, natriuretic peptides, adrenomedullin, and insulin can all alter blood volume and thus blood pressure.

15. The tissue renin-angiotensin system is activated in response to tissue injury. Studies examining the relationship between this system and maladaptive alterations, such as ventricular and vascular remodeling, alterations in renal function, and atherosclerosis, are gaining importance.

16. Particularly significant is an increased recognition of the role of angiotensin II for causing the systemic effects of vasoconstriction, hypertension, activation of the sympathetic nervous system, and retention of sodium and fluids.

17. Venous blood pressure is influenced by blood volume within the venous system and compliance of the venous walls.

18. Blood flow through the coronary circulation is governed not only by the same principles as flow through other vascular beds but also by adaptations dictated by cardiac dynamics. First, blood flows into the coronary arteries during diastole rather than systole, because during systole, the cusps of the aortic semilunar valve block the openings of the coronary arteries. Second, systolic contraction inhibits coronary artery flow by compressing the coronary arteries.

19. Autoregulation enables the coronary vessels to maintain optimal perfusion pressure despite systolic effects, and myoglobin in heart muscle stores oxygen for use during the systolic phase of the cardiac cycle.

The Lymphatic System

1. The vessels of the lymphatic system run in the same sheaths with the arteries and veins.

2. Lymph (interstitial fluid) is absorbed by lymphatic venules in the capillary beds and travels through ever larger lymphatic veins until it is emptied through the right lymphatic duct or thoracic duct into the right or left subclavian vein, respectively.

3. As lymph travels toward the thoracic ducts, it is filtered by thousands of lymph nodes clustered around the lymphatic veins. The lymph nodes are sites of immune function.

KEY TERMS

- Actin   561
- Adipokines   576
- Adrenomedullin (ADM)   576
- Afferent lymphatic vessel   580
- Afterload   564
- Angiotensin I (Ang I)   574
- Angiotensin II (Ang II)   574
- Anisotropic band (A band)   561
- Anterior interatrial myocardial band (Bachmann bundle)   557
- Anterior internodal pathway   557
- Antidiuretic hormone (ADH)   574
- Aorta   554
- Aortic semilunar valve   554
- Arteriole   567
- Artery   567
- AT_1 receptor   576
- AT_2 receptor   576
- Atrial natriuretic peptide (ANP)   576
- Atrioventricular node (AV node)   557
- Atrioventricular valve   553
- Automatic cell   559
- Automaticity   559
- Autoregulation   578
- Bainbridge reflex   565
- Baroreceptor reflex   565
- Blood flow   570
- Blood velocity   573
- Brain natriuretic peptide (BNP)   576
- Bundle of His (atrioventricular bundle)   557
- Calcium channel–blocking drug   562
- Capillary   567
- Cardiac action potential   557
- Cardiac cycle   554

- Cardiac output   563
- Cardiac vein   556
- Cardioexcitatory center   565
- Cardioinhibitory center   565
- Cardiovascular control center   565
- Chordae tendineae cordis   554
- Conduction system   557
- Coronary artery   556
- Coronary circulation   556
- Coronary ostium (pl., ostia)   556
- Coronary perfusion pressure   578
- Coronary sinus   556
- Cross-bridge theory of muscle contraction   562
- Depolarization   558
- Diastole   554
- Diastolic blood pressure   573
- Diastolic depolarization   560
- Efferent lymphatic vessel   580
- Ejection fraction   563
- Elastic artery   569
- Endocardium   553
- Endothelial cell   569
- Endothelium   569
- Excitation-contraction coupling   562
- Fenestration   569
- Frank-Starling law of the heart   563
- Great cardiac vein   557
- Heart rate   560
- Inferior vena cava (pl., cavae)   554
- Inotropic agent   564
- Insulin   576
- Intercalated disk   560
- Isotropic band (I band)   561
- Laminar flow   573

- Laplace law   563
- Left atrium   563
- Left bundle branch (LBB)   557
- Left coronary artery   556
- Left heart   551
- Left ventricle   553
- Length   570
- Lumen   569
- Lymph   579
- Lymph node   580
- Lymphatic vein   580
- Lymphatic venule   580
- M line   561
- Mean arterial pressure (MAP)   573
- Mediastinum   551
- Metabolic hypothesis   579
- Metarteriole   569
- Microcirculation   570
- Middle internodal pathway   557
- Mitral and tricuspid complex   554
- Mitral valve (left atrioventricular valve, bicuspid valve)   554
- Muscle pump   570
- Muscular artery   569
- Myocardial contractility   562
- Myocardial oxygen consumption ($M\dot{V}O_2$)   561
- Myocardium   552
- Myogenic hypothesis   579
- Myoglobin   578
- Myosin   561
- Natriuretic peptide (NP)   576
- Node   557
- P wave   559
- Papillary muscle   554

KEY TERMS—cont'd

- Perfusion 573
- Pericardial cavity 552
- Pericardial fluid 552
- Pericardium 552
- Peripheral vascular resistance (PVR) 564
- Peripheral vascular system 567
- Poiseuille law 570
- Posterior internodal pathway 557
- PR interval 559
- Precapillary sphincter 569
- Preload 563
- Pressure 570
- Pulmonary artery 554
- Pulmonary circulation 551
- Pulmonary vein 554
- Pulmonic semilunar valve 554
- Purkinje fiber 558
- QRS complex 559
- QT interval 559
- Radius (diameter) 570
- Refractory period 559
- Renin 574
- Repolarization 558

- Resistance 570
- Rhythmicity 560
- Right atrium 553
- Right bundle branch (RBB) 557
- Right coronary artery 556
- Right heart 551
- Right lymphatic duct 580
- Right ventricle 553
- Semilunar valve 554
- Sinoatrial node (SA node, sinus node) 557
- ST interval 559
- Stroke volume 564
- Superior vena cava (pl., cavae) 554
- Systemic circulation 551
- Systole 554
- Systolic blood pressure 573
- Systolic compressive effect 578
- Thoracic duct 580
- Total peripheral resistance (TPR) 564
- Total resistance 570
- Tricuspid valve (right atrioventricular valve) 554
- Tropomyosin 561

- Troponin C 561
- Troponin I 561
- Troponin T 561
- Troponin-tropomyosin complex 561
- Tunica externa (adventitia; external layer) 567
- Tunica intima (intimal layer) 567
- Tunica media (medial layer) 567
- Turbulent flow 573
- Vasa vasorum 569
- Vascular compliance 573
- Vasoconstriction 569
- Vasodilation 569
- Vein 570
- Ventricular end-diastolic pressure (VEDP) 563
- Ventricular end-diastolic volume (VEDV) 563
- Venule 567
- Viscosity 570
- Z line 561

REFERENCES

1. Mohrman DE, Heller JA, editors: *Cardiovascular physiology*, ed 6, Philadelphia, 2006, McGraw-Hill.
2. Kastrup J: Gene therapy and angiogenesis in patients with coronary artery disease, *Exp Rev Cardiovasc Ther* 8(8):1127–1138, 2010.
3. Ganong W: *Review of medical physiology*, ed 23, New York, 2010, McGraw-Hill.
4. Libby P, et al: *Braunwald's heart disease: a textbook of cardiovascular medicine*, ed 8, Philadelphia, 2008, Saunders.
5. Ho SY, Sánchez-Quintana D: The importance of atrial structure and fibers, *Clin Anat* 22(1):52–63, 2009.
6. Benitah JP, Alvarez JL, Gómez AM: L-type Ca(2+) current in ventricular cardiomyocytes, *J Mol Cell Cardiol* 48(1):26–36, 2010.
7. Ono K, Iijima T: Cardiac T-type Ca(2+) channels in the heart, *J Mol Cell Cardiol* 48(1):65–70, 2010.
8. Ferreira-Martins J, Leite-Moreira AF: Physiologic basis and pathophysiologic implications of the diastolic properties of the cardiac muscle, *J Biomed Biotechnol* 807084, 2010. [E-pub 2010 Jun 2.].
9. Patton KT, Thibodeau GA: *Anatomy & physiology*, ed 7, St Louis, 2010, Mosby Elsevier.
10. Berne RM, Levy MN, editors: *Cardiovascular physiology*, ed 8, St Louis, 2001, Mosby.
11. Omland T, Hagve TA: Natriuretic peptides: physiologic and analytic considerations, *Heart Fail Clin* 5(4):471–487, 2009.
12. Freestone B, Krishnamoorthy S, Lip GY: Assessment of endothelial dysfunction, *Exp Rev Cardiovasc Ther* 8(4):557–571, 2010.
13. Bie P, Damkjaer M: Renin secretion and total body sodium: pathways of integrative control, *Clin Exp Pharmacol Physiol* 37(2):e34–e42, 2010.
14. Vanderheyden PM: From angiotensin IV binding site to AT4 receptor, *Mol Cell Endocrinol* 302(2):159–166, 2009.
15. Benigni A, Cassis P, Remuzzi G: Angiotensin II revisited: new roles in inflammation, immunology and aging, *EMBO Mol Med* 2(7):247–257, 2010.
16. Bader M: Tissue renin-angiotensin-aldosterone systems: targets for pharmacological therapy, *Annu Rev Pharmacol Toxicol* 50:439–465, 2010.
17. Sata M, Fukuda D: Crucial role of renin-angiotensin system in the pathogenesis of atherosclerosis, *J Med Invest* 57(1–2):12–25, 2010.
18. Sun Y: Intracardiac renin-angiotensin system and myocardial repair/remodeling following infarction, *J Mol Cell Cardiol* 48(3):483–489, 2010.
19. Siragy HM, Carey RM: Role of the intrarenal renin-angiotensin-aldosterone system in chronic kidney disease, *Am J Nephrol* 31(6):541–550, 2010.
20. Briet M, Schiffrin EL: Aldosterone: effects on the kidney and cardiovascular system, *Nat Rev Nephrol* 6(5):261–273, 2010.
21. Miura S, et al: Molecular mechanisms of the antagonistic action between AT$_1$ and AT$_2$ receptors, *Biochem Biophys Res Commun* 391(1):85–90, 2010.
22. Calò LA, et al: Angiotensin II signaling via type 2 receptors in a human model of vascular hyporeactivity: implications for hypertension, *J Hypertens* 28(1):111–118, 2010.
23. Zhong J, et al: Angiotensin-converting enzyme 2 suppresses pathological hypertrophy, myocardial fibrosis, and cardiac dysfunction, *Circulation* 122(7):717–728, 2010:18 p following 728.
24. Lee CY, Burnett JC Jr: Natriuretic peptides and therapeutic applications, *Heart Fail Rev* 12(2):131–142, 2007.
25. Menon SG, et al: Clinical implications of defective B-type natriuretic peptide, *Clin Cardiol* 32(12):E36–E41, 2009.
26. O'Donoghue M, Braunwald E: Natriuretic peptides in heart failure: should therapy be guided by BNP levels? *Nat Rev Cardiol* 7(1):13–20, 2010.
27. Palmer SC, et al: Regional release and clearance of C-type natriuretic peptides in the human circulation and relation to cardiac function, *Hypertension* 54(3):612–618, 2009.
28. Lanfear DE: Genetic variation in the natriuretic peptide system and heart failure, *Heart Fail Rev* 15(3):219–228, 2010.
29. Yanagawa B, Nagaya N: Adrenomedullin: molecular mechanisms and its role in cardiac disease, *Amino Acids* 32(1):157–164, 2007.
30. Ribatti D, et al: The role of adrenomedullin in angiogenesis, *Peptides* 26(9):1670–1675, 2005.
31. Dai X, et al: Adrenomedullin and its expression in cancers and bone. A literature review, *Front Biosci* 2:1073–1080, 2010.
32. Duckles SP, Miller VM: Hormonal modulation of endothelial NO production, *Pflugers Arch* 459(6):841–851, 2010.
33. Richards OC, Raines SM, Attie AD: The role of blood vessels, endothelial cells, and vascular pericytes in insulin secretion and peripheral insulin action, *Endocr Rev* 31(3):343–363, 2010.
34. Yiannikouris F, et al: Adipokines and blood pressure control, *Curr Opin Nephrol Hypertens* 19(2):195–200, 2010.
35. Kotsis V, et al: Mechanisms of obesity-induced hypertension, *Hypertens Res* 33(5):386–393, 2010.

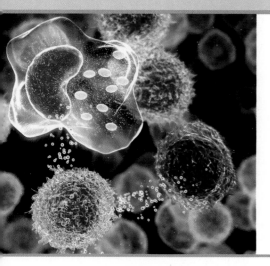

Alterations of Cardiovascular Function

Valentina L. Brashers

evolve WEBSITE

CHAPTER OUTLINE

Our understanding of the pathophysiology of cardiovascular diseases is evolving rapidly. The role of genetics and its interaction with the environment in the etiology and progression of all forms of cardiovascular disease is just one example of new information that is leading to improvements in prevention and treatment.

DISEASES OF THE VEINS

Varicose Veins and Chronic Venous Insufficiency

A **varicose vein** is a vein in which blood has pooled, producing distended, tortuous, and palpable vessels (Figure 23-1). Veins are thin-walled, highly distensible vessels with valves to prevent backflow and pooling of blood (see Figure 22-26). Varicose veins are caused by (1) trauma to the saphenous veins that damages one or more valves or (2) gradual venous distention caused by the action of gravity on blood in the legs.

If a valve is damaged, a section of the vein is subjected to the pressure of a larger volume of blood under the influence of gravity. The vein swells as it becomes engorged and surrounding tissue becomes edematous because increased hydrostatic pressure pushes plasma through the stretched vessel wall. Venous distention can develop over time in individuals who habitually stand for long periods, wear constricting garments, or cross the legs at the knees, which diminishes the action of the muscle pump (see Figure 22-27). Risk factors also include age, female gender, a family history of varicose veins, obesity, pregnancy, deep venous thrombosis, and previous leg injury. Eventually the pressure in the vein damages venous valves, rendering them incompetent and unable to maintain normal venous pressure.

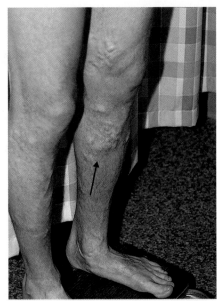

FIGURE 23-1 Varicose Veins of the Leg *(arrow).* (From Kumar V, Abbas A, Fausto N: *Robbins and Cotran pathologic basis of disease,* ed 8, Philadelphia, 2007, Saunders. Courtesy Dr. Magruder C. Donaldson, Brigham and Women's Hospital, Boston.)

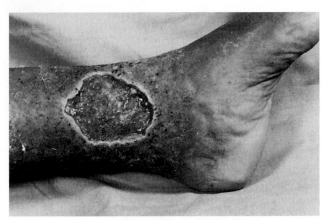

FIGURE 23-2 Venous Stasis Ulcer. (From Rosai J: *Ackerman's surgical pathology,* ed 7, vol 2, St Louis, 1989, Mosby.)

Varicose veins and valvular incompetence can progress to chronic venous insufficiency, especially in obese individuals.[1] **Chronic venous insufficiency (CVI)** is inadequate venous return over a long period. Venous hypertension, circulatory stasis, and tissue hypoxia cause an inflammatory reaction in vessels and tissue leading to fibrosclerotic remodeling of the skin and then to ulceration. Symptoms include edema of the lower extremities and hyperpigmentation of the skin of the feet and ankles. Edema in these areas may extend to the knees.

Circulation to the extremities can become so sluggish that the metabolic demands of the cells to obtain oxygen and nutrients and to remove wastes are barely met. Any trauma or pressure can therefore lower the oxygen supply and cause cell death and necrosis **(venous stasis ulcers)** (Figure 23-2). Infection can occur because poor circulation impairs the delivery of the cells and biochemicals necessary for the immune and inflammatory responses. This same sluggish circulation makes infection following reparative surgery a significant risk.

Treatment of varicose veins and CVI begins conservatively, and excellent wound healing results have followed noninvasive treatments such as elevating the legs, wearing compression stockings, and performing physical exercise.[2] Invasive management includes sclerotherapy or surgical ligation, conservative vein resection, and vein stripping.

Thrombus Formation in Veins

A **thrombus** is a blood clot that remains attached to a vessel wall (see Figure 20-17). A detached thrombus is a **thromboembolus.** Venous thrombi are more common than arterial thrombi because flow and pressure are lower in the veins than in the arteries. **Deep venous thrombosis (DVT)** occurs primarily in the lower extremity. Three factors (triad of Virchow) promote venous thrombosis: (1) venous stasis (e.g., immobility, age, congestive heart failure), (2) venous endothelial damage (e.g., trauma, intravenous medications), and (3) hypercoagulable states (e.g., inherited disorders, malignancy, pregnancy, use of oral contraceptives or hormone replacement therapy). Orthopedic trauma or surgery, spinal cord injury, and obstetric/gynecologic

conditions can be associated with up to a 100% likelihood of DVT. Numerous genetic abnormalities are associated with an increased risk for venous thrombosis primarily related to states of hypercoagulability. These inherited abnormalities include factor V Leiden mutation, prothrombin mutations, and deficiencies of protein C, protein S, and antithrombin; these abnormalities are commonly found in individuals who develop thrombi in the absence of the usual risk factors.[3]

Accumulation of clotting factors and platelets leads to thrombus formation in the vein, often near a venous valve. Inflammation around the thrombus promotes further platelet aggregation, and the thrombus propagates or grows proximally. This inflammation may cause pain and redness, but because the vein is deep in the leg, it is usually not accompanied by clinical symptoms or signs. If the thrombus creates significant obstruction to venous blood flow, increased pressure in the vein behind the clot may lead to edema of the extremity. Most thrombi will eventually dissolve without treatment; however, untreated DVT is associated with a high risk of embolization of a part of the clot to the lung (pulmonary embolism) (see Chapter 33). Persistent venous obstruction may lead to chronic venous insufficiency and post-thrombotic syndrome with associated pain, edema, and ulceration of the affected limb.[4]

Because DVT is usually asymptomatic and difficult to detect clinically, prevention is important in at-risk individuals and includes early ambulation, pneumatic devices, and prophylactic anticoagulation.[5] If thrombosis does occur, diagnosis is confirmed by a combination of serum D-dimer measurement and Doppler ultrasonography. Management consists of anticoagulation therapy using heparin (low-molecular-weight heparin) and warfarin. In selected individuals, thrombolytic therapy or placement of an inferior vena cava filter may be indicated.[6]

Superior Vena Cava Syndrome

Superior vena cava syndrome (SVCS) is a progressive occlusion of the superior vena cava (SVC) that leads to venous distention in the upper extremities and head. Causes include bronchogenic cancer (75% of cases), followed by lymphomas and metastasis of other cancers. Other less common causes include tuberculosis, mediastinal fibrosis, cystic fibrosis, and invasive therapies (pacemaker wires, central venous catheters, and pulmonary artery catheters). The SVC is a relatively low-pressure vessel that lies in the closed thoracic compartment; therefore tissue expansion can easily compress the SVC. The right main stem bronchus abuts the SVC so that cancers occurring in this bronchus may exert pressure on the SVC. Additionally, the SVC is surrounded by lymph nodes and lymph chains that commonly become involved in thoracic cancers and compress the SVC during tumor growth. Because onset of SVCS is slow, collateral venous drainage to the azygos vein usually has time to develop.

Clinical manifestations of SVCS are edema and venous distention in the upper extremities and face, including the ocular beds. Affected persons complain of a feeling of fullness in the head or tightness of shirt collars, necklaces, and rings. Cerebral edema may cause headache, visual disturbance, and impaired consciousness. The skin of the face and arms may become purple and taut, and capillary refill time is prolonged. Respiratory distress may be present because of edema of bronchial structures or compression of the bronchus by a carcinoma. In infants, SVCS can lead to hydrocephalus.

Diagnosis is made by chest x-ray, Doppler studies, computed tomography (CT), magnetic resonance imaging (MRI), and ultrasound. Because of its slow onset and the development of collateral venous drainage, SVCS is generally not a vascular emergency, but it is an oncologic emergency. Treatment for malignant disorders can include radiation therapy, surgery, chemotherapy, and the administration of diuretics, steroids, and anticoagulants, as necessary. Treatment for nonmalignant causes may include bypass surgery using various grafts, thrombolysis (both locally and systemically), balloon angioplasty, and placement of intravascular stents.[7]

✔ QUICK CHECK 23-1

1. What is chronic venous insufficiency, and how does it present clinically?
2. What are the major risk factors for DVT?
3. Name some causes of superior vena cava syndrome.

DISEASES OF THE ARTERIES

Hypertension

Hypertension is consistent elevation of systemic arterial blood pressure. Hypertension (HTN) is the most common primary diagnosis in the United States. One in three Americans has hypertension, and more than two thirds of those older than age 60 are affected.[8] The chance of developing primary hypertension increases with age. Although hypertension is usually considered an adult health problem, it is important to remember that hypertension does occur in children and is being diagnosed with increasing frequency (see Chapter 24). The prevalence of HTN is higher in blacks and in those with diabetes. Hypertension is defined by the Seventh Joint National Committee Report as a sustained systolic blood pressure of 140 mm Hg or greater or a diastolic pressure of 90 mm Hg or greater (Table 23-1).[9] Normal blood pressure is associated with the lowest cardiovascular risk, whereas those who fall into the prehypertension category (which includes between 25% and 37% of the U.S. population) are at risk for developing hypertension and many associated cardiovascular complications unless lifestyle modification and treatment are instituted.[8,10] All stages of hypertension are associated with increased risk for target organ disease events, such as myocardial infarction, kidney disease, and stroke; thus both stage I and stage II hypertension need effective long-term therapy.

Isolated systolic hypertension (ISH) is typically defined as a sustained systolic blood pressure (BP) reading that is ≥140 mm Hg and a diastolic BP measurement that is <90 mm Hg. ISH is becoming more prevalent in all age groups and is strongly associated with cardiovascular and cerebrovascular events.[11]

Most cases of hypertension are diagnosed as primary hypertension (also called essential or idiopathic hypertension). From 92% to 95% of hypertensive individuals have primary disease. Secondary

---

TABLE 23-1	CLASSIFICATION OF BLOOD PRESSURE FOR ADULTS AGE 18 YEARS AND OLDER			
CATEGORY	**SYSTOLIC (MM HG)**		**DIASTOLIC (MM HG)**	
Normal	<120	AND	<80	
Prehypertension	120-139	OR	80-89	
Stage 1 hypertension	140-159	OR	90-99	
Stage 2 hypertension	≥160	OR	≥100	

Data from Chobanian AV et al: The JNC 7 Report, *J Am Med Assoc* 289(19):2560–2572, 2003.

---

hypertension is caused by an underlying disorder such as renal disease. This form of hypertension accounts for only 5% to 8% of cases.

Factors Associated With Primary Hypertension

A specific cause for primary hypertension has not been identified, and a combination of genetic and environmental factors is thought to be responsible for its development.[12] Genetic predisposition to hypertension is believed to be polygenic. The inherited defects are associated with renal sodium excretion, insulin and insulin sensitivity, activity of the sympathetic nervous system (SNS) and the renin-angiotensin-aldosterone system (RAAS), and cell membrane sodium or calcium transport.[13] Factors associated with primary hypertension include (1) family history of hypertension; (2) advancing age; (3) gender (men younger than age 55 and women after age 70); (4) black race; (5) high dietary sodium intake; (6) glucose intolerance (insulin resistance and diabetes mellitus); (7) cigarette smoking; (8) obesity; (9) heavy alcohol consumption; and (10) low dietary intake of potassium, calcium, and magnesium (see *Risk Factors: Primary Hypertension*). Many of these factors are also risk factors for other cardiovascular disorders. In fact, obesity, hypertension, dyslipidemia, and glucose intolerance often are found together in a condition called the metabolic syndrome (see Chapter 18).

RISK FACTORS

Primary Hypertension

Family history
Advancing age
Cigarette smoking
Obesity
Heavy alcohol consumption
Gender (men > women before age 55, women > men after 55)
Black race
High dietary sodium intake
Low dietary intake of potassium, calcium, magnesium
Glucose intolerance

PATHOPHYSIOLOGY Hypertension results from a sustained increase in peripheral resistance (arteriolar vasoconstriction), an increase in circulating blood volume, or both.

Primary Hypertension

Primary hypertension is the result of an extremely complicated interaction of genetics and the environment mediated by a host of neurohumoral effects. Multiple pathophysiologic mechanisms mediate these effects, including the sympathetic nervous system (SNS), the renin-angiotensin-aldosterone system (RAAS), and natriuretic peptides.

Inflammation, endothelial dysfunction, obesity-related hormones, and insulin resistance also contribute to both increased peripheral resistance and increased blood volume. Increased vascular volume is related to a decrease in renal excretion of salt, often referred to as a shift in the **pressure-natriuresis relationship** (Figure 23-3). This means that for a given blood pressure, individuals with hypertension tend to secrete less salt in their urine.

The sympathetic nervous system has been implicated in both the development and the maintenance of elevated blood pressure and plays a role in hypertensive end-organ damage.[14] Increased SNS activity causes increased heart rate and systemic vasoconstriction, thus raising the blood pressure. Additional mechanisms of SNS-induced hypertension include structural changes in blood vessels (vascular remodeling), renal sodium retention (shift in natriuresis curve), insulin resistance, increased renin and angiotensin levels, and procoagulant effects.[15]

In hypertensive individuals, overactivity of the RAAS contributes to salt and water retention and increased vascular resistance (see Figure 22-32). High levels of angiotensin II contribute to endothelial dysfunction, insulin resistance, and platelet aggregation. Further, angiotensin II mediates arteriolar remodeling, which is structural change in the vessel wall that results in permanent increases in peripheral resistance[16] (see Figure 22-33). Angiotensin II is associated with end-organ effects of hypertension, including atherosclerosis, renal disease, and cardiac hypertrophy.[17] Finally, aldosterone not only contributes to sodium retention by the kidney but also has other deleterious effects on the cardiovascular system.[18] Medications, such as angiotensin-converting enzyme (ACE) inhibitors and angiotensin receptor blockers (ARBs), oppose the activity of the RAAS and are effective in reducing blood pressure and protecting against target organ damage[19] (see *Health Alert: The Renin-Angiotensin-Aldosterone System and Cardiovascular Disease*).

Populations with high dietary sodium intake have long been shown to have an increased incidence of hypertension. Low dietary potassium, calcium, and magnesium intakes also are risk factors because without their intake, sodium is retained. The natriuretic hormones modulate renal sodium (Na^+) excretion and require adequate potassium, calcium, and magnesium to function properly. The natriuretic hormones include atrial natriuretic peptide (ANP), brain natriuretic peptide (BNP), C-type natriuretic peptide (CNP), and urodilatin. Dysfunction

HEALTH ALERT
The Renin-Angiotensin-Aldosterone System and Cardiovascular Disease

The RAAS has multiple effects on the cardiovascular system. In recent years, it has been found that there are two primary RAA systems. The best known is described in Chapter 22 and includes the synthesis of angiotensin II via angiotensin-converting enzyme (ACE), stimulation of the AT_1 receptor (AT_1R), and secretion of aldosterone. In addition to causing systemic vasoconstriction and renal salt and water retention, this system has direct effects on blood vessel, heart, and kidney tissues. Angiotensin II is a vasoconstrictor, a growth factor, and an inflammatory mediator. When present in abnormal amounts, it contributes to inflammation and insulin resistance, remodeling of blood vessels with narrowing of blood vessel lumina, and decreased release of endothelial vasodilators and anticoagulants. In the heart angiotensin II and aldosterone contribute to hypertensive hypertrophy and fibrosis of heart muscle, remodeling of myocardial tissues after ischemia, decreased contractility, and an increased susceptibility to dysrhythmias and heart failure. In the kidney these hormones cause a shift in the pressure-natriuresis curve, inflammation, and glomerular remodeling and they are a major contributor to renal failure in individuals with hypertension and diabetes. Drugs that block this RAAS pathway include those that interfere with angiotensin II and aldosterone synthesis (angiotensin-converting enzyme [ACE] inhibitors and direct renin inhibitors), angiotensin II receptor blockers (ARBs), and aldosterone inhibitors. These medications are used widely in the management of hypertension, myocardial infarction, and heart failure to lower blood pressure and to protect and improve cardiovascular and renal function. In contrast, the second RAAS serves a counterregulatory system. Activation of a second ACE pathway (ACE_2) leads to the synthesis of angiotensin 1-7 from angiotensin II. Angiotensin 1-7 stimulates Mas receptors, which lower blood pressure, reduce inflammation, and prevent remodeling of target organ tissues. This pathway appears to be especially important in protecting renal tissue in those with diabetes and hypertension. New research is under way to develop genetic and pharmacologic interventions that will stimulate this second RAAS pathway.

Data from Bader M: *Annu Rev Pharmacol Toxicol* 50:439–465, 2010; Bakris G: *Am J Cardiol* 105(1 suppl):21A–29A, 2010; Ferreira AJ et al: *Hypertension* 55(2):207–213, 2010; Iwai M, Horiuchi M: *Hypertens Res* 32(7):533–536, 2009; Oudit GY et al: *Diabetes* 59(2):529–538, 2010; Wysocki J et al: *Hypertension* 55(1):90–98, 2010.

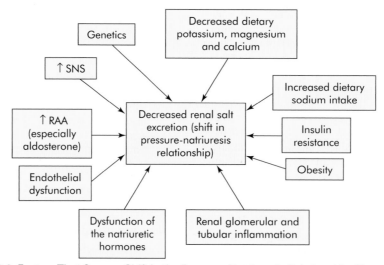

FIGURE 23-3 Factors That Cause a Shift in the Pressure-Natriuresis Relationship. Numerous factors have been implicated in the pathogenesis of sodium retention in individuals with hypertension. These factors cause less renal excretion of salt than would normally occur with increased blood pressure. This is called a shift in the pressure-natriuresis relationship and is believed to be a central process in the pathogenesis of primary hypertension. *RAA,* Renin-angiotensin-aldosterone; *SNS,* sympathetic nervous system.

of these hormones, along with alterations in the RAA system and the SNS, causes an increase in vascular tone and a shift in the pressure-natriuresis relationship. When there is inadequate natriuretic function, serum levels of the natriuretic peptides are increased. In hypertension, increased ANP and BNP levels are linked to an increased risk for ventricular hypertrophy, atherosclerosis, and heart failure.[20] Salt retention leads to water retention and increased blood volume, which contributes to an increase in blood pressure. Subtle renal injury results, with renal vasoconstriction and tissue ischemia. Tissue ischemia causes inflammation of the kidney and contributes to dysfunction of the glomeruli and tubules, which promotes additional sodium retention.

Inflammation plays a role in the pathogenesis of hypertension.[21] Endothelial injury and tissue ischemia result in the release of vasoactive inflammatory cytokines. Although many of these cytokines (e.g., histamine, prostaglandins) have vasodilatory actions in acute inflammatory injury, chronic inflammation contributes to vascular remodeling and smooth muscle contraction. Endothelial injury and dysfunction in primary hypertension is further characterized by a decreased production of vasodilators, such as nitric oxide, and an increased production of vasoconstrictors, such as endothelin.[22]

Obesity is recognized as an important risk factor for hypertension in both adults and children and contributes to many of the neurohumoral, metabolic, renal, and cardiovascular processes that cause hypertension.[23] Obesity causes changes in the adipokines (i.e., leptin and adiponectin) and also is associated with increased activity of the SNS and the RAAS. Obesity is linked to inflammation, endothelial dysfunction, and insulin resistance and an increased risk for cardiovascular complications from hypertension[24] (see *Health Alert: Obesity and Hypertension*).

Finally, insulin resistance is common in hypertension, even in individuals without clinical diabetes.[25] Insulin resistance is associated with decreased endothelial release of nitric oxide and other vasodilators. It also affects renal function and causes renal salt and water retention. Insulin resistance is associated with overactivity of the sympathetic nervous system and the renin-angiotensin-aldosterone system. It is interesting to note that in many individuals with diabetes treated with drugs that increase insulin sensitivity, blood pressure often declines, even in the absence of antihypertensive drugs. The interactions between

HEALTH ALERT

Obesity and Hypertension

Several hemodynamic and metabolic abnormalities have been implicated in the development of hypertension in obesity. These include increased inflammation, activation of the sympathetic nervous system and the renin-angiotensin-aldosterone system, insulin resistance, endothelial dysfunction, and renal function abnormalities. One of the major mechanisms leading to the development of obesity-induced hypertension appears to be leptin-mediated effects on blood vessels and the kidney. Leptin is a circulating peptide hormone that is primarily secreted by adipocytes. Although obesity is generally associated with resistance to the weight-reducing actions of leptin, the resultant increased levels of this peptide cause an increase in sympathetic nervous system activity and adversely shift the renal pressure-natriuresis curve, leading to sodium retention. Adiponectin is a protein that is produced by adipose tissue but is reduced in obesity. Decreased adiponectin is associated with insulin resistance, decreased endothelial-derived nitric oxide (vasodilator) production, and activation of both the sympathetic nervous and renin-angiotensin-aldosterone systems. Taken together, these obesity-related changes result in vasoconstriction, salt and water retention, and renal dysfunction; all of these factors may contribute to the development of hypertension. Further studies aimed at achieving a better understanding of **these mechanisms** may lead to new treatments for obesity-related hypertension.

Data from Bogaert YE, Linas S: *Nat Clin Pract Nephrol* 5(2):101–111, 2009; Kshatriya S et al: *Curr Opin Nephrol Hypertens* 19(1):72–78, 2010; Mathieu P et al: *Hypertension* 53(4):577–584, 2009; Papadopoulos DP et al: *J Clin Hypertens* 11(2):61–65, 2009; Patel JV et al: *Ann Med* 41(4):291–300, 2009; Rahmouni K: *Hypertension* 55(4):844–845, 2010; Sweeney G: *Nat Rev Cardiol* 7(1):22–29, 2010.

obesity, hypertension, insulin resistance, and lipid disorders in the metabolic syndrome result in a high risk of cardiovascular disease.[26,27]

It is likely that primary hypertension is an interaction between many of these factors leading to sustained increases in blood volume and peripheral resistance. The pathophysiology of primary hypertension is summarized in Figure 23-4.

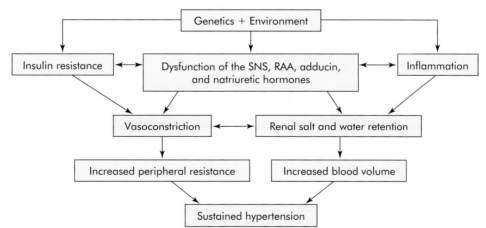

FIGURE 23-4 Pathophysiology of Hypertension. Numerous genetic vulnerabilities have been linked to hypertension and these, in combination with environmental risks, cause neurohumoral dysfunction (sympathetic nervous system *[SNS]*, renin-angiotensin-aldosterone *[RAA]* system, adducin (cytoskeleton protein involved with Na/K ATPase), and natriuretic hormones) and promote inflammation and insulin resistance. Insulin resistance and neurohumoral dysfunction contribute to sustained systemic vasoconstriction and increased peripheral resistance. Inflammation contributes to renal dysfunction, which, in combination with the neurohumoral alterations, results in renal salt and water retention and increased blood volume. Increased peripheral resistance and increased blood volume are two primary causes of sustained hypertension.

Secondary Hypertension

Secondary hypertension is caused by an underlying disease process or medication that raises peripheral vascular resistance or cardiac output. Examples include renal vascular or parenchymal disease, adrenocortical tumors, adrenomedullary tumors (pheochromocytoma), and drugs (oral contraceptives, corticosteroids, antihistamines). If the cause is identified and removed before permanent structural changes occur, blood pressure returns to normal.

Complicated Hypertension

As hypertension becomes more severe and chronic, tissue damage can occur in the blood vessels and tissues leading to target organ damage in the heart, kidney, brain, and eyes.[28] Cardiovascular complications of sustained hypertension include left ventricular hypertrophy, angina pectoris, heart failure, coronary artery disease, myocardial infarction, and sudden death. Myocardial hypertrophy in response to hypertension is mediated by several neurohormonal substances, including catecholamines from the SNS and angiotensin II. Hypertrophy is characterized by changes in the myocyte proteins, apoptosis of myocytes, and deposition of collagen in heart muscle, which causes it to become thickened, scarred, and less able to relax during diastole, leading to diastolic heart failure.[29,30] In addition, the increased size of the heart muscle increases demand for oxygen delivery over time, the contractility of the heart is impaired, and the individual is at increased risk for systolic heart failure. Vascular complications include the formation, dissection, and rupture of aneurysms (outpouchings in vessel walls) and atherosclerosis leading to vessel occlusion.

Renal complications of complicated hypertension include parenchymal damage, nephrosclerosis, renal arteriosclerosis, and renal insufficiency or failure. Microalbuminuria (small amounts of protein in the urine) occurs in 10% to 25% of individuals with primary hypertension and is now recognized as an early sign of impending renal dysfunction and significantly increased risk for cardiovascular events, especially in those who also have diabetes.[31] Complications specific to the retina include retinal vascular sclerosis, exudation, and hemorrhage. Cerebrovascular complications include transient ischemia, stroke, cerebral thrombosis, aneurysm, hemorrhage, and dementia.[32,33] The pathologic effects of complicated hypertension are summarized in Table 23-2.

Malignant hypertension is rapidly progressive hypertension in which diastolic pressure is usually greater than 140 mm Hg. High arterial pressure renders the cerebral arterioles incapable of regulating blood flow to the cerebral capillary beds. High hydrostatic pressures in the capillaries cause vascular fluid to exude into the interstitial space.

If blood pressure is not reduced, cerebral edema and cerebral dysfunction (encephalopathy) increase until death occurs. Organ damage resulting from malignant hypertension is life-threatening. Besides encephalopathy, malignant hypertension can cause papilledema, cardiac failure, uremia, retinopathy, and cerebrovascular accident.

CLINICAL MANIFESTATIONS The early stages of hypertension have no clinical manifestations other than elevated blood pressure; for this reason, hypertension is called a silent disease. Some hypertensive individuals never have signs, symptoms, or complications, whereas others become very ill, and hypertension can be a cause of death. Still other individuals have anatomic and physiologic damage caused by past hypertensive disease, despite current blood pressure measurements being within normal ranges. If elevated blood pressure is not detected and treated, it becomes established and may begin to accelerate its effects on tissues when the individual is 30 to 50 years of age. This sets the stage for the complications of hypertension that begin to appear during the fourth, fifth, and sixth decades of life.

Most clinical manifestations of hypertensive disease are caused by complications that damage organs and tissues outside the vascular system. Besides elevated blood pressure, the signs and symptoms therefore tend to be specific for the organs or tissues affected. Evidence of heart disease, renal insufficiency, central nervous system dysfunction, impaired vision, impaired mobility, vascular occlusion, or edema can all be caused by sustained hypertension.

EVALUATION AND TREATMENT A single elevated blood pressure reading does not mean that a person has hypertension. Diagnosis requires the measurement of blood pressure on at least two separate occasions, averaging two readings at least 2 minutes apart, with the following conditions: the person is seated, the arm is supported at heart level, the person must be at rest for at least 5 minutes, and the person should not have smoked or ingested any caffeine in the previous 30 minutes.[9] Diagnostic tests for further evaluation of hypertension include 24-hour blood pressure monitoring in selected individuals, complete blood count, urinalysis, biochemical blood profile (measures levels of plasma glucose, sodium, potassium, calcium, magnesium, creatinine, cholesterol, and triglycerides), and an electrocardiogram (ECG). Individuals who have elevated blood pressure are assumed to have primary hypertension unless their history, physical examination, or initial diagnostic screening indicates secondary hypertension. Once the diagnosis is made, a careful evaluation for other cardiovascular risk factors and for end-organ damage should be done.

TABLE 23-2	**PATHOLOGIC EFFECTS OF SUSTAINED, COMPLICATED PRIMARY HYPERTENSION**	
SITE OF INJURY	**MECHANISM OF INJURY**	**POTENTIAL PATHOLOGIC EFFECT**
Heart		
Myocardium	Increased workload combined with diminished blood flow through coronary arteries	Left ventricular hypertrophy, myocardial ischemia, heart failure
Coronary arteries	Accelerated atherosclerosis (coronary artery disease)	Myocardial ischemia, myocardial infarction, sudden death
Kidneys	Reduced blood flow, increased arteriolar pressure, RAAS and SNS stimulation, and inflammation	Glomerulosclerosis and decreased glomerular filtration, end-stage renal disease
Brain	Reduced blood flow and oxygen supply; weakened vessel walls, accelerated atherosclerosis	Transient ischemic attacks, cerebral thrombosis, aneurysm, hemorrhage, acute brain infarction
Eyes (retinas)	Retinal vascular sclerosis, increased retinal artery pressures	Hypertensive retinopathy, retinal exudates and hemorrhages
Aorta	Weakened vessel wall	Dissecting aneurysm (see p. 592)
Arteries of lower extremities	Reduced blood flow and high pressures in arterioles, accelerated atherosclerosis	Intermittent claudication, gangrene

Treatment of primary hypertension depends on its severity. Lifestyle modification is important for preventing hypertension (especially in those individuals with prehypertension) and for treating hypertension. Important lifestyle modifications include following an exercise program, making dietary modifications, stopping smoking, and losing weight. Pharmacologic treatment of hypertension reduces the risk of end-organ damage and prevents major diseases, such as myocardial infarction and stroke. Diuretics have been shown to be the safest and most effective medications for lowering blood pressure and preventing the cardiovascular complications of hypertension.[34] Some individuals will have "compelling indications" for choosing a particular antihypertensive as a first-line medication. For example, individuals with heart failure, chronic kidney disease, or who have a history of myocardial infarction or stroke should begin antihypertensive treatment with an ACE inhibitor, ARB, or aldosterone antagonist.[9] Some individuals require two drugs for blood pressure control, including combinations of diuretics and other antihypertensives, such as beta-blockers, calcium channel blockers, and ACE inhibitors.[35] Careful follow-up to support continued adherence, determine the response, and monitor for potential side effects of these medications is important.[36]

Orthostatic (Postural) Hypotension

The term orthostatic (postural) hypotension refers to a decrease in systolic blood pressure of at least 20 mm Hg or a decrease in diastolic blood pressure of at least 10 mm Hg within 3 minutes of moving to a standing position. The term *idiopathic*, or *primary*, orthostatic hypotension implies no known initial cause. Some define the disorder as a separate entity, whereas others suggest it is a part of a generalized degenerative central nervous system disease. It affects men more often than women and usually occurs between the ages of 40 and 70 years. Up to 18% of older adults may be affected by primary orthostatic hypotension, and it is a significant risk factor for falls and associated injury.[37]

Normally when an individual stands, the gravitational changes on the circulation are compensated by such mechanisms as reflex arteriolar and venous constriction and increased heart rate. Other compensatory mechanisms include mechanical factors, such as the closure of valves in the venous system, contraction of the leg muscles, and a decrease in intrathoracic pressure. The normally increased sympathetic activity during upright posture is mediated through a stretch receptor (baroreceptor) reflex that responds to shifts in volume caused by postural changes. This reflex promptly increases heart rate and constricts the systemic arterioles. Thus, arterial blood pressure is maintained. These mechanisms are dysfunctional or inadequate in individuals with orthostatic hypotension; consequently, upon standing, blood pools and normal arterial pressure cannot be maintained.

Orthostatic hypotension may be acute or chronic. Acute orthostatic hypotension is caused when the normal regulatory mechanisms are sluggish as a result of (1) altered body chemistry, (2) drug action (e.g., antihypertensives, antidepressants), (3) prolonged immobility caused by illness, (4) starvation, (5) physical exhaustion, (6) any condition that produces volume depletion (e.g., dehydration, diuresis, potassium or sodium depletion), or (7) any condition that results in venous pooling (e.g., pregnancy, extensive varicosities of the lower extremities). Elderly persons are particularly susceptible to this type of orthostatic hypotension.

Chronic orthostatic hypotension may be (1) secondary to a specific disease or (2) idiopathic or primary. The diseases that cause secondary orthostatic hypotension are endocrine disorders (e.g., adrenal insufficiency), metabolic disorders (e.g., porphyria), or diseases of the central or peripheral nervous systems (e.g., intracranial tumors, cerebral infarcts, Wernicke encephalopathy, peripheral neuropathies). Cardiovascular autonomic neuropathy is a common cause of orthostatic hypotension in persons with diabetes and is a serious and often overlooked complication. In addition to cardiovascular symptoms, associated impotence and bowel and bladder dysfunction are common.

Orthostatic hypotension is often accompanied by dizziness, blurring or loss of vision, and syncope or fainting caused by insufficient vasomotor compensation and reduction of blood flow through the brain. Although no curative treatment is available for idiopathic orthostatic hypotension, often it can be managed adequately with a combination of nondrug and drug therapies—increasing fluid and salt intake, wearing thigh-high stockings, and taking mineralocorticoids and vasoconstrictors.[37] Both acute and secondary forms of hypotension resolve when the underlying disorder is corrected.

> ✓ **QUICK CHECK 23-2**
> 1. What are the major risk factors for hypertension?
> 2. Summarize the pathophysiology of primary hypertension.
> 3. What is malignant hypertension?
> 4. What are the causes of orthostatic hypotension?

Aneurysm

An aneurysm is a localized dilation or outpouching of a vessel wall or cardiac chamber (Figure 23-5). The law of Laplace (discussed in detail in Chapter 22) can provide an understanding of the hemodynamics of an aneurysm. True aneurysms involve all three layers of the arterial wall and are best described as a weakening of the vessel wall (Figure 23-6, *A*). Most are fusiform and circumferential, whereas

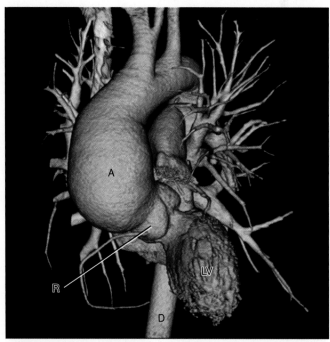

FIGURE 23-5 Aneurysm. A three dimensional CT scan shows the aneurysm *(A)* involves the ascending thoracic aorta. *D,* descending aorta; *LV,* left ventricle.

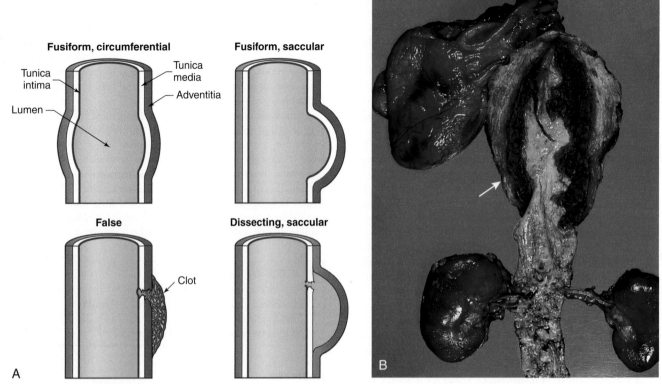

FIGURE 23-6 Longitudinal Sections Showing Types of Aneurysms. **A,** The fusiform circumferential and fusiform saccular aneurysms are true aneurysms, caused by weakening of the vessel wall. False and saccular aneurysms involve a break in the vessel wall, usually caused by trauma. **B,** Dissecting aneurysm of thoracic aorta *(arrow).* (**B** from Damjanov I, Linder J, editors: *Anderson's pathology,* ed 10, St Louis, 1996, Mosby.)

saccular aneurysms are basically spherical in shape. **False aneurysm** is an extravascular hematoma that communicates with the intravascular space. A common cause of this type of lesion is a leak between a vascular graft and a natural artery.

The aorta is particularly susceptible to aneurysm formation because of constant stress on the vessel wall and the absence of penetrating vasa vasorum in the media layer. Three fourths of all aneurysms occur in the abdominal aorta. Atherosclerosis is the most common cause of arterial aneurysms because plaque formation erodes the vessel wall and contributes to inflammation and release of proteinases that can further weaken the vessel. Hypertension also contributes to aneurysm formation by increasing wall stress. Collagen-vascular disorders (e.g., Marfan syndrome), syphilis, and other infections that affect arterial walls also can cause aneurysms.

Cardiac aneurysms most commonly form after myocardial infarction when intraventricular tension stretches the noncontracting infarcted muscle. The stretching produces infarct expansion, a weak and thin layer of necrotic muscle, and fibrous tissue that bulges with each systole.

Clinical manifestations depend upon where the aneurysm is located. Aortic aneurysms often are asymptomatic until they rupture, and then cause severe pain and hypotension. Thoracic aortic aneurysms can cause dysphagia (difficulty swallowing) and dyspnea (breathlessness). An aneurysm that impairs flow to an extremity causes symptoms of ischemia. Cerebral aneurysms, which often occur in the circle of Willis, are associated with signs and symptoms of increased intracranial pressure. Signs and symptoms of stroke occur when cerebral aneurysms

leak. (Cerebral aneurysms are described in Chapter 15.) Aneurysms in the heart present with dysrhythmias, heart failure, and embolism of clots to the brain or other vital organs.

Aortic aneurysms can be complicated by the acute aortic syndromes, which include aortic dissection, hemorrhage into the vessel wall, or vessel rupture. Dissection of the layers of the arterial wall occurs when there is a tear in the intima and blood enters the wall of the artery (see Figure 23-6, *B*). Dissections can involve any part of the aorta (ascending, arch, or descending) and can disrupt flow through arterial branches, thus creating a surgical emergency.

The diagnosis of an aneurysm is usually confirmed by ultrasonography, computed tomography, magnetic resonance imaging, or angiography. Medical treatment is indicated for slow-growing aortic aneurysms, particularly in early stages, and includes cessation of smoking, reduction of blood pressure and blood volume, and implementation of beta-adrenergic blockade. For those aneurysms that are dilating rapidly or have become large, surgical treatment is indicated and usually includes replacement with a prosthetic graft. New endovascular surgical techniques make aneurysm repair possible for more individuals.[38]

Thrombus Formation

As in venous thrombosis, arterial thrombi tend to develop when intravascular conditions promote activation of coagulation, or when there is stasis of blood flow. These conditions include those in which there is intimal irritation or roughening (such as in surgical procedures), inflammation, traumatic injury, infection, low blood pressures, or obstructions that cause blood stasis and pooling within the vessels. (Mechanisms of coagulation are described in Chapter 19.) Inflammation of the endothelium leads to activation of the clotting cascade, causing platelets to adhere readily. An anatomic change in an artery (such as an aneurysm) can contribute to thrombus formation, particularly if the change results in a pooling of arterial blood. Thrombi also form on heart valves altered by calcification or bacterial vegetation. Valvular thrombi are most commonly associated with inflammation of the endocardium (endocarditis) and rheumatic heart disease. Widespread arterial thrombus formation can occur in shock, particularly shock resulting from septicemia. In septic shock, systemic inflammation activates the intrinsic and extrinsic pathways of coagulation, resulting in microvascular thrombosis throughout the systemic arterial circulation.

Arterial thrombi pose two potential threats to the circulation. First, the thrombus may grow large enough to occlude the artery, causing ischemia in tissue supplied by the artery. Second, the thrombus may dislodge, becoming a thromboembolus that travels through the vascular system until it occludes flow into a distal systemic vascular bed.

Diagnosis of arterial thrombi is usually accomplished through the use of Doppler ultrasonography and angiography. Pharmacologic treatment involves the administration of heparin, warfarin derivatives, thrombin inhibitors, or thrombolytics. A balloon-tipped catheter also can be used to remove or compress an arterial thrombus. Various combinations of drug and catheter therapies are sometimes used concurrently.

Embolism

Embolism is the obstruction of a vessel by an **embolus**—a bolus of matter circulating in the bloodstream. The embolus may consist of a dislodged thrombus; an air bubble; an aggregate of amniotic fluid; an aggregate of fat, bacteria, or cancer cells; or a foreign substance. An embolus travels in the bloodstream until it reaches a vessel through which it cannot fit. No matter how tiny it is, an embolus will eventually lodge in a systemic or pulmonary vessel determined by its source. Pulmonary emboli originate on the venous side (mostly from the deep veins of the legs) of the systemic circulation or in the right heart; arterial emboli most commonly originate in the left heart and are associated with thrombi after myocardial infarction, valvular disease, left heart failure, endocarditis, and dysrhythmias.

Embolism causes ischemia or infarction in tissues distal to the obstruction, causing organ dysfunction and pain. Infarction and subsequent necrosis of a central organ are life-threatening. For example, occlusion of a coronary artery will cause a myocardial infarction, whereas occlusion of a cerebral artery causes a stroke (see Chapter 15). The types of emboli are summarized in Table 23-3.

QUICK CHECK 23-3
1. How does the law of Laplace function in aneurysms?
2. What is a thrombus?
3. Why are emboli dangerous?

Peripheral Vascular Disease
Thromboangiitis Obliterans (Buerger disease)

Thromboangiitis obliterans (Buerger disease) is an inflammatory disease of the peripheral arteries. It is strongly associated with smoking, and there is some evidence for a link with severe periodontal disease.[39] Thromboangiitis obliterans is characterized by the formation of thrombi filled with inflammatory and immune cells and accompanying

TABLE 23-3	**TYPES OF EMBOLI**
TYPE	**CHARACTERISTICS**
Arteries	
Arterial thromboembolism	Dislodged thrombus; source is usually from heart; most common sites of obstruction are lower extremities (femoral and popliteal arteries), coronary arteries, and cerebral vasculature
Veins	
Venous thromboembolism	Dislodged thrombus; source is usually from lower extremities; obstructs branches of pulmonary artery
Air embolism	Bolus of air displaces blood in vasculature; source usually room air entering circulation through IV lines; trauma to chest also may allow air from lungs to enter vascular space
Amniotic fluid embolism	Bolus of amniotic fluid; extensive intra-abdominal pressure attending labor and delivery can force amniotic fluid into bloodstream of mother; introduces antigens, cells, and protein aggregates that trigger inflammation, coagulation, and immune responses
Bacterial embolism	Aggregates of bacteria in bloodstream; source is subacute bacterial endocarditis or abscess
Fat embolism	Globules of fat floating in bloodstream associated with trauma to long bones; lungs in particular are affected
Foreign matter	Small particles or fibers introduced during trauma or through an IV or intra-arterial line; coagulation cascade is initiated and thromboemboli form around particles

vasospasm. Over time, these thrombi become organized and fibrotic and result in permanent occlusion and obliteration of portions of small- and medium-sized arteries in the feet and sometimes in the hands.[39] Although collateral vessels develop in Buerger disease, they are inadequate to supply the extremities with blood. These collateral vessels have a characteristic corkscrew shape, believed to be a result of dilated vasa vasorum in the affected artery.

The chief symptom of thromboangiitis obliterans is pain and tenderness of the affected part, usually affecting more than one extremity. Clinical manifestations are caused by sluggish blood flow and include rubor (redness of the skin), which is caused by dilated capillaries under the skin, and cyanosis, which is caused by tissue ischemia. Chronic ischemia causes the skin to thin and become shiny and the nails to become thickened and malformed. In advanced disease, profound ischemia of the extremities resulting from vessel obliteration can cause gangrene necessitating amputation. Buerger disease has also been associated with cerebrovascular disease (stroke), mesenteric disease, and rheumatic symptoms (joint pain).

Diagnosis of thromboangiitis obliterans is made by identification of the following common features—age <45 years, smoking history, evidence of peripheral ischemia—and by exclusion of other causes of arterial insufficiency. The most important part of treatment is cessation of cigarette smoking. If the person continues to smoke, the likelihood of recurrence of the disease and gangrene requiring amputation is high. Other measures are aimed at improving circulation to the foot or hand. Vasodilators are prescribed to alleviate vasospasm, and the individual receives instruction in exercises that use gravity to improve

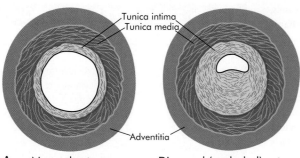

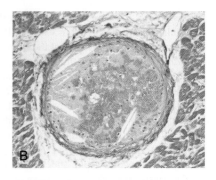

FIGURE 23-7 Arteriosclerosis. **A,** Cross section of a normal artery and an artery altered by disease. **B,** A small artery in the myocardium is occluded by a mass of blue-staining platelets, yellow-staining red cells, and cholesterol bodies. (**B** from Damjanov I, Linder J, editors: *Anderson's pathology,* ed 10, St Louis, 1996, Mosby.)

blood flow.[39] Recently, stem cell therapy to induce angiogenesis has shown promising results to treat severe ischemia.[40]

Raynaud Phenomenon and Disease

Both Raynaud phenomenon and Raynaud disease are characterized by attacks of vasospasm in the small arteries and arterioles of the fingers and, less commonly, the toes. Although the clinical manifestations of the phenomenon and the disease are the same, their causes differ.

Raynaud phenomenon is secondary to systemic diseases, particularly collagen vascular disease (scleroderma), vasculitis, malignancy, pulmonary hypertension, chemotherapy, cocaine use, hypothyroidism, thoracic outlet syndrome, trauma, serum sickness, or long-term exposure to environmental conditions, such as cold or vibrating machinery in the workplace.[41] Raynaud disease is a common primary vasospastic disorder of unknown origin. Blood vessels in affected individuals demonstrate endothelial dysfunction with an imbalance in endothelium-derived vasodilators (e.g., nitric oxide) and vasoconstrictors (e.g., endothelin-1). Platelet activation also may play a role. It tends to affect young women and to consist of vasospastic attacks triggered by brief exposure to cold or by emotional stress. Genetic predisposition may play a role in its development.

The clinical manifestations of the vasospastic attacks of either disorder are changes in skin color and sensation caused by ischemia. Vasospasm occurs with varying frequency and severity and causes pallor, numbness, and the sensation of coldness in the digits. Attacks tend to be bilateral, and manifestations usually begin at the tips of the digits and progress to the proximal phalanges. Sluggish blood flow resulting from ischemia may cause the skin to appear cyanotic. Rubor, throbbing pain, and paresthesias follow as blood flow returns. Skin color returns to normal after the attack, but frequent, prolonged attacks interfere with cellular metabolism, causing the skin of the fingertips to thicken and the nails to become brittle. In severe, chronic Raynaud phenomenon or disease, ischemia can eventually cause ulceration and gangrene.

Treatment for Raynaud phenomenon consists of removing the stimulus or treating the primary disease process. Treatment of Raynaud disease begins with avoidance of stimuli that trigger attacks (e.g., cold, emotional stress) and cessation of cigarette smoking to eliminate the vasoconstricting effects of nicotine. If attacks of vasospasm become frequent or prolonged, vasodilators, such as calcium channel blockers, nitric oxide agonists, alpha-blockers, prostaglandin analogs, or endothelin antagonists, are administered.[42] Sympathectomy may be indicated in severe cases, but may not be effective. If ischemia leads to ulceration and gangrene, amputation may be necessary.

> ✔ **QUICK CHECK 23-4**
> 1. What is Buerger disease and why does it occur?
> 2. Compare the physical manifestations of Buerger disease and Raynaud disease.

Atherosclerosis

Atherosclerosis is a form of arteriosclerosis characterized by thickening and hardening of the vessel wall. It is caused by the accumulation of lipid-laden macrophages within the arterial wall, which leads to the formation of a lesion called a plaque. Atherosclerosis is not a single disease entity but rather a pathologic process that can affect vascular systems throughout the body, resulting in ischemic syndromes that can vary widely in their severity and clinical manifestations. It is the leading cause of coronary artery and cerebrovascular disease. (Atherosclerosis of the coronary arteries is described later in this chapter, and atherosclerosis of the cerebral arteries is described in Chapter 15.)

PATHOPHYSIOLOGY   Atherosclerosis begins with injury to the endothelial cells that line artery walls. Pathologically, the lesions progress from endothelial injury and dysfunction to fatty streak to fibrotic plaque to complicated lesion (Figures 23-7 and 23-8). Possible causes of endothelial injury include the common risk factors for atherosclerosis, such as smoking, hypertension, diabetes, increased levels of low-density lipoprotein (LDL), decreased levels of high-density lipoprotein (HDL), and autoimmunity. Other "nontraditional" risk factors include elevated levels of highly-sensitive C-reactive protein (hs-CRP), increased serum fibrinogen level, insulin resistance, oxidative stress, infection, and periodontal disease. These risk factors are discussed in more detail in the following section on coronary artery disease (see p. 598).

Injured endothelial cells become inflamed. Inflammation plays a fundamental role in mediating the steps in the initiation and progression of atherogenesis.[43,44] Inflamed endothelial cells cannot make normal amounts of antithrombic and vasodilating cytokines (see Figures 22-24 and 22-25). Recent evidence indicates that individuals with a defect in the production of precursor endothelial cells in the bone marrow are at greater risk for atherosclerotic disease because these precursor cells are not available to repair injured endothelium.[45]

The next step in atherogenesis occurs when inflamed endothelial cells express adhesion molecules that bind macrophages and other inflammatory and immune cells. Macrophages adhere to the injured endothelium and release numerous inflammatory cytokines (e.g.,

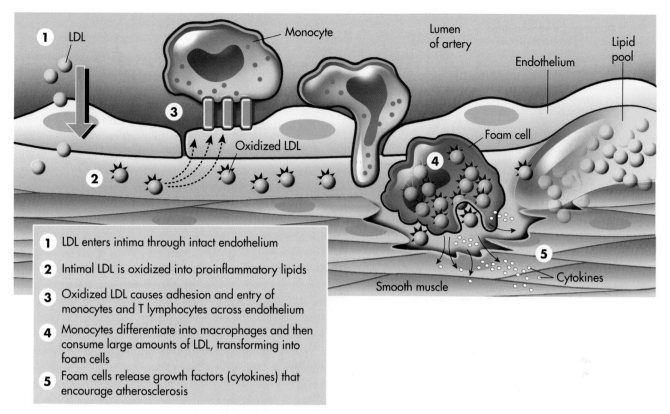

1 LDL enters intima through intact endothelium

2 Intimal LDL is oxidized into proinflammatory lipids

3 Oxidized LDL causes adhesion and entry of monocytes and T lymphocytes across endothelium

4 Monocytes differentiate into macrophages and then consume large amounts of LDL, transforming into foam cells

5 Foam cells release growth factors (cytokines) that encourage atherosclerosis

FIGURE 23-8 Low-Density Lipoprotein Oxidation. Low-density lipoprotein (LDL) enters the arterial intima through an intact endothelium. In hypercholesterolemia, the influx of LDL exceeds the eliminating capacity and an extracellular pool of LDL is formed. This is enhanced by association of LDL with the extracellular matrix. Intimal LDL is oxidized through the action of free oxygen radicals formed by enzymatic or nonenzymatic reactions. This generates proinflammatory lipids that induce endothelial expression of the adhesion molecule (i.e., vascular cell adhesion molecule-1), activate complement, and stimulate chemokine secretion. All of these factors cause adhesion and entry of mononuclear leukocytes, particularly monocytes and T lymphocytes. Monocytes differentiate into macrophages. Macrophages up-regulate and internalize oxidized LDL and transform into foam cells. Macrophage uptake of oxidized LDL also leads to presentation of its fragments to antigen-specific T cells. This induces an autoimmune reaction that leads to production of proinflammatory cytokines. Such cytokines include interferon-γ, tumor necrosis factor-alpha, and interleukin-1, which act on endothelial cells to stimulate expression of adhesion molecules and procoagulant activity; on macrophages to activate proteases, endocytosis, nitric oxide (NO), and cytokines; and on smooth muscle cells (SMCs) to induce NO production and inhibit growth and collagen and actin expression. *LDL,* Low-density lipoprotein. (Modified from Crawford MH, DiMarco JP, editors: *Cardiology,* London, 2001, Mosby.)

tumor necrosis factor-alpha [TNF-α], interferons, interleukins, and C-reactive protein) and enzymes that further injure the vessel wall.[46] Toxic oxygen radicals generated by the inflammatory process cause oxidation (i.e., addition of oxygen) of LDL that has accumulated in the vessel intima. Hyperlipidemia, diabetes, smoking, and hypertension contribute to LDL oxidation and its accumulation in the vessel wall.[47] Oxidized LDL causes additional adhesion molecule expression with the recruitment of monocytes that differentiate into macrophages. These macrophages penetrate into the intima where they engulf oxidized LDL. These lipid-laden macrophages are now called foam cells, and when they accumulate in significant amounts, they form a lesion called a fatty streak (see Figures 23-8 and 23-9).[48] These lesions can be found in the walls of arteries of most people, even young children. Once formed, fatty streaks produce more toxic oxygen radicals, recruit T cells leading to autoimmunity, and secrete additional inflammatory mediators resulting in progressive damage to the vessel wall.[49] Treatment that lowers LDL levels may reverse this process.

Macrophages also release growth factors that stimulate smooth muscle cell proliferation.[50] Smooth muscle cells in the region of endothelial injury proliferate, produce collagen, and migrate over the fatty streak, forming a fibrous plaque (Figure 23-10). The fibrous plaque may calcify, protrude into the vessel lumen, and obstruct blood flow to distal tissues (especially during exercise), which may cause symptoms (e.g., angina or intermittent claudication).

Many plaques, however, are "unstable," meaning they are prone to rupture even before they affect blood flow significantly and are clinically silent until they rupture.[51] Plaque rupture occurs because of the inflammatory activation of proteinases, such as the matrix metalloproteinases and the cathepsins, and can be accelerated by bleeding within the lesion (plaque hemorrhage).[52] Plaques that have ruptured are called complicated plaques (see Figure 23-9). Once rupture occurs, exposure of underlying tissue results in platelet adhesion, initiation of the clotting cascade, and rapid thrombus formation. The thrombus may suddenly occlude the affected vessel, resulting in ischemia and

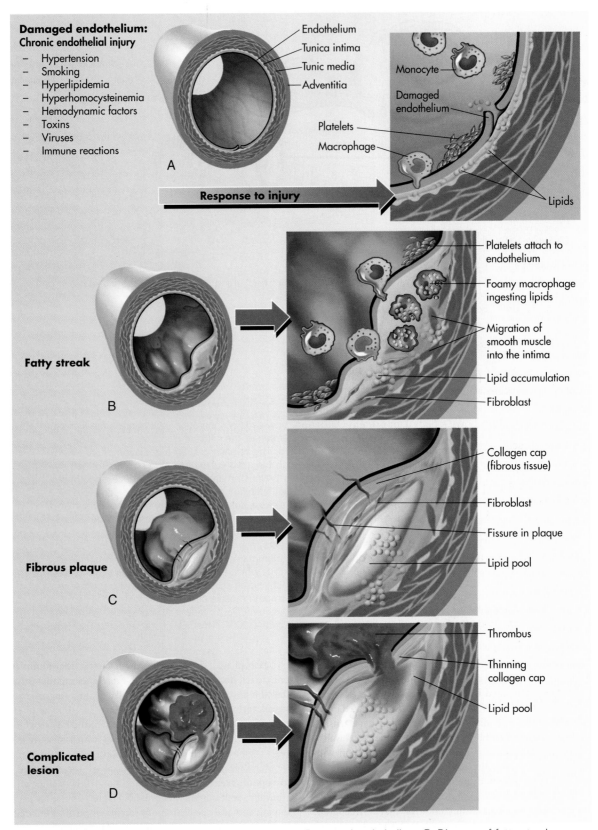

Damaged endothelium:
Chronic endothelial injury

- Hypertension
- Smoking
- Hyperlipidemia
- Hyperhomocysteinemia
- Hemodynamic factors
- Toxins
- Viruses
- Immune reactions

Endothelium
Tunica intima
Tunic media
Adventitia

Monocyte
Damaged endothelium
Platelets
Macrophage
Lipids

A

Response to injury

Fatty streak

B

Platelets attach to endothelium
Foamy macrophage ingesting lipids
Migration of smooth muscle into the intima
Lipid accumulation
Fibroblast

Fibrous plaque

C

Collagen cap (fibrous tissue)
Fibroblast
Fissure in plaque
Lipid pool

Complicated lesion

D

Thrombus
Thinning collagen cap
Lipid pool

FIGURE 23-9 Progression of Atherosclerosis. **A,** Damaged endothelium. **B,** Diagram of fatty streak and lipid core formation (see Figure 23-8 for a diagram of oxidized low-density lipoprotein [LDL]). **C,** Diagram of fibrous plaque. Raised plaques are visible: some are yellow; others are white. **D,** Diagram of complicated lesion; thrombus is red; collagen is blue. Plaque is complicated by red thrombus deposition.

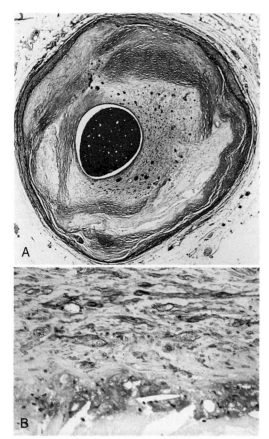

FIGURE 23-10 Atherosclerosis. **A,** Concentric coronary plaque. The lumen is central. There are multiple, new small blood vessels within the plaque, the late result of disruption. **B,** Cell types in fibro-lipid plaque. The plaque cap (brownish color) contains numerous elongated, smooth muscle cells; some contain lipid. Macrophages are clustered on the edge of the core. (From Damjanov I, Linder J, editors: *Anderson's pathology,* ed 10, St Louis, 1996, Mosby.)

infarction. Aspirin or other antithrombotic agents are used to prevent this complication of atherosclerotic disease.

CLINICAL MANIFESTATIONS Atherosclerosis presents with symptoms and signs that result from inadequate perfusion of tissues because of obstruction of the vessels that supply them. Partial vessel obstruction may lead to transient ischemic events, often associated with exercise or stress. As the lesion becomes complicated, increasing obstruction with superimposed thrombosis may result in tissue infarction. Obstruction of peripheral arteries can cause significant pain and disability. Coronary artery disease (CAD) caused by atherosclerosis is the major cause of myocardial ischemia and is one of the most important health issues in the United States. Atherosclerotic obstruction of the vessels supplying the brain is the major cause of stroke. Similarly, any part of the body may become ischemic when its blood supply is compromised by atherosclerotic lesions. Often, more than one vessel will become involved with this disease process such that an individual may present with symptoms from several ischemic tissues at the same time, and disease in one area may indicate that the individual is at risk for ischemic complications elsewhere.

EVALUATION AND TREATMENT In evaluating individuals for the presence of atherosclerosis, a complete health history (including risk factors and symptoms of ischemia) is essential. Physical examination

may reveal arterial bruits and evidence of decreased blood flow to tissues. Laboratory data that include measurement of levels of lipids, blood glucose, and hs-CRP are also indicated. Judicious use of x-ray films, electrocardiography, ultrasonography, nuclear scanning, CT, MRI, and angiography may be necessary to identify affected vessels, particularly coronary vessels.[53] New modalities aimed at identifying vulnerable plaques before the rupture are being evaluated.[51,54]

Current management of atherosclerosis is focused on detection and treatment of preclinical lesions with drugs aimed at stabilizing and reversing plaques before they rupture.[55] Once a lesion obstructs blood flow, the primary goal in the management of atherosclerosis is to restore adequate blood flow to the affected tissues. If an individual has presented with acute ischemia (e.g., myocardial infarction, stroke), interventions are specific to the diseased area and are discussed further under those topics. In situations where the disease process does not require immediate intervention, management focuses on reduction of risk factors and prevention of plaque progression. This includes implementation of an exercise program, cessation of smoking, and control of hypertension and diabetes where appropriate while reducing LDL cholesterol level by diet or medications, or both. Management of atherosclerotic risk factors is discussed further starting on p. 601.

Peripheral Artery Disease

Peripheral artery disease (PAD) refers to atherosclerotic disease of arteries that perfuse the limbs, especially the lower extremities. PAD affects up to 20% of Americans ages 65 or older.[8] The risk factors for PAD are the same as those previously described for atherosclerosis, and it is especially prevalent in individuals with diabetes.

Lower extremity ischemia resulting from arterial obstruction in PAD can be gradual or acute. In most individuals, gradually increasing obstruction to arterial blood flow to the legs caused by atherosclerosis in the iliofemoral vessels results in pain with ambulation called intermittent claudication. If a thrombus forms over the atherosclerotic lesion, complete obstruction of blood flow can occur acutely, causing severe pain, loss of pulses, and skin color changes in the affected extremity.

PAD is often asymptomatic in its early stages; therefore evaluation for PAD requires a careful history and physical examination that focuses on finding evidence of atherosclerotic disease (e.g., bruits), determining the ankle-brachial index, and measuring blood flow using noninvasive Doppler. Treatment includes risk factor reduction (smoking cessation and treatment of diabetes, hypertension, and dyslipidemia) and antiplatelet therapy. Symptomatic PAD should be managed with vasodilators in combination with antiplatelet or antithrombotic medications (aspirin, cilostazol, ticlopidine, or clopidogrel), cholesterol-lowering medications, and exercise rehabilitation.[56] If acute or refractory symptoms occur, emergent percutaneous or surgical revascularization may be indicated. Newer treatment modalities that are being explored include autologous stem cell therapies and angiogenesis.[57,58]

Coronary Artery Disease, Myocardial Ischemia, and Acute Coronary Syndromes

Coronary artery disease, myocardial ischemia, and myocardial infarction form a pathophysiologic continuum that impairs the pumping ability of the heart by depriving the heart muscle of blood-borne oxygen and nutrients. The earliest lesions of the continuum are those of coronary artery disease (CAD), which is usually caused by atherosclerosis (see Figure 23-10). CAD can diminish the myocardial blood supply until deprivation impairs myocardial metabolism enough to cause ischemia, a local state in which the cells are temporarily deprived of blood supply. They remain alive but cannot function normally. Persistent ischemia or the complete occlusion of a coronary artery causes the acute coronary syndromes including infarction, or irreversible myocardial damage. Infarction constitutes the often-fatal event known as a *heart attack*.

Development of Coronary Artery Disease

Coronary heart disease causes approximately one of every six deaths in the United States. In 2010 an estimated 785,000 Americans will have a new coronary attack. An American will have a coronary event every 25 seconds, and approximately every minute someone will die of one.[8] Risk factors for CAD are the same as those for atherosclerosis and can be categorized as conventional (major) versus nontraditional (novel) and as modifiable versus nonmodifiable. The plethora of new information obtained about the conventional risk factors has markedly improved prevention and management of CAD. In addition, nontraditional risk factors have been identified that have provided insight into the pathogenesis of CAD and may lead to future more effective interventions.

Conventional or major risk factors for CAD that are nonmodifiable include: (1) advanced age, (2) male gender or women after menopause, and (3) family history. Aging and menopause are associated with increased exposure to risk factors and poor endothelial healing. Family history may contribute to CAD through genetics and shared environmental exposures. Many gene polymorphisms have been associated with CAD and its risk factors.[59] Modifiable major risks include (1) dyslipidemia, (2) hypertension, (3) cigarette smoking, (4) diabetes and insulin resistance, (5) obesity, (6) sedentary lifestyle, and (7) atherogenic diet (see *Health Alert*: The Basics on Fats). Fortunately, modification of these factors can dramatically reduce the risk for CAD.

Dyslipidemia. The link between CAD and abnormal levels of lipoproteins is well documented.[60] The term lipoprotein refers to lipids, phospholipids, cholesterol, and triglycerides bound to carrier proteins. Lipids (cholesterol in particular) are required by most cells for the manufacture and repair of plasma membranes. Cholesterol is also a necessary component for the manufacture of such essential substances as bile acids and steroid hormones. Although cholesterol can easily be obtained from dietary fat intake, most body cells also can manufacture cholesterol.

The cycle of lipid metabolism is complex. Dietary fat is packaged into particles known as chylomicrons in the small intestine. Chylomicrons are required for absorption of fat; they function by transporting exogenous lipid from the intestine to the liver and peripheral cells. Chylomicrons are the least dense of the lipoproteins and primarily contain triglyceride. Some of the triglyceride may be removed and either stored by adipose tissue or used by muscle as an energy source. The chylomicron remnants, composed mainly of cholesterol, are taken up by the liver. A series of chemical reactions in the liver results in the production of several lipoproteins that vary in density and function. These include very-low-density lipoproteins (VLDLs), primarily triglyceride and protein; low-density lipoproteins (LDLs), mostly

cholesterol and protein; and high-density lipoproteins (HDLs), mainly phospholipids and protein.

Dyslipidemia (or dyslipoproteinemia) refers to abnormal concentrations of serum lipoproteins as defined by the Third Report of the National Cholesterol Education Program[60] (Table 23-4). An estimated

TABLE 23-4	CRITERIA FOR DYSLIPIDEMIA						
	OPTIMAL	NEAR OPTIMAL	DESIRABLE	LOW	BORDERLINE	HIGH	VERY HIGH
Total cholesterol			<200		200-239	≥240	
LDL	<100	100-129			130-159	160-189	≥190
Triglycerides			<150		150-199	200-499	≥500
HDL				<40		≥60	

Data from Expert Panel on Detection, Evaluation, and Treatment of High Blood Cholesterol in Adults, *JAMA* 285:2486–2497, 2001.

16% of adults ages 20 years or older have total serum cholesterol levels greater than 240 mg/dl.[8] These abnormalities are the result of a combination of genetic and dietary factors. Primary or familial dyslipoproteinemias result from genetic defects that cause abnormalities in lipid-metabolizing enzymes and abnormal cellular lipid receptors. Secondary causes of dyslipidemia include the existence of several common systemic disorders, such as diabetes, hypothyroidism, pancreatitis, and renal nephrosis, as well as the use of certain medications, such as some diuretics, glucocorticoids, interferons, and antiretrovirals.

An increased serum concentration of LDL is a strong indicator of coronary risk.[60] Serum levels of LDL are normally controlled by hepatic receptors that bind LDL and limit liver synthesis of this lipoprotein. High dietary intake of cholesterol and fats, often in combination with a genetic predisposition to accumulations of LDL in the serum (e.g., dysfunction of the hepatic LDL receptor), results in high levels of LDL in the bloodstream. The term LDL actually describes several types of LDL molecules of which the "small dense" LDL particles are the most atherogenic. LDL migration into the vessel wall, oxidation, and phagocytosis by macrophages are key steps in the pathogenesis of atherosclerosis (see Figure 23-8). LDL also plays a role in endothelial injury, inflammation, and immune responses that have been identified as being important in atherogenesis. Aggressive reduction of LDL levels by implementing a reduced fat diet and using cholesterol-lowering drugs such as the statins is associated with a decrease in risk for CAD.[61,62]

Low levels of HDL cholesterol also are a strong indicator of coronary risk, and high levels of HDL may be more protective for the development of atherosclerosis than low levels of LDL.[63,64] HDL is responsible for "reverse cholesterol transport," which returns excess cholesterol from the tissues to the liver for processing or elimination in the bile. HDL also participates in endothelial repair and decreases thrombosis. It can be fractionated into several particle densities (HDL-2 and HDL-3) that have different effects on vascular function. Exercise, weight loss, fish oil consumption, and moderate alcohol use result in modest increases in HDL level. Niacin, fibrates, and statins are drugs that can cause modest increases in HDL level. Newer drugs aimed at directly increasing HDL activity include recombinant apolipoprotein A-I (ApoA-I) mimetics, thiazolidinediones, and cholesterol transferase protein inhibitors, although the safety of these medications is still being evaluated.[65,66] Other lipoproteins associated with increased cardiovascular risk include elevated levels of serum VLDLs (triglycerides) and increased lipoprotein(a) levels. Triglycerides are associated with an increased risk for CAD, especially in combination with other risk factors such as diabetes. Lipoprotein(a) (Lp[a]) is a genetically determined molecular complex between LDL and a serum glycoprotein called apolipoprotein A and has been shown to be an important risk factor for atherosclerosis, especially in women.[67]

Hypertension. Hypertension is responsible for a twofold to threefold increased risk of atherosclerotic cardiovascular disease. It contributes to endothelial injury, a key step in atherogenesis (see p. 594). It also can cause myocardial hypertrophy, which increases myocardial demand for coronary flow. Overactivity of the SNS and RAAS commonly found in hypertension also contributes to the genesis of CAD.

Cigarette smoking. Both direct and passive (environmental) smoking increase the risk of CAD. Nicotine stimulates the release of catecholamines (epinephrine and norepinephrine), which increase heart rate and peripheral vascular constriction. As a result, blood pressure increases, as do cardiac workload and oxygen demand. Cigarette smoking is associated with an increase in LDL level, a decrease in HDL level, and generation of toxic oxygen radicals, which contribute to vessel inflammation and thrombosis. The risk of CAD increases with heavy smoking and decreases when smoking is stopped.

Diabetes mellitus. Diabetes mellitus is an extremely important risk factor for CAD. Insulin resistance and diabetes have multiple effects on the cardiovascular system including endothelial damage, thickening of the vessel wall, increased inflammation, increased thrombosis, glycation of vascular proteins, and decreased production of endothelial-derived vasodilators such as nitric oxide (see Chapter 18). Diabetes is also associated with dyslipidemia.

Obesity/sedentary lifestyle. It is estimated that 65% of the adult population in the United States is overweight or obese, and an estimated 47 million U.S. residents have a combination of obesity, dyslipidemia, hypertension, and insulin resistance, called the metabolic syndrome, which is associated with an even higher risk for CAD events.[8] Abdominal obesity has the strongest link with increased CAD risk and is related to inflammation, insulin resistance, decreased HDL level, increased blood pressure, and fewer changes in hormones called adipokines (leptin and adiponectin).[68,69] A sedentary lifestyle not only increases the risk of obesity but also has an independent effect on increasing CAD risk. Physical activity and weight loss offer substantial reductions in risk factors for CAD.

Nontraditional risk factors. Nontraditional, or novel, risk factors for CAD include (1) increased serum markers for inflammation and thrombosis, (2) hyperhomocysteinemia, (3) adipokines, and (4) infection. The amount of risk conferred by these relatively newly identified factors is still being explored.

Markers of inflammation and thrombosis. Of the numerous markers of inflammation that have been linked to an increase in CAD risk (hs-CRP, fibrinogen, protein C, plasminogen activator inhibitor), the relationship between serum levels of hs-CRP and CAD has been explored in the greatest depth. **Highly-sensitive C-reactive protein (hs-CRP)** is a protein mostly synthesized in the liver and is used as an indirect measure of atherosclerotic plaque–related inflammation. An elevated serum level of hs-CRP is correlated with an increased risk for coronary events, but is a nonspecific measure of inflammation and may indicate the presence of other inflammatory conditions. The primary use of hs-CRP is as an aid to decision-making about pharmacologic interventions for individuals with other risk factors for coronary disease.[70] Other markers of inflammation associated with CAD include the erythrocyte sedimentation rate and concentrations of von Willebrand factor, interleukin-6, interleukin-18, tumor necrosis factor, fibrinogen, and CD 40 ligand (see *Health Alert:* Inflammatory Markers for Cardiovascular Risk).[71]

Hyperhomocysteinemia. Hyperhomocysteinemia occurs because of a genetic lack of the enzyme that metabolizes homocysteine (an amino acid) or because of a nutritional deficiency of folate, cobalamin (vitamin B_{12}), or pyridoxine (vitamin B_6). It has been identified as a risk factor for CAD, although the effectiveness of treatments aimed at reducing homocysteine levels to lessen CAD has not been shown. Therefore the significance of hyperhomocysteinemia as a risk factor for CAD and stroke continues to be explored.[72]

Adipokines. Adipokines are a group of hormones released from adipose cells. The two that are the most studied are leptin and adiponectin. Obesity causes increased levels of leptin, which is implicated in hypertension and diabetes.[69] Obesity also causes decreased levels of adiponectin, which is a hormone that functions to protect the vascular endothelium and is anti-inflammatory.[73,74] A less well-studied adipokine is called resistin, which has been linked to inflammation in endothelial cells. Weight loss, exercise, and healthy diet improve adipokine levels.

Infection. Infection may play a role in atherogenesis and CAD risk, although cause and effect has not been proved. Several microorganisms, especially *Chlamydia pneumoniae* and *Helicobacter pylori*, are

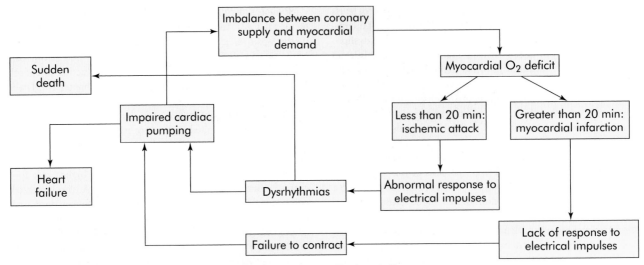

FIGURE 23-11 Cycle of Ischemic Events.

Data from Corrado E et al: *J Atheroscler Thromb* 17(1):1–11, 2010;
Ferri C et al: *Curr Pharm Des* 13(16):1631–1645, 2007; Menzaghi C
et al: *Diabetes* 56(5):1198–1209, 2007; Palazzuoli A et al: *Minerva
Cardioangiol* 55(4):491–496, 2007; Selcuk MT et al: *Coron Artery
Dis* 19(2):79–84, 2008; Singh SK et al: *Ann Med* 40:110–120, 2008;
Steffens S et al: *Circulation Res* 102(2):140–142, 2008; Virani SS et al:
Curr Atheroscler Rep 10(2):164–170, 2008.

HEALTH ALERT

Inflammatory Markers for Cardiovascular Risk

New Serum Markers of Cardiovascular Risk
A number of serum markers of inflammation have been found to be excellent predictors of cardiovascular risk, especially highly-sensitive C-reactive protein (hs-CRP). Other inflammatory markers determined to be predictive of cardiovascular risk include fibrinogen, erythrocyte sedimentation rate, von Willebrand factor, interleukin-6, interleukin-1, tumor necrosis factor-alpha, uric acid, adhesion molecules (selectins, intercellular adhesion molecules [ICAMs]), and serum amyloid A. hs-CRP is made by the liver in response to inflammatory stimuli and has been demonstrated convincingly to be a good predictor of coronary artery disease. However, several problems remain in determining its use in clinical practice. hs-CRP must be measured by a high-sensitivity technique and it is a nonspecific marker of inflammation. It can, therefore, be elevated in many other inflammatory states and its use for the diagnosis of CAD is limited to helping identify high-risk individuals and for following disease progression in individuals with known coronary disease. It should not be used to screen the general population. The HMG-CoA reductase drugs (statins) reduce hs-CRP levels. Another group of serum markers of cardiovascular risk are the adipokines, especially adiponectin. This hormone is secreted by fat cells and has anti-inflammatory and antiatherogenic properties. It is decreased in obesity and low levels have been linked to coronary artery disease. Other adipokines being evaluated for their association with atherosclerotic disease include leptin, resistin, visfatin, apelin, vaspin, and hepcidin. Brain natriuretic peptide also is linked with increased cardiovascular risk, especially in those with known coronary artery disease. A better understanding of the role of these serum biomarkers in cardiovascular disease may lead to earlier detection and more effective therapies.

often present in atherosclerotic lesions. Serum antibodies to microorganisms have been linked to an increased risk for CAD as has the presence of periodontal disease. Unfortunately, the use of antibiotics for the prevention and treatment of CAD has not yielded consistently positive results.

Myocardial Ischemia

PATHOPHYSIOLOGY The coronary arteries normally supply blood flow sufficient to meet the demands of the myocardium as it labors under varying workloads. Oxygen is extracted from these vessels with maximal efficiency. If demand increases, healthy coronary arteries can dilate to increase the flow of oxygenated blood to the myocardium. Narrowing of a major coronary artery by more than 50% impairs blood flow enough to hamper cellular metabolism when myocardial demand increases.

Myocardial ischemia develops if the flow or oxygen content of coronary blood is insufficient to meet the metabolic demands of myocardial cells (Figure 23-11). Imbalances between coronary blood supply and myocardial demand can result from a number of conditions. The most common cause of decreased coronary blood flow and resultant myocardial ischemia is the formation of atherosclerotic plaques in the coronary circulation. As the plaque increases in size, it may partially occlude the vessel lumina, thus limiting coronary flow and causing ischemia especially during exercise. Some plaques are "unstable," meaning they are prone to ulceration or rupture. When this ulceration or rupture occurs, underlying tissues of the vessel wall are exposed, resulting in platelet adhesion and thrombus formation (see Figures 23-9 and 23-17). Thrombus formation can suddenly stop blood supply to the heart muscle, resulting in acute myocardial ischemia, and if the vessel obstruction cannot be reversed rapidly, ischemia will progress to infarction. Myocardial ischemia also can result from other causes of decreased blood and oxygen delivery to the myocardium, such as coronary spasm, hypotension, dysrhythmias, and decreased oxygen-carrying capacity of the blood (e.g., anemia, hypoxemia). Common causes of increased myocardial demand for blood include tachycardia, exercise, hypertension (hypertrophy), and valvular disease.

Myocardial cells become ischemic within 10 seconds of coronary occlusion, thus hampering pump function and depriving the myocardium of a glucose source necessary for aerobic metabolism. Anaerobic

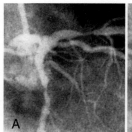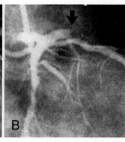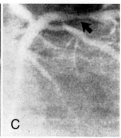

FIGURE 23-12 Angiogram of Coronary Arteries. **A,** Baseline. **B,** Transient total occlusion of left anterior descending branch of the left coronary artery after mental stress. **C,** After nitrates and nifedipine, artery reopened to same diameter as baseline. (Modified from Stern S, editor: *Silent myocardial ischemia*, St Louis, 1998, Mosby.)

processes take over, and lactic acid accumulates. After several minutes, the heart cells lose the ability to contract and cardiac output decreases. Cardiac cells remain viable for approximately 20 minutes under ischemic conditions. If blood flow is restored, aerobic metabolism resumes, contractility is restored, and cellular repair begins. If perfusion is not restored, then myocardial infarction occurs (see Figure 23-11).

CLINICAL MANIFESTATIONS Individuals with reversible myocardial ischemia present clinically in several ways. Chronic coronary obstruction results in recurrent predictable chest pain called *stable angina.* Abnormal vasospasm of coronary vessels results in unpredictable chest pain called *Prinzmetal angina.* Myocardial ischemia that does not cause detectable symptoms is called *silent ischemia.*

1. **Stable angina pectoris.** Angina is chest pain caused by myocardial ischemia. Stable angina is caused by gradual luminal narrowing and hardening of the arterial walls, so that affected vessels cannot dilate in response to increased myocardial demand associated with physical exertion or emotional stress. With rest, blood flow is restored and no necrosis of myocardial cells results. Angina pectoris is typically experienced as transient substernal chest discomfort, ranging from a sensation of heaviness or pressure to moderately severe pain. Individuals often describe the sensation by clenching a fist over the left sternal border. The discomfort may be mistaken for indigestion. The pain is caused by the buildup of lactic acid or abnormal stretching of the ischemic myocardium that irritates myocardial nerve fibers. These afferent sympathetic fibers enter the spinal cord from levels C3 to T4, accounting for a variety of locations and radiation patterns of anginal pain. Discomfort may radiate to the neck, lower jaw, left arm, and left shoulder, or occasionally to the back or down the right arm. Pallor, diaphoresis, and dyspnea may be associated with the pain.[75] The pain is usually relieved by rest and nitrates; lack of relief indicates an individual may be developing infarction.

   Myocardial ischemia in women may not present with typical anginal pain. Common symptoms in women include atypical chest pain, palpitations, sense of unease, and severe fatigue. Similarly, in individuals with autonomic nervous system dysfunction, such as older adults or those with diabetes, angina may be mild, atypical, or silent.[76]

2. **Prinzmetal angina.** Prinzmetal angina (also called variant angina) is chest pain attributable to transient ischemia of the myocardium that occurs unpredictably and often at rest. Pain is caused by vasospasm of one or more major coronary arteries with or without associated atherosclerosis. The pain often occurs at night during rapid eye movement sleep and may have a cyclic pattern of occurrence. The angina may result from decreased vagal activity, hyperactivity of the sympathetic nervous system, or decreased nitric oxide

activity.[77] Other causes include altered calcium channel function in arterial smooth muscle or impaired production or release of inflammatory mediators, such as serotonin, histamine, endothelin, or thromboxane. Serum markers of inflammation, such as CRP and interleukin-6 (IL-6), are elevated in individuals with this form of angina.[75] Prinzmetal angina is usually a benign condition, but can occasionally cause serious dysrhythmias.

3. **Silent ischemia** and **mental stress–induced ischemia.** Myocardial ischemia may not cause detectable symptoms such as angina. Ischemia can be totally asymptomatic and referred to as silent ischemia, or individuals may complain of fatigue, dyspnea, or a feeling of unease.[78] Silent ischemia and atypical symptoms are more common in women (see *Health Alert:* Women and Coronary Artery Disease). Some individuals only have silent ischemia, and episodes of silent ischemia are common in individuals who also experience angina. One proposed mechanism for the absence of angina in silent myocardial ischemia is the presence of a global or regional abnormality in left ventricular sympathetic afferent innervation. The most common cause of autonomic dysfunction leading to silent ischemia is diabetes mellitus. Other causes include surgical denervation during coronary artery bypass grafting (CABG) or cardiac transplantation, or following ischemic local nerve injury by myocardial infarction.

   Also of interest is silent ischemia occurring in some individuals during mental stress (Figures 23-12, 23-13, and 23-14). Chronic stress has been linked to an increase in the number of inflammatory cytokines and a hypercoagulable state that may contribute to acute ischemic events.[79] Silent ischemia can be detected by stress radionucleotide imaging. Detection and management of silent ischemia caused by coronary disease is important because it is an indicator of increased risk for serious cardiovascular events[80] (see *Health Alert:* Women and Coronary Artery Disease).

EVALUATION AND TREATMENT Many individuals with reversible myocardial ischemia will have a normal physical examination between events. Physical examination of those experiencing myocardial ischemia may disclose rapid pulse rate or extra heart sounds (gallops or murmurs), and pulmonary congestion indicating impaired left ventricular function. The presence of xanthelasmas (small fat deposits) around the eyelids or arcus senilis of the eyes (a yellow lipid ring around the cornea) suggests dyslipidemia and possible atherosclerosis. The presence of peripheral or carotid artery bruits suggests probable atherosclerotic disease and increases the likelihood that CAD is present.

Electrocardiography is a critical tool for the diagnosis of myocardial ischemia. Because many individuals have normal electrocardiograms

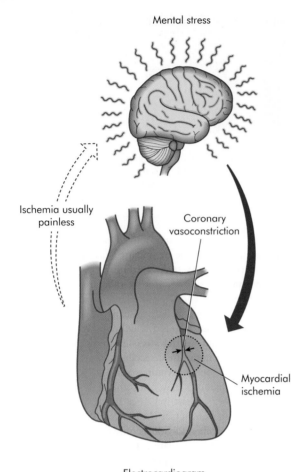

Mental stress

Ischemia usually
painless

Coronary
vasoconstriction

Myocardial
ischemia

Electrocardiogram

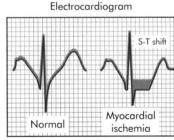

S-T shift

Normal

Myocardial
ischemia

FIGURE 23-13 Ischemic Cost of Aggravation. Linkages among daily mental and emotional stimuli, brain activity, and coronary and myocardial physiology. (Modified from Papodemetrion V et al: *Am Heart J* 132:1299, 1996.)

Data from Bugiardini R et al: Gender bias in acute coronary syndromes, *Curr Vasc Pharmacol* 8(2):276–284, 2010; Bukkapatnam RN, Gabler NB, Lewis WR: Statins for primary prevention of cardiovascular mortality in women: a systematic review and meta-analysis, *Prev Cardiol* 13(2):84–90, 2010; Collins P: HDL-C in post-menopausal women: an important therapeutic target, *Int J Cardiol* 124(3):275–282, 2008; Leuzzi C, Modena MG: Coronary artery disease: clinical presentation, diagnosis and prognosis in women, *Nutr Metab Cardiovasc Dis* 20(6):426–435, 2010; Miracle VA: Coronary artery disease in women: the myth still exists, unfortunately, *Dimens Crit Care Nurs* 29(5): 215–221, 2010; Szerlip M, Grines CL: Sex differences in response to treatments for chronic coronary artery disease, *Rev Cardiovasc Med* 10(suppl 2):S14–S23, 2009.

when there is no pain, diagnosis requires that electrocardiography be performed during an attack of angina or during exercise stress testing. The ST segment and the T wave segments of the electrocardiogram correlate with ventricular contraction and relaxation (see Figure 22-10). Transient ST segment depression and T wave inversion are characteristic signs of subendocardial ischemia. ST elevation, indicative of transmural ischemia, is seen in individuals with Prinzmetal angina, but is more common in transmural myocardial infarction (Figure 23-15). The electrocardiogram also can identify the coronary artery that is involved.

Exercise stress testing is indicated to detect ischemic changes in asymptomatic individuals with multiple risk factors for coronary disease, such as diabetes and dyslipidemia, and for older individuals who plan to start a vigorous exercise regimen. Stress testing is made more sensitive when radioisotope imaging is added to the ECG as an indicator of myocardial ischemia. Currently, the diagnostic modality of choice for the diagnosis of myocardial ischemia is single photon emission computerized tomography (SPECT), which is effective at identifying ischemia and estimating coronary risk. Radioisotope imaging with thallium-201 and stress echocardiography are other techniques used to diagnose CAD. Unfortunately, although all of these tests are helpful in documenting coronary obstruction, they cannot detect the presence of vulnerable plaques, which are the cause of the majority of acute coronary syndromes. Noninvasive tests for evaluating coronary atherosclerotic lesions include measurement of coronary artery calcium concentration by computed tomography (CT), noninvasive coronary angiography using electron beam CT, protein-weighted magnetic resonance imaging, and intravascular ultrasound; however, the sensitivity and specificity of these tests vary widely and are not recommended for routine evaluation of CAD.[75] Coronary angiography helps determine

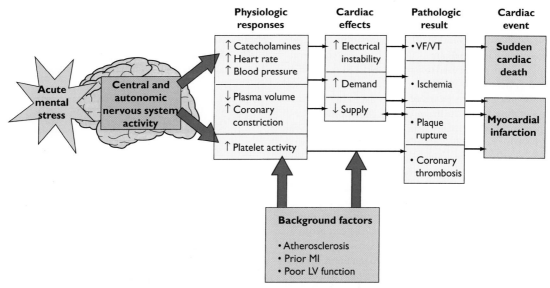

FIGURE 23-14 Pathophysiologic Model of the Effects of Acute Stress as a Trigger of Cardiac Clinical Events. Acting via the central and autonomic nervous systems, stress can produce a cascade of physiologic responses that may lead to myocardial ischemia, especially in persons with coronary artery disease; potentially fatal dysrhythmia; plaque rupture; or coronary thrombosis. *LV,* Left ventricular; *MI,* myocardial infarction; *VF,* ventricular fibrillation; *VT,* ventricular tachycardia. (From Krantz DS et al: Mental stress as a trigger of myocardial ischemia and infarction. In Deedwania PC, Tofler GH, editors: *Triggers and timing of cardiac events,* ed 2, London, 1996, Saunders.)

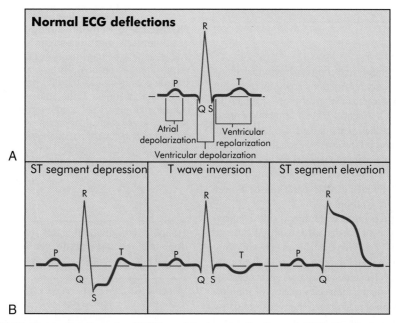

FIGURE 23-15 Electrocardiogram (ECG) and Ischemia. A, Normal ECG. **B,** Electrocardiographic alterations associated with ischemia.

the anatomic extent of CAD, but the procedure is expensive and carries some risk. It is used primarily to determine whether possible percutaneous coronary intervention (PCI) or coronary artery bypass graft (CABG) surgery is warranted for individuals whose noninvasive studies suggest severe disease.

The primary aims of therapy for myocardial ischemia and angina are to increase coronary blood flow and to reduce myocardial oxygen consumption. Coronary blood flow is improved by reversing

vasoconstriction, reducing plaque growth and rupture, and preventing clotting. Myocardial oxygen demand is reduced by manipulation of blood pressure, heart rate, contractility, and left ventricular volume. Several classes of drugs are useful for increasing coronary flow and decreasing myocardial demand, especially nitrates, beta-blockers, and calcium channel blockers.[81,82] Ranolazine represents a relatively new class of antianginal drugs known as sodium ion channel inhibitors and has been found to improve exercise tolerance, lessen anginal symptoms, and reduce the need for nitrates in many individuals with chronic stable angina.[83]

Percutaneous coronary intervention (PCI) is a procedure whereby stenotic (narrowed) coronary vessels are dilated with a catheter. Several different types of catheters can be used to open the blocked vessel. PCI most often is used to treat single-vessel disease, but it can be effective with multiple-vessel disease or restenosis of a coronary artery bypass graft.[82] Restenosis of the artery is the major complication of the procedure; however, placement of a coronary stent can reduce this risk. (See Box 23-2 for PCI-related myocardial infarction.) Pharmacologic treatment with antithrombotics, such as aspirin, clopidogrel, or glycoprotein IIb/IIIa receptor antagonists, after stenting also can improve outcomes.

Severe CAD can be surgically treated by a coronary artery bypass graft (CABG), usually using the saphenous vein from the lower leg. In selected individuals, a modified CABG procedure called minimally invasive direct coronary artery bypass (MIDCAB) can be used with much less surgical morbidity and more rapid recovery. In those individuals with refractory angina not amenable to standard bypass surgery, new techniques, such as laser revascularization, enhanced external counterpulsation, and myocardial gene therapy, are providing promising results.[75,84]

✔ **QUICK CHECK 23-5**
1. Define atherosclerosis, and briefly describe how it develops.
2. Why do hypertension and increased cholesterol level increase the likelihood of developing coronary artery disease?
3. Discuss the relationships among myocardial ischemia, angina, and silent ischemia.

Acute Coronary Syndromes

The process of atherosclerotic plaque progression can be gradual. However, when there is sudden coronary obstruction caused by thrombus formation over a ruptured or ulcerated atherosclerotic plaque, the acute coronary syndromes result (Figure 23-16). Unstable angina is the result of reversible myocardial ischemia and is a harbinger of impending infarction. Myocardial infarction (MI) results when there is prolonged ischemia causing irreversible damage to the heart muscle. MI can be further subdivided into non-ST elevation MI (non-STEMI) and ST elevation MI (STEMI). Sudden cardiac death can occur as a result of any of the acute coronary syndromes.

An atherosclerotic plaque that is prone to rupture is called "unstable" and has a core that is especially rich in deposited oxidized LDL and a thin fibrous cap[51] (Figure 23-17). These unstable plaques may not extend into the lumen of the vessel and may be clinically silent until they rupture. Plaque disruption (ulceration or rupture) occurs because of the effects of shear forces, inflammation with release of multiple inflammatory mediators, secretion of macrophage-derived degradative enzymes, and apoptosis of cells at the edges of the lesions. Exposure of the plaque substrate activates the clotting cascade. In addition, platelet activation results in the release of coagulants and exposure of platelet glycoprotein IIb/IIIa surface receptors, resulting in further platelet aggregation and adherence. The resulting thrombus can form very quickly (Figure 23-18, A). Vessel obstruction is further exacerbated by the release of vasoconstrictors, such as thromboxane A_2 and endothelin. The thrombus may shatter before permanent myocyte damage has occurred (unstable angina) or it may cause prolonged ischemia with infarction of the heart muscle (myocardial infarction) (Figure 23-18, B). Diagnostic tests aimed at identifying unstable plaques before they rupture include intravascular ultrasound or MRI, angioscopy, and

spectroscopy.[51,85] Medications such as statins, angiotensin-converting enzyme inhibitors, and beta-blockers can be used to help stabilize plaques and prevent rupture.[51]

Unstable angina. Unstable angina is a form of acute coronary syndrome that results from reversible myocardial ischemia. It is important

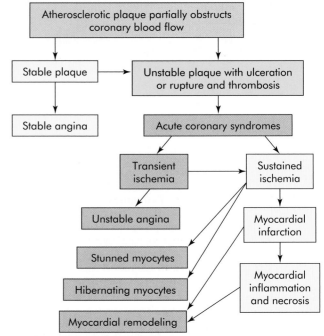

FIGURE 23-16 Pathophysiology of Acute Coronary Syndromes. The atherosclerotic process can lead to stable plaque formation and stable angina or can result in unstable plaques that are prone to rupture and thrombus. Thrombus formation on a ruptured plaque that disperses in less than 20 minutes leads to transient ischemia and unstable angina. If the vessel obstruction is sustained, myocardial infarction with inflammation and necrosis of the myocardium results. In addition, myocardial infarction is associated with other structural and functional changes, including myocyte stunning and hibernation and myocardial remodeling (see Figure 23-35).

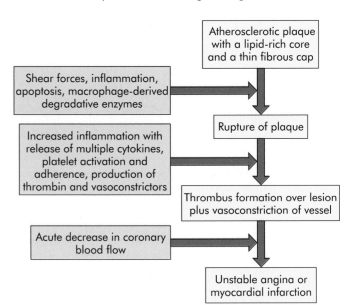

FIGURE 23-17 Pathogenesis of Unstable Plaques and Thrombus Formation.

to recognize this syndrome because it signals that the atherosclerotic plaque has become complicated, and infarction may soon follow. Unstable angina occurs when a fairly small fissuring or superficial erosion of the plaque leads to transient episodes of thrombotic vessel occlusion and vasoconstriction at the site of plaque damage. This thrombus is labile and occludes the vessel for no more than 10 to 20 minutes, with return of perfusion before significant myocardial necrosis occurs. Unstable angina presents as new-onset angina, angina that is occurring at rest, or angina that is increasing in severity or frequency (Box 23-1). Individuals may experience increased dyspnea, diaphoresis, and anxiety as the angina worsens. Physical examination may reveal evidence of ischemic myocardial dysfunction such as tachycardia, or pulmonary congestion. The ECG most commonly shows ST segment depression and T wave inversion during pain that resolve as the pain is relieved. The concentrations of serum cardiac biomarkers (troponins, creatine phosphokinase-myocardial bound [CPK-MB], and lactate dehydrogenase [LDH$_1$]) remain normal.[86] Approximately 20% of persons with unstable angina will progress to myocardial infarction or death. Management of unstable angina requires immediate hospitalization with administration of oxygen, aspirin (if not contraindicated), nitrates, and morphine if pain is still present.[87] Additional antithrombotic therapy with clopidogrel or glycoprotein IIb/IIIa platelet receptor antagonists may be indicated. Beta-blockers and ACE inhibitors also may be used. Anticoagulants (such as low-molecular-weight heparin) or direct thrombin inhibitors (e.g., fondaparinux) also can be given. Individuals with refractory angina and those with electrical or hemodynamic instability require immediate intervention with percutaneous coronary intervention (PCI) or coronary artery bypass grafting (CABG).

Myocardial infarction. When coronary blood flow is interrupted for an extended period of time, myocyte necrosis occurs. This results in myocardial infarction (MI). Plaque progression, disruption, and subsequent clot formation are the same for myocardial infarction as they are for unstable angina (see Figures 23-16, 23-17, and 23-18). In this case, however, the thrombus is less labile and occludes the vessel for a prolonged period, such that myocardial ischemia progresses to myocyte necrosis and death. Pathologically, there are two major types of myocardial infarction: subendocardial infarction and transmural infarction. Clinically, however, myocardial infarction is categorized as non-ST segment elevation myocardial infarction (non-STEMI) or ST segment elevation MI (STEMI).

If the thrombus disintegrates before complete distal tissue necrosis has occurred, the infarction will involve only the myocardium directly beneath the endocardium (subendocardial MI). This infarction will usually present with ST segment depression and T wave inversion without Q waves; therefore it is termed non-STEMI. It is especially important to recognize this form of acute coronary syndrome because recurrent clot formation on the disrupted atherosclerotic plaque is likely. If the thrombus lodges permanently in the vessel, the infarction will extend through the myocardium all the way from endocardium to epicardium, resulting in severe cardiac dysfunction (transmural MI). Transmural myocardial infarction will usually result in marked elevations in the ST segments on ECG and these individuals are categorized as having ST segment elevation MI, or STEMI. Clinically, it is important to identify those individuals with STEMI because they are at highest risk for serious complications and should receive definitive intervention without delay.

PATHOPHYSIOLOGY

Cellular injury. After 8 to 10 seconds of decreased blood flow, the affected myocardium becomes cyanotic and cooler. Myocardial oxygen reserves are used quickly (within about 8 seconds) after complete

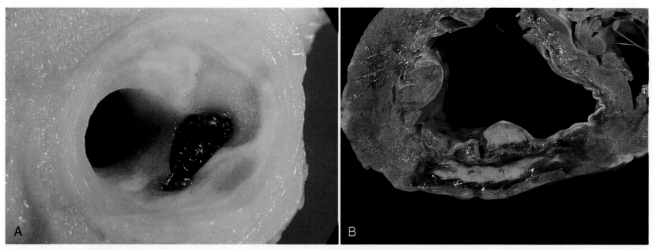

FIGURE 23-18 Plaque Disruption and Myocardial Infarction. **A,** Plaque disruption. The cap of the lipid-rich plaque has become torn with the formation of a thrombus, mostly inside the plaque. **B,** Myocardial infarction. This infarct is 6 days old. The center is yellow and necrotic with a hemorrhagic red rim. The responsible arterial occlusion is probably in the right coronary artery. The infarct is on the posterior wall. (From Damjanov I, Linder J, editors: *Anderson's pathology,* ed 10, St Louis, 1996, Mosby.)

cessation of coronary flow. Glycogen stores decrease as anaerobic metabolism begins. Unfortunately, glycolysis can supply only 65% to 70% of the total myocardial energy requirement and produces much less adenosine triphosphate (ATP) than aerobic processes. Hydrogen ions and lactic acid accumulate. Because myocardial tissues have poor buffering capabilities and myocardial cells are sensitive to low cellular pH, accumulation of these products further compromises the myocardium. Acidosis may make the myocardium more vulnerable to the damaging effects of lysosomal enzymes and may suppress impulse conduction and contractile function, thereby leading to heart failure.

Oxygen deprivation also is accompanied by electrolyte disturbances, specifically the loss of potassium, calcium, and magnesium from cells. Myocardial cells deprived of necessary oxygen and nutrients lose contractility, thereby diminishing the pumping ability of the heart. Ischemia causes the myocardial cells to release catecholamines, predisposing the individual to serious imbalances of sympathetic and parasympathetic function, irregular heartbeats (dysrhythmia), and heart failure. Catecholamines mediate the release of glycogen, glucose, and stored fat from body cells. Therefore plasma concentrations of free fatty acids and glycerol rise within 1 hour after the onset of acute myocardial infarction. Excessive levels of free fatty acids can have a harmful detergent effect on cell membranes. Norepinephrine elevates blood glucose levels through stimulation of liver and skeletal muscle cells and suppresses pancreatic beta-cell activity, which reduces insulin secretion and elevates blood glucose further. Hyperglycemia is noted approximately 72 hours after an acute myocardial infarction and is associated with an increased risk of death; therefore careful glucose monitoring and control after MI is essential.[88]

Angiotensin II is released during myocardial ischemia and contributes to the pathogenesis of myocardial infarction in several ways. First, it results in the systemic effects of peripheral vasoconstriction and fluid retention, which increase myocardial workload. Second, it is a growth factor for vascular smooth muscle cells, myocytes, and cardiac fibroblasts resulting in structural changes in the myocardium called "remodeling."[89] Finally, angiotensin II promotes catecholamine release and causes coronary artery spasm.

Cellular death. Cardiac cells can withstand ischemic conditions for about 20 minutes before irreversible hypoxic injury causes cellular death (apoptosis) and tissue necrosis.[90] This results in the release of intracellular enzymes such as creatine phosphokinase MB (CPK-MB) and myocyte proteins such as the troponins through the damaged cell membranes into the interstitial spaces. The lymphatics absorb the enzymes and transport them into the bloodstream, where they can be detected by serologic tests.

Structural and functional changes. Myocardial infarction results in both structural and functional changes of cardiac tissues (Figure 23-19). Gross tissue changes at the area of infarction may not become apparent for several hours, despite almost immediate onset (within 30 to 60 seconds) of electrocardiographic changes. Cardiac tissue surrounding the area of infarction also undergoes changes that can be categorized into (1) myocardial stunning—a temporary loss of contractile function that persists for hours to days after perfusion has been restored;[91] (2) hibernating myocardium—tissue that is persistently ischemic and undergoes metabolic adaptation to prolong myocyte survival until perfusion can be restored;[92] and (3) myocardial remodeling—a process mediated by angiotensin II, aldosterone, catecholamines, adenosine, and inflammatory cytokines that causes myocyte hypertrophy and loss of contractile function in the areas of the heart distant from the site of infarction.[89] All of these changes can be limited through rapid restoration of coronary flow and the use of ACE inhibitors or ARBs and beta-blockers after MI.

The severity of functional impairment depends on the size of the lesion and the site of infarction. Functional changes can include (1) decreased cardiac contractility with abnormal wall motion, (2) altered left ventricular compliance, (3) decreased stroke volume, (4) decreased ejection fraction, (5) increased left ventricular end-diastolic pressure, and (6) sinoatrial node malfunction. Life-threatening dysrhythmias and heart failure often follow myocardial infarction.

With infarction, ventricular function is abnormal and the ejection fraction falls, resulting in increases in ventricular end-diastolic volume (VEDV). If the coronary obstruction involves the perfusion to the left ventricle, pulmonary venous congestion ensues; if the right ventricle is ischemic, increases in systemic venous pressures occur.

Repair. Myocardial infarction causes a severe inflammatory response that ends with wound repair (see Chapter 5). Damaged cells undergo degradation, fibroblasts proliferate, and scar tissue is synthesized.[93] Many cell types, hormones, and nutrient substrates must be available for optimal healing to proceed. Within 24 hours, leukocytes infiltrate the necrotic area, and proteolytic enzymes from scavenger neutrophils degrade necrotic tissue. The collagen matrix that is deposited is initially weak, mushy, and vulnerable to reinjury. Unfortunately,

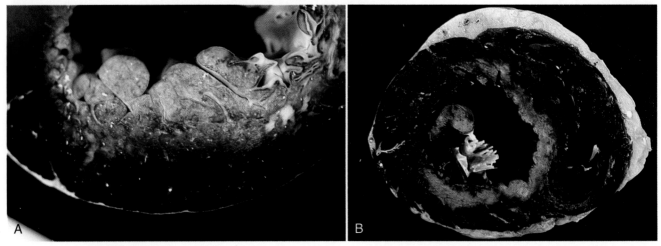

FIGURE 23-19 Myocardial Infarction. A, Local infarct confined to one region. **B,** Massive large infarct caused by occlusion of three coronary arteries. (From Damjanov I, Linder J, editors: *Anderson's pathology,* ed 10, St Louis, 1996, Mosby.)

it is at this time in the recovery period (10 to 14 days after infarction) that individuals feel more like increasing activities and may stress the newly formed scar tissue. After 6 weeks, the necrotic area is completely replaced by scar tissue, which is strong but cannot contract and relax like healthy myocardial tissue.

CLINICAL MANIFESTATIONS   The first symptom of acute myocardial infarction is usually sudden, severe chest pain. The pain is similar to that of angina pectoris but more severe and prolonged. It may be described as heavy and crushing, such as a "truck sitting on my chest." Radiation to the neck, jaw, back, shoulder, or left arm is common. Some individuals, especially those who are elderly or have diabetes, experience no pain, thereby having a "silent" infarction. Infarction often simulates a sensation of unrelenting indigestion. Nausea and vomiting may occur because of reflex stimulation of vomiting centers by pain fibers. Vasovagal reflexes from the area of the infarcted myocardium also may affect the gastrointestinal tract.

Various cardiovascular changes are found on physical examination:
1. The sympathetic nervous system is reflexively activated to compensate, resulting in a temporary increase in heart rate and blood pressure.
2. Abnormal extra heart sounds reflect left ventricular dysfunction.
3. Pulmonary findings of congestion including dullness to percussion and inspiratory crackles at the lung bases can occur if the individual develops heart failure.
4. Peripheral vasoconstriction may cause the skin to become cool and clammy.

Complications. The number and severity of postinfarction complications depend on the location and extent of necrosis, the individual's physiologic condition before the infarction, and the availability of swift therapeutic intervention. Sudden cardiac death can occur in individuals with myocardial ischemia even if infarction is absent or minimal and is a multifactorial problem. Risk factors for sudden death are related to three factors: ischemia, left ventricular dysfunction, and electrical instability. These factors interact with each other (Figure 23-20). Table 23-5 lists the most common complications.

EVALUATION AND TREATMENT   The diagnosis of acute myocardial infarction is made on the basis of history, physical examination, ECG, and serial cardiac biomarker alterations (Box 23-2).[94] The cardiac troponins (troponin I and troponin T) are the most specific indicators of MI.[70] A transient rise in these plasma enzyme levels can confirm the occurrence of MI and indicate its severity. Other enzymes released by myocardial cells include CPK-MB and LDH. These enzymes exist in several different active molecular forms called *isoenzymes*, which are present in different amounts within particular tissues. Blood is drawn for troponin and isoenzyme determinations as soon as possible after the onset of symptoms, and serial serum levels of these markers are assessed for several days. If serologic tests show abnormally high levels of troponin and isoenzymes, acute myocardial infarction probably has occurred. CK-MB is less specific than troponins and may increase in individuals with certain other conditions (e.g., muscular dystrophy, hypothermia, chronic obstructive pulmonary disease [COPD] associated with left heart failure and pulmonary embolism, extensive

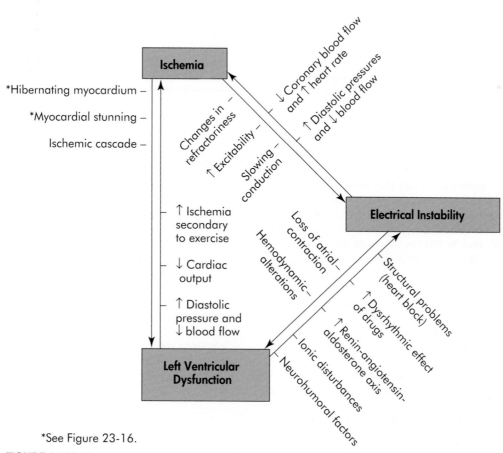

*See Figure 23-16.

FIGURE 23-20   Three Interacting Factors Related to Sudden Cardiac Death. The three factors are ischemia, left ventricular dysfunction, and electrical instability.

TABLE 23-5 COMPLICATIONS WITH MYOCARDIAL INFARCTIONS

TYPE	CHARACTERISTICS
Dysrhythmias	Disturbances of cardiac rhythm that affect 90% of persons with cardiac infarction Caused by ischemia, hypoxia, autonomic nervous system imbalances, lactic acidosis, electrolyte abnormalities, alterations of impulse conduction pathways or conduction abnormalities, drug toxicity, or hemodynamic abnormalities
Left ventricular failure (congestive heart failure)	Characterized by pulmonary congestion, reduced myocardial contractility, and abnormal heart wall motion Cardiogenic shock can develop
Inflammation of pericardium (pericarditis)	Includes pericardial friction rubs Often noted 2 to 3 days later and associated with anterior chest pain that worsens with respiratory effort
Dressler postinfarction syndrome	Essentially a delayed form of pericarditis that occurs 1 week to several months after acute MI syndrome Thought to be immunologic response to necrotic myocardium marked by pain, fever, friction rub, pleural effusion, and arthralgias
Organic brain syndrome	Occurs if blood flow to brain is impaired secondary to MI
Transient ischemic attacks or cerebrovascular accident	Occur if thromboemboli detach from clots that form in cardiac chambers or on cardiac valves
Rupture of heart structures	Caused by necrosis of tissue in or around papillary muscles Affects papillary muscles of chordae tendineae cordis Predisposing factors include thinning of wall, poor collateral flow, shearing effect of muscular contraction against stiffened necrotic area, marked necrosis at terminal end of blood supply, and aging of myocardium with laceration of myocardial microstructure
Rupture of wall of infarcted ventricle	Can be caused by aneurysm formation when pressure becomes too great
Left ventricular aneurysm	Late (month to years) complication of MI that can contribute to heart failure and thromboemboli
Infarctions around septal structures	Occur in those structures that separate heart chambers and lead to septal rupture Associated with audible, harsh cardiac murmurs; increased left ventricular end-diastolic pressure; and decreased systemic blood pressure
Systemic thromboembolism	May disseminate from debris and clots that collect inside dilated aneurysmal sacs or from infarcted endocardium
Pulmonary thromboembolism	Usually from deep venous thrombi of legs Reduced incidence associated with early mobilization and prophylactic anticoagulation therapy
Sudden death	Dysrhythmias frequently causative, particularly ventricular fibrillation Risk of death increased by age more than 65 years, previous angina pectoris, hypotension or cardiogenic shock, acute systolic hypertension at time of admission, diabetes mellitus, dysrhythmias, and previous MI

MI, Myocardial infarction.

BOX 23-2 UNIVERSAL DEFINITION OF MYOCARDIAL INFARCTION

The term myocardial infarction should be used when there is evidence of myocardial necrosis in a clinical setting with myocardial ischemia. Under these conditions any one of the following criteria meets the diagnosis for myocardial infarction:

- Detection of rise and/or fall of cardiac biomarkers (preferably troponin) with at least one value above the 99th percentile of the upper reference limit (URL) together with evidence of myocardial ischemia with at least one of the following:
  - Symptoms of ischemia
  - ECG changes indicative of new ischemia (new ST-T changes or new left bundle branch block [LBBB])
  - Development of pathologic Q waves in the ECG
  - Imaging evidence of new loss of viable myocardium or new regional wall motion abnormality
- Sudden, unexpected cardiac death, involving cardiac arrest, often with symptoms suggestive of myocardial ischemia, and accompanied by presumably new ST elevation, or new LBBB, and/or evidence of fresh thrombus by coronary angiography and/or at autopsy; but death occurring before blood samples could be obtained, or at a time before the appearance of cardiac biomarkers in the blood.

- For percutaneous coronary interventions (PCI) in persons with normal baseline troponin values, elevations of cardiac biomarkers above the 99th percentile URL are indicative of peri-procedural myocardial necrosis. By convention, increases of biomarkers greater than $3 \times$ 99th percentile URL have been designated as defining PCI-related myocardial infarction. A subtype related to a documented stent thrombosis is recognized.
- For coronary artery bypass grafting (CABG) in persons with normal baseline troponin values, elevations of cardiac biomarkers above the 99th percentile URL are indicative of peri-procedural myocardial necrosis. By convention, increases of biomarkers greater than $5 \times$ 99th percentile URL plus either new pathologic Q waves or new LBBB, or angiographically documented new graft or native coronary artery occlusion, or imaging evidence of new loss of viable myocardium have been designated as defining CABG-related myocardial infarction.
- Pathologic findings of an acute myocardial infarction.

Data from Thygesen K, Alpert J, White H: *J Am Coll Cardiol* 50:2173–2195, 2007.

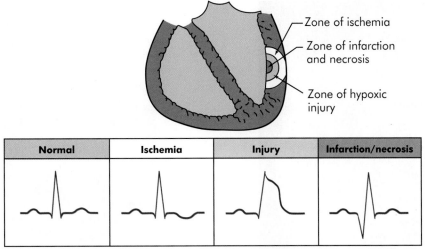

FIGURE 23-21 Electrocardiographic Alterations Associated With the Three Zones of Myocardial Infarction.

third-degree burns, small bowel infarction). Elevation of troponin, CK-MB, and LDH₁ levels may not occur immediately after infarction and laboratory confirmation that an infarction has occurred may be delayed up to 12 hours.

Myocardial infarction can occur in various regions of the heart wall and may be described as anterior, inferior, posterior, lateral, subendocardial, or transmural, depending on the anatomic location and extent of tissue damage from infarction. Twelve-lead electrocardiograms (ECGs) help to localize the affected area through identification of Q waves and changes in ST segments and T waves (Figure 23-21). The infarcted myocardium is surrounded by a zone of hypoxic injury, which may progress to necrosis or return to normal condition. Adjacent to this zone of hypoxic injury is a zone of reversible ischemia. Ischemic and injured myocardial tissue causes ST and T wave changes. Myocardial infarction documented by elevated levels of troponins and isoenzymes but with no elevation of the ST segment on electrocardiogram (ECG) is termed non-STEMI. It is especially important to recognize this form of acute coronary syndrome because recurrent clot formation on the disrupted atherosclerotic plaque is likely, with resultant infarct expansion. Transmural infarction presents with significant ST segment elevation on ECG (STEMI). A characteristic Q wave often will develop on ECG several hours later (Q wave MI). STEMI requires rapid intervention to prevent serious complications and sequelae, such as dysrhythmias and heart failure.

Acute myocardial infarction requires admission to the hospital, often directly into a coronary care unit. The individual should be placed on supplemental oxygen and given an aspirin immediately (ticlopidine if allergic to aspirin). Pain relief is of utmost importance and involves the use of sublingual nitroglycerin and morphine sulfate. Continuous monitoring of cardiac rhythms and enzymatic changes is essential, because the first 24 hours after onset of symptoms is the time of highest risk for sudden death. Both non-STEMI and STEMI are managed with the urgent administration of thrombolytics or by PCI along with antithrombotics. Further management may include ACE inhibitors and beta-blockers. Individuals who are in shock require aggressive fluid resuscitation, ionotropic drugs, and possible emergent invasive procedures.[87]

Bed rest, followed by gradual return to activities of daily living, reduces the myocardial oxygen demands of the compromised heart. Individuals not receiving thrombolytic or heparin infusion must receive deep venous thrombosis prophylaxis as long as their activity is significantly limited. Stool softeners are given to eliminate the need for straining, which can precipitate bradycardia and can be followed by increased venous return to the heart, causing possible cardiac overload. Hyperglycemia is treated with insulin.

Treatment of dyslipidemia with hydroxymethylglutaryl coenzyme A (HMG Co-A) reductase inhibitors (statins) can reduce the risk of future cardiovascular events.[87,95] Education regarding appropriate diet and caffeine intake, smoking cessation, exercise, and other aspects of risk factor reduction is crucial for secondary prevention of recurrent myocardial ischemia.

> ✔ **QUICK CHECK 23-6**
> 1. Describe the coronary artery disease–myocardial ischemia continuum.
> 2. Describe the pathophysiology of myocardial infarction.
> 3. What complications are associated with the period after infarction?

DISORDERS OF THE HEART WALL

Disorders of the Pericardium

Pericardial disease is a localized manifestation of another disorder, such as infection (bacterial, viral, fungal, rickettsial, or parasitic); trauma or surgery; neoplasm; or a metabolic, immunologic, or vascular disorder (uremia, rheumatoid arthritis, systemic lupus erythematosus, periarteritis nodosa). The pericardial response to injury from these diverse causes may consist of acute pericarditis, pericardial effusion, or constrictive pericarditis.[96]

Acute Pericarditis

Acute pericarditis is acute inflammation of the pericardium. The etiology of acute pericarditis is most often idiopathic or caused by viral infection by coxsackie, influenza, hepatitis, measles, mumps, or varicella viruses. It also is the most common cardiovascular complication of human immunodeficiency virus (HIV) infection. Other causes include myocardial infarction, trauma, neoplasm, surgery, uremia, bacterial infection (especially tuberculosis), connective tissue disease (especially systemic lupus erythematosus and rheumatoid arthritis), or radiation therapy.[97] The pericardial membranes become inflamed and roughened, and a pericardial effusion may develop that can be serous,

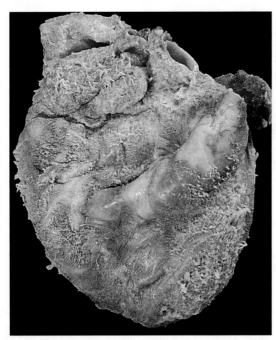

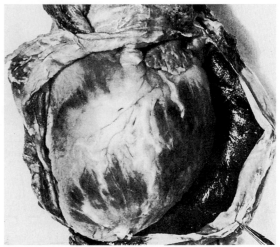

FIGURE 23-23 Exudate of Blood in the Pericardial Sac from Rupture of Aneurysm. (From Damjanov I, Linder J: *Pathology: a color atlas,* St Louis, 2000, Mosby.)

FIGURE 23-22 Acute Pericarditis. Note shaggy coat of fibers covering the surface of heart. (From Damjanov I, Linder J: *Pathology: a color atlas,* St Louis, 2000, Mosby.)

purulent, or fibrinous (Figure 23-22). Possible sequelae of pericarditis include recurrent pericarditis, pericardial constriction, and cardiac tamponade.

Symptoms may follow several days of fever and usually begin with the sudden onset of severe retrosternal chest pain that worsens with respiratory movements and when assuming a recumbent position. The pain may radiate to the back as a result of irritation of the phrenic nerve (innervates the trapezius muscles) as it traverses the pericardium. Individuals with acute pericarditis also report dysphagia, restlessness, irritability, anxiety, weakness, and malaise.

Physical examination often discloses low-grade fever (<38° C) and sinus tachycardia. A friction rub—a scratchy, grating sound—may be heard at the cardiac apex and left sternal border and is highly suggestive of pericarditis. The rub is caused by the roughened pericardial membranes rubbing against each other. Friction rubs are not always present and may be intermittently heard and transient. Hypotension or the presence of a pulsus paradoxus (a decrease in systolic blood pressure of >10 mm Hg with inspiration) is suggestive of cardiac tamponade, which can be life-threatening. Electrocardiographic changes may reflect inflammatory processes through PR segment depression and diffuse ST segment elevation without Q waves, and they may remain abnormal for days or even weeks. CT scanning and MRI may be used as diagnostic modalities.[97]

Treatment for uncomplicated acute pericarditis consists of relieving symptoms and includes administration of anti-inflammatory agents, such as salicylates and nonsteroidal anti-inflammatory drugs.[98] Colchicine may be added to prevent fibrosis. Exploration of the underlying cause is important. If pericardial effusion develops, aspiration of the excessive fluid may be necessary.

Pericardial Effusion

Pericardial effusion is the accumulation of fluid in the pericardial cavity and can occur in all forms of pericarditis. The fluid may be a transudate, such as the serous effusion that develops with left heart failure, overhydration, or hypoproteinemia. More often, however, the fluid is an exudate, which reflects pericardial inflammation like that seen with acute pericarditis, heart surgery, some chemotherapeutic agents, infections, and autoimmune disorders such as systemic lupus erythematosus. (Types of exudate are described in Chapter 5.) If the fluid is serosanguineous, the underlying cause is likely to be tuberculosis, neoplasm, uremia, or radiation. Idiopathic serosanguineous (cause unknown) effusion is possible, however. Effusions of frank blood are generally related to aneurysms, trauma, or coagulation defects (Figure 23-23). If chyle leaks from the thoracic duct, it may enter the pericardium and lead to cholesterol pericarditis.

Pericardial effusion, even in large amounts, is not necessarily clinically significant, except that it indicates an underlying disorder. If an effusion develops gradually, the pericardium can stretch to accommodate large quantities of fluid without compressing the heart. If the fluid accumulates rapidly, however, even a small amount (50 to 100 ml) may create sufficient pressure to cause cardiac compression, a serious condition known as tamponade. The danger is that pressure exerted by the pericardial fluid eventually will equal diastolic pressure within the heart chambers, which will interfere with right atrial filling during diastole. This causes increased venous pressure, systemic venous congestion, and signs and symptoms of right heart failure (distention of the jugular veins, edema, hepatomegaly). Decreased atrial filling leads to decreased ventricular filling, decreased stroke volume, and reduced cardiac output. Life-threatening circulatory collapse may occur.

An important clinical finding is pulsus paradoxus, in which arterial blood pressure during expiration exceeds arterial pressure during inspiration by more than 10 mm Hg. Pulsus paradoxus in the setting of a pericardial effusion indicates tamponade and reflects impairment of diastolic filling of the left ventricle plus reduction of blood volume within all four cardiac chambers. The presence of a large pericardial effusion or tamponade magnifies the normally insignificant effect of inspiration on intracardiac flow and volume.

Other clinical manifestations of pericardial effusion are distant or muffled heart sounds, poorly palpable apical pulse, dyspnea on exertion, and dull chest pain. A chest x-ray film may disclose a "water-bottle configuration" of the cardiac silhouette. An echocardiogram can detect an effusion as small as 20 ml and is a reliable and accurate diagnostic test, although CT scans also may be done.

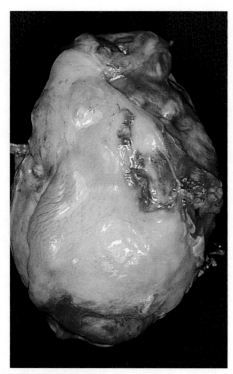

FIGURE 23-24 Constrictive Pericarditis. The fibrotic pericardium encases the heart in a rigid shell. (From Damjanov I, Linder J: *Pathology: a color atlas,* St Louis, 2000, Mosby.)

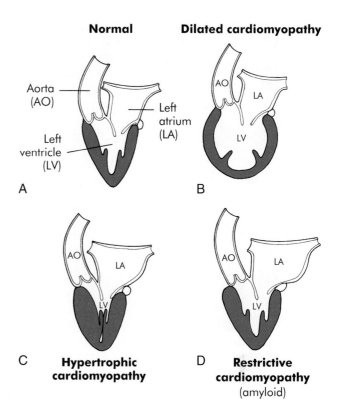

FIGURE 23-25 Diagram Showing Major Distinguishing Pathophysiologic Features of the Three Types of Cardiomyopathy. **A,** The normal heart. **B,** In the dilated type of cardiomyopathy, the heart has a globular shape and the largest circumference of the left ventricle is not at its base but midway between apex and base. **C,** In the hypertrophic type, the wall of the left ventricle is greatly thickened; the left ventricular cavity is small, but the left atrium may be dilated because of poor diastolic relaxation of the ventricle. **D,** In the restrictive (constrictive) type, the left ventricular cavity is of normal size, but, again, the left atrium is dilated because of the reduced diastolic compliance of the ventricle. (From Kissane JM, editor: *Anderson's pathology,* ed 9, St Louis, 1990, Mosby.)

Treatment of pericardial effusion or tamponade generally consists of pericardiocentesis (aspiration of excessive pericardial fluid) and treatment of the underlying condition. Persistent pain may be treated with analgesics, anti-inflammatory medications, or steroids. Surgery may be required if the underlying cause of tamponade is trauma or aneurysm. A pericardial "window" may be surgically created to prevent tamponade.[96]

Constrictive Pericarditis

Constrictive pericarditis, or restrictive pericarditis (chronic pericarditis), was synonymous with tuberculosis years ago, and tuberculosis continues to be an important cause of pericarditis in immunocompromised individuals. Currently in the United States, this form of pericardial disease is more commonly idiopathic or associated with radiation exposure, rheumatoid arthritis, uremia, or coronary artery bypass graft surgery.[96] In constrictive pericarditis, fibrous scarring with occasional calcification of the pericardium causes the visceral and parietal pericardial layers to adhere, obliterating the pericardial cavity. The fibrotic lesions encase the heart in a rigid shell (Figure 23-24). Like tamponade, constrictive pericarditis compresses the heart and eventually reduces cardiac output. Unlike tamponade, however, constrictive pericarditis always develops gradually.

Symptoms tend to be exercise intolerance, dyspnea on exertion, fatigue, and anorexia.[99] Clinical assessment shows edema, distention of the jugular vein, and hepatic congestion. Restricted ventricular filling may cause a pericardial knock (early diastolic sound).

ECG findings include T wave inversions and atrial fibrillation. Chest x-ray films often disclose prominent pulmonary vessels and calcification of the pericardium. CT, MRI, and transesophageal echocardiography are used to detect pericardial thickening and constriction and to distinguish constrictive pericarditis from restrictive cardiomyopathy. Pericardial biopsy may be needed to determine the etiology.

Initial treatment for constrictive pericarditis consists of restriction of dietary sodium intake and administration of digitalis glycosides and diuretics to improve cardiac output. Management also may include use of anti-inflammatory drugs and treatment of any underlying disorder. If these modalities are unsuccessful, surgical excision of the restrictive pericardium is indicated (pericardial decortication).[100]

Disorders of the Myocardium: The Cardiomyopathies

The cardiomyopathies are a diverse group of diseases that primarily affect the myocardium itself. Most are the result of remodeling caused by the effect of the neurohumoral responses to ischemic heart disease or hypertension on the heart muscle. They may, however, be secondary to infectious disease, exposure to toxins, systemic connective tissue disease, infiltrative and proliferative disorders, or nutritional deficiencies. Many cases are idiopathic—that is, their cause is unknown. The cardiomyopathies are categorized as dilated (formerly, congestive), hypertrophic, or restrictive, depending on their physiologic effects on the heart (Figure 23-25).

Dilated cardiomyopathy is usually the result of ischemic heart disease, valvular disease, diabetes, renal failure, alcohol or drug toxicity, peripartum complications, genetic disorder, or infection.[101] It is characterized by impaired systolic function leading to increases in

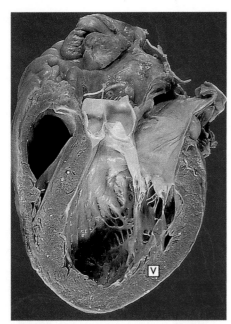

FIGURE 23-26 Dilated cardiomyopathy. The dilated left ventricle has a thin wall *(V)*. (From Stevens A, Lowe J: *Pathology,* St Louis, 1995, Mosby.)

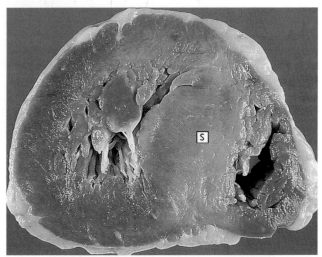

FIGURE 23-27 Hypertrophic cardiomyopathy. There is marked left ventricular hypertrophy. This often affects the septum *(S)*. (From Stevens A, Lowe J: *Pathology,* St Louis, 1995, Mosby.)

intracardiac volume, ventricular dilation, and systolic heart failure (Figure 23-26) (see p. 622). Individuals complain of dyspnea, fatigue, and pedal edema. Findings on examination include a displaced apical pulse, S$_3$ gallop, peripheral edema, jugular venous distention, and pulmonary congestion. Diagnosis is confirmed by chest x-ray and echocardiogram, and management is focused on reducing blood volume, increasing contractility, and reversing the underlying disorder if possible.[101] Heart transplant is required in severe cases.

Hypertrophic cardiomyopathy refers to two major categories of thickening of the myocardium: (1) hypertrophic obstructive cardiomyopathy (asymmetric septal hypertrophic cardiomyopathy or subaortic stenosis) and (2) hypertensive or valvular hypertrophic cardiomyopathy. Hypertrophic obstructive cardiomyopathy is the most commonly inherited cardiac disorder. It is characterized by thickening of the septal wall (Figure 23-27), which may cause outflow obstruction to the left ventricle outflow tract.[102] Obstruction of left ventricular outflow can occur when heart rate is increased and intravascular volume is decreased. This type of hypertrophic cardiomyopathy is a significant risk factor for serious ventricular dysrhythmias and sudden death, and has been implicated in more than 33% of sudden deaths in young athletes.[8,103] Hypertensive or valvular hypertrophic cardiomyopathy occurs because of increased resistance to ventricular ejection, which is commonly seen in individuals with hypertension or valvular stenosis (usually aortic). In this case, hypertrophy of the myocytes is an attempt to compensate for increased myocardial workload. Long-term dysfunction of the myocytes develops over time, with first diastolic dysfunction leading eventually to systolic dysfunction of the ventricle (see "Heart Failure," p. 622). Individuals with hypertrophic cardiomyopathy may be asymptomatic or may complain of angina, syncope, dyspnea on exertion, and palpitations. Examination may reveal extra heart sounds and murmurs. Echocardiography and cardiac catheterization can confirm the diagnosis.

Restrictive cardiomyopathy is characterized by restrictive filling and increased diastolic pressure of either or both ventricles with normal or near-normal systolic function and wall thickness. It may occur idiopathically or as a cardiac manifestation of systemic diseases, such as scleroderma, amyloidosis, sarcoidosis, lymphoma, and hemochromatosis, or a number of inherited storage diseases. The myocardium becomes rigid and noncompliant, impeding ventricular filling and raising filling pressures during diastole. The overall clinical and hemodynamic picture mimics and may be confused with that of constrictive pericarditis.

> ✔ **QUICK CHECK 23-7**
> 1. Why does pericarditis develop?
> 2. What are the cardiomyopathies? List the major disorders.
> 3. Briefly describe the pathophysiologic effects of the cardiomyopathies.

Disorders of the Endocardium
Valvular Dysfunction
Disorders of the endocardium (the innermost lining of the heart wall) damage the heart valves, which are composed of endocardial tissue. Endocardial damage can be either congenital or acquired. The acquired forms result from inflammatory, ischemic, traumatic, degenerative, or infectious alterations of valvular structure and function. One of the most common causes of acquired valvular dysfunction is degeneration or inflammation of the endocardium secondary to rheumatic heart disease (Table 23-6). Structural alterations of the heart valves are caused by remodeling changes in the valvular extracellular matrix and lead to stenosis, incompetence, or both.

In valvular stenosis, the valve orifice is constricted and narrowed, so blood cannot flow forward and the workload of the cardiac chamber proximal to the diseased valve increases (Figure 23-28). Pressure (intraventricular or atrial) rises in the chamber to overcome resistance to flow through the valve, necessitating greater exertion by the myocardium and producing myocardial hypertrophy.

Although all four heart valves may be affected, in adults those of the left heart (mitral and aortic valves) are far more commonly affected than those of the right heart (tricuspid and pulmonic valves). In valvular regurgitation (also called insufficiency or incompetence), the valve leaflets, or cusps, fail to shut completely, permitting blood flow to continue even when the valve is presumably closed (see Figure 23-28).

TABLE 23-6 CLINICAL MANIFESTATIONS OF VALVULAR STENOSIS AND REGURGITATION

MANIFESTATION	AORTIC STENOSIS	MITRAL STENOSIS	AORTIC REGURGITATION	MITRAL REGURGITATION	TRICUSPID REGURGITATION
Most common cause	Congenital bicuspid valve, degenerative (calcific) changes with aging, rheumatic heart disease	Rheumatic heart disease	Infective endocarditis; aortic root disease (connective tissue diseases, Marfan syndrome); dilation of aortic root from hypertension and aging	Myxomatous degeneration (mitral valve prolapse)	Congenital
Cardiovascular outcome (untreated)	Left ventricular hypertrophy followed by left heart failure; decreased coronary blood flow with myocardial ischemia	Left atrial hypertrophy and dilation with fibrillation, followed by right ventricular failure	Left ventricular hypertrophy and dilation, followed by left heart failure	Left atrial hypertrophy and dilation, followed by left heart failure	Right heart failure
Pulmonary effects	Pulmonary edema: dyspnea on exertion	Pulmonary edema: dyspnea on exertion, orthopnea, paroxysmal nocturnal dyspnea, predisposition to respiratory tract infections, hemoptysis, pulmonary hypertension	Pulmonary edema with dyspnea on exertion	Pulmonary edema with dyspnea on exertion	Dyspnea
Central nervous system effects	Syncope, especially on exertion	Neural deficits only associated with emboli (e.g., hemiparesis)	Syncope	None	None
Pain	Angina pectoris	Atypical chest pain	Angina pectoris	Atypical chest pain	Palpitations
Heart sounds	Systolic murmur heard best at right parasternal second intercostal space and radiating to neck	Low rumbling diastolic murmur heard best at apex and radiating to axilla, accentuated first heart sound, opening snap	Diastolic murmur heard best at right parasternal second intercostal space and radiating to neck	Murmur throughout systole heard best at apex and radiating to axilla	Murmur throughout systole heard best at left lower sternal border

With data from Braunwald E, editor: *Heart disease: a textbook of cardiovascular medicine,* ed 5, Philadelphia, 1997, Saunders; Carabello BA, Paulus WJ: Valvular heart disease. In Crawford MH, DiMarco JP, editors: *Cardiology,* London, 2001, Mosby.

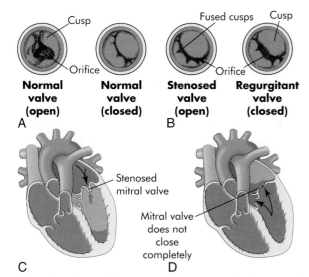

FIGURE 23-28 Valvular Stenosis and Regurgitation. **A,** Normal position of the valve leaflets, or cusps, when the valve is open and closed. **B,** Open position of a stenosed valve (left) and open position of a closed regurgitant valve (right). **C,** Hemodynamic effect of mitral stenosis. The stenosed valve is unable to open sufficiently during left atrial systole, inhibiting left ventricular filling. **D,** Hemodynamic effect of mitral regurgitation. The mitral valve does not close completely during left ventricular systole, permitting blood to reenter the left atrium.

During systole or diastole, some blood leaks back into the chamber proximal to the diseased valve, which increases the volume of blood the heart must pump and increases the workload of both atrium and ventricle. Increased volume leads to chamber dilation, and increased workload leads to hypertrophy, both of which are compensatory mechanisms intended to increase the pumping capability of the heart but that lead to cardiac dysfunction over time. Eventually, myocardial contractility diminishes, ejection fraction is reduced, diastolic pressure increases, and the ventricles fail from being overworked. Depending on the severity of the valvular dysfunction and the capacity of the heart to compensate, valvular alterations cause a range of symptoms and some degree of incapacitation (see Table 23-6).

In general, valvular disease is diagnosed by echocardiography, which can be used to assess the severity of valvular obstruction or regurgitation before the onset of symptoms. Management almost always includes careful fluid management, valvular repair, or valve replacement with a prosthetic valve followed by long-term anticoagulation therapy and prophylaxis for endocarditis as needed.[104,105]

Stenosis

Aortic stenosis. Aortic stenosis is the most common valvular abnormality, affecting nearly 2% of adults older than 65 years of age.[8] It has three common causes: (1) congenital bicuspid valve, (2) degeneration with aging, and (3) inflammatory damage caused by rheumatic heart disease. Numerous gene abnormalities have been associated with aortic stenosis. Aortic stenosis is also associated with many risk factors for coronary artery disease.[8] Aortic valve degeneration with aging is associated with chronic inflammation, lipoprotein deposition in the

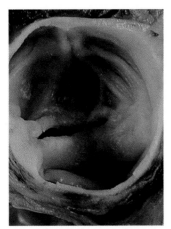

FIGURE 23-29 Aortic Stenosis. Mild stenosis in valve leaflets of a young adult. (From Damjanov I, Linder J: *Pathophysiology: a color atlas*, St Louis, 2000, Mosby.)

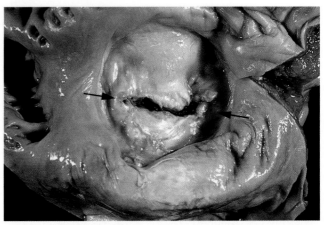

FIGURE 23-30 Mitral Stenosis With Classic "Fish Mouth" Orifice. (From Kumar V, Abbas A, Fausto N et al: *Pathologic basis of disease*, ed 8, St Louis, 2010, Mosby.)

tissue, and leaflet calcification. The orifice of the aortic valve narrows, causing resistance to blood flow from the left ventricle into the aorta (Figure 23-29). Outflow obstruction increases pressure within the left ventricle as it tries to eject blood through the narrowed opening. Left ventricular hypertrophy develops to compensate for the increased workload. Eventually, hypertrophy increases myocardial oxygen demand, which the coronary arteries may not be able to supply. If this occurs, ischemia may cause attacks of angina. In addition, aortic stenosis is frequently accompanied by atherosclerotic coronary disease, further contributing to inadequate coronary perfusion. Untreated aortic stenosis can lead to hypertrophic cardiomyopathy, dysrhythmias, myocardial infarction, and heart failure.[105]

Aortic stenosis usually develops gradually. Classic symptoms include angina, syncope, and dyspnea. Clinical manifestations include decreased stroke volume and narrowed pulse pressure (the difference between systolic and diastolic pressure). Heart rate is often slow, and pulses are delayed. Resistance to flow leads to a crescendo-decrescendo systolic heart murmur heard best at the right parasternal second intercostal space and may radiate to the neck. Echocardiography can be used to assess the severity of valvular obstruction before the onset of symptoms, and management almost always includes valve replacement with a prosthetic valve followed by long-term anticoagulation therapy and prophylaxis for endocarditis as needed. Percutaneous placement of a prosthetic valve avoids major heart surgery in selected individuals.[106] Once individuals become symptomatic from aortic stenosis, the prognosis is poor.

Mitral stenosis. **Mitral stenosis** impairs the flow of blood from the left atrium to the left ventricle. Mitral stenosis is more common in women and occurs in 40% of individuals with a history of rheumatic heart disease.[8] Autoimmunity in response to group A β-hemolytic streptococcal M protein antigens leads to inflammation and scarring of the valvular leaflets. Scarring causes the leaflets to become fibrous and fused, and the chordae tendineae cordis become shortened (Figure 23-30).

Impedance to blood flow results in incomplete emptying of the left atrium and elevated atrial pressure as the chamber tries to force blood through the stenotic valve. Continued increases in left atrial volume and pressure cause atrial dilation and hypertrophy. The risk of developing atrial dysrhythmias (especially fibrillation) and dysrhythmia-induced thrombi is high. As mitral stenosis progresses, symptoms of decreased cardiac output occur, especially during exertion. Continued elevation of left atrial pressure and volume causes pressure to rise in

the pulmonary circulation. If untreated, chronic mitral stenosis develops into pulmonary hypertension, pulmonary edema, and right ventricular failure.

Blood flow through the stenotic valve results in a rumbling decrescendo diastolic murmur heard best over the cardiac apex and radiating to the left axilla. If the mitral valve is forced open during diastole, it may make a sharp noise called an opening snap. The first heart sound (S_1) is often accentuated and somewhat delayed because of increased left atrial pressure. Other signs and symptoms are generally those of pulmonary congestion and right heart failure. Atrial enlargement and valvular obstruction are demonstrated by chest x-ray films, electrocardiography, and echocardiography. Management includes anticoagulation therapy and endocarditis prophylaxis along with beta-blockers or calcium channel blockers to slow the heart rate. Mitral stenosis can often be repaired surgically but may require valve replacement (usually porcine) in advanced cases.[105]

Regurgitation

Aortic regurgitation. Aortic regurgitation results from an inability of the aortic valve leaflets to close properly during diastole because of abnormalities of the leaflets, the aortic root and annulus, or both. It can be congenital (bicuspid valve) or acquired. Acquired aortic regurgitation may be idiopathic, or it can be caused by rheumatic heart disease, bacterial endocarditis, syphilis, hypertension, connective tissue disorders (e.g., Marfan syndrome and ankylosing spondylitis), appetite-suppressing medications, trauma, or atherosclerosis. During systole, blood is ejected from the left ventricle into the aorta. During diastole, some of the ejected blood flows back into the left ventricle through the leaking valve. Volume overload occurs in the ventricle because it receives blood both from the left atrium and from the aorta during diastole. The hemodynamic abnormalities depend on the amount of regurgitation. As the end-diastolic volume of the left ventricle increases, myocardial fibers stretch to accommodate the extra fluid. Compensatory dilation permits the left ventricle to increase its stroke volume and maintain cardiac output. Ventricular hypertrophy also occurs as an adaptation to the increased volume and because of increased afterload created by the high stroke volume and resultant systolic hypertension. Over time, ventricular dilation and hypertrophy eventually cannot compensate for aortic incompetence, and heart failure develops.

Clinical manifestations include widened pulse pressure resulting from increased stroke volume and diastolic backflow. Turbulence across the aortic valve during diastole produces a decrescendo murmur

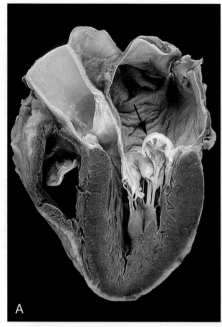
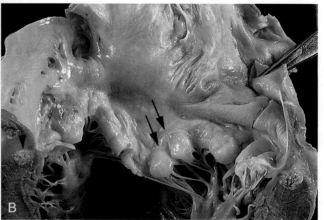

FIGURE 23-31 Mitral Valve Prolapse. **A,** Prolapsed mitral valve. Prolapse permits the valve leaflets to billow back *(arrow)* into the atrium during left ventricular systole. The billowing causes the leaflets to part slightly, permitting regurgitation into the atrium. **B,** Looking down into the mitral valve, the ballooning *(arrows)* of the leaflets is seen. (From Kumar V: *Pathologic basis of disease,* ed 8, St Louis, 2010, Mosby.)

in the second, third, or fourth intercostal spaces parasternally and may radiate to the neck. Large stroke volume and rapid runoff of blood from the aorta cause prominent carotid pulsations and bounding peripheral pulses (Corrigan pulse). Other symptoms are usually associated with heart failure that occurs when the ventricle can no longer pump adequately. Dysrhythmias are a common complication of aortic regurgitation. The severity of regurgitation can be estimated by echocardiography, and valve replacement may be delayed for many years through careful use of vasodilators and inotropic agents.[105]

Mitral regurgitation. Mitral regurgitation has many possible causes, including mitral valve prolapse, rheumatic heart disease, infective endocarditis, MI, connective tissue diseases (Marfan syndrome), and dilated cardiomyopathy. Mitral regurgitation permits backflow of blood from the left ventricle into the left atrium during ventricular systole, producing a holosystolic (throughout systole) murmur heard best at the apex, which radiates into the back and axilla. Because of increased volume from the left atrium, the left ventricle becomes dilated and hypertrophied to maintain adequate cardiac output. The volume of backflow reentering the left atrium gradually increases, causing atrial dilation and associated atrial fibrillation. As the left atrium enlarges, the valve structures stretch and become deformed, leading to further backflow. As mitral valve regurgitation progresses, left ventricular function may become impaired to the point of failure. Eventually, increased atrial pressure leads to pulmonary hypertension and failure of the right ventricle.[105] Mitral incompetence is usually well tolerated—often for years—until ventricular failure occurs. Most clinical manifestations are caused by heart failure. The severity of regurgitation can be estimated by echocardiography, and surgical repair or valve replacement may become necessary. In acute mitral regurgitation due to MI, surgical repair must be done emergently.

Tricuspid regurgitation. Tricuspid regurgitation is more common than tricuspid stenosis and is usually associated with failure and

dilation of the right ventricle secondary to pulmonary hypertension (see p. 700). Rheumatic heart disease and infective endocarditis are less common causes. Tricuspid valve incompetence leads to volume overload in the right atrium and ventricle, increased systemic venous blood pressure, and right heart failure. Pulmonic valve dysfunction can have the same consequences as tricuspid valve dysfunction.

Mitral Valve Prolapse Syndrome

In **mitral valve prolapse syndrome (MVPS),** one or both of the cusps of the mitral valve billow upward (prolapse) into the left atrium during systole (Figure 23-31). The most common cause of mitral valve prolapse is myxomatous degeneration of the leaflets in which the cusps are redundant, thickened, and scalloped because of changes in tissue proteoglycans, increased levels of proteinases, and infiltration by myofibroblasts. Mitral regurgitation occurs if the ballooning valve permits blood to leak into the atrium.[107]

Mitral valve prolapse is the most common valve disorder in the United States, with a prevalence of 2.4% of adults.[8] Studies suggest an autosomal dominant inheritance pattern. Because mitral valve prolapse can be associated with other inherited connective tissue disorders (Marfan syndrome, Ehlers-Danlos syndrome, osteogenesis imperfecta), it has been suggested that it results from a genetic or environmental disruption of valvular development during the fifth or sixth week of gestation. There also may be a relationship between symptomatic mitral valve prolapse and hyperthyroidism.

Many cases of mitral valve prolapse are completely asymptomatic. Cardiac auscultation on routine physical examination may disclose a regurgitant murmur or midsystolic click in an otherwise healthy individual, or echocardiography may demonstrate the condition in the absence of auscultatory findings. Symptomatic mitral valve prolapse can cause palpitations related to dysrhythmias, tachycardia, lightheadedness, syncope, fatigue (especially in the morning), lethargy,

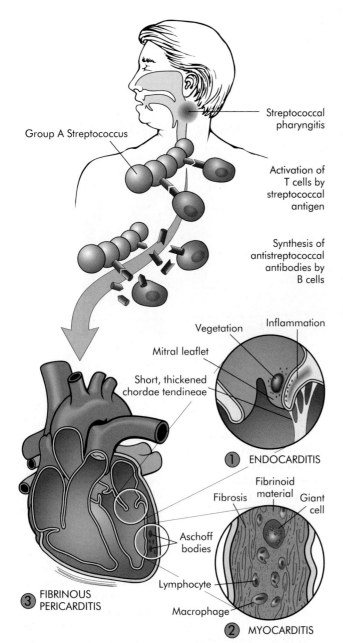

FIGURE 23-32 Pathogenesis and Structural Alterations of Acute Rheumatic Heart Disease. Beginning usually with a sore throat, rheumatic fever can develop only as a sequel to pharyngeal infection by group A β-hemolytic streptococcus. Suspected as a hypersensitivity reaction, it is proposed that antibodies directed against the M proteins of certain strains of streptococci cross-react with tissue glycoproteins in the heart, joints, and other tissues. The exact nature of cross-reacting antigens has been difficult to define, but it appears that the streptococcal infection causes an autoimmune response against self-antigens. Inflammatory lesions are found in various sites; the most distinctive within the heart are called Aschoff bodies. The chronic sequelae result from progressive fibrosis because of healing of the inflammatory lesions and the changes induced by valvular deformities. (From Damjanov I: *Pathology for the health professions,* ed 3, St Louis, 2006, Saunders.)

weakness, dyspnea, chest tightness, hyperventilation, anxiety, depression, panic attacks, and atypical chest pain. Many symptoms are vague and puzzling and are unrelated to the degree of prolapse. Most individuals with mitral valve prolapse have an excellent prognosis, do not develop symptoms, and do not require any restriction in activity or medical management. Occasionally, beta-blockers are needed to alleviate syncope, severe chest pain, or palpitations. A subset of individuals have an increased risk for complications such as infective endocarditis, cardioembolic stroke, and sudden death. These high-risk individuals can be identified by clinical and echocardiographic findings.[105]

Acute Rheumatic Fever and Rheumatic Heart Disease

Rheumatic fever is a systemic, inflammatory disease caused by a delayed exaggerated immune response to infection by the group A β-hemolytic streptococcus in genetically predisposed individuals. In its acute form, rheumatic fever is a febrile illness characterized by inflammation of the joints, skin, nervous system, and heart.[108] If untreated, rheumatic fever can cause scarring and deformity of cardiac structures, resulting in **rheumatic heart disease (RHD).**

The incidence of acute rheumatic fever declined in the United States during the 1960s, 1970s, and early 1980s because of medical and socioeconomic improvements. More recent outbreaks in the United States and abroad corresponded to the reappearance of highly virulent strains of the streptococcal microorganisms. The acute disease occurs most often in children between the ages of 5 and 15 years. Appropriate antibiotic therapy given within the first 9 days of infection usually prevents rheumatic fever.

PATHOPHYSIOLOGY Acute rheumatic fever can develop only as a sequel to pharyngeal infection by group A β-hemolytic streptococcus. Streptococcal skin infections do not progress to acute rheumatic fever, although both skin and pharyngeal infections can cause acute glomerulonephritis. This is because the strains of the microorganism that affect the skin do not have the same antigenic molecules in their cell membranes as those that cause pharyngitis and, therefore, do not elicit the same kind of immune response. Acute rheumatic fever is the result of an abnormal humoral and cell-mediated immune response to group A streptococcal cell membrane antigens called *M proteins* (Figure 23-32). This immune response cross-reacts with molecularly similar self-antigens in heart, muscle, brain, and joints, causing an autoimmune response that results in diffuse, proliferative, and exudative inflammatory lesions in these tissues.[108] The inflammation may subside before treatment, leaving behind damage to the heart valves. Repeated attacks of acute rheumatic fever cause chronic proliferative changes in the previously mentioned organs with resultant tissue scarring, granuloma formation, and thrombosis.

Approximately 10% of individuals with rheumatic fever develop rheumatic heart disease (RHD). In developed countries, the peak incidence of the development of RHD occurs in adults between the ages of 25 and 34. Although rheumatic fever can cause carditis in all three layers of the heart wall, the primary lesion usually involves the endocardium. Endocardial inflammation causes swelling of the valve leaflets, with secondary erosion along the lines of leaflet contact. Small, beadlike clumps of vegetation containing platelets and fibrin are deposited on eroded valvular tissue and on the chordae tendineae cordis. These lesions can become progressively adherent. Scarring and shortening of the involved structures occur over time. The valves lose their elasticity, and the leaflets may adhere to each other.

TABLE 23-7	JONES CRITERIA (UPDATED) USED FOR DIAGNOSIS OF INITIAL ATTACK OF RHEUMATIC FEVER
CRITERIA	**DESCRIPTION**
Major Manifestations	
Carditis	Previously undetected murmur, chest pain, pericardial effusion with audible friction rub, extra heart sounds, conduction delays, atrial fibrillation, and prolonged PR interval; valvular diseases (stenosis and regurgitation); recurrent infective endocarditis
Polyarthritis	Migratory polyarthritis (especially large joints of extremities); each joint simultaneously or in succession symptomatic for approximately 2 to 3 days; polyarthritis continued for up to 3 weeks; exudative synovitis (heat, redness, swelling, severe pain)
Chorea	Sudden, aimless, irregular, involuntary movements; more common in females than in males; may occur several months after streptococcal infection; self-limiting, lasting weeks or months; no permanent neural sequelae
Erythema marginatum	Nonpruritic, pink, erythematous macules on trunk that do not occur on face or hands; transitory and may change in appearance within minutes or hours; heat darkens rash; macules may fade in center and be mistaken for ringworm
Subcutaneous nodules	Palpable subcutaneous nodes over bony prominences and along extensor tendons
Minor Manifestations	
Arthralgias	Pain and stiffness in joints without heat, redness, or swelling
Fever	>39° C
Elevated CRP	Indicates inflammation
Prolonged PR interval	Change in ECG consistent with abnormal conduction
Supporting evidence of streptococcal infection	Increased titer of streptococcal antibodies: antistreptolysin O (ASO), positive throat streptococcal infection culture for group A *Streptococcus*

Data from Guidelines for the diagnosis of rheumatic fever: Jones Criteria, 1992 update; Special Writing Group of the Committee on Rheumatic Fever, Endocarditis, and Kawasaki Disease of the Council on Cardiovascular Disease in the Young of the American Heart Association, *JAMA* 268(15):2069–2073, 1992.

If inflammation penetrates the myocardium, called myocarditis, localized fibrin deposits develop that are surrounded by areas of necrosis. These fibrinoid necrotic deposits are called Aschoff bodies. Pericardial inflammation is usually characterized by serofibrinous effusion within the pericardial cavity. Cardiomegaly and left heart failure may occur during episodes of untreated acute or recurrent rheumatic fever. Conduction defects and atrial fibrillation often are associated with rheumatic heart disease.

CLINICAL MANIFESTATIONS   The common symptoms of acute rheumatic fever are fever, lymphadenopathy, arthralgia, nausea, vomiting, epistaxis (nosebleed), abdominal pain, and tachycardia. The major clinical manifestations of acute rheumatic fever usually occur singly or in combination 1 to 5 weeks after streptococcal infection of the pharynx. They are carditis, acute migratory polyarthritis, chorea, erythema marginatum, and subcutaneous nodules. Criteria for the diagnosis of rheumatic fever have been developed and updated by both the American Heart Association (Jones criteria; Table 23-7) and the World Health Organization (WHO).[109,110]

EVALUATION AND TREATMENT   As described in Table 23-7, supportive evidence for group A β-hemolytic streptococci includes positive throat cultures and measurement of serum antibodies against the hemolytic factor *streptolysin O*. Cultures may be negative when the rheumatic attack begins, however. Several other antibody tests are sensitive prognosticators of streptococcal infection, including antideoxyribonuclease B (anti-DNase B), antihyaluronidase, and antistreptozyme (ASTZ). Elevated measurements of white blood cell count, erythrocyte sedimentation rate, and C-reactive protein indicate inflammation. All three are usually increased at the time cardiac or joint symptoms begin to appear.

Therapy for acute rheumatic fever is aimed at eradicating the streptococcal infection and involves a 10-day regimen of oral penicillin or erythromycin administration. Nonsteroidal anti-inflammatory drugs are used as anti-inflammatory agents for both rheumatic carditis and arthritis. Serious carditis may require corticosteroids and diuretics. Because recurrent rheumatic fever occurs in more than half of affected children, continuous prophylactic antibiotic therapy may be necessary for as long as 5 years. Several potential group A streptococcus vaccines are being developed.[111] RHD may require surgical repair of damaged valves.

> **✓ QUICK CHECK 23-8**
> 1. Compare the effect of aortic stenosis with mitral stenosis on the left ventricle and atrium.
> 2. Describe aortic regurgitation, mitral regurgitation, and tricuspid regurgitation.
> 3. What are the common symptoms of mitral prolapse?
> 4. What is the cause of rheumatic heart disease?

Infective Endocarditis

Infective endocarditis is a general term used to describe infection and inflammation of the endocardium—especially the cardiac valves. There are approximately 15,000 new cases of infective endocarditis per year in the United States and it accounts for approximately 1 in 1000 admissions to the hospital.[112] Bacteria are the most common cause of infective endocarditis, especially streptococci, staphylococci, and enterococci. Other causes include viruses, fungi, rickettsia, and parasites. Infective endocarditis was once a lethal disease, but morbidity and mortality diminished significantly with the advent of antibiotics and improved diagnostic techniques (see *Risk Factors:* Infective Endocarditis).

PATHOPHYSIOLOGY The pathogenesis of infective endocarditis requires at least three critical elements (Figure 23-33):

1. *Endocardial damage.* Trauma, congenital heart disease, valvular heart disease, and the presence of prosthetic valves are the most common risk factors for endocardial damage that leads to infective endocarditis. Turbulent blood caused by these abnormalities usually affects the atrial surface of atrioventricular valves or the ventricular surface of semilunar valves.[112] Endocardial damage exposes the endothelial basement membrane, which contains a type of collagen that attracts platelets and thereby stimulates sterile thrombus formation on the membrane. This causes an inflammatory reaction (nonbacterial thrombotic endocarditis).

2. *Adherence of blood-borne microorganisms to the damaged endocardial surface.* Bacteria may enter the bloodstream during injection drug use, trauma, dental procedures that involve manipulation of the gingiva, cardiac surgery, genitourinary procedures and

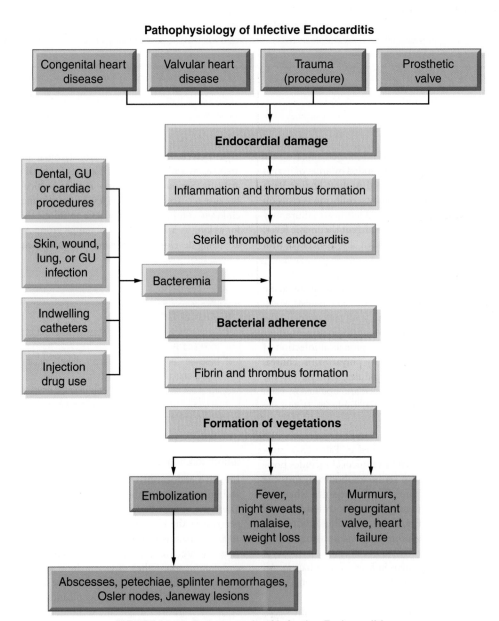

FIGURE 23-33 Pathogenesis of Infective Endocarditis.

indwelling catheters in the presence of infection, or gastrointestinal instrumentation, or they may spread from uncomplicated upper respiratory tract or skin infections. Bacteria adhere to the damaged endocardium using adhesins.[112]

3. *Formation of infective endocardial vegetations* (Figure 23-34). Bacteria infiltrate the sterile thrombi and accelerate fibrin formation by activating the clotting cascade. These vegetative lesions can form anywhere on the endocardium but usually occur on heart valves and surrounding structures. Although endocardial tissue is constantly bathed in antibody-containing blood and is surrounded by scavenging monocytes and polymorphonuclear leukocytes, bacterial colonies are inaccessible to host defenses because they are embedded in the protective fibrin clots. Embolization from these vegetations can lead to abscesses and characteristic skin changes, such as petechiae, splinter hemorrhages, Osler nodes, and Janeway lesions.

CLINICAL MANIFESTATIONS Infective endocarditis may be acute, subacute, or chronic. It causes varying degrees of valvular dysfunction and may be associated with manifestations involving several organ systems (respiratory [lungs], sensory [eyes], genitourinary [kidneys], musculoskeletal [bones, joints], and central nervous systems), making diagnosis exceedingly difficult. Signs and symptoms of infective endocarditis are caused by infection and inflammation, systemic spread of microemboli, and immune complex deposition. The "classic" findings are fever; new or changed cardiac murmur; and petechial lesions of the skin, conjunctiva, and oral mucosa. Characteristic physical findings include Osler nodes (painful erythematous nodules on the pads of the fingers and toes) and Janeway lesions (nonpainful hemorrhagic lesions on the palms and soles).[113] Other manifestations include weight loss, back pain, night sweats, and heart failure. Central nervous system, splenic, renal, pulmonary peripheral arterial, coronary, and ocular emboli may lead to a wide variety of signs and symptoms.

EVALUATION AND TREATMENT The criteria for the diagnosis of infective endocarditis include recognized risk factors, fever, repetitive blood cultures positive for bacteria, appropriate physical examination findings (murmur, skin findings), vascular complications, and echocardiographic documentation.[112] If infective endocarditis extends into the heart wall and invades the conduction system, electrocardiography may show significant conduction delays. If emboli to other organs are

suggested, scans can be performed to confirm their presence. Antimicrobial therapy is generally given for several weeks, beginning with intravenous and ending with oral administration. In some cases, two different antibiotics are given simultaneously to eliminate the offending microorganism and prevent the development of drug resistance. Other drugs may be necessary to treat left heart failure secondary to valvular dysfunction.[114]

Surgery that involves excision of infected tissue with or without valve replacement improves outcomes in many persons with infective endocarditis, especially those with severe heart failure or persistent bacteremia despite antibiotic therapy.[115] Unfortunately, valve failure and valve-induced embolization are known consequences of prosthetic valve placement, and the presence of an artificial valve is itself a significant risk factor for infective endocarditis.

In the past, individuals with valvular heart disease received prophylactic antibiotics for dental, genitourinary, or gastrointestinal procedures to prevent infective endocarditis. However, in 2008 the recommendations were changed such that only "high risk" individuals (history of infective endocarditis, prosthetic valves, cyanotic congenital heart disease, heart transplant with valvular defect) receive antibiotic prophylaxis, and only in the setting of gingival procedures or in the presence of documented acute gastrointestinal or genitourinary infection.[116]

Cardiac Complications in Acquired Immunodeficiency Syndrome (AIDS)

Individuals with HIV infection and AIDS are at risk for cardiac complications including dilated cardiomyopathy, myocarditis, pericardial effusion, endocarditis, pulmonary hypertension, and nonantiretroviral drug–related cardiotoxicity. In addition, cardiac involvement may be induced by various bacterial, viral, protozoal, mycobacterial, and fungal pathogens that complicate AIDS. Malignancies, such as lymphoma and Kaposi sarcoma, are seen often in individuals with AIDS and can affect the heart. Furthermore, treatment with highly active antiretroviral therapy (HAART) can cause hyperlipidemia and atherosclerotic disease.

Left heart failure is the most common complication of HIV infection and is related to left ventricular dilation and dysfunction. Pericardial effusion, ventricular dysrhythmias, electrocardiographic changes, and right ventricular dilation and hypertrophy are other less common findings.

> ✔ **QUICK CHECK 23-9**
> 1. What three critical elements are required for the pathogenesis of infective endocarditis?
> 2. Why does infective endocarditis involve several organ systems?
> 3. What effect does AIDS have on the heart?

MANIFESTATIONS OF HEART DISEASE

Dysrhythmias

A **dysrhythmia,** or **arrhythmia,** is a disturbance of heart rhythm. Normal heart rhythms are generated by the sinoatrial (SA) node and travel through the heart's conduction system, causing the atrial and ventricular myocardium to contract and relax at a regular rate that is appropriate to maintain circulation at various levels of physical activity (see Chapter 22). Dysrhythmias range in severity from occasional "missed" or rapid beats to serious disturbances that impair the pumping ability of the heart, contributing to heart failure and death. Dysrhythmias can be caused either by an abnormal rate of impulse generation (Table 23-8) from the SA node or other pacemaker or by the abnormal conduction of impulses (Table 23-9) through the heart's conduction system, including the myocardial cells themselves.

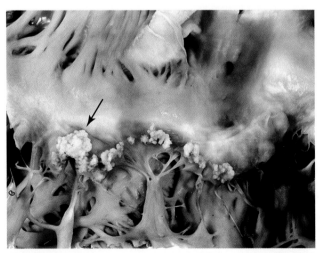

FIGURE 23-34 Bacterial Endocarditis of Mitral Valve. The valve is covered with large, irregular vegetations *(arrow).* (From Damjanov I, Linder J: *Pathology: a color atlas,* St Louis, 2000, Mosby.)

TABLE 23-8 DISORDERS OF IMPULSE FORMATION

TYPE	ELECTROCARDIOGRAM	EFFECT	PATHOPHYSIOLOGY	TREATMENT
Sinus bradycardia	P rate 60 or less PR interval normal QRS for each P	Increased preload Decreased mean arterial pressure	Hyperkalemia: slows depolarization Vagal hyperactivity: unknown Digoxin toxicity common Late hypoxia: lack of adenosine triphosphate (ATP)	If hypotensive, treat cause Sympathomimetics, anticholinergics Pacemaker placement
Simple sinus tachycardia	P rate 100-150 PR interval normal QRS for each P	Decreased filling times Decreased mean arterial pressure Increased myocardial demand	Catecholamines: rise in resting potential and calcium influx Fever: unknown Early heart failure: compensatory response to decreased stroke volume Lung disease: hypoxic cell metabolism Hypercalcemia	Oxygen, bed rest Calcium blockers
Premature atrial contractions (PACs) or beats*	Early P waves that may have morphologic changes PR interval normal QRS for each P	Occasional decreased filling time and mean arterial pressure	Electrolyte disturbances (especially hypercalcemia): alter action potentials Hypoxia and elevated preload: cell membrane disturbances	Treat underlying cause Digoxin
Sinus dysrhythmias	Rate varies P-P regularly irregular, short with inspiration, long with exhalation PR interval normal QRS for each P	Variable filling times Variable mean arterial pressure Variable oxygen demand	Unknown Common in young children and young adults	None
Atrial tachycardia (includes premature atrial tachycardia if onset is abrupt)	P rate 151-250 P morphology may differ from sinus P PR interval normal P/QRS ratio variable	Decreased filling time Decreased mean arterial pressure Increased myocardial demand	Same as PACs: leads to increased atrial automaticity, atrial reentry Digoxin toxicity: common Aging	Control ventricular rate Digoxin, calcium channel blockers, vagus stimulation Pacemaker to override atrial conduction Cardioversion
Atrial flutter*	P rate 251-300, morphology may vary from sinus P PR interval usually not observable P/QRS ratio variable	Decreased filling time Decreased mean arterial pressure	Same as atrial tachycardia	Same as atrial tachy- cardia
Atrial fibrillation*	P rate >300 and usually not observable No PR interval QRS rate variable and rhythm irregular	Same as atrial flutter	Same as atrial tachycardia	Same as atrial tachycardia
Idiojunctional rhythm	P absent or independent QRS normal, rate 41-59, regular	Decreased cardiac output from loss of atrial contribu- tion to ventricular preload	Atrial and sinus bradycardia, standstill, or block	Same as sinus bradycardia
Junctional bradycardia	P absent or independent QRS normal, rate 40 or less	Same as idiojunctional rhythm	Same as idiojunctional rhythm Vagal hyperactivity	Same as sinus bradycardia
Premature junctional contractions (PJCs) or beats	Early beats without P waves QRS morphology normal	Decreased cardiac output from loss of atrial contribution to ventricular preload for that beat	Hyperkalemia (5.4-6 mEq/L) Hypercalcemia, hypoxia, and elevated preload (see PACs)	Same as PAC
Accelerated junctional rhythm	P absent or independent QRS morphology normal, rate 60-99	Decreased cardiac output from loss of atrial contribu- tion to ventricular preload	Same as PJCs	Same as PAC
Junctional tachycardia	P absent or independent QRS morphology normal, rate 100 or more	Decreased cardiac output from loss of atrial contribu- tion to ventricular preload Increased myocar- dial demand because of tachycardia	Same as PJCs	Same as PAC

TABLE 23-8   DISORDERS OF IMPULSE FORMATION—cont'd

TYPE	ELECTROCARDIOGRAM	EFFECT	PATHOPHYSIOLOGY	TREATMENT
Idioventricular rhythm†	P absent or independent QRS >0.11 and rate 20-39	Same as idiojunctional rhythm	Sinus, atrial, and junctional bradycardia, standstill, or block	Same as sinus bradycardia
Ventricular bradycardia†	P absent or independent QRS >0.11 and rate 60-<60	Same as idiojunctional rhythm	Same as idiojunctional rhythm	Same as sinus bradycardia
Agonal rhythm/electromechanical dissociation†	P absent or independent QRS >0.11 and rate 20 or less	Absent or barely present cardiac output and pulse Not compatible with life	Depolarization and contraction not coupled: electrical activity present with little or no mechanical activity Usually caused by profound hypoxia	Vigorous pharmacologic treatment aimed at restoring rate and force Usually ineffective May attempt to use pacemaker
Ventricular standstill or asystole†	P absent or independent QRS absent	No cardiac output Not compatible with life	Profound ischemia, hyperkalemia, acidosis	Same as agonal rhythm, plus electrical defibrillation
Premature ventricular contractions (PVCs) or depolarizations*	Early beats with P waves QRS occasionally opposite in deflection from usual QRS	Same as premature junctional contractions	Same as PJCs, aging and induction of anesthesia Impulse originates in cell outside normal conduction system and spreads through intercalated disks	Pharmacologic interventions to change thresholds, refractory periods; reduce myocardial demand, increase supply
Accelerated ventricular rhythm	P absent or independent QRS >0.11 and rate of 41–99	Same as accelerated junctional rhythm	Same as PVCs	Removal of cause Same as PVCs
Ventricular tachycardia†	P absent or independent QRS >0.11 and rate 100 or more	Same as junctional tachycardia	Same as PVCs	Same as PVCs, plus electrical cardioversion
Ventricular fibrillation†	P absent QRS >300 and usually not observable	Same as ventricular standstill	Same as PVCs Rapid infusion of potassium	Same as PVCs, plus electrical cardioversion

*Most common in adults.
†Life-threatening in adults.

TABLE 23-9   DISORDERS OF IMPULSE CONDUCTION

TYPE	ECG	EFFECT	PATHOPHYSIOLOGY	TREATMENT
Sinus block	Occasionally absent P, with loss of QRS for that beat	Occasional decrease in cardiac output Increase in preload for following beat	Local hypoxia, scarring of intra-atrial conduction pathways, electrolyte imbalances Increased atrial preload	Conservative Usually do not progress in severity Pharmacologic treatment includes vagolytics, sympathomimetics, pacing
First-degree block*	PRI >0.2 sec	None	Same as sinus block Hyperkalemia (>7 mEq/L) Hypokalemia (<3.5 mEq/L) Formation of myocardial abscess in endocarditis	Conservative Discovery and correction of cause
Second-degree block, Mobitz I, or Wenckebach*	Progressive prolongation of PRI until one QRS is dropped Pattern of prolongation resumes	Same as sinus block	Hypokalemia (<3.5 mEq/L) Faulty cell metabolism in AV node Severity increases as heart rate increases Supports theory that AV node is fatiguing Digoxin toxicity, beta blockade CAD, MI, hypoxia, increased preload, valvular surgery and disease, diabetes	Same as sinus block
Second-degree block or Mobitz II	Same as sinus block	Same as sinus block	Hypokalemia (<3.5 mEq/L) Faulty cell metabolism below AV node Antidysrhythmics, tricyclic antidepressants CAD, MI, hypoxia, increased preload, valvular surgery and disease, diabetes	More aggressively than Mobitz I, because can progress to type III Pacemaker after pharmacologic treatment

Continued

TABLE 23-9   DISORDERS OF IMPULSE CONDUCTION—cont'd

TYPE	ECG	EFFECT	PATHOPHYSIOLOGY	TREATMENT
Third-degree block[†]	P waves present and independent of QRS. No observed relationship between P and QRS. Always AV dissociation	Same as idiojunctional rhythm	Hypokalemia (<3.5 mEq/L). Faulty cell metabolism low in bundle of His MI, especially inferior wall, as nodal artery interrupted; results in ischemia of AV node	Pacemaker after pharmacologic treatment. Temporary pacing if caused by inferior MI, because ischemia usually resolves
Atrioventricular dissociation	P waves present and independent of QRS, but not always because of block (e.g., ventricular tachycardia). AV dissociation not always third-degree block	Decreased cardiac output from loss of atrial contribution to ventricular preload. Variable effect on myocardial demand, depending on ventricular rate	May result from third-degree block or accelerated junctional or ventricular rhythm or be caused by sinus, atrial, and junctional bradycardias	Treat according to cause. Pacemaker or reducing rate of AV or ventricular discharge, or increasing rate of sinus or AV node discharge
Ventricular block	QRS >0.11 sec. R-S-R′ in V_1, V_2, V_5, V_6	None	Faulty cell metabolism in right and left bundle branches. RBBB more common than LBBB because of dual blood supply to left bundle branch. CHF, MR, especially anterior MI, because of infarct of fascicles. Left anterior hemiblock more common than left posterior hemiblock because posterior fascicles have dual blood supply	Isolated RBBB or LBBB or hemiblock not treated. If acute and/or associated with acute anterior MI, treated with permanent pacer and vigorous pharmacologic therapy
Aberrant conduction	QRS >0.11 sec	None, unless ventricular rate abnormalities present	Conduction of impulse through intercalated disks because conduction system transiently blocked as a result of hypoxia, electrolyte imbalances, digoxin toxicity, excessively rapid rate of discharge	Correct underlying cause
Preexcitation syndromes (Wolff-Parkinson-White and Lown-Ganong-Levine)	P present with QRS for each P. PRI <0.12 sec and QRS <0.11 sec because of delta wave in PRI	None	Congenital presence of accessory pathways (bundle of Kent and fiber of Mahaim) that conduct very rapidly and bypass AV node, causing early ventricular depolarization in relation to atrial depolarization. Prone to tachycardias and atrial fibrillation that can result in very rapid ventricular rates (reason unknown)	Aimed at aligning refractory periods of accessory pathway and AV node to prevent reentry. May slow rate with drug therapy. May surgically cut pathways

*Most common in adults.
†Life-threatening in adults.
AV, Atrioventricular; *CAD,* coronary artery disease; *CHF,* congestive heart failure; *LBBB,* left bundle branch block; *MI,* myocardial infarction; *MR,* mitral regurgitation; *PRI,* PR interval; *RBBB,* right bundle branch block.

Heart Failure

Heart failure is when the heart is unable to generate an adequate cardiac output, causing inadequate perfusion of tissues or increased diastolic filling pressure of the left ventricle, or both, so that pulmonary capillary pressures are increased. It affects nearly 10% of individuals older than age 65 and is the most common reason for admission to the hospital in that age group. Ischemic heart disease and hypertension are the most important predisposing risk factors.[8] Other risk factors include age, obesity, diabetes, renal failure, valvular heart disease, cardiomyopathies, myocarditis, congenital heart disease, and excessive alcohol use. Numerous genetic polymorphisms have been linked to an increased risk for heart failure, including genes for cardiomyopathies, myocyte contractility, and neurohumoral receptors. Recently, genetic changes in kinases, phosphatases, and cellular calcium cycling are being explored.[117] Most causes of heart failure result from dysfunction of the left ventricle (systolic and diastolic heart failure). The right ventricle also may be dysfunctional, especially in pulmonary disease (right ventricular failure). Finally, some conditions cause inadequate perfusion despite normal or elevated cardiac output (high-output failure).

Left Heart Failure (Congestive Heart Failure)

Left heart failure is commonly called *congestive heart failure* and can be further categorized as systolic heart failure or diastolic heart failure. It is possible for these two types of heart failure to occur simultaneously in one individual.

Systolic heart failure is defined as an inability of the heart to generate an adequate cardiac output to perfuse vital tissues. Cardiac output depends on the heart rate and stroke volume. Stroke volume is influenced by three major determinants: contractility, preload, and afterload (see Chapter 22).

Contractility is reduced by diseases that disrupt myocyte activity. Myocardial infarction is the most common primary cause of decreased contractility, and other causes include myocarditis and cardiomyopathies. Secondary causes of decreased contractility, such as recurrent myocardial ischemia and increased myocardial workload, contribute to inflammatory, immune, and neurohumoral changes (activation of the SNS and RAAS) that mediate a process called ventricular remodeling (Box 23-3).[89,118] Ventricular remodeling results in disruption of the normal myocardial extracellular structure with resultant dilation of the myocardium and causes progressive myocyte contractile dysfunction over time (Figure 23-35).[119] When contractility is decreased,

---

BOX 23-3 INFLAMMATION, IMMUNITY, AND HUMORAL FACTORS IN THE PATHOGENESIS OF HEART FAILURE

The treatment of the hemodynamic abnormalities of heart failure (HF) can provide short-term improvement in symptoms but will not prevent the progression of myocardial dysfunction over time. Studies have shown that the neurohumoral responses to heart failure (including changes in the renin-angiotensin-aldosterone system, catecholamines, natriuretic peptides, and vasopressin) exert direct cardiotoxicity that results in progressive damage to the heart muscle. Drugs such as ACE inhibitors, angiotensin receptor blockers, spironolactone, and beta-blockers can slow disease progression and are now the standard of care for HF. More recently, inflammatory cytokines such as tumor necrosis factor-alpha (TNF-α) and interleukins have been implicated in the pathogenesis of heart failure and its systemic complications (such as cachexia and malaise). Early trials with anticytokine drugs are under way.

Data from McMurray JJ: *N Engl J Med* 362:228–238, 2010; Picano E et al: *Ann N Y Acad Sci* 1207:107–115, 2010; Rehsia NS, Dhalla NS: *Heart Failure Rev* 15(1):85–101, 2010; Sciarretta S et al: *Clin Sci* 116(6):467–477, 2009; Sun Y: *Cardiovasc Res* 81(3):482–490, 2009; Triposkiadis F et al: *J Am Coll Cardiol* 54(19):1747–1762, 2009.

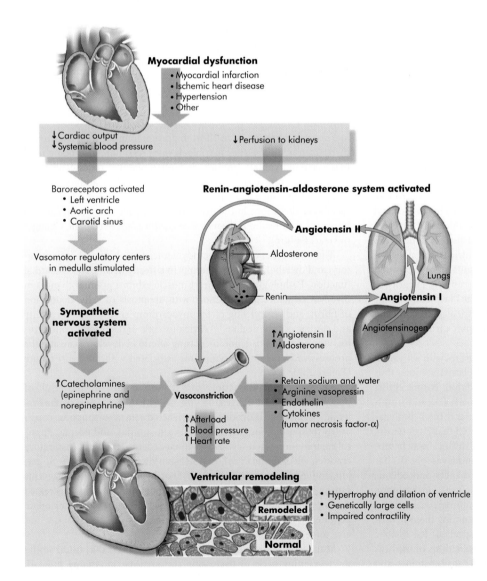

FIGURE 23-35 Pathophysiology of Ventricular Remodeling. Myocardial dysfunction activates the renin-angiotensin-aldosterone and sympathetic nervous systems, releasing neurohormones (angiotensin II, aldosterone, catecholamines, and cytokines). These neurohormones contribute to ventricular remodeling. (Redrawn from Carelock J, Clark AP: Heart failure: pathophysiologic mechanisms, *Am J Nurs* 101[12]:27, 2001.)

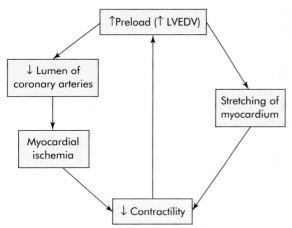

FIGURE 23-36 Effect of Elevated Preload on Myocardial Oxygen Supply and Demand. *LVEDV,* Left ventricular end-diastolic volume.

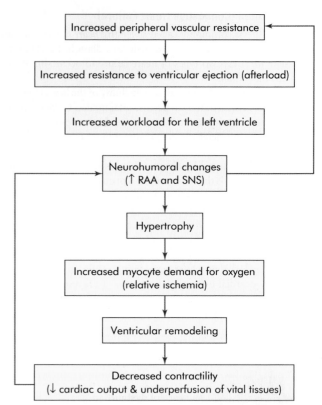

FIGURE 23-37 Role of Increased Afterload in the Pathogenesis of Heart Failure.

stroke volume falls and left ventricular end-diastolic volume (LVEDV) increases. This causes dilation of the heart and an increase in preload.

Preload, or LVEDV, increases with decreased contractility or an excess of plasma volume (intravenous fluid administration, renal failure, mitral valvular disease). Increases in LVEDV can actually improve cardiac output up to a certain point, but as preload continues to rise, it causes a stretching of the myocardium that eventually can lead to dysfunction of the sarcomeres and decreased contractility. This relationship is described by the Frank-Starling law of the heart (see Figure 22-16). Decreased contractility leads to further increases in preload (Figure 23-36).

Increased afterload is most commonly a result of increased peripheral vascular resistance (PVR), such as that seen with hypertension. It also can be the result of aortic valvular disease. With increased afterload, there is resistance to ventricular emptying and more workload for the ventricle, which responds with hypertrophy of the myocardium. Hypertrophy is mediated by angiotensin II and catecholamines and results in an increase in oxygen demand by the thickened myocardium. A state of relative ischemia develops that further contributes to changes in the myocytes themselves and ventricular remodeling (Figure 23-37).[118,120] In addition, hypertrophy results in the deposition of collagen between the myocytes, which can disrupt the integrity of the muscle, decrease contractility, and increase the likelihood that the ventricle will dilate and fail. These changes in ventricular structure and function are referred to as hypertensive hypertrophic cardiomyopathy (see p. 612).

As cardiac output falls, renal perfusion diminishes with activation of the RAAS, which acts to increase PVR and plasma volume, thus further increasing afterload and preload. In addition, baroreceptors in the central circulation detect the decrease in perfusion and stimulate the SNS to cause yet more vasoconstriction and the hypothalamus to produce antidiuretic hormone. It is believed that angiotensin, aldosterone, and the catecholamines not only disturb cardiac hemodynamics but also are directly cardiotoxic. Arginine vasopressin has been implicated in worsening electrolyte disturbances and edema, which are common complications of heart failure. Furthermore, natriuretic peptides are released in an effort to improve renal salt and water excretion but are inadequate to compensate for these neurohumoral perturbations. These neurohumoral aspects of left systolic heart failure have led to the routine use of combinations of medications that inhibit angiotensin, aldosterone, and catecholamines and

increase salt excretion in an effort to prevent long-term damage to the myocardium.[181,121] Drugs that block vasopressin are also being used in selected individuals. Immune and inflammatory processes also play an important role in the pathogenesis of heart failure and its systemic complications, such as weakness and cachexia (see Box 23-3). Other metabolic alterations in the myocardium include changes in calcium transport and insulin resistance (see *Health Alert:* Metabolic Changes in Heart Failure).

The interaction of these hemodynamic, neurohumoral, inflammatory, and metabolic processes results in a steady decline in myocardial function. Pathologically, the heart muscle exhibits gradual changes in myocyte structure and function, with apoptosis of cells, deposition of fibrin, and remodeling of the myocardium such that contractility and cardiac output decline.[118] A vicious cycle of decreasing contractility, increasing preload, and increasing afterload develops, causing the progressive worsening of symptoms associated with left heart failure (Figure 23-38).

The clinical manifestations of left heart failure are the result of pulmonary vascular congestion and inadequate perfusion of the systemic circulation. Individuals experience dyspnea, orthopnea, cough of frothy sputum, fatigue, decreased urine output, and edema. Physical examination often reveals pulmonary edema (cyanosis, inspiratory crackles, pleural effusions), hypotension or hypertension, an S_3 gallop, and evidence of underlying CAD or hypertension. The diagnosis can be further confirmed with echocardiography showing decreased cardiac output and cardiomegaly. The level of serum brain natriuretic peptide (BNP) can also help make the diagnosis of heart failure and give some insight into its severity.[122]

Management of systolic left heart failure is aimed at interrupting the worsening cycle of decreasing contractility, increasing preload,

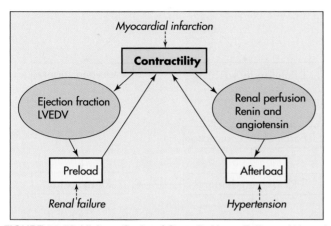

FIGURE 23-38 Vicious Cycle of Systolic Heart Failure. Although the initial insult may be one of primary decreased contractility (e.g., myocardial infarction), increased preload (e.g., renal failure), or increased afterload (e.g., hypertension), all three factors play a role in the progression of left heart failure (LHF). *LVEDV,* Left ventricular end-diastolic volume.

and increasing afterload. The acute onset of left heart failure is most often the result of acute myocardial ischemia and must be managed in conjunction with management of the underlying coronary disease (see p. 601). Oxygen, nitrate, and morphine administration improves myocardial oxygenation and helps relieve coronary spasm while lowering preload through systemic venodilation. Intravenous inotropic drugs, such as dopamine or dobutamine, increase contractility and can help raise the blood pressure in hypotensive individuals, and new inotropic drugs (e.g., levosimendan) are being evaluated. Diuretics reduce preload. ACE inhibitors, ARBs, and aldosterone blockers reduce both preload and afterload by decreasing aldosterone levels and reducing PVR. Short-acting intravenous beta-blockers also have been found to reduce mortality in selected people. Intravenous human recombinant brain natriuretic peptide (BNP) also may be used in acute heart failure, although the benefits of this therapy continue to be debated.[123] Finally, individuals with severe systolic failure may benefit from acute coronary bypass or percutaneous coronary intervention (PCI). These people often are supported with the intra-aortic balloon pump (IABP) until surgery can be performed. The IABP is positioned in the aorta just distal to the aortic valve and is inflated during diastole to improve coronary perfusion and deflated during systole to reduce afterload.

Management of chronic left heart failure relies on reducing preload and afterload. Salt restriction and diuretics (especially spironolactone) are effective in reducing preload. ACE inhibitors (or Ang II receptor blockers) reduce preload and afterload and have been shown to significantly reduce mortality in individuals with chronic left heart failure. Aldosterone blockers are also associated with improved outcomes. Beta-blockers improve symptoms and increase survival but must be used carefully to avoid hypotension.[121,124] The inotropic drug digoxin may be considered in selected individuals, especially those with atrial fibrillation. Although many individuals with left heart failure die suddenly from dysrhythmias, prophylactic administration of antidysrhythmics has not been shown to improve survival. In individuals with sustained ventricular tachycardia, amiodarone or implantable cardioverter-defibrillators should be considered. Cardiac resynchronization therapy is proving to be an important modality in selected individuals. For those individuals with coronary artery disease, coronary bypass surgery or PCI may

HEALTH ALERT
Metabolic Changes in Heart Failure

The heart is the largest consumer of energy in the body and relies on the efficient production of adenosine triphosphate (ATP). The heart has very little capacity for energy storage. In the failing heart, increased demand for oxygen and energy is coupled with a decreased ability to utilize fatty acids as an energy source. As a result, several genes are activated that alter the ability of myocytes to use lipids and glucose as fuel sources, the most studied of which are the peroxisome proliferator-activated receptor (PPAR) family of genes. These genes control fatty acid oxidation and are of particular importance in heart failure associated with insulin resistance and diabetes. Energy starvation and high levels of catecholamines associated with heart failure lead to altered fatty acid oxidation and decreased effective ATP generation and utilization. This results in decreased myocardial contractility and structural changes in the myocardium (remodeling). Increasing knowledge of these mechanisms has led to the exploration of potential new therapies for heart failure. For example, although currently available PPAR-γ agonists (thiazolidinediones) are contraindicated in worsening heart failure because of increased fluid retention at the renal tubule, new insulin sensitizers are being explored that may improve myocardial metabolic function. In addition, inhibitors of fatty acid oxidation (e.g., trimetazidine) have been tried in several small studies with some improvement in cardiac function. Many new potential pharmacologic interventions are under investigation, but in the meantime most researchers agree that exercise and a healthy diet can improve myocardial metabolic function.

Data from Abozguia K et al: *Curr Pharm Des* 15(8):827–835, 2009; Adachi T: *Adv Pharmacol* 59:165–195, 2010; Ashrafian H et al: *Circulation* 116(4):434–448, 2007; Boudina S et al: *Circulation* 115(25): 3213–3223, 2007; Lehnart SE, Maier LS, Hasenfuss G: *Heart Fail Rev* 14(4):213–224, 2009; Neubauer S: *N Engl J Med* 356(11):1140–1151, 2007; Mudd JO et al: *Nature* 451(7181):919–928, 2008; Nass RD et al: *Nat Clin Pract Cardiovasc Med* 5(4):196–207, 2008; Tang WH et al: *Diabetes Obes Metab* 9(4):447–454, 2007.

improve perfusion to ischemic myocardium (hibernating myocardium) and improve cardiac output. Surgical interventions that improve ventricular geometry or heart transplantation may need to be considered. Experimental therapies including gene and stem cell therapies are being explored.

Diastolic heart failure is also known as heart failure with preserved systolic function or heart failure with normal ejection fraction (HFNEF). Diastolic heart failure can occur singly or along with systolic heart failure. Isolated diastolic heart failure is defined as pulmonary congestion despite a normal stroke volume and cardiac output. It is the cause of 40% to 50% of all cases of left heart failure and is more common in women. It results from decreased compliance of the left ventricle and abnormal diastolic relaxation such that a normal left ventricular end-diastolic volume (LVEDV) results in an increased left ventricular end-diastolic pressure (LVEDP). This pressure is reflected back into the pulmonary circulation and results in pulmonary edema. The major causes of diastolic dysfunction include hypertension-induced myocardial hypertrophy and myocardial ischemia–induced ventricular remodeling. Hypertrophy and ischemia cause a decreased ability of the myocytes to actively pump calcium from the cytosol, resulting in impaired relaxation. Other causes include aortic valvular disease, mitral valve disease, pericardial diseases, and cardiomyopathies. Diabetes also increases the risk for diastolic dysfunction. Like systolic heart failure, diastolic failure is characterized by sustained activation of the RAAS and the SNS.

Individuals with diastolic dysfunction present with dyspnea on exertion, fatigue, and evidence of pulmonary edema (inspiratory crackles on auscultation, pleural effusions). There also may be evidence of underlying coronary disease, hypertension, or valvular disease. Diagnosis is based upon three factors: signs and symptoms of heart failure, normal left ventricular (LV) ejection fraction, and evidence of diastolic dysfunction. The diagnosis is made initially by echocardiography, which demonstrates poor ventricular filling with normal ejection fractions. Management is aimed at improving ventricular relaxation and prolonging diastolic filling times to reduce diastolic pressure. Calcium channel blockers, beta-blockers, ACE inhibitors, and ARBs have been used with varying success. Treatment with the HMG Co-A reductase inhibitors (statins) has consistently resulted in improvements in LV diastolic function.[125] Inotropic drugs are not indicated in isolated diastolic heart failure because contractility and ejection fraction are not affected; however, digoxin may be used to slow the heart rate in individuals with atrial fibrillation. Outcomes for individuals with diastolic heart failure are as poor as those with systolic heart failure, and there has been no improvement in prognosis despite numerous new treatment trials.[125]

Right Heart Failure

Right heart failure is defined as the inability of the right ventricle to provide adequate blood flow into the pulmonary circulation at a normal central venous pressure. It can result from left heart failure when an increase in left ventricular filling pressure is reflected back into the pulmonary circulation. As pressure in the pulmonary circulation rises, the resistance to right ventricular emptying increases (Figure 23-39). The right ventricle is poorly prepared to compensate for this increased afterload and will dilate and fail. When this happens, pressure will rise in the systemic venous circulation, resulting in peripheral edema and hepatosplenomegaly. Treatment relies on management of the left ventricular dysfunction as just outlined. When right heart failure occurs in the absence of left heart failure, it is typically attributable to diffuse hypoxic pulmonary disease such as chronic obstructive pulmonary disease (COPD), cystic fibrosis, and acute respiratory distress syndrome (ARDS). These disorders result in an increase in right ventricular afterload. The mechanisms for this type of right ventricular failure (cor pulmonale) are discussed in Chapter 26. Finally, myocardial infarction, cardiomyopathies, and pulmonic valvular disease interfere with right ventricular contractility and can lead to right heart failure.

High-Output Failure

High-output failure is the inability of the heart to adequately supply the body with blood-borne nutrients, despite adequate blood volume and normal or elevated myocardial contractility. In high-output failure, the heart increases its output but the body's metabolic needs are still not met. Common causes of high-output failure are anemia, septicemia, hyperthyroidism, and beriberi (Figure 23-40).

Anemia decreases the oxygen-carrying capacity of the blood. Metabolic acidosis occurs as the body's cells switch to anaerobic metabolism (see Chapter 4). In response to metabolic acidosis, heart rate and stroke volume increase in an attempt to improve tissue perfusion. If anemia is severe, however, even maximum cardiac output does not supply the cells with enough oxygen for metabolism.

In septicemia, disturbed metabolism, bacterial toxins, and the inflammatory process cause systemic vasodilation and fever. Faced with a lowered systemic vascular resistance (SVR) and an elevated metabolic rate, cardiac output increases to maintain blood pressure and prevent metabolic acidosis. In overwhelming septicemia, however, the heart may not be able to raise its output enough to compensate

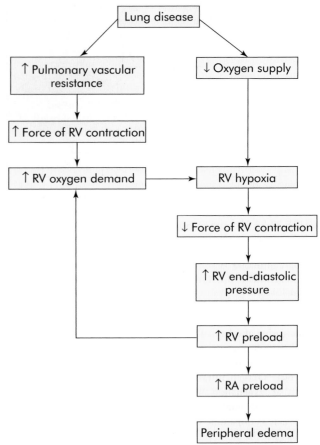

FIGURE 23-39 Right Heart Failure. *RA,* Right atrial; *RV,* right ventricular.

for vasodilation. Body tissues show signs of inadequate blood supply despite a high cardiac output.

Hyperthyroidism accelerates cellular metabolism through the actions of elevated levels of thyroxine from the thyroid gland. This may occur chronically (thyrotoxicosis) or acutely (thyroid storm). Because the body's increased demand for oxygen threatens to cause metabolic acidosis, cardiac output increases. If blood levels of thyroxine are high and the metabolic response to thyroxine is vigorous, even an abnormally elevated cardiac output may be inadequate.

In the United States, beriberi (thiamine deficiency) usually is caused by malnutrition secondary to chronic alcoholism. Beriberi actually causes a mixed type of heart failure. Thiamine deficiency impairs cellular metabolism in all tissues, including the myocardium. In the heart, impaired cardiac metabolism leads to insufficient contractile strength. In blood vessels, thiamine deficiency leads to peripheral vasodilation, which decreases SVR. Heart failure ensues as decreased SVR triggers increased cardiac output, which the impaired myocardium is unable to deliver. The strain of demands for increased output in the face of impaired metabolism may deplete cardiac reserves until low-output failure begins.

QUICK CHECK 23-10
1. Why are changes in LVEDV important for left heart failure?
2. What is ventricular remodeling?
3. What is the vicious cycle of systolic heart failure?

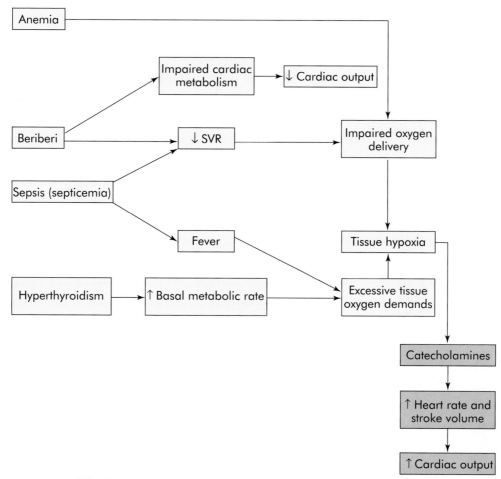

FIGURE 23-40 High-Output Failure. *SVR,* Systemic vascular resistance.

SHOCK

In shock the cardiovascular system fails to perfuse the tissues adequately, resulting in widespread impairment of cellular metabolism. Because tissue perfusion can be disrupted by any factor that alters heart function, blood volume, or blood pressure, shock has many causes and various clinical manifestations. Ultimately, however, shock progresses to organ failure and death, unless compensatory mechanisms reverse the process or clinical intervention succeeds. Untreated severe shock overwhelms the body's compensatory mechanisms through positive feedback loops that initiate and maintain a downward physiologic spiral.

The term multiple organ dysfunction syndrome (MODS) describes the failure of two or more organ systems after severe illness and injury and is a frequent complication of severe shock. The disease process is initiated and perpetuated by uncontrolled inflammatory and stress responses. It is progressive and is associated with significant mortality.

Impairment of Cellular Metabolism

The final common pathway in shock of any type is impairment of cellular metabolism. Figure 23-41 illustrates the pathophysiology of shock at the cellular level.

Impairment of Oxygen Use

In all types of shock, the cell either is not receiving an adequate amount of oxygen or is unable to use oxygen. Without oxygen, the cell shifts from aerobic to anaerobic metabolism. Anaerobic metabolism is a less efficient method of extracting energy from carbon bonds, and the cell begins to use its stores of adenosine triphosphate (ATP) faster than stores can be replaced. Without ATP, the cell cannot maintain an electrochemical gradient across its selectively permeable membrane. Specifically, the cell cannot operate the sodium-potassium pump. Sodium and chloride accumulate inside the cell, and potassium exits the cell. Cells of the nervous system and myocardium are profoundly and immediately affected. The resting potentials of these cells are reduced, and action potentials decrease in amplitude. Various clinical manifestations of impaired central nervous system and myocardial function result.

As sodium moves into the cell, water follows. Throughout the body, the water drawn from the interstitium into the cells is "replaced" by water that is, in turn, drawn out of the vascular space. This decreases circulatory volume. Within the cells, water causes cellular edema that disrupts cellular membranes, releasing lysosomal enzymes that injure the cells internally and then leak into the interstitium. Three positive feedback loops further impair oxygen use: (1) activation of the clotting cascade, (2) decreased circulatory volume, and (3) lysosomal enzyme release. The clotting cascade activates the inflammatory response and also accounts for typical complications of shock, such as acute tubular necrosis (ATN), acute respiratory distress syndrome (ARDS), and disseminated intravascular coagulation (DIC).[126]

Decreased circulatory volume causes the second positive feedback loop and magnifies decreased tissue perfusion in all types of shock. Lysosomal enzymes, the third positive feedback loop, not only injure the cell that released them but also injure adjacent cells. By damaging

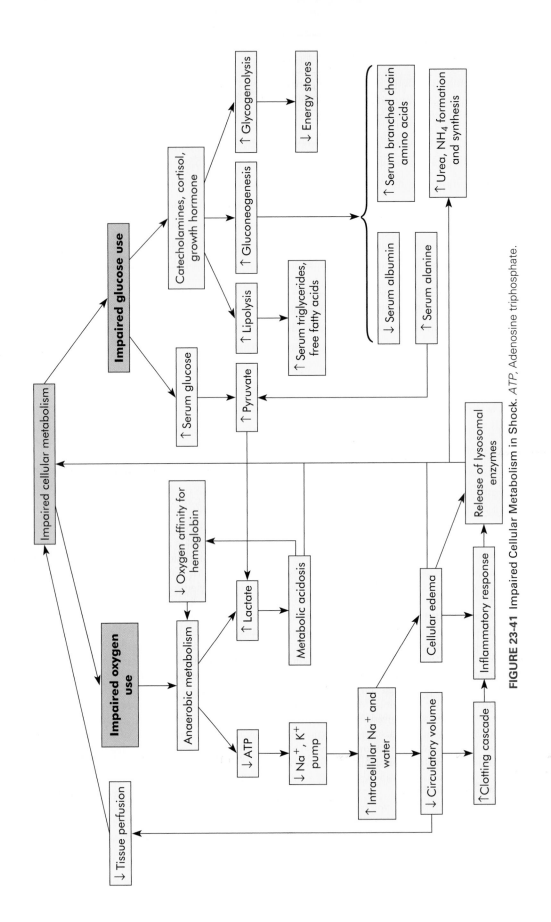

FIGURE 23-41 Impaired Cellular Metabolism in Shock. *ATP,* Adenosine triphosphate.

the mechanisms of surrounding cells, lysosomal enzymes extend areas of impaired metabolism and cellular injury.

In addition to decreasing ATP stores, anaerobic metabolism affects the pH of the cell, and metabolic acidosis develops. A compensatory mechanism enables cardiac and skeletal muscles to use lactic acid as a fuel source, but only for a limited time. The decreasing pH of the cell that is functioning anaerobically has serious consequences. Enzymes necessary for cellular function dissociate under acid conditions. Enzyme dissociation stops cell function, repair, and division. As lactic acid is released systemically, blood pH drops, reducing the oxygen-carrying capacity of the blood (see Chapter 4). Therefore less oxygen is delivered to the cells. Further acidosis triggers the release of more lysosomal enzymes because the low pH disrupts lysosomal membrane integrity.

Impairment of Glucose Use

Impaired glucose use can be caused by either impaired glucose delivery or impaired glucose uptake by the cells (see Figure 23-43). The reasons for inadequate glucose delivery are the same as those enumerated for inadequate oxygen delivery. In addition, in septic and anaphylactic shock, glucose metabolism may be increased or disrupted because of fever or bacteria, and glucose uptake can be prevented by the presence of vasoactive toxins, endotoxins, histamine, and kinins.

Some compensatory mechanisms activated by shock contribute to decreased glucose uptake by the cells. High serum levels of cortisol, thyroid hormone, and catecholamines account for hyperglycemia and insulin resistance, tachycardia, increased SVR, and increased cardiac contractility. Cells shift to glycogenolysis, gluconeogenesis, and lipolysis to generate fuel for survival (see Chapter 1). Except in the liver, kidneys, and muscles, the body's cells have extremely limited stores of glycogen. In fact, total body stores can fuel the metabolism for only about 10 hours. The depletion of fat and glycogen stores is not itself a cause of organ failure, but the energy costs of glycogenolysis and lipolysis are considerable and contribute to cell failure.

The depletion of protein also is a cause of organ failure. When gluconeogenesis causes proteins to be used for fuel, these proteins are no longer available to maintain cellular structure, function, repair, and replication. The breakdown of protein occurs in starvation states, hyperdynamic metabolic states, and septic shock. The metabolism of protein into amino acids that occurs with septicemia is called septic autocannibalism. During anaerobic metabolism, protein metabolism liberates alanine, which is converted to pyruvate. In sepsis, pyruvic acid is changed into lactic acid, and a positive feedback loop is formed.

As proteins are broken down anaerobically, ammonia and urea are produced. Ammonia is toxic to living cells. Uremia develops, and uric acid further disrupts cellular metabolism. Serum albumin and other plasma proteins are consumed for fuel first. Serum protein consumption decreases capillary osmotic pressure and contributes to the development of interstitial edema, creating another positive feedback loop that decreases circulatory volume. In septic shock, plasma protein breakdown includes metabolism of immunoglobulins, thereby impairing immune system function when it is most needed.

Muscle wasting caused by protein breakdown weakens skeletal and cardiac muscle. Skeletal muscle wasting impairs the muscles that facilitate breathing. Muscle wasting therefore alters the actions of both the heart and the lungs. The delivery of oxygen and glucose to the cells is directly reduced, as is the removal of waste products, forming another positive feedback loop.

A final outcome of impaired cellular metabolism is the buildup of metabolic end products in the cell and interstitial spaces. Waste products are toxic to the cells and further disrupt cellular function and membrane integrity. Once a sufficiently large number of cells from

vital organs have damage to cellular membranes, leakage of lysosomal enzymes, and ATP depletion, shock can be irreversible.

Clinical Manifestations of Shock

The clinical manifestations of shock are variable depending on the type of shock, and observable and measurable signs and symptoms are often conflicting in nature. Subjective complaints in shock are usually nonspecific. The individual may report feeling sick, weak, cold, hot, nauseated, dizzy, confused, afraid, thirsty, and short of breath. Hypotension, characterized by a mean arterial pressure below 60 mm Hg, is common to almost all shock states; however, it is a late sign of decreased tissue perfusion. Cardiac output and urinary output are usually variable early in shock states but generally become decreased as the shock syndrome progresses. Respiratory rate is usually increased, and a respiratory alkalosis may be an important early indicator of impending shock. Other variable indicators of shock include alterations of heart rate, core body temperature, skin temperature, systemic vascular resistance (SVR), and skin color. Altered sensorium may be another indicator of poor tissue perfusion. A decreased, mixed venous oxygen saturation indicates poor tissue oxygenation and an alteration in cellular oxygen extraction and can be used to monitor response to therapy.

Treatment for Shock

The first treatment for shock is to discover and correct or remove the underlying cause. General supportive treatment includes intravenous fluid administered to expand intravascular volume, vasopressors, and supplemental oxygen. Further treatment depends on the cause and severity of the shock syndrome, which is discussed with each type of shock. Once positive feedback loops are established, intervention in shock is difficult. Prevention and very early treatment offer the best prognosis.

Types of Shock

Shock is classified by cause as cardiogenic (caused by heart failure), hypovolemic (caused by insufficient intravascular fluid volume), neurogenic (caused by neural alterations of vascular smooth muscle tone), anaphylactic (caused by immunologic processes), or septic (caused by infection). As described previously, each of these share similar effects on tissues and cells but can vary in their clinical manifestations and severity.

Cardiogenic Shock

Cardiogenic shock is defined as decreased cardiac output and evidence of tissue hypoxia in the presence of adequate intravascular volume. Most cases of cardiogenic shock follow myocardial infarction, but shock also can follow left heart failure, dysrhythmias, acute valvular dysfunction, ventricular or septal rupture, myocardial or pericardial infections, massive pulmonary embolism, cardiac tamponade, and drug toxicity. The pathophysiology of cardiogenic shock is illustrated in Figure 23-42.

The clinical manifestations of cardiogenic shock are caused by widespread impairment of cellular metabolism. They include impaired mentation, dyspnea and tachypnea, systemic venous and pulmonary edema, dusky skin color, marked hypotension, oliguria, and ileus. Management of cardiogenic shock includes careful fluid and pressor administration followed by early angiography, intra-aortic balloon pump counterpulsation, ventricular assist devices, and early revascularization (PCI or bypass surgery).[127] Cardiogenic shock is often unresponsive to treatment, with a mortality of more than 70% reported. New therapies being explored include anti-inflammatory drugs and nitric oxide synthetase inhibitors.[127]

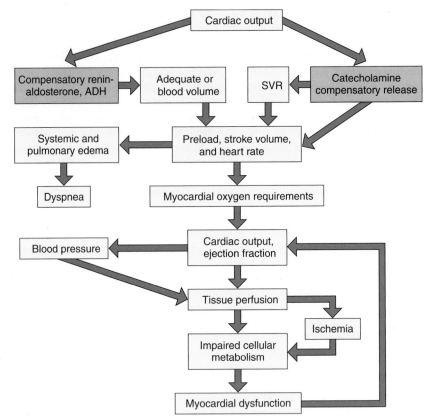

FIGURE 23-42 Cardiogenic Shock. Shock becomes life-threatening when compensatory mechanisms (in blue) cause increased myocardial oxygen requirements. Renal and hypothalamic adaptive responses (i.e., renin-angiotensin-aldosterone and antidiuretic hormone [ADH]) maintain or increase blood volume. The adrenal gland releases catecholamines (e.g., mostly epinephrine, some norepinephrine), causing vasoconstriction and increases in contractility and heart rate. These adaptive mechanisms, however, increase myocardial demands for oxygen and nutrients. These demands further strain the heart, which can no longer pump an adequate volume, resulting in shock and impaired metabolism. *SVR,* Systemic vascular resistance.

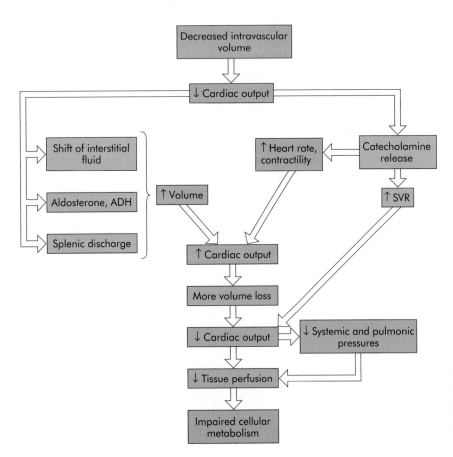

FIGURE 23-43 Hypovolemic Shock. This type of shock becomes life-threatening when compensatory mechanisms (in purple) are overwhelmed by continued loss of intravascular volume. *ADH,* Antidiuretic hormone; *SVR,* systemic vascular resistance.

Hypovolemic Shock

Hypovolemic shock is caused by loss of whole blood (hemorrhage), plasma (burns), or interstitial fluid (diaphoresis, diabetes mellitus, diabetes insipidus, emesis, diarrhea, or diuresis) in large amounts. Hypovolemic shock begins to develop when intravascular volume has decreased by about 15%.

Hypovolemia is offset initially by compensatory mechanisms (Figure 23-43). Heart rate and SVR increase, boosting both cardiac output and tissue perfusion pressures. Interstitial fluid moves into the vascular compartment. The liver and spleen add to blood volume by disgorging stored red blood cells and plasma. In the kidneys, renin stimulates aldosterone release and the retention of sodium (and hence water), whereas antidiuretic hormone (ADH) from the posterior pituitary gland increases water retention. However, if the initial fluid or blood loss is great or if loss continues, compensation fails, resulting in decreased tissue perfusion. As in cardiogenic shock, oxygen and nutrient delivery to the cells is impaired and cellular metabolism fails. Anaerobic metabolism and lactate production result in lactic acidosis and serum and cellular electrolyte abnormalities.

The clinical manifestations of hypovolemic shock include high SVR, poor skin turgor, thirst, oliguria, low systemic and pulmonary preloads, rapid heart rate, thready pulse, and mental status deterioration. The differences between the signs and symptoms of hypovolemic shock and those of cardiogenic shock are mainly caused by differences in fluid volume and cardiac muscle health. Management begins with rapid fluid replacement with crystalloids and blood products. For hemorrhagic hypovolemic shock, the administration of pharmacologic doses of ADH can improve blood pressure.[128] Hypothermia and coagulopathies frequently complicate treatment. If adequate tissue perfusion cannot be restored promptly, systemic inflammation and multiple organ dysfunction are likely.

Neurogenic Shock

Neurogenic shock (sometimes called vasogenic shock) is the result of widespread and massive vasodilation that results from parasympathetic overstimulation and sympathetic understimulation (Figure 23-44) (see Chapter 22). This type of shock can be caused by any factor that stimulates parasympathetic or inhibits sympathetic stimulation of vascular smooth muscle. Trauma to the spinal cord or medulla and conditions that interrupt the supply of oxygen or glucose to the medulla can cause neurogenic shock by interrupting sympathetic activity. Depressive drugs, anesthetic agents, and severe emotional stress and pain are other causes. The loss of vascular tone results in "relative hypovolemia," in which blood volume has not changed but SVR decreases drastically so that the amount of space containing the blood has increased. The pressure in the vessels falls below that which is needed to drive nutrients across capillary membranes to the cells. In addition, neurologic insult may cause bradycardia, which decreases cardiac output and further contributes to hypotension and underperfusion of tissues. As with other types of shock, this leads to impaired cellular metabolism. Management includes the careful use of fluids and pressors until blood pressure stabilizes.[129]

Anaphylactic Shock

Anaphylactic shock results from a widespread hypersensitivity reaction known as anaphylaxis. The lifetime prevalence of anaphylaxis is 0.5% to 2%.[130] The basic physiologic alteration is the same as that of neurogenic shock: vasodilation and relative hypovolemia, leading to decreased tissue perfusion and impaired cellular metabolism (Figure 23-45). Anaphylactic shock is characterized by other effects that rapidly involve the entire body.

Anaphylactic shock begins with exposure of a sensitized individual to an allergen. Common allergens known to cause these reactions

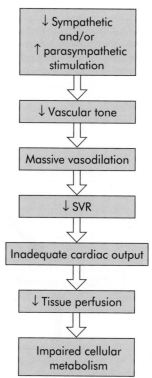

FIGURE 23-44 Neurogenic Shock. *SVR*, Systemic vascular resistance.

are insect venoms, shellfish, peanuts, latex, and medications such as penicillin. In genetically predisposed individuals, these allergens initiate a vigorous humoral immune response (type I hypersensitivity) that results in the production of large quantities of immunoglobulin E (IgE) antibody (see Chapter 6). Allergen bound to IgE causes degranulation of mast cells. Mast cells release a large number of vasoactive and inflammatory cytokines. This provokes an extensive immune and inflammatory response, including vasodilation and increased vascular permeability, resulting in peripheral pooling and tissue edema.[130] Extravascular effects include constriction of extravascular smooth muscle, often causing laryngospasm and bronchospasm (see Chapter 26) and cramping abdominal pain with diarrhea.

The onset of anaphylactic shock is usually sudden, and progression to death can occur within minutes unless emergency treatment is given. The primary clinical manifestations of anaphylaxis include anxiety, dizziness, difficulty breathing, stridor, wheezing, pruritus with hives (urticaria), swollen lips and tongue, and abdominal cramping.[130] A precipitous fall in blood pressure occurs, followed by impaired mentation. Other signs include decreased SVR, with high or normal cardiac output, and oliguria. Treatment begins with removal of the antigen (if possible). Epinephrine is administered intramuscularly to cause vasoconstriction and reverse airway constriction. Fluids are given intravenously to reverse the relative hypovolemia, and antihistamines and corticosteroids are administered to stop the inflammatory reaction. Vasopressors and inhaled β-adrenergic agonist bronchodilators may also be necessary.[130,131]

> **✓ QUICK CHECK 23-11**
> 1. Describe the mechanisms operative in shock.
> 2. Why does myocardial infarction often cause cardiogenic shock?
> 3. How is hypovolemic shock manifested?
> 4. Why is anaphylactic shock considered a medical emergency?

Septic Shock

Septic shock begins with an infection that progresses to bacteremia, then **systemic inflammatory response syndrome (SIRS)** with sepsis, then severe sepsis, then septic shock, and finally multiple organ dysfunction syndrome (MODS). Consensus about definitions of each component was achieved in 1992 and revised in 2001; these definitions are presented in Table 23-10.[132]

Septic shock, a common cause of death in intensive care units, has an overall mortality in the United States of 28% to 60% and can be caused by any class of microorganism. Although 2 decades ago gram-negative bacteria were by far the microorganisms most often responsible for causing septic shock, gram-positive bacteria now have become the most common isolates. Septic shock also can be caused by fungi and viruses, and in almost one third of cases, the infectious organism is

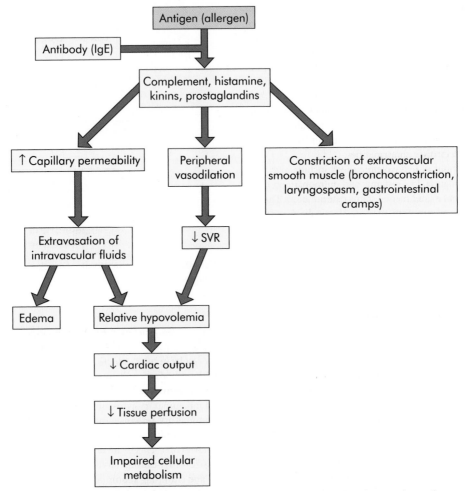

FIGURE 23-45 Anaphylactic Shock. *IgE,* Immunoglobulin E; *SVR,* systemic vascular resistance.

TABLE 23-10   CAUSES AND DEFINITIONS OF SEPTIC SHOCK

CAUSE	DEFINITION
Infection	Microbial phenomenon characterized by inflammatory response to presence of microorganisms or invasion of normally sterile host tissue by those microorganisms
Bacteremia	Presence of viable bacteria in blood
Systemic inflammatory response syndrome (SIRS)	Systemic inflammatory response to a variety of severe clinical insults manifested by two or more of following signs: Temperature >38° C or <36° C Heart rate >90 beats/min Respiratory rate >20 breaths/min or arterial blood carbon dioxide level <32 mm Hg White blood cell count >12,000 cells/mm³, <4000 cells/mm³, or containing <10% immature forms (bands)
Sepsis	Systemic response to infection characterized by 2 or more of SIRS criteria
Severe sepsis	Sepsis associated with organ dysfunction
Septic shock	Severe sepsis complicated by persistent hypotension refractory to early fluid therapy
Multiple organ dysfunction syndrome	Presence of altered organ function in an acutely ill individual such that homeostasis cannot be maintained without intervention

Data adapted from American College of Chest Physicians/Society of Critical Care Medicine Consensus Conference: *Crit Care Med* 20(6):864–874, 1992; Levy MM et al: SCCM/ES/CM/ACCP/ATS/SIS International Sepsis Definitions Conference, *Crit Care Med* 31(4):1250–1256, 2003.

never identified. The most common sources of infection are the lungs, urinary tract, gastrointestinal tract, wounds, and indwelling vascular catheters. The source and virulence of the infectious microorganism, as well as the underlying health of the affected individual, significantly affect prognosis.

Most septic shock begins when bacteria enter the bloodstream to produce bacteremia. These bacteria may directly stimulate an inflammatory response or they may release toxic substances into the bloodstream. Gram-negative microorganisms release endotoxins, and gram-positive microorganisms release exotoxins, lipoteichoic acids, and peptidoglycans. These substances trigger the septic syndrome by interacting with Toll-like receptors on macrophages and activate complement, coagulation, kinins, and inflammatory cells (Figure 23-46).[133]

The release of inflammatory mediators triggers intense cellular responses and the subsequent release of secondary mediators, including cytokines, complement fragments, prostaglandins, platelet-activating factor, oxygen free radicals, nitric oxide, and proteolytic enzymes. Chemotaxis, activation of granulocytes, and reactivation of the phagocytic cells and inflammatory cascades result (see *Risk Factors: Inflammatory Mediators Contributing to Septic Shock*). Chapter 5 discusses the description and function of inflammatory cells and mediators. This systemic inflammation, especially through the action of nitric oxide, leads to widespread vasodilation with compensatory tachycardia and increased cardiac output in the early stages of septic

shock (hyperdynamic phase) (see *Health Alert:* The Role of Nitric Oxide in Severe Sepsis).[133] Later in the course of disease, inflammatory mediators, such as complement and interleukins, depress myocardial contractility such that cardiac output falls and tissue perfusion decreases.[134] Tissue perfusion and cellular oxygen extraction also are affected by activation of the clotting cascade through the action of platelet-activating factor and depletion of the endogenous anticoagulant protein C. Furthermore, unresponsiveness to or depletion of vasoactive factors such as vasopressin contributes to hypotension and tissue hypoperfusion. The inflammatory response can become overwhelming, leading to the systemic inflammatory response syndrome (SIRS), which can progress to widespread tissue hypoxia, necrosis, and apoptosis, leading to septic shock and MODS. It has been determined that there is a parallel release of anti-inflammatory mediators that accompanies SIRS, causing a depression in the immune response to infection that contributes to the overall shock syndrome.[133]

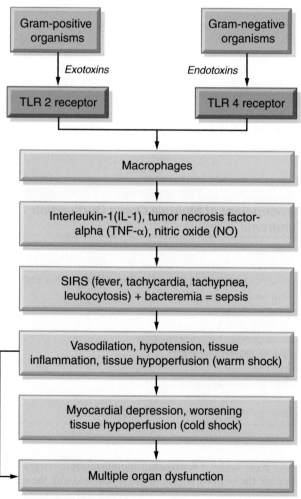

FIGURE 23-46 Septic Shock. *TLR,* Toll-like receptor.

RISK FACTORS

Inflammatory Mediators Contributing to Septic Shock

More than 100 inflammatory mediators have been implicated in the pathogenesis of septic shock. The following are some of the most important contributors:

Interleukin-1β (IL-1β)
Released by macrophages and lymphocytes in septic shock in response to bacterial toxins
Net effect: produces fever, vasodilation and hypotension, edema, myocardial depression, and elevated white blood count

Tumor Necrosis Factor-alpha (TNF-α)
Produced from macrophages, natural killer cells, and mast cells in response to endotoxin and interleukins
Net effect: generates same symptoms of septic shock as those seen with interleukins; thus is redundant

Platelet-Activating Factor (PAF)
Released from mononuclear phagocytes, platelets, and some endothelial cells in response to endotoxin
Net effect: contributes to widespread clotting, generates same symptoms of shock as those seen with interleukins and tumor necrosis factor-alpha, and may initiate multiple organ failure

High-Mobility Group Box 1 (HMGB1)
Released from mononuclear phagocytes, endothelial cells, neurons, and smooth muscle cells in response to endotoxin and exotoxins
Net effect: induces the release of interleukins and tumor necrosis factor

Clinical manifestations of septic shock are the result of inflammation, decreased perfusion of vital tissues attributable to low SVR from vasodilation, and an alteration in oxygen extraction by all cells. In early shock, tachycardia causes cardiac output to remain normal or become elevated, although myocardial contractility is reduced. Temperature instability is present, ranging from hyperthermia to hypothermia. Effects on other organ systems may result in deranged renal function, jaundice, clotting abnormalities with disseminated intravascular coagulation (DIC), deterioration of mental status, and ARDS. Gastrointestinal mucosa changes cause the translocation of bacteria from the gut

The Role of Nitric Oxide in Severe Sepsis

Nitric oxide (NO) is a free radical generated from L-arginine by a family of enzymes known as NO synthetases. The most important enzyme in sepsis is called iNOS (inducible NOS), which responds to immune/inflammatory insult and mediates tissue damage. In sepsis, iNOS is activated, and NO and OONO– (peroxynitrite) are produced in large quantities. In septic shock, nitric oxide has been shown to cause refractory peripheral vascular vasodilation, increase vascular permeability, and depress myocardial function. Nitric oxide contributes to the development of MODS because its effects include decreased cellular protein synthesis, oxidized cell membranes, damaged DNA, decreased glucose and glycogen production, and competition for cytochrome oxidase in the mitochondria, thus decreasing tissue oxygen utilization. Methylene blue, a selective inhibitor of guanylate cyclase (an enzyme involved in nitric oxide–mediated vasodilation), has shown promise in improving blood pressure in individuals with septic shock but has adverse effects on the pulmonary circulation. Studies are aimed at finding new treatments (such as antioxidants) to prevent the negative impact of this toxic free radical in sepsis.

Data from Azevedo LC: Mitochondrial dysfunction during sepsis, *Endocr Metab Immune Disord Drug Targets* 10(3):214–223, 2010; Fortin CF et al: Sepsis, leukocytes, and nitric oxide (NO): an intricate affair, *Shock* 33(4):344–352, 2010; Paciullo CA et al: Methylene blue for the treatment of septic shock, *Pharmacother* 30(7):702–715, 2010; Szabo C, Modis K: Pathophysiological roles of peroxynitrite in circulatory shock, *Shock* 34(suppl 1):4–14, 2010; Zhang T, Feng Q: Nitric oxide and calcium signaling regulate myocardial tumor necrosis factor-α expression and cardiac function in sepsis, *Can J Physiol Pharmacol* 88(2):92–104, 2010.

into the bloodstream. Increased permeability of the gut also can lead to increased inflammation and immune reactions attributable to toxins carried by the intestinal lymphatics.

The diagnosis of septic shock rests on the recognition of the systemic manifestations of overwhelming inflammation (SIRS) in individuals with suspected or documented infection. Determining the cause and severity of septic shock can be aided by measurement of levels of serum lactate, C-reactive protein, and procalcitonin.[135] The management of septic shock following the "surviving sepsis guidelines" has improved outcomes.[136] These guidelines include support of the respiratory system (including mechanical ventilation if needed), placement of a central venous catheter, the rapid administration of broad-spectrum antibiotics, removal of the source of infection if one is found, administration of intravenous fluids and vasopressors, and careful monitoring.[137] Selected individuals with severe refractory hypotension are given systemic corticosteroids and vasopressin. Individuals with refractory septic shock may respond to human recombinant activated protein C[138] (see *Health Alert:* The Role of Activated Protein C in Sepsis and DIC). Control of hyperglycemia with insulin, treatment of complications associated with MODS, careful nutritional support, and prevention of stress ulcers and deep venous thrombosis are also essential. Because the septic syndrome is incompletely understood, recommended treatment continues to evolve.

> ✔ **QUICK CHECK 23-12**
> 1. What are some of the important causes of septic shock?
> 2. What is the systemic inflammatory response syndrome?
> 3. Why is correction of the underlying problem the most important treatment for all kinds of shock?

The Role of Activated Protein C in Sepsis and DIC

Activated protein C is an endogenous anticoagulant that regulates the activity of factors VIIIa and Va. It is also anti-inflammatory and inhibits nitric oxide–induced vascular dysfunction. In sepsis and disseminated intravascular coagulation (DIC), activated protein C levels are decreased. The amount of decrease is associated with mortality. Human recombinant activated protein C is effective for the treatment of sepsis-associated DIC. Controversies remain, however, about the use of this treatment for sepsis. Current evidence suggests that administration of activated protein C improves outcomes in individuals with severe sepsis, and numerous trials continue to explore how best to use this important new treatment.

Data from Levi M, Lowenberg E, Meijers JC: *Sem Thromb Hemost* 36(5):550–557, 2010; Lindenauer PK et al: *Crit Care Med* 38(4):1101–1107, 2010; Neyrinck AP et al: *Br J Pharmacol* 158(4):1034–1047, 2009; Sanchez B et al: *J Crit Care* 25(2):343–347, 2010; Toussaint S, Gerlach H: *N Engl J Med* 361(27):2646–2652, 2009.

Multiple Organ Dysfunction Syndrome

Multiple organ dysfunction syndrome (MODS) is the progressive dysfunction of two or more organ systems resulting from an uncontrolled inflammatory response to a severe illness or injury. The organ dysfunction can progress to organ failure and death (Figure 23-47). Although sepsis and septic shock are the most common causes, any severe injury or disease process that activates a massive systemic inflammatory response in the host can initiate MODS. These triggers include severe trauma, burns, acute pancreatitis, obstetric complications, major surgery, circulatory shock, some drugs, and gangrenous or necrotic tissue.

MODS is the most common cause of mortality in intensive care units. Mortality for individuals increases to 100% if there is failure of five or more organs. People at greatest risk for developing MODS are elderly individuals and persons with significant tissue injury or preexisting disease (see *Risk Factors:* Development of Multiple Organ Dysfunction Syndrome).

Development of Multiple Organ Dysfunction Syndrome

Age >65 years
Major trauma
Baseline organ dysfunction (e.g., renal insufficiency, hepatic insufficiency)
Bowel infarction
Acute pancreatitits
Coma on admission
Immunosuppression (e.g., corticosteroids)
Inadequate, delayed resuscitation
Malnutrition
Multiple blood transfusions (>6 units/12 hr)
Persistent infectious focus
Preexisting chronic disease (e.g., cancer, diabetes)

PATHOPHYSIOLOGY   As a result of the initiating insult (sepsis, injury, or disease), the neuroendocrine system is activated with the release of the stress hormones cortisol, epinephrine, and norepinephrine into the

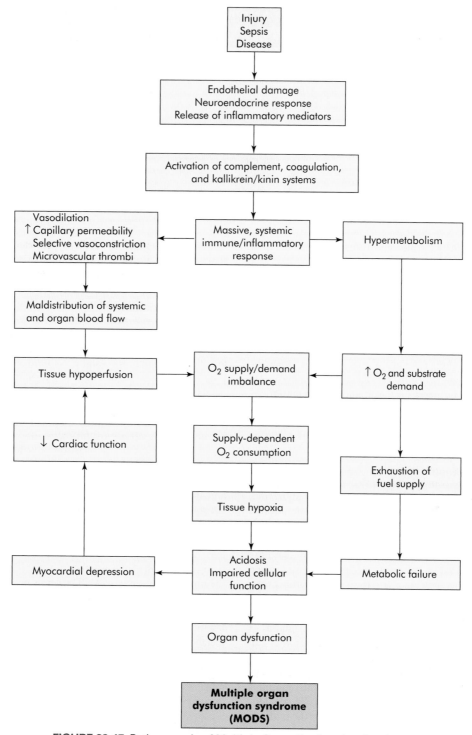

FIGURE 23-47 Pathogenesis of Multiple Organ Dysfunction Syndrome.

bloodstream (see Chapter 8). Vascular endothelial damage occurs as a direct result of injury or from damage by bacterial toxins and inflammatory mediators released into the circulation. The vascular endothelium becomes permeable, allowing fluid and protein to leak into the interstitial spaces, contributing to hypotension and hypoperfusion. When the endothelium is damaged, platelets and tissue thromboplastin are activated, resulting in systemic microvascular coagulation that may lead to DIC (see Chapter 20).[133,139]

Because of the release of inflammatory mediators, three major plasma enzyme cascades are activated: complement, coagulation, and kallikrein/kinin. The overall effect of the activation of these cascades is a hyperinflammatory and hypercoagulant state that maintains the interstitial edema formation, cardiovascular instability, endothelial damage, and clotting abnormalities characteristic of MODS. A massive systemic immune/inflammatory response then develops involving neutrophils, macrophages, and mast cells (Table 23-11). The

TABLE 23-11		CELLS OF INFLAMMATION AND MULTIPLE ORGAN DYSFUNCTION
CELL	**ACTIVATORS**	**CONTRIBUTION TO MULTIPLE ORGAN DYSFUNCTION**
Neutrophils	Complement, kinins, endotoxin, clotting factors	Release of phagocytic products: toxic oxygen free radicals, superoxide ion, hydrogen peroxide, hydroxyl radicals, proteases, platelet-activating factor (PAF), arachidonic acid metabolites (prostaglandins, thromboxane, leukotrienes)
		Endothelial damage, vasodilation, vasopermeability, microvascular coagulation, selective vasoconstriction, hypotension, shock
Macrophages	Complement, endotoxin, chemotactic factors	Release of same phagocytic products as neutrophils
		Release of monokines: tumor necrosis factor (TNF), interleukin-1 (IL-1)
		TNF produces fever, anorexia, hyperglycemia, weight loss
Mast cells	Direct injury, endotoxin, complement	Release of histamine, PAF, arachidonic acid metabolites
		Vasodilation, vasopermeability, hypotension, shock

inflammatory process initiated is the same as that described in septic shock and SIRS (see p. 632) and sets the stage for MODS.

The numerous inflammatory and clotting processes operating in MODS cause maldistribution of blood flow and hypermetabolism. Oxygen delivery to the tissues decreases despite the supranormal systemic blood flow for several reasons:

1. Shunting of blood past selected regional capillary beds is caused when inflammatory mediators override the normal vascular tone.
2. Interstitial edema, resulting from microvascular changes in permeability, contributes to decreased oxygen delivery by creating a relative hypovolemia and by increasing the distance oxygen must travel to reach the cells.[140]
3. Capillary obstruction occurs because of formation of microvascular thrombi and the aggregation of white blood cells.

Hypermetabolism in MODS with accompanying alterations in carbohydrate, fat, and lipid metabolism is initially a compensatory measure to meet the body's increased demands for energy. The alterations in metabolism affect all aspects of substrate utilization. The net result of hypermetabolism is depletion of oxygen and fuel supplies.

Decreased oxygen delivery to the cells caused by the maldistribution of blood flow, coagulation, myocardial depression, and the hypermetabolic state combine to create an imbalance in oxygen supply and demand. This imbalance is critical in the pathogenesis of MODS because it results in a pathologic condition known as supply-dependent oxygen consumption.[140] Ordinarily, the amount of oxygen consumed by the cells depends only on the demands of the cells, because there is an adequate reserve of oxygen that can be delivered if needed. The reserve, however, has been exhausted in MODS, and the amount of oxygen consumed becomes dependent on the amount the circulation is able to deliver; this amount is inadequate in MODS. Therefore tissue hypoxia with cellular acidosis and impaired cellular function ensue and result in the multiple organ failure.

CLINICAL MANIFESTATIONS There is often a predictable clinical pattern in the development of MODS, although there is certainly some individual variation. After the inciting event and aggressive resuscitation for approximately 24 hours, the individual develops a low-grade fever, tachycardia, dyspnea, altered mental status, and hyperdynamic and hypermetabolic states. The lung is often the first organ to fail, resulting in acute respiratory distress syndrome (ARDS) (see Chapter 26). Respiratory failure is characterized by tachypnea, pulmonary edema with crackles and diminished breath sounds, use of accessory muscles, and hypoxemia.

Between 7 and 10 days, the hypermetabolic and hyperdynamic states intensify, bacteremia with enteric microorganisms is common, and signs of liver and kidney failure appear. Liver failure, although developing early, is not clinically detectable until later stages of MODS, at which time jaundice, abdominal distention, liver tenderness, muscle wasting, and hepatic encephalopathy appear. All facets of metabolism, substance detoxification, and immune response are impaired; albumin and clotting factor synthesis decreases; protein wastes accumulate; and liver tissue macrophages (Kupffer cells) no longer function effectively. Progressive oliguria, azotemia, and edema mark the development of renal failure. Anuria, hyperkalemia, and metabolic acidosis may occur if renal shutdown is severe.

During days 14 to 24, renal and liver failure becomes more severe and the gastrointestinal system shows evidence of dysfunction. The gastrointestinal system is sensitive to ischemic and inflammatory injury. Clinical manifestations of bowel involvement are hemorrhage, ileus, malabsorption, diarrhea or constipation, vomiting, anorexia, and abdominal pain. Compounding the damage caused by injury to the bowel is the phenomenon of bacterial translocation. When mediators and severe ischemia injure the mucosal epithelium, bacteria and toxins pass from the gut into the portal circulation. The overwhelmed liver is unable to clear these products and they move into the systemic circulation. Thus, whether infection or some other injury was the precipitating cause of MODS, sepsis occurs once the gut barrier is damaged.

Hematologic failure and myocardial failure are usually later manifestations. The signs and symptoms of cardiac failure in the hypermetabolic, hyperdynamic phase of MODS are similar to those of septic shock: tachycardia, bounding pulse, increased cardiac output, decreased systemic vascular resistance, and hypotension. In the terminal stages, hypodynamic circulation with bradycardia, profound hypotension, and ventricular dysrhythmias may develop. Encephalopathy, characterized by mental status changes ranging from confusion to deep coma, may occur at any time. Ischemia and inflammation are responsible for the central nervous system manifestations, which include apprehension, confusion, disorientation, restlessness, agitation, headache, decreased cognitive ability and memory, and decreased level of consciousness. When ischemia is severe, seizures and coma can occur. Death may occur as early as 14 days or after a period of several weeks.

EVALUATION AND TREATMENT Early detection of organ failure is extremely important so that supportive measures can be initiated immediately. Frequent assessment of the clinical status of individuals at known risk is essential. The Acute Physiology and Chronic Health

Evaluation (APACHE) II and III systems assess for severity and progression of MODS. Once organ failure develops, monitoring of laboratory values and hemodynamic parameters also can be used to assess the degree of impairment.

Therapeutic management of MODS consists of prevention and support. First, if the initial insult is known, it is aggressively treated and sources of infection are removed. The second priority is restoration and maintenance of tissue oxygenation and cardiovascular function. Third, nutritional support must be provided (see *Health Alert:* Nutritional Support to Prevent and Treat MODS). Last, individual organs must be supported. Activated protein C (drotrecogin alfa) has been shown to improve outcomes in those with DIC and may be useful for the general management of septic shock with multiple organ dysfunction syndrome.[138,141]

QUICK CHECK 23-13

1. Why can MODS be initiated by either a septic or a nonseptic insult?
2. Why are inflammation and clotting triggered when the vascular endothelium is injured?
3. Describe the mechanisms that result in decreased oxygen delivery to the tissues in MODS.

HEALTH ALERT

Nutritional Support to Prevent and Treat MODS

Critical illness is associated with overgrowth of bacteria in the gut and increased permeability of the gut for microorganisms and toxins. These factors contribute to endotoxemia, sepsis, multiple organ failure, and death. The liver is also affected and contributes to metabolic, nutritional, and hemostatic dysfunction. Maintaining the integrity of the gastrointestinal tract is an important step in preventing and managing sepsis and multiple organ dysfunction. Nutritional support not only prevents malnutrition but also helps maintain adequate functioning of the gut and improves immunity. Enteral nutrition (EN) has advantages over parenteral nutrition (PN) for postoperative/post-trauma individuals. Immediate and early EN improves mucosal blood flow, reduces intramucosal acidosis and permeability problems, and decreases the need for stress ulcer prophylaxis. EN also maintains the protective role of the gut by decreasing inflammatory cytokine production and improving mucosal IgA levels, which helps prevent infection. EN should be given as soon as is practical. Jejunal tube feedings have advantages over gastric tube feedings, including faster metabolic recovery, less vomiting, and less risk of regurgitation and aspiration.

Data from Marla R, Dahn MS, Lange MP: *Surg Infect* 5(4):357–363, 2004; McClave SA, Heyland DK: *Nutr Clin Pract* 24(3):305–315, 2009; Moore FA, Moore EE: *Nutr Clin Pract* 24(3):297–304, 2009; Oz HS, Chen TS, Neuman M: *JPEN J Parenter Enteral Nutr* 33(4):380–389, 2009.

DID YOU UNDERSTAND?

Diseases of the Veins and Arteries

1. Varicosities are areas of veins in which blood has pooled, usually in the saphenous veins. Varicosities may be caused by damaged valves as a result of trauma to the valve or by chronic venous distention involving gravity and venous constriction.
2. Chronic venous insufficiency is inadequate venous return over a long period of time that causes pathologic ischemic changes in the vasculature, skin, and supporting tissues.
3. Venous stasis ulcers follow the development of chronic venous insufficiency and probably develop as a result of the borderline metabolic state of the cells in the affected extremities.
4. Deep venous thrombosis results from stasis of blood flow, endothelial damage, or hypercoagulability. The most serious complication of deep venous thrombosis is pulmonary embolism.
5. Superior vena cava syndrome is a progressive occlusion of the superior vena cava that leads to venous distention in the upper extremities and head. Because this syndrome is usually caused by bronchogenic cancer, it is generally considered an oncologic emergency rather than a vascular emergency.
6. Hypertension is the elevation of systemic arterial blood pressure resulting from increases in cardiac output (blood volume), total peripheral resistance, or both.
7. Hypertension can be primary, without a known cause, or secondary, caused by an underlying disease.
8. The risk factors for hypertension include a positive family history; male gender; advancing age; black race; obesity; high sodium intake; low magnesium, potassium, or calcium intake; diabetes mellitus; cigarette smoking; and heavy alcohol consumption.
9. The exact cause of primary hypertension is unknown, although several hypotheses are proposed, including overactivity of the sympathetic nervous system; overactivity of the renin-angiotensin-aldosterone system; sodium and water retention by the kidneys; hormonal inhibition of sodium-potassium transport across cell walls; and complex interactions involving insulin resistance, inflammation, and endothelial function.
10. Clinical manifestations of hypertension result from damage of organs and tissues outside the vascular system. These include retinal changes, heart disease, renal disease, and central nervous system problems, such as stroke and dementia.
11. Hypertension is managed with both pharmacologic and nonpharmacologic methods that lower the blood volume and the total peripheral resistance.
12. Orthostatic hypotension is a drop in blood pressure that occurs on standing. The compensatory vasoconstriction response to standing is replaced by a marked vasodilation and blood pooling in the muscle vasculature.
13. The clinical manifestations of orthostatic hypotension include fainting and may involve cardiovascular symptoms, as well as impotence and bowel and bladder dysfunction.
14. An aneurysm is a localized dilation of a vessel wall; the aorta is particularly susceptible.
15. A thrombus is a clot that remains attached to a vascular wall. An embolus is a mobile aggregate of a variety of substances that occludes the vasculature. Sources of emboli include clots, air, amniotic fluid, bacteria, fat, and foreign matter. These emboli cause ischemia and necrosis when a vessel is totally blocked.
16. The most common source of arterial thrombotic emboli is the heart as a result of mitral and aortic valvular disease and atrial fibrillation, followed by myxomas. Tissues affected include the lower extremities, the brain, and the heart.
17. Emboli to the central organs cause tissue death in lungs, kidneys, and mesentery.
18. Peripheral vascular diseases include Buerger disease and Raynaud disease, involving arterioles of the extremities.
19. Atherosclerosis is a form of arteriosclerosis and is the leading contributor to coronary artery disease (CAD) and cerebrovascular disease (CVD).
20. Atherosclerosis is an inflammatory disease that begins with endothelial injury.
21. Important steps in atherogenesis include vasoconstriction, adherence of macrophages, release of inflammatory mediators, oxidation of LDL, formation of foam cells and fatty streaks, and development of fibrous plaque.

Continued

DID YOU UNDERSTAND?—cont'd

22. Once a plaque has formed, it can rupture, resulting in clot formation and instability and vasoconstriction, which lead to obstruction of the lumen and inadequate oxygen delivery to tissues.

23. Peripheral artery disease is the result of atherosclerotic plaque formation in the arteries that supply the extremities, and it causes pain and ischemic changes in the nerves, muscles, and skin of the affected limb.

24. Coronary artery disease (CAD) is the result of an atherosclerotic plaque that gradually narrows the coronary arteries or that ruptures and causes sudden thrombus formation.

25. Many risk factors contribute to the onset and escalation of CAD, including traditional risk factors such as dyslipidemia, smoking, hypertension, diabetes mellitus (insulin resistance), and obesity/sedentary lifestyle and nontraditional risk factors such as elevated C-reactive protein levels, hyperhomocysteinemia, and changes in adipokines.

26. Ischemic heart disease is most commonly the result of coronary artery disease and the ensuing decrease in myocardial blood supply.

27. Atherosclerotic plaque progression can be gradual and cause stable angina pectoris, which is predictable chest pain caused by myocardial ischemia in response to increased demand (e.g., exercise) without infarction.

28. Prinzmetal angina results from coronary artery vasospasm.

29. Myocardial ischemia may be asymptomatic, which is called silent ischemia, and is a risk factor for the development of the acute coronary syndromes.

30. Sudden coronary obstruction due to thrombus formation causes the acute coronary syndromes. These include unstable angina, non-ST elevation myocardial infarction (non-STEMI), and ST elevation myocardial infarction (STEMI).

31. Unstable angina results in reversible myocardial ischemia.

32. Myocardial infarction is caused by prolonged, unrelieved ischemia that interrupts blood supply to the myocardium. After about 20 minutes of myocardial ischemia, irreversible hypoxic injury causes cellular death and tissue necrosis.

33. Myocardial infarction is clinically classified as non-STEMI or STEMI based on electrocardiographic findings that suggest the extent of myocardial damage (subendocardial versus transmural).

34. An increase in plasma enzyme levels is used to diagnose the occurrence of myocardial infarction as well as indicate its severity. Elevations of the isoenzymes creatine kinase-myocardial bound (CK-MB), troponins, and lactate dehydrogenase (LDH-1) are most predictive of a myocardial infarction.

35. Treatment of a myocardial infarction includes revascularization (thrombolytics or PCI) and administration of antithrombotics, ACE inhibitors, and beta-blockers. Pain relief and fluid management also are key components of care. Dysrhythmias and cardiac failure are the most common complications of acute myocardial infarction.

Disorders of the Heart Wall

1. Inflammation of the pericardium, or pericarditis, may result from several sources (infection, drug therapy, tumors). Pericarditis presents with symptoms that are physically troublesome, but in and of themselves they are not life-threatening.

2. Fluid may collect within the pericardial sac (pericardial effusion). Cardiac function may be severely impaired if the accumulation of fluid occurs rapidly and involves a large volume.

3. Cardiomyopathies are a diverse group of primary myocardial disorders that are usually the result of remodeling, neurohumoral responses, and hypertension. The cardiomyopathies are categorized as dilated (congestive), restrictive (rigid and noncompliant), and hypertrophic (asymmetric). The size of the cardiac muscle walls and chambers may increase or decrease depending on the type of cardiomyopathy, thereby altering contractile activity.

4. The hemodynamic integrity of the cardiovascular system depends to a great extent on properly functioning cardiac valves. Congenital or acquired disorders that result in stenosis, regurgitation, or both can structurally alter the valves.

5. Characteristic heart sounds, cardiac murmurs, and systemic complaints assist in identification of an abnormal valve. If severely compromised function exists, a prosthetic heart valve may be surgically implanted to replace the faulty one.

6. Mitral valve prolapse (MVP) describes the condition in which the mitral valve leaflets do not position themselves properly during systole. Mitral valve prolapse may be a completely asymptomatic condition or can result in unpredictable symptoms. Afflicted valves are at greater risk for developing infective endocarditis.

7. Rheumatic fever is an inflammatory disease that results from a delayed immune response to a streptococcal infection in genetically predisposed individuals. The disorder usually resolves without sequelae if treated early.

8. Severe or untreated cases of rheumatic fever may progress to rheumatic heart disease, a potentially disabling cardiovascular disorder.

9. Infective endocarditis is a general term for infection and inflammation of the endocardium, especially the cardiac valves. In the mildest cases, valvular function may be slightly impaired by vegetations that collect on the valve leaflets. If left unchecked, severe valve abnormalities, chronic bacteremia, and systemic emboli may occur as vegetations detach from the valve surface and travel through the bloodstream. Antibiotic therapy can limit the extension of this disease.

10. Human immunodeficiency virus (HIV) infection and AIDS are associated with cardiac abnormalities, including myocarditis, endocarditis, pericarditis, and cardiomyopathy.

Manifestations of Heart Disease

1. A dysrhythmia (arrhythmia) is a disturbance of heart rhythm. Dysrhythmias range in severity from occasional missed beats or rapid beats to disturbances that impair myocardial contractility and are life-threatening.

2. Dysrhythmias can occur because of an abnormal rate of impulse generation or an abnormal conduction of impulses.

3. Heart failure (HF) is an inability of the heart to supply the metabolism with adequate circulatory volume and pressure.

4. Left heart failure (congestive heart failure) can be divided into systolic and diastolic heart failure.

5. The most common causes of left ventricular failure are myocardial infarction and hypertension.

6. Systolic heart failure is caused by increased preload, decreased contractility, or increased afterload. These processes result in an increased left ventricular end-diastolic volume and an increased left ventricular end-diastolic pressure that cause increased pulmonary venous pressures and pulmonary edema.

7. In addition to the hemodynamic changes of left ventricular failure, there is a neuroendocrine response that tends to exacerbate and perpetuate the condition.

8. The neuroendocrine mediators of HF include the sympathetic nervous system and the renin-angiotensin-aldosterone system; thus diuretics, betablockers, and angiotensin-converting enzyme (ACE) inhibitors are important components of the pharmacologic therapy.

9. Diastolic heart failure is a clinical syndrome characterized by the symptoms and signs of heart failure, a preserved ejection fraction, and abnormal diastolic function.

10. Diastolic dysfunction means that the left ventricular end-diastolic pressure is increased, even if volume and cardiac output are normal.

11. Right heart failure can result from left heart failure or pulmonary disease.

DID YOU UNDERSTAND?—cont'd

Shock

1. Shock is a widespread impairment of cellular metabolism involving positive feedback loops that places the individual on a downward physiologic spiral leading to multiple organ dysfunction syndrome.

2. Types of shock are cardiogenic, hypovolemic, neurogenic, anaphylactic, and septic. Multiple organ dysfunction syndrome can develop from all types of shock.

3. The final common pathway in all types of shock is impaired cellular metabolism—cells switch from aerobic to anaerobic metabolism. Energy stores drop, and cellular mechanisms relative to membrane permeability, action potentials, and lysozyme release fail.

4. Anaerobic metabolism results in activation of the inflammatory response, decreased circulatory volume, and decreasing pH.

5. Impaired cellular metabolism results in cellular inability to use glucose because of impaired glucose delivery or impaired glucose intake, resulting in a shift to glycogenolysis, gluconeogenesis, and lipolysis for fuel generation.

6. Glycogenolysis is effective for about 10 hours. Gluconeogenesis results in the use of proteins necessary for structure, function, repair, and replication that leads to more impaired cellular metabolism.

7. Gluconeogenesis contributes to lactic acid, uric acid, and ammonia buildup, interstitial edema, and impairment of the immune system, as well as general muscle weakness, leading to decreased respiratory function and cardiac output.

8. Cardiogenic shock is decreased cardiac output, tissue hypoxia, and the presence of adequate intravascular volume.

9. Hypovolemic shock is caused by loss of blood or fluid in large amounts. The use of compensatory mechanisms may be vigorous, but tissue perfusion ultimately decreases and results in impaired cellular metabolism.

10. Neurogenic shock results from massive vasodilation, causing a relative hypovolemia even though cardiac output may be high, and leads to impaired cellular metabolism.

11. Anaphylactic shock is caused by physiologic recognition of a foreign substance. The inflammatory response is triggered, and a massive vasodilation with fluid shift into the interstitium follows. The relative hypovolemia leads to impaired cellular metabolism.

12. Septic shock begins with impaired cellular metabolism caused by uncontrolled septicemia. The infecting agent triggers the inflammatory and immune responses. This inflammatory response is accompanied by widespread changes in tissue and cellular function.

13. Multiple organ dysfunction syndrome (MODS) is the progressive failure of two or more organ systems after a severe illness or injury. It can be triggered by chronic inflammation, necrotic tissue, severe trauma, burns, adult respiratory distress syndrome, acute pancreatitis, and other severe injuries.

14. MODS involves the stress response; changes in the vascular endothelium resulting in microvascular coagulation; release of complement, coagulation, and kinin proteins; and numerous inflammatory processes. Consequences of all these mediators are a maldistribution of blood flow, hypermetabolism, hypoxic injury, and myocardial depression.

15. Clinical manifestations of MODS include inflammation, tissue hypoxia, and hypermetabolism. All organs can be affected including the kidney, lung, liver, gastrointestinal tract, and central nervous system.

KEY TERMS

- Acute coronary syndrome   598
- Acute pericarditis   609
- Anaphylactic shock   631
- Anaphylaxis   631
- Aneurysm   591
- Aortic regurgitation   614
- Aortic stenosis   613
- Arteriosclerosis   594
- Atherosclerosis   594
- Bacterial translocation
- Cardiogenic shock   629
- Cardiomyopathy   611
- Chronic left heart failure   625
- Chronic orthostatic hypotension   591
- Chronic venous insufficiency (CVI)   586
- Chylomicron   598
- Complicated plaque   595
- Constrictive pericarditis (restrictive pericarditis [chronic pericarditis])   611
- Coronary artery disease (CAD)   597
- Deep venous thrombosis (DVT)   586
- Diastolic heart failure   625
- Dilated cardiomyopathy   611
- Dyslipidemia (dyslipoproteinemia)   598
- Dysrhythmia (arrhythmia)   619
- Embolism   593
- Embolus   593
- False aneurysm   592

- Fatty streak   595
- Fibrous plaque   595
- Foam cell   595
- Heart failure   622
- Hibernating myocardium   606
- High-density lipoprotein (HDL)   590
- Highly-sensitive C-reactive protein (hs-CRP)   599
- High-output failure   626
- Hyperhomocysteinemia   599
- Hypertension   587
- Hypertensive hypertrophic cardiomyopathy   612
- Hypertrophic cardiomyopathy   612
- Hypertrophic obstructive cardiomyopathy   612
- Hypovolemic shock   631
- Infarction   598
- Infective endocarditis   617
- Intermittent claudication   597
- Ischemia   597
- Isolated systolic hypertension (ISH)   587
- Left heart failure   623
- Lipoprotein   598
- Lipoprotein(a) (Lp[a])   599
- Low-density lipoprotein (LDL)   594
- Malignant hypertension   590
- Mental stress–induced ischemia   601

- Metabolic syndrome   599
- Mitral regurgitation   615
- Mitral stenosis   614
- Mitral valve prolapse syndrome (MVPS)   615
- Multiple organ dysfunction syndrome (MODS)   634
- Myocardial infarction (MI)   604
- Myocardial remodeling   606
- Myocardial stunning   606
- Myocarditis   617
- Neurogenic shock (vasogenic shock)   631
- Nonbacterial thrombotic endocarditis   618
- Non-ST elevation MI (non-STEMI)   604
- Orthostatic (postural) hypotension   591
- Percutaneous coronary intervention (PCI)   604
- Pericardial effusion   610
- Peripheral artery disease (PAD)   597
- Peripheral pooling   631
- Plaque   594
- Pressure-natriuresis relationship   588
- Primary hypertension (essential hypertension, idiopathic hypertension)   587
- Prinzmetal angina   601
- Raynaud disease   594
- Raynaud phenomenon   594

Continued

KEY TERMS—cont'd

REFERENCES

1. Kostas TI, et al: Chronic venous disease progression and modification of predisposing factors, *J Vasc Surg* 51(4):900–907, 2010.
2. Brown A: Managing chronic venous leg ulcers: time for a new approach? *J Wound Care* 19(2):70–74, 2010.
3. Kovac M, et al: Type and location of venous thromboembolism in carriers of Factor V Leiden or prothrombin G20210A mutation versus patients with no mutation, *Clin Appl Thromb Hemost* 16(1):66–70, 2010.
4. Prandoni P, Kahn SR: Post-thrombotic syndrome: prevalence, prognostication and need for progress, *Br J Haematol* 145(3):286–295, 2009.
5. Eppsteiner RW, et al: Mechanical compression versus subcutaneous heparin therapy in postoperative and posttrauma patients: a systematic review and meta-analysis, *World J Surg* 34(1):10–19, 2010.
6. Young T, Tang H, Hughes R: Vena caval filters for the prevention of pulmonary embolism, *Cochrane Database Syst Rev* (2), 2010:CD006212.
7. Wan JF, Bezjak A: Superior vena cava syndrome, *Emerg Med Clin North Am* 27(2):243–255, 2009.
8. Lloyd-Jones D, et al: Writing Group for the Heart Disease and Stroke Statistics—2010 update: a report from the American Heart Association, *Circulation* 121:E46–E215, 2010.
9. Chobanian AV: The Seventh Report of the Joint National Committee on prevention, detection, evaluation, and treatment of high blood pressure: the JNC report, *J Am Med Assoc* 289(19):2560–2572, 2003.
10. Pimenta E, Oparil S: Prehypertension: epidemiology, consequences and treatment, *Nat Rev Nephrol* 6(1):21–30, 2010.
11. Grebla RC, et al: Prevalence and determinants of isolated systolic hypertension among young adults: the 1999–2004 US National Health and Nutrition Examination Survey, *J Hypertens* 28(1):15–23, 2010.
12. Kunes J, Zicha J: The interaction of genetic and environmental factors in the etiology of hypertension, *Physiol Res* 58(Suppl 2):S33–S41, 2009.
13. Conen D, et al: Association of 77 polymorphisms in 52 candidate genes with blood pressure progression and incident hypertension: the women's genome health study, *J Hypertens* 27(3):476–483, 2009.
14. Fink GD: Arthur C Corcoran Memorial Lecture. Sympathetic activity, vascular capacitance, and long-term regulation of arterial pressure, *Hypertension* 53(2):307–312, 2009.
15. Grassi G: Assessment of sympathetic cardiovascular drive in human hypertension: achievements and perspectives, *Hypertension* 54(4):690–697, 2009.
16. Steckelings UM, et al: The evolving story of the RAAS in hypertension, diabetes and CV disease: moving from macrovascular to microvascular targets, *Fundam Clin Pharmacol* 23(6):693–703, 2009.
17. Probstfield JL, O'Brien KD: Progression of cardiovascular damage: the role of renin-angiotensin system blockade, *Am J Cardiol* 105 (Suppl 1):A10–A20, 2010.
18. Tomaschitz A, et al: Aldosterone and arterial hypertension, *Nat Rev Endocrinol* 6(2):83–93, 2010.
19. Iwanami J, et al: Inhibition of the renin-angiotensin system and target organ protection, *Hypertens Res* 32(4):229–237, 2009.
20. Woodard GE, Rosado JA: Natriuretic peptides in vascular physiology and pathology, *Rev Cell Mol Biol* 268:59–93, 2008.
21. Androulakis ES, et al: Essential hypertension: is there a role for inflammatory mechanisms? *Cardiol Rev* 17(5):216–221, 2009.
22. Duan SZ, Usher MG, Mortensen RM: PPARs: the vasculature, inflammation and hypertension, *Curr Opin Nephrol Hypertens* 18(2):128–133, 2009.
23. Bogaert YE, Linas S: The role of obesity in the pathogenesis of hypertension, *Nat Clin Prac Nephrol* 5(2):101–111, 2009.
24. Grassi G, Diez J: Obesity-related cardiac and vascular structural alterations: beyond blood pressure overload, *J Hypertens* 27(9):1750–1752, 2009.
25. Barrios V, Escobar C: Diabetes and hypertension. What is new? *Minerva Cardioangiol* 57(6):705–722, 2009.
26. Redon J: Mechanisms of hypertension in the cardiometabolic syndrome, *J Hypertens* 27(3):441–451, 2009.
27. Reynolds K, Wildman RP: Update on the metabolic syndrome: hypertension, *Curr Hypertens Rep* 11(2):150–155, 2009.
28. Re RN: New insights into target organ involvement in hypertension, *Med Clin North Am* 93(3):559–567, 2009.
29. Gradman AH, Wilson JT: Hypertension and diastolic heart failure, *Curr Cardiol Rep* 11(6):422–429, 2009.
30. Verma A, Solomon SD: Diastolic dysfunction as a link between hypertension and heart failure, *Med Clin North Am* 93(3):647–664, 2009.
31. Waeber B, de la Sierra A, Ruilope LM: Target organ damage: how to detect it and how to treat it? *J Hypertens* 27(Suppl 3):S13–S18, 2009.
32. Nagai M, Hoshide S, Kario K: Hypertension and dementia, *Am J Hypertens* 23(2):116–124, 2010.
33. Veglio F, et al: Hypertension and cerebrovascular damage, *Atherosclerosis* 205(2):331–341, 2009.
34. Ernst ME, Moser M: Use of diuretics in patients with hypertension, *N Eng J Med* 361(22):2153–2164, 2009.
35. Williams B: The changing face of hypertension treatment: treatment strategies from the 2007 ESH/ESC hypertension guidelines, *J Hypertens* 27(suppl 3):S19–S26, 2009.
36. Glynn LG, et al: Interventions used to improve control of blood pressure in patients with hypertension: Update of *Cochrane Database Syst Rev* (4)CD005182, 2006:PMID: 17054244. *Cochrane Database Syst Rev* (3):CD005182, 2010.
37. Medow MS, et al: Pathophysiology, diagnosis, and treatment of orthostatic hypotension and vasovagal syncope, *Cardiol Rev* 16(1):4–20, 2008.
38. Mustafa ST, et al: Endovascular repair of nonruptured thoracic aortic aneurysms: systematic review, *Vascular* 18(1):28–33, 2010.
39. Piazza G, Creager MA: Thromboangiitis obliterans, *Circulation* 121 (16):1858–1861, 2010.
40. Boda Z, et al: Stem cell therapy: a promising and prospective approach in the treatment of patients with severe Buerger's disease, *Clin Appl Thromb Hemost* 15(5):552–560, 2009.
41. Gayraud M: Raynaud's phenomenon, *Joint Bone Spine* 74(1):E1–E8, 2007.
42. Lambova SN, Muller-Ladner U: New lines in therapy of Raynaud's phenomenon, *Rheumatol Int* 29(4):355–363, 2009.

43. Libby P, et al: Inflammation in atherosclerosis: transition from theory to practice, *Circ J* 74(2):213–220, 2010.

44. Lundberg AM, Hansson GK: Innate immune signals in atherosclerosis, *Clin Immunol* 134(1):5–24, 2010.

45. Steinmetz M, Nickenig G, Werner N: Endothelial-regenerating cells: an expanding universe, *Hypertension* 55(3):593–599, 2010.

46. Woollard KJ, Geissmann F: Monocytes in atherosclerosis: subsets and functions, *Nat Rev Cardiol* 7(2):77–86, 2010.

47. Miller Y, et al: Lipoprotein modification and macrophage uptake: role of pathologic cholesterol transport in atherogenesis, *Sub-Cell Biochem* 51:229–251, 2010.

48. Libby P, DiCarli M, Weissleder R: The vascular biology of atherosclerosis and imaging targets, *J Nuclear Med* 51(Suppl 1):S33–S37, 2010.

49. Andersson J, Libby P, Hansson GK: Adaptive immunity and atherosclerosis, *Clin Immunol* 134(1):33–46, 2010.

50. Orr AW, et al: Complex regulation and function of the inflammatory smooth muscle cell phenotype in atherosclerosis, *J Vasc Res* 47(2):168–180, 2010.

51. Moreno PR: Vulnerable plaque: definition, diagnosis, and treatment, *Cardiol Clin* 28(1):1–30, 2010.

52. Back M, Ketelhuth DF, Agewall S: Matrix metalloproteinases in athero-thrombosis, *Prog Cardiovas Dis* 52(5):410–428, 2010.

53. Hermus L, van Dam GM, Zeebregts CJ: Advanced carotid plaque imaging, *Eur J Vasc Endovasc Surg* 39(2):125–133, 2010.

54. Schafers M, Schober O, Hermann S: Matrix-metalloproteinases as imaging targets for inflammatory activity in atherosclerotic plaques, *J Nuclear Med* 51(5):663–666, 2010.

55. Lavoie A, et al: Findings of clinical trials that evaluate the impact of medical therapies on progression of atherosclerosis, *Curr Med Res Opin* 26(3):745–751, 2010.

56. Ferreira AC, Macedo FY: A review of simple, non-invasive means of assessing peripheral arterial disease and implications for medical management, *Ann Med* 42(2):139–150, 2010.

57. Fadini GP, Agostini C, Avogaro A: Autologous stem cell therapy for peripheral arterial disease: meta-analysis and systematic review of the literature, *Atherosclerosis* 209(1):10–17, 2010.

58. Pacilli A, et al: An update on therapeutic angiogenesis for peripheral vascular disease, *Ann Vasc Surg* 24(2):258–268, 2010.

59. Ding K, Kullo IJ: Genome-wide association studies for atherosclerotic vascular disease and its risk factors, *Circ Cardiovasc Genet* 2(1):63–72, 2009.

60. Expert Panel on Detection: Evaluation, and Treatment of High Blood Cholesterol in Adults: Executive summary of the third report of the National Cholesterol Education Program (NCEP) expert panel on detection, evaluation, and treatment of high blood cholesterol in adults (Adult Treatment Panel III), *J Am Med Assoc* 285(19):2486–2497, 2001.

61. Karalis DG: Intensive lowering of low-density lipoprotein cholesterol levels for primary prevention of coronary artery disease, *Mayo Clin Proc* 84(4):345–352, 2009.

62. Preiss D, Sattar N: Lipids, lipid modifying agents and cardiovascular risk: a review of the evidence, *Clin Endocrinol* 70(6):815–828, 2009.

63. Smith JD: Dysfunctional HDL as a diagnostic and therapeutic target, *Arterioscler Thromb Vasc Biol* 30(2):151–155, 2010.

64. Tsompanidi EM, et al: HDL biogenesis and functions: role of HDL quality and quantity in atherosclerosis, *Atherosclerosis* 208(1):3–9, 2010.

65. Mendez AJ: The promise of apolipoprotein A-I mimetics, *Curr Opin Endocrinol Diabetes Obes* 17(2):171–176, 2010.

66. Natarajan P, Ray KK, Cannon CP: High-density lipoprotein and coronary heart disease: current and future therapies, *J Am Coll Cardiol* 55(13):1283–1299, 2010.

67. Spence JD: The role of lipoprotein(a) in the formation of arterial plaques, stenoses and occlusions, *Can J Cardiol* 26(Suppl A):A37–A40, 2010.

68. Mathieu P, Lemieux I, Despres JP: Obesity, inflammation, and cardiovascular risk, *Clin Pharmacol Ther* 87(4):407–416, 2010.

69. Sweeney G: Cardiovascular effects of leptin, *Nat Rev Cardiol* 7(1):22–29, 2010.

70. Mohammed AA, Januzzi JL: Clinical applications of highly sensitive troponin assays, *Cardiol Rev* 18(1):12–19, 2010.

71. Corrado E, et al: An update on the role of markers of inflammation in atherosclerosis, *J Atheroscler Thromb* 17(1):1–11, 2010.

72. Di Minno MN, et al: Homocysteine and arterial thrombosis: challenge and opportunity, *Thromb Haemost* 103(5):942–961, 2010.

73. El-Menyar A, et al: Total and high molecular weight adiponectin in patients with coronary artery disease, *J Cardiovasc Med* 10(4):310–315, 2009.

74. Nanasato M, Murohara T: Role of adiponectin in cardiovascular protection, *Circul* 74(3):432–433, 2010.

75. Agarwal M, Mehta PK, Bairey Merz CN: Nonacute coronary syndrome anginal chest pain, *Med Clin North Am* 94(2):201–216, 2010.

76. Zbierajewski-Eischeid SJ, Loeb SJ: Myocardial infarction in women: promoting symptom recognition, early diagnosis, and risk assessment, *Dimens Crit Care Nurs* 28(1):1–6, 2009.

77. Stern S, Bayes de Luna A: Coronary artery spasm: a 2009 update, *Circulation* 119(18):2531–2534, 2009.

78. D'Antono B, et al: Silent ischemia: silent after all? *Can J Cardiol* 24(4):285–291, 2008.

79. Kop WJ, et al: Effects of acute mental stress and exercise on inflammatory markers in patients with coronary artery disease and healthy controls, *Am J Cardiol* 101(6):767–773, 2008.

80. Madsen JK, et al: DANAMI study group. Revascularization compared to medical treatment in patients with silent vs. symptomatic residual ischemia after thrombolyzed myocardial infarction—the DANAMI study, *Cardiology* 108(4):243–251, 2007.

81. Fraker T, Fihn S: 2007 chronic angina focused update of the ACC/AHA 2002 guidelines for the management of patients with chronic stable angina: a report of the American College of Cardiology/American Heart Association Task Force on Practice Guidelines Writing Group to develop the focused update of the 2002 guidelines for the management of patients with chronic stable angina, *J Am Coll Cardiol* 50:2264–2274, 2007.

82. Pfisterer ME, Zellweger MJ, Gersh BJ: Management of stable coronary artery disease, *Lancet* 375(9716):763–772, 2010.

83. Reffelmann T, Kloner RA: Ranolazine: an anti-anginal drug with further therapeutic potential, *Exp Rev Cardiovas Ther* 8(3):319–329, 2010.

84. Cassar A, et al: Chronic coronary artery disease: diagnosis and management, *Mayo Clin Proc* 84(12):1130–1146, 2009.

85. Ambrose JA, Srikanth S: Vulnerable plaques and patients: improving prediction of future coronary events, *Am J Med* 123(1):10–16, 2010.

86. Kumar A, Cannon CP: Acute coronary syndromes: diagnosis and management, part I, *Mayo Clin Proc* 84(10):917–938, 2009.

87. Anderson J, et al: ACC/AHA 2007 guidelines for the management of patients with unstable angina/non–ST-elevation myocardial infarction: a report of the American College of Cardiology/American Heart Association Task Force on Practice Guidelines, *J Am Coll Cardiol* 50:E1–E157, 2007.

88. Ceriello A, Zarich SW, Testa R: Lowering glucose to prevent adverse cardiovascular outcomes in a critical care setting, *J Am Coll Cardiol* 53 (Suppl 5):S9–S13, 2009.

89. Sun Y: Intracardiac renin-angiotensin system and myocardial repair/remodeling following infarction, *J Mol Cell Cardiol* 48(3):483–489, 2010.

90. Whelan RS, Kaplinskiy V, Kitsis RN: Cell death in the pathogenesis of heart disease: mechanisms and significance, *Annu Rev Physiol* 72:19–44, 2010.

91. Pomblum VJ, et al: Cardiac stunning in the clinic: the full picture, *Interact Cardiovasc Thorac Surg* 10(1):86–91, 2010.

92. Slezak J, et al: Hibernating myocardium: pathophysiology, diagnosis, and treatment, *Can J Physiol Pharmacol* 87(4):252–265, 2009.

93. van den Borne SW, et al: Myocardial remodeling after infarction: the role of myofibroblasts, *Nat Rev Cardiol* 7(1):30–37, 2010.

94. Thygesen K, Alpert J, White H: ESC/ACCF/AHA/WHF expert consensus document: universal definition of myocardial infarction, *J Am Coll Cardiol* 50:2173–2195, 2007.

95. Bavry AA, et al: Long-term benefit of statin therapy initiated during hospitalization for an acute coronary syndrome: a systematic review of randomized trials, *Am J Cardiovas Drugs* 7(2):135–141, 2007.

96. Khandaker MH, et al: Pericardial disease: diagnosis and management, *Mayo Clin Proc* 85(6):572–593, 2010.

97. Imazio M, et al: Aetiological diagnosis in acute and recurrent pericarditis: when and how, *J Cardiovasc Med* 10(3):217–230, 2009.

98. Imazio M, et al: Controversial issues in the management of pericardial diseases, *Circulation* 121(7):916–928, 2010.

99. Novik J, Weekes AJ: An unusual cause of severe dyspnea: diastolic dysfunction due to calcific constrictive pericarditis, *J Emerg Med* 38(2): 208–213, 2010.

100. Schwefer M, et al: Constrictive pericarditis, still a diagnostic challenge: comprehensive review of clinical management, *Eur J Cardiothorac Surg* 36(3):502–510, 2009.

101. Jefferies JL, Towbin JA: Dilated cardiomyopathy, *Lancet* 375:752–762, 2010.

102. Wang L, Seidman JG, Seidman CE: Narrative review: harnessing molecular genetics for the diagnosis and management of hypertrophic cardiomyopathy, *Ann Intern Med* 152(8):513–520, 2010:W181.

103. Maron BJ: Contemporary insights and strategies for risk stratification and prevention of sudden death in hypertrophic cardiomyopathy, *Circulation* 121(3):445–456, 2010.

104. Bonow RO, et al: ACC/AHA 2006 guidelines for the management of patients with valvular heart disease: a report of the American College of Cardiology/American Heart Association Task Force on Practice Guidelines (Writing Committee to Revise the 1998 Guidelines for the Management of Patients With Valvular Heart Disease), *J Am Coll Cardiol* 48:E1–E148, 2006.

105. Maganti K, et al: Valvular heart disease: diagnosis and management, *Mayo Clin Proc* 85(5):483–500, 2010.

106. Coeytaux RR, et al: Percutaneous heart valve replacement for aortic stenosis: state of the evidence, *Ann Intern Med* 153(5):314–324, 2010.

107. Foster E: Clinical practice. Mitral regurgitation due to degenerative mitral-valve disease, *N Engl J Med* 363(2):156–165, 2010.

108. Guilherme L, Kalil J: Rheumatic fever and rheumatic heart disease: cellular mechanisms leading to autoimmune reactivity and disease, *J Clin Immunol* 30(1):17–23, 2010.

109. Ferrieri P: Jones Criteria Working Group: Proceedings of the Jones Criteria Workshop, *Circulation* 106(19):2521–2523, 2002.

110. World Health Organization: *Rheumatic fever and rheumatic heart disease: report of a WHO expert consultation*, Geneva, 2004, Author.

111. Dale JB: Current status of group A streptococcal vaccine development, *Adv Exp Med Biol* 609:53–63, 2008.

112. McDonald JR: Acute infective endocarditis, *Infect Dis Clin North Am* 23(3):643–664, 2009.

113. Marrie TJ: Osler's nodes and Janeway lesions, *Am J Med* 121(2):105–106, 2008.

114. Chopra T, Kaatz GW: Treatment strategies for infective endocarditis, *Exp Opin Pharmacother* 11(3):345–360, 2010.

115. Prendergast BD, Tornos P: Surgery for infective endocarditis: who and when? *Circulation* 121(9):1141–1152, 2010.

116. Nishimura RA, et al: ACC/AHA 2008 guideline update on valvular heart disease: focused update on infective endocarditis: a report of the American College of Cardiology/American Heart Association Task Force on Practice Guidelines: endorsed by the Society of Cardiovascular Anesthesiologists, Society for Cardiovascular Angiography and Interventions, and Society of Thoracic Surgeons, *Circulation* 118(8):887–896, 2008.

117. Nass RD, et al: Mechanisms of disease: ion channel remodeling in the failing ventricle, *Nat Clin Pract Cardiovasc Med* 5(4):196–207, 2008.

118. McMurray JJ: Systolic heart failure, *N Engl J Med* 362:228–238, 2010.

119. Jourdan-Lesaux C, Zhang J, Lindsey ML: Extracellular matrix roles during cardiac repair, *Life Sci* 87(13–14):391–400, 2010.

120. Rohini A, et al: Molecular targets and regulators of cardiac hypertrophy, *Pharmacol Res* 61(4):269–280, 2010.

121. Ramani GV, Uber PA, Mehra MR: Chronic heart failure: contemporary diagnosis and management, *Mayo Clin Proc* 85:180–195, 2010.

122. O'Donoghue M, Braunwald E: Natriuretic peptides in heart failure: should therapy be guided by BNP levels? *Nat Rev Cardiol* 7(1):13–20, 2010.

123. DeWald TA, Hernandez AF: Efficacy and safety of nesiritide in patients with acute decompensated heart failure, *Exp Rev Cardiovasc Ther* 8(2):159–169, 2010.

124. Hunt SA, et al: 2009 focused update incorporated into the ACC/AHA 2005 Guidelines for the Diagnosis and Management of Heart Failure in Adults: a report of the American College of Cardiology Foundation/American Heart Association Task Force on Practice Guidelines: developed in collaboration with the International Society for Heart and Lung Transplantation, *Circulation* 119(14):E391–E479, 2009.

125. Paulus WJ: Novel strategies in diastolic heart failure, *Heart* 96(14): 1147–1153, 2010.

126. Gando S: Microvascular thrombosis and multiple organ dysfunction syndrome, *Crit Care Med* 38(Suppl 2):S35–S42, 2010.

127. den Uil CA, et al: Management of cardiogenic shock: focus on tissue perfusion, *Curr Prob Cardiol* 34(8):330–349, 2009.

128. Rajani RR, et al: Vasopressin in hemorrhagic shock: review article, *Am Surgeon* 75(12):1207–1212, 2009.

129. McMahon D, Tutt M, Cook AM: Pharmacological management of hemodynamic complications following spinal cord injury, *Orthopedics* 32(5):331, 2009.

130. Simons FE: Anaphylaxis, *J Allergy Clin Immunol* 125(2) (Suppl 2): S161–S181, 2010.

131. Worth A, Soar J, Sheikh A: Management of anaphylaxis in the emergency setting, *Exp Rev Clin Immunol* 6(1):89–100, 2010.

132. Levy MM, et al: 2001 SCCM/ES/CM/ACCP/ATS/SIS International Sepsis Definitions Conference, *Crit Care Med* 31(4):1250–1256, 2003.

133. Nduka OO, Parrillo JE: The pathophysiology of septic shock, *Crit Care Clin* 25(4):677–702, 2009:vii.

134. Zanotti-Cavazzoni SL, Hollenberg SM: Cardiac dysfunction in severe sepsis and septic shock, *Curr Opin Crit Care* 15(5):392–397, 2009.

135. Anderson R, Schmidt R: Clinical biomarkers in sepsis, *Front Biosci* 2:504–520, 2010.

136. Levy MM, et al: The surviving sepsis campaign: results of an international guideline-based performance improvement program targeting severe sepsis, *Crit Care Med* 38(2):367–374, 2010.

137. Dellinger RP, et al: Surviving Sepsis Campaign: international guidelines for management of severe sepsis and septic shock, *Crit Care Med* 36:296–327, 2008.

138. Toussaint S, Gerlach H: Activated protein C for sepsis, *N Engl J Med* 361(27):2646–2652, 2009.

139. Levi M, Schultz M, van der Poll T: Disseminated intravascular coagulation in infectious disease, *Sem Thromb Hemost* 36(4):367–377, 2010.

140. Mohammed I: Mechanisms, detection, and potential management of microcirculatory disturbances in sepsis, *Crit Care Clin* 26(2):393–408, 2010.

141. Levi M, Lowenberg E, Meijers JC: Recombinant anticoagulant factors for adjunctive treatment of sepsis, *Sem Thromb Hemost* 36(5):550–557, 2010.

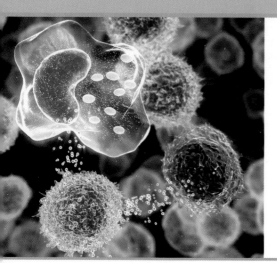

Alterations of Cardiovascular Function in Children

Nancy L. McDaniel and Valentina L. Brashers

evolve WEBSITE

http://evolve.elsevier.com/Huether/
- Review Questions and Answers
- Animations
- Quick Check Answers

- Key Terms Exercises
- Critical Thinking Questions with Answers
- Algorithm Completion Exercises
- WebLinks

CHAPTER OUTLINE

Cardiovascular disorders in children are classified as congenital or acquired. Congenital heart disease is the most common. The diagnosis and management of congenital heart disease continues to improve with the use of fetal echocardiography and early interventional catheterization or surgical repair. Acquired heart disease in children continues to present challenges to the practitioner. Although guidelines for diagnosing acquired diseases are available, work is still needed in developing standards of treatment and long-term follow-up protocols.

CONGENITAL HEART DISEASE

The incidence of congenital heart disease (CHD) varies from 4 to 8 per 1000 live births and is the major cause of death in the first year of life other than prematurity. Several environmental and genetic risk factors are associated with the incidence of different types of CHD. Among the environmental factors are (1) maternal conditions, such as intrauterine viral infections (especially rubella), diabetes mellitus, phenylketonuria, alcoholism, hypercalcemia, drugs (e.g., thalidomide, phenytoin), and complications of increased age; (2) antepartal bleeding; and (3) prematurity (Table 24-1).[1,2]

Genetic factors also have been implicated in the incidence of CHD, although the mechanism of causation is often unknown (Table 24-2).

The incidence of CHD is three to four times higher in siblings of affected children, and chromosomal defects account for about 6% of all cases of CHD. Down syndrome, trisomies 13 and 18, Turner syndrome, and cri du chat syndrome (chromosome 5p deletion syndrome) have been associated with a relatively high incidence of heart defects. Only a small percentage of cases of CHD are clearly linked solely to genetic or environmental factors. The cause of most defects is multifactorial.[1,2]

Congenital heart defects can be categorized according to (1) whether they cause cyanosis, (2) whether they increase or decrease blood flow into the pulmonary circulation, and (3) whether they obstruct blood flow from the ventricles (Figure 24-1). The normal movement of blood through the right side of the heart and into the pulmonary system is separate from the blood flow through the left side of the heart into the systemic circulation (Figure 24-2, *A*). Abnormal movement from one side of the heart to the other is termed a shunt. Shunting of blood flow from the left heart into the right heart is called a left-to-right shunt and occurs in conditions such as atrial septal defect and ventricular septal defect (see Figure 24-2, *B*). This increases blood flow into the pulmonary circulation. Because blood continues to flow through the lungs before passing into the systemic circulation, there is no decrease in tissue oxygenation or cyanosis. Thus defects that cause left-to-right shunt are termed acyanotic heart

TABLE 24-1	**MATERNAL CONDITIONS AND ENVIRONMENTAL EXPOSURES AND THE ASSOCIATED CONGENITAL HEART DEFECTS**
CAUSE	**TYPE OF CONGENITAL HEART DEFECT**
Infection	
Intrauterine	Patent ductus arteriosus (PDA), pulmonary stenosis, coarctation of aorta
Systemic viral	PDA, pulmonary stenosis, coarctation of aorta
Rubella	PDA, pulmonary stenosis, coarctation of aorta
Coxsackie B5	Endocardial fibroelastosis
Radiation	Specific cardiovascular effect not known
Metabolic Disorders	
Diabetes	Ventricular septal defect (VSD), cardiomegaly, transposition of the great vessels
Phenylketonuria (PKU)	Coarctation of aorta, PDA
Hypercalcemia	Supravalvular aortic stenosis, pulmonic stenosis; aortic hyperplasia
Drugs	
Thalidomide	No specific lesion
Dextroamphetamine	One case of reported transposition
Alcohol	Tetralogy of Fallot, atrial septal defect, VSD
Peripheral Conditions	
Increased maternal age	VSD, tetralogy of Fallot (relationship unclear)
Antepartal bleeding	Various defects (relationship unclear)
Prematurity	PDA, VSD
High altitude	PDA, atrial septal defect (increased incidence)

TABLE 24-2	**CONGENITAL HEART DISEASE IN SELECTED FETAL CHROMOSOMAL ABERRATIONS**	
CONDITIONS	**INCIDENCE OF CHD (%)**	**COMMON DEFECTS (IN DECREASING ORDER OF FREQUENCY)**
5p (cri du chat syndrome)	25	VSD, PDA, ASD
Trisomy 13 syndrome	90	VSD, PDA, dextrocardia
Trisomy 18 syndrome	99	VSD, PDA, PS
Trisomy 21 (Down syndrome)	50	AVSD, VSD
Turner syndrome (XO)	35	COA, AS, ASD
Klinefelter variant (XXXXY)	15	PDA, ASD

From Park MK: *Pediatric cardiology for practitioners*, ed 5, St Louis, 2008, Mosby.
AS, Aortic stenosis; *ASD*, atrial septal defect; *AVSD*, atrioventricular septal defect; *COA*, coarctation of the aorta; *PDA*, patent ductus arteriosus; *PS*, pulmonary stenosis; *VSD*, ventricular septal defect.

Obstructive Defects
Coarctation of the Aorta

PATHOPHYSIOLOGY Coarctation of the aorta (COA) is an abnormal localized narrowing of the aorta just proximal to the insertion of the ductus arteriosus. Before birth, the ductus arteriosus bypasses this obstruction and allows for blood to flow from the pulmonary artery into the distal aorta. However, once the ductus closes after birth, blood flow to the lower extremities is restricted by the coarctation. Clinically, there is increased blood pressure proximal to the defect (head and upper extremities, right greater than left) and decreased blood pressure distal to the obstruction (torso and lower extremities) (Figure 24-3).

CLINICAL MANIFESTATIONS The location and severity of the COA determine whether an infant will become symptomatic after the ductus arteriosus closes. If the COA is severe, infants will present with low cardiac output, poor tissue perfusion, acidosis, and hypotension. Physical examination of the infant will reveal weak or absent femoral pulses. Some infants with COA will remain asymptomatic after the closure of the ductus arteriosus. As they age, children with undiagnosed COA will present with unexplained upper extremity hypertension. Children may complain of leg pain or cramping with exercise. They also may rarely experience dizziness, headaches, fainting, or epistaxis from hypertension.[1,2]

EVALUATION AND TREATMENT Physical examination and measurement of upper and lower extremity blood pressures will often suggest the diagnosis. Echocardiography, magnetic resonance imaging (MRI), and cardiac catheterization may be needed to confirm the diagnosis. Initial treatment in the symptomatic newborn consists of continuous intravenous infusion of prostaglandin E_1 to maintain the patency of the ductus arteriosus. Once the symptomatic newborn is stabilized, surgical correction is indicated.[3]

Surgical correction consists of either resection of the narrowed portion of the aorta with an end-to-end anastomosis or enlargement of the constricted section using a graft taken from a portion of the left subclavian artery. Because this defect is outside the heart and pericardium, cardiopulmonary bypass usually is not required and a thoracotomy

defects. Other types of acyanotic heart defects obstruct blood flow from the ventricles but do not cause shunting. Cyanotic heart defects frequently cause shunting of blood from the right side of the heart directly into the left side of the heart (right-to-left shunt). This type of shunt decreases blood flow through the pulmonary system, causing less than normal oxygen delivery to the tissues and resultant cyanosis (see Chapter 26). The most common cyanotic heart defect is tetralogy of Fallot (TOF); in this condition, narrowing of the pulmonary outflow tract increases right heart pressures, thus forcing blood through a defect in the ventricular septum into the left heart (see Figure 24-2, C). Cyanosis, a bluish discoloration of the skin indicating that tissues are not receiving normal amounts of oxygen, also can be caused by other types of heart defects that result in the mixing of venous and arterial blood.

Most congenital heart defects are named to describe the underlying defect (for example, valvular abnormalities; abnormal openings in the septa, including persistence of the foramen ovale; continued patency of the ductus arteriosus; and malformation or abnormal placement of the great vessels). A description of the most common defects follows.

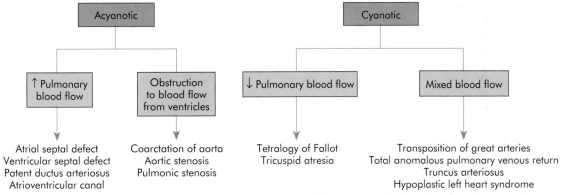

FIGURE 24-1 Comparison of Acyanotic-Cyanotic and Hemodynamic Classification Systems of Congenital Heart Disease. (From Hockenberry MJ et al: *Wong's nursing care of infants and children,* ed 9, St Louis, 2011, Mosby.)

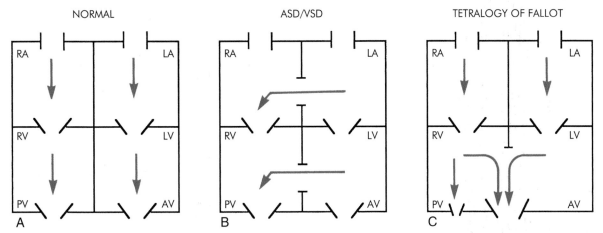

FIGURE 24-2 Shunting of Blood in Congenital Heart Disease. **A,** Normal. **B,** Acyanotic defect. **C,** Cyanotic defect. *ASD,* Atrial septal defect; *AV,* aortic valve; *LA,* left atrium; *LV,* left ventricle; *PV,* pulmonic valve; *RA,* right atrium; *RV,* right ventricle; *VSD,* ventricular septal defect. (Modified from Hockenberry MJ et al: *Wong's nursing care of infants and children,* ed 8, St Louis, 2009, Mosby.)

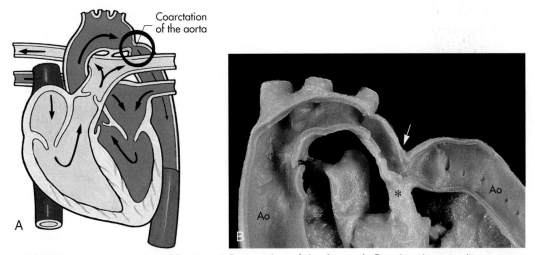

FIGURE 24-3 Postductal and Preductal Coarctation of the Aorta. **A,** Postductal coarctation occurs distal to ("after") the insertion of the closed ductus arteriosus into the aortic arch. Preductal coarctation occurs proximal to ("before") the insertion of the patent ductus arteriosus. The coarctation consists of a flap of tissue that protrudes from the tunica media of the aortic wall. **B,** Coarctation of the aorta with typical indentation of the aortic wall *(arrow)* opposite the ductal arterial ligament *(asterisk)*. *Ao,* Aorta. (**A** from Hockenberry MJ et al: *Wong's essentials of pediatric nursing,* ed 8, St Louis, 2009, Mosby; **B** from Damjanov I, Linder J, editors: *Anderson's pathology,* ed 10, St Louis, 1996, Mosby.)

incision is used. However, coarctation repair may be part of a more complex operation, which might require a sternotomy incision and cardiopulmonary bypass. Postoperative hypertension is treated with intravenous medication, often a short-acting beta-blocker, followed by oral medications, such as an angiotensin-converting enzyme inhibitor. Residual hypertension after repair of COA seems to be related to age and time of repair.

Studies have shown that percutaneous balloon angioplasty has been effective in reducing residual postoperative coarctation in most children.[1,2] Balloon angioplasty of COA as an initial intervention can also be considered. However, in infants younger than 7 months of age, most will experience recoarctation in only a short period of time after primary angioplasty. Other complications include aneurysm formation and blood vessel injury from arterial access. Data exist that support balloon angioplasty as an effective therapy in selected infants older than 7 months of age with a decreased risk of aneurysm formation as compared to younger infants.[4]

Aortic Stenosis

PATHOPHYSIOLOGY Aortic stenosis (AS) is a narrowing or stricture of the left ventricular outlet, causing resistance of blood flow from the left ventricle into the aorta (Figure 24-4). The physiologic consequence of severe AS is hypertrophy of the left ventricular wall, which eventually leads to increased end-diastolic pressure, resulting in pulmonary venous and pulmonary arterial hypertension. If severe, there may be decreased cardiac output and pulmonary vascular congestion. Left ventricular hypertrophy impedes coronary artery perfusion and may result in subendocardial ischemia and associated papillary muscle dysfunction that cause mitral insufficiency.

There are three types of AS. **Valvular AS** occurs as a consequence of malformed or fused cusps, resulting in a unicuspid or bicuspid valve. Valvular AS is a serious defect because (1) the obstruction tends to be progressive; (2) there may be sudden episodes of myocardial ischemia or low cardiac output that, on rare occasions, can result in sudden death in late childhood or adolescence; and (3) surgical repair will not result in a normal valve. This is one of the rare forms of congenital

heart disease in which strenuous physical activity may be curtailed because of the cardiac condition.[1,2]

Subvalvular AS is a stricture caused by a fibrous ring below a normal valve. It can also be caused by a narrowed left ventricular outflow tract in combination with a small aortic valve annulus. **Supravalvular AS,** a narrowing of the aorta just above the valve, occurs infrequently. It can occur as a single defect (familial supravalvular stenosis syndrome) or as a part of Williams-Beuren syndrome, which also is characterized by unusual facial appearance and mental disability.[5]

CLINICAL MANIFESTATIONS Infants with significant AS demonstrate signs of decreased cardiac output with faint pulses, hypotension, tachycardia, and poor feeding. A loud, harsh systolic ejection murmur is expected. Older children also may have complaints of exercise intolerance and, rarely, chest pain. Children are at risk for bacterial endocarditis, although prophylaxis with antibiotics is no longer routinely recommended (see *Health Alert:* Endocarditis Risk). Aortic stenosis, when severe, also can be complicated by coronary insufficiency, ventricular dysfunction, and, rarely, sudden death.

HEALTH ALERT

Endocarditis Risk

Children with congenital heart disease are at risk for developing endocarditis. Although the risk is low, a transient bacteremia has been noted to follow dental and surgical procedures and instrumentation involving mucosal surfaces. A blood-borne pathogen can inhabit areas of the heart where there is high turbulence (such as an abnormal valve or vessel) or reside on artificial material (such as a valve or homograft). *Streptococcus viridans* (α-hemolytic streptococci) is the most commonly found pathogen following dental or oral procedures. *Enterococcus faecalis* (enterococci) is the most common bacterium found following genitourinary and gastrointestinal tract surgery or instrumentation. The American Heart Association has provided updated guidelines for the prevention of bacterial endocarditis. The type and dose of antibiotic prophylaxis recommended depend on the procedure and the cardiac classification of risk for endocarditis. Good dental hygiene with daily brushing and flossing is critically important.

Data from the American Heart Association: available at www.americanheart.org.

EVALUATION AND TREATMENT

Valvular aortic stenosis. Valvular AS diagnosis is confirmed by echocardiography. Mild to moderate valvular AS does not usually require intervention or restriction of activity. Treatment of severe valvular AS varies, with nonsurgical palliation the initial treatment of choice by many interventional cardiologists. Dilation of the stenotic valve with balloon angioplasty, which is performed in the cardiac catheterization laboratory, still carries a high morbidity and mortality in the critically ill neonate; however, in older infants and children it compares favorably with surgical valvotomy.[4,6] Balloon angioplasty is, however, associated with the risk of aortic regurgitation (insufficiency). Children undergoing this procedure almost always require surgical intervention at some time to relieve recurrent narrowing or worsening regurgitation.[4,6]

Surgical treatment for valvular AS depends on the severity of the stenosis, previous interventions, and age of the child. Aortic valve commissurotomy or valvotomy may be used as an early intervention. Aortic valve replacement may be required if the valve is severely dysplastic. The Ross procedure, which involves moving the native pulmonary valve into the aortic position and replacing the pulmonary valve with a graft, has become an option. The advantage of the Ross procedure over

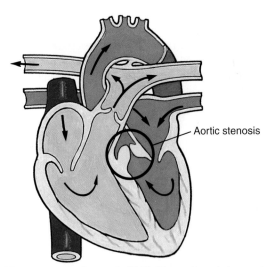

FIGURE 24-4 Aortic Stenosis (AS). Narrowing of the aortic valve causing resistance to blood flow in the left ventricle, decreased cardiac output, left ventricular hypertrophy, and pulmonary congestion. (From Hockenberry MJ et al: *Wong's essentials of pediatric nursing,* ed 8, St Louis, 2009, Mosby.)

— Aortic stenosis

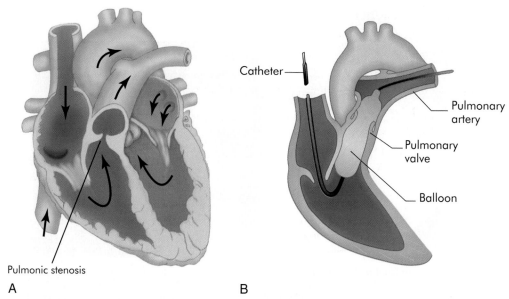

FIGURE 24-5 Pulmonic Stenosis (PS). A, The pulmonary valve narrows at the entrance of the pulmonary artery. **B,** Balloon angioplasty is used to dilate the valve. A catheter is inserted across the stenotic pulmonic valve into the pulmonary artery, and a balloon at the end of the catheter is inflated while it is positioned across the narrowed valve opening. (**A** from James SR, Ashwill JW: *Nursing care of children: principles and practice,* ed 3, St Louis, 2007, Saunders.)

mechanical valve replacement, especially in a young child, is that there is no requirement for long-term anticoagulation therapy; however, the valve may fail with time. Mechanical valve replacement is usually deferred as long as possible. Aortic stenosis requires lifelong evaluation and treatment. Multiple surgical or catheterization interventions are expected. Mortality for sick infants and young children is higher than that for older children.

Subvalvular aortic stenosis. Surgical correction for subvalvular AS involves incising the constricting fibromuscular ring. If the obstruction results from a narrow left ventricular outflow tract and a small aortic valve annulus, a patch may be required to enlarge the entire left ventricular outflow tract and annulus and replace the aortic valve, an approach known as the Konno procedure. An aortic homograft with a valve also may be used (extended aortic root replacement).

Supravalvular aortic stenosis. Surgery is usually required for management of moderate-to-severe supravalvular aortic stenoses. Balloon angioplasty and stent insertion have been successful but carry a higher risk of rupture.[5] An extended graft with coronary reimplantation may be needed if narrowing is severe.

Pulmonic Stenosis

PATHOPHYSIOLOGY Pulmonic stenosis (PS) is a narrowing or stricture of the pulmonary valve that causes resistance to blood flow from the right ventricle to the pulmonary artery (Figure 24-5). Generally moderate to severe stenosis causes right ventricular hypertrophy. Pulmonary atresia is an extreme form of PS with total fusion of the valve leaflets (blood cannot flow to the lungs); the right ventricle may be hypoplastic. In some cases of right ventricular outflow obstruction, the narrowing is below the valve (infundibular or subvalve PS).

CLINICAL MANIFESTATIONS Most infants are asymptomatic if the PS is mild to moderate. Newborns with severe PS or pulmonary atresia will be cyanotic (from a right-to-left shunt through an atrial septal defect [ASD]) and may have signs of decreased cardiac output. A harsh

systolic murmur is expected with PS. Pulmonary atresia produces a continuous murmur.

EVALUATION AND TREATMENT Echocardiography confirms the diagnosis and determines the severity of the PS. The treatment of choice for infants with moderate to severe pulmonary stenosis is balloon angioplasty (see Figure 24-5, *B*). A catheter with a special balloon device is used to dilate the area of narrowing. The procedure has proved highly effective, with a 50% to 75% reduction in pressure gradient across the pulmonic valve and a low rate of complications.[6] In rare cases, surgical valvotomy may be required. Pulmonary blood flood is supported with prostaglandin E_1 infusion to maintain the patency of the ductus arteriosus in cases of pulmonary atresia in the neonatal period until surgery is performed to supply pulmonary blood flow.[3,4]

Both balloon dilation and surgical valvotomy leave the pulmonary valve incompetent (insufficient); however, children are usually able to tolerate pulmonary valve incompetence and are asymptomatic. Long-term problems with restenosis or clinically significant valve incompetence may occur, but reintervention for uncomplicated PS is rarely necessary.[1,2]

Defects With Increased Pulmonary Blood Flow
Patent Ductus Arteriosus

PATHOPHYSIOLOGY Patent ductus arteriosus (PDA) is failure of the fetal ductus arteriosus (artery connecting the aorta and pulmonary artery) to close within the first weeks of life (Figure 24-6). The continued patency of this vessel allows blood to flow from the higher-pressure aorta to the lower-pressure pulmonary artery, causing a left-to-right shunt.

CLINICAL MANIFESTATIONS Infants may be asymptomatic or show signs of pulmonary overcirculation, such as dyspnea, fatigue, and poor feeding. There is a characteristic machinery-like murmur in both systole and diastole. Aortic flow (run-off) into the lower pressure

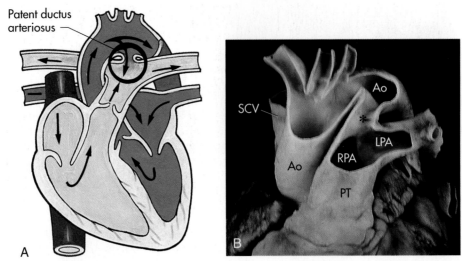

FIGURE 24-6 Patent Ductus Arteriosus (PDA). **A,** PDA with left-to-right shunt. **B,** PDA in an adult with pulmonary hypertension. *Ao,* Aorta; *LPA,* left pulmonary artery; *RPA,* right pulmonary artery; *SCV,* subclavian vein. (**A** from Hockenberry MJ et al: *Wong's essentials of pediatric nursing,* ed 8, St Louis, 2009, Mosby; **B** from Damjanov I, Linder J, editors: *Anderson's pathology,* ed 10, St Louis, 1996, Mosby.)

pulmonary circulation produces low diastolic blood pressure, widened pulse pressure, and bounding pulses. Children are at risk for bacterial endocarditis and, rarely, may develop pulmonary hypertension in later life from chronic excessive pulmonary blood flow.

EVALUATION AND TREATMENT Diagnosis is confirmed with echocardiography. Administration of indomethacin (a prostaglandin inhibitor) has proved successful in closing a PDA in premature infants and some newborns. Surgical division of the PDA through a left thoracotomy also may be done; in some cases the procedure can be performed with thoracoscopy. Closure with an occlusion device during cardiac catheterization is performed for most older children. Both surgical and nonsurgical procedures can be considered low risk.[6]

Atrial Septal Defect

PATHOPHYSIOLOGY An atrial septal defect (ASD) is an opening in the septal wall between the two atria. This opening allows blood to shunt from the left atrium to the right atrium. There are three types of ASDs. An ostium primum ASD is an opening low in the atrial septum and may be associated with abnormalities of the mitral valve. An ostium secundum ASD is an opening in the middle of the atrial septum and is the most common type. A sinus venosus ASD is an opening usually high in the atrial wall and may be associated with partial anomalous pulmonary venous connection.[7] Left-to-right shunting of blood can occur with a large ASD.

CLINICAL MANIFESTATIONS Children with an ASD are usually asymptomatic. Infants with a large ASD may, in rare cases, develop pulmonary overcirculation and slow growth. Some older children and adults will experience shortness of breath with activity as the right ventricle becomes less compliant with age. Pulmonary hypertension and stroke are associated rare complications. A systolic ejection murmur and a widely split second heart sound are the expected findings on physical exam.

EVALUATION AND TREATMENT Diagnosis is confirmed by echocardiography. The ASD may be closed surgically with primary repair (sutured closed) or with a patch. Surgical repair involves open-heart

surgery with cardiopulmonary bypass. Interventional catheterization closure involves placement of a closure device.[8] All options have low morbidity and mortality. Atrial dysrhythmias persist in about 10% of individuals in both groups after closure.

Ventricular Septal Defect

PATHOPHYSIOLOGY A ventricular septal defect (VSD) is an opening of the septal wall between the ventricles. VSDs are the most common type of congenital heart defect. VSDs are classified by location. Perimembranous VSDs are located high in the septal wall of the ventricle underneath the aortic valve. Muscular VSDs are located low in the septal wall. VSDs also can be located in the inlet or outlet portion of the ventricle. VSDs are similar to ASDs in that blood will shunt from left to right. Left-to-right shunting of blood can occur with a large VSD. Depending on the size and location, many VSDs close spontaneously, most often within the first 2 years of life.

CLINICAL MANIFESTATIONS Depending on the size, location, and degree of shunting and pulmonary vascular resistance, children may have no symptoms or have clinical effects from excessive pulmonary blood flow. In the infant, excessive pulmonary blood flow from left-to-right shunting causes dyspnea and tachypnea and is commonly called congestive heart failure (CHF), although the heart muscle functions well in VSD. A holosystolic (pansystolic) murmur is expected.

If the degree of shunting is significant and not corrected, the child is at risk for developing pulmonary hypertension. Irreversible pulmonary hypertension can result in Eisenmenger syndrome, a condition in which shunting of blood is reversed because of high pulmonary pressure and resistance (right-to-left shunt with cyanosis). Children with VSD are at risk for endocarditis.

EVALUATION AND TREATMENT Diagnosis is confirmed by echocardiogram. Cardiac catheterization may be needed to calculate the degree of shunting and to directly measure the pressures in the heart. Smaller VSDs require minimal treatment and may close completely or become small enough that surgical closure is not required. If the infant has severe CHF or failure to thrive that is unmanageable with medical

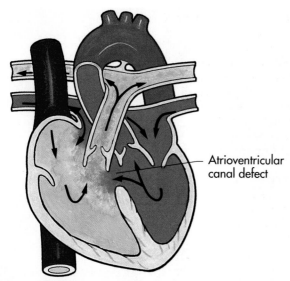

FIGURE 24-7 Atrioventricular Canal (AVC) Defect. (From Hockenberry MJ et al: *Wong's essentials of pediatric nursing*, ed 8, St Louis, 2009, Mosby.)

therapy, early surgical repair is performed. Surgical repair involves open-heart surgery with cardiopulmonary bypass. The opening is sutured closed primarily or with a patch. Nonsurgical intervention is available but only under restricted conditions.[6,9-11]

Atrioventricular Canal Defect

PATHOPHYSIOLOGY Atrioventricular canal (AVC) defect, also known as atrioventricular septal defect (AVSD) or by the traditional term endocardial cushion defect (ECD), is the result of incomplete fusion of endocardial cushions (Figure 24-7). AVC defect consists of an ostium primum ASD and inlet VSD with associated abnormalities of the atrioventricular valve tissue. These valve abnormalities range from a cleft in the mitral valve to a common mitral and tricuspid valve. The directions and pathways of flow are determined by pulmonary and systemic resistance, left and right ventricular pressures, and the compliance of each chamber. Flow is generally from left to right. AVC is a common cardiac defect in children with Down syndrome. However, most children with this defect have normal karyotype.

CLINICAL MANIFESTATIONS Infants with this defect often display moderate to severe heart failure attributable to left-to-right shunting and pulmonary overcirculation. Infants with pulmonary hypertension and high pulmonary resistance have less shunting and therefore minimal signs of CHF. There may be mild cyanosis that increases with crying. Those with a large left-to-right shunt will have a murmur, and those with minimal shunt may not have a murmur. Children with AVC are at risk for developing irreversible pulmonary hypertension if left surgically untreated.

EVALUATION AND TREATMENT AVC is one of the most frequent diagnoses made with fetal echocardiography. Cardiac catheterization usually is not needed. Initial treatment goals include aggressive medical management of CHF and nutritional supplementation. Infants are followed closely for signs or symptoms of failure to thrive. Complete surgical repair is performed between 3 and 6 months of age to prevent irreversible pulmonary hypertension. This procedure consists of patch closure of the septal defects and reconstruction of the AV valve tissue

(either repair of the mitral valve cleft or fashioning of two AV valves). If the mitral valve defect is severe, valve replacement may be needed. A potential problem following repair is mitral regurgitation, which may later require valve replacement.

Defects With Decreased Pulmonary Blood Flow
Tetralogy of Fallot

PATHOPHYSIOLOGY The classic form of tetralogy of Fallot (TOF) includes four defects: (1) ventricular septal defect, (2) pulmonic stenosis, (3) overriding aorta, and (4) right ventricular hypertrophy (Figure 24-8). The pathophysiology varies widely, depending not only on the degree of pulmonary stenosis but also on the pulmonary and systemic vascular resistance to flow. If total resistance to pulmonary flow is greater than systemic resistance, the shunt is from right to left. If systemic resistance is more than pulmonary resistance, the shunt is from left to right. Pulmonic stenosis decreases blood flow to the lungs and, consequently, the amount of oxygenated blood that returns to the left heart. Physiologic compensation to chronic, severe hypoxia includes production of more red blood cells (polycythemia), development of collateral bronchial vessels, and enlargement of the nail beds (clubbing).

CLINICAL MANIFESTATIONS Some infants may be acutely cyanotic at birth. In others, progression of hypoxia and cyanosis may be more gradual over the first year of life as the pulmonary stenosis worsens. Acute episodes of cyanosis and hypoxia can occur, called *hypercyanotic spells, blue spells,* or *"tet" spells.* These spells (increased right-to-left shunt) may occur during crying or after feeding. If prolonged or frequent, these spells are an indication for emergent evaluation and surgical treatment.

Chronic cyanosis may cause clubbing of the fingers and poor growth in children. Squatting can help with cyanosis in these children because it increases peripheral resistance in the systemic circulation, which causes an increase in pressures in the left heart and consequent reduction in right-to-left shunting and improvement in pulmonary perfusion. Children with unrepaired TOF are at risk for emboli, stroke, brain abscess, seizures, and loss of consciousness or sudden death following a tet spell.

EVALUATION AND TREATMENT Diagnosis is confirmed with echocardiography. Elective surgical repair is usually performed in the first year of life. Indications for earlier repair include increasing cyanosis or the development of hypercyanotic spells. Complete repair involves closure of the VSD, resection of the infundibular stenosis, and enlargement of the right ventricular outflow tract.

In very small infants who cannot undergo primary repair, a palliative procedure to increase pulmonary blood flow and increase oxygen saturation may be performed. This systemic artery to pulmonary artery anastomosis is the *Blalock-Taussig* or modified *Blalock-Taussig shunt,* which provides blood flow to the pulmonary arteries.

Tricuspid Atresia

PATHOPHYSIOLOGY Tricuspid atresia is failure of the tricuspid valve to develop; consequently, there is no communication from right atrium to right ventricle (Figure 24-9). Blood flows through an atrial septal defect or a patent foramen ovale to the left atrium and through a ventricular septal defect to the right ventricle. This condition is often associated with pulmonic stenosis or transposition of the great arteries. There is complete mixing of unoxygenated and oxygenated blood in the left side of the heart, resulting in systemic desaturation and mild

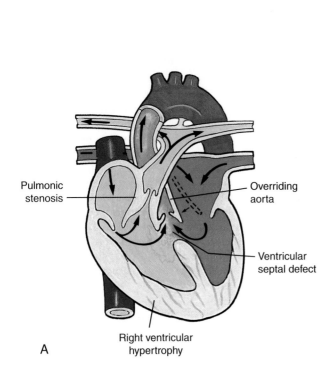

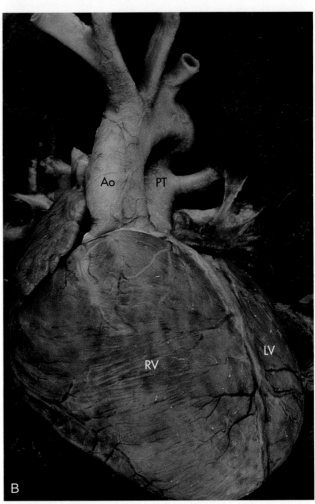

Pulmonic stenosis

Overriding aorta

Ventricular septal defect

Right ventricular hypertrophy

A

B

FIGURE 24-8 Tetralogy of Fallot (TOF). A, TOF hemodynamics. **B,** Right ventricular (RV) hypertrophy and AO. (**A** from Hockenberry MJ et al: *Wong's essentials of pediatric nursing,* ed 8, St Louis, 2009, Mosby; **B** from Damjanov I, Linder J, editors: *Anderson's pathology,* ed 10, St Louis, 1996, Mosby.)

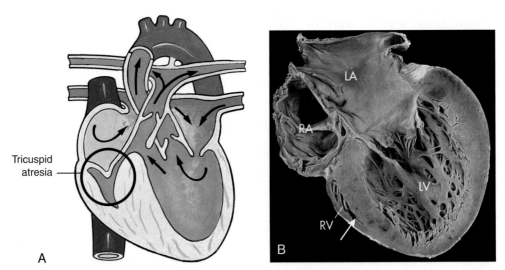

Tricuspid atresia

A

B

FIGURE 24-9 Tricuspid Atresia. A, Tricuspid atresia hemodynamics. **B,** Small right ventricle (RV) slit of VSD; left ventricle (LV) is enlarged. (**A** from Hockenberry MJ et al: *Wong's essentials of pediatric nursing,* ed 8, St Louis, 2009, Mosby; **B** from Damjanov I, Linder J, editors: *Anderson's pathology,* ed 10, St Louis, 1996, Mosby.)

cyanosis. The physiologic process that causes lesion development is variable, depending on the great vessel anatomy and amount of pulmonary stenosis.

CLINICAL MANIFESTATIONS   A murmur is noted, and cyanosis is usually seen in the newborn period. Tachycardia, dyspnea, fatigue, and poor feeding may be noted with excessive pulmonary blood flow. Older children may have signs of chronic hypoxemia with clubbing. Children are at risk for bacterial endocarditis, brain abscess, and stroke.

EVALUATION AND TREATMENT   After diagnosis is confirmed by echocardiography, the neonate with decreased pulmonary blood flow is treated with a continuous infusion of prostaglandin E_1 to maintain the patency of the ductus arteriosus until surgical intervention. If the ASD is restrictive, an atrial septostomy is done during cardiac catheterization.[10] Treatment is accomplished in staged procedures. Once the infant is stabilized, a Blalock-Taussig shunt (systemic to pulmonary artery anastomosis) is placed to increase blood flow to the lungs.

Further surgery is undertaken between 6 months and 2 years of age, depending on the child's growth and degree of pulmonary blood flow. The next step is usually a Glenn shunt in which the superior vena cava is anastomosed to the pulmonary artery. At that time, the pulmonary artery may be ligated or the Blalock-Taussig shunt may be removed. The final separation of the pulmonary circulation from the systemic circulation is the *Fontan procedure.* In this stage, the inferior vena caval blood flow is routed to the pulmonary artery using a tube graft or baffle. The infant must have normal ventricular function and low pulmonary vascular resistance for the procedure to be successful.

Postoperative complications that increase hospital stay include pleural and pericardial effusions, elevated pulmonary vascular resistance, and ventricular dysfunction. Exercise tolerance is limited in many children with the Fontan procedure, but general health is considered good.

Mixing Defects
Transposition of the Great Arteries or Transposition of the Great Vessels

PATHOPHYSIOLOGY   In transposition of the great arteries (TGA) or transposition of the great vessels (TGV), the pulmonary artery leaves the left ventricle and the aorta exits the right ventricle (Figure 24-10). Associated defects, such as ASD, VSD, or PDA, permit mixing of saturated and desaturated blood, which maintains adequate tissue oxygenation for a limited time.

CLINICAL MANIFESTATIONS   Clinical manifestations depend on the type and size of the associated defects. Children with limited communication between cardiac chambers are severely cyanotic, acidotic, and ill at birth. Those with large septal defects or a patent ductus arteriosus may be less severely cyanotic but may have symptoms of pulmonary overcirculation. Classically no murmur is heard unless there is an associated VSD.

EVALUATION AND TREATMENT   Diagnosis is suspected by physical examination and confirmed with echocardiography. Administration of intravenous prostaglandin E_1 to maintain the patency of the ductus arteriosis may be initiated to temporarily increase oxygen delivery. Enlargement of the patent foramen ovale by balloon atrial septostomy may be performed during cardiac catheterization to increase mixing and maintain cardiac output.[9,10]

The most preferred type of surgical repair for TGA performed in the first weeks of life is the *arterial switch procedure.* It involves transecting the great arteries and anastomosing the main pulmonary artery to the native proximal aorta (just above the aortic valve) and anastomosing the ascending aorta to the native proximal pulmonary artery. The coronary arteries are moved with a "button" of tissue from the proximal aorta to the proximal pulmonary artery, creating a new aorta. Reimplantation of the coronary arteries is critical to the infant's survival, and the arteries must be reattached without torsion or kinking to provide the heart with its supply of oxygen. The advantage of the

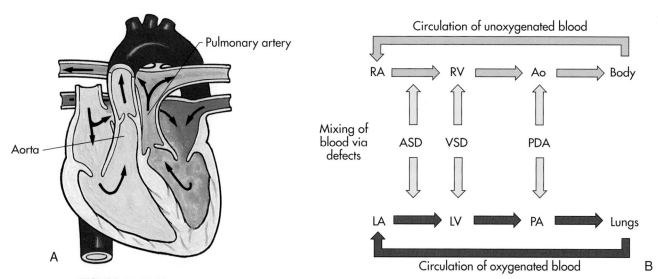

FIGURE 24-10 Hemodynamics in Transposition of the Great Vessels (TGV). **A,** Complete transposition of the great vessels with an intact interventricular septum. The aorta arises from the right ventricle and the pulmonary artery from the left ventricle. **B,** Oxygen saturation in the two, parallel circuits. *Ao,* Aorta; *ASD,* atrial septal defect; *LA,* left atrium; *LV,* left ventricle; *PA,* pulmonary artery; *PDA,* patent ductus arteriosus; *RA,* right atrium; *RV,* right ventricle; *VSD,* ventricular septal defect. (A from Hockenberry MJ et al: *Wong's essentials of pediatric nursing,* ed 8, St Louis, 2009, Mosby.)

arterial switch procedure is the reestablishment of normal circulation with the left ventricle acting as the systemic pump. Potential complications of the arterial switch include narrowing at the great artery anastomoses or coronary artery insufficiency. Long-term results for the arterial switch operation are usually good.

Total Anomalous Pulmonary Venous Connection

PATHOPHYSIOLOGY Total anomalous pulmonary venous connection (TAPVC) is a rare defect characterized by failure of the pulmonary veins to join the left atrium during cardiac development. TAPVC is also called *total anomalous pulmonary venous return (TAPVR)* or *total anomalous pulmonary venous drainage (TAPVD)* (Figure 24-11). The pulmonary venous return is connected to the right side of the circulation rather than to the left atrium. The type of TAPVC is classified according to the pulmonary venous point of attachment:

- *Supracardiac:* Attachment above the diaphragm, usually to the superior vena cava (most common form)
- *Cardiac:* Direct attachment to the heart, usually to the right atrium or coronary sinus
- *Infracardiac:* Attachment below the diaphragm, such as to the inferior vena cava (most severe and least common form)

The right atrium receives all the blood that normally would flow into the left atrium. As a result, the right side of the heart is enlarged and the left side, especially the left atrium, is smaller than normal. An associated ASD or patent foramen ovale allows systemic venous blood to shunt from the right atrium to the left side of the heart. As a result, the oxygen saturation of the blood in both sides of the heart (and, ultimately, in the systemic arterial circulation) is the same. If the pulmonary blood flow is increased, pulmonary venous return is also large, and the amount of saturated blood is relatively high. However, if there is obstruction to pulmonary venous drainage, the infant has severe cyanosis and low cardiac output. Infracardiac TAPVC often is associated with obstruction of pulmonary venous drainage and is a surgical emergency with high mortality.

CLINICAL MANIFESTATIONS Most infants develop cyanosis early in life. The degree of cyanosis is inversely related to the amount of pulmonary blood flow. Children with unobstructed TAPVC may be asymptomatic until pulmonary vascular resistance decreases during infancy, increasing pulmonary blood flow, with resulting signs of pulmonary overcirculation. Cyanosis becomes worse with pulmonary vein obstruction; once obstruction occurs, the infant's condition usually deteriorates rapidly. Without intervention, cardiac failure will progress to death. Murmur is not a common feature of TAPVC.

EVALUATION AND TREATMENT Diagnosis is suspected with echocardiography but may require confirmative angiography. Corrective repair is usually required in early infancy. The surgical approach varies with the anatomic defect. In general, however, the common pulmonary vein (venous confluence) is sutured to the left atrium, the ASD is closed, and the anomalous pulmonary venous connection may be ligated.

Truncus Arteriosus

PATHOPHYSIOLOGY Truncus arteriosus (TA) is failure of normal septation and division of the embryonic outflow track into a pulmonary artery and an aorta, resulting in a single vessel that exits the heart. There is always an associated VSD with mixing of the systemic and arterial circulations (Figure 24-12) causing some degree of cyanosis. Blood ejected from the heart flows preferentially to the lower-pressure pulmonary arteries, causing increased pulmonary blood flow. The three types are as follows:

- *Type I:* A single pulmonary trunk arises near the base of the truncus and divides into the left and right pulmonary arteries.
- *Type II:* The left and right pulmonary arteries arise separately from the posterior aspect of the truncus.
- *Type III:* The pulmonary arteries arise independently and from the lateral aspect of the truncus.

CLINICAL MANIFESTATIONS Most infants are symptomatic with moderate heart failure and variable cyanosis, poor growth, and activity intolerance. Children are at risk for brain abscess and bacterial endocarditis.

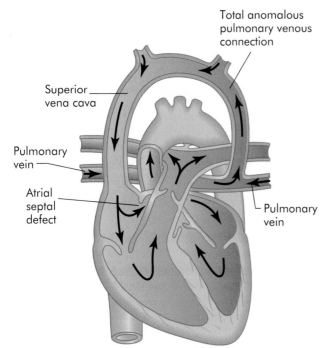

FIGURE 24-11 Total Anomalous Pulmonary Venous Connection (TAPVC).

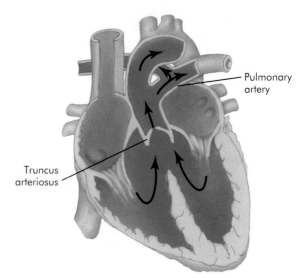

FIGURE 24-12 Truncus Arteriosus (TA). (From James SR, Ashwill JW: *Nursing care of children: principles and practice*, ed 3, St Louis, 2007, Saunders.)

EVALUATION AND TREATMENT Diagnosis is made by echocardiography. Corrective repair is a modification of the Rastelli procedure and is performed in the first few weeks or months of life. It involves closing the VSD so that the truncus arteriosus receives the outflow from the left ventricle, excising the pulmonary arteries from the aorta and attaching them to the right ventricle by means of a homograft. These children require additional procedures to replace the conduit as its size becomes inadequate in relation to growth.

Hypoplastic Left Heart Syndrome

PATHOPHYSIOLOGY Hypoplastic left heart syndrome (HLHS) is underdevelopment of the left side of the heart. Features include small left atrium, small or absent mitral valve, small or absent left ventricle, and a small or absent aortic valve. Coarctation also is expected (Figure 24-13). Most blood from the left atrium flows across the patent foramen ovale to the right atrium, to the right ventricle, and out the pulmonary artery. The descending aorta receives blood from the patent ductus arteriosus supplying systemic blood flow and filling the aorta and coronary arteries as well.

CLINICAL MANIFESTATIONS HLHS presents in the early newborn period as mild cyanosis, tachypnea, and low cardiac output if not already detected by fetal echocardiogram. Support of the systemic circulation is accomplished with prostaglandin E_1 infusion. If HLHS is not suspected and the patent ductus arteriosus closes, there is progressive deterioration with cyanosis and decreased cardiac output, leading to cardiovascular collapse. If untreated, HLHS is usually fatal in the first months of life.

EVALUATION AND TREATMENT Echocardiography shows all of the features of HLHS. Cardiac catheterization is rarely required. A multi-stage repair approach is used. The first stage is the *Norwood procedure,* which is anastomosis of the main pulmonary artery to the aorta to create a new aorta, construction of a shunt to provide pulmonary blood flow, creation of a large atrial septal defect, and repair of the coarctation. The second stage is a *bidirectional Glenn shunt* done at 6 to 9 months of age to relieve cyanosis and reduce the volume load on the right ventricle. The final repair is a *Fontan procedure.* Some centers perform heart transplantation in the newborn period rather than the staged procedure

(Norwood, Glenn, Fontan). Disadvantages of neonatal transplantation include shortage of newborn organ donors, risk of rejection, long-term problems with chronic immunosuppression, and infection.

Long-term (>10 years) outcome from both procedures has improved. The survival continues to improve and quality of life for the children is generally good.[7,9,10,12-14] No treatment is recommended for infants with little hope of surgical survival. The family is then offered palliative care.

✔ **QUICK CHECK 24-1**
1. What are the three principal classifications of congenital heart disease?
2. Describe the different characteristics that determine whether the defects are cyanotic or acyanotic.
3. What is the most common type of congenital heart defect?

Congestive Heart Failure

Congestive heart failure (CHF) is a common complication of many congenital heart defects. CHF occurs when the heart is unable to maintain sufficient cardiac output to meet the metabolic demands of the body. The most common congenital causes of CHF in infancy and childhood are listed in Table 24-3. Classic CHF in children also can be acquired, usually resulting from cardiomyopathies. Pulmonary overcirculation from large left-to-right shunt is often called CHF but is not usually associated with

---

TABLE 24-3 CAUSES OF CONGESTIVE HEART FAILURE RESULTING FROM CONGENITAL HEART DISEASE

AGE OF ONSET	CAUSE
At birth	HLHS
	Volume overload lesions
	Severe tricuspid or pulmonary insufficiency
	Large systemic AV fistula
First week	TGA
	PDA in small premature infants
	HLHS (with more favorable anatomy)
	TAPVR, particularly those with pulmonary venous obstruction
	Others
	Systemic AV fistula
	Critical AS or PS
1-4 weeks	COA with associated anomalies
	Critical AS
	Large left-to-right shunt lesions (VSD, PDA) in premature infants
	All other lesions previously listed
4-6 weeks	Some left-to-right shunt lesions, such as AVSD
6 weeks to 4 months	Large VSD
	Large PDA
	Others, such as anomalous left coronary artery from PA

From Park MK: *Pediatric cardiology for practitioners,* ed 5, St Louis, 2008, Mosby.
AS, Aortic stenosis; *AVSD,* atrioventricular septal defect; *AV,* atrioventricular; *COA,* coarctation of the aorta; *HLHS,* hypoplastic left heart syndrome; *PA,* pulmonary artery; *PDA,* patent ductus arteriosus; *PS,* pulmonic stenosis; *TAPVR,* total anomalous pulmonary venous return; *TGA,* transposition of great arteries; *VSD,* ventricular septal defect.

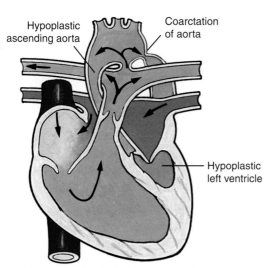

FIGURE 24-13 Hypoplastic Left Heart Syndrome (HLHS). (From Hockenberry MJ et al: *Wong's essentials of pediatric nursing,* ed 8, St Louis, 2009, Mosby.)

Hypoplastic ascending aorta
Coarctation of aorta
Hypoplastic left ventricle

decreased ventricular function and failure to meet metabolic demands. However, the clinical manifestations are similar, such as failure to thrive, tachypnea, tachycardia, and respiratory tract infections.[2]

In general, the pathophysiologic mechanisms of CHF in infants and children are similar to those in adults. It is most often a result of decreased left ventricular systolic function and the associated left atrial and pulmonary venous hypertension and pulmonary venous congestion. The same compensatory mechanisms are activated in the face of inadequate cardiac output (see Figure 23-38). Right ventricular failure is rare in childhood.

Left heart failure in infants is manifested as poor feeding and sucking, often leading to failure to thrive. In left heart failure, dyspnea, tachypnea, and diaphoresis may be accompanied by retractions, grunting, and nasal flaring. Wheezing, coughing, and rales are rare in childhood CHF.[1,12,13] Common skin changes, such as pallor or mottling, are often present (Box 24-1). Systemic venous congestion is rare in childhood. The presence of peripheral edema and weight gain suggests renal disease or nutritional disease much more often than cardiac dysfunction.

A thorough physical examination with emphasis on cardiac and pulmonary findings will often reveal the degree of CHF. Plotting a child's growth (height, weight, head circumference) is an important method of assessing a child's health. Infants with CHF or pulmonary overcirculation usually have low weight with normal length and head circumference measurements. The failure to thrive is usually the result of increased metabolic expenditure relative to caloric intake. An electrocardiogram (ECG) also should be performed to determine the presence of dysrhythmia or hypertrophy. A chest x-ray is useful in assessing the presence of cardiomegaly and signs of increased pulmonary circulation or pulmonary edema.

BOX 24-1   CLINICAL MANIFESTATIONS OF CONGESTIVE HEART FAILURE

Impaired Myocardial Function
Tachycardia
Sweating (inappropriate)
Decreased urinary output
Fatigue
Weakness
Restlessness
Anorexia
Pale, cool extremities
Weak peripheral pulses
Decreased blood pressure
Gallop rhythm
Cardiomegaly

Pulmonary Congestion
Tachypnea
Dyspnea
Retractions (infants)
Flaring nares
Exercise intolerance
Orthopnea
Cough, hoarseness
Cyanosis
Wheezing
Grunting

Excerpted from Hockenberry MJ et al: *Wong's nursing care of infants and children*, ed 9, St Louis, 2011, Mosby.

Treatment is aimed at decreasing cardiac workload and increasing the efficiency of heart function. Severe congenital heart disease is managed with surgical repair. Medical management initially consists of diuretics, such as furosemide. Depending on the degree of CHF, other diuretics can be used in combination with furosemide to counteract potassium losses. Agents that reduce afterload, such as captopril or enalapril and beta-blockers, are employed to further manage severe CHF.[1,2]

ACQUIRED CARDIOVASCULAR DISORDERS

Acquired heart diseases refer to disease processes or abnormalities that occur after birth. They result from various causes, such as infection, genetic disorders, autoimmune processes in response to infection, environmental factors, or autoimmune diseases. Examples of acquired heart diseases include Kawasaki disease, myocarditis, rheumatic heart disease, cardiomyopathy, and systemic hypertension. This chapter discusses Kawasaki disease and systemic hypertension. Myocarditis, rheumatic heart disease, and cardiomyopathy are discussed in Chapter 23.

Kawasaki Disease

Kawasaki disease (KD), formerly known as mucocutaneous lymph node syndrome, is an acute, usually self-limiting systemic vasculitis that may result in cardiac sequelae. It was first identified in 1967. Although KD occurs throughout the world, the greatest number of cases are seen in Japan.[1,2] This reflects the genetic component of KD, with the case rate being highest among Asians, less among white children, and rare in black children.

Kawasaki disease is primarily a condition of young children. Eighty percent of cases are seen in children younger than 5 years of age, with the incidence peaking in the toddler age group. Males are affected slightly more than females. The peak incidence is in the winter and spring.[1,2]

The etiology of Kawasaki disease remains unknown. Current etiologic theories center on an immunologic response to an infectious, toxic, or antigenic substance.[14]

PATHOPHYSIOLOGY Kawasaki disease progresses pathologically and clinically in the following stages. In the early or acute phase, small capillaries, arterioles, and venules become inflamed, as does the heart itself. In the subacute state, inflammation spreads to larger vessels and aneurysms of the coronary arteries may develop. In the convalescent stage, medium-sized arteries begin the granulation process and may cause coronary artery thickening with increased risk for thrombosis. After the convalescent stage, inflammation wanes with potential scarring of the affected vessels, calcification, and stenosis.

CLINICAL MANIFESTATIONS The clinical course of the disease progresses in three stages: acute, subacute, and convalescent. In the acute phase, the child with classic or typical KD has fever, conjunctivitis, oral changes ("strawberry" tongue), rash, and lymphadenopathy and is often irritable. During this phase, myocarditis may develop. The subacute phase begins when the fever ends and continues until the clinical signs have resolved. It is at this time that the child is most at risk for coronary artery aneurysm development. Desquamation of the palms and soles occurs at this time, as well as marked thrombocytosis. The convalescent phase is marked by the elevation of the erythrocyte sedimentation rate and C-reactive protein level, as well as by an increased platelet count. Arthritis may be present. This phase continues until all laboratory values return to normal—usually about 6 to 8 weeks after onset.[1] Atypical KD is now described with the presentation of infants as young as 6 weeks who have fever and coronary aneurysms without the "classic" physical findings or typical time course. Recognition is difficult and may delay treatment.[14]

EVALUATION AND TREATMENT The diagnosis is based on the diagnostic criteria for Kawasaki disease, which state that the child must exhibit five of six criteria, including fever (Box 24-2). These children usually have leukocytosis, increased erythrocyte sedimentation rates, thrombocytosis, and elevated levels of liver enzymes. An echocardiogram is obtained at the time of diagnosis as a baseline measurement to assess for coronary aneurysms or inflammation. Serial echocardiograms are obtained after treatment to assess for development of coronary aneurysms or regression of those present early in the course of the disease. Treatment includes oral administration of aspirin and intravenous infusion of gamma globulin (most often only one dose). Aspirin is continued until the manifestations of inflammation are resolved.

Treatment with aspirin and intravenous immunoglobulin during the acute phase has decreased the morbidity of Kawasaki disease and has reduced the incidence of coronary abnormalities from approximately 20% to less than 10% at 6 to 8 weeks after initiation of therapy. Most children recover completely from Kawasaki disease, including regression of aneurysms. The most common cardiovascular sequela is coronary thrombosis.[14]

Systemic Hypertension

Systemic hypertension in children is defined as systolic and diastolic blood pressure levels greater than the 95th percentile for age and gender on at least three occasions (Tables 24-4 and 24-5). The Fourth Task Force on Blood Pressure Control in Children uses height as an additional criterion to the blood pressure guidelines.[1,15]

BOX 24-2 DIAGNOSTIC CRITERIA FOR KAWASAKI DISEASE

The child must exhibit five of the following six criteria, including fever:

1. Fever for 5 or more days (often diagnosed with shorter duration of fever if other symptoms are present)
2. Bilateral conjunctival infection without exudation
3. Changes in the oral mucous membranes, such as erythema, dryness, and fissuring of the lips; oropharyngeal reddening; or "strawberry tongue"
4. Changes in the extremities, such as peripheral edema, peripheral erythema, and desquamation of palms and soles, particularly periungual peeling
5. Polymorphous rash, often accentuated in the perineal area
6. Cervical lymphadenopathy

Data from Hockenberry MJ et al: *Wong's nursing care of infants and children,* ed 9, St Louis, 2011, Mosby.

TABLE 24-4 NORMATIVE BLOOD PRESSURE LEVELS (SYSTOLIC/DIASTOLIC [MEAN]) BY DINAMAP MONITOR IN CHILDREN 5 YEARS OLD AND YOUNGER

AGE	MEAN BP LEVELS (mm Hg)	90TH PERCENTILE	95TH PERCENTILE
1-3 days	64/41 (50)	75/49 (50)	78/52 (62)
1 month to 2 years	95/58 (72)	106/68 (83)	110/71 (86)
2-5 years	101/57 (74)	112/66 (82)	115/68 (85)

Data from Park MK: *Pediatric cardiology for practitioners,* ed 5, St Louis, 2008, Mosby; modified from Park MK, Menard SM: *Am J Dis Children* 143:860, 1989.
BP, Blood pressure.

Hypertension is classified into two categories: primary, or essential, hypertension, in which a specific cause cannot be identified, and secondary hypertension, in which a cause *can* be identified (see Box 24-3). Hypertension (HTN) in children differs from adult hypertension in etiology and presentation. Children, when diagnosed with HTN, are often found to have secondary hypertension caused by some underlying disease, such as renal disease or coarctation of the aorta (see Box 24-3). An increased prevalence of primary HTN in older children has been noted. Researchers are now focusing on primary HTN in older children in relation to morbidity and the presence of early atherosclerotic disease. Certain factors influence blood pressure in children. Children who are overweight are often hypertensive (see *Health Alert: U.S. Childhood Obesity and Its Association With Cardiovascular Disease*). Smoking also is associated with an increased risk for HTN.[16-18]

HEALTH ALERT

U.S. Childhood Obesity and Its Association With Cardiovascular Disease

Childhood obesity is epidemic in the United States. The number of overweight children has doubled since the 1970s, and obesity has been called the most serious and prevalent nutritional disorder in the United States. Obesity is linked to insulin resistance and diabetes and increases cardiovascular risk, especially atherosclerosis, hypertension, and lipid abnormalities. The mechanisms by which insulin resistance and diabetes cause cardiovascular diseases include endothelial dysfunction, structural changes in arterial walls, abnormal vasoconstriction, and changes in renal function and salt transport. Research into genetics and insulin-regulated transcription factors suggests that obesity, insulin resistance, diabetes, and cardiovascular disease share important molecular etiologies and processes. These findings may lead investigators to important new treatments. For now, helping children develop good exercise and dietary habits has been shown to significantly improve arterial function and reduce cardiovascular risk.

Content and update references and statistics can be found at www. cdc.gov/obesity/childhood/index.html.

TABLE 24-5 SUGGESTED NORMAL BP VALUES (MM HG) BY AUSCULTATORY METHOD (SYSTOLIC/DIASTOLIC K5)

AGE (YR)	MEAN BP LEVELS	90TH PERCENTILE	95TH PERCENTILE
6-7	104/55	114/73	117/78
8-9	106/58	117/76	120/82
10-11*	108/60	120/77	124/82
12-13*	112/62	124/78	128/83
14-15			
Boys	116/66	132/80	138/86
Girls	112/68	126/80	130/83
16-18			
Boys	121/70	136/82	140/86
Girls	110/68	125/81	127/84

From Park MK: *Pediatric cardiology for practitioners,* ed 4, St Louis, 2002, Mosby; modified from Goldring D et al: *J Pediatr* 91:884, 1977; Prineas RJ et al: *Hypertension* 1(suppl):18, 1980.
BP, Blood pressure; *K5,* phase V of Korotkoff sound.
*Values for ages 10 to 13 years have been extrapolated from these two studies using age-related increments from other studies.

BOX 24-3 CONDITIONS ASSOCIATED WITH SECONDARY HYPERTENSION IN CHILDREN

Renal Disorders
Congenital defects
  Polycystic kidney, ectopic kidney, horseshoe kidney, etc.
  Obstructive anomalies
  Hydronephrosis
Renal tumor
  Wilms tumor
Renovascular disease
  Abnormalities of renal arteries
  Renal vein thrombosis
Acquired disorders
  Glomerulonephritis—acute or chronic
  Pyelonephritis
  Nephritis associated with collagen disease

Cardiovascular Disease
Coarctation of aorta
Arteriovenous fistulae
Patent ductus arteriosus
Aortic or mitral insufficiency

Metabolic and Endocrine Diseases
Adrenal tumors
  Adenoma
  Pheochromocytoma
  Neuroblastoma

Cushing syndrome
Adrenogenital syndrome
Hyperthyroidism
Aldosteronism
Hypercalcemia
Diabetes mellitus

Neurologic Disorders
Space-occupying lesions of cranium (increased intracranial pressure)
  Tumors
  Cysts
  Hematoma
Cerebral edema
Encephalitis (including Guillain-Barré and Reye syndromes)

Miscellaneous Causes
Drugs (corticosteroids, oral contraceptives, pressor agents, amphetamines)
Burns
Genitourinary surgery
Trauma (e.g., stretching of femoral nerve with leg traction)
Insect bites (e.g., scorpion)
Intravascular overload (blood, fluid)
Hypernatremia
Toxemia of pregnancy
Heavy metal poisoning

Modified from Hockenberry MJ et al: *Wong's nursing care of infants and children,* ed 9, St Louis, 2011, Mosby.

PATHOPHYSIOLOGY In infants and children, a cause of HTN is almost always found. In general, the younger the child with significant hypertension, the more likely a correctable cause can be determined. Therefore a thorough evaluation needs to be performed.[2,16]

The pathophysiology of primary HTN in children is not clearly understood but may result from a complex interaction of a strong predisposing genetic component with disturbances in sympathetic vascular smooth muscle tone, humoral agents (angiotensin, catecholamines), renal sodium excretion, and cardiac output. Ultimately these factors impair the ability of the peripheral vascular bed to relax.

CLINICAL MANIFESTATIONS Most children with systemic HTN are asymptomatic. It is necessary that a thorough history and physical examination be obtained. The examination should include an accurate blood pressure measurement on three separate occasions using an appropriate-size cuff.[16-18]

EVALUATION AND TREATMENT In children, the history and physical examination should be directed at determining the etiology of HTN, such as coarctation of the aorta or renal disease (Table 24-6). A complete blood count, serum chemistry levels, urinalysis, urine culture, lipid profile, and renal ultrasound are part of the routine evaluation for renal disease (Table 24-7). If coarctation of the aorta is found, surgical correction is initiated. If HTN is determined to be essential, or primary, in nature, nonpharmacologic therapy is used initially. Moderate weight loss and exercise can decrease systolic and diastolic pressures in many children. Appropriate diet, regular physical activity, and avoidance of smoking have been shown to be effective in reducing blood pressure.[18] Ambulatory blood pressure monitoring (ABPM) has the potential to become an important tool in the evaluation and management of childhood hypertension.[19]

TABLE 24-6 MOST COMMON CAUSES OF CHRONIC SUSTAINED HYPERTENSION

AGE GROUP	CAUSES
Newborn	Renal artery thrombosis, renal artery stenosis, congenital renal malformation, COA, bronchopulmonary dysplasia
<6 yr	Renal parenchymal disease, COA, renal artery stenosis
6-10 yr	Renal artery stenosis, renal parenchymal disease, primary hypertension
>10 yr	Primary hypertension, renal parenchymal disease

COA, Coarctation of the aorta.
From Park MK: *Pediatric cardiology for practitioners,* ed 5, St Louis, 2008, Mosby.

Medication therapy is controversial in children with primary hypertension; however, when nonpharmacologic therapy fails, the approach is similar to the treatment of hypertension in adults with the use of angiotensin-converting enzyme inhibitors or angiotensin receptor blocker medications.[2] The current emphasis on preventive cardiology, especially for children, is significant because many investigators believe signs of atherosclerosis are present during childhood.[1,18]

✔ **QUICK CHECK 24-2**
1. Why are the infant's height and weight important in the assessment of congestive heart failure?
2. Why is it of critical importance to recognize and treat children during the acute phase of Kawasaki disease?
3. Discuss the causes of the recent epidemic of obesity in children and the cardiovascular effects.

TABLE 24-7 ROUTINE AND SPECIAL LABORATORY TESTS FOR HYPERTENSION

LABORATORY TESTS	SIGNIFICANCE OF ABNORMAL RESULTS
Urinalysis, urine culture, blood urea nitrogen, and creatinine levels	Renal parenchymal disease
Serum electrolyte levels (hypokalemia)	Hyperaldosteronism, primary or secondary
	Adrenogenital syndrome
	Renin-producing tumors
ECG, chest x-ray studies	Cardiac cause of hypertension, also baseline function
Intravenous pyelography (or ultrasonography, radionuclide studies, computed tomography of kidneys)	Renal parenchymal diseases
	Renovascular hypertension
	Tumors (neuroblastoma, Wilms tumor)
Plasma renin activity, peripheral	High-renin hypertension
	Renovascular hypertension
	Renin-producing tumors
	Some caused by Cushing syndrome
	Some caused by essential hypertension
	Low-renin hypertension
	Adrenogenital syndrome
	Primary hyperaldosteronism
24-hr urine collection for 17-ketosteroids and 17-hydroxycorticosteroids	Cushing syndrome
	Adrenogenital syndrome
24-hr urine collection for catecholamine levels and vanillylmandelic acid	Pheochromocytoma
	Neuroblastoma
Aldosterone	Hyperaldosteronism, primary or secondary
	Renovascular hypertension
	Renin-producing tumors
Renal vein plasma renin activity	Unilateral renal parenchymal disease
	Renovascular hypertension
Abdominal aortogram	Renovascular hypertension
	Abdominal COA
	Unilateral renal parenchymal diseases
	Pheochromocytoma

From Park MK: *Pediatric cardiology for practitioners,* ed 6, St Louis, 2008, Mosby.
COA, Coarctation of the aorta; *ECG,* electrocardiogram.

DID YOU UNDERSTAND?

Congenital Heart Disease

1. Most congenital heart defects have begun to develop by the eighth week of gestation, and some have associated causes, both environmental and genetic.
2. Environmental risk factors associated with the incidence of congenital heart defects typically are maternal conditions. Maternal conditions include viral infections, diabetes, drug intake, and advanced maternal age.
3. Genetic factors associated with congenital heart defects include but are not limited to Down syndrome, trisomy 13, trisomy 18, cri du chat syndrome, and Turner syndrome.
4. Classification of congenital heart defects is based on (a) whether they cause blood flow to the lungs to increase, decrease, or remain normal; (b) whether they cause cyanosis; and (c) whether they cause obstruction to flow.
5. Cyanosis, a bluish discoloration of the skin, indicates that the tissues are not receiving normal amounts of oxygenated blood. Cyanosis can be caused by defects that (a) restrict blood flow into the pulmonary circulation; (b) overload the pulmonary circulation, causing pulmonary overcirculation, pulmonary edema, and respiratory difficulty; or (c) cause large amounts of unoxygenated blood to shunt from the pulmonary to the systemic circulation.
6. Congenital defects that maintain or create direct communication between the pulmonary and systemic circulatory systems cause blood to shunt from one system to another, mixing oxygenated and unoxygenated blood and increasing blood volume and, occasionally, pressure on the receiving side of the shunt.
7. The direction of shunting through an abnormal communication depends on differences in pressure and resistance between the two systems. Flow is always from an area of high pressure to an area of low pressure.
8. Obstruction of ventricular outflow is commonly caused by pulmonary stenosis (right ventricle) or aortic stenosis (left ventricle).
9. In less severe obstruction, ventricular outflow remains normal because of compensatory ventricular hypertrophy stimulated by increased afterload and, in postductal coarctation of the aorta, development of collateral circulation around the coarctation.
10. Acyanotic congenital defects that increase pulmonary blood flow consist of abnormal openings (atrial septal defect, ventricular septal defect, patent ductus arteriosus, or atrioventricular septal defect) that permit blood to shunt from left (systemic circulation) to right (pulmonary circulation). Cyanosis does not occur because the left-to-right shunt does not interfere with the flow of oxygenated blood through the systemic circulation.

Continued

DID YOU UNDERSTAND?—cont'd

11. If the abnormal communication between the left and right circuits is large, volume and pressure overload in the pulmonary circulation lead to left heart failure.
12. Cyanotic congenital defects in which saturated and desaturated blood mix within the heart or great arteries include truncus arteriosus, tricuspid atresia, tetralogy of Fallot, transposition of the great vessels, total anomalous pulmonary venous connection, and hypoplastic left heart syndrome.
13. In cyanotic heart defects that decrease pulmonary blood flow (tetralogy of Fallot), myocardial hypertrophy cannot compensate for restricted right ventricular outflow. Flow to the lungs decreases, and cyanosis is caused by an insufficient volume of oxygenated blood and right-to-left shunt.
14. Initial treatment for congenital heart disease, depending on the defect, is aimed at controlling the level of congestive heart failure or cyanosis. Interventional procedures in the cardiac catheterization laboratory and surgical palliation or repair are performed to restore circulation to as normal as possible.

15. Congestive heart failure is usually the result of congenital heart defects that increase blood volume in the pulmonary circulation. A clinical manifestation of CHF unique to children is failure to thrive.

Acquired Cardiovascular Disorders in Children

1. Two examples of acquired heart disease in children are Kawasaki disease and systemic hypertension.
2. Kawasaki disease is an acute systemic vasculitis that also may result in the development of coronary artery aneurysms and thrombosis.
3. Systemic hypertension in children differs from HTN in adults in etiology and presentation. When significant hypertension is found in a child, the examiner should evaluate for the presence of renal disease or coarctation.

KEY TERMS

- Acyanotic heart defect 643
- Aortic stenosis (AS) 646
- Atrial septal defect (ASD) 648
- Atrioventricular canal (AVC) defect (atrioventricular septal defect [AVSD], endocardial cushion defect [ECD]) 649
- Coarctation of the aorta (COA) 644
- Congenital heart disease (CHD) 643
- Congestive heart failure (CHF) 653
- Cyanosis 644
- Cyanotic heart defect 644
- Eisenmenger syndrome 648
- Hypoplastic left heart syndrome (HLHS) 653

- Kawasaki disease (KD) 654
- Left-to-right shunt 643
- Muscular VSD 648
- Ostium primum ASD 648
- Ostium secundum ASD 648
- Patent ductus arteriosus (PDA) 647
- Perimembranous VSD 648
- Pulmonary atresia 647
- Pulmonic stenosis (PS) 647
- Right-to-left shunt 644
- Shunt 643
- Sinus venosus ASD 648
- Subvalvular AS 646
- Supravalvular AS 646

- Systemic hypertension 655
- Tetralogy of Fallot (TOF) 649
- Total anomalous pulmonary venous connection (TAPVC) 652
- Transposition of the great arteries (TGA; transposition of the great vessels [TGV]) 651
- Tricuspid atresia 649
- Truncus arteriosus (TA) 652
- Valvular AS 646
- Ventricular septal defect (VSD) 648

REFERENCES

1. Allen HD, editor: *Moss and Adams' heart disease in infants, children, and adolescents including the fetus and young adults*, ed 7, Philadelphia, 2008, Lippincott Williams & Wilkins.
2. Park MK: *Pediatric cardiology for practitioners*, ed 5, St Louis, 2008, Mosby. Available at http://mdconsult/book.
3. Sadowski SL: Congenital cardiac disease in the newborn infant: past, present, and future, *Crit Care Nurs Clin North Am* 21:7–48, 2009.
4. Hijazi ZM, Awad SM: Pediatric cardiac interventions, *JACC Cardiovasc Interv* 1(6):603–611, 2008.
5. Pober BR: Williams-Beuren syndrome, *N Engl J Med* 362(3):239–252, 2010.
6. Hollinger I, Mittnacht A: Cardiac catheterization, interventional cardiology, and ablation techniques for children, *Int Anesthesiol Clin* 47(3):63–99, 2009.
7. Wong D, et al: *Whaley and Wong's nursing care of infants and children*, ed 7, St Louis, 2003, Mosby.
8. Gervasi L, Basu S: Atrial septal defect devices used in the cardiac catheterization laboratory, *Prog Cardiovasc Nurs* 24(3):86–89, 2009.
9. Barron DJ, et al: Hypoplastic left heart syndrome, *Lancet* 374(9589):551–564, 2009.
10. Kutty S, Zahn EM: Interventional therapy for neonates with critical congenital heart disease, *Catheter Cardiovasc Interv* 72(5):663–674, 2008.
11. Mehta R, et al: Complications of pediatric cardiac catheterization: a review in the current era, *Catheter Cardiovasc Interv* 72(2):278–285, 2008.
12. Federspiel MC: Cardiac assessment in the neonatal population, *Neonatal Netw* 29(3):135–142, 2010.
13. Hartas GA, Emmanouil T, Gupta-Malhotra M: Approach to diagnosing congenital cardiac disorders, *Crit Care Nurs Clin North Am* 21:27–36, 2009.
14. Newberger JW, et al: Diagnosis, treatment and long-term management of Kawasaki disease: a statement for health professionals from The Committee on Rheumatic Fever, Endocarditis and Kawasaki Disease, Council on Cardiovascular Disease in the Young, American Heart Association, *Circulation* 110:2747–2771, 2004.
15. National High Blood Pressure Education Program Working Group on High Blood Pressure in Children and Adolescents: The fourth report on the diagnosis, evaluation and treatment of high blood pressure in children and adolescents, *Pediatrics* 114(suppl 2, 4th rep):555–576, 2004.
16. Brady TM, Feld LG: Pediatric approach to hypertension, *Semin Nephrol* 29(4):379–388, 2009.
17. Nguyen M: Mitsnefes: Evaluation of hypertension by the general pediatrician, *Curr Opin Pediatr* 19(2):165–169, 2007.
18. Seikaly MG: Hypertension in children; an update on treatment strategies, *Curr Opin Pediatr* 19(2):170–177, 2007.
19. Urbina E, et al: Ambulatory blood pressure monitoring in children and adolescents: recommendations for standard assessment: a scientific statement from the American Heart Association Atherosclerosis, Hypertension and Obesity in Youth Committee of the Council on Cardiovascular Disease in the Young and the Council for High Blood Pressure Research, *Hypertension* 52(3):433–451, 2008.

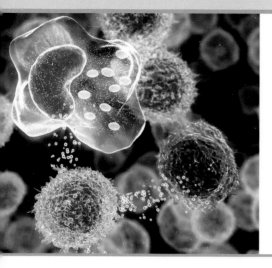

Structure and Function of the Pulmonary System

Valentina L. Brashers

The pulmonary system consists of the lungs, airways, chest wall, and pulmonary circulation. Its primary function is the exchange of gases between the environmental air and the blood. The three steps in this process are (1) ventilation, the movement of air into and out of the lungs; (2) diffusion, the movement of gases between air spaces in the lungs and the bloodstream; and (3) perfusion, the movement of blood into and out of the capillary beds of the lungs to body organs and tissues. The first two functions are carried out by the pulmonary system and the third by the cardiovascular system (see Chapter 22). Normally the pulmonary system functions efficiently under a variety of conditions and with little energy expenditure.

STRUCTURES OF THE PULMONARY SYSTEM

The pulmonary system consists of two lungs and their airways, the blood vessels that serve these structures (Figure 25-1), and the chest wall, or thoracic cage. The lungs are divided into lobes: three in the right lung (upper, middle, lower) and two in the left lung (upper, lower). Each lobe is further divided into segments and lobules. The space between the lungs, which contains the heart, great vessels, and esophagus, is called the *mediastinum*. A set of conducting airways, or bronchi, delivers air to each section of the lung. The lung tissue that surrounds the airways supports them, preventing their distortion or collapse as gas moves in and out during ventilation.

The lungs are protected from exogenous contaminants by a series of mechanical barriers (Table 25-1). These defense mechanisms are so effective that contamination of the lung tissue itself, particularly by infectious agents, is rare.

Conducting Airways

The conducting airways allow air into and out of the gas-exchange structures of the lung. The **nasopharynx, oropharynx,** and related structures are often called the *upper airway* (Figure 25-2). These structures are lined with a ciliated mucosa that warms and humidifies inspired air and removes foreign particles from it. The mouth and oropharynx are used for ventilation when the nose is obstructed or when increased flow is required, for example, during exercise. Filtering and humidifying are not as efficient with mouth breathing.

The **larynx** connects the upper and lower airways and consists of the endolarynx and its surrounding triangular-shaped bony and cartilaginous structures. The endolarynx encompasses two pairs of folds: the false vocal cords (supraglottis) and the true vocal cords. The slit-shaped space between the true cords forms the glottis (see Figure 25-2).

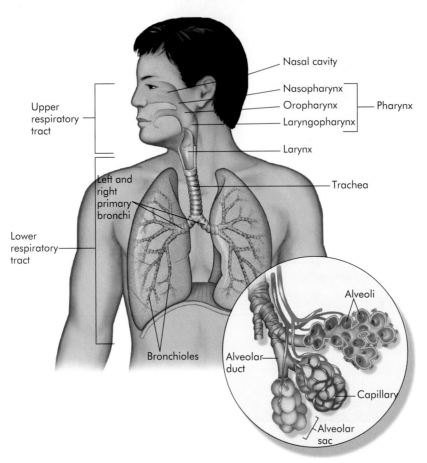

FIGURE 25-1 Structure of the Pulmonary System. The enlargement in the circle depicts the acinus, where oxygen and carbon dioxide are exchanged. (From Patton KT, Thibodeau GA: *Anatomy & physiology*, ed 7, St Louis, 2010, Mosby.)

TABLE 25-1	PULMONARY DEFENSE MECHANISMS
STRUCTURE OR SUBSTANCE	**MECHANISM OF DEFENSE**
Upper respiratory tract mucosa	Maintains constant temperature and humidification of gas entering lungs; traps and removes foreign particles, some bacteria, and noxious gases from inspired air
Nasal hairs and turbinates	Trap and remove foreign particles, some bacteria, and noxious gases from inspired air
Mucous blanket	Protects trachea and bronchi from injury; traps most foreign particles and bacteria that reach lower airways
Cilia	Propel mucous blanket and entrapped particles toward oropharynx, where they can be swallowed or expectorated
Alveolar macrophages	Ingest and remove bacteria and other foreign material from alveoli by phagocytosis (see Chapters 5 and 6)
Irritant receptors in nares (nostrils)	Stimulation by chemical or mechanical irritants triggers sneeze reflex, which results in rapid removal of irritants from nasal passages
Irritant receptors in trachea and large airways	Stimulation by chemical or mechanical irritants triggers cough reflex, which results in removal of irritants from lower airways

The vestibule is the space above the false vocal cords. The laryngeal box is formed of three large cartilages (epiglottis, thyroid, cricoid) and three smaller cartilages (arytenoid, corniculate, cuneiform) connected by ligaments. The supporting cartilages prevent collapse of the larynx during inspiration and swallowing. The internal laryngeal muscles control vocal cord length and tension, and the external laryngeal muscles move the larynx as a whole. Both sets of muscles are important to swallowing, ventilation, and vocalization.[1] The internal muscles contract during swallowing to prevent aspiration into the trachea. These muscles also contribute to voice pitch.

The **trachea,** which is supported by U-shaped cartilage, connects the larynx to the bronchi, the conducting airways of the lungs. The trachea branches into two main airways, or **bronchi** (sing., **bronchus**), at the **carina** (see Figure 25-1). The right and left main bronchi enter the lungs at the **hila** (sing., **hilum**), or "roots" of the lungs, along with the pulmonary blood and lymphatic vessels. From the hila the main bronchi branch farther, as shown in Figure 25-3.

The bronchial walls have three layers: an epithelial lining, a smooth muscle layer, and a connective tissue layer. The epithelial lining of the bronchi contains single-celled exocrine glands—the mucus-secreting **goblet cells**—and ciliated cells. The goblet cells produce a mucous blanket that protects the airway epithelium, and the ciliated epithelial cells rhythmically beat this mucous blanket toward the trachea and pharynx where it can be swallowed or expectorated by coughing. The layers of epithelium that line the bronchi become thinner with each successive branching (Figure 25-4).

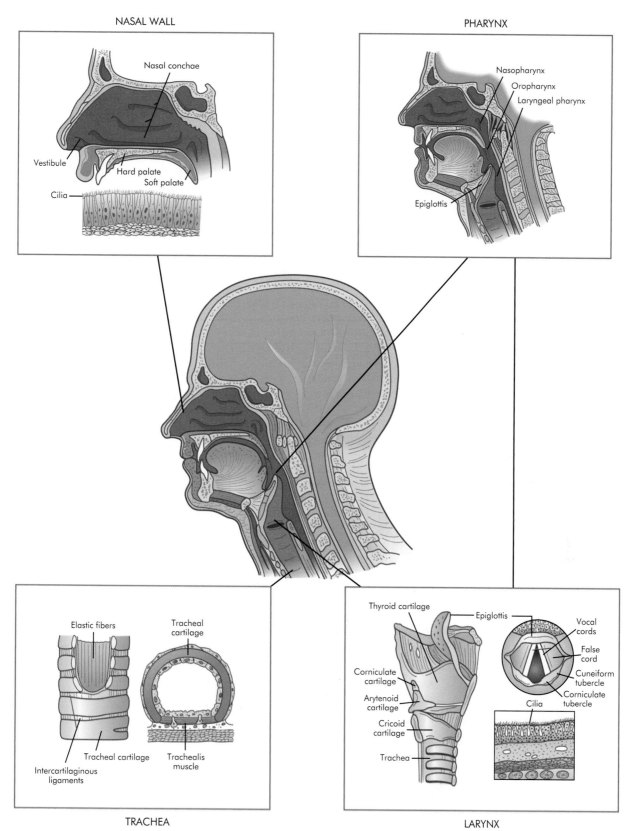

FIGURE 25-2 Structures of the Upper Airway. (Redrawn from Thompson JM et al: *Mosby's clinical nursing,* ed 5, St Louis, 2002, Mosby.)

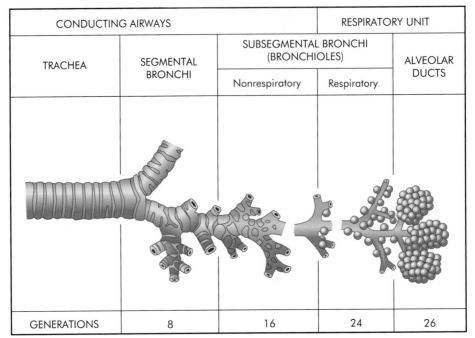

CONDUCTING AIRWAYS				RESPIRATORY UNIT
TRACHEA	SEGMENTAL BRONCHI	SUBSEGMENTAL BRONCHI (BRONCHIOLES)		ALVEOLAR DUCTS
		Nonrespiratory	Respiratory	
GENERATIONS	8	16	24	26

FIGURE 25-3 Structures of the Lower Airway. (Redrawn from Thompson JM et al: *Mosby's clinical nursing,* ed 5, St Louis, 2002, Mosby.)

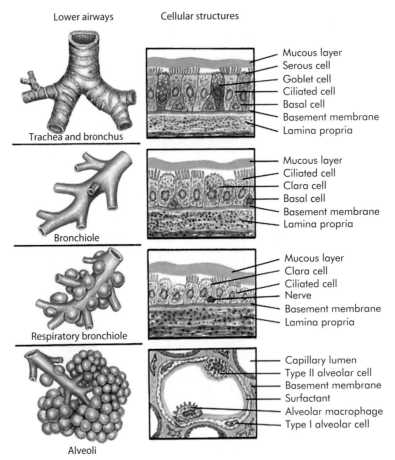

Lower airways   Cellular structures

Trachea and bronchus
— Mucous layer
— Serous cell
— Goblet cell
— Ciliated cell
— Basal cell
— Basement membrane
— Lamina propria

Bronchiole
— Mucous layer
— Ciliated cell
— Clara cell
— Basal cell
— Basement membrane
— Lamina propria

Respiratory bronchiole
— Mucous layer
— Clara cell
— Ciliated cell
— Nerve
— Basement membrane
— Lamina propria

Alveoli
— Capillary lumen
— Type II alveolar cell
— Basement membrane
— Surfactant
— Alveolar macrophage
— Type I alveolar cell

FIGURE 25-4 Changes in the Bronchial Wall With Progressive Branching. (From Wilson SF, Thompson JM: *Respiratory disorders,* St Louis, 1990, Mosby.)

Gas-Exchange Airways

The conducting airways terminate in the respiratory bronchioles, alveolar ducts, and alveoli (sing., alveolus). These thin-walled structures together are sometimes called the acinus (see Figures 25-1 and 25-3), and all of them participate in gas exchange.[2]

The alveoli are the primary gas-exchange units of the lung, where oxygen enters the blood and carbon dioxide is removed (Figure 25-5). Tiny passages called *pores of Kohn* permit some air to pass through the septa from alveolus to alveolus, promoting collateral ventilation and even distribution of air among the alveoli. The lungs contain approximately 25 million alveoli at birth and 300 million by adulthood.

Two major types of epithelial cells appear in the alveolus. Type I alveolar cells provide structure, and type II alveolar cells secrete surfactant, a lipoprotein that coats the inner surface of the alveolus and lowers alveolar surface tension at end-expiration, thereby preventing lung collapse.[1-4]

Like the bronchi, alveoli contain cellular components of inflammation and immunity, particularly the mononuclear phagocytes (called *alveolar macrophages*). These cells ingest foreign material that reaches the alveolus and prepare it for removal through the lymphatics. (Phagocytosis and the mononuclear phagocyte system are described in Chapters 5 and 6.)

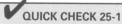

✔ **QUICK CHECK 25-1**
1. List the major components of the pulmonary system.
2. What are conducting airways?
3. Describe an alveolus.

Pulmonary and Bronchial Circulation

The pulmonary circulation facilitates gas exchange, delivers nutrients to lung tissues, acts as a reservoir for the left ventricle, and serves as a filtering system that removes clots, air, and other debris from the circulation.

Although the entire cardiac output from the right ventricle goes into the lungs, the pulmonary circulation has a lower pressure and resistance than the systemic circulation. Pulmonary arteries are exposed to about one fifth the pressure of the systemic circulation. Usually about one third of the pulmonary vessels are filled with blood (perfused) at any given time. More vessels become perfused when right ventricular cardiac output increases. Therefore increased delivery of blood to the lungs does not normally increase mean pulmonary artery pressure.

The pulmonary artery divides and enters the lung at the hila, branching with each main bronchus and with all bronchi at every division. Therefore every bronchus and bronchiole has an accompanying artery or arteriole. The arterioles divide at the terminal bronchioles to form a network of pulmonary capillaries around the acinus. Capillary walls consist of an endothelial layer and a thin basement membrane, which often fuses with the basement membrane of the alveolar septum. Consequently, very little separation exists between blood in the capillary and gas in the alveolus.

The shared alveolar and capillary walls compose the alveolocapillary membrane (Figure 25-6). Gas exchange occurs across this membrane. With normal perfusion, approximately 100 ml of blood in the pulmonary capillary bed is spread very thinly over 70 to 100 m[2] of alveolar surface area. Any disorder that thickens the membrane impairs gas exchange.

Each pulmonary vein drains several pulmonary capillaries. Unlike the pulmonary arteries, pulmonary veins are dispersed randomly throughout the lung and then leave the lung at the hila and enter the left atrium. They have no valves.

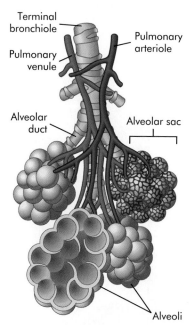

FIGURE 25-5 Alveoli. Bronchioles subdivide to form tiny tubes called *alveolar ducts,* which end in clusters of alveoli called *alveolar sacs*. (From Patton KT, Thibodeau GA: *Anatomy & physiology,* ed 7, St Louis, 2010, Mosby.)

The bronchial circulation is part of the systemic circulation, and it supplies nutrients to the conducting airways, large pulmonary vessels, and membranes (pleurae) that surround the lungs. Not all of its capillaries drain into its own venous system. Some empty into the pulmonary vein and contribute to the normal venous mixture of oxygenated and deoxygenated blood or right-to-left shunt (right-to-left shunts are described in Chapter 26). The bronchial circulation does not participate in gas exchange.[1]

Lung vasculature also includes deep and superficial lymphatic capillaries. Fluid and alveolar macrophages migrate from the alveoli to the terminal bronchioles, where they enter the lymphatic system. Both deep and superficial lymphatic vessels leave the lung at the hilum. The lymphatic system plays an important role in keeping the lung free of fluid. (The lymphatic system is described in Chapter 22.)

Chest Wall and Pleura

The chest wall (skin, ribs, intercostal muscles) protects the lungs from injury, and its muscles, along with the diaphragm, perform the muscular work of breathing. The thoracic cavity is contained by the chest wall and encases the lungs (Figure 25-7). A serous membrane called the pleura adheres firmly to the lungs and then folds over itself and attaches firmly to the chest wall. The membrane covering the lungs is the *visceral pleura;* that lining the thoracic cavity is the *parietal pleura*. The area between the two pleurae is called the pleural space, or pleural cavity. Normally, only a thin layer of fluid secreted by the pleura (pleural fluid) fills the pleural space, lubricating the pleural surfaces and allowing the two layers to slide over each other without separating. Pressure in the pleural space is usually negative or subatmospheric (−4 to −10 mm Hg).

FUNCTION OF THE PULMONARY SYSTEM

The pulmonary system (1) ventilates the alveoli, (2) diffuses gases into and out of the blood, and (3) perfuses the lungs so that the organs and tissues of the body receive blood that is rich in oxygen and low in

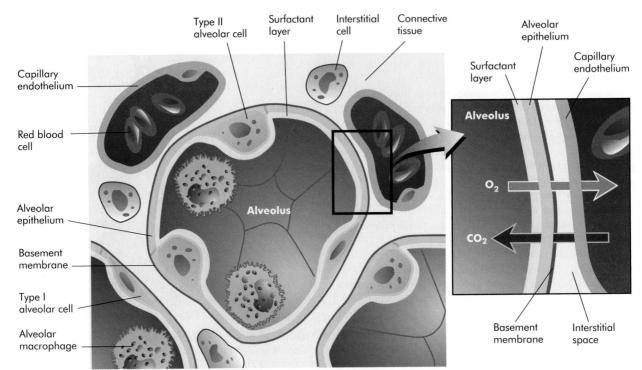

FIGURE 25-6 Section Through the Alveolar Septum (Gas-Exchange Membrane). Inset shows a magnified view of the respiratory membrane composed of the alveolar wall (fluid coating, epithelial cells, basement membrane), interstitial fluid, and wall of a pulmonary capillary (basement membrane, endothelial cells). The gases CO_2 (carbon dioxide) and O_2 (oxygen) diffuse across the respiratory membrane.

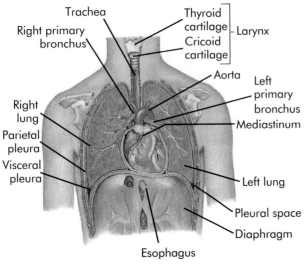

FIGURE 25-7 Thoracic (Chest) Cavity and Related Structures. The thoracic (chest) cavity is divided into three subdivisions (left and right pleural divisions and mediastinum) by a partition formed by a serous membrane called the *pleura*. (From Thibodeau GA, Patton KT: *Anatomy & physiology*, ed 3, St Louis, 1996, Mosby.)

carbon dioxide. Each component of the pulmonary system contributes to one or more of these functions (Figure 25-8).

Ventilation

Ventilation is the mechanical movement of gas or air into and out of the lungs. It is often misnamed *respiration*, which is actually the exchange of oxygen and carbon dioxide during cellular metabolism. "Respiratory rate" is actually the ventilatory rate, or the number of

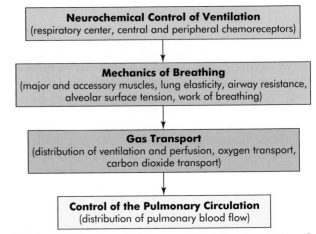

FIGURE 25-8 Functional Components of the Respiratory System. The central nervous system responds to neurochemical stimulation of ventilation and sends signals to the chest wall musculature. The response of the respiratory system to these impulses is influenced by several factors that impact the mechanisms of breathing and, therefore, affect the adequacy of ventilation. Gas transport between the alveoli and pulmonary capillary blood depends on a variety of physical and chemical activities. Finally, the control of the pulmonary circulation plays a role in the appropriate distribution of blood flow.

times gas is inspired and expired per minute. The amount of effective ventilation is calculated by multiplying the ventilatory rate (breaths per minute) by the volume or amount of air per breath (liters per breath or tidal volume). This is called the minute volume (or minute ventilation) and is expressed in liters per minute.

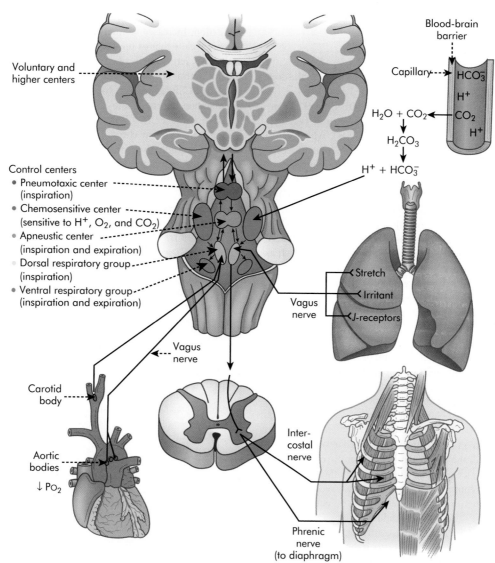

FIGURE 25-9 Neurochemical Respiratory Control System.

Carbon dioxide (CO_2), the gaseous form of carbonic acid (H_2CO_3), is produced by cellular metabolism. The lung eliminates about 10,000 milliequivalents (mEq) of carbonic acid per day in the form of CO_2, which is produced at the rate of approximately 200 ml/min. Carbon dioxide is eliminated to maintain a normal arterial CO_2 pressure ($Paco_2$) of 40 mm Hg and normal acid-base balance. Adequate ventilation is necessary to maintain normal $Paco_2$ levels. Diseases that limit ventilation result in CO_2 retention. The adequacy of alveolar ventilation *cannot* be accurately determined by observation of ventilatory rate, pattern, or effort. If a healthcare professional needs to determine the adequacy of ventilation, an arterial blood gas analysis must be performed to measure $Paco_2$.

✔ QUICK CHECK 25-2
1. List the major components of the pulmonary circulation.
2. What are the visceral and parietal pleurae?

Neurochemical Control of Ventilation

Breathing is usually involuntary, because homeostatic changes in ventilatory rate and volume are adjusted automatically by the nervous system to maintain normal gas exchange. Voluntary breathing is necessary for talking, singing, laughing, and deliberately holding one's breath. The mechanisms that control respiration are complex (Figure 25-9).

The respiratory center in the brain stem controls respiration by transmitting impulses to the respiratory muscles, causing them to contract and relax. The respiratory center is composed of several groups of neurons: the dorsal respiratory group (DRG), the ventral respiratory group (VRG), the pneumotaxic center, and the apneustic center.[1-4] The basic automatic rhythm of respiration is set by the DRG, which receives afferent input from peripheral chemoreceptors in the carotid and aortic bodies and from several different types of receptors in the lungs. The VRG contains both inspiratory and expiratory neurons and is almost inactive during normal, quiet respiration, becoming active when increased ventilatory effort is required. The pneumotaxic center and apneustic center, situated in the pons, do not generate primary rhythm but, rather, act as modifiers of the rhythm established by the medullary centers. The pattern of breathing can be influenced by emotion, pain, and disease.

Lung Receptors

Three types of lung receptors send impulses from the lungs to the dorsal respiratory group:

1. **Irritant receptors** (C-fibers) are found in the epithelium of all conducting airways. They are sensitive to noxious aerosols (vapors), gases, and particulate matter (e.g., inhaled dusts), which cause them to initiate the cough reflex.[5] When stimulated, irritant receptors also cause bronchoconstriction and increased ventilatory rate.

2. **Stretch receptors** are located in the smooth muscles of airways and are sensitive to increases in the size or volume of the lungs. They decrease ventilatory rate and volume when stimulated, an occurrence sometimes referred to as the Hering-Breuer expiratory reflex. This reflex is active in newborns and assists with ventilation. In adults, this reflex is active only at high tidal volumes (such as with exercise) and may protect against excess lung inflation. Stretch receptors called rapidly adapting receptors (RARs) have been found to be an important mediator of cough.[5]

3. **J-receptors** (juxtapulmonary capillary receptors) are located near the capillaries in the alveolar septa. They are sensitive to increased pulmonary capillary pressure, which stimulates them to initiate rapid, shallow breathing, hypotension, and bradycardia.[4]

The lung is innervated by the autonomic nervous system (ANS). Fibers of the sympathetic division in the lung branch from the upper thoracic and cervical ganglia of the spinal cord. Fibers of the parasympathetic division of the ANS travel in the vagus nerve to the lung. (Structures and function of the ANS are discussed in detail in Chapter 12.) The parasympathetic and sympathetic divisions control airway caliber (interior diameter of the airway lumen) by stimulating bronchial smooth muscle to contract or relax. The parasympathetic receptors cause smooth muscle to contract, whereas sympathetic receptors cause it to relax. Bronchial smooth muscle tone depends on equilibrium—that is, equal stimulation of contraction and relaxation. The parasympathetic division of the ANS is the main controller of airway caliber under normal conditions. Constriction occurs if the irritant receptors in the airway epithelium are stimulated by irritants in inspired air, by inflammatory mediators (e.g., histamine, serotonin, prostaglandins, leukotrienes), by many drugs, and by humoral substances.

Chemoreceptors

Chemoreceptors monitor the pH, $Paco_2$, and Pao_2 (arterial pressure of oxygen) of arterial blood.[6] **Central chemoreceptors** monitor arterial blood indirectly by sensing changes in the pH of cerebrospinal fluid (CSF) (see Figure 25-9, p. 665). They are located near the respiratory center and are sensitive to hydrogen ion concentration in the CSF. (Chapter 4 describes the relationship between ions and the pH, or acid-base status, of body fluids.) The pH of the CSF reflects arterial pH because carbon dioxide in arterial blood can diffuse across the blood-brain barrier (the capillary wall separating blood from cells of the central nervous system) into the CSF until the partial pressure of carbon dioxide (Pco_2) is equal on both sides. Carbon dioxide that has entered the CSF combines with H_2O to form carbonic acid, which subsequently dissociates into hydrogen ions that are capable of stimulating the central chemoreceptors. In this way, $Paco_2$ regulates ventilation through its impact on the pH (hydrogen ion content) of the CSF.[1-4,6]

If alveolar ventilation is inadequate, $Paco_2$ increases. Carbon dioxide diffuses across the blood-brain barrier until Pco_2 values in blood

and CSF reach equilibrium. As the central chemoreceptors sense the resulting decrease in pH (increase in hydrogen ion concentration), they stimulate the respiratory center to increase the depth and rate of ventilation. Increased ventilation causes the Pco_2 of arterial blood to decrease below that of the CSF, and carbon dioxide diffuses back out of the CSF, returning its pH to normal.

The central chemoreceptors are sensitive to very small changes in the pH of CSF (equivalent to a 1 to 2 mm Hg change in Pco_2) and can maintain a normal $Paco_2$ under many different conditions, including strenuous exercise.[6] If inadequate ventilation, or hypoventilation, is long term (e.g., in chronic obstructive pulmonary disease), these receptors become insensitive to small changes in $Paco_2$ ("reset") and regulate ventilation poorly (see *Health Alert:* Changes in the Chemical Control of Breathing During Sleep).

HEALTH ALERT

Changes in the Chemical Control of Breathing During Sleep

There are multiple sites of central carbon dioxide chemosensitivity in the brain stem, and there are specialized chemosensory sites that function only during certain sleep states. Chemical control of ventilation, related to both hypercapnia and hypoxia, appears to be blunted during sleep. The orexins are neurohormones that control feeding, vigilance, and sleep. It is postulated that changes in orexin activity contribute to the blunting of chemoreceptor sensitivity seen in many states, including obesity and sleep apnea. Congestive heart failure, chronic obstructive pulmonary disease, and hypertension also are associated with abnormal breathing responses during sleep. Changes in the chemical control of breathing during sleep may contribute to morbidity and mortality seen in individuals with these disorders.

Data from Brown LK: Hypoventilation syndromes, *Clin Chest Med* 31(2):249–270, 2010; Kuwaki T, Li A, Nattie E: State-dependent central chemoreception: a role of orexin, *Respir Physiol Neurobiol* 173(3):223–229, 2010; Nattie E, Li A: Central chemoreception in wakefulness and sleep: evidence for a distributed network and a role for orexin, *J Appl Physiol* 108(5):1417–1424, 2010; Pacchia CF: Sleep apnea and hypertension: role of chemoreflexes in humans, *Exp Physiol* 92(1):45–50, 2007; Pinna GD et al: Long-term time-course of nocturnal breathing disorders in heart failure patients, *Eur Respir J* 35(2):361–367, 2010; Piper AJ: The highs and lows of gas exchange during sleep, *Respirology* 15(2):191–193, 2010.

The peripheral chemoreceptors are somewhat sensitive to changes in $Paco_2$ and pH but are sensitive primarily to oxygen levels in arterial blood (Pao_2).[7] As Pao_2 and pH decrease, peripheral chemoreceptors, particularly in the carotid bodies, send signals to the respiratory center to increase ventilation. However, the Pao_2 must drop well below normal (to approximately 60 mm Hg) before the peripheral chemoreceptors have much influence on ventilation. If $Paco_2$ is elevated as well, ventilation increases much more than it would in response to either abnormality alone. The peripheral chemoreceptors become the major stimulus to ventilation when the central chemoreceptors are reset by chronic hypoventilation.[8]

> ✓ **QUICK CHECK 25-3**
> 1. Describe three functions of the respiratory center in the brain stem.
> 2. What are the three types of lung receptors?
> 3. How do the functions of central and peripheral chemoreceptors differ?

Mechanics of Breathing

The mechanical aspects of inspiration and expiration are known collectively as the mechanics of breathing and involve (1) major and accessory muscles of inspiration and expiration, (2) elastic properties of the lungs and chest wall, and (3) resistance to airflow through the conducting airways. Alterations in any of these properties increase the work of breathing or the metabolic energy needed to achieve adequate ventilation and oxygenation of the blood.

Major and Accessory Muscles

The major muscles of inspiration are the diaphragm and the external intercostal muscles (muscles between the ribs) (Figure 25-10). The diaphragm is a dome-shaped muscle that separates the abdominal and thoracic cavities. When it contracts and flattens downward, it increases the volume of the thoracic cavity, creating a negative pressure that draws gas into the lungs through the upper airways and trachea. Contraction of external intercostal muscles elevates the anterior portion of the ribs and increases the volume of the thoracic cavity by increasing its front-to-back (anterior-posterior [AP]) diameter. Although the

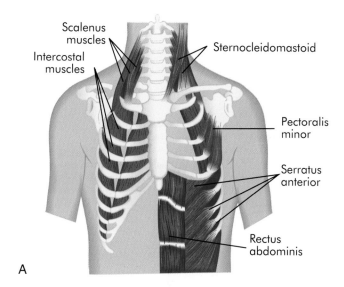

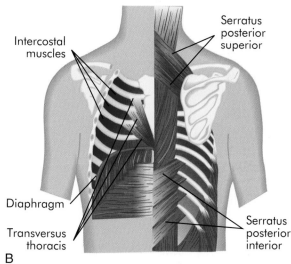

FIGURE 25-10 Muscles of Ventilation. A, Anterior view. **B,** Posterior view. (Modified from Thompson JM et al: *Mosby's clinical nursing*, ed 5, St Louis, 2002, Mosby.)

external intercostals may contract during quiet breathing, inspiration at rest is usually assisted by the diaphragm only.

The accessory muscles of inspiration are the sternocleidomastoid and scalene muscles. Like the external intercostals, these muscles enlarge the thorax by increasing its AP diameter. The accessory muscles assist inspiration when minute volume (volume of air inspired and expired per minute) is high, as during strenuous exercise, or when the work of breathing is increased because of disease. The accessory muscles do not increase the volume of the thorax as efficiently as the diaphragm does.

There are no major muscles of expiration because normal, relaxed expiration is passive and requires no muscular effort. The accessory muscles of expiration, the abdominal and internal intercostal muscles, assist expiration when minute volume is high, during coughing, or when airway obstruction is present. When the abdominal muscles contract, intra-abdominal pressure increases, pushing up the diaphragm and decreasing the volume of the thorax. The internal intercostal muscles pull down the anterior ribs, decreasing the AP diameter of the thorax.

Alveolar Surface Tension

Surface tension occurs at any gas-liquid interface and refers to the tendency for liquid molecules that are exposed to air to adhere to one another. This phenomenon can be seen in the way liquids "bead" when splashed on a waterproof surface.

Within a sphere, such as an alveolus, surface tension tends to make expansion difficult. According to the law of Laplace, the pressure (P) required to inflate a sphere is equal to two times the surface tension ($2T$) divided by the radius (r) of the sphere, or $P = 2T/r$. As the radius of the sphere (or alveolus) decreases, more and more pressure is required to inflate it. If the alveoli were lined only with a water-like fluid, taking breaths would be extremely difficult.

Alveolar ventilation, or distention, is made possible by surfactant, which lowers surface tension by coating the air-liquid interface in the alveoli. Surfactant, a lipoprotein produced by type II alveolar cells, includes two groups of *surfactant* proteins. One group consists of small hydrophobic molecules that have a detergent-like effect that separates the liquid molecules, thereby decreasing alveolar surface tension.[2,9] As the radius of a surfactant-lined sphere (alveolus) shrinks the surface tension decreases, and as the radius expands the surface tension increases. This occurs because the smaller radius causes surfactant molecules to crowd together and then repel one another strongly. A larger radius spreads them apart, decreasing their mutual repellence. Therefore normal alveoli are much easier to inflate at low lung volumes (i.e., after expiration) than at high volumes (i.e., after inspiration). The decrease in surface tension caused by surfactant also is responsible for keeping the alveoli free of fluid. If surfactant is not produced in adequate quantities, alveolar surface tension increases, causing alveolar collapse, decreased lung expansion, increased work of breathing, and severe gas-exchange abnormalities. The second group of surfactant proteins consists of large hydrophilic molecules called **collectins** that are capable of inhibiting foreign pathogens (see Chapter 5).[9]

Elastic Properties of the Lung and Chest Wall

The lung and chest wall have elastic properties that permit expansion during inspiration and return to resting volume during expiration. Elastin fibers in the alveolar walls and surrounding the small airways and pulmonary capillaries, as well as surface tension at the alveolar air-liquid interface, produce this effect. The elasticity of the chest wall is the result of the configuration of its bones and musculature.

Elastic recoil is the tendency of the lungs to return to the resting state after inspiration. Normal elastic recoil permits passive expiration, eliminating the need for major muscles of expiration. Passive elastic recoil may be insufficient during labored breathing (high minute volume), when the accessory muscles of expiration may be needed. The accessory muscles are used also if disease compromises elastic recoil (e.g., in emphysema) or blocks the conducting airways.

Normal elastic recoil depends on an equilibrium between opposing forces of recoil in the lungs and chest wall. Under normal conditions, the chest wall tends to recoil by expanding outward. The tendency of the chest wall to recoil by expanding is balanced by the tendency of the lungs to recoil or inward collapse around the hila. The opposing forces of the chest wall and lungs create the small negative intrapleural pressure.

Balance between the outward recoil of the chest wall and inward recoil of the lungs occurs at the resting level, the end of expiration, where the functional residual capacity (FRC) is reached. During inspiration, the diaphragm and intercostal muscles contract, air flows into the lungs, and the chest wall expands. Muscular effort is needed to overcome the resistance of the lungs to expansion. During expiration, the muscles relax and the elastic recoil of the lungs causes the thorax to decrease in volume until, once again, balance between the chest wall and lung recoil forces is reached (Figure 25-11).

Compliance is the measure of lung and chest wall distensibility and is defined as volume change per unit of pressure change. It represents the relative ease with which these structures can be stretched and is, therefore, the opposite of elasticity. Compliance is determined by alveolar surface tension and the elastic recoil of the lung and chest wall.

Increased compliance indicates that the lungs or chest wall is abnormally easy to inflate and has lost some elastic recoil. A decrease indicates that the lungs or chest wall is abnormally stiff or difficult to inflate. Compliance increases with normal aging and with disorders such as emphysema; it decreases in individuals with acute respiratory distress syndrome, pneumonia, pulmonary edema, and fibrosis. (These disorders are described in Chapter 26.)

Airway Resistance

Airway resistance, which is similar to resistance to blood flow (described in Chapter 22), is determined by the length, radius, and cross-sectional area of the airways and by the density, viscosity, and velocity of the gas (Poiseuille law). Resistance (R) is computed by dividing change in pressure (P) by rate of flow (F), or $R = P/F$ (Ohm law). Airway resistance is normally very low. One half to two thirds of total airway resistance occurs in the nose. The next highest resistance is in the oropharynx and larynx. There is very little resistance in the conducting airways of the lungs because of their large cross-sectional area. Airway resistance increases when the diameter of the airways decreases.

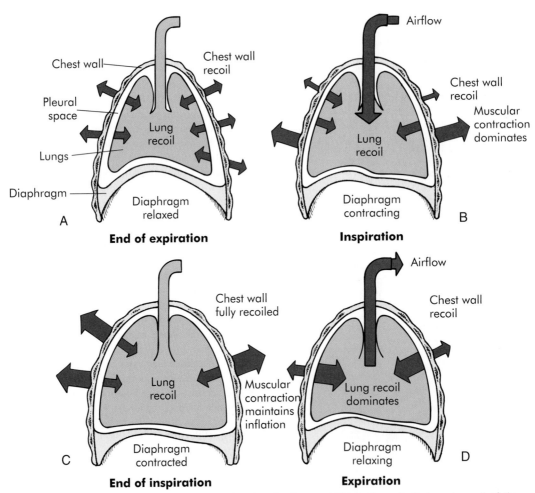

FIGURE 25-11 Interaction of Forces During Inspiration and Expiration. **A,** Outward recoil of the chest wall equals inward recoil of the lungs at the end of expiration. **B,** During inspiration, contraction of respiratory muscles, assisted by chest wall recoil, overcomes the tendency of lungs to recoil. **C,** At the end of inspiration, respiratory muscle contraction maintains lung expansion. **D,** During expiration, respiratory muscles relax, allowing elastic recoil of the lungs to deflate the lungs.

Bronchoconstriction, which increases airway resistance, can be caused by stimulation of parasympathetic receptors in the bronchial smooth muscle and by numerous irritants and inflammatory mediators.[2] Airway resistance can also be increased by edema of the bronchial mucosa and by airway obstructions such as mucus, tumors, or foreign bodies. Bronchodilation, which decreases resistance to airflow, is caused by β_2-adrenergic receptor stimulation.

Work of Breathing

The work of breathing is determined by the muscular effort (and therefore oxygen and energy) required for ventilation. Normally very low, the work of breathing may increase considerably in diseases that disrupt the equilibrium between forces exerted by the lung and chest wall. More muscular effort is required when lung compliance decreases (e.g., in pulmonary edema), chest wall compliance decreases (e.g., in spinal deformity or obesity), or airways are obstructed by bronchospasm or mucous plugging (e.g., in asthma or bronchitis). Pulmonary function tests (PFTs) measure lung volumes and flow rates and can be used to diagnose lung disease (Figure 25-12).

An increase in the work of breathing can result in a marked increase in oxygen consumption and an inability to maintain adequate ventilation.

Gas Transport

Gas transport, the delivery of oxygen to the cells of the body and the removal of carbon dioxide, has four steps: (1) ventilation of the lungs, (2) diffusion of oxygen from the alveoli into the capillary blood, (3) perfusion of systemic capillaries with oxygenated blood, and (4) diffusion of oxygen from systemic capillaries into the cells. Steps in the transport of carbon dioxide occur in reverse order: (1) diffusion of carbon dioxide from the cells into the systemic capillaries, (2) perfusion of the pulmonary capillary bed by venous blood, (3) diffusion of carbon dioxide into the alveoli, and (4) removal of carbon dioxide from the lung by ventilation. If any step in gas transport is impaired by a respiratory or cardiovascular disorder, gas exchange at the cellular level is compromised.

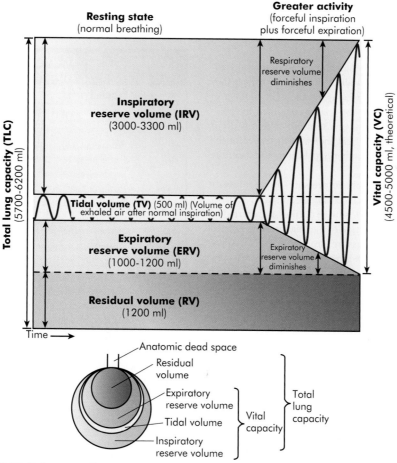

FIGURE 25-12 Spirogram. During normal, quiet respirations, the atmosphere and lungs exchange about 500 ml of air (V$_T$). With a forcible inspiration, about 3300 ml more air can be inhaled (IRV). After a normal inspiration and normal expiration, approximately 1000 ml more air can be forcibly expired (ERV). Vital capacity (VC) is the amount of air that can be forcibly expired after a maximal inspiration and indicates, therefore, the largest amount of air that can enter and leave the lungs during respiration. Residual volume (RV) is the air that remains trapped in the alveoli. (From Patton KT, Thibodeau GA: *Anatomy & physiology*, ed 7, St Louis, 2010, Mosby.)

A   B   C

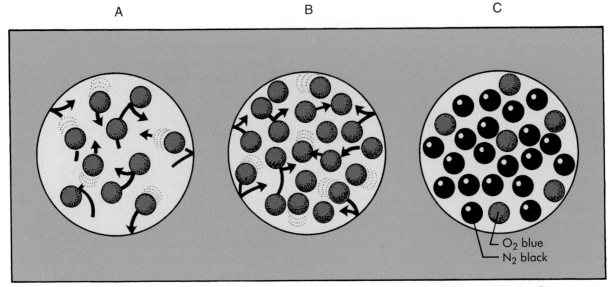

FIGURE 25-13 Relationship Between Number of Gas Molecules and Pressure Exerted by the Gas in an Enclosed Space. **A,** Theoretically, 10 molecules of the same gas exert a total pressure of 10 within the space. **B,** If the number of molecules is increased to 20, total pressure is 20. **C,** If there are different gases in the space, each gas exerts a partial pressure: here the partial pressure of nitrogen (N_2) is 20, that of oxygen (O_2) is 6, and the total pressure is 26.

Measurement of Gas Pressure

A gas is composed of millions of molecules moving randomly and colliding with each other and with the wall of the space in which they are contained. These collisions exert pressure. If the same number of gas molecules is contained in a small and a large container, the pressure is greater in the small container because more collisions occur in the smaller space (Figure 25-13). Heat increases the speed of the molecules, which also increases the number of collisions and therefore the pressure.

Barometric pressure (P_B) (atmospheric pressure) is the pressure exerted by gas molecules in air at specific altitudes. At sea level, barometric pressure is 760 mm Hg and is the sum of the pressure exerted by each gas in the air at sea level. The portion of the total pressure exerted by any individual gas is its **partial pressure** (see Figure 25-13). At sea level the air consists of oxygen (20.9%), nitrogen (78.1%), and a few other trace gases. The partial pressure of oxygen is equal to the percentage of oxygen in the air (20.9%) times the total pressure (760 mm Hg), or 159 mm Hg ($760 \times 0.209 = 158.84$ mm Hg). (Symbols used in the measurement of gas pressures and pulmonary ventilation are defined in Table 25-2.)

The amount of water vapor contained in a gas mixture is determined by the temperature of the gas and is unrelated to barometric pressure. Gas that enters the lungs becomes saturated with water vapor (humidified) as it passes through the upper airway. At body temperature (37° C), water vapor exerts a pressure of 47 mm Hg regardless of total (barometric) pressure. The partial pressure of water vapor must be subtracted from the barometric pressure before the partial pressure of other gases in the mixture can be determined. In saturated air at sea level, the partial pressure of oxygen is therefore $(760 - 47) \times 0.209 = 149$ mm Hg. All pressure and volume measurements made in pulmonary function laboratories specify the temperature and humidity of a gas at the time of measurement.

Many pressure measurements are stated as variations from barometric pressure, rather than percentages of it. On such scales,

TABLE 25-2	COMMON PULMONARY ABBREVIATIONS
SYMBOL	**DEFINITION**
V	Volume or amount of gas
Q	Perfusion or blood flow
P	Pressure (usually partial pressure) of a gas
Pa_{O_2}	Partial pressure of oxygen in arterial blood
$P_{A_{O_2}}$	Partial pressure of oxygen in alveolar gas
Pa_{CO_2}	Partial pressure of carbon dioxide in arterial blood
Pv_{O_2}	Partial pressure of oxygen in mixed venous or pulmonary artery blood
$P_{(A-a)O_2}$	Difference between alveolar and arterial partial pressure of oxygen (A–a gradient)
P_B	Barometric or atmospheric pressure
Sa_{O_2}	Saturation of hemoglobin (in arterial blood) with oxygen
Sv_{O_2}	Saturation of hemoglobin (in mixed venous blood) with oxygen
V_A	Alveolar ventilation
V_D	Dead-space ventilation
V_E	Minute capacity
V_T	Tidal volume or average breath
$\dot{V}/\dot{Q}^*$	Ratio of ventilation to perfusion
Fi_{O_2}	Fraction of inspired oxygen
FRC	Functional residual capacity
FVC	Forced vital capacity
FEV_1	Forced expiratory volume in 1 second

*An overhead dot means measurement over time, usually 1 minute.

barometric pressure is considered zero, and pressure varies up or down from zero. Physiologic pressure measurements that involve fluids, rather than gases, are measured as variations from barometric pressure. For example, a systolic blood pressure of 120 mm Hg indicates that systolic pressure is 120 mm Hg above barometric pressure.

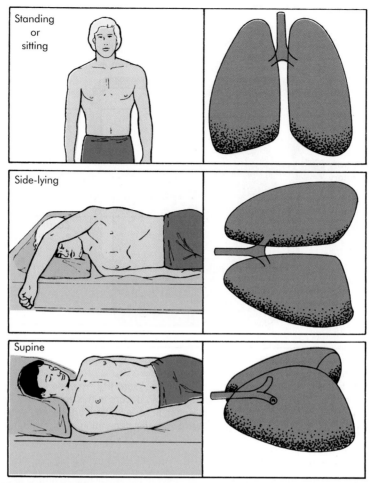

FIGURE 25-14 Pulmonary Blood Flow and Gravity. The greatest volume of pulmonary blood flow normally will occur in the gravity-dependent areas of the lung. Body position has a significant effect on the distribution of pulmonary blood flow.

Distribution of Ventilation and Perfusion

Effective gas exchange depends on an approximately even distribution of gas (ventilation) and blood (perfusion) in all portions of the lungs.[1] The lungs are suspended from the hila in the thoracic cavity. When an individual is in an upright position (sitting or standing), gravity pulls the lungs down toward the diaphragm and compresses their lower portions or bases. The alveoli in the upper portions, or apices, of the lungs contain a greater residual volume of gas and are larger and less numerous than those in the lower portions. Because surface tension increases as the alveoli become larger, the larger alveoli in the upper portions of the lung are more difficult to inflate (less compliant) than the smaller alveoli in the lower portions of the lung. Therefore, during ventilation most of the tidal volume is distributed to the bases of the lungs, where compliance is greater.

The heart pumps against gravity to perfuse the pulmonary circulation. As blood is pumped into the lung apices of a sitting or standing individual, some blood pressure is dissipated in overcoming gravity. As a result, blood pressure at the apices is lower than that at the bases. Because greater pressure causes greater perfusion, the bases of the lungs are better perfused than the apices (Figure 25-14). Thus ventilation and perfusion are greatest in the same lung portions—the lower lobes—and depend on body position. If a standing individual assumes a supine or side-lying position, the areas of the lungs that are then most dependent become the best ventilated and perfused.

Distribution of perfusion in the pulmonary circulation also is affected by alveolar pressure (gas pressure in the alveoli). The pulmonary capillary bed differs from the systemic capillary bed in that it is surrounded by gas-containing alveoli. If the gas pressure in the alveoli exceeds the blood pressure in the capillary, the capillary collapses and flow ceases. This is most likely to occur in portions of the lung where blood pressure is lowest and alveolar gas pressure is greatest—that is, at the apex of the lung.

The lungs are divided into three zones on the basis of relationships among all the factors affecting pulmonary blood flow. Alveolar pressure and the forces of gravity, arterial blood pressure, and venous blood pressure affect the distribution of perfusion, as shown in Figure 25-15.

In zone I, alveolar pressure exceeds pulmonary arterial and venous pressures. The capillary bed collapses, and normal blood flow ceases. Normally zone I is a very small part of the lung at the apex. In zone II, alveolar pressure is greater than venous pressure but not arterial pressure. Blood flows through zone II, but it is impeded to a certain extent by alveolar pressure. Zone II is normally above the level of the left atrium. In zone III, both arterial and venous pressures are greater than alveolar pressure and blood flow is not affected by alveolar pressure. Zone III is in the base of the lung. Blood flow through the pulmonary capillary bed increases in regular increments from the apex to the base.

Although both blood flow and ventilation are greater at the base of the lungs than at the apices, they are not perfectly matched in any zone.

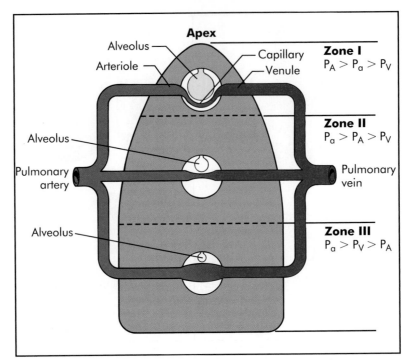

FIGURE 25-15 Gravity and Alveolar Pressure. Effects of gravity and alveolar pressure on pulmonary blood flow in the three lung zones. In zone I, alveolar pressure (P_A) is greater than arterial and venous pressures, and no blood flow occurs. In zone II, arterial pressure (P_a) exceeds alveolar pressure, but alveolar pressure exceeds venous pressure (P_V). Blood flow occurs in this zone, but alveolar pressure compresses the venules (venous ends of the capillaries). In zone III, both arterial and venous pressures are greater than alveolar pressure and blood flow fluctuates depending on the difference between arterial pressure and venous pressure.

Perfusion exceeds ventilation in the bases, and ventilation exceeds perfusion in the apices of the lung. The relationship between ventilation and perfusion is expressed as a ratio called the ventilation-perfusion ratio ($\dot{V}/\dot{Q}$).[1] The normal $\dot{V}/\dot{Q}$ ratio is 0.8. This is the amount by which perfusion exceeds ventilation under normal conditions.

Oxygen Transport

Approximately 1000 ml (1 L) of oxygen is transported to the cells of the body each minute. Oxygen is transported in the blood in two forms: a small amount dissolves in plasma, and the remainder binds to hemoglobin molecules. Without hemoglobin, oxygen would not reach the cells in amounts sufficient to maintain normal metabolic function. (Hemoglobin is discussed in detail in Chapter 19, and cellular metabolism is explored in Chapter 1.)

Diffusion across the alveolocapillary membrane. The alveolocapillary membrane is ideal for oxygen diffusion because it has a large total surface area (70 to 100 m^2) and is very thin (0.5 micrometer [μm]). In addition, the partial pressure of oxygen molecules in alveolar gas (P_AO_2) is much greater than that in capillary blood, a condition that promotes rapid diffusion down the concentration gradient from the alveolus into the capillary. The partial pressure of oxygen (oxygen tension) in mixed venous or pulmonary artery blood ($P\bar{v}O_2$) is approximately 40 mm Hg as it enters the capillary, and alveolar oxygen tension (P_AO_2) is approximately 100 mm Hg at sea level. Therefore, a pressure gradient of 60 mm Hg facilitates the diffusion of oxygen from the alveolus into the capillary (Figure 25-16).

Blood remains in the pulmonary capillary for about 0.75 second, but only 0.25 second is required for oxygen concentration to equilibrate (equalize) across the alveolocapillary membrane. Therefore

oxygen has ample time to diffuse into the blood, even during increased cardiac output, which speeds blood flow and shortens the time the blood remains in the capillary.

Determinants of arterial oxygenation. As oxygen diffuses across the alveolocapillary membrane, it dissolves in the plasma, where it exerts pressure (the partial pressure of oxygen in arterial blood, or PaO_2). As the PaO_2 increases, oxygen moves from the plasma into the red blood cells (erythrocytes) and binds with hemoglobin molecules. Oxygen continues to bind with hemoglobin until the hemoglobin-binding sites are filled or *saturated*. Oxygen then continues to diffuse across the alveolocapillary membrane until the PaO_2 (oxygen dissolved in plasma) and P_AO_2 (oxygen in the alveolus) equilibrate, eliminating the pressure gradient across the alveolocapillary membrane. At this point, diffusion ceases (see Figure 25-16).

The majority (97%) of the oxygen that enters the blood is bound to hemoglobin. The remaining 3% stays in the plasma and creates the partial pressure of oxygen (PaO_2). The PaO_2 can be measured in the blood by obtaining an arterial blood gas measurement. The oxygen saturation (SaO_2) is the percentage of the available hemoglobin that is bound to oxygen and can be measured using a device called an oximeter.

Because hemoglobin transports all but a small fraction of the oxygen carried in arterial blood, changes in hemoglobin concentration affect the oxygen content of the blood. Decreases in hemoglobin concentration below the normal value of 15 g/dl of blood reduce oxygen content, and increases in hemoglobin concentration may increase oxygen content, minimizing the impact of impaired gas exchange. In fact, increased hemoglobin concentration is a major compensatory mechanism in pulmonary diseases that impair gas exchange. For this reason, measurement of hemoglobin concentration is important in assessing

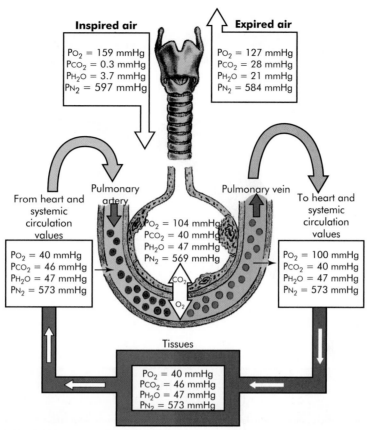

Inspired air

$PO_2 = 159$ mmHg
$PCO_2 = 0.3$ mmHg
$PH_2O = 3.7$ mmHg
$PN_2 = 597$ mmHg

Expired air

$PO_2 = 127$ mmHg
$PCO_2 = 28$ mmHg
$PH_2O = 21$ mmHg
$PN_2 = 584$ mmHg

From heart and systemic circulation values

$PO_2 = 40$ mmHg
$PCO_2 = 46$ mmHg
$PH_2O = 47$ mmHg
$PN_2 = 573$ mmHg

Pulmonary artery

$PO_2 = 104$ mmHg
$PCO_2 = 40$ mmHg
$PH_2O = 47$ mmHg
$PN_2 = 569$ mmHg

Pulmonary vein

To heart and systemic circulation values

$PO_2 = 100$ mmHg
$PCO_2 = 40$ mmHg
$PH_2O = 47$ mmHg
$PN_2 = 573$ mmHg

Tissues

$PO_2 = 40$ mmHg
$PCO_2 = 46$ mmHg
$PH_2O = 47$ mmHg
$PN_2 = 573$ mmHg

FIGURE 25-16 Partial Pressure of Respiratory Gases in Normal Respiration. The numbers shown are average values near sea level. The values of PO_2, PCO_2, and PN_2 fluctuate from breath to breath. (Modified from Thompson JM et al: *Mosby's clinical nursing,* ed 5, St Louis, 2002, Mosby.)

individuals with pulmonary disease. If cardiovascular function is normal, the body's initial response to low oxygen content is to accelerate cardiac output. In individuals who also have cardiovascular disease, this compensatory mechanism is ineffective, making increased hemoglobin concentration an even more important compensatory mechanism. (Hemoglobin structure and function are described in Chapter 19.)

Oxyhemoglobin association and dissociation. When hemoglobin molecules bind with oxygen, oxyhemoglobin (HbO$_2$) forms. Binding occurs in the lungs and is called *oxyhemoglobin association* or *hemoglobin saturation with oxygen* (SaO$_2$). The reverse process, where oxygen is released from hemoglobin, occurs in the body tissues at the cellular level and is called *hemoglobin desaturation*. When hemoglobin saturation and desaturation are plotted on a graph, the result is a distinctive S-shaped curve known as the oxyhemoglobin dissociation curve (Figure 25-17).

Several factors can change the relationship between PaO$_2$ and SaO$_2$, causing the oxyhemoglobin dissociation curve to shift to the right or left (see Figure 25-17). A shift to the right depicts hemoglobin's decreased affinity for oxygen or an increase in the ease with which oxyhemoglobin dissociates and oxygen moves into the cells. A shift to the left depicts hemoglobin's increased affinity for oxygen, which promotes association in the lungs and inhibits dissociation in the tissues.

The oxyhemoglobin dissociation curve is shifted to the right by acidosis (low pH) and hypercapnia (increased PaCO$_2$). In the tissues, the increased levels of carbon dioxide and hydrogen ions produced by metabolic activity decrease the affinity of hemoglobin for oxygen. The curve is shifted to the left by alkalosis (high pH) and hypocapnia (decreased PaCO$_2$). In the lungs, as carbon dioxide diffuses from the blood into the alveoli, the blood carbon dioxide level is reduced and the affinity of hemoglobin for oxygen is increased. The shift in the oxyhemoglobin dissociation curve caused by changes in carbon dioxide and hydrogen ion concentrations in the blood is called the Bohr effect.

The oxyhemoglobin curve is also shifted by changes in body temperature and increased or decreased levels of 2,3-diphosphoglycerate (2,3-DPG), a substance normally present in erythrocytes. Hyperthermia and increased 2,3-DPG levels shift the curve to the right. Hypothermia and decreased 2,3-DPG levels shift the curve to the left.

Carbon Dioxide Transport

Carbon dioxide is carried in the blood in three ways: (1) dissolved in plasma (PCO$_2$), (2) as bicarbonate, and (3) as carbamino compounds (including binding to hemoglobin). As CO$_2$ diffuses out of the cells into the blood, it dissolves in the plasma. Approximately 10% of the total CO$_2$ in venous blood and 5% of the CO$_2$ in arterial blood are transported dissolved in the plasma (PvCO$_2$ and PaCO$_2$, respectively). As CO$_2$ moves into the blood, it diffuses into the red blood cells. Within the red blood cells, CO$_2$, with the help of the enzyme carbonic anhydrase, combines with water to form carbonic acid and then quickly dissociates into H$^+$ and HCO$_3^-$. As carbonic acid dissociates, the H$^+$ binds to hemoglobin, where it is buffered, and the HCO$_3^-$ moves out of the red blood cell into the plasma. Approximately 60% of the CO$_2$ in venous blood and 90% of the CO$_2$ in arterial blood are carried in the form of bicarbonate. The remainder combines with blood proteins, hemoglobin in particular, to form carbamino compounds. Approximately 30% of the CO$_2$ in venous blood and 5% of the CO$_2$ in arterial blood are carried as carbamino compounds.

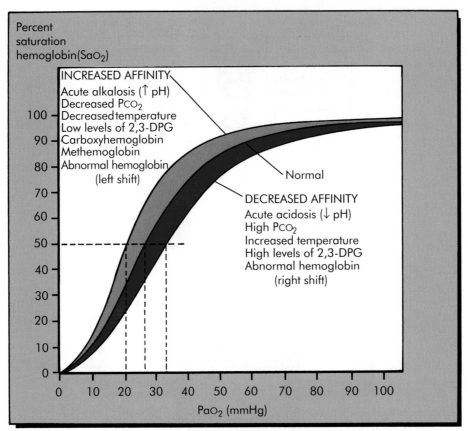

FIGURE 25-17 Oxyhemoglobin Dissociation Curve. The horizontal or flat segment of the curve at the top of the graph is the arterial or association portion, or that part of the curve where oxygen is bound to hemoglobin and occurs in the lungs. This portion of the curve is flat because partial pressure changes of oxygen between 60 and 100 mm Hg do not significantly alter the percentage saturation of hemoglobin with oxygen and allow adequate hemoglobin saturation at a variety of altitudes. If the relationship between SaO_2 and PaO_2 was linear (in a downward sloping straight line) instead of flat between 60 and 100 mm Hg, there would be inadequate saturation of hemoglobin with oxygen. The steep part of the oxyhemoglobin dissociation curve represents the rapid dissociation of oxygen from hemoglobin that occurs in the tissues. During this phase there is rapid diffusion of oxygen from the blood into tissue cells. The P_{50} is the PaO_2 at which hemoglobin is 50% saturated, normally 26.6 mm Hg. A lower than normal P_{50} represents increased affinity of hemoglobin for O_2; a high P_{50} is seen with decreased affinity. Note that variation from the normal is associated with decreased (low P_{50}) or increased (high P_{50}) availability of O_2 to tissues *(dashed lines)*. The shaded area shows the entire oxyhemoglobin dissociation curve under the same circumstances. *2,3-DPG*, 2,3-Diphosphoglycerate. (From Lane EE, Walker JF: *Clinical arterial blood gas analysis*, St Louis, 1987, Mosby.)

CO_2 is 20 times more soluble than O_2 and diffuses quickly from the tissue cells into the blood. The amount of CO_2 able to enter the blood is enhanced by diffusion of oxygen out of the blood and into the cells. Reduced hemoglobin (hemoglobin that is dissociated from oxygen) can carry more CO_2 than can hemoglobin saturated with O_2. Therefore the drop in SO_2 at the tissue level increases the ability of hemoglobin to carry CO_2 back to the lung.

The diffusion gradient for CO_2 in the lung is only approximately 6 mm Hg (venous PCO_2 = 46 mm Hg; alveolar PCO_2 = 40 mm Hg) (see Figure 25-16). Yet CO_2 is so soluble in the alveolocapillary membrane that the CO_2 in the blood quickly diffuses into the alveoli, where it is removed from the lung with each expiration. Diffusion of CO_2 in the lung is so efficient that diffusion defects that cause hypoxemia (low oxygen content of the blood) do not as readily cause hypercapnia (excessive carbon dioxide in the blood).

The diffusion of CO_2 out of the blood is also enhanced by oxygen binding with hemoglobin in the lung. As hemoglobin binds with O_2,

the amount of CO_2 carried by the blood decreases. Thus, in the tissue capillaries, O_2 dissociation from hemoglobin facilitates the pickup of CO_2, and the binding of O_2 to hemoglobin in the lungs facilitates the release of CO_2 from the blood. This effect of oxygen on CO_2 transport is called the Haldane effect.

✔ **QUICK CHECK 25-5**

1. What are the eight steps of gas transport?
2. Describe the relationship between ventilation and pulmonary blood flow.
3. What is the alveolocapillary membrane? How does it function in ventilation and perfusion?
4. Describe the process of oxyhemoglobin association and dissociation.
5. What is barometric pressure? How is it related to physiologic pressure measurements?

Control of the Pulmonary Circulation

The caliber of pulmonary artery lumina decreases as smooth muscle in the arterial walls contracts. Contraction increases pulmonary artery pressure. Caliber increases as these muscles relax, decreasing blood pressure. Contraction (vasoconstriction) and relaxation (vasodilation) primarily occur in response to local humoral conditions, even though the pulmonary circulation is innervated by the ANS as is the systemic circulation.

The most important cause of pulmonary artery constriction is a low alveolar P_{O_2} ($P_{A}O_2$). Vasoconstriction caused by alveolar and pulmonary venous hypoxia, often termed **hypoxic pulmonary vasoconstriction,** can affect only one portion of the lung (i.e., one lobe that is obstructed, decreasing its $P_{A}O_2$) or the entire lung.[10] If only one segment of the lung is involved, the arterioles to that segment constrict, shunting blood to other, well-ventilated portions of the lung. This reflex improves the lung's efficiency by better matching ventilation and perfusion. If all segments of the lung are affected, however, vasoconstriction occurs throughout the pulmonary vasculature and pulmonary hypertension (elevated pulmonary artery pressure) can result. The pulmonary vasoconstriction caused by low alveolar P_{O_2} is reversible if the alveolar P_{O_2} is corrected. Chronic alveolar hypoxia can result in permanent pulmonary artery hypertension, which eventually leads to right heart failure (cor pulmonale).

Acidemia also causes pulmonary artery constriction. If the acidemia is corrected, the vasoconstriction is reversed. (Respiratory acidosis and metabolic acidosis are described in Chapter 4.) An elevated $Paco_2$ value without a drop in pH does not cause pulmonary artery constriction. Other biochemical factors that affect the caliber of vessels in pulmonary circulation are histamine, prostaglandins, serotonin, nitric oxide, and bradykinin (see *Geriatric Considerations:* Aging & the Pulmonary System).

> ✔ **QUICK CHECK 25-6**
> 1. What is the most important factor causing pulmonary artery constriction? What other factors are involved?

GERIATRIC CONSIDERATIONS

Aging & the Pulmonary System

Elasticity/Chest Wall

Chest wall compliance decreases because ribs become ossified and joints are stiffer, which results in increased work of breathing.

Kyphoscoliosis may curve the vertebral column, decreasing lung volumes.

Respiratory muscle strength decreases.

Elastic recoil diminishes, possibly the result of loss of elastic fibers.

Result: Lung compliance increases and ventilatory capacity (VC) declines, residual volume (RV) increases, total lung capacity (TLC) is unchanged, ventilatory reserves decline, ventilation-perfusion ratios fall.

Gas Exchange

Pulmonary capillary network decreases.

Alveoli dilate, and peripheral airways lose supporting tissues.

Surface area for gas exchange decreases.

pH and P_{CO_2} do not change much, but P_{O_2} declines.

Sensitivity of respiratory centers to hypoxia or hypercapnia decreases.

Ability to initiate an immune response against infection decreases.

NOTE: Maximum Pao_2 at sea level can be estimated by multiplying person's age by 0.3 and subtracting the product from 100.

Exercise

Decreased Pao_2 and diminished ventilatory reserve lead to decreased exercise tolerance.

Early airway closure inhibits expiratory flow.

Changes depend on activity and fitness levels earlier in life.

An active, physically fit individual has fewer changes in function at any age than does a sedentary individual.

Respiratory muscle strength and endurance decrease but can be enhanced by exercise.

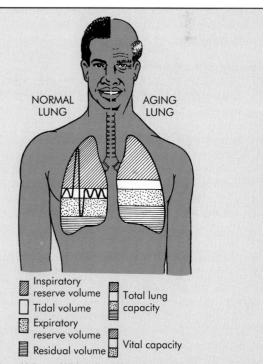

Legend:
- ▨ Inspiratory reserve volume
- ☐ Tidal volume
- ▦ Expiratory reserve volume
- ▥ Residual volume
- ▧ Total lung capacity
- ▨ Vital capacity

Changes in Lung Volumes With Aging. With aging, note particularly the dense vital capacity and the increase in residual volume. (See also Lee J, Sandford A, Man P, Sin DD: Is the aging process accelerated in chronic obstructive pulmonary disease? *Curr Opin Pulm Med* 17(2):90–97, 2011; Preston ME et al: Effect of menopause on the chemical control of breathing and its relationship with acid-base status, *Am J Physiol Regul Integr Comp Physiol* 296(3):R722–R727, 2009; Sharma G, Goodwin J: Effect of aging on respiratory system physiology and immunology, *Clin Interven Aging* 1(3):253–260, 2006; Smolej Narancic N et al: New reference equations for forced spirometry in elderly persons, *Respir Med* 103(4):621–628, 2009; Weiss CO et al: Relationships of cardiac, pulmonary, and muscle reserves and frailty to exercise capacity in older women, *J Gerontol A Biol Sci Med Sci* 65(3):287–294, 2010; Miller MR: Structural and physiological age-associated changes in aging lungs, *Semin Respir Crit Care Med* 31(5):521–527, 2010.)

DID YOU UNDERSTAND?

Structures of the Pulmonary System

1. The pulmonary system consists of the lungs, airways, chest wall, and pulmonary and bronchial circulation.
2. Air is inspired and expired through the conducting airways, which include the nasopharynx, oropharynx, trachea, bronchi, and bronchioles to the sixteenth division.
3. Gas exchange occurs in structures beyond the sixteenth division: the respiratory bronchioles, the alveolar ducts, and the alveoli. Together these structures compose the acinus.
4. The chief gas-exchange units of the lungs are the alveoli. The membrane that surrounds each alveolus and contains the pulmonary capillaries is called the *alveolocapillary membrane*.
5. The gas-exchange airways are served by the pulmonary circulation, a separate division of the circulatory system. The bronchi and other lung structures are served by a branch of the systemic circulation called the *bronchial circulation*.
6. The chest wall, which contains and protects the contents of the thoracic cavity, consists of the skin, ribs, and intercostal muscles, which lie between the ribs.
7. The chest wall is lined by a serous membrane called the *parietal pleura;* the lungs are encased in a separate membrane called the *visceral pleura.* The area where these two pleurae contact and slide over one another is called the *pleural space*.

Function of the Pulmonary System

1. The pulmonary system enables oxygen to diffuse into the blood and carbon dioxide to diffuse out of the blood.
2. Ventilation is the process by which air flows into and out of the gas-exchange airways.
3. Most of the time, ventilation is involuntary. It is controlled by the sympathetic and parasympathetic divisions of the autonomic nervous system, which adjust airway caliber (by causing bronchial smooth muscle to contract or relax) and control the rate and depth of ventilation.
4. Neuroreceptors in the lungs (lung receptors) monitor the mechanical aspects of ventilation. Irritant receptors sense the need to expel unwanted substances, stretch receptors sense lung volume (lung expansion), and J-receptors sense pulmonary capillary pressure.
5. Chemoreceptors in the circulatory system and brain stem sense the effectiveness of ventilation by monitoring the pH status of cerebrospinal fluid and the oxygen content (P_{O_2}) of arterial blood.
6. Successful ventilation involves the mechanics of breathing: the interaction of forces and counterforces involving the muscles of inspiration and expiration, alveolar surface tension, elastic properties of the lungs and chest wall, and resistance to airflow.
7. The major muscle of inspiration is the diaphragm. When the diaphragm contracts, it moves downward in the thoracic cavity, creating a vacuum that causes air to flow into the lungs.
8. The alveoli produce surfactant, a lipoprotein that lines the alveoli. Surfactant reduces alveolar surface tension and permits the alveoli to expand as air enters.
9. Compliance is the ease with which the lungs and chest wall expand during inspiration. Lung compliance is ensured by an adequate production of surfactant, whereas chest wall expansion depends on elasticity.
10. Elastic recoil is the tendency of the lungs and chest wall to return to their resting state after inspiration. The elastic recoil forces of the lungs and chest wall are in opposition and pull on each other, creating the normally negative pressure of the pleural space.
11. Gas transport depends on ventilation of the alveoli, diffusion across the alveolocapillary membrane, perfusion of the pulmonary and systemic capillaries, and diffusion between systemic capillaries and tissue cells.
12. Efficient gas exchange depends on an even distribution of ventilation and perfusion within the lungs. Both ventilation and perfusion are greatest in the bases of the lungs because the alveoli in the bases are more compliant (their resting volume is low) and perfusion is greater in the bases as a result of gravity.
13. Almost all the oxygen that diffuses into pulmonary capillary blood is transported by hemoglobin, a protein contained within red blood cells. The remainder of the oxygen is transported dissolved in plasma.
14. Oxygen enters the body by diffusing down the concentration gradient, from high concentrations in the alveoli to lower concentrations in the capillaries. Diffusion ceases when alveolar and capillary oxygen pressures equilibrate.
15. Oxygen is loaded onto hemoglobin by the driving pressure exerted by Pa_{O_2} in the plasma. As pressure decreases at the tissue level, oxygen dissociates from hemoglobin and enters tissue cells by diffusion, again down the concentration gradient.
16. Compared to oxygen, carbon dioxide is more soluble in plasma. Therefore carbon dioxide diffuses readily from tissue cells into plasma. Carbon dioxide returns to the lungs dissolved in plasma, as bicarbonate, or in carbamino compounds (e.g., bound to hemoglobin).
17. The pulmonary circulation is innervated by the autonomic nervous system (ANS), but vasodilation and vasoconstriction are controlled mainly by local and humoral factors, particularly arterial oxygenation and acid-base status.

GERIATRIC CONSIDERATIONS: Aging & the Pulmonary System

1. Aging affects the mechanical aspects of ventilation by decreasing chest wall compliance and elastic recoil of the lungs. Changes in these elastic properties reduce ventilatory reserve.
2. Aging causes the Pa_{O_2} to decrease.

KEY TERMS

- Acinus   663
- Alveolar duct   663
- Alveolar ventilation   665
- Alveolocapillary membrane   663
- Alveolus (pl. alveoli)   663
- Bohr effect   673
- Bronchus (pl. bronchi)   660
- Carina   660
- Central chemoreceptor   666
- Collectin   667
- Compliance   668
- Elastic recoil   667
- Goblet cell   660

- Haldane effect   674
- Hilum (pl. hila)   660
- Hypoxic pulmonary vasoconstriction   675
- Irritant receptor   666
- J-receptor   666
- Larynx   659
- Minute volume (minute ventilation)   664
- Nasopharynx   659
- Oropharynx   659
- Oxygen saturation (Sao_2)   672
- Oxyhemoglobin (HbO_2)   673
- Oxyhemoglobin dissociation curve   673

- Partial pressure (of a gas)   670
- Peripheral chemoreceptor   665
- Pleura (pl. pleurae)   663
- Pleural space (pleural cavity)   663
- Respiratory bronchiole   663
- Respiratory center   665
- Stretch receptor   666
- Surface tension   667
- Surfactant   663
- Thoracic cavity   663
- Trachea   660
- Ventilation   664
- Ventilation-perfusion ratio ($\dot{V}/\dot{Q}$)   672

REFERENCES

1. Levitsky MG: *Nunn's applied respiratory physiology*, ed 6, St Louis, 2007, Mosby.
2. Barrett KE, et al: *Gannong's review of medical physiology*, ed 23, New York, 2010, McGraw-Hill.
3. Clouter M, Thrall R: The respiratory system. In Koeppen BM, Stanton BA, editors: *Berne and Levy physiology*, ed 6, St Louis, 2010, Mosby, (updated addition).
4. West JB: *Respiratory physiology: the essentials*, ed 8, Philadelphia, 2008, Lippincott Williams & Wilkins.
5. Woodcock A, Young EC, Smith JA: New insights in cough, *Br Med Bull* 96:61–73, 2010.
6. Nattie E, Julius H, Comroe Jr: Distinguished lecture: central chemoreception: then…and now, *J Appl Physiol* 110(1):1–8, 2011.
7. Blain GM, et al: Peripheral chemoreceptors determine the respiratory sensitivity of central chemoreceptors to CO(2), *J Physiol* 588(Pt 13):2455–2471, 2010.
8. Brown LK: Hypoventilation syndromes, *Clin Chest Med* 31(2):249–270, 2010.
9. Orgeig S, et al: Recent advances in alveolar biology: evolution and function of alveolar proteins, *Respir Physiol Neurobiol* 173(suppl):S43–S54, 2010.
10. Ward JP, McMurtry IF: Mechanisms of hypoxic pulmonary vasoconstriction and their roles in pulmonary hypertension: new findings for an old problem, *Curr Opin Pharmacol* 9(3):287–296, 2009.

26

Alterations of Pulmonary Function

Valentina L. Brashers

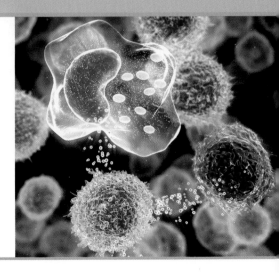

evolve WEBSITE

- Review Questions and Answers
- Animations
- Quick Check Answers

- Key Terms Exercises
- Critical Thinking Questions with Answers
- Algorithm Completion Exercises
- WebLinks

CHAPTER OUTLINE

The lungs, with their large surface area, are constantly exposed to the external environment. Therefore lung disease is greatly influenced by conditions of the environment, occupation, and personal and social habits. Pulmonary disease is often classified as acute or chronic, obstructive or restrictive, or infectious or noninfectious and is caused by alterations in the lung or heart. Symptoms of lung disease are common and associated not only with primary lung disorders but also with diseases of other organ systems.

CLINICAL MANIFESTATIONS OF PULMONARY ALTERATIONS

Signs and Symptoms of Pulmonary Disease

Pulmonary disease is associated with many signs and symptoms, the most common of which are dyspnea and cough. Others include abnormal sputum, hemoptysis, altered breathing patterns, hypoventilation and hyperventilation, cyanosis, clubbing, and chest pain.

Dyspnea

Dyspnea is defined as "a subjective experience of breathing discomfort that is comprised of qualitatively distinct sensations that vary in intensity. The experience derives from interactions among multiple

physiological, psychological, social, and environmental factors, and it may induce secondary physiological and behavioral responses."[1] It is often described as breathlessness, air hunger, shortness of breath, labored breathing, and preoccupation with breathing. Dyspnea may be the result of pulmonary disease, or many other conditions such as pain, heart disease, trauma, and anxiety.[2]

In pulmonary conditions, the severity of the experience of dyspnea may not directly correlate with the severity of underlying disease. Either diffuse or focal disturbances of ventilation, gas exchange, or ventilation-perfusion relationships can cause dyspnea, as can increased work of breathing or any disease that damages lung tissue (lung parenchyma). One proposed mechanism for dyspnea involves an impaired sense of effort where the perceived work of breathing is greater than the actual motor response that is generated. Stimulation of many receptors can contribute to the sensation of dyspnea, including mechanoreceptors in the chest wall, upper airway receptors, and central and peripheral chemoreceptors.[3]

The signs of dyspnea include flaring of the nostrils, use of accessory muscles of respiration, and retraction (pulling back) of the intercostal spaces. In dyspnea caused by parenchymal disease (e.g., pneumonia), retractions of tissue between the ribs (subcostal and intercostal retractions) may be observed, more commonly in children. In upper airway obstruction, supercostal retractions (retractions of tissues above the ribs) predominate. Dyspnea can be quantified by the use of both ordinal rating scales and visual analog scales and is frequently associated with significant anxiety.

Dyspnea may occur transiently or can become chronic. Often the first episode occurs with exercise and is called *dyspnea on exertion*. This type of dyspnea is common to many pulmonary disorders. Orthopnea is dyspnea that occurs when an individual lies flat and is common in individuals with heart failure. The recumbent position redistributes body water, causes the abdominal contents to exert pressure on the diaphragm, and decreases the efficiency of the respiratory muscles. Sitting in a forward-leaning posture or supporting the upper body on several pillows generally relieves orthopnea. Some individuals with pulmonary or cardiac disease awake at night gasping for air and have to sit or stand to relieve the dyspnea (paroxysmal nocturnal dyspnea [PND]).

Cough

Cough is a protective reflex that helps clear the airways by an explosive expiration. Inhaled particles, accumulated mucus, inflammation, or the presence of a foreign body initiates the cough reflex by stimulating the irritant receptors in the airway. There are few such receptors in the most distal bronchi and the alveoli; thus it is possible for significant amounts of secretions to accumulate in the distal respiratory tree without cough being initiated. The cough reflex consists of inspiration, closure of the glottis and vocal cords, contraction of the expiratory muscles, and reopening of the glottis, causing a sudden, forceful expiration that removes the offending matter. The effectiveness of the cough depends on the depth of the inspiration and the degree to which the airways narrow, increasing the velocity of expiratory gas flow. Cough occurs frequently in healthy individuals; however, those with an inability to cough effectively are at greater risk for pneumonia.

Acute cough is cough that resolves within 2 to 3 weeks of the onset of illness or resolves with treatment of the underlying condition. It is most commonly the result of upper respiratory tract infections, allergic rhinitis, acute bronchitis, pneumonia, congestive heart failure, pulmonary embolus, or aspiration. *Chronic cough* is defined as cough that has persisted for more than 3 weeks, although 7 or 8 weeks may be a more appropriate timeframe because acute cough and bronchial hyperreactivity can be prolonged in some cases of viral infection. In individuals who do not smoke, chronic cough is commonly caused by postnasal drainage syndrome, nonasthmatic eosinophilic bronchitis, asthma, or gastroesophageal reflux disease. In persons who smoke, chronic bronchitis is the most common cause of chronic cough, although lung cancer must always be considered. Up to 33% of individuals taking angiotensin-converting enzyme inhibitors for cardiovascular disease develop chronic cough that resolves with discontinuation of the drug.

Abnormal Sputum

Changes in the amount, color, and consistency of sputum provide information about progression of disease and effectiveness of therapy. The gross and microscopic appearances of sputum enable the clinician to identify cellular debris or microorganisms, which aids in diagnosis and choice of therapy.

Hemoptysis

Hemoptysis is the expectoration of blood or bloody secretions. This is sometimes confused with hematemesis, which is the vomiting of blood. Blood produced with coughing is usually bright red, has an alkaline pH, and is mixed with frothy sputum. Blood that is vomited is dark, has an acidic pH, and is mixed with food particles.

Hemoptysis usually indicates infection or inflammation that damages the bronchi (bronchitis, bronchiectasis) or the lung parenchyma (pneumonia, tuberculosis, lung abscess). Other causes include cancer and pulmonary infarction. The amount and duration of bleeding provide important clues about its source. Bronchoscopy, combined with chest computed tomography (CT), is used to confirm the site of bleeding.

Abnormal Breathing Patterns

Normal breathing (eupnea) is rhythmic and effortless. The resting ventilatory rate is 8 to 16 breaths per minute, and tidal volume ranges from 400 to 800 ml. A short expiratory pause occurs with each breath, and the individual takes an occasional deeper breath, or sighs. Sigh breaths, which help to maintain normal lung function, are usually 1.5 to 2 times the normal tidal volume and occur approximately 10 to 12 times per hour.

The rate, depth, regularity, and effort of breathing undergo characteristic alterations in response to physiologic and pathophysiologic conditions. Patterns of breathing automatically adjust to minimize the work of respiratory muscles. Strenuous exercise or metabolic acidosis induces Kussmaul respiration (hyperpnea), which is characterized by a slightly increased ventilatory rate, very large tidal volumes, and no expiratory pause.

Labored breathing occurs whenever there is an increased work of breathing, especially if the airways are obstructed. In large airway obstruction, a slow ventilatory rate, large tidal volume, increased effort, prolonged inspiration and expiration, and stridor or audible wheezing (depending on the site of obstruction) are typical. In small airway obstruction such as that seen in asthma and chronic obstructive pulmonary disease, a rapid ventilatory rate, small tidal volume, increased effort, prolonged expiration, and wheezing are often present.

Restricted breathing is commonly caused by disorders such as pulmonary fibrosis that stiffen the lungs or chest wall and decrease compliance. Small tidal volumes, rapid ventilatory rate (tachypnea), and rapid expiration are characteristic.

Shock and severe cerebral hypoxia (insufficient oxygen in the brain) contribute to gasping respirations that consist of irregular, quick inspirations with an expiratory pause. Anxiety can cause sighing respirations, which consist of irregular breathing characterized by frequent, deep sighing inspirations.

Cheyne-Stokes respirations are characterized by alternating periods of deep and shallow breathing. Apnea lasting from 15 to 60 seconds is followed by ventilations that increase in volume until a peak is reached; then ventilation (tidal volume) decreases again to apnea. Cheyne-Stokes respirations result from any condition that reduces blood flow to the brain stem, which in turn slows impulses sending information to the respiratory centers of the brain stem. Neurologic impairment above the brain stem is also a contributing factor (see Figure 14-1).

Hypoventilation/Hyperventilation

Hypoventilation is inadequate alveolar ventilation in relation to metabolic demands. Hypoventilation occurs when minute volume (tidal volume times respiratory rate) is reduced. It is caused by alterations in pulmonary mechanics or in the neurologic control of breathing.[4] When alveolar ventilation is normal, carbon dioxide (CO_2) is removed from the lungs at the same rate as it is produced by cellular metabolism; therefore arterial and alveolar Pco_2 values remain at normal levels (40 mm Hg). With hypoventilation, CO_2 removal is slower than CO_2 production and the level of CO_2 in the arterial blood ($Paco_2$) increases, causing hypercapnia ($Paco_2$ greater than 44 mm Hg) (see

Table 25-2 for a definition of gas partial pressures and other pulmonary abbreviations). This results in respiratory acidosis that can affect the function of many tissues throughout the body. Hypoventilation is often overlooked until it is severe because breathing pattern and ventilatory rate may appear to be normal and changes in tidal volume can be difficult to detect clinically. Blood gas analysis (i.e., measurement of the Paco$_2$ of arterial blood) reveals the hypoventilation.[3] Pronounced hypoventilation can cause somnolence or disorientation.

Hyperventilation is alveolar ventilation exceeding metabolic demands. The lungs remove CO$_2$ faster than it is produced by cellular metabolism, resulting in decreased Paco$_2$, or hypocapnia (Paco$_2$ less than 36 mm Hg). Hypocapnia results in a respiratory alkalosis that also can interfere with tissue function. Like hypoventilation, hyperventilation can be determined by arterial blood gas analysis. Increased respiratory rate or tidal volume can occur with severe anxiety, acute head injury, pain, and in response to conditions that cause insufficient oxygenation of the blood.

Cyanosis

Cyanosis is a bluish discoloration of the skin and mucous membranes caused by increasing amounts of desaturated or reduced hemoglobin (which is bluish) in the blood. It generally develops when 5 g of hemoglobin is desaturated, regardless of hemoglobin concentration.

Peripheral cyanosis (slow blood circulation in fingers and toes) is most often caused by poor circulation resulting from intense peripheral vasoconstriction, such as that observed in persons who have Raynaud disease, are in cold environments, or are severely stressed. Peripheral cyanosis is best observed in the nail beds. *Central cyanosis* is caused by decreased arterial oxygenation (low Pao$_2$) from pulmonary diseases or pulmonary or cardiac right-to-left shunts. Central cyanosis is best detected in buccal mucous membranes and lips.

Lack of cyanosis does not necessarily indicate that oxygenation is normal. In adults, cyanosis is not evident until severe hypoxemia is present and, therefore, is an insensitive indication of respiratory failure. Severe anemia (inadequate hemoglobin concentration) and carbon monoxide poisoning (in which hemoglobin binds to carbon monoxide instead of to oxygen) can cause inadequate oxygenation of tissues without causing cyanosis. Individuals with polycythemia (an abnormal increase in numbers of red blood cells), however, may have cyanosis when oxygenation is adequate. Therefore, cyanosis must be interpreted in relation to the underlying pathophysiologic condition. If cyanosis is suggested, the Pao$_2$ should be measured.

Clubbing

Clubbing is the selective bulbous enlargement of the end (distal segment) of a digit (finger or toe) (Figure 26-1); its severity can be graded from 1 to 5 based on the extent of nail bed hypertrophy and the amount of changes in the nails themselves or as early, moderate or severe. It is usually painless. Clubbing is commonly associated with diseases that cause chronic hypoxemia, such as bronchiectasis, cystic fibrosis, pulmonary fibrosis, lung abscess, and congenital heart disease. It can sometimes be seen in individuals with lung cancer even without hypoxemia because of the effects of inflammatory cytokines and growth factors (*hypertrophic osteoarthropathy*).[5]

Pain

Pain caused by pulmonary disorders originates in the pleurae, airways, or chest wall.[6] Infection and inflammation of the parietal pleura cause sharp or stabbing pain (pleurodynia) when the pleura stretches during inspiration. The pain is usually localized to a portion of the chest wall, where a unique breath sound called a *pleural friction rub* may be heard

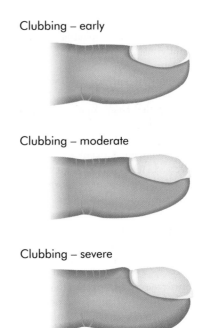

FIGURE 26-1 Clubbing of Fingers Caused by Chronic Hypoxemia. (Modified from Seidel HM et al: *Mosby's guide to physical examination,* ed 7, St Louis, 2011, Mosby.)

over the painful area. Laughing or coughing makes pleural pain worse. Pleural pain is common with pulmonary infarction (tissue death) caused by pulmonary embolism and emanates from the area around the infarction.

Pulmonary pain can be central chest pain that is pronounced after coughing and occurs in individuals with infection and inflammation of the trachea or bronchi (tracheitis or tracheobronchitis, respectively). It can be difficult to differentiate from cardiac pain. High blood pressure in the pulmonary circulation (pulmonary hypertension) can cause pain during exercise that is often mistaken for cardiac pain (angina pectoris).

Pain in the chest wall is muscle pain or rib pain. Excessive coughing (which makes the muscles sore) and rib fractures produce such pain. Inflammation of the costochondral junction (costochondritis) also can cause chest wall pain. Chest wall pain can often be reproduced by pressing on the sternum or ribs.

Conditions Caused by Pulmonary Disease or Injury
Hypercapnia

Hypercapnia, or increased carbon dioxide concentration in the arterial blood (increased Paco$_2$), is caused by hypoventilation of the alveoli. As discussed in Chapter 25, carbon dioxide is easily diffused from the blood into the alveolar space; thus, minute volume (respiratory rate times tidal volume) determines not only alveolar ventilation but also Paco$_2$. Hypoventilation is often overlooked because the breathing pattern and ventilatory rate may appear to be normal; therefore it is important to obtain blood gas analysis to determine the severity of hypercapnia and resultant respiratory acidosis (acid-base balance is described in Chapter 4).

There are many causes of hypercapnia. Most are a result of decreased drive to breathe or an inadequate ability to respond to ventilatory stimulation. Some of these causes include (1) depression of the respiratory center by drugs; (2) diseases of the medulla, including infections of the central nervous system or trauma; (3) abnormalities of the spinal conducting pathways, as in spinal cord disruption or poliomyelitis; (4) diseases of the neuromuscular junction or of the respiratory muscles themselves, as in myasthenia gravis or muscular dystrophy; (5) thoracic cage abnormalities, as in chest injury or congenital deformity; (6) large airway obstruction, as in tumors or sleep apnea; and (7) increased work of breathing or physiologic dead space, as in emphysema.

Hypercapnia and the associated respiratory acidosis result in electrolyte abnormalities that may cause dysrhythmias. Individuals also may present with somnolence and even coma because of changes in intracranial pressure associated with high levels of arterial carbon dioxide, which causes cerebral vasodilation. Alveolar hypoventilation with increased alveolar CO_2 concentration limits the amount of oxygen available for diffusion into the blood, thereby leading to secondary hypoxemia.

Hypoxemia

Hypoxemia, or reduced oxygenation of arterial blood (reduced Pao_2), is caused by respiratory alterations, whereas hypoxia, or reduced oxygenation of cells in tissues, may be caused by alterations of other systems as well. Although hypoxemia can lead to tissue hypoxia, tissue hypoxia can result from other abnormalities unrelated to alterations of pulmonary function, such as low cardiac output or cyanide poisoning.

Hypoxemia results from problems with one or more of the major mechanisms of oxygenation:

1. Oxygen delivery to the alveoli
   a. Oxygen content of the inspired air (Fio_2)
   b. Ventilation of the alveoli
2. Diffusion of oxygen from the alveoli into the blood
   a. Balance between alveolar ventilation and perfusion ($\dot{V}/\dot{Q}$ match)
   b. Diffusion of oxygen across the alveolar capillary barrier
3. Perfusion of pulmonary capillaries

The amount of oxygen in the alveoli is called the P_Ao_2 and is dependent on two factors. The first factor is the presence of adequate oxygen content of the inspired air. The amount of oxygen in inspired air is expressed as the percentage or fraction of air that is composed of oxygen, called the Fio_2. The Fio_2 of air at sea level is approximately 21% or 0.21. Anything that decreases the Fio_2 (such as high altitude) decreases the P_Ao_2. The second factor is the amount of alveolar minute volume (tidal volume times respiratory rate). Hypoventilation results in an increase in P_Aco_2 and a decrease in P_Ao_2 such that there is less oxygen available in the alveoli for diffusion into the blood. This type of hypoxemia can be completely corrected if alveolar ventilation is improved by increases in the rate and depth of breathing. Hypoventilation causes hypoxemia in unconscious persons; in persons with neurologic, muscular, or bone diseases that restrict chest expansion; and in individuals who have chronic obstructive pulmonary disease.

Diffusion of oxygen from the alveoli into the blood is also dependent on two factors. The first is the balance between the amount of air that enters alveoli ($\dot{V}$) and the amount of blood perfusing the capillaries around the alveoli ($\dot{Q}$). An abnormal ventilation-perfusion ratio ($\dot{V}/\dot{Q}$) is the most common cause of hypoxemia (Figure 26-2). The normal $\dot{V}/\dot{Q}$ is 0.8 because perfusion is somewhat greater than ventilation in the lung bases and because some blood is normally shunted to the bronchial circulation. $\dot{V}/\dot{Q}$ mismatch refers to an abnormal distribution of ventilation and perfusion. Hypoxemia can be caused by inadequate ventilation of well-perfused areas of the lung (low $\dot{V}/\dot{Q}$). Mismatching of this type, called shunting, occurs in atelectasis, in asthma as a result of bronchoconstriction, and in pulmonary edema and pneumonia when alveoli are filled with fluid. When blood passes through portions of the pulmonary capillary bed that receive

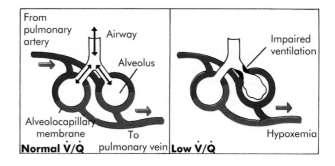

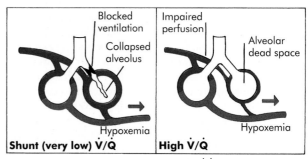

FIGURE 26-2 Ventilation-Perfusion ($\dot{V}\dot{Q}$) Abnormalities.

no ventilation, the pulmonary capillaries in that area constrict and a right-to-left shunt occurs, resulting in decreased systemic Pao_2 and hypoxemia. Hypoxemia also can be caused by poor perfusion of well-ventilated portions of the lung (high $\dot{V}/\dot{Q}$), resulting in wasted ventilation. The most common cause of high $\dot{V}/\dot{Q}$ is a pulmonary embolus that impairs blood flow to a segment of the lung. An area where alveoli are ventilated but not perfused is termed alveolar dead space.

The second factor affecting diffusion of oxygen from the alveoli into the blood is the alveolocapillary membrane. Diffusion of oxygen through the alveolocapillary membrane is impaired if the membrane is thickened or the surface area available for diffusion is decreased. Thickened alveolocapillary membranes, as occur with edema (tissue swelling) and fibrosis (formation of fibrous lesions), increase the time required for oxygen to diffuse from the alveoli into the capillaries. If diffusion is slowed enough, the Po_2 levels of alveolar gas and capillary blood do not have time to equilibrate during the fraction of a second that blood remains in the capillary. Destruction of alveoli, as in emphysema, decreases the surface area available for diffusion. Hypercapnia is seldom produced by impaired diffusion because carbon dioxide diffuses so easily from capillary to alveolus that the individual with impaired diffusion would die from hypoxemia before hypercapnia could occur.

Finally, hypoxemia can result from blood flow bypassing the lungs. This can occur because of intracardiac defects that cause right-to-left shunting or because of intrapulmonary arteriovenous malformations.

Hypoxemia is often associated with a compensatory hyperventilation and the resultant respiratory alkalosis (i.e., decreased $Paco_2$ and increased pH). However, in individuals with associated ventilatory difficulties, hypoxemia may be complicated by hypercapnia and respiratory acidosis. Hypoxemia results in widespread tissue dysfunction and, when severe, can lead to organ infarction. In addition, hypoxic pulmonary vasoconstriction can contribute to increased pressures in the pulmonary artery (pulmonary artery hypertension) and lead to right heart failure or *cor pulmonale*. Clinical manifestations of acute hypoxemia may include cyanosis, confusion, tachycardia, edema, and decreased renal output.

✔ QUICK CHECK 26-1
1. List the primary signs and symptoms of pulmonary disease.
2. What abnormal breathing patterns are seen with pulmonary disease?
3. What mechanisms produce hypercapnia?
4. What mechanisms produce hypoxemia?

Acute Respiratory Failure

Respiratory failure is defined as inadequate gas exchange such that $Pao_2 \leq 50$ mm Hg or $Paco_2 \geq 50$ mm Hg with pH ≤ 7.25. Respiratory failure can result from direct injury to the lungs, airways, or chest wall or indirectly because of injury to another body system, such as the brain or spinal cord. It can occur in individuals who have an otherwise normal respiratory system or in those with underlying chronic pulmonary disease. Most pulmonary diseases can cause episodes of acute respiratory failure. If the respiratory failure is primarily hypercapnic, it is the result of inadequate alveolar ventilation and the individual must receive ventilatory support, such as with a bag-valve mask or mechanical ventilator. If the respiratory failure is primarily hypoxemic, it is the result of inadequate exchange of oxygen between the alveoli and the capillaries and the individual must receive supplemental oxygen therapy. Many people will have combined hypercapnic and hypoxemic respiratory failure and will require both kinds of support.

Respiratory failure is an important potential complication of any major surgical procedure, especially those that involve the central nervous system, thorax, or upper abdomen. The most common postoperative pulmonary problems are atelectasis, pneumonia, pulmonary edema, and pulmonary emboli. People who smoke are at risk, particularly if they have preexisting lung disease. Limited cardiac reserve, chronic renal failure, chronic hepatic disease, and infection also increase the tendency to develop postoperative respiratory failure.

Prevention of postoperative respiratory failure includes frequent position changes, deep-breathing exercises, and early ambulation to prevent atelectasis and accumulation of secretions. Humidification of inspired air can help loosen secretions. Incentive spirometry gives individuals immediate feedback about tidal volumes, which encourages them to breathe deeply. Supplemental oxygen is given for hypoxemia, and antibiotics are given as appropriate to treat infection. If respiratory failure develops, the individual may require mechanical ventilation for a time.

DISORDERS OF THE CHEST WALL AND PLEURA

There are many conditions that can affect the chest wall and/or pleura that impact the function of the respiratory system. Chest wall disorders primarily affect tidal volume and, therefore, result in hypercapnia. Pleural diseases impact both ventilation and oxygenation.

Chest Wall Restriction

If the chest wall is deformed, traumatized, immobilized, or heavy from the accumulation of fat, the work of breathing increases and ventilation may be compromised because of a decrease in tidal volume. The degree of ventilatory impairment depends on the severity of the chest wall abnormality. Grossly obese individuals are often dyspneic on exertion or when recumbent. Individuals with severe kyphoscoliosis (lateral bending and rotation of the spinal column, with distortion of the thoracic cage) often present with dyspnea on exertion that can progress to respiratory failure. Such individuals also are susceptible to lower respiratory tract infections. Both obesity and kyphoscoliosis are risk factors for respiratory disease in individuals admitted to the hospital for other problems, particularly those who require surgery. Other

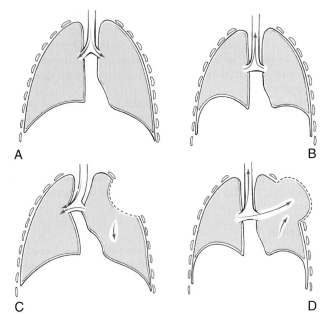

FIGURE 26-3 Flail Chest. Normal respiration: **A,** inspiration; **B,** expiration. Paradoxical motion: **C,** inspiration, area of lung underlying unstable chest wall flattens on inspiration; **D,** expiration, unstable area inflates. Note movement of mediastinum toward opposite lung during inspiration.

musculoskeletal abnormalities that can impair ventilation are ankylosing spondylitis (see Chapter 37) and pectus excavatum (a deformity characterized by depression of the sternum).

Impairment of respiratory muscle function caused by neuromuscular disease also can restrict the chest wall and impair pulmonary function. Muscle weakness can result in hypoventilation, inability to remove secretions, and hypoxemia. Respiratory difficulty is the most common cause of hospital admission for individuals with neuromuscular diseases such as poliomyelitis, muscular dystrophy, myasthenia gravis, and Guillain-Barré syndrome (see Chapter 15).

Trauma to the thorax or upper abdomen can restrict chest expansion because of pain. Trauma to the chest also can cause structural and mechanical changes that impair the ability of the chest to expand normally. **Flail chest** results from the fracture of several consecutive ribs in more than one place or fracture of the sternum and several consecutive ribs. These multiple fractures result in instability of a portion of the chest wall, causing paradoxic movement of the chest with breathing. During inspiration the unstable portion of the chest wall moves inward and during expiration it moves outward, impairing movement of gas in and out of the lungs (Figure 26-3).

Chest wall restriction results in a decrease in tidal volume. An increase in respiratory rate can compensate for small decreases in tidal volume, but many individuals will progress to hypercapnic respiratory failure. Diagnosis of chest restriction is made by pulmonary function testing (reduction in forced vital capacity [FVC]), arterial blood gas measurement (hypercapnia), and radiographs. Treatment is aimed at any reversible underlying cause but is otherwise supportive. In severe cases, mechanical ventilation may be indicated.

Pleural Abnormalities

Pneumothorax. Pneumothorax is the presence of air or gas in the pleural space caused by a rupture in the visceral pleura (which surrounds the lungs) or the parietal pleura and chest wall. As air separates the visceral and parietal pleurae, it destroys the negative pressure of the

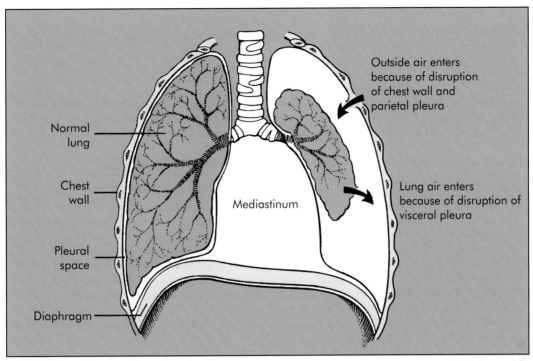

FIGURE 26-4 Pneumothorax. Air in the pleural space causes the lung to collapse around the hilus and may push mediastinal contents (heart and great vessels) toward the other lung.

TABLE 26-1	MECHANISM OF PLEURAL EFFUSION*	
TYPE OF FLUID/EFFUSION	**SOURCE OF ACCUMULATION**	**PRIMARY OR ASSOCIATED DISORDER**
Transudate (hydrothorax)	Watery fluid that diffuses out of capillaries beneath pleura (i.e., capillaries in lung or chest wall)	Cardiovascular disease that causes high pulmonary capillary pressures; liver or kidney disease that disrupts plasma protein production, causing hypoproteinemia (decreased oncotic pressure in blood vessels)
Exudate	Fluid rich in cells and proteins (leukocytes, plasma proteins of all kinds; see Chapter 5) that migrates out of capillaries	Infection, inflammation, or malignancy of pleura that stimulates mast cells to release biochemical mediators that increase capillary permeability
Pus (empyema)	Microorganisms and debris of infection (leukocytes, cellular debris) accumulate in pleural space	Pulmonary infections, such as pneumonia; lung abscesses; infected wounds
Blood (hemothorax)	Hemorrhage into pleural space	Traumatic injury, surgery, rupture, or malignancy that damages blood vessels
Chyle (chylothorax)	Chyle (milky fluid containing lymph and fat droplets) that moves from lymphatic vessels into pleural space instead of passing from gastrointestinal tract to thoracic duct	Traumatic injury, infection, or disorder that disrupts lymphatic transport

*The principles of diffusion are described in Chapter 1; mechanisms that increase capillary permeability and cause exudation of cells and proteins are discussed in Chapter 5.

pleural space and disrupts the equilibrium between elastic recoil forces of the lung and chest wall. The lung then tends to recoil by collapsing toward the hilum (Figure 26-4).

Primary (spontaneous) pneumothorax, which occurs unexpectedly in healthy individuals (usually men) between 20 and 40 years of age, is caused by the spontaneous rupture of blebs (blister-like formations) on the visceral pleura. Bleb rupture can occur during sleep, rest, or exercise. The ruptured blebs are usually located in the apices of the lungs. The cause of bleb formation is not known, although more than 80% of these individuals have been found to have emphysema-like changes in their lungs even if they have no history of smoking or no known genetic disorder. Approximately 10% of affected individuals

have a significant family history of primary pneumothorax that has been linked to mutations in the folliculin gene.[7]

A *secondary pneumothorax* can be caused by chest trauma (such as a rib fracture or stab and bullet wounds that tear the pleura; rupture of a bleb or bulla [larger vesicle], as occurs in emphysema; or mechanical ventilation, particularly if it includes positive end-expiratory pressure [PEEP]).

Both primary pneumothorax and secondary pneumothorax can present as either open or tension. In open (communicating) pneumothorax, air pressure in the pleural space equals barometric pressure because air that is drawn into the pleural space during inspiration (through the damaged chest wall and parietal pleura or through the lungs and damaged visceral pleura) is forced back out during expiration. In **tension pneumothorax,** however, the site of pleural rupture acts as a one-way valve, permitting air to enter on inspiration but preventing its escape by closing during expiration. As more and more air enters the pleural space, air pressure in the pneumothorax begins to exceed barometric pressure. Air pressure in the pleural space pushes against the already recoiled lung, causing compression atelectasis, and against the mediastinum, compressing and displacing the heart and great vessels. The pathophysiologic effects of tension pneumothorax are life-threatening.

Clinical manifestations of spontaneous or secondary pneumothorax begin with sudden pleural pain, tachypnea, and dyspnea. Manifestations depend on the size of the pneumothorax. Physical examination may reveal absent or decreased breath sounds and hyperresonance to percussion on the affected side. Tension pneumothorax may be complicated by severe hypoxemia, tracheal deviation away from the affected lung, and hypotension (low blood pressure). Deterioration occurs rapidly and immediate treatment is required. Diagnosis of pneumothorax is made with chest radiographs and computed tomography (CT). Pneumothorax is treated with insertion of a chest tube that is attached to a water-seal drainage system with suction. After the pneumothorax is evacuated and the pleural rupture is healed, the chest tube is removed. For individuals with persistent air leaks, other interventions may be needed including surgery, pleurodesis, endobronchial embolization, or thoracoscopic gluing techniques.[8,9]

Pleural effusion. **Pleural effusion** is the presence of fluid in the pleural space. The most common mechanism of pleural effusion is migration of fluids and other blood components through the walls of intact capillaries bordering the pleura. Pleural effusions that enter the pleural space from intact blood vessels can be **transudative** (watery) or **exudative** (high concentrations of white blood cells and plasma proteins). Other types of pleural effusion are characterized by the presence of microorganisms (empyema), blood (hemothorax), or chyle (chylothorax). Mechanisms of pleural effusion are summarized in Table 26-1.

Small collections of fluid may not affect lung function and may remain undetected. Most will be removed by the lymphatic system once the underlying condition is resolved. Dyspnea, compression atelectasis with impaired ventilation, and pleural pain are common. Mediastinal shift and cardiovascular manifestations occur in a large, rapidly developing effusion. Physical examination shows decreased breath sounds and dullness to percussion on the affected side. A pleural friction rub can be heard over areas of inflamed pleura.

Diagnosis is confirmed by chest x-ray and thoracentesis (needle aspiration), which can determine the type of effusion and provide symptomatic relief. If the effusion is large, drainage usually requires the placement of a chest tube and surgical interventions may be needed to prevent recurrence of the effusion.[10]

Empyema. **Empyema (infected pleural effusion)** is the presence of microorganisms and cellular debris (pus) in the pleural space. Empyema occurs most commonly in older adults and children and usually develops as a complication of pneumonia, surgery, trauma, or bronchial obstruction from a tumor. Commonly documented infectious organisms include *Staphylococcus aureus, Escherichia coli,* anaerobic bacteria, and *Klebsiella pneumoniae.*

Individuals with empyema present clinically with cyanosis, fever, tachycardia (rapid heart rate), cough, and pleural pain. Breath sounds are decreased directly over the empyema. Diagnosis is made by chest radiographs, thoracentesis, and sputum culture. The treatment for empyema includes the administration of appropriate antimicrobials and drainage of the pleural space with a chest tube. In severe cases,

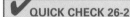

QUICK CHECK 26-2
1. How does chest wall restriction affect ventilation?
2. How does pneumothorax differ from pleural effusion?
3. What causes empyema?

ultrasound-guided pleural drainage, instillation of fibrinolytic agents, or introduction of deoxyribonuclease (DNase) into the pleural space is needed for adequate drainage.[11]

PULMONARY DISORDERS

Restrictive Lung Diseases

Restrictive lung diseases are characterized by decreased compliance of the lung tissue. This means that it takes more effort to expand the lungs during inspiration, which increases the work of breathing. Individuals with lung restriction complain of dyspnea and have an increased respiratory rate and decreased tidal volume. Pulmonary function testing discloses a decrease in forced vital capacity (FVC). Restrictive lung diseases commonly cause $\dot{V}/\dot{Q}$ mismatch and affect the alveolocapillary membrane, which reduces the diffusion of oxygen from the alveoli into the blood and leads to hypoxemia. Some of the most common restrictive lung diseases in adults are aspiration, atelectasis, bronchiectasis, bronchiolitis, pulmonary fibrosis, inhalational disorders, pneumoconiosis, allergic alveolitis, pulmonary edema, and acute respiratory distress syndrome.

Aspiration

Aspiration is the passage of fluid and solid particles into the lung. It tends to occur in individuals whose normal swallowing mechanism and cough reflex are impaired by central or peripheral nervous system abnormalities. Predisposing factors include an altered level of consciousness caused by substance abuse, sedation, or anesthesia; seizure disorders; cerebrovascular accident; and neuromuscular disorders that cause dysphagia. Elderly individuals also are at increased risk for aspiration.[12] The right lung, particularly the right lower lobe, is more susceptible to aspiration than the left lung because the branching angle of the right main stem bronchus is straighter than the branching angle of the left main stem bronchus.

The aspiration of large food particles or foreign bodies can obstruct a bronchus, resulting in bronchial inflammation and collapse of airways distal to the obstruction. Clinical manifestations include the sudden onset of choking, coughing, vomiting, dyspnea, and wheezing. If the aspirated solid is not identified and removed by bronchoscopy, a chronic, local inflammation develops that may lead to recurrent infection and bronchiectasis (permanent dilation of the bronchus). Once the pathologic process has progressed to bronchiectasis, surgical resection of the affected area is usually required.

Aspiration of acidic gastric fluid (pH <2.5) may cause severe pneumonitis (lung inflammation). Bronchial damage includes inflammation, loss of ciliary function, and bronchospasm. In the alveoli, acidic fluid damages the alveolocapillary membrane, allowing plasma and blood cells to move from capillaries into the alveoli, resulting in hemorrhagic pneumonitis. The lung becomes stiff and noncompliant as surfactant production is disrupted, leading to further edema and collapse.

Preventive measures for individuals at risk are more effective than treatment of known aspiration. The most important preventive measures include employment of the semirecumbent position, surveillance of enteral feeding, use of promotility agents, and avoidance of excessive sedation. Nasogastric tubes, which are often used to remove stomach

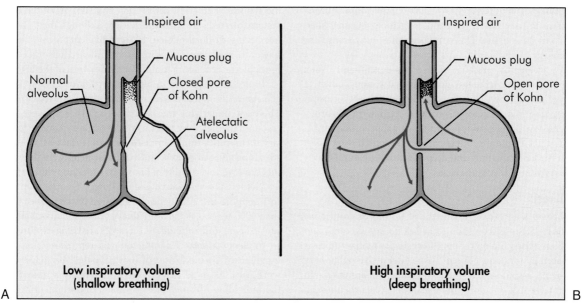

FIGURE 26-5 Pores of Kohn. **A,** Absorption atelectasis caused by lack of collateral ventilation through pores of Kohn. **B,** Restoration of collateral ventilation during deep breathing.

contents, are used to prevent aspiration but also can cause aspiration if fluid and particulate matter are regurgitated as the tube is being placed. Treatment of aspiration includes use of supplemental oxygen and mechanical ventilation with positive end-expiratory pressure (PEEP), restriction of fluid intake, and administration of corticosteroids. Bacterial pneumonia may develop as a complication of aspiration pneumonitis and must be treated with broad-spectrum antimicrobials.

Atelectasis

Atelectasis is the collapse of lung tissue. There are three types of atelectasis:

1. Compression atelectasis is caused by external pressure exerted by tumor, fluid, or air in pleural space or by abdominal distention pressing on a portion of lung, causing alveoli to collapse.
2. Absorption atelectasis results from removal of air from obstructed or hypoventilated alveoli or from inhalation of concentrated oxygen or anesthetic agents.
3. Surfactant impairment results from decreased production or inactivation of surfactant, which is necessary to reduce surface tension in the alveoli and thus prevent lung collapse during expiration. Surfactant impairment can occur because of premature birth, acute respiratory distress syndrome, anesthesia induction, or mechanical ventilation.

Atelectasis tends to develop after surgery and is estimated to occur in more than 90% of individuals administered a general anesthetic.[13] Postoperative persons are often in pain, breathe shallowly, are reluctant to change position, and produce viscous secretions that tend to pool in dependent portions of the lung.

Clinical manifestations of atelectasis are similar to those of pulmonary infection including dyspnea, cough, fever, and leukocytosis. Prevention and treatment of postoperative atelectasis usually include deep-breathing exercises, frequent position changes, and early ambulation. Deep breathing and the use of an incentive spirometer help open connections between patent and collapsed alveoli, called *pores of Kohn* (Figure 26-5). This allows air to flow into the collapsed alveoli (collateral ventilation) and aids in the expulsion of intrabronchial obstructions.

Bronchiectasis

Bronchiectasis is persistent abnormal dilation of the bronchi. Hospitalizations for bronchiectasis have steadily increased in the United States over the past two decades and most commonly occur in women older than 60 years.[14] Cystic fibrosis is the most common cause of bronchiectasis in children. In adults it usually occurs in conjunction with other respiratory conditions that cause chronic inflammation of the bronchial wall, such as obstruction of an airway with mucous plugs, atelectasis, aspiration of a foreign body, infection, tuberculosis, congenital weakness of the bronchial wall, or impaired defense mechanisms. Chronic inflammation of the bronchi leads to destruction of elastic and muscular components of their walls and permanent dilation. Bronchiectasis also is associated with a number of systemic disorders, such as rheumatologic disease, inflammatory bowel disease, and immunodeficiency syndromes (e.g., acquired immunodeficiency syndrome [AIDS]).

The primary symptom of bronchiectasis is a chronic productive cough that may date back to a childhood illness or infection. The disease is commonly associated with recurrent lower respiratory tract infections and expectoration of voluminous amounts of foul-smelling purulent sputum (measured in cupfuls). Hemoptysis and clubbing of the fingers (from chronic hypoxemia) are common. Pulmonary function studies show decreased vital capacity (VC) and expiratory flow rates. Hypoxemia eventually leads to cor pulmonale (see p. 700). Diagnosis is usually confirmed by the use of high-resolution computed tomography. Bronchiectasis is treated with antibiotics, bronchodilators, chest physiotherapy, and supplemental oxygen.

Bronchiolitis

Bronchiolitis is a diffuse, inflammatory obstruction of the small airways or bronchioles occurring most commonly in children. In adults it usually accompanies chronic bronchitis but can occur in otherwise healthy individuals in association with an upper or lower respiratory tract viral infection or with inhalation of toxic gases. Bronchiolitis also is a serious complication of stem cell and lung transplantation and can progress to **bronchiolitis obliterans,** a fibrotic process that occludes airways and causes permanent scarring of the lungs.[15] Bronchiolitis obliterans organizing pneumonia (BOOP) is a complication of bronchiolitis obliterans in which the alveoli and bronchioles become filled with plugs of connective tissue. This complication of lung transplant has a high morbidity.

Bronchiolitis frequently presents with a rapid ventilatory rate; marked use of accessory muscles; low-grade fever; dry, nonproductive cough; and hyperinflated chest. A decrease in the ventilation-perfusion ratio results in hypoxemia. Diagnosis is made by spirometry and bronchoscopy with biopsy. Bronchiolitis is treated with appropriate antibiotics, corticosteroids, immunosuppressive agents, and chest physical therapy (humidified air, coughing and deep breathing, postural drainage) as indicated by the underlying cause.

Pulmonary Fibrosis

Pulmonary fibrosis is an excessive amount of fibrous or connective tissue in the lung. The most common form has no known cause and therefore is called idiopathic pulmonary fibrosis. Pulmonary fibrosis also can be caused by formation of scar tissue after active pulmonary disease (e.g., acute respiratory distress syndrome, tuberculosis), in association with a variety of autoimmune disorders (e.g., rheumatoid arthritis, progressive systemic sclerosis, sarcoidosis), or by inhalation of harmful substances (e.g., coal dust, asbestos).

Fibrosis causes a marked loss of lung compliance. The lung becomes stiff and difficult to ventilate, and the diffusing capacity of the alveolocapillary membrane may decrease, causing hypoxemia. Diffuse pulmonary fibrosis has a poor prognosis.

Idiopathic pulmonary fibrosis. Idiopathic pulmonary fibrosis (IPF) is the most common idiopathic interstitial lung disorder. It is more common in men than in women and most cases occur after age 60. Although IPF is characterized by chronic inflammation, recent studies suggest that it results from aberrant healing responses to epithelial cell injury, which probably occurs in response to a combination of environmental insults and genetic predispositions.[16,17] Fibroproliferation of the interstitial lung tissue around the alveoli causes decreased oxygen diffusion across the alveolocapillary membrane and hypoxemia. As the disease progresses, decreased lung compliance leads to increased work of breathing, decreased tidal volume, and resultant hypoventilation with hypercapnia.

The primary symptom of IPF is increasing dyspnea on exertion. Physical examination reveals diffuse inspiratory crackles. The diagnosis is confirmed by pulmonary function testing (decreased FVC), high-resolution computed tomography, and lung biopsy. Treatment includes corticosteroids and cytotoxic drugs, although success rates are low and toxicities are high. Newer therapies include antifibrotic drugs (such as *N*-acetylcysteine and pirfenidone), interferon, and anticoagulation therapy.[16] Selected individuals may benefit from lung transplantation.

Inhalation Disorders

Exposure to toxic gases. Inhalation of gaseous irritants can cause significant respiratory dysfunction. Commonly encountered toxic gases include smoke, ammonia, hydrogen chloride, sulfur dioxide, chlorine, phosgene, and nitrogen dioxide. Inhalation injuries in burns can include toxic gases from household or industrial combustants, heat, and smoke particles. Inhaled toxic particles cause damage to the airway epithelium, mucus secretion, inflammation, mucosal edema, ciliary damage, pulmonary edema, and surfactant inactivation. The cellular effects of toxic gases are described in Chapter 2. Acute toxic inhalation is frequently complicated by acute respiratory distress syndrome (ARDS) and pneumonia. Initial symptoms include burning of the eyes, nose, and throat; coughing; chest tightness; and dyspnea. Hypoxemia is common. Treatment includes supplemental oxygen,

mechanical ventilation with PEEP, and support of the cardiovascular system. Steroids are sometimes used, although their effectiveness has not been well documented. Most individuals recover quickly. Some, however, may improve initially and then deteriorate as a result of bronchiectasis or bronchiolitis (inflammation of the bronchioles).

Prolonged exposure to high concentrations of supplemental oxygen can result in a relatively rare condition known as oxygen toxicity. The basic underlying mechanism of injury is a severe inflammatory response mediated by toxic oxygen radicals. Damage to alveolocapillary membranes results in disruption of surfactant production, interstitial and alveolar edema, and a decrease in lung compliance. In infants this can lead to a condition known as bronchopulmonary dysplasia in which there is severe scarring of the lung.[18] Treatment involves ventilatory support and a reduction of inspired oxygen concentration to less than 60% as soon as the individual can tolerate this change. Surfactant replacement and antioxidant therapies are being explored.[19]

Pneumoconiosis. Pneumoconiosis represents any change in the lung caused by inhalation of inorganic dust particles, usually in the workplace. As in all cases of environmentally acquired lung disease, the individual's history of exposure is important in determining the diagnosis. Pneumoconiosis often occurs after years of exposure to the offending dust, with progressive fibrosis of lung tissue.

The dusts of silica, asbestos, and coal are the most common causes of pneumoconiosis. Others include talc, fiberglass, clays, mica, slate, cement, cadmium, beryllium, tungsten, cobalt, aluminum, and iron. Deposition of these materials in the lungs cause the release of proinflammatory cytokines, such as interleukin-1 beta (IL-1β).[20] This leads to chronic inflammation with scarring of the alveolar capillary membrane resulting in pulmonary fibrosis and progressive pulmonary deterioration. Clinical manifestations with advancement of disease include cough, chronic sputum production, dyspnea, decreased lung volumes, and hypoxemia. Diagnosis is confirmed by chest x-ray and computed tomography (CT). Treatment is usually palliative and focuses on preventing further exposure, particularly in the workplace. New therapies being investigated include blockers of inflammatory cytokines, such as IL-1β.[20]

Allergic alveolitis. Inhalation of organic dusts can result in an allergic inflammatory response called extrinsic allergic alveolitis, or hypersensitivity pneumonitis.[21] Many allergens can cause this disorder, including grains, silage, bird droppings or feathers, wood dust (particularly redwood and maple), cork dust, animal pelts, coffee beans, fish meal, mushroom compost, and molds that grow on sugarcane, barley, and straw. The lung inflammation, or pneumonitis, occurs after repeated, prolonged exposure to the allergen. Lymphocytes and inflammatory cells infiltrate the interstitial lung tissue, releasing a variety of autoimmune and inflammatory cytokines. Recent studies suggest an important role for interleukin-17, which promotes epithelial cell injury.[21]

Allergic alveolitis can be acute, subacute, or chronic. The acute form causes fever, cough, and chills a few hours after exposure. In the subacute form, coughing and dyspnea are common and sometimes necessitate hospital care. Diagnosis is made by history of exposure, chest x-ray, and serologic testing. Treatment consists of removal of the offending agent and administration of corticosteroids. Recovery is complete if the offending agent can be avoided in the future. With continued exposure, the disease becomes chronic and pulmonary fibrosis develops.

Pulmonary Edema

Pulmonary edema is excess water in the lung. The normal lung is kept dry by lymphatic drainage and a balance among capillary hydrostatic pressure, capillary oncotic pressure, and capillary permeability.

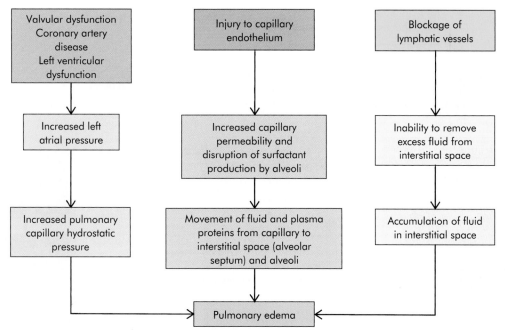

FIGURE 26-6 Pathogenesis of Pulmonary Edema.

In addition, surfactant lining the alveoli repels water, keeping fluid from entering the alveoli. Predisposing factors for pulmonary edema include heart disease, acute respiratory distress syndrome, and inhalation of toxic gases. The pathogenesis of pulmonary edema is shown in Figure 26-6.

The most common cause of pulmonary edema is left-sided heart disease. When the left ventricle fails, filling pressures on the left side of the heart increase. Vascular volume redistributes into the lungs, causing an increase in pulmonary capillary hydrostatic pressure. When the hydrostatic pressure exceeds oncotic pressure (which holds fluid in the capillary), fluid moves out into the interstitial space (the space within the alveolar septum between alveolus and capillary). When the flow of fluid out of the capillaries exceeds the lymphatic system's ability to remove it, pulmonary edema develops.

Another cause of pulmonary edema is capillary injury that increases capillary permeability, as in cases of acute respiratory distress syndrome or inhalation of toxic gases, such as ammonia. Capillary injury and inflammation causes water and plasma proteins to leak out of the capillary and move into the interstitial space, increasing the interstitial oncotic pressure (which is usually very low). As the interstitial oncotic pressure begins to exceed capillary oncotic pressure, water moves out of the capillary and into the lung. (This phenomenon is discussed in Chapter 4, Figures 4-1 and 4-2.) Pulmonary edema also can result from obstruction of the lymphatic system. Drainage can be blocked by compression of lymphatic vessels by edema, tumors, and fibrotic tissue and by increased systemic venous pressure.

Clinical manifestations of pulmonary edema include dyspnea and increased work of breathing. Physical examination may disclose inspiratory crackles (rales) and dullness to percussion over the lung bases. $\dot{V}/\dot{Q}$ mismatch leads to hypoxemia. In severe edema, pink frothy sputum is expectorated and lung compliance decreases, leading to decreased tidal volume and hypercapnia.

The treatment of pulmonary edema depends on its cause. If the edema is caused by increased hydrostatic pressure that results from

heart failure, therapy is geared toward improving cardiac output with diuretics, vasodilators, and drugs that improve the contraction of the heart muscle. If edema is the result of increased capillary permeability resulting from injury, the treatment is focused on removing the offending agent and implementing supportive therapy to maintain adequate ventilation and circulation. Individuals with either type of pulmonary edema require supplemental oxygen. Positive-pressure mechanical ventilation may be needed if edema significantly impairs ventilation and oxygenation.

Acute Respiratory Distress Syndrome

Acute respiratory distress syndrome (ARDS) is characterized by acute lung inflammation and diffuse alveolocapillary injury. Acute lung injury (ALI) is a less severe form of lung inflammation. Both ARDS and ALI are defined as (1) the acute onset of bilateral infiltrates on chest radiograph, (2) a low ratio of partial pressure of arterial oxygen to the fraction of inhaled oxygen, and (3) the absence of clinical evidence of left atrial hypertension.[22] In the United States more than 30% of intensive care unit (ICU) admissions are complicated by ARDS. Advances in therapy have decreased overall mortality in people younger than 60 years to approximately 40%, although mortality in older adults and those with severe infections remains much higher. The most common predisposing factors are sepsis and multiple trauma; however, there are many other causes, including pneumonia, burns, aspiration, cardiopulmonary bypass surgery, pancreatitis, blood transfusions, drug overdose, inhalation of smoke or noxious gases, fat emboli, high concentrations of supplemental oxygen, radiation therapy, and disseminated intravascular coagulation.

PATHOPHYSIOLOGY All disorders causing ARDS cause massive pulmonary inflammation that injures the alveolocapillary membrane and produces severe pulmonary edema, $\dot{V}/\dot{Q}$ mismatch (shunting), and hypoxemia (Figure 26-7). Most commonly, this occurs indirectly because of the effects of inflammatory mediators released in response

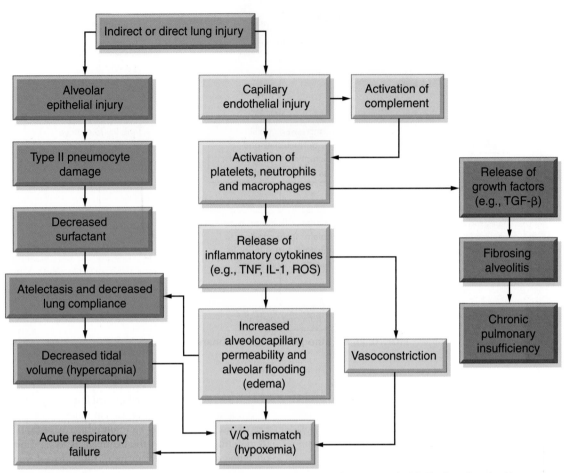

FIGURE 26-7 Pathogenesis of Acute Respiratory Distress Syndrome (ARDS). *IL-1,* Interleukin-1; *ROS,* reactive oxygen species; *TGF-β,* transforming growth factor-beta; *TNF,* tumor necrosis factor.

to systemic disorders, such as sepsis and trauma. The damage also can occur directly, because of the aspiration of highly acidic gastric contents or the inhalation of toxic gases. Injury to the pulmonary capillary endothelium stimulates platelet aggregation and intravascular microthrombus formation. Endothelial damage also initiates the complement cascade, stimulating neutrophil and macrophage activity and the inflammatory response.[23]

Once activated, macrophages produce toxic mediators such as tumor necrosis factor (TNF) and interleukin 1 (IL-1). The role of neutrophils is central to the development of ARDS. Activated neutrophils release a battery of inflammatory mediators, including proteolytic enzymes, toxic oxygen products, arachidonic acid metabolites (prostaglandins, thromboxanes, leukotrienes), and platelet-activating factor.[23,24] These mediators extensively damage the alveolocapillary membrane and greatly increase capillary membrane permeability. This allows fluids, proteins, and blood cells to leak from the capillary bed into the pulmonary interstitium and alveoli. The resulting pulmonary edema severely reduces lung compliance and impairs alveolar ventilation. Because this form of pulmonary edema is not secondary to heart failure, ARDS is often referred to as *noncardiogenic pulmonary edema*. Mediators released by neutrophils and macrophages also cause pulmonary vasoconstriction, which leads to worsening $\dot{V}/\dot{Q}$ mismatch and hypoxemia.

The initial lung injury also damages the alveolar epithelium. This type II alveolar cell injury increases alveolocapillary permeability,

increases susceptibility to bacterial infection and pneumonia, and decreases surfactant production.[24] Alveoli and respiratory bronchioles fill with fluid or collapse. The lungs become less compliant, the work of breathing increases, ventilation of alveoli decreases, and hypercapnia develops. The end result is acute respiratory failure.

Approximately 24 to 48 hours after the acute phase of ARDS, hyaline membranes form. Inflammatory cells release growth factors and, after approximately 7 days, fibrosis progressively obliterates the alveoli, respiratory bronchioles, and interstitium (fibrosing alveolitis), which can result in chronic pulmonary insufficiency.[25] Functional residual capacity declines, and more severe right-to-left shunting is evident.

The chemical mediators responsible for the alveolocapillary damage of ARDS often cause widespread inflammation, endothelial damage, and capillary permeability throughout the body resulting in the systemic inflammatory response syndrome (SIRS), which then leads to multiple organ dysfunction syndrome (MODS). In fact, death may not be caused by respiratory failure alone but by MODS associated with ARDS. (MODS is discussed in Chapter 23.)

CLINICAL MANIFESTATIONS The classic signs and symptoms of ARDS are marked dyspnea; rapid, shallow breathing; inspiratory crackles; respiratory alkalosis; decreased lung compliance; hypoxemia unresponsive to oxygen therapy (refractory hypoxemia); and diffuse alveolar infiltrates seen on chest radiographs, without evidence of cardiac disease. Symptoms develop progressively, as follows:

Dyspnea and hypoxemia
↓
Hyperventilation and respiratory alkalosis
↓
Decreased tissue perfusion, organ dysfunction, and metabolic acidosis
↓
Increased work of breathing, decreased tidal volume, and hypoventilation
↓
Respiratory acidosis and worsening hypoxemia
↓
Hypotension, decreased cardiac output, death

EVALUATION AND TREATMENT Diagnosis is based on physical examination, analysis of blood gases, and radiologic examination. Measurement of serum biomarkers, such as TNF, brain natriuretic peptide (BNP), and IL-8, may aid in the diagnosis of ARDS in cases of trauma.[26] Treatment is based on early detection, supportive therapy, and prevention of complications. Supportive therapy is focused on maintaining adequate oxygenation and ventilation while preventing infection. This often requires alternative modes of mechanical ventilation. Pharmacologic therapy continues to be explored.[27] Low-dose corticosteroids may improve survival in selected individuals, and surfactant can be given to improve lung compliance. Anticoagulant therapy with recombinant human activated protein C improves outcomes in sepsis associated with ARDS and continues to be evaluated.

✔ **QUICK CHECK 26-3**
1. Contrast aspiration and atelectasis.
2. What are some of the causes of pulmonary fibrosis?
3. What symptoms are produced by inhalation of toxic gases?
4. Describe pneumoconiosis, and give two examples.
5. Briefly describe the role of neutrophils in acute respiratory distress syndrome (ARDS).

Obstructive Lung Diseases

Obstructive lung disease is characterized by airway obstruction that is worse with expiration. More force (i.e., use of accessory muscles of expiration) is required to expire a given volume of air and emptying of the lungs is slowed. In adults the major obstructive lung diseases are asthma, chronic bronchitis, and emphysema. Asthma is one of the most common lung disorders in the United States. Because many individuals have both chronic bronchitis and emphysema, these diseases together are often called *chronic obstructive pulmonary disease (COPD)*. Asthma is more acute and intermittent than COPD, even though it can be chronic (Figure 26-8). The unifying symptom of obstructive lung diseases is dyspnea, and the unifying sign is wheezing. Individuals have an increased work of breathing, ventilation-perfusion mismatching, and a decreased forced expiratory volume in 1 second (FEV_1).

Asthma

Asthma is a chronic inflammatory disorder of the bronchial mucosa that causes hyperresponsiveness and constriction of the airways.[28] Asthma occurs at all ages, with approximately half of all cases developing during childhood (see Chapter 27) and another third before age 40. In the United States asthma has been diagnosed in more than 34 million persons.[29] Death rates have declined since 1995 in the United

States but the incidence of asthma has increased, especially in urban areas.

Asthma is a familial disorder, and more than 100 genes have been identified that may play a role in the susceptibility and pathogenesis of asthma, including those that influence the production of interleukin-4 (IL-4) and interleukin-5 (IL-5), immunoglobulin E (IgE), eosinophils, mast cells, and β-adrenergic receptors as well as those that increase bronchial hyperresponsiveness.[30] The expression of these genetic factors is influenced by other risk factors including age at onset of disease; levels of allergen exposure; urban residence; exposure to air pollution, tobacco smoke, and environmental tobacco smoke; recurrent respiratory tract viral infections; gastroesophageal reflux disease; and obesity.[28,31,32] There is considerable evidence that exposure to high levels of certain allergens during childhood increases the risk for asthma. Furthermore, decreased exposure to certain infectious organisms appears to create an immunologic imbalance that favors the development of allergy and asthma. This complex relationship has been called the *hygiene hypothesis*.[33] Urban exposure to pollution and cockroaches, decreased exercise, and increased obesity play a role in the increasing prevalence of asthma, particularly in children.

PATHOPHYSIOLOGY Many cells and cellular elements contribute to the persistent inflammation of the bronchial mucosa and hyperresponsiveness of the airways, including mast cells, eosinophils, basophils, macrophages (dendritic cells), neutrophils, and lymphocytes. Inflammatory mediators released by these cells increase capillary permeability and stimulate smooth muscle contraction and increased secretion of mucus. Airway epithelial exposure to antigen initiates both an innate and an adaptive immune response (type I hypersensitivity) in sensitized individuals (see Chapter 7).[34,35] There is both an immediate (acute asthmatic response) and a late (delayed) response.

During the *early asthmatic response* antigen exposure to the bronchial mucosa activates B cells (plasma cells) to produce antigen-specific IgE. Cross-linking of IgE molecules with the antigen on the surface of mast cells causes mast cell degranulation with the release of inflammatory mediators including histamine, bradykinins, leukotrienes and prostaglandins, platelet activating factor, and interleukins (see Figures 5-8 and 7-9 for additional details).[35] These mediators cause vasodilation, increased capillary permeability, mucosal edema, bronchial smooth muscle contraction (bronchospasm), and mucus secretion from mucosal goblet cells with narrowing of the airways and obstruction to airflow (see Figures 26-8 and 27-7, A).[36] Other inflammatory cytokines, such as TNF and IL-1, have been found to alter muscarinic receptor function and lead to increased levels of acetylcholine, which cause bronchial smooth muscle contraction and mucus secretion. The *late asthmatic response* begins 4 to 8 hours after the early response (see Figure 27-7, B). Chemotactic recruitment of neutrophils, eosinophils, and lymphocytes during the acute response causes a latent release of inflammatory mediators, again inciting bronchospasm, edema, and mucus secretion with obstruction to airflow. Synthesis of leukotrienes contributes to prolonged smooth muscle contraction. Eosinophils cause direct tissue injury with fibroblast proliferation and airway scarring. Release of toxic neuropeptides contributes to increased bronchial hyperresponsiveness. Damage to ciliated epithelial cells contributes to impaired mucociliary function, with the accumulation of mucus and cellular debris forming plugs in the airways (see Figures 26-9 and 27-7 for additional details).[35,37] Untreated inflammation can lead to long-term airway damage that is irreversible, known as *airway remodeling* (subepithelial fibrosis, smooth muscle hypertrophy).[38]

Airway obstruction increases resistance to airflow and decreases flow rates, especially expiratory flow. Impaired expiration causes air

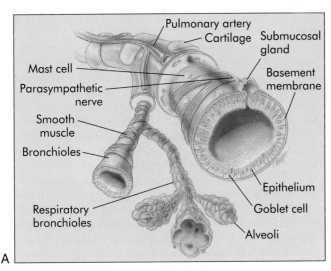

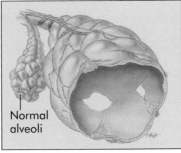

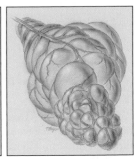

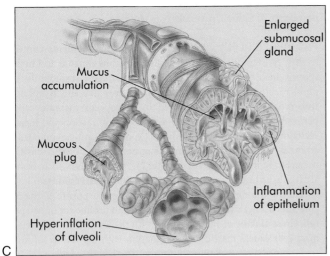

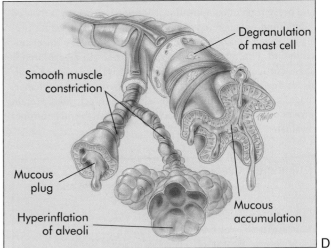

FIGURE 26-8 Airway Obstruction Caused by Emphysema, Chronic Bronchitis, and Asthma. **A,** The normal lung. **B,** Emphysema: enlargement and destruction of alveolar walls with loss of elasticity and trapping of air; *(left)* panlobular emphysema showing abnormal weakening and enlargement of all air spaces distal to the terminal bronchioles (normal alveoli shown for comparison only); *(right)* centrilobular emphysema showing abnormal weakening and enlargement of the respiratory bronchioles in the proximal portion of the acinus. **C,** Chronic bronchitis: inflammation and thickening of mucous membrane with accumulation of mucus and pus leading to obstruction; characterized by cough. **D,** Bronchial asthma: thick mucus, mucosal edema, and smooth muscle spasm causing obstruction of small airways; breathing becomes labored, and expiration is difficult. (Modified from Des Jardins T, Burton GG: *Clinical manifestations and assessment of respiratory disease,* ed 5, St Louis, 2006, Mosby.)

trapping, hyperinflation distal to obstructions, and increased work of breathing. Changes in resistance to airflow are not uniform throughout the lungs and the distribution of inspired air is uneven, with more air flowing to the less resistant portions. Continued air trapping increases intrapleural and alveolar gas pressures and causes decreased perfusion of the alveoli. Increased alveolar gas pressure, decreased ventilation, and decreased perfusion lead to variable and uneven ventilation-perfusion relationships within different lung segments. Hyperventilation is triggered by lung receptors responding to increased lung volume and obstruction. The result is early hypoxemia without CO_2 retention. Hypoxemia further increases hyperventilation through stimulation of the respiratory center, causing $Paco_2$ to decrease and pH to increase (respiratory alkalosis). With progressive obstruction of expiratory airflow, air trapping becomes more severe and the lungs and thorax become hyperexpanded, positioning the respiratory muscles at a mechanical disadvantage. This leads to a fall in tidal volume with

increasing CO_2 retention and respiratory acidosis. Respiratory acidosis signals respiratory failure, especially when left ventricular filling, and thus cardiac output, becomes compromised because of severe hyperinflation.

CLINICAL MANIFESTATIONS Between attacks, individuals are asymptomatic and pulmonary function tests are normal. At the beginning of an attack, the individual experiences chest constriction, expiratory wheezing, dyspnea, nonproductive coughing, prolonged expiration, tachycardia, and tachypnea. Severe attacks involve the accessory muscles of respiration and wheezing is heard during both inspiration and expiration. A **pulsus paradoxus** (decrease in systolic blood pressure during inspiration of more than 10 mm Hg) may be noted. Peak flow measurements should be obtained. Because the severity of blood gas alterations is difficult to evaluate by clinical signs alone, arterial blood gas tensions should be measured if oxygen saturation

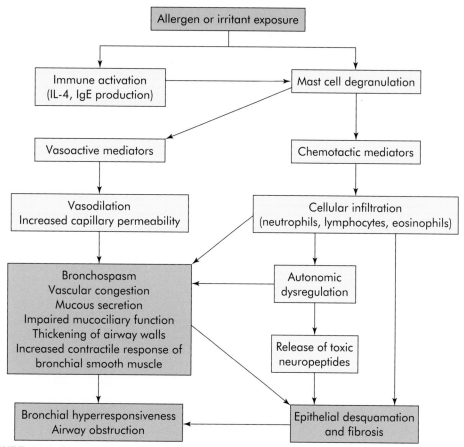

FIGURE 26-9 Pathophysiology of Asthma. Allergen or irritant exposure results in a cascade of inflammatory events leading to acute and chronic airway dysfunction (also see Figure 27-7).

falls below 90%. Usual findings are hypoxemia with an associated respiratory alkalosis. In the *late asthma response,* symptoms can be even more severe than the initial attack.

If bronchospasm is not reversed by usual measures, the individual is considered to have severe bronchospasm or status asthmaticus. If status asthmaticus continues, hypoxemia worsens, expiratory flows and volumes decrease further, and effective ventilation decreases. Acidosis develops as $Paco_2$ level begins to rise. Asthma becomes life-threatening at this point if treatment does not reverse this process quickly. A silent chest (no audible air movement) and a $Paco_2$ >70 mm Hg are ominous signs of impending death.

EVALUATION AND TREATMENT The diagnosis of asthma is supported by a history of allergies and recurrent episodes of wheezing, dyspnea, and cough or exercise intolerance. Further evaluation includes spirometry, which may document reversible decreases in FEV_1 during an induced attack.

The evaluation of an acute asthma attack requires the rapid assessment of arterial blood gases and expiratory flow rates (using a peak flow meter) and a search for underlying triggers, such as infection. Hypoxemia and respiratory alkalosis are expected early in the course of an acute attack. The development of hypercapnia with respiratory acidosis signals the need for mechanical ventilation. Management of the acute asthma attack requires immediate administration of oxygen and inhaled beta-agonist bronchodilators. In addition, oral corticosteroids should be administered early in the course of management. Careful monitoring of gas exchange and airway obstruction in response to therapy provides information necessary to determine whether

hospitalization is necessary. Antibiotics are not indicated for acute asthma unless there is a documented bacterial infection.[39]

Management of asthma begins with avoidance of allergens and irritants. Individuals with asthma tend to underestimate the severity of their asthma and extensive education is important, including use of a peak flow meter and adherence to an action plan should symptoms worsen. In the mildest form of asthma (intermittent), short-acting beta-agonist inhalers are prescribed. For all categories of persistent asthma, anti-inflammatory medications are essential and inhaled corticosteroids are the mainstay of therapy. In individuals who are not adequately controlled with inhaled corticosteroids, leukotriene antagonists can be considered. In more severe asthma, long-acting beta agonists can be used to control persistent bronchospasm; however, these agonists can actually worsen asthma in some individuals with certain genetic polymorphisms (see *Health Alert:* Pharmacogenetics and Beta Agonists in the Treatment of Asthma). Immunotherapy has been shown to be an important tool in reducing asthma exacerbations and can now be given sublingually.[40] Monoclonal antibodies to IgE (omalizumab) have been found to be helpful in selected individuals. The National Asthma Education and Prevention Program offers step-wise guidelines for the diagnosis and management of chronic asthma based on clinical severity and they may be reviewed at www.nhlbi.nih.gov/guidelines/asthma/asthgdln.htm.[28]

Chronic Obstructive Pulmonary Disease

Chronic obstructive pulmonary disease (COPD) is defined as a preventable and treatable disease with some significant extrapulmonary effects that may contribute to the severity in individual patients.

HEALTH ALERT

Pharmacogenetics and Beta Agonists in the Treatment of Asthma

Long-acting beta agonists (LABAs) (salmeterol and formoterol) are recommended by the National Asthma Education and Prevention Program (NAEPP) to be used in conjunction with inhaled corticosteroids as step 3 therapy for asthma. LABAs have been found to improve symptoms in many individuals and exert both a bronchodilatory and an anti-inflammatory effect on the airways. However, the safety of LABAs has been questioned because of increased mortality in some populations using these drugs. Recent evidence suggests that the reason for this increased mortality is that those individuals who exhibited worsening symptoms while taking LABAs used these medications alone, instead of in conjunction with inhaled steroids as recommended. Thus they were simply masking ongoing inflammation and airway damage. There also is some evidence to suggest that persons who have a polymorphism of the beta-adrenergic receptor gene *(ADRβ2)* are at risk for complications if they use LABAs. This polymorphism is known as the Arg16Arg genotype and is associated with an increased risk for worsening bronchospasm, increased hospitalizations, and increased mortality when using LABAs. This genotype occurs more frequently in blacks and may explain some of the differences in asthma mortality among these individuals. Studies continue to evaluate other genes and their relationship to medication response, a field of study now known as pharmacogenetics.

Data from Ducharme FM, Lasserson TJ, Cates CJ: Addition to inhaled corticosteroids of long-acting beta2-agonists versus anti-leukotrienes for chronic asthma, *Cochrane Database Syst Rev* 5:CD003137, 2011; Schachter EN: New β₂-adrenoceptor agonists for the treatment of chronic obstructive pulmonary disease, *Drugs Today (Barc)* 6(12):911–918, 2010; Sears MR: The addition of long-acting beta-agonists to inhaled corticosteroids in asthma, *Curr Opin Pulm Med* 17(1):23–28, 2011; Hodgson D, Mortimer K, Harrison T: Budesonide/formoterol in the treatment of asthma, *Expert Rev Respir Med* 4(5):557–566, 2010; Chung LP, Waterer G, Thompson PJ: Pharmacogenetics of β2 adrenergic receptor gene polymorphisms, long-acting β-agonists and asthma, *Clin Exp Allergy* 41(3):312–326, 2011.

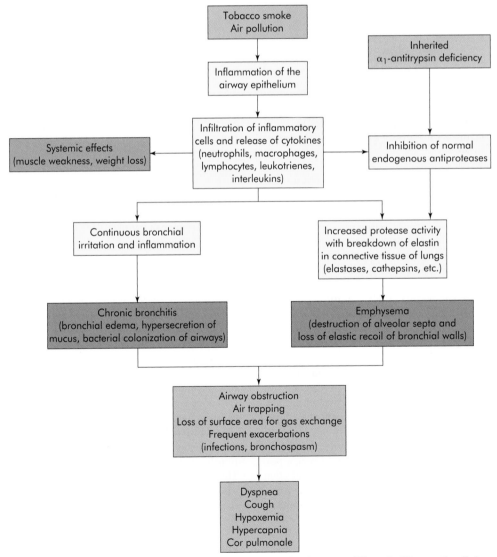

FIGURE 26-10 Pathogenesis of Chronic Bronchitis and Emphysema (Chronic Obstructive Pulmonary Disease [COPD]).

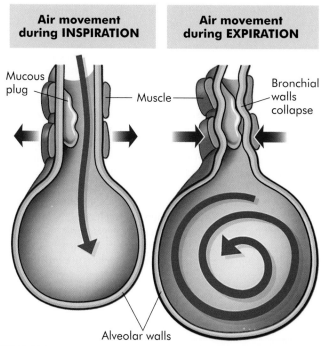

Air movement during INSPIRATION

Air movement during EXPIRATION

Mucous plug — Muscle — Bronchial walls collapse

Alveolar walls

FIGURE 26-11 Mechanisms of Air Trapping in COPD. Mucous plugs and narrowed airways cause air trapping and hyperinflation of alveoli on expiration. During inspiration, the airways are pulled open, allowing gas to flow past the obstruction. During expiration, decreased elastic recoil of the bronchial walls results in collapse of the airways and prevents normal expiratory airflow.

Its pulmonary component is characterized by airflow limitation that is not fully reversible. The airflow limitation is usually progressive and associated with an abnormal inflammatory response of the lung to noxious particles or gases.[41] COPD is the fourth leading cause of death in the United States and is the sixth leading cause of death worldwide. Overall mortality from COPD has increased in the United States over the past 30 years; however, COPD mortality in women has increased more than twice that amount.[42] Risk factors for COPD include tobacco smoke (cigarette, pipe, cigar, and environmental tobacco smoke), occupational dusts and chemicals (vapors, irritants, and fumes), indoor air pollution from biomass fuel used for cooking and heating (in poorly vented dwellings), outdoor air pollution, and any factor that affects lung growth during gestation and childhood (low birthweight, respiratory tract infections).[41] Genetic susceptibilities have been identified including polymorphisms of genes that code for tumor necrosis factor, surfactant, proteases, and antiproteases.[43] An inherited mutation in the α_1-antitrypsin gene results in the development of COPD at an early age, even in individuals who do not smoke.

Chronic Bronchitis

COPD includes the pathologic lung changes consistent with emphysema or chronic bronchitis. Chronic bronchitis is defined as hypersecretion of mucus and chronic productive cough for at least 3 months of the year (usually the winter months) for at least 2 consecutive years.

PATHOPHYSIOLOGY Inspired irritants result in airway inflammation with infiltration of neutrophils, macrophages, and lymphocytes into the bronchial wall. Continual bronchial inflammation causes bronchial edema and increases the size and number of mucous glands and goblet cells in the airway epithelium. Thick, tenacious mucus is produced and cannot be cleared because of impaired ciliary function.[44]

CLINICAL MANIFESTATIONS	BRONCHITIS	EMPHYSEMA
Productive cough	Classic sign	Late in course with infection
Dyspnea	Late in course	Common
Wheezing	Intermittent	Common
History of smoking	Common	Common
Barrel chest	Occasionally	Classic
Prolonged expiration	Always present	Always present
Cyanosis	Common	Uncommon
Chronic hypoventilation	Common	Late in course
Polycythemia	Common	Late in course
Cor pulmonale	Common	Late in course

TABLE 26-2 CLINICAL MANIFESTATIONS OF CHRONIC OBSTRUCTIVE LUNG DISEASE

The lung's defense mechanisms are, therefore, compromised, increasing susceptibility to pulmonary infection and injury. Frequent infectious exacerbations are complicated by bronchospasm with dyspnea and productive cough.[45] The pathogenesis of chronic bronchitis is shown in Figure 26-10.

Initially this process affects only the larger bronchi, but eventually all airways are involved. The thick mucus and hypertrophied bronchial smooth muscle constrict the airways and lead to obstruction, particularly during expiration when the airways are narrowed (Figure 26-11). Obstruction eventually leads to ventilation-perfusion mismatch with hypoxemia. The airways collapse early in expiration, trapping gas in the distal portions of the lung. Air trapping expands the thorax and positions the respiratory muscles at a mechanical disadvantage. This leads to decreased tidal volume, hypoventilation, and hypercapnia.

CLINICAL MANIFESTATIONS Table 26-2 lists the common clinical manifestations of chronic obstructive lung disease, chronic bronchitis, and emphysema.

EVALUATION AND TREATMENT Diagnosis is based on physical examination, chest radiograph, pulmonary function tests, and blood gas analyses; these tests reflect the progressive nature of the disease. Prevention of chronic bronchitis is essential because pathologic changes are not reversible. By the time an individual seeks medical care for symptoms, considerable airway damage is present. If the individual stops smoking, disease progression can be halted.

Bronchodilators and expectorants are prescribed as needed to control cough and reduce dyspnea. Chest physical therapy may be helpful and includes deep breathing and postural drainage.[41] During acute exacerbations (infection and bronchospasm), individuals require treatment with antibiotics and steroids and may need mechanical ventilation.[45] Chronic use of oral steroids may be needed late in the course of the disease but should be considered a last resort. Individuals with severe hypoxemia will require home oxygen therapy. Teaching includes nutritional counseling, respiratory hygiene, recognition of the early signs of infection, and techniques that relieve dyspnea, such as pursed-lip breathing.

Emphysema

Emphysema is abnormal permanent enlargement of gas-exchange airways (acini) accompanied by destruction of alveolar walls without obvious fibrosis. Obstruction results from changes in lung tissues,

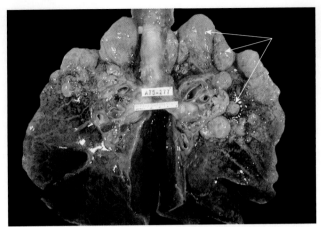

FIGURE 26-12 Bullous Emphysema with Large Apical and Sub-pleural Bullae (see arrows). (From Kumar V et al, editors: *Robbins basic pathology*, ed 8, Philadelphia, 2007, Saunders/Elsevier.)

rather than mucus production and inflammation as in chronic bronchitis. The major mechanism of airflow limitation is loss of elastic recoil (see Figure 26-11).

Primary emphysema, which accounts for 1% to 3% of all cases of emphysema, is commonly linked to an inherited deficiency of the enzyme α_1-antitrypsin, which is a major component of α_1-globulin, a plasma protein. Normally α_1-antitrypsin inhibits the action of many proteolytic enzymes; therefore α_1-antitrypsin deficiency (an autosomal recessive trait) produces an increased likelihood of developing emphysema because proteolysis in lung tissues is not inhibited. α_1-Antitrypsin deficiency is suggested in individuals who develop emphysema before 40 years of age and in individuals who do not smoke but still develop the disease. The major cause of secondary emphysema is the inhalation of cigarette smoke, although air pollution, occupational exposures, and childhood respiratory tract infections are known to be contributing factors.

PATHOPHYSIOLOGY Emphysema begins with destruction of alveolar septa, which eliminates portions of the pulmonary capillary bed and increases the volume of air in the acinus. It is postulated that inhaled oxidants in tobacco smoke and air pollution inhibit the activity of endogenous antiproteases and stimulate inflammation with increased activity of the proteases (e.g., elastase). Thus the balance is tipped toward alveolar destruction and loss of the normal elastic recoil of the bronchi (see Figure 26-10). Cellular apoptosis and early cellular senescence contribute to loss of alveolar cells and reduced surface area for gas exchange.[46] Alveolar destruction also produces large air spaces within the lung parenchyma (bullae) and air spaces adjacent to pleurae (blebs) (Figure 26-12). Bullae and blebs are not effective in gas exchange and result in significant ventilation-perfusion ($\dot{V}/\dot{Q}$) mismatching and hypoxemia. Expiration becomes difficult because loss of elastic recoil reduces the volume of air that can be expired passively and air is trapped in the lungs (see Figure 26-11). Air trapping causes hyperexpansion of the chest, placing the muscles of respiration at a mechanical disadvantage. This results in increased workload of breathing, so that late in the course of disease, many individuals will develop hypoventilation and hypercapnia. Persistent inflammation in the airways can result in hyperreactivity of the bronchi with bronchoconstriction, which may be partially reversible with bronchodilators. Chronic inflammation also can have significant systemic effects including weight loss, muscle weakness, and increased susceptibility to comorbidities, such as infection.

CLINICAL MANIFESTATIONS The clinical manifestations of emphysema are listed in Table 26-2.

EVALUATION AND TREATMENT Pulmonary function testing, chest x-ray, high-resolution computed tomography (CT), and arterial blood gas measurements are used to diagnose emphysema. Pulmonary function measurements, especially FEV_1 values, also are helpful in determining the stage of disease, appropriate treatment, and prognosis. Chronic management of emphysema begins with smoking cessation. Pharmacologic management is based on clinical severity (mild, moderate, severe, or very severe).[41] Inhaled anticholinergic agents and beta agonists should be prescribed.[47] Inhaled corticosteroids are indicated for severe COPD, although long-term therapy with oral steroids should be avoided if possible. Pulmonary rehabilitation, improved nutrition, and breathing techniques all can improve symptoms. Progressive pulmonary dysfunction with hypoxemia and hypercapnia may require long-term oxygen therapy and ventilation if indicated.[41] A class of drugs called *phosphodiesterase E4 (PDE4)* inhibitors are proving to be effective in selected individuals with severe COPD.[48] Selected individuals with severe emphysema can benefit from lung reduction surgery or lung transplantation.

 QUICK CHECK 26-4
1. What mechanisms cause airway obstruction in asthma?
2. How does emphysema affect oxygenation and ventilation?
3. Define chronic bronchitis.

Respiratory Tract Infections

Respiratory tract infections are the most common cause of short-term disability in the United States. Most of these infections—the common cold, pharyngitis (sore throat), and laryngitis—involve only the upper airways. Although the lungs have direct contact with the atmosphere, they usually remain sterile. Infections of the lower respiratory tract occur most often in individuals whose normal defense mechanisms are impaired.

Pneumonia

Pneumonia is infection of the lower respiratory tract caused by bacteria, viruses, fungi, protozoa, or parasites. It is the sixth leading cause of death in the United States. The incidence and mortality of pneumonia are highest in the elderly. Risk factors for pneumonia include advanced age, compromised immunity, underlying lung disease, alcoholism, altered consciousness, impaired swallowing, smoking, endotracheal intubation, malnutrition, immobilization, underlying cardiac or liver disease, and residence in a nursing home. Individuals who live in poverty also are at significantly increased risk for pneumonia.[49] The causative microorganism influences how the individual presents clinically, how the pneumonia should be treated, and the prognosis. Community-acquired pneumonia (CAP) tends to be caused by different microorganisms as compared with those infections acquired in the hospital (nosocomial). In addition, the characteristics of the individual are important in determining which etiologic microorganism is likely; for example, immunocompromised individuals tend to be susceptible to opportunistic infections that are uncommon in normal adults. In general, nosocomial infections and those affecting immunocompromised individuals have a higher mortality than CAPs. Some of the most common causal microorganisms are included in the list at the top of p. 695.

COMMUNITY-ACQUIRED PNEUMONIA (CAP)	NOSOCOMIAL PNEUMONIA	IMMUNO-COMPROMISED INDIVIDUALS
Streptococcus pneumoniae	*Pseudomonas aeruginosa*	*Pneumocystis jiroveci*
Mycoplasma pneumoniae	*Staphylococcus aureus*	*Mycobacterium tuberculosis*
Haemophilus influenzae	*Klebsiella pneumoniae*	Atypical mycobacteria
Oral anaerobic bacteria	*Escherichia coli*	Fungi
Influenza virus Respiratory syncytial virus		Respiratory viruses
Staphylococcus aureus		Protozoa
Chlamydia pneumoniae		Parasites
Moraxella catarrhalis		

The most common community-acquired pneumonia is caused by *Streptococcus pneumoniae* (also known as *pneumococcus*), which results in hospitalization in more than half of affected individuals and an overall hospital mortality of 10%.[50] *Mycoplasma pneumoniae* is a common cause of pneumonia in young people, especially those living in group housing such as dormitories and army barracks. Community-acquired methicillin-resistant *Staphylococcus aureus* (MRSA) is becoming more common.[51,52] Influenza and respiratory syncytial virus are the most common causes of viral community-acquired pneumonia in adults.[53] Nosocomial pneumonia is a frequent complication in the intensive care unit, most often in persons placed on mechanical ventilation (ventilator-associated pneumonia [VAP]) (see *Health Alert:* Ventilator-Associated Pneumonia [VAP]). *Pseudomonas aeruginosa*, other gram-negative microorganisms, and *Staphylococcus aureus* (including MRSA) are the most common etiologic agents in nosocomial pneumonia. Immunocompromised individuals (e.g., those with human immunodeficiency virus [HIV] or those undergoing organ transplantation) are especially susceptible to *Pneumocystis jiroveci* (formerly called *P. carinii*), mycobacterial infections, and fungal infections of the respiratory tract. These infections can be difficult to treat and have a high mortality.

PATHOPHYSIOLOGY Aspiration of oropharyngeal secretions is the most common route of lower respiratory tract infection; thus, the nasopharynx and oropharynx constitute the first line of defense for most infectious agents. Another route of infection is through the inhalation of microorganisms that have been released into the air when an infected individual coughs, sneezes, or talks, or from aerosolized water such as that from contaminated respiratory therapy equipment. This route of infection is most important in viral and mycobacterial pneumonias and in *Legionella* outbreaks. Pneumonia also can occur when bacteria are spread to the lung in the blood from bacteremia that can result from infection elsewhere in the body or from IV drug abuse.

In healthy individuals, pathogens that reach the lungs are expelled or controlled by mechanisms of self-defense (see Chapters 5, 6, and 7). If a microorganism evades the upper airway defense mechanisms, such as the cough reflex and mucociliary clearance, the next line of defense is the airway epithelial cell. Airway epithelial cells can recognize some pathogens directly (e.g., *Pseudomonas aeruginosa* and *Staphylococcus*

HEALTH ALERT

Ventilator-Associated Pneumonia (VAP)

Ventilator-associated pneumonia (VAP) is a common complication of mechanical ventilation and is the most serious infection in the intensive care unit. Mortality ranges from 15% to 70% depending on the underlying condition of the affected individual. Risk factors include age greater than 65 years, presence of comorbidities, length of intubation time, use of sedation, supine posture, poor oral hygiene, and immunocompromised status. Common etiologic microorganisms include *Staphylococcus aureus*, *Pseudomonas aeruginosa*, *Klebsiella* species, *Escherichia coli*, *Acinetobacter* species, and *Enterobacter* species. Multidrug-resistant strains are common. Bacterial colonization of the oropharynx occurs soon after placement of the endotracheal (ET) tube with subsequent aspiration and pooling of bacteria near the ET tube cuff. Many bacteria are capable of forming a protective coating, called a biofilm, on the surface of the ET tube that contributes to bacterial replication and makes microorganisms less vulnerable to antibiotics. Injury to the tracheal mucosa and decreased mucociliary clearance contribute to lower airway infection. Implementation of certain treatment protocols has shown improved outcomes regarding VAP prevention and mortality reduction, especially the use of a "bundle" of techniques including raising the head of the bed, improving oral hygiene, providing continuous suction of subglottic secretions by antimicrobial-impregnated ET tubes, instilling saline before suctioning and rapidly instituting antibiotic therapy, using checklists, and encouraging effective team communication.

Data from Blamoun J et al: Efficacy of an expanded ventilator bundle for the reduction of ventilator-associated pneumonia in the medical intensive care unit, *Am J Infect Control* 37:172–175, 2009; Lipitz-Snyderman A et al: Impact of a statewide intensive care unit quality improvement initiative on hospital mortality and length of stay: retrospective comparative analysis, *Br Med J* 342:d219, 2011; Lorente L, Blot S, Rello J: New issues and controversies in the prevention of ventilator-associated pneumonia, *Am J Respir Crit Care Med* 182(7):870–876, 2010; Palmer LB: Ventilator-associated infection, *Curr Opin Pulmon Med* 15(3):230–235, 2009; Jones RN: Microbial etiologies of hospital-acquired bacterial pneumonia and ventilator-associated bacterial pneumonia, *Clin Infect Dis* 51(suppl 1):S81–S87, 2010; Vincent JL et al: Diagnosis, management and prevention of ventilator-associated pneumonia: an update, *Drugs* 70(15):1927–1944, 2010.

aureus). The most important guardian cell of the lower respiratory tract is the alveolar macrophage; it recognizes pathogens through its pattern-recognition receptors (e.g., Toll-like receptors) and then activates both innate and adaptive immune responses. Release of tumor necrosis factor-alpha (TNF-α) and interleukin-1 (IL-1) from macrophages contributes to widespread inflammation in the lung and recruitment of neutrophils from the capillaries of the lungs into the alveoli. Macrophages also present infectious antigens to the adaptive immune system, activating T cells and B cells with the induction of both cellular and humoral immunity. The resulting inflammatory mediators and immune complexes can damage bronchial mucous membranes and alveolocapillary membranes, causing the acini and terminal bronchioles to fill with infectious debris and exudate. In addition, some microorganisms release toxins from their cell walls that can cause further lung damage and consolidation of lung tissue. The accumulation of exudate in the acinus leads to dyspnea and to $\dot{V}/\dot{Q}$ mismatching and hypoxemia.

Pneumococcal pneumonia. Pneumococci can infect the lungs through inhalation of aerosolized bacteria or more commonly by aspiration of colonized oropharyngeal secretions. These bacteria have several virulence factors; most importantly, they have capsules that make

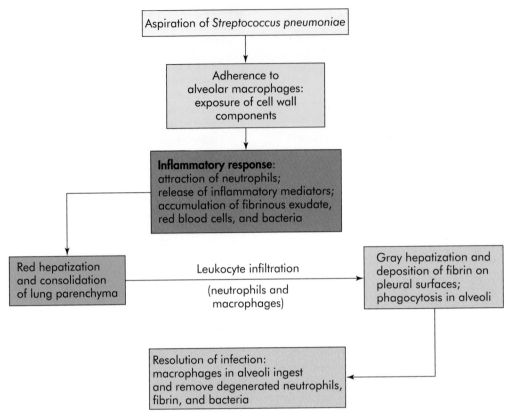

FIGURE 26-13 Pathophysiologic Course of Pneumococcal Pneumonia.

phagocytosis by alveolar macrophages more difficult and they have the ability to release a variety of toxins, including pneumolysin, which damages airway and alveolar cells.[54] An intense inflammatory response is initiated with release of TNF-α and IL-1. Neutrophils and inflammatory exudates cause alveolar edema, which leads to the other changes shown in Figure 26-13.

Viral pneumonia. Viral pneumonia is usually mild and self-limiting but can set the stage for a secondary bacterial infection by damaging ciliated epithelial cells, which normally prevent pathogens from reaching the lower airways. Influenza pneumonia can be severe, especially influenza A of the H1N1 type.[55] Immunocompromised individuals are at risk for very serious viral infections, such as pneumonia caused by cytomegalovirus. Viral pneumonia also can be a complication of another viral illness, such as chickenpox or measles (spread from the blood). Viruses destroy the ciliated epithelial cells and invade the goblet cells and bronchial mucous glands. Sloughing of destroyed bronchial epithelium occurs throughout the respiratory tract, preventing mucociliary clearance. Bronchial walls become edematous and infiltrated with leukocytes. In severe cases, the alveoli are involved with decreased compliance and increased work of breathing.

CLINICAL MANIFESTATIONS Many cases of pneumonia are preceded by a viral upper respiratory tract infection. Individuals then develop fever, chills, productive or dry cough, malaise, pleural pain, and sometimes dyspnea and hemoptysis. Physical examination may show signs of pulmonary consolidation, such as dullness to percussion, inspiratory crackles, increased tactile fremitus, egophony, and whispered pectoriloquy. Individuals also may demonstrate symptoms and signs of underlying systemic disease or sepsis.

EVALUATION AND TREATMENT Diagnosis is made on the basis of physical examination, white blood cell count, chest x-ray, stains and cultures of respiratory tract secretions, and blood cultures. The white blood cell count is usually elevated, although it may be low if the individual is debilitated or immunocompromised. Serum biologic markers are increasingly being used to differentiate bacterial from other causes of pneumonia (see *Health Alert:* Serum Biomarkers for the Diagnosis of Pneumonia). Chest radiographs show infiltrates that may involve a single lobe of the lung or may be more diffuse. Once the diagnosis of pneumonia has been made, the pathogen is identified by means of sputum characteristics (Gram stain, color, odor) and cultures or, if sputum is absent, blood cultures. Because many pathogens exist in the normal oropharyngeal flora, the specimen may be contaminated with pathogens from oral secretions. If sputum studies fail to identify the pathogen, the individual is immunocompromised, or the individual's condition worsens, further diagnostic studies may include bronchoscopy or lung biopsy. Positive identification of viruses can be difficult. Blood cultures often help to identify the virus if systemic disease is present.

Prevention of pneumonia includes prevention of aspiration, respiratory isolation of immunocompromised individuals, and vaccination for appropriate populations. The first step in the management of pneumonia is establishing adequate ventilation and oxygenation. Adequate hydration and good pulmonary hygiene (e.g., deep breathing, coughing, chest physical therapy) also are important. Antibiotics are used to treat bacterial pneumonia; however, resistant strains of pneumococci, staphylococci, and gram-negative bacteria are becoming more prevalent.[56,57] Empiric antibiotics are chosen based on the likely causative microorganism, although the toxicity of using multiple broad-spectrum antibiotics must be considered.[58] Viral pneumonia is usually treated with supportive therapy alone; however, antivirals

Serum Biomarkers for the Diagnosis of Pneumonia

Measurement of serum biomarkers can help to determine the infectious etiology of pneumonia. The two most widely used biomarkers are procalcitonin (PCT) and C-reactive protein (CRP). PCT is produced by the liver, kidneys, and monocytes after stimulation by proinflammatory cytokines and by bacterial products. CRP is produced by the liver in response to proinflammatory cytokines. In individuals with pneumonia, low levels of PCT (<0.1 mcg/L) or CRP (<40 mg/L) make bacterial infection unlikely, suggesting either viral, fungal, or noninfectious causes for the individual's symptoms. An increase in the levels of serum PCT (>1.0 mcg/L) or CRP (>200 mg/L) makes bacterial infection highly likely. Recent studies suggest that measurement of low procalcitonin levels prevents the inappropriate use of antibiotics for nonbacterial pneumonia. Other serum biomarkers, such as interleukin-1β, interleukin-8, proadrenomedullin, pro-atrial natriuretic peptide, pro-vasopressin, and copeptin, are being explored.

Data from Bellmann-Weiler R et al: Clinical potential of C-reactive protein and procalcitonin serum concentrations to guide differential diagnosis and clinical management of pneumococcal and Legionella pneumonia, *J Clin Microbiol* 48(5):1915–1917, 2010; Brown JS: Biomarkers and community-acquired pneumonia, *Thorax* 64(7):556–558, 2009; Conway Morris A et al: Diagnostic importance of pulmonary interleukin-1beta and interleukin-8 in ventilator-associated pneumonia, *Thorax* 65(3):201–207, 2010; Heppner HJ et al: Procalcitonin: inflammatory biomarker for assessing the severity of community-acquired pneumonia—a clinical observation in geriatric patients, *Gerontology* 56(4):385–389, 2010; Kruger S et al: Pro-atrial natriuretic peptide and pro-vasopressin for predicting short-term and long-term survival in community-acquired pneumonia: results from the German Competence Network CAPNETZ, *Thorax* 65(3):208–214, 2010; Torres A, Rello J: Update in community-acquired and nosocomial pneumonia 2009, *Am J Respir Crit Care Med* 181(8):782–787, 2010.

may be needed in severe cases. Infections with opportunistic microorganisms may be polymicrobial and require multiple drugs, including antifungals.

Tuberculosis

Tuberculosis (TB) is an infection caused by *Mycobacterium tuberculosis,* an acid-fast bacillus that usually affects the lungs but may invade other body systems. Tuberculosis is the leading cause of death from a curable infectious disease in the world. TB cases increased greatly during the mid-1990s as a result of acquired immunodeficiency syndrome (AIDS). Emigration of infected individuals from high-prevalence countries, transmission in crowded institutional settings, homelessness, substance abuse, and lack of access to medical care also have contributed to the spread of TB.

PATHOPHYSIOLOGY Tuberculosis is highly contagious and is transmitted from person to person in airborne droplets.[59] In immunocompetent individuals, the microorganism is usually contained by the inflammatory and immune response systems. This results in latent TB infection (LTBI) and is associated with no clinical evidence of disease. Microorganisms lodge in the lung periphery, usually in the upper lobe. Some bacilli migrate through the lymphatics and become lodged in the lymph nodes, where they encounter lymphocytes and initiate the immune response.

Once the bacilli are inspired into the lung, they multiply and cause localized nonspecific pneumonitis (lung inflammation). Inflammation in the lung causes activation of alveolar macrophages and neutrophils.

These phagocytes engulf the bacilli and begin the process by which the body's defense mechanisms isolate the bacilli, preventing them from spreading. The neutrophils and macrophages seal off the colonies of bacilli, forming a granulomatous lesion called a *tubercle* (see Chapter 5). Infected tissues within the tubercle die, forming cheeselike material called *caseation necrosis.* Collagenous scar tissue then grows around the tubercle, completing isolation of the bacilli. The immune response is complete after about 10 days, preventing further multiplication of the bacilli.

Once the bacilli are isolated in tubercles and immunity develops, tuberculosis may remain dormant for life. If the immune system is impaired, reactivation with progressive disease occurs and may spread through the blood and lymphatics to other organs. Infection with human immunodeficiency virus (HIV) is the single greatest risk factor for reactivation of tuberculosis infection. Cancer, immunosuppressive medications (e.g., corticosteroids), poor nutritional status, and renal failure can also reactivate disease.[59]

CLINICAL MANIFESTATIONS LTBI is asymptomatic. Symptoms of active disease often develop so gradually that they are not noticed until the disease is advanced. Common clinical manifestations include fatigue, weight loss, lethargy, anorexia (loss of appetite), and a low-grade fever that usually occurs in the afternoon. A cough that produces purulent sputum develops slowly and becomes more frequent over several weeks or months. Night sweats and general anxiety are often present. Dyspnea, chest pain, and hemoptysis may occur as the disease progresses. Extrapulmonary TB disease is common in HIV-infected individuals and may cause neurologic deficits, meningitis symptoms, bone pain, and urinary symptoms.

EVALUATION AND TREATMENT Tuberculosis is diagnosed by a positive tuberculin skin test (TST; purified protein derivative [PPD]), sputum culture, immunoassays, and chest radiographs.[60] A positive skin test indicates the need for yearly chest radiographs to detect active disease. When active pulmonary disease is present, the tubercle bacillus can be cultured from the sputum and may be seen with an acid-fast stain. However, sputum culture can take up to 6 weeks to become positive.

Treatment consists of antibiotic therapy to control active disease or prevent reactivation of LTBI. Recommended treatment includes a combination of as many as four different drugs to which the organism is susceptible. Side effects are common and new drugs are being explored.[61] Two worrisome treatment categories of TB have become more prevalent in recent years. "Multidrug-resistant TB" now accounts for approximately 5% of cases worldwide. Even more concerning is the emergence of "extensively drug-resistant TB" for which finding effective treatment is even more difficult.[62,63]

Acute Bronchitis

Acute bronchitis is acute infection or inflammation of the airways or bronchi and is usually self-limiting. In the vast majority of cases, acute bronchitis is caused by viruses. Bacterial bronchitis is rare in healthy adults but is common in individuals with COPD. Although many of the clinical manifestations are similar to those of pneumonia (i.e., fever, cough, chills, malaise), chest radiographs show no infiltrates. Individuals with viral bronchitis present with a nonproductive cough that often occurs in paroxysms and is aggravated by cold, dry, or dusty air. In some cases, purulent sputum is produced. Chest pain often develops from the effort of coughing. Treatment consists of rest, aspirin, humidity, and a cough suppressant, such as codeine. Bacterial bronchitis is treated with rest, antipyretics, humidity, and antibiotics.

Abscess Formation and Cavitation

An abscess is a circumscribed area of suppuration and destruction of lung parenchyma. Abscess formation follows consolidation of lung tissue, in which inflammation causes alveoli to fill with fluid, pus, and microorganisms. Aspiration abscess can occur from aspiration of anaerobes, such as those found in individuals who have pneumonia or who are infected with *Klebsiella* or *Staphylococcus*. Aspiration abscess is usually associated with alcohol abuse, seizure disorders, general anesthesia, and swallowing disorders. Necrosis (death and decay) of consolidated tissue may progress proximally until it communicates with a bronchus. Cavitation is the process of the abscess emptying into a bronchus and cavity formation. Abscess communication with a bronchus causes production of copious amounts of often foul-smelling sputum, and occasionally hemoptysis. Other clinical manifestations include fever, cough, chills, and pleural pain. The diagnosis is made by chest radiography. Treatment includes appropriate antibiotics and chest physical therapy (chest percussion and postural drainage). Bronchoscopy may be performed to drain the abscess.

> ✔ **QUICK CHECK 26-5**
> 1. Compare pneumococcal and viral pneumonia as to severity of disease.
> 2. Describe the pathophysiologic features of tuberculosis.
> 3. How does lung abscess present clinically?

Pulmonary Vascular Disease

Blood flow through the lungs can be disrupted by disorders that occlude the vessels, increase pulmonary vascular resistance, or destroy the vascular bed. Effects of altered pulmonary blood flow may range from insignificant dysfunction to severe and life-threatening changes in ventilation-perfusion ratios. Major disorders include pulmonary embolism, pulmonary hypertension, and cor pulmonale.

Pulmonary Embolism

Pulmonary embolism (PE) is occlusion of a portion of the pulmonary vascular bed by an embolus. PE most commonly results from embolization of a clot from deep venous thrombosis involving the lower leg (see Chapter 23). Other less common emboli include tissue fragments, lipids (fats), a foreign body, or an air bubble. Risk factors for PE include conditions and disorders that promote blood clotting as a result of venous stasis (immobilization, heart failure), hypercoagulability (inherited coagulation disorders, malignancy, hormone replacement therapy, oral contraceptives), and injuries to the endothelial cells that line the vessels (trauma, caustic intravenous infusions). Genetic risks include factor V Leiden, antithrombin II, protein S, protein C, and prothrombin gene mutations. No matter its source, a blood clot becomes an embolus when all or part of it detaches from the site of formation and begins to travel in the bloodstream.

PATHOPHYSIOLOGY The impact or effect of the embolus depends on the extent of pulmonary blood flow obstruction, the size of the affected vessels, the nature of the embolus, and the secondary effects. Pulmonary emboli can occur as any of the following:
1. *Embolus with infarction:* an embolus that causes infarction (death) of a portion of lung tissue
2. *Embolus without infarction:* an embolus that does not cause permanent lung injury (perfusion of the affected lung segment is maintained by the bronchial circulation)
3. *Massive occlusion:* an embolus that occludes a major portion of the pulmonary circulation (i.e., main pulmonary artery embolus)
4. *Multiple pulmonary emboli:* multiple emboli may be chronic or recurrent

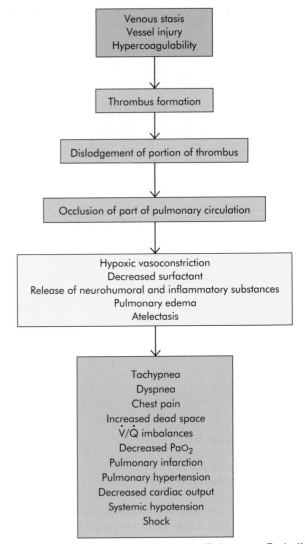

FIGURE 26-14 Pathogenesis of Massive Pulmonary Embolism Caused by a Thrombus (Pulmonary Thromboembolism).

Significant obstruction of the pulmonary vasculature leads to increased pulmonary artery pressures (pulmonary hypertension). The pathogenesis of pulmonary embolism caused by a thrombus is summarized in Figure 26-14.

If the embolus does not cause infarction, the clot is dissolved by the fibrinolytic system and pulmonary function returns to normal. If pulmonary infarction occurs, shrinking and scarring develop in the affected area of the lung.

CLINICAL MANIFESTATIONS In most cases, the clinical manifestations of PE are nonspecific, so evaluation of risk factors and predisposing factors is an important aspect of diagnosis. Although most emboli originate from clots in the lower extremities, deep vein thrombosis is often asymptomatic, and clinical examination has low sensitivity for the presence of clot, especially in the thigh.

An individual with PE usually presents with the sudden onset of pleuritic chest pain, dyspnea, tachypnea, tachycardia, and unexplained anxiety. Occasionally syncope (fainting) or hemoptysis occurs. With large emboli, a pleural friction rub, pleural effusion, fever, and leukocytosis may be noted. Recurrent small emboli may not be detected until progressive incapacitation, precordial pain, anxiety, dyspnea, and right ventricular enlargement are exhibited. Massive occlusion causes severe pulmonary hypertension and shock.

EVALUATION AND TREATMENT   Routine chest radiographs and pulmonary function tests are not definitive for pulmonary embolism. Arterial blood gas analyses usually demonstrate hypoxemia and hyperventilation (respiratory alkalosis). The diagnosis is made by measuring elevated levels of D-dimer in the blood in combination with scanning using spiral computed tomography (CT). Serum brain natriuretic peptide levels are increased in PE and levels are correlated with the severity of associated hemodynamic complications.[64]

Prevention of PE depends on elimination of predisposing factors for individuals at risk. Venous stasis in hospitalized persons is minimized by leg elevation, bed exercises, position changes, early postoperative ambulation, and pneumatic calf compression. Clot formation is also prevented by prophylactic low-dose anticoagulant therapy usually with low-molecular-weight heparin or warfarin. Newer medications such as the antithrombotics fondaparinux, idraparinux, and ximelagatran are superior to standard prevention in high-risk individuals undergoing orthopedic surgery.

Anticoagulant therapy is the primary treatment for pulmonary embolism. Initial anticoagulant therapy usually includes low-molecular-weight heparins (e.g., enoxaparin), fondaparinux, or unfractionated heparin.[64,65] If a massive life-threatening embolism occurs, a fibrinolytic agent, such as streptokinase, is sometimes used, and some individuals will require surgical thrombectomy. After stabilization, coumadin or low-molecular-weight heparin is continued for several months.

Pulmonary Hypertension

Pulmonary hypertension is defined as a mean pulmonary artery pressure >25 mm Hg. Pulmonary hypertension is classified into several categories[66]:

1. Pulmonary arterial hypertension (PAH) that is idiopathic, heritable, drug or toxin induced (weight loss medications, amphetamines, cocaine), or associated with other conditions, such as HIV infection and collagen vascular diseases
2. Pulmonary hypertension associated with left heart diseases (discussed in Chapters 23 and 24)
3. Pulmonary hypertension associated with lung respiratory disease or hypoxia, or both
4. Chronic thromboembolic pulmonary hypertension
5. Pulmonary hypertension with unclear and/or multifactorial mechanisms

PATHOPHYSIOLOGY   *Idiopathic pulmonary arterial hypertension (IPAH)* is a rare condition and usually occurs in women between the ages of 20 and 40. IPAH is characterized by endothelial dysfunction with overproduction of vasoconstrictors, such as thromboxane and endothelin, and decreased production of vasodilators, such as prostacyclin. Vascular growth factors are released that cause changes in the vascular smooth wall called *remodeling*. Angiotensin II, serotonin, electrolyte transporter mechanisms, and nitric oxide also play a role in the pathogenesis of this disorder. Together, this results in fibrosis and thickening of vessel walls (arteriopathy) with luminal narrowing and abnormal vasoconstriction.[67] These changes cause resistance to pulmonary artery blood flow, thus increasing the pressure in the pulmonary arteries. As resistance and pressure increase, the workload of the right ventricle increases and subsequent right ventricular hypertrophy, followed by failure, may occur (*cor pulmonale*).

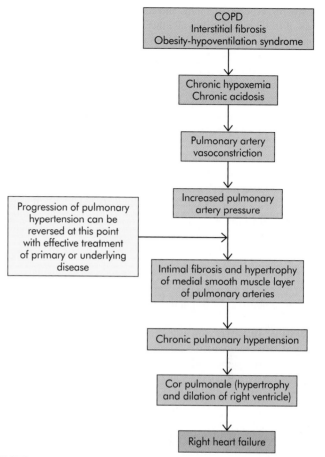

FIGURE 26-15 Pathogenesis of Pulmonary Hypertension and Cor Pulmonale.

Pulmonary hypertension associated with lung respiratory disease or hypoxia, or both, is a serious complication of many acute and chronic pulmonary disorders, such as COPD, fibrosis, and hypoventilation associated with obesity. These conditions are complicated by hypoxic pulmonary vasoconstriction that further increases pulmonary artery pressures. Acute pulmonary hypertension will resolve if the underlying condition can be reversed quickly. In chronic conditions where hypertension persists, hypertrophy occurs in the medial smooth muscle layer of the arterioles. The larger arteries stiffen and hypertension progresses, causing right ventricular hypertrophy and eventually cor pulmonale. The pathogenesis of pulmonary hypertension and cor pulmonale resulting from disease of the respiratory system is shown in Figure 26-15.

CLINICAL MANIFESTATIONS   Pulmonary hypertension may not be detected until it is quite severe. The symptoms are often masked by other forms of pulmonary or cardiovascular disease. The first indication of pulmonary hypertension may be an abnormality seen on a chest radiograph (enlarged right heart border) or an electrocardiogram that shows right ventricular hypertrophy. Manifestations of fatigue, chest discomfort, tachypnea, and dyspnea (particularly with exercise) are common. Examination may reveal peripheral edema, jugular venous distention, a precordial heave, and accentuation of the pulmonary component of the second heart sound.

EVALUATION AND TREATMENT   Definitive diagnosis of pulmonary hypertension can be made only with right heart catheterization. Common diagnostic modalities used to determine the cause include chest x-ray, echocardiography, and computed tomography. The diagnosis of IPAH is made when all other causes of pulmonary hypertension have been ruled out. Individuals with IPAH should be advised to continue physical activity within symptom limits, and oxygen therapy should be used for advanced stages. Diuretics, anticoagulants, digitalis, and calcium channel blockers may be used as general supportive therapy. Prostacyclin analogs (epoprostenol, beraprost, iloprost) and endothelin-receptor antagonists (ambrisentan, sitaxsentan, bosentan) have been shown to reduce pulmonary artery pressures and improve symptoms.[66] Recent studies suggest that hydroxymethylglutaryl-coenzyme A (HMG-CoA) reductase inhibitors (statins) may also be helpful.[67] Those individuals who do not achieve adequate clinical remission may require lung transplantation.

The most effective treatment for pulmonary hypertension associated with lung respiratory disease or hypoxia, or both, is treatment of the primary disorder. Supplemental oxygen may be indicated to reverse hypoxic vasoconstriction.

Cor Pulmonale

Cor pulmonale is defined as right ventricular enlargement (hypertrophy, dilation, or both) caused by pulmonary hypertension (see Figure 26-15).

PATHOPHYSIOLOGY Cor pulmonale develops as pulmonary hypertension exerts chronic pressure overload in the right ventricle. Pressure overload increases the work of the right ventricle and causes hypertrophy of the normally thin-walled heart muscle. This eventually progresses to dilation and failure of the ventricle.

CLINICAL MANIFESTATIONS The clinical manifestations of cor pulmonale may be obscured by underlying respiratory or cardiac disease and appear only during exercise testing. The heart may appear normal at rest, but with exercise, cardiac output falls. The electrocardiogram may show right ventricular hypertrophy. The pulmonary component of the second heart sound, which represents closure of the pulmonic valve, may be accentuated, and a pulmonic valve murmur also may be present. Tricuspid valve murmur may accompany the development of right ventricular failure. Increased pressures in the systemic venous circulation cause jugular venous distention, hepatosplenomegaly, and peripheral edema.

EVALUATION AND TREATMENT Diagnosis is based on physical examination, radiologic examination, electrocardiogram, and echocardiography. The goal of treatment for cor pulmonale is to decrease the workload of the right ventricle by lowering pulmonary artery pressure. Treatment is the same as that for pulmonary hypertension, and its success depends on reversal of the underlying lung disease.

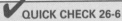

QUICK CHECK 26-6
1. What factors influence the impact of an embolus?
2. List three causes of pulmonary hypertension.
3. What is cor pulmonale?

Malignancies of the Respiratory Tract
Lip Cancer

Cancer of the lip is more prevalent in men, with 3000 new cases per year.[68] Long-term exposure to sun, wind, and cold over a period of years results in dryness, chapping, hyperkeratosis, and predisposition to malignancy. In addition, immunosuppression, such as that seen in individuals with renal transplants, increases the risk for lip cancer. The lower lip is the most common site.

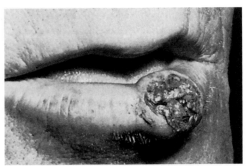

FIGURE 26-16 Lip Cancer. Carcinoma of lower lip with central ulceration and raised, rolled borders. (From del Regato JA, Spjut HJ, Cox JD: *Ackerman and del Regato's cancer*, ed 2, St Louis, 1985, Mosby.)

BOX 26-1 STAGING OF LIP CANCER

Stage I
Primary tumor less than 2 cm: no palpable nodes

Stage II
Primary tumor 2 to 4 cm; no palpable nodes

Stage III
Primary tumor >4 cm; metastasis to lymph nodes

Stage IV
Large primary tumors; nodes fixed to mandible or distant metastases

---

PATHOPHYSIOLOGY The most common form of lower lip cancer is termed *exophytic*. The lesion usually develops in the outer part of the lip along the vermilion border. The lip becomes thickened and evolves to an ulcerated center with a raised border (Figure 26-16). Verrucous-type lesions are less common. They have an irregular surface, follow cracks in the lip, and tend to extend toward the inner surface. Squamous cell carcinoma is the most common cell type. Basal cell carcinoma does not develop unless there is extension from the mucous membrane or vermilion border of the lip.

CLINICAL MANIFESTATIONS Malignant lesions are often preceded by the development of a blister that evolves into a superficial ulceration that may bleed. Metastases to the cervical lymph nodes have a low rate of occurrence (2% to 8%) and are more likely when the primary lesion is larger and exists for a longer period.

EVALUATION AND TREATMENT Diagnosis is commonly made by clinical history and examination of the lesion. Biopsy confirms the presence of malignant cells. The staging for lip cancer is summarized in Box 26-1. Surgical excision is usually effective for smaller lesions. Larger lesions that require extensive resection may need subsequent cosmetic surgeries. Interstitial irradiation and radioactive implants have proven effective for control of primary lesions. The prognosis for recovery is excellent.

Laryngeal Cancer

Cancer of the larynx represents approximately 2% to 3% of all cancers in the United States, with more than 12,000 new cases diagnosed in 2010.[68] The primary risk factor for laryngeal cancer is tobacco smoking; risk is further heightened with the combination of smoking and alcohol consumption. The human papillomavirus (HPV) also has been

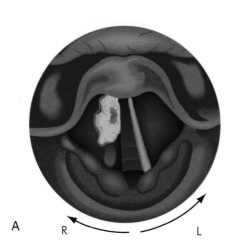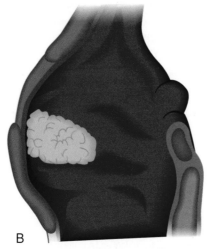

FIGURE 26-17 Laryngeal Cancer. **A,** Mirror view of carcinoma of the right false cord partially hiding the true cord. **B,** Lateral view. (Redrawn from del Regato JA, Spjut HJ, Cox JD: *Ackerman and del Regato's cancer,* ed 2, St Louis, 1985, Mosby.)

linked to both benign and malignant disease of the larynx.[69] The highest incidence is in men between 50 and 75 years of age.

PATHOPHYSIOLOGY Carcinoma of the true vocal cords (glottis) is more common than that of the supraglottic structures (epiglottis, aryepiglottic folds, arytenoids, false cords). Tumors of the subglottic area are rare. Squamous cell carcinoma is the most common cell type, although small cell carcinomas also occur (Figure 26-17). Metastasis develops by spread to the draining lymph nodes, and distant metastasis is rare.

CLINICAL MANIFESTATIONS The presenting symptoms of laryngeal cancer include hoarseness, dyspnea, and cough. Progressive hoarseness can result in voice loss. Dyspnea is rare with supraglottic tumors but can be severe in subglottic tumors. Cough may follow swallowing. Laryngeal pain is likely with supraglottic lesions.

EVALUATION AND TREATMENT Evaluation of the larynx includes external inspection and palpation of the larynx and the lymph nodes of the neck. Indirect laryngoscopy provides a stereoscopic view of the structure and movement of the larynx. A biopsy also can be obtained during this procedure. Direct laryngoscopy provides more thorough visualization of the tumor. Computed tomography facilitates the identification of tumor boundaries and the degree of extension to surrounding tissue.

Combined chemotherapy and radiation can result in cure in selected cases; however, sequelae such as swallowing and speech difficulties may result. Endoscopic laser for partial laryngectomies is emerging as the preferred treatment for small supraglottic and subglottic malignancies.[70] Total laryngectomy is required when lesions are extensive and involve the cartilage. Swallowing and speech therapy after treatment can significantly improve recovery.

Lung Cancer

Lung cancers (bronchogenic carcinomas) arise from the epithelium of the respiratory tract. Therefore the term *lung cancer* excludes other pulmonary tumors, including sarcomas, lymphomas, blastomas, hematomas, and mesotheliomas. There were an estimated 222,000 new cases of lung cancer in the United States in 2010.[68] It is the most common cause of cancer death in the United States and is responsible for 31% of all cancer deaths in men and 26% of all cancer deaths in women. Overall 5-year survival remains low at 20%.

The most common cause of lung cancer is tobacco smoking. Smokers with obstructive lung disease (low FEV_1 measurements) are at even greater risk. Other risk factors for lung cancer include secondhand (environmental) smoke, occupational exposures to certain workplace toxins, radiation, and air pollution. Genetic risks include polymorphisms of the genes responsible for growth factor receptors, DNA repair, and detoxification of inhaled smoke.[71]

Types of lung cancer. Primary lung cancers arise from cells that line the bronchi within the lungs and are therefore called *bronchogenic carcinomas*. It is now believed that most of these cancers arise from mutated epithelial stem cells.[72] Although there are many types of lung cancer, they can be divided into two major categories: non–small cell lung carcinoma (NSCLC) and neuroendocrine tumors of the lung. The category of non–small cell lung carcinoma accounts for 75% to 85% of all lung cancers and can be subdivided into three types of lung cancer: squamous cell carcinoma, adenocarcinoma, and large cell undifferentiated carcinoma. Neuroendocrine tumors of the lung arise from the bronchial mucosa and include: small cell carcinoma, large cell neuroendocrine carcinoma, typical carcinoid and atypical carcinoid tumors.[73] Small cell carcinoma is the most common of these neuroendocrine tumors, accounting for 15% to 20% of all lung cancers. Characteristics of these tumors, including clinical manifestations, are listed in Table 26-3. Many cancers that arise in other organs of the body metastasize to the lungs; however, these are not considered lung cancers and are categorized by their primary site of origin.

Non–small cell lung cancer. Squamous cell carcinoma accounts for about 30% of bronchogenic carcinomas. These tumors are typically located near the hila and project into bronchi (Figure 26-18, *A*). Because of this central location, symptoms of nonproductive cough or hemoptysis are common. Pneumonia and atelectasis are often associated with squamous cell carcinoma (see Figure 26-18, *A*). Chest pain is a late symptom associated with large tumors. These tumors are often fairly well localized and tend not to metastasize until late in the course of the disease.

Adenocarcinoma (tumor arising from glands) of the lung constitutes 35% to 40% of all bronchogenic carcinomas (Figure 26-18, *B*).

TABLE 26-3   CHARACTERISTICS OF LUNG CANCERS

TUMOR TYPE	GROWTH RATE	METASTASIS	MEANS OF DIAGNOSIS	CLINICAL MANIFESTATIONS AND TREATMENT
Non–Small Cell Carcinoma				
Squamous cell carcinoma	Slow	Late; mostly to hilar lymph nodes	Biopsy, sputum analysis, bronchoscopy, electron microscopy, immunohistochemistry	Cough, hemoptysis, sputum production, airway obstruction, hypercalcemia; treated surgically, chemotherapy and radiation as adjunctive therapy
Adenocarcinoma	Moderate	Early; to lymph nodes, pleura, bone, adrenal glands, and brain	Radiography, fiberoptic bronchoscopy, electron microscopy	Pleural effusion; treated surgically, chemotherapy as adjunctive therapy
Large cell carcinoma	Rapid	Early and widespread	Sputum analysis, bronchoscopy, electron microscopy (by exclusion of other cell types)	Chest wall pain, pleural effusion, cough, sputum production, hemoptysis, airway obstruction resulting in pneumonia; treated surgically
Neuroendocrine Tumors of the Lung				
Small cell carcinoma	Very rapid	Very early; to mediastinum, lymph nodes, brain, bone marrow	Radiography, sputum analysis, bronchoscopy, electron microscopy, immunohistochemistry	Cough, chest pain, dyspnea, hemoptysis, localized wheezing, airway obstruction, signs and symptoms of excessive hormone secretion; treated by chemotherapy and ionizing radiation to thorax and central nervous system

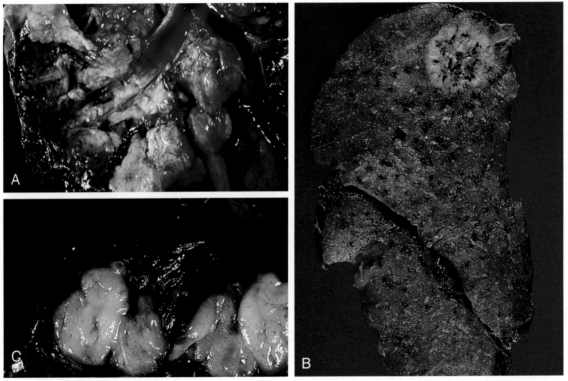

FIGURE 26-18 Lung Cancer. A, Squamous cell carcinoma. This hilar tumor originates from the main bronchus. **B,** Peripheral adenocarcinoma. The tumor shows prominent black pigmentation, suggestive of having evolved in an anthracotic scar. **C,** Small cell carcinoma. The tumor forms confluent nodules. On cross section, the nodules have an encephaloid appearance. (From Damjanov I, Linder J, editors: *Anderson's pathology,* ed 10, St Louis, 1996, Mosby.)

Pulmonary adenocarcinoma develops in a stepwise fashion through atypical adenomatous hyperplasia, adenocarcinoma in situ, and minimally invasive adenocarcinoma to invasive carcinoma.[74] These tumors, which are usually smaller than 4 cm, more commonly arise in the peripheral regions of the pulmonary parenchyma. They may be asymptomatic and discovered by routine chest roentgenogram in the early stages, or the individual may present with pleuritic chest pain and shortness of breath from pleural involvement by the tumor.

Included in the category of adenocarcinoma is bronchioloalveolar cell carcinoma. These tumors arise from terminal bronchioles and alveoli. They are slow-growing tumors with an unpredictable pattern of metastasis through the pulmonary arterial system and mediastinal lymph nodes.

Large cell carcinomas constitute 10% to 15% of bronchogenic carcinomas. This cell type has lost all evidence of differentiation and is therefore sometimes referred to as undifferentiated large cell anaplastic cancer. The cells are large and contain darkly stained nuclei. These tumors commonly arise centrally and can grow to distort the trachea and cause widening of the carina.

Small cell lung cancer. Small cell carcinomas are the most common type of neuroendocrine lung tumors. Most of these tumors are central in origin (Figure 26-18, C). Cell sizes range from 6 to 8 μm. Because these tumors show a rapid rate of growth and tend to metastasize early and widely, small cell carcinomas have the worst prognosis. Small cell carcinoma arises from neuroendocrine cells that contain neurosecretory granules; thus small cell carcinoma is often associated with ectopic hormone production. Ectopic hormone production is important to the clinician because resulting signs and symptoms (called *paraneoplastic syndromes*) may be the first manifestation of the underlying cancer. Small cell carcinomas most commonly produce antidiuretic hormone, resulting in the syndrome of inappropriate antidiuretic hormone secretion (SIADH). In other tumors, adrenocorticotropic hormone (ACTH) secretion leads to the development of Cushing syndrome. Signs and symptoms related to this condition include muscular weakness, facial edema, hypokalemia, alkalosis, hyperglycemia, hypertension, and increased pigmentation. Small cell lung cancer cells also can produce gastrin-releasing peptide and calcitonin.

PATHOPHYSIOLOGY Tobacco smoke contains more than 30 carcinogens and is responsible for causing 80% to 90% of lung cancers. These carcinogens, along with probable inherited genetic predisposition to cancers, result in multiple genetic abnormalities in bronchial cells including deletions of chromosomes, activation of oncogenes, and inactivation of tumor-suppressor genes. The most common genetic abnormality associated with lung cancer is loss of the tumor-suppressor gene *p53*.[71] Once lung cancer is initiated by these carcinogen-induced mutations, further tumor development is promoted by growth factors such as epidermal growth factor.

Repetitive exposure of the bronchial mucosa to tobacco smoke leads to epithelial cell changes that progress from metaplasia to carcinoma in situ, and finally to invasive carcinoma. Further tumor progression includes invasion of surrounding tissues and finally metastasis to distant sites including the brain, bone marrow, and liver.

CLINICAL MANIFESTATIONS Table 26-3 summarizes the characteristic clinical manifestations according to tumor type. By the time these symptoms are severe enough to motivate the individual to seek medical advice, the disease is usually advanced.

EVALUATION AND TREATMENT Diagnostic tests for the evaluation of lung cancer include chest x-ray, sputum cytologic studies, chest computed tomography, fiberoptic bronchoscopy, and biopsy. Low-dose helical computed tomography is emerging as a sensitive and specific diagnostic test. Biopsy determines the cell type, and the evaluation of lymph nodes and other organ systems is used to determine the stage of the cancer. The histologic cell type and the stage of the disease are the major factors that influence choice of therapy. The current accepted system for the staging of non–small cell cancer is the TNM classification (*T* denotes the extent of the primary tumor, *N* indicates the nodal involvement, *M* describes the extent of metastasis).[75]

The only proven way of reducing the risk for lung cancer is the cessation of smoking, although chemopreventive measures are being explored. Routine early screening modalities such as chest x-ray and computed tomography in asymptomatic individuals have not resulted in a decrease in lung cancer mortality. Serum biomarkers are being explored as a means for detecting lung cancer at earlier stages and for helping to choose appropriate treatments.[76]

For all types of early-stage lung carcinoma, the preferred treatment is surgical resection. Once metastasis has occurred, total surgical resection is more difficult and survival rates dramatically decrease. For individuals with non–small cell carcinoma, adjunctive radiation and chemotherapy may improve outcomes.[77] New treatment modalities, such as dose-intensified radiation radiofrequency ablation and microwave ablation, may be available as primary or palliative treatment for those for whom surgical removal is not an option.[78] In advanced disease, palliative procedures (comfort measures) may be used to relieve obstructive pneumonitis or prevent recurrence of pleural effusion.

Only about 20% of individuals with small cell lung cancer present at an early stage and can be cured of their disease. The outcome for the remainder of affected individuals is extremely poor, and treatment is usually palliative.[79] Chemotherapy and radiation can significantly prolong life and relieve symptoms, but relapse is inevitable.[80] Research is in progress to improve treatment options (see *Health Alert:* Genetic and Immunologic Advancements in Lung Cancer Treatment).

HEALTH ALERT

Genetic and Immunologic Advancements in Lung Cancer Treatment

Although new chemotherapeutic agents have improved outcomes slightly in the management of lung cancer, overall survival rates remain poor and the toxicities of these regimens limit their use. New understandings of the genetic and immunologic features of lung cancer cells have led to new treatment options. Gene therapy is emerging as a way of restoring normal tumor-suppressor gene function (e.g., *p53*) and increasing tumor responsiveness to chemoradiation through gene transfer, restoring normal DNA methylation patterns, and altering microRNA function. Immunologic therapies include antibodies to epidermoid growth factor receptors (erlotinib, gefitinib, and cetuximab) and antiangiogenesis drugs. The effectiveness of these strategies is still being evaluated, but new knowledge is leading to opportunities for innovative treatment.

Data from Kotsakis A, Georgoulias V: Targeting epidermal growth factor receptor in the treatment of non-small-cell lung cancer, *Exp Opin Pharmacol* 11(14):2363–2389, 2010; Lin PY, Yu SL, Yang PC: MicroRNA in lung cancer, *Br J Cancer* 103(8):1144–1148, 2010; MacKinnon AC, Kopatz J, Sethi T: The molecular and cellular biology of lung cancer: identifying novel therapeutic strategies, *Br Med Bull* 95:47–61, 2010; Pao W, Chmielecki J: Rational, biologically based treatment of EGFR-mutant non-small-cell lung cancer, *Nat Rev Cancer* 10(11):760–774, 2010; Suzuki M, Yoshino I: Aberrant methylation in non-small cell lung cancer, *Surg Today* 40(7):602–607, 2010; Triano LR, Deshpande H, Gettinger SN: Management of patients with advanced non-small cell lung cancer: current and emerging options, *Drugs* 70(2):167–179, 2010; Tufman A, Huber RM: Biological markers in lung cancer: a clinician's perspective, *Cancer Biomark* 6(3–4):123–135, 2010; Vachani A et al: Gene therapy for mesothelioma and lung cancer, *Am J Respir Cell Mol Biol* 42(4):385–393, 2010.

✔ **QUICK CHECK 26-7**
1. What are the principal features of lip cancer?
2. Describe squamous cell carcinoma of the vocal cords.
3. Compare the causes and survival statistics of three types of lung cancer.

DID YOU UNDERSTAND?

Clinical Manifestations of Pulmonary Alterations

1. Dyspnea is the feeling of breathlessness and increased respiratory effort.
2. Coughing is a protective reflex that expels secretions and irritants from the lower airways.
3. Changes in the sputum volume, consistency, or color may indicate underlying pulmonary disease.
4. Hemoptysis is expectoration of bloody mucus.
5. Abnormal breathing patterns are adjustments made by the body to minimize the work of respiratory muscles. They include Kussmaul, obstructed, restricted, gasping, Cheyne-Stokes respirations, and sighing.
6. Hypoventilation is decreased alveolar ventilation caused by airway obstruction, chest wall restriction, or altered neurologic control of breathing and results in increased Pa_{CO_2} (hypercapnia).
7. Hyperventilation is increased alveolar ventilation produced by anxiety, head injury, or severe hypoxemia and causes decreased Pa_{CO_2} (hypocapnia).
8. Cyanosis is a bluish discoloration of the skin caused by desaturation of hemoglobin, polycythemia, or peripheral vasoconstriction.
9. Clubbing of the fingertips is associated with diseases that interfere with oxygenation of the tissues.
10. Chest pain can result from inflamed pleurae, trachea, bronchi, or respiratory muscles.
11. Hypoxemia is a reduced Pa_{O_2} caused by (a) decreased oxygen content of inspired gas, (b) hypoventilation, (c) diffusion abnormality, (d) ventilation-perfusion mismatch, or (e) shunting.

Disorders of the Chest Wall and Pleura

1. Chest wall compliance is diminished by obesity and kyphoscoliosis, which compress the lungs, and by neuromuscular diseases that impair chest wall muscle function.
2. Flail chest results from rib or sternal fractures that disrupt the mechanics of breathing.
3. Pneumothorax is the accumulation of air in the pleural space. It can be caused by spontaneous rupture of weakened areas of the pleura or can be secondary to pleural damage caused by disease, trauma, or mechanical ventilation.
4. Tension pneumothorax is a life-threatening condition caused by trapping of air in the pleural space.
5. Pleural effusion is the accumulation of fluid in the pleural space resulting from disorders that promote transudation or exudation from capillaries underlying the pleura or from blockage or injury to lymphatic vessels that drain into the pleural space.
6. Empyema is the presence of pus in the pleural space (infected pleural effusion) usually from lymphatic drainage from sites of bacterial pneumonia.

Pulmonary Disorders

1. Atelectasis is the collapse of alveoli resulting from compression of lung tissue or absorption of gas from obstructed alveoli.
2. Bronchiectasis is abnormal dilation of the bronchi secondary to another pulmonary disorder, usually infection or inflammation.
3. Inhalation of noxious gases or prolonged exposure to high concentrations of oxygen can damage the bronchial mucosa or alveolocapillary membrane and cause inflammation or acute respiratory failure.
4. Pneumoconiosis, which is caused by inhalation of dust particles in the workplace, can cause pulmonary fibrosis, increase susceptibility to lower airway infection, and initiate tumor formation.
5. Allergic alveolitis is an allergic or hypersensitivity reaction to many allergens.
6. Bronchiolitis is the inflammatory obstruction of small airways. It is most common in children.
7. Pulmonary fibrosis is excessive connective tissue in the lung that diminishes lung compliance; it may be idiopathic or caused by disease.
8. Pulmonary edema is excess water in the lung caused by increased capillary hydrostatic pressure, decreased capillary oncotic pressure, or increased capillary permeability. A common cause is left heart failure that increases capillary hydrostatic pressure in the pulmonary circulation.
9. Acute respiratory distress syndrome (ARDS) results from an acute, diffuse injury to the alveolocapillary membrane and decreased surfactant production, which increases membrane permeability and causes edema and atelectasis.
10. Obstructive lung disease is characterized by airway obstruction that causes difficult expiration. Obstructive disease can be acute or chronic and includes asthma, chronic bronchitis, and emphysema.
11. Asthma is an inflammatory disease of the airways resulting from a type I hypersensitivity immune response involving the activity of antigen, IgE, mast cells, eosinophils, and other inflammatory cells and mediators.
12. In asthma, airway obstruction is caused by episodic attacks of bronchospasm, bronchial inflammation, mucosal edema, and increased mucus production.
13. Chronic obstructive pulmonary disease (COPD) is the coexistence of chronic bronchitis and emphysema and is an important cause of hypoxemic and hypercapnic respiratory failure.
14. Chronic bronchitis causes airway obstruction resulting from bronchial smooth muscle hypertrophy and production of thick, tenacious mucus.
15. In emphysema, destruction of the alveolar septa and loss of passive elastic recoil lead to airway collapse and obstruct gas flow during expiration.
16. Pneumococcal pneumonia is an acute lung infection resulting in an inflammatory response with four phases: (a) consolidation, (b) red hepatization, (c) gray hepatization, and (d) resolution.
17. Viral pneumonia can be severe, but is more often an acute, self-limiting lung infection usually caused by the influenza virus.
18. Tuberculosis is a lung infection caused by *Mycobacterium tuberculosis* (tubercle bacillus). In tuberculosis, the inflammatory response proceeds to isolate colonies of bacilli by enclosing them in tubercles and surrounding the tubercles with scar tissue.
19. Pulmonary vascular diseases are caused by embolism or hypertension in the pulmonary circulation.
20. Pulmonary embolism is most often the result of embolism of part of a clot from deep venous thrombosis and causes $\dot{V}/\dot{Q}$ mismatch, hypoxemia, and pulmonary hypertension.
21. Pulmonary hypertension (pulmonary artery pressure >25 mm Hg) can be idiopathic or associated with left heart failure, lung disease, or recurrent pulmonary emboli.
22. Cor pulmonale is right ventricular enlargement or failure caused by pulmonary hypertension.
23. Laryngeal cancer occurs primarily in men and represents 2% to 3% of all cancers. Squamous cell carcinoma of the true vocal cords is most common and presents with a clinical symptom of progressive hoarseness.
24. Lung cancer, the most common cause of cancer death in the United States, is commonly caused by tobacco smoking.
25. Lung cancer cell types include non–small cell carcinoma (squamous cell, adenocarcinoma, and large cell) and neuroendocrine tumors (small cell carcinoma, large cell neuroendocrine carcinoma, typical carcinoid and atypical carcinoid tumors). Each type arises in a characteristic site or type of tissue, causes distinctive clinical manifestations, and differs in likelihood of metastasis and prognosis.

KEY TERMS

- Abscess 698
- Absorption atelectasis 685
- Acute bronchitis 697
- Acute lung injury (ALI) 687
- Acute respiratory distress syndrome (ARDS) 687
- Adenocarcinoma 701
- Alveolar dead space 681
- Aspiration 684
- Asthma 689
- Atelectasis 685
- Bronchiectasis 685
- Bronchiolitis 685
- Bronchiolitis obliterans 685
- Bronchiolitis obliterans organizing pneumonia (BOOP) 686
- Cavitation 698
- Cheyne-Stokes respiration 679
- Chronic bronchitis 693
- Chronic obstructive pulmonary disease (COPD) 691
- Clubbing 680
- Compression atelectasis 685
- Consolidation 695

- Cor pulmonale 700
- Cough 679
- Cyanosis 680
- Dyspnea 678
- Emphysema 693
- Empyema (infected pleural effusion) 684
- Extrinsic allergic alveolitis (hypersensitivity pneumonitis) 686
- Exudative effusion 684
- Flail chest 682
- Hemoptysis 679
- Hypercapnia 680
- Hyperventilation 680
- Hypocapnia 680
- Hypoventilation 679
- Hypoxemia 681
- Hypoxia 681
- Idiopathic pulmonary fibrosis (IPF) 686
- Kussmaul respiration (hyperpnea) 679
- Large cell carcinoma 702
- Laryngeal cancer 700
- Latent TB infection (LTBI) 697
- Lip cancer 700
- Lung cancer 701

- Open pneumothorax (communicating pneumothorax) 683
- Orthopnea 679
- Oxygen toxicity 686
- Paroxysmal nocturnal dyspnea (PND) 679
- Pleural effusion 684
- Pneumoconiosis 686
- Pneumonia 694
- Pneumothorax 682
- Pulmonary edema 686
- Pulmonary embolism (PE) 698
- Pulmonary fibrosis 686
- Pulmonary hypertension 699
- Pulsus paradoxus 690
- Respiratory failure 682
- Shunting 681
- Small cell carcinoma 703
- Squamous cell carcinoma 701
- Status asthmaticus 691
- Surfactant impairment 685
- Tension pneumothorax 684
- TNM classification 703
- Transudative effusion 684
- Tuberculosis (TB) 697

REFERENCES

1. American Thoracic Society: Dyspnea. Mechanisms, assessment, and management: a consensus statement, *Am J Respir Crit Care Med* 159:321–340, 1999.
2. Lepor NE, McCullough PA: Differential diagnosis and overlap of acute chest discomfort and dyspnea in the emergency department, *Rev Cardiovasc Med* 11(suppl 2):S13–S23, 2010.
3. Mason RJ, et al, editors: *Murray and Nadal's textbook of respiratory medicine*, ed 5, Philadelphia, 2010, Saunders.
4. Guyton AC, Hall JE, editors: *Textbook of medical physiology*, ed 12, Philadelphia, 2011, Saunders.
5. Ito T, et al: Hypertrophic pulmonary osteoarthropathy as a paraneoplastic manifestation of lung cancer, *J Thoracic Oncol* 5(7):976–980, 2010.
6. Brims FJ, Davies HE, Lee YC: Respiratory chest pain: diagnosis and treatment, *Med Clin North Am* 94(2):217–232, 2010.
7. Sundaram S, Tasker AD, Morrell NW: Familial spontaneous pneumothorax and lung cysts due to a Folliculin exon 10 mutation, *Eur Respir J* 33(6):1510–1512, 2009.
8. Kurihara M, et al: Latest treatments for spontaneous pneumothorax, *Gen Thoracic Cardiovasc Surg* 58(3):113–119, 2010.
9. Nakajima J: Surgery for secondary spontaneous pneumothorax, *Curr Opin Pulmon Med* 16(4):376–380, 2010.
10. Christie NA: Management of pleural space: effusions and empyema, *Surg Clin North Am* 90(5):919–934, 2010.
11. Lee SF, et al: Thoracic empyema: current opinions in medical and surgical management, *Curr Opin Pulmon Med* 16(3):194–200, 2010.
12. Sue Eisenstadt E: Dysphagia and aspiration pneumonia in older adults, *J Am Acad Nurse Pract* 22(1):17–22, 2010.
13. Hedenstierna G, Edmark L: Mechanisms of atelectasis in the perioperative period, *Best Pract Res Clin Anaesthesiol* 24(2):157–169, 2010.
14. Seitz AE, et al: Trends and burden of bronchiectasis-associated hospitalizations in the United States, 1993–2006, *Chest* 138(4):944–949, 2010.
15. Pandya CM, Soubani AO: Bronchiolitis obliterans following hematopoietic stem cell transplantation: a clinical update, *Clin Transplant* 24(3): 291–306, 2010.

16. du Bois RM: Strategies for treating idiopathic pulmonary fibrosis, *Nat Rev Drug Discov* 9(2):129–140, 2010.
17. Harari S, Caminati A: IPF: new insight on pathogenesis and treatment, *Allergy* 65(5):537–553, 2010.
18. Hayes D Jr, et al: Pathogenesis of bronchopulmonary dysplasia, *Respiration* 79(5):425–436, 2010.
19. Auten RL, Davis JM: Oxygen toxicity and reactive oxygen species: the devil is in the details, *Pediatr Res* 66(2):121–127, 2009.
20. Hoffman HM, Wanderer AA: Inflammasome and IL-1beta-mediated disorders, *Curr Allergy Asthma Rep* 10(4):229–235, 2010.
21. Girard M, Cormier Y: Hypersensitivity pneumonitis, *Curr Opin Allergy Clin Immunol* 10(2):99–103, 2010.
22. Bernard GR, et al: The American-European Consensus Conference on ARDS. Definitions, mechanisms, relevant outcomes, and clinical trial coordination, *Am J Respir Crit Care Med* 149:818–824, 1994.
23. Ware LB, Matthay MB: The acute respiratory distress syndrome, *N Engl J Med* 342(18):1334–1349, 2000.
24. Cehovic GA, Hatton KW, Fahy BG: Adult respiratory distress syndrome, *Int Anesthesiol Clin* 47(1):83–95, 2009.
25. Rocco PR, Dos Santos C, Pelosi P: Lung parenchyma remodeling in acute respiratory distress syndrome, *Minerva Anesthesiol* 75(12):730–740, 2009.
26. Fremont RD, et al: Acute lung injury in patients with traumatic injuries: utility of a panel of biomarkers for diagnosis and pathogenesis, *J Trauma-Injury* 68(5):1121–1127, 2010.
27. Frank AJ, Thompson BT: Pharmacological treatments for acute respiratory distress syndrome, *Curr Opin Crit Care* 16(1):62–68, 2010.
28. National Heart, Lung, and Blood Institute: National Asthma Education and Prevention Program Expert Panel Report 3: *Guidelines for the diagnosis and management of asthma*, 2007. Accessed March 13, 2011. Available at www.nhlbi.nih.gov/guidelines/asthma/asthgdln.pdf.
29. Centers for Disease Control and Prevention: *FastStatsL asthma* (updated Oct 27, 2010). Available at www.cdc.gov/nchs/fastats/asthma.htm.
30. Meyers DA: Genetics of asthma and allergy: what have we learned? *J Allergy Clin Immunol* 126(3):439–446, 2010.
31. Ho SM: Environmental epigenetics of asthma: an update, *J Allergy Clin Immunol* 126(3):453–465, 2010.

32. Long A: Aeroallergen sensitization in asthma: Genetics, environment, and pathophysiology, *Allergy Asthma Proc* 31(2):89–95, 2010.

33. Okada H, et al: The 'hygiene hypothesis' for autoimmune and allergic diseases: an update, *Clin Exp Immunol* 160(1):1–9, 2010.

34. Holt PG, Strickland DH: Interactions between innate and adaptive immunity in asthma pathogenesis: new perspectives from studies on acute exacerbations, *J Allergy Clin Immunol* 125(5):963–972, 2010.

35. Murphy DM, O'Byrne PM: Recent advances in the pathophysiology of asthma, *Chest* 137(6):1417–1426, 2010.

36. Busse WW: The relationship of airway hyperresponsiveness and airway inflammation: airway hyperresponsiveness in asthma: its measurement and clinical significance, *Chest* 138(suppl 2):4S–10S, 2010.

37. Alcorn JF, Crowe CR, Kolls JK: TH17 cells in asthma and COPD, *Annu Rev Physiol* 72:495–516, 2010.

38. Bai TR: Evidence for airway remodeling in chronic asthma, *Curr Opin Allergy Clin Immunol* 10(1):82–86, 2010.

39. Lazarus SC: Clinical practice. Emergency treatment of asthma, *N Engl J Med* 363(8):755–764, 2010.

40. Penagos M, et al: Metaanalysis of the efficacy of sublingual immunotherapy in the treatment of allergic asthma in pediatric patients, 3 to 18 years of age, *Chest* 133(3):599–609, 2008.

41. Global Strategy for the Diagnosis, Management, and Prevention of COPD: *Scientific information and recommendations for COPD programs* (updated 2010). Accessed March 13, 2011. Available at http://goldcopd.com/.

42. Ben-Zaken Cohen S, et al: The growing burden of chronic obstructive pulmonary disease and lung cancer in women: examining sex differences in cigarette smoke metabolism, *Am J Resp Crit Care Med* 176(2):113–120, 2007.

43. Wan ES, Silverman EK: Genetics of COPD and emphysema, *Chest* 136(3):859–866, 2009.

44. Voynow JA, Rubin BK: Mucins, mucus, and sputum, *Chest* 135(2):505–512, 2009.

45. Sethi S: Antibiotics in acute exacerbations of chronic bronchitis, *Exp Rev Antiinfect Ther* 8(4):405–417, 2010.

46. Aoshiba K, Nagai A: Senescence hypothesis for the pathogenetic mechanism of chronic obstructive pulmonary disease, *Proc Am Thoracic Soc* 6(7):596–601, 2009.

47. Lee TA, et al: Outcomes associated with tiotropium use in patients with chronic obstructive pulmonary disease, *Arch Intern Med* 169(15):1403–1410, 2009.

48. Barnes PJ: New therapies for chronic obstructive pulmonary disease, *Med Princ Pract* 19(5):330–338, 2010.

49. Burton DC, et al: Socioeconomic and racial/ethnic disparities in the incidence of bacteremic pneumonia among US adults, *Am J Public Health* 100(10):1904–1911, 2010.

50. Torres A, Rello J: Update in community-acquired and nosocomial pneumonia 2009, *Am J Resp Crit Care Med* 181(8):782–787, 2010.

51. Hidron AI, et al: Emergence of community-acquired methicillin-resistant *Staphylococcus aureus* strain USA3 00 as a cause of necrotising community-onset pneumonia, *Lancet Infect Dis* 9(6):384–392, 2009.

52. Klevens RM, et al: Invasive methicillin-resistant *Staphylococcus aureus* infections in the United States, *J Am Med Assoc* 298:1763–1771, 2007.

53. Lieberman D, et al: Respiratory viruses in adults with community-acquired pneumonia, *Chest* 138(4):811–816, 2010.

54. Van der Poll T, Opal SM: Pathogenesis, treatment, and prevention of pneumococcal pneumonia, *Lancet* 374:1543–1556, 2009.

55. Rothberg MB, Haessler SD: Complications of seasonal and pandemic influenza, *Crit Care Med* 38(suppl 4):e91–e97, 2010.

56. Falcone M, et al: Role of multidrug-resistant pathogens in health-care-associated pneumonia, *Lancet Infect Dis* 11:11–12, 2011.

57. Song JH, Chung DR: Respiratory infections due to drug-resistant bacteria, *Infect Dis Clin North Am* 24(3):639–653, 2010.

58. Kett DH, et al: Implementation of guidelines for management of possible multidrug-resistant pneumonia in intensive care: an observational, multicentre cohort study, *Lancet Infect Dis* 11(2):1–9, 2011.

59. Schlossberg D: Acute tuberculosis, *Infect Dis Clin North Am* 24(1):139–146, 2010.

60. Pai M, et al: New and improved tuberculosis diagnostics: evidence, policy, practice, and impact, *Curr Opin Pulmon Med* 16(3):271–284, 2010.

61. Leibert E, Rom WN: New drugs and regimens for treatment of TB, *Expert Rev Anti Infect Ther* 8(7):801–813, 2010.

62. Caminero JA, et al: Best drug treatment for multidrug-resistant and extensively drug-resistant tuberculosis, *Lancet Infect Dis* 10(9):621–629, 2010.

63. Dheda K, et al: Extensively drug-resistant tuberculosis: epidemiology and management challenges, *Infect Dis Clin North Am* 24(3):705–725, 2010.

64. Agnelli G, Becattini C: Acute pulmonary embolism, *N Engl J Med* 363(3):266–274, 2010.

65. Bounameaux H: Contemporary management of pulmonary embolism: the answers to ten questions, *J Intern Med* 268(3):218–231, 2010.

66. Galie N, et al: Guidelines for the diagnosis and treatment of pulmonary hypertension: the task force for the diagnosis and treatment of pulmonary hypertension of the European Society of Cardiology (ESC) and the European Respiratory Society (ERS), endorsed by the International Society of Heart and Lung Transplantation (ISHLT), *Eur Heart J* 30:2493–2537, 2009.

67. Firth AL, Mandel J, Yuan JX: Idiopathic pulmonary arterial hypertension, *Dis Models Mech* 3(5–6):268–273, 2010.

68. American Cancer Society: *Cancer facts and figures*, 2010. Available at http://www.cancer.org/acs/groups/content/@nho/documents/document/acspc-024113.pdf. Accessed May 18, 2011.

69. Stelow EB, et al: Human papillomavirus-associated squamous cell carcinoma of the upper aerodigestive tract, *Am J Surg Pathol* 34(7):e15–e24, 2010.

70. Grant DG, et al: Transoral laser microsurgery for early laryngeal cancer, *Expert Rev Anticancer Ther* 10(3):331–338, 2010.

71. Varella-Garcia M: Chromosomal and genomic changes in lung cancer, *Cell Adh Migr* 4(1):100–106, 2010.

72. Kratz JR, Yagui-Beltran A, Jablons DM: Cancer stem cells in lung tumorigenesis, *Ann Thorac Surg* 89(6):S2090–S2095, 2010.

73. Travis WD, et al: in collaboration with Sobin LH and Pathologists from 14 Countries: *World Health Organization international histological classification of tumours. Histological typing of lung and pleural tumours*, ed 3, Berlin, Heidelberg, New York, 1999, Springer-Verlag.

74. Noguchi M: Stepwise progression of pulmonary adenocarcinoma—clinical and molecular implications, *Cancer Metastasis Rev* 29(1):15–21, 2010.

75. Lababede O, Meziane M, Rice T: Seventh edition of the cancer staging manual and stage grouping of lung cancer, *Chest* 139(1):183–189, 2011.

76. Van't Westeinde SC, van Klaveren RJ: Screening and early detection of lung cancer, *Cancer J* 17(1):3–10, 2011.

77. Triano LR, Deshpande H, Gettinger SN: Management of patients with advanced non-small cell lung cancer: current and emerging options, *Drugs* 70(2):167–179, 2010.

78. Das M, et al: Alternatives to surgery for early stage non-small cell lung cancer-ready for prime time? *Curr Treat Options Oncol* 11(1-2):24–35, 2010.

79. Dowell JE: Small cell lung cancer: are we making progress? *Am J Med Sci* 339(1):68–76, 2010.

80. Ganti AK, et al: Current concepts in the diagnosis and management of small-cell lung cancer, *Oncology (Williston Park)* 24(11):1034–1039, 2010.

Alterations of Pulmonary Function in Children

Kristi K. Gott and Valentina L. Brashers

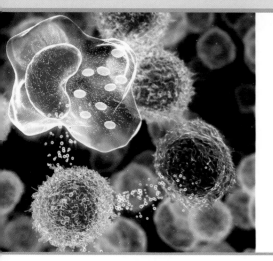

evolve WEBSITE

http://evolve.elsevier.com/Huether/
- Review Questions and Answers
- Animations
- Quick Check Answers

- Key Terms Exercises
- Critical Thinking Questions with Answers
- Algorithm Completion Exercises
- WebLinks

CHAPTER OUTLINE

Alterations of respiratory function in children are influenced by physiologic maturation, which is determined by age, genetics, and environmental conditions. Infants, especially premature infants, may present special problems because of incomplete development of the airways, circulation, chest wall, and immune system. A variety of upper and lower airway infections can cause respiratory compromise or play a role in the pathogenesis of more chronic pulmonary disease. Pulmonary dysfunction can be categorized into disorders of either the upper or the lower airways.

DISORDERS OF THE UPPER AIRWAYS

Disorders of the upper airways can cause significant obstruction to airflow. Common causes of upper airway obstruction in children are infections, foreign body aspiration, and obstructive sleep apnea.

Infections of the Upper Airways

Table 27-1 compares some of the more common upper airway infections.

Croup

Croup illnesses can be divided into three categories: (1) acute laryngotracheobronchitis (croup), (2) spasmodic croup, and (3) bacterial laryngotracheitis.[1] Diphtheria can also be considered a croup illness but is now rare because of vaccinations. Croup illnesses are all characterized by infection and obstruction of the upper airways.

Croup is an acute laryngotracheobronchitis and almost always occurs in children between 6 months and 5 years of age with a peak incidence at 2 years of age. In 85% of cases, croup is caused by a virus, most commonly parainfluenza and in other instances by influenza A, rhinovirus, or respiratory syncytial virus.[2,3] The incidence of croup is higher in males and is most common during the winter months. Approximately 15% of affected children have a strong family history of croup.[2] Spasmodic croup usually occurs in older children. The etiology is unknown although association with viruses, allergies, asthma, and gastroesophageal reflux disease (GERD) is being investigated.[2,3] Bacterial laryngotracheitis is the most common potentially life-threatening upper airway infection in children. It is most often caused by *Staphylococcus aureus (S. aureus)* (including methicillin-resistant

TABLE 27-1	COMPARISON OF UPPER AIRWAY INFECTIONS				
CONDITION	**AGE**	**ONSET**	**ETIOLOGY**	**PATHOPHYSIOLOGY**	**SYMPTOMS**
Acute laryngotracheo-bronchitis	6 mos to 3 yr	Usually gradual	Viral	Inflammation from larynx to bronchi	Harsh cough; stridor; low-grade fever; may have nasal discharge, conjunctivitis
Acute tracheitis	1 to 12 yr	Abrupt or following viral illness	*Staphylococcus aureus*	Inflammation of upper trachea	High fever; toxic appearance; harsh cough; purulent secretions
Acute epiglottitis	2 to 6 yr	Abrupt	*Haemophilus influenzae* group A streptococcus	Inflammation of supraglottic structures	Severe sore throat; dysphagia; high fever; toxic appearance; muffled voice; may drool; dyspnea; sits erect and quietly

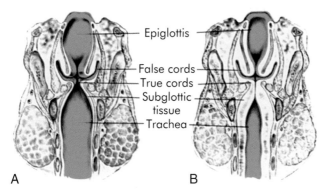

FIGURE 27-1 The Larynx and Subglottic Trachea. **A,** Normal trachea. **B,** Narrowing and obstruction from edema caused by croup. (From Hockenberry MJ et al: *Wong's nursing care of infants and children,* ed 9, St Louis, 2010, Mosby.)

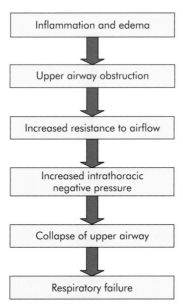

FIGURE 27-2 Upper Airway Obstruction With Croup.

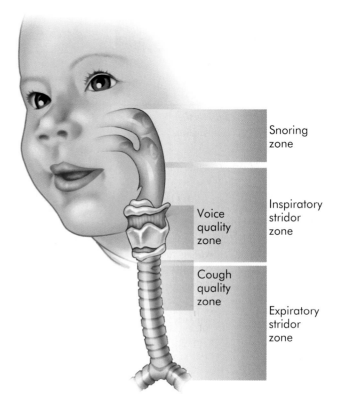

FIGURE 27-3 Listening Can Help Locate the Site of Airway Obstruction. A loud, gasping snore suggests enlarged tonsils or adenoids. In inspiratory stridor, the airway is compromised at the level of the supraglottic larynx, vocal cords, subglottic region, or upper trachea. Expiratory stridor results from a narrowing or collapse in the trachea or bronchi. Airway noise during both inspiration and expiration often represents a fixed obstruction of the vocal cords or subglottic space. Hoarseness or a weak cry is a by-product of obstruction at the vocal cords. If a cough is croupy, suspect constriction below the vocal cords. (Redrawn from Eavey RD: *Contemp Ped* 3[6]:79, 1986; original illustration by Paul Singh-Roy.)

S. aureus [MRSA] strains), *Haemophilus influenzae (H. influenzae),* or group A beta-hemolytic *Streptococcus* (GABHS).[1,4]

PATHOPHYSIOLOGY The pathophysiology of viral croup is caused primarily by subglottic inflammation and edema from the infection.[5] The mucous membranes of the larynx are tightly adherent to the underlying cartilage, whereas those of the subglottic space are looser and thus allow accumulation of mucosal and submucosal edema (Figure 27-1). Furthermore, the cricoid cartilage is structurally the narrowest point of the airway, making edema in this area critical. Spasmodic croup also causes obstruction but with less inflammation and edema. As illustrated in Figure 27-2, increased resistance to airflow leads to increased work of breathing, which generates more negative intrathoracic pressure that, in turn, may exacerbate dynamic collapse of the upper airway. In cases of bacterial laryngotracheitis, the presence of airway edema and copious purulent secretions leads to airway obstruction that can be worsened by the formation of a tracheal pseudomembrane and mucosal sloughing.[1,4]

CLINICAL MANIFESTATIONS Typically, the child experiences rhinorrhea, sore throat, and low-grade fever for a few days, and then develops a harsh (seal-like) barking cough, inspiratory stridor, and hoarse voice. The quality of voice, cough, and stridor may suggest the location of the obstruction (Figure 27-3). Most cases resolve spontaneously within 24 to 48 hours and do not warrant hospital admission. A child with severe croup usually displays deep retractions (Figure 27-4), stridor, agitation, tachycardia, and sometimes pallor or cyanosis.

Spasmodic croup is characterized by similar hoarseness, barking cough, and stridor. It is of sudden onset and usually occurs at night and without prodromal symptoms. It usually resolves quickly. Children with bacterial laryngotracheitis present with high fever, stridor, and increased secretions from the mouth and nose that progress over hours to days.

EVALUATION AND TREATMENT The degree of symptoms determines the level of treatment. The most common tool for estimating croup severity is the Westley croup score.[6] Most children with croup require no treatment; however, some cases require outpatient treatment. These children usually have only mild stridor or retractions and appear alert, playful, and able to eat. There has been much debate about the most effective outpatient treatments for croup. Common nonpharmacologic treatments include steam inhalation and ice masks, although there is no scientific evidence to support their use. Glucocorticoids—either injected, oral (dexamethasone), or nebulized (budesonide)—have been shown to improve symptoms. The presence of stridor at rest, moderate or severe retractions of the chest, or agitation suggests more severe disease and does require inpatient observation and treatment. For acute respiratory distress, nebulized epinephrine stimulates α- and β-adrenergic receptors and decreases mucosal edema and airway secretions.[7] Oxygen should be administered. Heliox (helium-oxygen mixture) also can be used in severe cases although it is not yet considered a mainstay of routine treatment. This works by improving gas flow and thus decreasing the flow resistance of the narrowed airway.[8] In rare cases croup and spasmodic croup may require placement of an endotracheal tube. Bacterial tracheobronchitis is treated with immediate administration of antibiotics and endotracheal intubation to prevent total upper airway obstruction.[1]

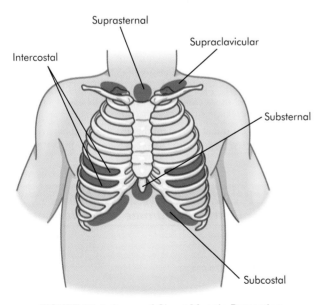

FIGURE 27-4 Areas of Chest Muscle Retraction.

Acute Epiglottitis

Historically, acute epiglottitis was caused by *H. influenzae* type B. Since the advent of *H. influenzae* vaccine, the overall incidence of acute epiglottitis has been reduced by 80% to 90%; however, up to 25% of epiglottitis cases are still caused by nontypeable strains of *H. influenzae*.[9] Current cases in children usually are related to vaccine failure or are caused by other pathogens, such as GABHS, *Streptococcus pneumoniae, Candida* species, *S. aureus*, MRSA, or viral pathogens.

PATHOPHYSIOLOGY The epiglottis arises from the posterior tongue base and covers the laryngeal inlet during swallowing. Bacterial invasion of the mucosa with associated inflammation leads to the rapid development of edema causing severe, life-threatening obstruction of the upper airway.[10]

CLINICAL MANIFESTATIONS In the classic form of the disease, a child between 2 and 7 years of age suddenly develops high fever, irritability, sore throat, inspiratory stridor, and severe respiratory distress. The child appears anxious and has a voice that sounds muffled ("hot potato" voice). Drooling and dysphagia (inability to swallow) are common. In addition to appearing ill, the child will generally adopt a position of leaning forward (tripoding) to try to improve breathing. Death can occur in a few hours. Nasotracheal intubation or tracheotomy is mandatory in instances of rapidly increasing obstruction. Pneumonia, cervical lymph node inflammation, otitis, and, rarely, meningitis or septic arthritis may occur concomitantly because of bacterial sepsis.

EVALUATION AND TREATMENT Acute epiglottitis is a life-threatening emergency. Efforts should be made to keep the child calm and undisturbed. Examination of the throat should not be attempted because it may trigger laryngospasm and cause respiratory collapse.[10] With severe airway obstruction, the airway may be secured with intubation and antibiotics are administered promptly. Racemic epinephrine and corticosteroids may be given until definitive management of the airway can be achieved.[10,11] Resolution with treatment is usually rapid. Postexposure prophylaxis with rifampin is recommended for all household contacts after a child is diagnosed.

Tonsillar Infections

Tonsillar infections (tonsillitis) are occasionally severe enough to cause upper airway obstruction. As with other infections of the upper airway, the incidence of tonsillitis secondary to GABHS (group A beta-hemolytic *Streptococcus*) and MRSA has risen in the past 15 years. Upper airway obstruction because of tonsillitis is a well-known complication of infectious mononucleosis, especially in a young child. Tonsillitis may be complicated by formation of a tonsillar abscess, which can further contribute to airway obstruction. The development of significant obstruction in tonsillar infections may require the use of corticosteroids, especially in the case of mononucleosis. The management of severe bacterial tonsillitis requires the use of antibiotics. Some children with recurrent tonsillitis benefit from tonsillectomy.[12]

Aspiration of Foreign Bodies

Aspiration of foreign bodies (FBs) into the airways usually occurs in children 1 to 3 years of age. More than 100,000 cases occur each year.[13] Most objects are expelled by the cough reflex, but some objects may lodge in the larynx, trachea, or bronchi. Large objects (e.g., a bite of hot dog, nuts, popcorn, grapes, beans, toy pieces, fragments of popped balloons, or coins) may occlude the airway and become life-threatening. Items of particular concern would be batteries and magnets. The aspiration event commonly is not witnessed or is not recognized when it happens because the coughing, choking, or gagging symptoms may resolve quickly. Foreign bodies lodged in the larynx or upper trachea cause cough, stridor, hoarseness or inability to speak, respiratory distress, and agitation or panic; the presentation is often dramatic and frightening. If the child is acutely hypoxic and unable to move air, immediate action such as sweeping the oral airway or performing abdominal thrusts (formerly called the Heimlich maneuver) may be required to prevent tragedy. Otherwise, bronchoscopic removal should be performed urgently. If an aspirated foreign body is small enough, it will be transferred to a bronchus before becoming lodged. If the foreign body is lodged in the airway for a notable period of time, local irritation, granulation, obstruction, and infection will ensue. Thus children may present with cough or wheezing, atelectasis, pneumonia, lung abscess, or blood-streaked sputum. These children are treated by prompt bronchoscopic removal of the object and administration of antibiotics as necessary.[14]

Obstructive Sleep Apnea

Obstructive sleep apnea syndrome (OSAS) is defined by partial or intermittent complete upper airway obstruction during sleep with disruption of normal ventilation and sleep patterns. Childhood OSAS is quite common, with an estimated prevalence of 2% to 3% of children 12 to 14 years of age and up to 13% of children between 3 and 6 years of age.[15,16] Prevalence is estimated to be two to four times higher in vulnerable populations (blacks, Hispanics, and preterm infants).[17] In children, unlike adults, OSAS occurs equally among girls and boys. Possible influences early in life may include passive smoke inhalation, socioeconomic status, and snoring together with genetic modifiers that promote airway inflammation. OSAS also is more likely to occur in children who have a history of a clinically significant episode of respiratory syncytial virus (RSV) bronchiolitis in infancy; this is believed to change the neuroimmunomodulatory pathways in the upper airway.[18]

PATHOPHYSIOLOGY By far the most common predisposing factor to OSAS in children is adenotonsillar hypertrophy, which causes physical impingement on the nasopharyngeal airway. OSAS also may occur in children who are overweight or obese, and in those with craniofacial anomalies (with structurally small nasopharyngeal airways) or reduced motor tone of the upper airways (as may be seen in neurologic disorders, cerebral palsy, and Down syndrome). Allergy and asthma also may contribute to this condition. Current research links sleep disordered breathing (SDB) with airway inflammation and elevated levels of C-reactive protein.[19] In addition, there are neuroimmunomodulatory responses that are changed in this condition, such as greater expression of nerve growth factor (NGF) and neurokinin 1 (NK1) receptor mRNA linked with protein concentrations.[16,20] Lastly, genetics may indeed play a role in the neurocognitive dysfunction associated with the condition.

CLINICAL MANIFESTATIONS There usually is a history of snoring and labored breathing during sleep, which may be continuous or intermittent. The child may also experience restlessness and sweating. There may be episodes of increased respiratory effort but no audible airflow, often terminated by snorting, gasping, repositioning, or arousal. Daytime sleepiness/napping is occasionally reported, as well as nocturnal enuresis. Often the child is a chronic mouth breather and has large tonsils. There is no correlation between sleep position and OSAS in children, except for those children who are notably obese. Obese children may adopt the prone position to attempt improved ventilation. Significant morbidity can result from the effects of OSAS, including cognitive and neurobehavioral impairment, excessive daytime sleepiness,

impaired school performance, and poor quality of life.[17] Left untreated OSAS also may cause cardiovascular and pulmonary disease, as well as insulin resistance and reduced somatic growth.

EVALUATION AND TREATMENT All parents should be asked if their child exhibits snoring, a symptom that is often not spontaneously reported to the healthcare provider. History and physical examination are key to diagnosis and a variety of screening tools are available. Radiographs of the upper airway may be used to rule out adenoidal hypertrophy.[21] The most definitive evaluation is the polysomnographic sleep study, which documents obstructed breathing and physiologic impairment. If obstructive sleep apnea is documented or strongly suspected clinically, children are most often referred for tonsillectomy and adenoidectomy (T & A) on the basis of described symptoms and physical findings, such as enlarged tonsils, adenoidal facies, and mouth breathing.[22] For severely affected children who do not respond to T & A or who have different problems, such as obesity, that cannot be remedied rapidly, continuous positive airway pressure (CPAP) may be delivered through a tight-fitting nasal mask used during sleep. Treatment is important to minimize associated morbidities.

> ✔ **QUICK CHECK 27-1**
> 1. Compare and contrast pathology, clinical presentations, and severity of croup and epiglottitis.
> 2. What symptoms indicate aspiration of a foreign body?
> 3. What signs and symptoms suggest obstructive sleep apnea?

DISORDERS OF THE LOWER AIRWAYS

A number of disorders of the lower respiratory tract are specific to children, such as newborn respiratory distress syndrome, bronchopulmonary dysplasia, and congenital malformations. Lower airway infections, such as viral bronchiolitis and bacterial pneumonia, occur fairly often in children. Chronic pulmonary conditions, such as asthma and cystic fibrosis, frequently first present clinically in childhood.

Respiratory Distress Syndrome of the Newborn

Respiratory distress syndrome (RDS) of the newborn (previously also called *hyaline membrane disease [HMD]*) is a significant cause of neonatal morbidity and mortality.[23] It occurs almost exclusively in premature infants and the incidence has increased in the United States over the past 2 decades.[24] RDS occurs in 50% to 60% of infants born at 29 weeks' gestation and decreases significantly by 36 weeks. Infants of diabetic mothers and those with cesarean delivery (especially elective C-section) also are more likely to develop RDS. It is more common in boys than girls and more common in whites than non-whites. Death rates have declined significantly since the introduction of antenatal steroid therapy and postnatal surfactant therapy. Risk factors are summarized in *Risk Factors:* Respiratory Distress Syndrome of the Newborn.

> **RISK FACTORS**
> ### *Respiratory Distress Syndrome of the Newborn*
> - Premature birth
> - Male gender
> - Cesarean delivery without labor
> - Diabetic mother
> - Perinatal asphyxia

PATHOPHYSIOLOGY   RDS is caused by surfactant deficiency, which decreases the alveolar surface area available for gas exchange. Surfactant is a lipoprotein with a detergent-like effect that separates the liquid molecules inside the alveoli, thereby decreasing alveolar surface tension. Without surfactant, alveoli collapse at the end of each exhalation. Surfactant normally is not secreted by the alveolar cells until approximately 30 weeks' gestation. In addition to surfactant deficiency, premature infants are born with underdeveloped and small alveoli that are difficult to inflate and have thick walls and inadequate capillary blood supply such that gas exchange is significantly impaired. Furthermore, the infant's chest wall is weak and highly compliant and, thus, the rib cage tends to collapse inward with respiratory effort. The net effect of all these adverse factors is *atelectasis* (collapsed alveoli), resulting in significant hypoxemia. Atelectasis is difficult for the neonate to overcome because it requires a significant negative inspiratory pressure to open the alveoli with each breath. This increased work of breathing may result in hypercapnia. Hypoxia and hypercapnia cause pulmonary vasoconstriction and increase intrapulmonary resistance and shunting. This results in hypoperfusion of the lung and a decrease in effective pulmonary blood flow. Increased pulmonary vascular resistance may even cause a partial return to fetal circulation, with right-to-left shunting of blood through the ductus arteriosus and foramen ovale. Inadequate perfusion of tissues and hypoxemia contribute to metabolic acidosis.

Inadequate alveolar ventilation can be further complicated by increased pulmonary capillary permeability. Many premature infants with RDS will require mechanical ventilation, which damages alveolar epithelium. Together these conditions result in the leakage of plasma proteins into the alveoli. Fibrin deposits in the airspaces create the appearance of *"hyaline membranes,"* for which the disorder was originally named. The plasma proteins leaked into the airspace have the additional adverse effect of inactivating any surfactant that may be present. The pathogenesis of RDS is summarized in Figure 27-5.

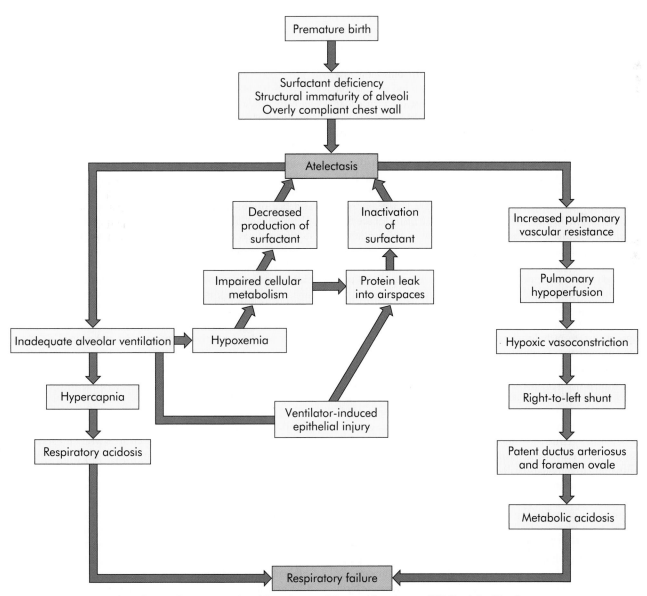

FIGURE 27-5 Pathogenesis of Respiratory Distress Syndrome (RDS) of the Newborn.

CLINICAL MANIFESTATIONS Signs of RDS appear within minutes of birth. Some neonates require immediate resuscitation because of asphyxia or severe respiratory distress. Severity tends to increase over the first 2 days of life. Characteristic signs are tachypnea (respiratory rate greater than 60 breaths/min), expiratory grunting, intercostal and subcostal retractions, nasal flaring, and cyanosis. The natural course is characterized by progressive hypoxemia and dyspnea. Apnea and irregular respirations occur as the infant tires. Severity of hypoxemia and difficulty in providing supplemental oxygenation have resulted in the Vermont Oxford Neonatal Network definition of RDS: a Pao_2 less than 50 mm Hg in room air, central cyanosis in room air, or a need for supplemental oxygen to maintain Pao_2 greater than 50 mm Hg, as well as classic chest film appearance.[25] The typical chest radiograph shows diffuse, fine granular densities within the first 6 hours of life. This "ground glass" appearance is associated with alveolar flooding. Ventilatory support is often required. In most cases the clinical manifestations reach a peak within 3 days, after which there is gradual improvement.

EVALUATION AND TREATMENT Diagnosis is made on the basis of premature birth or other risk factors, chest radiographs, and, if needed, analysis of amniotic fluid or tracheal aspirates to estimate lung maturity (lecithin/sphingomyelin ratio [L/S ratio]). The ultimate treatment for RDS would be prevention of premature birth. For women in preterm labor, antenatal treatment with glucocorticoids induces a significant and rapid acceleration of lung maturation and stimulation of surfactant production in the fetus. There is extensive evidence that maternal antenatal corticosteroid therapy significantly reduces the incidence of RDS and death, although it is unclear whether repeated courses of steroids are safe in this setting.[25,26]

Current recommendations for infants weighing less than 1000 g include prophylaxis beginning within 15 to 30 minutes of birth by administration of exogenous surfactant (either synthetic or natural) through nebulizer or nasal continuous positive airway pressure (CPAP) ventilation. Repeat doses are given every 12 hours for the first few days. There is usually a dramatic improvement in oxygenation as well as a decreased incidence of RDS death, pneumothorax, and pulmonary interstitial emphysema.[27] For infants weighing more than 1000 g, surfactant replacement is based on clinical need. Surfactant therapy should be considered complementary to antenatal glucocorticoids. The two therapies together appear to have an additive effect on improving lung function.

Supportive care includes oxygen administration and often such measures as mechanical ventilation. Mechanical ventilation can result in a proinflammatory state that may contribute to the development of chronic lung disease, such as bronchopulmonary dysplasia (BPD). Strategies that are lung protective, such as greater reliance on nasal CPAP, permissive hypercapnia, lower oxygen saturation targets, modulation of tidal volume (V_t) settings, and use of high-frequency oscillation, are being evaluated.[28] Inhaled nitric oxide (iNO) resulted in lowered O_2 levels and fewer days of ventilation in some trials, although its utility in preterm infants has been questioned.[29] Most infants survive RDS and, in many cases, recovery may be complete within 10 to 14 days. However, the incidence of subsequent chronic lung disease is significant among very-low-birthweight infants.[24]

Bronchopulmonary Dysplasia

Bronchopulmonary dysplasia (BPD), also known as *chronic lung disease (CLD) of infancy*, is the term used to describe persisting lung disease following neonatal lung injury, usually associated with premature birth and perinatal respiratory support. There are approximately 60,000 U.S.

RISK FACTORS
Bronchopulmonary Dysplasia (BPD)

- Premature birth (especially ≤28 weeks)
- Positive-pressure ventilation
- Supplemental oxygen administration
- Antenatal chorioamnionitis
- Postnatal sepsis or pneumonia
- Patent ductus arteriosus
- Nutritional deficiencies
- Early adrenal insufficiency

infants born weighing less than 1500 g on an annual basis. About 20% to 30% of these infants develop BPD.[30] Risk factors for BPD are summarized in the *Risk Factors: Bronchopulmonary Dysplasia (BPD)* box.

In the current era of neonatology, the widespread use of antenatal glucocorticoids and postnatal surfactant has lessened the incidence and severity of RDS, and BPD is occurring primarily in the smallest premature infants (23 to 28 weeks' gestation) who have received mechanical ventilation. Surprisingly, some of these tiny infants who develop BPD have shown few or no clinical signs of RDS at birth or have initially received only low levels of supplemental oxygen or ventilatory support, sometimes for other reasons such as apnea.

PATHOPHYSIOLOGY *Classic BPD* evolves over several weeks, with an early exudative inflammatory phase followed by a fibroproliferative phase. However, this severe form, resulting in evidence of marked airway injury and cyst formation, is no longer common. Instead, the predominant histopathologic findings in the "*new BPD*" are those of disrupted lung development with poor formation of the alveolar architecture. Alveoli are large and fewer in number, thereby presenting decreased surface area for gas exchange.[31] Furthermore, there is evidence of abnormal vascular endothelial growth factor signaling, with resultant abnormal pulmonary capillary development, leading to impaired gas exchange, ventilation-perfusion mismatch, and poor capacity to exercise.[32] Genetic influences on inflammatory regulation have been documented in association with the "new BPD."[33] Concentrations of proinflammatory cytokines, such as tumor necrosis factor-alpha, interleukin-1, interleukin-6, and interleukin-8, are all elevated in the amniotic fluid or tracheal aspirates, or both, of preterm infants who later develop BPD. Inflammation invites neutrophils and macrophages to release reactive oxygen species and proteolytic enzymes.[34] In more severe cases of BPD, pulmonary hypertension may develop because of abnormal muscularization of the primary vasculature in response to recurrent hypoxemia or inflammatory stimuli. Figure 27-6 illustrates the pathophysiology of BPD.

CLINICAL MANIFESTATIONS The current definition of BPD includes need for supplemental oxygen at 36 weeks for at least 28 days after birth. It also details a graded severity dependent on required respiratory support at term (mild, moderate, and severe based on oxygen requirements and ventilatory needs). Clinically, the infant exhibits hypoxemia and hypercapnia caused by ventilation-perfusion mismatch and diffusion defects. The work of breathing increases and the ability to feed may be impaired. Intermittent bronchospasm, mucus plugging, and pulmonary hypertension characterize the clinical course. Of the most severely affected infants, dusky spells may occur with agitation, feeding, or gastroesophageal reflux. Infants with mild BPD may demonstrate only mild tachypnea and difficulty handling respiratory tract infections.

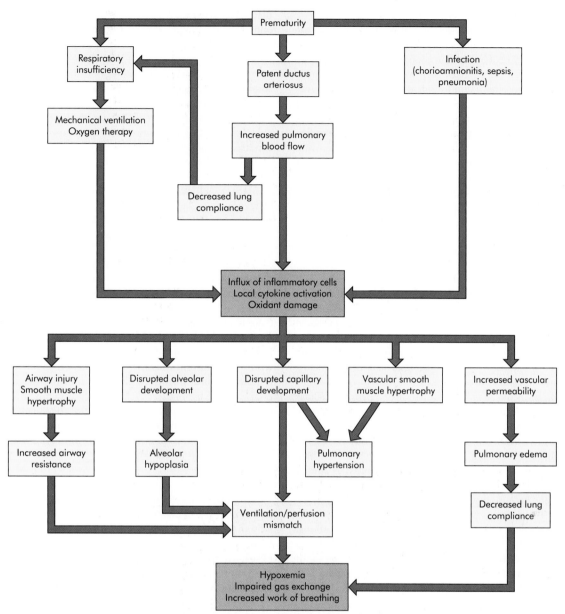

FIGURE 27-6 Pathophysiology of Bronchopulmonary Dysplasia (BPD).

EVALUATION AND TREATMENT Infants with severe BPD require prolonged assisted ventilation. Prevention of lung damage with "gentle ventilation" or early nasal CPAP, or both, is used in clinical situations when permitted. When compared to mechanical ventilation, use of CPAP has resulted in fewer days of oxygen and ventilator requirement by reducing the amount of lung injury.[35] Diuretics are used to control pulmonary edema. Bronchodilators reduce airway resistance. Inhaled corticosteroids improve the rate of extubation and reduce the time that mechanical ventilation is required.[36] Caffeine citrate administration, vitamin A supplementation, and careful nutritional support are routinely used and have resulted in improved outcomes.[30]

Death from BPD is usually caused by infection, cor pulmonale, or respiratory failure. However, most infants with BPD improve substantially during the first 2 to 3 years of life. Nevertheless, there is an increased incidence of asthma during childhood, and pulmonary function abnormalities (significant airflow limitation with bronchodilator responsiveness) may persist for many years.[37] Children who survive BPD also have increased rates of cognitive, educational, and behavioral impairments.[38]

> ✔ **QUICK CHECK 27-2**
> 1. Why are premature infants susceptible to RDS?
> 2. Describe the pathologic findings of "new BPD."

Respiratory Tract Infections

Respiratory tract infections are common in children and are a frequent cause for emergency department visits and hospitalizations. Clinical presentation, age of the child, and season of the year can often provide clues to the etiologic agent, even when the agent cannot be proven.

Bronchiolitis

Bronchiolitis is a common, viral lower respiratory tract infection that occurs almost exclusively in infants and young toddlers and is a major reason for hospitalization of infants and young children.[39] It has a seasonal, yearly incidence, from approximately November to April, and is the leading cause of hospitalization for infants during the winter season. The most common associated pathogen is respiratory syncytial virus (RSV), which accounts for up to 75% of cases,[39] but bronchiolitis also may be associated with adenoviruses, influenza, parainfluenza, and mycoplasma. Healthy infants usually make a full recovery from RSV bronchiolitis, but infants who were premature (birthweight <2500 g) or who have underlying BPD or heart disease may have a much higher risk for a more severe or even deadly course. Bronchiolitis has been linked to an increased risk for asthma later in childhood.[40] Associations with rhinovirus and low vitamin D levels also are being investigated because they appear to correlate with the increased likelihood that children develop asthma after they have experienced bronchiolitis.[41]

PATHOPHYSIOLOGY Viral infection causes necrosis of the bronchial epithelium and destruction of ciliated epithelial cells. There is infiltration with lymphocytes around the bronchioles and a cell-mediated hypersensitivity to viral antigens with release of lymphokines causing inflammation, as well as activation of eosinophils, neutrophils, and monocytes. The submucosa becomes edematous and cellular debris and fibrin form plugs within the bronchioles.

Edema of the bronchiolar wall, accumulation of mucus and cellular debris, and, perhaps, bronchospasm narrow many peripheral airways. Other airways become partially or completely occluded. Atelectasis occurs in some areas of the lung and hyperinflation in others.

The mechanics of breathing are disrupted by bronchiolitis. There is air trapping, and functional residual capacity (FRC) is greatly increased. Compliance is decreased because the lungs are already highly inflated and because airway resistance within the lung is uneven and increased. The decrease in compliance and the increase in airway resistance result in a substantial increase in the work of breathing. Serious alterations in gas exchange occur because of airway obstruction and patchy atelectasis. Hypoxemia develops because of ventilation-perfusion mismatch (see Chapter 26), and hypercapnia may occur in severe cases.

CLINICAL MANIFESTATIONS Symptoms usually begin with significant rhinorrhea followed by a tight cough over the next several days, along with systemic signs of decreased appetite, lethargy, and fever. Infants typically have tachypnea, variable degrees of respiratory distress, and abnormal auscultatory findings of the chest. Wheezing is most common, but rales or rhonchi also may be present. Chest radiographs often reveal hyperexpanded lungs, patchy or peribronchial infiltrates, and, sometimes, atelectasis of the right upper lobe. Very young infants may present with severe apnea before lower respiratory tract symptoms appear, and these apneas frequently require mechanical ventilation. Many children also may present with conjunctivitis or otitis media.

EVALUATION AND TREATMENT Diagnosis of bronchiolitis is made by review of signs and symptoms (e.g., rhinitis, cough, wheezing, chest retractions, tachypnea) and radiologic examination. Nasal washings may be tested for specific viral agents, such as RSV. RSV swabs are positive in 70% of these cases.

Treatment for bronchiolitis is determined by the severity of the disease and the age of the child. Most cases are mild and require no specific treatment and may be monitored as outpatients. When treatment is indicated, it is primarily supportive in nature. Supplemental oxygen and increased hydration are commonly used. Inhaled hypertonic saline has been found to decrease clinical severity and length of hospital stay.[40,42] Inhaled bronchodilators and steroids benefit infants with underlying lung disease, but have not been found to be effective in otherwise healthy infants. Mechanical ventilation is occasionally necessary and the use of nasal CPAP and heliox (a mixture of helium and oxygen) is being explored.[43,44] Preventive treatment with RSV-specific monoclonal antibody, provided as a monthly injection through the RSV season, is recommended for high-risk infants younger than 2 years who meet specific criteria.

Pneumonia

Pneumonia is infection and inflammation in the terminal airways and alveoli. It is a major cause of morbidity and mortality, particularly in developing countries. The most common agents are viruses, followed by bacteria and atypical microorganisms (e.g., mycoplasma) (Table 27-2). Community-acquired pneumonia (CAP) is one of the most common childhood infections and one of the leading causes of hospitalization. Risk factors for developing CAP are age younger than

TABLE 27-2	COMMON TYPES OF PNEUMONIA IN CHILDREN			
TYPE	**CAUSAL AGENT**	**AGE**	**ONSET**	**SIGNS/SYMPTOMS**
Viral pneumonia	Respiratory syncytial virus (RSV), influenza, adenovirus, others	Infants for RSV, all ages for others	Acute or gradual, winter and early spring	Mild to high fever, cough, rhinorrhea, malaise, rales, rhonchi, or wheezing, apnea, variable radiographic pattern
Pneumococcal pneumonia	Pneumococci (*Streptococcus pneumoniae*)	Usually 1 to 4 yr	Acute, follows an upper respiratory tract infection, winter and early spring	High fever, productive cough, pleuritic pain, increased respiration rate, decreased breath sounds in area of consolidation; lobar infiltrate or "round pneumonia" on radiograph
Staphylococcal pneumonia	*Staphylococcus aureus* (including methicillin-resistant strains)	1 wk to 2 yr	Acute, winter	High fever, cough, respiratory distress, empyema or pneumatoceles common
Streptococcal pneumonia	Group A beta-hemolytic streptococci	All ages	Acute, any season	High fever, chills, respiratory distress, sepsis, or shock
Mycoplasmal and chlamydophilal pneumonia	*Mycoplasma pneumoniae, Chlamydophila pneumoniae*	School-age and adolescents	Gradual	Low-grade fever, cough

2 years, overcrowded living conditions, winter season, recent antibiotic treatment, day-care attendance, and passive smoke exposure. Nutritional status, age, and underlying disease process influence morbidity and mortality rates related to CAP.

Viral pneumonia is more common than bacterial pneumonia and children are two to three times more likely than adults to acquire these viruses. Mortality in the developed world is rare but morbidity is significant. The incidence of viral pneumonia generally follows a seasonal pattern. The most common viral pneumonia in young children is RSV (respiratory syncytial virus). A number of other viruses are important, including parainfluenza, influenza, and adenoviruses. Certain serotypes of adenovirus can cause necrotizing disease, sometimes leading to bronchiolitis obliterans and significant lung disability.

Acquisition of these viruses is by direct contact, droplet transmission, or aerosol.[45] There is initial destruction of ciliated epithelium of the distal airway with sloughing of cellular material. A mononuclear-predominant inflammatory response occurs, in the interstitium initially, and later may involve the alveoli as well. Early in the course of the disease, it is often difficult to determine whether the pneumonia is viral or bacterial. Differences in the clinical presentation can help to determine origin, such as degree of elevation of temperature, absolute neutrophil counts, and percentage of bands. Ultimately diagnosis requires laboratory confirmation using immunofluorescence tests. Development of safe agents to treat and prevent viral pneumonia continues to be a focus of much research.[45]

Bacterial pneumonia usually begins with inhalation of microbes dispersed in ambient air or in secretion droplets (person-to-person spread) or by aspiration of one's own nasopharyngeal bacteria.[46] A preceding viral infection sometimes sets the stage for bacterial infection by causing epithelial damage and reduced mucociliary clearance in the trachea and major bronchi. Once in the alveolar region, bacteria encounter local host defenses, such as antibodies, complement, and cytokines, which prepare bacteria for ingestion by alveolar macrophages. Alveolar macrophages recognize bacteria with their surface receptors and phagocytose them. If these mechanisms fail, macrophages release numerous inflammatory cytokines and neutrophils will be recruited into the lung.[47] An intense, cytokine-mediated inflammation will ensue. Vascular engorgement, edema, and a fibrinopurulent exudate occur. Alveolar filling precludes gas exchange and, if extensive, can lead to respiratory failure. If sepsis occurs at the same time, shock and end-organ hypoperfusion will cause metabolic acidosis.

Beyond the neonatal period, infection with streptococci and staphylococci microorganisms is most common for this diagnosis. Pneumococcal (*Streptococcus pneumoniae*) pneumonia is the most common cause of community-acquired bacterial pneumonia and presents acutely and with variable severity.[48] In 2000 a polyvariant pneumococcal conjugate vaccine (PCV7) was incorporated into routine childhood immunizations and appears to have lessened the incidence of pneumococcal pneumonia in children younger than 2 years of age.[48] Staphylococcal pneumonia and group A streptococcal pneumonia can be particularly fulminant (sudden, severe) and necrotizing (causing cell death) with a high incidence of accompanying empyema, pneumatocele, and sepsis. *H. influenzae* pneumonia has become rare because of widespread immunization.

The clinical presentation of bacterial pneumonia, particularly pneumococcal, may include a preceding viral illness followed by fever with chills and rigors, shortness of breath, and an increasingly productive cough. Occasionally, there is blood streaking of the sputum. Respiratory rate and oxygen saturation also are important clinical indicators. Auscultation usually shows such abnormalities as crackles or decreased breath sounds. Other less specific findings may include malaise, emesis, abdominal pain, and chest pain. Chest film will usually present with a lobar pattern in older children and adolescents but may appear patchier with a bronchopneumonic pattern in younger children.

Atypical pneumonia (*Mycoplasma pneumoniae, Chlamydophila pneumoniae*) is the most common cause of community-acquired pneumonia for school-age children and young adults. *Chlamydophila* pneumonia is clinically indistinguishable from and is typically grouped with *Mycoplasma* as "atypical pneumonia." Transmission is from person-to-person with a 2- to 3-week incubation period.

Mycoplasmic microorganisms lack cell walls but have a limiting membrane and a specialized receptor for attaching to ciliated respiratory epithelial cells. Local sloughing of cells occurs. Peribronchial lymphocytic infiltration develops, along with neutrophil recruitment to the airway lumen. The pattern resembles bronchitis or bronchopneumonia.

Onset is usually gradual, resembling a typical upper respiratory tract infection but with low-grade fever and prominent cough. Mycoplasma can cause a wide spectrum of disease and is more extensive as a cause of complications than previously noted. It also is occurring more frequently in infants and younger children.[49] Most cases are not clinically severe and full recovery should be expected. Complications, when they do occur, can include bronchopneumonia, parapneumonic effusions, and necrotizing pneumonitis.

EVALUATION AND TREATMENT Diagnosis of pneumonia is based on clinical and laboratory findings and chest radiograph confirmation; the etiologic agent can sometimes be inferred from the age of the child and clinical scenario.[50] Guidelines have been developed but often are very difficult to apply in practice and thus there is lack of consensus regarding their use.[51] Although laboratory testing is available, it is again often difficult to apply with children because they may have an overlapping clinical picture (viral versus bacterial). Measurement of serum levels of highly-sensitive C-reactive protein (hs-CRP) may help discern between the two entities. Several microbiologic tests are available, such as PCR (polymerase chain reaction) and nucleic acid amplification tests (NAATs). A bacterial pneumonia will initially produce a patchy infiltration and later cause a segmental or lobar disease. A unilateral lobar consolidation on a chest x-ray film is often associated with *Streptococcus pneumoniae*. The formation of small areas of airway dilation (called pneumatoceles) most commonly suggests *Staphylococcus pneumoniae*. Pleural effusions are rarely seen with viral pneumonias or atypical pneumonias.

Some pneumonias may be treated on an outpatient basis; however, many children require oxygen supplementation and, occasionally, assisted ventilation. This is particularly true with infants who have a viral interstitial pneumonia, such as RSV. In addition, adequate hydration, proper nutrition, and supportive pulmonary therapy are required to reduce the duration and severity of illness. Many infants are markedly tachypneic and unable to coordinate their breathing with swallowing; they may require enteral feeding. Aspiration is always a risk with infants in respiratory distress.

Appropriate antibiotic administration for bacterial pneumonias should be instituted.[52,53] Local patterns of resistance must be considered when choosing appropriate antibiotics.[54,55] Both pneumococcal and mycoplasmal pneumonias present some unique treatment obstacles and often need a multifaceted approach to care, including vaccine antigens, antibiotic combinations, and immunoadjuvant therapies.[47,55,56]

Aspiration Pneumonitis

Aspiration pneumonitis is caused by a foreign substance, such as food, meconium, secretions (saliva or gastric), or environmental compounds, entering the lung and resulting in inflammation of the lung tissue. The aspiration of meconium from amniotic fluid can occur at birth. Neurologically compromised children or children with chronic lung disease may have chronic pulmonary aspiration (CPA), which can cause progressive lung disease, bronchiectasis, and respiratory failure. This is the leading cause of death in children who are neurologically compromised.[57] Children undergoing sedation or anesthesia also may aspirate oral secretions contaminated with anaerobic bacteria or acidic stomach contents. The severity of lung injury after an aspiration incident is determined by the volume and pH of the material aspirated and the presence of pathogenic bacteria. Very low pH or extremely high pH will cause a significant inflammatory response. With hydrocarbon ingestions, lung injury is determined by the volatility and viscosity of the aspirated substance. A low-viscosity substance, such as gasoline or lighter fluid, is the most toxic, and high-viscosity hydrocarbons, such as petroleum jelly or mineral oil, are much less likely to cause a pneumonitis. Treatment for aspiration pneumonitis depends on the material aspirated but generally includes broad-spectrum antibiotic coverage. Children with CPA and a large amount of upper respiratory tract secretions may benefit from salivary gland injection with botulinum toxin A (BTX-A) to suppress secretion.[58]

Bronchiolitis Obliterans

Bronchiolitis obliterans (BO) is relatively rare in children. It is characterized by fibrotic obstruction of the respiratory bronchioles and alveolar ducts secondary to intense inflammation. Two types are noted in the literature, proliferative and constrictive, with the latter being the more common form. BO most often occurs as a sequela of a severe viral pulmonary infection (e.g., influenza, adenovirus, pertussis [whooping cough], or measles). Other cases may be secondary to parainfluenza, RSV, human immunodeficiency virus (HIV), or *M. pneumoniae* infection. It also may occur after lung, heart-lung, or bone marrow transplantation, or be associated with collagen vascular disease, toxic fume inhalation, chronic hypersensitivity pneumonitis, Crohn disease, and Stevens-Johnson syndrome.[59] Although the child may initially improve after the acute insult, the progression of disease is then reflected by increasing tachypnea, dyspnea, cough, sputum production, crackles, wheezing, increased chest anteroposterior diameter (APD), and hypoxemia.

There is no specific treatment for bronchiolitis obliterans. Some children deteriorate rapidly and die within weeks, whereas others follow a more chronic course. Antiviral agents may assist in blunting the initial viral response but otherwise have limited effect on the illness. Anti-inflammatory agents are showing promise in reducing airway inflammation and improving pulmonary function. For those children having undergone lung transplantation, increased immunosuppressive regimens are sometimes helpful and new research is showing promise with improved understanding of leukocyte trafficking and matrix metalloproteinase-8.[60]

Asthma

Asthma is a chronic inflammatory disease characterized by bronchial hyperreactivity and reversible airflow obstruction, usually in response to an allergen (see Chapter 26). It is the most prevalent chronic disease in childhood, affecting 10% of U.S. children between 5 and 17 years of age with boys more often affected than girls.[61] Populations most affected include black and Hispanic children, those living in an urban setting, ethnic minorities, and those of low socioeconomic status.[62]

Childhood asthma results from a complex interaction between *genetic* susceptibility and *environmental* factors, including early exposure to allergens (e.g., air pollution, dust mites, cockroach antigen, cat exposure, and tobacco smoke) and infections, particularly viral respiratory tract infections (e.g., rhinovirus and RSV).[63] Vitamin D insufficiency may be a risk factor for wheezing in children.[64]

PATHOPHYSIOLOGY The pathophysiology of asthma in children is similar to that for adults and is described in Chapter 26. It is initiated by a type I hypersensitivity reaction (see Chapter 7). The *early asthmatic response* is summarized in Figure 26-9 and Figure 27-7, *A*). The *late asthmatic response* begins 4 to 8 hours after the acute response and is summarized in Figure 27-7, *B*. In *chronic asthma,* some of these mechanisms may be operational on an ongoing basis.

CLINICAL MANIFESTATIONS In a typical acute asthma attack in children, the major complaints are coughing, wheezing, and shortness of breath. There may or may not have been signs of a preceding upper respiratory tract infection, such as rhinorrhea or low-grade fever. In children, about 70% to 80% of acute wheezing episodes are associated with viral respiratory tract infections. In infants and toddlers less than 2 years old, the most common of these is respiratory syncytial virus (RSV). In older children and adults, the major viral trigger is rhinovirus (the "common cold" virus).[65]

On physical examination, there is expiratory wheezing that is often described as high pitched and musical, and there is prolongation of the expiratory phase of the respiratory cycle. Breath sounds may become faint when air movement is poor. The child may speak in clipped sentences or not at all because of dyspnea. Sometimes hyperinflation (barrel chest) is visible. Respiratory rate and heart rate are elevated. Nasal flaring and use of accessory muscles with retractions in the substernal, subcostal, intercostal, suprasternal, or sternocleidomastoid areas are evident. Infants may appear to be "head bobbing" because of sternocleidomastoid muscle use. Pulsus paradoxus (decrease in systolic blood pressure of more than 10 mm Hg during inspiration) may be present. The child may appear anxious or diaphoretic, important signs of respiratory compromise.

Findings in chronic asthma may include hyperinflation of the thorax or pectus excavatum. Clubbing should not be seen with asthma and, if present, should trigger evaluation for other conditions such as cystic fibrosis. Exercise intolerance may indicate underlying asthma (see *Health Alert:* Exercise-Induced Bronchoconstriction).

EVALUATION AND TREATMENT Asthma is often underdiagnosed and undertreated, especially in preschool-age children because asthma symptoms overlap with other respiratory illnesses, such as bronchitis or upper respiratory tract infections. Diagnosis of asthma is based on episodes of wheezing as well as a variety of risk factors including parental history of asthma, atopic dermatitis, sensitization to aeroallergens or foods, blood eosinophilia, or wheezing not associated with upper respiratory tract illnesses. The modified Asthma Predictive Index (API) can be used to help with asthma diagnosis and is recommended by the National Institutes of Health (NIH) guidelines.[66]

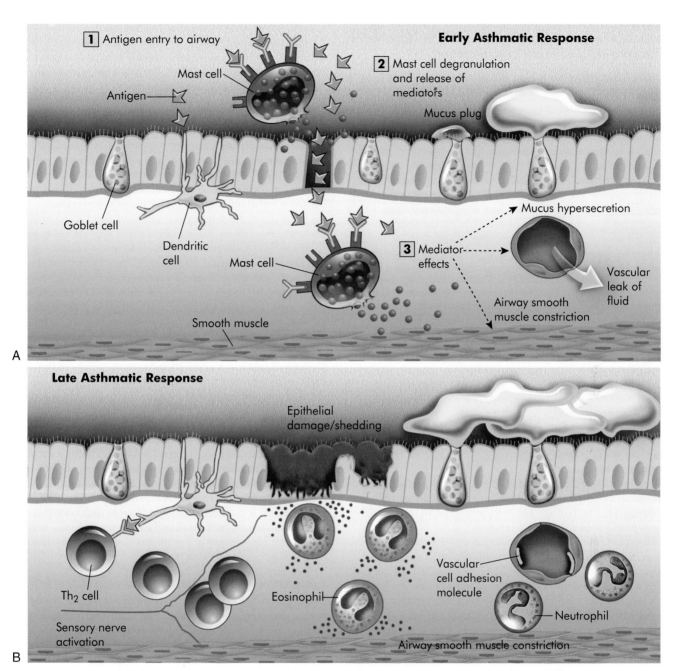

FIGURE 27-7 Asthmatic Responses. A, In the early asthmatic response, inhaled antigen *(1)* binds to preformed IgE on mast cells. Mast cells degranulate *(2)* and release mediators such as histamine, leukotrienes, prostaglandin D_2, platelet activating factor, and others. Acute inflammation opens intercellular tight junctions, allowing allergen to penetrate and activate submucosal mast cells. Secreted mediators *(3)* induce active bronchospasm, edema, and mucus secretion causing airway obstruction. Inflammatory responses are triggered by chemotactic factors and up-regulation of adhesion molecules (not shown). At the same time, as shown on the left, antigen may be received by dendritic cells and later presented, either to regional lymph nodes of naïve (Th_0) T lymphocytes or locally to memory Th_2 cells in the airway mucosa (see **B**). **B,** In the late asthmatic response, there are areas of epithelial damage and shedding caused at least in part by toxicity of eosinophil products (major basic protein, eosinophilic cationic protein, eosinophil-derived neurotoxin, and eosinophil peroxidase). Many inflammatory cells are recruited by chemokines and up-regulation of vascular cell adhesion molecules. Local T lymphocytes display a predominant Th_2 cytokine profile. They produce IL-4 and IL-13, which promote switching of B cells to favor IgE production; and IL-3, IL-5, and granulocyte-macrophage colony-stimulating factor, which encourage eosinophil differentiation and survival. Inflammatory mediators also activate sensory nerves, further stimulating bronchoconstriction (also see Figure 26-9).

Exercise-Induced Bronchoconstriction

Exercise-induced bronchoconstriction (EIB) occurs in 90% of children diagnosed with asthma. It is estimated to occur in 12% of the population without diagnosed asthma and is surprisingly common among young, elite athletes. In the 2008 Olympics, nearly 50% of tested elite athletes had EIB, with swimmers demonstrating some of the highest prevalence rates. A proposed mechanism for EIB is epithelial injury and inflammation from the inhalation of particles and toxins at high flow rates. This results in increased type I hypersensitivity and airway hyperresponsiveness (AHR) in those with asthma and is associated with an increase in leukotriene release. In nonasthmatics, bronchoconstriction with exercise may be a protective reflex; however, repetitive exposure to high-flow inhaled air has been found to cause AHR and EIB over time. Although bronchodilators remain the most commonly used medications for EIB, studies suggest that inhaled corticosteroids or leukotriene inhibitors are more effective and safer in children.

Data from Bikov A et al: Exercise increases exhaled breath condensate cysteinyl leukotriene concentration in asthmatic patients, *J Asthma* 47(9):1057–1062, 2010; Bougault V, Turmel J, Boulet LP: Bronchial challenges and respiratory symptoms in elite swimmers and winter sport athletes: airway hyperresponsiveness in asthma: its measurement and clinical significance, *Chest* 138(2 suppl):31S–37S, 2010; Kersten ET et al: Pilot study: the effect of reducing treatment on exercise induced bronchoconstriction, *Pediatr Pulmonol* 45(9):927–933, 2010; Randolph C: The challenge of asthma in adolescent athletes: exercise induced bronchoconstriction (EIB) with and without known asthma, *Adolesc Med State Art Rev* 21(1):44–56, viii, 2010; Szefler SJ: Advances in pediatric asthma in 2008: where do we go now? *J Allergy Clin Immunol* 123(1):28–34, 2009.

Confirmation of the diagnosis of asthma relies on pulmonary function testing using spirometry, which can be accomplished only after the child is 5 to 6 years of age. For younger children, an empiric trial of asthma medications is commonly initiated.

The goal of asthma therapy is to achieve long-term control by reduction in impairment and risk.[66] Child/family education and appropriate allergen avoidance techniques should begin immediately. Care providers need to periodically assess asthma control in children. Key features for assessment include nighttime awakenings, interference with normal activities, use of short-acting β_2-agonists, pulmonary function testing, and exacerbations requiring steroids. Peak flow meters are often used to help guide treatment. Before therapy is augmented, care providers need to assess medication administration techniques, environmental controls, and comorbidities. For reduction in therapy, the asthma needs to be under good control for a minimum of 3 months.[66]

The pharmacologic treatment of asthma in children is essentially the same as that for adults and is initiated in a stepwise sequence based on asthma severity and response to treatment (see Chapter 26).

✔ QUICK CHECK 27-4
1. What are the key features of the early and late asthmatic responses?
2. Explain the full progression of blood gas abnormalities in a severe asthma attack.

Acute Respiratory Distress Syndrome

Acute respiratory distress syndrome (ARDS) is a dramatic, life-threatening condition resulting from a direct pulmonary insult (such as pneumonia, aspiration, near drowning, or smoke inhalation) or a systemic insult (such as sepsis or multiple trauma), either of which activates an inflammatory response that causes alveolocapillary injury. ARDS accounts for approximately 10% of total patient days and one third of all deaths in pediatric intensive care units. Mortality in pediatric ARDS remains high, at approximately 40%.[67]

PATHOPHYSIOLOGY The hallmark of ARDS is lung inflammation. Activation of the inflammatory response (see Chapter 26, Figure 26-7) includes polymorphonucleocytes, complement, cytokines, arachidonic acid metabolites, and reactive oxygen species. Injury to pulmonary capillary endothelium results in capillary leakage and noncardiogenic pulmonary edema. Edema fluid contains plasma proteins that can inactivate surfactant, contributing further to alveolar collapse. During the acute phase, the pulmonary microcirculation is compromised by the formation of thrombi composed of fibrin, platelets, and leukocytes.

The early accumulation of edema fluid in the airspaces results in decreased lung compliance, decreased functional residual volume, and increased dead space. There is ventilation-perfusion mismatching, intrapulmonary shunting, and hypoxemia. In the fibroproliferative phase, type II alveolar cells proliferate, and alveolar septal thickening and collagen deposition occur. Interstitial fibrosis can be evident as early as 10 days after the initial insult. Similarly, vascular changes may occur, including obliteration of the microcirculation and thickening of the walls of pulmonary arterioles and arteries, which can then lead to chronic pulmonary hypertension in survivors.

CLINICAL MANIFESTATIONS ARDS develops acutely after the initial insult, usually within 24 hours, though occasionally it is delayed up to a few days. ARDS is characterized by progressive respiratory distress, severe hypoxemia, decreased pulmonary compliance, and diffuse densities on chest radiograph. Initially, hyperventilation occurs, but CO_2 retention may ultimately occur as well because of inadequate functional airspace and respiratory muscle fatigue. The severity of the overall picture is modified by comorbid factors, such as the presence of sepsis or multiorgan failure, and by the presence or absence of complications, such as nosocomial pneumonia. Some children who recover have residual pulmonary abnormalities.

EVALUATION AND TREATMENT Treatment for ARDS remains supportive in nature, and the goals are to maintain adequate tissue oxygenation, minimize acute lung injury, and avoid iatrogenic pulmonary complications. Most individuals with ARDS require mechanical ventilation and often relatively high levels of positive end-expiratory pressure (PEEP) to promote alveolar ventilation and stabilization, and redistribution of alveolar edema fluid into the interstitium. Lung-protective ventilation strategies may include low tidal volume, permissive hypercapnia, prone positioning, and high-frequency oscillation. Systemic steroids remain a mainstay of treatment to decrease postextubation stridor and reduce reintubation rates.[68] Inhaled nitric oxide and prostacyclins are under investigation although results have not been encouraging to date.[69,70]

Cystic Fibrosis

Cystic fibrosis (CF) is an autosomal recessive inherited disease that results from defective epithelial chloride ion transport. The CF gene is located on chromosome 7. There are more than 1500 known mutations of this gene divided into 5 classes.[71] These mutations result in abnormal expression of the protein cystic fibrosis transmembrane conductance regulator (CFTR), which is a chloride channel present on the surface of many types of epithelial cells including airways, bile ducts, pancreas, sweat ducts, and vas deferens.[72,73] CF affects primarily whites (approximately 1 in 3500 in North America and Europe). There are approximately 1000 new cases of CF diagnosed each year and the median age at diagnosis is 6 months. The projected life expectancy for those with CF has increased from 31 years to 37 years over the past decade. The estimated carrier frequency is high, 1 in 29 whites in the United States. Carriers are not affected by the mutation.

PATHOPHYSIOLOGY   Although CF is a multiorgan disease, its most important effects are on the lungs, and respiratory failure is almost always the cause of death. The typical features of CF lung disease are mucus plugging, chronic inflammation, and chronic infection. The mucus plugging seen in CF results from both increased production and altered physicochemical properties of the mucus. Mucus-secreting airway cells (goblet cells and submucosal glands) are increased in number and size. CF mucus is dehydrated and viscous because of defective chloride secretion and excess sodium absorption. The periciliary fluid layer is depleted in volume, impairing the mobility of the cilia and thereby allowing mucus to adhere to the airway epithelium, along with bacteria and injurious by-products from neutrophils.[71-73] Neutrophils are present in great excess in the airways and release damaging oxidants and proteases that cause direct damage to lung structural proteins, induce airway cells to produce interleukin-8 (IL-8) (which attracts more neutrophils and stimulates mucus secretion), and destroy immunoglobulin G (IgG) and complement components important for opsonization and phagocytosis of pathogens.[71]

The CF airway microenvironment favors bacterial colonization. *Pseudomonas aeruginosa* ultimately colonizes airways in at least 75% of children with CF and *Staphylococcus aureus* is common. Persistence of these microorganisms incites chronic local inflammation and airway damage with microabscess formation, bronchiectasis, patchy consolidation and pneumonia, peribronchial fibrosis, and cyst formation (Figure 27-8).[71,73] The pathogenesis for these changes is outlined in Figure 27-9. Peripheral bullae may develop and pneumothorax may occur. Hemoptysis, sometimes life-threatening, may occur because of the erosion of enlarged bronchial arteries. Over time, pulmonary vascular remodeling occurs because of localized hypoxia and arteriolar vasoconstriction. Pulmonary hypertension and cor pulmonale may develop in the late stages of disease.

CLINICAL MANIFESTATIONS   The most common presenting symptoms of CF are respiratory or gastrointestinal (see Chapter 35). Respiratory symptoms include persistent cough or wheeze and recurrent or severe pneumonia. Physical signs that develop over time include barrel chest and digital clubbing. More subtle presentations include chronic sinusitis and nasal polyps. Newborn screening for CF has expanded rapidly throughout the United States and will increase the numbers of early, presymptomatic diagnosis (see *Health Alert:* Newborn Screening for Cystic Fibrosis).[74]

EVALUATION AND TREATMENT   The standard method of diagnosis is the sweat test, which reveals sweat chloride concentration in excess of 60 mEq/L. Genotyping for CFTR mutations is available as an alternative or supplemental method.[72,73] Treatment is primarily focused on nutrition (see Chapter 35) and pulmonary health.

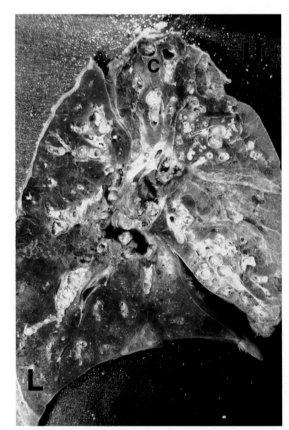

FIGURE 27-8 Pathology of the Lung in End-Stage Cystic Fibrosis. Key features are widespread mucus impaction of airways and bronchiectasis (especially from the upper lobe *[U]*), with hemorrhagic pneumonia in the lower lobe *(L)*. Small cysts *(C)* are present at the apex of the lung. (From Kleinerman J, Vauthy P: *Pathology of the lung in cystic fibrosis,* Atlanta, 1976, Cystic Fibrosis Foundation.)

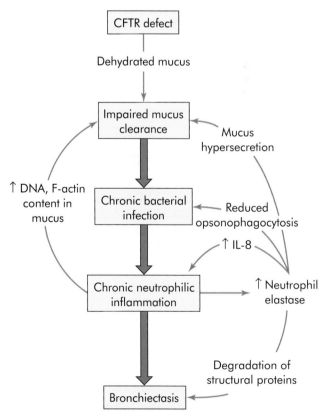

FIGURE 27-9 Pathogenesis of Cystic Fibrosis Lung Disease. *CFTR,* Cystic fibrosis transmembrane conductance regulator.

Common pulmonary therapies include techniques to promote mucus clearance, such as chest physical therapy and related mechanical devices, bronchodilators, and aerosolized DNase and hypertonic saline, which liquefy mucus.[75,76] Inhaled maintenance can be used to suppress *Pseudomonas aeruginosa* or other bacteria, resulting in beneficial clinical impact.[73] Oral antibiotics or intravenous antibiotics are used to treat exacerbations of pulmonary infection. Macrolide antibiotics, such as azithromycin and clarithromycin, have shown improvement in lung function as they target the chronic inflammatory component of the disease. Recombinant human growth hormone has been shown to improve lung function, height, and weight in children with severe CF.[77] Individuals with end-stage lung disease may consider lung transplantation. Newer approaches to gene therapy are being explored (see *Health Alert:* Gene Therapies for Cystic Fibrosis).[71]

SUDDEN INFANT DEATH SYNDROME

Sudden infant death syndrome (SIDS) remains a disease of unknown cause and is the most common cause of unexplained infant death in Western countries.[78,79] It is defined as "sudden death of an infant under 1 year of age which remains unexplained after a thorough case investigation, including performance of a complete autopsy, examination of the death scene, and review of the clinical history."[80]

The incidence of SIDS is low during the first month of life but sharply increases in the second month of life and peaks at 3 to 4 months of age, then gradually declines. It is more common in male (60%) than female (40%) infants. The incidence of SIDS in the United States is 0.54/1000 live births.[81] SIDS almost always seems to occur during nighttime sleep, when infants are least likely to be observed. A seasonal variation has been noted, with higher frequencies during the winter months. This has been related to a higher rate of respiratory tract infection during those months, which likely decreases sleep arousal. In fact, such infections are often reported to have preceded the death. Clinical risk groups include babies who were preterm or low birthweight, who were one of simultaneous multiple births, and who were siblings of prior SIDS victims

(fivefold increase in risk for these infants). Nevertheless, about 75% of all SIDS victims have no known predisposing clinical risk factor.

Additional risk factors fall into the categories of socioeconomic or maternal factors, and factors in the baby's sleeping situation. Maternal factors that predict increased SIDS risk are young maternal age (under 20 years), unmarried mothers, less prenatal care, poverty, and illicit drug use or binge-drinking. Pre- and postnatal exposure to cigarette smoke doubles the risk of SIDS. Risk factors that relate to the baby's sleeping situation are prone positioning, sleeping on a soft surface, and overheating. Prone sleeping was concluded to be a major and modifiable risk factor (see *Risk Factors:* Sudden Infant Death Syndrome [SIDS]). Epidemiologic studies have now shown lowering of SIDS rates by 50% to 90% in countries, including the United States, where massive public campaigns warned against prone sleeping for infants. Infants should sleep on their backs, even in preference over side sleeping.

RISK FACTORS

Sudden Infant Death Syndrome (SIDS)

- Prone and side-lying sleeping position
- Overheated sleeping environment
- Lower socioeconomic status
- Mothers younger than 20
- Low birthweight
- Preterm delivery
- Multiple birth
- Sibling who died of SIDS
- Smoking during pregnancy
- Exposure to tobacco smoke
- Lack of prenatal care
- Illicit drug use or binge-drinking
- Sleeping on soft bedding
- Larger family size

The etiology of SIDS remains unknown. There is a combination of factors including a vulnerable infant, environmental stressor, and predesignated developmental period, usually noted in these cases.[82] A leading hypothesis is that there may be developmental immaturity or anomalies of ventilatory and arousal responses, particularly those regulated by the hypoglossal nucleus (HGN), to hypoxemia or hypercarbia.[83] Alternative theories involve airway obstruction events, such as control of tongue movements related to inspiratory activity; increased vagal tone; sudden intrapulmonary shunting because of abnormalities of surfactant or pulmonary vessels; or exaggerated inflammation, eosinophil degranulation, and massive cytokine release causing pulmonary edema in response to either bacterial pathogens from the nasopharynx or viral respiratory tract infections. Even genetic factors may be linked including those for congenital cardiac conduction abnormalities and cardiomyopathies (e.g., long QT syndrome or viral cardiomyopathies).[84]

Currently, the best strategies for reducing SIDS seem to be avoidance of all the controllable risk factors. Parents of infants with clinical risk should be taught cardiopulmonary resuscitation (CPR) as a precaution. Although home monitoring has not been proven to decrease the incidence of SIDS, some at-risk infants may warrant cardiorespiratory monitoring after careful consideration of the individual situation.

> **✓ QUICK CHECK 27-5**
> 1. How are the alveoli and capillaries affected by the inflammation of acute respiratory distress syndrome (ARDS)?
> 2. What aspects of lung disease in cystic fibrosis are the focus of current therapies?
> 3. What are the risk factors for SIDS?

DID YOU UNDERSTAND?

Disorders of the Upper Airways

1. Croup is an acute laryngotracheobronchitis, usually caused by parainfluenza virus. This infection causes swelling of the upper trachea. The typical sign is a seal-like barking cough, which appears after a few days of rhinorrhea, sore throat, and low-grade fever.
2. Spasmodic croup is characterized by a similar barking cough but occurs in older children, is of sudden onset at night, without fever, and has unknown etiology.
3. Bacterial laryngotracheitis (croup) is the most common potentially life-threatening upper airway infection in children.
4. Acute epiglottitis is a potentially life-threatening airway infection whose incidence has decreased dramatically since the advent of *H. influenzae* vaccine. Now other pathogens, such as group A beta-hemolytic *Streptococcus*, *Candida* species, *S. aureus*, MRSA, or viral pathogens, are usually the causative agents.
5. Aspiration of foreign bodies that lodge in the airways may cause cough, hoarseness, stridor or wheezing, and dyspnea. The severity of the situation depends on the location of the foreign body within the airway and the degree of obstruction. Blockage of the larynx or trachea can be fatal, whereas bronchial obstruction may not even be diagnosed immediately.
6. Obstructive sleep apnea syndrome (OSAS) is defined by partial or intermittent upper airway obstruction during sleep with disruption of normal ventilation and normal sleep patterns. The most common cause in children is adenotonsillar hypertrophy.

Disorders of the Lower Airways

1. Respiratory distress syndrome (RDS) of the newborn usually occurs in premature infants who are born before surfactant production and alveolocapillary development are complete. Atelectasis and hypoventilation cause shunting, hypoxemia, and hypercapnia. Prenatal steroids and postnatal surfactant are beneficial therapies.
2. Bronchopulmonary dysplasia (BPD) is the result of tissue injury and repair and disrupted alveolar development in the lungs of infants who required ventilatory support during a time when their lungs were underdeveloped because of their prematurity. Infants with BPD may require oxygen and additional therapies for many months.
3. Bronchiolitis is a viral lower respiratory tract infection that presents with runny nose, wheezing, cough, and tachypnea in infants and is usually caused by infection with respiratory syncytial virus (RSV). Infants with risk factors of prematurity or underlying lung or heart disease are at high risk and may receive immunizations to prevent RSV disease.
4. Viral pneumonia and bacterial pneumonia cause varying degrees of illness in children and viral pneumonia frequently precedes bacterial pneumonia. Community-acquired bacterial pneumonia is one of the leading causes of hospitalization.
5. Aspiration pneumonitis is caused by inhalation of a foreign substance, such as food, milk, secretions, or environmental compounds, into the lung, and results in inflammation.
6. Bronchiolitis obliterans is a rare postinflammatory condition in which the bronchioles and some small bronchi are partially or completely obliterated by fibrous tissue, causing pulmonary impairment and disability.
7. Asthma is a chronic inflammatory disease characterized by bronchial hyperreactivity and reversible airflow obstruction, and is usually a type I hypersensitivity response to an antigen. Its origins are probably multifactorial, including genetic, allergic, and viral-triggered mechanisms.
8. Acute respiratory distress syndrome (ARDS) can occur when there is an insult to the lung that activates an inflammatory response causing alveolar capillary injury, usually within 24 hours. There is progressive respiratory distress with severe hypoxemia and respiratory failure.
9. Cystic fibrosis is an autosomal recessive genetic disease that affects many organ systems, especially the lungs and digestive system. Airway secretions are particularly thick and tenacious, and the airways develop chronic bacterial infection with pathogens such as *Pseudomonas aeruginosa* and *Staphylococcus aureus*. Chronic infection, plugged airways, and severe inflammation cause long-term lung damage and ultimately death. However, the prognosis is improving, and most children with CF now survive to adulthood.

Sudden Infant Death Syndrome (SIDS)

1. Sudden infant death syndrome is the leading cause of postnatal death for infants outside of the hospital setting and is associated with low birthweight, prone sleeping position, and other environmental factors. There has been a significant reduction in SIDS since widespread adoption of recommendations for supine positioning of infants during sleep.

REFERENCES

1. Cherry JD: Clinical practice. Croup, *N Engl J Med* 358(4):384–391, 2008.
2. Arslan Z, et al: Evaluation of allergic sensitization and gastroesophageal reflux disease in children with recurrent croup, *Pediatr Int* 51(5):661–665, 2009.
3. Wall S, et al: The viral aetiology of croup and recurrent croup, *Arch Dis Child* 94(5):359–360, 2009.
4. Sammer M, Pruthi S: Membranous croup (exudative tracheitis or membranous laryngotracheobronchitis), *Pediatr Radiol* 40:781, 2010.
5. Everard M: Acute bronchiolitis and croup, *Pediatr Clin North Am* 56:119–133, 2009.
6. Li SF: The Westley croup score, *Acad Emerg Med* 10(3):289, 2003:author reply 289.
7. Bjornson C, et al: Nebulized epinephrine for croup in children, *Cochrane Database Syst Rev* 2:CD006619, 2011.
8. Vorwerk C, Coats T: Heliox for croup in children (review), *Cochrane Database Syst Rev* (2):CD006822, 2010.
9. Rogers D, Sie K, Manning S: Epiglottitis due to nontypeable *Haemophilus influenzae* in a vaccinated child, *Int J Pediatr Otorhinlaryngol* 74:218–220, 2010.
10. Sobol S, Zapata S: Epiglottitis and croup, *Otolaryngol Clin North Am* 41:551–566, 2008.
11. Acevedo J, et al: Airway management in pediatric epiglottitis: a national perspective, *Otolaryngol Head Neck Surg* 140:548–551, 2009.
12. Burton MJ, Glasziou PP: Tonsillectomy or adeno-tonsillectomy versus non-surgical treatment for chronic/recurrent acute tonsillitis, *Cochrane Database Syst Rev* (1): CD001802, 2009.
13. Kay M, Wyllie R: Pediatric foreign bodies and their management, *Curr Gastroenterol Rep* 7(3):212–218, 2005.
14. Shlizerman L, et al: Foreign body aspiration in children: the effects of delayed diagnosis, *Am J Otolaryngol* 31(5):320–324, 2010.
15. Katz E, D'Ambrosio C: Pediatric obstructive sleep apnea syndrome, *Clin Chest Med* 31:221–234, 2010.
16. Snow A, et al: Pediatric obstructive sleep apnea: a potential late consequence of respiratory syncitial virus bronchiolitis, *Pediatr Pulmonol* 44:1186–1191, 2009.
17. Katz ES, D'Ambrosio CM: Pediatric obstructive sleep apnea syndrome, *Clin ChestMed* 31(2):221–234, 2010.
18. Snow A, et al: Catecholamine alterations in pediatric obstructive sleep apnea: effect on obesity, *Pediatr Pulmonol* 44:559–567, 2009.
19. Goldbart A, et al: Inflammatory mediators in exhaled breath condensate of children with obstructive sleep apnea syndrome, *Chest* 130:143–148, 2006.
20. Kheirandish-Gozal L, Bhattacharjee R, Gozal D: Autonomic alterations and endothelial dysfunction in pediatric obstructive sleep apnea, *Sleep Med* 11:714–720, 2010.
21. Fauroux B, Aubertin G, Clement A: What's new in paediatric sleep in 2007? *Paediatr Respir Rev* 9:139–143, 2008.
22. Friedman M, et al: Updates systematic review of tonsillectomy and adenoidectomy for treatment of pediatric obstructive sleep apnea/hypopnea syndrome, *Otolaryngol Head Neck Surg* 140:800–808, 2009.
23. Fraser M, Walls M, McGuire W: Respiratory complications of preterm birth, *Br Med J* 329:962–965, 2004.
24. Colin A, McEvoy C, Castile R: Respiratory morbidity and lung function in preterm infants of 32 to 36 weeks' gestational age, *Pediatrics* 126:115–128, 2010.
25. Sweet D, et al: European consensus guidelines on the management of neonatal respiratory distress syndrome, *J Perinatal Med* 35:175–186, 2007.
26. Waters T, Mercer B: Impact of timing of antenatal corticosteroid exposure on neonatal outcomes, *J Matern Fetal Neonatal Med* 22(4):311–314, 2009.
27. Verder H, et al: Nasal CPAP and surfactant for treatment of respiratory distress syndrome and prevention of bronchopulmonary dysplasia, *Acta Paediatr* 98(9):1400–1408, 2009.
28. Soll RF: Current trials in the treatment of respiratory failure in preterm infants, *Neonatol* 95(4):368–372, 2009.
29. Donohue PK, et al: Inhaled nitric oxide in preterm infants: a systematic review, *Pediatrics* 127(2):e414–e422, 2011.
30. Van Marter LJ: Epidemiology of bronchopulmonary dysplasia, *Semin Fetal Neonatal Med* 14(6):358–366, 2009.
31. Hayes D Jr, et al: Pathogenesis of bronchopulmonary dysplasia, *Respiration* 79(5):425–436, 2010.
32. Abman SH: Impaired vascular endothelial growth factor signaling in the pathogenesis of neonatal pulmonary vascular disease, *Adv Exp Med Biol* 661:323–335, 2010.
33. Baraldi E, Filippone M: Chronic lung disease after premature birth, *N Eng J Med* 357(19):1946–1955, 2007.
34. Davies P, et al: Relationship of proteinases and proteinase inhibitors with microbial presence in chronic lung disease of prematurity, *Thorax* 65:246–251, 2010.
35. Gupta S, Sinha SK, Donn SM: Ventilatory management and bronchopulmonary dysplasia in preterm infants, *Semin Fetal Neonatal Med* 14(6):367–373, 2009.
36. SUPPORT Study Group of the Eunice Kennedy Shriver NICHD Neonatal Research Network: early CPAP versus surfactant in extremely preterm infants, *N Engl J Med* 362(21):1970–1979, 2010.
37. Kwinta P, Pietrzyk JJ: Preterm birth and respiratory disease in later life, *Exp Rev Respir Med* 4(5):593–604, 2010.
38. Doyle LW, Anderson PJ: Long-term outcomes of bronchopulmonary dysplasia, *Semin Fetal Neonatal Med* 14(6):391–395, 2009.
39. Wainwright C: Acute viral bronchiolitis in children—a very common condition with few therapeutic options, *Paediatr Respir Rev* 11(1):39–45, 2010:quiz 45.
40. Jartti T, et al: Bronchiolitis: age and previous wheezing episodes are linked to viral etiology and atopic characteristics, *Pediatr Infect Dis J* 28(4):311–317, 2009.
41. Mansbach J, Camargo C: Respiratory viruses in bronchiolitis and their link to recurrent wheezing and asthma, *Clin Lab Med* 29:741–755, 2009.
42. Grewal S, et al: A randomized trial of nebulized 3% hypertonic saline with epinephrine in the treatment of acute bronchiolitis in the emergency department, *Arch Pediatr Adolesc Med* 163(11):1007–1012, 2009.
43. Liet J, et al: Heliox inhalation therapy for bronchiolitis in infants (review), *Cochrane Database Syst Rev* (4): CD006915, 2010.
44. Martinon-Torres F, et al: Nasal continuous positive airway pressure with heliox versus air oxygen in infants with acute bronchiolitis: a crossover study, *Pediatrics* 121:e1190–e1195, 2008.
45. Kesson AM: Respiratory virus infections, *Paediatr Respir Rev* 8(3):240–248, 2007.

46. Nohynek H, Madhi S, Grijalva CG: Childhood bacterial respiratory diseases: past, present, and future, *Pediatr Infect Dis J* 28(suppl 10): S127–S132, 2009.

47. Van Der Poll T, Opal S: Pathogenesis, treatment and prevention of pneumococcal pneumonia, *Lancet* 374:1543–1556, 2009.

48. Lynch JP III, Zhanel GG: *Streptococcus pneumoniae*: epidemiology and risk factors, evolution of antimicrobial resistance, and impact of vaccines, *Curr Opin Pulmon Med* 16(3):217–225, 2010.

49. Bradley J, et al: Comparative study of levofloxacin in the treatment of children with community-acquired pneumonia, *Pediatr Infect Dis J* 26(10):868–878, 2007.

50. Craig J, et al: The accuracy and clinical symptoms and signs for the diagnosis of serious bacterial infection in young febrile children: prospective cohort study of 15781 febrile illnesses, *Br Med J* 340:c1594, 2010:(online).

51. Lynch T, et al: A systematic review on the diagnosis of pediatric bacterial pneumonia: when gold is bronze, *PLoS ONE* 5(8):e11989, 2010:[electronic resource].

52. Kabra SK, Lodha R, Pandey RM: Antibiotics for community-acquired pneumonia in children (Review), *Cochrane Database Syst Rev* (3): CD004874, 2010.

53. Nascimento-Carvalho C: Pharmacotherapy of childhood pneumonia, *Exp Opin Pharmacother* 11(2):225–231, 2010.

54. Fontoura M, et al: Clinical failure among children with nonsevere community-acquired pneumonia treated with amoxicillin, *Exp Opin Pharmacother* 11(9):1–8, 2010.

55. Li X, et al: Emerging macrolide resistance in *Mycoplasma pneumoniae* in children, *Pediatr Infect Dis J* 28(8):693–696, 2009.

56. Mulholland S, Gavranich JB, Chang AB: Antibiotics for community-acquired lower respiratory tract infections secondary to *Mycoplasma pneumoniae* in children, *Cochrane Database Syst Rev* (7):CD004875, 2010.

57. Boesch RP, et al: Advances in the diagnosis and management of chronic pulmonary aspiration in children, *Eur Respir J* 28:847–861, 2006.

58. Pena A, et al: Botulinum toxin A injection of salivary glands in children with drooling and chronic aspiration, *J Vasc Interv Radiol* 20(3):368–373, 2009.

59. Colom A, et al: Risk factors for the development of bronchiolitis obliterans in children with bronchiolitis, *Thorax* 61:503–506, 2006.

60. Grasemann H, Ratjen F: Leukocyte trafficking and matrix metalloproteinase-8 in obliterative bronchiolitis, *J Leukoc Biol* 87:23–24, 2010.

61. American Lung Association: *Trends in asthma morbidity and mortality*. Available at www.lungusa.org/finding-cures/our-research/trend-reports/asthma-trend-report.pdf. Accessed Feb 2010.

62. Clement L, Jones C, Cole J: Health disparities in the United States: childhood asthma, *Am J Med Sci* 335(4):260–265, 2008.

63. Ho SM: Environmental epigenetics of asthma: an update, *J Allergy Clin Immunol* 126(3):453–465, 2010.

64. Brehm J, et al: Serum vitamin D levels and severe asthma exacerbations in the Childhood Asthma Management Program Study, *J Allergy Clin Immunol* 126(1):52–58, 2010.

65. Brownlee J, Turner R: New developments in the epidemiology and clinical spectrum of rhinovirus infections, *Curr Opin Pediatr* 20:67–71, 2008.

66. National Heart, Lung, and Blood Institute: *National Asthma Education and Prevention Program Expert Panel Report 3: guidelines for the diagnosis and management of asthma*, 2007. Available at www.nhlbi.nih.gov/guidelines.

67. Willson DF, Chess PR, Notter RH: Surfactant for pediatric acute lung injury, *Pediatr Clin North Am* 55(3):545–575, 2008:ix.

68. Randolph AG: Management of acute lung injury and acute respiratory distress syndrome in children, *Crit Care Med* 37(8):2448–2454, 2009.

69. Afshari A, et al: Inhaled nitric oxide for acute respiratory distress syndrome (ARDS) and acute lung injury in children and adults, *Cochrane Database Syst Rev* (7): CD002787, 2010.

70. Afshari A, et al: Aerosolized prostacyclin for acute lung injury (ALI) and acute respiratory distress syndrome (ARDS), *Cochrane Database Syst Rev* (8): CD007733, 2010.

71. O'Sullivan BP, Freedman SD: Cystic fibrosis, *Lancet* 373(9678):1891–1904, 2009.

72. Messick J: A 21st-century approach to cystic fibrosis: optimizing outcomes across the disease spectrum, *J Pediatr Gastroenterol Nutr* 51(suppl 7):S1–S7, 2010:quiz 3 p following S7.

73. Mogayzel PJ Jr, Flume PA: Update in cystic fibrosis 2009, *Am J Respir Crit Care Med* 181(6):539–544, 2010.

74. Castellani C, Massie J: Emerging issues in cystic fibrosis newborn screening, *Curr Opin Pulm Med* 16(6):584–590, 2010.

75. Flume PA, et al: Cystic fibrosis pulmonary guidelines: airway clearance therapies, *Respir Care* 54:522–537, 2009.

76. Jones AP, Wallis C: Dornase alfa for cystic fibrosis, *Cochrane Database Syst Rev* (3):CD001127, 2010.

77. Phung OJ, et al: Recombinant human growth hormone in the treatment of patients with cystic fibrosis, *Pediatrics* 126(5):e1211–e1226, 2010.

78. Dwyer T, Ponsonby AL: Sudden infant death syndrome and prone sleeping position, *Ann Epidemiol* 19(4):245–249, 2009.

79. Mitchell EA: SIDS: past, present and future, *Acta Paediatr* 98(11): 1712–1719, 2009.

80. Randall B, et al: A practical classification schema incorporating consideration of possible asphyxia in cases of sudden unexpected infant death, *Forensic Sci Med Pathol* 5:254–260, 2009.

81. Poetsch M, et al: Impact of sodium/proton exchanger 3 gene variants on sudden infant death syndrome, *J Pediatr* 156(1):44–48, 2010.

82. Ostfeld B, et al: Concurrent risks in sudden infant death syndrome, *Pediatrics* 125:447–453, 2010.

83. Lavezzi AM, et al: Study of the human hypoglossal nucleus: normal development and morpho-functional alterations in sudden unexplained late fetal and infant death, *Brain Develop* 32:275–284, 2010.

84. Dettmeyer RB, Kandolf R: Cardiomyopathies-misdiagnosed as sudden infant death syndrome (SIDS), *Forensic Sci Inter* 194:e21–e24, 2010.

Structure and Function of the Renal and Urologic Systems

Sue E. Huether

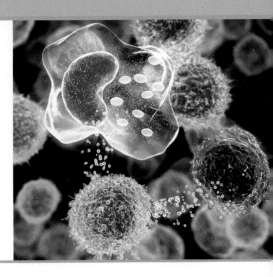

CHAPTER OUTLINE

The primary function of the kidney is to maintain a stable internal environment for optimal cell and tissue metabolism. The kidneys accomplish these life-sustaining tasks by balancing solute and water transport, excreting metabolic waste products, conserving nutrients, and regulating acids and bases. The kidney also has an endocrine function and secretes the hormones renin, erythropoietin, and 1,25-dihydroxyvitamin D_3 for regulation of blood pressure, erythrocyte production, and calcium metabolism, respectively. In times of severe fasting, the kidney also can synthesize glucose from amino acids, performing the process of gluconeogenesis. The formation of urine is achieved through the processes of glomerular filtration, and tubular reabsorption, and secretion within the kidney. The bladder stores the urine that it receives from the kidney by way of the ureters. Urine is then released from the bladder through the urethra.

STRUCTURES OF THE RENAL SYSTEM

Structures of the Kidney

The **kidneys** are paired organs located on the posterior abdominal wall outside the peritoneal cavity. They lie on either side of the vertebral column with their upper and lower poles extending from the twelfth thoracic vertebra to the third lumbar vertebra (Figure 28-1). Each kidney is approximately 11 cm long, 5 to 6 cm wide, and 3 to 4 cm thick. A tightly adhering capsule (the **renal capsule**) surrounds each kidney, and the kidney then is embedded in a mass of fat. The capsule and fatty layer are covered with a double layer of **renal fascia,** fibrous tissue that attaches the kidney to the posterior abdominal wall. The cushion of fat and the position of the kidney between the abdominal organs and muscles of the back protect it from trauma.

The right kidney is slightly lower than the left; it is displaced downward by the overlying liver. A medial indentation (the **hilum**) in the kidney is the location of the entry and exit for the renal blood vessels, nerves, lymphatic vessels, and ureter.

The outer layer of the kidney is called the **cortex** and it contains all of the glomeruli, most of the proximal tubules, and some segments of the distal tubule. The **medulla** forms the inner part of the kidney and consists of regions call **pyramids.** Columns of renal cortex (renal columns) extend down between the pyramids. The pyramids extend into the renal pelvis and contain the loops of Henle and collecting ducts. The **calyces** are chambers that receive urine from the collecting ducts and form the entry into the renal pelvis, an extension of the upper ureter.

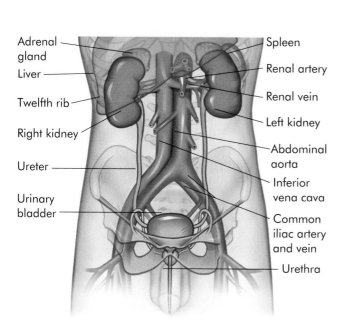

FIGURE 28-1 Organs of the Urinary System. (From Thibodeau GA, Patton KT: *Anatomy & physiology,* ed 6, St Louis, 2007, Mosby.)

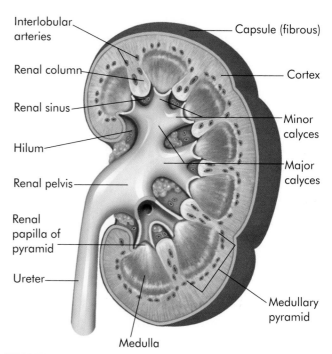

FIGURE 28-2 Kidney Structure. (From Thibodeau GA, Patton KT: *Anatomy & physiology,* ed 6, St Louis, 2007, Mosby.)

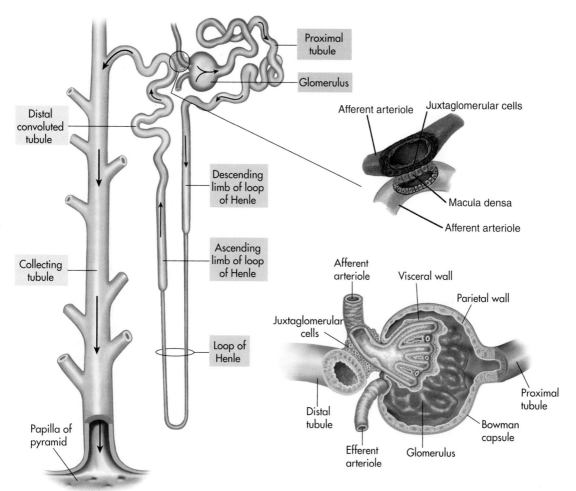

FIGURE 28-3 Components of Nephron. (From Patton KT, Thibodeau GA: *Anatomy & physiology,* ed 7, St Louis, 2010, Mosby; Damjanov I: *Pathology for the health professions,* St Louis, 2006, Mosby.)

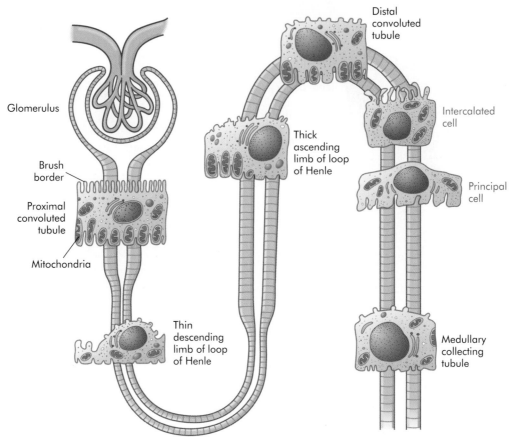

FIGURE 28-4 Epithelial Cells of the Various Segments of Nephron Tubules. The brush border and high number of mitochondria in cells of the proximal tubule promote reabsorption of 50% of the glomerular filtrate. Intercalated cells secrete H^+ (through K^+ exchange) or reabsorb HCO_3^-. Principal cells are influenced by aldosterone and reabsorb Na^+ and water and secrete K^+.

The structural unit of the kidney is the lobe. Each **lobe** is composed of a pyramid and the overlying cortex. There are about 14 lobes in each kidney. The gross structure of the kidney can be reviewed in Figure 28-2.

Nephron

The **nephron** is the functional unit of the kidney. Each kidney contains approximately 1.2 million nephrons. The nephron is a tubular structure with subunits that include the renal corpuscle, proximal convoluted tubule, loop of Henle, distal convoluted tubule, and collecting duct, all of which contribute to the formation of final urine (Figure 28-3). The different structures of the epithelial cells lining various segments of the tubule facilitate the special functions of secretion and reabsorption (Figure 28-4).

The kidney has three kinds of nephrons: (1) superficial **cortical nephrons** (85% of all nephrons), which extend partially into the medulla; (2) **midcortical nephrons** with short or long loops; and (3) **juxtamedullary nephrons,** which lie close to and extend deep into the medulla and are important for the concentration of urine (Figure 28-5). The **glomerulus** is a tuft of capillaries that loop into Bowman capsule, like fingers pushed into bread dough. Together, the glomerulus and Bowman capsule are called the **renal corpuscle.** **Mesangial cells** (shaped like smooth muscle cells) and the mesangial matrix lie between and support the capillaries (Figure 28-6). Mesangial cells have phagocytic ability similar to monocytes, release inflammatory cytokines, and can contract to regulate glomerulus

capillary blood flow.[1,2] The space inside Bowman capsule is called **Bowman space.**

The **glomerular filtration membrane** filters blood components through its three layers: (1) an inner capillary endothelium, (2) a middle basement membrane, and (3) an outer layer of capillary epithelium. The capillary endothelium is composed of cells in continuous contact with the basement membrane and contains pores. The middle basement membrane is a selectively permeable network of glycoproteins and mucopolysaccharides. The epithelium has specialized cells called **podocytes** from which pedicles (foot projections) radiate and adhere to the basement membrane. The pedicles interlock with the pedicles of adjacent podocytes, forming an elaborate network of intercellular clefts (**filtration slits,** or slit membranes). The endothelium, basement membrane, and podocytes are covered with protein molecules bearing anionic (negative) charges that retard the filtration of anionic proteins and prevent proteinuria. The glomerular filtration membrane separates the blood of the glomerular capillaries from the fluid in Bowman space. The glomerular filtrate passes through the three layers of the glomerular membrane and forms the primary urine.[3,4]

The glomerulus is supplied by the afferent arteriole and drained by the efferent arteriole. A group of specialized cells known as **juxtaglomerular cells** (renin-releasing cells) are located around the afferent arteriole where it enters the glomerulus (see Figure 28-3). Between the afferent and efferent arterioles is the **macula densa** (sodium-sensing cells) of the distal tubule (see Figure 28-6). Together the juxtaglomerular cells and macula densa cells form the **juxtaglomerular apparatus**

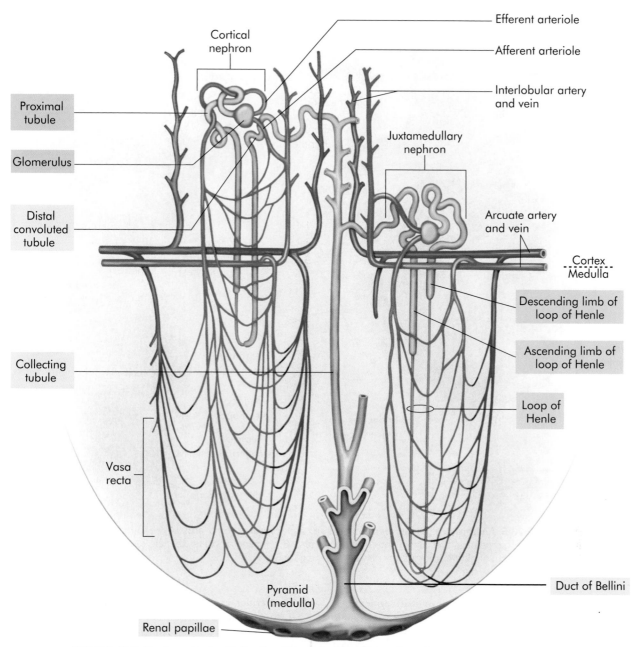

FIGURE 28-5 Nephron Unit with Its Blood Vessels. Blood flows through nephron vessels as follows: interlobular artery, afferent arteriole, glomerulus, efferent arteriole, peritubular capillaries (around the tubules), venules, interlobular vein. The vasa recta capillaries distribute along the long loops of Henle of the juxtamedullary nephrons. (From Thibodeau GA, Patton KT: *Anatomy & physiology,* ed 6, St Louis, 2007, Mosby.)

(see Figure 28-3). Control of renal blood flow, glomerular filtration, and renin secretion occurs at this site.[5,6]

The proximal tubule continues from Bowman space and has an initial convoluted segment (pars convoluta) and then a straight segment (pars recta) that descends toward the medulla (see Figure 28-3). The proximal tubular lumen consists of one layer of cuboidal cells. This is the only surface inside the nephron where the cells are covered with microvilli (a brush border). This greatly expands the surface area of the tubule and enhances its reabsorptive function (see Figure 28-4). The proximal tubule joins the loop of Henle, which extends into the medulla. The tube then loops and becomes a thickening

ascending segment that extends toward the cortex. A thin segment is composed of thin squamous cells with no active transport function. The cells of the thick segment are cuboidal and actively transport several solutes.

The major structural difference between the glomeruli in the types of nephrons is the length of the loop of Henle. In cortical nephrons, the loop is short and may not extend into the medulla. The loops of Henle for the juxtamedullary nephrons, however, may extend the whole length of the medulla (40 mm). Juxtamedullary nephrons represent about 12% of the total number of nephrons and are important for the concentration and dilution of urine.

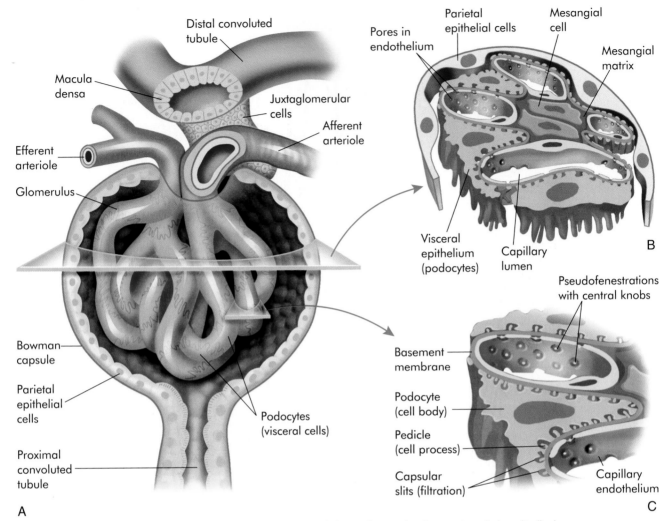

FIGURE 28-6 Anatomy of the Glomerulus and Juxtaglomerular Apparatus. A, Longitudinal cross section of glomerulus and juxtaglomerular apparatus. **B,** Horizontal cross section of glomerulus. **C,** Enlargement of glomerular capillary filtration membrane.

The **distal tubule** has straight and convoluted segments. It extends from the macula densa to the **collecting duct,** a large tubule that descends down the cortex, through the renal pyramids of the inner and outer medullae, and into the minor calyx. In the distal tubule, **principal cells** reabsorb sodium and secrete potassium and **intercalated cells** reabsorb potassium and bicarbonate and secrete hydrogen.

Blood Vessels of the Kidney

The blood vessels of the kidney closely parallel nephron structure. The major vessels are as follows:

1. **Renal arteries.** Arise as the fifth branches of the abdominal aorta, divide into anterior and posterior branches at the renal hilum, and then subdivide into lobar arteries supplying blood to the lower, middle, and upper thirds of the kidney.
2. **Interlobar arteries.** Further subdivisions travel down renal columns and between pyramids; form afferent glomerular arteries.
3. **Arcuate arteries.** Consist of branches of interlobar arteries at the cortical-medullary junction; arch over the base of the pyramids and run parallel to the surface.

4. **Glomerular capillaries.** Four to eight vessels are arranged in a fistlike structure; arise from the afferent arteriole and empty into the efferent arteriole, which carries blood to the peritubular capillaries.
5. **Peritubular capillaries.** Surround convoluted portions of the proximal and distal tubules and the loop of Henle; adapted for cortical and juxtamedullary nephrons.
6. **Vasa recta.** Network of capillaries forms loops and closely follows the loops of Henle; is only blood supply to the medulla.
7. **Renal veins.** Follow arterial path and have same names as the corresponding arteries; eventually empty into the inferior vena cava.

Note that the lymphatic vessels tend also to follow the distribution of the blood vessels.

✔ QUICK CHECK 28-1

1. What is the major structural difference between the cortex and medulla of the kidney?
2. What is the function of the nephron?
3. Why are proteins not filtered at the glomerulus?

Urinary Structures

Ureters

The urine formed by the nephrons flows from the distal tubules and collecting ducts through the duct of Bellini and the renal papillae (projections of the ducts) into the calyces, where it is collected in the renal pelvis (see Figures 28-2 and 28-5), and then funneled into the ureters. Each adult ureter is approximately 30 cm long and is composed of long, intertwining muscle bundles. The lower ends pass obliquely through the posterior aspect of the bladder wall. The close approximation of muscle cells permits the direct transmission of electrical stimulation, and the resulting peristaltic activity propels urine into the bladder. Peristaltic activity is affected by urine volume. When urine flow is slow, the contraction is segmented, with downward propulsion of urine. Increasing flow rates increase peristalsis. Peristalsis is maintained even when the ureter is denervated; therefore ureters can be transplanted. The upper part of the ureter is innervated by the tenth thoracic nerve roots, with referred pain to the umbilicus. The innervation of lower segments of the ureter arises from the sacral nerves with referred pain to the vulva or penis. The distal end of the ureter passes through the detrusor muscle and enters the submucosal tunnel terminating at the ureteral orifice. Contraction of the bladder during micturition (urination) compresses the distal end of the ureter, preventing reflux. The ureters have a rich blood supply from the kidney with contributions by the lumbar and superior vesical arteries.

Bladder and Urethra

The bladder is a bag of smooth muscle fibers that forms the detrusor muscle and its smooth lining of uroepithelium. While the bladder fills with urine, it distends and the layers of uroepithelium slide past each other and become thinner. The uroepithelium forms the interface between the urinary space and underlying vasculature and connective, nervous, and muscle tissue. The uroepithelium maintains an important barrier function to prevent movement of water and solutes between the urine and the blood and communicates information about urine pressure and composition to surrounding nerve and muscle cells.[7] The detrusor is the smooth muscle coat of the bladder, and the trigone is a smooth triangular area between the openings of the two ureters and the urethra (Figure 28-7). The position of the bladder varies with age and gender. The bladder has a profuse blood supply, accounting for the bleeding that readily occurs with trauma, surgery, or inflammation.

The urethra extends from the inferior side of the bladder to the outside of the body. A ring of smooth muscle forms the internal urethral sphincter at the junction of the urethra and bladder. The external urethral sphincter is composed of striated muscles and is under voluntary control. The entire urethra is lined with mucus-secreting glands. The female urethra is short (3 to 4 cm). The male urethra is long (18 to 20 cm) and has three segments: prostatic, membranous, and cavernous. The prostatic urethra is closest to the bladder. It passes through the prostate gland and contains the openings of the ejaculatory ducts. The membranous urethra passes through the floor of the pelvis. The cavernous segment forms the remainder of the tube. It is surrounded by erectile tissue and contains the openings of the bulbourethral mucous glands.

The innervation of the bladder and internal urethral sphincter is supplied by parasympathetic fibers of the autonomic nervous system. The reflex arc required for micturition is stimulated by mechanoreceptors that respond to stretching of tissue, sensing bladder fullness and sending impulses to the sacral level of the cord. When the bladder accumulates 250 to 300 ml of urine, the bladder contracts and the internal urethral sphincter relaxes through activation of the spinal

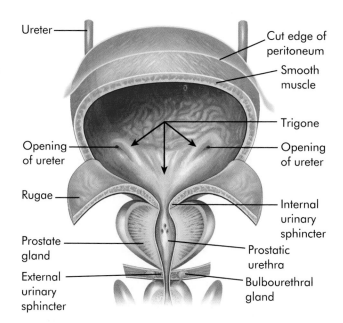

FIGURE 28-7 **Structure of the Urinary Bladder.** Frontal view of a dissected urinary bladder (male) in a fully distended position. (From Thibodeau GA, Patton KT: *Anatomy & physiology,* ed 6, St Louis, 2007, Mosby.)

reflex arc (known as the *micturition reflex*). At this time, a person feels the urge to void. In older children and adults, the reflex can be inhibited or facilitated by impulses coming from the brain, resulting in voluntary control of micturition by the relaxation or contraction of the external sphincter.

RENAL BLOOD FLOW

The kidneys are highly vascular organs and usually receive 1000 to 1200 ml of blood per minute, or about 20% to 25% of the cardiac output. With a normal hematocrit of 45%, about 600 to 700 ml of blood flowing through the kidney per minute is plasma. From the renal plasma flow (RPF), 20% (approximately 120 to 140 ml/min) is filtered at the glomerulus and passes into Bowman capsule. The filtration of the plasma per unit of time is known as the glomerular filtration rate (GFR), which is directly related to the perfusion pressure of the glomerular capillaries.

The remaining 80% (about 480 ml) of plasma flows through the efferent arterioles to the peritubular capillaries. The ratio of glomerular filtrate to renal plasma flow per minute (125/600 = 0.20) is called the *filtration fraction*. Normally all but 1 to 2 ml of the glomerular filtrate is reabsorbed from nephron tubules and returned to the circulation by the peritubular capillaries.

The GFR is directly related to renal blood flow (RBF), which is regulated by intrinsic autoregulatory mechanisms, by neural regulation, and by hormonal regulation. In general, blood flow to any organ is determined by the arteriovenous pressure differences across the vascular bed. If mean arterial pressure decreases or vascular resistance increases, RBF declines.

Autoregulation of Intrarenal Blood Flow

In the kidney, a local mechanism tends to keep the rate of intrarenal blood flow and therefore the GFR fairly constant over a range of arterial pressures between 80 and 180 mm Hg (Figure 28-8). Changes in

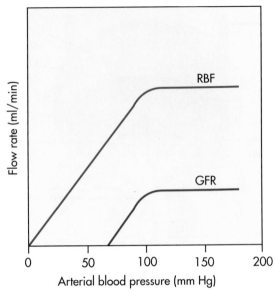

FIGURE 28-8 Renal Autoregulation. Blood flow and glomerular filtration rate are stabilized in the face of changes in perfusion pressure. (From Levy MN, editor: *Berne & Levy principles of physiology,* ed 4, Philadelphia, 2006, Mosby.)

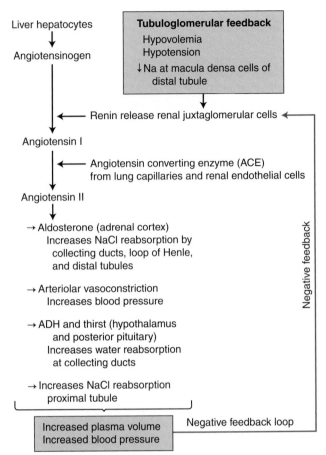

FIGURE 28-9 Renin-Angiotensin-Aldosterone System. Activation of tubuloglomerular feedback mechanisms stimulates the release of renin with activation of the renin-angiotensin-aldosterone cascade. Plasma volume and blood pressure are increased with the reabsorption of sodium chloride and water from the renal tubules. The restoration of plasma volume and blood pressure then decreases the release of renin, forming a negative feedback loop.

afferent arteriolar resistance and arteriolar pressure occur in the same direction. Therefore, RBF and GFR are relatively constant, a relationship maintained by an intrinsic autoregulatory mechanism. The purpose of autoregulation of blood flow is to prevent large changes in GFR when there are increases or decreases in systemic blood pressure. Solute and water excretion and thus blood volume are regulated when arterial pressure changes.[8]

A mechanism that keeps RBF and GFR constant and stable is tubuloglomerular feedback. Because the glomerular filtration rate in an individual nephron increases or decreases, the macula densa cells in the distal tubule sense the increasing or decreasing amounts of filtered sodium. When GFR and sodium concentration increase, the macula densa cells stimulate afferent arteriolar vasoconstriction and decrease GFR. The opposite occurs with decreases in GFR and sodium concentration at the macula densa.[9]

Neural Regulation of Renal Blood Flow

The blood vessels of the kidney are innervated by the autonomic nervous system through sympathetic fibers that cause vasoconstriction and decrease renal blood flow. There is no significant parasympathetic innervation. The innervation of the kidney arises primarily from the celiac ganglion and greater splanchnic nerve (see Figure 12-26). The afferent and efferent arterioles are richly innervated, but nerves have not been observed in the glomerular capillaries.

When systemic arterial pressure decreases, increased renal sympathetic nerve activity is mediated reflexively through the carotid sinus and the baroreceptors of the aortic arch. This stimulates renal arteriolar vasoconstriction and decreases both RBF and GFR. The decreased RBF also diminishes excretion of sodium and water, promoting an increase in blood volume and thus an increase in systemic pressure.

Exercise, body position, and hypoxia also influence RBF. Exercise and change of body position activate renal sympathetic neurons and cause mild vasoconstriction. Severe hypoxia stimulates the chemoreceptors of the carotid and aortic bodies and decreases RBF by means of sympathetic stimulation. Hemorrhage induces intense sympathetic stimulation and vasoconstriction, and both GFR and blood flow are

reduced. The sympathetic nervous system also participates in hormonal regulation of renal blood flow.

Hormonal Regulation of Renal Blood Flow

A major hormonal regulator of renal blood flow is the renin-angiotensin-aldosterone system, which can increase systemic arterial pressure and change RBF. Renin is an enzyme formed and stored in the cells of the arterioles of the juxtaglomerular apparatus (see Figure 28-3). Several complex physiologic mechanisms stimulate its release, including decreased blood pressure in the afferent arterioles, which reduces the stretch of the juxtaglomerular cells, decreased sodium chloride concentration in the distal convoluted tubule, and sympathetic nerve stimulation of β-adrenergic receptors on the juxtaglomerular cells and prostaglandins.[10] Numerous physiologic effects of the renin-angiotensin-aldosterone system stabilize systemic blood pressure and preserve the extracellular fluid volume during hypotension or hypovolemia, including sodium reabsorption, systemic vasoconstriction, sympathetic nerve stimulation, and thirst stimulation with increased fluid intake. The effects of aldosterone combine with those of antidiuretic hormone in regulating blood volume. The effects are summarized in Figures 28-9, 22-32, and 22-33 (also see *Health Alert:* Multiple Effects of the Renin-Angiotensin-Aldosterone System in Chapter 22, p. 577).

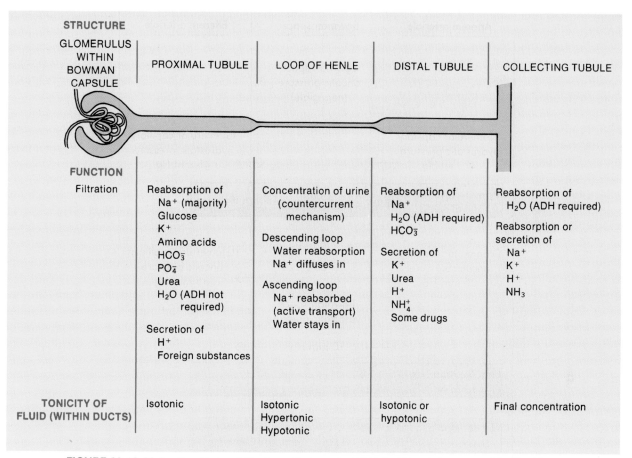

FIGURE 28-10 Major Functions of Nephron Segments. *ADH*, Antidiuretic hormone. (Modified from Hockenberry MJ et al: *Wong's nursing care of infants and children*, ed 8, St Louis, 2007, Mosby.)

KIDNEY FUNCTION

Nephron Function

The nephron can perform many functions simultaneously, as follows:
1. Filters plasma at glomerulus.
2. Reabsorbs and secretes different substances along tubular structures.
3. Forms a filtrate of protein-free fluid (ultrafiltration).
4. Regulates the filtrate to maintain body fluid volume, electrolyte composition, and pH within narrow limits.

Glomerular filtration is the movement of fluid and solutes across the glomerular capillary membrane and into the Bowman space. **Tubular reabsorption** is the movement of fluids and solutes from the tubular lumen to the peritubular capillary plasma. **Tubular secretion** is the transfer of substances from the plasma of the peritubular capillary to the tubular lumen. The transport mechanisms are both active and passive (processes defined in Chapter 1). **Excretion** is the elimination of a substance in the final urine (Figure 28-10).

Glomerular Filtration

The fluid filtered by the glomerular capillary filtration membrane is protein free but contains electrolytes (such as sodium, chloride, and potassium) and organic molecules (such as creatinine, urea, and glucose) in the same concentrations as found in plasma. Like other capillary membranes, the glomerulus is freely permeable to water and relatively impermeable to large colloids, such as plasma proteins. The molecule's size and electrical charge affect the permeability of substances crossing the glomerulus.

Capillary pressure also affects glomerular filtration. The hydrostatic pressure within the capillary is the major force for moving water and solutes across the filtration membrane and into Bowman capsule. Two forces oppose the filtration effects of the glomerular capillary hydrostatic pressure (P_{GC}): (1) the hydrostatic pressure in Bowman space (P_{BC}) and (2) the effective oncotic pressure of the glomerular capillary blood (π_{GC}). Because the fluid in Bowman space normally contains only minute amounts of protein, it does not usually have an oncotic influence on the plasma of the glomerular capillary (Figure 28-11).

The combined effect of forces favoring and forces opposing filtration determines the filtration pressure. The **net filtration pressure (NFP)** is the sum of forces favoring and opposing filtration. The estimated values contributing to the forces of net filtration are presented in Table 28-1.

While the protein-free fluid is filtered into Bowman capsule, the plasma oncotic pressure increases and the hydrostatic pressure decreases. The increase in glomerular capillary oncotic pressure is great enough to reduce the net filtration pressure to zero at the efferent end

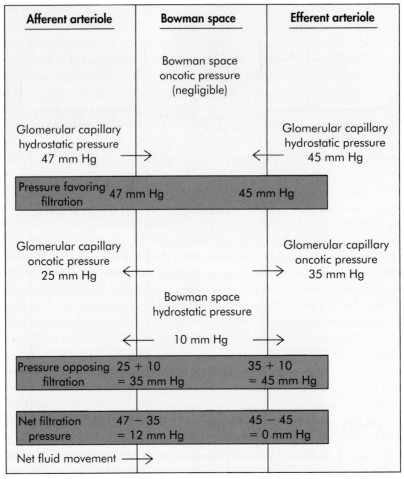

FIGURE 28-11 Glomerular Filtration Pressures.

TABLE 28-1 GLOMERULAR FILTRATION PRESSURES

		PRESSURES (mm Hg)	
FORCES	PRESSURES	BEGINNING OF CAPILLARY	END OF CAPILLARY
Promoting Filtration			
Glomerular capillary hydrostatic pressure	P_{GC}	47	45
Bowman capsule oncotic pressure	π_{BC}	Negligible effect	Negligible effect
Opposing Filtration			
Bowman capsule hydrostatic pressure	P_{BC}	10	10
Glomerular capillary oncotic pressure	π_{GC}	25	35
Net filtration pressure		12	0

of the capillary and to stop the filtration process effectively. The low hydrostatic pressure and the increased oncotic pressure in the efferent arteriole then are transferred to the peritubular capillaries and facilitate reabsorption of fluid from the proximal tubules.

Filtration rate. The total volume of fluid filtered by the glomeruli averages 180 L/day, or approximately 120 ml/min, a phenomenal amount considering the size of the kidneys. Because only 1 to 2 L of urine is excreted per day, 99% of the filtrate is reabsorbed into the peritubular capillaries and returned to the blood. The factors determining the GFR are directly related to the pressures that favor or oppose filtration. For example, if the afferent arteriole constricts, blood flow decreases with a corresponding drop in glomerular pressure. The GFR then decreases, and body fluids are conserved. Conversely, constriction of the efferent arteriole increases the net filtration pressure and the GFR increases. When both afferent and efferent arterioles constrict, little change occurs in filtration pressure but RBF is reduced and so is the GFR.

Obstruction to the outflow of urine (caused by strictures, stones, or tumors along the urinary tract) can cause a retrograde increase in pressure at Bowman capsule and a decrease in GFR. Excessive loss of protein-free fluid from vomiting, diarrhea, use of diuretics, or excessive sweating can increase glomerular capillary oncotic pressure and decrease the GFR. Renal disease also can cause changes in pressure relationships by altering capillary permeability and the surface area available for filtration (see Chapter 29).

Tubular Transport

By the end of the proximal tubule, approximately 60% to 70% of filtered sodium and water and about 50% of urea have been actively reabsorbed, along with 90% or more of potassium, glucose, bicarbonate, calcium, phosphate, amino acids, and uric acid. Chloride, water, and urea are reabsorbed passively but linked to the active transport of sodium (co-transport). Active transport in the renal tubules can be limited as the carrier molecules become saturated, a phenomenon known as transport maximum (Tm). For example, when the carrier molecules for glucose become saturated (i.e., with the development of hyperglycemia) the excess will be excreted in the urine.

Proximal tubule. Active reabsorption of sodium is the primary function of the proximal tubule. Water, most electrolytes, and organic substances are co-transported with sodium. The osmotic force generated by active sodium transport promotes the passive diffusion of water out of the tubular lumen and into the peritubular capillaries. Passive transport of water is further enhanced by the elevated oncotic pressure of the blood in the peritubular capillaries, which is created by the previous filtration of water at the glomerulus. The reabsorption of water leaves an increased concentration of urea within the tubular lumen, creating a gradient for its passive diffusion to the peritubular plasma.

While the positively charged sodium ions leave the tubular lumen, negatively charged chloride ions passively follow to maintain electroneutrality. Because the proximal tubular cell has a limited permeability to chloride, chloride reabsorption lags behind sodium. Hydrogen ions are actively exchanged for sodium ions. The hydrogen ions (H^+) then combine with bicarbonate (HCO_3^-). Bicarbonate is completely filtered at the glomerulus, and approximately 90% is reabsorbed in the proximal tubule. In the tubular lumen, hydrogen and bicarbonate ions form carbonic acid (H_2CO_3), which rapidly breaks down, or dissociates, to carbon dioxide (CO_2) and water (H_2O). These then diffuse into the tubular cell, where carbonic anhydrase again catalyzes the CO_2 and H_2O to form HCO_3^- and H^+. The H^+ is secreted again, and HCO_3^- combines with sodium and is transported to the peritubular capillary blood. Bicarbonate is thus conserved, and the hydrogen is reabsorbed as water. Therefore, these ions normally do not contribute to the urinary excretion of acid or the addition of acid to the blood.

In addition to the proximal tubular secretion of hydrogen ions, secretory transport mechanisms exist for creatinine, other organic bases, and endogenous and exogenous organic acids including *para*-aminohippurate (PAH) and penicillin (Box 28-1). These secretory mechanisms eliminate drugs and other exogenous chemical products from the body, often after first conjugating them with sulfate and glucuronic acid in the liver. Many drugs and their metabolites are eliminated from the body in this way. When the renal tubules are damaged, metabolic by-products and drugs may accumulate, causing toxic levels.

Glomerulotubular balance. Normally, 99% of the glomerular filtrate is reabsorbed. When the GFR spontaneously decreases or increases, the renal tubules, primarily the proximal tubules, automatically adjust their rate of reabsorption of sodium and water to balance the change in GFR. This prevents wide fluctuations in the excretion of sodium and water into the urine and is known as glomerulotubular balance.

Loop of Henle and distal tubule. Urine can be hypotonic, isotonic, or hypertonic. Urine concentration or dilution occurs principally in the loop of Henle, distal tubules, and collecting ducts. The structural features of the medullary hairpin loops allow the kidney to concentrate urine and conserve water for the body. The transition of the filtrate into the final urine reflects the concentrating ability of the loops. Final adjustments in urine composition are made by the distal tubule and collecting duct according to body needs.

BOX 28-1	**SUBSTANCES TRANSPORTED BY RENAL TUBULES**
REABSORPTION	**SECRETION**
Albumin	Choline
Ascorbate	Creatinine
Fructose	Histamine
Galactose	Methylguanidine
Glutamate	*para*-Aminohippurate
Glucose	Penicillin and many other drugs
Phosphate	Steroid glucuronides
Sulfate	Thiamine
Xylose	

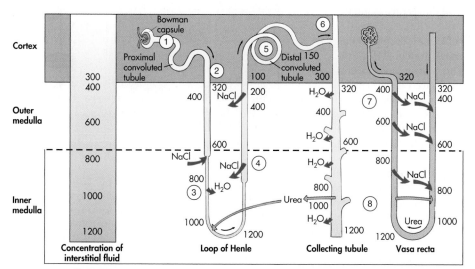

FIGURE 28-12 Countercurrent Mechanism for Concentrating and Diluting Urine. *ADH,* Antidiuretic hormone. (NOTE: Numbers on illustration represent milliosmoles [mOsm].)

Producing a concentrated urine involves a **countercurrent exchange system**, in which fluid flows in opposite directions through the parallel tubes of the loop of Henle. A concentration gradient causes fluid to be exchanged across the parallel pathways. The longer the loop, the greater the concentration gradient and the concentration gradient increases from the cortex to the tip of the medulla. The loops of Henle multiply the concentration gradient, and the vasa recta act as a countercurrent exchanger for maintaining the gradient.[11] The process is initiated in the thick ascending limb of the loop of Henle with the active transport of chloride and sodium out of the tubular lumen and into the medullary interstitium (Figure 28-12). Because the lumen of the ascending limb is impermeable to water, water cannot follow the sodium-chloride transport. This causes the ascending tubular fluid to become hypoosmotic and the medullary interstitium to become hyperosmotic. The descending limb of the loop, which receives fluid from the proximal tubule, is highly permeable to water but it is the only place in the nephron that does not actively transport either sodium or chloride. Sodium and chloride may, however, diffuse into the descending tubule from the interstitium. The hyperosmotic medullary interstitium causes water to move out of the descending limb, and the remaining fluid in the descending tubule becomes increasingly concentrated while it flows toward the tip of the medulla. While the tubular fluid rounds the loop and enters the ascending limb, sodium and chloride are removed and water is retained. The fluid then becomes more and more dilute as it encounters the distal tubule.

The slow rate of blood flow and the hairpin structure of the vasa recta allow blood to flow through the medullary tissue without disturbing the osmotic gradient. While blood flows into the descending limb of the vasa recta, it encounters the increasing osmotic concentration gradient of the medullary interstitium. Water moves out and sodium and chloride diffuse into the descending vasa recta. The plasma becomes increasingly concentrated as it flows toward the tip of the medulla.

While the blood flow passes into the ascending limb and back toward the cortex, the surrounding interstitial fluid becomes comparatively more dilute. Water then moves back into the vasa recta, and sodium and chloride diffuse out. The net result is a preservation of the medullary osmotic gradient. If blood were to flow rapidly through the vasa recta, as occurs in some renal diseases, the medullary concentration gradient would be washed away and the ability to concentrate urine and conserve water would be lost. The efficiency of water conservation is related to the length of the loops: the longer the loops, the greater the ability to concentrate the urine.

Another important function of the loop of Henle is the production of **uromodulin** (also known as **Tamm-Horsfall protein [THP]**), the most abundant protein in human urine. This protein binds to uropathogens to prevent urinary tract infection, protects the uroepithelium from injury, and protects against kidney stone formation.[12]

The convoluted portion of the distal tubule is poorly permeable to water but readily reabsorbs ions and contributes to the dilution of the tubular fluid. The later, straight segment of the distal tubule and the collecting duct are permeable to water as controlled by antidiuretic hormone (ADH). Sodium is readily reabsorbed by the later segment of the distal tubule and collecting duct under the regulation of the hormone aldosterone (see Chapter 17). Potassium is actively secreted in these segments and is also controlled by aldosterone and other factors related to the concentration of potassium in body fluids.

Acidification of urine. Hydrogen is secreted by the distal tubule and combines with non–bicarbonate buffers (i.e., ammonium and phosphate) for the elimination of acids in the urine. The distal tubule

thus contributes to the regulation of acid-base balance by excreting hydrogen ions into the urine and by adding new bicarbonate to the plasma. The mechanism is similar to the conservation of bicarbonate by the proximal tubule, except that the hydrogen ion is excreted in the urine and influences acid-base balance (Figure 28-13). (The specific mechanisms of acid-base balance and acid excretion are described in Chapter 4.)

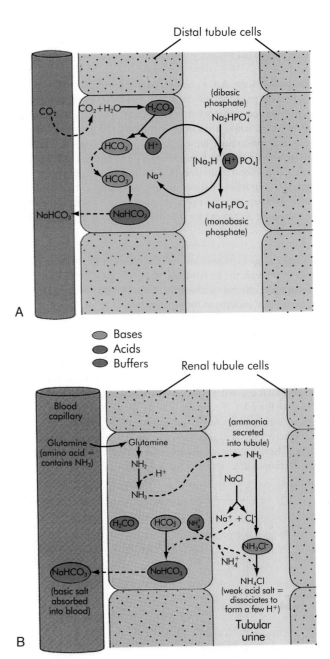

FIGURE 28-13 Acidification of Urine by Tubule Excretion of Phosphate and Ammonia (NH_3). **A,** Acidification of urine and conservation of base by distal renal tubule excretion of H^+ via phosphate buffers. **B,** An amino acid (glutamine) moves into the tubule cell and forms ammonia (NH_3), which is secreted into the urine and combines with H^+ to form ammonium ion (NH_4^+) and an ammonium salt (NH_4Cl). In exchange, the tubule cell absorbs a basic salt (mainly $NaHCO_3$) into blood from urine. (From Thibodeau GA, Patton KT: *Anatomy & physiology,* ed 4, St Louis, 1999, Mosby.)

Urea is the major constituent of urine along with water. The glomerulus freely filters urea, and tubular reabsorption depends on urine flow rate, with less reabsorption at higher flow rates. Approximately 50% of urea is excreted in the urine, and 50% is recycled within the kidney. This recycling contributes to the osmotic gradient within the medulla and is necessary for the concentration and dilution of urine (see Figure 28-12). Because urea is an end product of protein metabolism, individuals with protein deprivation cannot maximally concentrate their urine.

Urine

Urine is normally clear yellow or amber in color. Cloudiness may indicate the presence of bacteria, cells, or high solute concentration. The pH ranges from 4.6 to 8.0, but it is normally acidic, providing protection against bacteria. Specific gravity ranges from 1.001 to 1.035. Normal urine does not contain glucose or blood cells and only occasionally contains traces of protein, usually in association with rigorous exercise (see *Health Alert:* Cranberry Juice and Urinary Tract Infection).

HEALTH ALERT

Cranberry Juice and Urinary Tract Infection

Cranberry juice (CBJ) has long been used to prevent and treat uncomplicated urinary tract infections (UTIs). Although CBJ is nonbacteriostatic and incapable of urine acidification, it does inhibit bacterial adhesion to uroepithelial cells by the action of epicatechin, a proanthocyanidin. Randomized trials of cranberry extract or powder ingestion show a significant effect in preventing *E. coli* uropathogenic adherence and UTIs in women, and it is not likely to alter the pharmacokinetics of oral antibiotics. Randomized controlled trials are needed to determine the effectiveness of CBJ for treatment of recurrent UTIs in children. CBJ has not proven to be effective in preventing UTIs in individuals with spinal cord injury. The cost of CBJ for prophylaxis also may be more expensive than antibiotic prophylaxis and other preventive measures.

Data from Howell AB et al: Dosage effect on uropathogenic *Escherichia coli* anti-adhesion activity in urine following consumption of cranberry powder standardized for proanthocyanidin content: a multicentric randomized double blindstudy, *BMC Infect Dis* 10:94, 2010; Li M et al: Effects of cranberry juice on pharmacokinetics of beta-lactam antibiotics following oral administration, *Antimicrob Agents Chemother* 53(7):2725–2732, 2009; Opperman EA: Cranberry is not effective for the prevention or treatment of urinary tract infections in individuals with spinal cord injury, *Spinal Cord* 48(6):451–456, 2010; Rossi R et al: Overview on cranberry and urinary tract infections in females, *J Clin Gastroenterol* 44(suppl 1):S61–S62, 2010.

Hormones and Nephron Function
Antidiuretic Hormone

The distal tubule in the cortex receives the hypoosmotic urine from the ascending limb of the loop of Henle. The concentration of the final urine is controlled by antidiuretic hormone (ADH), which is secreted from the posterior pituitary or neurohypophysis. ADH increases water permeability and reabsorption in the last segment of the distal tubule and along the entire length of the collecting ducts, which pass through the inner and outer zones of the medulla. The water diffuses into the ascending limb of the vasa recta and returns to the systemic circulation. The excreted urine can have a high osmotic concentration, up to 1400 mOsm. The volume is normally reduced to about 1% of the amount that was filtered at the glomerulus.

ADH secretion is therefore one cause of oliguria—diminished excretion of urine, less than 400 ml/day or 30 ml/hr. Fluid imbalance may be related to the syndrome of inappropriate secretion of ADH, which is a cause of water excess (see Chapter 4). Inadequate secretion of ADH results in diabetes insipidus, the excretion of a large volume of dilute urine (see Chapter 18).

In the absence of ADH, water diuresis, an increase in excretion of a highly dilute urine, takes place. The distal tubules and collecting ducts become impermeable to water. Water remains in the tubular lumen and is excreted as a dilute and large volume of urine. Because ADH has no effect on sodium reabsorption, it continues to be actively transported from the distal tubule. (The mechanism for the regulation of ADH and plasma osmolality is described in Chapters 4 and 17.)

Aldosterone

Aldosterone is synthesized and secreted by the adrenal cortex under the regulation of the renin-angiotensin-aldosterone system (see Chapter 17, and the previous discussion of the renin-angiotensin-aldosterone system on p. 730). Aldosterone stimulates the epithelial cells of the distal tubule and collecting duct to reabsorb sodium (promoting water reabsorption) and increases the excretion of potassium and hydrogen ion.

Atrial Natriuretic Peptide

Atrial natriuretic peptide (ANP) is secreted from cells in the right atrium of the heart. When right atrial pressure rises, ANP inhibits secretion of renin, inhibits angiotensin-induced secretion of aldosterone, relaxes vascular smooth muscle, and inhibits sodium and water absorption by kidney tubules. The result is decreased blsood volume and blood pressure. Natriuretic hormones are also produced by other tissues including the brain and vascular system and have effects on heart tissue, vasodilation, and bone growth.[13]

Diuretics as a Factor in Urine Flow

A diuretic is any agent that enhances the flow of urine. Clinically, diuretics interfere with renal sodium reabsorption and reduce extracellular fluid volume. Diuretics are commonly used to treat hypertension and edema caused by heart failure, cirrhosis, and nephrotic syndrome.

Diuretics are divided into five general categories: (1) osmotic diuretics, (2) carbonic anhydrase inhibitors (inhibitors of urinary acidification), (3) inhibitors of loop sodium or chloride transport, (4) aldosterone antagonists (potassium sparing), and (5) aquaretics. (The physiologic mechanism related to each category is summarized in Table 28-2.)

Renal Hormones

Certain hormones are either activated or synthesized by the kidney. These hormones have significant systemic effects and include urodilatin, the active form of vitamin D, and erythropoietin.

Urodilatin

Urodilatin, a natriuretic peptide, is produced by the distal tubule and collecting ducts when there is increased circulating volume and increased blood pressure. It inhibits sodium and water resorption from the medullary part of the collective duct, producing diuresis.

Vitamin D

Vitamin D is a hormone that can be obtained in the diet or synthesized by the action of ultraviolet radiation on cholesterol in the skin. These forms of vitamin D_3 (cholecalciferol) are inactive and require

TABLE 28-2 ACTION OF DIURETICS

DIURETIC	SITE OF ACTION	ACTION	COMMON SIDE EFFECTS
Osmotic Diuretics			
Mannitol	Proximal tubule	Freely filtered but not reabsorbed; osmotically attract water and diminish sodium reabsorption	Hypokalemia, dehydration
Glycerol			
Urea			
Carbonic Anhydrase Inhibitors			
Acetazolamide	Proximal tubule	Inhibits carbonic anhydrase; blocks hydrogen ion secretion and reabsorption of sodium and bicarbonate	Hypokalemia, systemic acidosis, alkaline urine
Inhibitors of Sodium/Chloride Reabsorption			
Thiazides	Distal convoluted tubules	Inhibit sodium and chloride reabsorption; mildly suppress carbonic anhydrase; reduce calcium excretion	Hypokalemia, metabolic alkalosis
Furosemide	Thick ascending limb of loop of Henle	Inhibit active transport of chloride, sodium, and potassium	Hypokalemia, uric acid retention
Ethacrynic acid			
Torsemide	Cortical vasodilation	Increase rate of urine formation	Hypokalemia, uric acid retention
Bumetanide			
Potassium-Sparing Diuretics			
Spironolactone	Distal tubule/collecting duct	Inhibits aldosterone, blocks sodium reabsorption, and results in potassium retention	Hyperkalemia, nausea, confusion, gynecomastia
Triamterene and amiloride	Distal tubule/collecting duct	Inhibit sodium reabsorption and inhibit potassium excretion	Nausea, vomiting, headache, granulocytopenia, skin rash
Aquaretics			
Vasopressin (V₂) blockers (i.e., Conivaptan)	Distal tubule/collecting ducts	Block action of antidiuretic hormone	Dehydration

two hydroxylations to establish a metabolically active form. The first step occurs in the liver and the second in the kidneys.

Vitamin D is necessary for the absorption of calcium and phosphate by the small intestine. The renal hydroxylation step is stimulated by parathyroid hormone (see Chapter 17). A decreased plasma calcium level (less than 10 mg/dl) stimulates the secretion of parathyroid hormone. Parathyroid hormone then stimulates a sequence of events that help restore plasma calcium toward normal levels:

1. Calcium mobilization from bone
2. Synthesis of 1,25-dihydroxyvitamin D_3
3. Absorption of calcium from the intestine
4. Increased renal calcium reabsorption
5. Decreased renal phosphate reabsorption

Serum phosphate fluctuations also influence the renal hydroxylation of vitamin D. Decreased levels stimulate active 1,25-dihydroxyvitamin D_3 formation, and increased levels inhibit formation. This results in compensatory changes in phosphate absorption from bone and intestine. Individuals with renal disease have a deficiency of 1,25-dihydroxyvitamin D_3 (1,25-OH_2D_3) and manifest symptoms of disturbed calcium and phosphate balance (see Chapters 4 and 29).

Erythropoietin

Oxygen-sensing erythropoietin-producing cells are located in the juxtamedullary cortex.[14] **Erythropoietin** stimulates the bone marrow to produce red blood cells in response to tissue hypoxia and may have tissue protective effects.[14a] (Erythrocyte production is discussed in Chapter 19.) The stimulus for erythropoietin release is decreased oxygen delivery in the kidneys. The anemia of chronic renal failure, in which kidney cells have become nonfunctional, can be related to the lack of this hormone.[15]

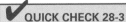

QUICK CHECK 28-3
1. Outline the process of glomerular filtration.
2. What types of absorption/reabsorption take place in the proximal tubule, the loops of Henle, and the distal tubule?
3. What is the countercurrent exchange system? What substances are involved?
4. What hormones are activated or synthesized by the kidney?

TEST OF RENAL FUNCTION

The Concept of Clearance

A number of specific renal functions can be measured by renal clearance. Renal clearance techniques determine how much of a substance can be cleared from the blood by the kidneys per given unit of time. The application of this principle permits an indirect measure of GFR, tubular secretion, tubular reabsorption, and RBF.

Clearance and Glomerular Filtration Rate

The GFR provides the best estimate of functioning renal tissue. Loss or damage to nephrons leads to a corresponding decrease in GFR. The measurement of GFR requires the use of a substance that has a stable plasma concentration, is freely filtered at the glomerulus, and is not secreted, reabsorbed, or metabolized by the tubules. *Inulin* (a fructose polysaccharide) is one substance that meets the criteria for measurement of GFR.

The accurate determination of inulin clearance requires constant infusion to maintain a stable plasma level. This is time-consuming and inconvenient. Therefore the clearance of creatinine, a natural substance produced by muscle and released into the blood at a relatively constant rate, is commonly used as an estimate clinically. It is freely filtered at the glomerulus, but a small amount is secreted by the renal tubules. Therefore creatinine clearance overestimates the GFR but within tolerable limits. Creatinine clearance provides a good measure of GFR because only one blood sample is required in addition to a 24-hour volume of urine. Cystatin C, a stable protein in serum, is also a marker for estimating GFR, particularly for mild to moderate impaired renal function.[16]

The GFR can also be estimated using formulas. The Cockcroft and Gault creatinine-based formula is one that is commonly used and considers age, body weight, and plasma creatinine (P_{cr}) values: The National Kidney Foundation recommends the Modification of Diet in Renal Disease (MDRD) equation.[17] The Chronic Kidney Disease Epidemiology Collaboration (CKD-EPI) equation has been developed as a more precise estimate of GFR than the MDRD and considers age, gender, and race.[18] Calculators for estimates of GFR using these formulas are readily available on the Internet.

Substances freely filtered at the glomerulus but with a clearance less than inulin or creatinine have been reabsorbed along the tubules. For example, glucose is completely reabsorbed and has a clearance rate of nearly zero. Conversely, substances secreted by the tubules have a clearance rate greater than inulin or creatinine (i.e., greater than 1.0).

Plasma Creatinine Concentration

A chronic decline in the GFR over weeks or months is reflected in the plasma creatinine (P_{cr}) concentration (normal value = 0.7 to 1.2 mg/dl). The P_{cr} concentration has a stable value when the GFR is stable, because creatinine has a constant rate of production as a product of muscle metabolism. The amount filtered is approximately equal to the amount excreted. When the GFR declines, the P_{cr} increases proportionately. Thus the GFR and P_{cr} are inversely related. If the GFR were to decrease by 50%, the filtration and excretion of creatinine would be reduced by 50% and creatinine would accumulate in plasma to twice the normal value. Therefore elevated P_{cr} values represent decreasing GFR. In the new steady state, however, the total amount of creatinine excreted in the urine would remain the same because of the proportionate decrease in GFR and increase in P_{cr}.

The application of this principle is simple and useful for monitoring progressive changes in renal function. The test is most valuable for monitoring the progress of chronic rather than acute renal disease because it takes 7 to 10 days for the plasma creatinine level to stabilize when GFR declines. Serial measures can be obtained over a long time and plotted as a curve of glomerular function. The P_{cr} also becomes elevated during trauma or the breakdown of muscle tissue. In such instances, the value is then not useful for estimating GFR.

Blood Urea Nitrogen

The concentration of urea nitrogen in the blood reflects glomerular filtration and urine-concentrating capacity. Because urea is filtered at the glomerulus, blood urea nitrogen (BUN) levels increase as glomerular filtration drops. Because urea is reabsorbed by the blood through the permeable tubules, the BUN value rises in states of dehydration and acute and chronic renal failure when passage of fluid through the tubules slows. BUN value also changes as a result of altered protein intake and protein catabolism. The normal range for BUN level in the adult is 10 to 20 mg/dl of blood.

Urinalysis

Urinalysis is a noninvasive and relatively inexpensive diagnostic procedure. The best results are obtained from a fresh, cleanly voided specimen because decay permits changes in the composition of urine. Urinalysis includes evaluation of color, turbidity, protein, pH, specific gravity, sediment, and supernatant. Urine tests are listed in Table 28-3 and bladder function tests are listed in Table 28-4.

TABLE 28-3	NORMAL RENAL FUNCTION TESTS	
TEST	**NORMAL VALUE**	**INTERPRETATION**
Urine		
Color	Amber-yellow	Drugs and foods may change color
Turbidity	Clear	Purulent matter will make cloudy
pH	4.6-8.0	Bacteria create an alkaline urine
Specific gravity (density of water = 1.000)		Represents concentrating ability or density of urine in relation to density of water (i.e., higher when contains glucose or protein; lower with dilute urine)
Adults	1.010-1.025	
Infants	1.010-1.018	
Blood	Negative	Bleeding along urinary tract
Microscopic Urine		
Bacteria	None	Infection
Red blood cells	Negative	Bleeding along urinary tract
White blood cells	Negative	Urinary tract infection
Crystals	Negative	May have potential for stones
Fat	Negative	Can be associated with nephrosis
Casts	Occasional	A few are normal; may represent renal disease
Urinary Chemistry		
Bilirubin	Negative	Increases may cause dark orange color
Urobilinogen	Less than 4 mg/24 hr	Increases may indicate red blood cell hemolysis
Ketones	Negative	Represents an increase in fat metabolism
Glucose	Negative	Usually signifies hyperglycemia
Sodium	100-260 mEq/24 hr	Can increase or decrease with renal disease
Potassium	25-100 mEq/24 hr	Can increase or decrease with renal disease, potassium intake, aldosteronism, or diuretic use
Protein	Negative-trace	Dysfunction of glomerulus
Normal Serum Values		
BUN	7-18 mg/dl	Elevated with diseased kidneys
Creatinine	Elevated with decreased GFR	
Male	0.6-1.5 mg/dl	
Female	0.6-1.1 mg/dl	
Cystatin C	0.8-2.1 mg/L	Early detection of decreased GFR
Potassium		Elevated in renal failure

TABLE 28-4 BLADDER FUNCTION TESTS

PROCEDURE	DESCRIPTION
Urodynamic Tests	
Cystometry (cystometrogram)	Measurement of bladder pressure determined using a pressure-measuring catheter; fluid volume and pressures are measured as bladder is filled with fluid; simultaneous pressures may be measured in rectum; sensations of bladder fullness are also recorded; coughing or straining can lead to involuntary bladder contractions
	Bladder capacity: Male 350-750 ml; female 350-550 ml
	Intrabladder pressure with empty bladder: 40 cm H_2O
	Detrusor pressure: <10 cm H_2O
	Residual urine: <30 ml
Uroflowmetry	Measures time it takes to empty a full bladder of urine; flow rates may be faster with urge incontinence or slower with prostatic obstruction
Postvoid residual urine	Measures residual urine in bladder after voiding; urine can be removed with catheter or by use of ultrasound imaging; postvoid residual of more than 200 ml is abnormal and requires further evaluation
Measurement of leak point pressure	Pressure at which bladder fluid will leak from bladder without warning
Pressure flow study	Measures pressure required to empty bladder; pressure flow study identifies bladder outlet obstruction such as that occurring with prostate enlargement
Electromyography	Measures nerve impulses and muscle activity in urethral sphincter by placing sensors on skin near urethra and rectum or by placing sensors on catheter placed in urethra or rectum
Video urodynamics	Imaging of x-rays or ultrasound waves during fluid filling of bladder; shows size and shape of urinary tract
Direct Visualization Diagnostic Procedure	
Cystoscopy	Cystoscope (a type of endoscope) is inserted through urethra and is used to visualize inside of bladder
Ureteroscopy	Ureteroscope is inserted through urethra and bladder and directly into ureter and upper urinary tract to visualize upper urinary tract

PEDIATRIC CONSIDERATIONS

Pediatrics & Renal Function

Glomerular filtration rate in infants does not reach adult levels until 1 to 2 years of age, and newborns have a decreased ability to efficiently remove excess water and solutes. Their shorter loops of Henle also decrease concentrating ability and produce a more dilute urine than that produced by adults. Risks for metabolic acidosis are increased during the first few months of life while the mechanisms for excreting acid and retaining bicarbonate are maturing. These normal developmental processes result in a narrow safety margin for fluid and electrolyte balance when there is any disturbance such as diarrhea, infection, fever, fasting for diagnostic tests, improper feeding, or fluid replacement. An increased risk of toxicity accompanies drug administration. Low-birthweight infants are at greater risk for low nephron numbers and chronic kidney disease as adults.

Data from Luyckx VA, Brenner BM: The clinical importance of nephron mass, *J Am Soc Nephrol* 21(6):898–910, 2010; Schwartz GJ, Work DF: Measurement and estimation of GFR in children and adolescents, *Clin J Am Soc Nephrol* 4(11):1832–1843, 2009.

QUICK CHECK 28-4
1. Why is creatinine clearance a good estimate of glomerular filtration rate?
2. What is the relationship between plasma creatinine concentration and glomerular filtration rate?

GERIATRIC CONSIDERATIONS

Aging & Renal Function

- Structural changes commonly occur in the kidney with aging, including loss of renal mass, arterial sclerosis, an increased number of sclerotic glomeruli, loss of tubules, and interstitial fibrosis. These changes contribute to a slow decline in GFR in most individuals, but generally it is not significant enough to lead to severe loss of renal function. As the number of nephrons decreases and degenerative changes occur, nephrons are less able to concentrate urine and less able to tolerate dehydration or excessive water loads.
- The presence of comorbid conditions, such as hypertension and diabetes mellitus, accelerates the decline of renal function. Obesity does not accelerate a decline in GFR.
- Response to acid-base changes and reabsorption of glucose may be delayed.
- Drugs eliminated by the kidney can accumulate in the plasma, causing toxic reactions; GFR and drug dosage should be carefully evaluated.
- Decreased thirst sensation and diminished water intake may alter water balance.
- Impairment in renal blood flow, hormonal regulatory systems, and metabolism of medications may alter sodium and water balance.

Data from Aymanns C et al: Review on pharmacokinetics and pharmacodynamics and the aging kidney, *Clin J Am Soc Nephrol* 5(2):314–327, 2010; Esposito C, Dal Canton A: Functional changes in the aging kidney, *J Nephrol* 23(suppl 15):S41–S45, 2010; Pannarale G et al: The aging kidney: structural changes, *J Nephrol* 23(suppl 15):S37–S40, 2010; Peters AM et al: Obesity does not accelerate the decline in glomerular filtration rate associated with advancing age, *Int J Obes (Lond)* 33(3):379–381, 2009; Weinstein JR, Anderson S: The aging kidney: physiological changes, *Adv Chronic Kidney Dis* 17(4):302–307, 2010.

DID YOU UNDERSTAND?

Structures of the Renal System

1. The kidneys are paired structures lying bilaterally between the twelfth thoracic and third lumbar vertebrae.
2. The kidney is composed of an outer cortex and an inner medulla.
3. The calyces join to form the renal pelvis, which is continuous with the upper end of the ureter.
4. The nephron is the urine-forming unit of the kidney and is composed of the glomerulus, proximal tubule, hairpin loops of Henle, distal tubule, and collecting duct.
5. The glomerulus contains loops of capillaries. The capillary walls serve as a filtration membrane for the formation of the primary urine.
6. The proximal tubule is lined with microvilli to increase surface area and enhance reabsorption.
7. The hairpin loops of Henle transport solutes and water, contributing to the hypertonic state of the medulla.
8. The distal tubule adjusts acid-base balance by excreting acid into the urine and forming new bicarbonate ions.
9. The ureters extend from the renal pelvis to the posterior wall of the bladder. Urine flows through the ureters by means of peristaltic contraction of the ureteral muscles.
10. The bladder is a bag composed of the detrusor and trigone muscles and innervated by parasympathetic fibers. When accumulation of urine reaches 250 to 300 ml, mechanoreceptors, which respond to stretching of tissue, stimulate the micturition reflex.

Renal Blood Flow

1. Renal blood flows at about 1000 to 1200 ml/min, or 20% to 25% of the cardiac output.
2. Blood flow through the glomerular capillaries is maintained at a constant rate in spite of a wide range of arterial pressures.
3. The glomerular filtration rate (GFR) is the filtration of plasma per unit of time and is directly related to the perfusion pressure of renal blood flow.
4. Autoregulation of renal blood flow and neural regulation of vasoconstriction maintain a constant GFR.
5. Renin is an enzyme secreted from the juxtaglomerular apparatus and causes the generation of angiotensin, a potent vasoconstrictor. The renin-angiotensin-aldosterone system is thus a regulator of renal blood flow.

Kidney Function

1. The major function of the nephron is urine formation, which involves the processes of glomerular filtration, tubular reabsorption, and tubular secretion and excretion.
2. Glomerular filtration is favored by capillary hydrostatic pressure and opposed by oncotic pressure in the capillary and hydrostatic pressure in Bowman capsule. The balance of favoring and opposing filtration forces is known as net filtration pressure (NFP).

3. The GFR is approximately 120 ml/min, and 99% of the filtrate is reabsorbed.
4. The proximal tubule reabsorbs about 60% to 70% of the filtered sodium and water and 90% of other electrolytes.
5. Because most molecules are reabsorbed by active transport, the carrier mechanism can become saturated at a point known as the transport maximum (T_m). Molecules not reabsorbed are excreted with the urine.
6. The distal tubules actively reabsorb sodium and secrete potassium and hydrogen for the regulation of electrolyte and acid-base balance.
7. The concentration of the final urine is a function of the level of antidiuretic hormone (ADH) that stimulates the distal tubules and collecting ducts to reabsorb water. The countercurrent exchange system of the long loops of Henle and their accompanying capillaries establishes a concentration gradient within the renal medulla to facilitate the reabsorption of water from the collecting duct.
8. The distal nephron regulates acid-base balance by excreting hydrogen ions and forming new bicarbonate.
9. The kidney secretes or activates a number of hormones that have systemic effects, including 1,25-dihydroxyvitamin D_3, erythropoietin, and natriuretic hormone.

Tests of Renal Function

1. Creatinine, a substance produced by muscle, is measured in both plasma and urine to calculate a commonly used clinical measurement of GFR.
2. Plasma creatinine concentration, cystatin C level, and blood urea nitrogen (BUN) level are estimates of glomerular function. BUN value also is an indicator of hydration status.
3. Formulas for estimating GFR can be helpful clinical indicators.
4. Urinalysis involves evaluation of color, turbidity, protein, pH, specific gravity, sediment, and supernatant. Presence of bacteria, red blood cells, white blood cells, casts, or crystals in the urine sediment may indicate a renal or bladder disorder.

PEDIATRIC CONSIDERATIONS: Pediatrics & Renal Function

1. Compared to adults, infants and children have more dilute urine because of higher blood flow and shorter loops of Henle.
2. Children are more affected than adults by fluid imbalances resulting from diarrhea, infection, or improper feeding because of their limited ability to quickly regulate changes in pH or osmotic pressure.

GERIATRIC CONSIDERATIONS: Aging & Renal Function

1. Older adults have a decreased ability to concentrate urine and are less able to tolerate dehydration or water loads because they have fewer nephrons.
2. Response to acid-base changes and reabsorption of glucose are delayed in older adults.
3. In older adults, drugs eliminated by the kidney can accumulate in the plasma, causing toxic reactions.

KEY TERMS

- Aldosterone   735
- Antidiuretic hormone (ADH)   735
- Arcuate artery   728
- Atrial natriuretic peptide (ANP)   735
- Autoregulation of blood flow   730
- Bladder   729
- Bowman capsule   726
- Bowman space   726
- Calyx (pl., calyces)   724
- Collecting duct   728
- Cortex   724
- Cortical nephron   726
- Countercurrent exchange system   734
- Detrusor   729
- Distal tubule   728
- Diuretic   735
- Erythropoietin   736
- Excretion   731
- External urethral sphincter   729
- Filtration slit   726
- Glomerular capillary   728
- Glomerular filtration   731
- Glomerular filtration membrane   726
- Glomerular filtration rate (GFR)   729
- Glomerulotubular balance   733
- Glomerulus   726
- Hilum   724
- Intercalated cell   728
- Interlobar artery   728
- Internal urethral sphincter   729
- Juxtaglomerular apparatus   726
- Juxtaglomerular cell   726
- Juxtamedullary nephron   726
- Kidney   724
- Lobe   726
- Loop of Henle   727
- Macula densa   726
- Medulla   724
- Mesangial cell   726
- Micturition   729
- Midcortical nephron   726
- Nephron   726
- Net filtration pressure (NFP)   731
- Oliguria   735
- Peritubular capillary   728
- Plasma creatinine (P_{cr}) concentration   737
- Podocyte   726
- Principal cell   728
- Proximal tubule   727
- Pyramid   724
- Renal artery   728
- Renal capsule   724
- Renal corpuscle   726
- Renal fascia   724
- Renal papilla (pl., papillae)   729
- Renal vein   728
- Renin-angiotensin-aldosterone system   730
- Tamm-Horsfall protein (THP)   734
- Transport maximum (T_m)   733
- Trigone   729
- Tubular reabsorption   731
- Tubular secretion   731
- Tubuloglomerular feedback   730
- Urea   735
- Ureter   729
- Urethra   729
- Urinalysis   737
- Urine concentration   733
- Urine dilution   733
- Urodilatin   735
- Uromodulin   734
- Vasa recta   728
- Vitamin D   735
- Water diuresis   735

REFERENCES

1. Schlöndorff D, Banas B: The mesangial cell revisited: no cell is an island, *J Am Soc Nephrol* 20(6):1179–1187, 2009.
2. Vaughan MR, Quaggin SE: How do mesangial and endothelial cells form the glomerular tuft? *J Am Soc Nephrol* 19(1):24–33, 2008.
3. Jarad G, Miner JH: Update on the glomerular filtration barrier, *Curr Opin Nephrol Hypertens* 18(3):226–232, 2009.
4. Haraldsson B, Jeansson M: Glomerular filtration barrier, *Curr Opin Nephrol Hypertens* 18(4):331–335, 2009.
5. Peti-Peterdi J, Harris RC: Macula densa sensing and signaling mechanisms of renin release, *J Am Soc Nephrol* 21(7):1093–1096, 2010.
6. Kurtz A: Renin release: sites, mechanisms, and control, *Annu Rev Physiol* 73:377–399, 2011.
7. Birder LA, et al: Is the urothelium intelligent? *Neurourol Urodyn* 29(4):598–602, 2010.
8. Loutzenhiser R, et al: Renal autoregulation: new perspectives regarding the protective and regulatory roles of the underlying mechanisms, *Am J Physiol Regul Integr Comp Physiol* 290(5):R1153–R1167, 2006.
9. Singh P, Thomson SC: Renal homeostasis and tubuloglomerular feedback, *Curr Opin Nephrol Hypertens* 19(1):59–64, 2010.
10. Castrop H, et al: Physiology of kidney renin, *Physiol Rev* 90(2):607–673, 2010.
11. Koeppen BM, Stanton BA: *Renal physiology*, ed 4, St Louis, 2007, Mosby, pp 81–83.
12. Saemann MD, et al: Tamm-Horsfall protein: a multilayered defence molecule against urinary tract infection, *Eur J Clin Invest* 35(4):227–235, 2005.
13. Nishikimi T, Kuwahara K, Nakao K: Current biochemistry, molecular biology, and clinical relevance of natriuretic peptides, *J Cardiol* 57(2):131–140, 2011.
14. Wenger RH, Hoogewijs D: Regulated oxygen sensing by protein hydroxylation in renal erythropoietin-producing cells, *Am J Physiol Renal Physiol* 298(6):F1287–F1296, 2010.
14a. Moore EM, Bellomo R, Nichol AD: Erythropoietin as a novel brain and kidney protective agent, *Anaesth Intensive Care* 39(3):356–372, 2011.
15. Lankhorst CE, Wish JB: Anemia in renal disease: diagnosis and management, *Blood Rev* 24(1):39–47, 2010.
16. Peralta CA, et al: Detection of chronic kidney disease with creatinine, cystatin C, and urine albumin-to-creatinine ratio and association with progression to end-stage renal disease and mortality, *JAMA* 305(15):1545–1552, 2011.
17. Botev R, et al: Estimating glomerular filtration rate: Cockcroft-Gault and modification of diet in renal disease formulas compared to renal insulin clearance, *Clin J Am Soc Nephrol* 4(5):899–906, 2009.
18. Levey AS, et al: A new equation to estimate glomerular filtration rate, *Ann Intern Med* 150(9):604–612, 2009.

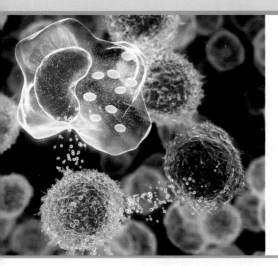

Alterations of Renal and Urinary Tract Function

Sue E. Huether

⊖volve WEBSITE

http://evolve.elsevier.com/Huether/
- Review Questions and Answers
- Animations
- Quick Check Answers
- Key Terms Exercises
- Critical Thinking Questions with Answers
- Algorithm Completion Exercises
- WebLinks

CHAPTER OUTLINE

Renal and urinary function can be affected by a variety of disorders. The most common type of urinary dysfunction is infection of the bladder. Stones, tumors, or inflammation also can obstruct the urinary tract. Renal function can be impaired by disorders of the kidney itself or by systemic diseases and may ultimately result in acute kidney injury or chronic kidney disease. Because the kidney filters the blood, it is directly linked to every other organ system. Renal failure, whether acute or chronic, is therefore a life-threatening condition.

URINARY TRACT OBSTRUCTION

Urinary tract obstruction is an interference with the flow of urine at any site along the urinary tract (Figure 29-1). An obstruction may be anatomic or functional; it impedes flow proximal to the blockage, dilates the urinary system, increases the risk for infection, and compromises renal function. Anatomic changes in the urinary system caused by obstruction are referred to as **obstructive uropathy.** The severity of an obstructive uropathy is determined by (1) the location of the obstructive lesion, (2) the involvement of one or both upper urinary tracts, (3) the severity (completeness) of the blockage, (4) the duration of the blockage, and (5) the nature of the obstructive lesion.[1,2]

Obstructions may be relieved or partially alleviated by correction of the obstruction, although permanent impairments occur if a complete or partial obstruction persists over a period of weeks to months or longer.

Upper Urinary Tract Obstruction

Common causes of upper urinary tract obstruction include stricture or congenital compression of a calyx or the ureteropelvic or ureterovesical junction (e.g., stones [calculi]); compression from an aberrant vessel, tumor, or abdominal inflammation and scarring (retroperitoneal fibrosis); or ureteral blockage from stones or a malignancy of the renal pelvis or ureter.

Obstruction of the upper urinary tract causes dilation of the ureter, renal pelvis, calyces, and renal parenchyma proximal to the site of urinary blockage. Dilation of the ureter is referred to as **hydroureter** (accumulation of urine in the ureter), and dilation of the renal pelvis and calyces proximal to a blockage leads to **hydronephrosis** (enlargement of the renal pelvis and calyces) or **ureterohydronephrosis** (dilation of both the ureter and the pelvicaliceal system) (Figure 29-2). Dilation of the upper urinary tract is an early response to obstruction. It reflects smooth muscle hypertrophy and accumulation of urine above the level of blockage (urinary stasis). Unless the obstruction is relieved,

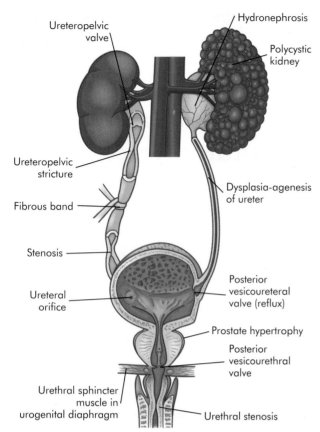

FIGURE 29-1 Major Sites of Urinary Tract Obstruction.

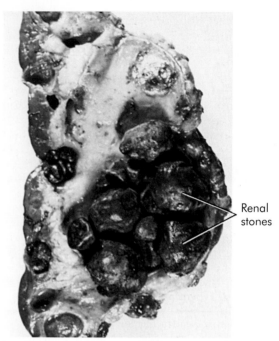

FIGURE 29-2 Hydronephrosis. Hydronephrosis with renal stones in renal pelvis and calyces. (From Kissane JM, editor: *Anderson's pathology*, ed 9, St Louis, 1990, Mosby.)

this dilation leads to enlargement and tubulointerstitial fibrosis affecting the distal nephron and renal function within approximately 7 days. By 14 days, obstruction has adversely affected both distal and proximal aspects of the nephron. Within 28 days, the glomeruli of the kidney have been damaged and the renal cortex and medulla are reduced in size (thinned). Tubular damage initially decreases the kidney's ability to concentrate urine, causing an increase in urine volume despite a decrease in glomerular filtration rate (GFR). The affected kidney is unable to conserve sodium, bicarbonate, and water or to excrete hydrogen or potassium, leading to metabolic acidosis and dehydration. The magnitude of this damage, and the kidney's ability to recover normal homeostatic function, is affected by the severity and duration of the obstruction. With complete obstruction and compression of the renal vasculature, damage to the renal tubules occurs in a matter of hours, and irreversible damage occurs within 4 weeks. Nevertheless, even in the face of a complete obstruction, the human kidney may recover at least partial homeostatic function provided the blockage is removed within 56 to 69 days.[3] This recovery requires a period of approximately 4 months. Partial obstruction, in the absence of renal infection, leads to subtler but ultimately permanent impairments including loss of the kidney's ability to concentrate urine, reabsorb bicarbonate, excrete ammonia, or regulate metabolic acid-base balance.

The body is able to partially counteract the negative consequences of unilateral obstruction by a process called **compensatory hypertrophy** and **hyperfunction**.[4] Compensatory response is the result of two growth processes: obligatory growth occurs under the influence of somatomedins, and compensatory growth occurs under the influence of still unidentified hormone(s). These processes cause the unobstructed kidney to increase the size of individual glomeruli and tubules but not the total number of functioning nephrons. The ability of the body to engage in compensatory hypertrophy and hyperfunction diminishes with age, and the process is reversible when relief of obstruction results in recovery of function by the obstructed kidney.

Relief of bilateral, partial urinary tract obstruction or complete obstruction of one kidney is usually followed by a brief period of diuresis (commonly called **postobstructive diuresis**).[5] It is a physiologic response and is typically mild, representing a restoration of fluid and electrolyte imbalance caused by the obstructive uropathy. Occasionally, relief of obstruction will cause rapid excretion of large volumes of water, sodium, or other electrolytes, resulting in a urine output of 10 L/day or more. Rapid postobstructive diuresis causes dehydration and fluid and electrolyte imbalances that must be promptly corrected. Risk factors for severe postobstructive diuresis include chronic, bilateral obstruction, impairment of one or both kidneys' ability to concentrate urine or reabsorb sodium *(nephrogenic diabetes insipidus)*, hypertension, edema and weight gain, congestive heart failure, and uremic encephalopathy.

Kidney Stones

Calculi, or **urinary stones**, are masses of crystals, protein, or other substances that are a common cause of urinary tract obstruction in adults. They can be located in the kidneys, ureters, and urinary bladder. The prevalence of stones in the United States is approximately 6% in women and 15% in men.[6] The recurrence rate is approximately 30% to 50% within 5 years.[7] Most renal stones are unilateral. The risk of urinary calculi formation is influenced by a number of factors, including age, gender, race, geographic location, seasonal factors, fluid intake, diet, and occupation. Most persons develop their first stone before age 50 years. Geographic location influences the risk of stone formation because of indirect factors, including average temperature, humidity, and rain fall, and their influence on fluid intake and dietary patterns. Persons who regularly consume an adequate volume of water and those who are physically active are at reduced risk when compared to persons who are inactive or consume lower volumes of fluid.

Urinary calculi can be classified according to the primary minerals (salts) that make up the stones. The most common stone types include calcium oxalate or phosphate (70% to 80%), struvite (magnesium-ammonium-phosphate) (15%), and uric acid (7%). Cystine stones are rare (<1%).

PATHOPHYSIOLOGY Calculus formation is complex and related to (1) supersaturation of one or more salts in the urine, (2) precipitation of the salts from a liquid to a solid state, (3) growth through crystallization or agglomeration (sometimes called *aggregation*), and (4) the presence or absence of stone inhibitors (e.g., Tamm-Horsfall protein). *Supersaturation* is the presence of a higher concentration of a salt within a fluid (in this case, the urine) than the volume is able to dissolve to maintain equilibrium.

Human urine contains many ions capable of *precipitating* from solution and forming a variety of salts. The salts form crystals that are retained and grow into stones. *Crystallization* is the process by which crystals grow from a small *nidus* or nucleus to larger stones in the presence of supersaturated urine. Although supersaturation is essential for stone formation, the urine need not remain continuously supersaturated for a calculus to grow once its nidus has precipitated from solution. Intermittent periods of supersaturation after the ingestion of a meal or during times of dehydration are sufficient for stone growth in many individuals. In addition, the renal tubules and papillae have many surfaces that may attract a crystalline nidus and add biologic material (matrix) to the forming stone.[8] *Matrix* is an organic material that is formed in the presence of urea-splitting pathogens and occurs in stones associated with infection.

The temperature and pH of the urine also influence the risk of precipitation and calculus formation, and pH is most important. An alkaline urinary pH significantly increases the risk of calcium phosphate stone formation, whereas acidic urine increases the risk of uric acid stone formation. Cystine and xanthine precipitate more readily in acidic urine.

Stone or *crystal growth inhibiting substances,* such as potassium citrate, Tamm-Horsfall protein, pyrophosphate, and magnesium, are capable of crystal growth inhibition, thereby reducing the risk of calcium phosphate or calcium oxalate precipitation in the urine and preventing subsequent stone formation.

The size of a stone determines the likelihood that it will pass through the urinary tract and be excreted through micturition.[9] Stones smaller than 5 mm have about a 50% chance of spontaneous passage, whereas stones that are 1 cm have almost no chance of spontaneous passage.

Retention of *crystal particles* occurs primarily at the papillary collecting ducts. Although most crystals are flushed from the tract through antegrade urine flow, urinary stasis, anatomic abnormalities, or inflamed epithelium within the urinary tract may prevent prompt flushing of crystals from the system, thus increasing the risk of calculus formation.

Calcium stones (calcium phosphate or calcium oxalate) account for 70% to 80% of all stones requiring treatment. Most individuals have *idiopathic calcium urolithiasis (ICU),* a condition whose exact etiology has not yet been defined. However, hypercalciuria, hyperoxaluria, hyperuricosuria, hypocitraturia, mild renal tubular acidosis, or crystal growth inhibitor deficiencies and alkaline urine are associated with calcium stones. Hypercalciuria is usually attributable to intestinal hyperabsorption of dietary calcium. Hyperparathyroidism and bone demineralization associated with prolonged immobilization are also known to cause hypercalciuria. Although oxalate in the diet influences the risk of calcium stones, primary hyperoxaluria is a rare, inherited disorder.

Struvite stones primarily contain magnesium-ammonium-phosphate as well as varying levels of matrix. Matrix forms in an alkaline urine and during infection with a urease-producing bacterial pathogen, such as a *Proteus, Klebsiella,* or *Pseudomonas.* Struvite calculi may grow quite large and branch into a staghorn configuration (staghorn calculus) that approximates the pelvicaliceal collecting system.

Uric acid stones occur in persons who excrete excessive uric acid in the urine, such as those with gouty arthritis. Uric acid is primarily a product of biosynthesis of endogenous purines and is secondarily affected by consumption of purines in the diet. A consistently acidic urine greatly increases this risk. Cystine and xanthine are amino acids that precipitate more readily in acidic urine. *Cystinuria* and *xanthinuria* are both genetic disorders of amino acid metabolism, and excess of these amino acids in urine can cause cystinuric, or xanthine, stone formation in the presence of a low urine pH of 5.5 or less.

CLINICAL MANIFESTATIONS Renal colic, described as moderate to severe pain often originating in the flank and radiating to the groin, usually indicates obstruction of the renal pelvis or proximal ureter.[10] Colic that radiates to the lateral flank or lower abdomen typically indicates obstruction in the midureter, and bothersome lower urinary tract symptoms (urgency, frequent voiding, urge incontinence) indicate obstruction of the lower ureter or ureterovesical junction. The pain can be severe and incapacitating and may be accompanied by nausea and vomiting. Gross or microscopic hematuria may be present.

EVALUATION AND TREATMENT The evaluation and diagnosis of urinary calculi is based on presenting symptoms and history combined with a focused physical assessment. Imaging studies determine the location of the calculi, the severity of obstruction, and associated obstructive uropathy.[11] The history queries dietary habits, the age of the first stone episode, stone analysis, and presence of complicating factors including hyperparathyroidism or recent gastrointestinal or genitourinary surgery. Urinalysis (including pH) is obtained and a 24-hour urine is completed to identify calcium oxalate, citrate, and other significant constituents. In addition, every effort is made to retrieve and analyze calculi that are passed spontaneously or retrieved through aggressive intervention. To diagnose and manage underlying metabolic disorders, additional tests are completed for those with suspected hyperparathyroidism or cystine or uric acid stones.

The components of treatment include (1) managing pain, (2) reducing the concentration of stone-forming substances by increasing urine flow rate with high fluid intake, (3) implementing medical therapy that promotes stone passage, (4) decreasing the amount of stone-forming substances in the urine by decreasing dietary intake or endogenous production or by altering urine pH,[12] and (5) removing stones using percutaneous nephrolithotomy, ureteroscopy, or ultrasonic or laser lithotripsy to fragment stones for excretion in the urine.[11]

Lower Urinary Tract Obstruction

Obstructive disorders of the lower urinary tract (LUT) are primarily related to storage of urine in the bladder or emptying of urine through the bladder outlet. The causes of obstruction include both neurogenic and anatomic alterations or, in some instances, a combination of both. Incontinence is a common symptom and types of incontinence are reviewed in Table 29-1.

Neurogenic Bladder

Neurogenic bladder is a general term for bladder dysfunction caused by neurologic disorders (Table 29-2). The types of dysfunction are related to the sites in the nervous system that control sensory and motor bladder function. Lesions that develop in upper motor neurons of the brain and spinal cord result in dyssynergia (loss of coordinated neuromuscular contraction) and overactive or hyperreflexive bladder function. Lesions in the sacral area of the spinal cord or peripheral nerves result in underactive, hypotonic, or atonic (flaccid) bladder function, often with loss of bladder sensation.

Neurologic disorders that develop above the pontine micturition center result in detrusor hyperreflexia, also known as an uninhibited or reflex bladder. This is an upper motor neuron disorder in which the bladder empties automatically when it becomes full and the external sphincter functions normally. Because the pontine micturition center remains intact, there is coordination between detrusor muscle contraction and relaxation of the urethral sphincter. Stroke, traumatic brain injury, dementia, and brain tumors are examples of disorders that result in detrusor hyperreflexia. Symptoms include urine leakage and incontinence.

Neurologic lesions that occur below the pontine micturition center but above the sacral micturition center (between C2 and S1) are also upper motor neuron lesions and result in detrusor hyperreflexia with vescicosphincter dyssynergia. There is loss of pontine coordination of detrusor muscle contraction and external sphincter relaxation, so both the bladder and the sphincter are contracting at the same time causing a functional obstruction of the bladder outlet.[13] Spinal cord injury, multiple sclerosis, Guillain-Barré syndrome, and vertebral disk problems are causes of this disorder. There is diminished bladder relaxation during storage with small urine volumes and high intravesicular (inside the bladder) pressures. This results in an overactive bladder syndrome with symptoms of frequency, urgency, urge incontinence, and increased risk for urinary tract infection.

Lesions that involve the sacral micturition center (below S1; may also be termed *cauda equina syndrome*) or peripheral nerve lesions result in detrusor areflexia (acontractile detrusor), a lower motor neuron disorder. The result is an acontractile detrusor or atonic bladder with retention of urine and distention. If the sensory innervation of the bladder is intact, the full bladder will be sensed but the detrusor may not contract. This is an *underactive bladder syndrome* and may have symptoms of stress and overflow incontinence. Myelodysplasia, multiple sclerosis, tabes dorsalis, and peripheral polyneuropathies are associated with this disorder.

Overactive Bladder Syndrome

Overactive bladder syndrome (OAB) is a syndrome of detrusor overactivity characterized by urgency with involuntary detrusor contractions during the bladder filling phase that may be spontaneous or provoked.[14] There is coordination between the contracting bladder and the external sphincter, but the detrusor is too weak to empty the bladder, resulting in urinary retention with overflow or stress incontinence. Overactive bladder is defined by the International Continence Society as a *symptom syndrome* of urgency, with or without urge incontinence and usually associated with frequency and nocturia.[15] Overactive bladder syndrome affects millions of adults and children. Adults are often reluctant to discuss this syndrome with their healthcare provider. Diagnosis is usually made by evaluation of symptoms. Urodynamic evaluation confirms the diagnosis. Antimuscarinics are the most common treatment and in intractable cases surgery is recommended.[16] Untreated OAB impairs health and quality of life, causes depression, and leads to social isolation; in the elderly it may cause risk for falls and urinary tract infection.[17]

TABLE 29-1 TYPES OF INCONTINENCE

TYPE	DESCRIPTION
Urge incontinence (most common in older adults)	Involuntary loss of urine associated with abrupt and strong desire to void (urgency); often associated with involuntary contractions of detrusor; when associated with neurologic disorder, this is called detrusor hyperreflexia; when no neurologic disorder exists, this is called detrusor instability; may be associated with decreased bladder wall compliance
Stress incontinence (most common in women <60 years and men who have had prostate surgery)	Involuntary loss of urine during coughing, sneezing, laughing, or other physical activity associated with increased abdominal pressure
Overflow incontinence	Involuntary loss of urine with overdistention of bladder; associated with neurologic lesions below S1, polyneuropathies, and urethral obstruction (e.g., enlarged prostate)
Mixed incontinence (most common in older women)	Combination of both stress and urge incontinence
Functional incontinence	Involuntary loss of urine attributable to dementia or immobility

Data from Agency for Health Care Policy and Research: *Overview: urinary incontinence in adults, clinical practice guideline update*, Rockville, Md, 1996, www.ahrq.gov/clinic/uiovervw.htm.

TABLE 29-2 NEUROGENIC BLADDER

SITE OF LESION	CAUSE (SYMPTOMS)	DISEASES
Lesions above C2 involve pontine micturition center	Detrusor hyperreflexia (urgency and urine leakage)	Stroke, traumatic brain injury, multiple sclerosis (MS), hydrocephalus, cerebral palsy, Alzheimer disease, brain tumors
Lesions between C2 and S1	Detrusor sphincter dyssynergia with detrusor hyperreflexia (functional bladder outlet obstruction)	Spinal cord injury C2-T12, MS, transverse myelitis, Guillain-Barré syndrome, disk problems
Lesions below S1 (cauda equina syndrome)	Acontractile detrusor, with or without urethral sphincter incompetence (stress urinary incontinence)	Myelodysplasia, peripheral polyneuropathies, MS, tabes dorsalis, spinal injury T12-S1, cauda equina syndrome, herpes simplex/zoster

Obstructions to Urine Flow

Anatomic causes of resistance to urine flow include urethral stricture, prostatic enlargement in men, and pelvic organ prolapse in women. Symptoms of obstruction are more common in men and include (1) frequent daytime voiding (urination more than every 2 hours while awake); (2) nocturia (awakening more than once each night to urinate for adults less than 65 years of age or more than twice for older adults); (3) poor force of stream; (4) intermittency of urinary stream; (5) bothersome urinary urgency, often combined with hesitancy; and (6) feelings of incomplete bladder emptying despite micturition.

A urethral stricture is a narrowing of its lumen. It occurs when infection, injury, or surgical manipulation produces a scar that reduces the caliber of the urethra.[18] The vast majority of urethral strictures occur in men; they are rare in women.[19] The severity of obstruction is influenced by its location within the urethra, its length, and the minimum caliber of urethral lumen within the stricture. Specifically, proximal urethral strictures cause more severe obstruction than do strictures of the distal urethra, longer strictures tend to be more obstructive, and the magnitude of blockage is *inversely* proportional to the urethral caliber.

Prostate enlargement is caused by acute inflammation, benign prostatic hyperplasia, or prostate cancer (see Chapter 32). Each of these disorders can cause encroachment on the urethra with obstruction to urine flow and the symptoms summarized previously.

Severe pelvic organ prolapse (see Chapter 32) in a woman causes bladder outlet obstruction when a cystocele (the downward protrusion of the bladder into the vagina) descends below the level of the urethral outlet. Cystoceles that reach or protrude beyond the vaginal introitus create the greatest risk for obstruction, particularly if the bladder neck has been surgically repaired without simultaneous repair of the cystocele. In men the bladder may rarely herniate into the scrotum, causing a similar type of obstruction.

Partial obstruction of the bladder outlet or urethra initially causes an increase in the force of detrusor contraction. If the blockage persists, afferent nerves within the bladder wall are adversely affected, leading to urinary urgency and, in some cases, overactive detrusor contractions (a myogenic cause of overactive bladder). When obstruction persists, there is an increased deposition of collagen within the smooth muscle bundles of the detrusor muscle (*trabeculation*), possibly in an attempt to increase the force of its contraction strength. Ultimately, the bladder wall loses its ability to stretch and accommodate urine, a condition called low bladder wall compliance, and the detrusor loses its ability to contract efficiently. Low bladder wall compliance chronically elevates intravesicular pressure, greatly increasing the likelihood of hydroureter, hydronephrosis, and impaired renal function.

EVALUATION AND TREATMENT   Although the history and physical examination are critical to the evaluation of lower urinary tract disorders, it must be remembered that no symptom or cluster of symptoms has been identified that accurately differentiates the various causes of these disorders. For example, symptoms such as urgency, urge incontinence, frequent urination, and nocturia may develop because of overactive bladder or either increased or decreased bladder outlet resistance. Reduced resistance is associated with the symptom

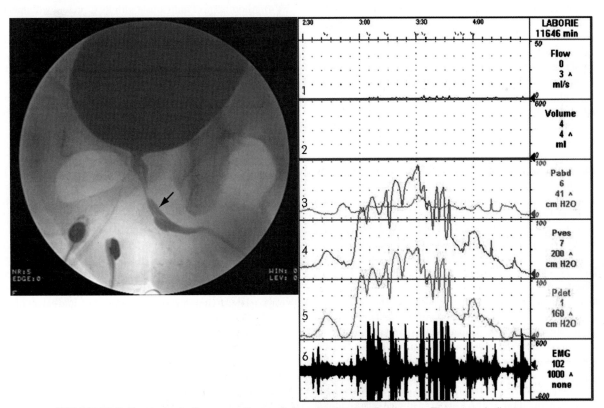

FIGURE 29-3 Neurogenic Detrusor Overactivity with Vesico-Sphincter. The arrow indicates narrowing of the striated sphincter consistent with electromyographic activity *(line 6)* noted on the urodynamic tracing. Note the characteristic poor flow pattern *(line 1)* with elevated voiding pressures *(lines 4 and 5)* indicating obstruction. *Line 1,* Urine flow rate; *line 2,* urine volume; *line 3,* abdominal pressure (Pabd); *line 4,* intravesicular (inside bladder) pressure (Pves); *line 5,* detrusor muscle pressure (Pdet); *line 6,* bladder electromyelogram (EMG).

of stress incontinence (incontinence with coughing or sneezing) and symptoms of increased resistance are similar to bladder outlet obstruction, including poor force of urinary stream, hesitancy, and feelings of incomplete bladder emptying.

Various diagnostic tests assist with evaluation. The *postvoid urine* is measured by catheterization within 5 to 15 minutes of urination or through a bladder ultrasound machine that measures bladder height and width to provide an approximation of urine within the vesicle. This measurement may be combined with *uroflowmetry*, a graphic representation of the force of the urinary stream expressed as milliliters voided per second. Each of these measurements assesses the lower urinary tract's efficiency in evacuating urine through micturition but neither differentiates poor detrusor contraction strength from obstruction as a cause of urinary retention. Instead, *multichannel urodynamic testing* is used to identify obstruction, quantify its severity, and measure detrusor contraction strength (Figure 29-3). *Video-urodynamic recordings* can also demonstrate overactive bladder and detrusor sphincter dyssynergia. An evaluation of renal function, including functional imaging studies and measurement of serum creatinine level, is completed particularly when obstruction is severe and associated with elevated residuals or urinary tract infection.

Because the bladder neck consists of circular smooth muscle with adrenergic innervation, detrusor sphincter dyssynergia may be managed by α-adrenergic blocking (antimuscarinic) medications. Obstruction that is not adequately managed by pharmacotherapy may require bladder neck incision. Detrusor sphincter dyssynergia may be managed by intermittent catheterization in combination with higher dose antimuscarinic drugs to prevent overactive detrusor contractions and associated dyssynergia while ensuring regular, complete bladder evacuation by catheterization. Alternatively, men with dyssynergia may be managed by condom catheter containment, supplemented by an α-adrenergic-blocking drug or transurethral sphincterotomy (surgical incision of the striated sphincter) to relieve obstruction. Low bladder wall compliance may be managed by antimuscarinic drugs and intermittent catheterization; however, more severe cases may require augmentation enterocystoplasty (enlargement of the low compliant bladder wall using a detubularized piece of small bowel), urinary diversion, or long-term indwelling catheterization.

Prostate enlargement is managed by treating the underlying cause of the prostate enlargement with medication or surgery. Urinary retention may require transient placement of a suprapubic catheter. Urethral stricture is treated with urethral dilation accomplished by using a steel instrument shaped like a catheter (urethral sound) or a series of incrementally increasing catheter-like tubes (filiforms and followers). Long, dense strictures typically require surgical repair to prevent recurrence.

Tumors

Renal Tumors

Renal tumors account for about 58,240 (3.8%) of new cancer cases and 13,040 deaths each year,[19] and there are a number of different types of kidney tumors. Renal adenomas (benign tumors) are uncommon but are increasing in number. The tumors are encapsulated and are usually located near the cortex of the kidney. Because they can become malignant, they are usually surgically removed. Renal cell carcinoma (RCC) is the most common renal neoplasm (85% of all renal neoplasms) and represents about 2% of cancer deaths. Renal transitional cell carcinoma (RTCC) is rare and primarily arises in the renal parenchyma and renal pelvis. Renal cell carcinoma usually occurs in men (two times more often than in women) between 50 and 60 years of age. Risk factors include cigarette smoking, obesity, and uncontrolled hypertension. With surgical resection five-year survival is about 90% for stage I cancer.[19]

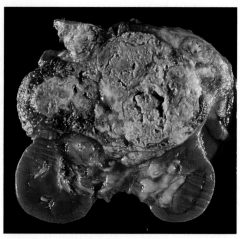

FIGURE 29-4 Renal Cell Carcinoma. Renal cell carcinomas usually are spheroidal masses composed of yellow tissue mottled with hemorrhage, necrosis, and fibrosis. (From Damjanov I, Linder J, editors: *Anderson's pathology,* ed 10, St Louis, 1996, Mosby.)

PATHOGENESIS Renal cell carcinomas are adenocarcinomas that usually arise from tubular epithelium commonly in the renal cortex. The etiology is unknown. They are classified according to cell type and extent of metastasis. *Clear cell tumors,* the most common, present a better prognosis than granular cell or spindle tumors. Confinement within the renal capsule, together with treatment, is associated with a better survival rate. The tumors usually occur unilaterally (Figure 29-4). About 25% of individuals with RCC present with metastasis.[20]

CLINICAL MANIFESTATIONS The classic clinical manifestations of renal tumors are hematuria, dull and aching flank pain, palpable flank mass, and weight loss, but all of these symptoms occur in fewer than 10% of cases. Further, they represent an advanced stage of disease, whereas earlier stages are often silent. The most common sites of distant metastasis are the lung, lymph nodes, liver, bone, thyroid, and central nervous system.[21]

EVALUATION AND TREATMENT Diagnosis is based on the clinical symptoms, plain x-ray films of the abdomen, intravenous pyelography, renal angiography, and computed tomography (CT). (Staging of renal cell carcinoma is presented in Table 29-3.) Staging systems using molecular tumor markers are rapidly advancing.[22] Treatment for localized disease is surgical removal of the affected kidney (radical nephrectomy) or partial nephrectomy for smaller tumors, with combined use of chemotherapeutic agents. Radiation therapy also may be used. Immunotherapy (i.e., interferon-alpha and interleukin-2) is promising in selected cases and new targeted therapies are being developed.[23] Survival is related to tumor grade, tumor cell type, and extent of metastasis.

Bladder Tumors

Bladder tumors are the fifth most common malignancy[24] and represent about 1% of all malignant tumors with 70,530 new cases each year and 14,680 deaths.[19] The development of bladder cancer is most common in men older than 60 years. *Transitional cell carcinoma* is the most common bladder malignancy and tumors are usually superficial.

PATHOGENESIS The risk of primary bladder cancer is greater among people who smoke or are exposed to metabolites of aniline dyes or other aromatic amines. Bladder cancer results from a genetic alteration in normal bladder epithelium.[25] Metastasis is usually to lymph

TABLE 29-3 STAGING OF RENAL CELL CARCINOMA

STAGE	METASTASIS
I	Tumor confined within kidney capsule; ≤7 cm in diameter
II	Invasion through renal capsule and renal vein but within surrounding fascia; >7 cm in diameter
III	Involvement of one lymph node, or vena cava, or adrenal glands
IV	Distant metastases (e.g., liver and lung) and more than one lymph node

Adapted from American Cancer Society: *Detailed guide: kidney cancer. How is kidney cancer (renal cell carcinoma) staged?* Accessed July 2011. Available at www.cancer.org/Cancer/BladderCancer/Detailed Guide/bladder_cancer_staging.

TABLE 29-4 STAGING OF BLADDER CARCINOMA (TNM SYSTEM)

STAGE	DESCRIPTION
Primary Tumor	
T0	No primary tumor identified
Ta	Noninvasive papillary carcinoma—not in bladder muscle
Tis	Carcinoma in situ (CIS)
T1	Tumor invades connective tissue
T2	Tumor invades detrusor muscle
T3	Invasion of fatty tissue around bladder
T4	Tumor has invaded adjacent structures
Region of Lymph Nodes	
N0	No lymph node involvement
N1 to N3	Lymph node metastasis to pelvic or adjacent region
Distant Metastasis	
M0	No metastasis
M1	Distant metastasis

Adapted from American Cancer Society: *Detailed guide: bladder cancer. How is bladder cancer staged?* Accessed July 2011. Available at www.cancer.org/Cancer/BladderCancer/DetailedGuide/bladder_cancer_staging.
T, Tumor; *N*, node; *M*, metastasis.

nodes, liver, bones, or lungs. Staging for bladder carcinoma is presented in Table 29-4. Secondary bladder cancer develops by invasion of cancer from bordering organs, such as cervical carcinoma in women or prostatic carcinoma in men.

CLINICAL MANIFESTATIONS Gross painless hematuria is the archetypal clinical manifestation of bladder cancer. Episodes of hematuria tend to recur, and they are often accompanied by bothersome lower urinary tract symptoms including daytime voiding frequency, nocturia, urgency, and urge urinary incontinence, particularly for carcinoma in situ. Flank pain may occur if tumor growth obstructs one or both ureterovesical junctions.

EVALUATION AND TREATMENT Urinalysis for evidence of hematuria in the absence of infection provides a useful screening tool for high-risk individuals. Several bladder tumor antigen-testing systems

have been developed for screening, but they have proved more useful in monitoring individuals with known cancer as compared to being used for primary screening. Urine cytologic study (pathologic analysis of sloughed cells within the urine) is completed in individuals with evidence of hematuria from unknown causes; cystoscopy with tissue biopsy confirms the diagnosis. Use of biologic markers for the diagnosis of bladder cancer is under investigation.[26]

Transurethral resection or laser ablation, combined with intravesical chemotherapy or immunotherapy, is effective for superficial tumors, but radical cystectomy with urinary diversion and adjuvant chemotherapy is required for locally invasive tumors.

> ✓ **QUICK CHECK 29-1**
> 1. List two typical complications of urinary tract obstruction, and briefly describe them.
> 2. How do kidney stones form?
> 3. Which population group is at greatest risk for bladder tumors?

URINARY TRACT INFECTION

Causes of Urinary Tract Infection

A **urinary tract infection (UTI)** is an inflammation of the urinary epithelium usually caused by bacteria from gut flora. A UTI can occur anywhere along the urinary tract including the urethra, prostate, bladder, ureter, or kidney. At risk are premature newborns; prepubertal children; sexually active and pregnant women; women treated with antibiotics that disrupt vaginal flora; spermicide users; estrogen-deficient postmenopausal women; individuals with indwelling catheters; and persons with diabetes mellitus, neurogenic bladder, or urinary tract obstruction. Cystitis is more common in women because of the shorter urethra and the closeness of the urethra to the anus (increasing the possibility of bacterial contamination). Up to 50% of women may have a lower UTI at some time in their life.[27] Generally, UTIs are mild, without complications, and occur in individuals with a normal urinary tract; these infections are termed *uncomplicated UTI*. A *complicated UTI* develops when there is an abnormality in the urinary system or a health problem that compromises host defenses or response to treatment. UTI may occur alone or in association with pyelonephritis, prostatitis or kidney stones.

Several factors normally combine to protect against UTIs. Most bacteria are washed out of the urethra during micturition. The low pH and high osmolality of urea, the presence of Tamm-Horsfall protein, and secretions from the uroepithelium provide a bactericidal effect. The ureterovesical junction closes during bladder contraction, preventing reflux of urine to the ureters and kidneys. Both the longer urethra and prostatic secretions decrease the risk of infection in men.

Types of Urinary Tract Infection
Acute Cystitis

Acute cystitis is an inflammation of the bladder and is the most common site of UTI. The morphologic appearance of the bladder through cystoscopy describes different types of cystitis. With mild inflammation, the mucosa is hyperemic (red). More advanced cases may show diffuse hemorrhage (termed *hemorrhagic cystitis*), pus formation, or suppurative exudates (termed *suppurative cystitis*) on the epithelial surface of the bladder. Prolonged infection may lead to sloughing of the bladder mucosa with ulcer formation (termed *ulcerative cystitis*). The most severe infections may cause necrosis of the bladder wall (termed *gangrenous cystitis*).

PATHOPHYSIOLOGY The most common infecting microorganisms are uropathic strains of *Escherichia coli* and the second most common is *Staphylococcus saprophyticus*. Less common microorganisms include *Klebsiella, Proteus, Pseudomonas* fungi, viruses, parasites, or tubercular bacilli. Schistosomiasis is the most common cause of parasitic invasion of the urinary tract on a global basis; it infects over 200 million people and has a strong association with bladder cancer.[28]

Bacterial contamination of the normally sterile urine usually occurs by retrograde movement of gram-negative bacilli into the urethra and bladder and then to the ureter and kidney. Uropathic strains of *E. coli* have *type-1 fimbriae* that bind to latex catheters and receptors on uroepithelium. They resist flushing during normal micturition. These strains also have *P fimbriae* (pyelonephritis-associated fimbriae) that bind to uroepithelial P-blood group antigen which is present in most of the human population and readily ascends the urinary tract.[29] Some women may be genetically susceptible to certain strains of *E. coli* attachment.[30] Hematogenous infections are uncommon and often preceded by septicemia. Infection initiates an inflammatory response and the symptoms of cystitis. The inflammatory edema in the bladder wall stimulates discharge of stretch receptors initiating symptoms of bladder fullness with small volumes of urine and producing the urgency and frequency of urination associated with cystitis.

CLINICAL MANIFESTATIONS Many individuals with bacteriuria are asymptomatic and the elderly have the highest risk. Clinical manifestations of cystitis, however, usually include frequency, urgency, dysuria (painful urination), and suprapubic and low back pain. Hematuria, cloudy urine, and flank pain are more serious symptoms. Approximately 10% of individuals with bacteriuria have no symptoms, and 30% of individuals with symptoms are abacteriuric. Elderly persons with cystitis may be asymptomatic or demonstrate confusion or vague abdominal discomfort. The elderly with recurrent UTI and other concurrent illness have a higher risk of mortality.[27]

EVALUATION AND TREATMENT Infections are diagnosed by urine culture of specific microorganisms with counts of 10,000/ml or more from freshly voided urine. Urine dipstick testing that is positive for leukocyte esterase or nitrite reductase is used for the diagnosis of uncomplicated UTI.[31] Risk factors, such as urinary tract obstruction, should be identified and treated. Evidence of bacteria from urine culture and antibiotic sensitivity warrants treatment with a microorganism-specific antibiotic. A 3-day course may be effective for uncomplicated UTI. Three to 7 days of treatment is most common; complicated UTI requires 7 to 14 days of treatment. From 20% to 25% of women have relapsing infection within 7 to 10 days requiring prolonged antibiotic treatment.[32] Follow-up urine cultures should be obtained 1 week after initiation of treatment and at monthly intervals for 3 months. Clinical symptoms are frequently relieved, but bacteriuria may still be present. Repeat cultures should be obtained every 3 to 4 months until 1 year after treatment for evaluation of recurrent infection.[31] See *Health Alert:* Urinary Tract Infection and Antibiotic Resistance.

Painful Bladder Syndrome/Interstitial Cystitis

Painful bladder syndrome/interstitial cystitis (PBS/IC) is a condition that includes **nonbacterial infectious cystitis** (viral, mycobacterial, chlamydial, fungal), **noninfectious cystitis** (radiation, chemical, autoimmune, hypersensitivity), and interstitial cystitis. It occurs most commonly in women ages 20 to 30 years who have symptoms of cystitis, such as frequency, urgency, dysuria and, nocturia, but with negative urine cultures and no other known etiology. Nonbacterial infectious

HEALTH ALERT

Urinary Tract Infection and Antibiotic Resistance

Uncomplicated urinary tract infection (UTI) is one of the most common bacterial infections. The leading cause of UTI is *Escherichia coli (E. coli)*, and antibiotics are the mainstay of treatment. Of major concern is the worldwide emergence of bacterial strains resistant to specific antibiotics in both hospital- and community-acquired infections. The resistance is caused in part by high human use of antibiotics and antibiotics in animal feed. Rates of resistance are highest in regions with the highest rates of prescription; ampicillin and trimethoprim-sulfamethoxazole (TMP-SMX) have a high rate of resistance and fluoroquinolone resistance is increasing worldwide. In more complicated UTIs treated with carbapenem, bacteria are emerging that produce carbapenemases. Risks for resistance include TMP-SMX treatment within last 3 months, diabetes mellitus, recent hospitalization, and specific antibiotic resistance rates in a community of greater than 20%. However, reliable data regarding the true prevalence of resistance in a community are often lacking. First time uncomplicated UTI can be treated empirically with a 3-day regimen. Complicated infection requires treatment based on history, physical examination, urine culture, and sensitivity and possible radiologic evaluation. Asymptomatic bacteriuria only requires treatment in exceptional cases. Cranberry products can be useful for prophylaxis.

Data from Chakupurakal R et al: Urinary tract pathogens and resistance pattern, *J Clin Pathol* 63(7):652–654, 2010; National Guideline Clearinghouse (NGC): *Guideline synthesis: diagnosis and management of uncomplicated lower urinary tract infection,* Rockville, Md, revised 2009, National Guideline Clearinghouse (NGC) website. Available at www.guideline.gov. Accessed July 9, 2011; Pallett A, Hand K: Complicated urinary tract infections: practical solutions for the treatment of multiresistant gram-negative bacteria, *J Antimicrob Chemother* 65(suppl 3):iii25–33, 2010; Pfeifer Y, Cullik A, Witte W: Resistance to cephalosporins and carbapenems in gram-negative bacterial pathogens, *Int J Med Microbiol* 300(6):371–379, 2010; Rossi R, Porta S, Canovi B: Overview on cranberry and urinary tract infections in females, *J Clin Gastroenterol* 44(suppl 1):S61–S62, 2010; Walsh C, Fanning S: Antimicrobial resistance in foodborne pathogens—a cause for concern? *Curr Drug Targets* 9(9):808–815, 2008; Yamamoto S, Higuchi Y, Nojima M: Current therapy of acute uncomplicated cystitis, *Int J Urol* 17(5):450–456, 2010.

cystitis is most common among those who are immunocompromised. Noninfectious cystitis is associated with radiation or chemotherapy treatment for pelvic and urogenital cancers.

The cause of painful bladder syndrome/interstitial cystitis is unknown. An autoimmune reaction may be responsible for the inflammatory response, which includes mast cell activation, altered epithelial permeability, and increased sensory nerve sensitivity. Inflammation and fibrosis of the bladder wall are accompanied by the presence of hemorrhagic ulcers (Hunner ulcers), and bladder volume may decrease as a result of fibrosis. The derangement of the bladder mucosa makes it more susceptible to penetration by bacteria. More recently, the identification of antiproliferative factor (APF), a protein expressed by the bladder uroepithelium in those with IC, is important. APF appears to block the normal growth of cells that line the inside wall of the bladder and indirectly increases bladder sensation.[33] Characteristic symptoms of PBS/IC include bladder fullness, frequency (including nocturia), small urine volume, and chronic pelvic pain with symptoms lasting longer than 9 months. Diagnosis of PBS/IC requires the exclusion of other diagnoses, and extensive evaluations are completed. No single treatment is effective, and different approaches are used for symptom relief.[34]

TABLE 29-5 COMMON CAUSES OF PYELONEPHRITIS

PREDISPOSING FACTOR	PATHOLOGIC MECHANISMS
Kidney stones	Obstruction and stasis of urine contributing to bacteriuria and hydronephrosis; irritation of epithelial lining with entrapment of bacteria
Vesicoureteral reflux	Chronic reflux of urine up the ureter and into kidney during micturition, contributing to bacterial infection
Pregnancy	Dilation and relaxation of ureter with hydroureter and hydronephrosis; partly caused by obstruction from enlarged uterus and partly from ureteral relaxation caused by higher progesterone levels
Neurogenic bladder	Neurologic impairment interfering with normal bladder contraction with residual urine and ascending infection
Instrumentation	Introduction of organisms into urethra and bladder by catheters and endoscopes introduced into urinary tract for diagnostic purposes
Female sexual trauma	Movement of organisms from urethra into bladder with infection and retrograde spread to kidney

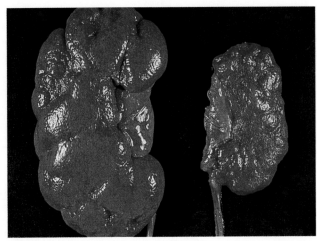

FIGURE 29-5 Pyelonephritis. *(Right)* Small, shrunken, irregularly scarred kidney of an individual with chronic pyelonephritis. *(Left)* Kidney is of normal size but also shows scarring on the upper pole. (From Damjanov I: *Pathology for the health professions,* ed 3, St Louis, 2006, Saunders.)

Acute Pyelonephritis

Pyelonephritis is an infection of one or both upper urinary tracts (ureter, renal pelvis, and interstitium). Common causes are summarized in Table 29-5. Urinary obstruction and reflux of urine from the bladder (vesicoureteral reflux) are the most common underlying risk factors. One or both kidneys may be involved. Most cases occur in women. The responsible microorganism is usually *E. coli, Proteus,* or *Pseudomonas.* The latter two microorganisms are more commonly associated with infections after urethral instrumentation or urinary tract surgery. These microorganisms also split urea into ammonia, making alkaline urine that increases the risk of stone formation.

PATHOPHYSIOLOGY The infection is probably spread by ascending uropathic microorganisms along the ureters, but spread also may occur by way of the bloodstream. The inflammatory process is usually focal and irregular, primarily affecting the pelvis, calyces, and medulla. The infection causes medullary infiltration of white blood cells with renal inflammation, renal edema, and purulent urine. In severe infections, localized abscesses may form in the medulla and extend to the cortex. Primarily affected are the tubules; the glomeruli usually are spared. Necrosis of renal papillae can develop. After the acute phase, healing occurs with fibrosis and atrophy of affected tubules (Figure 29-5). The number of bacteria decreases until the urine again becomes sterile. Acute pyelonephritis rarely causes renal failure.[35]

CLINICAL MANIFESTATIONS The onset of symptoms is usually acute, with fever, chills, and flank or groin pain. Symptoms characteristic of a UTI, including frequency, dysuria, and costovertebral tenderness, may precede systemic signs and symptoms. Older adults may have nonspecific symptoms, such as low grade fever and malaise.

EVALUATION AND TREATMENT Differentiating symptoms of cystitis from those of pyelonephritis by clinical assessment alone is difficult. The specific diagnosis is established by urine culture, urinalysis, and clinical signs and symptoms. White blood cell casts indicate pyelonephritis, but they are not always present in the urine. Complicated pyelonephritis requires blood cultures and urinary tract imaging.[36]

Uncomplicated acute pyelonephritis responds well to 2 to 3 weeks of microorganism-specific antibiotic therapy. Follow-up urine cultures are obtained at 1 and 4 weeks after treatment if symptoms recur. Antibiotic-resistant microorganisms or reinfection may occur in cases of urinary tract obstruction or reflux. Intravenous pyelography and voiding cystourethrography identify surgically correctable lesions.

Chronic Pyelonephritis

Chronic pyelonephritis is a persistent or recurrent infection of the kidney leading to scarring of one or both kidneys. The specific cause of chronic pyelonephritis is difficult to determine. Recurrent infections from acute pyelonephritis may be associated with chronic pyelonephritis. Generally, chronic pyelonephritis is more likely to occur in individuals who have renal infections associated with some type of obstructive pathologic condition, such as renal stones and vesicoureteral reflux.

PATHOPHYSIOLOGY Chronic urinary tract obstruction starts a process of progressive inflammation, altered renal pelvis and calyces, destruction of the tubules, atrophy or dilation and diffuse scarring, and finally impaired urine-concentrating ability, leading to chronic kidney failure.

The lesions of chronic pyelonephritis are sometimes termed *chronic interstitial nephritis* because the inflammation and fibrosis are located in the interstitial spaces between the tubules (see Figure 29-5). Causes other than chronic pyelonephritis include drug toxicity from analgesics such as phenacetin, aspirin, and acetaminophen; ischemia; irradiation; and immune complex diseases.

CLINICAL MANIFESTATIONS The early symptoms of chronic pyelonephritis are often minimal and may include hypertension, frequency, dysuria, and flank pain. Progression leads to kidney failure, particularly in the presence of obstructive uropathy or diabetes mellitus.[35]

EVALUATION AND TREATMENT   Urinalysis, intravenous pyelography, and ultrasound are used diagnostically. Treatment is related to the underlying cause. Obstruction must be relieved. Antibiotics may be given, with prolonged antibiotic therapy for recurrent infection.

> ✔ **QUICK CHECK 29-2**
> 1. Why is cystitis more common in women?
> 2. What is interstitial cystitis?
> 3. How does pyelonephritis differ from cystitis?

GLOMERULAR DISORDERS

Glomerulonephritis

Glomerulonephritis is an inflammation of the glomerulus caused by *primary glomerular injury,* including immunologic responses, ischemia, free radicals, drugs, toxins, vascular disorders, and infection. *Secondary glomerular injury* is a consequence of systemic diseases, including diabetes mellitus, systemic lupus erythematosus, congestive heart failure, and human immunodeficiency virus (HIV)-related kidney disease.

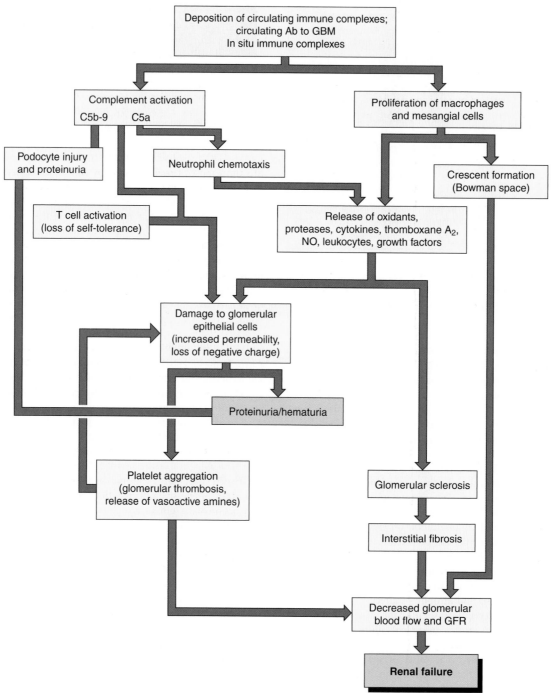

FIGURE 29-6 Mechanisms of Glomerular Injury. *Ab,* Antibody; *GBM,* glomerular basement membrane; *GFR,* glomerular filtration rate; *NO,* nitric oxide.

PATHOPHYSIOLOGY Immune mechanisms are a major cause of injury for both primary and secondary causes of glomerulonephritis (Figure 29-6). The most common types of immune injury are (1) deposition of circulating antigen-antibody immune complexes into the glomerulus (type III hypersensitivity) and (2) antibodies reacting in situ against planted antigens within the glomerulus (type II hypersensitivity, cytotoxic) (see Chapter 7). Nonimmune glomerular injury is related to ischemia, toxin exposure, drugs, vascular disorders, and infection with direct injury to glomerular cells. Different causes of injury may result in more than one type of glomerular lesion; thus lesions are not necessarily disease specific (Table 29-6).

Immune injury is caused by activation of biochemical mediators of inflammation (i.e., complement and cytokines from leukocytes) and begins after the antigen-antibody complexes have deposited or formed in the glomerular capillary wall. Complement is deposited with the antibodies and activation can cause cell lysis or serve as a chemotactic stimulus for attraction of neutrophils, monocytes, and T lymphocytes.[37] These phagocytes, along with activated platelets, further the inflammatory reaction by releasing mediators that injure the glomerular filtration membrane, including epithelial cells, glomerular basement membrane, and endothelial cells (podocytes and filtration slits).[38] The injury increases glomerular membrane permeability and reduces glomerular membrane surface area. The GFR decreases. There also may be swelling and proliferation of mesangial cells and expansion of the extracellular matrix in the Bowman space contributing to crescent formation (deposition of substances in the Bowman space, forming the shape of a crescent moon). The result is a decrease in glomerular blood flow, decreased driving hydrostatic pressure, decreased GFR, and hypoxic injury.[39]

Loss of negative electrical charge across the glomerular filtration membrane and increase in filtration pore size enhance movement of proteins into the urine. Proteins are normally repelled because they also have a negative charge. Red blood cells also escape if pore size is large enough. Proteinuria or hematuria, or both, develops. The severity of glomerular damage and decline in glomerular function is related to the size, number, and location (focal or diffuse) of cells injured, duration of exposure, and type of antigen-antibody complexes.

CLINICAL MANIFESTATIONS The onset of glomerulonephritis may be sudden or insidious and significant loss of nephron function can occur before symptoms develop. Glomerulonephritis may be silent, mild, moderate, or severe in symptom presentation. Severe or progressive glomerular disease causes oliguria (urine output of 30 ml/hour or less), hypertension, and renal failure. Focal lesions tend to produce less severe clinical symptoms. Salt and water are reabsorbed, contributing to fluid volume expansion, edema, and hypertension. Major life-threatening problems during the first few weeks are acute renal insufficiency with fluid and electrolyte alterations, and metabolic acidosis. Acute severe hypertension may cause hypertensive encephalopathy, circulatory failure, and pulmonary edema.

Two major symptoms distinctive of more severe glomerulonephritis are (1) hematuria with red blood cell casts and (2) proteinuria exceeding 3 to 5 g/day with albumin (macroalbuminuria) as the major protein. Gross proteinuria is associated with nephrotic syndrome (see p. 753). Red blood cells escaping through the glomerular membrane produce a smoky brown–tinged urine, red blood cell casts, and an accompanying proteinuria, and is associated with nephritic syndrome (see p. 754). Glomerular bleeding provides prolonged contact with the acidic urine and transforms hemoglobin to methemoglobin, which has a brownish color and no blood clots. Bleeding from sites lower in the urinary tract produces pink- or red-colored urine. The history and physical examination may disclose findings that differentiate glomerular disease from another source of urinary tract bleeding.

Different types of glomerulonephritis may be associated with different patterns of urinary sediment. Urine with a nephritic sediment is characterized by the presence of blood with red cell casts, white cell casts, and varying degrees of protein, which usually is not severe. Urine with nephrotic sediment contains massive amounts of protein and lipids and either a microscopic amount of blood or no blood. The sediment of chronic glomerular disease has waxy casts, granular casts, and less protein and blood than found in nephrotic or nephritic sediment.

EVALUATION AND TREATMENT The diagnosis of glomerular disease is confirmed by the progressive development of clinical manifestations and laboratory findings of abnormal urinalysis with proteinuria, red blood cells, white blood cells, and casts. Microscopic evaluation from renal biopsy provides a specific determination of renal injury and type of pathologic condition.

Patterns of antigen-antibody complex deposition within the glomerular capillary filtration membrane have been established using light, electron, and immunofluorescent microscopy for different disease processes. The findings with light microscopy provide information about the distribution and extent of immune response injury (Table 29-7). Electron microscopy differentiates morphologic changes within the glomerular capillary wall. Staining with fluorescein identifies different antibodies (i.e., immunoglobulin G [IgG] or immunoglobulin A [IgA]) and their configurations when viewed under ultraviolet (black) light with a microscope.

Reduced GFR during glomerulonephritis is evidenced by elevated plasma urea, cystatin C, and creatinine concentrations, or by reduced creatinine clearance (see Chapter 28). Edema, caused by excessive sodium and water retention, may require the use of diuretics or dialysis.

TABLE 29-6	**TYPES OF GLOMERULAR LESIONS**
LESION	**CHARACTERISTICS**
Glomerular Lesions	
Diffuse	Relatively uniform involvement of most or all glomeruli; most common form of glomerulonephritis
Focal	Changes in only some glomeruli, whereas others are normal
Segmental-local	Changes in one part of glomerulus with other parts unaffected
Lesion Characteristics	
Mesangial	Deposits of immunoglobulins in mesangial matrix, mesangial cell proliferation
Membranous	Thickening of glomerular capillary wall with immune deposits
Proliferative	Increase in number of glomerular cells
Sclerotic	Glomerular scarring from previous glomerular injury
Crescentic	Accumulation of proliferating cells within Bowman space, making crescent appearance
Interstitial fibrosis	Scarring between glomerulus and tubules

TABLE 29-7	IMMUNOLOGIC PATHOGENESIS OF GLOMERULONEPHRITIS
GLOMERULAR INJURY	**MECHANISM**
Soluble immune-complex glomerulonephritis (90%)	Formation of antibodies stimulated by presence of endogenous or exogenous antigens results in circulating soluble antigen-antibody complexes, which are deposited in glomerular capillaries; glomerular injury occurring with complement activation and release of immunologic substances that lyse cells and increase membrane permeability; severity of glomerular injury related to number of complexes formed; type III hypersensitivity reaction
Anti–glomerular basement membrane glomerulonephritis (5%)	Antibodies are formed and act directly against glomerular basement membrane; immune response causes accumulation of inflammatory cells in Bowman space (in shape of a crescent moon) surrounding and compressing glomerular capillaries; generally associated with rapidly progressive renal failure, such as Goodpasture syndrome; type II hypersensitivity reaction
Alternative complement pathway	Relatively obscure mechanism associated with low levels of complement and membranoproliferative glomerulonephritis; type III hypersensitivity reaction
Cell-mediated immunity	Delayed hypersensitivity response that damages glomerulus; actual cellular mechanism not clearly understood; type IV hypersensitivity reaction

Management principles for treating glomerulonephritis are related to treating the primary disease, preventing or minimizing immune responses, and correcting accompanying problems, such as edema, hypertension, and hyperlipidemia. Specific treatment regimens are necessary for particular types of glomerulonephritis. Antibiotic therapy is essential for the management of underlying infections that may be contributing to ongoing antigen-antibody responses. Corticosteroids decrease antibody synthesis and suppress inflammatory responses. Cytotoxic agents (e.g., cyclophosphamide) may be used to suppress the immune response. Anticoagulants may be useful for controlling fibrin crescent formation in rapidly progressive glomerulonephritis.

Types of Glomerulonephritis

The classification of glomerulonephritis can be described according to cause, pathologic lesions, disease progression (acute, rapidly progressive, chronic), or clinical presentation (nephrotic syndrome, nephritic syndrome, acute or chronic renal failure). In nearly all types of glomerulonephritis, the epithelial or podocyte layer of the glomerular capillary membrane is disturbed with loss of negative charges and changes in membrane permeability; the mesangial matrix may be expanded or the basement membrane thickened. Features of the patterns of glomerular injury are summarized in Table 29-8. Many types of glomerular injury occur most often in children or young adults, including acute postinfectious glomerulonephritis and minimal change nephropathy (lipoid nephrosis). Details of these diseases are presented in Chapter 30.

Complications of diabetic nephropathy and systemic lupus erythematosus can affect the entire nephron and glomerular injury is significant. Different patterns of injury develop over the course of these diseases. Diabetic nephropathy develops from metabolic and vascular complications (see Chapter 18). Changes in the glomerulus are characterized by progressive thickening and fibrosis of the glomerular basement membrane and expansion of the mesangial matrix with proteinuria and progression to chronic renal failure.[40] Diabetic nephropathy is the most common cause of chronic kidney disease and end-stage renal failure. Lupus nephritis is caused by the formation of autoantibodies against double-stranded DNA with glomerular deposition of the immune complexes. There is complement activation and a cascade of inflammatory events resulting in damage to the glomerular membrane with mesangial expansion.[41]

IgA nephropathy (Berger disease) is the most common form of acute glomerulonephritis in developed countries, especially Asia. The cause is unknown and more commonly affects adults 20 to 30 years of age. Abnormal glycosylated IgA-1 (galactose-deficient IgA-1) and complement molecules bind to glomerular mesangial cells, stimulating them to proliferate and release oxidants and proteases, thereby contributing to diffuse mesangioproliferative glomerular injury and glomerulosclerosis. The disease manifests with gross or microscopic (30% to 40%) hematuria 24 to 48 hours after an upper respiratory tract or gastrointestinal mucosal viral infection.[42]

Membranous Nephropathy

Membranous nephropathy, also known as membranous glomerulonephritis, is one of the most common causes of glomerulonephritis. It is caused by deposition either of circulating antibodies or of antibodies formed in situ to antigens expressed by podocytes on the glomerular membrane. The antigen-antibody complexes activate C5b-C9 fragments of complement (the membrane attack complex) on glomerular epithelial cells with injury and release of inflammatory mediators by mesangial and epithelial cells, resulting in increased membrane permeability, thickening of the glomerular membrane, and, ultimately, glomerular sclerosis. Proteinuria and nephrotic syndrome are common manifestations.[43]

Rapidly progressive glomerulonephritis (RPGN) is a severe form of membranous glomerulonephritis that develops over a period of days to weeks.[44] By the time RPGN is diagnosed, renal insufficiency is apparent. Anti–glomerular basement membrane disease (Goodpasture syndrome) is a type of autoimmune RPGN. The disease is rare and associated with antibody formation against both pulmonary capillary and glomerular basement membranes. Pulmonary hemorrhage and renal failure can occur.

Chronic Glomerulonephritis

Chronic glomerulonephritis encompasses several glomerular diseases with a progressive course leading to chronic kidney failure. There may be no history of kidney disease before the diagnosis. Hypercholesterolemia and proteinuria have been associated with progressive glomerular and tubular injury. The proposed mechanism is related to those observed in glomerulosclerosis and interstitial injury.[45] The primary cause may be difficult to establish because advanced pathologic changes may obscure specific disease characteristics (Figure 29-7). Diabetes mellitus and lupus erythematosus are examples of secondary causes of chronic glomerular injury.[46] Renal insufficiency usually begins to develop after 10 to 20 years, followed by nephrotic syndrome and an accelerated progression to end-stage renal failure. Symptom patterns vary depending on the underlying

TABLE 29-8   FEATURES OF THE COMMON TYPES OF GLOMERULONEPHRITIS

TYPE AND CAUSE	PATHOPHYSIOLOGY
Associated with Nephritic Syndrome	
Acute postinfectious glomerulonephritis (Group A β-hemolytic streptococcus)	Diffuse deposits of immune complexes (IgG and complement) in glomerular capillary wall; infiltration of leukocytes; mesangial proliferation
	Decreased capillary blood flow and GFR
Crescentic or rapidly progressive glomerulonephritis	Accumulation of immune deposits and inflammatory cells and debris that proliferate into Bowman space and form crescent-shaped lesions
In situ formation of anti–glomerular basement membrane antibodies or immune complex deposition	Decreased capillary blood flow and GFR
Nonspecific response to glomerular injury; can occur in any severe glomerular disease	Can result in renal failure
Mesangial proliferative glomerulonephritis	Deposits of immune complexes in mesangium with mesangial proliferation
Usually associated with IgA nephropathy	Decreased glomerular blood flow and GFR
Associated with nephrotic syndrome	
Minimal change disease (lipoid nephrosis)	Uniform diffuse thinning of epithelial (podocyte) foot processes; loss of negative charge in basement membrane and increased permeability
Glomerular basement membrane appears normal	
Usually idiopathic	Severe proteinuria and nephrotic syndrome
No immune deposits	
Focal segmented glomerulosclerosis	Similar to minimal change disease
Usually idiopathic	
Membranous nephropathy (autoimmune response to unknown renal antigen)	Thickening of glomerular capillary wall caused by antibody and complement deposition and release of inflammatory cytokines with increased permeability, proteinuria, and nephrotic syndrome
Usually idiopathic	
Can be associated with systemic diseases (i.e., hepatitis B virus, systemic lupus erythematous, solid malignant tumors)	
Membranoproliferative glomerulonephritis	Mesangial cell proliferation; thickening of basement membrane; subendothelial deposits of immune complex occlude glomerular capillary blood flow
Usually idiopathic; associated with low complement levels	
	Decreased GFR
IgA nephropathy (Berger disease)	Mesangial deposits of IgA and proliferation of inflammatory cells into Bowman space with sclerosis and fibrosis of glomerulus and crescent formation
Usually idiopathic; elevated IgA plasma levels	
	Decreased GFR and hematuria; usually focal, some diffuse lesions
Chronic glomerulonephritis	Glomerular fibrosis and scarring, interstitial and tubular fibrosis and vascular sclerosis; original glomerular lesions may not be definable; progression to end-stage kidney disease with uremia
Can be a consequence of any type of glomerulonephritis; more common with crescentic or rapidly progressive glomerulonephritis	

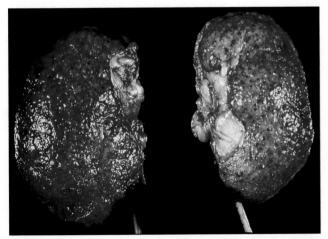

FIGURE 29-7 Chronic Glomerulonephritis. The kidneys appear small, are uniformly shrunken, and have a finely granular external surface. (From Damjanov I: *Pathology for the health professions,* ed 3, St Louis, 2006, Saunders.)

cause. Use of steroids usually does not change the course of chronic glomerular disease, and dialysis or kidney transplantation ultimately may be needed.

Nephrotic and Nephritic Syndromes

Nephrotic syndrome is the excretion of 3.5 g or more of protein in the urine per day and is characteristic of glomerular injury. *Primary causes of nephrotic syndrome* include minimal change disease (lipoid nephrosis) (see Chapter 30), membranous glomerulonephritis, and focal segmental glomerulosclerosis.[47] *Secondary forms of nephrotic syndrome* occur in systemic diseases, including diabetes mellitus, amyloidosis, systemic lupus erythematosus, and Henoch-Schönlein purpura (see Chapter 30). Nephrotic syndrome also is associated with certain drugs, infections, malignancies, and vascular disorders. When present as a secondary complication with renal diseases, nephrotic syndrome often signifies a more serious prognosis.[47] Nephrotic syndrome is more common in children than adults (see Chapter 30).

PATHOPHYSIOLOGY Disturbances in the glomerular basement membrane and podocyte injury lead to increased permeability to protein and loss of electrical negative charge. Loss of plasma proteins, particularly albumin and some immunoglobulins, occurs across the injured glomerular filtration membrane. Hypoalbuminemia results from urinary loss of albumin combined with a diminished synthesis of replacement albumin by the liver. Albumin is lost in the greatest quantity because of its high plasma concentration and low molecular weight. Decreased dietary intake of protein from anorexia or malnutrition or accompanying liver disease may also contribute to lower levels of plasma albumin. Loss of albumin stimulates lipoprotein synthesis by the liver and hyperlipidemia. Loss of immunoglobulins may increase susceptibility to infections. Sodium retention is common.

CLINICAL MANIFESTATIONS Many clinical manifestations of nephrotic syndrome are related to loss of serum proteins and associated sodium retention (Table 29-9). They include edema, hyperlipidemia, lipiduria, vitamin D deficiency, and hypothyroidism.[48,49] Vitamin D deficiency is related to loss of serum transport proteins and decreased vitamin D activation by the kidney. Hypothyroidism can result from urinary loss of thyroid-binding protein and thyroxine. Alterations in coagulation factors can cause hypercoagulability and may lead to thromboembolic events.[50]

EVALUATION AND TREATMENT Nephrotic syndrome is diagnosed when the protein level in a 24-hour urine collection is greater than 3.5 g. Serum albumin level decreases (to less than 3 g/dl), and concentrations of serum cholesterol, phospholipids, and triglycerides increase. Fat bodies may be present in the urine. The specific pathologic condition is identified by renal biopsy.

Nephrotic syndrome is commonly treated by adhering to a normal-protein (i.e., 1 g/kg body weight/day), low-fat, salt-restricted diet and by prescribing diuretics, immunosuppressive drugs, and heparinoids. When diuretics are used, care must be taken to observe for hypovolemia and hypokalemia or potassium toxicity in the presence of renal insufficiency. Aldactone may be combined with loop diuretics to suppress aldosterone activity to conserve potassium. Steroids or cyclophosphamide may be effective for the initial treatment of steroid-dependent nephrotic syndrome in children.[51] Immunosuppressive drugs and angiotensin-converting enzyme (ACE) inhibitors are used with steroid-resistant nephrotic syndrome.[52]

In nephritic syndrome, hematuria (usually microscopic) is present and red blood cell casts are present in the urine in addition to proteinuria, which is not severe. It is caused by increased permeability of the glomerular filtration membrane with pore sizes large enough to allow the passage of red blood cells and protein. Nephritic syndrome is associated with postinfectious glomerulonephritis, rapidly progressive (crescentic) glomerulonephritis, IgA nephropathy, lupus nephritis,

and diabetic nephropathy. The pathophysiology is related to immune injury of the glomerulus as previously described. Hypertension and uremia occur in advanced stages of disease. The symptoms and treatment are similar to those described for nephrotic syndrome.[53]

QUICK CHECK 29-3
1. What is glomerulonephritis? List two types.
2. What immune mechanisms are operative in glomerulonephritis?
3. Why is edema present in individuals with nephrotic syndrome?

ACUTE KIDNEY INJURY

Classification of Kidney Dysfunction

Acute kidney injury (AKI) is a sudden decline in kidney function with a decrease in glomerular filtration and accumulation of nitrogenous waste products in the blood as demonstrated by an elevation in plasma creatinine and blood urea nitrogen levels. The term *acute kidney injury* is preferred to the term *acute renal failure* because it captures the spectrum of this syndrome, which ranges from minimal or subtle changes in renal function to complete renal failure requiring renal replacement therapy. Classification criteria have been developed to guide the diagnosis of renal injury and are described by the acronym RIFLE (R = risk, I = injury, F = failure, L = loss, and E = end-stage kidney disease [ESKD]), representing three levels of renal dysfunction of increasing severity (Table 29-10).[54]

Renal insufficiency generally refers to a decline in renal function to about 25% of normal or a GFR of 25 to 30 ml/min. Levels of serum creatinine and urea are mildly elevated. Renal failure refers to significant loss of renal function requiring dialysis. End-stage renal failure (ESRF) refers to a renal function of less than 10% requiring dialysis or transplant.

PATHOPHYSIOLOGY AKI commonly results from extracellular volume depletion, decreased renal blood flow, or toxic/inflammatory injury to kidney cells resulting in alterations in renal function that may be minimal or severe. Acute kidney injury can be classified as prerenal (renal hypoperfusion), intrarenal (disorders involving renal parenchymal or interstitial tissue), or postrenal (urinary tract obstructive disorders) (Table 29-11).[55]

Prerenal acute kidney injury is the most common reason for AKI and is caused by renal hypoperfusion. The GFR declines because of the decrease in filtration pressure. Poor perfusion can result from renal vasoconstriction, hypotension, hypovolemia, hemorrhage, or inadequate cardiac output. AKI may occur during chronic renal failure if

TABLE 29-9	CLINICAL MANIFESTATIONS OF NEPHROTIC SYNDROME	
MANIFESTATION	**CONTRIBUTING FACTORS**	**RESULT**
Proteinuria	Increased glomerular permeability, decreased proximal tubule reabsorption	Edema, increased susceptibility to infection from loss of immunoglobulins
Hypoalbuminemia	Increased urinary losses of protein	Edema
Edema	Hypoalbuminemia (decreased plasma oncotic pressure, sodium and water retention, increased aldosterone and antidiuretic hormone [ADH] secretion), unresponsiveness to atrial natriuretic peptides	Soft, pitting, generalized edema
Hyperlipidemia	Decreased serum albumin level; increased hepatic synthesis of very-low-density lipoproteins; increased levels of cholesterol, phospholipids, triglycerides	Increased atherogenesis
Lipiduria	Sloughing of tubular cells containing fat (oval fat bodies); free fat from hyperlipidemia	Fat droplets that may float in urine

a sudden stress is imposed on already marginally functioning kidneys. Failure to restore blood volume or blood pressure and oxygen delivery can cause cell injury and acute tubular necrosis or acute interstitial necrosis, a more severe form of AKI.

Intrarenal (intrinsic) acute kidney injury usually results from ischemic **acute tubular necrosis (ATN)** related to prerenal AKI, nephrotoxic ATN (i.e., exposure to radiocontrast media), acute glomerulonephritis, vascular disease (malignant hypertension, disseminated intravascular coagulation, and renal vasculitis), allograft rejection, or interstitial disease (drug allergy, infection, tumor growth). ATN caused by ischemia occurs most often after surgery (40% to 50% of cases) but also is associated with sepsis, obstetric complications, and severe trauma, including severe burns. Hypotension associated with hypovolemia produces ischemia, generating toxic oxygen free radicals that cause cellular swelling, injury, and necrosis.[56] Ischemic necrosis tends to be patchy and may be distributed along any part of the nephron.

Nephrotoxic ATN can be produced by radiocontrast media and numerous antibiotics, particularly the aminoglycosides (neomycin, gentamicin, tobramycin) because these drugs accumulate in the renal cortex. Other substances, such as excessive myoglobin (oxygen-transporting substance from muscles), carbon tetrachloride, heavy metals (mercury, arsenic), or methoxyflurane anesthetic, and bacterial toxins may promote renal failure. Dehydration, advanced age, concurrent renal insufficiency, and diabetes mellitus tend to enhance nephrotoxicity. Necrosis caused by nephrotoxins is usually uniform and limited to the proximal tubules.

Postrenal acute kidney injury is rare and usually occurs with urinary tract obstruction that affects the kidneys bilaterally (e.g., bladder outlet obstruction, prostatic hypertrophy, bilateral ureteral obstruction), tumors, or neurogenic bladder. A pattern of several hours of anuria with flank pain followed by polyuria is a characteristic finding. The obstruction causes an increase in intraluminal pressure upstream from the site of obstruction with a gradual decrease in GFR. This type of renal failure can occur after diagnostic catheterization of the ureters, a procedure that may cause edema of the tubular lumen.

Oliguria can occur in AKI and three mechanisms have been proposed to account for the decrease in urine output.[57,58] All three mechanisms probably contribute to oliguria in varying combinations and degrees throughout the course of the disease (Figure 29-8). These mechanisms are as follows:

1. *Alterations in renal blood flow.* Efferent arteriolar vasoconstriction may be produced by intrarenal release of angiotensin II or there may be redistribution of blood flow from the cortex to the medulla. Autoregulation of blood flow may be impaired, resulting in decreased GFR. Changes in glomerular permeability and decreased GFR also may result from ischemia.
2. *Tubular obstruction.* Necrosis of the tubules causes sloughing of cells, cast formation, or ischemic edema that results in tubular obstruction, which in turn causes a retrograde increase in pressure and reduces the GFR. Renal failure can occur within 24 hours.
3. *Back leak.* Glomerular filtration remains normal, but tubular reabsorption of filtrate is accelerated as a result of permeability caused by ischemia.

CLINICAL MANIFESTATIONS The clinical progression of AKI with recovery of renal function occurs in three phases: initiation phase, maintenance phase, and recovery phase. The *initiation phase* is the phase of reduced perfusion or toxicity in which kidney injury is evolving. Prevention of injury is possible during this phase. The *maintenance phase* is the period of established kidney injury and dysfunction after the initiating event has been resolved and may last from weeks to months. Urine

---

TABLE 29-10 RIFLE CRITERIA FOR ACUTE KIDNEY DYSFUNCTION/FAILURE

CATEGORY	GFR CRITERIA	URINE OUTPUT (UO) CRITERIA
Risk	Increased creatinine × 1.5 or GFR decrease >25%	UO <0.5 ml/kg/hr × 6 hr
Injury	Increased creatinine × 2 or GFR decrease >50%	UO <0.5 ml/kg/hr × 12 hr
Failure	Increased creatinine × 3 or GFR decrease >75%	UO <0.3 ml/kg/hr × 24 hr or anuria × 12 hr
Loss	Persistent ARF = complete loss of kidney function >4 weeks	
ESKD	End-stage kidney disease (>3 months)	

Adapted from Bellomo R et al: Acute dialysis quality initiative II: the Vicenza conference, *Curr Opin Crit Care* 8(6):505–508, 2002; Bellomo R et al: Acute renal failure—definition, outcome measures, animal models, fluid therapy and information technology needs: the Second International Consensus Conference of the Acute Dialysis Quality Initiative (ADQI) Group, *Crit Care* 8(4):R204–R212, 2004. Available at www.medicalcriteria.com/criteria/neph_rifle.htm, Accessed Feb 2011. *ARF,* Acute renal failure; *ESKD,* end-stage kidney disease; *GFR,* glomerular filtration rate.

TABLE 29-11 CLASSIFICATION OF ACUTE KIDNEY INJURY

AREA OF DYSFUNCTION	POSSIBLE CAUSES
Prerenal	*Hypovolemia*
	Hemorrhagic blood loss (trauma, gastrointestinal bleeding, complications of childbirth)
	Loss of plasma volume (burns, peritonitis)
	Water and electrolyte losses (severe vomiting or diarrhea, intestinal obstruction, uncontrolled diabetes mellitus, inappropriate use of diuretics)
	Hypotension or hypoperfusion
	Septic shock
	Cardiac failure or shock
	Massive pulmonary embolism
	Stenosis or clamping of renal artery
Intrarenal	*Acute tubular necrosis (postischemic or nephrotoxic)*
	Glomerulopathies
	Acute interstitial necrosis (tumors or toxins)
	Vascular damage
	Malignant hypertension, vasculitis
	Coagulation defects
	Renal artery/vein occlusion
	Bilateral acute pyelonephritis
Postrenal	*Obstructive uropathies (usually bilateral)*
	Ureteral destruction (edema, tumors, stones, clots)
	Bladder neck obstruction (enlarged prostate)
	Neurogenic bladder

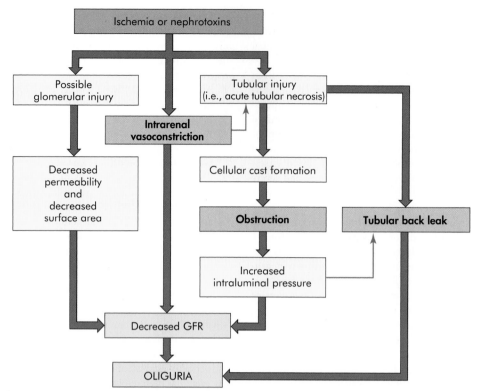

FIGURE 29-8 Mechanisms of Oliguria in Acute Kidney Failure. *GFR,* Glomerular filtration rate.

output is lowest during this phase and serum creatinine and blood urea nitrogen (BUN) levels both increase. The *recovery phase* is the interval when kidney injury is repaired and normal renal function is reestablished. Diuresis is common during this phase with a decline in serum creatinine and urea concentrations and an increase in creatinine clearance.

Oliguria begins within 1 day after a hypotensive event and lasts 1 to 3 weeks, but it may regress in several hours or extend for several weeks, depending on the duration of ischemia or the severity of injury or obstruction. Renal failure can present with nonoliguria, particularly with intrinsic kidney injury associated with nephrotoxins. The urine output may vary in volume, but the BUN and plasma creatinine concentrations increase (plasma creatinine concentration is inversely proportional to the GFR). Other early manifestations depend on the underlying cause of renal failure.

As renal function improves, increase in urine volume (diuresis) is progressive. The tubules are still damaged early in the recovery phase but are recovering function. Fluid and electrolyte balance must be carefully monitored and excessive urinary losses replaced.

Serial measurements of plasma creatinine concentration provide an index of renal function during the *recovery phase*. Return to normal status may take from 3 to 12 months, and some individuals do not have full recovery of a normal GFR or tubular function.

EVALUATION AND TREATMENT The diagnosis of AKI is related to the cause of the disease. A history of surgery, trauma, or cardiovascular disorders is common, and exposure to nephrotoxins and obstructive uropathies (e.g., an enlarged prostate) must be considered. The diagnostic challenge is to differentiate prerenal AKI from intrarenal AKI, and some evidence is available from urinalysis and measurement of plasma creatinine and BUN levels (Table 29-12). Biomarkers are being developed to assess the extent of kidney injury.[59] Prevention of AKI is a

major treatment factor and involves avoidance of hypotension, hypovolemia, and nephrotoxicity.

The primary goal of therapy is to maintain the individual's life until renal function has been recovered. Management principles directly related to physiologic alterations generally include (1) correcting fluid and electrolyte disturbances, (2) treating infections, (3) maintaining nutrition, and (4) remembering that drugs or their metabolites are not excreted. Continuous renal replacement therapy may be indicated. The mortality rate is greater than 50% with renal replacement therapy.[60]

CHRONIC KIDNEY DISEASE

Chronic kidney disease (CKD) is the progressive loss of renal function associated with systemic diseases, such as hypertension and diabetes mellitus, or with intrinsic kidney diseases, such as chronic glomerulonephritis, chronic pyelonephritis, obstructive uropathies, or vascular disorders. The National Kidney Foundation defines kidney damage as a glomerular filtration rate (GFR) <60 ml/min/1.73 m² for 3 months or more, irrespective of cause. *Chronic kidney disease* is the preferred terminology and refers to declining glomerular filtration rate (GFR). The terms *renal insufficiency* and *chronic renal failure* are still often used to describe declining renal function, but they do not have the specificity of the five stages recommended by the National Kidney Foundation (Table 29-13). CKD decreases GFR and tubular functions with changes manifested throughout all organ systems (Table 29-14 and Figure 29-9).[61]

PATHOPHYSIOLOGY The kidneys have a remarkable ability to adapt to loss of nephron mass.[62] Symptomatic changes resulting from increased levels of creatinine, urea, and potassium and from alterations

TABLE 29-12	DIFFERENTIATION OF ACUTE OLIGURIC KIDNEY FAILURE					
	URINE VOLUME	URINE SPECIFIC GRAVITY	URINE OSMOLALITY	URINE SODIUM CONCENTRATION	BUN/PLASMA CREATININE RATIO	FE$_{NA}$*
Prerenal failure	<400 ml	1.016-1.020	>500 mOsm	<10 mEq/L	>15:1	<1% (also seen in acute glomerulonephritis)
Intrarenal failure (i.e., acute tubular necrosis)	<400 ml	1.010-1.012	<400 mOsm	>30 mEq/L	<15:1	>1% (also seen in acute urinary tract obstruction and renal parenchymal disease)

$$*FE_{Na} = \frac{Urine\ Na\,/\,plasma\ Na}{Urine\ creatinine\,/\,plasma\ creatinine} = \times 100$$

TABLE 29-13	STAGES OF CHRONIC KIDNEY DISEASE	
STAGE	DESCRIPTION	SIGNS/SYMPTOMS
I	Normal kidney function Normal or high GFR (>90 ml/min)	*Usually none* Hypertension common
II	Mild kidney damage, mild reduction in GFR (60-89 ml/min)	*Subtle* Hypertension Increasing creatinine and urea levels
III	Moderate kidney damage GFR 30-59 ml/min	*Mild* As above
IV	Severe kidney damage GFR 15-29 ml/min	*Moderate* As above Erythropoietin deficiency anemia Hyperphosphatemia Increased triglycerides Metabolic acidosis Hyperkalemia Salt/water retention
V	End-stage kidney disease Established kidney failure GFR <15 ml/min	*Severe* As above

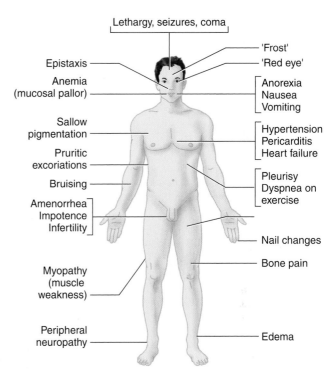

FIGURE 29-9 Common Signs and Symptoms of Kidney Failure (see text for reference site). (From Goldman L, Ausiello D: *Cecil medicine*, ed 23, Philadelphia, 2008, Saunders.)

in salt and water balance usually do not become apparent until renal function declines to less than 25% of normal when adaptive renal reserves have been exhausted.

Different theories have been proposed to account for the adaptation to loss of renal function. The *intact nephron hypothesis* proposes that loss of nephron mass with progressive kidney damage causes the surviving nephrons to sustain normal kidney function. These nephrons are capable of a compensatory hypertrophy and expansion or hyperfunction in their rates of filtration, reabsorption, and secretion and can maintain a constant rate of excretion in the presence of overall declining GFR. The intact nephron hypothesis explains adaptive changes in solute and water regulation that occur with advancing renal failure. Although the urine of an individual with chronic renal failure may contain abnormal amounts of protein and red and white blood cells or casts, the major end products of excretion are similar to those of normally functioning kidneys until the advanced stages of renal failure, when there is a significant reduction of functioning nephrons.[63,64]

However, the continued loss of functioning nephrons and the adaptive hyperfiltration (increased glomerular pressure) can result in further glomerulosclerosis, contributing to uremia and end-stage renal failure.[64] This is known as the *trade off hypothesis*. Factors involved in the progression of chronic kidney disease are outlined in Table 29-15.

Progression of chronic kidney disease is thought to be associated with common pathogenic processes regardless of the initial disease (Figure 29-10).[65] These processes include the following[66]:

- Glomerular hypertension, hyperfiltration, and hypertrophy
- Glomerulosclerosis
- Tubulointerstitial inflammation and fibrosis

The factors that contribute to the pathogenesis of chronic kidney disease are complex and involve the interaction of many cells, cytokines, and structural alterations. Two factors that have consistently been recognized to advance renal disease are the presence of proteinuria and increased angiotensin II activity.[67-69] Glomerular hyperfiltration and increased glomerular capillary permeability lead to proteinuria. Proteinuria contributes to tubulointerstitial injury by accumulating in the interstitial space and activating complement proteins and other mediators and cells, such as macrophages, that promote inflammation and progressive fibrosis. Angiotensin II activity is elevated with progressive nephron injury. Angiotensin II promotes glomerular hypertension and hyperfiltration caused by efferent arteriolar vasoconstriction and also promotes systemic hypertension. The chronically high intraglomerular pressure increases glomerular capillary permeability, contributing to proteinuria. Angiotensin II also may promote the activity of inflammatory cells and growth factors that participate in tubulointerstitial fibrosis and scarring.

CLINICAL MANIFESTATIONS The clinical manifestations of chronic kidney disease are often described using the terms *azotemia* and *uremia*. Azotemia is increased levels of serum urea and other nitrogenous compounds related to decreasing kidney function. Uremia, or uremic syndrome, is the systemic symptoms associated with the accumulation of nitrogenous wastes and accumulation of toxins in

TABLE 29-14 SYSTEMIC EFFECTS OF CHRONIC KIDNEY FAILURE

SYSTEM	MANIFESTATIONS	MECHANISMS	TREATMENT
Skeletal	Spontaneous fractures and bone pain Deformities of long bones	Osteitis fibrosa: bone inflammation with fibrous degeneration related to hyperparathyroidism Osteomalacia: bone resorption associated with vitamin D and calcium deficiency	Control of hyperphosphatemia to reduce hyperparathyroidism; administration of calcium and aluminum hydroxide antacids, which bind phosphate in the gut, together with a phosphate-restricted diet; vitamin D replacement; avoidance of magnesium antacids because of impaired magnesium excretion
Cardiopulmonary	Pulmonary edema, Kussmaul respirations	Fluid overload associated with pulmonary edema and metabolic acidosis leading to Kussmaul respirations	ACE inhibitors; combination of propranolol, hydralazine, and minoxidil for those with high levels of renin; bilateral nephrectomy with dialysis or transplantation
Cardiovascular	Left ventricular hypertrophy, cardiomyopathy, and ischemic heart disease; hypertension, dysrhythmias, accelerated atherosclerosis; pericarditis with fever, chest pain, and pericardial friction rub	Extracellular volume expansion and hypersecretion of renin associated with hypertension; anemia increases cardiac workload; hyperlipidemia promotes atherosclerosis; toxins precipitate into pericardium	Volume reduction with diuretics that are not potassium sparing (to avoid hyperkalemia); dialysis
Neurologic	Encephalopathy (fatigue, reduced attention span, difficulty with problem solving); peripheral neuropathy (pain and burning in legs and feet, loss of vibration sense and deep tendon reflexes); loss of motor coordination, twitching, fasciculations, stupor, and coma with advanced uremia	Progressive accumulation of uremic toxins associated with end-stage renal disease Stroke or intracerebral hemorrhage associated with chronic dialysis	Dialysis or successful kidney transplantation
Hematologic	Anemia, usually normochromic-normocytic; platelet disorders with prolonged bleeding times	Reduced erythropoietin secretion and reduced red cell production; uremic toxins shorten red blood cell survival and alter platelet function	Dialysis; recombinant human erythropoietin and iron supplementation; conjugated estrogens; DDAVP (1-desamino-8-D-arginine vasopressin); transfusion
Gastrointestinal	Anorexia, nausea, vomiting; mouth ulcers, stomatitis, urinous breath (uremic factor), hiccups, peptic ulcers, gastrointestinal bleeding, and pancreatitis associated with end-stage renal failure	Retention of metabolic acids and other metabolic waste products	Protein-restricted diet for relief of nausea and vomiting
Integumentary	Abnormal pigmentation and pruritus	Retention of urochromes, contributing to sallow, yellow color; high plasma calcium levels and neuropathy associated with pruritus	Dialysis with control of serum calcium levels
Immunologic	Increased risk of infection that can cause death; increased risk of carcinoma	Suppression of cell-mediated immunity; reduction in number and function of lymphocytes, diminished phagocytosis	Routine dialysis
Reproductive	Sexual dysfunction: menorrhagia, amenorrhea, infertility, and decreased libido in women; decreased testosterone levels, infertility, and decreased libido in men	Dysfunction of ovaries and testes; presence of neuropathies	No specific treatment

With data from Almeras C, Argilés A: The general picture of uremia, *Semin Dial* 22(4):329–333, 2009; Keane WF: *Kidney Int Suppl* 75:S27–S31, 2000; Thomas R, Kanso A, Sedor JR: Chronic kidney disease and its complications, *Prim Care* 35(2):329–344, 2008.

the plasma caused by the decline in renal function. Sources of toxins include end products of protein metabolism, alterations in electrolytes, metabolic acidosis, and intestinal absorption of toxins produced by gut bacteria. Uremia represents a proinflammatory state with many systemic effects.[70] The many systemic manifestations associated with chronic kidney disease are discussed in the following sections and summarized in Table 29-14 and Figure 29-9 (p. 757).

Creatinine and urea clearance. Creatinine is constantly released from muscle and excreted primarily by glomerular filtration. In chronic kidney disease (CKD), as glomerular filtration rate (GFR) declines, the plasma creatinine level increases by a reciprocal amount to maintain a constant rate of excretion. As GFR continues to decline, plasma creatinine concentration increases. The clearance of *urea* follows a similar pattern, but urea is both filtered and reabsorbed and its level varies with the state of hydration; therefore urea concentration is not a good index of GFR. However, as the GFR decreases, plasma urea concentration also increases.

Fluid and electrolyte balance. Fluid and electrolyte and acid-base balance is significantly disturbed with chronic kidney disease. When the GFR decreases to 25%, there is an obligatory loss of 20 to 40 mEq of *sodium* per day with osmotic loss of water. Dietary intake must be maintained to prevent sodium deficits and volume depletion. As GFR continues to decline, there also is loss of tubular function to dilute and concentrate the urine and urine specific gravity becomes fixed at about 1.010. Ultimately the kidney loses its ability to regulate sodium and water balance. Both sodium and water are retained, contributing to edema and hypertension.

In early kidney failure, tubular secretion of *potassium* is maintained and larger amounts of potassium are lost through the bowel. With the onset of oliguria, total body potassium can increase to life-threatening levels and must be controlled by dialysis.

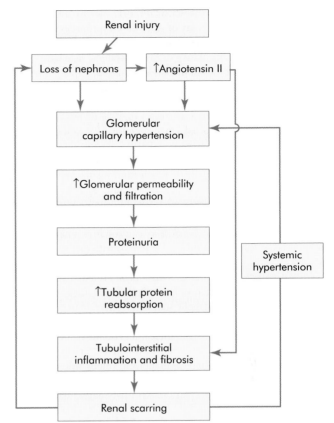

FIGURE 29-10 Mechanisms Related to the Progression of Chronic Kidney Disease.

TABLE 29-15	**FACTORS REPRESENTING PROGRESSION OF CHRONIC KIDNEY FAILURE**
FACTOR	**CHARACTERISTICS**
Proteinuria	Glomerular hyperfiltration of protein contributes to tubular interstitial injury by accumulating in interstitial space and promoting inflammation and progressive fibrosis.
Creatinine and urea clearance	In chronic renal failure, the GFR falls and the plasma creatinine concentration increases by a reciprocal amount; because there is no regulatory adjustment for creatinine, plasma levels continue to rise and serve as an index of changing glomerular function.
	As GFR declines, urea clearance increases. (NOTE: Urea is both filtered and reabsorbed and varies with state of hydration.)
Sodium and water balance	In chronic renal failure, sodium load delivered to nephrons exceeds normal, so excretion must increase; thus less is reabsorbed. Obligatory loss occurs, leading to sodium deficits and volume depletion. As GFR is reduced, ability to concentrate and dilute urine diminishes.
Phosphate and calcium balance	Changes in acid-base balance affect phosphate and calcium balance. Major disorders associated with chronic renal failure are reduced renal phosphate excretion, decreased renal synthesis of 1,25-dihydroxyvitamin D_3, and hypocalcemia.
	Hypocalcemia leads to secondary hyperparathyroidism, GFR falls, and progressive hyperphosphatemia, hypocalcemia, and dissolution of bone result.
Hematocrit	Because of anemia that accompanies chronic renal failure, lethargy, dizziness, and low hematocrit are common.
Potassium balance	In chronic renal failure, tubular secretion of potassium increases until oliguria develops.
	Use of potassium-sparing diuretics also may precipitate elevated serum potassium levels.
	As disease progresses, total body potassium levels can rise to life-threatening levels and dialysis is required.
Acid-base balance	In early renal insufficiency, acid excretion and bicarbonate reabsorption are increased to maintain normal pH. Metabolic acidosis begins when GFR reaches 30% to 40%.
	Metabolic acidosis and hyperkalemia may be severe enough to require dialysis when end-stage renal failure develops.
Dyslipidemia	Chronic hyperlipidemia may induce glomerular and tubulointerstitial injury, contributing to progression of chronic renal disease.

GFR, Glomerular filtration rate.

Metabolic acidosis develops when GFR decreases to less than 20% to 25% of normal. The causes of acidosis are primarily related to decreased hydrogen ion elimination and decreased bicarbonate reabsorption. With end-stage kidney disease, metabolic acidosis may be severe enough to require alkali therapy and dialysis.[71]

Calcium, phosphate, and bone. Bone and skeletal changes develop with alterations in calcium and phosphate metabolism. These changes begin when the GFR decreases to 25% or less. *Hypocalcemia* is accelerated by impaired renal synthesis of 1,25-dihydroxyvitamin D$_3$ (calcitiol) with decreased intestinal absorption of calcium. Renal phosphate excretion also decreases and the increased serum phosphate binds calcium, further contributing to hypocalcemia. Acidosis also contributes to a negative calcium balance. Decreased serum calcium level stimulates parathyroid hormone secretion with mobilization of calcium from bone. The combined effect of *hyperparathyroidism* and *vitamin D deficiency* can result in renal osteodystrophies (i.e., *osteomalacia* and *osteitis fibrosa*) with increased risk for fractures.[72]

Protein, carbohydrate, and fat metabolism. Protein, carbohydrate, and fat metabolism is altered in CKD. Proteinuria, metabolic acidosis, inflammation, and a catabolic state contribute to a negative nitrogen balance. Levels of serum proteins diminish, including albumin, complement, and transferrin, and there is loss of muscle mass. Insulin resistance and glucose intolerance are common and may be related to proinflammatory cytokines, and alterations in adipokines (high leptin and low adiponectin levels) that interfere with insulin action.[73] Hyperparathyroidism also decreases insulin sensitivity and impairs glucose tolerance.[74]

Dyslipidemia is common among individuals with CKD. There is a high ratio of low-density lipoprotein (LDL) to high-density lipoprotein (HDL), a high level of triglycerides, and an accumulation of LDL particles with accelerated atherosclerosis and vascular calcification. Uremia causes a deficiency in lipoprotein lipase and a decreased level of hepatic triglyceride lipase. Decreased lipolytic activity results in a reduction in HDL level. The concentration of apolipoprotein B is also elevated, thereby accelerating atherogenesis.[75]

Cardiovascular system. Cardiovascular disease is a major cause of morbidity and mortality in CKD. Proinflammatory cytokines, oxidative stress, and metabolic derangements are significant contributors.[76] *Hypertension* is the result of excess sodium and fluid volume. Elevated renin concentration also stimulates the secretion of aldosterone, increasing sodium reabsorption. *Dyslipidemia* promotes atheromatous plaque formation. Endothelial cell dysfunction and calcium deposits lead to a loss of vessel elasticity and vascular calcification. The resulting vascular disease increases the risk for *ischemic heart disease, left ventricular hypertrophy, congestive heart failure, stroke,* and *peripheral vascular disease* in individuals with uremia. Declining erythropoietin production causes anemia, thereby increasing demands for cardiac output and adding to the cardiac workload. *Pericarditis* can develop from inflammation caused by the presence of uremic toxins. Accumulation of fluid in the pericardial space can compromise ventricular filling and cardiac output.

Pulmonary system. Pulmonary complications are associated with fluid overload, congestive heart failure, and dyspnea. Pulmonary edema develops and metabolic acidosis can cause Kussmaul respirations.

Hematologic system. Hematologic alterations include *normochromic-normocytic anemia, impaired platelet function,* and *hypercoagulability.* Inadequate production of erythropoietin decreases red blood cell production and uremia decreases red blood cell life span. Lethargy, dizziness, and low hematocrit values are common findings.

Defective platelet aggregation and altered vascular endothelium promote an increased bleeding tendency, increased risk for bruising, epistaxis, gastrointestinal bleeding, or cerebrovascular hemorrhage. Alterations in thrombin and other clotting factors contribute to hypercoagulability; thus control of coagulation is essential during dialysis.

Immune system. Immune system dysregulation with immune suppression, deficient response to vaccination, and increased risk for infection develops with chronic renal failure (CRF). Chemotaxis, phagocytosis, antibody production, and cell-mediated immune responses are suppressed. Malnutrition, metabolic acidosis, and hyperglycemia may amplify immunosuppression.

Neurologic system. Neurologic symptoms are common and progressive with CKD. Symptoms may include headache, pain, drowsiness, sleep disorders, impaired concentration, memory loss, and impaired judgment. Neuromuscular irritation can cause hiccups, muscle cramps, and muscle twitching. In advanced stages of renal failure, symptoms may progress to seizures and coma. Peripheral neuropathies can also develop with impaired sensations particularly in the lower limbs.[77]

Gastrointestinal system. Gastrointestinal complications are common in individuals with CKD. Uremic gastroenteritis can cause bleeding ulcer and significant blood loss. Nonspecific symptoms include anorexia, nausea, vomiting, constipation, or diarrhea. Uremic fetor is a form of bad breath caused by the breakdown of urea by salivary enzymes. Malnutrition is common.

Endocrine and reproductive systems. Endocrine and reproductive alterations develop with progression of CKD. Both males and females have a decrease in levels of circulating sex steroids. Males often experience a reduction in testosterone levels and may be impotent. Oligospermia and germinal cell dysplasia can result in infertility. Females have reduced estrogen levels, amenorrhea, and difficulty maintaining a pregnancy to term. A decrease in libido occurs in both genders.

Insulin resistance is common in uremia, and as CKD progresses the ability of the kidney to degrade insulin is reduced and the half-life of insulin is prolonged. Individuals with diabetes mellitus and CRF need to carefully manage their insulin dosages. Low-protein diets and renal replacement therapy improve insulin sensitivity.[78]

CRF also causes alterations in thyroid hormone metabolism, known as nonthyroidal illness syndrome.[79] A low-protein, low-phosphorus diet may improve thyroid hormone function.[80]

Integumentary system. Skin changes are associated with other complications that develop with CKD. Anemia can cause pallor and bleeding into the skin and results in hematomas and ecchymosis. Retained urochromes manifest as a sallow skin color. Hyperparathyroidism and uremic skin residues (known as uremic frost) are associated with inflammation, irritation, and pruritus with scratching, excoriation, and increased risk for infection.[81]

EVALUATION AND TREATMENT Early screening and evaluation of CKD is based on the risk factors, history, presenting signs and symptoms, and diagnostic testing. Elevated serum creatinine and serum urea nitrogen concentrations are consistent with chronic renal failure. Markers of kidney damage include urine protein, particularly albumin, and examination of urine sediment. Ultrasound, CT scan, or plain x-ray films will show small kidney size. Renal biopsy confirms the diagnosis.

Management involves dietary control, including phosphate restriction, supplementation with vitamin D or vitamin D receptor activators, sodium and fluid maintenance, potassium restriction, adequate caloric intake, management of dyslipidemias, and use of erythropoietin as needed. Angiotensin-converting enzyme (ACE) inhibitors or angiotensin receptor blockers are often used to control systemic hypertension, reduce proteinuria, and provide renoprotection.[82] End-stage renal failure related to diabetic nephropathy can be significantly reduced with control of hyperglycemia by insulin therapy.[83] End-stage renal failure is treated with dialysis, supportive therapy, and renal transplantation.[84,85]

✔ **QUICK CHECK 29-4**
1. What mechanisms cause prerenal acute renal failure?
2. How does intrarenal acute renal failure differ from postrenal failure?
3. Briefly describe the causes of anemia, cardiovascular disease, and bone and neurologic changes associated with chronic renal failure.

DID YOU UNDERSTAND?

Urinary Tract Obstruction

1. Obstruction can occur anywhere in the urinary tract, and it may be anatomic or functional, including renal stones, an enlarged prostate gland, or urethral strictures. The most serious complications are hydronephrosis, hydroureter, ureterohydronephrosis, and infection caused by the accumulation of urine behind the obstruction.
2. Hypertrophy of the opposite kidney compensates for loss of function of the kidney with obstructive disease.
3. Relief of obstruction is usually followed by postobstructive diuresis and may cause fluid and electrolyte imbalance.
4. Persistent obstruction of the bladder outlet leads to residual urine volumes, low bladder wall compliance, and risk for vesicoureteral reflux and infection.
5. Kidney stones are caused by supersaturation of the urine with precipitation of stone-forming substances, changes in urine pH, or urinary tract infection.
6. The most common kidney stone is formed from calcium oxalate and most often causes obstruction by lodging in the ureter.
7. Obstructions of the bladder are a consequence of neurogenic or anatomic alteration of the bladder, or both.
8. A neurogenic bladder is caused by a neural lesion that interrupts innervation of the bladder.
9. Upper motor neuron lesions result in overactive or hyperreflexive bladder function and dyssynergia (lack of coordinated neuromuscular contraction).
10. Lower motor neuron lesions result in underactive, hypotonic, or atonic bladder function.
11. Overactive bladder (OAB) syndrome is an uncontrollable or premature contraction of the bladder that results in urgency with or without incontinence, frequency, and nocturia.
12. Underactive bladder (UAB) is a condition in which the duration or strength of contraction is inadequate to empty the bladder, resulting in distention and overflow incontinence.
13. Detrusor sphincter dyssynergia is failure of the urethrovesical junction smooth muscle to release urine during micturition and causes a functional obstruction.
14. Other causes of lower urinary tract obstruction include prostatic enlargement, urethral stricture, and pelvic organ prolapse in women.
15. Partial obstruction of the bladder can result in overactive bladder contractions with urgency. There is deposition of collagen in the bladder wall over time, resulting in decreased bladder wall compliance and ineffective detrusor muscle contraction.
16. Renal cell carcinoma is the most common renal neoplasm. The larger neoplasms tend to metastasize to the lung, liver, and bone.
17. Bladder tumors are commonly composed of transitional cells with a papillary appearance and a high rate of recurrence.

Urinary Tract Infection

1. Urinary tract infections (UTIs) are commonly caused by the retrograde movement of bacteria into the urethra and bladder. UTIs are uncomplicated when the urinary system is normal or complicated when there is an abnormality.
2. Cystitis is an inflammation of the bladder commonly caused by bacteria and may be acute or chronic.
3. Painful bladder syndrome/interstitial cystitis includes nonbacterial infectious cystitis (viral, mycobacterial, chlamydial, fungal), noninfectious cystitis (i.e., radiation injury), and interstitial cystitis, which is related to autoimmune injury.
4. Pyelonephritis is an acute or chronic inflammation of the renal pelvis often related to obstructive uropathies and may cause abscess formation and scarring with an alteration in renal function.

Glomerular Disorders

1. Glomerular disorders are a group of related diseases of the glomerulus that can be caused by immune responses, toxins or drugs, vascular disorders, and other systemic diseases.
2. Acute glomerulonephritis commonly results from inflammatory damage to the glomerulus as a consequence of immune reactions after a streptococcal infection.
3. The urine sediment may contain large amounts of protein (nephrotic sediment) or have red and white blood cells and protein (nephritic sediment).
4. Rapidly progressive glomerulonephritis (RPGN) is associated with injury that results in the proliferation of glomerular capillary endothelial cells and a rapid loss of renal function.
5. Chronic glomerulonephritis is related to a variety of diseases that cause deterioration of the glomerulus and a progressive loss of renal function.
6. Immune mechanisms in glomerulonephritis are the deposition of antigen-antibody complexes often with complement components and the formation of antibodies specific for the glomerular basement membrane.
7. Nephrotic syndrome is the excretion of at least 3.5 g of protein (primarily albumin) in the urine per day because of glomerular injury with increased capillary permeability and loss of membrane negative charge. Its principal signs are hypoproteinuria, hyperlipidemia, and edema. The liver cannot produce enough protein to adequately compensate for urinary loss.

Acute Kidney Injury

1. Acute kidney failure is classified as prerenal, intrarenal, or postrenal and is usually accompanied by oliguria with elevated plasma BUN and plasma creatinine levels.
2. Prerenal acute kidney failure is caused by decreased renal perfusion with a decreased GFR, ischemia, and tubular necrosis.
3. Intrarenal acute kidney failure is associated with several systemic diseases but is commonly related to acute tubular necrosis (ATN).
4. Postrenal kidney failure is associated with diseases that obstruct the flow of urine from the kidneys.

Chronic Kidney Disease

1. Chronic kidney failure represents a progressive loss of renal function. Plasma creatinine levels gradually become elevated as GFR declines; sodium is lost in the urine; potassium is retained; acidosis develops; calcium metabolism and phosphate metabolism are altered; and erythropoietin production is diminished. All organs systems are affected by CRF.

KEY TERMS

- Acute cystitis 747
- Acute kidney injury (AKI) 754
- Acute tubular necrosis (ATN) 755
- Angiotensin II 758
- Anti–glomerular basement membrane disease (Goodpasture syndrome) 752
- Azotemia 758
- Calcium stone 743
- Calculus (pl., calculi) (urinary stone) 742
- Chronic glomerulonephritis 752
- Chronic kidney disease (CKD) 756
- Chronic pyelonephritis 749
- Compensatory hypertrophy 742
- Cystinuric (xanthine) stone 743
- Detrusor areflexia 744
- Detrusor hyperreflexia with vesicosphincter dyssynergia 744
- Diabetic nephropathy 752
- Dyssynergia 744
- End-stage renal failure (ESRF) 754
- Glomerulonephritis 750
- Hydronephrosis 741
- Hydroureter 741
- Hyperfunction 742
- IgA nephropathy (Berger disease) 752
- Intrarenal (intrinsic) acute kidney injury 755
- Low bladder wall compliance 745
- Lupus nephritis 752
- Membranous nephropathy (membranous glomerulonephritis) 752
- Nephritic sediment 751
- Nephritic syndrome 754
- Nephrotic sediment 751
- Nephrotic syndrome 753
- Neurogenic bladder 743
- Nonbacterial infectious cystitis 748
- Noninfectious cystitis 748
- Obstructive uropathy 741
- Oliguria 755
- Overactive bladder syndrome (OAB) 744
- Painful bladder syndrome/interstitial cystitis (PBS/IC) 748
- Partial obstruction of the bladder outlet or urethra 745
- Pelvic organ prolapse 745
- Postobstructive diuresis 742
- Postrenal acute kidney injury 755
- Prerenal acute kidney injury 754
- Prostate enlargement 745
- Proteinuria 758
- Pyelonephritis 749
- Rapidly progressive glomerulonephritis (RPGN) 752
- Renal adenoma 746
- Renal cell carcinoma (RCC) 746
- Renal colic 743
- Renal failure 754
- Renal insufficiency 754
- Renal transitional cell carcinoma (RTCC) 746
- Staghorn calculus 743
- Struvite stone 743
- Uremia (uremic syndrome) 758
- Ureterohydronephrosis 741
- Urethral stricture 745
- Uric acid stone 743
- Urinary tract infection (UTI) 747

REFERENCES

1. Siddiqui MM, McDougal WS: Urologic assessment of decreasing renal function, *Med Clin North Am* 95(1):161–168, 2011.
2. Tseng TY, Stoller ML: Obstructive uropathy, *Clin Geriatr Med* 25(3):437–443, 2009.
3. Gillenwater JY: Hydronephrosis. In Gillenwater JY, et al: *Adult and pediatric urology*, ed 4, Philadelphia, 2002, Lippincott Williams & Wilkins.
4. Maarten TW, Brenner BM: Adaptation to nephron loss. In Brenner BM, editor: *Brenner and Rector's the kidney*, ed 8, Philadelphia, 2008, Saunders.
5. Frokiaer J, Zeidel ML: Urinary tract obstruction. In Brenner BM, editor: *Brenner and Rector's the kidney*, ed 8, Philadelphia, 2008, Saunders.
6. Porena M, Guggi P, Micheli C: Prevention of stone disease, *Urol Int* 79(suppl 1):37–46, 2007.
7. Chandhoke PS: Evaluation of the recurrent stone former, *Urol Clin North Am* 34(3):315–322, 2007.
8. Schade GR, Faerber GJ: Urinary tract stones, *Prim Care* 37(3):565–581, 2010.
9. Lingeman JE, Lifshitz DA, Evan AP: Surgical management of urinary lithiasis. In Walsh PC, et al: *Campbell's urology*, ed 8, Philadelphia, 2002, Saunders.
10. Teichman JMH: Acute renal colic from ureteral calculus, *N Engl J Med* 350:684–693, 2004.
11. Tseng TY, Stoller ML: Medical and medical/urologic approaches in acute and chronic urologic stone disease, *Med Clin North Am* 95(1):169–177, 2011.
12. Taylor EN, Curhan GC: Diet and fluid prescription in stone disease, *Kidney Int* 70(5):835–839, 2006.
13. Karsenty G, et al: Understanding detrusor sphincter dyssynergia—significance of chronology, *Urology* 66(4):763–768, 2005.
14. Ashok K, Wang A: Detrusor overactivity: an overview, *Arch Gynecol Obstet* 282(1):33–41, 2010.
15. Abrams P, et al: The standardisation of terminology of lower urinary tract function: report from the Standardisation Sub-committee of the International Continence Society, *Am J Obstet Gynecol* 187(1):116–126, 2002.
16. Smith AL, Wein AJ: Recent advances in the development of antimuscarinic agents for overactive bladder, *Trends Pharmacol Sci* 231(10):470–475, 2010.
17. Kraus SR, et al: Vulnerable elderly patients and overactive bladder syndrome, *Drugs Aging* 27(9):697–713, 2010.
18. Mundy AR, Andrich DE: Urethral strictures, *BJU Int* 107(1):6–26, 2011.
19. American Cancer Society: *Cancer facts & figures—2010*, Atlanta, 2010, Author.
20. Kane CJ, et al: Renal cell cancer stage migration: analysis of the national cancer data base, *Cancer* 113(1):78–83, 2008.
21. Tigrani VS, et al: Potential role of nephrectomy in the treatment of metastatic renal cell carcinoma: a retrospective analysis, *Urology* 55(1):36–40, 2000.
22. Truong LD, Shen SS: Immunohistochemical diagnosis of renal neoplasms, *Arch Pathol Lab Med* 135(1):92–109, 2011.
23. Hutson TE: Targeted therapies for the treatment of metastatic renal cell-carcinoma: clinical evidence, *Oncologist* 2(suppl 16):14–22, 2011.
24. Pelucchi C, et al: Mechanisms of disease: the epidemiology of bladder cancer, *Nat Clin Pract Urol* 3(6):327–340, 2006.
25. Volanis D, et al: Environmental factors and genetic susceptibility promote urinary bladder cancer, *Toxicol Lett* 193(2):131–137, 2010.
26. Proctor I, Stoeber K, Williams GH: Biomarkers in bladder cancer, *Histopathology* 57(1):1–13, 2010.
27. Dielubanza EJ, Schaeffer AJ: Urinary tract infections in women, *Med Clin North Am* 95(1):27–41, 2011.
28. World Health Organization (WHO): *Schistosomiasis*. Accessed Jan 19, 2011. Available at www.who.int/schistosomiasis/en/.
29. Dhakal BK, Kulesus RR, Mulvey MA: Mechanisms and consequences of bladder cell invasion by uropathogenic *Escherichia coli*, *Eur J Clin Invest* 38(suppl 2):2–11, 2008.
30. Zaffanello M, et al: Genetic risk for recurrent urinary tract infections in humans: a systematic review, *J Biomed Biotechnol*: 321082, 2010.
31. Litza JA, Brill JR: Urinary tract infections, *Prim Care* 37(3):491–507, 2010:viii.
32. Foster RT Sr: Uncomplicated urinary tract infections in women, *Obstet Gynecol Clin North Am* 35(2):235–248, 2008:viii.

33. Graham E, Chai TC: Dysfunction of bladder urothelium and bladder urothelial cells in interstitial cystitis, *Curr Urol Rep* 7(6):440–446, 2006.

34. Dasgupta J, Tincello DG: Interstitial cystitis/bladder pain syndrome: an update, *Maturitas* 64(4):212–217, 2009.

35. Funfstuck R, Ott U, Naber KG: The interaction of urinary tract infection and renal insufficiency, *Int J Antimicrob Agents* 28(suppl 1):S72–S77, 2006.

36. Norris DL, Young JD: Urinary tract infections: diagnosis and management in the emergency department, *Emerg Med Clin North Am* 23(2):413–430, 2008:ix.

37. Berger SP, Daha MR: Complement in glomerular injury, *Semin Immunopathol* 29(4):375–384, 2007.

38. Lizakowski S, et al: Plasma tissue factor and tissue factor pathway inhibitor in patients with primarily glomerulonephritis, *Scand J Urol Nephrol* 41(3):237–242, 2007.

39. Chadban SJ, Atkins RC: Glomerulonephritis, *Lancet* 365(9473):1797–1806, 2005.

40. Dronavalli S, Duka I, Bakris GL: The pathogenesis of diabetic nephropathy, *Nat Clin Pract Endocrinol Metab* 4(8):444–452, 2008.

41. Tucci M, et al: Cytokine overproduction, T-cell activation, and defective T-regulatory functions promote nephritis in systemic lupus erythematosus, *J Biomed Biotechnol*: 457146, 2010.

42. Glassock RJ: The pathogenesis of IgA nephropathy, *Curr Opin Nephrol Hypertens* 20(2):153–160, 2011.

43. Cybulsky AV: Membranous nephropathy, *Contrib Nephrol* 169:107–125, 2011.

44. Hotta O, et al: 2006 Improvements in treatment strategies for patients with antineutrophil cytoplasmic antibody-associated rapidly progressive glomerulonephritis, *Ther Apher Dial* 10(5):390–395, 2006.

45. Wolf G, Ziyadeh FN: Cellular and molecular mechanisms of proteinuria in diabetic nephropathy, *Nephron Physiol* 106(2):26–31, 2007.

46. Johnson DW: Evidence-based guide to slowing the progression of early renal insufficiency, *Intern Med J* 34(1–2):50–57, 2004.

47. Kodner C: Nephrotic syndrome in adults: diagnosis and management, *Am Fam Physician* 80(10):1129–1134, 2009.

48. de Seigneux S, Martin PY: Management of patients with nephrotic syndrome, *Swiss Med Wkly* 139(29–30):416–422, 2009.

49. Iglesias P, Díez JJ: Thyroid dysfunction and kidney disease, *Eur J Endocrinol* 160(4):503–515, 2009.

50. Schwartz JC, et al: The nephrotic syndrome: an unusual case of multiple embolic events, *Vasc Endovasc Surg* 43(2):207–210, 2009.

51. Chen SY, et al: Treatment course of steroid-dependent nephrotic syndrome: emphasized on treatment effect, *Nephrology* (Carlton) 15(3):336–339, 2010.

52. Gipson DS, et al: Management of childhood onset nephrotic syndrome, *Pediatrics* 124(2):747–757, 2009.

53. Khanna R: Clinical presentation & management of glomerular diseases: hematuria, nephritic & nephrotic syndrome, *Mo Med* 108(1):33–36, 2011.

54. Bellomo R, et al: Acute renal failure—definition, outcome measures, animal models, fluid therapy and information technology needs: the Second International Consensus Conference of the Acute Dialysis Quality Initiative (ADQI) Group, *Crit Care* 8(4):R204–R212, 2004.

55. Andreoli SP: Acute kidney injury in children, *Pediatr Nephrol* 24(2):253–263, 2009.

56. Munshi R, Hsu C, Himmelfarb J: Advances in understanding ischemic acute kidney injury, *BMC Med* 9:11, 2011.

57. Rimmelé T, Kellum JA: Oliguria and fluid overload, *Contrib Nephrol* 164:39–45, 2010.

58. Ronco C, et al: Oliguria, creatinine and other biomarkers of acute kidney injury, *ContribNephrol* 164:118–127, 2010.

59. Siew ED, Ware LB, Ikizler TA: Biological markers of acute kidney injury, *J Am Soc Nephrol* 22(5):810–820, 2011.

60. Kellum JA, Hoste EA: Acute kidney injury: epidemiology and assessment, *Scand J Clin Lab Invest* 241(suppl):6–11, 2008.

61. Thomas R, Kanso A, Sedor JR: Chronic kidney disease and its complications, *Prim Care* 35(2):329–344, 2008:vii.

62. Mene P, Polci R, Festuccia F: Mechanisms of repair after kidney injury, *J Nephrol* 16(2):186–195, 2003.

63. Bricker NS, Morrin PA, Kime SW Jr: The pathologic physiology of chronic Bright's disease: an exposition of the "intact nephron hypothesis," *J Am Soc Nephrol* 8(9):1470–1476, 1997.

64. Tall MW, Luychx VA, Brenner BM: Adaptation to nephron loss. In Brenner BM, editor: *Brenner and Rector's the kidney*, ed 8, Philadelphia, 2007, Saunders.

65. Schieppati A, Pisoni R, Remuzzi G: Pathophysiology and management of chronic kidney disease. In Greenberg A, editor: *Primer on kidney diseases*, ed 4, St Louis, 2005, Elsevier Saunders, pp 445–447.

66. Hewitson TD: Renal tubulointerstitial fibrosis: common but never simple, *Am J Physiol Renal Physiol* 296(6):F1239–F1244, 2009.

67. James MT, Hemmelgarn BR, Tonelli M: Early recognition and prevention of chronic kidney disease, *Lancet* 375(9722):1296–1309, 2010.

68. Kalaitzidis RG, Bakris GL: The current state of RAAS blockade in the treatment of hypertension and proteinuria, *Curr Cardiol Rep* 11(6):436–442, 2009.

69. Macconi D: Targeting the renin angiotensin system remission/regression of chronic kidney disease, *Histol Histopathol* 25(5):655–668, 2010.

70. Guarnieri G, et al: Chronic systemic inflammation in uremia: potential therapeutic approaches, *Semin Nephrol* 24(5):441–445, 2004.

71. Kraut JA, Madias NE: Consequences and therapy of the metabolic acidosis of chronic kidney disease, *Pediatr Nephrol* 26(1):19–28, 2011.

72. Sprague SM: Renal bone disease, *Curr Opin Endocrinol Diabetes Obes* 17(6):535–539, 2010.

73. Siew ED, Ikizler TA: Insulin resistance and protein energy metabolism inpatients with advanced chronic kidney disease, *Semin Dial* 23(4):378–382, 2010.

74. Procopio M, Borretta G: 2003 Derangement of glucose metabolism in hyperparathyroidism, *J Endocrinol Invest* 26(11):1136–1142, 2003.

75. Vaziri ND: Causes of dysregulation of lipid metabolism in chronic renal failure, *Semin Dial* 22(6):644–651, 2009.

76. Zyga S, Christopoulou G, Malliarou M: Malnutrition-inflammation-atherosclerosis syndrome in patients with end-stage renal disease, *J Ren Care* 37(1):12–15, 2011.

77. Krishnan AV, Kiernan MC: Neurological complications of chronic kidney disease, *Nat Rev Neurol* 5(10):542–551, 2009.

78. Rigalleau V, Gin H: Carbohydrate metabolism in uraemia, *Curr Opin Clin Nutr Metab Care* 8(4):463–469, 2005.

79. Iglesias P, Díez JJ: Thyroid dysfunction and kidney disease, *Eur J Endocrinol* 160(4):503–515, 2009.

80. Rosolowska-Huszcz D, Kozlowska L, Rydzewski A: Influence of low protein diet on nonthyroidal illness syndrome in chronic renal failure, *Endocrine* 27(3):283–288, 2005.

81. Kuypers DR: Skin problems in chronic kidney disease, *Nat Clin Pract Nephrol* 5(3):157–170, 2009.

82. Hou FF, Zhou QG: Optimal dose of angiotensin-converting enzyme inhibitor or angiotensin II receptor blocker for renoprotection, *Nephrology* (Carlton) 15(suppl 2):57–60, 2010.

83. Shrishrimal K, Hart P, Michota F: Managing diabetes in hemodialysis patients: observations and recommendations, *Cleve Clin J Med* 76(11):649–655, 2009.

84. Murphree DD, Thelen SM: Chronic kidney disease in primary care, *J Am Board Fam Med* 23(4):542–550, 2010.

85. Power A, Duncan N, Goodlad C: Advances and innovations in dialysis in the 21st century, *Postgrad Med J* 85(1000):102–107, 2009.

Alterations of Renal and Urinary Tract Function in Children

Patricia Ring and Sue E. Huether

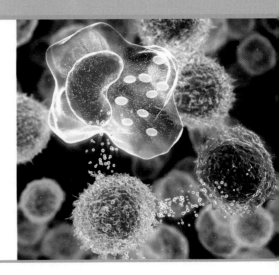

evolve WEBSITE

CHAPTER OUTLINE

The incidence and type of renal and urinary tract disorders experienced by children vary with age and maturation. Newborn disorders may involve congenital malformations. During childhood, the kidney and genitourinary structures continue to develop, so renal dysfunction may be associated with mechanisms and manifestations that differ from those found in adults.

STRUCTURAL ABNORMALITIES

Congenital abnormalities of the kidney and urinary tract occur in about 1 out of 500 newborns.[1] These abnormalities range from minor, nonpathologic, or easily correctable anomalies to those that are incompatible with life. For example, the kidneys may fail to ascend from the pelvis to the abdomen, causing ectopic kidneys—which usually function normally. The kidneys also may fuse as they ascend, causing a single, U-shaped horseshoe kidney. Approximately one third of individuals with horseshoe kidneys are asymptomatic, and the most

common problems are hydronephrosis, infection, stone formation, and, rarely, renal malignancies.[2,3] Collectively, structural anomalies of the renal system account for approximately 45% of cases of renal failure in children, and many are linked to gene defects.[4,5]

Certain structural anomalies are commonly associated with urinary tract malformations,[6] including:
    Low-set, malformed ears
    Chromosomal disorders, especially trisomy 13 (Patau syndrome) and trisomy 18
    Absent abdominal muscles (prune-belly syndrome)
    Anomalies of the spinal cord and lower extremities
    Imperforate anus or genital deviation
    Nephroblastoma (Wilms tumor)
    Congenital ascites
    Cystic disease of the liver
    Positive family history of renal disease (hereditary nephritis or cystic disease)

Hypospadias

Hypospadias is a congenital condition in which the urethral meatus is located on the ventral side or undersurface of the penis. The meatus can be located anywhere on the glans, on the penile shaft, at the base of the penis, at the penoscrotal junction, or in the perineum (Figure 30-1). This is the most common anomaly of the penis; it occurs in about 1 in 300[7] infant boys, and the incidence appears to be increasing.[8] The cause of this condition is multifactorial and includes genetic, endocrine, and environmental factors. Advanced maternal age and low birthweight also have been implicated.[7] **Chordee** or penile torsion may accompany cases of hypospadias. In chordee, skin tethering and shortening of subcutaneous tissue cause the penis to bend or "bow ventrally" (Figure 30-2). Penile torsion is rotation of the penile shaft to either the right or the left. Partial absence of the foreskin and cryptorchidism (undescended testes; see Chapter 32) are associated with the anomaly.[9]

The goals for corrective surgery on the child with hypospadias are (1) a straight penis when erect to facilitate intercourse as an adult, (2) a uniform urethra of adequate caliber to prevent spraying during urination, (3) a cosmetic appearance satisfactory to the individual, and (4) repair completed in as few procedures as possible. Surgery is most effective, psychologically as well as physically, when performed between 6 and 12 months of age.[10]

Epispadias and Exstrophy of the Bladder

Epispadias and exstrophy of the bladder are the same congenital defect expressed to differing degrees. In male epispadias, the urethral opening is on the dorsal surface of the penis. In females, a cleft along the ventral urethra usually extends to the bladder neck. The incidence of epispadias is 1 in 40,000 to 118,000 births. Twice as many boys as girls present with this defect.[11]

In boys, the urethral opening may be small and situated behind the glans (anterior epispadias), or a fissure may extend the entire length of the penis and into the bladder neck (posterior epispadias). Children with anterior epispadias may only have stress incontinence, but those with posterior epispadias will experience constant dribbling of urine.[12] Treatment is surgical reconstruction.

Exstrophy of the bladder is a rare extensive congenital anomaly of herniation of the bladder through the abdominal wall. The bony part of the pelvis remains open (Figure 30-3), and the posterior portion of the bladder mucosa is exposed through the abdominal opening and appears bright red. The incidence of bladder exstrophy in the United States is 2.15 per 100,000 live births and occurs equally in males and females.[13]

Exstrophy of the bladder is caused by intrauterine failure of the abdominal wall and the mesoderm of the anterior bladder to fuse. The rectus muscles below the umbilicus are separated, and the pubic rami (bony projections of the pubic bone) are not joined. This causes a waddling gait when the child first learns to walk, but most children quickly learn to compensate. The clitoris in girls is divided into two parts with the urethra between each half. The penis in boys is epispadiac. Urine seeps onto the abdominal wall from the ureters, causing a constant odor of urine and excoriation of the surrounding skin. Because the exposed bladder mucosa becomes hyperemic and edematous, it bleeds easily and is painful.

The unrepaired exstrophic bladder is prone to cancerous changes as soon as 1 year after birth. Ideally, the bladder and pubic defect should be closed before the infant is 72 hours old. Surgical reconstruction is usually

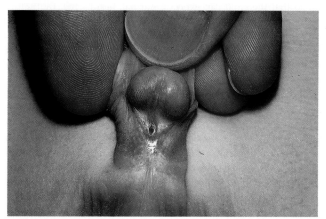

FIGURE 30-1 Hypospadias. (Courtesy H. Gil Rushton, MD, Children's National Medical Center, Washington, DC; from Hockenberry MJ, Wilson D: *Wong's nursing care of infants and children,* ed 8, St Louis, 2007, Mosby.)

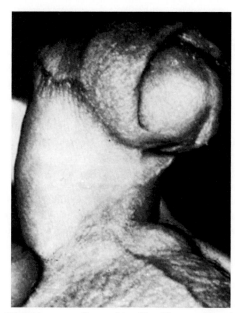

FIGURE 30-2 Hypospadias with Significant Chordee. (From Shirkey HC, editor: *Pediatric therapy,* ed 6, St Louis, 1980, Mosby.)

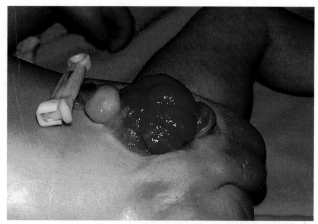

FIGURE 30-3 Exstrophy of Bladder. (Courtesy H. Gil Rushton, MD, Children's National Medical Center, Washington, DC; from Hockenberry MJ, Wilson D: *Wong's nursing care of infants and children,* ed 8, St Louis, 2007, Mosby.)

performed within the first year either as a complete primary repair or as staged procedures. Staged procedures may include bladder augmentation, bladder neck reconstruction, and epispadias repair.[14] Objectives of management include preservation of renal function, attainment of urinary control, prevention of infection, and improvement of sexual function.[15] Diagnosis is often made by prenatal ultrasound.

Cloacal exstrophy is the most rare and severe form of bladder exstrophy. The intestine and spine may be involved, and reconstruction with restored urine and fecal control is difficult.

Bladder Outlet Obstruction

Congenital causes of bladder outlet obstruction are rare and include urethral valves and polyps. A urethral valve is a thin membrane of tissue that occludes the urethral lumen and obstructs urinary outflow in males. Most valves occur in the posterior urethra, although a few arise from the embryologically distinct anterior urethra. Urethral polyps arising from the prostatic urethra are rare.[16] They often cause relatively severe obstruction and may impair renal embryogenesis and lead to renal failure.[17] Urethral valves or polyps are resected as soon as they are diagnosed.[18]

Ureteropelvic Junction Obstruction

Ureteropelvic junction (UPJ) obstruction is a blockage of the tapered point where the renal pelvis transitions into the ureter.[19] UPJ obstruction is the most common cause of hydronephrosis in neonates. An intrinsic malformation of smooth muscle or urothelial development produces obstruction in 90% of cases, and approximately 10% are caused by extrinsic compression.[19] During infancy or childhood, secondary ureteropelvic junction (UPJ) obstruction is caused by kinking or secondary scarring in the presence of high-grade vesicoureteral reflux (see p. 769). There is an increased risk of vesicoureteral reflux in children with UPJ obstruction in the obstructed or contralateral kidney, or both; whether this represents a sequela of the embryonic defect leading to the UPJ defect is not known. Diagnosis can be made by ultrasound. Obstruction of the distal ureter (ureterovesical junction obstruction) causes dilation of the entire ureter, renal pelvis, and caliceal system. An ureterocele is a cystic dilation of the intravesical ureter. Open or endoscopic surgery to relieve an obstruction occurs if there is decline of renal drainage or function.[20]

Hypoplastic/Dysplastic Kidneys

During embryologic development, the ureteric duct grows into the metanephric tissue, triggering the formation of the kidneys. If this growth does not occur, the kidney is absent—a condition called renal aplasia. A hypoplastic kidney is small with a decreased number of nephrons. These conditions may be unilateral or bilateral; the occurrence may be incidental or familial.[21] Bilateral hypoplastic kidneys are a common cause of chronic renal failure in children. Segmental hypoplasia—the Ask-Upmark kidney—may be congenital or secondary to vesicoureteral reflux. Systemic hypertension is a common presentation.[22]

Renal dysplasia usually results from abnormal differentiation of the renal tissues; for example, primitive glomeruli and tubules, cysts, and nonrenal tissue (such as cartilage) are found in the dysplastic kidney. Dysplasia may be secondary to antenatal obstruction of the urinary tract from ureteroceles, posterior urethral valves, or prune-belly syndrome (congenital absence of abdominal muscles).

Polycystic Kidney Disease

Polycystic kidney disease (PKD) is an autosomal dominant disease (*PDK1* or *PDK2* gene) occurring in 1 of 1000 live births,[23] or an autosomal recessive (*PKHD1* gene) inherited disorder. Affected kidneys have multiple cysts that interfere with renal function. Autosomal dominant PKD (ADPKD) usually presents in late childhood or adulthood. Defects in the formation of epithelial cells and their cilia result in cyst formation in all parts of the nephron. Cysts in other organs, including the liver, pancreas, and ovaries, may occur. Hypertension, aortic and intracranial aneurysms, and heart valve defects may develop. Autosomal recessive PKD (ARPKD) is often first suspected on a prenatal ultrasound. Epithelial hyperplasia and fluid secretion result in collecting duct cysts. Hepatic disease and hypertension typically accompany autosomal recessive PKD. No treatment is available.[24]

Renal Agenesis

Renal agenesis (the absence of one or both kidneys) may be unilateral or bilateral, and may occur randomly or be hereditary. It may be an isolated entity or be associated with anomalies in other organs.

Unilateral renal agenesis occurs in approximately 1 of 1000 live births. Males are more often affected, and it is usually the left kidney that is absent. The single remaining kidney is often completely normal so that the child can expect a normal, healthy life. By the time the child is several years old, the volume of this kidney may approach twice the normal size. In some instances, however, the single kidney is abnormally formed and associated with abnormalities of its collecting system. Extrarenal congenital abnormalities of the urogenital, skeletal, cardiac, and other systems may co-exist.[25]

Bilateral renal agenesis is a rare disorder incompatible with extrauterine life. Approximately 75% of affected children are males. Oligohydramnios (low amount of amniotic fluid) leads to underdeveloped lungs and Potter syndrome (wide-set eyes, parrot-beak nose, low-set ears, and receding chin). Approximately 40% of affected infants are stillborn. Infants with this condition rarely live more than 24 hours because of pulmonary insufficiency. Renal agenesis can be detected prenatally by ultrasound.[1]

> **QUICK CHECK 30-1**
> 1. Describe hypospadias.
> 2. Why does bladder exstrophy occur?
> 3. Contrast dysplastic kidney and hypoplastic kidney.

GLOMERULAR DISORDERS

Common glomerular disorders in children are glomerulonephritis, nephrotic syndrome, immunoglobulin A (IgA) nephropathy, and hemolytic uremic syndrome. Most glomerular diseases are acquired and immunologically mediated (see Chapter 29 and Tables 29-6 and 29-7 and Figure 29-6). The disease can be acute or chronic. The likelihood of developing renal failure depends on the specific condition.

Glomerulonephritis

Glomerulonephritis includes a number of renal disorders in which proliferation and inflammation of the glomeruli are secondary to an immune mechanism. Chronic glomerulonephritis accounts for about 53% of the cases of renal failure in children and is the causative factor for most school-age and teenage children that require dialysis and kidney transplantation.

Acute Poststreptococcal Glomerulonephritis

Acute poststreptococcal glomerulonephritis (APGN) is one of the most common immune complex–mediated renal diseases in children. It most commonly occurs after a throat or skin infection with a nephritogenic strain of group A β-hemolytic streptococci, although other bacteria and viruses also may be responsible.[26] Sporadic occurrences have been observed after bacterial endocarditis, which may be associated with streptococcal or staphylococcal microorganisms, or after viral diseases, such as varicella-zoster virus and hepatitides B and C. Glomerulonephritis develops with the deposition of antigen-antibody complexes in the glomerulus. The antigen-antibody complex activates complement and the release of inflammatory mediators that damage endothelial and epithelial cells lying on the glomerular basement membrane. Damage to the glomerular basement membrane leads to hematuria and proteinuria.

Symptoms usually begin 1 to 2 weeks after an upper respiratory tract infection (more common during cold weather) and up to 6 weeks after skin infections such as impetigo (more common during warm weather).

The onset of symptoms is abrupt, varying with disease severity. The child typically has gross or microscopic hematuria, proteinuria, edema, and renal insufficiency. Oliguria may be present. Hypertension occurs because of increased vascular volume. Acute hypertension may cause headache, vomiting, somnolence, and other central nervous system (CNS) manifestations. Cardiovascular symptoms are related to circulatory overload and are compounded by hypertension. These include dyspnea, tachypnea, and an enlarged, tender liver. The most severely affected children develop acute renal failure with oliguria. As many as half of children affected are asymptomatic.

The disease usually runs its course in 1 month, but urine abnormalities may be found for up to 1 year after the onset. Less than 1% of children develop rapidly progressive glomerulonephritis, characterized by rapid decline of renal function. Prolonged proteinuria and abnormal glomerular filtration rate (GFR) indicate an unfavorable prognosis. More than 95% recover completely. Treatment is supportive and symptom specific.[27]

Immunoglobulin A Nephropathy

Immunoglobulin A (IgA) nephropathy is the most common form of glomerulonephritis worldwide and occurs more often in males. It is characterized by deposition primarily of immunoglobulin A and complement proteins in the mesangium of the glomerulus. No systemic immunologic disease is evident.[28] Deposits of IgA cause immune injury to the glomerulus that is usually reversible. Henoch-Schönlein purpura nephritis is a particular form of IgA nephropathy that involves a systemic vasculitis. The pathogenesis is unknown.

Children with the disease have recurrent gross hematuria concurrent with a respiratory tract infection. Most continue to have microscopic hematuria between the attacks of gross hematuria and have a mild proteinuria as well. Treatment is supportive because kidney damage is generally insignificant. Approximately 25% of affected children develop the progressive form of the disease, however, with hypertension and decreasing renal function. These children eventually require dialysis and transplantation.[29]

Nephrotic Syndrome

Nephrotic syndrome is characterized by severe proteinuria, hypoalbuminemia, hyperlipidemia, and edema. The syndrome is more common in children than in adults. When no identifiable cause is found, the condition is primary (idiopathic) nephrotic syndrome. If it results from a systemic disease or other causes (e.g., drugs, toxins), it is called secondary nephrotic syndrome. Primary nephrotic syndrome is found predominantly in the preschool-age child, with a peak incidence of onset between 2 and 3 years of age. It is rare after 8 years of age. Boys are affected more often than girls. No prevalent racial or geographic distributions are evident. The incidence is approximately 3 per 100,000 children per year.

PATHOPHYSIOLOGY   The most common causes of primary nephrotic syndrome in children are minimal change nephropathy and focal segmental glomerulosclerosis. Minimal change nephropathy (MCN) (lipoid nephrosis) is characterized by fusion of the glomerular podocyte foot processes, which are seen by electron microscopy. The glomeruli appear normal by light microscopy. A systemic immune mechanism is a likely cause of the disease, but the true etiology is unknown. An unidentified circulating permeability factor released by T lymphocytes has been proposed.[30] Loss of the electrical negative charge and increased permeability within the glomerular capillary wall lead to albuminuria. Hyperlipidemia leads to hyperlipiduria and primarily results from increased hepatic lipid synthesis and decreased plasma lipid catabolism.

In idiopathic focal segmental glomerulosclerosis (FSGS) there is segmental loss of glomerular capillaries with proliferation of the mesangial matrix and adhesion of the capillaries to Bowman capsule. Hypoalbuminemia (causing decreased plasma oncotic pressure) and sodium retention contribute to edema.[31]

CLINICAL MANIFESTATIONS   Onset of nephrotic syndrome can be insidious with periorbital edema as the usual first sign. The edema is most noticeable in the morning and subsides during the day as fluid shifts to the abdomen, genitalia, and lower extremities. Parents may notice diminished, frothy, or foamy urine output; when edema becomes pronounced with ascites, respiratory difficulty from pleural effusion or labial or scrotal swelling may develop. Edema of the intestinal mucosa may cause diarrhea, anorexia, and poor absorption. Edema often masks the malnutrition caused by malabsorption and protein loss. Pallor, with shiny skin and prominent veins, also is common. Blood pressure is usually normal. The child has an increased susceptibility to infection, especially pneumonia, peritonitis, cellulitis, and septicemia. Irritability, fatigue, and lethargy are common. Congenital nephrotic syndrome (Finnish type) is caused by an autosomal recessive mutation of the NPHS1 gene that encodes an immunoglobulin-like protein, nephrin, at the podocyte slit membrane. Congenital nephrotic syndrome presents with heavy proteinuria in the first 3 months of life. These babies do not respond to steroid treatment. Babies with congenital nephrotic syndrome have widely separated cranial sutures and flexion deformities of the hips, knees, and elbows.[32]

EVALUATION AND TREATMENT   The diagnosis of nephrotic syndrome is evident from the findings of proteinuria, hyperlipidemia, and edema. Diagnostic testing, including kidney biopsy, may be required to determine whether the cause is an intrinsic renal disease or a consequence of systemic disease. Basic management of nephrotic syndrome includes administering glucocorticosteroids (prednisone); adhering to a low-sodium, well-balanced diet; performing good skin care; and, if edema becomes problematic, prescribing diuretics (furosemide, metolazone). Immunosuppressive agents (i.e., cyclophosphamide) may be used with children who have frequent relapses or who are resistant to steroid therapy. Long-term outcomes depend on the underlying cause of the nephrotic syndrome. Children with minimal change disease tend to do very well, whereas those with other conditions may develop end-stage kidney disease.

Hemolytic Uremic Syndrome

Hemolytic uremic syndrome (HUS) is an acute disorder characterized by hemolytic anemia, thrombocytopenia, and acute renal failure. HUS is the most common cause of acute renal failure in children. The disease occurs most often in infants and children younger than 4 years of age but has been known to occur in adolescents and adults.[33] The prognosis has improved dramatically, with more than 90% of children surviving and most regaining normal renal function.[34]

PATHOPHYSIOLOGY HUS has been associated with bacterial and viral agents, as well as endotoxins, especially that from *Escherichia coli* 0157:H7[35] and more recently *Escherichia coli* 0104:H4 (Shiga toxins).[35a] In HUS, the endothelial lining of the glomerular arterioles becomes swollen and occluded with platelets and fibrin clots. Narrowed vessels damage passing erythrocytes. These damaged red blood cells are removed by the spleen, causing acute hemolytic anemia. Fibrinolysis, the process of dissolution of a clot, acts on precipitated fibrin, causing the fibrin split products to appear in serum and urine. Platelet thrombi develop within damaged vessels, and platelet removal produces thrombocytopenia. Varying degrees of vascular occlusion cause altered renal perfusion and renal insufficiency or failure.[35]

CLINICAL MANIFESTATIONS A prodromal gastrointestinal illness (fever, vomiting, diarrhea) or, less frequently, an upper respiratory tract infection often precedes the onset of HUS by 1 to 2 weeks. After a symptom-free 1- to 5-day period, the sudden onset of pallor, bruising or purpura, irritability, and oliguria heralds the commencement of the disease. Slight fever, anorexia, vomiting, diarrhea (with the stool characteristically watery and blood stained), abdominal pain, mild jaundice, and circulatory overload are accompanying symptoms. Seizures and lethargy indicate CNS involvement. Renal failure is apparent within the first days of onset. The renal failure causes metabolic acidosis, azotemia, hyperkalemia, and often hypertension.

EVALUATION AND TREATMENT Clinical evaluation includes history of preexisting illness, presenting symptoms, and urine and blood analysis. Management is supportive. When renal failure occurs, early and frequent dialysis is indicated. Blood transfusions with packed red cells are needed to maintain reasonable hemoglobin levels. Most children recover but some will develop kidney failure.[36]

Other Renal Disorders

Other disorders of the kidney occurring in children include renal tubular acidosis and acute and chronic renal failure. The pathophysiology for these conditions is similar to that in adults and is described in Chapter 29.

BLADDER DISORDERS

Urinary Tract Infections

Urinary tract infections (UTIs) are rare in newborns; however, when they occur, they are usually caused by bacteria from the bloodstream that have settled in the urinary tract. Urinary tract infections in children are most common in 7- to 11-year-old girls (8.1%) as a result of perineal bacteria, especially *E. coli,* ascending the urethra.[37,38] Susceptibility, bacterial virulence, and the host's anatomy (presence of reflux, obstruction, stasis, or stones) affect the severity of the disease. An abnormal urinary tract is particularly susceptible to infection.[39] Sexually active female adolescents are at increased risk to have a UTI.

Cystitis, or infection of the bladder, results in mucosal inflammation and congestion. This causes detrusor muscle hyperactivity and a resulting decrease in bladder capacity, resulting in urgency and frequency. It may also cause distortion of the ureterovesical (UV) junction leading to transient reflux of infected urine up the ureters, causing acute or chronic pyelonephritis.[40]

Differentiating whether an infection is in the bladder or the kidneys is difficult based on symptoms alone. Infants may be asymptomatic or develop fever, lethargy, vomiting, diarrhea, or jaundice. Children may present with fever of undetermined origin, frequency, urgency, dysuria, enuresis or incontinence in a previously dry child, abdominal pain, and sometimes hematuria. Acute pyelonephritis usually causes chills, high fever, and flank or abdominal pain, along with enlarged kidney(s) caused by inflammatory edema. Chronic pyelonephritis may be asymptomatic.

Diagnosis of UTIs is by urine culture. Dipstick analyses for nitrite, leukocyte esterase, and blood may be used as a screening tool. Any positive or strong suspicion of a UTI requires urine culture.[41] Diagnostic imaging may be necessary to rule out obstructions, renal scarring, or functional abnormalities.[42] With treatment, UTI symptoms are usually relieved in 1 to 2 days, and the urine becomes sterile. A 2- to 4-day course of oral antibiotics is effective for uncomplicated UTI. Longer treatment may be required if the child has a history of recurrent UTIs or has congenital abnormalities of the urinary tract. If there is no improvement in 2 days, the child should be reevaluated[43] (see *Health Alert:* Childhood Urinary Tract Infections).

HEALTH ALERT
Childhood Urinary Tract Infections

Childhood urinary tract infections are often seen in primary care settings and can cause significant longer-term morbidity if not treated. Children younger than 2 years often have few, nonspecific signs of infection, including fever, irritability, poor feeding, failure to thrive, and diarrhea. Obtaining a proper urine sample and culture is vital because true infections require further examination. Antibiotic prophylaxis may be considered because of the link between vesicoureteral reflux, recurrent UTIs, and renal scarring and hypertension; however, administration of antibiotics to children is a controversial issue. Current recommendations are to *consider* prophylaxis for children less than 1 year of age with VUR and a history of febrile UTIs, and other children as indicated. Circumcision status is controversial; however, recent studies have shown a decreased rate of UTIs in circumcised boys. The position of the American Academy of Pediatrics is that scientific evidence shows medical benefits of neonatal circumcision, but data are insufficient to support routine neonatal circumcision. Abnormalities in bowel and bladder function must be addressed because they can impact the development of UTIs and affect the resolution of VUR. Surgical management of VUR is considered based on failure of medical management to prevent recurrent infections, VUR grade, and degree of renal scarring.

Data from American Academy of Pediatrics: Circumcision policy statement Task Force on Circumcision, *Pediatrics* 103(3):686–693, 1999; Chang SL, Shortliffe LD: Pediatric urinary tract infections, *Pediatr Clin North Am* 53(3):279–400, 2006; Peters CA et al: Summary of the AUA guideline on management of primary vesicoureteral reflux in children, *J Urol* 184(3):1134–1144, 2010.

Vesicoureteral Reflux

Vesicoureteral reflux (VUR) is the retrograde flow of urine from the bladder into the kidney or ureters, or both. This allows infected urine from the bladder to reach the kidneys. Vesicoureteral reflux occurs more often in girls by a ratio of 10:1 and is uncommon in blacks. The actual incidence is unknown because VUR is often undiagnosed. An estimated 30% to 40% of children under the age of 5 years who develop a UTI have VUR.[44] Siblings of those affected have about a 27% to 39% chance of having reflux,[1,45] but children with parents who had childhood reflux have almost a 70% chance of reflux.[46] Although reflux is considered abnormal at any age, the shortness of the submucosal tunnel of the ureter during infancy and childhood renders the antireflux mechanism relatively inefficient and delicate. Thus reflux is seen commonly in association with infections during early childhood but rarely in older children and adults.

PATHOPHYSIOLOGY   The normal distal ureter enters the bladder through the detrusor muscle and passes through a submucosal tunnel before opening into the bladder lumen via the ureteral orifice. As the bladder fills with urine the ureter is compressed within the bladder wall preventing reflux. Primary VUR results from a congenital abnormally short submucosal tunnel and ureter that permits reflux by the rising pressure of the filling bladder (Figure 30-4). Urine sweeps up into the ureter and then flows back into the empty bladder. The reflux perpetuates infection by preventing complete emptying of the bladder and providing a reservoir for infection. With the next bladder filling, the maximal intravesical pressure can be transmitted up the ureter to the renal pelvis and calyces. The combination of reflux and infection is an important cause of pyelonephritis. Renal parenchymal injury, scarring, hypertension, and chronic renal insufficiency can occur many years later making early diagnosis and treatment important. Secondary reflux develops in association with acquired conditions (e.g., neurogenic bladder dysfunction, ureteral obstruction, voiding disorders, or surgery on the UV junction). Reflux may be unilateral or bilateral, and can be graded using the International Reflux Grading System[47] (Figure 30-5):

Grade I: reflux into a nondilated distal ureter
Grade II: reflux into the upper collecting system without dilation
Grade III: reflux into a dilated ureter or blunting of calyceal fornices
Grade IV: reflux into a grossly dilated ureter and calyces
Grade V: massive reflux with urethral dilation and tortuosity and effacement of the calyceal details

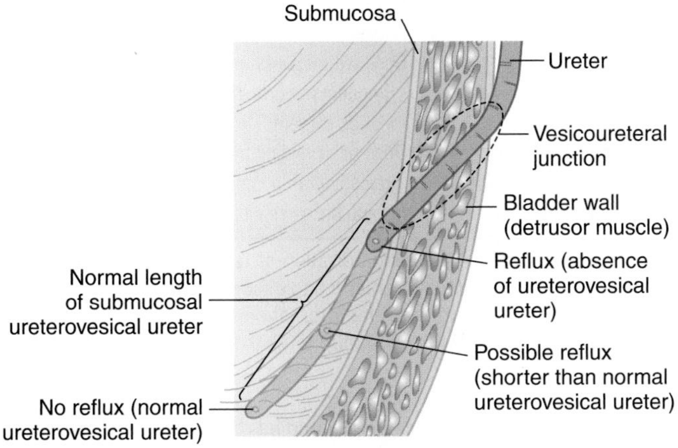

CLINICAL MANIFESTATIONS   Children with reflux may be asymptomatic or have recurrent urinary tract infections, unexplained fevers, poor growth and development, irritability, and feeding problems. The family history may reveal VUR or urinary tract infections.

EVALUATION AND TREATMENT   In addition to the history of recurrent urinary tract infection and other symptoms, a voiding cystourethrogram is the primary diagnostic procedure. Most children with vesicoureteral reflux respond to nonoperative management aimed at prevention and treatment of infection. Spontaneous remission of grades I and II reflux may occur in 30% to 60% of children younger than 5 years. Children with grades III and IV reflux need careful monitoring. Recurrent infection may require surgical intervention or endoscopic injection of a synthetic ureteral orfice valve. In cases of grade V reflux, early surgical intervention may be indicated to prevent renal scarring.[48]

> ✓ **QUICK CHECK 30-2**
> 1. What is the cause of proteinuria?
> 2. How does the cause of urinary tract infections (UTIs) in newborns differ from that in older children?
> 3. How does vesicoureteral reflux occur?

NEPHROBLASTOMA

Nephroblastoma (Wilms tumor) is a rare embryonal tumor of the kidney arising from undifferentiated mesoderm and represents 5% of childhood cancers in the United States.[49] Its incidence remains constant in the United States, with 7.8 cases per 1 million population ages 1 to 14 years. Approximately 500 children are diagnosed each year in the United States, most between 1 and 5 years of age.[50] The peak incidence occurs between 2 and 3 years of age. Nephroblastoma is the most common solid tumor occurring in children. Maternal preconception toxin exposure (e.g., pesticides) may be associated with increased risk

FIGURE 30-4 Normal and Abnormal Configurations of the Ureterovesical Ureter. A refluxing ureterovesical ureter has the same anatomic features as a nonrefluxing ureter, except for the shorter length of the intravesical ureter which allows reflux of urine during filling of the bladder.

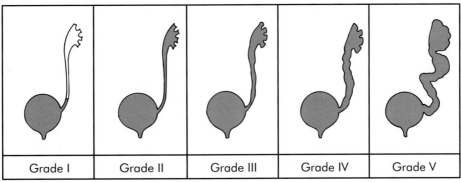

FIGURE 30-5 Grades of Vesicoureteral Reflux.

in offspring.[51] Nephroblastoma is slightly more common in black children than in white children.

PATHOGENESIS Nephroblastoma has both sporadic and inherited origins. The sporadic form occurs in children with no known genetic predisposition. Inherited cases, which are relatively rare, are transmitted in an autosomal dominant fashion. Nephroblastoma has been linked to mutation of several tumor-suppressor genes (i.e., *WT1* mutations).[52]

Eighteen percent of children who have nephroblastoma also have a number of congenital anomalies. The anomalies associated with nephroblastoma are aniridia (lack of an iris in the eye), hemihypertrophy (an asymmetry of the body), and genitourinary malformations (i.e., horseshoe kidneys, hypospadias, ureteral duplication, polycystic kidneys).[53] Children with both congenital anomalies and nephroblastoma are more likely to have the inherited bilateral form of the disease.

CLINICAL MANIFESTATIONS Most children with nephroblastoma present with an enlarging asymptomatic abdominal mass before the age of 5 years. Many tumors are actually discovered by the child's parent, who feels or notices an abdominal swelling, usually while dressing or bathing the child. The child appears healthy and thriving. Other presenting complaints include vague abdominal pain, hematuria, anemia, and fever.[54] Hypertension may be present, often as a result of excessive renin secretion by the tumor.[55]

Nephroblastoma may occur in any part of the kidney and varies greatly in size at the time of diagnosis. The tumor generally appears as a solitary mass surrounded by a smooth, fibrous external capsule and also may contain cystic or hemorrhagic areas. A pseudocapsule generally separates the tumor from the renal parenchyma.

EVALUATION AND TREATMENT On physical examination, the tumor feels firm, nontender, and smooth, and is generally confined to one side of the abdomen. If the tumor is palpable past the midline of the abdomen, it may be large or may be arising from a horseshoe or ectopic kidney. Once an abdominal mass is detected, diagnostic imaging demonstrates a solid intrarenal mass.

Diagnosis is based on surgical biopsy. Additional laboratory and radiologic studies are used to evaluate the presence or absence of metastasis. The most common sites of metastasis are regional lymph nodes and the lungs, and less commonly the liver, brain, and bone.

Several staging systems for nephroblastoma have been developed and serve as guides to treatment. The most widely accepted system was developed by the National Wilms Tumor Study Group (Table 30-1). Primary treatment is usually surgical exploration and resection or chemotherapy and then surgical resection. Radiation therapy may be used for children with higher stages of disease and metastases. Survival is greater than 90% for localized disease and up to 80% for higher stages.[52]

URINARY INCONTINENCE

Urinary incontinence refers to the involuntary passage of urine by a child who is beyond the age when voluntary bladder control should have been acquired. Bladder control is accomplished by most children before the age of 5 years, although this is largely influenced by cultural beliefs and parental toilet training practices.

Types of Incontinence

Wetness that occurs during the day is called **daytime incontinence.** Nighttime wetting is called **enuresis. Primary incontinence** (enuresis) means the child has never been continent, whereas **secondary**

STAGE	TUMOR CHARACTERISTICS
TABLE 30-1	**STAGING OF NEPHROBLASTOMA TUMOR***
I	Tumor limited to kidney; can be completely resected
II	Tumor ascending beyond kidney but is totally resected
III	Residual nonhematogenous tumor confined to abdomen
IV	Hematogenous metastases to organs such as lungs, liver, bone, or brain
V	Bilateral disease either at diagnosis or later, then staged for each kidney

*Staging system of the National Wilms Tumor Study Group.

TABLE 30-2	**CLASSIFICATION OF INCONTINENCE**
TYPE	**DEFINITION**
Daytime voiding frequency	Decreased: 3 or fewer voids per day Increased: 8 or more voids per day
Dysfunctional voiding	Habitual contraction of urethral sphincter during voiding; observed by uroflow measurements
Enuresis	Incontinence of urine while sleeping
Incontinence, continuous	Continuous leakage, not in discrete portions
Incontinence, stress	Leakage with raised intra-abdominal pressure
Urgency	Sudden, unexpected, immediate need to void
Overactive bladder	Child with urgency; increased voiding frequency and/or incontinence may or may not be present
Underactive bladder	Decreased voiding frequency with use of raised intra-abdominal pressure to void
Urge incontinence	Incontinence in children with urgency

From Neveus T et al: The standardization of terminology of lower urinary tract function in children and adolescents: report from the Standardization Committee of the International Children's Continence Society, *J Urol* 176(1):312–324, 2006.

incontinence (enuresis) means the child has been continent for at least 6 months before wetting recurs. A child may have daytime incontinence, enuresis, or a combination of both. (Types of incontinence are defined in Table 30-2.)

The incidence of incontinence (enuresis) is difficult to determine because it is not a problem that parents often discuss. Enuresis occurs in as many as 10% of 7-year-old males and resolves at a rate of 15% per year. Daytime incontinence occurs in up to 9% of early school age children.[56]

PATHOGENESIS A combination of factors is likely to be responsible for incontinence or enuresis. Organic causes account for 2% to 10% of cases and include UTIs; constipation and neurologic disturbances; congenital defects of the meatus, urethra, or bladder neck; and allergies. Disorders that increase the normal output of urine, such as diabetes mellitus and diabetes insipidus, or disorders that impair the concentrating ability of the kidney, such as chronic renal failure or sickle cell disease, should be considered during evaluation. Some incontinence or enuresis, in which no structural or neurologic abnormality is identified, is common in children. Other conditions that may be associated with incontinence include perinatal anoxia, CNS trauma, seizures, attention-deficit/hyperactivity disorder, developmental delay, imperforate anus, bladder trauma or surgery, and occult spinal dysraphism. Difficult sleep arousal and obstructive sleep apnea may be associated with enuresis. Stressful psychologic situations, such as a new sibling, may cause incontinence or enuresis to develop.[57,58]

Genetic factors contribute to some types of incontinence. At least four gene loci associated with enuresis have been identified. Enuresis occurs with high frequency among parents, siblings, and other near relatives of symptomatic children. There is a high concordance rate in monozygotic twins with enuresis.[59]

EVALUATION AND TREATMENT Diagnostic evaluation of childhood incontinence includes a thorough history, voiding diary, physical examination, and urinalysis. Urodynamic flow studies or imaging may be required based on the history and physical findings. Therapeutic management of incontinence or enuresis begins with education. If the child and family understand the probably etiology of the child's condition, they are better able to choose and participate in therapies that are most likely to succeed. Treatment of daytime incontinence includes behavioral therapy, including timed voiding; fluid management; treatment of constipation, urinary tract infections, and other coexisting conditions if present; and medication (anticholinergic or alpha-blocker medications). Enuresis treatment also may include enuresis alarms or other medications (e.g., desmopressin acetate).[60,61]

✔ **QUICK CHECK 30-3**
1. What is Wilms tumor, and what cellular components are involved?
2. What organic causes are operative in enuresis?

DID YOU UNDERSTAND?

Structural Abnormalities

1. Congenital renal disorders affect 10% to 15% of the population. These disorders range in severity from minor, easily correctable anomalies to those incompatible with life.
2. Hypospadias is a congenital condition in which the urethral meatus can be located anywhere on the ventral surface of the glans, the penile shaft, the midline of the scrotum, or the perineum.
3. Exstrophy of the bladder is a congenital malformation in which the pubic bones are separated, the lower portion of the abdominal wall and anterior wall of the bladder are missing, and the posterior wall of the bladder is everted through the opening.
4. Urethral valves and polyps are congenital formations of tissue that block the urethra.
5. Ureteropelvic junction obstruction is blockage where the renal pelvis joins the ureter and is often caused by smooth muscle or urothelial malformation or by scarring that leads to hydronephrosis.
6. A dysplastic kidney is the result of abnormal differentiation of renal tissues. A hypoplastic kidney is small with a decreased number of nephrons.
7. Polycystic kidney disease (ARPKD or ADPKD) is a cystic genetic disorder resulting in multiple, bilateral renal cysts.
8. Renal agenesis is the failure of a kidney to grow or develop. The condition may be unilateral or bilateral and may occur as an isolated entity or in association with other disorders.

Glomerular Disorders

1. Glomerulonephritis is an inflammation of the glomeruli characterized by hematuria, edema, and hypertension. The cause is unknown but is often immune mediated. Glomerulonephritis may follow infections, especially those of the upper respiratory tract caused by strains of group A β-hemolytic streptococcus. Increases in glomerular capillary permeability lead to hematuria and proteinuria.

2. IgA nephropathy occurs with deposition of IgA in the glomerulus, causing glomerular injury with gross hematuria.
3. *Nephrotic syndrome* is a term used to describe a symptom complex characterized by proteinuria, hypoproteinemia, hyperlipidemia, and edema. Metabolic, biochemical, or physiochemical disturbances in the glomerular basement membrane may lead to increased permeability to protein.
4. Hemolytic uremic syndrome is an acute disorder characterized by hemolytic anemia, acute renal failure, and thrombocytopenia.

Bladder Disorders

1. Urinary tract infections can result from general sepsis in the newborn but are caused by bacteria ascending the urethra in older children. The bladder alone is infected in cystitis. The infection ascends to one or both kidneys in pyelonephritis. Urinary tract anomalies must be surgically corrected to prevent frequent recurrent infections.
2. Vesicoureteral reflux is the retrograde flow of bladder urine into the kidney or ureter, or both, increasing the risk for polynephritis. It can be unilateral or bilateral; primary or secondary.

Nephroblastoma

1. Nephroblastoma (Wilms tumor) is an embryonal tumor of the kidney that usually presents between birth and 5 years of age. The tumor can be successfully treated by surgery, a combination of drugs, and, sometimes, radiation therapy.

Urinary Incontinence

1. Urinary incontinence is the involuntary passage of urine. It may occur during the day (incontinence) or at night (enuresis), or both. Maturational delay, UTIs, constipation, and many other factors may contribute.

KEY TERMS

- Acute poststreptococcal glomerulonephritis (APGN) 766
- Acute pyelonephritis 768
- Ask-Upmark kidney 766
- Chordee 765
- Chronic pyelonephritis 768
- Congenital nephrotic syndrome (Finnish type) 767
- Cystitis 768
- Daytime incontinence 770
- Enuresis 770
- Epispadias 765
- Exstrophy of the bladder 765
- Focal segmental glomerulosclerosis (FSGS) 767
- Glomerulonephritis 766
- Hemolytic uremic syndrome (HUS) 767
- Henoch-Schönlein purpura nephritis 767
- Horseshoe kidney 764
- Hypoplastic kidney 766
- Hypospadias 765
- Immunoglobulin A (IgA) nephropathy 767
- Minimal change nephropathy (MCN; lipoid nephrosis) 767
- Nephroblastoma (Wilms tumor) 769
- Oligohydramnios 766
- Polycystic kidney disease (PKD) 766
- Potter syndrome 766
- Primary incontinence 770
- Primary (idiopathic) nephrotic syndrome 767
- Renal agenesis 766
- Renal dysplasia 766
- Secondary incontinence 770
- Secondary nephrotic syndrome 767
- Secondary ureteropelvic junction (UPJ) obstruction 766
- Ureterocele 766
- Ureteropelvic junction (UPJ) obstruction 766
- Urethral polyp 766
- Urethral valve 766
- Urethrovesical junction obstruction 766
- Urinary incontinence 770
- Urinary tract infection (UTI) 768
- Vesicoureteral reflux (VUR) 768

REFERENCES

1. Schedl A: Renal abnormalities and their developmental origin, *Nat Rev Genet* 8(10):791–802, 2007.
2. Glodny B, et al: Kidney fusion anomalies revisited: clinical and radiological analysis of 209 cases of crossed fused ectopia and horseshoe kidney, *Br J Urol Int* 103(2):224–235, 2008.
3. Sawicz-Birkowska K, et al: Malignant tumours in a horseshoe kidney in children: a diagnostic dilemma, *Eur J Pediatr Surg* 15(1):48–52, 2005.
4. Glassberg KI: Normal and abnormal development of the kidney: a clinician's interpretation of current knowledge, *J Urol* 167(6):2339–2350, 2002:discussion 2350–2351.
5. Toka HR, et al: Congenital anomalies of kidney and urinary tract, *Semin Nephrol* 30(4):374–386, 2010.
6. Casas KA, Kamil ES, Rimoin DL: Congenital disorders of the urinary tract. In Rimoin DL, et al, editors: *Principles and practice of medical genetics*, ed 5, vol 2, Philadelphia, 2007, Churchill Livingstone, Elsevier.
7. Kalfa N, Philibert P, Sultan C: Is hypospadias a genetic, endocrine, or environmental disease, or still an unexplained malformation? *Int J Androl* 32(3):187–197, 2009.
8. Nelson CP, et al: The increasing incidence of congenital penile anomalies in the United States, *J Urol* 174(4 Pt 2):1573–1576, 2005.
9. Wan J, Rew KT: Common penile problems, *Prim Care* 37(3):627–642, x, 2010.
10. Roberts J: Hypospadias surgery past, present and future, *Curr Opin Urol* 20(6):483–489, 2010.
11. Surer I, et al: Continent urinary diversion and the exstrophy-epispadias complex, *J Urol* 169(3):1102–1105, 2003.
12. Frimberger D: Diagnosis and management of epispadias, *Semin Pediatr Surg* 20(2):85–90, 2011.
13. Nelson CP, Dunn RL, Wei JT: Contemporary epidemiology of bladder exstrophy in the United States, *J Urol* 173(5):1728–1731, 2005.
14. Borer JG, et al: Bladder growth and development after complete primary repair of bladder exstrophy in the newborn with comparison to staged approach, *J Urol* 174(4 Pt 2):1553–1557, 2005.
15. Ebert AK, et al: The exstrophy-epispadias complex, *Orphanet J Rare Dis* 4:23, 2009.
16. Levin TL, Han B, Little BP: Congenital anomalies of the male urethra, *Pediatr Radiol* 37(9):851–852, 2007.
17. Ruano R: Fetal surgery for severe lower urinary tract obstruction, *Prenat Diagn* 31(7):667–674, 2011.
18. Narasimhan KL, et al: Does mode of treatment affect outcome of neonatal posterior urethral valves? *J Urol* 171(6 Pt 1):2423–2426, 2004.
19. Zhang PL, Peters CA, Rosen S: Ureteropelvic junction obstruction: morphological and clinical studies, *Pediatr Nephrol* 14(8–9):820–826, 2000.
20. Mei H, et al: Laparoscopic versus open pyeloplasty for ureteropelvic junction obstruction in children: a systematic review and meta-analysis, *J Endourol* 25(5):727–736, 2011.
21. Woolf AS: Renal hypoplasia and dysplasia: starting to put the puzzle together, *J Am Soc Nephrol* 17(10):2647–2649, 2006.
22. Babin J, et al: The Ask-Upmark kidney: a curable cause of hypertension in young patients, *J Hum Hypertens* 19(4):315–316, 2005.
23. Chang M-Y, Ong ACM: Autosomal dominant polycystic kidney disease: recent advances in pathogenesis and treatment, *Nephron Physiol* 108(1):1–7, 2008.
24. Park EY, Woo YM, Park JH: Polycystic kidney disease and therapeutic approaches, *BMB Rep* 44(6):359–368, 2011.
25. Dursun H, et al: Associated anomalies in children with congenital solitary functioning kidney, *Pediatr Surg Int* 21(6):456–459, 2005.
26. Eison TM, et al: Post-streptococcal acute glomerulonephritis in children: clinical features and pathogenesis, *Pediatr Nephrol* 26(2):165–180, 2011.
27. Zaffanello M, et al: Evidence-based treatment limitations prevent any therapeutic recommendation for acute poststreptococcal glomerulonephritis in children, *Med Sci Monit* 16(4):RA79–84, 2010.
28. Glassock RJ: The pathogenesis of IgA nephropathy, *Curr Opin Nephrol Hypertens* 20(2):153–160, 2011.
29. Coppo R: Pediatric IgA nephropathy: clinical and therapeutic perspectives, *Semin Nephrol* 28(1):18–26, 2008.
30. Saha TC, Singh H: Minimal change disease: a review, *South Med J* 99(11):1264–1270, 2006.
31. Kim SW, Frøkiaer J, Nielsen S: Pathogenesis of oedema in nephrotic syndrome: role of epithelial sodium channel, *Nephrology (Carlton)* 12(Suppl 3):S8–S10, 2007.
32. Benoit G, Machuca E, Antignac C: Hereditary nephrotic syndrome: a systematic approach for genetic testing and a review of associated podocyte gene mutations, *Pediatr Nephrol* 25(9):1621–1632, 2010.
33. Miller DP, et al: Incidence of thrombotic thrombocytopenic purpura/hemolytic uremic syndrome, *Epidemiology* 15(2):208–215, 2004.
34. Franchini M, Zaffanello M, Veneri D: Advances in the pathogenesis, diagnosis and treatment of thrombotic thrombocytopenic purpura and hemolytic uremic syndrome, *Thromb Res* 118(2):177–184, 2006.
35. Zoja C, Buelli S, Morigi M: Shiga toxin-associated hemolytic uremic syndrome: pathophysiology of endothelial dysfunction, *Pediatr Nephrol* 25(11):2231–2240, 2010.
35a. Frank C, et al: Epidemic profile of shiga-toxin–producing *Escherichia coli* O104:H4 outbreak in Germany—preliminary report, *N Engl J Med*, June 22, 2010, pages 1-11. Available at http://www.nejm.org/doi/full/10.1056/NEJMoa1106483.

36. Michael M, et al: Interventions for hemolytic uremic syndrome and thrombotic thrombocytopenic purpura: a systematic review of randomized controlled trials, *Am J Kidney Dis* 53(2):259–272, 2009.

37. American Academy of Pediatrics, Committee on Quality Improvement, Subcommittee on Urinary Tract Infection: Practice parameter: the diagnosis, treatment, and evaluation of the initial urinary tract infection in febrile infants and young children, *Pediatrics* 103(4 Pt 1):843–852, 1999.

38. Bell LE, Mattoo TK: Update on childhood urinary tract infection and vesicoureteral reflux, *Semin Nephrol* 29(4):349–359, 2009.

39. Tanaka ST, Brock JW 3rd: Pediatric urologic conditions, including urinary infections, *Med Clin North Am* 95(1):1–13, 2011.

40. Chishti AS, et al: A guideline for the inpatient care of children with pyelonephritis, *Ann Saudi Med* 30(5):341–349, 2010.

41. Bauer R, Kogan BA: New developments in the diagnosis and management of pediatric UTIs, *Urol Clin North Am* 35(1):47–58, 2008.

42. Clak CJ, Kennedy WA 2nd, Shortliffe LD: Urinary tract infection in children: when to worry, *Urol Clin North Am* 37(2):229–241, 2010.

43. White B: Diagnosis and treatment of urinary tract infections in children, *Am Fam Physician* 83(4):409–415, 2011.

44. Cooper CS: Diagnosis and management of vesicoureteral reflux in children, *Nat Rev Urol* 6(9):481–489, 2009.

45. Skoog SJ, et al: Pediatric Vesicoureteral Reflux Guidelines Panel Summary Report: Clinical practice guidelines for screening siblings of children with vesicoureteral reflux and neonates/infants with prenatal hydronephrosis, *J Urol* 184(3):1145–1151, 2010.

46. Menezes M, Puri P: Familial vesicoureteral reflux—is screening beneficial? *J Urol* 182(4 suppl):1673–1677, 2009.

47. Lebowitz RL, et al: International system of radiographic grading of vesicoureteric reflux. International Reflux Study in Children, *Pediatr Radiol* 15(2):105–109, 1985.

48. Peters CA, et al: Summary of the AUA guideline on management of primary vesicoureteral reflux in children, *J Urol* 184(3):1134–1144, 2010.

49. American Cancer Society: *Detailed guide: Wilms' tumor: what are the key statistics for Wilms' tumor?* Available at http://www.cancer.org/Cancer/WilmsTumor/DetailedGuide/wilms-tumor-key-statistics. Accessed June 2011.

50. Bernstein L, et al: Renal tumors. In Ries LA, et al, editors: *Cancer incidence and survival among children and adolescents: United States SEER Program 1975-1995*, Bethesda, Md, 1999, National Cancer Institute (NIH Pub No. 99–4649).

51. Chu A, et al: Wilms' tumour: a systematic review of risk factors and meta-analysis, *Paediatr Perinat Epidemiol* 24(5):449–469, 2010.

52. Huff V: Wilms' tumours: about tumour suppressor genes, an oncogene and a chameleon gene, *Nat Rev Cancer* 11(2):111–121, 2011.

53. Scott RH, et al: Syndromes and constitutional chromosomal abnormalities associated with Wilms tumour, *J Med Genet* 43(9):705–715, 2006.

54. Sarhan OM, et al: Bilateral Wilms' tumors: single-center experience with 22 cases and literature review, *Urology* 76(4):946–951, 2010.

55. Mullen EA, Weldon C, Kreidberg JA: Pediatric renal tumors. In Avner ED, et al *Pediatric nephrology*, ed 6, vol 2, Berlin Heidelberg, 2009, Springer Verlag, pp 1431–1455.

56. Buckley BS, Lapitan MCM: Prevalence of urinary incontinence in men, women, and children—current evidence: findings of the Fourth International Consultation on Incontinence, *Urology* 76(2):265–270, 2010.

57. Herndon CD, Joseph DB: Urinary incontinence, *Pediatr Clin North Am* 53(3):366–377, 2006.

58. Schulman SL: Voiding dysfunction in children, *Urol Clin North Am* 31(3):481–490, 2004.

59. von Gontard A, Heron J, Joinson C: Family history of nocturnal enuresis and urinary incontinence: results from a large epidemiological study, *J Urol* 185(6):2303–2306, 2011.

60. Brown ML, Pope AW, Brown EJ: Treatment of primary nocturnal enuresis in children: a review, *Child Care Health Dev* 37(2):153–160, 2011.

61. Nevéus T, et al: Evaluation and treatment for monosymptomatic enuresis: a standardization document from the International Children's Continence Society, *J Urol* 183(2):441–447, 2010.

31

Structure and Function of the Reproductive Systems

Angela Deneris and Sue E. Huether

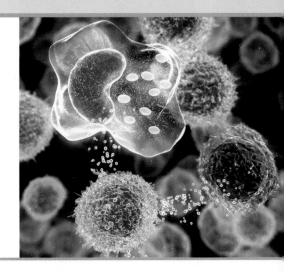

evolve WEBSITE

CHAPTER OUTLINE

The male and female reproductive systems have several anatomic and physiologic features in common. Most obvious is their major function—reproduction—through which a 23-chromosome female gamete, the ovum, and a 23-chromosome male gamete, the **spermatozoon (sperm cell),** unite to form a 46-chromosome zygote that is capable of developing into a new individual. The male reproductive system produces sperm that can be transferred to the female reproductive tract. The female reproductive system produces the **ovum** (pl., ova), and if the ovum is fertilized (then called the embryo and developing fetus), it can be nurtured and protected until it is expelled at birth. These functions are determined not only by anatomic structures but also by complex hormonal, neurologic, and psychogenic factors.[1]

DEVELOPMENT OF THE REPRODUCTIVE SYSTEMS

The structure and function of both male and female reproductive systems depend on steroid hormones called **sex hormones** and their precursors. Cholesterol is the precursor for steroid hormones, including

the sex hormones. Other hormones support reproduction. The actions of both sex and reproductive hormones are summarized in Table 31-1. Sex hormones, like all hormones, act on target tissues by binding with cellular receptors (see Chapter 17). Hormonal effects on the reproductive systems begin during embryonic development and continue in varying degrees throughout life.

Sexual Differentiation in Utero

Initially, in embryonic development, the reproductive structures of male and female embryos are homologous (the same), consisting of one pair of primary sex organs, or **gonads,** and two pairs of ducts: the mesonephric ducts (wolffian ducts) and the paramesonephric ducts (müllerian ducts) (Figure 31-1). Both pairs of ducts empty into the urogenital sinus.

Between 6 and 7 weeks' gestation, the male embryo will differentiate under the influence of testes-determining factor (TDF), a protein expressed by a gene in the sex-determining region on the Y chromosome *(SRY).* When the *SRY* gene is expressed, male gonadal

TABLE 31-1 SUMMARY OF FEMALE AND MALE SEX AND REPRODUCTIVE HORMONES

HORMONE (SOURCE)	ACTION FEMALES	ACTION MALES
Dehydroepiandrosterone (DHEA) (adrenal gland, ovary, other tissues)	Converted to androstenedione and then to estrogens, testosterone, or both	Converted to androstenedione and then to estrogens, testosterone, or both
Estrogens (estrone, estradiol, estriol) function through estrogen receptors alpha and beta (ovary and placenta, small amounts in other tissues)	Stimulates development of female sexual characteristics: maturation of breast, uterus, and vagina; promotes proliferative development of endometrium during menstrual cycle; during pregnancy promotes mammary gland development, fetal adrenal gland function, and uteroplacental blood flow (see Box 31-1)	Growth at puberty, growth plate fusion in bone, prevention of apoptosis of germ cells
Testosterone (adrenal glands from DHEA, ovaries)	Libido, learning, sleep, protein anabolism, growth of muscle and bone; growth of pubic and axillary hair; activation of sebaceous glands, accounting for some cases of acne during puberty	Stimulates spermatogenesis, stimulates development of primary and secondary sexual characteristics, promotes growth of muscle and bone (anabolic effect); growth of pubic and axillary hair; activates sebaceous glands, accounting for some cases of acne during puberty; maintains libido
Gonadotropin-releasing hormone (GnRH) (hypothalamus-neuroendocrine cells)	Stimulates secretion of gonadotropins (FSH and LH) from anterior pituitary	Stimulates secretion of gonadotropins (FSH and LH) from anterior pituitary
Follicle-stimulating hormone (FSH) (anterior pituitary, gonadotroph cells)	Gonadotropin; promotes development of ovarian follicle; stimulates estrogen secretion	Gonadotropin; promotes development of testes and stimulates spermatogenesis by Sertoli cells
Luteinizing hormone (LH) (anterior pituitary, gonadotroph cells)	Gonadotropin; triggers ovulation; promotes development of corpus luteum	Gonadotropin; stimulates testostertone production by Leydig cells of testis
Inhibin (ovary and testes)	Inhibits FSH production in anterior pituitary (perhaps by limiting GnRH)	Inhibits FSH production in anterior pituitary
Human chorionic gonadotropin (hCG) (placenta)	Supports corpus luteum, which secretes estrogen and progesterone during first 7 weeks of pregnancy	
Activin (ovary)	Stimulates secretion of FSH and pituitary response to GnRH and FSH binding in dominant granulosa cells	
Progesterone (ovary and placenta)	Promotes secretory changes in endometrium during luteal phase of menstrual cycle; quiets uterine myometrium (muscle) activity and prevents lactogenesis during pregnancy	
Relaxin (corpus luteum, myometrium and placenta)	Inhibits uterine contractions during pregnancy and softens pelvic joints and cervix to facilitate childbirth	

development prevails. TDF stimulates the male gonads to develop into the two testes and by 8 weeks' gestation testosterone secretion begins. By 9 months' gestation, the male gonads (testes) have descended into the scrotum. The testes produce sperm after puberty.[2,3]

Female gonadal development occurs in the absence of *SRY* expression and with the expression of other genes.[4] The presence of *estrogen* and the absence of *testosterone* cause a loss in the wolffian system, and at 6 to 8 weeks' gestation the two female gonads develop into ovaries, which will produce ova. In females the mesonephric ducts deteriorate, and the lower ends of the paramesonephric ducts join to become the uterus. The upper portions of the paramesonephric ducts unite to become the uterus, fallopian tubes, cervix, and upper two thirds of the vagina. The fallopian tubes will carry ova from the ovaries to the uterus during a woman's reproductive years.

Like the internal reproductive structures, the external structures develop from homologous embryonic tissues. During the first 7 to 8 weeks' gestation, both male and female embryos develop an elevated structure called the *genital tubercle* (Figure 31-2). Testosterone is necessary for the genital tubercle to differentiate into male genitalia; otherwise, female genitalia develop, which may occur even in the absence of ovaries, possibly because of the presence of placental estrogens.[1]

Anterior pituitary development begins between the fourth and fifth weeks of fetal life and the vascular connection between the hypothalamus and the pituitary is established by the twelfth week. Gonadotropin-releasing hormone (GnRH) is produced in the hypothalamus by 10 weeks' gestation and controls the production of two gonadotropins, luteinizing hormone (LH) and follicle-stimulating hormone (FSH), by the anterior pituitary gland. In the female fetus, high levels of FSH and LH are excreted. FSH and LH stimulate the production of estrogen and progesterone by the ovary. The production of FSH and LH increases until about 28 weeks' gestation, when the production of estrogen and progesterone by the ovaries and placenta is high enough to result in the decline of gonadotropin production.[1] Production of primitive female gametes (ova) occurs solely during fetal life. From puberty to menopause, one female gamete matures per menstrual cycle. Production of the male gametes (sperm) begins at puberty; after that, millions are produced daily, usually for life.

With a term pregnancy, a sensitive negative feedback system, which includes the gonadostat (also known as the gonadotropin-releasing

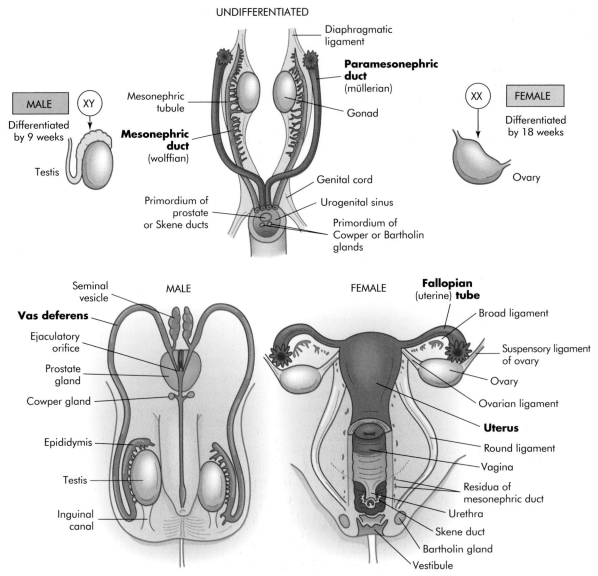

FIGURE 31-1 Internal Genitalia Development. Embryonic and fetal development of the internal genitalia.

hormone pulse generator), is operative in the human fetus. The gonadostat responds to high levels of placental estrogens by releasing low levels of GnRH. Soon after birth, steroid hormone levels drop because of the loss of maternal placental hormones. Hypothalamic pulsatile GnRH is secreted and gonadotropins LH and FSH are released; their levels peak at 3 to 6 months for boys and at 12 to 18 months for girls and then fall steadily. The gonadotropins will be suppressed until the onset of puberty.

Puberty and Reproductive Maturation

Puberty is the onset of sexual maturation and differs from adolescence. Adolescence is the stage of human development between childhood and adulthood and includes social, psychological, and biologic changes. In girls, puberty begins at about age 8 to 9 years with thelarche (breast development). In boys, it begins later—at about age 11 years. Genetics, environment, ethnicity, general health, and nutrition can influence the timing of puberty. Girls who are obese mature earlier, perhaps from higher estrogen levels related to leptin and gonadotropin secretion,[5] and girls who have low body fat, reduced

body weight, and perform intense exercise may experience delayed maturation.[6]

Reproductive maturation involves the hypothalamic-pituitary-gonadal axis, the central nervous system, and the endocrine system (Figure 31-3). There is a sequential series of hormonal events that promote sexual maturation as puberty approaches. About 1 year before puberty in girls, nocturnal pulses of gonadotropin secretion (i.e., LH and FSH) and an increased response in the pituitary to GnRH occur. This, in turn, stimulates gonadal maturation (gonadarche) with estradiol secretion in girls and testosterone secretion in boys. Estradiol causes breast development (thelarche), maturation of the reproductive organs (vagina, uterus, ovaries), and deposition of fat in the female's hips. Estrogen and increased production of growth factors cause rapid skeletal growth in both boys and girls. Testosterone causes growth of the testes, scrotum, and penis. A positive feedback loop is created with gonadotropins stimulating the gonads to produce more sex hormones. The most important hormonal effects occur in the gonads. In males, the testes begin to produce mature sperm that are capable of fertilizing an ovum. Male puberty

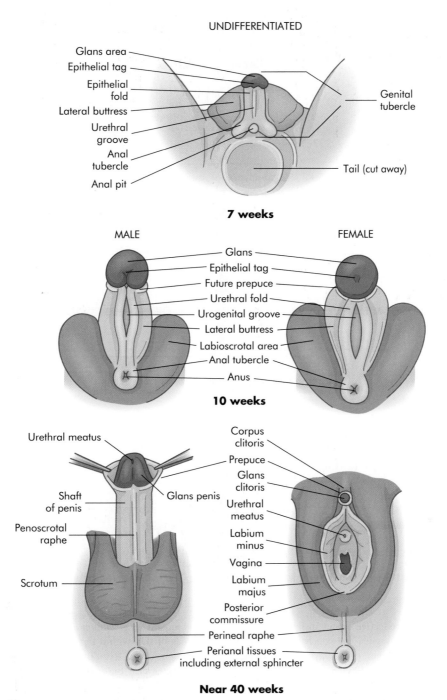

FIGURE 31-2 External Genitalia Development. Embryonic and fetal development of the external genitalia.

is complete with the first ejaculation that contains mature sperm. In females, the ovaries begin to release mature ova. Female puberty is complete at the time of the first ovulatory menstrual period; however, this can take up to 1 to 2 years after menarche. **Adrenarche** is the increased production of adrenal **androgens** (dehydroepiandrosterone and androstenedione, which are converted to testosterone and estrogen) before puberty, which occurs in both sexes and is manifested by growth of axillary and pubic hair and activation of sweat and sebaceous glands. Puberty is complete when an individual is capable of reproduction.

> ✓ **QUICK CHECK 31-1**
> 1. When do sex hormones first exhibit an effect on sexual development?
> 2. Why are sex hormones necessary for reproduction?

THE FEMALE REPRODUCTIVE SYSTEM

The function of the female reproductive system is to produce mature ova; if fertilization occurs, the female reproductive system provides protection and nourishment of the fetus until it is expelled at birth.

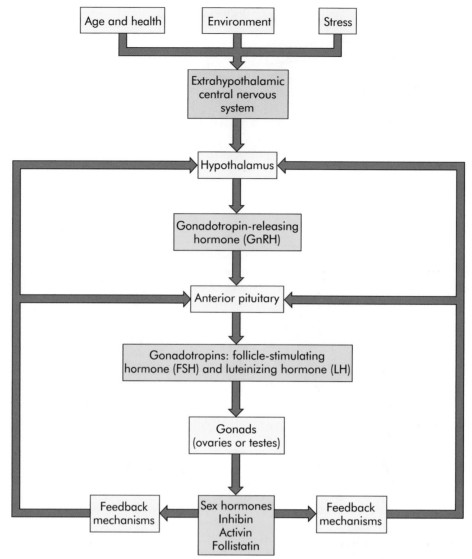

FIGURE 31-3 Hormonal Stimulation of the Gonads. The hypothalamic-pituitary-gonadal axis.

The most important internal reproductive organs in females are the ovaries, fallopian tubes, uterus, and vagina. The external genitalia protect body openings and play an important role in sexual functioning.

External Genitalia

Figure 31-4 shows the external female genitalia, known collectively as the vulva, or pudendum. The major structures are as follows:

Mons pubis: Fatty layer of tissue over pubic symphysis (joint formed by union of the pubic bones). During puberty it becomes covered with pubic hair, and sebaceous and sweat glands become more active. Estrogen causes fat to be deposited under the skin, gives the mons pubis a moundlike shape, and protects the pubic symphysis during sexual intercourse.

Labia majora (sing., labium majus): Two folds of skin arising at the mons pubis and extending back to the fourchette, forming a cleft. During puberty the amount of fatty tissue increases, pubic hair grows on lateral surfaces, and sebaceous glands on hairless medial surfaces secrete lubricants. This structure is highly sensitive to temperature, touch, pressure, and pain; it is homologous to the male scrotum; and it protects the inner structures of the vulva.

Labia minora (sing., labium minus): Two smaller, thinner, asymmetric folds of skin within the labia majora that form the clitoral hood (prepuce) and frenulum, then split to enclose the vestibule, and converge near the anus to form the fourchette. The labia minora are hairless, pink, and moist; they are well supplied by nerves, blood vessels, and sebaceous glands that secrete bactericidal fluid with a distinctive odor that lubricates and waterproofs vulvar skin. The labia swell with blood during sexual arousal.

Clitoris: Richly innervated erectile organ between the labia minora. It is a small, cylindric structure having a visible glans and a shaft that lies beneath the skin; the clitoris is homologous to the penis. It secretes smegma, which has a unique odor that may be sexually arousing to the male. Like the penis, the clitoris is a major site of sexual stimulation and orgasm. With sexual arousal, erectile tissue fills with blood, causing the clitoris to enlarge slightly.

Vestibule: An area protected by the labia minora that contains the external opening of the vagina, called the *introitus* or vaginal orifice. A thin, perforated membrane, the *hymen,* may cover the introitus. The vestibule also contains the opening of the urethra, or *urinary meatus* (orifice). These structures are lubricated by two

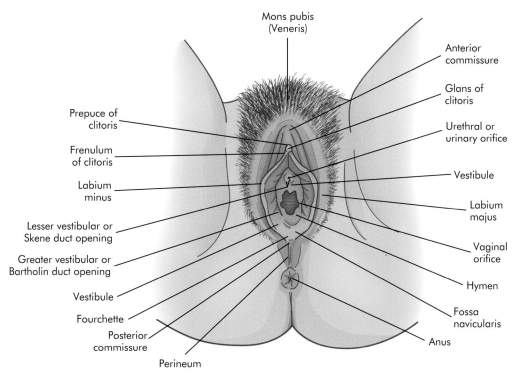

FIGURE 31-4 External Female Genitalia.

pairs of glands: Skene glands and Bartholin glands. The ducts of the *Skene glands* (also called the *lesser vestibular* or *paraurethral glands)* open on both sides of the urinary meatus. The ducts of the *Bartholin glands (greater vestibular* or *vulvovaginal glands)* open on either side of the introitus. In response to sexual stimulation, Bartholin glands secrete mucus that lubricates the inner labial surfaces, as well as enhances the viability and motility of sperm. Skene glands help lubricate the urinary meatus and the vestibule. Secretions from both sets of glands facilitate coitus. In response to sexual excitement, the highly vascular tissue just beneath the vestibule also fills with blood and becomes engorged.

Perineum: An area with less hair, skin, and subcutaneous tissue lying between the vaginal orifice and anus. Unlike the rest of the vulva, this area has little subcutaneous fat so the skin is close to the underlying muscles. The perineum covers the muscular *perineal body,* a fibrous structure that consists of elastic fibers and connective tissue and serves as the common attachment for the bulbocavernosus, external anal sphincter, and levator ani muscles. The perineum varies in length from 2 to 5 cm or more and has elastic properties. The length of the perineum and the elasticity of the perineal body influence tissue resistance and injury during childbirth.

Internal Genitalia
Vagina
The **vagina** is an elastic, fibromuscular canal that is 9 to 10 cm long in a reproductive-age female. It extends up and back from the introitus to the lower portion of the uterus. As Figure 31-5 shows, the vagina lies between the urethra (and part of the bladder) and the rectum. Mucosal secretions from the upper genital organs, menstrual fluids, and products of conception leave the body through the vagina, which also receives the penis during coitus. During sexual excitement, the vagina lengthens and widens and the anterior third becomes congested with blood.

The vaginal wall is composed of four layers:
1. Mucous membrane lining of squamous epithelial cells that thickens and thins in response to hormones, particularly estrogen. The squamous epithelial membrane is continuous with the membrane that covers the lower part of the uterus. In women of reproductive age, the mucosal layer is arranged in transverse wrinkles, or folds, called **rugae** (sing., ruga) that permit stretching during coitus and childbirth
2. Fibrous connective tissue containing numerous blood and lymphatic vessels
3. Smooth muscle
4. Connective tissue and a rich network of blood vessels

The upper part of the vagina surrounds the cervix, the lower end of the uterus (see Figure 31-5). The recessed space around the cervix is called the **fornix** of the vagina. The posterior fornix is "deeper" than the anterior fornix because of the angle at which the cervix meets the vaginal canal. In most women this angle is about 90 degrees. A pouch called the **cul-de-sac** separates the posterior fornix and the rectum.

Its elasticity and relatively sparse nerve supply enhance the vagina's function as the birth canal. During sexual arousal, the vaginal wall becomes engorged with blood, like the labia minora and clitoris. Engorgement pushes some fluid to the surface of the mucosa, enhancing lubrication. The vaginal wall does not contain mucus-secreting glands; rather, secretions drain into the vagina from the endocervical glands or from the Bartholin and Skene glands of the vestibule.

Two factors help to maintain the self-cleansing action of the vagina and to defend it from infection, particularly during the reproductive years. They are (1) an acid-base balance that discourages the proliferation of most pathogenic bacteria and (2) the thickness of the vaginal epithelium. Before puberty, vaginal pH is about 7.0 (neutral) and the vaginal epithelium is thin. At puberty, the pH becomes more acidic (4.0 to 5.0) and the squamous epithelial lining thickens. These changes are maintained until menopause (cessation of menstruation), when

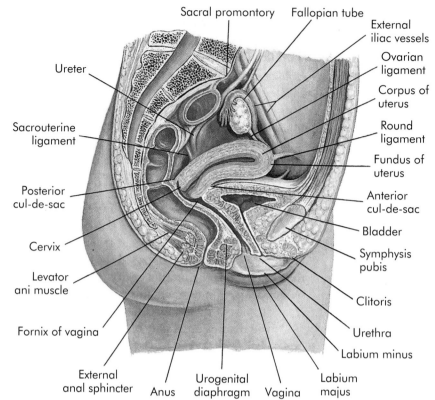

FIGURE 31-5 Internal Female Genitalia and Other Pelvic Organs. (From Seidel HM et al: *Mosby's guide to physical examination,* ed 7, St Louis, 2011, Mosby.)

the pH rises again to more alkaline levels and the epithelium thins. Therefore protection from infection is greatest during the years when a woman is most likely to be sexually active. Both defense factors are greatest when estrogen levels are high and the vagina contains a normal population of *Lactobacillus acidophilus,* a harmless resident bacterium that helps to maintain pH at acidic levels. Any condition that causes vaginal pH to rise, such as douching or use of vaginal sprays or deodorants, low estrogen levels, or destruction of *L. acidophilus* by antibiotics, lowers vaginal defenses against infection.

Uterus

The **uterus** is a hollow, pear-shaped organ whose lower end opens into the vagina. It anchors and protects a fertilized ovum, provides an optimal environment while the ovum develops, and pushes the fetus out at birth. In addition, the uterus plays an important role in sexual response and conception. During sexual excitement, the opening of the lower uterus (the cervix) dilates slightly. At the same time, the uterus increases in size and moves upward and backward, creating a tenting effect in the midvagina that results in the cervix "sitting" in a pool of semen. During orgasm, rhythmic contractions facilitate movement of sperm through the cervical os while also enhancing physical pleasure.

At puberty, the uterus attains its adult size and proportions and descends from the abdomen to the lower pelvis, between the bladder and the rectum (see Figure 31-5). The uterus of a mature, nonpregnant female is approximately 7 to 9 cm long and 6.5 cm wide, with muscular walls 3.5 cm thick.[1] It is held loosely in position by ligaments, peritoneal tissue folds, and the pressure of adjacent organs, especially the urinary bladder, sigmoid colon, and rectum. In most women, the uterus is tipped forward (anteverted) so that it rests on the urinary bladder;

however, it may be tipped backward (retroverted). Various degrees of flexion are normal (Figure 31-6).

The uterus has two major parts: the body, or **corpus,** and the cervix (Figure 31-7). The top of the corpus, above the insertion of the fallopian tubes, is called the **fundus.** The diameter of the uterine cavity is widest at the fundus and narrowest at the **isthmus,** just above the **cervix** (see Figure 31-5). The cervix, or "neck of the uterus," extends from the isthmus to the vagina. The passageway between the upper opening (the internal os) and the lower opening (the external os) of the cervix is called the **endocervical canal** (see Figure 31-7). The entire uterus, like the upper vagina, is innervated exclusively by motor and sensory fibers of the autonomic nervous system.

The uterine wall is composed of three layers (see Figure 31-7). The **perimetrium (parietal peritoneum)** is the outer serous membrane that covers the uterus. The **myometrium** is the thick, muscular middle layer. It is thickest at the fundus, apparently to facilitate birth. The **endometrium,** or uterine lining, is composed of a functional layer (superficial compact layer and spongy middle layer) and a basal layer. The functional layer of the endometrium responds to the sex hormones estrogen and progesterone. Between puberty and menopause, this layer proliferates and is shed monthly. The basal layer, which is attached to the myometrium, regenerates the functional layer after shedding (menstruation).

The endocervical canal does not have an endometrial layer but is lined with columnar epithelial cells. It is continuous with the lining of the outer cervix and vagina, which are lined with squamous epithelial cells. The point where the two types of cells meet is called the *transformation zone,* or **squamous-columnar junction.** The transformation zone is vulnerable to the human papillomavirus, which can lead to cervical dysplasia or carcinoma in situ (see Figure 32-13). Cells of the

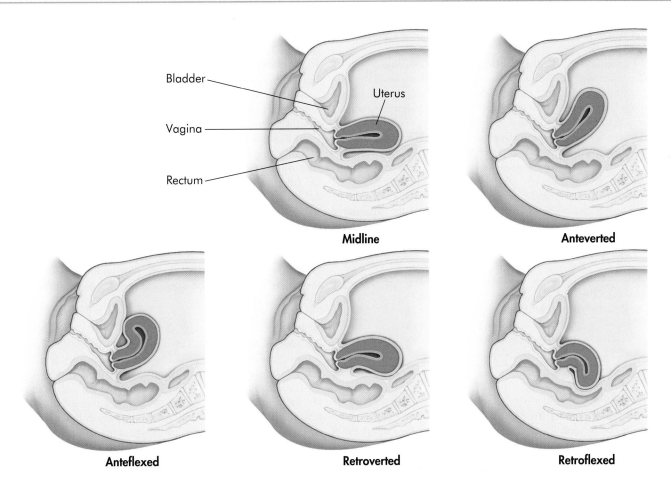

FIGURE 31-6 Uterine Positions.

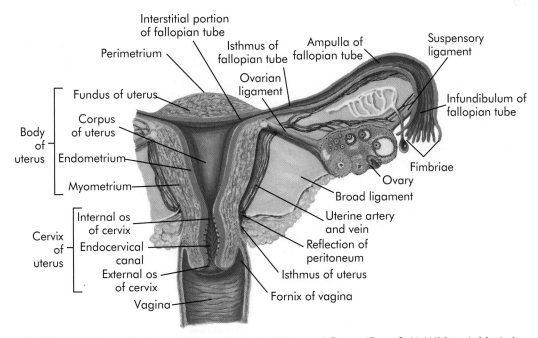

FIGURE 31-7 Cross Section of Uterus, Fallopian Tube, and Ovary. (From Seidel HM et al: *Mosby's guide to physical examination,* ed 7, St Louis, 2011, Mosby.)

transformation zone are removed for examination during a Papanicolaou (Pap) smear.[1]

The cervix acts as a mechanical barrier to infectious microorganisms from the vagina. The external cervical os is a very small opening that contains thick, sticky mucus (the mucous "plug") during the luteal phase of the menstrual cycle and throughout pregnancy. During ovulation, the mucus changes under the influence of estrogen and forms watery strands, or **spinnbarkeit mucus,** to facilitate the transport of sperm into the uterus. In addition, the downward flow of cervical secretions moves microorganisms away from the cervix and uterus. In women of reproductive age, the pH of these secretions is inhospitable to many bacteria. Further, mucosal secretions contain enzymes and antibodies (mostly immunoglobulin A [IgA]) of the secretory immune system. Uterine pathophysiologic disorders include infection, displacement of the uterus within the pelvis, benign growths of the uterine wall, and cancer.

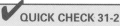

QUICK CHECK 31-2
1. Name three functions of the uterus.
2. Where are the Bartholin glands located? What is their function?
3. What is the name of the cells in which cervical cancer is most likely to grow?

Fallopian Tubes

The two **fallopian tubes** (oviducts, **uterine tubes**) enter the uterus bilaterally just beneath the fundus (see Figure 31-7). They direct the ova from the spaces around the ovaries to the uterus. From the uterus,

the fallopian tubes curve up and over the two ovaries. Each tube is 8 to 12 cm long and about 1 cm in diameter, except at its ovarian end, which resembles the bell of a trumpet and is fringed or fimbriated (**infundibulum**). The **fimbriae** (fringes) move, creating a current that draws the ovum into the infundibulum. Once the ovum enters the fallopian tube, cilia (hairlike structures) and peristalsis (muscle contractions) keep it moving toward the uterus.

The ampulla, or distal third, of the fallopian tube is the usual site of fertilization (see Figure 31-7). Sperm released into the vagina travel upward through the endocervical canal and uterine cavity and enter the fallopian tubes. If an ovum is present in either tube, fertilization can occur. Whether or not the ovum encounters sperm, it continues to travel through the fallopian tube to the uterus. If fertilized, the ovum (then called a *blastocyst*) implants itself in the endometrial layer of the uterine wall. If not fertilized, the ovum fragments and leaves the uterus with menstrual fluids. Disorders that affect the fallopian tubes (e.g., congenital malformations, infection, and inflammation) block the path of both sperm and ovum and may cause infertility or ectopic (tubal) pregnancy.

Ovaries

The **ovaries,** the female gonads, are the primary female reproductive organs (Figure 31-8). Their two main functions are secretion of female sex hormones and development and release of female gametes, or ova.

The almond-shaped ovaries are located on both sides of the uterus and are suspended and supported by the mesovarium portions of the broad ligament, ovarian ligaments, and suspensory ligaments (see Figure 31-7). The ovaries are smaller than their male homologs, the testes. In women of reproductive age, each ovary is 3 to 5 cm long, 2.5 cm

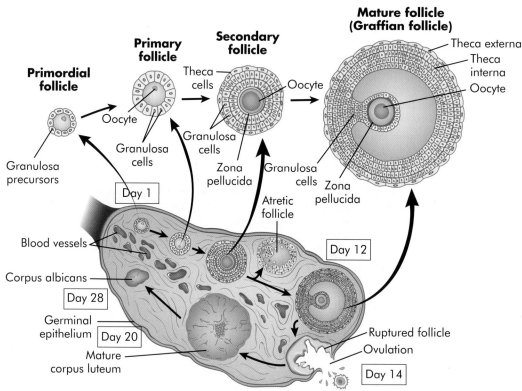

FIGURE 31-8 Cross Section of Ovary and Development of an Ovarian Follicle. Schematic representation (not to scale) of the structure of the ovary, showing the various stages in the development of the follicle and its successor structure, the corpus luteum. (Adapted from Berne RM, Levy MN, editors: *Physiology,* ed 5, St Louis, 2003, Mosby.)

wide, and 2 cm thick and weighs 4 to 8 g. Size and weight vary slightly during each phase of the menstrual cycle (see p. 784).

At birth, the cortex of each ovary contains approximately 1 million ova within primordial (immature) ovarian follicles. By puberty, the number ranges between 300,000 and 500,000, and some of the follicles and the ova within them begin to mature. Between puberty and menopause, the ovarian cortex always contains follicles and ova in various stages of development (primary and secondary follicles). Once every menstrual cycle (about every 28 days), one of the follicles reaches maturation and discharges its ovum through the ovary's outer covering, the germinal epithelium. During the reproductive years, 400 to 500 ovarian follicles mature completely and release an ovum (ovulation). The rest either fail to develop at all or degenerate without maturing completely and are known as atretic follicles[1] (see Figure 31-8).

Having ejected a mature ovum, the follicle develops into another structure, the corpus luteum (see Figure 31-8). If fertilization occurs, the corpus luteum enlarges and begins to secrete hormones that maintain and support pregnancy. If fertilization does not occur, the corpus luteum secretes these hormones for approximately 14 days and then degenerates, which triggers the maturation of another follicle. The ovarian cycle—the process of follicular maturation, ovulation, corpus luteum development, and corpus luteum degeneration—is continuous from puberty to menopause, except during pregnancy or hormonal contraceptive use. At menopause, this process ceases and the ovaries atrophy to the point that they cannot be felt during a pelvic examination.

Sex hormones are secreted by cells present within the ovarian cortex, including two types of cells in the ovarian follicle—theca cells (produce androgens that migrate to granulosa cells) and granulosa cells (convert androgens to estradiol)—and cells of the corpus luteum (secrete primarily progesterone and estrogen and inhibin) (see Figure 31-8). These cells all contain receptors for the gonadotropins (LH, FSH) or for the sex hormones, which are discussed in the next section.

Female Sex Hormones

The sex hormones are all steroid hormones and are synthesized from cholesterol (see Chapter 17). Both male and female sex hormones are present in all adults. However, the female body contains low levels of testosterone and other androgens, and the male body contains low levels of estrogen. Individual effects of sex hormones depend on the amount and concentration in the blood.

Estrogens and Androgens

Estrogen is a generic term for any of three similar hormones: estradiol, estrone, and estriol. Estradiol (E2) is the most potent and plentiful of the three and is principally produced (95%) by the ovaries (ovarian follicle and corpus luteum). Limited amounts are secreted by the cortices of the adrenal glands and the placenta during pregnancy. Androgens are converted to estrone in ovarian and peripheral adipose tissue; estriol is the peripheral metabolite of estrone and estradiol.

Estrogen has numerous biologic effects, many of which involve interactions with other hormones, and is needed for maturation of reproductive organs, development of secondary sex characteristics, growth, and maintenance of pregnancy, as well as the many nonreproductive effects of estrogen including maintenance of bone, skin and systemic organ function (see Table 31-1 and Box 31-1). After menopause, the ovaries dramatically reduce production of estradiol and secretion of estrone also is markedly diminished (see Aging and the Female Reproductive System p. 794). At this time, the majority of estrogen is derived from extraovarian and extraglandular production of estrones.[7] Disturbances of estrogen production can be

---

BOX 31-1	**SUMMARY OF NONREPRODUCTIVE EFFECTS OF ESTROGEN**

- Estrogens (including estrone, estradiol, estriol) function through estrogen receptors alpha and beta.
- Maintains bone density.
- Acts in liver to decrease cholesterol level, increase high-density lipoprotein (HDL) level, and decrease low-density lipoprotein (LDL) level (antiatherosclerotic); promotes fat deposition.
- Maintains nervous system (neurotrophic and neuroprotective); facilitates memory and cognition.
- Increases collagen content, dermal thickness, elasticity, water content, and healing ability of skin.
- Protects against chronic kidney disease in individuals without diabetes.
- Prevents vascular injury and early atheroma formation through endothelial mechanisms.
- Inhibits platelet adhesiveness.
- Promotes inflammation and has variable effects on immunity.
- Estrogen associated with pregnancy or use in contraceptive pills promotes clotting and increased risk of thromboembolism.

Data from Arevalo MA et al: Actions of estrogens on glial cells: implications for neuroprotection, *Biochim Biophys Acta* 1800(10):1106–1112, 2010; Arnal JF et al: Estrogen receptors and endothelium, *Arterioscler Thromb Vasc Biol* 30(8):1506–1512, 2010; Cunningham M, Gilkeson G: Estrogen receptors in immunity and autoimmunity, *Clin Rev Allergy Immunol* 40(1):66–73, 2011; Doublier S et al: Estrogens and progression of diabetic kidney damage, *Curr Diabetes Rev* 7(1):28–34, 2011; Farage MA, Neill S, MacLean AB: Physiological changes associated with the menstrual cycle: a review, *Obstet Gynecol Surv* 64(1):58–72, 2009; Gilliver SC: Sex steroids as inflammatory regulators, *J Steroid Biochem Mol Biol* 120(2–3):105–115, 2010; Komukai K, Mochizuki S, Yoshimura M: Gender and the renin-angiotensin-aldosterone system, *Fundam Clin Pharmacol* 24(6):687–698, 2010.

---

caused by abnormalities that affect (1) secretion of GnRH by the hypothalamus, (2) secretion of LH or FSH by the anterior pituitary, (3) mechanisms of hormonal feedback, or (4) structural integrity of the ovaries. Estrogen's role in the menstrual cycle is described on p. 786.

Although androgens are primarily male sex hormones produced in the testes, small amounts are produced in the adrenal cortex in both men and women, and in the ovaries in women. Some androgens (dehydroepiandrosterone and its metabolite androstenedione) are precursors of estrogens (estrone, estradiol) (see Table 31-1).

Progesterone

Luteinizing hormone (LH) from the anterior pituitary stimulates the corpus luteum to secrete progesterone, the second major female sex hormone. With estrogen, progesterone controls the ovarian-menstrual cycle. LH surge occurs when there is a peak level of estrogen, about 24 to 36 hours before ovulation. LH promotes luteinization of the granulosa in the dominant follicle, resulting in progesterone production and the development of blood vessels and connective tissue. During the follicular phase, the ovary and adrenal glands each contribute approximately 50% of the progesterone production. Conversely, large amounts are cyclically secreted from the ovary while the corpus luteum is active for about 9 to 13 days after ovulation. The complementary and opposing effects of progesterone and estrogen are listed in Table 31-2. Progesterone secreted by the corpus luteum stimulates the thickened

TABLE 31-2 COMPLEMENTARY AND OPPOSING EFFECTS OF ESTROGEN AND PROGESTERONE

STRUCTURE	EFFECT OF ESTROGEN	EFFECT OF PROGESTERONE
Vaginal mucosa	Proliferation of squamous epithelium; increase in glycogen content of cells; layering (cornification) of cells	Thinning of squamous epithelium; decornification
Cervical mucosa	Production of abundant fluid secretions that favor survival and enhance motility of sperm	Production of thick, sticky secretions that tend to plug cervical os
Fallopian tube	Increase of motility and ciliary action	Decrease of motility and ciliary action
Uterine muscle	Increase of blood flow; increase of contractile proteins; increase of uterine muscle and myometrial excitability to action potential; increase of sensitization to oxytocin	Relaxation of myometrium; decrease of sensitization to oxytocin
Endometrium	Stimulation of growth; increase in number of progesterone receptors	Activation of glands and blood vessels; decrease in number of estrogen receptors
Breasts	Growth of ducts; promotion of prolactin effects	Growth of lobules and alveoli; inhibition of prolactin effects

endometrium to become more complex in preparation for implantation of a blastocyte. If conception and implantation do occur, the corpus luteum persists and secretes progesterone (and estrogen) until the placenta is well established at approximately 8 to 10 weeks' gestation and undertakes progesterone production.

Progesterone is sometimes called the *hormone of pregnancy.* Progesterone's effects in pregnancy include: (1) maintaining the thickened endometrium; (2) relaxing smooth muscle in the myometrium, which prevents premature contractions and helps the uterus to expand; (3) thickening (hypertrophy) the myometrium, which prepares it for the muscular work of labor; (4) promoting growth of lobules and alveoli in the breast in preparation for lactation[8] but preventing lactation until the fetus is born; (5) preventing additional maturation of ova by suppressing FSH and LH, thereby stopping the menstrual cycle; and (6) providing immune modulation, allowing tolerance against fetal antigens (the mother's immune system does not attack the fetus).[9]

✔ QUICK CHECK 31-3

1. What hormones does the ovary produce?
2. Why is the ovary the most essential female reproductive organ?

Menstrual Cycle

In addition to pregnancy, the obvious manifestation of female reproductive functioning is menstrual bleeding (the menses), which starts with **menarche** (first menstruation) and ends with **menopause** (cessation of menstrual flow for 1 year). In the United States, the median age of first menstruation is 12.14 years in black females, 12.25 years in Latina or Hispanic females, and 12.6 years in white females, with a range from 9 to 13.5 years.[10] Menarche appears to be related to body weight, especially percentage of body fat (ratio of fat to lean tissue), which may trigger a change in the metabolic rate and lead to hormonal changes associated with early menarche.[11]

There is an increased sensitivity to leptin (regulates appetite and energy metabolism) during puberty and, in theory, the adolescent consumes more calories to meet the caloric needs of the pubertal growth spurt.[12] At first, cycles are anovulatory and may vary in length from 10 to 60 days or more. As adolescence proceeds, regular patterns of menstruation and ovulation are established at intervals ranging between 25 and 35 days.[13] Menstruation continues to recur in a recognizable and characteristic pattern during adulthood, with the length of the menstrual cycle varying considerably among women. The commonly accepted cycle average is 28 (25 to 30) days, with rhythmic intervals of 21 to 35 days considered normal (see Figure 31-9). Approximately 2 to 8 years before menopause, cycles begin to lengthen again. Menstrual cyclicity and regular ovulation are dependent on (1) the activity of GnRH; (2) the initial pituitary secretion of the gonadotropin FSH; and (3) the estrogen (estradiol) positive feedback mechanism for preovulatory FSH and LH surge, oocyte maturation, corpus luteum formation, and progesterone production.[14]

Phases of the Menstrual Cycle

The menstrual cycle (Figure 31-9) consists of ovulation, which occurs in three phases: the follicular/proliferative phase (postmenstrual); the luteal/secretory phase (premenstrual); and the ischemic phase (menstrual), known as *menstruation.* During ovulation, an ovum from a mature ovarian follicle is released.

During **menstruation (menses),** the functional layer of the endometrium disintegrates and is discharged through the vagina. Menstruation is followed by the **follicular/proliferative phase.** This phase is named for two simultaneous processes: maturation of an ovarian follicle and proliferation of the endometrium (see Figure 31-9). During this phase, GnRH and a balance between activin and inhibin levels from the granulosa cells contribute to the increase of FSH level, which stimulates a number of follicles. The pulsatile secretion of FSH from the anterior pituitary gland rescues a dominant ovarian follicle from apoptosis by days 5 to 7 of the cycle. Together estrogen and FSH increase the number of FSH receptors in the granulosa cells of the primary follicle, making them more sensitive to FSH. FSH and estrogen combine to induce production of LH receptors on the granulosa cells, thus promoting LH stimulation to combine with FSH stimulation and cause a more rapid secretion of follicular estrogen. As estrogen level increases, FSH level drops because of an increase in inhibin-B secreted by the granulosa cells in the dominant follicle. This drop in FSH concentration decreases the growth of less developed follicles (see Figure 31-8). Estrogen causes cells of the endometrium to proliferate and stimulates production of LH. A surge in the levels of both FSH and LH is required for final follicular growth and ovulation.

Ovulation marks the beginning of the **luteal/secretory phase** of the menstrual cycle. The ovarian follicle begins its transformation into a corpus luteum (see Figure 31-8), hence the name *luteal phase.* Pulsatile

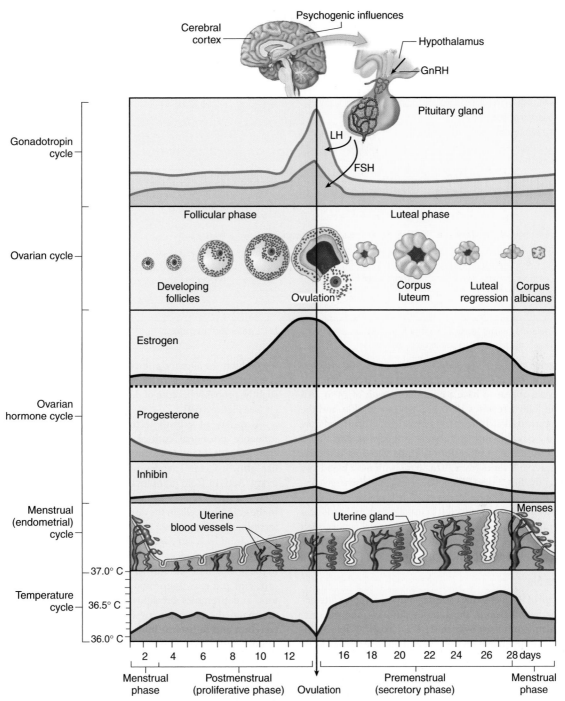

FIGURE 31-9 Female Reproductive Cycles. This figure illustrates the interrelationships among the cerebral, hypothalamic, pituitary, ovarian, and uterine functions throughout a standard 28-day menstrual cycle. The variations in basal body temperature are also illustrated. (From Patton KT, Thibodeau GA: *Anatomy & physiology*, ed 7, St Louis, 2010, Mosby.)

secretion of LH from the anterior pituitary stimulates the corpus luteum to secrete progesterone, which in turn initiates the secretory phase of endometrial development. Glands and blood vessels in the endometrium branch and curl throughout the functional layer, and the glands begin to secrete a thin, glycogen-containing fluid, hence the name *secretory phase*. If conception occurs, the nutrient-laden endometrium is ready for implantation. Human chorionic gonadotropin (hCG) is secreted 3 days after fertilization by the blastocytes and

maintains the corpus luteum once implantation occurs at about day 6 or 7. hCG can be detected in maternal blood and urine 8 to 10 days after ovulation. The production of estrogen and progesterone will continue until the placenta can adequately maintain hormonal production. If conception and implantation do not occur, the corpus luteum degenerates and ceases its production of progesterone and estrogen. Without progesterone or estrogen to maintain it, the endometrium enters the ischemic ("blood-starved") phase and disintegrates, hence the name

TABLE 31-3 HORMONAL FEEDBACK MECHANISM IN THE MENSTRUAL CYCLE

PHASE OF CYCLE AND OVARIAN HORMONE LEVELS	FEEDBACK TO HYPOTHALAMUS AND ANTERIOR PITUITARY	RESULTANT GNRH, FSH, AND LH LEVELS	OVARIAN AND MENSTRUAL EVENTS
Early follicular phase: estrogen levels low; minute amount of progesterone secreted	Negative and inhibitory	All low	Ovarian follicle develops; endometrium proliferates
Late follicular (preovulatory) phase: estrogen levels high; progesterone level increases with small surge before ovulation	Positive and stimulatory	All surge; LH dominates	Process of ovulation begins; endometrial proliferation complete
Ovulatory phase: estrogen levels dip; progesterone levels begin to rise	Negative and inhibitory	All fall sharply	Corpus luteum begins to develop; endometrium enters secretory phase
Early luteal phase: estrogen and progesterone levels high; progesterone dominates	Negative and inhibitory	All continue to decline, but gradually	Corpus luteum fully developed; endometrium ready for implantation
Late luteal phase: estrogen and progesterone levels fall sharply	Negative and inhibitory; feedback lessens slightly	All rise slightly	Corpus luteum regresses; endometrium disintegrates; menstruation begins
Menstrual phase: estrogens levels low; minute amount of progesterone secreted	Negative and inhibitory	All low	More ovarian follicles begin to develop; functional layer of endometrium is shed

FSH, Follicle-stimulating hormone; *GnRH,* gonadotropin-releasing hormone; *LH,* luteinizing hormone.

ischemic/menstrual phase. Then menstruation occurs, marking the beginning of another cycle.

Ovulatory cycles appear to have a minimum length of 24 to 26.5 days: the ovarian follicle requires 10 to 12.5 days to develop, and the luteal phase appears fixed at 14 days (±3 days). Menstrual blood flow usually lasts 3 to 7 days but may last as long as 8 days or stop after 2 days and still be considered within normal limits. Bleeding is consistently scant to heavy and varies from 30 to 80 ml, with most blood loss occurring during the first 3 days of menses. Menstrual discharge consists of blood, mucus, and desquamated endometrial tissue and does not clot under normal circumstances. It is usually dark and produces a characteristic musty odor on oxidation. Environmental factors, such as severe emotional stress, illness, malnutrition, obesity, and seasonal variation, may affect the length of the menstrual cycle.[15-17]

Hormonal Controls

Hormonal control of the menstrual cycle depends on complex interactions among the hypothalamus, the anterior pituitary, and the ovaries (or hypothalamic-pituitary-ovarian [H-P-O] axis)[18] (Table 31-3). Hormonal control is dependent on negative and positive ovarian feedback mechanisms. GnRH controls the gonadotropin production of FSH and LH, and the constant and pulsatile release of GnRH is critical to the timing of the menstrual cycle. GnRH is secreted by the hypothalamus into the hypophysial portal system and travels to the anterior pituitary, where it stimulates the secretion of FSH and LH. FSH and LH are released from the anterior pituitary in pulses that correspond to the secretion of GnRH.

During the early follicular phase, estrogen levels rise steadily and, through negative feedback, suppress FSH production and positively increase the production of LH. During the late follicular phase, the preovulatory rise in progesterone level facilitates a positive feedback loop whereby estrogen levels begin to increase, stimulating a surge of FSH and LH secretion from the anterior pituitary. The midcycle surge of LH and FSH induces ovulation. A nonsteroidal ovarian factor, gonadotropin surge-attenuating factor (GnSAF), may antagonize the effect of estrogen on the pituitary and regulate the surge of LH at midcycle.[19] Rising estrogen and progesterone levels during the luteal phase

may inhibit the anterior pituitary and thus reduce LH and FSH secretion. Just before menstruation, FSH and LH levels begin to increase slightly, probably because of declining estrogen and progesterone levels (see Figure 31-9).

A variety of growth factors and autocrine/paracrine peptides influence hormonal control and follicular response. During the early follicular stage, FSH stimulates FSH and LH receptors, insulin-like growth factor 1, and production of inhibin and activin in the ovary. Activin from granulosa cells stimulates the secretion of FSH, increases the pituitary response to GnRH, and increases FSH binding in the granulosa cells in the dominant follicle. FSH stimulates inhibin secretion from granulosa cells and it, in turn, suppresses FSH synthesis. Inhibin B is primarily secreted in the follicular phase of the cycle but sharply spikes when ovulation occurs. Inhibin A is secreted in the luteal phase and further suppresses FSH. Inhibin also restrains prolactin and growth hormone release, interferes with GnRH receptors, and promotes breakdown of intracellular gonadotropins. In summary, the balance between activin and inhibin regulates FSH secretion and follistatin inhibits activin and boosts inhibin activity. Inhibin and activin also regulate LH stimulation of androgen synthesis in theca cells.[20] Figure 31-9 depicts fluctuating estrogen, progesterone, gonadotropin, and inhibin levels. Research continues to advance understanding of the function and structural complexity of these polypeptides and their interaction with GnRH, gonadotropins, and sex hormones.

Ovarian Cycle

By stimulating follicles, gonadotropins initiate their growth and maturation. The most important hormonal event is a rise in FSH level. The decline in luteal phase estrogen, progesterone, and inhibin secretion allows FSH level to rise; concurrently there is a slight increase in LH levels (see Figure 31-9). FSH stimulates granulosa cell growth and initiates estrogen production in these cells. At this time, a group of ovarian follicles is recruited and begins to mature; the exact number depends on the remaining pool of inactive follicles. As the follicles mature, granulosa cells multiply, increasing estradiol secretion. Within a few days of the cycle, one follicle becomes dominant and the others atrophy.

The mechanism for follicular recruitment or dominance is unknown. The dominant follicle begins to secrete progressively larger amounts of estrogen (estradiol), which exerts an increase in GnRH receptor concentration and an increase in pituitary sensitivity to GnRH, creating a positive feedback effect that causes a FSH and LH surge. Ovulation occurs 1 to 2 hours before the final progesterone surge, or about 12 to 36 hours after the onset of the FSH and LH surge. Progesterone, proteolytic enzymes, and prostaglandins trigger mechanisms controlling follicular rupture and release of the ovum.[21]

The FSH and LH surge also transforms the granulosa cells of the ovulatory follicle into the corpus luteum. The corpus luteum secretes both estrogen and progesterone in amounts that depend, in part, on adequate development of the follicle before ovulation. Progesterone acts both centrally and locally within the ovary to suppress new follicular growth during the early to midluteal phases. If pregnancy does not occur, the corpus luteum persists for 11 to 14 days and then regresses and eventually disappears. An increase in pulse frequency of GnRH from a low level reactivates hormonal control of the menstrual cycle.

Uterine Phases

Uterine phases of the menstrual cycle—the proliferative phase, the secretory phase, and menstruation—involve the cyclic changes that occur in the endometrium controlled by estrogen and progesterone. Hormonal effects are influenced by the presence of receptors and numerous growth factors, peptides, and enzymes that act as intermediaries between the sex steroids and the endometrium.[22] During the midfollicular phase, increasing levels of estrogen contribute to endometrial repair and proliferation, thus increasing endometrial thickness. Once ovulation occurs and serum progesterone levels increase, the endometrial tissue develops secretory characteristics. If implantation of a fertilized ovum does not take place, endometrial tissue begins to break down approximately 11 days after ovulation (ischemic phase of menstruation; see Figure 31-9). Shedding of tissue (menstrual bleeding) begins about 14 days after ovulation.

Cervical mucus also undergoes cyclic changes. During the proliferative phase, the cervical mucus is thin and watery. Peak estrogen levels occur just before ovulation and maximally stimulate the cervical glands to produce mucus. Cervical mucus becomes abundant and more elastic (spinnbarkeit). Increasing estrogen levels apparently contribute to the development of tiny channels in cervical mucus, providing access for sperm into the interior of the uterus. Changes in the consistency of cervical mucus can be used to identify fertile intervals.[23]

Vaginal Response

The vaginal endothelium also responds to the cyclic hormonal changes of the menstrual cycle. Under the influence of estrogen, cells of the vaginal epithelium grow maximally during the follicular/proliferative phase. After ovulation, layers of keratinized cells overgrow the basal epithelium, a process known as **cornification.** Near the end of the luteal phase, leukocytes invade vaginal epithelium, removing the outer layers in a process termed **decornification.**

Body Temperature

Basal body temperature (BBT) undergoes characteristic biphasic changes during menstrual cycles in which ovulation occurs. During the follicular phase, the BBT fluctuates around 98° F (37° C). During the luteal phase, the average temperature increases by 0.4° to 1.0° F (0.2° to 0.5° C). At the end of the luteal phase, 1 to 3 days before the onset of menstruation, BBT declines to follicular-phase levels. The shift in temperature is related to ovulation, corpus luteum formation, and increased serum progesterone levels. Progesterone probably acts on the thermoregulatory center of the hypothalamus to increase body temperature. Changes in BBT are used to document ovulatory cycles but when used alone are not the best method to predict the exact timing of ovulation.[24]

> ✔ **QUICK CHECK 31-4**
> 1. Why does menstruation occur?
> 2. What event is associated with the luteal/secretory phase of the menstrual cycle?

STRUCTURE AND FUNCTION OF THE BREAST

The **breasts** are modified sebaceous glands that lie on the ventral surface of the thorax, within the superficial fascia of the chest wall. They extend vertically from the second rib to the sixth or seventh intercostal

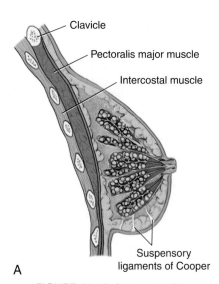
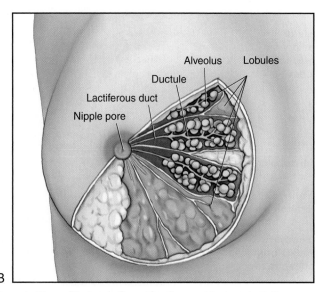

FIGURE 31-10 Schematic Diagram of Breast. (From Riodan J: *Breastfeeding and human lactation,* ed 4, Sudbury, Mass, 2010, Jones and Bartlett.)

space and laterally from the side of the sternum to the midaxillary line. Breast tissue also may extend into the axilla; this tissue is known as the *tail of Spence.*

Female Breast

The female breast is composed of 15 to 20 pyramid-shaped lobes that are separated and supported by Cooper ligaments (Figure 31-10). Each lobe contains 20 to 40 lobules (alveoli), which subdivide further into many functional units called **acini** (sing., acinus). Each acinus is lined with a layer of epithelial cells capable of secreting milk and a layer of subepithelial cells capable of contracting to squeeze milk from the acinus. The acini empty into a network of lobular collecting ducts, which empty into interlobular collecting and ejecting ducts. These ducts reach the skin through openings (pores) in the nipple. The lobes and lobules are surrounded and separated by muscle strands and fatty connective tissue. The amount of fatty connective tissue varies among individuals, depending on weight and genetic and endocrine factors, and contributes to the diversity of breast size and shape and the function of the mammary epithelium.[25]

An extensive capillary network surrounds the acini and is supplied by the internal and lateral thoracic arteries and the intercostal arteries. Venous return follows arterial supply, with relatively rapid emptying into the superior vena cava. The breasts receive sensory innervation from branches of the second through sixth intercostal nerves and the cervical plexus. This accounts for the fact that breast pain may be referred to the chest, back, scapula, medial arm, and neck. Lymphatic drainage of the breast occurs largely through axillary nodes, but there may be predominance of superficial mammary routes with asymmetry between breasts of each side[26] (Figure 31-11).

The **nipple** is a pigmented cylindric structure usually located at the fourth or fifth intercostal space. On its surface lie multiple openings, one from each lobe. It measures 0.5 to 1.3 cm in diameter and is approximately 10 to 12 mm in height when erect. The **areola** is the pigmented circular area around the nipple. It may be 15 to 60 mm in diameter. A number of sebaceous glands, the **glands of Montgomery,** are located within the areola and aid in lubrication of the nipple during lactation. The nipple and areola contain smooth muscles, which receive motor innervation from the sympathetic nervous system. Sexual stimulation, breast-feeding, and exposure to cold cause the nipple to become erect.

The fetal and early postnatal development of breast tissue does not depend on hormones, although fetal breast tissue does become progressively responsive to hormonal stimulation. During childhood, breast growth is latent and growth of the nipple and areola keeps pace with body surface growth. At the onset of puberty in the female, estrogen secretion stimulates mammary growth. Breast development, or thelarche, is usually the first sign of puberty in the female. Full differentiation and development of breast tissue are mediated by several hormones, including estrogen, progesterone, prolactin, growth hormone, thyroid and parathyroid hormones, insulin, and cortisol.

During the reproductive years, the breast undergoes cyclic changes in response to changes in the levels of estrogen and progesterone associated with the menstrual cycle. Estrogen promotes development of the lobular ducts; progesterone stimulates development of cells lining the acini. Lactation (milk production) occurs after childbirth in response to increased levels of prolactin. Prolactin secretion, in turn, increases by continued breast-feeding. **Oxytocin,** another hormone released after delivery, controls milk ejection (let down) from acini cells. During the follicular/proliferative phase of the menstrual cycle, high estradiol levels increase the vascularity of breast tissue and stimulate

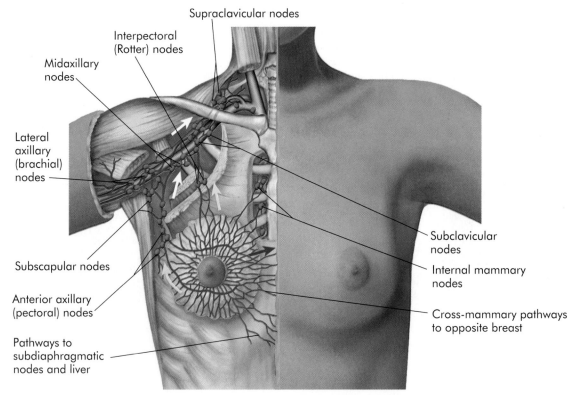

FIGURE 31-11 Lymphatic Drainage of the Female Breast. (From Seidel HM et al: *Mosby's guide to physical examination,* ed 7, St Louis, 2011, Mosby.)

proliferation of ductal and acinar tissue. This effect is sustained into the luteal/secretory phase of the cycle. During this phase, progesterone levels increase and contribute to the breast changes induced by estradiol. Specific effects of progesterone include dilation of the ducts and conversion of the acinar cells into secretory cells. Most women experience some degree of premenstrual breast fullness, tenderness, and increased breast nodularity. Breast volume may increase as much as 10 to 30 ml. Because the length of the menstrual cycle does not allow for complete regression of new cell growth, breast growth continues at a slow rate until approximately 35 years of age. Because of the cyclic changes that occur in breast tissue, breast examination should be conducted at the conclusion of or a few days after the menstrual cycle, when hormonal effects are minimal and breasts are at their smallest.

The function of the female breast is primarily to provide a source of nourishment for the newborn. Physiologically, breast milk is the most appropriate nourishment for newborns. Not only does its composition change over time to meet the changing digestive capabilities and nutritional requirements of the infant, but also breast milk contains specific immunoglobulins, especially IgA, and nonspecific antimicrobial factors, such as lysosomes and lactoferrin, that protect the infant against infection. During lactation, high prolactin levels interfere with hypothalamic-pituitary hormones that stimulate ovulation. This mechanism suppresses the menstrual cycle and can prevent ovulation.[27] In many parts of the world (underdeveloped or Third World countries), breast-feeding is the major means of contraception (lactational amenorrhea method.)[28] However, it is not absolute that ovulation will not occur, and this method will not assure that pregnancy will not occur. Breasts are also a source of pleasurable sexual sensation and in Western cultures have become a sexual symbol.

Male Breast

Until puberty, development of the male breast is similar to that of the female breast. In the absence of sufficiently high levels of estrogen and progesterone, the male breast does not develop any further. The normal male breast consists of a small, underdeveloped nipple; some fatty and fibrous tissue; and a few ductlike structures in the subareolar area. The male breast may appear enlarged in obese men because of accumulation of fatty tissue. During puberty, some males experience gynecomastia (benign proliferation of male breast glandular tissue), a condition in which the breasts enlarge temporarily as a result of hormonal fluctuations.[29]

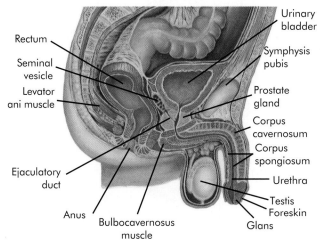

FIGURE 31-12 Structure of the Male Reproductive Organs. (From Seidel HM et al: *Mosby's guide to physical examination,* ed 7, St Louis, 2011, Mosby.)

THE MALE REPRODUCTIVE SYSTEM

In men, the external genitalia perform the major functions of reproduction. Sperm are produced in the male gonads and the testes, and delivered by the penis. The internal male genitalia have a more accessory function. They consist of conducting tubes and fluid-producing glands, all of which aid in the transport of sperm from the testes to the urethral opening of the penis. The male reproductive and urinary structures are shown in Figure 31-12.

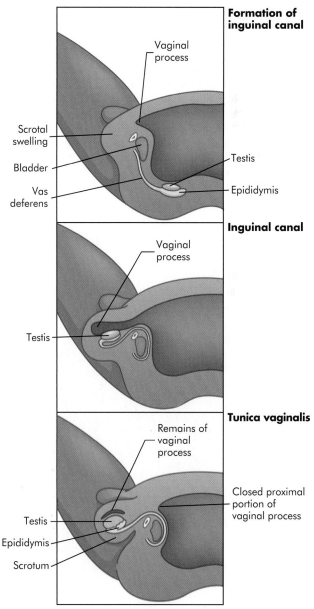

FIGURE 31-13 Descent of a Testis. The testes descend from the abdominal cavity to the scrotum during the last 3 months of fetal development.

External Genitalia
Testes

The testes are the essential organs of male reproduction. Like the ovaries, the testes have two functions: (1) production of gametes (i.e., sperm) and (2) production of sex hormones (i.e., androgens and testosterone).

During embryonic and fetal life, the testes develop within the abdomen (see Figure 31-1). About 3 months before birth, the testes start to descend toward the developing scrotum. About 1 month before birth, they enter twin passageways called **inguinal canals.** The inguinal canals are vaginal processes created by outpouchings of the peritoneum (lining of the abdominal cavity). The descent of a testis is shown in Figure 31-13. When descent is complete, the abdominal end of each vaginal process closes and the inguinal canal disappears. Failure of the testes to descend through the inguinal canal is known as cryptorchidism. The scrotal end of each vaginal process becomes the outer covering of the testis, the **tunica vaginalis.**

Figure 31-14 shows a sagittal section of a mature testis. The adult **testis** is oval and varies considerably in length (3 to 6 cm), width (2 to 3.5 cm), depth (3 to 4 cm), and weight (10 to 40 g). The testis is almost entirely surrounded by the tunica vaginalis, which separates the testis from the scrotal wall, and the **tunica albuginea.** Inward extensions of the tunica albuginea separate the testis into about 250 compartments, or lobules, each of which contains several tortuously coiled ducts called **seminiferous tubules.** Sperm are produced in these tubules. (Sperm production, termed *spermatogenesis,* is described on pp. 792-793.) Tissue surrounding these ducts contains **Leydig cells,** which occur in clusters and produce androgens, chiefly testosterone.

The two ends of each seminiferous tubule join and leave the lobule through the **tubulus rectus,** which leads to the central portion of the testis, the **rete testis.** The sperm then move through the **efferent tubules,** or vasa efferentia, to the epididymis, where they mature.

The testes are innervated by adrenergic fibers whose sole function apparently is to regulate blood flow to the Leydig cells. Arterial blood from the internal spermatic and differential arteries flows over the surface of the testes before entering the parenchyma (functional tissues). Surface flow cools the blood to temperatures that promote spermatogenesis, approximately 1° to 2° C below body core temperature.[30] Additionally, the testes are suspended outside the pelvic cavity to facilitate cooling.

Epididymis

The **epididymis** (pl., epididymides) is a comma-shaped structure that curves over the posterior portion of each testis (see Figure 31-14). It consists of a single, 60- to 70-cm, densely packed and markedly coiled duct measuring 5 cm in length. The epididymis has structural and physiologic functions. Its structural function is to conduct sperm from the efferent tubules to the vas deferens, whereas physiologic functions include sperm maturation, mobility, and fertility. When sperm enter the head of the epididymis, they are not fully mature or motile, nor can they fertilize an ovum. During the 12 days (or more) sperm take to travel the length of the epididymis, they receive nutrients and testosterone and their capacity for fertilization is enhanced.[31]

After traveling the length of the epididymis, sperm are stored in the epididymal tail and vas deferens. The **vas deferens** is a duct with muscular layers capable of powerful peristalsis that transports sperm toward the urethra. The vas deferens enters the pelvic cavity through the spermatic cord (see Figure 31-14).

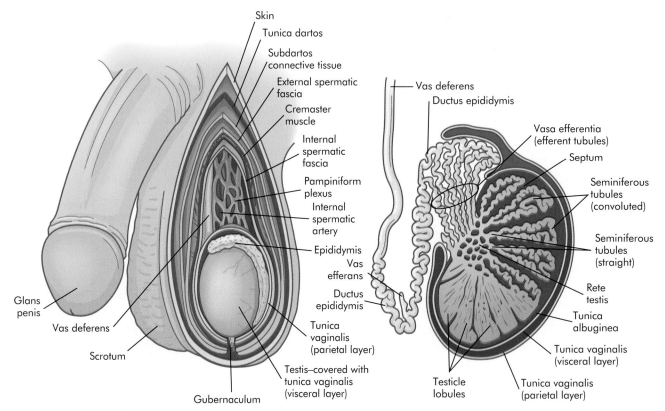

Skin
Tunica dartos
Subdartos connective tissue
External spermatic fascia
Cremaster muscle
Internal spermatic fascia
Pampiniform plexus
Internal spermatic artery
Epididymis
Vas efferans
Ductus epididymis
Tunica vaginalis (parietal layer)
Testis–covered with tunica vaginalis (visceral layer)
Gubernaculum
Scrotum
Vas deferens
Glans penis

Vas deferens
Ductus epididymis
Vasa efferentia (efferent tubules)
Septum
Seminiferous tubules (convoluted)
Seminiferous tubules (straight)
Rete testis
Tunica albuginea
Tunica vaginalis (visceral layer)
Tunica vaginalis (parietal layer)
Testicle lobules

FIGURE 31-14 The Testes. External and sagittal views showing interior anatomy. (Redrawn from Seidel HM et al: *Mosby's guide to physical examination,* ed 5, St Louis, 2003, Mosby.)

Scrotum

The testes, epididymides, and spermatic cord are enclosed and protected by the scrotum, a skin-covered, fibromuscular sac homologous to the female labia majora (see Figure 31-2). The skin of the scrotum is thin and has rugae (wrinkles or folds), which enable it to enlarge or relax away from the body. At puberty the scrotal skin darkens, develops active sebaceous glands, and becomes sparsely covered with hair. Just under the skin lies a layer of connective tissue (fascia) and smooth muscle, the tunica dartos (see Figure 31-14). The tunica dartos also forms a septum that separates the two testes. Exposure to cold temperatures causes the tunica dartos to contract, pulling the testes close to the warm body. In warm temperatures, the tunica dartos relaxes, suspending the testes away from body heat. These mechanisms promote optimal temperatures for spermatogenesis. In addition, scrotal sensitivity to touch, pressure, temperature, and pain protects the testes from potential harm. During sexual excitement, the scrotal skin and tunica thicken, the scrotum tightens and lifts, and the spermatic cords shorten, partially elevating the testes toward the body. As excitement plateaus, the engorged testes increase 50% in size, rotate anteriorly, and flatten against the body, signaling impending ejaculation.

Penis

The penis has two main functions: delivery of sperm and elimination of urine. (Urine formation and excretion are discussed in Chapter 28.) Embryonically, the penis is homologous to the female clitoris (see Figure 31-2).

Figure 31-15 shows a sagittal section of the adult penis and its anatomic relation to other urogenital structures. Externally, the penis consists of a shaft with a tip (the glans) that contains the opening of the urethra (see Figures 31-14 and 31-15). The skin of the glans folds over the tip of the penis, forming the prepuce, or foreskin. The skin of the penis is continuous with that of the groin, scrotum, and inner thighs. It is hairless, movable, and darker than surrounding skin.

Internally, the penis consists of the urethra and three compartments: two corpora cavernosa and the corpus spongiosum (see Figure 31-15) separated by Buck fascia; like the testes, the compartments are enclosed by a tunica albuginea. The urethra passes through the corpus spongiosum and ends at a sagittal slit in the glans.[32]

Penetration of the female vagina is made possible by the erectile reflex, a process in which erectile tissues within the corpora cavernosa and corpus spongiosum become engorged with blood. The erectile tissues consist of vascular spaces, or chambers, supplied with blood by arterioles (small arteries). Usually, the arterioles are constricted, so that not much blood flows through the erectile tissues. Sexual stimulation, however, causes the arterioles to dilate and fill with blood, expanding the erectile tissues and causing an erection. Erection apparently is maintained by compression or constriction of veins that drain the corpora cavernosa and corpus spongiosum. When sexual stimulation ceases or orgasm and ejaculation occur, these veins open, blood flows out of the arterioles, and the penis becomes flaccid (soft and pendulous). Erection is under the control of the autonomic nervous system but can be stimulated or inhibited by central nervous system input, such as stress, medications, and pictures.

Erections begin in utero and continue throughout life, but ejaculation does not occur until sperm production begins at puberty. Growth of the penis and scrotal contents continues well past puberty, however, and may not be complete until the late teens or early 20s. Penis size, when flaccid, varies considerably; with an erection, difference in penis size diminishes. Sexual excitement causes the corpora cavernosa to increase in length and width and become rigid; the penis becomes erect. Stimulation of the glans, which is endowed with copious sensitive nerve endings, provides maximum erotic sensation. With sexual arousal, skin color deepens, the glans doubles in size, and the urethral meatus dilates. Ejaculation occurs with frequent, strong contractions of the vas deferens, epididymis, seminal vesicles, prostate, urethra, and penis.

Internal Genitalia

Figure 31-12 shows the anatomy of the internal genitalia and their relation to other pelvic organs. The internal genitalia consist of ducts and glands, as follows:

Ducts—consist of two vasa deferentia, ejaculatory duct, and urethra; conduct sperm and glandular secretions from the testes to the urethral opening of the penis

Glands—consist of prostate gland, two seminal vesicles, and two Cowper (bulbourethral) glands; secrete fluids that serve as a vehicle for sperm transport and create nutritious alkaline medium that promotes sperm motility and survival

Together the sperm and the glandular fluids compose semen.

Sperm leave the epididymides and travel rapidly through the internal ducts (emission). Emission occurs just seconds before ejaculation, at the moment when sexual arousal peaks. It always leads to ejaculation.

Emission occurs as smooth muscle in the walls of the epididymides and vasa deferentia begins to contract rhythmically, pushing sperm and epididymal secretions through the vasa deferentia. Each vas deferens is a firm, elastic, fibromuscular tube that begins at the tail of the epididymis, enters the pelvic cavity within the spermatic cord, loops up and over the bladder, and ends in the prostate gland (see Figures 31-13 and 31-16). Sperm are conducted by peristaltic contractions of smooth muscle in the walls of the vas deferens.

As sperm leave the ampulla (wide portion) of the vas deferens, the seminal vesicles secrete a nutritive, glucose-rich fluid into the ejaculate (semen). The seminal vesicles are glands about 4 to 6 cm long that lie behind the urinary bladder and in front of the rectum. The ducts of the seminal vesicles join the ampulla of the vas deferens to become the ejaculatory duct, which contracts rhythmically during emission and ejaculation. As seen in Figures 31-13 and 31-16, the ejaculatory duct joins the urethra, where both pass through the prostate gland. During emission and ejaculation, a sphincter (muscle surrounding a duct) closes, preventing urine from entering the prostatic urethra.

The prostate gland is composed of alveoli and ducts embedded in fibromuscular tissue. It measures 4 cm in diameter and weighs approximately 20 g. While semen moves through the prostatic portion of the urethra, the prostate gland contracts rhythmically and secretes

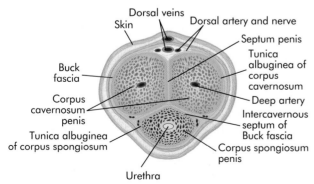

FIGURE 31-15 Cross Section of the Penis. (From Thompson JM et al, editors: *Mosby's clinical nursing*, ed 5, St Louis, 2002, Mosby.)

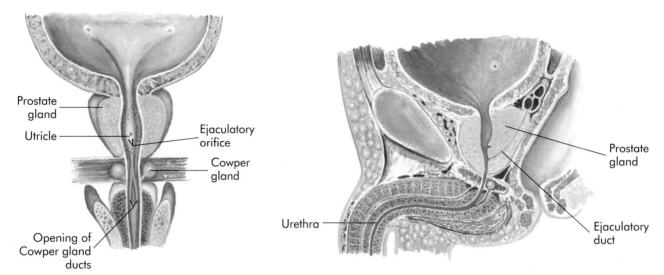

FIGURE 31-16 Anatomy of the Prostate Gland and Seminal Vesicles. (Modified from Seidel HM et al: *Mosby's guide to physical examination,* ed 7, St Louis, 2011, Mosby.)

prostatic fluid (a thin, milky substance with an alkaline pH that helps sperm to survive in the acid environment of the female reproductive tract) into the mixture. In addition, substances in seminal and prostatic fluids help to mobilize sperm after ejaculation.

Cowper glands (bulbourethral glands) are the last pair of glands to add fluid to the ejaculate; their ducts secrete mucus into the urethra near the base of the penis. Ejaculation occurs as semen reaches the base of the penis, where muscles rhythmically contract and expel semen. Normally a man ejaculates between 2 and 6 ml of semen, containing 75 million to 400 million sperm. About 98% of the ejaculate consists of glandular fluids; 60% to 70% of the volume originates from the seminal vesicles and 20% from the prostate. Therefore the ejaculate of a man who has undergone a vasectomy (a surgical procedure that prevents sperm from entering the vas deferens) is reduced by only about 2%.

Spermatogenesis

Spermatogenesis begins at puberty and continues for life. In this respect, spermatogenesis differs markedly from oogenesis (production of primordial ova), which occurs during fetal life only.

Spermatogenesis takes place within the seminiferous tubules of the testes (see Figure 31-14). The basement membrane of each seminiferous tubule is lined with diploid (46-chromosome) germ cells called spermatogonia (sing., spermatogonium). These cells undergo continuous mitotic division. (Mitotic division, in which a cell divides into two identical cells, is described in Chapter 1.) Some spermatogonia move away from the basement membrane and mature, becoming primary spermatocytes (Figure 31-17). These undergo meiosis, a type of cell division that results in two haploid (23-chromosome) cells called secondary spermatocytes. (Meiosis is described and illustrated in Chapter 2.) The secondary spermatocytes then undergo meiosis, resulting in four spermatids. The spermatids differentiate into spermatozoa, or sperm, each of which contains 23 chromosomes (Figure 31-18).

The development of spermatids into sperm depends on the presence of Sertoli cells (nondividing support cells) within the seminiferous tubules. Spermatids attach themselves to the Sertoli cells (see Figure 31-17) where they receive nutrients and hormonal signals necessary to develop into sperm.[33]

The process of spermatogenesis, from mitotic division of a spermatogonium to maturation of the spermatids, takes about 70 to 80 days. Mature sperm migrate from the seminiferous tubules to the epididymides, where their capacity for fertilization continues to develop. Although they are completely mature by the time they are ejaculated, the sperm do not become motile (capable of movement) until they are activated by biochemicals in semen and in the female reproductive tract.

Male Sex and Reproductive Hormones

The male sex hormones are androgens. Testosterone, the primary male sex hormone, and other androgens are produced mainly by Leydig cells of the testes, but they are also produced by the adrenal glands (see Table 31-1 and discussion about adrenarche under Puberty and Reproductive Maturation, p. 776). In men, sex hormone production is relatively constant and does not occur in a cyclic pattern, as it does in women.

The androgens' physiologic actions are related to the growth and development of male tissues and organs.[34,35] Androgens are responsible for the fetal differentiation and development of the male urogenital system and have some effects on the fetal brain. After birth, the Leydig cells become quiescent until activated by the gonadotropins during puberty. Then androgens cause the sex organs to grow and secondary sex characteristics to develop.

Testosterone affects nervous and skeletal tissues, bone marrow, skin and hair, and sex organs. It has an anabolic effect on skeletal muscle tissue, thereby contributing to the difference in body weight and composition between men and women. Testosterone also stimulates growth of the musculature and cartilage of the larynx, causing a permanent deepening of the voice. Testosterone directly stimulates the bone marrow and indirectly stimulates renal erythropoietin production to achieve increased hemoglobin and hematocrit levels. Because sebaceous gland activity is stimulated by testosterone, acne may develop. Hair becomes coarser in texture, and facial, axillary, and pubic hair grows in male patterns. Later in life, testosterone causes baldness in genetically susceptible individuals. Testosterone is required for spermatogenesis and for secretion of fluid by the prostate gland, seminal vesicles, and Cowper glands. Testosterone is also associated

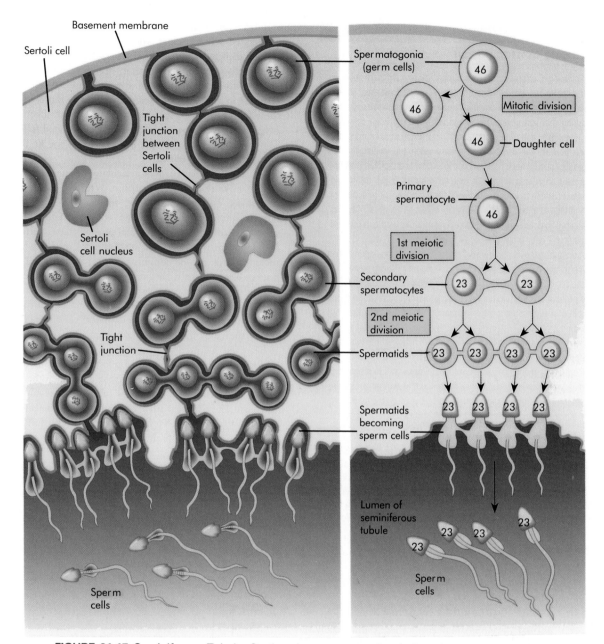

FIGURE 31-17 Seminiferous Tubule. Section shows process of meiosis and sperm cell formation (spermatogenesis). (From Thibodeau GA, Patton KT: *Anatomy & physiology,* ed 6, St Louis, 2007, Mosby.)

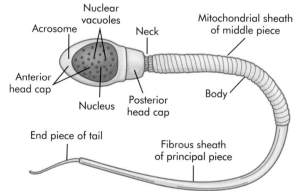

FIGURE 31-18 Mature Sperm Cell (Spermatozoon). Anatomy of mature sperm cell.

with libido (sex drive). Other, less-understood effects of testosterone include alterations in fatty acid and cholesterol metabolism.

The regulation of androgen production and spermatogenesis is achieved by a complex feedback system involving the extrahypothalamic central nervous system, the hypothalamus, the anterior pituitary, the testes, and the androgen-sensitive end organs (see *Health Alert: Male Hormone Contraception*). These relationships are essentially the same in women (see Figure 31-3).

> **✓ QUICK CHECK 31-6**
> 1. Which cells produce testosterone?
> 2. Why do sperm take 12 days to travel the length of the epididymis?
> 3. What is the purpose of prostatic secretion?

Male Hormone Contraception

There is an increasing interest and commitment by men to participate in sharing contraceptive responsibility for family planning. Extensive clinical trials have been completed in the development of male hormone contraception (MHC) during the past several years and their use has been shown to be effective, reversible, and well tolerated. Criteria for successful male hormone contraception are the same as those for women and include the following: the product should have high efficacy (universally effective); it should be reversible, safe (few side effects or long-term health risks), affordable, available, and acceptable to couples; it should have rapid onset of action, no interference with libido or sexual activity, and no effect on eventual offspring. Currently evaluated regimens include preparations of testosterone or preparations of testosterone with progestins added. East Asian men respond much better to the spermatogenesis-suppressing effect of testosterone agents than white men. White men require the addition of other agents, usually gestagens, to testosterone for effective suppression of spermatogenesis. Both preparations suppress follicle-stimulating hormone and luteinizing hormone to arrest sperm production in the testes while maintaining the peripheral effects of testosterone. Onset of MHC is usually delayed by 2 to 3 months. Most men will recover sperm output thresholds compatible with male fertility within 12 months of contraceptive discontinuation. The long-term effects of using hormone contraception for many years are unknown. Work is still in progress to introduce a male hormone contraceptive to the market, as well as to develop a nonhormonal form of male contraception.

Data from Cheng CY, Mruk DD: New frontiers in nonhormonal male contraception, *Contraception* 82(5):476–482, 2010; Glasier A: Acceptability of contraception for men: a review, *Contraception* 82(5):453–456, 2010; Liu PY, Swerdloff RS, Wang C: Recent methodological advances in male hormonal contraception, *Contraception* 82(5):471–475, 2010; Nieschlag E: The struggle for male hormonal contraception, *Best Pract Res Clin Endocrinol Metab* 25(2):369–375, 2011; Roth MY, Amory JK: Pharmacologic development of male hormonal contraceptive agents, *Clin Pharmacol Ther* 89(1):133–136, 2011.

AGING & REPRODUCTIVE FUNCTION

Aging and the Female Reproductive System

Menopause is a normal developmental event that is universally experienced by the average age of 50.5 to 51.4 years in North America.[36] It is not affected by age at menarche, childbearing history, weight, socioeconomic factors, oral contraception, or race. However, it is genetically predetermined, which has been documented by family history. It can occur 2 years sooner on average for smokers, and thinner women also tend to experience menopause at a slightly younger age.

Changes are caused primarily by declining ovarian function and a resulting decrease in ovarian hormone secretion. The primary changes of menopause are as follows:

Perimenopause: This is the transitional period between reproductive and nonreproductive years and can last 1 to 8 years. About 5 to 10 years before menopause, approximately 90% of women note mild to extreme variability in frequency and quality of menstrual flow. Symptoms usually begin with a shortening of the menstrual cycle, which correlates with a shorter follicular phase, followed by unpredictable or irregular ovulation and a lengthening of the menstrual cycle. The perimenopause varies between women and from cycle to cycle in the same woman.

Ovarian changes: Around 37 to 38 years of age, women experience accelerated follicular loss, which ends when the supply of follicles is depleted at menopause. This accelerated loss is correlated with increased FSH stimulation, declining inhibin production, and slightly elevated estradiol levels (Figure 31-19). The ovarian response to high FSH level recruits increasing numbers of follicles; these follicles only partially develop, with a net effect of irregular ovulation, lower progesterone levels, and depleted follicle reserve. The ovaries begin to decrease in size around age 30; this decrease accelerates after age 60.

Uterine changes: The increase in anovulatory cycles allows for proliferative growth of the endometrium. With this longer exposure to unopposed estrogen and greater thickness of the endometrium, 50% of perimenopausal women will experience dysfunctional uterine bleeding that is heavy and unpredictable. In the past, this has put women at high risk for hysterectomy. Newer treatment includes progesterone administration or endometrial ablation by laser or electrocautery. New methods of decreasing the function of the endometrial tissue are being developed.

Systemic changes: Vasomotor flushes are characterized by a rise in skin temperature, dilation of peripheral blood vessels, increased blood flow in the hands, increased skin conductance, and transient increase in heart rate followed by a temperature drop and profuse perspiration over the area of flush distribution. This usually occurs in the face and neck and may radiate into the chest and other parts of the body. Dizziness, nausea, headaches, or palpitations may accompany the flush. These flushes can vary in frequency, intensity, and duration and are experienced for 1 to 15 years (mean 1 to 5 years) by up to 85% of perimenopausal to postmenopausal women (see *Health Alert:* Symptoms of Menopause and Breast Cancer Risk). Flushes are believed to be caused by rapid change in estrogen levels, and estrogen replacement therapy can ameliorate these symptoms. Rapid changes in estrogen levels also can increase emotional stress with unpredictable mood swings, weight gain, migraine headaches, and insomnia. Lower estrogen levels will decrease skin thickness and diminish skin elasticity, thereby causing increased skin dryness and wrinkling.

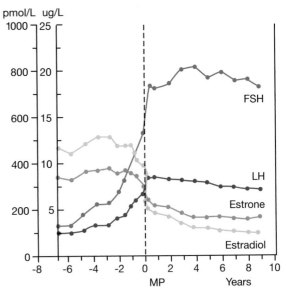

FIGURE 31-19 Perimenopausal Hormone Transition. Mean circulating hormone levels. *FSH,* Follicle-stimulating hormone; *LH,* luteinizing hormone.

Symptoms of Menopause and Breast Cancer Risk

The first study linking menopausal symptoms and breast cancer risk was reported in February 2011. Breast cancer is the second leading cause of cancer death among U.S. women. The study queried 1437 postmenopausal women between the ages of 55 and 74 years, 988 of whom had been diagnosed with breast cancer and 449 with no history of breast cancer. The menopausal symptoms included hot flashes, night sweats, insomnia, vaginal dryness, irregular or heavy menstrual bleeding, depression, and anxiety. Women who had the most frequent and severe hot flashes had a 50% lower average risk of invasive ductal and invasive lobular carcinoma (the two most common breast cancers) compared to women who reported no menopausal symptoms. The risk was not altered with the consideration of other factors, including obesity and use of hormone replacement therapy. The study proposes there is a possible association between high circulating levels of estrogen and breast cancer risk or low circulating levels of estrogen and less breast cancer risk. Levels of both estrogen and progesterone decline during the menopausal transition, but the specific biologic mechanism of hot flashes is unknown. More research is needed to confirm these findings and to better understand the association between menopause, hormone changes, and breast cancer (see Chapter 32, Breast Cancer section).

Data from Huang Y et al: Relationship between menopausal symptoms and risk of postmenopausal breast cancer, *Cancer Epidemiol Biomarkers Prev* 20:379–388, 2011.

Menopause: Menopause is defined by the point that marks 12 consecutive months of amenorrhea. This means that it is determined retrospectively after a woman has not had a menstrual period for 1 year. It is characterized by loss of ovarian function, low estrogen and progesterone levels, and high FSH and LH levels (see Figure 31-19).[37]

Breast tissue changes: Breast tissue becomes involuted; fat deposits and connective tissue increase; and breasts are reduced in size and firmness.

Urogenital tract changes: The ovaries shrink; the uterus atrophies; and the vagina shortens, narrows, and loses some elasticity. Lubrication of the vagina diminishes and vaginal pH increases, creating higher incidence of vaginitis. The cervix atrophies; the cervical os shrinks; vaginal epithelium atrophies; labia major and minora become less prominent; some pubic hair is lost; urethral tone declines along with muscle tone throughout the pelvic area; urinary frequency or urgency, urinary tract infections, and incontinence may occur. Regular sexual activity and orgasm may diminish some of these changes. Sexually active women have less vaginal atrophy.

Skeletal changes: Bone mass is lost, leading to increased brittleness and porosity and possibly osteoporosis.

Cardiac changes: The risk of coronary heart disease increases significantly.

Aging and the Male Reproductive System

No known discrete event, comparable to menopause, characterizes aging of the male reproductive system. Changes do occur, however, in testicular structure and function and sexual behavior. Emotional and physical changes associated with androgen deficiency in the aging male are known as **andropause,** but it occurs in only a small percentage of men.[38] Contributing factors include testicular failure and changes in the hypothalamus and pituitary gland.[39] Obesity also contributes to decreased testosterone production in aging men.[40] Primary changes are summarized as follows[41]:

Sexual drive (libido): Influenced by changes in health status with aging.

Erectile/ejaculatory capacity: Longer stimulation needed to achieve full erection, slower and less forceful ejaculation, less pelvic muscle involvement; decreased vasocongestive response; longer refractory time, up to 24 hours.

Testicular changes: Decreased weight, atrophy, softening of testes; seminiferous tubules thicken in basement membrane area, have germ cell arrest, decrease in spermatogenic activity, and collapse; then sclerosis and fibrosis cause complete obstruction; semen volume, sperm concentration, total sperm count, sperm motility, and number of motile sperm decrease; morphologic appearance of sperm changes.

Hormonal changes: Hormone synthesis decreases and target tissues decline in responsiveness; testosterone levels decline as number of Leydig cells decreases; gonadotropin levels increase.

Associated change: Functional deterioration of accessory sex organs; loss of muscle mass, strength, and endurance; decrease in libido.

 QUICK CHECK 31-7

1. What are the physical changes associated with menopausal decreases in estrogen level?
2. How does andropause affect muscle mass?

DID YOU UNDERSTAND?

Development of the Reproductive Systems

1. Differentiation of female and male genitalia begins around 7 to 8 weeks of embryonic development when the gonads of genetically male embryos begin to secrete male sex hormones, primarily testosterone, under the influence of *SRY* gene expression and testosterone-determining factor (TDF). Female gonadal development occurs in the absence of *SRY* gene expression. Until that time, the primitive reproductive organs of males and females are homologous (the same).

2. The structure and function of both male and female reproductive systems depend on interactions among the central nervous system (hypothalamus), the endocrine system (anterior pituitary), the gonads (ovaries, testes), and the hypothalamic-pituitary-gonadal (H-P-G) axis. A set of complex neurologic and hormonal interactions accelerate at puberty and lead to sexual maturation and reproductive capability.

3. Production of primitive female gametes (ova) occurs solely during fetal life. From puberty to menopause, one female gamete matures per menstrual cycle. Production of the male gametes (sperm) begins at puberty; after that, millions are produced daily, usually for life.

4. Puberty is the onset of sexual maturation. Adolescence is a stage of human development between childhood and adulthood and includes social, psychological, and biologic changes.

5. At puberty, extrahypothalamic factors cause the hypothalamus to secrete gonadotropin-releasing hormone (GnRH), which stimulates the anterior pituitary to secrete the gonadotropins follicle-stimulating hormone (FSH) and luteinizing hormone (LH) that stimulate the gonads (ovaries and testes) to secrete female (estrogen and progesterone) or male sex hormones (testosterone). Puberty is complete in females with the first ovulatory menstrual period and is complete in males with the first ejaculation that contains mature sperm.

Continued

DID YOU UNDERSTAND?—cont'd

The Female Reproductive System

1. The function of the female reproductive system is to produce mature ova and, when they are fertilized, to protect and nourish them through embryonic and fetal life and expel them at birth.

2. The external female genitalia are the mons pubis, labia majora, labia minora, clitoris, vestibule (urinary and vaginal openings), Bartholin glands, and Skene glands. They protect body openings and may play a role in sexual functioning.

3. The internal female genitalia are the vagina, uterus, fallopian tubes, and ovaries. Although all these organs are needed for reproduction, the ovaries are the most essential because they produce the female gametes and female sex hormones.

4. The vagina is a fibromuscular canal that receives the penis during sexual intercourse and is the exit route for menstrual fluids and products of conception. The vagina leads from the introitus (its external opening) to the cervical portion of the uterus.

5. The uterus is the hollow, muscular organ in which a fertilized ovum develops until birth. The uterine walls have three layers: the endometrium (lining), myometrium (muscular layer), and perimetrium (outer covering, which is continuous with the pelvic peritoneum). The endometrium proliferates (thickens) and is shed in response to cyclic changes in levels of female sex hormones. The cervix is the narrow, lower portion of the uterus that opens into the vagina.

6. The two fallopian tubes extend from the uterus to the ovaries. Their function is to conduct ova from the spaces around the ovaries to the uterus. Fertilization normally occurs in the distal third of the fallopian tubes.

7. From puberty to menopause, the ovaries are the site of (a) ovum maturation and release and (b) production of female sex hormones (estrogen, progesterone) and androgens. The female sex hormones are involved in sexual differentiation and development, the menstrual cycle, pregnancy, and lactation. Although they are primarily male sex hormones, androgens in women are precursors of female sex hormones and contribute to the prepubertal growth spurt, pubic and axillary hair growth, and activation of sebaceous glands.

8. Estrogen (primarily estradiol) is produced by cells in the developing ovarian follicle (structure that encloses the ovum). Progesterone is produced by cells of the corpus luteum, the structure that develops from the ruptured ovarian follicle after ovulation (ovum release). Androgens are produced within the ovarian follicle, adrenal glands, and adipose tissue.

9. The average menstrual cycle lasts 27 to 30 days and consists of three phases, which are named for ovarian and endometrial changes: the follicular/proliferative phase, the luteal/secretory phase, and menstruation.

10. Ovarian events of the menstrual cycle are controlled by gonadotropins and follicular secretion of inhibin. High follicle-stimulating hormone (FSH) levels stimulate follicle and ovum maturation (follicular phase); then a surge of luteinizing hormone (LH) causes ovulation, which is followed by development of the corpus luteum (luteal phase).

11. Uterine (endometrial) events of the menstrual cycle are caused by ovarian hormones. During the follicular phase of the ovarian cycle, estrogen produced by the follicle causes the endometrium to proliferate (proliferative phase). During the luteal phase, estrogen maintains the thickened endometrium, and progesterone causes it to develop blood vessels and secretory glands (secretory phase). During the ischemic/menstrual phase, the corpus luteum degenerates, production of both hormones drops sharply, and the "starved" endometrium degenerates and is shed, causing menstruation.

12. Cyclic changes in hormone levels also cause thinning and thickening of the vaginal epithelium, thinning and thickening of cervical secretions, and changes in basal body temperature.

Structure and Function of the Breast

1. Until puberty, the female and male breasts are similar, consisting of a small, underdeveloped nipple, some fatty and fibrous tissue, and a few ductlike structures under the areola. At puberty, however, a variety of hormones (estrogen, progesterone, prolactin, growth hormone, insulin, cortisol) cause the female breast to develop into a system of glands and ducts that is capable of producing and ejecting milk.

2. The basic functional unit of the female breast is the lobe, a system of ducts that branches from the nipple to milk-producing units called *lobules*. Each breast contains 15 to 20 lobes, which are separated and supported by Cooper ligaments. The lobules contain *acini cells*, which are convoluted spaces lined with epithelial cells. Contraction of the subepithelial cells of each acinus moves milk into the system of ducts that leads to the nipple.

3. Milk production occurs in response to prolactin, a hormone that is secreted in larger amounts after childbirth. Milk ejection is under the control of oxytocin, another hormone of pregnancy and lactation.

4. During the reproductive years, breast tissue undergoes cyclic changes in response to hormonal changes of the menstrual cycle. At menopause, the tissue involutes, fat deposits and connective tissue increase, and the breasts reduce in size and firmness.

The Male Reproductive System

1. The function of the male reproductive system is to produce male gametes (sperm) and deliver them to the female reproductive tract.

2. The external male genitalia are the testes, epididymides, scrotum, and penis. The internal genitalia are the vas deferens, ejaculatory duct, prostatic and membranous sections of the urethra, seminal vesicles, prostate gland, and Cowper glands.

3. The testes (male gonads) are paired glands suspended within the scrotum. The testes have two functions: spermatogenesis (sperm production) and production of male sex hormones (androgens, chiefly testosterone).

4. The epididymis is a long, coiled tube arranged in a comma-shaped compartment that curves over the top and rear of the testis. The epididymis receives sperm from the testis and stores them while they develop further. Sperm travel the length of the epididymis and then are ejaculated into the vas deferens, which transports sperm to the urethra.

5. The scrotum is a skin-covered, fibromuscular sac that encloses the testes and epididymides, which are suspended within the scrotum by the spermatic cord. The scrotum keeps these organs at optimal temperatures for sperm survival (about 1° to 2° C lower than body temperature) by contracting in cold environments and relaxing in warm environments.

6. The penis is a cylindric organ consisting of three longitudinal compartments (two corpora cavernosa and one corpus spongiosum) and the urethra. The urethra runs through the corpus spongiosum. The corpora cavernosa and corpus spongiosum consist of erectile tissue. Externally the penis consists of a shaft and a tip, which is called the *glans*.

7. The penis has two functions: delivery of sperm and elimination of urine.

8. Sexual intercourse is made possible by the erectile reflex, in which tactile or psychogenic stimulation of the parasympathetic nerves causes arterioles in the corpora cavernosa and corpus spongiosum to dilate and fill with blood, causing the penis to enlarge and become firm.

9. Emission, which occurs at the peak of sexual arousal, is the movement of semen from the epididymides to the penis. Ejaculation, which is a continuation of emission, is the pulsatile ejection of semen from the penis.

10. Spermatogenesis is a continuous process because spermatogonia, the primitive male gametes, undergo continuous mitosis within the seminiferous tubules of the testes. Some spermatogonia develop into primary spermatocytes, which divide meiotically into secondary spermatocytes and then spermatids. The spermatids develop into sperm with the help of nutrients and hormonal signals from Sertoli cells.

DID YOU UNDERSTAND?—cont'd

11. Production of the male sex hormones (androgens) is controlled by interactions among the hypothalamus, anterior pituitary, and gonads. The male hormones are produced steadily rather than cyclically, however.

Aging & Reproductive Function

1. Perimenopause is the transitional period between reproductive and nonreproductive years in women.

2. Menopause, the point that marks 12 consecutive months of amenorrhea, includes atrophic changes in the ovaries and vagina, loss of bone mass, and increased risk of cardiovascular disease.

3. Andropause is androgen deficiency in the aging male and occurs in about 1 in 200 men. There is a decrease in testosterone production with some loss of muscle mass and strength.

■ KEY TERMS

- Acinus (pl., acini) of breast 788
- Activin 786
- Adrenarche 777
- Androgen 777
- Andropause 795
- Areola 788
- Breast 787
- Cervix 780
- Cornification 787
- Corpus (body of uterus) 780
- Corpus cavernosum (pl., corpora cavernosa) 791
- Corpus luteum 783
- Corpus spongiosum 791
- Cowper gland (bulbourethral gland) 792
- Cul-de-sac 779
- Decornification 787
- Efferent tubule 790
- Ejaculatory duct 791
- Emission 791
- Endocervical canal 780
- Endometrium 780
- Epididymis (pl., epididymides) 790
- Erectile reflex 791
- Estradiol (E2) 783
- Estrogen 783
- Fallopian tube (uterine tube) 782
- Fimbriae 782
- Follicle-stimulating hormone (FSH) 775
- Follicular/proliferative phase 784
- Follistatin 786
- Fornix 779
- Fundus 780
- Glands of Montgomery 788
- Glans 791
- Gonad 774
- Gonadarche 776
- Gonadostat (gonadotropin-releasing hormone pulse generator) 775
- Gonadotropin-releasing hormone (GnRH) 775
- Granulosa cell 783
- Infundibulum 782
- Inguinal canal 790
- Inhibin 786
- Ischemic/menstrual phase 786
- Isthmus 780
- Leydig cell 790
- Libido 793
- Luteal/secretory phase 784
- Luteinizing hormone (LH) 775
- Menarche 784
- Menopause 784
- Menstruation (menses) 784
- Myometrium 780
- Nipple 788
- Ovarian cycle 783
- Ovarian follicle 783
- Ovary 782
- Ovulation 783
- Ovum (pl., ova) 774
- Oxytocin 788
- Penis 791
- Perimetrium (parietal peritoneum) 780
- Prepuce (foreskin) 791
- Primary spermatocyte 792
- Progesterone 783
- Prostate gland 791
- Rete testis 790
- Ruga (pl., rugae; pertains to vagina and testes) 779
- Scrotum 791
- Secondary spermatocyte 792
- Semen 791
- Seminal vesicle 791
- Seminiferous tubule 790
- Sertoli cell (nondividing support cell) 792
- Sex hormone 774
- Spermatid 792
- Spermatogenesis 792
- Spermatogonium (pl., spermatogonia) 792
- Spermatozoon (sperm cell) 774
- Spinnbarkeit mucus 782
- Squamous-columnar junction 780
- Testis 790
- Testosterone 775
- Theca cell 783
- Thelarche 776
- Tubulus rectus 790
- Tunica albuginea 790
- Tunica dartos 791
- Tunica vaginalis 790
- Urethra 791
- Uterine tubes 782
- Uterus 780
- Vagina 779
- Vas deferens 790
- Vasomotor flush 794
- Vulva 778

REFERENCES

1. Fritz MA, Speroff L: *Clinical gynecologic endocrinology and infertility,* ed 8, Philadelphia, 2011, Lippincott Williams & Wilkins.
2. Piprek RP: Molecular and cellular machinery of gonadal differentiation in mammals, *Int J Dev Biol* 54(5):779–786, 2010.
3. Schlessinger D, et al: Determination and stability of gonadal sex, *J Androl* 31(1):16–25, 2010.
4. Nef S, Vassalli JD: Complementary pathways in mammalian female sex determination, *J Biol* 8(8):74, 2009.
5. Jasik CB, Lustig RH: Adolescent obesity and puberty: the "perfect storm," *Ann N Y Acad Sci* 1135:265–279, 2008.
6. Burt Solorzano CM, McCartney CR: Obesity and the pubertal transition in girls and boys, *Reproduction* 140(3):399–410, 2010.
7. Clarke BL, Khosla S: Female reproductive system and bone, *Arch Biochem Biophys* 503(1):118–128, 2010.
8. Riordan J: *Breastfeeding and human lactation,* ed 3, Sudbury, Mass, 2005, Jones and Bartlett.
9. Kyurkchiev D, Ivanova-Todorova E, Kyurkchiev SD: New target cells of the immunomodulatory effects of progesterone, *Reprod Biomed Online* 21(3):304–311, 2010.
10. Euling SY, et al: Examination of US puberty-timing data from 1940 to 1994 for secular trends: panel findings, *Pediatrics* 121(Suppl 3):S172–S191, 2008.
11. Karapanou O, Papadimitriou A: Determinants of menarche, *Reprod Biol Endocrinol* 8:115, 2010.

12. Rogol AD: Sex steroids, growth hormone, leptin and the pubertal growth spurt, *Endocr Dev* 17:77–85, 2010.

13. World Health Organization Task Force on Adolescent Reproductive Health: World Health Organization multicenter study on menstrual and ovulatory patterns in adolescent girls. II: longitudinal study of menstrual patterns in the early postmenarcheal period, duration of bleeding episodes and menstrual cycles, World Health Organization Task Force on Adolescent Reproductive Health, *J Adolesc Health Care* 7(4):236–244, 1986.

14. Adams Hillard PJ, Deitch HR: Menstrual disorders in the college age female, *Pediatr Clin North Am* 52(1):179–197, ix–x, 2005.

15. Yamanoto K, et al: The relationship between premenstrual symptoms, menstrual pain, irregular menstrual cycles, and psychosocial stress among Japanese college students, *J Physiol Anthropol* 28(3):129–136, 2009.

16. Pandey S, Bhattacharya S: Impact of obesity on gynecology, *Womens Health (London)* 6(1):107–117, 2010.

17. Scheid JL, De Souza MJ: Menstrual irregularities and energy deficiency in physically active women: the role of ghrelin, PYY and adipocytokines, *Med Sport Sci* 55:82–102, 2010.

18. Richards JS, Pangas SA: The ovary: basic biology and clinical implications, *J Clin Invest* 120(4):963–972, 2010.

19. Messinis IE: Ovarian feedback, mechanism of action and possible clinical implications, *Hum Reprod Update* 12(5):557–571, 2006.

20. Thackray VG, Mellon PL, Coss D: Hormones in synergy: regulation of the pituitary gonadotropin genes, *Mol Cell Endocrinol* 314(2):192–203, 2010.

21. Robker RL, Akison LK, Russell DL: Control of oocyte release by progesterone receptor-regulated gene expression, *Nucl Recept Signal* 7:e012, 2009.

22. Critchley HO, Saunders PT: Hormone receptor dynamics in a receptive human endometrium, *Reprod Sci* 16(2):191–199, 2009.

23. Wolman I, Gal TB, Jaffa AJ: Cervical mucus status can be accurately estimated by transvaginal ultrasound during fertility evaluation, *Fertil Steril* 92(3):1165–1167, 2009.

24. Pallone SR, Bergus GR: Fertility awareness-based methods: another option for family planning, *J Am Board Fam Med* 22(2):147–157, 2009.

25. Hovey RC, Aimo L: Diverse and active roles for adipocytes during mammary gland growth and function, *J Mammary Gland Biol Neoplasia* 15(3):279–290, 2010.

26. Suami H, et al: The lymphatic anatomy of the breast and its implications for sentinel lymph node biopsy: a human cadaver study, *Ann Surg Oncol* 3:863–871, 2008.

27. Bachelot A, Binart N: Reproductive role of prolactin, *Reproduction* 133(2):361–369, 2007.

28. Romero-Gutiérrez G, et al: Actual use of the lactational amenorrhoea method, *Eur J Contracept Reprod Health Care* 12(4):340–344, 2007.

29. Ma NS, Geffner ME: Gynecomastia in prepubertal and pubertal men, *Curr Opin Pediatr* 20(4):465–470, 2008.

30. Jung A, Schuppe HC: Influence of genital heat stress on semen quality in humans, *Andrologia* 39(6):203–215, 2007.

31. Cornwall GA: New insights into epididymal biology and function, *Hum Reprod Update* 15(2):213–227, 2009.

32. Yiee JH, Baskin LS: Penile embryology and anatomy, *Scientific World J* 10:1174–1179, 2010.

33. Hogarth CA, Griswold MD: The key role of vitamin A in spermatogenesis, *J Clin Invest 1* 120(4):956–962, 2010.

34. Bain J: Testosterone and the aging male: to treat or not to treat? *Maturitas* 66(1):16–22, 2010.

35. Traish AM: Androgens play a pivotal role in maintaining penile tissue architecture and erection: a review, *J Androl* 30(4):363–369, 2009.

36. Palacios S, et al: Age of menopause and impact of climacteric symptoms by geographical region, *Climacteric* 13(5):419–428, 2010.

37. Su HI, Freeman EW: Hormone changes associated with the menopausal transition, *Minerva Gynecol* 61(6):483–489, 2009.

38. Pines A: Male menopause: is it a real clinical syndrome? *Climacteric* 14(1):15–17, 2011.

39. Wu FCW, et al: Hypothalamic–pituitary–testicular axis disruptions in older men are differentially linked to age and modifiable risk factors: the European Male Aging Study, *J Clin Endocrinol Metab* 93:2737–2745, 2008.

40. Mah PM, Wittert GA: Obesity and testicular function, *Mol Cell Endocrinol* 316(2):180–186, 2010.

41. Perheentupa A, Huhtaniemi I: Aging of the human ovary and testis, *Mol Cell Endocrinol* 299(1):2–13, 2009.

Alterations of the Reproductive Systems, Including Sexually Transmitted Infections

Gwen Latendresse and Kathryn L. McCance

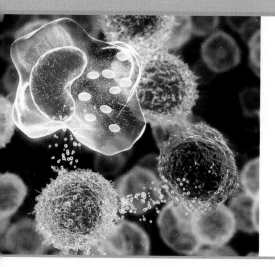

evolve WEBSITE

CHAPTER OUTLINE

Alterations of the reproductive system span a wide range of concerns from delayed sexual development and suboptimal sexual performance to structural and functional abnormalities. Many common reproductive disorders carry potentially serious physiologic or psychologic consequences. For example, sexual or reproductive dysfunction, such as impotence or infertility, can dramatically affect self-concept, relationships, and overall quality of life. Conversely, organic and psychosocial problems, such as alcoholism, depression, situational stressors, chronic illness, and medications, can affect ovulation and menstruation, sexual performance, and fertility and may be risk factors for the development of some types of reproductive tract cancers. Prostate cancer is the second leading cause of cancer deaths in men, and breast cancer is the second leading cause of cancer deaths in women.[1] Diagnosis and treatment of reproductive system disorders, however, are often complicated by the stigma and symbolism associated with the reproductive organs and emotion-laden beliefs and behaviors related to reproductive health. Treatment or diagnosis for any problem may be delayed because of embarrassment, guilt, fear, or denial.

ALTERATIONS OF SEXUAL MATURATION

The process of sexual maturation, or puberty, is marked by the development of secondary sex characteristics, rapid growth, and, ultimately, the ability to reproduce. A variety of congenital and endocrine disorders can disrupt the timing of puberty. Puberty that occurs too late (delayed puberty) or too early (precocious puberty) is caused by the inappropriate onset of sex hormone production.

The average age of pubertal onset appears to be decreasing for girls, primarily in breast development, not menarche.[2] The age of pubertal onset has remained essentially unchanged for boys.

Delayed or Absent Puberty

About 3% of children living in North America experience delayed development of secondary sex characteristics.[3] The first sign of puberty in girls is thelarche, or breast development; it should begin by 13 years of age. Normally, boys tend to mature later than girls, around 14 to 14.5 years of age. In boys, the first sign of maturity is enlargement of

---

BOX 32-1 CAUSES OF DELAYED PUBERTY

Hypergonadotropic Hypogonadism (Increased Follicle-Stimulating Hormone [FSH] and Luteinizing Hormone [LH])
1. Gonadal dysgenesis, most commonly Turner syndrome (45,X/46,XX; structural X or Y abnormalities; or mosaicism)
2. Klinefelter syndrome (47,XXY)
3. Bilateral gonadal failure
   a. Traumatic or infectious
   b. Postsurgical, postirradiation, or postchemotherapy
   c. Autoimmune
   d. Idiopathic empty-scrotum or vanishing-testes syndrome (congenital anorchia) or resistant-ovary syndrome

Hypogonadotropic Hypogonadism (Decreased LH, Depressed FSH)
1. Reversible
   a. Physiologic delay
   b. Weight loss/anorexia
   c. Strenuous exercise
   d. Severe obesity
   e. Illegal drug use, especially marijuana
   f. Primary hypothyroidism

g. Congenital adrenal hyperplasia
h. Cushing syndrome
i. Prolactinomas
2. Irreversible
   a. Gonadotropin-releasing hormone (GnRH) deficiency (Kallmann syndrome) or idiopathic hypogonadotropic hypogonadism (IHH)
   b. Hypopituitarism
   c. Congenital central nervous system (CNS) defects
   d. Other pituitary adenomas
   e. Craniopharyngioma
   f. Malignant pituitary tumors

Eugonadism
These conditions are associated with amenorrhea but may have otherwise normal pubertal development:
1. Congenital anomalies
   a. Müllerian agenesis
   b. Vaginal septum or imperforate hymen
2. Androgen insensitivity syndrome
3. Inappropriate positive feedback

BOX 32-2 PRIMARY FORMS OF PRECOCIOUS PUBERTY

Complete Precocious Puberty
Premature development of appropriate characteristics for the child's gender
Hypothalamic-pituitary-ovarian axis functioning normally but prematurely
In about 10% of cases, lethal central nervous system tumor may be the cause

Partial Precocious Puberty
Partial development of appropriate secondary sex characteristics
Premature thelarche (breast budding) seen in girls between 6 months and 2 years of age
Does not progress to complete puberty (ovulation and menstruation)

Premature adrenarche (growth of axillary and pubic hair) tends to occur between 5 and 8 years of age
Can progress to complete precocious puberty; may be caused by estrogen-secreting neoplasms or may be a variant of normal pubertal development

Mixed Precocious Puberty
Causes the child to develop some secondary sex characteristics of the opposite gender
Common causes: adrenal hyperplasia or androgen-secreting tumors

Data from Burchett MLR et al: Endocrine and metabolic diseases. In Burns CE et al, editors: *Pediatric primary care,* St Louis, 2009, Saunders; Jospe N: Disorders of pubertal development. In Osborn LM et al, editors: *Pediatrics,* Philadelphia, 2005, Mosby.

---

testes and thinning of the scrotal skin. In delayed puberty, these secondary sex characteristics develop later.

In about 95% of cases, delayed puberty is a normal physiologic event. Hormonal levels are normal, the hypothalamic-pituitary-gonadal axis is intact, and maturation is slowly occurring. Treatment is seldom needed unless the delayed puberty is causing psychosocial problems.[4]

The other 5% of cases are caused by the disruption of the hypothalamic-pituitary-gonadal axis or by the outcomes of a systemic disease. Treatment depends on the cause (Box 32-1), and referral to a pediatric endocrinologist is necessary.[5]

Precocious Puberty

Precocious puberty is a rare event, affecting about 1 in 10,000 girls and fewer than 1 in 50,000 boys. Precocious puberty has been defined as sexual maturation occurring before age 6 in African American girls or age 7 in Caucasian girls, with Mexican American girls falling between the two. Precocious puberty for boys of all ethnic/racial groups is

defined as sexual maturation occurring before age 9.[6] Precocious puberty may be caused by many conditions (Box 32-2), including lethal central nervous system tumors. All cases of precocious puberty require thorough evaluation.

All forms of precocious puberty are treated by identifying and removing the underlying cause or administering appropriate hormones. In many cases, precocious puberty can be reversed. However, complete precocious puberty (development consistent with the gender of the individual) is difficult to treat and can cause long bones to stop growing before the child has reached normal height.

QUICK CHECK 32-1
1. Why does puberty occur too late or too early in some individuals?
2. Why do all forms of precocious puberty require evaluation?

DISORDERS OF THE FEMALE REPRODUCTIVE SYSTEM

Hormonal and Menstrual Alterations

Dysmenorrhea

Primary dysmenorrhea is painful menstruation associated with the release of prostaglandins in ovulatory cycles but not with pelvic disease. Between 50% and 90% of women ages 15 to 25 years are affected—some (up to 15%)[7] are affected severely enough to cause missed work or school. Primary dysmenorrhea begins with the onset of ovulatory cycles. The incidence steadily rises, peaks in women in the late teens and early twenties, and decreases slowly thereafter.[8]

Secondary dysmenorrhea is related to pelvic pathologic conditions, manifests later in the reproductive years, and may occur any time in the menstrual cycle.[7]

PATHOPHYSIOLOGY   Primary dysmenorrhea results mostly from excessive prostaglandin $F_2\alpha$ ($PGF_2\alpha$) found in secretory endometrium. These lipid hormones increase myometrial contractions and constrict endometrial blood vessels, causing ischemia and endometrial shedding. In addition, prostaglandins and prostaglandin metabolites can cause gastrointestinal complaints, headache, and syncope.

Secondary dysmenorrhea results from disorders such as endometriosis, pelvic adhesions, inflammation, uterine fibroids, polyps, tumors, cysts, or intrauterine devices (IUDs).

CLINICAL MANIFESTATIONS   The chief symptom of dysmenorrhea is pelvic pain associated with the onset of menses. The severity is directly related to length and amount of menstrual flow. The pain often radiates into the groin and may be accompanied by backache, anorexia, vomiting, diarrhea, syncope, and headache. The discomfort commonly begins shortly before the onset of menstruation and rarely persists beyond the second day.

EVALUATION AND TREATMENT   Primary dysmenorrhea can be differentiated from secondary dysmenorrhea by a thorough medical history and pelvic examination. In women who desire contraception, dysmenorrhea may be relieved with hormonal contraceptives. Hormonal contraception stops ovulation and creates an atrophic endometrium, thereby decreasing prostaglandin synthesis and myometrial contractility. Nonsteroidal anti-inflammatory medications[9] are effective in a majority of women with primary dysmenorrhea and should be taken before or at the onset of bleeding or cramping. Regular exercise seems to prevent or reduce symptoms. Other palliative measures include local application of heat, massage, relaxation techniques, vitamin B and magnesium supplementation, and high-frequency transcutaneous electrical nerve stimulation (TENS).[10] Orgasm may relieve or worsen symptoms.

Primary Amenorrhea

Amenorrhea means lack of menstruation; the most common cause is pregnancy. Primary amenorrhea is defined as the failure of menarche and the absence of menstruation by age 14 years with no development of secondary sex characteristics or the absence of menstruation by age 16 years regardless of the presence of secondary sex characteristics. Causes include a diverse group of abnormalities, such as congenital defects of gonadotropin-releasing hormone (GnRH) production; genetic disorders (Turner syndrome); congenital central nervous system (CNS) defects (e.g., hydrocephalus); congenital anatomic malformations of the reproductive system (e.g., absence of

vagina or uterus); and acquired CNS lesions, including trauma, infection, and tumors.

PATHOPHYSIOLOGY   One approach to understanding the pathophysiology is to compartmentalize. Compartment I disorders are anatomic defects, including absence of the vagina and uterus. Compartment II disorders involve the ovary, primarily genetic disorders (such as Turner syndrome) and androgen insensitivity syndrome (AIS). In AIS the target organs (e.g., ovaries) are completely resistant to the action of androgens, resulting in lack of estrogen. Compartment III disorders are of the anterior pituitary gland, including tumors, and result in failure of signaling to the ovaries through follicle-stimulating hormone (FSH) and luteinizing hormone (LH) secretion. Compartment IV disorders primarily involve hypothalamic defects that prevent secretion of GnRH; thus there is no signaling to the pituitary to release FSH and LH.

CLINICAL MANIFESTATIONS   The major clinical manifestation of primary amenorrhea is the absence of menarche. The cause of the amenorrhea determines whether secondary sex characteristics and height are affected.

EVALUATION AND TREATMENT   Diagnosis of primary amenorrhea is based on history and physical examination. Laboratory studies may be required to document abnormal levels of gonadotropins or ovarian hormones, or the presence of genetic conditions. Diagnostic imaging is used to document structural abnormalities.

Treatment involves correction of any underlying disorders and hormone replacement therapy to induce the development of secondary sex characteristics. Although surgical alteration of the genitalia may be undertaken to correct abnormalities, it should be postponed until the individual can make a truly informed decision.

Secondary Amenorrhea

Secondary amenorrhea is the absence of menstruation for a time equivalent to three or more cycles or 6 months in women who have previously menstruated. Many disorders and physiologic conditions are associated with secondary amenorrhea. Secondary amenorrhea is common (normal) during early adolescence, pregnancy, lactation, and the perimenopausal period, primarily because of anovulation. Dramatic weight loss, malnutrition, and excessive exercise also are frequent contributors.

PATHOPHYSIOLOGY   The pathophysiology of secondary amenorrhea is summarized in Figure 32-1.

CLINICAL MANIFESTATIONS   The major manifestation of secondary amenorrhea is the absence of menses. Depending on the underlying cause of the amenorrhea, infertility, vasomotor flushes, vaginal atrophy, acne, and hirsutism (abnormal hairiness) also may be present.

EVALUATION AND TREATMENT   Pregnancy is the most common cause of secondary amenorrhea and must be ruled out before any further evaluation. Hypothyroidism also is a common cause and should be ruled out as well. Diagnosis of secondary amenorrhea involves identifying underlying hormonal or anatomic alterations. A complete history and physical examination are done. Evaluation of thyroid-stimulating hormone (TSH) or prolactin levels may be indicated. Depending on the cause of the amenorrhea, treatment may involve hormone replacement therapy or a corrective procedure, such as surgical removal of pituitary tumors.

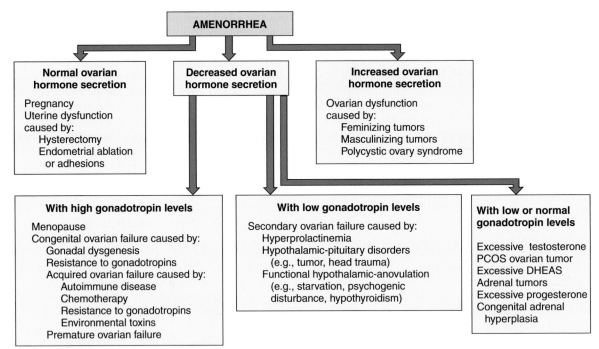

FIGURE 32-1 Causes of Secondary Amenorrhea. Of note, hypothyroidism is a relatively common condition and should be ruled out as the cause of hyperprolactinemia before more extensive evaluation (i.e., computed tomography or magnetic resonance imaging) occurs.

Abnormal Uterine Bleeding

Menstrual irregularity or abnormal bleeding patterns (Table 32-1) account for 33% of all gynecologic visits. The most common cause of cycle irregularity is failure to ovulate related to age, stress, or endocrinopathy. Common causes of abnormal bleeding based on age group and frequency are presented in Table 32-2.

Dysfunctional uterine bleeding (DUB) is heavy or irregular bleeding in the absence of disease (i.e., uterine fibrosis, polyps, or infection). DUB is a diagnosis of exclusion made only after other causes have been ruled out. DUB affects 15% to 20% of all women at some time during their menstrual life and accounts for 70% of all hysterectomies, and almost all endometrial ablation procedures.[11] Perimenopausal women are by far the most affected by DUB because of frequent anovulation.

PATHOPHYSIOLOGY More than 80% of DUB is associated with anovulatory cycles that occur more frequently in adolescents (20% of DUB cases) and perimenopausal women (50% of DUB cases). Polycystic ovary syndrome (PCOS), obesity, and thyroid disease also are common contributors.[12]

Progesterone is absent in anovulatory cycles, yet estrogen continues to be secreted. This results in excessive and irregular endometrial thickness, and subsequent excessive and irregular bleeding. Estrogen unopposed by progesterone creates a progression of endometrial responses, including proliferation and hyperplasia. Over many years, this pattern may end with atypia and carcinoma.[12]

Abnormal bleeding in ovulatory cycles is less common, and mechanisms underlying the bleeding are unclear. Excessive fibrinolytic activity and changes in prostaglandin production may be implicated. Infection or structural abnormalities also may be present.

CLINICAL MANIFESTATIONS DUB is characterized by unpredictable and variable bleeding in terms of amount and duration. Especially during perimenopause, dysfunctional bleeding also may involve flooding and the passing of large clots.[13] Although large clots often indicate excessive blood loss, it is difficult to estimate the severity of blood loss; healthy women usually do not become anemic until blood loss exceeds 1.6 L over a short time or with chronic heavy flow. Heavy bleeding may be preceded by episodes of amenorrhea and be perceived by individuals as a miscarriage.

EVALUATION AND TREATMENT DUB is diagnosed after other organic conditions that could cause abnormal bleeding are eliminated. Goals of therapy are to control bleeding, prevent hyperplasia, prevent or treat anemia, and treat concurrent endocrine problems if present. Usual therapy is hormonal and may consist of progestin-estrogen therapy, short-term estrogen, cyclic low-dose contraceptives, progestins, or progesterone.[14] Dilation and curettage (D&C) or hysterectomy

TABLE 32-1	ABNORMAL MENSTRUAL BLEEDING
TERM	**DEFINITION**
Polymenorrhea	Cycles shorter than 3 weeks; may indicate disturbance in endocrine control of ovulation
Oligomenorrhea	Cycles longer than 6-7 weeks; may indicate disturbance in endocrine control of ovulation
Metrorrhagia	Intermenstrual bleeding or bleeding of light character occurring irregularly between cycles; may be a sign of organic disease
Hypermenorrhea	Excessive flow; may be a sign of organic disease
Menorrhea	Increased amount and duration of flow
Menorrhagia	Increased amount and duration of flow
Menometrorrhagia	Prolonged flow associated with irregular and intermittent spotting between bleeding episodes

TABLE 32-2	COMMON CAUSES OF ABNORMAL (VAGINAL/GENITAL) BLEEDING IN DESCENDING ORDER OF FREQUENCY	
AGE GROUP	**CAUSE**	
Prepubescence	Sexual assault	
	Trauma	
	Foreign bodies	
	Precocious puberty	
Adolescence	Anovulation (immature hypothalamic-pituitary-ovarian axis)	
	Trauma and sexual abuse	
Reproductive years	Pregnancy	
	Pelvic inflammatory disease	
	Coagulation disorder	
	Hormonal contraceptives	
	Endometriosis	
	Anovulation	
	IUDs	
	Ovarian cysts	
	Uterine polyps/tumors	
	PCOS	
	Bleeding disorders (e.g., von Willebrand)	
	Trauma/rape	
Perimenopause	Anovulation	
	Malignancy	
	Pregnancy	
	Endometriosis	
	Benign neoplasms (myomas, adenomyosis)	
Postmenopause	Malignancy	
Other: non–age specific	Chronic conditions	
	Adrenal conditions	
	Thyroid disorders	
	Liver disease	
	Diabetes mellitus	
	Obesity	
	Hypertension	

IUD, Intrauterine device; *PCOS,* polycystic ovary syndrome.

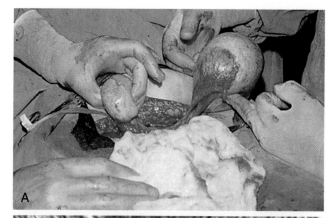
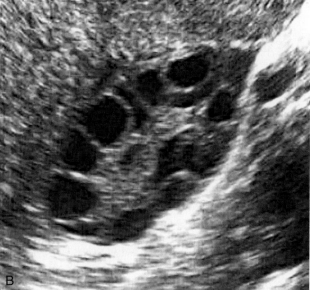

FIGURE 32-2 Polycystic Ovary. **A,** Surgical view of polycystic ovaries. **B,** Ultrasound of polycystic ovary. (**A** from Symonds EM, Macpherson MBA: *Diagnosis in color: obstetrics and gynecology,* London, 1997, Mosby-Wolfe; **B** from King J: Polycystic ovary syndrome: *J Midwifery Womens Health* 51[6]:415–422, 2006. Reprinted with permission.)

has been replaced with endometrial ablation as the treatment of choice for DUB not responsive to hormonal therapy. The levonorgestrel-intrauterine system (LNG-IUS), a contraceptive hormonal intrauterine device (IUD), also is being successfully used. The LNG-IUS results in an 86% to 97% reduction in blood loss by decreasing endometrial proliferation.

Polycystic Ovary Syndrome

Polycystic ovary syndrome (PCOS) remains one of the most common endocrine disturbances affecting women (Figure 32-2). PCOS has at least two of the following conditions: few or anovulatory menstrual cycles, elevated levels of androgens, and polycystic ovaries. Polycystic ovaries, however, do not have to be present to diagnose PCOS and their presence alone does not establish the diagnosis. Furthermore, PCOS should not be confused with benign ovarian cysts, which are common during the reproductive years and have a different etiology (see section titled Benign Ovarian Cysts). PCOS is a leading cause of infertility in the United States, where the prevalence rate is estimated between 4% and 12%. PCOS may be familial. Signs and symptoms of PCOS can vary over time, with metabolic syndrome becoming more prominent with age.[15] PCOS is often found in association with other endocrine disorders and several other conditions, such as Cushing syndrome, acromegaly, premature ovarian failure, simple obesity, congenital adrenal hyperplasia, thyroid disease, androgen-producing adrenal tumors or ovarian tumors (see Figure 32-2), and syndromes with hyperprolactinemia.[16]

PATHOPHYSIOLOGY The direct cause of PCOS is unknown but a genetic basis is suspected. A hyperandrogenic state is a cardinal feature in the pathogenesis of PCOS. However, glucose intolerance/insulin resistance (IR) and hyperinsulinemia often occur concurrently and markedly aggravate the hyperandrogenic state, thus contributing to the severity of signs and symptoms of PCOS.[15] Obesity worsens IR and, thus, can add to severity as well.

Insulin stimulates androgen secretion by the ovarian stroma and reduces serum sex hormone–binding globulin (SHBG) directly and independently. The net effect is an increase in free testosterone levels.

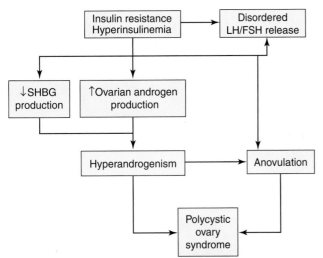

FIGURE 32-3 Insulin Resistance and Hyperinsulinemia in Polycystic Ovary Syndrome (PCOS). See text for explanation. *FSH,* Follicle-stimulating hormone; *LH,* luteinizing hormone; *SHBG,* sex hormone–binding globulin.

Excessive androgens affect follicular growth, and insulin affects follicular decline by suppressing apoptosis and enabling the survival of follicles that would normally disintegrate (Figure 32-3). Further, there seems to be a genetic ovarian defect in PCOS that makes the ovary either more susceptible to or more sensitive to insulin's stimulation of androgen production in the ovary.[17]

Inappropriate gonadotropin secretion triggers the beginning of a vicious cycle that perpetuates anovulation. Typically, levels of follicle-stimulating hormone (FSH) are low or below normal, and the luteinizing hormone (LH) level is elevated. Persistent LH level elevation causes an increase in androgens (dehydroepiandrosterone sulfate [DHEAS] from the adrenal glands and testosterone, androstenedione, and dehydroepiandrosterone [DHEA] from the ovary). Androgens are converted to estrogen in peripheral tissues, and increased testosterone levels cause a significant reduction (approximately 50%) in SHBG level, which, in turn, causes increased levels of free estradiol. Elevated estrogen levels trigger a positive feedback response in LH and a negative feedback response in FSH. Because FSH levels are not totally depressed, new follicular growth is continuously stimulated, but not to full maturation and ovulation (see Figure 32-3).[15,16]

CLINICAL MANIFESTATIONS Clinical manifestations of PCOS usually appear within 2 years of puberty, but may appear after a period of normal menstrual function and pregnancy. Symptoms are related to anovulation and hyperandrogenism and include dysfunctional uterine bleeding or amenorrhea, hirsutism, acne, and infertility (Box 32-3). Approximately 41% of women with PCOS are obese. Hypertension and dyslipidemia also are frequently found in association with PCOS.

EVALUATION AND TREATMENT Diagnosis of PCOS is based on evidence of androgen excess (hirsutism, male pattern hair distribution, acne), chronic anovulation (as evidenced by irregular menstrual patterns, amenorrhea, and infertility), insulin resistance (obesity may be an indication, as well as abnormal glucose tolerance testing), and inappropriate gonadotropin secretion (low serum FSH concentration, and elevated levels of LH and DHEA). Treatment of PCOS often includes use of combined oral contraceptives to control irregular menstrual cycles and to oppose estrogens and androgens. Insulin sensitizers, such

---

BOX 32-3 CLINICAL MANIFESTATIONS OF POLYCYSTIC OVARY SYNDROME

Presenting Signs and Symptoms (% of Women Affected)
Obesity (41%)
Menstrual disturbance (70% [e.g., dysfunctional uterine bleeding])
Oligomenorrhea (47%)
Amenorrhea (19%)
Regular menstruation (48%)
Hyperandrogenism (69-74%)
Infertility (73% of anovulatory infertility)
Asymptomatic (20% of those with polycystic ovary syndrome)

Hormonal Disturbances
Increased insulin (independent of obesity)
Decreased SHBG
Increased androgens (testosterone, androstenedione)
Increased DHEA (occurs in 50% of women)
Increased LH (genetic variant LH-β subunit)
Increased prolactin
Increased leptin, especially in obesity (independent of insulin)
Suggested decreased insulin-like growth factor 1 (IGF-1) receptors on theca cells
Possible decreased estrogen receptors (intraovarian and along hypothalamic-pituitary axis)

Possible Late Sequelae
Dyslipidemia: increased low-density lipoproteins, decreased high-density lipoproteins, increased triglycerides
Diabetes mellitus (30% of women with or without obesity will develop type 2 diabetes mellitus by age 30)
Cardiovascular disease; hypertension
Endometrial hyperplasia and carcinoma (anovulatory women are hyperestrogenic)

Other
Women with PCOS are at increased risk of gestational diabetes mellitus, pregnancy-induced hypertension, preterm birth, and perinatal mortality

Adapted from Azziz R et al: *Fertil Steril,* Oct 22, 2008 [Epub ahead of print]; Boomsma CM et al: *Semin Reprod Med* 26(1):72–84, 2008; Diamanti-Kandarakis E: *Expert Rev Mol Med* 10(2):e3, 2008; Simoni M et al: *Hum Reprod Update* 14(5):459–484, 2008.
DHEA, Dehydroepiandrosterone; *LH,* luteinizing hormone; *PCOS,* polycystic ovary syndrome; *SHBG,* sex hormone–binding globulin.

---

as metformin, may be used to decrease insulin resistance, prevent diabetes and heart disease, and restore fertility.[18] Insulin sensitizers combined with clomiphene citrate may be effective for ovulation induction for women who are trying to become pregnant.[19] Reductions in weight can dramatically improve insulin sensitivity and return of ovulatory cycles.[20]

Premenstrual Syndrome

Premenstrual syndrome (PMS) and **premenstrual dysphoric disorder (PMDD)** are the cyclic recurrence (in the luteal phase of the menstrual cycle) of distressing physical, psychologic, or behavioral changes that impair interpersonal relationships or interfere with usual activities.[12] PMDD is listed as a mood disorder in the American Psychiatric Association's *Diagnostic and Statistical Manual of Mental Disorders-IV (DSM-IV).* The prevalence of PMS and PMDD is difficult to determine. It has been estimated that 5% to 10% of menstruating women have severe to disabling premenstrual symptoms, 3% to 8% have cyclic dysphoria warranting treatment, and 20% or more have mild to moderately distressing symptoms.[21] To confuse matters, symptoms are experienced to some degree by most adolescent and adult women and can occur throughout all menstrual phases, the presence and severity of symptoms in any one woman may be inconsistent from month to month, the menstrual phase for peak symptom severity may differ depending on the population studies, and inconsistent and overlapping use of terminology and criteria are used to describe these syndromes. PMDD is the term often used to refer to the premenstrual disorder with a predominant psychosocial or functional impairment, similar to dysthymia and minor depression.[22]

PATHOPHYSIOLOGY   It is thought that PMS/PMDD is the result of abnormal tissue response to the normal changes of the menstrual cycle. Premenstrual disorders occur almost exclusively in ovulatory cycles, thus leading to the theory that symptoms are triggered by the preovulatory estrogen level peak or postovulatory progesterone level increase, or both.[23] However, the exact mechanisms are unknown. Furthermore, neurotransmitters, such as serotonin, may contribute to symptoms by interacting with estrogen and progesterone, both of which are known to have mood and behavioral effects, including irritability, aggression, impulse control, and negative mood.[12] This may explain why selective serotonin reuptake inhibitors often are effective in the treatment of PMS/PMDD.

A predisposition to PMS occurs in families, perhaps because of genetics or shared environment. A woman's menstrual experience is often similar to her mother's or her sister's experience. Evidence supports a relationship between severity and frequency of PMS/PMDD and reports of low well-being, major affective disorder, and personal characteristics such as increased stress, poor nutrition, lack of exercise, low self-esteem, perfectionism, history of sexual abuse, and family conflict. In turn, when PMS/PMDD is distressing, the quality of interpersonal relationships and self-image are negatively affected.

CLINICAL MANIFESTATIONS   The pattern of symptom frequency and severity is more important than specific complaints. Nearly 300 physical, emotional, and behavioral symptoms have been attributed to PMS/PMDD. Emotional symptoms, particularly depression, anger, irritability, and fatigue, have been reported as the most prominent and the most distressing, whereas physical symptoms seem to be the least prevalent and problematic. Approximately 6% of women have classic PMS/PMDD and 7% report premenstrual magnification of symptoms that are present during the entire cycle. The presence of underlying physical or psychologic disease may be aggravated premenstrually and must be diagnosed and treated independently of PMS/PMDD.

EVALUATION AND TREATMENT   Diagnosis of PMS/PMDD is based on health history and symptoms. Diagnostic criteria for PMDD are presented in Box 32-4. Current treatment is symptomatic because the cause is complex and cannot be reduced to a single biologic explanation and because the occurrence and severity are mediated by lifestyle, social, and psychologic factors. For many women, nonpharmacologic therapies, with or without medication, can be as effective in controlling symptoms as medication alone.[24]

Initial treatment focuses on validation of premenstrual experience, education about PMS/PMDD, self-help techniques, and elimination of contributing factors or coexisting disorders. Approaches may include stress reduction, exercise, family or individual counseling, biofeedback, imagery, and rest. Dietary changes—such as eating six small

---

BOX 32-4   AMERICAN COLLEGE OF OBSTETRICIANS AND GYNECOLOGISTS (ACOG) CRITERIA

A problem with premenstrual dysphoric disorder (PMDD) diagnosis is that many women with clinically relevant premenstrual syndrome/premenstrual dysphoric disorder (PMS/PMDD) symptoms do not meet the full criteria of the *Diagnostic and Statistical Manual of Mental Disorders-IV (DSM-IV)*. The ACOG attempts to rectify this problem by using the following definitions: "Presence of at least one psychological or physical symptom that causes significant impairment and is confirmed by means of prospective ratings (i.e., 2 cycles of a symptom diary)."

Data from American College of Obstetricians and Gynecologists: *ACOG Pract Bull* 15, 2000; Yonkers KA et al: *Lancet* 371(9619): 1200–1210, 2008.

---

meals each day; increasing intake of complex carbohydrates, fiber, and water; and decreasing consumption of caffeine, alcohol, sugar, and animal fat—can be beneficial.

After a trial of nonpharmacologic therapies, or if criteria for diagnosis of PMDD are met, medications may be added to the treatment regimen. Drugs often prescribed include vitamin and mineral supplements, selective serotonin reuptake inhibitors (SSRIs), antiprostaglandins, and antianxiolytics. SSRIs relieve symptoms in about 60% to 90% of women and may be given continuously or only during the premenstrual period. Edema associated with PMS is a result of local fluid shifts rather than fluid retention; therefore diuretics are not recommended. Combined hormonal treatment (i.e., oral contraceptives, vaginal rings, or patches) are often ineffective.[25]

However, in severe cases, menses can be abolished by eliminating cyclic ovarian hormones and perhaps the biologic trigger for PMS/PMDD. This is accomplished by the use of combined hormonal contraceptives, injectable or implantable progestins, or GnRH agonists.[26]

✔ QUICK CHECK 32-2
1. Why does amenorrhea occur?
2. Why do anovulatory cycles lead to dysfunctional uterine bleeding?
3. What other conditions are associated with PCOS?

Infection and Inflammation

Infections of the genital tract may result from exogenous or endogenous microorganisms. Exogenous pathogens are most often sexually transmitted. Endogenous causes of infection include microorganisms that are normally resident in the vagina, bowel, or vulva. Infection occurs if these microorganisms migrate to a new location or overproliferate when the immune system and other defense mechanisms are impaired.

Skin disorders that can affect the vulva include reactive dermatitis, contact dermatitis, psoriasis, and impetigo. (For a discussion of skin disorders, see Chapter 38.) Most infectious disorders that affect the vulva and vagina are sexually transmitted, however. These disorders are described in Table 32-16 on p. 858.

Pelvic Inflammatory Disease

Pelvic inflammatory disease (PID) is an acute inflammatory process caused by infection (Figure 32-4). PID may involve any organ, or combination of organs, of the upper genital tract—the uterus, fallopian

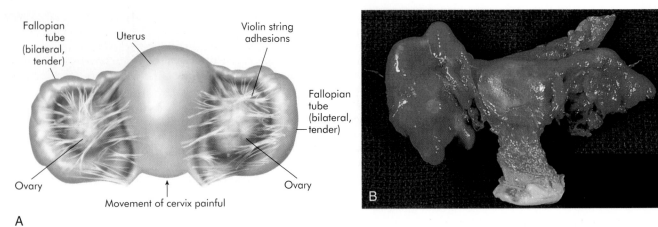

FIGURE 32-4 Pelvic Inflammatory Disease. **A,** Drawing depicting involvement of both ovaries and fallopian tubes. **B,** Total abdominal hysterectomy and bilateral salpingo-oophorectomy specimen showing unilateral pyosalpinx. (**A** from Seidel HM et al: *Mosby's guide to physical examination,* ed 6, St Louis, 2006, Mosby; **B** from Morse SA, Ballard RC, Holmes KK et al: *Atlas of sexually transmitted diseases and AIDS,* ed 3, Edinburgh, 2003, Mosby.)

tubes, or ovaries—and, in its most severe form, the entire peritoneal cavity. Inflammation of the fallopian tubes is termed **salpingitis** (Figure 32-5); inflammation of the ovaries is called **oophoritis.** Many cases of PID are caused by sexually transmitted microorganisms, such as chlamydia and gonorrhea that migrate from the vagina to the uterus, fallopian tubes, and ovaries.[27]

PATHOPHYSIOLOGY The development of upper genital tract infections is mediated by a number of defense mechanisms, including virulence of the microorganism, size of the inoculum, and immune defense status of the individual. PID develops when pathologic microbes ascend from an infected cervix to infect the uterus and adnexae. The resultant inflammatory response leads to necrosis with repeated infections and may predispose a woman to PID. PID is considered a polymicrobial infection. Although frequently initiated by gonorrhea or *Chlamydia,* the majority of cases (up to 84%) are caused by mixed nongonococcal/nonchlamydial bacteria, including anaerobes (*Bacteroides* species and *Peptostreptococci*), facultative microorganisms (*Gardnerella vaginalis, Haemophilus influenzae,* and *Streptococci*), and genital tract mycoplasmas (*Mycoplasma hominis, Mycoplasma genitalis,* and *Ureaplasma urealyticum*).[27] Identification of *Neisseria gonorrhoeae* (37% to 44%), or *Chlamydia trachomatis* (10% to 45%), or both (9% to 12%) is variable; however, facultative or anaerobic bacteria have been isolated in about 50% of women with acute PID. About 25% to 50% of the time, only facultative or anaerobic microorganisms are identified. Bacterial vaginosis (BV), a bacterial overgrowth of the vagina, and *M. genitalis* also have been linked to clinical findings of PID and endometritis.

After one episode of PID, 15% to 25% of women develop long-term sequelae, such as infertility, ectopic pregnancy, chronic pelvic pain, dyspareunia, pelvic adhesions, perihepatitis, and tubo-ovarian abscess. The incidence of complications increases markedly with repeated infections. Tubal infertility occurs in 8% to 11% of women after one episode, 20% to 30% after two episodes, and 40% to 50% after three episodes. In 2009, the mortality rate associated with PID was 0.20 deaths per 100,000 women ages 14 to 44. Most deaths resulting from PID are caused by septic shock.[28]

CLINICAL MANIFESTATIONS The clinical manifestations of PID vary from sudden, severe abdominal pain with fever to no symptoms

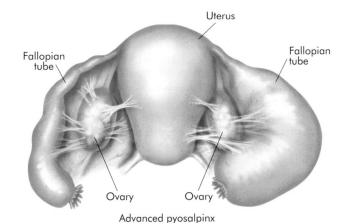

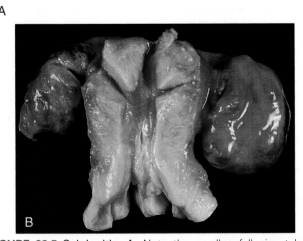

FIGURE 32-5 Salpingitis. **A,** Note the swollen fallopian tubes. **B,** Bilateral, retort-shaped, swollen sealed tubes and adhesions of ovaries are typical of salpingitis. (**A** from Seidel HM et al: *Mosby's guide to physical examination,* ed 6, St Louis, 2006, Mosby; **B** from Damjanov I, Linder J, editors: *Anderson's pathology,* ed 10, St Louis, 1996, Mosby.)

at all. An asymptomatic cervicitis may be present for some time before PID develops. Of women with salpingitis, 67% to 75% may have a subclinical infection. The first sign of the ascending infection may be the onset of low bilateral abdominal pain, often characterized as dull and steady with a gradual onset. Symptoms are more likely to develop during or immediately after menstruation. The pain of PID may worsen with walking, jumping, or intercourse. Other manifestations of PID include dysuria (difficult or painful urination) and irregular bleeding.

EVALUATION AND TREATMENT The diagnosis of PID is based on history, abdominal tenderness, presence of uterine and cervical movement tenderness on bimanual pelvic examination, mucopurulent discharge at the cervical os, white blood cells on Gram stain or wet mount of cervical discharge, leukocytosis, and increased erythrocyte sedimentation rate. To support the diagnosis, tests for chlamydia and gonorrhea are done; sonography, laparoscopy, and culdocentesis are indicated when a woman has recurrent symptoms or symptoms unresponsive to outpatient treatment regimens, a temperature greater than 38° C (100.4° F), or an adnexal mass. Other conditions that cause pelvic pain must be excluded, including ectopic pregnancy, threatened abortion, ovarian torsion, ovarian cyst, or appendicitis. Because of the significance of the complications of PID (septic shock and infertility), aggressive treatment is recommended with broad-spectrum antibiotics, and includes treatment of *N. gonorrhoeae* and *Chlamydia trachomatis*.[28] Follow-up appointments should occur within 72 hours of diagnosis and treatment. From 25% to 40% of women require hospitalization for intravenous administration of antibiotics and treatment of peritonitis or a tubo-ovarian abscess.[29] Recommendations for physical rest and avoidance of intercourse are often given as precautionary and comfort measures during initial recovery (i.e., 1 to 2 weeks). To prevent recurrence, sexual partners also are treated with antibiotic combinations.

Vaginitis

Vaginitis is infection of the vagina. The major causes are sexually transmitted pathogens, bacterial vaginosis, and *Candida albicans*. The incidence of sexually transmitted vaginitis remains highest in women 15 to 24 years of age.[27]

The development of vaginitis is related to complications with local defense mechanisms, such as skin integrity, immune reaction, and vaginal pH. The pH of the vagina (normally 4.0 to 4.5) depends on cervical secretions and the presence of normal flora that help maintain an acidic environment.[30] Variables that affect the vaginal pH, and therefore the bactericidal nature of secretions (see Chapter 30) and the predisposition to infection, include douching; use of soaps, spermicides, feminine hygiene sprays, deodorant menstrual pads or tampons; and conditions associated with increased glycogen content of vaginal secretions, such as pregnancy and diabetes.

Antibiotics often destroy normal vaginal flora, facilitating overgrowth of *C. albicans* and causing a yeast infection. Increased vaginal alkalinity also may enhance susceptibility to trichomoniasis and BV.

Normally, vaginal discharge is a clear, milky, or cloudy secretion with a slippery or clumpy texture. It is nonirritating, has a mild inoffensive odor, and turns yellow after drying. The amount and texture of a woman's discharge will change in response to hormonal fluctuation throughout the menstrual cycle. Vaginal secretions increase at the time of ovulation, during pregnancy, and with sexual arousal; just before menstruation, vaginal discharge becomes thick and sticky. Although the amount of vaginal discharge alone is not an indication of infection, any other change in discharge may indicate a problem. Infection is suggested with a marked change in color or if the discharge becomes copious, malodorous, or irritating.

Diagnosis is based on history, physical examination, and examination of the discharge by wet mount. Treatment involves developing and maintaining an acidic environment, relieving symptoms (usually pruritus and irritation), and administering antimicrobial or antifungal medications to eradicate the infectious organism. If the infection can be sexually transmitted, the woman's partner will also need to be treated.

Cervicitis

Cervicitis is a nonspecific term used to describe inflammation of the cervix before the identification of pathogens. Mucopurulent cervicitis (MPC) is usually caused by one or more sexually transmitted pathogens, such as *Trichomonas*, gonorrhea, *Chlamydia*, *Mycoplasma*, or *Ureaplasma*. Infection causes the cervix to become red and edematous. A mucopurulent (mucus- and pus-containing) exudate drains from the external cervical os, and the individual may report vague pelvic pain, bleeding, or dysuria. The infectious organisms are cultured or identified by immunoassay. Definitive diagnosis is followed by oral antibiotic therapy. Sexual partners are usually treated to prevent reinfection and transmission to other partners.[27]

Vulvovestibulitis

Vulvovestibulitis (VV) (also referred to as vulvitis, vestibulitis, or vulvodynia) is inflammation of the vulva or vaginal vestibule, or both. In many cases it may represent several disorders without an identifiable cause. VV is fairly common, affecting approximately 10% of women at some point in life.[31] While the inflammation of VV may be caused by contact dermatitis (i.e., exposure to soaps, detergents, lotions, sprays, shaving, menstrual pads/tampons, perfumed toilet paper, tight-fitting clothes), the condition may be more complex and represent abnormalities in three interdependent systems: vestibular mucosa, pelvic floor musculature, and central nervous system pain regulatory pathways. The condition also may represent an autoimmune reaction. The mechanisms of VV are poorly understood; thus VV is often a difficult condition to evaluate and treat. Many women suffer through years of misdiagnosis as a result.[32]

After ruling out and treating conditions that can contribute to or cause vulvar inflammation (e.g., *Candida*, sexually transmitted infections, dermatologic conditions, contact dermatitis), there are few treatment options. Suggested approaches include use of hydrocortisone cream; application of a water barrier (such as thick skin cream or solid vegetable shortening) during a period of healing; behavioral treatment (35% to 83% of women benefit); or vestibulectomy (61% to 94% success rate), a procedure that is understandably unacceptable to many women because of the invasiveness of the procedure. Women also are advised to avoid irritants, wear loose cotton clothing, and use appropriate antimicrobial/antifungal treatments for any recurrent vaginitis.[33]

Bartholinitis

Bartholinitis (Bartholin cyst) is inflammation of one or both of the ducts that lead from the introitus (vaginal opening) to the Bartholin glands (Figure 32-6). The usual causes are microorganisms that infect the lower female reproductive tract, such as streptococci, staphylococci, and sexually transmitted pathogens. Acute bartholinitis may be preceded by an infection, such as cervicitis, vaginitis, or urethritis.

Infection or trauma causes inflammatory changes that narrow the distal portion of the duct, leading to obstruction and stasis of glandular secretions. The obstruction, or cyst, varies from 1 to 8 cm in diameter and is located in the posterolateral portion of the vulva. The affected area is usually red and painful, and pus may be visible at the opening

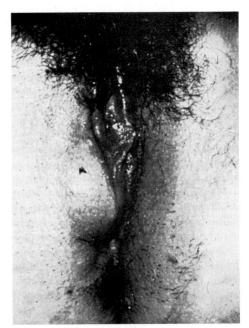

FIGURE 32-6 Inflammation of Bartholin Glands. (From Gardner HL, Kaufman RH: *Benign diseases of the vulva and vagina,* St Louis, 1969, Mosby.)

of the duct. This exudate should be cultured. The individual may have fever and malaise.

Chronic bartholinitis is characterized by the presence of a small cyst that is slightly tender but otherwise is asymptomatic. Most Bartholin cysts require no treatment. Symptoms only occur if an exacerbation of infection causes an abscess to form in the gland itself.

Diagnosis is based on the clinical manifestations and the identification of infectious microorganisms. Infection is treated with antibiotics, and pain is relieved with analgesics and warm sitz baths. If an abscess forms, it may be surgically drained.

Pelvic Organ Prolapse

The bladder, urethra, and rectum are supported by the endopelvic fascia and perineal muscles. This muscular and fascial tissue loses tone and strength with aging and may fail to maintain the pelvic organs in the proper position. Progressive descent of the pelvic support structures may cause pelvic floor disorders, such as urinary and fecal incontinence and pelvic organ prolapse. Pelvic organ prolapse (POP) is thought be caused by direct trauma (such as childbirth), pelvic floor surgery, or damage to pelvic innervation, particularly the pudendal nerve. However, nulliparous women with congenital weakness and relaxation of musculature also can experience these conditions. Prolapse of the bladder, urethra, rectum, or uterus may occur many years after an initial injury to the supporting structure, and a strong familial tendency/genetic component appears to be present.

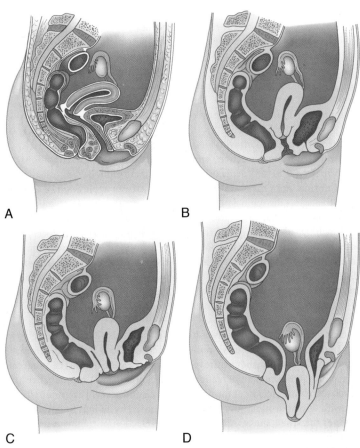

FIGURE 32-7 Degrees of Uterine Prolapse. **A,** Normal uterus (grade 0). **B,** Grade 1 prolapse: descent within the vagina. **C,** Grade 2 prolapse: descent into the hymen. **D,** Grade 4 prolapse: minimal possible descent of the uterus. Grade 3 (not shown) protrudes just beyond the introitus.

Pelvic organ prolapse is progressive and related to the inherent strength or weakness of the woman's musculofascial tissue. Heavy lifting and refractory constipation also may contribute. Nearly 24% of women experience at least one pelvic floor disorder during their lifetime. Descriptive terminology is often used to indicate the extent (degree or grade) and location (i.e., posterior or anterior vaginal wall and uterine, cervical, perineal, or rectal prolapse) of the pelvic organ prolapse.[34] Figure 32-7 illustrates the different degrees (grades) of uterine prolapse, showing descent of the cervix or the entire uterus into the vaginal canal. In severe cases, the uterus falls completely through the vagina and protrudes from the introitus, creating ulceration and obvious discomfort. Grade 1 prolapse is not treated unless it causes discomfort. Grades 2 and 3 prolapses usually cause feelings of fullness, heaviness, and collapse through the vagina. Symptoms of other pelvic floor disorders also may be present. Figure 32-8 shows pelvic organ prolapse associated with cystocele and rectocele. **Cystocele** is descent of the bladder and anterior vaginal wall into the vaginal canal. It is usually accompanied by **urethrocele,** or sagging of the urethra. In severe cases, the bladder and anterior vaginal wall bulge outside the introitus. Symptoms are usually insignificant in mild to moderate cases. Increased bulging and descent of the anterior vaginal wall and urethra can be aggravated by vigorous activity, prolonged standing, sneezing, coughing, or straining and can be relieved by rest or by assumption of a recumbent or prone position. If the prolapse is large, women may complain of vaginal pressure or the feeling of "sitting on a ball."[35]

Although commonly associated with urinary stress incontinence, cystocele does not cause it. **Stress incontinence** is likely the result of relaxation of the musculofascial support tissues of the urethra that also

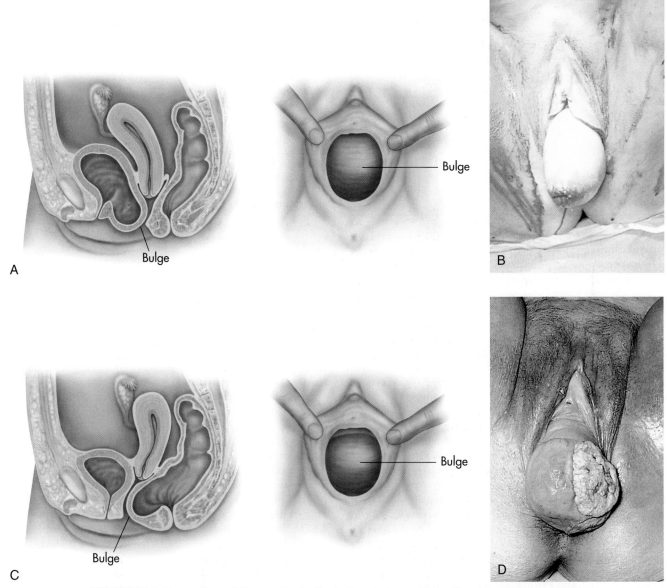

FIGURE 32-8 Cystocele and Rectocele. A, Grade 2: anterior vaginal wall prolapse (i.e., cystocele). **B,** Grade 4: prolapse. **C,** Grade 2: posterior wall prolapse (i.e., rectocele). **D,** Grade 4: associated with ulceration of vaginal wall. Grades 1 and 3 not shown. (**A** and **C** from Seidel HM et al: *Mosby's guide to physical examination,* ed 4, St Louis, 1999, Mosby; **B** and **D** from Symonds EM, Macpherson MBA: *Color atlas of obstetrics and gynecology,* London, 1994, Mosby-Wolfe.)

TABLE 32-3	PELVIC ORGAN PROLAPSE: SYMPTOMS AND TREATMENTS
SYMPTOMS	**TREATMENT**
Urinary Sensation of incomplete emptying of bladder Urinary incontinence Urinary frequency/urgency Bladder "splinting" to accomplish voiding	Depending on age of woman and cause and severity of condition: Isometric exercises to strengthen pubococcygeal muscles (Kegel exercises) Estrogen to improve tone and vascularity of fascial support (postmenopausal) Pessary (a removable device) to hold pelvic organs in place Surgical: Reconstructive: autologous grafts; synthetic mesh/sling Obliterative (most extreme) Weight loss Avoidance of constipation Treatment of cough/lung conditions
Bowel Constipation or feeling of rectal fullness or blockage Difficult defecation Stool or flatus incontinence Urgency Manual "splinting" of posterior vaginal wall to accomplish defecation	
Pain and Bulging Vaginal, bladder, rectum Pelvic pressure, bulging, pain Lower back pain	
Sexual Dyspareunia Decreased sensation, lubrication, arousal	

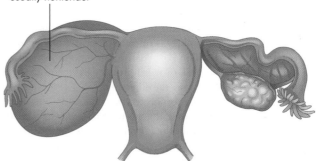

One or both sides, usually nontender

FIGURE 32-9 Depiction of Ovarian Cyst.

HEALTH ALERT

Dietary Interventions and Lifestyle Changes for Pelvic Prolapse

Constipation contributes to chronic straining and pelvic prolapse. Increasing fiber intake to 25 to 35 mg/day and water intake to 8 to 10 glasses per day will prevent constipation and consequently straining and prolapse. Other lifestyle changes may help also. These include achieving and maintaining ideal body weight, performing pelvic floor exercises, avoiding or reducing heavy lifting, avoiding high-impact aerobics or jogging, and quitting smoking.

Data from Jelovsek JE, Maher C, Barber MD: Pelvic organ prolapse, *Lancet* 369(9566):1027–1038, 2007; Forrest DE: Common gynecologic pelvic disorders. In Youngkin EQ, Davis MS, editors: *Women's health: a primary care clinical guide*, ed 3, Upper Saddle River, NJ, 2004, Prentice Hall.

contribute to the cystocele. Operative correction of a large cystocele may actually cause, rather than correct, stress incontinence. **Rectocele** is the bulging of the rectum and posterior vaginal wall into the vaginal canal. Lifelong chronic constipation and straining may produce or aggravate a rectocele. A large rectocele may cause vaginal pressure, rectal fullness, and incomplete bowel evacuation. Defecation may be difficult and can be facilitated by applying manual pressure to the posterior vaginal wall. An **enterocele** is a herniation of the rectouterine pouch into the rectovaginal septum (between the rectum and the posterior vaginal wall). It is usually associated with other pelvic organ prolapse and is more often found in grossly obese and older adults.

Table 32-3 summarizes the symptoms and treatment of pelvic organ prolapse. Treatment for pelvic organ prolapse may include the insertion of a **pessary,** which is a removable mechanical device that holds the uterus, bladder, or bowel in position. The pelvic fascia may be strengthened through Kegel exercises (repetitive isometric tightening and relaxing of the pubococcygeal muscles) or by a course of estrogen therapy in menopausal women. Maintaining a healthy body mass index, preventing constipation, and treating chronic cough may help prevent prolapse (see *Health Alert:* Dietary Interventions and Lifestyle Changes for Pelvic Prolapse). Surgical repair, with or without hysterectomy, is the treatment of last resort.[36]

Benign Growths and Proliferative Conditions
Benign Ovarian Cysts

Benign cysts of the ovary may occur at any time during the life span, but are most common during the reproductive years and, in particular, at the extremes of those years (Figure 32-9). An increase in benign ovarian cysts occurs when hormonal imbalances are more common, around puberty and menopause.[37] Benign ovarian cysts are quite common, comprising a third of gynecologic hospital admissions. Two common causes of benign ovarian enlargement in ovulating women are follicular cysts and corpus luteum cysts. These cysts are called **functional cysts** because they are caused by variations of normal physiologic events. Follicular and corpus luteum cysts are unilateral. They are typically 5 to 6 cm in diameter but can grow as large as 8 to 10 cm. Most women are asymptomatic.

Benign cysts of the ovary are produced when a follicle or a number of follicles are stimulated but no dominant follicle develops and completes the maturity process. Every month about 3 to 12 follicles are stimulated, but normally only 1 succeeds in ovulation of a mature ova.

Normally, in the early follicular phase of the menstrual cycle, follicles of the ovary respond to hormonal signals from the brain. The pituitary produces FSH to mature follicles in the ovary. As the follicles enlarge, granulosa cells in the follicle multiply and secrete estradiol. As a dominant follicle develops, it secretes higher levels of estradiol, which stimulates the LH surge that comes from the pituitary. The LH surge stimulates the follicle to rupture, releasing the ova and transforming the granulosa cells of the dominant follicle into the corpus luteum. If the dominant follicle develops properly before ovulation, the corpus luteum becomes vascularized and secretes progesterone. Progesterone arrests development of other follicles in both ovaries in that cycle. Progesterone, proteolytic enzymes, and prostaglandins trigger follicular rupture and release of the ovum.

Follicular cysts can be caused by a transient condition in which the dominant follicle fails to rupture or one or more of the nondominant follicles fail to regress. This disturbance is not well understood. It may be that the hypothalamus does not receive or send a message strong enough to increase FSH levels to the degree necessary to develop or mature a dominant follicle. The hypothalamus monitors blood levels of estradiol and progesterone; when FSH level is low, estradiol concentration does not increase enough to stimulate LH surge. Research indicates that when progesterone is not being produced, the hypothalamus releases gonadotropin-releasing hormone (GnRH) to increase the FSH level.[37] FSH continues to stimulate follicles to mature, and the granulosa cells grow and, presumably, estradiol level increases. This abnormal cycle continues to stimulate follicular size and causes follicular cysts to develop. Clinical symptoms of follicular cysts or even a single cyst are pelvic pain, a sensation of feeling bloated, or irregular menses. After several subsequent cycles in which hormone levels once again follow a regular cycle and progesterone levels are restored, cysts usually will be absorbed or will regress. Follicular cysts can be random or recurrent events.

A corpus luteum cyst may develop because there is an intracystic hemorrhage that occurs in the vascularization stage; the affected cyst then consists of blood. In normal cycles, the vascularization is replaced by a clear fluid that accumulates in the cavity of the corpus luteum.

Corpus luteum cysts are less common than follicular cysts, but luteal cysts typically cause more symptoms, particularly if they rupture. Manifestations include dull pelvic pain and amenorrhea or delayed menstruation, followed by irregular or heavier-than-normal bleeding. Rupture occasionally occurs and can cause massive bleeding with excruciating pain; immediate surgery may be required. Corpus luteum cysts usually regress spontaneously in nonpregnant women. Oral contraceptives may be used to prevent cysts from forming in the future.

Dermoid cysts are ovarian teratomas that contain elements of all three germ layers; they are common ovarian neoplasms. These growths may contain mature tissue including skin, hair, sebaceous and sweat glands, muscle fibers, cartilage, and bone. Dermoid cysts are usually asymptomatic and are found incidentally on pelvic examination. Dermoid cysts have malignant potential and should be removed.

Torsion of the ovary may occur as a complication of ovarian cysts or tumors or enlargement of the ovary associated with infertility treatments. Ovarian torsion is rare but is a gynecologic emergency when present. Individuals present with acute, severe unilateral abdominal or pelvic pain related to a change of position.

> **QUICK CHECK 32-3**
> 1. Why is prompt treatment of pelvic inflammatory disease (PID) critical to reproductive health?
> 2. Why do benign ovarian cysts develop in women who ovulate?
> 3. What is the difference between a follicular cyst and a corpus luteum cyst?

Endometrial Polyps

An **endometrial polyp** is a mass of endometrial tissue and contains a variable amount of glands, stroma, and blood vessels. Endometrial polyps are usually solitary and originate at the fundus but also may be multiple (20% of cases) or originate from the lower uterine segment or upper endocervix and contain mixed epithelium. Polyps are morphologically diverse and are usually classified as hyperplastic, atrophic (or inactive), or functional. In the latter case, the surface epithelium may be "out of phase" with other endometrial tissue. Hyperplastic polyps are often pedunculated and may be mistaken for endometrial

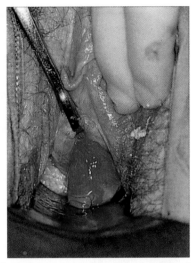

FIGURE 32-10 Endometrial Polyp. Polyp is protruding through the cervical os. (From Symonds EM, Macpherson MBA: *Color atlas of obstetrics and gynecology,* London, 1994, Mosby.)

hyperplasia or, if large, adenosarcoma (Figure 32-10). Although polyps most often develop in women between ages 40 and 50 years, they can occur at all ages.[38] Hyperestrogenic states, obesity, and hypertension are risk factors for developing polyps.

Most polyps are asymptomatic; however, they are a common cause of intermenstrual bleeding or even excessive menstrual bleeding. Diagnosis is made by hysteroscopy or ultrasonography. The lesions can be removed with small, curved forceps but there is a high rate of spontaneous resolution. Coexistence of a separate endometrial atypical hyperplasia or adenocarcinoma is possible, but malignancy is extremely rare (1% to 2%).

Leiomyomas

Leiomyomas, commonly called *myomas* or *uterine fibroids,* are benign tumors that develop from smooth muscle cells in the myometrium. Leiomyomas are the most common benign tumors of the uterus, affecting 70% to 80% of all women, and most remain small and asymptomatic. Prevalence increases in women ages 30 to 50 years but decreases with menopause.[39] The incidence of leiomyomas in black and Asian women is two to five times higher than that in white women.

The cause of uterine leiomyomas is unknown, although the size of the tumor appears to be related to hormonal fluctuations (particularly estrogen). Because leiomyomas are estrogen- and progesterone-sensitive, uterine leiomyomas are not seen before menarche, are common during the reproductive years, and generally shrink after menopause if present. Tumors in pregnant women enlarge rapidly but often decrease in size after termination of the pregnancy.[39] Risk factors include heredity, nulliparity, obesity, PCOS, diabetes, and hypertension.

PATHOPHYSIOLOGY Most leiomyomas occur in multiples in the fundus of the uterus, although often occurring singly and throughout the uterus. Leiomyomas are classified as subserous, submucous, or intramural, according to location within the various layers of the uterine wall (Figure 32-11). Uterine leiomyomas are usually firm and surrounded by a pseudocapsule composed of compressed but otherwise normal uterine myometrium. Degeneration and necrosis may occur when the leiomyoma outgrows its blood supply, which is more common in larger tumors and is frequently accompanied by pain.

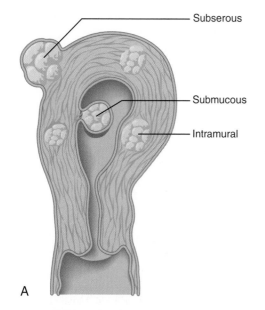

Subserous

Submucous

Intramural

A

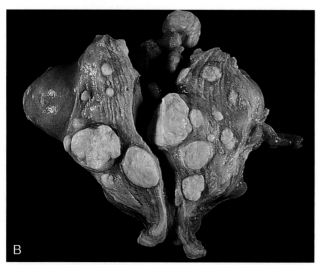

B

FIGURE 32-11 Leiomyomas. A, Uterine section showing whorl-like appearance and locations of leiomyomas, which are also called *uterine fibroids.* **B,** Multiple leiomyomas in sagittal section. Typical, well-circumscribed, solid, light gray nodules distort uterus. (**B** from Damjanov I, Linder J: *Pathology: a color atlas,* St Louis, 2000, Mosby.)

CLINICAL MANIFESTATIONS Although fibroids rarely present problems, pain, abnormal vaginal bleeding, and symptoms related to pressure on nearby structures are often experienced. Fibroids may also contribute to infertility and subfertility, as well as obstruction during birth if large enough. The leiomyoma can make the uterine cavity larger, thereby increasing the endometrial surface area. This may account for the increased menstrual bleeding associated with leiomyomas. Pain or cramping occurs with the devascularization of larger leiomyomas and is associated with blood vessel compression that limits blood supply to adjacent structures. Because the tumor is relatively slow growing, enabling adjacent structures to adapt to pressure, symptoms of abdominal pressure develop slowly. Pressure on the bladder may contribute to urinary frequency, urgency, and dysuria. Pressure on the ureter may cause it to become distended "upstream" from the pressure point; rectosigmoid pressure may lead to constipation. Larger tumors may cause a sensation of abdominal or genital heaviness.

EVALUATION AND TREATMENT Uterine leiomyomas are suspected when bimanual examination discloses irregular, nontender nodularity of the uterus. Pelvic sonography or magnetic resonance imaging (MRI) confirms the diagnosis. Treatment depends on symptoms, tumor size, and age, reproductive status, and overall health of the individual. Most myomas are asymptomatic and can be managed by observation only. Medical treatment is aimed at shrinking the myoma. Use of hormonal contraceptives may shrink or enhance growth and should be closely monitored. Mifepristone (formerly RU-486), an antiprogesterone, also may be useful as a conservative treatment, as well as GnRH agonists for temporary management.[40] Myomectomy may be undertaken and has been the surgical treatment of choice. Experimental treatments, such as embolization of uterine arteries, laser ablation, and levonorgestrel-intrauterine system (LNG-IUS), all hold promise.[41] Benefits and risks should be carefully considered, as well as a woman's desire for future pregnancy.

Adenomyosis

Adenomyosis is the presence of islands of endometrial glands surrounded by benign endometrial stroma within the uterine myometrium. It commonly develops during the late reproductive years, with the highest incidence among women in their forties and women taking tamoxifen. Adenomyosis has been found in 18% of hysterectomy specimens and 53% of specimens from women taking tamoxifen.[42] Adenomyosis may be asymptomatic or may be associated with abnormal menstrual bleeding, dysmenorrhea, uterine enlargement, and uterine tenderness during menstruation. Secondary dysmenorrhea becomes increasingly severe as disease progresses. On examination, the uterus is enlarged, globular, and most tender just before or after menstruation. Diagnosis is confirmed with ultrasonography or MRI. Treatment is asymptomatic, similar to dysmenorrhea (i.e., nonsteroidal anti-inflammatory drugs [NSAIDs], hormonal contraceptives, or levonorgestrel-intrauterine system [LNG-IUS]). Other options include surgical resection or hysterectomy.

Endometriosis

Endometriosis is the presence of functioning endometrial tissue or implants outside the uterus. Like normal endometrial tissue, the ectopic (out-of-place) endometrium responds to the hormonal fluctuations of the menstrual cycle. Endometriosis affects 2% to 22% of reproductive-age women and 2% to 4% of menopausal women. As many as 50% of women evaluated for pelvic pain, infertility, or pelvic mass are diagnosed with endometriosis. Theories of the cause of endometriosis are shown in Box 32-5, but the cause is unknown.

PATHOPHYSIOLOGY Endometrial implants can occur throughout the body but occur primarily in the abdominal and pelvic cavities. The most common sites of implantation are the ovaries, uterine ligaments, rectovaginal septum, and pelvic peritoneum (Figure 32-12). Less common sites include the sigmoid colon, small intestine, rectum, appendix, bladder, uterus, vulva, vagina, cervix, lymph nodes, extremities, pleural cavity, lungs, laparotomy scars, and hernial sacs.

If the blood supply is sufficient, the ectopic endometrium proliferates, breaks down, and bleeds in conjunction with the normal menstrual cycle. The bleeding causes inflammation and pain in surrounding tissues. The inflammation may lead to fibrosis, scarring, and adhesions.

CLINICAL MANIFESTATIONS The clinical manifestations of endometriosis vary in frequency and severity and can mimic other pelvic

BOX 32-5   THEORIES OF ENDOMETRIOSIS

- Implantation of endometrial cells during retrograde menstruation, in which menstrual fluids move through the fallopian tubes and empty into the pelvic cavity; occurs in most women, but few develop endometriosis as a result
- Spread of endometrial cells through the vascular or lymphatic systems— helps explain the rare sites
- Immunologic factors that may include depressed cytotoxic T cell response and natural killer (NK) cell activity
- Stimulation of multipotential epithelial cells covering the reproductive organs that develop into endometrial cells
- Genetic predisposition based on familial tendencies
- Dioxin and dioxin-like compounds may stimulate endometriosis formation and block normal progesterone effects

Data from Caserta DL et al: Impact of endocrine disruptor chemicals in gynaecology, *Hum Reprod Update* 14(1):59–72, 2008; Fritz M, Speroff L, editors: *Clinical gynecologic endocrinology and fertility,* ed 8, Philadelphia, 2011, Lippincott Williams & Wilkins.

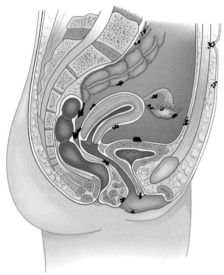

FIGURE 32-12 Pelvic Sites of Endometrial Implantation in Endometriosis. Endometrial cells may enter the pelvic cavity during retrograde menstruation.

disease (i.e., pelvic inflammatory disease, ovarian cysts, irritable bowel, dysmenorrhea). Symptoms include infertility, pelvic pain, dyschezia (pain on defecation), dyspareunia, and, less commonly, constipation and abnormal vaginal bleeding. If implants are located within the pelvis, an asymptomatic pelvic mass having irregular, movable nodules and a fixed, retroverted uterus are found on examination. Most symptoms can be explained by the proliferation, breakdown, and bleeding of the ectopic endometrial tissue with subsequent formation of adhesions. In most instances, however, the degree of endometriosis is not related to the frequency or severity of symptoms. Dysmenorrhea, for example, does not appear to be related to the degree of endometriosis. With involvement of the rectovaginal septum or the uterosacral ligaments, dyspareunia develops. Dyschezia, a hallmark symptom of endometriosis, occurs with bleeding of ectopic endometrium in the rectosigmoid musculature and subsequent fibrosis.

Up to 25% to 40% of women with infertility have endometriosis. However, the degree of disease is not closely associated with infertility. Infertility may be the result of (1) mechanical interference with ovulation or ovum transport, (2) effects of inflammation and cytotoxic activity, (3) phagocytosis of spermatozoa by macrophages, (4) impairment of follicle development, (5) defects in implantation, and (6) oxidative stress effects. However, the exact mechanism is not known.[43]

EVALUATION AND TREATMENT   A presumptive diagnosis is based on the previously described symptoms, but pelvic laparoscopy is required for a definitive diagnosis.[44] The American Fertility Society has proposed that endometriosis be classified by the extent of the disease as stage I, mild; stage II, moderate; stage III, severe; and stage IV, extensive. All treatment is based on the stage of the disease and aimed toward preventing progression of the disease, alleviating pain, and/or restoring fertility. Medical therapies include suppression of ovulation with various medications, such as combined hormonal contraceptives, depot medroxyprogesterone acetate, danazol, GnRH agonists, mifepristone, or levonorgestrel-containing IUD. Conservative surgical treatment includes laparoscopic removal of endometrial implants with conventional or laser techniques and presacral neurectomy for severe dysmenorrhea. All treatments have risks or side effects, and recurrent symptoms will develop in as many as 74% of women within a few years.

Cancer

Malignant tumors of the female reproductive system are common. Endometrial carcinoma accounts for approximately 5.8% of all cancers in women; ovarian tumors, 3.1%; and cervical tumors, 1.6%.[1] Malignant neoplasms of the female reproductive tract account for about 1 of 8 diagnosed cancers and 1 of 10 cancer deaths in women in the United States.[1]

Cervical Cancer

Cancer of the cervix is the most common cancer in women worldwide; however, in the United States, it is the fourteenth most common type of cancer in women.[1] In the United States, the rates of invasive cancer have steadily decreased (a 75% reduction since the 1960s) and mortality rates caused by cervical cancer have declined (more than 45% since the early 1970s) largely because of the increased prevalence and frequency of cervical cancer screening with the Pap smear. The incidence rate in black women (11.1 per 100,000) exceeds the rate in white women (7.9 per 100,000); the mortality rate is more than double (4.6 per 100,000) for black women compared to the mortality rate for white women (2.2 per 100,000). In 2010 the American Cancer Society estimated 12,200 new cases of cervical invasive cancer and 4210 cervical cancer deaths.[1]

It is now widely known that cervical cancer is almost exclusively caused by cervical human papillomavirus (HPV) infection. Infection with "high-risk" (oncogenic) types of HPV (predominantly 16 and 18) is a necessary precursor to development of the precancerous dysplasia of the cervix that leads to invasive cancer. Precancerous dysplasia, also called *cervical intraepithelial carcinoma (CIN)* or *cervical carcinoma in situ (CIS)*, occurs more often in younger women. Fifty percent of adolescents and young women acquire HPV (predominantly high-risk types) within 3 years of initiation of sexual intercourse; half of these are within 3 months.[45] However, most of these infections are spontaneously cleared by the immune system; the vast majority of these cases do not progress into CIS or invasive cervical cancer.[46] Vaccination against HPV is currently being promoted as a promising preventive approach (see *Health Alert:* Cervical Cancer Primary Prevention). Smoking, immunosuppression, and poor nutrition are considered cofactors, perhaps explaining why some HPV infections do progress to cervical cancer.

PATHOGENESIS   Cervical cancer is a slowly progressive disease and moves from normal cervical epithelial cells to dysplasia to CIS to invasive cancer (Figure 32-13). Table 32-4 summarizes the staging of

Normal CIN 1 CIN 2 CIN 3

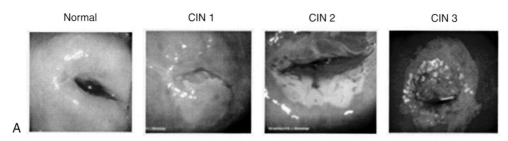

A

Cervical Disease Progression[1-6]

Most HPV infections will clear, and most cervical lesions will not progress[1-3]

Months Years

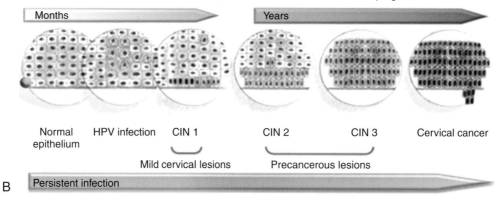

Normal epithelium — HPV infection — CIN 1 — CIN 2 — CIN 3 — Cervical cancer

Mild cervical lesions — Precancerous lesions

B Persistent infection

- CIN 2/3 lesions are more likely to progress to cervical cancer than CIN 1 lesions[1]

1. Oster A. Int J of Gynecol Path, 1993, 12:186-92. 2. Moscicki A et al, Vaccine, 2006, 2453:42-51. 3. Einstein M. Cancer Immunol Immunother, 2008, 57:443-51. 4. Winer R. et al. J Int Dis, 2005, 191:731-38. 5. Holowaty P. et al. J Natl Cancer Inst, 1999, 91:252-58. 6. Solomon D. et al. JAMA, 2002, 287:2114-19.

FIGURE 32-13 Cervical Intraepithelial Neoplasia (CIN). **A,** Normal multiparous cervix including the transformation zone *(TZ)* where precancerous and cancerous changes occur (see next photos). CIN stage 1, note the white appearance of part of the anterior lip of the cervix associated with neoplastic changes; CIN stage 2, lesions also are reflected in distant capillaries; CIN stage 3, lesions predominantly around the external os. **B,** Normal epithelium, HPV infection progressing to CIN stage 1, and then with more time persistent HPV infections progressing to precancerous lesions CIN 2 and CIN 3 and eventually cervical cancer. Most cervical lesions do not progress to cervical cancer. (**A** from Ostör AG: Natural history of cervical intraepithelial neoplasia: a critical review, *Int J Gynecol Pathol* 23:186–192, 1993; **B** from Symonds EM, Macpherson MBA: *Color atlas of obstetrics and gynecology,* London, 1994, Mosby.)

TABLE 32-4		CLINICAL STAGING FOR CANCER OF THE CERVIX
STAGE		**CHARACTERISTICS**
0	IA	Cancer in situ, intraepithelial carcinoma; earliest stage of cancer; cancer confined to its original site
I	IA1	Carcinoma confined to cervix (extension to corpus disregarded)
	IA2	Earliest form of stage I; there is very small amount of cancer, which is visible only under a microscope
		Area of invasion is <3 mm (about ⅛ inch) deep and <7 mm (about ⅓ inch) wide
		Area of invasion is between 3 and 5 mm (about ⅕ inch) deep and <7 mm (about ⅓ inch) wide
IB		Includes cancers that can be seen without a microscope; also includes cancers seen only with a microscope that have spread deeper than 5 mm (about ⅕ inch) into connective tissue of cervix or are wider than 7 mm
	IB1	A IB cancer that is no longer than 4 cm (about 1⅗ inches)
	IB2	A IB cancer that is >4 cm
II		Cancer has spread beyond cervix to upper part of vagina; cancer does not involve lower third of vagina
	IIA	Cancer has spread beyond cervix to upper part of vagina; cancer does not involve lower third of vagina
	IIB	Cancer has spread to tissue next to cervix, called *parametrial tissue*
III		Cancer has spread to lower part of vagina or pelvic wall; cancer may be blocking ureters (tubes that carry urine from kidneys to bladder)
	IIIA	Cancer has spread to lower third of vagina but not to pelvic wall
	IIIB	Cancer extends to pelvic wall or blocks urine flow to bladder
IV		Most advanced stage of cervical cancer; cancer has spread to other parts of body
	IVA	Cancer has spread to bladder or rectum, which are organs close to cervix
	IVB	Cancer has spread to distant organs beyond pelvic area, such as lungs

Excerpted from the American Cancer Society: *Detailed guide: cervical cancer: how is cervical cancer staged?*

Cervical Cancer Primary Prevention

The Food and Drug Administration licensed two vaccines against human papillomavirus (HPV) for girls ages 9 to 26 years—Gardasil (Merck & Company) in 2002 and Cervarix (GlaxoSmithKline) in 2009. Both vaccines are effective in preventing HPV "high risk" types 16 and 18, which are responsible for 70% of all cervical cancers. Gardasil also provides protection against HPV types 6 and 11, which are responsible for 90% of all benign genital warts. The Advisory Committee on Immunization Practices (ACIP) recommends routine vaccination of females 11 or 12 years of age with a three-dose series of either vaccine. The vaccination series can be started at 9 years of age. Ideally, vaccination should occur before potential exposure to HPV through sexual contact. In clinical trials, vaccine efficacy was as high as 97% in the prevention of HPV16- or HPV18-related cervical intraepithelial neoplasia grade 2 or 3 or adenocarcinoma in situ. Studies now suggest that vaccination of boys and men 9 to 26 years of age against all HPV6-, HPV11-, HPV16-, and HPV18-associated diseases also may provide substantial cost-effective public health benefits (i.e., reduction in cervical cancer in women). The controversial practice of male circumcision also my reduce transmission of HPV to their sex partners. In observational studies in Uganda, a 28% reduction in the prevalence of high-risk HPV was noted in women with partners who were circumcised.

Data from Centers for Disease Control and Prevention: FPA licensure of bivalent human papillomavirus vaccine (HPV2, Cervarix) for use in females and updated HPV vaccination recommendations from the Advisory Committee on Immunization Practices (ACIP), *MMWR Morb Mortal Wkly Rep* 59(20):626–629, 2010; Elbasha EH, Dasbach EJ: Impact of vaccinating boys and men against HPV in the United States, *Vaccine* 28(42):6856–6867, 2010; Wawer MJ et al: Effect of circumcision of HIV-negative men on transmission of human papillomavirus to HIV-negative women: a randomized trial in Rakai, Uganda, *Lancet* 377(9761):209–218, 2011.

cervical cancer. Testing for high-risk HPV is often positive for many years (10 years or more) before dysplasia progresses to high-grade squamous intraepithelial lesions (HSILs) that can develop into invasive cervical cancer. The genetics of cervical cancer remain poorly understood. Like other cancers, cervical cancer requires the accumulation of genetic alterations for carcinogenesis to occur.

CLINICAL MANIFESTATIONS   Because cervical neoplasms are often asymptomatic, regular Pap smear, HPV screening, or both is necessary. About 90% of cervical cancers can be detected early through the use of Pap and HPV testing. If symptoms exist, they may include a change in vaginal discharge or bleeding. Bleeding varies and may occur after intercourse or between menstrual periods. At times, women will complain of abnormal menses or postmenopausal bleeding. A less common symptom may be a serosanguineous or yellowish vaginal discharge. A new or foul odor also may be present. Pelvic or epigastric pain is experienced only with large lesions. Advanced disease may cause urinary or rectal symptoms and pelvic or back pain.

EVALUATION AND TREATMENT   When dysplasia is detected, colposcopy is usually indicated to identify lesions and obtain biopsies of the ectocervix and endocervix. If invasive carcinoma is found, lymphangiography, computed tomography (CT) scan, ultrasonography, or radioimmunodetection methods are used to assess lymphatic involvement.

The treatment depends on the degree of neoplastic change, the size and location of the lesion, and the extent of metastatic spread. With

TABLE 32-5	RECOMMENDED TREATMENT BASED ON CLINICAL STAGING FOR CANCER OF THE CERVIX
STAGE	**TREATMENT**
0	Cryosurgery, laser surgery, loop electrosurgical excision procedure (LEEP), electrocautery
I	LEEP, laser surgery, conization, cryosurgery, radiation without surgery, total hysterectomy with or without bilateral pelvic lymphadenectomy
II	Radiation, radical hysterectomy and pelvic lymphadenectomy often followed by radiation
III	Radiation with external beam or implant(s) with or without hydroxyurea
IV	Radiation with external beam or implant(s) with or without hydroxyurea, chemotherapy (cisplatin or ifosfamide with distant site involvement)

early detection and treatment (cryosurgery, loop conization, or electrosurgical excision), the prognosis for invasive cervical cancer is excellent. The overall 5-year survival rate is 71% and 95% for stage IA or lower. A cure rate of 100% is possible for women with dysplasia or carcinoma in situ.[1] The prevention of HPV infection may be the key to substantially reducing the risk of cervical cancer (see *Health Alert: Cervical Cancer Primary Prevention*). Table 32-5 contains recommended treatment based on staging of disease.

Vaginal Cancer

Cancer of the vagina is the rarest of the female genital cancers. It can occur at any age but is found predominantly in women 50 years of age and older. More than 90% of women with vaginal cancer have squamous cell carcinoma, although rare melanomas, sarcomas, and adenocarcinomas are also found. (Types of tumors are described in Chapter 9.) Metastatic cancers are more common than primary lesions in older women.

Vaginal and cervical cancers are thought to have similar etiology. Both start as intraepithelial lesions and occur in sexually active women. HPV infection and prior carcinoma of the cervix place a woman at higher risk for developing vaginal cancer.[47] In addition, exposure in utero to nonsteroidal estrogens (diethylstilbestrol [DES]) also has been identified as a risk factor. DES was given to millions of women between 1938 and 1971 to prevent miscarriage. Between 0.14 and 1.4 cases of vaginal cancer develop per 1000 women at risk. The average age at which clear cell carcinoma develops as a result of DES exposure is 19 years.

Like cervical neoplasms, vaginal cancers are classified as intraepithelial neoplasia (dysplasia), carcinoma in situ, or invasive carcinoma. The lesion usually is not invasive, and it most often occurs in the upper third of the vagina.

Vaginal cancer is generally asymptomatic. Therefore, regular pelvic examinations, particularly for women with a history of intrauterine DES exposure, are extremely important. Clinical manifestations that occur include abnormal vaginal bleeding or discharge. Pain, rectal or bladder symptoms, vulvar pruritus, and leg edema are symptoms of advanced disease.

Biopsy techniques confirm the tumor type and determine its size, location, and extent. Treatment depends on these findings and on the age of the individual. Surgery may be followed by radiation and chemotherapy.

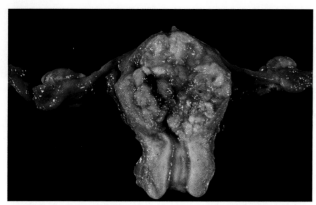

FIGURE 32-14 Endometrial Cancer. Tumor fills the endometrial cavity. Obvious myometrial invasion is shown. (From Damjanov I, Linder J, editors: *Anderson's pathology,* ed 10, St Louis, 1996, Mosby.)

Vulvar Cancer

Cancer of the vulva was responsible for approximately 3% to 5% of all gynecologic cancers; an incidence of 3900 new cases was estimated for 2010.[1] The majority (90%) are squamous cell carcinomas, although melanoma (5%), Bartholin gland carcinoma (2%), sarcoma (2%), and adenosquamous carcinoma (1%) may occur. Squamous dysplasia of the vagina or cervix is a major risk factor, as are smoking and coffee use.[1] Early detection is critical, and all suspicious lesions should be biopsied. Treatment includes surgery, radiation, and chemotherapy. Prognosis depends on lesion size, location, histologic studies, and lymph involvement.[48]

Endometrial Cancer

Carcinoma of the endometrium is the most prevalent gynecologic malignancy (Figure 32-14). It accounts for about 6% of cancers affecting women and more than 51% of gynecologic cancers. Estimates include 43,470 new cases in 2010, with approximately 7950 deaths.[1] The primary risk factor is unopposed estrogen exposure with resultant hyperplasia. However, other risk factors have been identified (see *Risk Factors: Estrogen-Related Exposures*). Ninety-five percent of endometrial cancers occur in postmenopausal women, with the peak incidence occurring in the late fifties to early sixties. Although incidence rates are

higher in white than black women, mortality rates in black women are nearly twice as high.

Delayed menarche, pregnancy, and the use of combined hormonal contraception have a protective effect, as do progestin-containing IUDs. After 12 months' use of combined hormonal contraception, a 50% reduction in risk continues for at least 10 to 12 years after discontinuation.

Abnormal vaginal bleeding is the most common clinical manifestation of endometrial cancer. Postmenopausal women, obese women, and women with unopposed estrogenic conditions (i.e., anovulatory cycles) should be evaluated in the event of unscheduled or persistent, irregular vaginal bleeding. Diagnosis is made by direct cytologic sampling of the endometrium. This may be accomplished by endometrial biopsy or measurement of endometrial thickness, or both, by transvaginal ultrasound. An endometrial depth of less than 5 mm established by ultrasonography rules out proliferation. Evaluation for metastasis includes routine blood work, metabolic studies, chest x-ray films, intravenous pyelography (IVP), barium enema, ultrasonography, and lymphangiography.

Treatment is based on the extent of the disease, and may include curettage for carcinoma in situ, total abdominal hysterectomy, chemotherapy, radiation, and progestins. The 5-year survival rate is 95% with early diagnosis and 64% if diagnosis occurred in the late stage.

Ovarian Cancer

The American Cancer Society (ACS) estimated 21,880 new cases of ovarian cancer and 13,150 ovarian cancer deaths in 2010 (Figure 32-15).[1] Ovarian cancer causes more deaths than any other cancer of the female reproductive system.[49]

Multiple epidemiologic studies agree that an increased risk of epithelial ovarian cancer has been linked to advancing age; family history of breast, colon, or ovarian cancer; and frequency of ovulation.[49] Despite study limitations, several factors related to ovulation have been consistently associated with increased or decreased risk of developing ovarian cancer (see *Risk Factors: Ovarian Cancer*). Risk is reduced by factors that suppress ovulation (pregnancy, breastfeeding, and combined hormonal contraceptive use).[49] Ovarian cancer has been a very difficult disease to diagnose and treat. Because symptoms in the early stage are often vague, the disease is usually not diagnosed until the late stage when prognosis is poor and treatment is largely ineffective. Only 20% of all ovarian cancers are found in the early stage.

RISK FACTORS

Estrogen-Related Exposures

- Unopposed estrogen replacement therapy
- Tamoxifen
- Early menarche
- Late menopause
- Anovulatory cycles (PCOS, perimenopause)
- Nulliparity
- Obesity (androgenous source of estrogen)

Other Risk Factors
- Diabetes
- Gallbladder disease
- Physical inactivity
- High-fat, low-fiber diet
- Hypertension
- Family history of colon, endometrial, or ovarian cancer

Data from American Cancer Society: *Cancer facts and figures—2010,* New York, 2010, Author.

RISK FACTORS

Ovarian Cancer

- Family history of ovarian, breast, uterine, pancreatic, or colon cancer
- Personal history of breast and colorectal cancer
- Obesity
- Age: postmenopausal
- Infertility or prolonged use of fertility drugs without achieving pregnancy
- Early menarche, late menopause, or no children or first child after age 30 years (uninterrupted ovulation)
- Genetic predisposition, especially *BRCA1, BRCA2, HNPCC, ARID1A* mutations

Data from American Cancer Society: *Cancer facts and figures—2010,* New York, 2010, Author; American Cancer Society: *Overview: ovarian cancer,* New York, 2010, Author.
HNPCC, Hereditary nonpolyposis colon cancer.

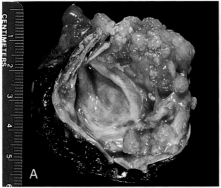
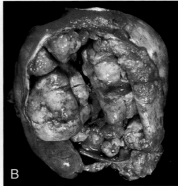
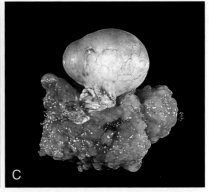

FIGURE 32-15 Ovarian Tumors. A serous borderline tumor displays a cyst cavity lined by papillary tumor growths **(A)**. The cyst is opened **(B)** to reveal a large bulky tumor mass called cystadenocarcinoma **(C)**, a tumor on the ovarian surface. Bilaterality of tumors is common, occurring in 20% of benign tumors, 30% of serous borderline tumors, and approximately 66% of serous carcinomas. A significant proportion of both borderline malignant and malignant tumors involve the surface of the ovary **(C)**. (From Kumar et al: *Robbins and Cotran pathologic basis of disease*, ed 8, St. Louis, 2010, Saunders.)

PATHOGENESIS Etiology is largely unknown but may be related to mechanisms involved in ovulation, as well as exposure to cancer-causing substances that pass through the vagina to reach the fallopian tubes and ovaries. More than 90% of ovarian cancers arise from epithelial cells—the ovarian surface epithelium.[12] Cancers also can arise from germ cells (2%) or theca cells (1%) of the ovarian stroma. Germ cell tumors occur in younger women, whereas those from epithelial tissue primarily occur in women more than 50 years of age. Ovarian cancers exhibit a distinctive pattern of progression spreading intra-abdominally over the surface of the peritoneum. Loss of tumor-suppressor genes and activation of oncogenes have both been described. Most ovarian cancers are sporadic and not associated with any pattern of inheritance. Of the approximately 10% that are inherited, the majority are associated with mutations of the breast cancer susceptibility gene (*BRCA1*, *BRCA2*, and hereditary nonpolyposis colon cancer [HNPCC]).[12] Breast, ovarian, and colon cancers appear to share common genetic markers or genes, or both. Recent data also implicate *ARID1A*, a tumor-suppressor gene that is frequently disrupted in ovarian clear cell and endometrioid carcinomas. This is considered to confirm a link between endometriosis and increased ovarian cancer risk.[50]

CLINICAL MANIFESTATIONS Ovarian cancer is generally considered a silent disease, meaning that by the time the individual experiences symptoms and seeks treatment, the disease has spread beyond the primary site. The most obvious symptoms are pelvic pain and abdominal swelling (ascites) that arise from the primary ovarian mass. Gastrointestinal symptoms are common, such as anorexia, early satiety, upset stomach, and constipation. Other symptoms include fatigue, urinary urgency or frequency, back pain, dyspareunia, and pelvic pressure.[49] Abnormal vaginal bleeding may occur if the postmenopausal endometrium is stimulated by a hormone-secreting tumor. The tumor also may cause ulcerations through the vaginal wall that result in bleeding.

Tumor obstruction of vascular channels can cause venous and, occasionally, arterial thrombosis. Alterations in coagulability also occur, contributing to clot formation. Metastasis often causes pleural effusion (Figure 32-16).

EVALUATION AND TREATMENT Because ovarian cancer has no early symptoms and there are no effective screening techniques to detect it, the disease is usually advanced by the time treatment is

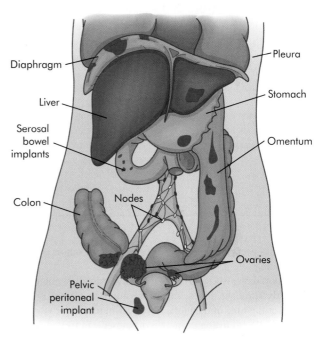

FIGURE 32-16 Metastasis of Ovarian Cancer. Pattern of spread for epithelial cancer of the ovary.

sought. Transvaginal ultrasound and a tumor marker (CA-125) may assist diagnosis but are not recommended for routine screening. Research is ongoing to develop more effective screening in high-risk women. Diagnosis is made after ultrasound, CT scan, magnetic resonance imaging (MRI), or other imaging techniques that enable clinicians to localize the tumor mass. The International Federation of Gynecologists and Obstetricians (FIGO) staging system is described in Table 32-6.

The initial approach to treatment is surgery, which is performed to determine the stage of disease and to remove as much of the tumor as possible. Radiation therapy may follow if the tumor is smaller than 2 cm in size and is confined to the abdominopelvic area without involvement of the kidneys or liver. The success of chemotherapy depends on the extent of disease, whether the tumor is a discrete mass, and whether there has been prior exposure to chemotherapeutic agents.

TABLE 32-6 FIGO* STAGING OF CARCINOMA OF THE OVARY

STAGE	CHARACTERISTICS
I	Growth limited to ovaries
II	Growth involving one or both ovaries and involvement of other organs (i.e., uterus, bladder, colon)
III	Cancer involves one or both ovaries, and one or both of following are present: (1) cancer has spread beyond pelvis to lining of abdomen, (2) cancer has spread to lymph nodes
IV	Growth involving one or both ovaries with distant metastases to lungs, liver, or other organs outside peritoneal cavity
Recurrent	Cancer recurred after completion of treatment

*The International Federation of Gynecologists and Obstetricians.

TABLE 32-7 POSSIBLE EFFECTS OF CHRONIC DISEASE ON SEXUAL FUNCTIONING IN WOMEN

DISEASE	SEXUAL FUNCTION
Cerebral palsy	Intact genital sensations, decreased lubrication; difficulty with sexual activity/positioning because of muscle spasticity, rigidity, or weakness; pain with positioning caused by contracture of knees and hips or because of increased spasms with arousal
Cerebrovascular accident (CVA)	Difficulties in sexual positioning and sensitivity because of impaired motor strength, coordination, or paralysis; decreased libido with stroke on dominant side of brain
Diabetes	Diminished intensity of orgasm and gradual decline in ability to achieve orgasm; decreased lubrication or recurrent vaginal infections with resultant dyspareunia
Chronic renal failure	Decreased arousal; increasingly rare and less intense orgasms; decreased lubrication
Rheumatoid arthritis (RA)	Painful sexual activity/positions because of swollen, painful joints, muscular atrophy, and joint contracture; decreased libido because of pain, fatigue, or medication; genital sensations remain intact
Systemic lupus erythematosis (SLE)	Similar to RA; decreased lubrication and vaginal lesions result in painful penetration
Myocardial infarction (MI)	Most literature male-oriented; problems related to medications
Multiple sclerosis (MS)	Diminished genital sensitivity; decreased lubrication; declining orgasmic ability; difficulty with sexual activity because of muscle weakness, pain, or incontinence
Spinal cord injury	Reflex sexual response with injury above sacral area; disrupted response with lesion at or below sacrum; loss of sensation, decreased lubrication; spasticity, incontinence, or pain with arousal; continued orgasmic sensations or sensations diffused in general or to specific body parts, such as breast or lips

Research into prevention and treatment of ovarian cancer is ongoing and expanding.

The mortality associated with ovarian cancer has not changed significantly since the 1980s, mainly because the disease is already advanced at the time of diagnosis. Five-year mortality for women for all stages is 53%.[1] If ovarian cancer is diagnosed and treated early, the survival rate is 94%; however, only 20% of cases are detected at earlier stages (see *Health Alert: Recovery After Cancer Treatment*).

HEALTH ALERT

Recovery After Cancer Treatment

- Stop tobacco use.
- Limit alcohol to less than 1 drink per day.
- Improve nutrition—increase intake of fruits, vegetables, whole grains, and high-fiber foods; limit fat, especially animal fats.
- Exercise daily.
- Rest frequently.
- Join a support group and attend meetings (family members should attend support groups also).
- Communicate openly, honestly, and frequently with members of the cancer care team.

See American Cancer Society: www.cancer.org/Treatment/Survivorship DuringandAfterTreatment/BeHealthyafterTreatment/index.

Sexual Dysfunction

Increased awareness of female sexual dysfunction is relatively new; most information in this area is derived from clinical observations and anecdotal reports from women, and adequate research is lacking. Both organic and psychosocial disorders can be implicated in sexual dysfunction. Organic problems may be the underlying cause in 10% to 20% of cases and may contribute to another 15% of cases. Chronic illness can affect sexual functioning and response. Table 32-7 outlines possible effects of specified chronic diseases on female sexual functioning.

Disorders of desire (inhibited sexual desire, decreased libido) may be a biologic manifestation of depression, alcohol or other substance abuse, prolactin-secreting pituitary tumors, or testosterone deficiency. β-Adrenergic blockers used for heart disease also may inhibit sexual desire.

Vaginismus is an involuntary muscle spasm of the pubococcygeal muscle in response to attempted penetration. Common psychologic causes include prior sexual trauma and fear of sex. Organic causes are similar to those that cause dyspareunia, including vulvovestibulitis. Even after the underlying organic problem is detected and successfully treated, vaginismus may persist.

Anorgasmia (orgasmic dysfunction) is the inability of a woman to reach or achieve orgasm. Specific disorders that may block orgasm are diabetes, alcoholism, neurologic disturbances, hormonal deficiencies, and pelvic disorders, such as infections, trauma, and surgical scarring.

Other inhibitors include drugs, such as narcotics, tranquilizers, antidepressants, and antihypertensive medications.

Dyspareunia (painful intercourse) is common. Women may experience pain at any time from the beginning of arousal to after intercourse. The pain may have a burning, sharp, searing, or cramping quality and may be described as external, vaginal, deep abdominal, or pelvic. A variety of psychosocial and organic causes have been identified. Inadequate lubrication may make penetration or intercourse difficult or painful. Drugs with a drying effect, such as antihistamines, certain tranquilizers, and marijuana, and disorders such as diabetes, vaginal infections, and estrogen deficiency can decrease lubrication. Other causes include skin problems around the introitus or affecting the vulva; irritation or infection of the clitoris; disorders of the vaginal opening, such as scarring from episiotomy or chronically infected hymenal remnants; intact hymen; bartholinitis; disorders of the urethra or anus; disorders of the vagina, such as infections, thinning of the walls caused by aging or decreased estrogen level, or irritation caused by spermicides or douches; and pelvic disorders, such as infection, tumors, cervical or uterine abnormalities, or torn uterine ligaments.

Sexual dysfunction may develop as a coping mechanism. Women with a history of sexual trauma—rape, incest, or molestation—often have problems with desire, arousal, or orgasm or experience pain with sexual activity. In extreme cases, total sexual aversion may develop. At other times, sexual dysfunction may be a symptom of marital or relationship problems. Often, unresolved anger manifests as inhibited desire or diminished arousal. Relationship factors may be more important in decreasing libido than age of menopause. Physiologic and psychologic factors are more prominent in genital arousal with decreased organic functioning.

Impaired Fertility

Infertility affects approximately 15% of all couples and is defined as the inability to conceive after 1 year of unprotected intercourse. Fertility can be impaired by factors in the man or in the woman or in both partners. Male factors include diminished quality and production of sperm. Causes include infections or inflammation, endocrine or hormonal disorders, immunologic problems in which men produce antibodies to their own sperm, and environmental or lifestyle factors.[51] Female infertility factors are associated with malfunctions of the fallopian tubes, the ovaries, reproductive hormones, and thyroid disorders. Adhesions from pelvic infection may cause blockage of one or both fallopian tubes, preventing access of the sperm to the ovum. Hormonal or local factors may disrupt ovulation or prevent a fertilized egg from implantation. Endometriosis also may contribute to infertility. A number of diagnostic procedures are required in the routine investigation of the infertile couple. Initial workup includes semen analysis and determination of ovulation. In many instances, no cause may be identified.

Treatment of infertility is aimed toward correcting problems identified during the diagnostic workup. The best treatment for infertility is prevention of sexually transmitted infection that can result in scarring and adhesion formation in the reproductive tract of either the man or the woman.

> ✔ **QUICK CHECK 32-4**
> 1. Why is cervical cancer considered a sexually transmitted infection?
> 2. Why does the American Cancer Society recommend screening for cervical cancer?
> 3. What are the risk factors for endometrial cancer?
> 4. What factors reduce the risk of ovarian cancer?

DISORDERS OF THE MALE REPRODUCTIVE SYSTEM
Disorders of the Urethra

Urethritis and urethral strictures are common disorders of the male urethra. Urethral carcinoma, an extremely rare form of cancer, can occur in men older than 60 years.

Urethritis

Urethritis is an inflammatory process that is usually, but not always, caused by a sexually transmitted microorganism. Infectious urethritis caused by *N. gonorrhoeae* is often called *gonococcal urethritis (GU);* urethritis caused by other microorganisms is called *nongonococcal urethritis (NGU).* Nonsexual origins of urethritis include inflammation or infection as a result of urologic procedures, insertion of foreign bodies into the urethra, anatomic abnormalities, or trauma.

Noninfectious urethritis is rare and is associated with the ingestion of wood or ethyl alcohol or turpentine. It is also seen with reactive arthritis.[52]

Symptoms of urethritis include urethral tingling or itching or a burning sensation, and frequency and urgency with urination. The individual may note a purulent or clear mucous-like discharge from the urethra. Nucleic acid detection amplification tests allow early detection of *N. gonorrhoeae* and *C. trachomatis* in urine tests. Treatment consists of appropriate antibiotic therapy for infectious urethritis and avoidance of future exposure or mechanical irritation.

Urethral Strictures

A urethral stricture is a narrowing of the urethra caused by scarring. The scars may be congenital but are more likely to result from trauma (e.g., injury or urologic instrumentation) or untreated or severe urethral infections. Infections also can occur from long-term use of indwelling catheters. Prostatitis and infection secondary to urinary stasis are common complications. Severe and prolonged obstruction can result in hydronephrosis and renal failure.

The clinical manifestations of uretheral stricture are caused by bladder outlet obstruction. The primary symptom is diminished force and caliber of the urinary system; other symptoms include urinary frequency and hesitancy, mild dysuria, double urinary stream or spraying, and dribbling after voiding. Urethral stricture is diagnosed on the basis of history, physical examination, flow rates, and cystoscopy. Treatment is usually surgical and may involve urethral dilation, urethrotomy, or a variety of open surgical techniques. The choice of surgical intervention depends on the age of the individual and the severity of the problem.

Disorders of the Penis
Phimosis and Paraphimosis

Phimosis and paraphimosis are both disorders in which the foreskin (prepuce) is "too tight" to move easily over the glans penis. Phimosis is a condition in which the foreskin cannot be retracted back over the glans, whereas paraphimosis is the opposite: the foreskin is retracted and cannot be moved forward (reduced) to cover the glans (Figure 32-17). Both conditions can cause penile pathologic conditions.

The inability to retract the foreskin is normal in infancy and is caused by congenital adhesions. During the first 3 years of life, congenital adhesions (between the foreskin and glans) separate naturally with penile erections and are not an indication for circumcision. Phimosis can occur at any age and is most commonly caused by poor hygiene and chronic infection. It rarely occurs with normal foreskin.

Reasons for seeking treatment include edema, erythema, and tenderness of the prepuce and purulent discharge; inability to retract the foreskin is a less common complaint. Circumcision, if needed, is

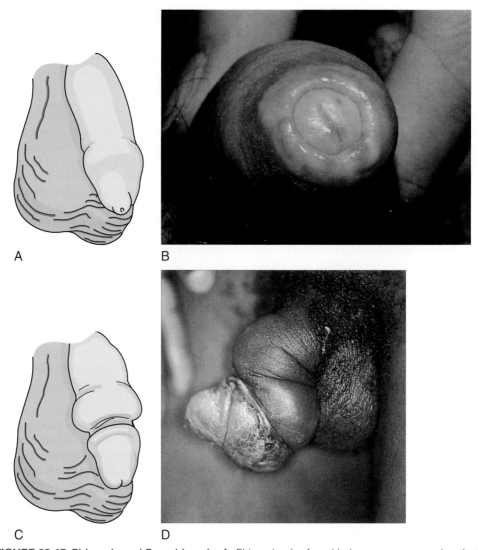

A   B

C   D

FIGURE 32-17 Phimosis and Paraphimosis. A, Phimosis: the foreskin has a narrow opening that is not large enough to permit retraction over the glans. **B,** Lesions on the prepuce secondary to infection cause swelling, and retraction of foreskin may be impossible. Circumcision is usually required. **C,** Paraphimosis: the foreskin is retracted over the glans but cannot be reduced to its normal position. Here it has formed a constricting band around the penis. **D,** Ulcer on the retracted prepuce with edema. (**A** and **C** from Monahan FD et al: *Phipps' medical-surgical nursing: health and illness perspectives,* ed 8, St Louis, 2007, Mosby; **B** from Taylor PK: *Diagnostic picture tests in sexually transmitted diseases,* St Louis, 1995, Mosby; **D** from Morse SA, Ballard RC, Holmes KK et al: *Atlas of sexually transmitted diseases and AIDS,* ed 3, Edinburgh, 2003, Mosby.)

performed after infection has been eradicated. Complications of phimosis include inflammation of the glans (balanitis) or prepuce (posthitis) and paraphimosis. There is a higher incidence of penile carcinoma in uncircumcised males, but chronic infection and poor hygiene are usually the underlying factors in such cases.

Paraphimosis, in which the foreskin is retracted, can constrict the penis, causing edema of the glans. If the foreskin cannot be reduced manually, surgery must be performed to prevent necrosis of the glans caused by constricted blood vessels. Severe paraphimosis is a surgical emergency.

Peyronie Disease

Peyronie disease ("bent nail syndrome") is a fibrotic condition that causes lateral curvature of the penis during erection (Figure 32-18). Peyronie disease develops slowly and is characterized by tough fibrous

thickening of the fascia in the erectile tissue of the corpora cavernosa. A dense, fibrous plaque is usually palpable on the dorsum of the penile shaft. The problem usually affects middle-aged men and is associated with painful erection, painful intercourse (for both partners), and poor erection distal to the involved area. In some cases, impotence or unsatisfactory penetration occurs. When the penis is flaccid, there is no pain.

A local vasculitis-like inflammatory reaction occurs, and decreased tissue oxygenation results in fibrosis and calcification. The exact cause is unknown. Peyronie disease is associated with Dupuytren contracture (a flexion deformity of the fingers or toes caused by shortening or fibrosis of the palmar or plantar fascia), diabetes, tendency to develop keloids, and, in rare cases, use of beta-blocker medications.[53]

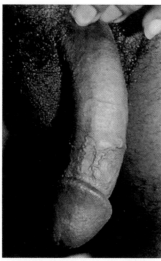

FIGURE 32-18 Peyronie Disease. This person complained of pain and deviation of his penis to one side on erection. (From Taylor PK: *Diagnostic picture tests in sexually transmitted diseases,* London, 1995, Mosby.)

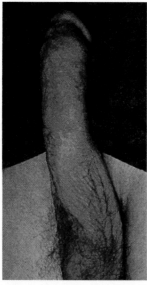

FIGURE 32-19 Priapism. (From Lloyd-Davies RW et al: *Color atlas of urology,* ed 2, London, 1994, Wolfe Medical.)

There is no definitive treatment for Peyronie disease; however, treatment can include pharmacologic agents and surgery. Spontaneous remissions occur in as many as 50% of individuals.

Priapism

Priapism is an uncommon condition of prolonged penile erection. It is usually painful and is not associated with sexual arousal (Figure 32-19). Priapism is idiopathic in 60% of cases; the remaining 40% of cases can be associated with spinal cord trauma, sickle cell disease, leukemia, pelvic tumors, infections, or penile trauma.

Priapism must be considered a urologic emergency. Treatment within hours is effective and prevents impotence. Conservative approaches include iced saline enemas, ketamine administration, and spinal anesthesia. Needle aspiration of blood from the corpus through the dorsal glans is often effective and is followed by catheterization

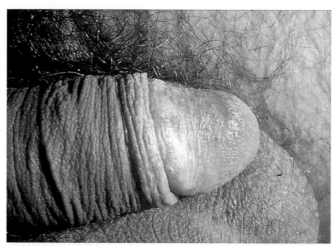

FIGURE 32-20 Balanitis. (From Taylor PK: *Diagnostic picture tests in sexually transmitted diseases,* London, 1995, Mosby.)

and pressure dressings to maintain decompression. More aggressive surgical treatments include the creation of vascular shunts to maintain blood flow. Erectile dysfunction results in up to 50% of prolonged cases.

Balanitis

Balanitis is an inflammation of the glans penis (Figure 32-20) and usually occurs in conjunction with posthitis, an inflammation of the prepuce. (Inflammation of the glans and the prepuce is called *balanoposthitis.*) It is associated with poor hygiene and phimosis. The accumulation under the foreskin of glandular secretions (smegma), sloughed epithelial cells, and *Mycobacterium smegmatis* can irritate the glans directly or lead to infection. Skin disorders (e.g., psoriasis, lichen planus, eczema) and candidiasis must be differentiated from inflammation resulting from poor hygienic practices. Balanitis is most commonly seen in men with poorly controlled diabetes mellitus and candidiasis. The infection is treated with antimicrobials. After the inflammation has subsided, circumcision can be considered to prevent recurrences.

Tumors of the Penis

Tumors of the penis are not common. The most frequent are the benign epithelial tumor condyloma acuminatum and penile carcinomas.

Condyloma acuminatum is a benign tumor caused by human papillomavirus (HPV), a sexually transmitted infection. HPV type 6 and, less often, type 11 are the most frequent types and can cause a common wart and moist surface of the external genitalia.

Penile Cancer

Carcinoma of the penis is rare in the United States, constituting about 1 in 100,000 men. It does account, however, for about 10% of cancers in African and South American men. It can affect men 40 to 70 years of age, with two thirds of men diagnosed at 65 years of age and older. The disease occurs almost twice as often in blacks as in whites in the United States. Although the exact cause is unknown, major risk factors include HPV infection, smoking, and psoriasis. Circumcision at birth decreases the risk of penile cancer and penile cancer is more common in men with phimosis and those with acquired immunodeficiency syndrome (AIDS).[54]

Squamous cell carcinoma accounts for 95% of invasive penile cancers. Other premalignant lesions, or in situ forms of epidermal carcinoma, that occur on the penis include leukoplakia (white plaque), Paget disease (red, inflamed areas), erythroplasia of Queyrat (raised red areas), and Buschke-Löwenstein patches (large venous areas). HPV6 and HPV11 associated with genital warts (condylomata acuminata) have low cancer risks.[55] At times, the penis might be the site of metastatic spread of solid tumors from the bladder, prostate, rectum, or kidney. Early squamous cell carcinoma and premalignant epidermal lesions are easily treated, but delays in seeking treatment are attributed to denial, embarrassment, failure to detect lesions under a phimotic foreskin, fear, guilt, and ignorance.

Squamous cell carcinoma usually begins as a small, flat, ulcerative or papillary lesion on the glans or foreskin that grows to involve the entire penile shaft. Extensive lesions are associated with metastases and a poor prognosis. The regional femoral and iliac lymph nodes are common metastatic sites; the urethra and bladder are rarely involved. Weight loss, fatigue, and malaise accompany chronic suppurative lesions.

The specific diagnosis is made by biopsy after examination to document the location, size, and fixation of the lesion. After a positive biopsy, the extent of cancer spread is determined by imaging studies. Distant metastases are uncommon. Stages of carcinoma of the penis are presented in Box 32-6.

Penile carcinoma is managed primarily with surgery. Newer, innovative surgical techniques can preserve as much penile tissue as possible without compromising cancer control. A multimodal approach with chemotherapy is under study.[56] Palliative treatment with radiation or chemotherapy may be used when the disease is inoperable and bulky inguinal metastases have occurred. Options for individuals with carcinoma in situ include local excision, radiation, laser surgery, cryosurgery, chemosurgery, or chemotherapy with topical (5%) 5-fluorouracil. The 5-year survival rate for stage I disease is more than 80%; the average 5-year survival rate for all stages is 50%.[1,54,57]

BOX 32-6   STAGING FOR PENILE CANCER

Stage 0: Tis or Ta, N0, M0
The cancer has not grown into tissue below the top layers of skin and has not spread to lymph nodes or distant sites.

Stage I: T1a, N0, M0
The cancer has grown into tissue just below the superficial layer of skin but has not grown into blood or lymph vessels. It is a grade 1 or 2. It has not spread to lymph nodes or distant sites.

Stage II: Any of the following:
   T1b, N0, M0
The cancer has grown into tissue just below the superficial layer of skin and is high grade or has grown into blood or lymph vessels. It has not spread to lymph nodes or distant sites.
   Or
   T2, N0, M0
The cancer has grown into one of the internal chambers of the penis (the corpus spongiosum or corpora cavernosa). The cancer has not spread to lymph nodes or distant sites.
   Or
   T3, N0, M0
The cancer has grown into the urethra. It has not spread to lymph nodes or distant sites.

Stage IIIA: T1 to T3, N1, M0
The cancer has grown into tissue below the superficial layer of skin (T1). It also may have grown into the corpus spongiosum, the corpora cavernosa, or the urethra (T2 or T3). The cancer has spread to a single groin lymph node (N1). It has not spread to distant sites.

Stage IIIB: T1 to T3, N2, M0
The cancer has grown into the tissues of the penis and may have grown into the corpus spongiosum, the corpora cavernosa, or the urethra (T1 to T3). It has spread to two or more groin lymph nodes. It has not spread to distant sites.

Stage IV: Any of the following:
   T4, any N, M0
The cancer has grown into the prostate or other nearby structures. It may or may not have spread to groin lymph nodes. It has not spread to distant sites.
   Or
   Any T, N3, M0
The cancer has spread to lymph nodes in the pelvis or spread in the groin lymph nodes and grown through the lymph nodes' outer covering and into surrounding tissue. The cancer has not spread to distant sites.
   Or
   Any T, any N, M1
The cancer has spread to distant sites.

T, Primary tumor size; *N,* regional lymph nodes; *M,* distant metastasis.

✔ QUICK CHECK 32-5
1. Why are priapism and severe paraphimosis considered urologic emergencies?
2. What are the risk factors for cancer of the penis?

Disorders of the Scrotum, Testis, and Epididymis
Disorders of the Scrotum

Men may seek treatment for painful or painless scrotal masses. Masses may be serious (cancer or torsion) or benign (hydrocele or cyst), and may require immediate surgical intervention or allow for careful observation. Varicocele, hydrocele, and spermatocele are common intrascrotal disorders. A **varicocele** is an abnormal dilation of the testicular vein and the pampiniform plexus within the scrotum, and is classically described as a "bag of worms" (Figure 32-21). Varicoceles are one of the most commonly identified scrotal abnormalities and abnormal

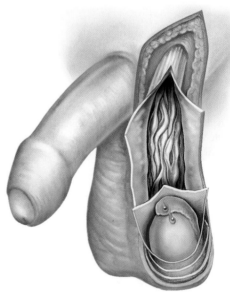

FIGURE 32-21 Depiction of a Varicocele. Dilation of veins within the spermatic cord. (From Seidel HM et al: *Mosby's guide to physical examination,* ed 6, St Louis, 2006, Mosby.)

finding among infertile men. Advancements in diagnostic techniques indicate that the incidence of varicoceles is significantly greater than previously reported.[58] Most (90%) occur on the left side because of discrepancies in venous drainage and may be painful or tender. Varicocele occurs in 10% to 15% of males and is seen most often after puberty.[58] Because most develop in adolescence, physiologic changes in testosterone level may contribute to increasing blood flow to the testicle, causing venous dilation.[58] Unilateral right-sided varicoceles are rare and result from compression or obstruction of the inferior vena cava by a tumor or thrombus. Varicoceles may be less likely to be diagnosed among obese men.[58]

The cause of varicocele is poorly understood.[58] Blood pools in the veins rather than flowing into the venous system. Varicocele decreases blood flow through the testis, interfering with spermatogenesis and causing infertility. Varicoceles can alter testosterone and follicle-stimulating hormone levels, cause oxidative stress, decrease sperm count, and affect sperm quality.[58] Varicocele surgical repair is generally done when the male has a grade II or III varicocele and an abnormal semen analysis and the female has no known cause of infertility.[58] If varicocele is mild and fertility is not an issue, a scrotal support is usually sufficient to relieve symptoms of scrotal heaviness or "dragging." Color Doppler ultrasonography is used to confirm diagnosis.

A hydrocele is a collection of fluid between the layers of the tunica vaginalis (Figure 32-22). It is the most common cause of scrotal swelling. Hydroceles occur in 6% of male newborns and are congenital malformations that often resolve spontaneously in the first year of life. In North America, common infectious causes include epididymitis and viruses. Worldwide, however, filariasis is a major cause especially with recent travel to tropical countries.[58] Other causes include trauma, torsion of the testicle or testicular appendage, and recent scrotal surgery.[58] A man presenting with a hydrocele in his third or fourth decade needs careful evaluation for testicular cancer.[58]

Hydroceles vary in size and most are asymptomatic. The most important feature on physical examination is a tense, smooth, scrotal mass that easily transluminates. Translumination or holding a light behind the scrotum can help distinguish a hydrocele from a hernia or a solid mass.[58] Treatment includes watchful waiting in infants and for those older than 1 year; 75% resolve within 6 months.[58] Symptomatic or communicating hydroceles need definitive treatment. Treatment includes surgical resection, aspiration, and sclerotherapy (injection of a sclerosing agent into the scrotal sac [cystic dilation]) to excise the tunica vaginalis.[58]

Spermatoceles (epididymal cysts) are benign cystic collections of fluid of the epididymis located between the head of the epididymis and the testis. Spermatoceles are filled with a milky fluid containing sperm and are usually painless (Figure 32-23). Spermatoceles that cause significant pain or discomfort are excised. Both spermatoceles and epididymal cysts present clinically as discrete, firm, freely mobile masses distinct from the testis that may be transilluminated. Usually, however, spermatoceles are asymptomatic or produce mild discomfort that is relieved by scrotal support. Neither hydroceles nor spermatoceles are associated with infertility.

Cryptorchidism and Ectopy

Cryptorchidism is a group of abnormalities in which the testis fails to descend completely, whereas an ectopic testis has strayed from the normal pathway of descent. Ectopy may be caused by an abnormal connection at the distal end of the gubernaculum testis that leads the gonad to an abnormal position, usually at the superficial inguinal site. In cryptorchidism, the descent of one or both testes is arrested with unilateral arrest occurring more often than bilateral arrest. The testes may remain in the abdomen, or testicular descent may be arrested in the inguinal canal or the puboscrotal junction. About 3% to 6% of full-term and 20% to 30% of premature male infants have undescended testes at birth.[58] Half of such testes descend in the first month of life and a few more at puberty. The incidence of cryptorchidism in adults is 0.7% to 0.8%.[58] Cryptorchidism is commonly associated with vasal or epididymal abnormalities. These congenital anomalies affect about 33% to 66% of newborns with cryptorchidism. Other structural anomalies include posterior urethral valves (less than 5%), upper genital tract abnormalities (less than 5%), and hypospadias. The

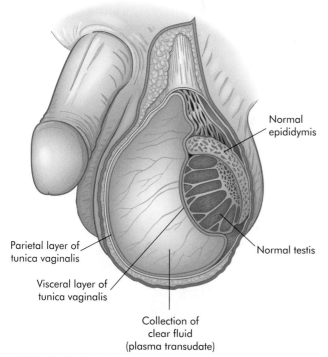

FIGURE 32-22 Depiction of a Hydrocele. Accumulation of clear fluid between the visceral (inner) and parietal (outer) layers of the tunica vaginalis.

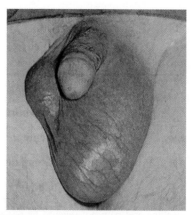

FIGURE 32-23 Spermatocele. Retention cyst of the head of the epididymis or of an aberrant tubule or tubules of the rete testis. The spermatocele lies outside the tunica vaginalis; therefore, on palpation it can be readily distinguished and separated from the testis. (From Lloyd-Davies RW et al: *Color atlas of urology,* ed 2, London, 1994, Wolfe Medical.)

presence of both hypospadias and cryptorchidism raises the suspicion of mixed gonadal dysgenesis (intersex infant). It has been hypothesized that cryptorchidism may result from an absence or abnormality of the gubernaculum, a cordlike structure that extends from the lower pole of the testis to the scrotum; a congenital gonadal or dysgenetic defect that makes the testis insensitive to gonadotropins (a likely explanation for unilateral cryptorchidism); or lack of maternal gonadotropins (a likely explanation for bilateral cryptorchidism of prematurity).

Mechanical possibilities include a short spermatic cord, fibrous bands or adhesions in the normal path of the testes, or a narrowed inguinal canal. Chromosomal studies do not support a genetic component. Physiologic cryptorchidism, also called *retractile* or *migratory testis,* is an involuntary retraction of the testes out of the scrotum that occurs with excitement, physical activity, or exposure to cold and is caused by the small mass of prepubertal testis and the strength of the cremaster muscle. This is a common phenomenon that is self-limiting (descent occurs at puberty).

Physical examination discloses the absence of one or both testes in the scrotum and an atrophic scrotum on the affected side. If the undescended testis is in a vulnerable position, over the pubic bone for example, an individual may complain of severe pain secondary to trauma. The adult male with bilateral cryptorchidism may be infertile.

Undescended testes are susceptible to neoplastic processes: the risk of testicular cancer is 35 to 50 times greater for men with cryptorchidism or a history of cryptorchidism than for the general male population. Because definite histologic change occurs in the cryptorchid testis by 1 year of age, surgical correction is recommended around that age.[58,59] Treatment often begins with administration of GnRH or human chorionic gonadotropin (hCG), hormones that may initiate descent and make surgery unnecessary. GnRH is available as a nasal spray in Europe and may enhance germ cell counts even when the testis does not descend.[59] If hormonal therapy is not successful (success rates range from 6% to 75%), the testis is located and moved surgically (orchiopexy) in young children or removed (orchiectomy) in adults and children more than 10 years of age.[59,60] The testis that is properly placed in the scrotum provides adequate hormonal function and gives the scrotum a normal appearance. A successful operation does not ensure fertility if the testis is congenitally defective. Approximately 20% of males with unilateral undescended testis remain infertile even though orchiopexy is performed by age 1 year; most individuals with treated or untreated bilateral testicular maldescent have poor fertility.

Torsion of the Testis and Testicular Appendages

In torsion of the testis, the testis rotates on its vascular pedicle, interrupting its blood supply (Figure 32-24). Torsion of the testis is one of several conditions that cause an acute scrotum, which is testicular pain and swelling. Testicular appendages include the appendix testis (a remnant of the müllerian duct) and the appendix epididymis (a remnant of the wolffian duct). Torsion of the appendages can also cause acute scrotum and be confused with testicular torsion, a urologic emergency.

Torsion of the testis can occur at any age but is most common among neonates and adolescents, particularly at puberty. Onset may be spontaneous or follow physical exertion or trauma. Torsion twists the arteries and veins in the spermatic cord, reducing or stopping circulation to the testis. Vascular engorgement and ischemia develop, causing scrotal swelling and pain not relieved by rest or scrotal support. Diagnostic testing includes urinalysis (for infection) and color Doppler ultrasonography. Torsion of the testis is a surgical emergency. If it cannot be reduced manually (scrotal elevation), surgery must be performed within 6 hours after the onset of symptoms to preserve normal testicular function.

Orchitis

Orchitis is an acute inflammation of the testes (Figure 32-25) and is uncommon except as a complication of systemic infection or as an extension of an associated epididymitis (see p. 826). Infectious organisms may reach the testes through the blood or the lymphatics or, most commonly, by ascent through the urethra, vas deferens, and epididymis. Most cases of orchitis are actually cases of epididymo-orchitis (inflammation of both the epididymis and testis). Occasionally in

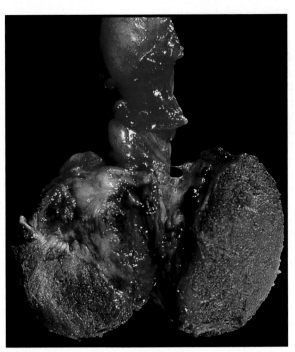

FIGURE 32-24 Torsion of the Testis. The testes appear dark red and partially necrotic as a result of hemorrhagic infarction. (From Damjanov I, Linder J, editors: *Anderson's pathology,* ed 10, St Louis, 1996, Mosby.)

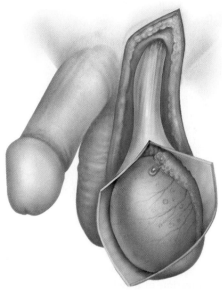

FIGURE 32-25 Depiction of Orchitis. (From Seidel HM et al: *Mosby's guide to physical examination,* ed 6, St Louis, 2006, Mosby.)

middle-aged men, a nonspecific, apparently noninfectious, inflammatory process (called *granulomatous orchitis*) can occur, presumably a granulomatous response to spermatozoa.

Mumps is the most common infectious cause of orchitis and usually affects postpubertal males. The onset is sudden, occurring 3 to 4 days after the onset of parotitis. Signs and symptoms include high fever, reaching 40° C (104° F), marked prostration, bilateral or unilateral erythema, edema and tenderness of the scrotum, and leukocytosis. An acute hydrocele may develop. Urinary signs and symptoms, which accompany epididymitis, are absent. Atrophy with irreversible damage to spermatogenesis may result in 30% of affected testes. Bilateral orchitis does not affect hormonal function but may cause permanent sterility.

Treatment is supportive and includes bed rest, scrotal support, elevation of the scrotum, hot or cold compresses, and analgesic agents for relief of pain. If an acute hydrocele develops, it is aspirated. Testicular abscess usually requires orchiectomy (removal of the testis). Appropriate antimicrobial drugs should be used for bacterial orchitis, and corticosteroids are indicated in proven cases of nonspecific granulomatous orchitis.

Cancer of the Testis

Testicular cancer is among the most curable of cancers, with cure rates greater than 95%. Overall, testicular cancers are uncommon, accounting for approximately 1% of all male cancers and 0.13% of cancer deaths in men; yet they are the most common solid tumor of young adult men.[1] Cancer of the testis occurs most commonly in men between the ages of 15 and 35 years.[1] In the United States, the lifetime probability of developing testicular cancer is 0.3% for white men, an incidence that is 4.5 times higher than in blacks. Testicular tumors are slightly more common on the right side than on the left, a pattern that parallels the occurrence of cryptorchidism, and they are bilateral in 1% to 3% of cases (Figure 32-26).

PATHOPHYSIOLOGY   Ninety percent of testicular cancers are germ cell tumors, arising from the male gametes. Germ cell tumors include

seminomas (most common), embryonal carcinomas, teratomas, and choriosarcomas. Testicular tumors also can arise from specialized cells of the gonadal stroma (Leydig, Sertoli, granulosa, theca cells).

The cause of testicular neoplasms is unknown (see *Risk Factors: Cancer of the Testis*). A genetic predisposition is suggested by the fact that the incidence is higher among brothers, identical twins, and other close male relatives. Genetic predisposition is supported statistically showing that the disease is relatively rare among Africans, black Americans, Asians, and native New Zealanders. Risk factors include history of cryptorchidism, abnormal testicular development, HIV and AIDS, Klinefelter syndrome, and history of testicular cancer.[61]

RISK FACTORS
Cancer of the Testis

- HIV and AIDS
- History of cryptorchidism
- Abnormal testicular development
- Klinefelter syndrome
- History of testicular cancer

CLINICAL MANIFESTATIONS   Painless testicular enlargement commonly is the first sign of testicular cancer. Occurring gradually, it may be accompanied by a sensation of testicular heaviness or a dull ache in the lower abdomen. Occasionally acute pain occurs because of rapid growth resulting in hemorrhage and necrosis. Ten percent of affected men have epididymitis, 10% have hydroceles, and 5% have breast enlargement (gynecomastia). The testicular mass is usually discovered by the individual or by his sexual partner. At the time of initial diagnosis, approximately 10% of individuals already have symptoms related to metastases. Lumbar pain also may be present and usually is caused by retroperitoneal node metastasis. Signs of metastasis to the lungs include cough, dyspnea, and bloody sputum (hemoptysis). Supraclavicular node involvement may cause difficulty swallowing (dysphagia) and neck swelling. With metastasis to the central nervous system (CNS), alterations in vision or mental status, papilledema, and seizures may be experienced.

EVALUATION AND TREATMENT   An incorrect diagnosis at the initial examination occurs in as many as 25% of men with testicular cancer. Epididymitis and epididymo-orchitis are the most common misdiagnoses; others include hydrocele and spermatocele. Evaluation begins with careful physical examination, including palpation of the scrotal contents with the individual in the erect and supine positions. Signs of testicular cancer include abnormal consistency, induration, nodularity, or irregularity of the testis. The abdomen and lymph nodes are palpated to seek evidence of metastasis, and tumor type is identified after orchiectomy. Although testicular self-examination has not been studied enough to be recommended by the American Cancer Society, many physicians recommend monthly examinations after puberty. Testicular biopsy is not recommended because it may cause dissemination of the tumor and increase the risk of local recurrence. Primary testicular cancer can be assessed rapidly and accurately by scrotal ultrasonography. Tumor markers are higher than normal in the presence of a tumor and may help detect a tumor that is too small to be palpated during physical examination or to be visualized on imaging. Radiologic imaging and measurement of serum markers are used in clinical staging of the disease. Besides surgery, treatment involves radiation and chemotherapy singly or in combination. Factors influencing the prognosis include histologic studies of the tumor stage of the disease

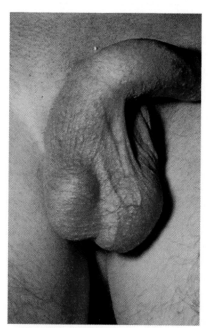

FIGURE 32-26 Testicular Tumor. (From *400 Self-assessment picture tests in clinical medicine,* London, 1984, Wolfe Medical.)

and selection of appropriate treatment. Most individuals treated for cancer of the testis can expect a normal life span; some have persistent paresthesias, Raynaud phenomenon, or infertility. Approximately 10% of men treated for testicular cancer will experience a relapse; if the relapse is discovered early and treated, 99% can be cured. Orchiectomy does not affect sexual function.

Epididymitis

Epididymitis, or inflammation of the epididymis, generally occurs in sexually active young males (younger than 35 years) and is rare before puberty (Figure 32-27). In young men, the usual cause is a sexually transmitted microorganism, such as *N. gonorrhoeae* or *C. trachomatis*. Coliform bacteria are the common pathogens in other age groups.[62] Men who practice unprotected anal intercourse may acquire sexually transmitted epididymis that results from infection with *E. coli*, *H. influenzae*, tuberculosis, or *Cryptococcus* or *Brucella* species. In men older than 35 years, *Enterobacteriaceae* (intestinal bacteria) and *Pseudomonas aeruginosa* associated with urinary tract infections and prostatitis also may cause epididymitis. Epididymitis also may result from a chemical inflammation caused by the reflux of sterile urine into the ejaculatory ducts and is then called chemical epididymitis.[54] It is associated with urethral strictures, congenital posterior valves, and excessive physical straining in which increased abdominal pressure is transmitted to the bladder. Chemical epididymitis is usually self-limiting and does not require evaluation or intervention unless it persists.

PATHOPHYSIOLOGY The pathogenic microorganism usually reaches the epididymis by ascending the vasa deferentia from an already infected urethra or bladder. The resulting inflammatory response causes symptoms of bacterial epididymitis. Epididymitis caused by heavy lifting or straining results from reflux of urine from the bladder into the vas deferens and epididymis. Urine is extremely irritating to the epididymis and initiates the inflammatory response called *chemical epididymitis.*

CLINICAL MANIFESTATIONS The main symptom of epididymitis is scrotal or inguinal pain caused by inflammation of the epididymis and surrounding tissues. The pain is usually acute and severe. Flank

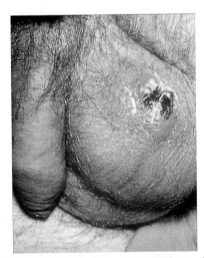

FIGURE 32-27 Epididymitis Secondary to Gonorrhea or Nongonococcal Urethritis. This infection spread to the testes, and rupture through the scrotal wall is threatened. (From Taylor PK: *Diagnostic picture tests in sexually transmitted disease,* London, 1995, Mosby.)

pain may occur if, as the urethra passes over the spermatic cord, edematous swelling of the cord obstructs the urethra. The individual may have pyuria, bacteriuria, and a history of urinary symptoms, including urethral discharge. The scrotum on the involved side is red and edematous. The tail of the epididymis near the lower pole of the testis usually swells first; then swelling ascends to the head of the epididymis. The spermatic cord also may be swollen and tender.

Complications include abscess formation, infarction of the testis, recurrent infection, and infertility. Infarction is probably caused by thrombosis (obstruction by blood clots) of the prostatic vessels secondary to severe inflammation. Recurrent epididymitis may result from inadequate initial treatment or failure to identify or treat predisposing factors. Chronic epididymitis can cause scarring of the epididymal endothelium and infertility. Once scarring has occurred, treatment with antibiotics is ineffective because adequate antibiotic levels cannot be achieved within the epididymis.

EVALUATION AND TREATMENT A history of recent urinary tract infection or urethral discharge suggests the diagnosis of epididymitis. Common physical findings include a swollen, tender epididymis or testis located in the normal anatomic position with an intact same-side cremasteric reflex.[62] The relief of pain when the inflamed testis and epididymis are elevated (Prehn sign) is also diagnostic. Definitive diagnosis is based on culture or Gram stain of a urethral swab. Epididymal aspiration may be necessary to obtain a specimen, especially if the individual has been taking antibiotics and has sterile urine.

Treatment includes antibiotic therapy for the infection itself and various measures to provide symptomatic relief. Complete resolution of swelling and pain may take several weeks to months. The individual's sexual partner should be treated with antibiotics if the causative microorganism is a sexually transmitted pathogen.

 QUICK CHECK 32-6

1. Why is a genetic predisposition suggested for testicular cancer?
2. Why is epididymitis rare in prepubescent males?
3. Why is testicular torsion considered a urologic emergency?

Disorders of the Prostate Gland
Benign Prostatic Hyperplasia

Benign prostatic hyperplasia (BPH), also called benign prostatic hypertrophy, is the enlargement of the prostate gland (Figure 32-28). (Because the major prostatic changes are caused by hyperplasia, not hypertrophy, benign prostatic hyperplasia is the preferred term.) This condition becomes problematic when prostatic tissue compresses the urethra, where it passes through the prostate, resulting in frequency of lower urinary tract symptoms. Similar to prostate cancer, BPH occurs more often in Westernized countries (e.g., United States, United Kingdom, and Canada). BPH appears to be more common in black men than white men and family history may increase the risk. Being overweight or obese with central fat distribution (i.e., around the abdomen) increases the risk of developing BPH. BPH is common and involves a complex pathophysiology with several endocrine and local factors and remodeled microenvironment. Its relationship to aging is well documented. At birth, the prostate is pea sized, and growth of the gland is gradual until puberty. At that time, there is a period of rapid development that continues until the third decade of life when the prostate reaches adult size (see Chapter 30). Around 40 to 45 years of age, benign hyperplasia begins and continues slowly until death. Although androgens, such as dihydrotestosterone (DHT), are necessary for

Prostate zones

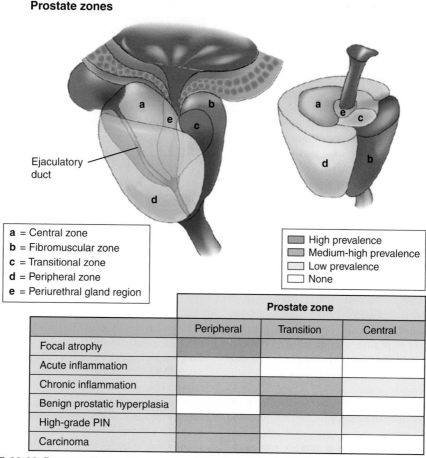

a = Central zone
b = Fibromuscular zone
c = Transitional zone
d = Peripheral zone
e = Periurethral gland region

High prevalence
Medium-high prevalence
Low prevalence
None

	Prostate zone		
	Peripheral	Transition	Central
Focal atrophy			
Acute inflammation			
Chronic inflammation			
Benign prostatic hyperplasia			
High-grade PIN			
Carcinoma			

FIGURE 32-28 Prostate Zones, Benign Prostatic Hyperplasia (BPH), and Prostate Cancer Locations. Benign prostatic hyperplasia (BPH) occurs in the peripheral zone of the prostate gland that can enlarge (not shown). BPH nodules and atrophy are associated with inflammation in the transition zone. Most cancer lesions occur in the peripheral zone. Carcinoma can involve the central zone but rarely occurs in isolation, suggesting that prostatic intraepithelial neoplasia (PIN) lesions do not easily progress to carcinoma in this region. (Adapted from De Marzo AM et al: Inflammation in prostate carcinogenesis, *Nat Rev Cancer* 7:256–269, 2007.)

normal prostatic development, their role in BPH remains unclear. Among all the androgen-metabolizing enzymes within the prostate, 5α-reductase is the most powerful. This reductase corresponds to an age-dependent DHT level. Therefore, although levels of 5α-reductase and DHT in the epithelium decrease with age, they remain constant in the stroma (microenvironment) of the prostate gland.

PATHOGENESIS Current causative theories of BPH focus on aging and levels and ratios of endocrine factors such as androgens and estrogens (androgen/estrogen ratio), the role of chronic inflammation, and autocrine/paracrine growth-stimulating and growth-inhibiting factors. These factors include insulin-like growth factors (IGFs), epidermal growth factors, fibroblast factors, as well as several others. Recent data show that human prostate stromal cells can actively contribute to the inflammatory process from the induction of inflammatory cytokines and chemokines.[63]

With aging, circulating androgens are associated with BPH and enlargement. Other effects related to estrogens include apoptosis, aromatase expression, and paracrine regulation that may be important for stimulating inflammation.[64] Early data showed 17β-estradiol increased the accumulation of collagen in the prostate.[65] The hormonal imbalance with aging may cause mechanical tension changes (especially with collagen changes) consistent with prostate growth in pathologic states.[66] Altogether, these factors are proposed as disrupting the balance of growth factor signaling pathways and stromal epithelial interactions, creating a growth-promoting (and increase in prostate volume) and tissue-remodeling microenvironment.[67] The remodeled stroma promotes local inflammation with altered cytokine, reactive oxygen/nitrogen species, and chemoattractants.[67,68] The resultant increased oxygen demands of proliferating cells cause a local hypoxia that induces angiogenesis and changes to fibroblasts. Functional and phenotypic changes of fibroblasts are a "hallmark" of the remodeled microenvironment.[67] Investigators are also studying whether abnormal blood flow patterns in the aging prostate gland might lead to hypoxia-stimulated prostate growth.[69,70] This hypothesis seems important with the new understanding that in most men symptoms result from a combination of BPH *and* age-related bladder dysfunction.[71,72] Conflicting data relate BPH to anthropometric measurements (height, weight, waist and/or hip circumference) or metabolic syndrome, or both.[73,74]

BPH begins in the periurethral glands, which are the inner glands or layers of the prostate. The prostate enlarges as nodules form and grow (nodular hyperplasia) and glandular cells enlarge (hypertrophy). The development of BPH occurs over a prolonged period of time, and changes within the urinary tract are slow and insidious.

CLINICAL MANIFESTATIONS As nodular hyperplasia and cellular hypertrophy progress, tissues that surround the prostatic urethra compress it, usually, but not always, causing bladder outflow obstruction. These symptoms are sometimes called the spectrum of lower urinary tract symptoms (LUTS). Symptoms include the urge to urinate often, some delay in starting urination, and decreased force of the urinary stream. As the obstruction progresses, often over several years, the bladder cannot empty all the urine, and the increasing volume leads to long-term urine retention. The volume of urine retained may be great enough to produce uncontrolled "overflow incontinence" with any increase in intra-abdominal pressure. At this stage, the force of the urinary stream is significantly reduced, and much more time is required to initiate and complete voiding. Acute urinary retention may be associated with an increased risk for recurrent urinary tract infections and bladder stones (calculi).

Progressive bladder distention causes diverticular outpouchings of the bladder wall. The ureters may be obstructed where they pass through the hypertrophied detrusor muscle, potentially causing hydroureter, hydronephrosis, and bladder or kidney infection.

EVALUATION AND TREATMENT Diagnosis is made from a medical history, physical examination, and laboratory tests, including urinalysis. Careful review of symptoms is necessary. Digital rectal examination (DRE) and measurement of prostate-specific antigen (PSA) are conducted to determine hyperplasia. PSA level alone, however, cannot confirm symptoms are attributable to BPH because PSA level is elevated in both BPH and prostate cancer.

Treatment depends on the severity of symptoms, including post-void residual urine (PVR), pressure-flow study, creatinine and blood urea nitrogen (BUN) values, and subjective symptom scores. Thirty percent of men with mild to moderate symptoms improve with watchful waiting. Those with moderately elevated symptom scores or severe symptom scores without large PVR levels can be treated with medications, such as 5α-reductase inhibitors (e.g., finasteride) or selective α_1-blocking agents (e.g., prazosin, tamsulosin).[75,76] Candidates for surgical intervention include those with severe symptoms, large PVR, or complications, or those men who fail to improve with medical therapy or newer minimally invasive procedures. Newer minimally invasive treatments include interstitial laser treatment, transurethral radiofrequency procedures (such as transurethral needle ablation [TUNA]), and cooled ThermoTherapy.

Prostatitis

Prostatitis is an inflammation of the prostate. Some degree of prostatic inflammation is present in 4% to 36% of the male population, increasing to 50% in older men. Inflammation is usually limited to a few of the gland's excretory ducts.

Prostatitis syndromes have been classified by the National Institutes of Health as (1) acute bacterial prostatitis (ABP), (2) chronic bacterial prostatitis (CBP), (3) chronic pelvic pain syndrome (CPPS), and (4) asymptomatic inflammatory prostatitis (Box 32-7). ABP and CBP are mostly caused by gram-negative *Enterobacteriaceae* and enterococci species that originate in the gastrointestinal flora. The most common organism is *Escherichia coli*, which is identified in the majority of infections.[77] *Klebsiella* species, *Pseudomonas aeruginosa,* and *Serratia* species are common gram-negative cultured microorganisms. Nonbacterial prostatitis (CP/CPPS) syndromes are caused by a cascade of inflammatory, immunologic, neuroendocrine, and neuropathic mechanisms whereby the initiating cause is unknown.

Bacterial prostatitis. Acute bacterial prostatitis (ABP, category I) is an ascending infection of the urinary tract that tends to occur in men

---

BOX 32-7 NIH CLASSIFICATION OF THE PROSTATITIS SYNDROME

This system, developed for clinical research purposes, can be simplified for use in primary care practice (see text).

Category I, or acute bacterial prostatitis (ABP), is an acute infection of the prostate and is manifested by systemic signs of infection and positive urine culture.

Category II, or chronic bacterial prostatitis (CBP), is a chronic bacterial infection in which bacteria are received in significant numbers from a purulent prostatic fluid. These bacteria are thought to be the most common cause of recurrent urinary tract infection in men.

Category III, or chronic pelvic pain syndrome (CPPS), is diagnosed when no pathologic bacteria can be localized to the prostate (culture of expressed prostatic fluid or postprostatic massage urine specimen) and is further divided into IIIa and IIIb. Category IIIa refers to the inflammatory CPPS where a significant number of white blood cells (WBCs) are localized to the prostate, whereas category IIIb is noninflammatory.

Category IV refers to asymptomatic inflammatory prostatitis in which bacteria or WBCs are localized to the prostate, but individuals are asymptomatic.

---

between the ages of 30 and 50 years but is also associated with BPH in older men. Infection stimulates an inflammatory response in which the prostate becomes enlarged, tender, firm, or boggy. The onset of prostatitis may be acute and unrelated to previous illnesses, or it may follow catheterization or cystoscopy.

Clinical manifestations of acute bacterial prostatitis are those of urinary tract infection or pyelonephritis. Sudden onset of malaise, low back and perineal pain, high fever (up to 40° C [104° F]), and chills is common, as are dysuria, inability to empty the bladder, nocturia, and urinary retention. The individual also may have symptoms of lower urinary tract obstruction, such as slow, small, "narrowed" urinary stream, which may be a medical emergency. Acute inflammatory prostatic edema can compress the urethra, causing urinary obstruction. Systemic signs of infection include sudden onset of a high fever, fatigue, arthralgia, and myalgia. Prostatic pain may occur, especially when the individual is in an upright position, because the pelvic floor muscles tighten with standing and compression of the prostate gland occurs. Some individuals experience low back pain, painful ejaculation, and rectal or perineal pain. Palpation discloses an enlarged, extremely tender and swollen prostate that is firm, indurated, and warm to the touch.

Because acute bacterial prostatitis is usually associated with a bladder infection caused by the same microorganism, urine cultures disclose its identity. Prostatic massage may express enough secretions from the urethra for direct bacterial examination, but massage may be painful and increases the risk that the infection will ascend to adjacent structures or enter the bloodstream and cause septicemia.

To resolve the infection and control its spread, individuals may require antibiotics. In severe cases, the individual is hospitalized and treated with intravenous antibiotics, followed by oral antibiotics. Analgesics, antipyretics, bed rest, and adequate hydration are also therapeutic. Complications include urinary retention that resolves with antibiotic therapy; prostatic abscess that may rupture into the urethra, rectum, or perineum; epididymitis; bacteremia; and septic shock. Urinary retention requiring drainage is best managed with a suprapubic catheter; Foley catheterization is contraindicated during acute infection.

Chronic bacterial prostatitis (CBP, category II) is characterized by recurrent urinary tract symptoms and persistence of pathogenic bacteria (usually gram negative) in urine or prostatic fluid. This form of prostatitis is the most common recurrent urinary tract infection in men. Symptoms may be similar to those of an acute bladder infection: frequency, urgency, dysuria, perineal discomfort, low back pain, myalgia, arthralgia, and sexual dysfunction. The prostate may be only slightly enlarged or boggy, but it may be fibrotic because repeated infections can cause it to be firm and irregular in shape.

When the initial urine sample is bacteria-free, prostatic massage is used to express secretions. Subsequently, the first 10 ml of voided urine is collected and examined microscopically. Prostatic secretions showing more than 10 white blood cells (WBCs) per high-power field (hpf) and macrophages containing fat are indicative of bacterial infection; diagnosis is confirmed by culture. A pelvic x-ray or transurethral ultrasound (TRUS) may show prostatic calculi.

Treatment of chronic bacterial prostatitis is difficult because it is often caused by prostatic calculi. Calculi are silent and are found in up to 50% of men with prostatitis, and infected calculi can serve as a source of bacterial persistence and relapsing urinary tract infection.[78] Calculi harbor pathogens within the stone and, consequently, pathogens cannot be eradicated from the urinary tract. Permanent cure is achieved by surgical intervention.

Chronic prostatitis/chronic pelvic pain syndrome. Chronic prostatitis/chronic pelvic pain syndrome (CP/CPPS, category III) is diagnosed when no pathogenic bacteria can be localized to the prostate, and is further subdivided into categories IIIa and IIIb (see Box 32-7). Category IIIa refers to inflammatory chronic pelvic pain syndrome in which white blood cell count is elevated and localized to the prostate. Compared to category III, symptoms tend to be milder but are persistent and annoying. Presumably, noninfectious prostatitis or pain is caused by reflux of sterile urine into the ejaculatory ducts because of high-pressure voiding.[78] Reflux may be triggered by spasms of the external or internal sphincters. Category IIIb is noninflammatory. Category IV exists when individuals are asymptomatic but have

an increase in bacteria and white blood cells localized to the prostate. Microorganisms suspected of causing CP/CPPS include *Escherichia coli, Enterobacter, Pseudomonas aeruginosa,* and, a new suspect, *Helicobacter pylori.*[79]

Men with nonbacterial prostatitis may complain of pain or a dull ache that is continuous or spasmodic in the suprapubic, infrapubic, scrotal, penile, or inguinal area. Other symptoms are pain on ejaculation and urinary symptoms, such as frequency of urination. The prostate gland generally feels normal on palpation.

Nonbacterial prostatitis is a diagnosis of exclusion. Digital examination of the prostate, bacterial cultures of the urogenital tract, microscopic examination of expressed prostatic fluid, urethroscopy, and urodynamic studies are used to verify the diagnosis of nonbacterial prostatitis.

There is no generally accepted treatment for nonbacterial prostatitis. Hot sitz baths, bed rest, and pharmacologic therapies, including anti-inflammatory drugs, can relieve symptoms.

Cancer of the Prostate

Prostate cancer is among the most common male cancers, but the incidence varies greatly worldwide. It is the most common cancer in American males but the third most common cancer worldwide. Figure 32-29 shows the remarkable worldwide variation. Understanding worldwide variations for diseases is important because it demonstrates that the disease is influenced by cultural lifestyle (i.e., dietary practices) and environmental differences. Prostate cancer is the second most frequently diagnosed cancer and the sixth leading cause of death worldwide.[80] More than half of these cases and deaths are expected to occur in more developed countries.[80] Among countries with reliable cancer statistics, prostate cancer rates are highest in Westernized countries such as the United States and Western Europe and lowest in Asian countries. More than any other cancer, prostate cancer incidence warrants interpretation in the context of diagnostic

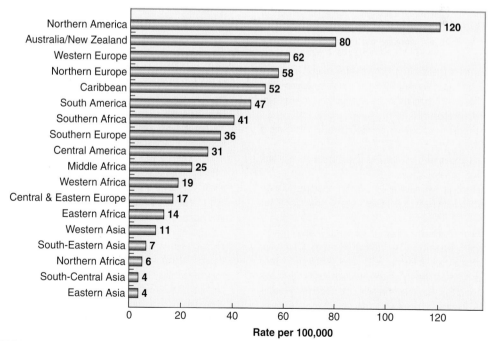

FIGURE 32-29 Selected World Population Age-Standardized (to the World Population) Incidence Rates of Prostate Cancer. *ASR,* Age-standardized rate. (From Jemal A et al: Global patterns of cancer incidence and mortality rates and trends in cancer epidemiology, *Biomark Prev* 19:1893, 2010.)

intensity and screening behavior. Screening according to PSA value can amplify the incidence of prostate cancer by allowing the detection of prostatic lesions that meet pathologic criteria for malignancy but have low potential for growth and metastasis. This screening method is considered controversial. Thus screening can amplify the incidence of prostate cancer (e.g., overdiagnosis) by allowing the detection of these localized lesions. Therefore, incidence rates in some countries, such as the United States, reflect both clinical and latent (or preclinical) disease compared to other countries with only clinical disease. Recent estimates are that 23% to 42% of prostate cancer cases in the United States and Europe may be caused by overdiagnosis through PSA testing.[80-82] Comparing data in the pre-PSA era, however, reflects less extreme incidence rates; however, country ranking reveals the United States as still being in the lead. In the United States and other parts of the world (e.g., Jamaica, Trinidad and Tobago), prostate incidence and mortality rates among black populations may reflect differences in genetic susceptibility.[80]

Prostate cancer death rates have been declining in most Western countries including the United States, Canada, Finland, France, Israel, Italy, Netherlands, Norway, Portugal, Sweden, and Australia.[83] These declines may reflect improved treatment and early detection.[84,85] Two recent randomized trials on PSA testing showed that it reduced deaths from prostate cancer in Europe; however, the trial in the United States failed to show this benefit.[86,87]

In contrast to the incidence rates in Western countries the incidence of prostate cancer is rising in some Asian and eastern European countries, including Japan, Singapore, and Poland, where PSA testing is uncommon.[80] The increase in incidence in these countries is reported to reflect the Westernized lifestyle with high consumption of animal fat, obesity, and lack of physical activity.[83]

The overall mortality rates are predominantly in men over the age of 65; within younger age groups, mortality has been stable across decades. Incidence increases with advancing age, with more than 75% of all prostate cancers diagnosed in men older than 65 years. By age 85 years, about one in six American men will develop prostate cancer in their lifetime, and approximately 3% will die from it. Most of the androgen-metabolizing enzymes undergo significant alteration with aging. Age is the strongest risk factor and other established factors include family history of prostate cancer, a Western lifestyle, obesity, and an African-American heritage. Expanding literature suggests a possible link between chronic inflammation and prostate cancer. The molecular pathogenesis of prostate cancer has shown several alterations of genes involved in defenses against inflammatory damage and tissue recovery (see the Pathogenesis section presented later in the chapter).

Dietary factors. The worldwide distribution of prostate cancer and the increased risk in migrants who relocate from low-risk to high-risk countries provide evidence that diet plays a role in the development of prostate cancer, especially if the diet affects hormone levels.[88] Those factors linked with protection or the development and aggressiveness of prostate cancer include dietary fat, red and processed meat, vitamin E, selenium, tomatoes, cruciform vegetables, and green tea.[88] Box 32-8 contains a summary of diet and additional references.

BOX 32-8   SUMMARY OF DIET FOR PROSTATE CANCER

- Total fat intake, animal and saturated fat, red meat, and dairy products increase prostate cancer risk.
- Obesity is linked to advanced and aggressive prostate cancer.
- High BMI is associated with more aggressive disease and a worse outcome.
- Calorie-dense or excessive carbohydrate intake and obesity, independent of dietary fat intake, may increase the risk of developing prostate cancer.
- Dietary fat may increase androgens, increase oxidative stress, and increase reactive oxygen species (ROS).
- Monounsaturated fats may decrease the risk of prostate cancer.
- High levels of linoleic acid (found in corn oil) act as a proinflammatory eicosanoid, which is implicated in promotion of cell proliferation and angiogenesis as well as inhibition of apoptosis.
- The Western diet has increased omega-6 to omega-3 ratios and therefore is proinflammatory.
- Cooking meat at high temperatures produces heterocyclic amines and aromatic hydrocarbons that are carcinogenic.
- Carcinogenic nitrosamines are formed after consumption of processed meat that contains nitrites and from heme iron present in large quantities of red meat.
- Vitamin E has been long considered a candidate for prostate cancer prevention from in vitro and in vivo animal studies. Vitamin E belongs to the family of tocopherols and tocotrienols that exist as α, β, γ, and δ isoforms. Among these, δ-tocopherol is the major dietary isoform, whereas supplements contain α-tocopherol. Vitamin E is a fat-soluble vitamin obtained from vegetable oils, nuts, and egg yolk. It is a potent intracellular antioxidant known to inhibit peroxidation and DNA damage. The Alpha-Tocopherol, Beta-Carotene Cancer Prevention study (ATBC) showed supplementation with vitamin E could reduce the incidence of prostate cancer among men who smoked. in vitro studies demonstrate that α-tocopherol succinate induces cell cycle arrest in human prostate cancer cells (i.e., induces apoptosis) and inhibits the androgen receptor. Mouse studies show vitamin E can inhibit the growth-promoting effects of a high-fat diet; however, vitamin E in combination with selenium does not reduce the incidence of prostate cancer in Lady mice models. In the prospective large clinical trial SELECT, the study found no apparent benefit of administering vitamin E.
- Selenium is a trace mineral and exists in food as selenomethionine and selenocysteine. It is essential for the functioning of many antioxidant enzymes and proteins in the body. Humans receive selenium in their diet through plant (dependent on soil concentrations) and animal products. Several large prospective studies reported 50% to 65% reductions in prostate cancer risk with high levels versus low levels of selenium as measured in toenails and plasma. The NPC trial reported a 50% reduction in risk of developing prostate cancer. No potential benefit was found in the SELECT trial, whereas a small insignificant increase was noted for type 2 diabetes. From these two trials two different forms of selenium were used—the NPC trial used selenized yeast and the SELECT trial used selenomethionine. Selenium has several modes of action depending on its form. Selenomethionine inhibits cell proliferation and induces cell cycle arrest of human prostate cells (i.e., apoptosis) and inhibits angiogenesis mediated in part by the androgen receptor. This also is true of methylselenic acid. Sodium selenite's anticancer effects are mediated through cellular antioxidants leading to increased apoptosis and sensitizing cells to radiation-induced killing. Selenium and its derivatives can activate both intrinsic and extrinsic pathways of apoptosis. Selenium intervention may depend on individual genotype.
- Vitamin D may play an important role in prostate cancer prevention.
- Soy anticancer properties include inhibition of cell proliferation and angiogenesis and reduction in PSA and androgen receptor levels.

BOX 32-8 SUMMARY OF DIET FOR PROSTATE CANCER—cont'd

- Tomatoes or tomato products ingested daily seem to reduce prostate cancer risk. in vitro studies show lycopene inhibits DNA strand breaks. Unresolved is whether lycopene itself or a metabolic product is responsible for its biologic effect. In clinical studies tomato paste, which is high in lycopene, reduced plasma PSA levels in those men with benign prostatic hyperplasia. Lycopene administration is associated with cell cycle arrest (apoptosis) and growth factor signaling. In 2007 the FDA evaluated 13 available studies and found the relationship between lycopene and reduced risk of prostate cancer inadequate.

- Vegetables including broccoli, cabbage, cauliflower, brussels sprouts, Chinese cabbage, and turnips (all crucifers) may be protective (several epidemiologic studies) against prostate cancer. In particular, a diet high in broccoli reduced cancer risk. By contrast, four studies revealed no cancer preventive effects. Cruciforms have anticancer properties mediated by the phytochemicals phenethyl isothiocyanate, sulforaphane, and indole-3-carbinol. Sulforaphane is a naturally occurring isothiocyanate that was first isolated in broccoli. It protects against carcinogen-induced cancer in many rodents. Mice given 240 mg of broccoli sprouts per day showed a significant reduction in growth of prostate cancer cells. Sulforaphane treatment lowered androgen receptor protein and gene expression.

- Green tea contains polyphenols, including epigallocatechin gallate (EGCG). Green tea consumption has been associated with a reduced incidence of several cancers including prostate cancer. Green tea consumed within a balanced controlled diet in humans improved overall antioxidant potential. The anticancer effect potential of green tea from in vitro and experimental studies shows these compounds bind directly to carcinogens and induce phase II enzymes that inhibit heterocyclic amines. EGCG administration decreased NF-κB activity. Green tea was shown to inhibit IGF-1 and increase IGFBP3, leading to inhibition of prostate cancer development and progression. Yet, in two small randomized studies in individuals with high-grade prostatic neoplasia, it showed no effects.

- Curcumin has anticarcinogenic potential with well-characterized anti-inflammatory, antiangiogenic, and antioxidant properties. Recent studies report curcumin modulates the Wingless signaling pathway (Wnt) that supports its antiproliferative potential.

- Overall, multiple signaling pathways are involved in prostate cancer development and progression, many of which are affected by dietary and lifestyle factors.

General References

Astorg P: Dietary N-6 and N-3 polyunsaturated fatty acids and prostate cancer risk: a review of epidemiological and experimental evidence, *Cancer Causes Control* 15:367–386, 2004.

Beier R, et al: Induction of cyclin E-cdk2 kinase activity, E2F-dependent transcription and cell growth by Myc are genetically separable events, *EMBO J* 19(21):5813–5823, 2000.

Dagnelie PC, et al: Diet, anthropometric measures and prostate cancer risk: a review of prospective cohort and intervention studies, *BJ Int* 93(8):1139–1150, 2004.

Demark-Wahnefried W, Moyad MA: Dietary intervention in the management of prostate cancer, *Curr Opin Urol* 17:168–174, 2007. 737–743, 2001.

Freedland SJ, Aronson WJ: Obesity and prostate cancer, *Urology* 65:433–439, 2005.

Giovannucci E, et al: Risk factors for prostate cancer incidence and progression in the health professionals follow-up study, *Int J Cancer* 121:1571–1578, 2007.

Greenwald P: Clinical trials in cancer prevention: current results and perspectives for the future, *J Nutr* 134(12 suppl):3507S–3512S, 2004.

Hill P, et al: Diet and urinary steroids in black and white North American men and black South African men, *Cancer Res* 39:5101–5105, 1979.

Kim DJ, et al: Premorbid diet in relation to survival from prostate cancer (Canada), *Cancer Causes Control* 11:65–77, 2000.

Kobayashi N, et al: Effect of altering dietary omega-6/omega-3 fatty acid ratios on prostate cancer membrane composition, cyclooxygenase-2, and prostaglandin E$_2$, *Clin Cancer Res* 12(15):4660–4670, 2006.

Kolonel LN: Fat, meat, and prostate cancer, *Epidemiol Rev* 23:72–81, 2001.

Lloyd JC, et al: Effect of isocaloric low fat diet on prostate cancer xenograft progression in a hormone deprivation model, *J Urol* 183:1619–1624, 2010.

Matsumura K, et al: Involvement of the estrogen receptor beta in genistein-induced expression of p21 (waf1/cip1) in PC-3 prostate cancer cells, *Anticancer Res* 28:709–714, 2008.

Ngo TH, et al: Effect of diet and exercise on serum insulin, IGF-1, and IGFBP-1 levels and growth of LNCaP cells in vitro (United States), *Cancer Causes Control* 13:929–935, 2002.

Ngo TH, et al: Effect of isocaloric low-fat diet on human LAPC-4 prostate cancer xenografts in severe combined immunodeficient mice and the insulin-like growth factor axis, *Clin Cancer Res* 9:2734–2743, 2003.

Ni J, Yeh S: The roles of alpha-vitamin E and its analogues in prostate cancer, *Vitam Horm* 76:493–518, 2007.

Rodriguez C, et al: Body mass index, weight change, and risk of prostate cancer in the Cancer Prevention Study II Nutrition Cohort, *Cancer Epidemiol Biomarkers Prev* 16:63–69, 2007.

Sinha R, et al: Meat and meat-related compounds and risk of prostate cancer in a large prospective cohort study in the United States, *Am J Epidemiol* 170:1165–1177, 2009.

Teiten M, et al: Anti-proliferative potential of curcumin in androgen dependent prostate cancer cells occurs through modulation of the Wingless signaling pathway, *Int J Oncol* 38:603–611, 2011.

Migration of individuals from low-risk geographic areas of the world, such as Japan, to high-risk countries, such as the United States, increases risk considerably. These changes in risk probably reflect differences in lifestyle and dietary habits. Geographically, individuals who reside in regions with less sunlight have a higher risk of prostate cancer. The highest rates of mortality from prostate cancer in the world are in Scandinavian countries, where exposure to ultraviolet light is low; the possible link is less vitamin D induced by less sun exposure. Vitamin D (1,25-dihydroxyvitamin D$_3$) inhibited the growth of certain human prostate cancer cell lines through the function of an androgen-dependent mechanism.[89] The Cure of Cancer of the Prostate (CaP CURE) report states that of all the risk factors for prostate cancer, only nutrition seems to explain the differences in global distribution of prostate cancer.[90]

Hormones. Prostate cancer develops in an androgen-dependent epithelium and is usually androgen sensitive. Androgens are synthesized not only in the testis, accounting for 50% to 60% of the total testosterone in the prostate, but also in the prostate gland itself. In a process called intraprostatic conversion, the hormone DHEA produced by the adrenal glands[91,92] is converted to testosterone and then into DHT in the prostate (Figure 32-30). Additionally, prostate cancer

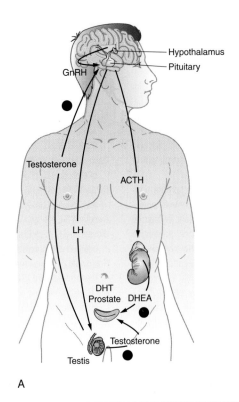

A

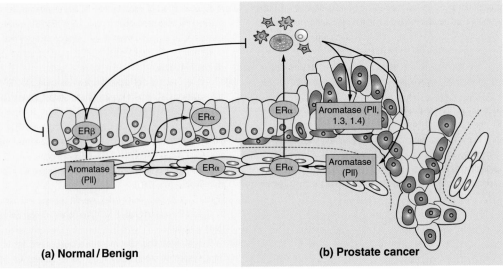

B

FIGURE 32-30 Sources of Androgens and Aromatase and Estrogen Signaling in the Prostate.
A, Body sources of androgens in the prostate gland. Hypothalamic GnRH causes the release of LH from
the anterior pituitary gland. LH stimulates the testes to produce testosterone, which then accumulates
in the blood. Pituitary ACTH release stimulates the adrenal glands, which secrete the androgen precursor DHEA into the blood. DHEA is converted into testosterone and then into DHT in the prostate.
B, Aromatase and estrogen signaling in the prostate. In normal and benign tissue, aromatase is expressed
within the stroma and regulated by promoter PII. Estrogen then exerts its effects in an autocrine fashion
through the stromal ER-α receptor and also in a paracrine fashion through both ER-α and ER-β receptors. With prostate cancer, aromatase is now expressed within the tumor cells and in stromal cells, and
regulated by aromatase promoters 1.3, 1.4, and PII. Thus estrogen exerts its effects in an autocrine
way through stromal and epithelial ER-α and ER-β. Consequently, the increased levels of estrogen and
abnormal ER-α signaling promote inflammation, which increases aromatase expression and the development of a positive feedback cycle. Inflammation drives aromatase expression, thus increasing estrogen,
which in turn promotes further inflammation. *ACTH,* Adrenocorticotropic hormone; *DHEA,* dehydroepiandrosterone; *DHT,* dihydrotestosterone; *GnRH,* gonadotropin-releasing hormone; *LH,* luteinizing
hormone. (**A** adapted from Labrie F: Blockage of testicular and adrenal androgens in prostate cancer
treatment, *Nat Rev Urol* 8:73–80, 2011. **B** from Ellem SJ, Risbridger GP: Aromatase and regulating the
estrogen:androgen ratio in the prostate gland, *J Steroid Biochem Mol Biol* 118[4–5]:246–251, 2010.)

cells have been reported to make androgens from cholesterol (i.e., de novo).[93] However, these overall relative contributions from intratumoral sources remain to be determined. Population studies have not, however, provided clear and convincing patterns involving associations between circulating (e.g., not tissue concentrations) hormone concentrations and prostate cancer risk.[94,95] Thus, there is universal agreement that androgens are important for prostatic growth, development, and maintenance of tissue balance but their role in cancer is controversial.[96] Evidence for involvement of 5α-reductase activity, which is critical in androgen activity in the prostate, is contradictory and inconsistent[94,95] (see Figure 32-30). A prevention study has provided some of the strongest hormonal data with the drug finasteride, which inhibits 5α-reductase. The 7-year intervention study reduced prostate cancer risk in healthy men by about 25%.[97] Important, however, was that more high-grade tumors were found in those men who developed prostate cancer while on the drug. In men younger than 50 years, circulating levels of androgens and estrogens appear to be higher in men of African descent than in European-American men.

Despite the well-documented importance of androgens, their pathophysiologic process in prostate diseases is incomplete.[96] Androgens also are metabolized to estrogens (see Figure 32-30, *B*) through the action of the enzyme aromatase, and a growing body of evidence implicates estrogens in the etiology of prostate disease (see Pathogenesis section). Importantly, the aberrant expression of aromatase has been implicated in other tissues, such as the breast and endometrium.[96]

Investigations directed at understanding the hormonal basis of prostate (as well as breast) carcinogenesis have numerous problems. The complexities of interacting hormones and separating the effects of a single hormone are profound. In addition, only single *blood* samples are generally available, *tissue* hormone samples important for paracrine signaling are not consistently measured, and within-subject variations over time and differences in circadian rhythms cannot be adequately measured. The results of several animal studies do support elevation in levels of bioavailable and bioactive androgens in the circulation and in target tissue as an important risk factor. Animal studies also indicate that increased biologic activity of the androgen receptor may be associated with prostate cancer. A more thorough discussion of the role of hormones in the pathogenesis of prostate cancer is in the Pathogenesis section.

Vasectomy. Vasectomy has been identified as a possible risk factor for prostate cancer in both case-controlled studies and cohort studies.[98,99] Three mechanisms by which vasectomy could increase risk are (1) elevation of circulating androgens; (2) activation of immunologic mechanisms involving antisperm antibodies; and (3) reduction of seminal fluid levels of 5α-dihydrotestosterone, the active metabolite of testosterone in the prostate, in vasectomized men. Other investigators reported a decrease in sex hormone–binding globulin (SHBG) level and an increase in the ratio of testosterone to SHBG.[100] These results suggest an elevation of circulating free testosterone after vasectomy.[94] The epidemiologic literature, however, is consistent with no appreciable association of vasectomy and prostate cancer or a weak positive association.[101]

Chronic inflammation. The results of a 5-year longitudinal study of the influence of chronic inflammation and prostate cancer have been reported.[102] The study included 144 men, 33 of whom presented with chronic inflammation in their initial biopsy. Biopsies revealed prostatic hyperplasia and proliferative inflammatory atrophy in those with chronic inflammation. Upon repeat biopsy, 29 new cancers were diagnosed, representing a new cancer incidence of 20%.[102] In contrast, of the 33 men initially showing no inflammation, 2 (6%) were found to have adenocarcinoma. The causes of chronic inflammation are unknown (possible causes are shown in Figure 32-31). Thus,

chronic inflammation may be an important risk factor for prostatic adenocarcinoma.

Genetic and epigenetic factors. Other possible causes are those of genetic predisposition (familial and hereditary forms). Genetic studies suggest that strong familial predisposition may be responsible for 5% to 10% of prostate cancers.[54] Compared to men with no family history, those with one first-degree relative with prostate cancer have twice the risk and those with two-first degree relatives have five times the risk.[103] Men with *BRCA2* (tumor suppressor) germline mutations have a 20-fold increase in risk of prostate cancer. The most common epigenetic alteration in prostate cancer is hypermethylation of the glutathione S-transferase *(GSTPl)* gene located on chromosome 11. Other epigenetic modifications have been reported.[103] The hereditary form constitutes about 9% of all prostate cancers and approximately 43% of cancers in men younger than 55 years of age.[104] There is no clear evidence of a causal link between BPH and prostate cancer, even though they may often occur together. Variations in several other genes related to inflammatory pathways might affect the probability of developing prostate cancer.

PATHOGENESIS   More than 95% of prostatic neoplasms are adenocarcinomas,[105] and most occur in the periphery of the prostate (Figures 32-28 and 32-32). Prostatic adenocarcinoma is a heterogeneous group of tumors with a diverse spectrum of molecular and pathologic characteristics and therefore clinical behaviors and challenges.[106] The biologic aggressiveness of the neoplasm appears to be related to the degree of differentiation rather than the size of the tumor (Box 32-9).

Hormonal factors. Just as the testicles are the male equivalent of the female ovaries, the prostate is the male equivalent of the female uterus; in both situations they originate from the same embryonic cells. This may be important in understanding the role of the associated hormones testosterone (T), dihydrotestosterone (DHT), and estrogens in prostate cancer development. Testicular testosterone synthesis and serum testosterone levels fall as men age, but the levels of estradiol do not decline, remaining unchanged or increasing with age.[107,108] The relationship between hormones and the pathophysiology of prostate carcinogenesis is incomplete and controversial. The main issues and controversies include (1) sources of androgen production outside of the testes, or extratesticular sources (e.g., from adrenal DHEA and from prostate cholesterol [de novo] itself); (2) the role of prostatic androgen receptor (AR); (3) the role of estrogens, aromatase enzyme, and the estrogen receptors ER-α and ER-β; and (4) the role of the surrounding microenvironment or stroma.

Testicular testosterone provides the main source of androgens in the prostate (see Figure 32-30) and is the major *circulating* androgen, whereas DHT predominates in prostate tissue and binds to the androgen receptor (AR) with greater affinity than does T.[109] The adrenal cortex contributes the far less potent dehydroepiandrosterone (DHEA) that promotes synthesis of androgens in the prostate. In the target tissues and, to a lesser extent, in the testes themselves, testosterone is converted to dihydrotestosterone (DHT) by the enzyme 5α-reductase (Figure 32-33). Thus, DHT is the most potent intraprostatic androgen.

Normally, a small amount of estrogen is produced daily—estrone and estradiol—by the aromatization of androstenedione and testosterone, respectively. This reaction is catalyzed by the enzyme aromatase. A small quantity of estradiol is released by the testes (see Figure 32-33); the rest of the estrogens in males are produced by adipose tissue, liver, skin, brain, and other nonendocrine tissue. Thus, testosterone is a precursor of two hormones—DHT and estradiol.

Recent studies show aromatase is expressed in stromal tissue in the benign human prostate gland.[110] Thus it appears that both normal

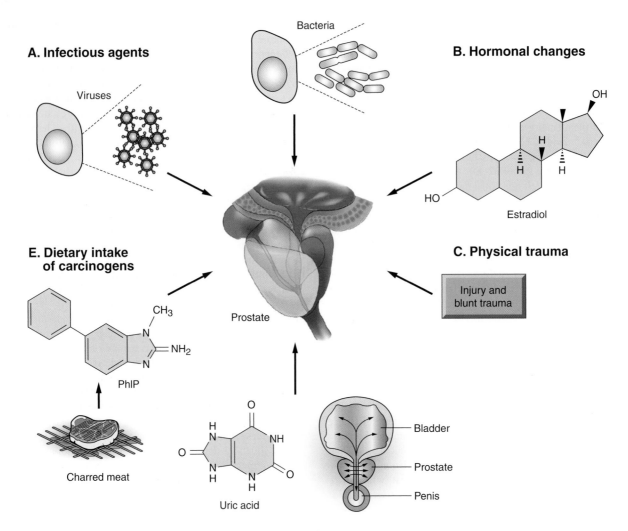

A. Infectious agents

Viruses

Bacteria

B. Hormonal changes

Estradiol

E. Dietary intake of carcinogens

PhIP

Charred meat

Prostate

Uric acid

C. Physical trauma

Injury and blunt trauma

Bladder

Prostate

Penis

D. Urine reflux

FIGURE 32-31 Possible Causes of Prostate Inflammation. *A,* Infection, including viruses, bacteria, fungi, and parasites. *B,* Hormones, for example, estrogen at key times during development. *C,* Physical trauma, any type of blunt physical injury. *D,* Urine reflex. *E,* Certain dietary factors (see text).

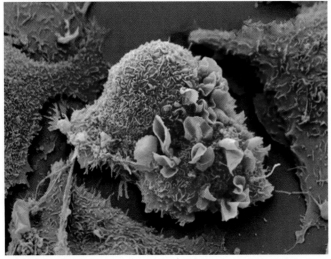

FIGURE 32-32 Photomicrograph of Prostate Cancer Cells. Pink ruffled cells are prostate cancer cells. (From Cancer Research UK, London Research Institute, Electron Microscopy Unit.)

BOX 32-9 DETERMINING THE GRADE OF PROSTATE CANCER WITH THE GLEASON SCORE

Grade 1. The cancer cells closely resemble normal cells. They are small, uniform in shape, evenly spaced, and well differentiated (i.e., they remain separate from one another).

Grade 2. The cancer cells are still well differentiated, but they are arranged more loosely and are irregular in shape and size. Some of the cancer cells have invaded the neighboring prostate tissue.

Grade 3. This is the most common grade. The cells are less well differentiated (some have fused into clumps) and are more variable in shape.

Grade 4. The cells are poorly differentiated and highly irregular in shape. Invasion of the neighboring prostate tissue has progressed further.

Grade 5. The cells are undifferentiated. They have merged into large masses that no longer resemble normal prostate cells. Invasion of the surrounding tissue is extensive.

prostate and benign prostate have the capacity to locally metabolize androgens to estrogens through aromatase. This leads to the following question: How does aromatase gene expression contribute to the etiology and progression of prostate cancer? Investigators have demonstrated altered aromatase expression in prostate cancer[108,110] (see Figure 32-30, *B*, p. 832).

The effect of estrogen is determined by the two receptors ER-α and ER-β. ER-α leads to abnormal proliferation, inflammation, and the development of premalignant lesions.[108] In contrast, ER-β leads to antiproliferative, anti-inflammatory, and potentially anticarcinogenic effects that act in concert or balance the actions of ER-α and androgens.[108] Increased expression of ER-α has been found to be associated with prostate cancer progression, metastasis, and the so-called castration-resistant (medical treatment that suppresses androgens) phenotype.[111] A specific oncogene is regulated by ERs, and those hormones that stimulate the ER-α receptor-like (i.e., agonists) endogenous estrogens can stimulate oncogene expression.[112]

Most of the androgen-metabolizing enzymes undergo a significant age-dependent alteration. In epithelium, both the blood levels of 5α-reductase activity and the DHT level decrease with age, whereas in stroma (prostate), not only the 5α-reductase activity but also the stromal DHT level is rather constant over the lifetime. In contrast to the relatively unaltered DHT level over time, the estrogen concentration follows an age-dependent increase. Thus the age-dependent decrease of the DHT accumulation in epithelium and the concomitant increase of the estrogen accumulation in stroma lead to a tremendous increase with age of the estrogen/androgen ratio in the human prostate. In animal studies, chronic exposure to testosterone plus estradiol is strongly carcinogenic, whereas testosterone alone is weakly carcinogenic.[95] In mice studies, elevated testosterone level in the absence of estrogen leads to the development of hypertrophy and hyperplasia but not malignancy.[108] High estrogen and low testosterone levels have been shown to lead to inflammation with aging and the emergence of precancerous lesions.[108] The mechanism is not clearly understood and may involve estrogen-generated oxidative stress and DNA toxicity, and it requires androgen-mediated and estrogen receptor–mediated processes, such as changes in sex steroid metabolism and receptor status.[95] In addition, there are changes in the balance between autocrine/paracrine growth-stimulatory and growth-inhibitory factors, such as the insulin growth factors (IGFs).

Androgen receptor signaling. The androgenic hormone responses in the normal prostate and prostate cancer are mediated by **androgen receptor (AR) signaling.**[113] Exactly how AR drives the growth of prostate cancer cells is not fully known. Several mechanisms have been suggested[113] and specific pathways of signaling are important because they can provide novel therapeutic targets.

Prostate epithelial neoplasia. A precursor lesion, **prostatic epithelial neoplasia (PIN),** has been described. PIN may be more concentrated in prostates containing cancer and is noted in proximity to cancer.[103] However, the final fate of PIN is unknown, including the possibilities of latency, invasion, and even regression. The current working model of prostate carcinogenesis suggests that repeated cycles of injury and cell death occur to the prostate epithelium as a result of damage (i.e., from oxidative stress) from inflammatory responses.[114] The direct injury is hypothesized as a response to infections; autoimmune disease; circulating carcinogens or toxins, or both, from the diet; or urine that has refluxed into the prostate (see Figure 32-31). The resultant manifestation of this injury is focal atrophy or prostate intraepithelial atrophy (PIA). Biologic responses cause an increase in proliferation and a massive increase in epithelial cells that possess a phenotype intermediate between basal cells and mature luminal cells (Figure 32-34).[114] In a small subset of cells, some may contain "stem cell" or tumor–initiating properties and telomere shortening (see Chapter 9). A subset of PIN cells may activate telomerase enzyme, causing the cells to become immortal.[115] Molecular genetic and epigenetic changes can increase genetic instability that might progress to high-grade PIN and early prostate cancer formation. This model of prostate carcinogenesis needs much more research.

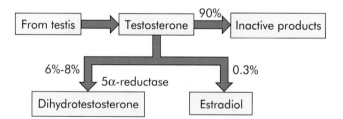

FIGURE 32-33 Testosterone and Conversion to Dihydrotestosterone (DHT).

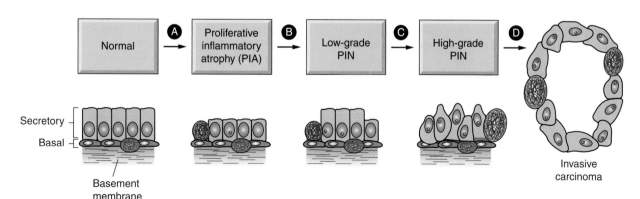

FIGURE 32-34 Cellular and Molecular Model of Early Prostate Neoplasia Progression. A, This stage includes infiltration of lymphocytes, macrophages, and neutrophils caused by repeated infections, dietary factors, urine reflux, injury, onset of autoimmunity (which triggers inflammation), and wound healing. **B,** Epigenetic alterations mediate telomere shortening. **C,** Genetic instability and accumulation of genetic alterations. **D,** Continued proliferation of genetically unstable cells leading to cancer progression. *PIN,* Prostatic intraepithelial neoplasia.

Stromal environment. The prostate gland is composed of secretory luminal epithelium, basal epithelium, neuroendocrine cells, and various cell types comprising supportive tissue or stroma. **Stroma,** or tissue microenvironment, produces autocrine/paracrine factors as well as structural supporting molecules that help regulate normal cell behavior and organ homeostasis.[66] **Fibroblasts** are the most important cells during the reconstructive phase of wound healing (see Chapter 5). The collagen and connective tissue proteins produced by fibroblasts are deposited in wounded areas after fibroblasts have entered the lesion. Thus, their presence is a signature of alterations in the stroma. Reactive tumor stroma is associated with an increased number of fibroblasts, increased capillary density, and collagen and fibrin deposition. These findings suggest that alteration in the prostate microenvironment, mediated by changes associated with aging or senescence, or both, promote epithelial responses that contribute to diseases.[66] In animal studies, investigators have noted that the microenvironment has an increased number of cells that promote inflammation and a collapsed appearance of the smooth muscle cells within adjacent glandular stroma.[66] Fibroblast spreading has been proposed as indicative of decreased mechanical tension because of a lack of direct association of the fibroblasts with aged fragmented collagen fibrils.[116,117] These alterations in mechanical tension and cell shape are suggested as determinants in altering gene expression and cellular function. These alterations in aged prostate stroma for mice and men include significant enhancement for inflammation pathways (e.g., NF-κβ, collagens).[116,117] Inflammation can induce cell stress and stressed mesenchymal cells can secrete inflammatory mediators (chemoattractants); however, it remains to be determined whether inflammatory infiltrates are a cause of or response to the alterations of aged stroma.[118] There is supporting evidence that inflammation has a role in the pathogenesis of prostate cancer.[114,119] Investigators recently found that disruption of fibroblast growth factor signaling pathways leads to strongly activated and atypical stroma that preceded the development of mice PIN (mPIN).[120]

Epithelial-mesenchymal transition (EMT) was first described in embryonic development, and is observed in a number of solid tumors[121] (also see p. 851). Cells that undergo EMT become more migratory and invasive and gain access to vascular vessels.[122] Numerous studies have shown that these transition states (EMT and mesenchymal-epithelial transition [MET]) are a consequence of tumor-stromal interactions.[122,123]

Investigators studying prostate cancer cells in vitro correlated EMT with increased growth, migration, and invasion.[124] These investigators demonstrated that the microenvironment is a critical site for the transition of human prostate cancer cells from epithelial to mesenchymal structure, resulting in increased metastatic potential for bone and adrenal gland.[124]

Prostate cancer is known to be diverse and composed of multiple genetically distinct cancer cell clones. Recent studies, however, indicate that most metastatic cancers arise from a single precursor cancer cell.[125]

From all of these observations, the following multifactorial general hypothesis of prostate carcinogenesis emerges: (1) androgens act as strong tumor promoters through androgen receptor–mediated mechanisms to enhance the carcinogenic activity of strong endogenous DNA toxic carcinogens, including reactive estrogen metabolites and estrogen, and prostate-generated reactive oxygen species; (2) alterations in autocrine/paracrine growth-stimulating and growth-inhibiting factors between the prostate tumor cells and microenvironment influence cancer pathogenesis; and (3) possibly unknown environmental-lifestyle carcinogens may contribute to prostate cancer. All of these factors are modulated by diet and genetic determinants, such as

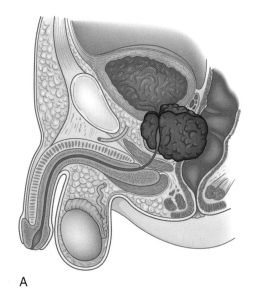

A

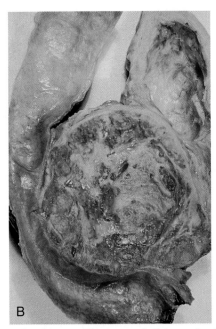

B

FIGURE 32-35 Carcinoma of Prostate. **A,** Schematic of carcinoma of the prostate. **B,** Carcinoma of the prostate extending into the rectum and urinary bladder. (B from Damjanov I, Linder J, editors: *Pathology: a color atlas,* St Louis, 2000, Mosby.)

hereditary susceptibility genes and polymorphic genes, which encode receptors and enzymes involved in the metabolism and action of steroid hormones.[95]

The most common sites of distant metastasis are the lymph nodes, bones, lungs, liver, and adrenals. The pelvis, lumbar spine, femur, thoracic spine, and ribs are the most common sites of bone metastasis. Local extension is usually posterior, although late in the disease the tumor may invade the rectum or encroach on the prostatic urethra and cause bladder outlet obstruction (Figure 32-35). The spread of cancer through blood vessels is illustrated in Figure 32-36.

CLINICAL MANIFESTATIONS Prostatic cancer often causes no symptoms until it is far advanced. The first manifestations of disease

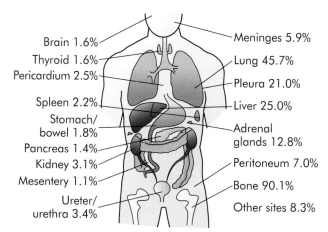

FIGURE 32-36 Distribution of Hematogenous Metastases in Prostate Cancer. Study of 556 individuals with metastatic prostate cancer. (Adapted from Budendorf L et al: Metastatic patterns of prostate cancer: an autopsy study of 1,589 patients, *Hum Pathol* 31:578, 2000.)

are those of bladder outlet obstruction: slow urinary stream, hesitancy, incomplete emptying, frequency, nocturia, and dysuria. Unlike the symptoms of obstruction caused by BPH, the symptoms of obstruction caused by prostatic cancer are progressive and do not remit. Local extension of prostatic cancer can obstruct the upper urinary tract ureters as well. Rectal obstruction also may occur, causing the individual to experience large bowel obstruction or difficulty in defecation. Symptoms of late disease include bone pain at sites of bone metastasis, edema of the lower extremities, enlargement of lymph nodes, liver enlargement, pathologic bone fractures, and mental confusion associated with brain metastases. Prostatic cancer and its treatment can affect sexual functioning.

EVALUATION AND TREATMENT Screening for prostatic cancer includes digital rectal examination (DRE), prostate-specific antigen (PSA) blood tests, and transrectal ultrasound (TRUS). Researchers at Memorial Sloan-Kettering Cancer Center have found that change in PSA levels over time—known as PSA velocity—is a poor predictor of prostate cancer and may lead to many unnecessary biopsies.[126] The controversy about PSA velocity is whether it adds any additional predictive accuracy to PSA alone or other standard measures such as, a positive digital rectal exam. Cancer diagnosis is confirmed through tissue biopsy and microscopic examination of tissue. Lymphography, bone scans, MRI, and CT scans also may be used to determine metastasis to lymph, bone, or other adjacent tissue. Important for treatment is to accurately measure the size of the index (longest) tumor and its percentage Gleason grade of differentiation.[127]

Treatment of prostatic cancer depends on the stage of the disease (see Box 32-9), the anticipated effects of treatment, and the age, general health, and life expectancy of the individual. Options range from hormonal or radiation therapy or chemotherapy to surgery (contemporary nerve sparing or robotic surgery), any combination of these, or no treatment. Palliative treatment is aimed at relieving urinary, bladder outlet, or colon obstruction; spinal cord compression; and pain.

Prognosis and survival rates have improved steadily since the 1950s. Currently, 85% of all prostate cancers are discovered in the local and regional stages; in these stages, the 5-year survival rate is 100%.[1] For those men whose cancer has spread to distant tissue when it is found, the 5-year survival is 34%.[1]

Treatment for prostate cancer may lead to loss of urinary control, which can return to normal after several weeks or months. Mild stress incontinence can occur after surgery and mild urge incontinence after radiation therapy. Prostate cancer and its treatment can affect sexual functioning. Most men will need assistance (medication) with obtaining an erection for 3 to 12 months after surgery. Sensation of orgasm is not usually affected, but smaller amounts of ejaculate will be produced or men may experience a "dry" ejaculate because of retrograde ejaculation.

Sexual Dysfunction

In males, the normal sexual response involves erection, emission, and ejaculation. Sexual dysfunction is the impairment of any or all of these processes and can be caused by various physiologic, psychologic, and emotional factors.

Until the late 1970s, most cases of male sexual dysfunction were considered psychogenic. Now there is evidence that 89% to 90% of cases involve organic factors and include (1) vascular, endocrine, and neurologic disorders; (2) chronic disease, including renal failure and diabetes mellitus; (3) penile diseases and penile trauma; and (4) iatrogenic factors, such as surgery and pharmacologic therapies. Most of these disorders cause erectile dysfunction.[128]

PATHOPHYSIOLOGY Sexual dysfunction can have a specific physiologic cause, can be associated with many chronic diseases and their treatment, or may be related to low energy levels, stress, or depression. For example, vascular disease may cause impotence, and endocrine disorders or conditions that cause decreased testosterone levels or testicular atrophy can diminish sexual functioning or libido. In addition, neurologic disorders and spinal cord injuries can interfere with sympathetic, parasympathetic, and CNS mechanisms required for erection, emission, and ejaculation.

Drug-induced sexual dysfunction consists of decreased desire, decreased erectile ability, or decreased ejaculatory ability. Alcohol and other CNS depressants, antihypertensives, antidepressants, antihistamines, and hormonal preparations are commonly used drugs that affect sexual functioning. Other pharmacologic agents may diminish the quality or quantity of sperm or cause priapism.

CLINICAL MANIFESTATIONS AND TREATMENT Evaluation of sexual dysfunction includes a thorough history and physical examination. Particular attention is given to drug history and examination of the genitalia, prostate, and nervous system. Basic laboratory tests are used to identify the presence of endocrinopathies or other underlying disorders that can cause dysfunction. Psychologic evaluation is indicated for younger men with a sudden onset of sexual dysfunction or men of any age who can achieve but not maintain an erection. If no physiologic cause is found and the condition does not improve with psychotherapy, the man is referred for further investigation of organic causes.

Treatments for organic sexual dysfunction include both medical and surgical approaches. The drug Viagra (sildenafil) has created much enthusiasm over its ability to help a man maintain an erection. For a small percentage of men (1%), however, this improvement in sexual function is accompanied by heart attacks and death. Whether these effects are the result of sexual performance or Viagra has been controversial. Research has shown that Viagra increases blood concentrations of the enzyme cGMP-dependent protein kinase (PKG), which increases blood flow to the penis. PKG, however, plays a dual role: first it increases platelet aggregation and then, minutes later, it decreases clot size. The initial clot could cause some men with heart disease to experience cardiac arrest.[129] Nonsurgical approaches include correction of underlying disorders, particularly drug-induced dysfunction and endocrinopathy-related (e.g., reduced testosterone level associated with chronic renal failure) dysfunction. Use of vasodilators and cessation of smoking can benefit individuals with vasculogenic erectile dysfunction. Surgical approaches include penile implants, penile revascularization, and correction of other anatomic defects contributing to sexual dysfunction.

Impairment of Sperm Production and Quality

Spermatogenesis requires adequate secretion of follicle-stimulating hormone (FSH) and luteinizing hormone (LH) by the pituitary and sufficient secretion of testosterone by the testes. Inadequate secretion of gonadotropins may be caused by numerous alterations (e.g., hypothyroidism, hyperadrenocortisolism, hyperprolactinemia, or hypogonadotropic hypogonadism). In the absence of adequate gonadotropin levels, the Leydig cells are not stimulated to secrete testosterone, and sperm maturation is not promoted in the Sertoli cells. Spermatogenesis also depends on an appropriate response by the testes. Defects in testicular response to the gonadotropins result in decreased secretion of testosterone and inhibin B and occur as a result of normal feedback mechanisms and high levels of circulating gonadotropins. In the absence of adequate testosterone levels, spermatogenesis is impaired. Newer studies demonstrate the importance of inhibin B as a valuable marker of the competence of Sertoli cells and spermatogenesis.[130] Impaired spermatogenesis also can be caused by testicular trauma, infection, atrophy of the testes, systemic illness involving high fever, ingestion of various drugs, exposure to environmental toxins, and cryptorchidism.

Fertility is adversely affected if spermatogenesis is normal but the sperm are chromosomally or morphologically abnormal or are produced in insufficient quantities. Chromosomal abnormalities are caused by genetic factors and by external variables, such as exposure to radiation or toxic substances. Because the Y chromosome plays a key role in testis determination and control of spermatogenesis, understanding how the genes interact can elucidate exact causes of infertility. The most common mutations are microdeletion of the Y chromosome (AZ [azoospermia] a, b, and c).[131] Research related to mapping the critical genes and gene pathways is the current focus of male infertility. Common mechanisms may be involved in infertility and testicular cancer. In utero environmental exposure to endocrine disruptors modulates the genetic makeup of the gonad and may result in both infertility and testicular cancer.[131-136]

Sperm motility also may affect fertility. Motility appears to be affected by characteristics of semen. Prostatic dysfunction, excessive semen viscosity, presence of drugs or toxins in the semen, and presence of antisperm antibodies are associated with impaired sperm motility. However, new data show that motile density may not be a good indicator of infertility.[137] Approximately 17% of infertile males have antisperm antibodies in their semen. These antibodies may be (1) cytotoxic antibodies, which attack sperm and reduce their number in the semen, or (2) sperm-immobilizing antibodies, which impair sperm motility and reduce their ability to traverse the endocervical canal.

Treatment for impaired spermatogenesis involves correcting any underlying disorders, avoiding radiation and possibly electromagnetic radiation (hypothesis from cell phones) and toxins, and using hormones to enhance spermatogenesis. In addition, semen can be modified to improve sperm motility; modifications are followed by artificial insemination.

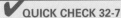

✔ QUICK CHECK 32-7
1. What is the current understanding of hormones in the pathophysiology of prostate cancer?
2. Why is the worldwide variation of prostate cancer incidence important?
3. Describe what is meant by prostate cancer cell and stromal interactions for carcinogenesis.
4. What causes impaired spermatogenesis?

DISORDERS OF THE BREAST

Disorders of the Female Breast

Galactorrhea

Galactorrhea (inappropriate lactation) is the persistent and sometimes excessive secretion of a milky fluid from the breasts of a woman who is not pregnant or nursing an infant. Galactorrhea, which also can occur in men, may involve one or both breasts and is not associated with breast cancer.[138]

The incidence of galactorrhea is difficult to estimate because of differences among definitions of the condition, examination techniques, and populations of women who have been studied. Prevalence has been documented as 0.1% to 32% of all women.

PATHOPHYSIOLOGY Galactorrhea is not a breast disorder but, rather, a manifestation of pathophysiologic processes elsewhere in the body. These processes are chiefly hormone imbalances caused by hypothalamic-pituitary disturbances, pituitary tumors, or neurologic damage. Exogenous causes include drugs, estrogen (e.g., in oral contraceptives), and manipulation of the nipples.

The most common cause of galactorrhea is nonpuerperal hyperprolactinemia, or excessive amounts of prolactin in the blood not related to pregnancy or childbirth. Nonpuerperal hyperprolactinemia can be caused by any factor that (1) stimulates or overstimulates the prolactin-secreting units of the pituitary gland; (2) interferes with production of prolactin-inhibiting factor (PIF), a neurotransmitter (probably dopamine) that inhibits prolactin secretion; or (3) interferes with pituitary receptors for PIF.

Certain drugs can cause nonpuerperal hyperprolactinemia. They include the phenothiazines, reserpine, and methyldopa; exogenous estrogens, particularly in oral contraceptives; morphine; and the tricyclic antidepressants.

Hypothyroidism causes increased secretion of hypothalamic thyroid-releasing hormone (TRH), which stimulates prolactin release from the pituitary. Hypothyroidism also is associated with reduced metabolic clearance of prolactin, which prolongs its effects.

Many types of pituitary tumors cause hyperprolactinemia, particularly prolactinoma. Prolactinomas cause hyperprolactinemia by secreting prolactin, decreasing production of PIF, or applying pressure to the pituitary stalk, thus preventing delivery of PIF to the anterior pituitary. Growth hormone–secreting pituitary tumors may cause galactorrhea through the intrinsic lactogenic effect that growth hormone appears to have on mammary tissue. Prolactin-secreting lung and kidney tumors also cause hyperprolactinemia.

Galactorrhea can be induced by persistent and repeated sucking or squeezing of the nipples and has been documented in women who manipulate their breasts and nipples daily. Monthly examination of the breasts for nipple discharge usually is not associated with the development of galactorrhea.

CLINICAL MANIFESTATIONS Inappropriate lactation is manifested by the appearance of a milky breast secretion from one or both breasts of nonpregnant, nonlactating women. Most women with galactorrhea experience menstrual abnormality. If a pituitary process is involved, the woman usually experiences hirsutism and infertility; if a hypothalamic lesion is present, she may report CNS symptoms, such as intractable headache, visual field disturbances, sleep disturbances, and abnormal temperature, thirst, or appetite.[139]

EVALUATION AND TREATMENT Galactorrhea in nulliparous women (women who have never been pregnant) or in parous women who have not breast-fed for 12 months must be thoroughly evaluated. Serum prolactin levels are measured, and at least two positive results are needed to diagnose hyperprolactinemia. Prolactin levels higher than 25 to 30 ng/ml (measured by radioimmunoassay) are considered elevated. Those in the range of 75 to 100 ng/ml are considered to be caused by a pituitary tumor until proven otherwise. Serum thyroxine (T_4) and thyroid-stimulating hormone (TSH) levels are measured to rule out hypothyroidism, and LH and FSH levels are obtained if the individual is menorrheic. CT, MRI, and carotid angiography may assist in the localization of adenomas.

Treatment for galactorrhea consists of identification and treatment of the cause. Medical and surgical therapies may be involved.

Benign Breast Disease/Conditions

Benign breast disease (BBD) is a condition of noncancerous changes in the breast. Numerous benign alterations in ducts and lobules occur in the breast. These changes include irregular lumps, cysts, sensitive nipples, and pruritus. The most common symptoms reported by women are pain, palpable mass, or nipple discharge; the majority of these prove to have a benign cause. Recently, however, histologic features, age at biopsy, and degree of family history were found as major determinants of the risk of breast cancer after a diagnosis of BBD.[140] Benign epithelial lesions can be broadly classified according to their future risk of developing breast cancer as (1) nonproliferative breast lesions, (2) proliferative breast disease, and (3) atypical (atypia) hyperplasia.

Nonproliferative breast lesions. The term *nonproliferative* has been used to discriminate from the "proliferative" changes commonly associated with increased risk for development of breast cancer. This nonproliferative group includes fibrocystic changes (FCC)—the most widely accepted term for physiologic nodularity and breast tenderness that waxes and wanes with the menstrual cycle. On palpation, breasts are lumpy or bumpy and, from radiology studies, breast tissue appears dense with cysts. These lesions mimic carcinoma and women seek medical attention because they produce palpable lumps or nipple discharge. Cysts, fluid-filled sacs, are a specific type of lump that commonly occurs in women in their thirties, forties, and early fifties. Cysts do not increase the risk of breast cancer. Cysts feel squishy when they occur close to the surface of the breast but when deeply embedded they can feel hard. It has become increasingly clear that FCC is a heterogeneous group of lesions that should be diagnosed separately. An estimated 50% to 80% of women normally experience some of these changes. The prevalence of fibrocystic lesions is probably related to hormonal changes, which in turn are affected by genetic background, age, parity, history of lactation, and use of caffeine and exogenous hormones.[141] Cystic changes can be induced in experimental animals by altering ratios of estrogens and progesterone. It is assumed, therefore, that breast cysts are the result of ovarian alterations, but the exact mechanism is unknown. Calcifications (found in cysts and adenosis) or an increase in the number of acini per lobule can produce mammographically suspicious alterations.[142] Cysts also can be associated with unilateral nipple discharge. Cysts often rupture with release of

secretory material into the adjacent tissue. The resulting chronic inflammation and scarring fibrosis contribute to the palpable firmness of the breast.[142] Fibrous tissue increases progressively until menopause and regresses thereafter.

The College of American Pathologists has classified biopsy tissue according to breast cancer risk. These classifications are listed in Box 32-10. In addition to FCC, many women experience several other types of benign breast tumors (Table 32-8). In general, the frequency of chromosome abnormalities is lower in benign lesions than in breast cancer. Genetic aberrations are more common in proliferative than in nonproliferative lesions.[142] The *multiplicity* of benign breast lesions in a biopsy, sometimes called *heterogeneous benign breast disease (HBBD)*, appears to be a factor for progression to breast cancer.[143]

Proliferative breast lesions without atypia. These disorders are characterized by proliferation of ductal epithelium or stroma, or both, without cellular signs of malignancy. The following structurally diverse lesions are included: (1) moderate or florid epithelial hyperplasia, (2) sclerosing adenosis, (3) complex sclerosing lesions (radial scar), (4) papillomas, and (5) fibroadenoma with complex features[142]:
1. Epithelial hyperplasia is defined by the presence of *more* than two cell layers above the basement membrane. In the normal breast, only myoepithelial cells and a single layer of luminal cells are present above the basement membrane.[142] Moderate to florid hyperplasia is more than four cell layers above the basement membrane. The proliferating epithelium fills and distends the ducts and lobules by both luminal and myoepithelial cells.
2. Sclerosing adenosis is present when the number of acini per terminal duct is greater than twice the number found in uninvolved lobules.[142] Calcification is commonly present within the lumens; however, the normal lobular arrangement is maintained. The acini are structurally altered, and myoepithelial cells are prominent. Occasionally, stromal fibrosis may mimic the appearance of invasive carcinoma.[142]
3. Complex sclerosing lesion (radial scar) refers to an irregular, radial proliferation of ductlike small tubules entrapped in a dense central fibrosis. The term *scar* refers to the structural appearance only because these lesions are not associated with prior injury or surgery. Radial scar also has been called *radial sclerosing lesions* and *sclerosing papillary proliferation*. Radial scars have been implicated

---

BOX 32-10 | **CLASSIFICATION OF BREAST BIOPSY TISSUE ACCORDING TO RISK FOR BREAST CANCER**

No Increased Risk
Adenosis (sclerosing or florid)
Apocrine metaplasia
Macrocysts or microcysts
Fibroadenoma
Fibrosis
Mild hyperplasia (3-4 cells deep)
Mastitis or periductal mastitis
Squamous metaplasia

Slightly Increased Risk (1½ to 2 Times)
Moderate or florid hyperplasia
Papilloma

Moderately Increased Risk (3 to 5 Times)
Atypical hyperplasia (ductal or lobular)

TABLE 32-8 EXAMPLES OF BENIGN BREAST DISORDERS

BENIGN BREAST DISEASE	PERIOD OF GREATEST RISK	PATHOPHYSIOLOGY	CLINICAL MANIFESTATIONS OF LESION	TREATMENT
Fibroadenoma	Puberty, early adulthood, rare after menopause	Unknown but thought to be associated with exposure to increased estrogen levels	Painless, firm, solitary, well-circumscribed mobile mass; usually in upper outer quadrant of breast	Surgical excision of mass or careful observation
Mammary duct ectasia (comedomastitis)	Menopause, postmenopause, during pregnancy and lactation	Subareolar ducts become dilated and fill with cellular debris, initiating inflammatory reaction; rupture of ducts may occur	Blood-stained, sticky, thick, spontaneous, multiple-duct discharge; ductal rupture creates palpable mass; burning pain, swelling of areolar area may occur	Condition usually resolves 7-10 days after onset with or without antibiotic therapy
Solitary intraductal papilloma	Age 40-50 years	Unknown	Lesion is slow-growing and cauliflower-like and extends length of involved duct; nipple discharge from one or two ductal openings may be watery, serous, serosanguineous, or sanguineous	Surgical excision of involved duct
Multiple papillomas	Age 35-40 years	Unknown	Similar to solitary intraductal papilloma, except that discharge is from multiple ductal openings	Depends on extent of involvement; if lesion is small, excision of that breast segment; total mastectomy if disease is widespread
Fat necrosis	Age 14-80 years, average age 50 years	Breast trauma, including silicone injections and breast biopsy, cause hemorrhage and induration, leading to formation of a palpable mass	Unilateral, fairly immobile breast mass, located close to surface; mass is usually tender and painful	Mass may be reabsorbed spontaneously or local excision

as a risk factor for hyperplasias and carcinoma.[144] A retrospective study of 9556 women found that although radial scar mildly elevates the risk of invasive breast cancer, the risk was largely attributed to coexisting proliferative disease.[145] Invasive breast cancer risk was further increased in women with atypia hyperplasia.[145,146] The appearance in mammograms of radial scar, as well as the gross and microscopic appearance, can cause it to be confused with infiltrating ductal carcinoma.[147]

4. **Papillomas** consist of multiple, finger-like projections or a branching axis lined by myoepithelial cells and luminal cells. Hyperplasia and metaplasia are often present within the ducts. Small duct papillomas increase the risk of subsequent carcinoma; it is unknown whether large duct papillomas do as well. Multiple papillomas even without identified atypia hyperplasia (next section) increase breast cancer risk significantly.[148]

Proliferative breast lesions with atypia. Proliferative breast lesions with some abnormal structure, or *atypia*, include atypical ductal hyperplasia (ADH) and atypical lobular hyperplasia (ALH).[142] Overall, proliferative disease, unlike nonproliferative changes, is correlated with increases in breast cancer risk.

Atypical hyperplasia (AH) is an increase in the number of cells, and the cells have some variation in structure. Recent studies continue to indicate that women with AH have an increased risk (about fourfold) of breast cancer compared with women who have nonproliferative lesions.[149] From the Nurses' Health Study, time of benign breast biopsy appeared to influence the degree of later breast cancer risk among women with AH.[149] Among women who were premenopausal at the time of their benign biopsy, the risk of breast cancer was substantially increased among women with AH (odds ratio [OR], 7.3) than among women with ADH (OR, 2.72). With women who were postmenopausal at the time of benign biopsy, the risks were similar for women with ALH and those with ADH.[149] In this same Nurses' Health Study, among women with AH who developed breast cancer, 59% of cancers occurred in the same breast as the benign biopsy that revealed AH.[149] In those women with ADH who developed breast cancer, 56% of cancers occurred on the same side (ipsilateral) as the biopsy. Among women with ALH, 61% of subsequent breast cancers occurred in the same breast as the biopsy. Other investigators have reported similar findings.[150,151]

Ductal hyperplasia is an increased number of cells mostly within the lumen of the terminal ducts. It includes a continuum of changes—cell structure and placement—ranging from an increase in cellularity to features of ductal carcinoma in situ (DCIS; see p. 851). In ADH, the cells fail to completely fill ductal spaces as compared to DCIS. Lobular hyperplasia refers to proliferation of small, uniform cells in the lumen of lobular units. The abnormal cells of atypical lobular hyperplasia (ALH) and lobular carcinoma in situ (LCIS) are identical, but the cells in ALH do not distend more than 50% of the acini within a lobule.[142] ALH can extend into ducts, and this is associated with an increased risk of invasive carcinomas.[142]

EVALUATION AND TREATMENT Breast problems are diagnosed from a mutimodal approach that combines physical examination, mammography, ultrasonography, thermography, possibly MRI, and needle biopsy. The dense breast tissue often seen in young women can make mammographic interpretation extremely difficult (see Chapter 9 *Health Alert:* Screening Mammograms: Far from Perfect, p. 243). Ultrasonography (ultrasound) is used to differentiate a solid mass from a cystic (fluid-filled) mass, which is generally benign.

Treatment consists largely of relieving symptoms. Reduction in the consumption of caffeinated beverages (e.g., cola, root beer) and chocolate, which can cause overstimulation for some women, may reduce pain and nodularity. Given time, the cysts may disappear without treatment.

Although still controversial, isoflavone exposure was associated with a decreased risk of proliferative benign fibrocystic changes, non-proliferative changes, and breast cancer.[152] Genistein, a soy isoflavone, has been reported to down-regulate an enzyme important in cancer progression (i.e., telomerase) and contributes to inhibition in both breast benign and cancer cells.[153] Although quite controversial, another preventive factor may be iodine[154] (see *Health Alert:* Iodine and Breast Diseases Including Breast Cancer).

Breast Cancer

Breast cancer, the most common cancer in American women, is the leading cause of death in women 40 to 44 years of age and the second most common killer of women of all ages after lung cancer. The incidence of breast cancer has risen steadily since 1950 and is leveling off at about 124 cases per 100,000 women per year. Table 32-9 presents breast cancer risk by age. Surveillance Epidemiology and End Results (SEER) data revealed approximately 0.0% of breast cancers were diagnosed under the age of 20; 0.9% between 20 and 34; 6.0% between 35 and 44; 15% between 45 and 54; 20.8% between 55 and 64; 19.7% between 65 and 74; 22.6% between 75 and 84; and 15.1% 85 years and older.[155] In women younger than 45 or even 50 years of age, blacks experience a higher incidence of early-onset breast cancer and higher breast cancer mortality.[156] Black women in all age groups experience the highest mortality rates for breast cancer although the reason for this disparity is not clearly understood.[157] It was estimated that about 207,090 women will be diagnosed with breast cancer and 39,840 women will die in 2010.[155] More than two thirds of breast cancer cases occur in women older than age 55. The median age for breast cancer diagnosis is 61 years of age. The median age at death for breast cancer was 69 years of age.[157] Because ductal carcinoma in situ (DCIS)

HEALTH ALERT

Iodine and Breast Diseases Including Breast Cancer

The last national nutritional survey revealed that 15% of the U.S. adult female population is iodine deficient according to the standards of the World Health Organization (WHO)—that is, less than 0.05 mg/L of urine. Recommendations by the WHO, the United Nations International Children's Emergency Fund, and the International Council for the Control of Iodine Deficiency Disorders set 10 mcg/dl as the minimum urinary iodine concentration for iodine sufficiency. This amount corresponds to a daily intake of 150 mcg of iodine. Large segments of Europe continue to have iodine deficiency. Significant deficiency is present in 45 countries in Africa, 15 in the Americas, 24 in Europe and Central Asia, 11 in Southeast Asia, 10 in the Middle East, and 9 in the Far East. Iodine deficiency is a common endocrine problem, presumably easy to correct, and the most preventable cause of mental retardation in many underdeveloped countries. Iodine, as well as selenium, is found in abundance in marine plants (e.g., seaweed). Iodine also is found in animals, in deposits of organic origin, in certain natural mineral waters, in phosphate rock, and in association with mineral deposits. A small fraction is from drinking water. The addition of chlorine during water purification for drinking water may be a contributor to iodine deficiency. Important factors in the depletion of iodine have been glaciation, which removes old soil and scrapes virgin rocks; the substitution of bromine for iodine in bread manufacturing; and decreases in iodinated salt intake.

Several studies have shown the beneficial potential of molecular iodine (I_2) in breast pathologies (e.g., fibrocystic disease and breast cancer) in both animals and humans. In mammary glands, I_2 decreased or alleviated breast pain (mastalgia) and exerted a potent antineoplastic effect on carcinogen-induced cancer progression in rats. Iodine deficiency, either dietary or pharmacologic, can lead to breast atypia and increased cancer development in animal models. Iodine treatment in animals can reverse dysplasia that resulted from iodine deficiency.

Recently, investigators found that breast tumors contain higher concentrations of arachidonic acid than normal mammary tissue and that iodine treatment (I_2) is accompanied by a 12-fold increase in interleukin-6 (IL-6) formation. These findings add to other findings that the antiproliferative effect of I_2 is mediated by the formation of IL-6. In the thyroid gland, the apoptotic effect of iodine excess is mediated by IL-6 and/or iodohexadecanal, both of which are generated by the oxidation and organification of iodide (I^-) by thyroperoxidase (TPO). Importantly, this finding indicates that I_2 can bind with organic components and thereby inhibit gene expression. Other investigators have provided the first gene array profiling of an estrogen-responsive breast cancer cell line demonstrating that the combination of iodine and iodide alters gene expression. Some of the altered genes found were estrogen responsive. Thus, the protective effects of iodine/iodide on breast alterations may be in part through the initiation or modulation of estrogen pathways. Altogether, these data support the notion that I_2 supplementation could be an adjuvant in the therapy of breast cancer, and the mechanisms involved may be apoptosis and/or activation of anti-invasive molecular pathways, including decreasing the levels of estrogen-responsive genes. Understanding iodine's mechanism of action is of crucial importance. Verifying the protective effects of iodine on breast tissue physiology will lead researchers toward the development of novel treatments or enhancements of current therapies.

Data from Aceves C et al: Antineoplastic effect of iodine in mammary cancer: participation of 6-iodolactone (IL-6) and peroxisome proliferator-activated receptors (PPAR), *Mol Cancer* 8:33, 2009; Arroyo-Helguera O et al: Signaling pathways involved in the antiproliferative effect of molecular iodine in normal and tumoral breast cells: evidence that 6-iodolactone mediates apoptotic effects, *Endocr Relat Cancer* 15(4):1003–1011, 2008; Eskin BA et al: Different tissue responses for iodine and iodide in rat thyroid and mammary glands, *Biol Trace Elem Res* 49:9–19, 1995; Funahashi H et al: Suppressive effect of iodine on DMBA-induced breast tumor growth in the rat, *J Surg Oncol* 61(3):209–213, 1996; Garcia-Solis et al: Inhibition of N-methyl-N-nitrosourea-induced mammary carcinogenesis by molecular iodine (I_2) but not by iodide (I^-) treatment. Evidence that I_2 prevents cancer promotion, *Mol Cell Endocrinol* 236:49–57, 2005; Ghent WR et al: Iodine replacement in fibrocystic disease of the breast, *Can J Surg* 36:453–460, 1993; Hollowell JG et al: Iodine nutrition in the United States. Trends and public health implications: iodine excretion data from National Health and Nutrition Examination Surveys I and II (1971-1974 and 1988-1994), *J Clin Endocrinol Metab* 83(10):3401–3408, 1998; Kessler J: The effect of supraphysiologic levels of iodine on patients with cyclic mastalgia, *Breast J* 10:328–336, 2004; Samson L et al: Addition of chlorine during water purification reduces iodine content of drinking water and contributes to iodine deficiency, *J Endocrinol Invest* 2011 May 27 [Epub ahead of print]; Stoddard FR et al: Iodine alters gene expression in the MCF7 breast cancer cell line: evidence for an anti-estrogen effect of iodine, *Int J Med Sci* 5(4):189–196, 2008; Strum JM: Effect of iodide-deficiency on rat mammary gland, *Virchows Arch B Cell Pathol Incl Mol Pathol* 30(2):209–220, 1979; World Health Organization, United Nations Children's Emergency Fund, International Council for the Control of Iodine Deficiency Disorders: *Indicators for assessing iodine deficiency disorders and their control through salt iodination,* Geneva, 1994, World Health Organization.

TABLE 32-9	CHANCE OF BEING DIAGNOSED WITH BREAST CANCER*
BY AGE (YEARS)	**BY RATIO**
30-39	1 in 238
40-49	1 in 69
50-59	1 in 38
60-69	1 in 27
Ever†	1 in 8
Never	7 in 8

Data from Reis LAG et al: *Cancer statistics review, 1975-2005*, Bethesda, Md, 2008, National Cancer Institute. Available at http://seer.cancer.gov/csr/1975_2005. Based on Nov 2007 SEER data, posted SEER website, 2008.

*NOTE: These calculations are averages. An individual's risk may be higher or lower depending on several factors (e.g., family history, reproductive history, race, ethnicity, and others).

†Absolute lifetime risk.

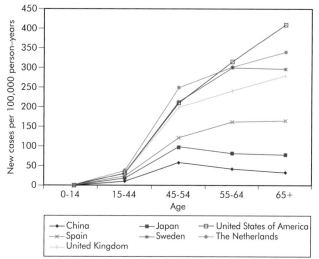

FIGURE 32-37 Age-Specific Incidence Rates of Breast Cancer Among Women. (Data from Ferlay J et al: *GLOBOCAN 2000: cancer incidence, mortality, and prevalence worldwide*, Lyon, 2001, International Agency for Research on Cancer.)

is almost exclusively detected by mammography, the large increase in incidence of DCIS over the past 20 years can be attributed to screening.

Age-specific incidence and mortality rates vary internationally (Figure 32-37). Data reveal that death rates declined 1.4% per year from 1989 to 1995 and 3.2% thereafter, with the largest decreases in younger women—both whites and blacks. The causes for the decline are unknown. Breast cancers account for about 30% of all cancer cases found in women and 16% of cancer deaths. The highest rates of breast cancer are in North America and Europe, and the lowest rates are in Asia.

Although breast cancer is a multifactorial disease involving a complex web of interacting factors, risk is related to timing, duration, and pattern of exposures. Risk factors and possible causes of breast cancer can be classified broadly as reproductive, hormonal, environmental, and familial (Table 32-10). However, two factors emerging as important are involution of the mammary gland and breast density, which are not as easily classified (see following discussion).

TABLE 32-10	ESTABLISHED RISK FACTORS FOR BREAST CANCER	
RELATIVE RISK (RR)	**RISK FACTOR**	
>4.0	Female	
	Age	
	Family history of breast cancer	
	Personal history of breast cancer	
	Inherited genetic mutations (*BRCA1/2* and others)	
	High breast density	
	Atypical hyperplasia	
2.1-4.0	Family history (one first-degree relative)	
	High-dose radiation to chest/breast	
	Prior benign breast disease	
1.1-2.0	No full-term pregnancies	
	Late age at first full-term pregnancy (>30 years)	
	Early menarche (<12 years)	
	Late menopause (>55 years)	
	Never breast-fed children	
	High alcohol consumption	
	Smoking	
	Recent oral contraceptive use	
	Recent or current use of combined hormone replacement therapy	
	Physical inactivity	
	Obesity or adult weight gain (postmenopausal)	

Data from American Cancer Society: *Cancer facts & figures 2010*, Atlanta, 2010, Author.

Reproductive factors: pregnancy. A clearer understanding of mammary gland structure (morphology) and function from fetal development to puberty, pregnancy, and aging will help elucidate fundamental changes to breast development and disease. A key element in that process is "branching morphogenesis," in which the mammary gland fulfills its function by producing and delivering copious amounts of milk by forming a rootlike network of branched ducts from a rudimentary epithelial bud[158] (see Figure 32-39, p. XXX). Branching morphogenesis begins in fetal development, pauses after birth, starts again in response to estrogens at puberty, and is modified by cyclic ovarian hormonal action. This systemic hormonal action elicits local paracrine interactions between the developing epithelial ducts and their adjacent mesenchyme (embryonic) or postnatal stroma.[158] The local cellular cross-talk then directs the tissue remodeling, ultimately producing a mature ductal tree.[158]

A woman's age when her first child is born affects her risk for developing breast cancer—the younger she is, the lower the risk. A complete pregnancy before age 20 reduces the risk of breast cancer by 20% to 50%.[159-161] The protective factor is especially observed in the years of peak incidence, the postmenopausal years.[162] Paradoxically, however, a transient *increase* in breast cancer risk lasting 3 to 5 years after pregnancy is reported in women 25 years of age or older during pregnancy.[159,163,164] In addition, pregnancy induces a *lifelong*, not *transient, increase* in breast cancer risk in women who are more than 30 years of age at the time of first pregnancy.[165] Why age affects this transient increase in breast cancer risk is unknown. Possibilities reported for these risks include failure to induce full mammary differentiation, possibly related to familial history, and those women exposed to the highest levels of estrogen during pregnancy are at greatest risk.[159] A recent hypothesis for risk at any age is that gland *involution* after pregnancy and lactation uses some of the same tissue remodeling pathways activated during wound healing (i.e., proinflammatory pathways).[166] The proinflammatory environment, although physiologically normal, promotes tumor progression. The presence of macrophages in the involuting mammary gland may be contributing to carcinogenesis.[166] (Involution is a new and important topic discussed below.)

The main mechanisms for the *protective* effect of pregnancy are controversial, including (1) induction of breast differentiation with lasting protective phenotypic (morphologic) changes; (2) altered cell fate with removal or modification of vulnerable cells (for example, stem cells prone to facilitate breast cancer); (3) enhancement of the ability for DNA repair or apoptosis, or both; (4) altered systemic hormonal regulation and possible persistent changes in intracellular pathways regulating proliferation; (5) decreased proliferation in the parous involuted gland; and (6) effect of early-life hormonal and dietary exposures on subsequent breast cancer risk.[162]

Lobular involution and age. Part of the uniqueness of the mammary gland is its profound physiologic changes throughout the phases of a woman's life. These phases include puberty, pregnancy, lactation, postlactational involution, and aging. The human breast is organized into 15 to 20 major lobes, each with lobules containing milk-forming acini (see Figure 31-10). With aging, breast lobules regress or involute with a decrease in the number and size of acini per lobule and with replacement of the intralobular stroma with the denser collagen of connective tissue.[167] Over time, the glandular elements and collagen are replaced with fatty tissue, a process called **lobular involution.** During lobular involution, the parenchymal elements progressively atrophy and disappear over the course of many years. The first study of its kind found lobular involution was associated with reduced risk of breast cancer.[167-169] Breast cancer risk decreased with increasing extent of involution in both high- and low-risk subgroups defined by family history of breast cancer, epithelial atypia, reproductive history, and age.[167] Based on pathologic and epidemiologic factors, these investigators propose that delayed involution (persistent glandular epithelium) is a major risk factor for breast cancer.[167-170]

Investigators suggest that the effect of lobular involution on breast cancer risk is a reduction in tissue from the involuting process, or the issue may be aging. Widely appreciated is that as women age, their risk of breast cancer increases. But, the *rate* of increase of breast cancer *slows* at about 50 years of age.[171,172] This decline has been attributed to a reduction in ovarian hormone production. Milanese and colleagues[167] observed a definite increase in the process of involution at about 50 years of age with complete involution present in 5.8% of women ages 40 to 49 years and 21.6% of women ages 50 to 59 years. Investigators propose that involution may contribute to this slowing in the rate of increase of breast cancer among women older than 50 years.[169] Importantly, investigators found an inverse association between lobular involution and parity.[167] Other investigators have reported the more children a woman has, the more likely she is to have persistent lobular tissue,[173,174] which Milanese and colleagues[167] found was associated with increased risk of breast cancer. However, multiparity also has been found to reduce risk of breast cancer.[175,176] This apparent contradiction may be explained by studies documenting that full-term pregnancies after 35 years of age are correlated with an increased risk of breast cancer.[177] In the Milanese study, the age of the mother at each child's birth was unknown.

Henson and colleagues[178] proposed that after the initiation of involution, late pregnancy with its concomitant increase in the proliferation of the ductal-alveolar epithelium is likely to interrupt the process

of involution. Involution typically begins between 30 and 40 years of age. The processes of involution include massive cell death (i.e., apoptosis) of secretory epithelia requiring recruitment and activation of fibroblasts; immune cells, especially macrophages (i.e., proinflammatory); and other stromal effectors.[158] Thus, the activated stromal environment is similar to that present in invasive breast cancer. The long-term protective effects of pregnancy from hormones released during pregnancy affect remodeling of the stromal microenvironment by causing apoptosis and involution. However, a short-term increase in breast cancer risk following pregnancy may be caused by the process of mammary gland involution, which returns the tissue to its prepregnant state, and is co-opted by the process of wound healing, resulting in a proinflammatory environment that although physiologically normal can promote carcinogenesis.[166]

Interestingly, oophorectomy, which is associated with a decrease in risk of breast cancer, leads to atrophy of breast parenchyma in young women as is noted in older women.[178] Thus the risk reduction of oophorectomy may be caused by an accelerated involution.[178]

Investigators have shown that a benign biopsy demonstrating histologic changes consistent with incomplete or nonexistent involution or a mammogram classified as high density is independently associated with breast cancer risk, and that these factors combined are associated with an even greater risk.[170] The assessment of these "phenotypes" shows promise for improving risk prediction, particularly because they reflect the cumulative interaction of numerous genetic and environmental breast cancer risk factors over time; however, this work is just beginning.

Hormonal factors. The link between breast cancer and hormones is based on six factors that affect risk: (1) the protective effect of an early (i.e., in the twenties) first pregnancy; (2) the protective effect of removal of the ovaries and pituitary gland; (3) the increased risk associated with early menarche, late menopause, and nulliparity; (4) the relationship between types of fat, free estrogen levels, and oxidative changes in estrogen metabolism; (5) the hormone-dependent development and differentiation of mammary gland structures; and (6) the efficacy of anti–hormone therapies for treatment and prevention of breast cancer. Throughout its existence, the mammary gland epithelium proceeds through critical "exposure periods" of rapid growth or cycles of proliferation, including neonatal growth, pubertal development, pregnancy lactation, and involution after pregnancy and postmenopause.[157,166]

The understanding of the role of systemic hormones as powerful regulators of mammary gland development is shifting. Evidence is pointing to the wide-ranging effects of systemic hormones as possibly not due to their *direct* hormone action but rather their *induced* actions from multiple secondary paracrine effectors—thus the term *hierarchical.*[158,179] Unraveling is a complex model of hormone, paracrine, and adhesion molecule signaling pathways affecting both epithelial and stromal cell fate in both breast development and carcinogenesis (Figure 32-38). Despite differences between the organized process of development and the less organized, even chaotic, environment of invasive cancer, both processes share many identical mechanisms and signaling pathways. Key is *tissue remodeling* that applies not only to pubertal growth but also immediately after pregnancy and during involution (see previous section).[166,180-182]

The female reproductive hormones (estrogens, progesterone, and prolactin) have a major role and impact on mammary gland development and breast cancer[179] (Figure 32-39). Experiments in animals showed the major sources of hormones that cause developmental changes in the breast.[179] A vast majority of breast cancers are *initially* hormone dependent (estrogen positive [ER+] and/or progesterone positive [PR+]), with estrogens playing a crucial role in their development.[183] Estrogens control processes critical for cellular functions by regulating activities and expression of key signaling molecules. These processes include regulation of receptor activity and receptor interaction with other intracellular proteins and DNA.[183] Estrogens thus play prominent roles in cellular proliferation, differentiation, and apoptosis.[183-185] Estrogens affect microtubules that are essential for establishing cell shape and cell polarity, processes necessary for epithelial gland organization.[183]

It is possible to consider four major hormonal hypotheses for breast cancer: (1) ovarian androgen excess (testosterone, for example); (2) elevated estrogen and progesterone levels (ovarian and hormonal

replacement); (3) elevated estrogen levels alone (ovarian and hormone replacement); and (4) local biosynthesis of estrogens in breast tissue. These hypotheses, however, may not be mutually exclusive. Hormone replacement therapy is discussed later in a separate section; the present discussion is concerned with endogenous levels of hormones.

The first hypothesis that breast cancer risk is increased among women who have an ovarian androgen excess also includes chronic anovulation and reduction of luteal-phase (menstrual cycle) progesterone production. Therefore, it is also called the "ovarian hyperandrogenism/luteal inadequacy hypothesis." This hypothesis, actually proposed by Grattarola in the 1960s, was based on the observation that women with breast cancer also reveal hyperplasia of the endometrium—a common symptom of ovarian androgen excess chronic anovulation and progesterone deficiency.[186] From a pooled analysis of nine prospective studies of postmenopausal women, all the androgens were positively (significantly) associated with breast cancer risk.[187] The majority of data from this pooled analysis were for testosterone. Similar findings were observed in the EPIC cohort study.[186] Four prospective studies have reported a positive association for premenopausal women between testosterone level and risk of breast cancer.[188] A prospective Italian study showed a significant increase in breast cancer risk for premenopausal women who had elevated levels of testosterone and lower levels of progesterone.[189] Unclear is whether the association with testosterone is direct or indirect (i.e., enzyme conversion by aromatase of testosterone to estradiol) (Figure 32-40). Overall, the association between circulating testosterone in postmenopausal women and subsequent risk of breast cancer is now well established.[190]

The second hypothesis is breast cancer risk is increased among women with elevations of both estrogens and progesterone. These observations revealed increased proliferation rates of breast epithelium during the luteal phase of the menstrual cycle when the ovaries produce both estradiol and progesterone. Data supporting the "estrogen-plus-progesterone hypothesis" suggest hormone replacement therapy (HRT) with estrogen plus progestin increases breast cancer risk to a greater degree than estrogen alone.[191,192] (see Hormone Replacement Therapy section, p. 846). Although this hypothesis is for combined estrogen and progesterone (see HRT section), data on progesterone also will be discussed here (also see previous discussion and following discussion on estrogen and estrogen alone, respectively). Only one prospective study[193] has evaluated the association of postmenopausal circulating progesterone level and breast cancer risk. No association

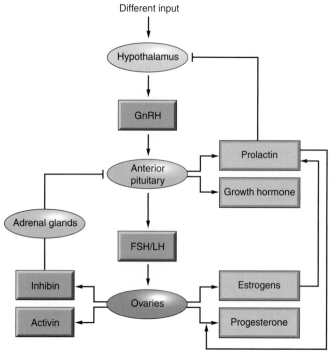

FIGURE 32-38 Female Endocrine System. The different mammary growth (mammotropic) hormone sites are shown in ovals, hormones are noted in blue boxes, and mammotropic hormones are noted in red boxes.

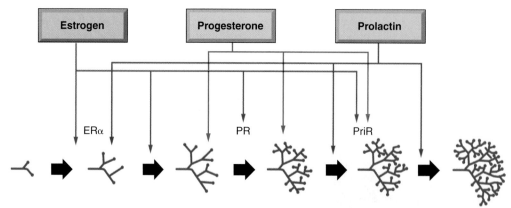

FIGURE 32-39 Factors Involved in Mammary Gland Development. Work of many laboratories led to the identification of many genes important in mammary gland development that are summarized in the scheme. (Adapted from Brisken C, O'Malley B: Hormone action in the mammary gland, *Cold Spring Harb Perspect Biol* 2[12]:a003178. [Epub 2010 Aug 25.])

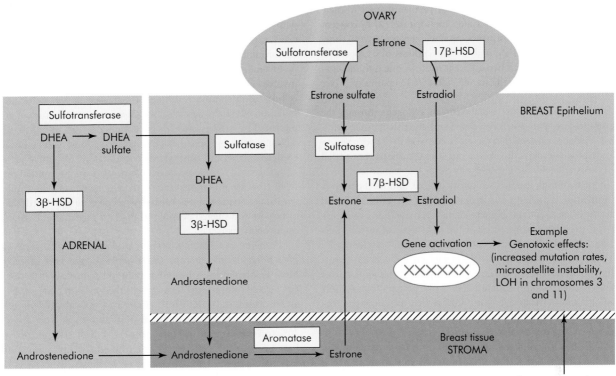

FIGURE 32-40 Local Biosynthesis of Estrogens. Three main enzyme complexes *(yellow)* involved in estrogen formation in breast tissue, including aromatase, sulfatase, and 17β-estradiol hydroxysteroid dehydrogenase (17β-HSD). Thus, despite low levels of circulating estrogens in postmenopausal women with breast cancer, the tissue levels are several-fold higher than those in plasma, suggesting tumor accumulation of these estrogens. Data suggest that most abundant is sulfatase in both premenopausal and postmenopausal women with breast cancer. Numerous agents can block the aromatase action, exploration of progesterone, and various progestins to inhibit sulfatase and 17β-HSD or stimulate sulfotransferase (i.e., breast cancer cells cannot inactivate estrogens because they lack sulfotransferase) may provide new possibilities for treatment. *LOH,* Loss of heterozygosity (see Chapter 8). (Adapted from Russo J, Russo I: *Molecular basis of breast cancer: prevention and treatment,* Germany, 2004, Springer-Verlag, Berlin Heidelberg.)

was observed. To date, 6 prospective studies have investigated progesterone levels and breast cancer risk in premenopausal women; however, 4 of the 6 studies included 65 or fewer cases.[188,190] Overall, these data are too limited to draw any *firm* conclusions.[190] Depending on the experimental model system used, progesterone in animal and progesterone in vitro studies show both an increase and a decrease in breast cancer risk.[194-196] New data identify mammary stem cells (MaSCs) as critical targets for ovarian hormones, especially during the normal reproductive cycle when progesterone levels surge and during pregnancy when the proliferation of mammary stem cells is increased.[197,198]

The third hypothesis is often called the "estrogen-alone hypothesis." Substantial prospective data have accrued on the relationship between levels of circulating estrogens and breast cancer risk in postmenopausal women.[187,190,199] From the EPIC study,[186] increasing blood levels of estradiol also increased the risks for breast cancer (relative risks 1.4, 1.2, 1.8, 2.0). Updated analyses from two cohorts of the pooled analysis of nine prospective studies provide strong evidence that levels of circulating hormones are an important marker of increased risk in postmenopausal women and not a result of the production of hormones by a tumor.[200] Positive associations with urinary estrogen levels also were similar from two prospective studies.[201,202] EPIC and other studies, however, observed no clear relationship between plasma estrogen

levels and breast cancer risk in *premenopausal* women.[186] Yet, investigators had difficulty evaluating the relationships between hormone levels and phases of the menstrual cycle. In premenopausal women, the Nurses' Health Study II (NHS II) found that in the follicular phase of the menstrual cycle, but not the luteal phase, levels of circulating total and free estradiol were significantly associated with breast cancer risk.[203] Experimental studies have also provided strong and consistent evidence that estrogens can promote and possibly *initiate* breast tumor development and growth[204] (see the Pathogenesis section).

Overall, the positive association between levels of circulating estrogens in postmenopausal women and subsequent risk of breast cancer is now well established. The association appears strongest for estrogen-positive tumors and is statistically robust across groups of women at varying risk of breast cancer.[190] Relatively few studies on circulating sex steroids and breast cancer have been conducted in premenopausal women, possibly because of the difficulty of accurately assessing hormone levels during the menstrual cycle.

The fourth hypothesis suggests that *local* (in situ; paracrine) formation of estrogens in breast tumors may be more significant than circulating estrogens in *plasma* for the growth and survival of estrogen-dependent breast cancer in postmenopausal women.[183] The rationale is based on the following evidence: (1) estradiol (E$_2$) levels in breast tumors are equivalent to those of premenopausal women, despite plasma E_2 levels being lower after menopause; (2) E_2 concentrations in breast tumors of postmenopausal women are 10 to 40 times higher than serum levels of E_2; and (3) biosynthesis of estrogens in breast tumors occurs through two different routes—one is the aromatase pathway and the other is the steroid sulfate (STS) pathway[183] (see Figure 32-40).

Breast tissue (endogenous) metabolism of estrogens through the aromatase-mediated pathway is correlated with the risk of breast carcinogenesis. Evidence suggests that the site of conversion of androgens to estrogens in breast cancer is the stroma and not the malignant epithelial cells.[205] Consistent evidence also suggests either that tumor location is related to areas of high aromatase activity or that tumors themselves induce aromatase expression in surrounding adipose tissue.[205] Breast tissue, however, may contain higher sulfatase activity than aromatase activity and produce estrone through the hydrolysis of estrone sulfate[183] (see Figure 32-40). Thus, quantitatively estrone sulfate may be the most important circulating estrogen in women; it increases the reservoir for the production of estrone and, ultimately, estradiol. It was found that E_2, itself, has anti-sulfatase action.[206] This paradoxical effect of estradiol could be related to some studies that have found estrogen replacement therapy (ERT) either to have no effect or to decrease breast cancer mortality in postmenopausal women[206] (see p. 847). In summary, the blockage of estradiol through both the aromatase and sulfatase pathways, as well as the stimulation of sulfotransferase activity (i.e., sulfation is important to estrogens because the addition of the charged sulfonate group protects the hormones [estrogens] from binding to their receptors and, consequently, inhibiting cell growth), can provide new and potentially powerful applications in breast cancer.

Although experimental, clinical, and epidemiologic research have implicated endogenous estrogens in the etiology of breast and endometrial cancer and, possibly, ovarian cancer, the role of individual *patterns* of estrogen metabolism is a new focus, especially for epidemiology.[204] Estrogen metabolism from oxidation of the parent estrogens, estrone, and estradiol occurs at either the 2-, the 4-, or the 16-position of the carbon skeleton to yield 2-hydroxylated, 4-hydroxylated, or 16-hydroxylated estrogens, respectively. The 4- and 16-hydroxylated pathways are tumor promoting; conversely, the 2-hydroxylated pathway has been demonstrated to be less tumor promoting and, possibly, tumor inhibiting.[207]

Overall, two main mechanisms of carcinogenicity of estrogens involve (1) a receptor-mediated hormonal activity shown to stimulate cellular proliferation, resulting in increased opportunities for accumulation of genetic damage, and (2) oxidative catabolism of estrogens mediated by various cytochrome complexes (e.g., P450) that eventually activate and generate reactive oxygen species (ROS) that can cause oxidative stress and genomic damage directly. Oxidative metabolites of estrogens, if found, can develop ultimate carcinogens that react with DNA to cause mutations leading to carcinogenesis. Thus, imbalances in estrogen metabolites in breast tissue correlate with the development of tumors and suggest possible biomarkers related to the risk of developing breast cancer.

Hormone replacement therapy and breast cancer risk: estrogen plus progesterone therapy (HRT) and estrogen only therapy (ERT). Most epidemiologic studies have found an increase in breast cancer risk related to hormone replacement therapy with combined estrogen and progestogens (HRT)[208,209] (Table 32-11). Evidence is derived from observational studies and clinical trials and suggests an approximate 30% to 70% increase in breast cancer risk with HRT current use and breast cancer risk disappearing after treatment discontinuation.[210-212] Additional support for HRT to increase breast cancer risk was the *reduction* in risk reported by several countries with discontinuation of HRT use.[209,213]

Evidence on the route of administration of HRT, oral versus transdermal (gel or patch), and the risk of breast cancer has limited research. To date, epidemiologic data suggest that route has no impact on the risk of breast cancer and hip fracture.[214] Results comparing route of HRT and risk of coronary heart disease (CHD) and colorectal cancer are inconsistent. Studies on the risks of diabetes and stroke are too limited for clinical evidence. Additionally, there is a suggestion, that needs research confirmation, that oral route versus transdermal HRT may increase the risk of thromboembolism.[215]

TABLE 32-11	**HORMONAL TREATMENTS ASSESSED BY THE IARC MONOGRAPH WORKING GROUP**			
GROUP 1 AGENT	**CANCER ON WHICH SUFFICIENT EVIDENCE IN HUMANS IS BASED**	**SITES WHERE CANCER RISK IS REDUCED**	**ESTABLISHED MECHANISTIC EVENTS**	**OTHER LIKELY MECHANISTIC EVENTS**
Diethylstilbestrol	Breast (exposure during pregnancy), vagina and cervix (exposure in utero); limited evidence: testis (exposure in utero), endometrium	—	Estrogen receptor–mediated events (vagina, cervix), genotoxicity	Epigenetic programming
Estrogen only menopausal therapy	Endometrium, ovary; limited evidence: breast	—	Estrogen receptor–mediated events	Genotoxicity
Combined estrogen-progestagen menopausal therapy	Endometrium (risk decreases with number days/month of progestagen use), breast	—	Receptor-mediated events	Estrogen genotoxicity
Combined estrogen-progestagen oral contraceptives	Breast, cervix, liver	Endometrium, ovary	Receptor-mediated events	Estrogen genotoxicity, hormone-stimulated expression of human papillomavirus genes
Tamoxifen	Endometrium	Breast	Estrogen receptor–mediated events, genotoxicity	—

From IARC Special Report: Policy: a review of human carcinogens—Part A: pharmaceuticals, *Lancet* 10:13–14, 2009.

HRT use has been associated with a greater breast cancer risk than ERT. Whether ERT use is associated with a greater increase in breast cancer risk compared with women who have *never used* hormone therapy continues to be intensely debated. Use of ERT was associated with a *decreased* risk in the Women's Health Initiative (WHI) randomized trial even after cessation of treatment,[216,217] but not in observational studies.[211,212,218,219] From the recent WHI report, women with a prior hysterectomy who were followed for 10.7 years and who used conjugated equine estrogen (CEE) for an average of 3.5 years (median of 5.9 years) were not associated with an increased or decreased risk of CHD, deep vein thrombosis, stroke, hip fracture, colorectal cancer, or total mortality and the previous finding of a decrease in breast cancer risk persisted.[216] According to investigators, this decrease in risk is neither perplexing nor contradictory to other findings where estrogen increases risk because of the underlying biology of breast cancer and estrogen. Laboratory data support a protective effect of estrogen under the right environment—that is, after a period of long-term natural (endogenous) estrogen deprivation. If this environment exists, then exogenous estrogen will induce apoptosis or cell death of the occult breast cancer cells.[220] Nonetheless, careful debate has continued. These issues include (1) a potential age effect (younger versus older women) on the risk-to-benefit profile of hormone therapy (HT), (2) overall duration and safety (short- and long-term) of HT use, (3) differential effects of HT in slender or overweight/obese women, and (4) estrogen decline or deprivation (menopause) for a specified time (length unknown) and then followed by ERT replacement leading to apoptosis of lingering breast cancer cells. Thus, because the use of ERT in the WHI in ≥80% (of study pills) was 3.5 years, longer use may still increase breast cancer risk. Longer use in animal studies has been linked with increased cell proliferation, angiogenesis, and inhibition of apoptosis.[221] Longer use of ERT that may increase breast cancer risk was found in combined data of 16 studies and another analysis of 52,705 women with breast cancer.[218,219] In these studies and the Million Women Study, leaner women had an even higher risk of breast cancer.[222] Women in the WHI do not represent the typical woman who might be prescribed hormone therapy for menopausal symptoms.[223] For example, 68% of the women in the WHI were older than age 60 when enrolled in the study, thus an older population than the average woman entering menopause.

Insulin and insulin-like growth factors. Insulin-like growth factors (IGFs) regulate cellular functions involving cell proliferation, differentiation, and apoptosis. Insulin-like growth factor 1 (IGF-1) is a protein hormone with a structure similar to that of insulin. The growth hormone–IGF-1 axis can stimulate proliferation of both breast cancer and normal breast epithelial cells.[224] A pooled analysis of 17 studies showed a significant association of IGF-1 level and breast cancer risk.[225] Interestingly, no significant difference was found according to menopausal status. Joint associations of IGF-1 and estradiol together showed they were related to risk and those women in the top thirds of estradiol and IGF-1 levels had the highest risk. Estradiol increases IGF-1 activity in the breast.[226]

Tumor growth (in vivo) can be accelerated by light at night in part from continuous activation of IGF-1 receptor (IGF-1R) signaling.[227] A recent case-control study of 1679 women exposed to light at night during sleep was significantly associated with breast cancer risk.[227] This study was the first to identify bedroom light intensity and breast cancer risk. Although inconclusive, shift-work and its disruptive effects on circadian rhythms and sleep deprivation at night have been suggested as a risk factor for breast cancer.[228]

Prolactin and growth hormone. Growth hormone (GH) injected in mice acted on mammary stroma.[229] GH induces the production of IGFs in the liver; IGF signaling is important for breast development and is implicated in breast carcinogenesis. Two studies, however,

have reported a link between growth hormone level and breast cancer risk.[230,231] In the largest prospective analysis comparing circulating prolactin levels and breast cancer risk, those with the highest levels had the highest risk.[232]

Human chorionic gonadotropin. Human chorionic gonadotropin (hCG) level increases during the first trimester of pregnancy and then rapidly declines to a steady state throughout pregnancy. Data from rat studies indicate that hCG may be useful in developing new therapies because it has antiproliferative and anti-invasive effects.[233] However, insufficient data exist on the safety of hCG; its role in carcinogenesis is complex and much research needs to be done.[234]

Oral contraceptives. The International Agency for Research on Cancer (IARC) Group confirmed that combined estrogen-progestagen oral contraceptives (OCs) increase the risk for breast, cervix, and liver cancers.[209] However, the efficacy of OCs in protecting against ovarian cancer and endometrial cancer is well established. Hormones are discussed further in the Pathogenesis section.

Mammographic breast density. Mammographic density (MD) is the radiologic appearance of the breast, reflecting variations in breast composition (Figure 32-41). Mammographic breast density (MBD) appears white or dense on a mammogram and is a strong and consistent risk factor for breast cancer.[170] MBD decreases with age and is associated with body mass index (BMI), family history, and postmenopausal hormone use.[235,236] Investigators are studying if MBD is related to reduced lobular involution of breast tissue in dense breasts (reduced involution increases cancer risk). A recent study found that having a combination of dense breasts and no lobular involution was associated with higher breast cancer risk than having nondense or fatty breasts and complete involution.[170] Women with dense breasts occupying more than 60% to 75% of the breast have a fourfold to sixfold increased risk of breast cancer compared to those with little or no density.[236,237] Mammographic dense tissue has been thought to represent both epithelial and stromal components. One hypothesis is that the stromal-rich environment in MBD may have an abundance of growth factors that could stimulate the epithelium in a noninvoluted breast, thereby increasing the risk of malignant transformation.[170,238] Finding tumors

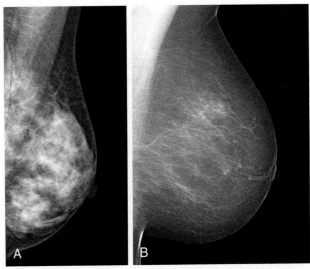

FIGURE 32-41 Breast Density Varies Among Women. The sensitivity of mammography for detecting malignancy is significantly reduced if the breast consists of a high proportion of fibroglandular (dense) breast tissue **(A)** compared to a breast that is fatty **(B)**. (From O'Malley FP, Pinder SE, editors: *Breast pathology*, New York, 2006, Churchill Livingstone.)

- The USPSTF recommends against routine screening mammography in women in their forties who are not at increased risk for breast cancer. The decision to start mammography before age 50 should be based on a woman's risk for breast cancer and personal preferences about the benefits and harms.
- The USPSTF recommends mammography every 2 years for women ages 50 to 74.
- Current evidence is not sufficient to assess the effectiveness of clinical breast exam in addition to screening mammography.
- The USPST recommends against clinicians teaching women breast self-examination.
- Current evidence is not sufficient to assess the additional effectiveness of digital mammography or breast MRI instead of film mammography for breast cancer screening.

Data from U.S. Preventive Services Task Force: Screening for breast cancer, *Ann Intern Med* 716–726, 2009.

in women with MBD is a challenge because they both appear white; as Dr. Susan Love states, "like trying to find a polar bear in a snow storm."

Environmental factors. The environmental causes of breast cancer possibly affect the breast the most during critical phases or "windows" of development including early differential stages—that is, undifferentiated cells to alveolar buds and then lobules, puberty, pregnancy and lactation, involution, and menopause. During these early phases, mitotic activity and cell division are greater than later in life.

Radiation. High doses of ionizing radiation are associated with an increased risk of breast cancer, especially if exposure occurs during adolescence or pregnancy, when breast cells are proliferating rapidly. Radiologic exposure of the upper spine, heart, ribs, lungs, shoulders, and esophagus also exposes breast tissue to radiation. A hot topic currently is the effect of low-dose ionizing radiation. The debate is that low-energy x-rays may be more hazardous per unit dose than previously reported. The scientific community is working hard to estimate the risks of low doses of radiation; however, the risks are largely unknown and uncertainties associated with the best estimates are great.[239,240] New biologic understandings of low doses of radiation are presented in Chapter 10. The United States Preventive Services Task Force (USPSTF) has updated the recommendations for mammography because of overdiagnosis and overtreatment issues related to screening mammography (see *Health Alert:* Screening Mammograms: Far from Perfect in Chapter 9, p. 243) for women 40 to 49 years of age and Box 32-11).

Diet. Prospective epidemiologic studies on diet and breast cancer risk fail to show an association that is consistent, strong, and statistically significant except for alcohol intake, being overweight, and weight gain after menopause (see following discussion).[241] Diet has been postulated as important for breast cancer risk because of the international correlations of consumption of specific dietary factors (e.g., fats) and breast cancer incidence and mortality and because of migrant studies showing greater incidence of breast cancer among descendants who relocated to another country compared to those in the country of origin. International variations also can occur because of differences in reproductive history, physical activity, obesity, and other factors.

Dietary fat and breast cancer risk is the subject of much study, controversy, and debate. Potential biologic mechanisms between fat intake and breast cancer risk include the following: (1) fat may stimulate endogenous steroid hormone production (also affects weight gain, age of menarche); (2) fat interferes with immune or inflammatory function; and (3) fat influences gene expression. Although prospective studies and case-control studies on fat and breast cancer risk have been inconsistent, concern has been that any association with fat intake may be because of total energy intake. Moreover, there is limited evidence that modest reductions in fat intake (less than 20% of caloric intake) reduce breast cancer risk.[242] Overall, despite extensive investigation, there is no conclusive evidence that *adult* consumption of macronutrients including fat, carbohydrate, or fiber is strongly related to breast cancer incidence.[243] This null result could be because breast cancer risk is determined earlier in life, before the period of investigation, and adult dietary exposures have little influence on carcinogenesis. The hypothesis that exposures that occur between menarche and first pregnancy are especially important in determining subsequent risk of breast cancer is supported by several lines of evidence. Animal studies demonstrate increased susceptibility to mammary carcinogens before first pregnancy compared to administration at a later age,[244,245] and epidemiologic investigations of women who survived the atomic bomb in Hiroshima and Nagasaki show no increase in risk among women older than 35 at the time of the bombing but increased breast cancer risk among women younger than 20 years when exposed.[246] A recent and first prospective study of 39,268 premenopausal women observed a modest direct association between adolescent intake of fat and breast cancer.[247] This association persisted after adjusting for adult fat intake. Subtypes of fat were not significantly related to invasive breast cancer. Additionally, from this same study, milk, dairy, and total carbohydrate intake in adolescence, as well as the quality of carbohydrate as assessed by glycemic load, glycemic index, and dietary fiber, was not associated with breast cancer. Frequent consumption of fat, especially saturated fat, during adolescence was positively related to the incidence of hormone receptor negative breast tumors.

The association between individual foods and breast cancer is inconsistent, and new data on *dietary patterns* are emerging. The Mediterranean diet includes high intake of vegetables, legumes, fruits, nuts, and minimally processed cereals; moderately high intake of fish; and high intake of monounsaturated lipids coupled with low intake of saturated fat, low to moderate intake of dairy products, low intake of meat products, and moderate intake of alcohol. The Mediterranean pattern was recently reported (EPIC study) to lower overall cancer risk.[248] The Western pattern includes higher intake of red and processed meats, refined grains, sweets and desserts, and high-fat dairy products. Nutrition remains an important area of study.

Obesity. Obesity, measured as BMI, has been associated with a *reduced* risk of *premenopausal* breast cancer. Recently reported (from the Nurses' Health Study I and II), however, was that weight gain or weight loss since age 18 did not significantly decrease the risk of premenopausal breast cancer.[249] Other data measuring adiposity using waist/hip ratio (WHR) have not found a reduced risk but rather no association (null) or an increased risk.[250,251] Further research is needed to understand if central adiposity versus general adiposity is more important for breast cancer risk.

In 2002 the International Agency for Research into Cancer (IARC) concluded that excess body weight (EBW) increased the risk of developing postmenopausal breast, colorectum, endometrium, kidney, and esophageal adenocarcinoma.[252] The World Cancer Research Fund (WCRF) used a more standardized approach to evaluate studies and concluded that evidence is convincing and that a probable association exists between body fat and postmenopausal breast cancer.[253]

Despite strong links with endogenous estrogen levels, body fat has been consistently but *weakly* related to increased postmenopausal risk.[254] This observation (i.e., weakly) has been surprising because obese postmenopausal women have endogenous estrogen levels (estrone and estradiol) nearly double those of lean women.[254,255] This weak association is possibly related to two factors. First, the premenopausal reduction in breast cancer risk related to being overweight possibly persists, opposing the adverse effect of elevated levels of estrogens after menopause. Thus, *weight gain* should be more strongly related to postmenopausal breast cancer risk than attained weight. In two case-control studies and prospective studies, this was indeed true.[256-259] Premenopausal and postmenopausal weight gain is also associated with higher estradiol and estrone levels and lower levels of sex hormone–binding globulin (SHBG) available as a transporter protein; low levels of SHBG cause higher levels of bioavailable estrogen.[260] The increase in estrogens, particularly estradiol, is from aromatization in the adipose tissue. Second, use of exogenous hormones postmenopausally obscures the variation in endogenous estrogens and can modify the association between BMI and breast cancer risk.[261]

Obesity is associated with poor survival among women with breast cancer and the association of obesity with mortality from breast cancer appears to be stronger than its association with incidence.[254,258] The increase in breast cancer risk with increasing BMI among postmenopausal women is possibly the result of increases in levels of estrogens, especially estradiol.[262,263] However, studies of hormones secreted by adipose tissue, *leptin* and *adiponectin*, may underlie the association between obesity and breast cancer risk. Because increasing BMI and central fat deposition are associated with increased risk for breast cancer in prospective studies, increased leptin exposure associated with obesity and central adiposity could explain the greater incidence of breast cancer in overweight or obese postmenopausal women. in vitro studies have shown leptin stimulated breast carcinogenesis.[264,265] Leptin stimulates tumor growth in animal models.[266] From molecular mechanism studies, leptin enhances breast cancer cell proliferation by inhibiting cell death (pro-apoptosis) signaling pathways and by increasing in vitro sensitivity to estrogens.[266] Adiponectin has been shown to exert antiproliferative effects in vitro of human breast cancer cells.[264,266,267]

Age at menarche also indicates childhood energy balance. Prospective studies document weight, height, and body fat as predictors of age at menarche.[268,269] Age at menarche is 12 to 13 years in Western countries; in rural China (where the risk of breast cancer is low) the typical age of menarche has been 17 to 18.[270]

Most prospective studies have not supported a link between fiber intake and breast cancer.[271,272] Carbohydrate quality, however, rather than absolute amount, may be important for breast cancer risk, especially for premenopausal women.

Evidence exists that alcohol consumption increases breast cancer risk. In a pooled analysis of the six largest cohort studies, the risk of breast cancer increased incrementally with increasing intake of alcohol.[273] A more recent analysis of observational studies with a large population reported women who drank alcohol had a 22% higher relative risk of breast cancer than those who did not.[274] Beer, wine, and liquor all contributed to the positive association and risks did not differ by menopausal status. In large prospective studies, high intake of folic acid appeared to decrease the enhanced risk for breast cancer caused by alcohol.[275-277] The mechanisms by which alcohol intake increases the risk of breast cancer are unknown; however, physiologic studies have reported an estrogen level increase in women taking hormone replacement therapy (HRT) and IGF-1 level increases with alcohol intake. It is not known whether reducing or discontinuing alcohol consumption in midlife decreases the risk of breast cancer. The relationship between fruit and vegetable intake and reduction in breast cancer risk has been studied over three decades. No protective effects have been firmly established to date.[278]

Soy products are a hot topic because of their consumption in Asian countries that have low rates of cancer. However, no consensus has emerged regarding the protective aspects of soy. Soybeans are the main source of isoflavones. The isoflavone compounds, including diadzein and genistein, can bind estrogen receptors but are far less potent than estradiol. Soy may act like other antiestrogens (e.g., tamoxifen) by blocking the action of endogenous estrogens to reduce breast cancer risk. Thus, depending on the estradiol concentration, soy exhibits weak estrogenic or antiestrogenic activity. Isoflavones can influence transcription and cell proliferation. They modulate enzyme activities as well as signal transduction and have antioxidant properties.[279,280] Results of clinical studies on the effects of soy products or isolated isoflavones on vasomotor symptoms are contradictory. Concerns, however, are that soy or isoflavones may increase proliferating cells. Soy may cause breast cells to grow; however, in vitro properties of soy for blocking invasion and antiangiogenesis may be more important in preventing breast cancer. Other factors may modify the association between soy and breast cancer, including amount, form of isoflavones, timing of exposure (e.g., age), estrogen receptor status of tumors, and hormonal profile.[280] in vitro and animal studies show soy to inhibit breast cancer growth, and additional research showed this effect occurred on both ER-positive and ER-negative cancer cells.[281]

Iodine deficiency is hypothesized as contributing to the development of breast pathology and cancer.[154,282,283] Iodine plays a significant role in breast health[283-286] (see *Health Alert:* Iodine and Breast Diseases Including Breast Cancer, p. 841). Evidence reveals that iodine is an antioxidant and antiproliferative agent contributing to the integrity of normal mammary tissue.[287] Seaweed, which is iodine-rich, is an important dietary item in Asian communities and has been associated with the *low* incidence of benign and breast cancer disease in Japanese women.[287] Molecular iodine (I_2) supplementation exerts an inhibitory effect on the development and size of benign and cancerous tissue.[288]

Environmental chemicals. Evidence for linking chemicals to the cause of breast cancer is difficult. It is challenging because it is a life history of exposure that is important—not just a single chemical but complex mixtures of chemicals and their interaction with endogenous hormones. In addition, newer investigative models with epigenetic alterations may increase understanding. The highest rates of breast cancer are found in superindustrialized countries—North America and Europe—and the lowest rates in Central Africa and Asia. With industrial development, breast cancer rates increase. An estimated 85,000 synthetic chemicals are registered for use in the United States, another 1000 or more are added each year, and toxicologic screening for these chemicals is minimal. In fact, toxicologic screening is only available for about 7% of these chemicals.[289] Chemicals persist in the environment, accumulate in adipose tissue, interact with local adipose tissue physiology in an endocrine/paracrine manner, and remain in breast tissue for decades. Some of these chemicals are known human carcinogens and have been linked to breast tumors in animals. Women who immigrate to the United States from Asian countries experience an enormous percent increase in risk within one generation. A generation later, the rate of their daughter's risk approaches that of women born in the United States. This change in risk suggests that in utero exposures affect subsequent disease risk. It is difficult to know whether these changes in risk emanate from nutritional content, pollutants, food additives, or other factors.

Xenoestrogens are synthetic chemicals that mimic the actions of estrogens and are found in many pesticides, fuels, plastics, detergents, and drugs.[147] Because many factors correlated with breast cancer (e.g., early menarche, delayed pregnancy and breast-feeding, late menopause) are associated with lifetime exposure to estrogens, investigators reasoned that environmental chemicals affect estrogen metabolism and contribute to breast cancer. The most significant chemicals may be polychlorinated biphenyls (PCBs) such as dichloro-diphenyltrichloroethane (DDT), pesticides (Dieldrin, aldrin, heptachlor, and others), Bisphenol A (pervasive in polycarbonate plastics), tobacco smoke (active and passive), dioxins (vehicle exhaust, incineration, contaminated food supply), alkylphenols (detergents and cleaning products), metals, phthalates (makes plastics flexible, some cosmetics), parabens (antimicrobials), food additives (recombinant bovine somatotropin [rBST] and zeranol, to enhance growth in cattle and sheep), HRT, and others. Some chemicals are fat soluble, and the estrogenic effect would require either that they bind to the nuclear estrogen receptor and then cause cell division or gene transcription or that they activate ROS through oxidative catabolism of estrogens (see p. 843).

Physical activity. Regular physical activity may reduce overall risk of breast cancer, especially in premenopausal or young postmenopausal women.[290-292] Activity also may reduce the invasiveness of breast cancer.[293] A recent large, prospective study found that both walking for 1 hour per day and following an additional weekly exercise regimen seemed to be protective against breast cancer regardless of menopausal status.[294] Mechanisms for this protective effect are not known but include alterations in endogenous free radical formation and oxidative damage, effects on DNA repair capacity, alteration in carcinogen-metabolizing enzymes, increased intestinal transit times (i.e., reduced exposures to carcinogens), weight loss, and changes in endogenous sex hormone levels.[291,292]

Familial factors and tumor-related genes. Genetically, breast cancer can be divided into three main groups: (1) sporadic (the majority or 40% of women with breast cancer have no known family history); (2) inherited autosomal dominant cancer gene syndromes; and (3) probably polygenic—there is family history but it is not passed on to future generations as a dominant gene. Unknown are the genes in the polygenic model that could be involved, the nature of the interactions among these genes, and the interactions of these genes with environmental factors.

A history of breast cancer in first-degree relatives (mother or sister) increases a woman's risk two to three times. Risk increases even more if two first-degree relatives are involved, especially if the disease occurred before menopause and was bilateral. A small total

TABLE 32-12	TYPES OF BREAST CARCINOMAS AND MAJOR DISTINGUISHING FEATURES
HISTOLOGIC TYPE	**DISTINGUISHING FEATURES**
Carcinoma of Mammary Ducts	
Papillary	Well-delineated cystic masses in multiple areas; hemorrhage often present; majority appear in 40- to 60-year age group; often involves skin
Intraductal (comedo)	Often accompanied by evidence of inflammation; well-circumscribed tumors within duct; well-differentiated tumor cells; rarely ulcerates skin
Infiltrating Carcinoma	
Ductal (no specific type [NST])	Fibrous, firm, glistening, gray-tan mass with chalky streaks, mixture of patterns; may cause discharge from nipple; represents about 79% of all breast cancers
Mucinous	Usually large (>3 cm in diameter), circumscribed, and encapsulated, glistening appearance, varies in color; two types: pure and mixed; pure tumor is surrounded by mucin; infrequent; found in lateral half of breast; tends to occur in women after age 70 years
Medullary	Encapsulated and grows very large (7-8 cm in diameter); commonly surrounded by lymphocytic inflammatory infiltrate; occurs after age 50 years
Tubular	Well-differentiated with orderly tubules in center (stroma) of mass; can be associated with noninfiltrating ductal carcinoma; occurs in women about 50 years of age; nodal metastasis infrequent; occurrence rare
Adenoid cystic	Very rare; well-circumscribed, painless mass arising from nipple and areola
Metaplastic	Involves cartilage or bone, mixed tumors or osteogenic sarcomas
Squamous cell	Frequent in blacks; originates in ductal epithelium
Carcinoma of Mammary Lobules	
Lobular carcinoma in situ	Found in individuals with fibrocystic disease; localized to upper breast quadrants; 15-35% risk of becoming invasive; occurs frequently in mid-40s; infiltrating variety occurs in early 50s
Infiltrating lobular	Infiltrates from duct; firm mass with chalky streaks
Paget disease	Eczema of nipple that extends to areola; cancer usually found underneath nipple; poorly circumscribed; large Paget cells arise from duct and directly invade nipple; history of scaly, red rash spreading from nipple; lesion palpable beneath nipple, often bilateral; occurs in middle age
Inflammatory carcinoma	Not a histologic type; fairly diffuse within breast tissue, diffuse edema of overlying skin; extremely undifferentiated, very rare; most metastasize to axilla
Sarcoma of the Breast	
Cystosarcoma phyllodes	Usually large (>17 cm in diameter); mostly localized but can rupture through skin; rarely metastasizes to lymph nodes; history of painless nodule present for years before it forms a large mass; ulceration and bleeding of skin often present; occurs in wide age range (13-77 years)
Fibrosarcoma	Well-circumscribed, firm, and usually does not involve skin or nipple; well-differentiated to extremely undifferentiated; arises from connective tissue; extremely rare (e.g., liposarcoma, angiosarcoma)

proportion of breast cancers (5% to 10%, although the prevalence is significant) are the result of highly penetrant dominant genes (i.e., hereditary breast cancers). The most important of the dominant genes are the breast cancer susceptibility genes (*BRCA1*, *BRCA2*). *BRCA1* is located on chromosome 17 and *BRCA2* is located on chromosome 13. A family history of both breast cancer and ovarian cancer increases the risk that an individual with breast cancer carries a *BRCA1* mutation. Up to age 40, a woman with *BRCA1* mutation is estimated to have a 20 times greater risk of breast cancer compared to the general population and a lifetime risk of 60% to 85%.[292] Race is also an important distinction for genetic risk. A population-based study showed that whereas 3.3% of white women with breast cancer had *BRCA1* mutations, none of the 88 black women with breast cancer had a *BRCA1* mutation.[295] Carriers of the *BRCA1* gene are also at higher risk for ovarian cancer. *BRCA1* is a tumor-suppressor gene; therefore any mutation in the gene may inhibit or retard its suppressor function, leading to uncontrolled cell proliferation.[296] Men who develop breast cancer are more likely to have a *BRCA2* mutation than a *BRCA1* mutation.

Another suppressor gene, *p53*, is mutated in approximately 20% to 40% of individuals with breast cancer.[297] *p53* is a regulatory gene (i.e., a "policeman") that increases DNA repair, and if damage is extensive cell death (i.e., apoptosis) occurs in mutated cells. Thus *p53* helps to eliminate cancer proliferating cells. When *p53* is mutated, its regulatory properties are radically altered, conferring a loss of tumor-suppressor activity and, possibly, even a gain of tumor-promotion function. *Her-2/neu*, another oncogene, is overexpressed in 25% to 30% of breast cancer cells. It transmits a growth signal to the nucleus. The drug trastuzumab (Herceptin) blocks the signal in about 35% of those affected, thereby decreasing the growth of the tumor.

C-myc is a proto-oncogene expressed in cells and is one of the immediate, early growth response genes that are rapidly induced when quiet cells receive a signal to divide. Mutation of *c-myc* is amplified in breast, colon, lung, and many other cancers.

PATHOGENESIS Most breast cancers arise from the ductal epithelium. Tumors of the infiltrating ductal type do not grow to a large size, but they metastasize early. This type accounts for 70% of breast cancers. Table 32-12 lists the different types of breast carcinomas and summarizes their major characteristics.

Breast cancer is a heterogeneous disease with diverse molecular, phenotypic, and pathologic changes. Despite heroic efforts, this diversity has greatly challenged the understanding of breast cancer evolution. Recent research suggests that breast cancer is heterogeneous from its initial preinvasive stages.[298] Heterogeneity is an important concept because the biologic attributes of a tumor as a whole are strongly influenced by its subpopulation of cells as well as the tumor's surrounding neighborhood or microenvironment.[299] The two models (i.e., hypotheses) that account for breast carcinogenesis are the sporadic clonal evolution model and the cancer stem cell (CSC) model.[300] The sporadic clonal evolution model stipulates that *any* breast epithelial cell can be the target of random mutations.[300] According to this model both genetic and epigenetic alterations can contribute over time to breast cancer progression. The second, or CSC, model postulates that only stem and progenitor cells (representing a small population of cells within the tumor) can initiate and maintain tumor progression. Normal breast stem cells are long-lived and remain in breast tissue; they are capable of self-renewal activity and differentiation of several different kinds of cells (i.e., lineages) that collectively can reconstitute breast architecture.[301,302,303] Many of the biologic traits of high-grade malignancy have been traced to subpopulations of CSCs

within carcinomas.[304,305] Traits, such as motility, invasiveness, and self-renewal, are central to the pathogenesis and malignancy of neoplastic cells and may be a function of the CSCs.[303] Another important trait for pathogenesis is the resistance to apoptosis. Thus several lines of evidence suggest multiple molecular genetic pathways of complex crosstalking networks that progress toward malignancy.

Recently, two groups of investigators provided evidence that progesterone indirectly controls the number and function of breast stem cells through paracrine signaling from neighboring progesterone-positive (PR+) breast epithelial cells.[197,198] Importantly, these hormone findings further our understanding of steroid control of normal breast development and may provide a novel mechanism for therapy of breast cancer. Hormones may act as accelerators, as well as initiators, and influence the susceptibility of the breast epithelium to environmental carcinogens because hormones control the differentiation of the mammary gland epithelium and, thereby, regulate the rate of stem cell division.

Three decades of research have defined a cell-biologic program, called the **epithelial-to-mesenchymal transition (EMT)**, important for embryologic development and wound healing. This program is also referred to as a transdifferentiation program, employing many transcription factors that enable cells of epithelial origin to transition to mesenchymal phenotypes. Therefore EMT is prominently implicated as a means by which the transformed epithelial cells can acquire the abilities to invade, resist apoptosis, and disseminate.[306] Activation of an EMT program during cancer development often requires signaling between cancer cells and neighboring stromal cells.[303] In advanced primary carcinomas, cancer cells recruit a variety of cell types into the surrounding stroma, including fibroblasts, myofibroblasts, granulocytes, macrophages, mesenchymal stem cells, and lymphocytes (Figure 32-42).

These recruited cells create a "reactive stroma"—an inflammatory microenvironment that appears to result in the release of EMT-inducing signals.[303] Overall, increasing evidence suggests that interactions of cancer cells with adjacent tumor-associated stromal cells induce malignant cell phenotypes (Figure 32-43).

Ductal and lobular carcinoma in situ. The ductal and lobular subtypes constitute the majority of all breast cancers worldwide with the ductal type accounting for 40% to 75% of all diagnosed individuals.[307] Ductal carcinoma in situ (DCIS) refers to a heterogeneous group of proliferations limited to ducts and lobules (LCIS) (Figure 32-44, *B*). DCIS occurs predominantly in females but can occur in males. The cells sometimes extend to the overlying skin without crossing the basement membrane and mistakenly appear as Paget disease[308] (see Table 32-12). Before 1980, DCIS was a rare disease and usually presented as a palpable lesion, nipple discharge, or Paget disease (eczema-like lesions of the nipple). Since 1980, with the increased use of mammography, the incidence and presentation have changed dramatically.[309] DCIS presents as microcalcifications (low grade) (see Figure 32-44, *B*) or rod-shaped branching (high grade) on a mammogram (Figure 32-44, *A*).

Still controversial, DCIS does not appear to progress from sequential steps of low grade or risk types to higher grades or risk types en route to cancer or recurrence.[298,300] This property, therefore, suggests a stable population.[298] Emerging evidence suggests that DCIS may have programmed potential for phenotype, including progression to invasion, metastasis, hormone receptor expression, and treatment resistance.[298] The main issue and challenge concern which lesions of the category DCIS become invasive, why, and how soon this occurs.[309] In a study of 110 autopsies of young and middle-aged women (20 to 54 years), 14% were found to have DCIS,[310] suggesting that the preclinical prevalence (subtle histologic distortion and/or nonpalpable mass) is

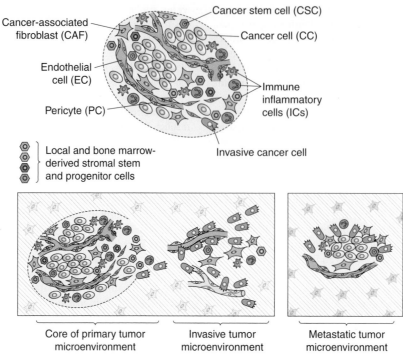

FIGURE 32-42 Cells of the Tumor Microenvironment. A, Distinct cell types constitute most solid tumors including breast tumors. Both the main cellular tissue, called parenchyma, and the surrounding tissue, or stroma, of tumors contain cell types that enable tumor growth and progression. For example, the immune-inflammatory cells present in tumors can include both tumor-promoting and tumor-killing subclasses of cells. **B,** The microenvironment of tumors. Multiple stromal cell types create a succession of tumor microenvironments that change as tumors invade normal tissue, eventually seeding and colonizing distant tissues. The organization, numbers, and phenotypic characteristics of the stromal cell types and the extracellular matrix (hatched background) evolve during progression and enable primary, invasive, and metastatic growth. (Not shown are the premalignant stages.) (Data from Hanahan D, Weinberg R: Hallmarks of cancer: the next generation, *Cell* 144:646–674, 2011.)

significantly higher than the clinical expression. Other autopsy series show that not all DCIS lesions progress to invasion or become clinically significant.[310,311] DCIS is detected more often in younger women than in older women.

Lobular carcinoma in situ (LCIS) originates from the terminal duct-lobular unit. Unlike DCIS, LCIS has a uniform appearance in which the cells occur in noncohesive (discohesive) clusters primarily in lobules. The model of lobular neoplasia proposes a multistep progression from normal epithelium to atypical lobular hyperplasia (ALH), lobular carcinoma in situ (LCIS), and invasive lobular carcinoma (ILC).[300] LCIS is fairly uncommon (up to 3.8% of all specimens).[312] LCIS is bilateral in 20% to 40% of women and the majority (80% to 90%) of cases occur before menopause. Invasive carcinoma develops in 25% to 35% of women with LCIS and the contralateral (opposite) breast also is at risk.[313]

The majority of carcinomas of the breast occur in the upper outer quadrant, where most of the glandular tissue of the breast is located. The lymphatic spread of cancer to the opposite breast, to lymph nodes in the base of the neck, and to the abdominal cavity is caused by obstruction of the normal lymphatic pathways or destruction of lymphatic vessels by surgery or radiotherapy (see Figure 31-11). The less common inner quadrant tumors may spread to mediastinal nodes or Rotter nodes, which are located between the pectoral muscles (see Figure 31-11).

Internal mammary chain nodes are also common sites of metastasis. Metastases from the vertebral veins can involve the vertebrae, pelvic bones, ribs, and skull. The lungs, kidneys, liver, adrenal glands, ovaries, and pituitary gland are also sites of metastasis.

CLINICAL MANIFESTATIONS The first sign of breast cancer is usually a painless lump. Lumps caused by breast tumors do not have any classic characteristics. Other presenting signs include palpable nodes in the axilla, retraction of tissue (dimpling) (Figure 32-45), or bone pain caused by metastasis to the vertebrae. Table 32-13 summarizes the clinical manifestations of breast cancers. Manifestations vary according to the type of tumor and stage of disease.

EVALUATION AND TREATMENT Clinical breast examination, mammography, ultrasound, thermography, MRI, percutaneous needle aspiration, biopsy or minimally invasive biopsy, hormone receptor assays, and gene expression profiling are used in evaluating breast alterations and cancer.

Treatment is based on the extent or stage of the cancer (Box 32-12). The extent of the tumor at the primary site, the presence and extent of lymph node metastasis, and the presence of distant metastases are all evaluated to determine the stage of disease. Treatment includes surgery, radiation, chemotherapy, hormone therapy, and biologic therapy.

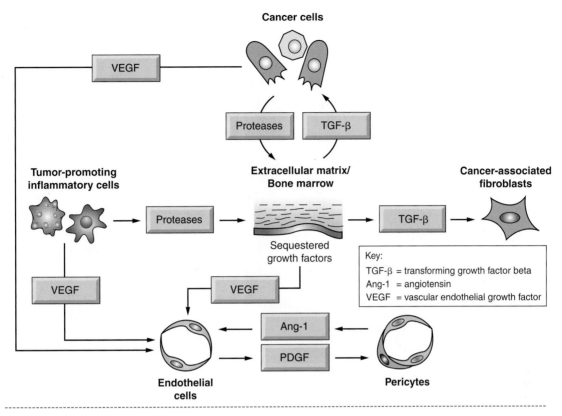

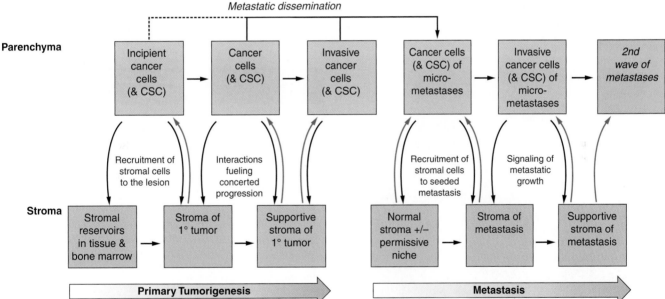

FIGURE 32-43 Signaling Interactions in the Tumor Microenvironment During Malignant Progression. *Upper panel:* Numerous cell types constitute the tumor microenvironment and are orchestrated and maintained by reciprocal interactions. *Lower panel:* The reciprocal interactions between the breast main tissue or parenchyma and the surrounding stroma are important for cancer progression and growth. Certain organ sites of "fertile soil" or "metastasis niches" facilitate metastatic seeding and colonization. Cancer stem cells are involved in some or all stages of tumor development and progression. (Adapted from Hanahan D, Weinberg R: Hallmarks of cancer: the next generation, *Cell* 144:646–674, 2011.)

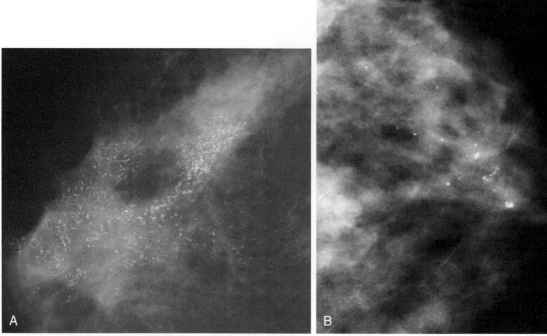

FIGURE 32-44 Ductal Carcinoma in Situ (DCIS). **A,** Malignant microcalcifications. Extensive area of pleomorphic microcalcifications; granular, rod-shaped, and branching microcalcifications can be identified. The appearances are typical of high-grade DCIS. **B,** Craniocaudal mammography reveals fine and coarse granular calcifications. Histopathologic analysis revealed low-grade DCIS. (**A** from O'Malley FP, Pinder SE, editors: *Breast pathology,* New York, 2006, Churchill Livingstone/Elsevier. **B** from Donegan WL, Spratt JS: *Cancer of the breast,* ed 5, Philadelphia, 2002, Saunders.)

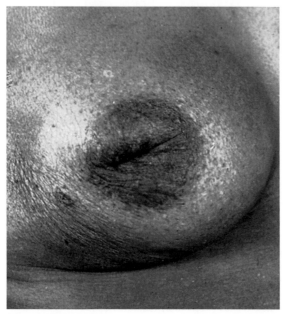

FIGURE 32-45 Retraction of Nipple Caused by Carcinoma. (From del Regato JA, Spjut HJ, Cox JD: *Ackerman and del Regato's cancer: diagnosis, treatment, and prognosis,* ed 6, St Louis, 1985, Mosby.)

TABLE 32-13	CLINICAL MANIFESTATIONS OF BREAST CANCER
CLINICAL MANIFESTATION	**PATHOPHYSIOLOGY**
Local pain	Local obstruction caused by tumor
Dimpling of skin	Can occur with invasion of dermal lymphatics because of retraction of Cooper ligament or involvement of pectoralis fascia
Nipple retraction	Shortening of mammary ducts
Skin retraction	Involvement of suspensory ligament
Edema	Local inflammation or lymphatic obstruction
Nipple/areolar eczema	Paget disease
Pitting of skin (similar to surface of an orange [peau d'orange])	Obstruction of subcutaneous lymphatics, resulting in accumulation of fluid
Reddened skin, local tenderness, and warmth	Inflammation
Dilated blood vessels	Obstruction of venous return by a fast-growing tumor; obstruction dilates superficial veins
Nipple discharge in a nonlactating woman	Spontaneous and intermittent discharge caused by tumor obstruction
Ulceration	Tumor necrosis
Hemorrhage	Erosion of blood vessels
Edema of arm	Obstruction of lymphatic drainage in axilla
Chest pain	Metastasis to lung

BOX 32-12 STAGING OF BREAST CANCER

Stage 0: Tis, N0, M0
This is *ductal carcinoma in situ (DCIS)*, the earliest form of breast cancer. In DCIS, cancer cells are still within a duct and have not invaded deeper into the surrounding fatty breast tissue. *Lobular carcinoma in situ (LCIS)* is sometimes also classified as Stage 0 breast cancer but most oncologists believe it is not a true breast cancer. In LCIS, normal cells grow within the lobules or milk-producing glands but they do not penetrate through the walls of these lobules. Paget disease of the nipple (without an underlying tumor mass) also is Stage 0. In all cases the cancer has not spread to lymph nodes or distant sites.

Stage IA: T1, N1mi, M0
The tumor is 2 cm (about ¾ of an inch) or less across (T1) and has not spread to lymph nodes (N0) or distant sites (M0).

Stage 1B: T0 or T1, N1mi, M0
The tumor is 2 cm or less across (or is not found) (T0 or T1) with micrometastases (mic) in 1 to 3 axillary lymph nodes (the cancer in the lymph nodes is greater than 0.2 mm across and/or more than 200 cells but is not larger than 2 mm) (N1mic). The cancer has not spread to distant sites (M0).

Stage IIA
One of the following applies:

T0 or T1, N1 (but not N1mi), M0
The tumor is 2 cm or less across (or is not found) (T1 or T0) and either:
It has spread to 1 to 3 axillary lymph nodes, with the cancer in the lymph nodes larger than 2 mm across (N1a); *or*
Tiny amounts of cancer are found in internal mammary lymph nodes on sentinel lymph node biopsy (N1b); *or*
It has spread to 1 to 3 axillary lymph nodes and to internal mammary lymph nodes (found on sentinel lymph node biopsy) (N1c).

Or

T2, N0, M0
The tumor is larger than 2 cm across and less than 5 cm (T2) but has not spread to the lymph nodes (N0). The cancer has not spread to distant sites (M0).

Stage IIB
One of the following applies:

T2, N1, M0
The tumor is larger than 2 cm and less than 5 cm across (T2). It has spread to 1 to 3 axillary lymph nodes and/or tiny amounts of cancer are found in internal mammary lymph nodes on sentinel lymph node biopsy (N1). The cancer has not spread to distant sites (M0).

Or

T3, N0, M0
The tumor is larger than 5 cm across but does not grow into the chest wall or skin and has not spread to lymph nodes (T3, N0). The cancer has not spread to distant sites (M0).

Stage IIIA
One of the following applies:

T0 to T2, N2, M0
The tumor is not more than 5 cm across (or cannot be found) (T0 to T2). It has spread to 4 to 9 axillary nodes or it has enlarged the internal mammary lymph nodes (N2). The cancer has not spread to distant sites (M0).

Or

T3, N1 or N2, M0
The tumor is larger than 5 cm across but does not grow into the chest wall or skin (T3). It has spread to 4 to 9 axillary nodes or to internal mammary nodes (N1 or N2). The cancer has not spread to distant sites (M0).

Stage IIIB: T4, N0 to N2, M0
The tumor has grown into the chest wall or skin (T4) and one of the following applies:
• It has not spread to the lymph nodes (N0); *or*
• It has spread to 1 to 3 axillary lymph nodes and/or tiny amounts of cancer are found in internal mammary lymph nodes on sentinel lymph node biopsy (N1); *or*
• It has spread to 4 to 9 axillary lymph nodes or it has enlarged the internal mammary lymph nodes (N2).
• The cancer has not spread to distant sites (M0). Inflammatory breast cancer is classified as T4 and is Stage IIIB unless it has spread to distant lymph nodes or organs, in which case it would be Stage IV.

Stage IIIC: Any T, N3, M0
The tumor is any size (or cannot be found) and one of the following applies:
• The cancer has spread to 10 or more axillary lymph nodes (N3); *or*
• The cancer involves axillary lymph nodes and has enlarged the internal mammary lymph nodes (N3); *or*
• The cancer has spread to 4 or more axillary lymph nodes and tiny amounts of cancer are found in internal mammary lymph nodes on sentinel lymph node biopsy (N3).
• The cancer has not spread to distant sites (M0).

Stage IV: Any T, Any N, M1
The cancer can be any size (any T) and may or may not have spread to nearby lymph nodes (any N). It has spread to distant organs or to lymph nodes far from the breast (M1). The most common sites of spread are to the bone, liver, brain, or lung.

Data from American Cancer Society: *Learn about cancer, breast cancer staging.* Accessed Feb 1, 2011. Available at www.cancer.org/cancer/breast cancer/detailedguide/breast-cancer-staging.
T, Primary tumor size; *N*, regional lymph nodes; *M*, distant metastasis.

✔ **QUICK CHECK 32-8**

1. What types of fibrocystic breast changes increase the risk of breast cancer?
2. What is the role of hormones and growth factors in the pathophysiology of breast cancer?
3. Why are reproductive factors, such as early menarche and late menopause, important for the pathogenesis of breast cancer?
4. Why is complete breast involution important for reducing risk of breast cancer?
5. Discuss the role of the microenvironment or stromal tissue on breast cancer development.

Disorders of the Male Breast

Gynecomastia

Gynecomastia is the overdevelopment of breast tissue in a male. Gynecomastia accounts for approximately 85% of all masses that develop in the male breast and affects 32% to 40% of the male population. If only one breast is involved, it is typically the left. Incidence is greatest among adolescents and men older than 50 years.

Gynecomastia results from hormonal alterations, which may be idiopathic or caused by systemic disorders, drugs, or neoplasms. Gynecomastia usually involves an imbalance of the estrogen/testosterone ratio. The normal estrogen/testosterone ratio can be altered in one of two ways. First, estrogen levels may be excessively high, although testosterone levels are normal. This is the case in drug-induced and tumor-induced hyperestrogenism. Second, testosterone levels may be extremely low, although estrogen levels are normal, as is the case in hypergonadism. Gynecomastia also can be caused by alterations in breast tissue responsiveness to hormonal stimulation. Breast tissue may have increased responsiveness to estrogen or decreased responsiveness to androgen. Alterations of responsiveness may cause many cases of idiopathic gynecomastia.

Besides puberty and aging, estrogen/testosterone imbalances are associated with hypogonadism, Klinefelter syndrome, and testicular neoplasms. Hormone-induced gynecomastia is usually bilateral. Pubertal gynecomastia is a self-limiting phenomenon that usually disappears within 4 to 6 months. Senescent gynecomastia usually regresses spontaneously within 6 to 12 months.

Systemic disorders associated with gynecomastia include cirrhosis of the liver, infectious hepatitis, chronic renal failure, chronic obstructive lung disease, hyperthyroidism, tuberculosis, and chronic malnutrition. It may be that these disorders ultimately alter the estrogen/testosterone ratio, initiating the gynecomastia.

Gynecomastia is often seen in males receiving estrogen therapy, either in preparation for a gender-change operation or in the treatment of prostatic carcinoma. Other drugs that can cause gynecomastia include digitalis, cimetidine, spironolactone, reserpine, thiazide, isoniazid, ergotamine, tricyclic antidepressants, amphetamines, vincristine, and busulfan. Gynecomastia is usually unilateral in these instances.

Malignancies of the testes, adrenals, or liver can cause gynecomastia if they alter the estrogen/testosterone ratio. Pituitary adenomas and lung cancer also are associated with gynecomastia.

PATHOPHYSIOLOGY The enlargement of the breast consists of hyperplastic stroma and ductal tissue. Hyperplasia results in a firm, palpable mass that is at least 2 cm in diameter and located beneath the areola.

EVALUATION AND TREATMENT The diagnosis of gynecomastia is based on physical examination. Identification and treatment of the cause are likely to be followed by resolution of the gynecomastia. The man should be taught to perform breast self-examination and is reexamined at 6- and 12-month intervals if the gynecomastia persists.

Carcinoma

Breast cancer in males accounts for 0.26% of all male cancers and 1.1% of all breast cancers. About 1970 new cases of breast cancer in men were estimated in 2010.[1] It is seen most commonly after the age of 60 years, with the peak incidence between 60 and 69 years. It has, however, been reported in males as young as 6 years old and in adolescents. Risk factors for men include age, race, radiation exposure, and family history of breast cancer. Inconclusive risk factors include gynecomastia, hormonal factors, previous breast cancer, obesity, and environmental exposures.[314] At all ages black men have a higher incidence than white men. Approximately 15% to 20% of men with breast cancer report a family history of breast or ovarian cancer.[314] The effects of inheritance of the breast cancer susceptibility gene (BRCA1) in men are unclear. Although the risk of developing breast cancer is almost nonexistent, men with this gene may have a slight increase in prostate cancer; this is still under investigation. Male carriers of the BRCA1 gene, however, can pass the gene on to their children.[1] In terms of breast cancer susceptibility genes, men who develop breast cancer are more likely to have a BRCA2 mutation than a BRCA1 mutation.[314]

Male breast tumors often resemble carcinoma of the breast in women. The majority of male breast cancers express estrogen and progesterone receptors.[314] Because of small sample sizes, however, all data need careful review and more data are needed. The majority of tumors were ductal carcinoma followed by DCIS.[314] The malignant male breast lesion is usually a unilateral solid mass located near the nipple. Because the nipple is commonly involved, crusting and nipple discharge are typical clinical manifestations. Other findings include skin retraction, ulceration of the skin over the tumor, and axillary node involvement. Patterns of metastasis are similar to those in females.

The diagnosis of cancer is confirmed by biopsy. Because of delays in seeking treatment, male breast cancer tends to be advanced at the time of diagnosis and therefore has a poor prognosis. Treatment protocols are similar to those for female breast cancer, but endocrine therapy (e.g., tamoxifen) is used more often for males because a higher percentage of male tumors are hormone dependent. Orchiectomy is performed to treat metastatic disease.

SEXUALLY TRANSMITTED INFECTIONS

Sexually contracted infections affect approximately 19 million Americans per year[28] and account for about one third of the reproductive mortality in the United States[28] (Table 32-14). Untreated or undertreated chlamydial infections are the primary cause of preventable infertility and ectopic pregnancy. Reportable infections do not include some of the most prevalent sexually transmitted infections (STIs), including human papillomavirus (HPV) or herpes simplex virus (HSV). Complications of STIs include pelvic inflammatory disease (PID), infertility, ectopic pregnancy, chronic pelvic pain, neonatal morbidity and mortality, genital cancer, and epidemiologic synergy with HIV transmission. Long-term sequelae of untreated or undertreated STIs may be disastrous and can impact a person's physical, emotional, and financial well-being. (STIs are described and illustrated in Table 32-16, pp. 858–859.)

TABLE 32-14 ESTIMATED NEW CASES OF REPORTABLE AND NONREPORTABLE STIs EACH YEAR

INFECTION	NUMBER OF CASES
Reportable STIs (New Cases Each Year)	
Chlamydia	1,244,180
Gonorrhea	301,174
Syphilis	44,828
Nonreportable STIs (Estimated Prevalence)	
Herpes	16.2%
Human papillomavirus (low- and high-risk types	26.8%
Trichomonas	3.1%

Data from Centers for Disease Control and Prevention: *Sexually transmitted disease surveillance 2009*, Atlanta, 2010, U.S. Department of Health and Human Services.

TABLE 32-15 CURRENTLY RECOGNIZED SEXUALLY TRANSMITTED INFECTIONS

CAUSAL MICROORGANISM	DISEASE
Bacteria	
Campylobacter	*Campylobacter* enteritis
Calymmatobacterium granulomatis	Granuloma inguinale
Chlamydia trachomatis	Urogenital infections; lymphogranuloma venereum
Polymicrobial Organisms	
Haemophilus ducreyi	Chancroid
Mycoplasma	Mycoplasmosis
Neisseria gonorrhoeae	Gonorrhea
Shigella	Shigellosis
Treponema pallidum	Syphilis
Viruses	
Cytomegalovirus	Cytomegalic inclusion disease
Hepatitides A, B, and C virus	Hepatitis
Herpes simplex virus (HSV)	Genital herpes
Human immunodeficiency virus (HIV)	Acquired immunodeficiency syndrome (AIDS)
Human papillomavirus (HPV)	Condylomata acuminata
Molluscum contagiosum virus	Molluscum contagiosum
Protozoa	
Entamoeba histolytica	Amebiasis; amebic dysentery
Giardia lamblia	Giardiasis
Trichomonas vaginalis	Trichomoniasis
Ectoparasites	
Phthirus pubis	Pediculosis pubis
Sarcoptes scabiei	Scabies

Sexually transmitted diseases are infections contracted by intimate as well as sexual contact and include systemic infections, such as tuberculosis and hepatitis, that can spread to a sexual partner. The etiology of an STI may be bacterial, viral, or parasitic (Table 32-15). Although the majority of STIs can be treated, viral-induced STIs are considered incurable. Of note, bacterial vaginosis (BV) is sexually associated but is no longer considered an STI (see *Health Alert:* Bacterial Vaginosis).

HEALTH ALERT
Bacterial Vaginosis

Bacterial vaginosis (BV) is a sexually associated condition but is not considered an STI. BV occurs almost exclusively in women who are sexually active. The exact etiology is unknown but an overgrowth of various anaerobes, including *Gardnerella vaginalis*, *Mycoplasma hominis*, *Bacteroides*, and *Mobiluncus*, occurs when normal vaginal flora (i.e., lactobacilli) are decreased or absent. BV is characterized by increased, thin, gray-white vaginal discharge with a strong "fishy" odor. BV is diagnosed by wet mount of vaginal secretions and treated with antibiotics. Treatment of sex partners is not necessary.

Data from Donders G: Diagnosis and management of bacterial vaginosis and other types of abnormal vaginal bacterial flora: a review, *Obstet Gynecol Surv* 65(7):462–473, 2010.

An increased incidence of STIs can be attributed to (1) earlier onset of sexual activity, (2) a greater number of lifetime sexual partners, and (3) high-risk sexual behavior (i.e., failure to use a condom in nonmonogamous or new sexual relationships, illicit drug use, prostitution, selection of high-risk sexual partners). Many infected individuals do not seek treatment because symptoms are absent, minor, or transient, thus contributing to ongoing transmission to others. Perhaps partly as a result of risk-taking behavior, adolescents tend to be at highest risk for STI exposure and infection. Victims of sexual assault can receive prophylactic treatment against potential STI transmission (see *Health Alert:* Anti-Infective Treatment for Victims of Sexual Assault). Table 32-16 summarizes the major STIs.

HEALTH ALERT
Anti-Infective Treatment for Victims of Sexual Assault

Victims of sexual assault are given prophylaxis against gonorrhea, trichomoniasis, bacterial vaginosis, and chlamydia using the current recommended treatment based on Centers for Disease Control and Prevention (CDC) guidelines. Hepatitis B vaccination is highly recommended, and emergency contraception is also available.

Centers for Disease Control and Prevention: Sexually transmitted diseases treatment guidelines, *MMWR Morb Mortal Wkly Rep* 59 (RR-12):1–110, 2010.

✔ QUICK CHECK 32-9
1. What is the cause of male gynecomastia?
2. What are the risk factors for male breast cancer?
3. What factors increase the incidence of STIs?

TABLE 32-16 MAJOR SEXUALLY TRANSMITTED INFECTIONS

SOURCE OF INFECTION	EPIDEMIOLOGY/CLINICAL MANIFESTATIONS	EVALUATION AND TREATMENT
Bacteria		
Chancroid *(Haemophilus ducreyi)*	Incidence is low in United States; women are generally asymptomatic, whereas men develop inflamed, painful genital ulcer	Definitive diagnosis is from cultured specimens
	Secondary infections can occur	Treat with antibiotics
Chlamydial infections *(Chlamydia trachomatis)*	Most common bacterial STI in United States; leading cause of infertility for both men and women; cause of ectopic pregnancy; leading cause of blindness worldwide; frequently asymptomatic, particularly in women	Diagnosed by amplified DNA or fluorescent monoclonal antibody screening of urethral or vaginal discharge; urine assay
	Infections in men can cause urethritis and epididymitis; infection in women may cause urethritis and mucopurulent cervical discharge; newborns can be infected; perinatal exposure involves eye, oropharynx, urogenital tract, and rectum	Treatment of both sexual partners with antibiotics
Gonorrhea *(Neisseria gonorrhoeae)*	Adolescents 15-19 years at highest risk; transmitted by oral, anal, or vaginal intercourse; mother-to-child transmission during vaginal delivery	Amplified DNA or culture of endocervical, pharyngeal, anal, and urethral secretions; concomitant screening for chlamydia
	Manifestations include urethral, renal, vaginal, and oral infections; vaginal discharge; bleeding or spotting and heavy menses; painful urination; up to 50% are asymptomatic	Treat both sexual partners with antibiotics
Lymphogranuloma venereum (LGV)	Often confused with syphilis, herpes, or chancroid	Diagnosed through LGV complement-fixation tests, tissue culture, and monoclonal antibody tests
	Begins as skin lesion, spreads to lymphatic tissue; appears as multivesicular ulcer on penis or scrotum in men and appears on vaginal wall, cervix, or labia in women; anorectal lesions, from anal intercourse, can appear in both men and women	Treated with antibiotics
Syphilis *(Treponema pallidum)*	Higher incidence among men who have sex with men; in urban and poverty stricken areas and prison populations; transmitted during first few years of infection; can be transmitted to fetus during pregnancy	Dark-field or fluorescent antibody examination of fluid from syphilitic chancre; VDRL or RPR
	Hard chancre develops in primary stage; systemic symptoms include low-grade fever, malaise, sore throat, hoarseness, anorexia, headache, joint pain, skin rashes; latent (tertiary) stages usually asymptomatic	Treatment includes penicillin injections for primary or secondary infections
	Neurosyphilis and life-threatening hypersensitivities can develop without treatment	
Viruses*		
Condylomata acuminata (human papillomavirus [HPV])	Most common viral STI in United States	Diagnosis based on clinical manifestations; Pap smears and HPV DNA tests
	Risk factors include multiple sexual partners, early onset of sexual activity (16-25 years of age); HPV is associated with cervical and vulvar cancer in females and with anorectal and squamous cell carcinoma of penis in men; genital warts contagious; infants can be infected during delivery; HPV is frequently asymptomatic	Treated with topical acids, cryosurgery or immune system modifiers; cervical and extensive vaginal lesions treated with 5-FU or surgical excision
	Warts are soft, skin-colored, whitish pink to reddish brown; may occur singly or in clusters	Treatment is not curative; follow-up for progression to cervical cancer is important
Genital herpes (type 1 [HSV-1] or type 2 [HSV-2])	Most common cause of genital ulceration in United States; reaching epidemic status	Diagnosis based on clinical manifestations, tissue culture, or serologic antibody testing
	Neonatal infections can occur primarily intrapartum and postpartum; virus undergoes local replication in dermis and epidermis leading to vesicles; can remain in latent stage until reactivated; cause of reactivation unknown but may be related to stress, sun exposure, hormonal fluctuations, or illness; small, scattered vesicles are quite painful, lasting 5-21 days	No curative treatment; oral antivirals (i.e., acyclovir, famciclovir, or valacyclovir) may be used; IV acyclovir reserved for severely immunocompromised persons

TABLE 32-16	MAJOR SEXUALLY TRANSMITTED INFECTIONS—cont'd	
SOURCE OF INFECTION	**EPIDEMIOLOGY/CLINICAL MANIFESTATIONS**	**EVALUATION AND TREATMENT**
Parasites		
Pediculosis pubis (*Phthirus pubis* [crab louse])	Primarily transmitted sexually, causes "crabs;" most common in single persons ages 15-25 years	Definitive diagnosis by examination (lice and nits are visible to unaided eye)
	Ranges from mild pruritus to severe, intolerable pruritus in pubic area	Treated with lotion, cream, or shampoo
Scabies *(Sarcoptes scabiei)*	First human disease with known cause; worldwide distribution; most recent outbreak in United States began in 1971, subsided in 1981; transmitted by close skin-to-skin contact, typically occurring within families or between sexual partners	Diagnosed from clinical manifestations, microscopic identification of mites, eggs, or larvae
	Predominant manifestation is intense pruritus	Treated with lotion, cream, or shampoo
Trichomoniasis *(Trichomonas vaginalis)*	Common cause of lower genital tract infection; found in both partners; urethra most common site of infection in men, primarily involves vagina in women	Definitive diagnosis through microscopic confirmation of trichomonads in vaginal secretions
	Manifestations range from none to severe, including pain on intercourse, dysuria, copious frothy vaginal discharge, and internal pruritus; most men remain asymptomatic	Treat with antibiotics for both sexual partners

DNA, Deoxyribonucleic acid; *5-FU,* 5-fluorouracil; *IV,* intravenous; *RPR,* rapid plasma reagin test; *STI,* sexually transmitted infection; *VDRL,* Venereal Disease Research Laboratory test.

NOTE: AIDS is discussed extensively in Chapter 7.

BACTERIAL SOURCES

Gonococcal infections

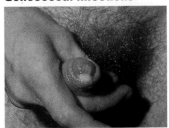

Symptomatic gonococcal urethritis.

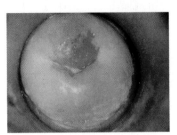

Endocervical gonorrhea.

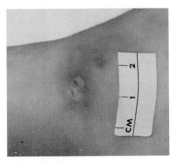

Skin lesions of disseminated gonococcal infection.

Bacterial vaginosis

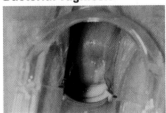

Vaginal examination showing mild bacterial vaginosis.

Syphilis

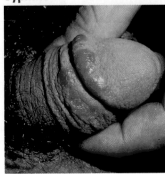

Erythematous penile plaques of secondary syphilis.

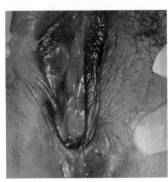

Multiple primary syphilitic chancres of labia and perineum.

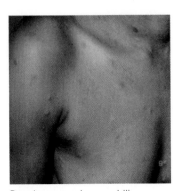

Papular secondary syphilis.

Lymphogranuloma

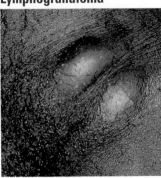

"Groove sign" in man with lymphogranuloma venereum (LV).

Chlamydial infections

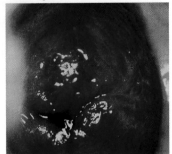

Beefy red mucosa in chlamydial infection.

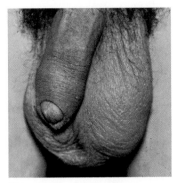

Chlamydial epididymitis.

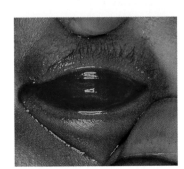

Chlamydial ophthalmia: erythematous conjunctiva in infant.

From Morse SA, Moreland AA, Holmes KK: *Atlas of sexually transmitted diseases and AIDS*, ed 2, London, 1996, Mosby.

VIRAL SOURCES

Genital herpes

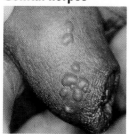

Early lesions of primary genital herpes.

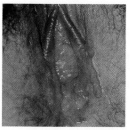

Primary vulvar herpes.

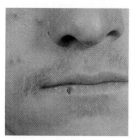

Generalized herpes simplex in patient with atopic dermatitis.

PARASITE SOURCES

Trichomonisasis

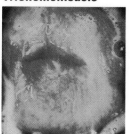

"Strawberry cervix" seen with trichomoniasis.

Human papillomavirus (HPV)

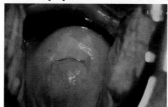

Human papillomavirus (HPV) infection of the cervix.

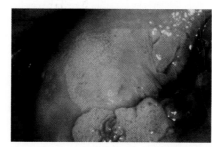

Subclinical HPV infection
Cervical os
Cervical intraepithelial neoplasia
Exophytic condyloma

Exophytic (outward-growing) condyloma, subclinical human papillomavirus (HPV) infection, and high-grade cervical intraepithelial neoplasia (CIN).

Condylomata acuminata

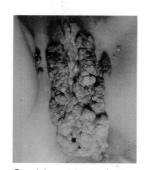

Condylomata acuminata: vulva and perineum.

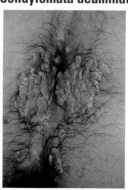

Condylomata acuminata: perianal.

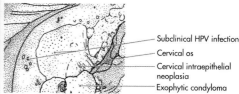

Condylomata acuminata: penile.

Scabies

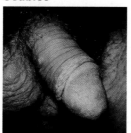

Nodular lesions of scabies on male genitalia.

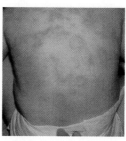

Urticaria associated with scabies.

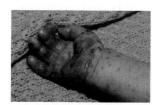

Scabies of palm with secondary pyoderma in infant.

Pediculosis pubis (*Phthirus pubis* [crablouse])

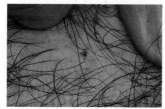

Phthirus pubis feeding on its host.

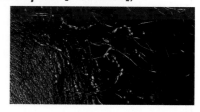

Pubic hair with multiple nits.

DID YOU UNDERSTAND?

Alterations of Sexual Maturation

1. Sexual maturation, or puberty, should begin in girls between the ages of 8 and 13 years and in boys between the ages of 9 and 14 years.
2. Delayed puberty is the onset of sexual maturation after these ages; precocious puberty is the onset before these ages. Treatment depends on the cause.

Disorders of the Female Reproductive System

1. The female reproductive system can be altered by hormonal imbalances, infectious microorganisms, inflammation, structural abnormalities, and benign or malignant proliferative conditions.
2. Primary dysmenorrhea is painful menstruation not associated with pelvic disease. It results from excessive synthesis of prostaglandin F. Secondary dysmenorrhea results from endometriosis, pelvic adhesions, inflammatory disease, uterine fibroids, or adenomyosis.
3. Primary amenorrhea is the continued absence of menarche and menstrual function by 14 years of age without the development of secondary sex characteristics or by 16 years of age if these changes have occurred.
4. Secondary amenorrhea is the absence of menstruation for a time equivalent to more than 3 cycles or 6 months in women who have previously menstruated. Secondary amenorrhea is associated with anovulation.
5. Dysfunctional uterine bleeding (DUB) is heavy or irregular bleeding caused by a disturbance of the menstrual cycle.
6. Polycystic ovary syndrome (PCOS) is a condition in which excessive androgen production is triggered by inappropriate secretion of gonadotropins. This hormonal imbalance prevents ovulation and causes enlargement and cyst formation in the ovaries, excessive endometrial proliferation, and often hirsutism. Hyperinsulinemia plays a key role in androgen excess.
7. Premenstrual syndrome (PMS) is the cyclic recurrence of physical, psychologic, or behavioral changes distressing enough to disrupt normal activities or interpersonal relationships. Emotional symptoms, particularly depression, anger, irritability, and fatigue, are reported as the most distressing symptoms; physical symptoms tend to be less problematic. Treatment is symptomatic and includes self-help techniques, lifestyle changes, counseling, and medication.
8. Infection and inflammation of the female genitalia can result from microorganisms from the environment or overproliferation of microorganisms that normally populate the genital tract.
9. Pelvic inflammatory disease (PID) is an acute ascending infection of the upper genital tract caused by a sexually transmitted pathogen. Untreated PID can lead to infertility.
10. Vaginitis, or vaginal infection, is usually caused by sexually transmitted pathogens or *Candida albicans,* which causes candidiasis.
11. Cervicitis, which is infection of the cervix, can be acute (mucopurulent cervicitis) or chronic. Its most common cause is a sexually transmitted pathogen.
12. Vulvitis is an inflammation of the skin of the vulva. It can be caused by chemical irritants, allergens, skin disorders, irritation from tight-fitting clothing, or the dissemination of vaginal infections, such as candidiasis.
13. Bartholinitis, also called Bartholin cyst, is an infection of the ducts that lead from the Bartholin glands to the surface of the vulva. Infection blocks the glands, preventing the outflow of glandular secretions.
14. The pelvic relaxation disorders—uterine displacement, uterine prolapse, cystocele, rectocele, and urethrocele—are caused by the relaxation of muscles and fascial supports, usually a result of advancing age or following childbirth or other trauma, and are more likely to occur in women with a familial or genetic predisposition.

15. Benign ovarian cysts develop from mature ovarian follicles that do not release their ova (follicular cysts) or from a corpus luteum that persists abnormally instead of degenerating (corpus luteum cyst). Cysts usually regress spontaneously.
16. Endometrial polyps consist of overgrowths of endometrial tissue and often cause abnormal bleeding in the premenopausal woman.
17. Leiomyomas, also called *uterine fibroids,* are benign tumors arising from the smooth muscle layer of the uterus, the myometrium.
18. Adenomyosis is the presence of endometrial glands and stroma within the uterine myometrium.
19. Endometriosis is the presence of functional endometrial tissue (i.e., tissue that responds to hormonal stimulation) at sites outside the uterus. Endometriosis causes an inflammatory reaction at the site of implantation and is a cause of infertility.
20. Most cancers of the female genitalia involve the uterus (particularly the endometrium), the cervix, and the ovaries. Cancer of the vagina is rare.
21. Cervical cancer arises from the cervical epithelium and is triggered by human papillomavirus (HPV). The progressively serious neoplastic alterations are cervical intraepithelial neoplasia (cervical dysplasia), cervical carcinoma in situ, and invasive cervical carcinoma. Smoking is a cofactor.
22. Most vaginal cancers are not invasive. Like cervical cancers, they arise from the epithelium and are identified as intraepithelial neoplasia (dysplasia), carcinoma in situ, or invasive carcinoma.
23. Risk factors for endometrial cancer include exposure to unopposed estrogen, obesity, high-fat diet, infertility or no pregnancies, late menopause, diabetes, and hypertension. Hormonal contraception protects against endometrial and ovarian cancers. The incidence of endometrial cancer is greatest among women in their fifties and early sixties.
24. Risk factors for ovarian cancer include family history, residence in an industrialized country, prior breast or endometrial cancer, infertility, early menopause, obesity, a high-fat diet, and exposure to asbestos or talc. Ovarian cancer causes more deaths than any other genital cancer in women.
25. Infertility, or the inability to conceive after 1 year of unprotected intercourse, affects approximately 15% of all couples. Fertility can be impaired by factors in the male, female, or both partners.
26. Chronic illness, medications, infection, sexual trauma, and a variety of psychosocial concerns have been implicated as causes of female sexual dysfunction.

Disorders of the Male Reproductive System

1. Disorders of the urethra include urethritis (infection of the urethra) and urethral strictures (narrowing or obstruction of the urethral lumen caused by scarring).
2. Most cases of urethritis result from sexually transmitted pathogens. Urologic instrumentation, foreign body insertion, trauma, or an anatomic abnormality can cause urethral inflammation with or without infection.
3. Urethritis causes urinary symptoms, including a burning sensation during urination (dysuria), frequency, urgency, urethral tingling or itching, and clear or purulent discharge.
4. The scarring that causes urethral stricture can be caused by trauma or by severe untreated urethritis.
5. Manifestations of urethral stricture include those of bladder outlet obstruction: urinary frequency and hesitancy, diminished force and caliber of the urinary stream, dribbling after voiding, and nocturia.
6. Phimosis and paraphimosis are penile disorders involving the foreskin (prepuce). In phimosis, the foreskin cannot be retracted over the glans. In paraphimosis, the foreskin is retracted and cannot be reduced (returned to its normal anatomic position over the glans). Phimosis is caused by poor hygiene and chronic infection and can lead to paraphimosis. Paraphimosis can constrict the penile blood vessels, preventing circulation to the glans.

DID YOU UNDERSTAND?—cont'd

7. Peyronie disease consists of fibrosis affecting the corpora cavernosa, which causes penile curvature during erection. Fibrosis prevents engorgement on the affected side, causing a lateral curvature that can prevent intercourse.

8. Priapism is a prolonged, painful erection that is not stimulated by sexual arousal. The corpora cavernosa (but not the corpus spongiosum) fill with blood will not drain from the area, probably because of venous obstruction. Priapism is associated with spinal cord trauma, sickle cell disease, leukemia, and pelvic tumors. It can also be idiopathic.

9. Balanitis is an inflammation of the glans penis. It is associated with phimosis, inadequate cleansing under the foreskin, skin disorders, and pathogens (e.g., *Candida albicans*).

10. Cancer of the penis is rare. Penile carcinoma in situ tends to involve the glans; invasive carcinoma of the penis involves the shaft as well.

11. A varicocele is an abnormal dilation of the veins within the spermatic cord caused either by congenital absence of valves in the internal spermatic vein or by acquired valvular incompetence.

12. A hydrocele is a collection of fluid between the testicular and scrotal layers of the tunica vaginalis. Hydroceles can be idiopathic or caused by trauma or infection of the testes.

13. A spermatocele is a cyst located between the testis and epididymis that is filled with fluid and sperm.

14. Cryptorchidism is a congenital condition in which one or both testes fail to descend into the scrotum. Uncorrected cryptorchidism is associated with infertility and significantly increased risk of testicular cancer.

15. Testicular torsion is the rotation of a testis, which twists blood vessels in the spermatic cord. This interrupts the blood supply to the testis, resulting in edema and, if not corrected within 6 hours, necrosis and atrophy of testicular tissues.

16. Orchitis is an acute infection of the testes. Complications of orchitis include hydrocele and abscess formation.

17. Testicular cancer is the most common malignancy in males 15 to 35 years of age. Although its cause is unknown, high androgen levels, genetic predisposition, and history of cryptorchidism, trauma, or infection may contribute to tumorigenesis.

18. Spermatogenesis (sperm production by the testes) can be impaired by disruptions of the hypothalamic-pituitary-testicular axis that reduce testosterone secretion and by testicular trauma, infection, or atrophy from any cause. Sperm production is also impaired by neoplastic disease, cryptorchidism, or any factor that causes testicular temperature to rise (e.g., circulatory impairment, wearing tight clothing).

19. Epididymitis, an inflammation of the epididymis, is usually caused by a sexually transmitted pathogen that ascends through the vasa deferentia from an already infected urethra or bladder.

20. Benign prostatic hyperplasia (BPH), also called benign prostatic hypertrophy, is the enlargement of the prostate gland. This condition becomes symptomatic as the enlarging prostate compresses the urethra, causing symptoms of bladder outlet obstruction and urine retention.

21. Prostatitis is inflammation of the prostate. Prostatitis syndromes have been classified by the National Institutes of Health as (a) acute bacterial prostatitis (ABP), (b) chronic bacterial prostatitis (CBP), (c) chronic pelvic pain syndrome (CPPS), and (d) asymptomatic inflammatory prostatitis.

22. Prostate cancer is the most common cancer in American males, and the incidence varies greatly worldwide. Possible causes include genetic predisposition, environmental and dietary factors, inflammation, and alterations in levels of hormones (testosterone, dihydrotestosterone, and estradiol) and growth factors. Incidence is greatest among northwestern European and North American men (particularly blacks) older than 65 years.

23. Most cancers of the prostate are adenocarcinomas that develop at the periphery of the gland.

24. Sexual dysfunction in males can be caused by any physical or psychologic factor that impairs erection, emission, or ejaculation.

Disorders of the Breast

1. Most disorders of the breast are disorders of the mammary gland—that is, the female breast.

2. Galactorrhea, or inappropriate lactation, is the persistent secretion of a milky substance by the breasts of a woman who is not in the postpartum state or nursing an infant. Its most common cause is nonpuerperal hyperprolactinemia, a rise in serum prolactin levels.

3. Benign breast conditions are numerous and involve both ducts and lobules. Benign epithelial lesions can be broadly classified according to their future risk of developing breast cancer as (a) nonproliferative breast lesions, (b) proliferative breast disease, and (c) atypical (atypia) hyperplasia.

4. Nonproliferative lesions include fibrocystic changes (FCC). In addition to FCC, many women experience several other types of benign breast tumors.

5. Proliferative breast lesions without atypia are characterized by proliferation of ductal epithelium or stroma, or both, without cellular signs of malignancy.

6. Proliferative breast lesions with atypia include atypical ductal hyperplasia (ADH) and atypical lobular hyperplasia (ALH).

7. Ductal carcinoma in situ (DCIS) refers to a heterogeneous group of lesions, presumably malignant epithelial cells, within the ductal system. Because not all DCIS lesions progress to invasion or become clinically significant, the main concern is which DCIS lesions become invasive. Lobular carcinoma in situ (LCIS) originates from the duct-lobular unit.

8. Breast cancer is the most common form of cancer in women and second to lung cancer as the most common cause of cancer death. It is a heterogeneous disease with diverse molecular, phenotypic, and pathologic changes.

9. The major risk factors for breast cancer are reproductive factors, such as nulliparity; hormonal factors and growth factors, such as excessive estradiol and IGF-1; familial factors, such as a family history of breast cancer; and environmental factors, such as ionizing radiation. Physical activity and lack of postmenopausal weight gain may be risk-reducing factors.

10. A dominating movement in the field of cancer research is that epithelial function depends on the *entire* tissue including the stroma or microenvironment. Breast cancer and other types of cancer are becoming known as tissue-based diseases with a possible abnormal, aberrant wound healing and inflammatory stromal (reactive stroma) component.

11. The exact molecular events leading to breast invasion are complex and not completely understood. These events involve genetic and epigenetic alterations and cancer cell and stromal interactions. Approximately one third of breast cancers are hormone dependent (progesterone receptor positive or estrogen receptor positive).

12. Most breast cancers arise from the ductal epithelium and then may metastasize to the lymphatics, opposite breast, abdominal cavity, lungs, bones, kidneys, liver, adrenal glands, ovaries, and pituitary glands.

13. The first clinical manifestation of breast cancer is usually a small, painless lump in the breast. Other manifestations include palpable lymph nodes in the axilla, dimpling of the skin, nipple and skin retraction, nipple discharge, ulcerations, reddened skin, and bone pain associated with bony metastases.

14. Gynecomastia is the overdevelopment (hyperplasia) of breast tissue in a male. It is first seen as a firm, palpable mass at least 2 cm in diameter and is located in the subareolar area.

Continued

DID YOU UNDERSTAND?—cont'd

15. Gynecomastia affects 32% to 40% of the male population. The incidence is greatest among adolescents and men older than 50 years of age.
16. Gynecomastia is caused by hormonal or breast tissue alterations that cause estrogen to dominate. These alterations can result from systemic disorders, drugs, neoplasms, or idiopathic causes.
17. Breast cancer is relatively uncommon in males, but it has a poor prognosis because men tend to delay seeking treatment until the disease is advanced. The incidence is greatest in men in their sixties.
18. Most breast cancers in men are estrogen receptor positive.

Sexually Transmitted Infections

1. Sexually transmitted diseases are infections contracted by intimate as well as sexual contact and include systemic infections, such as tuberculosis and hepatitis, that can spread to a sexual partner.
2. The etiology of an STI may be bacterial, viral, protozoan, parasitic, or fungal.
3. Although the majority of STIs can be treated, viral-induced STIs are considered incurable.

KEY TERMS

- Acute bacterial prostatitis (ABP, category I) 828
- Adenomyosis 812
- Amenorrhea 801
- Androgen receptor (AR) signaling 835
- Anorgasmia (orgasmic dysfunction) 818
- Atypical hyperplasia (AH) 840
- Balanitis 821
- Bartholinitis (Bartholin cyst) 807
- Benign breast disease (BBD) 839
- Benign prostatic hyperplasia (BPH, benign prostatic hypertrophy) 826
- Bladder outflow obstruction 828
- Cervicitis 807
- Chemical epididymitis 826
- Chronic bacterial prostatitis (CBP, category II) 828
- Chronic prostatitis/chronic pelvic pain syndrome (CPPS, category III) 829
- Complete precocious puberty 800
- Complex sclerosing lesion (radial scar) 839
- Condyloma acuminatum 821
- Corpus luteum cyst 811
- Cryptorchidism 823
- Cyst 839
- Cystocele 809
- Delayed puberty 800
- Dermoid cyst 811
- Ductal carcinoma in situ (DCIS) 851
- Ductal hyperplasia 840
- Dysfunctional uterine bleeding (DUB) 802
- Dyspareunia (painful intercourse) 819
- Ectopic testis 823
- Endometrial polyp 811
- Endometriosis 812
- Enterocele 810
- Epididymitis 826
- Epithelial hyperplasia 839
- Epithelial-to-mesenchymal transition (EMT) 851
- Fibroblast 836
- Fibrocystic change (FCC) 839
- Florid hyperplasia 839
- Follicular cyst 811
- Functional cyst 810
- Galactorrhea (inappropriate lactation) 838
- Gynecomastia 856
- Hydrocele 823
- Infertility 819
- Intraprostatic conversion 831
- Leiomyoma 811
- Lobular carcinoma in situ (LCIS) 852
- Lobular hyperplasia 840
- Lobular involution 843
- Mammographic density (MD) 847
- Mucopurulent cervicitis (MPC) 807
- Nonbacterial prostatitis 829
- Nonpuerperal hyperprolactinemia 838
- Oophoritis 806
- Orchitis 824
- Ovarian torsion 811
- Papilloma 840
- Paraphimosis 819
- Pelvic inflammatory disease (PID) 805
- Pelvic organ prolapse (POP) 808
- Pessary 810
- Peyronie disease ("bent nail syndrome") 820
- Phimosis 819
- Polycystic ovary syndrome (PCOS) 803
- Precocious puberty 800
- Premenstrual dysphoric disorder (PMDD) 804
- Premenstrual syndrome (PMS) 804
- Priapism 821
- Primary amenorrhea 801
- Primary dysmenorrhea 801
- Prolactin-inhibiting factor (PIF) 838
- Prostatic epithelial neoplasia (PIN) 835
- Prostatitis 828
- Rectocele 810
- Salpingitis 806
- Sclerosing adenosis 839
- Secondary amenorrhea 801
- Secondary dysmenorrhea 801
- Sexual dysfunction 837
- Spermatocele (epididymal cyst) 823
- Stress incontinence 809
- Stroma 836
- Testicular appendage 824
- Torsion of the testis 824
- Urethral stricture 819
- Urethritis 819
- Urethrocele 809
- Vaginismus 818
- Vaginitis 807
- Varicocele 822
- Vulvovestibulitis (VV) 807
- Xenoestrogen 849

REFERENCES

1. American Cancer Society: *Cancer facts & figures 2010*, Atlanta, 2010, Author.
2. Slyper AH: The pubertal timing controversy in the USA and a review of possible causative factors for the advance in timing of onset of puberty, *Clin Endocrinol* 65(1):1–8, 2006.
3. Jospe N: Disorders of pubertal development. In Osborn LM, et al, editors: *Pediatrics*, Philadelphia, 2005, Mosby.
4. Burchett MLR, et al: Endocrine and metabolic diseases. In Burns CE, et al, editors: *Pediatric primary care*, St Louis, 2009, Saunders.
5. Foster DL, et al: Programming of GnRH feedback controls timing puberty and adult reproductive activity, *Mol Cell Endocrinol* 254–255:109–119, 2006.
6. Euling SY, et al: Examination of US puberty-timing data from 1940 to 1994 for secular trends: panel findings, *Pediatrics* 12(suppl 3):S172–S191, 2008.
7. Fritz MA, Speroff L: *Clinical gynecologic endocrinology and infertility*, ed 8, Philadelphia, 2011, Lippincott Williams & Wilkins.

8. Dawood MY: Primary dysmenorrhea: advances in pathogenesis and management, *Obstet Gynecol* 108(2):428–441, 2006.

9. Harel Z: Dysmenorrhea in adolescents and young adults: from pathophysiology to pharmacological treatments and management strategies, *Exp Opin Pharmacother* 9(15):2661–2672, 2008.

10. Proctor ML, et al: Transcutaneous electrical nerve stimulation and acupuncture for primary dysmenorrhea, *Cochrane Database Syst Rev* (1):CD002123, 2002.

11. Pitkin J: Dysfunctional uterine bleeding, *Br Med J* 334(7603):1110–1111, 2007.

12. Schorge JO, et al, editors: *William's gynecology*, New York, 2008, McGraw-Hill.

13. Faucher MA, Schuiling KD: Normal and abnormal uterine bleeding. In Schuiling KD, et al, editors: *Women's gynecologic health*, Sudbury, Mass, 2006, Jones and Bartlett.

14. Hickey M, et al: Progesterones versus oestrogens and progestogens for irregular uterine bleeding associated with anovulation, *Cochrane Database Syst Rev* (4):CD001895, 2007.

15. Azziz R, et al: The Androgen Excess and PCOS Society criteria for the polycystic ovary syndrome: the complete task force reports, *Fertil Steril* 91(2):456–488, 2009.

16. Diamanti-Kandarakis E: Polycystic ovarian syndrome: pathophysiology, molecular aspects and clinical implications, *Exp Rev Mol Med* 10(2):e3, 2008.

17. Legro RS: Polycystic ovarian syndrome. In Leung PC, Adashi EY, editors: *The ovary*, ed 2, St Louis, 2004, Elsevier Academic Press.

18. Palomba S, et al: Role of metformin in patients with polycystic ovary syndrome: the state of the art, *Minerva Ginecol* 60(1):77–82, 2008.

19. Sinawat S, et al: Long versus short term course treatment with metformin and clomiphene citrate for ovulation induction in women with PCOS, *Cochrane Database Syst Rev* (1):CD006226, 2008.

20. Moran LJ, et al: Dietary therapy in polycystic ovary syndromes, *Semin Reprod Med* 26(1):85–92, 2008.

21. Yonkers KA, et al: Premenstrual syndrome, *Lancet* 371(9619):1200–1210, 2008.

22. Halbreich U: The etiology, biology, and evolving pathology of premenstrual syndromes, *Psychoneuroendocrinol* 28(3):55–99, 2003.

23. Halbreich U, Monacelli E: Some clues to the etiology of premenstrual syndrome/premenstrual dysphoric disorder, *Prim Psychiatry* 11:33–40, 2004.

24. Jarvis CI, Lynch AM, Morin AK: Management strategies for premenstrual syndrome/premenstrual dysphoric disorder, *Ann Pharmacother* 42(7):967–978, 2008.

25. Rapkin AJ: Premenstrual symptoms: current concepts in diagnosis and treatment, *J Reprod Med* 51(4):337–338, 2006.

26. Wyatt KM, et al: The effectiveness of GnRH with and without 'add-back' therapy in treating premenstrual syndrome: a meta-analysis, *BJOG* 111(6):585–593, 2004.

27. Centers for Disease Control and Prevention: *Sexually transmitted disease surveillance 2009*, Atlanta, 2010, U.S. Department of Health and Human Services.

28. Centers for Disease Control and Prevention: Sexually transmitted diseases treatment guidelines, *MMWR Morb Mortal Wkly Rep* 59(RR-12):1–110, 2010.

29. Jaiyeoba O, Lazenby G, Soper DE: Recommendations and rationale for the treatment of pelvic inflammatory disease, *Exp Rev Anti Infect Ther* 9(1):61–70, 2011.

30. Hainer B, Gibson M: Vaginitis: diagnosis and treatment, *Am Fam Physician* 83(7):807–815, 2011.

31. Goldstein AT, Burrows L: Vulvodynia, *J Sex Med* 5(1):5–14, 2008. quiz 15.

32. Gunter J: Vulvodynia: new thoughts on a devastating condition, *Obstet Gynecol Surv* 62(12):812–819, 2007.

33. Landry TS, et al: The treatment of provoked vestibulodynia: a critical review, *Clin J Pain* 24(2):155–171, 2008.

34. Nygaard I, et al: Prevalene of symptomatic pelvic floor disorders in US women, *J Am Med Assoc* 300(11):1311–1316, 2008.

35. Hughes D: Pelvic organ prolapse. In Schorge JO, et al, editors: *Williams gynecology*, New York, 2008, McGraw-Hill, pp 532–555.

36. Jelovsek JE, et al: Pelvic organ prolapse, *Lancet* 369(9566):1027–1038, 2007.

37. Hoffman BL: Pelvic mass. In Schorge JO, et al: *Williams gynecology*, New York, 2008, McGraw-Hill, pp 187–224.

38. Silberstein T, et al: Endometrial polyps in reproductive-age fertile and infertile women, *Isr Med Assoc J* 8(3):192–195, 2006.

39. Okolo S: Incidence, aetiology, and epidemiology of uterine fibroids, *Best Pract Res Clin Obstet Gynaecol* 22(4):571–588, 2008.

40. Tropeano G, Amoroso S, Scambia G: Non-surgical management of uterine fibroids, *Hum Reprod Update* 14(3):259–274, 2008.

41. Viswanathan M, et al: Management of uterine fibroids: an update of the evidence, *Evid Rep Technol Assess* (154):1–122, 2007.

42. Fong K, et al: Transvaginal US and hysterosonography in postmenopausal women with breast cancer receiving tamoxifen: correlation with hysteroscopy and pathologic study, *Radiographics* 23(1):137–150, 2003. discussion 151–155.

43. Carr BR: Endometriosis. In Schorge JO, et al: *Williams gynecology*, New York, 2008, McGraw-Hill, pp 225–254.

44. Forrest DE: Common gynecologic pelvic disorders. In Youngkin EQ, Davis MS, editors: *Women's health: a primary care clinical guide*, ed 3, Stamford, Conn, 2004, Appleton & Lange.

45. Widdice LE, Moscicki AB: Updated guidelines for Papanicolaou tests, colposcopy, and human papillomavirus testing in adolescents, *J Adolesc Health* 43(suppl 4):S41–S51, 2008.

46. Griffith WF: Preinvasive lesions of the lower genital tract. In Scorge JO, et al, editors: *Williams gynecology*, New York, 2008, McGraw-Hill Medical, pp 617–645.

47. Nishida KJ: Vaginal cancer. In Schorge JO, et al, editors: *Williams gynecology*, New York, 2008, McGraw-Hill, pp 677–686.

48. Lea JS: Invasive cancer of the vulva. In Schorge JO, et al, editors: *Williams gynecology*, New York, 2008, McGraw-Hill, pp 665–676.

49. American Cancer Society: *Overview: ovarian cancer*, New York, 2010, Author.

50. Wiegand KC, et al: *ARID1A* mutations in endometriosis-associated ovarian carcinomas, *N Engl J Med* 363(16):1532–1543, 2010.

51. Olshansky E: Infertility. In Schuiling KD, Likis FE, editors: *Women's gynecologic health*, Sudbury, Mass, 2006, Jones & Bartlett.

52. Kwiatkowska B, Filipowicz-Sosnowska A: Reactive arthritis, *Pol Arch Med Wewn* 119(1–2):60–65, 2009.

53. Montorsi F, et al: Summary of the recommendations on sexual dysfunctions in men, *J Sex Med* 7:3572–3588, 2010.

54. American Cancer Society: *Penile cancer resource center*, 2008. Available at www.cancer.org.

55. Trottler H, Burchell AN: Epidemiology of mucosal human papillomavirus infection and associated diseases, *Public Hlth Genomics* 12(5–6):291–307, 2009.

56. Pagliaro LC, et al: Neoadjuvant paclitaxel, ifosfamide, and cisplatin chemotherapy for metastatic penile cancer: a phase II study, *J Clin Oncol* 28:3851, 2010.

57. American Cancer Society: *Penile cancer*, New York, 2008, Author.

58. Wampler SM, Llanes M: Common scrotal and testicular problems, *Prim Care* 37(3):613–626, 2010.

59. Walsh TJ, et al: Prepubertal orchiopexy for crytorchidism may be associated with lower risk of testicular cancer, *J Urol* 178(4 pt 1):1440–1446, 2007.

60. Esosito C, et al: Management of boys with nonpalpable undescended testis, *Nat Clin Pract Urol* 5(5):252–260, 2008.

61. CancerNet: *Cancer facts: questions and answers about testicular cancer*, 2000, National Cancer Institute. Available at www.cancernet.nci.nih.gov/.

62. Trojian TH, Lishnak TS, Heiman D: Epididymitis and orchitis: an overview, *Am Fam Physician* 79(7):583–587, 2009.

63. Penna G, et al: Human benign hyperplasia stromal cells as inducers and targets of chronic immune-mediated inflammation, *J Immunol* 182(7):4056–4064, 2009.

64. Ho CK, Habib FK: Estrogen and androgen signaling in the pathogenesis of BPH, *Nat Rev Urol* 8:29–41, 2011.

65. Suzuki H, Nakada T: Alteration of collagen biosynthesis and analysis of type I and type III collagens of prostate in young rats following sex hormone treatments, *Arch Androl* 36:205–216, 1996.

66. Bianchi-Frias D, et al: The effects of aging on the molecular and cellular composition of the prostate microenvironment, *PLoS* 5(9):e12501, 2010.

67. Sampson N, Madersbacher S, Berger P: Pathophysiology and therapy of benign prostatic hyperplasia, *Wien Klin Wochenscher* 120(13–14):390–401, 2008.

68. Schauer IG: Elevated epithelial expression to interleukin-8 correlates with a myoblast reactive stroma in benign prostatic hyperplasia, *Urology* 72(1):205–213, 2008.

69. Ghafar MA, et al: Does the prostatic vascular system contribute to the development of benign prostatic hyperplasia? *Curr Urol Rep* 3(4):292–296, 2002. review.

70. Semenza GL: Regulation of vascularization by hypoxia-inducible factor 1, *Ann N Y Acad Sci* 1177:2–8, 2009.

71. Roehrborn CG, Rosen RC: Medical therapy options for aging men with benign prostatic hyperplasia: focus with afuzosin 10 mg once daily, *Clin Interv Aging* 3(30):511–524, 2008.

72. Sampson N, et al: The ageing male reproductive tract, *J Pathol* 211(2):206–218, 2007.

73. Burke JP, et al: Association of anthropometric measures with the presence and progression of benign prostatic hyperplasia, *Am J Epidemiol* 164(1):41–46, 2006.

74. Kasturi S, Russell S, McVary KT: Metabolic syndrome and lower urinary tract symptoms secondary to benign prostatic hyperplasia, *Curr Urol Rep* 7(4):288–292, 2006.

75. Garg G, et al: Management of benign prostate hyperplasia: an overview of alpha-adrenergic antagonist, *Biol Pharm Bull* 29(8):1554–1558, 2006.

76. Wilt TJ, Mac Donald R, Rutks I: Tamsulosin for benign prostatic hyperplasia, *Cochrane Database Syst Rev* (1):CD002081, 2003.

77. Touma NJ, Nickel JC: Prostatitis and chronic pelvic pain in men, *Med Clin North Am* 95:75–86, 2011.

78. LaRock DR, Sant GR: Lower urinary tract infections. In Nseyo UO, Weinman E, Lamm DL, editors: *Urology for primary care physicians*, Philadelphia, 1999, Saunders.

79. Karatas OF, et al: *Helicobacter pylori* seroprevalence in patients with chronic prostatitis: a pilot study, *Scand J Urol Nephrol* 44(2):91–94, 2010.

80. Jemal A, et al: Global patterns of cancer incidence and mortality rates and trends, *Cancer Epidemiol Biomarkers Prev* 19:1893–1907, 2010.

81. Draisma G: Lead time and overdiagnosis in prostate-specific antigen screening: importance of methods and context, *J Natl Cancer Inst* 101:347–383, 2009.

82. Etzioni R, et al: Overdiagnosis due to prostate-specific antigen screening: lessons from U.S. prostate cancer incidence trends, *J Natl Cancer Inst* 94:981–990, 2002.

83. Baade PD, Youlden DR, Krnjacki LJ: International epidemiology of prostate cancer: geographical distribution and secular trends, *Mol Nutr Food Res* 53:171–184, 2009.

84. Collin SM, et al: Prostate-cancer mortality in the USA and UK in 1975–2004: an ecological study, *Lancet Oncol* 9:445–452, 2008.

85. Etzioni R, et al: Quantifying the role of PSA screening in the US prostate cancer mortality decline, *Cancer Causes Control* 19:175–181, 2008.

86. Andriole GL, et al: Mortality results from a randomized prostate-cancer screening trial, *N Engl J Med* 360:1310–1319, 2009.

87. Schroder FH, et al: Screening and prostate-cancer mortality in a randomized European study, *N Engl J Med* 360:1320–1328, 2009.

88. Venkateswaran V, Klotz LH: Diet and prostate cancer: mechanisms of action and implications for chemoprevention, *Nat Rev Urol* 7:442–453, 2010.

89. Zhao XY, et al: 1-alpha,25-Dihydroxyvitamin D3 inhibits prostate cancer cell growth by androgen-dependent and androgen-independent mechanisms, *Endocrinol* 141(7):2548–2556, 2000.

90. CaP CURE Nutrition Project: *Nutrition and prostate cancer a monograph from the CaP CURE Nutrition Project* ed 3, 1999, Santa Monica Calif, p 4.

91. Belanger B, et al: Comparison of residual C-19 steroids in plasma and prostatic tissue of human, rat, guinea pig after castration: unique importance of extratesticular androgens in men, *J Steroid Biochem* 32:695–698, 1989.

92. Labrie F: Blockage of testicular and adrenal androgens in prostate cancer treatment, *Nat Rev Urol* 8:73–80, 2011.

93. Montgomery RB: Maintenance of intratumoral androgens in metastatic prostate cancer: a mechanism for castration-resistant tumor growth, *Cancer Res* 68(11):4447–4454, 2008.

94. Bosland MC: The role of steroid hormones in prostate carcinogenesis, *J Natl Cancer Inst Mongr* (27):39–66, 2000.

95. Bosland MC: Sex steroids and prostate carcinogenesis: integrated, multifactorial working hypothesis, *Ann N Y Acad Sci* 1089:168–176, 2006.

96. Ellem SJ, Risbridger GP: The dual, opposing roles of estrogen in the prostate, *Ann N Y Acad Sci* 1155:174–186, 2009.

97. Thompson IM, et al: The influence of finasteride on the development of prostate cancer, *N Engl J Med* 349:215–224, 2003.

98. Meinbach DS, Lokeshwar BL: Insulin-like growth factors and their binding proteins in prostate cancer: cause of consequence? *Urol Oncol* 24(4):294–306, 2006.

99. Peterson DE, et al: Vasectomy and the risk of prostate cancer, *Am J Epidemiol* 135(3):324–325, 1992.

100. Ferris-Tortajada J, et al: Constitutional risk factors in prostate cancer, *Actas Urol Esp* 35(5):289–295, 2011.

101. Giovannucci E, et al: Insulin-like growth factors and colon cancer: a review of the evidence, *J Nutr* 131(suppl 11):3109S–3120S, 2001. review.

102. MacLennan GT, et al: The influence of chronic inflammation in prostatic carcinogenesis: a 5-year follow-up study, *J Urol* 176(3):1012–1016, 2006.

103. Epstein JI: The lower urinary tract and male genital system. In Kumar V, Abbas AK, Fausto N, editors: *Robbins and Cotran pathologic basis of disease*, ed 8, Philadelphia, 2009, Saunders.

104. Narayan P: Neoplasms of the prostate gland. In Tanagho EA, McAninch JW, editors: *Smith's general urology*, ed 14, Norwalk, Conn, 1995, Appleton & Lange.

105. Brown SL, Resnick MI: Transrectal ultrasound and the prostate biopsy: clinical and pathologic issues. In Lepor H, editor: *Prostatic diseases*, Philadelphia, 2000, Saunders.

106. Mackinnon AC, et al: Molecular biology underlying the clinical heterogeneity of prostate cancer: an update, *Arch Pathol Lab Med* 133(7):1033–1040, 2009.

107. Bonkoff H, Berges R: The evolving role of oestrogens and their receptors in the development and progression of prostate cancer, *Euro Urology* 55:533–542, 2009.

108. Ellem SJ, Risbridger GP: Aromatase and regulating the estrogen: androgen ratio in the prostate gland, *J Steroid Biochem Mol Biol* 118(4–5):246–251, 2010.

109. Parnes HL, Thompson IM, Ford LG: Review article: prevention of hormone-related cancers: prostate cancer, *J Clin Oncol* 23(2):368–377, 2005.

110. Ellem SJ, et al: Local aromatase expression in human prostate is altered in malignancy, *J Clin Endocrinol Metab* 89(5):2434–2441, 2004.

111. Bonkhoff H, et al: Progesterone receptor expression in human prostate cancer: correlation with tumor progression, *Prostate* 48(4):285–291, 2001.

112. Setlur SR, et al: Estrogen-dependent signaling in a molecularly distinct subclass of aggressive prostate cancer, *J Natl Cancer Inst* 100:815–825, 2008.

113. Vander Griend DJ, et al: Cell autonomous intracellular androgen signaling drives the growth of human prostate cancer-initiating cells, *Prostate* 70(1):90–99, 2010.

114. DeMarzo AM, et al: Inflammation in prostate carcinogenesis, *Nat Rev Cancer* 7:256–269, 2007.

115. Marian CO, Shay JW: Prostate tumor initiating cells: a new target for telomerase inhibition therapy? *Biochim Biophys Acta* 1792:289–296, 2009.

116. DeMagalhaes JP, Curado J, Church GM: Meta-analysis of age-related gene expression profiles identifies common signatures of aging, *Bioinformatics* 25:875–881, 2009.

117. Kim SK: Common aging pathways in worms, flies, mice and humans, *J Exp Biol* 210:1607–1612, 2007.

118. Kuilman T, et al: Oncogene-induced senescence relayed by an interleukin-dependent inflammatory network, *Cell* 133:1019–1031, 2008.

119. Paapatto GS, et al: Prostate carcinogenesis and inflammation: emerging insights, *Carcinogenesis* 26:1170–1181, 2005.

120. Elo TD, et al: Stromal activation associated with development of prostate cancer in prostate-targeted fibroblast growth factor 8b transgenic mice, *Neoplasia* 12(11):915–927, 2010.

121. Thiery JP: Epithelial-mesenchymal transitions in tumor progression, *Nat Rev Cancer* 2(6):442–454, 2002.

122. Josson S, et al: Tumor-stromal interaction influence radiation sensitivity in epithelial versus mesenchymal-like prostate cancer cell, *J Oncol* pii: 232831, 2010.

123. Bhowmick NA, Moses HL: Tumor-stroma interactions, *Curr Opin Genet Develop* 15(1):97–101, 2005.

124. Xu J, et al: Prostate cancer metastasis: role of the host microenvironment in promoting epithelial to mesenchymal transition and increase bone adrenal gland metastasis, *Prostate* 66:1664–1673, 2006.

125. Liu W, et al: Copy number analysis indicates monoclonal origin of lethal metastatic prostate cancer, *Nat Med* 15(5):559–565, 2009.

126. Vickers A, et al: An empirical evaluation of guidelines on prostate-specific antigen velocity in prostate cancer detection, *J Natl Cancer Inst* 103(6):462–469, 2011.

127. Stamey TA: The era of serum prostate specific antigens as a marker for biopsy of the prostate and detecting prostate cancer is now over in the USA, *BJU Int* 94(7):963–964, 2004.

128. Jefferson Health System, Men's Health: *Overview of impotence,* 1997. Available at www.jeffersonhealth.orgdiseases/mens_health/impotenc.htm.

129. Carson CC: Long-term use of sildenafil, *Exp Opin Pharmacother* 4(3):397–405, 2003.

130. Raivio T, Wikstrom AM, Dunkel L: Treatment of gonadotropin-deficient boys with recombinant human FSH: long term observation and outcome, *Eur J Endocrinol* 156(1):105–111, 2007.

131. Ferlin A, et al: The human Y chromosome azoospermia factor b (AZFb) region: sequence, structure, and deletion analysis in infertile men, *J Med Genet* 40(1):18–24, 2003.

132. BrughIII VM, Maduro MR, Lamb DJ: Genetic disorders and infertility, *Urol Clin North Am* 30(1):143–152, 2003.

133. Lewis-Jones I, et al: Sperm chromosomal abnormalities are linked to sperm morphologic deformities, *Fertil Steril* 79(1):212–215, 2003.

134. Padrich DA: Testicular cancer and male infertility, *Curr Opin Urol* 16(6):419–427, 2006.

135. Pagani R, BrughIII VM, Lamb DJ: Y chromosome genes and male infertility, *Urol Clin North Am* 29(4):745–753, 2002. review.

136. Turek PJ, Pera RA: Current and future genetic screening for male infertility, *Urol Clin North Am* 29(4):767–792, 2002.

137. Check JH: The infertile male: diagnosis, *Clin Exp Obstet Gynecol* 33(3):133–139, 2006.

138. Speroff L, Glass RH, Kase NG: *Clinical gynecologic endocrinology and infertility,* ed 6, Baltimore, 1999, Williams & Wilkins.

139. Kase N, Weingold AB, Gershenon DM, editors: *Principles and practice of clinical gynecology,* ed 2, New York, 1990, Churchill Livingstone.

140. Hartmann LC, et al: Benign breast disease and risk of breast cancer, *N Engl J Med* 353(3):229–237, 2005.

141. Lester SC: The breast. In Kumar V, Abbas AK, Fausto N, editors: *Robbins & Cotran pathologic basis of disease,* ed 7, Philadelphia, 2005, Elsevier-Saunders.

142. Jacobs TW: Radial scars in benign breast-biopsy specimens and the risk of breast cancer, *N Engl J Med* 340(6):430, 1999.

143. Warsham MJ, et al: Multiplicity of benign lesions is a risk factor for progression to breast cancer, *Clin Cancer Res* 13(18 pt 1):5474–5479, 2007.

144. Perry N, Bartella L, Morrison I: The radial scar. In Rovere GQD, Warren R, Benson JR, editors: *Early breast cancer: from screening to multidisciplinary management,* New York, 2006, Taylor & Francis.

145. Sanders ME, et al: Interdependence of radial scar and proliferative disease with respect to invasive breast carcinoma risk to patients with benign breast biopsies, *Cancer* 106(7):1453–1461, 2006.

146. Berg JC, et al: Breast cancer risk in women with radial scars in benign breast biopsies, *Breast Cancer Res Treat* 108(2):167–174, 2008.

147. Berg JW: Clinical implications of risk factors for breast cancer, *Cancer* 53(suppl 3):589–591, 1984.

148. Lewis JT, et al: An analysis of breast cancer risk in women with single, multiple, and atypical papilloma, *Am J Surg Pathol* 30(6):665–672, 2006.

149. Collins LC, et al: Magnitude and laterality of breast cancer risk according to histologic type of atypical hyperphasia: results from the Nurses' Health Study, *Cancer* 109(2):180–187, 2006.

150. Page DL, et al: Atypical hyperplastic lesions of the female breast. A long-term follow-up study, *Cancer* 55:2698–2708, 1985.

151. Page DL, et al: Atypical lobular hyperplasia as a unilateral predictor of breast cancer risk: a retrospective cohort study, *Lancet* 361:125–129, 2003.

152. Hollowell JG, et al: Iodine nutrition in the United States. Trends and public health implications: iodine excretion data from National Health and Nutrition Examination Surveys I and II (1971–1974 and 1988–1994), *J Clin Endocrinol Metab* 83(10):3401–3408, 1998.

153. Li Y, et al: Genistein depletes telomerase activity through cross-talk between genetic and epigenetic mechanism, *Int J Cancer* 125(2):286–296, 2009.

154. Iodine monograph, *Altern Med Rev* 15(3):273–278, 2010.

155. Howlander N, et al: *SEER cancer statistics review, 1975–2008,* Bethesda, Md, 2010, National Cancer Institute. Available at http://seer.cancer.gov/csr1975-2008/2010.

156. Axelrod D, et al: Breast cancer in young women, *J Am Coll Surg* 206(3):1193–1203, 2008.

157. Reis LAG, et al: *Cancer statistics review, 1975–2005,* Bethesda, Md, 2008, National Cancer Institute. Available at http://seer.cancer.gov/csr/1975_2005/.

158. Sternlicht MD, et al: Hormonal and local control of mammary branching morphogenesis, *Differentiation* 74:365–381, 2006.

159. Clarke LH, et al: Differentiation of mammary gland as a mechanism to reduce breast cancer risk, *J Nutr* 136:2697S–2699S, 2006.

160. Trichopoulos D, et al: Age at any birth and breast cancer risk, *J Int Cancer* 321:701–704, 1983.

161. White E: Projected changes in breast cancer incidence due to the trend toward delayed childbearing, *Am J Public Health* 77:495–497, 1987.

162. Medina D: Breast cancer: the protective effect of pregnancy, *Clin Cancer Res* 10(1 pt 2):380S–384S, 2004.

163. Hsieh C, et al: Dual effect of parity on breast cancer risk, *Eur J Cancer* 30A:969–973, 1994.

164. Williams EM, et al: Short term increase in risk of breast cancer associated with full pregnancy, *BMJ* 300:578–579, 1990.

165. MacMahon B, et al: Age at first birth and breast cancer, *Bull World Health Organ* 43:209–221, 1970.

166. Schedin P, et al: Microenvironment of the involuting mammary gland mediates mammary cancer progression, *J Mammary Gland Biol Neoplasia* 12:71–82, 2007.

167. Milanese TR, et al: Age-related lobular involution and risk of breast cancer, *J Natl Cancer Inst* 98(2):1600–1607, 2006.

168. Henson DE, Tarone RE: On the possible role of involution in the natural history of breast cancer, *Cancer* 71(suppl 6):2154–2156, 1993.

169. Henson DE, Tarone RE: Involution and the etiology of breast cancer, *Cancer* 74(suppl 1):424–429, 1994.

170. Ghosh K, et al: Independent association of lobular involution and mammographic breast density with breast cancer risk, *J Natl Cancer Inst* 102(22):1716–1723, 2010.

171. Clemmesen J: The Danish cancer registry: problems and results, *Acta Pathol Microbiol Scand* 25:26–30, 1948.

172. Cutler SY, Young JL: Third National Cancer Survey: incidence data, *Natl Cancer Inst Monog* 41, 1975.

173. Vorrherr H, editor: *The breast: morphology, physiology, and lactation,* New York, 1974, Academic Press.

174. Geschickter CD: *Diseases of the breast*, ed 2, Philadelphia, 1945, Lippincott.

175. Kelsey JL, Gammon MD, John EM: Reproductive factors and breast cancer, *Epidemiol Rev* 15:36–47, 1993.

176. Ursin G, et al: Reproductive factors and subtypes of breast cancer defined by hormone receptor and histology, *Br J Cancer* 93:364–371, 2005.

177. Trichopoulos D, et al: Age at any birth and breast cancer risk, *Int J Cancer* 31:701–704, 1983.

178. Henson DE, Tarone RE, Nsouli H: Lobular involution: the physiologic prevention of breast cancer, *J Natl Cancer Inst* 98(22):1589–1590, 2006.

179. Brisken C, O'Malley B: Hormone action in the mammary gland, *Cold Spring Harb Perspect Biol* 2(12):a003178. (Epub 2010 Aug 25.)

180. Fenton SE: Endocrine-disrupting compounds and mammary gland development: early exposure and later life consequences, *Endocrinology* 147(6 suppl):S18–S24, 2006.

181. Khokha R, Werb Z: Mammary gland reprogramming: metalloproteinases couple form with function, *Cold Spring Harb Perspect Biol* 3(4):pii. a004333, 2011.

182. Lanigan F, et al: Molecular links between mammary gland development and breast cancer, *Cell Mol Life Sci* 64:3161–3184, 2007.

183. Russo J, Russo I: *Molecular basis of breast cancer: prevention and treatment*, Germany, 2004, Springer.

184. Cheskis BJ, et al: Signaling by estrogens: mini review, *J Cell Physiol* 213(3):610–617, 2007.

185. Cheskis BJ, et al: MNAR plays an important role in ERa activation of Src/MAPK and PI3K/Akt signaling pathways, *Steroids* 73(9–10):901–905, 2008.

186. Kaaks R, et al: Postmenopausal serum androgens, oestrogens, and breast cancer risk: the European prospective investigation into cancer and nutrition, *Endocr Relat Cancer* 12(4):1017–1082, 2005.

187. Key T, et al: Endogenous sex hormones and breast cancer in postmenopausal women; reanalysis of nine prospective studies, *J Natl Cancer Inst* 94:606–616, 2002.

188. Key TJ: Endogenous oestrogens and breast cancer risk in premenopausal and postmenopausal women, *Steroids* 2011 Apr 5. [Epub ahead of print.]

189. Micheli A, et al: Endogenous sex hormones and subsequent breast cancer in premenopausal women, *Int J Cancer* 112:213–218, 2004.

190. Hankinson SE, Eliassen H: Endogenous estrogen, testosterone, and progesterone levels in relation to breast cancer risk, *J Steroid Biochem Mol Biol* 106(1–5):24–30, 2007.

191. Beral V, et al: Breast cancer and hormone-replacement therapy in the Million Women Study, *Lancet* 362(9382):419–427, 2003.

192. Rossouw JE, et al: Risks and benefits of estrogen plus progestin in healthy postmenopausal women: principle results from the Women's Health Initiative randomized controlled trial, *J Am Med Assoc* 288(3):321–333, 2002.

193. Missmer SA, et al: Endogenous estrogen, androgen, and progesterone concentrations and breast cancer risk among postmenopausal women, *J Natl Cancer Inst* 96:1856–1865, 2004.

194. Campagnoli C, et al: Progestins and progesterone in hormone replacement therapy and the risk of breast cancer, *J Steroid Biochem Mol Biol* 96(B):95–108, 2005.

195. Lanaric C, Molinolo AA: Progesterone receptors—animal models and cell signaling in breast cancer. Diverse activation pathways for the progesterone receptor: possible implications for breast biology and cancer, *Breast Can Res* 4:240–243, 2002.

196. Rajkumar L, et al: Long-term hormonal overcomes genetic resistance to mammary cancer, *Steroids* 76:31–37, 2011.

197. Asselin-Labat M, et al: Control of mammary stem cell function by steroid hormone signaling, *Nature* 465(7299):798–802, 2010.

198. Joshi PA, et al: Progesterone induces adult mammary stem cell expansion, *Nature* 465(7299):803–807, 2010.

199. Manjer J, et al: Postmenopausal breast cancer risk in relation to sex steroid hormones, prolactin and SHBG (Sweden), *Cancer Causes Control* l4, 2003. 599–560.

200. Zeleniuch-Jacquotte A, et al: Postmenopausal levels of oestrogen, androgen, and SHBG and breast cancer: long-term results of a prospective study, *Br J Cancer* 90:153–159, 2004.

201. Key TJ, et al: A prospective study of urinary oestrogen excretion and breast cancer risk, *Br J Cancer* 73:1615–1619, 1996.

202. Onland-Moret NC, et al: Urinary endogenous sex hormone levels and the risk of postmenopausal breast cancer, *Br J Cancer* 88:1394–1399, 2003.

203. Eliassen AH, et al: Endogenous steroid hormone concentrations and risk of breast cancer among predominantly premenopausal women, *J Natl Cancer Inst* 98(19):1406–1415, 2006.

204. Yager JD, Davidson NE: Estrogen carcinogenesis in breast cancer, *N Engl J Med* 354:270–282, 2006.

205. Foster PA: Steroid metabolism in breast cancer, *Minerva Endocrinol* 33:27–37, 2008.

206. Pasqualini JR, Chetrite GS: Recent insight on the control of enzymes involved in estrogen formation and transformation in human breast cancer, *J Steroid Biochem Mol Biol* 93(2–5):221–236, 2005.

207. Cavalieri E, Rogan E: Catechol quinines of estrogen in the initiation of breast, prostate, and other cancers: keynote lecture, *Ann N Y Acad Sci* 1089:286–301, 2006.

208. Cogliano V, et al: Carcinogenicity of combined estrogen-progestogen contraceptives and menopausal treatment, *Lancet Oncol* 6:552–553, 2005.

209. IARC Special Report: Policy: a review of human carcinogens—Part A: pharmaceuticals, *Lancet* 10:13–14, 2009.

210. Chlebowski RT, et al: Breast cancer after use of estrogen plus progestin in postmenopausal women, *N Engl J Med* 360:573–587, 2009.

211. Collins JA, Blake JM, Crosinani PG: Breast cancer risk with postmenopausal hormone treatment, *Hum Repro Update* 11:545–560, 2005.

212. Shah NR, Borenstein J, Dubois RW: Postmenopausal hormone therapy and breast cancer: a systematic review and meta-analysis, *Menopause* 12:668–678, 2005.

213. Ringa V, Fournier A: Did the decrease in use of menopausal hormone therapy induce a decrease in the incidence of breast cancer in France (and elsewhere)? *Rev Epidemiol Sante Publique* 56:297–301, 2008.

214. Fournier A: Should transdermal rather than oral estrogens be used in menopausal hormone therapy? A review, *Menopause Int* 16(1):23–32, 2010.

215. Canonico M, et al: Postmenopausal hormone therapy and risk of idiopathic venous thromboembolism: results from the E3N cohort study, *Arterioscler Thromb Vasc Biol* 30:340–345, 2010.

216. Lacroix AZ, et al: Health outcomes after stopping conjugated equine estrogens among postmenopausal women with prior hysterectomy: a randomized controlled trial, *J Am Med Assoc* 305(13):1305–1314, 2011.

217. Stefanick ML, et al: Effects of conjugated equine estrogens on breast cancer and mammography screening in postmenopausal women with hysterectomy, *J Am Med Assoc* 295:1647–1657, 2006.

218. Collaborative Group on Hormonal Factors in Breast Cancer: Breast cancer and hormone replacement therapy: collaborative reanalysis of data from 51 epidemiological studies of 52,705 women with breast cancer and 108,411 women without breast cancer. Collaborative Group on Hormonal Factors in Breast Cancer, *Lancet* 350(9084):1047–1059, 1997.

219. Steinberg KK, et al: A meta-analysis of the effect of estrogen replacement therapy on the risk of breast cancer, *J Am Med Assoc* 265(15):1985–1990, 1991.

220. Jordan VC, Ford LG: Paradoxical clinical effect of estrogen on breast cancer risk: a "new biology of estrogen–induced apoptosis," *Cancer Prev Res (Phila)* 2011 Apr 11. [Epub ahead of print.]

221. Rajkumar L, et al: Long-term hormonal promotion overcomes genetic resistance to mammary cancer, *Steroids* 76(1–2):31–37, 2010.

222. Beral V, et al: Breast cancer risk in relation to the interval between menopause and starting hormone therapy, *J Natl Cancer Inst* 103(4):296–305, 2011.

223. Jungheim ES, Colditz GA: Short-term use of unopposed estrogen, *J Am Med Assoc* 305(13):1354–1355, 2011.

224. Pollack M: IGF-1 physiology and breast cancer, *Recent Results Cancer Res* 152:63–70, 1998.

225. Endogenous Hormones and Breast Cancer Collaborative Group, et al: Insulin-like growth factor-1(IGF1), IGF binding protein 3 (IGFBP3), and breast cancer risk: pooled individual data analysis of 17 prospective studies, *Lancet Oncol* 11:530–542, 2010.

226. Kleinberg DL, Feldman M, Ruan W: IGF-1: an essential factor in terminal end bud formation and ductal morphogenesis, *J Mammary Gland Biol Neoplasia* 5(1):7–17, 2000. review.

227. Wu J, et al: Light at night activates IGF-1R/PDK1 signaling and accelerates tumor growth in human breast cancer xenografts, *Cancer Res* 71(7):2622–2631, 2011.

228. Wang XS, et al: Shift work and chronic disease: the epidemiological evidence, *Occup Med (Lond)* 61(2):78–89, 2011.

229. Wennbo H, Tornell J: The role of prolactin and growth hormone in breast cancer, *Oncogene* 19(8):1072–1076, 2000.

230. Renehen AG, Brennan BM: Acromegaly, growth hormone and cancer risk, *Best Pract Res Clin Endocrinol Metab* 22:639–657, 2008.

231. Schernhammer ES, et al: Insulin-like growth factor-l, its binding protein (LGFBP-L and IBFBP-3), and growth hormone and breast cancer risk in The Nurses Health Study II, *Endocr Relat Cancer* 13:583–592, 2006.

232. Tworoger SS, et al: A prospective study of plasma prolactin concentrations and risk of premenopausal and postmenopausal breast cancer, *J Clin Oncol* 25:1482–1488, 2007.

233. Tanaka Y, et al: Gonadotropins stimulate growth of MCF-7 human breast cancer cells by promoting intercellular conversion of adrenal androgens to estrogens, *Oncol* 59(suppl 11):19–23, 2000.

234. IIes RK, Delves PJ, Butler SA: Does hCG or hCGβ play a role in cancer cell biology review? *Mol Cell Endocrinol* 329(1–2):62–70, 2010.

235. Boyd NF, et al: Mammographic breast density as an intermediate phenotype for breast cancer, *Lancet Oncol* 6(10):798–808, 2005.

236. Vachon CM, et al: Mammographic density, breast cancer risk and risk prediction breast, *Cancer Res* 9(6):217, 2007.

237. Boyd NF, et al: Mammographic density and the risk and detection of breast cancer, *N Engl J Med* 56(3):227–236, 2007.

238. Wiseman BS, Werb Z: Stromal effects on mammary gland development and breast cancer, *Science* 296(5570):1046–1049, 2002.

239. Brenner DJ: We don't know enough about low-dose radiation risk, *Nature*, 2011. doi.10.1038/news.2011.206.

240. Semelka R: Imaging x-rays cause cancer: a call to action for caregivers and patients, *Medscape*, Feb 13, 2006.

241. Michels KB, et al: Diet and breast cancer: a review of the prospective observational studies, *Cancer* 109(suppl 12):2712–2749, 2007.

242. Bartsch H, Nair J, Owen RW: Dietary polyunsaturated fatty acids and cancer of the breast and colorectum: emerging evidence for their role as risk modifiers, *Carcinogenesis* 20(12):2209, 1999.

243. Linos E, Holmes MD, Willett WC: Diet and breast cancer, *Curr Oncol Rep* 9(1):31–41, 2007.

244. Ariazi JL, et al: Mammary glands of sexually immature rats are more susceptible than those of mature rats to the carcinogenic, lethal, and mutagenic effects of N-nitroso-N-methylurea, *Mol Carcinog* 43(3):155–164, 2005.

245. Russo J, Russo IH: Cellular basis of breast cancer susceptibility, *Oncol Res* 11(4):169–178, 1999.

246. Land CE, et al: Incidence of female breast cancer among atomic bomb survivors, Hiroshima and Nagasaki, 1950–1990, *Radiat Res* 160(6):707–717, 2003.

247. Linos E, et al: Adolescent diet and risk of breast cancer among premenopausal women, *Cancer Epidemiol Biomarkers Prev* 19(3):689–696, 2010.

248. Couto E, et al: Mediterranean dietary pattern and cancer risk in the EPIC cohort, *Br J Cancer* 104:1493–1499, 2011.

249. Michels KB, et al: Adult weight change and incidence of premenopausal breast cancer, *Int J Cancer* 2011 Mar 16. [Epub ahead of print.]

250. Connolly BS, et al: A meta-analysis of published literature on waist-to-hip ratio and risk of breast cancer? *Lancet* 368(9536):624–625, 2006.

251. Harvie M, Hooper L, Howell AH: Central obesity and breast cancer risk: a systematic review, *Obes Rev* 4(3):157–173, 2003.

252. Vaino H, Bianchini F, editors: *IARC. International Agency for Research in Cancer. Weight control and physical activity*, Lyon, 2002, IARC Press.

253. World Cancer Research Fund (WCRF): *Food, nutrition, physical activity, and the prevention of cancer; a global perspective*, ed 2, Washington, DC, 2007, American Institute for Cancer Research.

254. Holmes MD, Willett WC: Does diet affect breast cancer risk? *Breast Cancer Res* 6(4):170–178, 2004.

255. Wenten M, et al: Associations of weight, weight change, and body mass with breast cancer risk in Hispanic and non-Hispanic white women, *Ann Epidemiol* 12(6):435–444, 2002.

256. Trentham-Diaz A, et al: Weight change and risk of postmenopausal breast cancer (United States), *Cancer Causes Control* 11(6):533–542, 2000.

257. Le Marchand L, et al: Body size at different periods of life and breast cancer risk, *Am J Epidemiol* 128(1):137–152, 1998.

258. Morimoto LM, et al: Obesity, body size, and risk of postmenopausal breast cancer: the Women's Health Initiative (United States), *Cancer Causes Control* 13(8):741–751, 2002.

259. Endogenous Hormones Breast Cancer Collaborative Group: Body mass index, serum sex hormones, and breast cancer risk in postmenopausal women, *J Natl Cancer Inst* 95(6):1218–1226, 2003.

260. Tretli S, Gaard M: Lifestyle changes during adolescence and risk of breast cancer: an ecologic study of the effect of World War II in Norway, *Cancer Causes Control* 7(5):507–512, 1996.

261. Renehan AG, Soerjomataram I, Leitzmann MF: Interpreting the epidemiological evidence linking obesity and cancer: a framework for population-attributable risk estimations in Europe, *Eur J Cancer* 46:2581–2592, 2010.

262. Byers T: Nutritional risk factors for breast cancer, *CA Cancer J Clin* 74(suppl 1):288, 1994.

263. Mahabir S, et al: Usefulness of body mass index as a sufficient adiposity measurement for sex hormone concentration associations in postmenopausal women, *Cancer Epidemiol Biomarkers Prev* 15(12):2502–2507, 2006.

264. Korner A, et al: Total and high molecular weight adiponectin in breast cancer: in vitro and in vivo studies, *J Clin Endocrinol Metab* 92(3):1041–1048, 2007.

265. Surmacz E: Obesity hormone leptin: a new target in breast cancer? *Breast Cancer Res* 9(1):301, 2007.

266. Jarde T, et al: Molecular mechanism of leptin and adiponectin in breast cancer, *Eur J Cancer* 47:33–43, 2011.

267. Arditi JD, et al: Antiproliferative effect of adiponectin on MCF7 breast cancer cells: a potential hormonal link between obesity and cancer, *Horm Metab Res* 39(1):9–13, 2007.

268. Merzenich H, Boeing H, Wahrendorf J: Dietary fat and sports activity as determinants of age at menarche, *Am J Epidemiol* 138(4):217–224, 1993.

269. Chen J, Campbell TC, Junyao L: *Diet, lifestyle, and mortality in China: a study of the characteristics of 65 Chinese counties*, Oxford, England, 1990, Oxford University Press.

270. Cho E, et al: *Premenopausal dietary carbohydrate, glycemic index, glycemic load, and fiber in relation to risk of breast cancer*, Toronto, Canada, 2003, American Association for Cancer Research.

271. Terry P, et al: No association among total dietary fiber, fiberfractions, and risk of breast cancer, *Cancer Epidemiol Biomarkers Prev* 11(11):1507–1508, 2002.

272. Witte JS, et al: Diet and premenopausal bilateral breast cancer: a case-control study, *Breast Cancer Res Treat* 42(3):243–251, 1997.

273. Kuller LH: The etiology of breast cancer: from epidemiology to prevention, *Public Health Rev* 23(2):157–213, 1995.

274. Key J, et al: Meta-analysis of studies of alcohol and breast cancer with consideration of the methodological issues, *Cancer Causes Control* 17(6):759–770, 2006.

275. Ginsburg ES, et al: The effect of acute ethanol ingestion on estrogen levels in postmenopausal women using transdermal estradiol, *J Soc Gynecol Investig* 2(1):26–29, 1995.

276. Sellers TA, et al: Dietary folate intake, alcohol, and risk of breast cancer in a prospective study of postmenopausal women, *Epidemiology* 12(4):420–428, 2001.

277. Zhang S, et al: A prospective study of folate intake and the risk of breast cancer, *JAMA* 281(17):1632–1637, 1999.

278. Key TJ: Minireview: fruit and vegetables and cancer risk, *Br J Cancer* 104:6–11, 2011.

279. Cross HS, et al: Phytoestrogens and vitamin D metabolism: a new concept for the prevention and therapy of colorectal, prostate, and mammary carcinomas, *J Nutr* 134(5):1207–1212S, 2004.

280. Nagata C: Factors to consider in the association between soy isoflavone intake and breast cancer risk, *J Epidemiol* 20(2):83–89, 2010.

281. Petrakis NL, et al: Stimulatory influence of soy protein isolate on breast secretion in pre- and postmenopausal women, *Cancer Epidemiol Biomarkers Prev* 5(10):785–794, 1996.

282. Venturi S: Is there a role for iodine in breast disease? *The Breast* 10:379–382, 2001.

283. Aceves C, Anguiano B, Delgado G: Is iodine a gatekeeper of the integrity of the mammary gland? *J Mammary Gland Biol Neoplasia* 10(2):189–196, 2005.

284. Cann SA, van Netten JP, van Netten C: Hypothesis: iodine, selenium and the development of breast cancer, *Cancer Causes Control* 11:121–127, 2000.

285. Eskin BA, et al: Different tissue responses for iodine and iodide in rat thyroid and mammary glands, *Biol Trace Elem Res* 49:9–19, 1995.

286. Ghent WR, et al: Iodine replacement in fibrocystic disease of the breast, *Can J Surg* 36:453–460, 1993.

287. Funahashi H, et al: Seaweed prevents breast cancer, *Jpn J Cancer Res* 92(5):483–487, 2001.

288. Smyth PP: Role of iodine in antioxidant defense in thyroid and breast disease, *Biofactors* 19(3–4):121–130, 2003.

289. Bennett LM, Davis BJ: Identification of mammary carcinogens in rodent bioassays, *Environ Mol Mutagen* 39(2–3):150–157, 2002.

290. Friedenreich CM, Orenstein MR: Physical activity and cancer prevention: etiologic evidence and biological mechanisms, *J Nutr* 132(suppl 11):3464–3465S, 2002.

291. Kaaks R, Lukanova A: Effects of weight control and physical activity in cancer prevention: role of endogenous hormone metabolism, *Ann N Y Acad Sci* 963:268–281, 2002.

292. Garber JE, Offit K: Hereditary cancer predisposition syndromes, *J Clin Oncol* 23(2):276–292, 2005.

293. Sprague BL, et al: Lifetime recreational and occupational physical activity and risk of in situ and invasive breast cancer, *Cancer Epidemiol Biomarkers Prev* 16(2):236–243, 2007.

294. Rennix CP, et al: Risk of breast cancer among enlisted army women occupationally exposed to volatile organic compounds, *Am J Ind Med* 48:157–167, 2005.

295. Newman B, et al: Frequency of breast cancer attributable to BRCA1 in population-based series of American women, *J Am Med Assoc* 279(12):915–921, 1998.

296. Miki Y, et al: A strong candidate for the breast and ovarian cancer susceptibility gene BRCA1, *Science* 266(5182):66–71, 1994.

297. Sullivan A, et al: Concomitant inactivation of p53 and ChK2 in breast cancer, *Oncogene* 21(9):1316–1324, 2002.

298. Damonte P, et al: Mammary carcinoma behavior is programmed in the precancer stem cell, *Breast Cancer Res* 10(3):R50, 2008.

299. Hanahan D, Weinberg R: Hallmarks of cancer: the next generation, *Cell* 144:646–674, 2011.

300. Bombonati A, Sgroi DC: The molecular pathology of breast cancer progression, *J Pathol* 223:307–317, 2011.

301. Stingl J, et al: Epithelial progenitors in the normal human mammary gland, *J Mammary Gland Biol Neoplasia* 10:49–59, 2005.

302. Villadsen R, et al: Evidence for a stem cell hierarchy in the adult human breast, *J Cell Biol* 177:87–101, 2007.

303. Chaffer CL, Weinberg RA: A perspective on cancer cell metastasis, *Science* 331(6024):1559–1564, 2011.

304. Charafe-Jauffret E, et al: Breast cancer cell lines contain functional cancer stem cells with metastatic capacity and a distinct molecular signature, *Cancer Res* 69(4):1302–1313, 2009.

305. Marcato P, et al: Aldehyde dehydrogenase activity of breast cancer stem cells is primarily due to isoform ALDH1A3 and its expression is predictive of metastasis, *Stem Cell* 29(1):32–45, 2011.

306. Polyak K, Weinber RA: Transitions between epithelial and mesenchymal states: acquisition of malignant and stem cell traits, *Nat Rev Cancer* 9(4):265–273, 2009.

307. Tavassoli F: *World Health Organization classification of tumours: pathology and genetics of tumours of the breast and female genital organs,* Geneva, 2003, World Health Organization, pp 9–19.

308. Lester SC: The breast. In Kumar V, Abbas AK, Fausto N, editors: *Robbins and Cotran pathologic basis of disease,* ed 7, Philadelphia, 2005, Saunders.

309. Silverstein MJ, Baril NB: In situ carcinoma of the breast. In Donegan WL, Spratt JS, editors: *Cancer of the breast,* Philadelphia, 2002, Saunders.

310. Nielsen M, et al: Breast cancer and atypia among young and middle-aged women: a study of 110 medicolegal autopsies, *Br J Cancer* 56(6):814–819, 1987.

311. Alpers CE, Wellings SR: The prevalence of carcinoma in situ in normal and cancer-associated breasts, *Hum Pathol* 16(8):796–807, 1985.

312. Reis-Filho JS, Lakhani SR: Molecular genetics of ADH/DCIS and ALH/LCIS. In O'Malley FP, Pinder SE, editors: *Breast pathology,* New York, 2006, Churchill Livingstone/Elsevier.

313. Page DL, et al: Atypical lobular hyperplasia as a unilateral predictor of breast cancer risk: a retrospective cohort study, *Lancet* 361(9352):125–129, 2003.

314. Korde L, et al: Multidisciplinary meeting on male breast cancer: summary and research recommendations, *J Clin Oncol* 28(12):2114–2122, 2010.

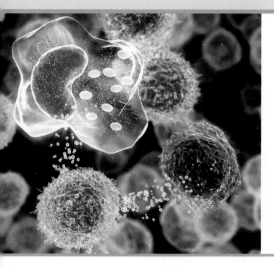

Structure and Function of the Digestive System

Sue E. Huether

evolve WEBSITE

CHAPTER OUTLINE

The digestive system includes the gastrointestinal tract and accessory organs of digestion: the salivary glands, liver, gallbladder, and exocrine pancreas. The digestive system breaks down ingested food, prepares it for uptake by the body's cells, provides body water, and eliminates wastes. Food breakdown begins in the mouth with chewing and continues in the stomach, where food is churned and mixed with acid, mucus, enzymes, and other secretions. From the stomach, the fluid and partially digested food pass into the small intestine, where biochemical agents and enzymes secreted by the intestinal cells, liver, gallbladder, and exocrine pancreas break it down into absorbable components of proteins, carbohydrates, and fats. These nutrients pass through the walls of the small intestine into blood vessels and lymphatics that carry them to the liver for storage or further processing.

Ingested substances and secretions that are not absorbed in the small intestine pass into the large intestine, where fluid continues to be absorbed. Fluid wastes travel to the kidneys and are eliminated in the urine. Solid wastes pass into the rectum and are eliminated from the body through the anus (Figure 33-1).

Except for chewing, swallowing, and defecation of solid wastes, the movements of the digestive system (gastrointestinal motility) are all controlled by hormones and the autonomic nervous system. The autonomic innervation, both sympathetic and parasympathetic, is controlled by centers in the brain and by local stimuli that are mediated at plexuses (networks of nerve fibers) within the gastrointestinal walls.

THE GASTROINTESTINAL TRACT

The alimentary canal, or gastrointestinal tract, consists of the mouth, esophagus, stomach, small intestine, large intestine, rectum, and anus (Figure 33-1). It carries out the following digestive processes:
1. Ingestion of food
2. Propulsion of food and wastes from the mouth to the anus
3. Secretion of mucus, water, and enzymes
4. Mechanical digestion of food particles
5. Chemical digestion of food particles
6. Absorption of digested food
7. Elimination of waste products by defecation

Histologically, the gastrointestinal tract consists of four layers. From the inside out they are the mucosa, submucosa, muscularis, and serosa or adventitia. These concentric layers vary in thickness, and each layer has sublayers (Figure 33-2). A network of intrinsic nerves that controls mobility, secretion, sensation, and blood flow is located solely within the gastrointestinal tract and controlled by local and autonomic nervous system stimuli through the enteric plexus located in different layers of the gastrointestinal walls (see Figure 33-2).

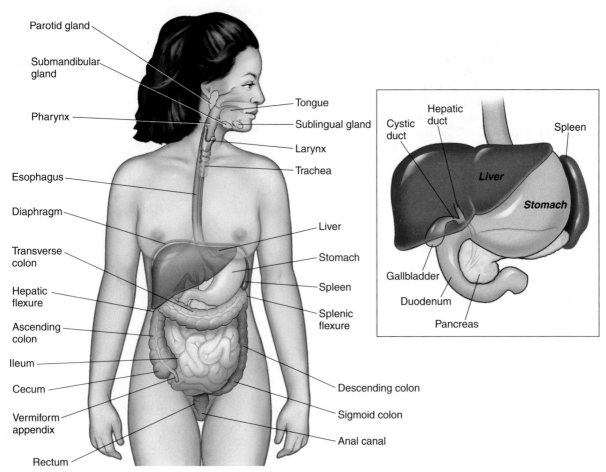

FIGURE 33-1 Structures of the Digestive System. (From Patton KT, Thibodeau GA: *Anatomy & physiology*, ed 7, St Louis, 2010, Mosby.)

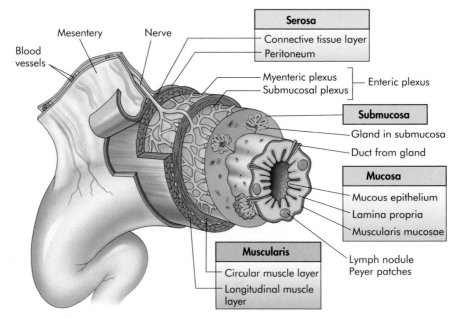

FIGURE 33-2 Wall of the Gastrointestinal Tract. The wall of the gastrointestinal tract is made up of four layers with a network of nerves between the layers. This generalized diagram shows a segment of the gastrointestinal tract. Note that the serosa is continuous with a fold of serous membrane called the *mesentery*. Note also that digestive glands may empty their products into the lumen of the gastrointestinal tract by way of ducts. (From Thibodeau GA, Patton KT: *Anatomy & physiology*, ed 6, St Louis, 2007, Mosby.)

Mouth and Esophagus

The **mouth** is a reservoir for the chewing and mixing of food with saliva. There are 32 permanent teeth in the adult mouth, and they are important for speech and mastication. As food particles become smaller and move around in the mouth, the taste buds and olfactory nerves are continuously stimulated, adding to the satisfaction of eating. The tongue's surface contains thousands of chemoreceptors, or taste buds, which can distinguish salty, sour, bitter, sweet, and savory (umami) tastes. Tastes and food odors help to initiate salivation and the secretion of gastric juice in the stomach.

Salivation

The three pairs of **salivary glands**—the submandibular, sublingual, and parotid glands (Figure 33-3)—secrete about 1 L of saliva per day. **Saliva** consists mostly of water with mucus, sodium, bicarbonate, chloride, potassium, and **salivary α-amylase (ptyalin)**, an enzyme that initiates carbohydrate digestion in the mouth and stomach.

Both sympathetic and parasympathetic divisions of the autonomic nervous system control salivation. Cholinergic parasympathetic fibers stimulate the salivary glands, and atropine (an anticholinergic agent) inhibits salivation and makes the mouth dry. β-Adrenergic stimulation from sympathetic fibers also increases salivary secretion. The salivary glands are not regulated by hormones.

The composition of saliva depends on the rate of secretion (Figure 33-4). Aldosterone can increase an exchange of sodium for potassium, increasing sodium conservation and potassium excretion. The bicarbonate concentration of saliva sustains a pH of about 7.4, which neutralizes bacterial acids and prevents tooth decay. Saliva also contains mucin, immunoglobulin A (IgA), and other antimicrobial substances, which helps prevent infection. Mucin provides lubrication. Exogenous fluoride (e.g., fluoride in drinking water) is also secreted in the saliva, providing additional protection against tooth decay.

Swallowing

The **esophagus** is a hollow, muscular tube approximately 25 cm long that conducts substances from the oropharynx to the stomach (see Figure 33-1). Swallowed food is moved to the stomach by **peristalsis,** the coordinated sequential contraction and relaxation of outer longitudinal and inner circular layers of muscles. The upper third of the esophagus contains striated muscle (voluntary) that is directly innervated by motor neurons. The lower two thirds contains smooth muscle (involuntary) that is innervated by preganglionic cholinergic fibers from the vagus nerve. The fibers are activated in a downward sequence and coordinated by the swallowing center in the medulla. Peristalsis is stimulated when afferent fibers distributed along the length of the esophagus sense changes in wall tension caused by stretching as food passes. The greater the tension, the greater the intensity of esophageal contraction. Occasionally, intense contractions cause pain similar to "heartburn" or angina.

Each end of the esophagus is opened and closed by a sphincter. The **upper esophageal sphincter** keeps air from entering the esophagus during respiration. The **lower esophageal sphincter (cardiac sphincter)** prevents regurgitation from the stomach and caustic injury to the esophagus.

Swallowing is coordinated primarily by the swallowing center in the medulla. During the **oropharyngeal (voluntary) phase**, the following steps occur:
1. Food is segmented into a bolus by the tongue and forced posteriorly toward the pharynx.
2. The superior constrictor muscle of the pharynx contracts so the food cannot move into the nasopharynx.
3. Respiration is inhibited, and the epiglottis slides down to prevent the food from entering the larynx and trachea.
   This entire sequence takes place in less than 1 second.

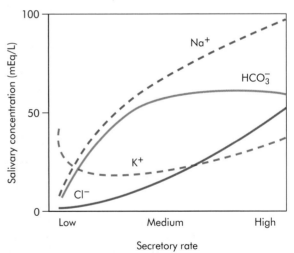

FIGURE 33-4 Salivary Electrolyte Concentrations and Flow Rate. Changes in concentrations of sodium (Na^+), potassium (K^+), chloride (Cl^-), and bicarbonate (HCO_3^-) increase flow rate of saliva. *Green line,* sodium; *orange line,* bicarbonate; *red line,* chloride; *blue line,* potassium. At low rates of salivary flow (i.e., between meals), sodium, chloride, and bicarbonate are reabsorbed in the collecting ducts of the salivary glands, and the saliva contains fewer of these electrolytes (i.e., is more hypotonic). At higher flow rates (i.e., stimulated by food), reabsorption decreases and saliva is hypertonic. By this mechanism, sodium, chloride, and bicarbonate are recycled until they are released to help with digestion and absorption.

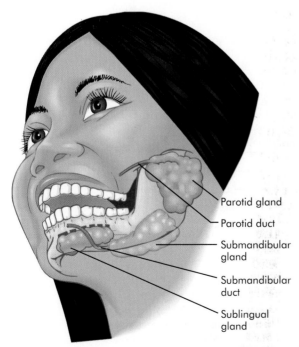

FIGURE 33-3 Salivary Glands. (From Thibodeau GA, Patton KT: *Anatomy & physiology,* ed 6, St Louis, 2007, Mosby.)

The **esophageal phase** proceeds as follows:

1. The bolus of food enters the esophagus.
2. Waves of relaxation travel the esophagus, preparing for the movement of the bolus.
3. Peristalsis, the sequential waves of muscular contractions that travel down the esophagus, transports the food to the lower esophageal sphincter, which is relaxed at that point.
4. The bolus enters the stomach, and the sphincter muscles return to their resting tone.

This phase takes 5 to 10 seconds, with the bolus moving 2 to 6 cm/sec.

Peristalsis that immediately follows the oropharyngeal phase of swallowing is called **primary peristalsis**. If a bolus of food becomes stuck in the esophageal lumen, **secondary peristalsis**—a wave of contraction and relaxation independent of voluntary swallowing—occurs. This is in response to stretch receptors stimulated by increased wall tension, which activate impulses from the swallowing center of the brain.

The lower esophageal sphincter is normally constricted and serves as a barrier between the stomach and esophagus. The muscle tone of the lower sphincter changes with neural and hormonal stimulation and relaxes with swallowing. Cholinergic vagal input and the digestive hormone gastrin increase sphincter tone. Nonadrenergic, noncholinergic vagal impulses relax the lower esophageal sphincter, as do the hormones progesterone, secretin, and glucagon.[1]

> ✔ **QUICK CHECK 33-1**
> 1. What are the functions of saliva?
> 2. What are the phases of swallowing and how are they controlled?

Stomach

The **stomach** is a hollow, muscular organ just below the diaphragm that stores food during eating, secretes digestive juices, mixes food with these juices, and propels partially digested food, called **chyme**, into the duodenum of the small intestine. The anatomy of the stomach is presented in Figure 33-5. Its major anatomic boundaries are the lower esophageal sphincter, where food passes through the **cardiac orifice** into the stomach; the greater and lesser curvatures; and the **pyloric sphincter**, which relaxes as food is propelled through the **pylorus (gastroduodenal junction)** into the duodenum. Functional areas are the **fundus** (upper portion), **body** (middle portion), and **antrum** (lower portion).

The stomach has three layers of smooth muscle: an outer, longitudinal layer; a middle, circular layer; and an inner, oblique layer (the most prominent) (see Figure 33-5). These layers become progressively thicker in the body and antrum where food is mixed and pushed into the duodenum. The glandular epithelium is discussed under Gastric Secretion (see p. 876).

The stomach's blood supply comes from a branch of the celiac artery (Figure 33-6) and is so abundant that nearly all arterial vessels must be occluded before ischemic changes occur in the stomach wall. The splenic vein drains the right side of the stomach, and the gastric vein drains the left side.

Sympathetic and parasympathetic divisions of the autonomic nervous system innervate the stomach. Some of the autonomic fibers are extrinsic—that is, they originate outside the stomach and are controlled by nerve centers in the brain. Others are intrinsic: they originate within the stomach and also respond to local stimuli. Extrinsic sympathetic fibers reach the stomach through the celiac plexus (solar plexus), whereas extrinsic parasympathetic fibers enter through the gastric branch of the vagus nerve.

Gastric Motility

In its resting state, the stomach is small and contains about 50 ml of fluid. There is no wall tension, and the muscle layers in the fundus contract very little. Swallowing causes the fundus to relax (receptive relaxation) to receive a bolus of food from the esophagus (see Swallowing, p. 873). Relaxation is coordinated by efferent, nonadrenergic,

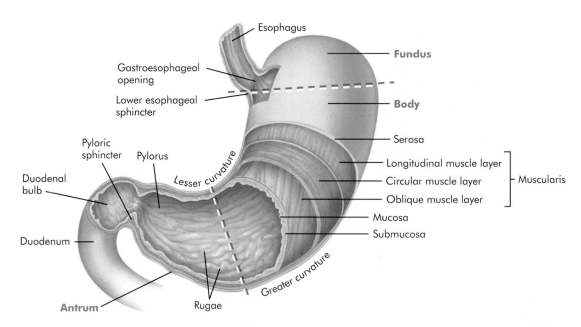

FIGURE 33-5 Stomach. A portion of the anterior wall has been excised to reveal the muscle layers of the stomach wall. Note that the mucosa lining the stomach forms folds called *rugae*. The dashed lines distinguish the fundus, body, and antrum of the stomach. (Modified from Thibodeau GA, Patton KT: *Anatomy & physiology*, ed 6, St Louis, 2007, Mosby.)

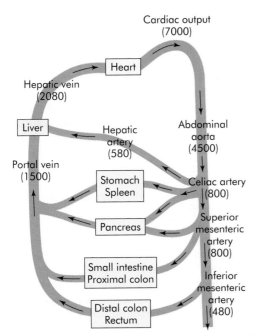

FIGURE 33-6 Major Blood Vessels and Organs Supplied with Blood in the Splanchnic Circulation. Numbers in parentheses reflect approximate blood flow values (ml/min) for each major vessel in an 80-kg normal, resting, adult human subject. Arrows indicate the direction of blood flow. (Modified from Johnson LR: *Gastrointestinal pathophysiology,* St Louis, 2001, Mosby.)

noncholinergic vagal fibers and is facilitated by gastrin and cholecystokinin—two polypeptide hormones secreted by the gastrointestinal mucosa. (The actions of digestive hormones are summarized in Table 33-1.) Food is stored in vertical or oblique layers as it arrives in the fundus, whereas fluids flow relatively quickly down to the antrum.

Gastric (stomach) motility increases with the initiation of peristaltic waves, which sweep over the body of the stomach toward the antrum. The rate of peristaltic contractions is approximately three per minute and is influenced by neural and hormonal activity. Gastrin, motilin (an intestinal hormone), and the vagus nerve increase contraction by lowering the threshold potential of muscle fibers. (The neural and biochemical mechanisms of muscle contraction are described in Chapter 36.) Sympathetic activity and secretin (another intestinal hormone) are inhibitory and raise the threshold potential. The rate of peristalsis is mediated by pacemaker cells that initiate a wave of depolarization (basic electrical rhythm), which moves from the upper part of the stomach to the pylorus.

The mixing and emptying of food (chyme) from the stomach take several hours. Mixing occurs as food is propelled toward the antrum. As food approaches the pylorus, the velocity of the peristaltic wave increases. This forces the contents back toward the body of the stomach. This retropulsion effectively mixes food with digestive juices, and the oscillating motion breaks down large food particles. With each peristaltic wave, a small portion of the gastric contents (chyme) passes through the pylorus and into the duodenum. The pylorus is about 1.5 cm long and is always open about 2.0 mm. It opens wider during antral contraction. Normally there is no regurgitation from the duodenum into the antrum.

	HORMONE/	STIMULUS	
SOURCE	NEUROTRANSMITTER	FOR SECRETION	ACTION
Mucosa of stomach	Gastrin	Presence of partially digested proteins in stomach	Stimulates gastric glands to secrete hydrochloric acid and pepsinogen; growth of gastric mucosa
	Histamine	Gastrin	Stimulates acid secretion
	Somatostatin	Acid in stomach	Inhibits acid and pepsinogen secretion and release of gastrin
	Acetylcholine	Vagus and local nerves in stomach	Stimulates release of pepsinogen and acid secretion
	Gastrin-releasing peptide (bombesin)	Vagus and local nerves in stomach	Stimulates gastrin and release of pepsinogen and acid secretion
Mucosa of small intestine	Motilin	Presence of acid and fat in duodenum	Increases gastrointestinal motility
	Secretin	Presence of chyme (acid, partially digested proteins, fats) in duodenum	Stimulates pancreas to secrete alkaline pancreatic juice and liver to secrete bile; decreases gastrointestinal motility; inhibits gastrin and gastric acid secretion
	Cholecystokinin	Presence of chyme (acid, partially digested proteins, fats) in duodenum	Stimulates gallbladder to eject bile and pancreas to secrete alkaline fluid; decreases gastric motility; constricts pyloric sphincter; inhibits gastrin
	Enteroglucagon	Intraluminal fats and carbohydrates	Weakly inhibits gastric and pancreatic secretion and enhances insulin release, lipolysis, ketogenesis, and glycogenolysis
	Gastric inhibitory peptide (GIP)	Fat and glucose in small intestine	Inhibits gastric secretion and emptying; stimulates insulin release
	Peptide YY	Intraluminal fat and bile acids	Inhibits postprandial gastric acid and pancreatic secretion and delays gastric and small bowel emptying
	Pancreatic polypeptide	Protein, fat, and glucose in small intestine	Decreases pancreatic HCO_3^- and enzyme secretion
	Vasoactive intestinal peptide	Intestinal mucosa and muscle	Relaxes intestinal smooth muscle

TABLE 33-1   SELECTED HORMONES* AND NEUROTRANSMITTERS OF THE DIGESTIVE SYSTEM

Modified from Johnson LR: *Gastrointestinal physiology,* ed 7, St Louis, 2007, Mosby. Data from Schubert ML, Peura DA: *Gastroenterology* 134(7):1842–1860, 2008; Wren AM, Bloom SR: *Gastroenterology* 132(6):2116–2130, 2007.
***NOTE:** The digestive hormones are not secreted into the gastrointestinal lumen but instead into the bloodstream, in which they travel to target tissues. There are more than 30 peptide hormone genes expressed in the gastrointestinal tract and more than 100 hormonally active peptides.

The rate of **gastric emptying** (movement of gastric contents into the duodenum) depends on the volume, osmotic pressure, and chemical composition of the gastric contents. Larger volumes of food increase gastric pressure, peristalsis, and rate of emptying. Solids, fats, and nonisotonic solutions (i.e., hypertonic or hypotonic gastric tube feedings) delay gastric emptying. (Osmotic pressure and tonicity are described in Chapters 1 and 4.) Products of fat digestion, which are formed in the duodenum by the action of bile from the liver and enzymes from the pancreas, stimulate the secretion of cholecystokinin. This hormone inhibits gastric motility and decreases gastric emptying so that fats are not emptied into the duodenum at a rate that exceeds the rate of bile and enzyme secretion. Osmoreceptors in the wall of the duodenum are sensitive to the osmotic pressure of duodenal contents. The arrival of hypertonic or hypotonic gastric contents activates the osmoreceptors, which delay gastric emptying to facilitate formation of an isosmotic duodenal environment. The rate at which acid enters the duodenum also influences gastric emptying. Secretions from the pancreas, liver, and duodenal mucosa neutralize gastric acid in the duodenum. The rate of emptying is adjusted to the duodenum's ability to neutralize the incoming acidity.[2]

Phases of Gastric Secretion

The secretion of gastric juice is influenced by numerous stimuli that together facilitate the process of digestion. The phases of gastric secretion are the *cephalic phase* (stimulated by the thought, smell, and taste of food), the *gastric phase* (stimulated by distention of the stomach), and the *intestinal phase* (stimulated by histamine and digested protein). All phases promote the secretion of acid by the stomach.

Gastric Secretion

Gastric secretion is stimulated by eating (gastric distention), by the hormone gastrin, paracrine pathways (histamine, ghrelin, somatostatin), by the neurotransmitter acetylcholine and chemicals (ethanol, coffee, protein). The stomach secretes large volumes of gastric juices or gastric secretions, including mucus, acid, enzymes, hormones, intrinsic factor, and gastroferrin. Intrinsic factor is necessary for the intestinal absorption of vitamin B_{12}, and gastroferrin facilitates small intestinal absorption of iron. The hormones are secreted into the blood and travel to target tissues. The other gastric secretions are released directly into the stomach lumen.[2a]

In the fundus and body of the stomach, the **gastric glands** of the mucosa are the primary secretory units (Figure 33-7). The composition of gastric juice depends on volume and flow rate (Figure 33-8). Potassium remains relatively constant, but its concentration is greater in gastric juice than in plasma. The rate of secretion varies with the time of day. Generally, the rate and volume of secretion are lowest in the morning and highest in the afternoon and evening. Loss of gastric juices through vomiting, drainage, or suction may decrease body stores of sodium and potassium and result in fluid, electrolyte (e.g., hyponatremia, hypokalemia, dehydration, and acid-base imbalances (e.g., metabolic alkalosis) (see Chapters 4 and 34).[3]

Gastric secretion is inhibited by somatostatin, by unpleasant odors and tastes, and by rage, fear, or pain. A discharge of sympathetic impulses inhibits parasympathetic impulses. Increased secretions are associated with aggression or hostility and may contribute to some forms of gastric pathology.

Acid. The major functions of gastric acid are to dissolve food fibers, act as a bactericide against swallowed microorganisms, and convert pepsinogen to pepsin. The production of acid by the parietal cells requires the transport of hydrogen and chloride from the parietal cells to the stomach lumen. Acid is formed in the parietal cells, primarily through the hydrolysis of water (Figure 33-9). At a high rate of gastric secretion, bicarbonate moves into the plasma, producing an "alkaline tide" in the venous blood, which also may result in a more alkaline urine.[3]

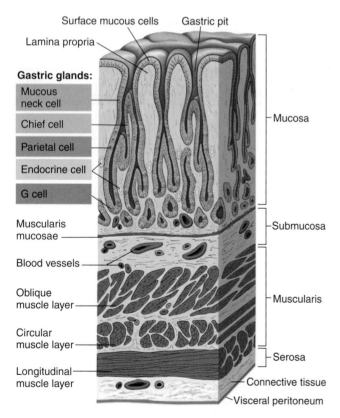

FIGURE 33-7 Gastric Pits and Gastric Glands. Gastric pits are depressions in the epithelial lining of the stomach. At the bottom of each pit are one or more tubular *gastric glands*. Chief cells produce pepsinogen, which is converted to pepsin (a proteolytic enzyme); parietal cells secrete hydrochloric acid and intrinsic factor; G cells produce gastrin; endocrine cells (enterochromaffin-like cells and D cells) secrete histamine and somatostatin. (From Thibodeau GA, Patton KT: *Anatomy & physiology*, ed 6, St Louis, 2007, Mosby.)

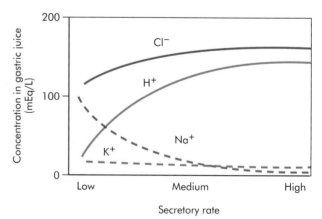

FIGURE 33-8 Relationship Between Secretory Rate and Electrolyte Composition of the Gastric Juice. Sodium (Na+) concentration is lower in the gastric juice than in the plasma, whereas hydrogen (H+), potassium (K+), and chloride (Cl−) concentrations are higher. *Red line,* chloride; *orange line,* hydrogen; *green line,* sodium; *blue line,* potassium.

Acid secretion is stimulated by the vagus nerve, which releases acetylcholine and stimulates the secretion of gastrin; then gastrin stimulates the release of histamine from enterochromaffin cells (mast cells; see Chapter 5) in the gastric mucosa. Histamine stimulates acid secretion by activating histamine receptors (H2 receptors) on acid-secreting parietal cells. Acid secretion is inhibited by somatostatin, secretin, and other intestinal hormones.[2a]

Pepsin. Acetylcholine, gastrin, and secretin stimulate the chief cells to release pepsinogen during eating. Pepsinogen is quickly converted to pepsin in the acidic gastric environment (optimum pH for pepsin activation = 2.0). Pepsin is a proteolytic enzyme—that is, it breaks down protein and forms polypeptides in the stomach. Once chyme has entered the duodenum, the alkaline environment of the duodenum inactivates pepsin.

Mucus. The gastric mucosa is protected from the digestive actions of acid and pepsin by intercellular tight junctions and a coating of mucus called the mucosal barrier. Prostaglandins protect the mucosal barrier by stimulating the secretion of mucus and bicarbonate and by inhibiting the secretion of acid. Mucosal blood flow is important to maintaining mucosal protective functions. A break in the protective barrier may occur from ischemia or by exposure to *Helicobacter pylori*, aspirin, nonsteroidal anti-inflammatory drugs (inhibit prostaglandin synthesis), ethanol, or regurgitated bile. Breaks cause inflammation and ulceration.

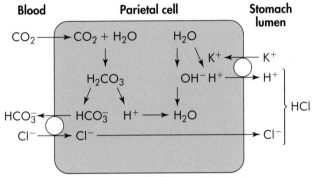

FIGURE 33-9 Hydrochloric Acid Secretion by Parietal Cell.

> **✓ QUICK CHECK 33-2**
> 1. Why are there three layers of stomach muscle?
> 2. What hormones are involved in gastric motility?
> 3. What are the phases of gastric secretion?

Small Intestine

The small intestine is about 5 to 6 meters long and is functionally divided into three segments: the duodenum, jejunum, and ileum (Figure 33-10). The duodenum begins at the pylorus and ends where it joins the jejunum at a suspensory ligament called the *Treitz ligament*. The end of the jejunum and beginning of the ileum are not distinguished by

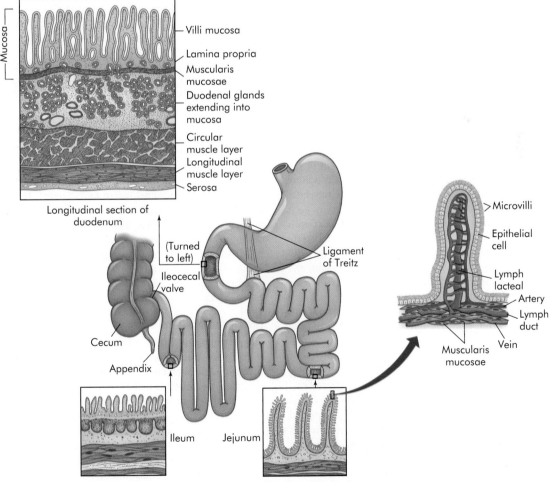

FIGURE 33-10 The Small Intestine.

an anatomic marker. These structures are not grossly different, but the jejunum has a slightly larger lumen than the ileum. The **ileocecal valve,** or **sphincter,** controls the flow of digested material from the ileum into the large intestine and prevents reflux into the small intestine.[4]

The **peritoneum** is the serous membrane surrounding the organs of the abdomen and pelvic cavity. It is analogous to the pericardium and pleura, which surround the heart and lungs, respectively. The visceral peritoneum is positioned over the organs, and the parietal peritoneum lines the wall of the abdominal cavity. The space between these two layers is called the **peritoneal cavity** and normally contains just enough fluid to lubricate the two layers and prevent friction during organ movement.

The duodenum lies behind the peritoneum, or retroperitoneally, and is attached to the posterior abdominal wall. The ileum and jejunum are suspended in loose folds from the posterior abdominal wall by a peritoneal membrane called the **mesentery.** The mesentery facilitates intestinal motility and supports blood vessels, nerves, and lymphatics.

The arterial supply to the duodenum arises primarily from the gastroduodenal artery. The jejunum and ileum are supplied by branches of the superior mesenteric artery. The superior mesenteric vein joins the splenic vein and empties into the portal circulation to the liver. The regional lymph nodes and lymphatics drain into the thoracic duct. Both divisions of the autonomic nervous system innervate the small intestine (enteric nerves). Secretion, motility, pain sensation, and intestinal reflexes (e.g., relaxation of the lower esophageal sphincter) are mediated by parasympathetic nerves. Sympathetic activity inhibits motility and produces vasoconstriction. Intrinsic motor innervation is mediated by the **myenteric plexus (Auerbach plexus)** and the **submucosal plexus (Meissner plexus).**

The smooth muscles of the small intestine are arranged in two layers: a longitudinal outer layer and a thicker inner circular layer (see Figures 33-2 and 33-10). Mucosal folds (plica) within the small intestine slow the passage of food, thereby providing more time for digestion and absorption. The folds are most numerous and prominent in the jejunum and upper ileum (see Figure 33-10).

Absorption occurs through **villi** (sing., **villus**), which cover the mucosal folds and are the functional units of the intestine. Each villus (see Figure 33-10) secretes some of the enzymes necessary for digestion and absorbs nutrients. A villus is composed of absorptive columnar cells (enterocytes) and mucus-secreting goblet cells of the mucosal epithelium. Near the surface, columnar cells closely adhere to each other at sites called *tight junctions.* Water and electrolytes are absorbed through these intercellular spaces. The surface of each columnar epithelial cell contains tiny projections called **microvilli** (sing., **microvillus**) (see Figure 33-10). Together the microvilli create a mucosal surface known as the **brush border.** The villi and microvilli greatly increase the surface area available for absorption. Coating the brush border is an "unstirred" layer of fluid that is important for the absorption of water-soluble substances including emulsified micelles of fat. The **lamina propria** (a connective tissue layer of the mucous membrane) lies beneath the epithelial cells of the villi and contains lymphocytes and plasma cells, which produce immunoglobulins (see the following section: The Gastrointestinal Tract and Immunity).

Central arterioles ascend within each villus and branch into a capillary array that extends around the base of the columnar cells and cascades down to the venules that lead to the portal circulation (see Figure 33-10). A central **lacteal,** or lymphatic channel, is also contained within each villus and is important for the absorption and transport of fat molecules. Contents of the lacteals flow to regional nodes and channels that eventually drain into the thoracic duct.[5]

Between the bases of the villi are the **crypts of Lieberkühn,** which extend to the submucosal layer. Undifferentiated cells arise from stem cells at the base of the crypt and move toward the tip of the villus, maturing to become columnar epithelial secretory cells (water, electrolytes, and enzymes) and goblet cells (mucus). After completing their migration to the tip of the villus, they function for a few days and then are shed into the intestinal lumen and digested. Discarded epithelial cells are an important source of endogenous protein. The entire epithelial population is replaced about every 4 to 7 days. Many factors can influence this process of cellular proliferation. Starvation, vitamin B_{12} deficiency, and cytotoxic drugs or irradiation suppress cell division and shorten the villi. Decreased absorption across the epithelial membrane can cause diarrhea and malnutrition. Nutrient intake and intestinal resection stimulate cell production.

The Gastrointestinal Tract and Immunity

The gastrointestinal tract plays a major role in immune defenses by killing many microorganisms. The mucosa of the intestine covers a large surface area and muscosal secretions produce antibodies, particularly IgA, and enzymes that provide defenses against microorganisms. **Paneth cells,** located near the crypts of Lieberkühn, produce defensins and other antibiotic peptides and proteins important to mucosal immunity.[6] **Peyer patches** (lymph nodes containing collections of lymphocytes, plasma cells, and macrophages) produce immunoglobulins as a component of the gut-associated lymph tissue in the small intestine (see Figures 33-2 and 6-11). Peyer patches are important for antigen processing and immune defense (see Chapter 6).

BOX 33-1 DIETARY FAT

Saturated Fatty Acids (e.g., Palmitic Acid [$C_{16}H_{32}O_2$])
Each carbon atom in the chain is linked by single bonds to adjacent carbon and hydrogen atoms:
1. Solid at room temperatures; include animal fat and tropical oils (coconut and palm oils).
2. Increase low-density lipoprotein (LDL) cholesterol ("bad" cholesterol) blood levels.
3. Increase the risk of coronary artery disease.

Unsaturated Fatty Acids
Soft or liquid at room temperature; omega-6 fatty acids are found in plants and vegetables (olive, canola, and peanut oils); omega-3 fatty acids are found in fish and shellfish.

Monounsaturated Fatty Acids (e.g., Oleic Acid [$C_{18}H_{34}O_2$])
Contain one double bond in the carbon chain:
1. Found in both plants and animals.
2. May be beneficial in reducing blood cholesterol level, glucose level, and systolic blood pressure.
3. Do not lower high-density lipoprotein (HDL) cholesterol ("good" cholesterol) level.
4. Low HDL levels have been associated with coronary heart disease.

Polyunsaturated Fatty Acids (e.g., Linoleic Acid [$C_{18}H_{32}O_2$])
Contain two or more double bonds in the carbon chain:
1. Found in plants and fish oils.
2. Omega-6 fatty acids lower total and LDL cholesterol blood levels.
3. High levels of polyunsaturated fatty acids may lower LDL levels; omega-3 fatty acids lower blood triglyceride levels and reduce platelet aggregation and therefore blood coagulation.
4. Necessary for growth and development and may prevent coronary artery disease, hypertension, and inflammatory and immune disorders.

Intestinal Digestion and Absorption

The process of digestion is initiated in the stomach by the actions of hydrochloric acid and pepsin. The chyme that passes into the duodenum is a liquid with small particles of undigested food. Digestion continues in the proximal portion of the small intestine by the action of pancreatic enzymes, intestinal enzymes, and bile salts. There carbohydrates are broken down to monosaccharides and disaccharides; proteins are degraded further to amino acids and peptides; and fats are emulsified and reduced to fatty acids (Box 33-1) and monoglycerides (Figure 33-11). These nutrients, along with water, vitamins, and electrolytes, are absorbed across the intestinal mucosa by active transport, diffusion, or facilitated diffusion. Products of carbohydrate and protein breakdown

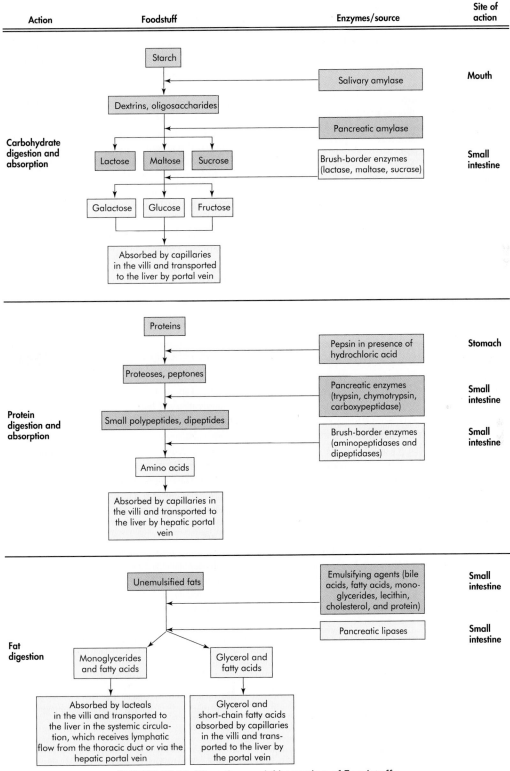

FIGURE 33-11 Digestion and Absorption of Foodstuffs.

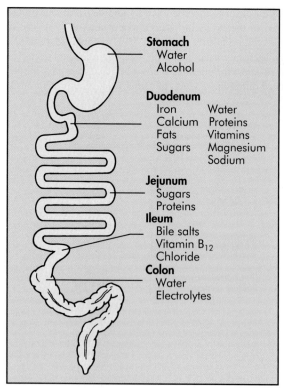

FIGURE 33-12 Sites of Absorption of Major Nutrients.

move into villus capillaries and then to the liver through the portal vein. Digested fats move into the lacteals and eventually reach the liver through the systemic circulation. Intestinal motility exposes nutrients to a large mucosal surface area by mixing chyme and moving it through the lumen. Different segments of the gastrointestinal tract absorb different nutrients. Digestion and absorption of all major nutrients and many drugs occur in the small intestine. Sites of absorption are shown in Figure 33-12. Box 33-2 outlines the major nutrients involved in this process.

Intestinal Motility

The movements of the small intestine facilitate both digestion and absorption. Chyme leaving the stomach and entering the duodenum stimulates intestinal movements that help blend secretions from the liver, pancreas, and intestinal glands. A churning motion brings the luminal contents into contact with the absorbing cells of the villi. Propulsive movements then advance the chyme toward the large intestine.

Intestinal motility is affected by the following two movements:

1. Haustral segmentation. Localized rhythmic contractions of circular smooth muscles divide and mix the chyme, enabling the chyme to have contact with digestive enzymes and the absorbent mucosal surface, and then propel it toward the large intestine.
2. Peristalsis. Waves of contraction along short segments of longitudinal smooth muscle allow time for digestion and absorption. The intestinal villi move with contractions of the muscularis mucosae, a thin layer of muscle separating the mucosa and submucosa, with absorption promoted by the swaying of the villi in the luminal contents.

BOX 33-2 MAJOR NUTRIENTS ABSORBED IN THE SMALL INTESTINE

Water and Electrolytes
- Approximately 85% to 90% of the water that enters the gastrointestinal tract is absorbed in the small intestine.
- Sodium passes through tight junctions and is actively transported across cell membranes; it is exchanged for bicarbonate to maintain electroneutrality in the ileum; sodium absorption is enhanced by glucose transport.
- Potassium moves passively across tight junctions with changes in the electrochemical gradient.

Carbohydrates
- Only monosaccharides are absorbed by intestinal mucosa, so complex carbohydrates must be hydrolyzed to simplest form.
- Salivary and pancreatic amylases break down starches to oligosaccharides (sucrose, maltose, lactose) in stomach and duodenum; brush-border enzymes hydrolyze them in intestine so they can pass through unstirred layer by diffusion.
- Fructose diffuses into the bloodstream; glucose and galactose diffuse or are actively transported.
- Cellulose remains undigested and stimulates large intestine motility.

Proteins
- From 90% to 95% of protein is absorbed; major hydrolysis is accomplished in the small intestine by the pancreatic enzymes trypsin, chymotrypsin, and carboxypeptidase.
- Brush-border enzymes break down proteins into smaller peptides that can cross cell membranes when the cytosol metabolizes them into amino acids, specifically neutral amino acids, basic amino acids, and proline and hydroxyproline.

Fats
Digestion and absorption occur in four phases:
1. Emulsification and lipolysis—agents cover small fat particles and prevent them from re-forming into fat droplets; then lipolysis divides them into diglycerides, monoglycerides, free fatty acids, and glycerol.
2. Micelle formation—products are made water soluble.
3. Fat absorption—move from micelle to absorbing surface of intestinal epithelium and diffuse through resynthesis.
4. Triglycerides and phospholipids—become chylomicrons that eventually enter the systemic circulation.

Minerals
- Calcium—absorbed by passive diffusion and transported actively across cell membranes bound to a carrier protein; absorption primarily in ileum.
- Magnesium—50% absorbed by active transport or passive diffusion in jejunum and ileum.
- Phosphate—absorbed by passive diffusion and active transport in small intestine.
- Iron—absorbed by epithelial cells of duodenum and jejunum; vitamin C facilitates.

Vitamins
- Absorbed mainly by sodium-dependent active transport, with vitamin B_{12} bound to intrinsic factor and absorbed in terminal ileum.

Neural reflexes along the length of the small intestine facilitate motility, digestion, and absorption. The ileogastric reflex inhibits gastric motility when the ileum becomes distended. This prevents the continued movement of chyme into an already distended intestine. The intestinointestinal reflex inhibits intestinal motility when one part of the intestine is overdistended. Both of these reflexes require extrinsic innervation. The gastroileal reflex, which is activated by an increase in gastric motility and secretion, stimulates an increase in ileal motility and relaxation of the ileocecal valve (sphincter). This empties the ileum and prepares it to receive more chyme. The gastroileal reflex is probably regulated by the hormones gastrin and cholecystokinin.

During prolonged fasting or between meals, particularly overnight, slow waves sweep along the entire length of the intestinal tract from the stomach to the terminal ileum. This interdigestive myoelectric complex appears to propel residual gastric and intestinal contents into the colon.

The ileocecal valve (sphincter) marks the junction between the terminal ileum and the large intestine. This valve is intrinsically regulated and is normally closed. The arrival of peristaltic waves from the last few centimeters of the ileum causes the ileocecal valve to open, allowing a small amount of chyme to pass through. Distention of the upper large intestine causes the sphincter to constrict, preventing further distention or retrograde flow of intestinal contents.

> ✔ **QUICK CHECK 33-3**
> 1. What cells arise from the crypts of Lieberkühn?
> 2. How are fats absorbed from the small intestine?
> 3. Which reflexes inhibit intestinal motility? Which promote it?

Large Intestine

The large intestine is approximately 1.5 meters long and consists of the cecum, appendix, colon (ascending, transverse, descending, and sigmoid), rectum, and anal canal (Figure 33-13). The cecum is a pouch that receives chyme from the ileum. Attached to it is the vermiform appendix, an appendage having little or no physiologic function. From the cecum, chyme enters the colon, which loops upward, traverses the abdominal cavity, and descends to the anal canal. The four parts of the colon are the ascending colon, transverse colon, descending colon, and sigmoid colon. Two sphincters control the flow of intestinal contents through the cecum and colon: the ileocecal valve, which admits chyme from the ileum to the cecum, and the O'Beirne sphincter, which controls the movement of wastes from the sigmoid colon into the rectum. A thick (2.5 to 3 cm) portion of smooth muscle surrounds the anal canal, forming the internal anal sphincter. Overlapping it distally is the striated muscle of the external anal sphincter.

In the cecum and colon, the longitudinal muscle layer consists of three longitudinal bands called teniae coli (see Figure 33-13). They are shorter than the colon and give it a gathered appearance. The circular muscles of the colon separate the gathers into outpouchings called haustra (sing., haustrum). The haustra become more or less prominent with the contractions and relaxations of the circular muscles. The mucosal surface of the colon has rugae (folds), particularly between the haustra, and Lieberkühn crypts but no villi. Columnar epithelial cells and mucus-secreting goblet cells form the mucosa throughout the large intestine. The columnar epithelium absorbs fluid and electrolytes, and the mucus-secreting cells lubricate the mucosa.

The myenteric plexus regulates motor and secretory activity independently of the extrinsic system. Extrinsic parasympathetic innervation occurs through the vagus and extends from the cecum up to the

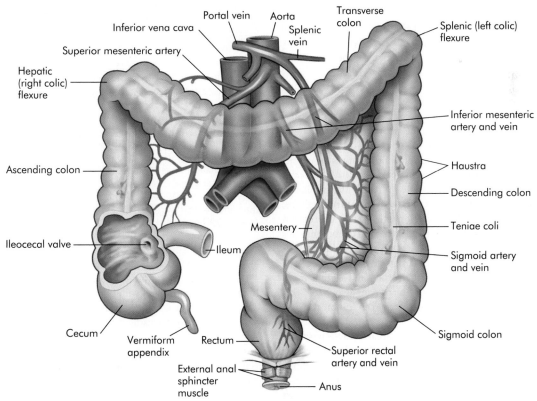

FIGURE 33-13 Division of the Large Intestine. (From Thibodeau GA, Patton KT: *Anatomy & physiology,* ed 6, St Louis, 2007, Mosby.)

first part of the transverse colon. Vagal stimulation increases rhythmic contraction of the proximal colon. Extrinsic parasympathetic fibers reach the distal colon through the pelvic nerves and can increase motility throughout the colon. The internal anal sphincter is usually contracted, and its reflex response is to relax when the rectum is distended. The intrinsic nerve plexuses innervate the internal anal sphincter, which also receives sympathetic innervation to maintain contraction and parasympathetic innervation that facilitates relaxation when the rectum is full. Branches of the sacral division of the spinal cord innervate the external anal sphincter. Sympathetic activity in the entire large intestine modulates intestinal reflexes, conveys somatic sensations of fullness and pain, participates in the defecation reflex, and constricts blood vessels. The blood supply of the large intestine and rectum is derived primarily from branches of the superior and inferior mesenteric arteries (see Figure 33-6)[7] and venous blood drains via the inferior mesenteric vein.

The primary colonic movement is segmental. The circular muscles contract and relax at different sites, shuttling the intestinal contents back and forth between the haustra, most commonly during fasting. The movements massage the intestinal contents, called the fecal mass at that point, and facilitate the absorption of water. Propulsive movement occurs with the proximal-to-distal contraction of several haustral units. Peristaltic movements also occur and promote the emptying of the colon. The gastrocolic reflex initiates propulsion in the entire colon, usually during or immediately after eating, when chyme enters from the ileum. The gastrocolic reflex causes the fecal mass to pass rapidly into the sigmoid colon and rectum, stimulating defecation. Gastrin may participate in stimulating this reflex.

Approximately 500 to 700 ml of chyme flows from the ileum to the cecum per day. Most of the water is absorbed in the colon by diffusion and active transport. Aldosterone increases membrane permeability to sodium, thereby increasing both the diffusion of sodium into the cell and the active transport of sodium to the interstitial fluid. (See Chapter 17 for a discussion of aldosterone secretion.) The colon does not absorb monosaccharides and amino acids, but some short-chain free fatty acids, which are produced by fermentation, are absorbed.

Absorption and epithelial transport occur in the cecum, ascending colon, transverse colon, and descending colon. By the time the fecal mass enters the sigmoid colon, the mass consists entirely of wastes and is called the *feces*, composed of food residue, unabsorbed gastrointestinal secretions, shed epithelial cells, and bacteria.

The movement of feces into the sigmoid colon and rectum stimulates the defecation reflex (rectosphincteric reflex). The rectal wall stretches, and the tonically constricted internal anal sphincter (smooth muscle with autonomic nervous system control) relaxes, creating the urge to defecate. The defecation reflex can be overridden voluntarily by contraction of the external anal sphincter and muscles of the pelvic floor. The rectal wall gradually relaxes, reducing tension, and the urge to defecate passes. Retrograde contraction of the rectum may displace the feces out of the rectal vault until a more convenient time for evacuation. Pain or fear of pain associated with defecation (e.g., rectal fissures or hemorrhoids) can inhibit the defecation reflex.

Squatting and sitting facilitate defecation because these positions straighten the angle between the rectum and anal canal and increase the efficiency of straining (increasing intra-abdominal pressure). Intra-abdominal pressure is increased by initiating the Valsalva maneuver—that is, inhaling and forcing the diaphragm and chest muscles against the closed glottis to increase both intrathoracic and intra-abdominal pressure, which is transmitted to the rectum.

✔ **QUICK CHECK 33-4**
1. What is the major arterial blood supply to the large intestine?
2. What are haustra?
3. What two functions does the large intestine play in relation to the fecal mass?

Intestinal Bacteria

The number of bacterial flora increases from the stomach to the distal colon. The stomach is relatively sterile because of the secretion of acid that kills ingested pathogens or inhibits bacterial growth (with the exception of *Helicobacter pylori*) (see *Health Alert: Helicobacter pylori and Gastric Cancer*). Bile acid secretion, intestinal motility, and antibody production suppress bacterial growth in the duodenum, and in the duodenum and jejunum there is a low concentration of aerobes (10^{-1} to 10^{-4}/ml), primarily streptococci, lactobacilli, staphylococci, and enterobacteria. Anaerobes are found distal to the ileocecal valve but not proximal to the ileum. They constitute about 95% of the fecal flora in the colon and contribute one third of the solid bulk of feces. *Bacteroides*, clostridia, anaerobic lactobacilli, and coliforms are the most common microorganisms from the ileum to the cecum.

HEALTH ALERT
Helicobacter Pylori and Gastric Cancer

Helicobacter pylori (H. pylori) is a gram-negative gastric pathogen that can survive in an acidic medium and infects about 50% of the world population. About 10% of infected individuals develop gastric and duodenal ulcers, and 1% develop gastric cancer and mucosa-associated lymphoid tissue B cell lymphoma. Risk is associated with the strain of *H. pylori;* the cytotoxin-associated antigen A (CagA) strain has been shown to cause gastric epithelial cell disruption, chronic inflammation, gastric atrophy, and activation of oncogenic pathways that lead to gastric cancer. Host genetic factors and exposure to a high-salt diet and nitrate preservatives amplify risk. Because gastric cancer has a poor prognosis and few treatment options, diagnosis and eradication of *H. pylori* infection are essential to gastric cancer prevention and risk reduction. Clinical trials are in progress for prophylactic and therapeutic vaccines against *H. pylori*.

Data from Ding SZ, Goldberg JB, Hatakeyama M: *Helicobacter pylori* infection, oncogenic pathways and epigenetic mechanisms in gastric carcinogenesis, *Future Oncol* 6(5):851–862, 2010; Peek RM Jr, Fiske C, Wilson KT: Role of innate immunity in *Helicobacter pylori*–induced gastric malignancy, *Physiol Rev* 90(3):831–858, 2010; Czinn SJ, Blanchard T: Vaccinating against *Helicobacter pylori* infection, *Nat Rev Gastroenterol Hepatol* 8(3):133–140, 2011; Kim SS, et al: *Helicobacter pylori* in the pathogenesis of gastric cancer and gastric lymphoma, *Cancer Lett* 305(2):228–238, 2011.

The intestinal tract is sterile at birth but becomes colonized with *Escherichia coli, Clostridium welchii,* and *Streptococcus* within a few hours. Within 3 to 4 weeks after birth, the normal flora are established. The normal flora do not have the virulence factors associated with pathogenic microorganisms, thus permitting immune tolerances.[8] The intestinal bacteria do not have major digestive or absorptive functions but do play a role both in metabolism of bile salts, estrogens, androgens, lipids, carbohydrates, various nitrogenous substances, and drugs and in protection against infection.

Endogenous infections of the gastrointestinal tract occur by three major mechanisms: proliferation or overgrowth of bacteria, perforation of the intestine, and contamination of neighboring structures.

Splanchnic Blood Flow

The splanchnic blood flow provides blood to the esophagus, stomach, small and large intestine, liver, gallbladder, pancreas, and spleen (see Figure 33-6). Blood flow is regulated by cardiac output and blood volume, the autonomic nervous system, hormones, and local autoregulatory blood flow mechanisms. The splanchnic circulation serves as an important reservoir of blood volume to maintain circulation to the heart and lungs when needed. The superior and inferior mesenteric arteries provide the blood supply to the large intestine (see Figures 33-6 and 33-13).

ACCESSORY ORGANS OF DIGESTION

The liver, gallbladder, and exocrine pancreas all secrete substances necessary for the digestion of chyme. These secretions are delivered to the duodenum through the sphincter of Oddi at the major duodenal papilla (of Vater) (Figure 33-14). The liver produces bile, which contains salts necessary for fat digestion and absorption. Between meals, bile is stored in the gallbladder. The exocrine pancreas produces (1) enzymes needed for the complete digestion of carbohydrates, proteins, and fats and (2) an alkaline fluid that neutralizes chyme, creating a duodenal pH that supports enzymatic action.

The liver also receives nutrients absorbed by the small intestine and metabolizes or synthesizes them into forms that can be absorbed by the body's cells. It then releases the nutrients into the bloodstream or stores them for later use.

Liver

The liver weighs 1200 to 1600 g. It is located under the right diaphragm and is divided into right and left lobes. The larger, right lobe is divided further into the caudate and quadrate lobes (Figure 33-15). The falciform ligament separates the right and left lobes and attaches the liver to the anterior abdominal wall. The round ligament (ligamentum teres) extends along the free edge of the falciform ligament,

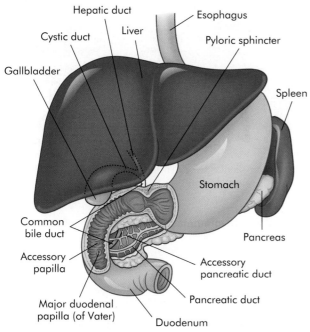

FIGURE 33-14 Location of the Liver, Gallbladder, and Exocrine Pancreas, Which Are the Accessory Organs of Digestion.

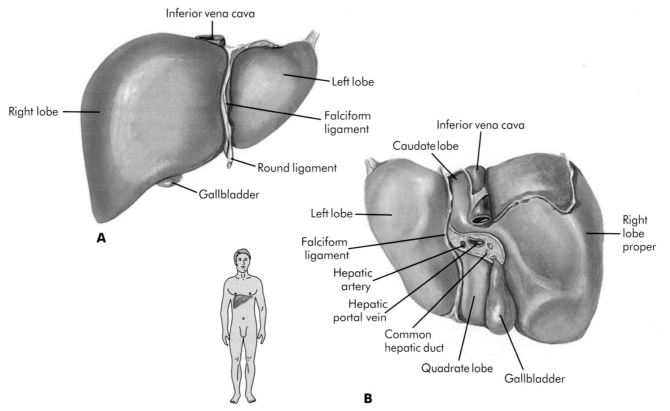

FIGURE 33-15 Gross Structure of the Liver. **A,** Anterior view. **B,** Inferior view. (From Thibodeau GA, Patton KT: *Anatomy & physiology*, ed 6, St Louis, 2007, Mosby.)

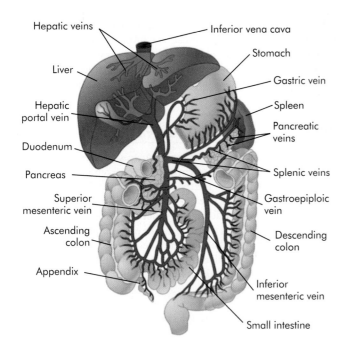

FIGURE 33-16 Hepatic Portal Circulation. In this unusual circulatory route, a vein is located between two capillary beds. The hepatic portal vein collects blood from capillaries in visceral structures located in the abdomen and empties into the liver. Hepatic veins return blood to the inferior vena cava. (Organs are not drawn to scale.) (From Thibodeau GA, Patton KT: *Anatomy & physiology*, ed 6, St Louis, 2007, Mosby.)

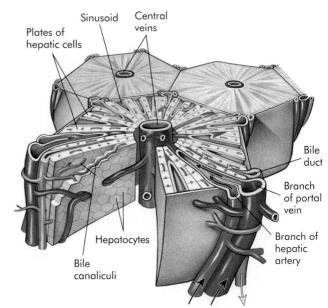

FIGURE 33-17 Diagrammatic Representation of a Liver Lobule. A central vein is located in the center of the lobule with plates of hepatic cells disposed radially. Branches of the portal vein and hepatic artery are located on the periphery of the lobule and blood from both perfuses the sinusoids. Peripherally located bile ducts drain the bile canaliculi that run between the hepatocytes. (Modified from Thibodeau GA, Patton KT: *Anatomy & physiology*, ed 6, St Louis, 2007, Mosby.)

extending from the umbilicus to the inferior surface of the liver. The coronary ligament branches from the falciform ligament and extends over the superior surface of the right and left lobes, binding the liver to the inferior surface of the diaphragm. The liver is covered by the **Glisson capsule,** which contains blood vessels, lymphatics, and nerves. When the liver is diseased or swollen, distention of the capsule causes pain and the lymphatics may ooze fluid into the peritoneal space.

The metabolic functions of the liver require a large amount of blood. The liver receives blood from both arterial and venous sources. The **hepatic artery** branches from the abdominal aorta and provides oxygenated blood at the rate of 400 to 500 ml/min (about 25% of the cardiac output). The **hepatic portal vein** receives deoxygenated blood from the inferior and superior mesenteric veins, the splenic vein, the gastric and esophageal veins, and delivers about 1000 to 1500 ml/min to the liver (Figure 33-16). Portal venous blood constitutes 70% of the blood supply to the liver. This blood carries some oxygen and is rich in nutrients absorbed from the digestive tract.

Within the liver lobes are multiple, smaller anatomic units called **liver lobules** (Figure 33-17). They are formed of cords or plates of **hepatocytes,** which are the functional cells of the liver. These cells can regenerate; therefore damaged or resected liver tissue can regrow. Small capillaries, or **sinusoids,** are located between the plates of hepatocytes. They receive a mixture of venous and arterial blood from branches of the hepatic artery and portal vein. Blood from the sinusoids drains to a central vein in the middle of each liver lobule. Venous blood from all the lobules then flows into the **hepatic vein,** which empties into the inferior vena cava. Small channels (**bile canaliculi**) conduct bile, which is produced by the hepatocytes, outward to bile ducts and eventually drain into the **common bile duct** (see Figure 33-17). This duct empties

bile into the ampulla of Vator, then into the duodenum through an opening called the **major duodenal papilla** (sphincter of Oddi).

The sinusoids of the liver lobules are lined with highly permeable endothelium. This permeability enhances the transport of nutrients from the sinusoids into the hepatocytes, where they are metabolized. The sinusoids are also lined with phagocytic **Kupffer cells (tissue macrophages),** and are part of the mononuclear phagocyte system. Kupffer cells are bacteriocidal and also are important for bilirubin production and lipid metabolism. Because the liver receives all the venous blood from the gut and pancreas, the Kupffer cells play an important role in destroying intestinal bacteria and preventing infections. Between the endothelial lining of the sinusoid and the hepatocyte is the **Disse space,** which drains interstitial fluid into the hepatic lymph system. Hepatic stellate cells are located here. They are contractile, help regulate sinusoidal blood flow, and participate in innate immunity.[9]

> ✓ **QUICK CHECK 33-5**
> 1. Where does blood in the portal vein originate?
> 2. What is the function of hepatocytes?
> 3. What are sinusoids?

Secretion of Bile

The liver assists intestinal digestion by secreting 700 to 1200 ml of bile per day. **Bile** is an alkaline, bitter-tasting, yellowish green fluid that contains bile salts (conjugated bile acids), cholesterol, bilirubin (a pigment), electrolytes, and water. It is formed by hepatocytes and secreted into the canaliculi. **Bile salts,** which are conjugated bile acids, are required for the intestinal emulsification and absorption of fats.

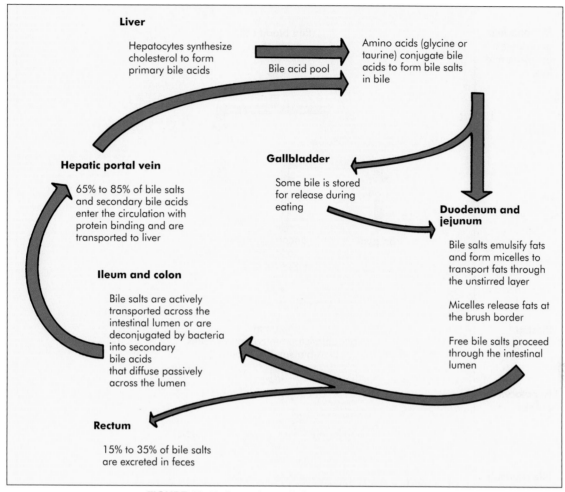

FIGURE 33-18 Enterohepatic Circulation of Bile Salts.

Having facilitated fat emulsification and absorption, most bile salts are actively absorbed in the terminal ileum and returned to the liver through the portal circulation for resecretion. The recycling of bile salts is termed the enterohepatic circulation (Figure 33-18).

Bile has two fractional components: the acid-dependent fraction and the acid-independent fraction. Hepatocytes secrete the bile acid–dependent fraction, which consists of bile acids, cholesterol, lecithin (a phospholipid), and bilirubin (a bile pigment). The bile acid–independent fraction, which is secreted by the hepatocytes and epithelial cells of the bile canaliculi, is a bicarbonate-rich aqueous fluid that gives bile its alkaline pH.

Bile salts are conjugated in the liver from primary and secondary bile acids. The primary bile acids are cholic acid and chenodeoxycholic (chenic) acid. These acids are synthesized from cholesterol by the hepatocytes. The secondary bile acids are deoxycholic and lithocholic acid. These acids are formed in the small intestine by intestinal bacteria, after which they are absorbed and flow to the liver (see Figure 33-18). Both forms of bile acids are conjugated with amino acids (glycine or taurine) in the liver to form bile salts. Conjugation makes the bile acids more water soluble, thus restricting their diffusion from the duodenum and ileum. The primary and secondary bile acids together form the bile acid pool.

Some bile salts are deconjugated by intestinal bacteria to secondary bile acids. These acids diffuse passively into the portal blood from both small and large intestines. An increase in the plasma concentration of

bile acids accelerates the uptake and resecretion of bile acids and salts by the hepatocytes. The cycle of hepatic secretion, intestinal absorption, and hepatic resecretion of bile acids completes the enterohepatic circulation.

Bile secretion is called choleresis. A choleretic agent stimulates the liver to secrete bile. One strong stimulus is a high concentration of bile salts. Other choleretics include cholecystokinin, vagal stimulation, and secretin, which increases the rate of bile flow by promoting the secretion of bicarbonate from canaliculi and other intrahepatic bile ducts.

Metabolism of Bilirubin

Bilirubin is a by-product of the destruction of aged red blood cells. It gives bile a greenish black color and produces the yellow tinge of jaundice. Aged red blood cells are absorbed and destroyed by macrophages (Kupffer cells) of the mononuclear phagocyte system (also called the reticuloendothelial system), primarily in the spleen and liver. Within these cells, hemoglobin is separated into its component parts: heme and globin (Figure 33-19). The globin component is further degraded into its constituent amino acids, which are recycled to form new protein. The heme moiety is converted to biliverdin by the enzymatic cleavage of iron. The iron attaches to transferrin in the plasma and can be stored in the liver or used by the bone marrow to make new red blood cells. The biliverdin is enzymatically converted to bilirubin in the macrophage and then is released into the plasma, where it binds

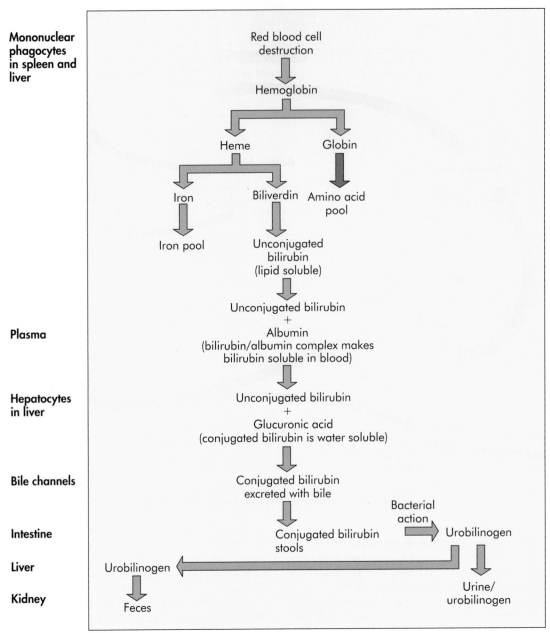

FIGURE 33-19 Bilirubin Metabolism.

to albumin and is known as unconjugated bilirubin, or free bilirubin, which is lipid soluble.

In the liver, unconjugated bilirubin moves from plasma in the sinusoids into the hepatocyte. Within hepatocytes, unconjugated bilirubin joins with glucuronic acid to form conjugated bilirubin, which is water soluble and is secreted in the bile. When conjugated bilirubin reaches the distal ileum and colon, it is deconjugated by bacteria and converted to urobilinogen. Most of the urobilinogen is then excreted in the urine as urobilin, and a small amount is eliminated in feces.

Vascular and Hematologic Functions

Because of its extensive vascular network, the liver can store a large volume of blood. The amount stored at any one time depends on pressure relationships in the arteries and veins. The liver also can release blood to maintain systemic circulatory volume in the event of hemorrhage.

The liver also has hemostatic functions. It synthesizes prothrombin, fibrinogen, and factors I, II, VII, IX, and X, all of which are necessary for effective clotting (see Chapter 19). Vitamin K, a fat-soluble vitamin, is essential for the synthesis of other clotting factors. Because bile salts are needed for reabsorption of fats, vitamin K absorption depends on adequate bile production in the liver.

Metabolism of Nutrients

Fats. Fat is synthesized from carbohydrate and protein, primarily in the liver. Ingested fat absorbed by lacteals in the intestinal villi enters the liver through the lymphatics, primarily as triglycerides. In the liver, the triglycerides can be hydrolyzed to glycerol and free fatty acids and used to produce metabolic energy (adenosine triphosphate [ATP]), or they can be released into the bloodstream as lipoproteins (lipids bound to proteins). Blood carries the lipoproteins to adipose cells for storage. The liver also synthesizes phospholipids and cholesterol, which

TABLE 33-2 IMPORTANCE OF PROTEINS IN THE BODY

FUNCTION	EXAMPLE
Contraction	Actin and myosin enable muscle contraction and cellular movement.
Energy	Proteins can be metabolized for energy.
Fluid balance	Albumin is a major source of plasma oncotic pressure.
Protection	Antibodies and complement protect against infection and foreign substances.
Regulation	Enzymes control chemical reactions; hormones regulate many physiologic processes.
Structure	Collagen fibers provide structural support to many parts of body; keratin strengthens skin, hair, and nails.
Transport	Hemoglobin transports oxygen and carbon dioxide in blood; plasma proteins, particularly albumin, serve as transport molecules (i.e., for hormones, cations, bilirubin, and drugs) and maintain plasma oncotic pressure; proteins in cell membranes control movement of materials into and out of cells.
Coagulation	Hemostasis is regulated by clotting factors and proteins that balance coagulation and anticoagulation.

are needed for the hepatic production of bile salts, steroid hormones, components of plasma membranes, and other special molecules.

Proteins. Protein synthesis requires the presence of all the essential amino acids (obtained only from food), as well as nonessential amino acids. Proteins perform many important roles in the body; these are summarized in Table 33-2.

Within hepatocytes, amino acids are converted to carbohydrates (keto acids) by the removal of ammonia (NH_3), a process known as deamination. The ammonia is converted to urea by the liver and passes into the blood to be excreted by the kidneys. Depending on the nutritional status of the body, the keto acids either are converted to fatty acids for fat synthesis and storage or are oxidized by the Krebs tricarboxylic acid cycle (see Chapter 1) to provide energy for the liver cells.

The plasma proteins, including albumins and globulins (with the exception of gamma globulin, which is formed in lymph nodes and lymphoid tissue), are synthesized by the liver. They play an important role in preserving blood volume and pressure by maintaining plasma oncotic pressure. The liver also synthesizes several nonessential amino acids and serum enzymes, including aspartate aminotransferase (AST; previously SGOT), alanine aminotransferase (ALT; previously SGPT), lactate dehydrogenase (LDH), and alkaline phosphatase.

Carbohydrates. The liver contributes to the stability of blood glucose levels by releasing glucose during hypoglycemia (low blood glucose level) and absorbing glucose during hyperglycemia (high blood glucose level) and storing it as glycogen (glyconeogenesis) or converting it to fat. When all glycogen stores have been used, the liver can convert amino acids and glycerol to glucose (gluconeogenesis).

Metabolic Detoxification

The liver alters exogenous and endogenous chemicals (e.g., drugs), foreign molecules, and hormones to make them less toxic or less biologically active. This process, called metabolic detoxification or biotransformation, diminishes intestinal or renal tubular reabsorption of potentially toxic substances and facilitates their intestinal and renal

excretion. In this way alcohol, barbiturates, amphetamines, steroids, and hormones (including estrogens, aldosterone, antidiuretic hormone, and testosterone) are metabolized or detoxified, preventing excessive accumulation and adverse effects. Although metabolic detoxification is usually protective, the end products of metabolic detoxification sometimes become toxins (see *Health Alert:* Paracetamol [Acetaminophen] and Acute Liver Failure) or active metabolites. Toxins of alcohol metabolism, for example, are acetaldehyde and hydrogen, which can damage the liver's ability to function (see Chapter 3 and Figure 3-10).

HEALTH ALERT

Paracetamol (Acetaminophen) and Acute Liver Failure

Paracetamol (acetaminophen) toxicity from chronic use or intentional overdose is the leading cause of acute liver failure in the developed world. Liver injury may occur with doses of 4 to 10 grams and hepatoxicity should be suspected when doses exceed 4 grams per day. Overdose is usually unintentional because individuals are not aware of toxicity hazards. The onset of toxicity is sudden and lasts for up to 24 hours. Symptoms include signs of gastrointestinal upset, nausea, vomiting, anorexia, diaphoresis, and pallor. Elevated levels of serum aminotransferase appear after 48 hours accompanied by hypoprothrombinemia, metabolic acidosis, and renal failure. Early treatment (within 8 hours) with *N*-acetylcysteine provides a 66% chance of recovery and there is 70% survival at 1 year after liver transplantation.

Data from Hinson JA, Roberts DW, James LP: Mechanisms of acetaminophen-induced liver necrosis, *Handb Exp Pharmacol* 19(6):369–405, 2010; Khandelwal N, et al: Unrecognized acetaminophen toxicity as a cause of indeterminate acute liver failure, *Hepatology* 53(2):567–576, 2011; Craig DG, et al: Overdose pattern and outcome in paracetamol-induced acute severe hepatotoxicity, *Br J Clin Pharmacol* 71(2):273–282, 2011.

Storage of Minerals and Vitamins

The liver stores certain vitamins and minerals, including iron and copper, in times of excessive intake and releases them in times of need. The liver can store vitamins B_{12} and D for several months and vitamin A for several years. The liver also stores vitamins E and K. Iron is stored in the liver as ferritin, an iron-protein complex, and is released as needed for red blood cell production. Common tests of liver function are listed in Table 33-3.

Gallbladder

The gallbladder is a saclike organ on the inferior surface of the liver (Figure 33-20). Its primary function is to store and concentrate bile between meals. Bile flows from the liver through the right or left hepatic duct into the common hepatic duct and meets resistance at the closed sphincter of Oddi, which controls flow into the duodenum and prevents backflow of duodenal contents into the pancreatobiliary system. Bile then flows through the cystic duct into the gallbladder, where it is concentrated and stored. The mucosa of the gallbladder wall readily absorbs water and electrolytes, leaving a high concentration of bile salts, bile pigments, and cholesterol. The gallbladder holds about 90 ml of bile.

Within 30 minutes after eating, the gallbladder begins to contract and the sphincter of Oddi relaxes, forcing bile into the duodenum through the major duodenal papilla. During the cephalic and gastric phases of digestion, gallbladder contraction is mediated by cholinergic branches of the vagus nerve. Hormonal regulation of gallbladder contraction is derived primarily from the release of cholecystokinin and motilin secreted by the duodenal mucosa in the presence of fat.

TABLE 33-3 SELECTED TESTS OF LIVER FUNCTION

TEST	NORMAL VALUE	CLINICAL SIGNIFICANCE
Serum Enzymes		
Alkaline phosphatase	20-125 units/L	Increases with biliary obstruction and cholestatic hepatitis
Aspartate aminotransferase (AST; previously SGOT)	6-21 units/L	Increases with hepatocellular injury
Alanine aminotransferase (ALT; previously SGPT)	0-48 units/L	Increases with hepatocellular injury
Lactate dehydrogenase (LDH)	0-250 units/L	Isoenzyme LD_5 is elevated with hypoxic and primary liver injury
5′-Nucleotidase	2-11 units/L	Increases with increase in alkaline phosphatase and cholestatic disorders
Bilirubin Metabolism		
Serum bilirubin		
Indirect (unconjugated)	0-1.0 mg/dl	Increases with hemolysis (lysis of red blood cells)
Direct (conjugated)	0-0.3 mg/dl	Increases with hepatocellular injury or obstruction
TOTAL	0-1.0 mg/dl	Increases with biliary obstruction
Urine bilirubin	0.2-1.3 mg/dl	Increases with biliary obstruction
Urine urobilinogen	0.3-2.1 mg/2 hr (male)	Increases with hemolysis or shunting of portal blood flow
	0.1-1.1 mg/2 hr (female)	
Serum Proteins		
Albumin	4.0-6.0 g/dl	Decreases with hepatocellular injury
Globulin	2.0-4.0 g/dl	Increases with hepatitis
TOTAL	6-8 g/dl	
A/G ratio	1.5:1 to 2.5:1	Ratio reverses with chronic hepatitis or other chronic liver disease
Transferrin	250-300 mcg/dl	Liver damage with decreased values; iron deficiency with increased values
α-Fetoprotein	<10 ng/ml	Elevated values in primary hepatocellular carcinoma
Blood Clotting Functions		
Prothrombin time (PT)	10-14 sec or 90%-100% of control	Increases with chronic liver disease (cirrhosis) or vitamin K deficiency
International Normalized Ratio (INR)	0.9-1.3	Increased values indicate high chance of bleeding; useful for monitoring effects of drugs such as warfarin
Partial thromboplastin time (PTT)	25-40 sec	Increases with severe liver disease or heparin therapy
Bromsulphalein (BSP) excretion	<6% retention in 45 min	Increased retention with hepatocellular injury

Vasoactive intestinal peptide, pancreatic polypeptide, and sympathetic nerve stimulation relax the gallbladder.

Exocrine Pancreas

The pancreas is approximately 20 cm long, with its head tucked into the curve of the duodenum and its tail touching the spleen. The body of the pancreas lies deep in the abdomen, behind the stomach (see Figure 33-20). The pancreas is unique in that it has both endocrine and exocrine functions. The endocrine pancreas secretes hormones: insulin, glucagon, somatostatin, and pancreatic polypeptide (see Chapter 17).

The exocrine pancreas is composed of acinar cells that secrete enzymes and networks of ducts that secrete alkaline fluids. Both have important digestive functions. The acinar cells are organized into spherical lobules around small secretory ducts (see Figure 33-20). Secretions drain into a system of ducts that leads to the pancreatic duct (Wirsung duct), which empties into the common bile duct at the ampulla of Vater, and then into the duodenum. In some individuals, an accessory duct (the duct of Santorini) branches off the pancreatic duct and drains directly into the duodenum at the minor duodenal papilla.

Arterial blood is supplied to the pancreas by branches of the celiac and superior mesenteric arteries. Venous blood leaves the head of the pancreas through the portal vein, with the body and tail being drained through the splenic vein. All hormonal pancreatic secretions also pass through the portal vein into the liver.

Pancreatic innervation arises from preganglionic parasympathetic fibers of the vagus nerve. These fibers activate postganglionic fibers, which stimulate enzymatic and hormonal secretion. Sympathetic postganglionic fibers from the celiac and superior mesenteric plexuses innervate the blood vessels, cause vasoconstriction, and inhibit pancreatic secretion.

The aqueous secretions of the exocrine pancreas are isotonic and contain potassium, sodium, bicarbonate, and chloride. The highly alkaline pancreatic juice neutralizes the acidic chyme that enters the duodenum from the stomach and provides the alkaline medium needed for the actions of digestive enzymes and intestinal absorption of fat.

In the pancreas, transport of water and electrolytes through the ductal epithelium involves both active and passive mechanisms. The ductal cells actively transport hydrogen into the blood and bicarbonate into the duct lumen. Potassium and chloride are secreted by diffusion according to changes in electrochemical potential gradients. As the secretion flows down the duct, water is osmotically transported into the juice until it becomes isosmotic. At low flow rates bicarbonate is exchanged passively for chloride, but at higher flow rates there is less time for this exchange and bicarbonate concentration increases.

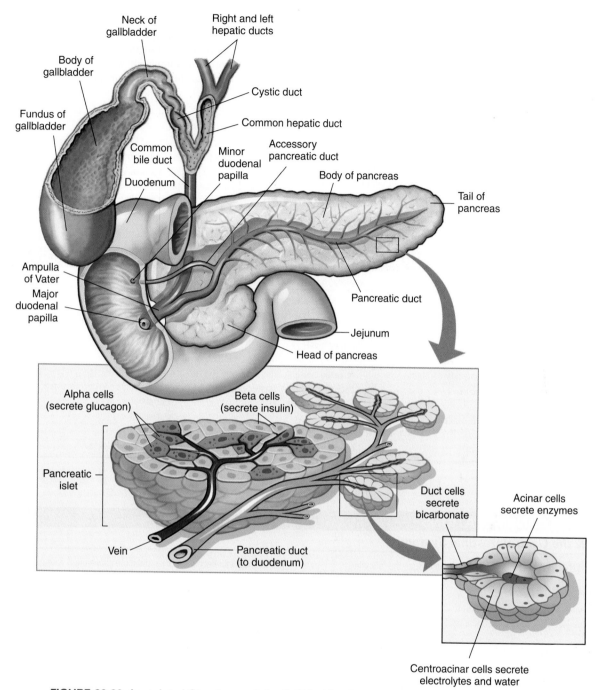

FIGURE 33-20 Associated Structures of the Gallbladder, Pancreas, and Pancreatic Acinar Cells and Duct. (Main illustration from Thibodeau GA, Patton KT: *Anatomy & physiology*, ed 6, St Louis, 2007, Mosby.)

Because eating stimulates the flow of pancreatic juice, the juice is most alkaline when it needs to be: during digestion.

The pancreatic enzymes can hydrolyze proteins (proteases), carbohydrates (amylases), and fats (lipases). The proteolytic (protein-digesting) enzymes include trypsin, chymotrypsin, carboxypeptidase, and elastase. These enzymes are secreted in their inactive forms—that is, as trypsinogen, chymotrypsinogen, procarboxypeptidase, and proelastase, respectively—to protect the pancreas from the digestive effects of its own enzymes. For further protection, the pancreas produces **trypsin inhibitor,** which prevents the activation of proteolytic enzymes while they are in the pancreas. Once in the duodenum, the

inactive forms (proenzymes) are activated by **enterokinase,** an enzyme secreted by the duodenal mucosa. Trypsinogen is the first proenzyme to be activated. Its conversion to trypsin stimulates the conversion of chymotrypsinogen to chymotrypsin and procarboxypeptidase to carboxypeptidase. Each of these enzymes cleaves specific peptide bonds to reduce polypeptides to smaller peptides.

Secretion of the aqueous and enzymatic components of pancreatic juice is controlled by hormonal and vagal stimuli. Secretin stimulates the acinar and duct cells to secrete the bicarbonate-rich fluid that neutralizes chyme and prepares it for enzymatic digestion. As chyme enters the duodenum, its acidity (pH of 4.5 or less) stimulates the

S cells (secretin-producing cells) of the duodenum to release secretin, which is absorbed by the intestine and delivered to the pancreas in the bloodstream. In the pancreas, secretin causes ductal and acinar cells to release alkaline fluid. Secretin also inhibits the actions of gastrin, thereby decreasing gastric acid secretion and motility. The overall effect is to neutralize the contents of the duodenum.

Enzymatic secretion follows, stimulated by cholecystokinin and acetylcholine. Cholecystokinin is released in the duodenum in response to the essential amino acids and fatty acids already present in chyme. Acetylcholine is liberated from pancreatic branches of the vagus nerve during the cephalic phase of digestion. Cholecystokinin and acetylcholine both act on the acinar cells, causing enzyme release. Once in the small intestine, the secretion of more cholecystokinin and acetylcholine is inhibited by the negative feedback of activated pancreatic enzymes. Pancreatic polypeptide is released after eating and inhibits postprandial pancreatic exocrine secretion. (See Table 33-1 for a summary of hormonal stimulation of pancreatic secretions.) Selected tests of pancreatic function are listed in Table 33-4.

✔ **QUICK CHECK 33-6**
1. Trace the route of bile salts and acids from formation to recycling.
2. What are the two types of bilirubin?
3. What is the function of the gallbladder?
4. How do pancreatic beta cells differ from acinar cells?

TABLE 33-4 SELECTED LABORATORY TESTS OF EXOCRINE PANCREATIC FUNCTION

TEST	NORMAL VALUE	CLINICAL SIGNIFICANCE
Serum amylase	27-131 units/L	Elevated levels with pancreatic inflammation
Serum lipase	20-180 units/L	Elevated levels with pancreatic inflammation (may be elevated with other conditions; differentiates with amylase isoenzyme study)
Urine amylase	2-19 units/hr	Elevated levels with pancreatic inflammation
Secretin test	Volume 1.8 ml/kg/hr	Decreased volume with pancreatic disease because a secretin stimulates pancreatic secretion
	Bicarbonate concentration: > 80 mEq/L	Decreased concentration or secretion or can occur with pancreatic injury related to pancreatitis. Lack of buffering of gastric acid can lead to intestinal ulcers and decrease activation of digestive enzymes and drugs that require a higher pH.
	Bicarbonate output: >10 mEq/L/30 sec	See above
Stool fat	2-5 g/24 hr	Measures fatty acids; decreased pancreatic lipase increases stool fat

GERIATRIC CONSIDERATIONS

Aging & the Gastrointestinal System

Age-related changes in gastrointestinal function include the following:

Oral Cavity and Esophagus
1. Tooth enamel and dentin deteriorate, so cavities are more likely.
2. Teeth are lost as a result of periodontal disease and brittle roots that break easily.
3. Taste buds decline in number.
4. Sense of smell diminishes.
5. Salivary secretion decreases.
6. Dysphagia is much more common.
Result: Eating is less pleasurable, appetite is reduced, and food is not sufficiently chewed or lubricated; therefore swallowing is difficult.

Stomach and Intestines
1. Gastric motility, blood flow, and volume and acid content of gastric juice may be reduced, particularly with gastric atrophy.
2. Protective mucosal barrier decreases.
3. There is a change in the composition of the microflora and resultant increased susceptibility to disease.

4. Intestinal villi become shorter and more convoluted, with diminished reparative capacity.
5. Intestinal absorption, motility, and blood flow decrease, impairing nutrient absorption.
6. Nutritive substances are absorbed more slowly and in smaller amounts.
7. Rectal muscle mass decreases, and the anal sphincter weakens.
8. Constipation is common and is related to immobility, low-fiber diet, and changes in enteric nervous system functions.

Liver
1. There is decreased hepatic regeneration; size and weight of liver decrease.
2. Ability to detoxify drugs decreases.
3. Blood flow decreases, influencing efficiency of drug metabolism.

Pancreas and Gallbladder
1. Fibrosis, fatty acid deposits, and pancreatic atrophy occur.
2. Secretion of digestive enzymes, particularly proteolytic enzymes, decreases.
3. No changes in gallbladder and bile ducts occur, but there is an increased prevalence of gallstones and cholecystitis.

Data from Bernard CE et al: Effect of age on the enteric nervous system of the human colon, *Neurogastroenterol Motil* 21(7):746–e46, 2009; Bouras EP, Tangalos EG: Chronic constipation in the elderly, *Gastroenterol Clin North Am* 38(3):463–480, 2009; Drozdowski L, Thomson AB: Aging and the intestine, *World J Gastroenterol* 12(47):7578–7584, 2006; Meier J, Sturm A: The intestinal epithelial barrier: does it become impaired with age? *Dig Dis* 27(3):240–245, 2009; Newton JL: Changes in upper gastrointestinal physiology with age, *Mech Ageing Dev* 125(12):867–870, 2004; Timchenko NA: Aging and liver regeneration, *Trends Endocrinol Metab* 20(4):171–176, 2009.

DID YOU UNDERSTAND?

The Gastrointestinal Tract

1. The major functions of the gastrointestinal tract are the mechanical and chemical breakdown of food and the absorption of digested nutrients.
2. The gastrointestinal tract is a hollow tube that extends from the mouth to the anus.
3. The walls of the gastrointestinal tract have several layers: mucosa, muscularis mucosae, submucosa, tunica muscularis (circular muscle and longitudinal muscle), and serosa.
4. The peritoneum is a double layer of membranous tissue. The visceral layer covers the abdominal organs, and the parietal layer extends along the abdominal wall.
5. Except for swallowing and defecation, which are controlled voluntarily, the functions of the gastrointestinal tract are controlled by extrinsic and intrinsic autonomic nerves and intestinal hormones.
6. Digestion begins in the mouth, with chewing and salivation. The digestive component of saliva is α-amylase, which initiates carbohydrate digestion.
7. The esophagus is a muscular tube that transports food from the mouth to the stomach. The tunica muscularis in the upper part of the esophagus is striated muscle, and that in the lower part is smooth muscle.
8. Swallowing is controlled by the swallowing center in the reticular formation of the brain. The two phases of swallowing are the oropharyngeal phase (voluntary swallowing) and the esophageal phase (involuntary swallowing).
9. Food is propelled through the gastrointestinal tract by peristalsis: waves of sequential relaxations and contractions of the tunica muscularis.
10. The lower esophageal sphincter opens to admit swallowed food into the stomach and then closes to prevent regurgitation of food back into the esophagus.
11. The stomach is a baglike structure that secretes digestive juices, mixes and stores food, and propels partially digested food (chyme) into the duodenum.
12. The vagus nerve stimulates gastric (stomach) secretion and motility.
13. The hormones gastrin and motilin stimulate gastric emptying; the hormones secretin and cholecystokinin delay gastric emptying.
14. Mucus is secreted throughout the stomach and protects the stomach wall from acid and digestive enzymes.
15. Gastric glands in the fundus and body of the stomach secrete intrinsic factor, which is needed for vitamin B_{12} absorption, and hydrochloric acid, which dissolves food fibers, kills microorganisms, and activates the enzyme pepsin.
16. Chief cells in the stomach secrete pepsinogen, which is converted to pepsin in the acidic environment created by hydrochloric acid.
17. Acid secretion is stimulated by the vagus nerve, gastrin, and histamine and is inhibited by sympathetic stimulation and cholecystokinin.
18. The three phases of acid secretion by the stomach are the cephalic phase (anticipation and swallowing), the gastric phase (food in the stomach), and the intestinal phase (chyme in the intestine).
19. The small intestine is 5 meters long and has three segments: the duodenum, jejunum, and ileum.
20. The duodenum receives chyme from the stomach through the pyloric valve. The presence of chyme stimulates the liver and gallbladder to deliver bile and the pancreas to deliver digestive enzymes. Bile and enzymes flow through an opening guarded by the sphincter of Oddi.
21. Bile is produced by the liver and is necessary for fat digestion and absorption. Bile's alkalinity helps to neutralize chyme, thereby creating a pH that enables the pancreatic enzymes to digest proteins, carbohydrates, and fats.
22. Enzymes secreted by the small intestine (maltase, sucrase, lactase), pancreatic enzymes, and bile salts act in the small intestine to digest proteins, carbohydrates, and fats.
23. Digested substances are absorbed across the intestinal wall and then transported to the liver, where they are metabolized further.
24. The ileocecal valve connects the small and large intestines and prevents reflux into the small intestine.
25. Villi are small fingerlike projections that extend from the small intestinal mucosa and increase its absorptive surface area.
26. Carbohydrates, amino acids, and fats are absorbed primarily by the duodenum and jejunum; bile salts and vitamin B_{12} are absorbed by the ileum. Vitamin B_{12} absorption requires the presence of intrinsic factor.
27. Bile salts emulsify and hydrolyze fats and incorporate them into water-soluble micelles, which are then transported through the unstirred layer to the brush border of the intestinal mucosa. The fat content of the micelles readily diffuses through the epithelium into lacteals (lymphatic ducts) in the villi. From there, fats flow into lymphatics and into the systemic circulation, which delivers them to the liver.
28. Minerals and water-soluble vitamins are absorbed by both active and passive transport throughout the small intestine.
29. Peristaltic movements created by longitudinal muscles propel the chyme along the intestinal tract, and contractions of the circular muscles (haustral segmentation) mix the chyme.
30. The ileogastric reflex inhibits gastric motility when the ileum is distended.
31. The intestinointestinal reflex inhibits intestinal motility when one intestinal segment is overdistended.
32. The gastroileal reflex increases intestinal motility when gastric motility increases.
33. The large intestine consists of the cecum, appendix, colon (ascending, transverse, descending, and sigmoid), rectum, and anal canal.
34. The teniae coli are three bands of longitudinal muscle that extend the length of the colon.
35. Haustra are pouches of colon formed with alternating contraction and relaxation of the circular muscles.
36. The mucosa of the large intestine contains mucus-secreting cells and mucosal folds, but no villi.
37. The large intestine massages the fecal mass and absorbs water and electrolytes.
38. Distention of the ileum with chyme causes the gastrocolic reflex, or the mass propulsion of feces to the rectum.
39. Defecation is stimulated when the rectum is distended with feces. The tonically contracted internal anal sphincter relaxes, and if the voluntarily regulated external sphincter relaxes, defecation occurs.
40. The largest number of intestinal bacteria is in the colon. They are anaerobes consisting of *Bacteroides,* clostridia, coliforms, and lactobacilli.
41. The intestinal tract is sterile at birth and becomes totally colonized within 3 to 4 weeks.
42. Endogenous infections of the gastrointestinal tract occur by excessive proliferation of bacteria, perforation of the intestine, or contamination from neighboring structures.
43. The splanchnic blood flow provides blood to the esophagus, stomach, small and large intestine, gallbladder, pancreas, and spleen.

Accessory Organs of Digestion

1. The liver is the second largest organ in the body. It has digestive, metabolic, hematologic, vascular, and immunologic functions.
2. The liver is divided into the right and left lobes and is supported by the falciform, round, and coronary ligaments.
3. Liver lobules consist of plates of hepatocytes, which are the functional cells of the liver.

Continued

DID YOU UNDERSTAND?—cont'd

4. The hepatocytes synthesize 700 to 1200 ml of bile per day and secrete it into the bile canaliculi, which are small channels between the hepatocytes. The bile canaliculi drain bile into the common bile duct and then into the duodenum through an opening called the *major duodenal papilla (sphincter of Oddi)*.

5. Sinusoids are capillaries located between the plates of hepatocytes. Blood from the portal vein and hepatic artery flows through the sinusoids to a central vein in each lobule and then to the hepatic vein and inferior vena cava.

6. Kupffer cells, which are part of the mononuclear phagocyte system, line the sinusoids and destroy microorganisms in sinusoidal blood.

7. The primary bile acids are synthesized from cholesterol by the hepatocytes. The primary acids are then conjugated to form bile salts. The secondary bile acids are the product of bile salt deconjugation by bacteria in the intestinal lumen.

8. Most bile salts and acids are recycled. The absorption of bile salts and acids from the terminal ileum and their return to the liver are known as the *enterohepatic circulation of bile*.

9. Bilirubin is a pigment liberated by the lysis of aged red blood cells in the liver and spleen. Unconjugated bilirubin is fat soluble and can cross cell membranes. Unconjugated bilirubin is converted to water-soluble, conjugated bilirubin by hepatocytes and is secreted with bile.

10. The gallbladder is a saclike organ located on the inferior surface of the liver. The gallbladder stores bile between meals and ejects it when chyme enters the duodenum.

11. Stimulated by cholecystokinin, the gallbladder contracts and forces bile through the cystic duct and into the common bile duct. The sphincter of Oddi relaxes, enabling bile to flow through the major duodenal papilla into the duodenum.

12. The pancreas is a gland located behind the stomach. The endocrine pancreas produces hormones (glucagon, insulin) that facilitate the formation and cellular uptake of glucose. The exocrine pancreas secretes an alkaline solution and the enzymes (trypsin, chymotrypsin, carboxypeptidase, α-amylase, lipase) that digest proteins, carbohydrates, and fats.

13. Secretin stimulates pancreatic secretion of alkaline fluid, and cholecystokinin and acetylcholine stimulate secretion of enzymes. Pancreatic secretions originate in acini and ducts of the pancreas and empty into the duodenum through the common bile duct or an accessory duct that opens directly into the duodenum.

KEY TERMS

- Alimentary canal (gastrointestinal tract)   871
- Ampulla of Vater   888
- Antrum of stomach   874
- Ascending colon   881
- Bile   884
- Bile acid pool   885
- Bile acid–dependent fraction   885
- Bile acid–independent fraction   885
- Bile canaliculi   884
- Bile salt   884
- Bilirubin   885
- Body of stomach   874
- Brush border   878
- Cardiac orifice   874
- Cecum   881
- Chief cell   877
- Cholecystokinin   875
- Choleresis   885
- Choleretic agent   885
- Chyme   874
- Colon   881
- Common bile duct   884
- Conjugated bilirubin   886
- Crypts of Lieberkühn   878
- Cystic duct   887
- Deamination   887
- Defecation reflex (rectosphincteric reflex)   882
- Descending colon   881
- Disse space   884
- Duodenum   877
- Enteric plexus   871
- Enterohepatic circulation   885
- Enterokinase   889
- Esophageal phase of swallowing   874
- Esophagus   873
- Exocrine pancreas   888
- External anal sphincter   881
- Fecal mass   882
- Fundus of stomach   874
- Gallbladder   887
- Gastric emptying   876
- Gastric gland   876
- Gastrin   875
- Gastrocolic reflex   882
- Gastroileal reflex   881
- Glisson capsule   884
- Haustral segmentation   880
- Haustrum (pl., haustra)   881
- Hepatic artery   884
- Hepatic portal vein   884
- Hepatic vein   884
- Hepatocyte   884
- Ileocecal valve (sphincter)   878
- Ileogastric reflex   881
- Ileum   877
- Internal anal sphincter   881
- Intestinointestinal reflex   881
- Jejunum   877
- Kupffer cell (tissue macrophage)   884
- Lacteal   878
- Lamina propria   878
- Large intestine   881
- Liver   883
- Liver lobule   884
- Lower esophageal sphincter (cardiac sphincter)   873
- Major duodenal papilla   884
- Mesentery   878
- Metabolic detoxification (biotransformation)   887
- Microvillus (pl., microvilli)   878
- Motilin   875
- Mouth   873
- Mucosal barrier   877
- Myenteric plexus (Auerbach plexus)   878
- O'Beirne sphincter   881
- Oropharyngeal (voluntary) phase of swallowing   873
- Pancreas   888
- Pancreatic duct (Wirsung duct)   888
- Paneth cell   878
- Pepsin   877
- Peristalsis   873
- Peritoneal cavity   878
- Peritoneum   878
- Peyer patch   878
- Primary bile acid   885
- Primary peristalsis   874
- Pyloric sphincter   874
- Pylorus (gastroduodenal junction)   874
- Rectum   882
- Reticuloendothelial system   885
- Retropulsion   875
- S cell   890

KEY TERMS—cont'd

- Saliva 873
- Salivary α-amylase (ptyalin) 873
- Salivary gland 873
- Secondary bile acid 885
- Secondary peristalsis 874
- Secretin 875
- Sigmoid colon 881
- Sinusoid 884

- Small intestine 877
- Sphincter of Oddi 887
- Splanchnic blood flow 883
- Stomach 874
- Submucosal plexus (Meissner plexus) 878
- Swallowing 873
- Teniae coli 881
- Transverse colon 881

- Trypsin inhibitor 889
- Unconjugated bilirubin 886
- Upper esophageal sphincter 873
- Urobilinogen 886
- Valsalva maneuver 882
- Vermiform appendix 881
- Villus (pl., villi) 878

REFERENCES

1. Goyal RK, Chaudhury A: Physiology of normal esophageal motility, *J Clin Gastroentrol* 42(5):610–619, 2008.
2. Hellström PM, Grybäck P, Jacobsson H: The physiology of gastric emptying, *Best Pract Res Clin Anaesthesiol* 20(3):397–407, 2006.
2a. Schubert ML: Gastric secretion, *Curr Opin Gastroenterol* 26(6):598–603, 2010.
3. Niv Y, Fraser GM: The alkaline tide phenomenon, *J Clin Gastroenterol* 35(1):5–8, 2002.
4. Malbert CH: The ileocolonic sphincter, *Neurogastroenterol Motil* 17(suppl 1):41–49, 2005.
5. Johnson LR: Gastrointestinal physiology. In Johnson LR, editor: *Mosby physiology monograph series*, ed 7, St Louis, 2007, Mosby.
6. Ouellette AJ: Paneth cells and innate mucosal immunity, *Curr Opin Gastroenterol* 26(6):547–553, 2010.
7. Horton KM, Fishman EK: CT angiography of the mesenteric circulation, *Radiol Clin North Am* 48(2):331–345, 2010:viii.
8. Sekirov I, et al: Gut microbiota in health and disease, *Physiol Rev* 90(3):859–904, 2010.
9. Dienes HP, Drebber U: Pathology of immune-mediated liver injury, *Dig Dis* 28(1):57–62, 2010.

Alterations of Digestive Function

Sharon Dudley-Brown and Sue E. Huether

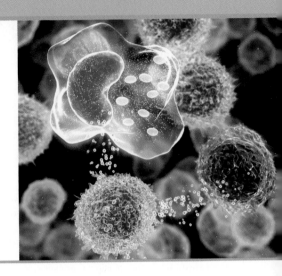

CHAPTER OUTLINE

The gastrointestinal (GI) tract is a continuous, hollow organ that extends from the mouth to the anus. It includes the esophagus, stomach, small intestine, large intestine, and rectum. The accessory organs of digestion include the salivary glands, liver, gallbladder, and pancreas.

Disorders of the gastrointestinal tract disrupt one or more of its functions. Structural and neural abnormalities can slow, obstruct, or accelerate the movement of intestinal contents at any level of the gastrointestinal tract. Inflammatory and ulcerative conditions of the gastrointestinal wall disrupt secretion, motility, and absorption. Inflammation or obstruction of the liver, pancreas, or gallbladder can alter metabolism and result in local and systemic symptoms. Many clinical manifestations of gastrointestinal tract disorders are nonspecific and can be caused by a variety of impairments.

DISORDERS OF THE GASTROINTESTINAL TRACT

Clinical Manifestations of Gastrointestinal Dysfunction

Anorexia

Anorexia is lack of a desire to eat despite physiologic stimuli that would normally produce hunger. This nonspecific symptom is often associated with nausea, abdominal pain, diarrhea, and psychologic stress.

Side effects of drugs and disorders of other organ systems, including cancer, heart disease, and renal disease, are often accompanied by anorexia. The eating disorder anorexia nervosa is discussed on p. 914.

Vomiting

Vomiting (emesis) is the forceful emptying of stomach and intestinal contents (chyme) through the mouth. Stimuli initiating the vomiting reflex include severe pain; distention of the stomach or duodenum; the presence of ipecac or copper salts in the duodenum; side effects of many drugs; torsion or trauma affecting the ovaries, testes, uterus, bladder, or kidney; motion; and activation of the chemoreceptor trigger zone (CTZ) (area postrema) in the medulla (e.g., morphine).[1]

Nausea and retching (dry heaves) usually precede vomiting. Nausea is a subjective experience associated with various conditions, including abnormal pain and labyrinthine stimulation (i.e., spinning movement). Specific neural pathways have not been identified, but hypersalivation and tachycardia are common associated symptoms. Retching begins with deep inspiration. The glottis closes, the intrathoracic pressure falls, and the esophagus becomes distended. Simultaneously, the abdominal muscles contract, creating a pressure gradient from abdomen to thorax. The lower esophageal sphincter (LES) and body of the stomach relax, but the duodenum and antrum of the stomach spasm. The reverse peristalsis and pressure gradient force chyme from the stomach and duodenum up into the esophagus. Because the upper esophageal sphincter is closed, chyme does not enter the mouth. As the abdominal muscles relax, the contents of the esophagus drop back into the stomach. This process may be repeated several times before vomiting occurs. A diffuse sympathetic discharge causes the tachycardia, tachypnea, and diaphoresis that accompany retching and vomiting. The parasympathetic system mediates copious salivation, increased gastric motility, and relaxation of the upper and lower esophageal sphincters.

Vomiting is usually associated with nausea and follows retching. The duodenum and antrum of the stomach produce reverse peristalsis, while the body of the stomach and the esophagus relax. When the stomach is full of gastric contents, the diaphragm is forced high into the thoracic cavity by strong contractions of the abdominal muscles. The higher intrathoracic pressure forces the upper esophageal sphincter to open, and chyme is expelled from the mouth. Then the stomach relaxes and the upper part of the esophagus contracts, forcing the remaining chyme back into the stomach. The lower esophageal sphincter then closes. The cycle is repeated if there is a volume of chyme remaining in the stomach.

Spontaneous vomiting not preceded by nausea or retching is called *projectile vomiting*. It is caused by direct stimulation of the vomiting center by neurologic lesions (e.g., increased intracranial pressure, tumors, or aneurysms) involving the brain stem or can be a symptom of gastrointestinal obstruction (pyloric stenosis). The metabolic consequences of vomiting are fluid, electrolyte, and acid-base disturbances including hyponatremia, hypokalemia, hypochloremia, and metabolic alkalosis (see Chapter 4).

Constipation

Constipation is difficult or infrequent defecation. It is a common problem and usually means a decrease in the number of bowel movements per week, hard stools, and difficult evacuation, but the definition must be individually determined. Normal bowel habits range from one to three evacuations per day to one per week. Constipation can occur as a primary or secondary condition.

PATHOPHYSIOLOGY Primary constipation is generally classified into three categories: *normal transit (functional) constipation* involves a normal rate of stool passage but there is difficulty with stool evacuation; *slow-transit constipation* involves impaired colonic motor activity with infrequent bowel movements, straining to defecate, mild abdominal distention, and palpable stool in the sigmoid colon; and *pelvic floor dysfunction* (pelvic floor dyssynergia) refers to an inability or difficulty expelling stool because of dysfunction of the pelvic floor muscles or anal sphincter.[1a]

Secondary constipation can be caused by neurogenic disorders (e.g., stroke, Parkinson disease, spinal cord lesions, multiple sclerosis, Hirschsprung disease) in which neural pathways or neurotransmitters are altered and colon transit time delayed.[2] A low-residue diet (the habitual consumption of highly refined foods) decreases the volume and number of stools and causes constipation. Activity stimulates peristalsis and a sedentary lifestyle and lack of regular exercise are common causes of constipation. Lack of access to toilet facilities, consistent suppression of the urge to empty the bowel, and dehydration are other causes. Opiates (particularly codeine), antacids containing calcium carbonate or aluminum hydroxide, anticholinergics, iron, and bismuth tend to inhibit bowel motility. Endocrine or metabolic disorders associated with constipation include hypothyroidism, diabetes mellitus, hypokalemia, and hypercalcemia. Pelvic hiatal hernia

(herniation of the bowel through the floor of the pelvis), diverticuli, irritable bowel syndrome–constipation predominant, and pregnancy are associated with constipation. Aging may result in decreased mobility, changes in neuromuscular function, use of medications, and comorbid medical conditions causing constipation.[3] Constipation as a notable change in bowel habits can be an indication of colorectal cancer.

CLINICAL MANIFESTATIONS Indicators of constipation include two of the following for at least 3 months: (1) straining with defecation at least 25% of the time; (2) lumpy or hard stools at least 25% of the time; (3) sensation of incomplete emptying at least 25% of the time; (4) manual maneuvers to facilitate stool evacuation for at least 25% of defecations; and (5) less than three bowel movements per week.[1a] Changes in bowel evacuation patterns, such as less frequent defecation, smaller stool volume, hard stools, difficulty passing stools (straining), or a feeling of bowel fullness and discomfort, require investigation. Fecal impaction (hard, dry stool retained in the rectum) is associated with rectal bleeding, abdominal or cramping pain, nausea and vomiting, weight loss, and episodes of diarrhea. Straining to evacuate stool may cause engorgement of the hemorrhoidal veins and hemorrhoidal disease or thrombosis with rectal pain, bleeding, and itching. Passage of hard stools can cause painful anal fissures.

EVALUATION AND TREATMENT The history, current use of medications, physical examination, and stool diaries provide precise clues regarding the nature of constipation. The individual's description of frequency, stool consistency, associated pain, and presence of blood or whether evacuation was stimulated by enemas or cathartics (laxatives) is important. Palpation may disclose colonic distention, masses, and tenderness. Digital examination of the rectum and anorectal manometry are performed to assess sphincter tone and detect anal lesions. Colonic transit time and imaging techniques can assist in identifying the cause of constipation. Colonoscopy is used to visualize the lumen directly.

The treatment for constipation is to manage the underlying cause or disease for each individual. Management of constipation usually consists of bowel retraining, in which the individual establishes a satisfactory bowel evacuation routine without becoming preoccupied with bowel movements. The individual also may need to engage in moderate exercise, drink more fluids, and increase fiber intake. Fiber supplements, stool softeners, and laxative agents are useful for some individuals. Enemas can be used to establish bowel routine, but they should not be used habitually. Biofeedback may be beneficial in some instances for forming new bowel evacuation habits. When there is failure to respond to dietary or medical therapies, surgery (colectomy) is considered as a last resort.[3a]

Diarrhea

Diarrhea is an increase in the frequency of defecation and in the fluid content and volume of feces. More than three stools per day are considered abnormal. Many factors determine stool volume and consistency, including water content of the colon and the presence of nonabsorbed food, nonabsorbable material, and intestinal secretions. Stool volume in the normal adult averages less than 200 g/day. Stool volume in children depends on age and size. An infant may pass up to 100 g/day. The adult intestine processes approximately 9 L of luminal contents per day: 2 L is ingested and the remaining 7 L consists of intestinal secretions. Of this volume, 99% of the fluid is absorbed: 90% (7 to 8 L) in the small intestine and 9% (1 to 2 L) in the colon. Normally, approximately 150 ml of water is excreted daily in the stool.

PATHOPHYSIOLOGY Diarrhea in which the volume of feces is increased is called *large-volume diarrhea.* It generally is caused by excessive amounts of water or secretions or both in the intestines. *Small-volume diarrhea,* in which the volume of feces is not increased, usually results from excessive intestinal motility.

The three major mechanisms of diarrhea are osmotic, secretory, and motile:

1. Osmotic diarrhea. A nonabsorbable substance in the intestine draws excess water into the intestine and increases stool weight and volume, producing large-volume diarrhea. Causes include lactase and pancreatic enzyme deficiency; excessive ingestion of synthetic, nonabsorbable sugars; full-strength tube-feeding formulas; or dumping syndrome associated with gastric resection (see p. 907).
2. Secretory diarrhea. Excessive mucosal secretion of fluid and electrolytes produces large-volume diarrhea. Infectious causes include viruses (e.g., rotavirus), bacterial enterotoxins (e.g., *Escherichia coli* and *Vibrio cholerae*), or exotoxins from overgrowth of *Clostridium difficile* following antibiotic therapy.[4] Small-volume diarrhea is usually caused by an inflammatory disorder of the intestine, such as ulcerative colitis or Crohn disease, but also can result from fecal impaction.
3. Motility diarrhea. Food is not mixed properly, digestion and absorption are impaired, and motility is increased. Causes include resection of the small intestine (short bowel syndrome), surgical bypass of an area of the intestine or fistula formation between loops of intestine, irritable bowel syndrome–diarrhea predominant, excessive motility of the intestine caused by diabetic neuropathy and hyperthyroidism, and laxative abuse.

CLINICAL MANIFESTATIONS Diarrhea can be acute or chronic, depending on its cause. Systemic effects of prolonged diarrhea are dehydration, electrolyte imbalance (hyponatremia, hypokalemia), and weight loss. Manifestations of acute bacterial or viral infection include fever, with or without cramping pain. Fever, cramping pain, and bloody stools accompany diarrhea caused by inflammatory bowel disease or dysentery. Steatorrhea (fat in the stools), bloating, and diarrhea are common signs of malabsorption syndromes. Anal and perineal skin irritation can occur.

EVALUATION AND TREATMENT A thorough history is taken to document the onset and frequency of diarrhea number and volume of stools. Exposure to contaminated food or water is indicated if the individual has traveled in foreign countries or areas where drinking water might be contaminated. Iatrogenic diarrhea is suggested if the individual has undergone abdominal radiation therapy, intestinal resection, or treatment with selected drugs (e.g., antibiotics, diuretics, antihypertensives, laxatives, or chemotherapy). Physical examination helps identify underlying systemic disease. Stool studies, abdominal imaging, and intestinal biopsies provide more specific data.

Treatment for diarrhea includes restoration of fluid and electrolyte balance, administration of antimotility (e.g., loperamide) and/or water absorbent (e.g., attapulgite and polycarbophil) medications, and treatment of causal factors. Nutritional deficiencies need to be corrected in cases of chronic diarrhea or malabsorption.[5]

Abdominal Pain

Abdominal pain is the presenting symptom of a number of gastrointestinal diseases and can be acute or chronic.[6] The causal mechanisms of abdominal pain are *mechanical, inflammatory,* or *ischemic.* Generally, the abdominal organs are not sensitive to mechanical stimuli, such as cutting, tearing, or crushing. These organs are, however, sensitive to stretching and distention, which activate nerve endings in both hollow and solid structures. Pain accompanies rapid distention rather than gradual distention. Traction on the peritoneum caused by adhesions, distention of the common bile duct, or forceful peristalsis resulting from intestinal obstruction causes pain because of increased tension. Capsules that surround solid organs, such as the liver and gallbladder, contain pain fibers that are stimulated by stretching if these organs swell. Abdominal pain may be generalized to the abdomen or localized to a particular abdominal quadrant. The nature of the pain is often described as sharp, dull, or colicky.

Abdominal pain is usually associated with tissue injury. Biochemical mediators of the inflammatory response, such as histamine, bradykinin, and serotonin, stimulate organic nerve endings and produce abdominal pain. The edema and vascular congestion that accompany chemical, bacterial, or viral inflammation also causes painful stretching. Hindrance of blood flow from the distention of bowel obstruction or mesenteric vessel thrombosis produces the pain of ischemia, and increased concentrations of tissue metabolites stimulate pain receptors.

Abdominal pain can be parietal (somatic), visceral, or referred. Parietal pain, from the parietal peritoneum, is more localized and intense than visceral pain, which arises from the organs themselves. Parietal pain lateralizes because, at any particular point, the parietal peritoneum is innervated from only one side of the nervous system.

Visceral pain arises from a stimulus (distention, inflammation, ischemia) acting on an abdominal organ. It is usually poorly localized with a radiating pattern and may be referred pain. Visceral pain is diffuse and vague because nerve endings in abdominal organs are sparse and multisegmented. Pain arising from the stomach, for example, is experienced as a sensation of fullness, cramping, or gnawing in the midepigastric area.

Referred pain is visceral pain felt at some distance from a diseased or affected organ. It is usually well localized and is felt in skin or deeper tissues that share a central afferent pathway with the affected organ. For example, acute cholecystitis may have pain referred to the right shoulder or scapula. Generally, referred pain develops as the intensity of a visceral pain stimulus increases.

Gastrointestinal Bleeding

Upper gastrointestinal bleeding is bleeding in the esophagus, stomach, or duodenum, and is characterized by frank, bright red bleeding or dark, grainy digested blood ("coffee ground") that has been affected by stomach acids[7] (see Table 34-1).

TABLE 34-1 PRESENTATIONS OF GASTROINTESTINAL BLEEDING

PRESENTATIONS	DEFINITION
Acute bleeding	
Hematemesis	Bloody vomitus; either fresh, bright red blood or dark grainy digested blood with "coffee grounds" appearance
Melena	Black, sticky, tarry, foul-smelling stools caused by digestion of blood in gastrointestinal tract; to be distinguished from black stools caused by dietary iron supplements, blackberries, or bismuth (e.g., Pepto-Bismol)
Hematochezia	Fresh, bright red blood passed from rectum
Occult bleeding	Trace amounts of blood in normal-appearing stools or gastric secretions; detectable only with positive fecal occult blood test (guaiac test)

Upper gastrointestinal bleeding is commonly caused by bleeding varices (varicose veins) in the esophagus, peptic ulcers, or a Mallory-Weiss tear at the esophageal/gastric junction caused by severe retching. **Lower gastrointestinal bleeding,** or bleeding from the jejunum, ileum, colon, or rectum, can be caused by polyps, diverticulitis, inflammatory disease, cancer, or hemorrhoids. **Occult bleeding** is usually caused by slow, chronic blood loss that is not obvious and results in iron deficiency anemia as iron stores in the bone marrow are slowly depleted. Acute, severe gastrointestinal bleeding is life-threatening, depending on the volume and rate of blood loss, associated disease and age of the affected individual, and effectiveness of treatment.[8]

Physiologic response to gastrointestinal bleeding depends on the amount and rate of the loss (Figure 34-1). Changes in blood pressure and heart rate are the best indicators of massive blood loss in the

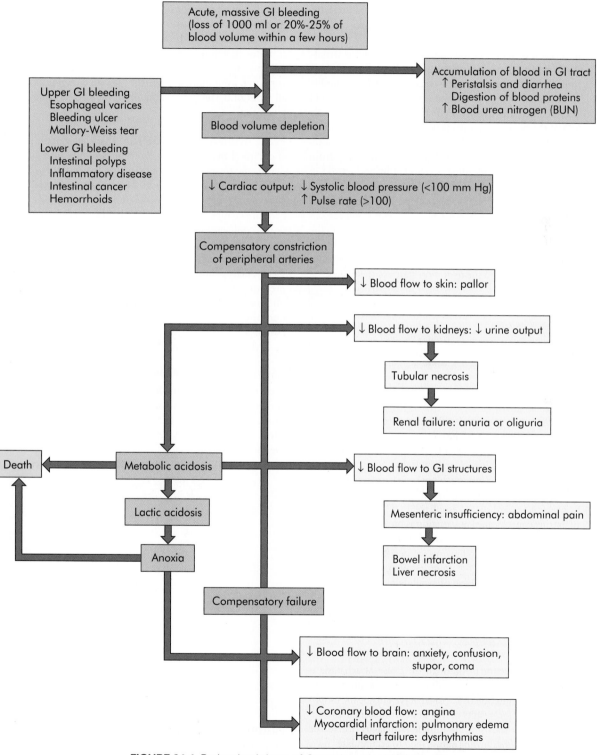

FIGURE 34-1 Pathophysiology of Gastrointestinal (GI) Bleeding.

gastrointestinal tract. During the early stages of blood volume depletion, the peripheral vascular compartment constricts to shunt blood to vital organs, including the brain. This is manifested as postural hypotension (a drop in blood pressure that occurs with a change from the recumbent position to a sitting or upright position), light-headedness, and loss of vision. Tachycardia develops as a compensatory response to maintain cardiac output and tissue perfusion. If blood loss continues, hypovolemic shock progresses (see Chapter 23). Diminished blood flow to the kidneys causes decreased urine output and may lead to oliguria (low urine output), tubular necrosis, and renal failure. Ultimately, insufficient cerebral and coronary blood flow causes irreversible anoxia and death.

The accumulation of blood in the gastrointestinal tract is irritating and increases peristalsis, causing vomiting or diarrhea, or both. If bleeding is from the lower gastrointestinal tract, the diarrhea is frankly bloody. Bleeding from the upper gastrointestinal tract also can be rapid enough to produce hematochezia (bright red stools), but generally some digestion of the blood components will have occurred, producing melena—black or tarry stools that are sticky and have a characteristic foul odor. The digestion of blood proteins originating from massive upper gastrointestinal bleeding is reflected by an increase in blood urea nitrogen (BUN) levels (see Figure 34-1).

The hematocrit and hemoglobin values are not the best indicators of acute gastrointestinal bleeding because plasma volume and red cell volume are lost proportionately. As the plasma volume is replaced, the hematocrit and hemoglobin values begin to reflect the extent of blood loss. The interpretation of these values is modified to account for exogenous replacement of fluids and the hydration status of the tissues.

✔ QUICK CHECK 34-1

1. How is visceral pain "referred"?
2. How does osmotic diarrhea differ from secretory diarrhea?
3. What are the best clinical indicators of acute GI bleeding blood loss?

Disorders of Motility
Dysphagia

PATHOPHYSIOLOGY Dysphagia is difficulty swallowing. It can result from *mechanical obstruction* of the esophagus or a functional disorder that impairs esophageal motility. Intrinsic obstructions originate in the wall of the esophageal lumen and include tumors, strictures, and diverticular herniations (outpouchings). Extrinsic mechanical obstructions originate outside the esophageal lumen and narrow the esophagus by pressing inward on the esophageal wall. The most common cause of extrinsic mechanical obstruction is tumor.

Functional dysphagia is caused by neural or muscular disorders that interfere with voluntary swallowing or peristalsis. Disorders that affect the striated muscles of the upper esophagus interfere with the oropharyngeal (voluntary) phase of swallowing. Typical causes are dermatomyositis (a muscle disease) and neurologic impairments caused by cerebrovascular accidents, Parkinson disease, or achalasia.

Achalasia is a rare form of dysphagia characterized by loss of esophageal peristalsis and failure of the lower esophageal sphincter (LES) to relax (functional obstruction). Although the cause of achalasia is unknown, it develops from autoimmune destruction of neurons in the myenteric plexus and dysfunction of the vagal nerve outside the esophagus.[9] Disrupted innervation results in loss of neuromuscular coordination and decreased peristalsis of the middle esophagus. Decreased relaxation of the LES after swallowing allows food to accumulate above the obstruction, which distends the esophagus and causes dysphagia

(Figure 34-2). As hydrostatic pressure increases, food is slowly forced past the obstruction into the stomach. Psychosocial achalasia has been documented and may be the result of life stressors.

CLINICAL MANIFESTATIONS Distention and spasm of the esophageal muscles during eating or drinking may cause a mild or severe stabbing pain at the level of obstruction. Discomfort occurring 2 to 4 seconds after swallowing is associated with upper esophageal obstruction. Discomfort occurring 10 to 15 seconds after swallowing is more common in obstructions of the lower esophagus. If obstruction results from a growing tumor, dysphagia begins with difficulty swallowing solids and advances to difficulty swallowing semisolids and liquids. If motor function is impaired, both solids and liquids are difficult to swallow. Regurgitation of undigested food, unpleasant taste sensation, vomiting, aspiration, and weight loss are common manifestations of all types of dysphagia. Aspiration of esophageal contents can lead to pneumonia.

EVALUATION AND TREATMENT Knowledge of the person's history and clinical manifestations contributes significantly to a diagnosis of dysphagia. Imaging is used to visualize the contours of the esophagus and identify structural defects. Manometry and intraluminal impedance monitoring documents the duration and amplitude of abnormal pressure changes associated with obstruction or loss of neural regulation. Esophageal endoscopy is performed to examine the esophageal mucosa and obtain biopsy specimens.

The individual is taught to manage symptoms by eating small meals slowly, taking fluid with meals, and sleeping with the head elevated to prevent regurgitation and aspiration. Anticholinergic drugs (e.g., botulinum toxin) may relieve symptoms of dysphagia. Mechanical dilation of the esophageal sphincter and surgical separation of the lower esophageal muscles with a longitudinal incision (myotomy) are the most effective treatments.[10]

Gastroesophageal Reflux Disease (GERD)

Gastroesophageal reflux disease (GERD) is the reflux of chyme (acid and pepsin) from the stomach through the lower esophageal sphincter to the esophagus. The LES may relax spontaneously and transiently 1 to 2 hours after eating, permitting gastric contents to regurgitate into the esophagus. The acid is usually neutralized and cleared from the esophagus by peristaltic action within 1 to 3 minutes, and sphincter

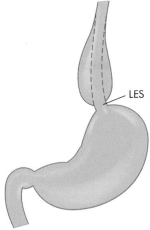

FIGURE 34-2 Achalasia. Increased LES muscle tone and loss of peristaltic function prevent food from entering the stomach, causing esophageal distention. *LES,* Lower esophageal sphincter.

tone is restored. Gastroesophageal reflux that does not cause symptoms is known as *physiologic reflux*. In nonerosive reflux disease (NERD),[11] individuals have symptoms of reflux disease but no visible esophageal mucosal injury. In some individuals, however, a combination of factors causes an inflammatory response to reflux called reflux esophagitis.[12]

PATHOPHYSIOLOGY Normally the resting tone of the LES maintains a zone of high pressure that prevents reflux. In individuals who develop reflux esophagitis, this pressure tends to be lower than normal. The severity of the esophagitis depends on the composition of the gastric contents and the length of time they are in contact with the esophageal mucosa. If the chyme is highly acidic or contains bile salts and pancreatic enzymes, reflux esophagitis can be severe. In individuals with weak esophageal peristalsis, refluxed chyme remains in the esophagus longer than usual. Vomiting, coughing, lifting, bending, obesity, or pregnancy increases abdominal pressure, contributing to the development of reflux esophagitis. Delayed gastric emptying contributes to reflux esophagitis by (1) lengthening the period during which reflux is possible and (2) increasing the acid content of chyme. Disorders that delay emptying include gastric or duodenal ulcers, which can cause pyloric edema; strictures that narrow the pylorus; and hiatal hernia, which can weaken the LES.[12] Reflux esophagitis causes inflammatory responses in the esophageal wall, such as hyperemia, increased capillary permeability, edema, tissue fragility, and erosion. Fibrosis and thickening may develop. Precancerous lesions (Barrett esophagus, see p. 925) can be a long-term consequence.[13] The association of *Helicobacter pylori* in the stomach and GERD is controversial. However, *H. pylori* may be protective by decreasing the potency of the gastric refluxate (gastritis leading to achlorhydria).[14]

CLINICAL MANIFESTATIONS The clinical manifestations of erosive reflux esophagitis are heartburn (pyrosis), acid regurgitation, dysphagia, chronic cough, asthma attacks (see Chapter 26), laryngitis, and upper abdominal pain within 1 hour of eating. The symptoms worsen if the individual lies down or if intra-abdominal pressure increases (e.g., as a result of coughing, vomiting, or straining at stool). Edema, strictures, esophageal spasm, or decreased esophageal motility may result in dysphagia with weight loss. Alcohol or acid-containing foods, such as citrus fruits, can cause discomfort during swallowing.

EVALUATION AND TREATMENT Diagnosis of reflux esophagitis is based on clinical manifestations, esophageal endoscopy that shows edema and erosion, and impedance/pH monitoring (measures the movement of stomach contents upward into the esophagus and the acidity of the refluxate). Esophageal endoscopy shows edema and erosion, and allows for evaluation of dysplastic changes (see Barrett esophagus, p. 925) and the development of esophageal carcinoma and associated conditions, such as hiatal hernia, gastric ulcers, and abnormal contours of the esophageal lumen. Because heartburn also may be experienced as chest pain, cardiac ischemia must be ruled out.

Proton pump inhibitors are the agents of choice for controlling symptoms and healing esophagitis.[15] Other therapies include H2-receptor antagonists or prokinetics, antacids, and alginate-antacids. Weight reduction, smoking cessation, and elevation of the head of the bed 6 inches also help to alleviate symptoms. If other treatments fail or if erosive esophagitis fails to heal, the LES may be narrowed with laparoscopic surgery (fundoplication).[13]

Hiatal Hernia

PATHOPHYSIOLOGY Hiatal hernia is a type of diaphragmatic hernia with protrusion (herniation) of the upper part of the stomach through the diaphragm and into the thorax (Figure 34-3).[16] The two most common types of hiatal hernia are as follows:

1. Sliding hiatal hernia (the most common). The stomach slides or moves into the thoracic cavity through the esophageal hiatus; a congenitally short esophagus, trauma, or weakening of the diaphragmatic muscles at the gastroesophageal junction is contributory. Coughing, bending, tight clothing, ascites, obesity, and pregnancy accentuate the hernia.
2. Paraesophageal hiatal hernia. The greater curvature of the stomach herniates through a secondary opening in the diaphragm and lies alongside the esophagus. Symptoms include congestion of mucosal blood flow leading to gastritis and ulcer formation. Strangulation of the hernia is a major complication.

Hiatal hernias of both types tend to occur in conjunction with several other diseases, including reflux esophagitis, peptic ulcer, cholecystitis (gallbladder inflammation), cholelithiasis (gallstones), chronic pancreatitis, and diverticulosis.

CLINICAL MANIFESTATIONS Hiatal hernias are often asymptomatic. Generally, a wide variety of symptoms develop later in life and are associated with other gastrointestinal disorders as well. Manifestations include gastroesophageal reflux, dysphagia, heartburn, vomiting, and epigastric pain. Regurgitation and substernal discomfort after eating are common.

EVALUATION AND TREATMENT Diagnostic procedures include barium swallow/upper GI series x-ray and endoscopy. A chest x-ray film often will show the protrusion of the stomach into the thorax, indicating paraesophageal hiatal hernia.

Treatment for sliding hiatal hernia is usually conservative. The individual can diminish reflux by eating small, frequent meals and avoiding the recumbent position after eating. Abdominal supports and tight clothing should be avoided, and weight control is recommended for obese individuals. Antacids alleviate reflux esophagitis. Individuals

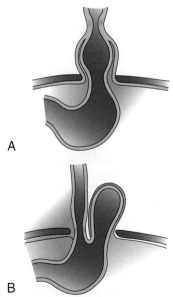

FIGURE 34-3 Types of Hiatal Hernia. **A,** Sliding hiatal hernia. **B,** Paraesophageal hiatal hernia.

who are uncomfortable at night benefit from sleeping with the head of the bed elevated 6 inches. Surgery (fundoplication) may be performed if medical management fails to control symptoms.[17]

Gastroparesis, or delayed gastric emptying in the absence of mechanical gastric outlet obstruction, is estimated to occur in 20%-40% of individuals with diabetes mellitus and may also be present in 25%-40% of individuals with functional (non-ulcer) dyspepsia, a condition affecting approximately 20% of the U.S. general population. The pathophysiology is not well understood but involves abnormalities of the autonomic nervous system, smooth muscle cells, enteric neurons, and gastrointestinal hormones. The major categories of gastroparesis are diabetic, postsurgical, and idiopathic. Diabetic gastroparesis represents a form of neuropathy involving the vagus nerve. Idiopathic gastroparesis is present in many patients with functional dyspepsia and may in some cases occur after an intestinal infection. Symptoms include nausea, vomiting, abdominal pain, and postprandial fullness or bloating. Treatment includes dietary management, prokinetic drugs, and in some cases, gastric electrical stimulation.

Pyloric Obstruction

PATHOPHYSIOLOGY Pyloric obstruction (gastric outlet obstruction) is the narrowing or blocking of the opening between the stomach and the duodenum. This condition can be congenital (e.g., infantile hypertrophic pyloric stenosis; see Chapter 35) or acquired. Acquired obstruction is caused by peptic ulcer disease or carcinoma near the pylorus. Duodenal ulcers are more likely than gastric ulcers to obstruct the pylorus. Ulceration causes obstruction resulting from inflammation, edema, spasm, fibrosis, or scarring. Tumors cause obstruction by growing into the pylorus.

CLINICAL MANIFESTATIONS Early in the course of pyloric obstruction, the individual experiences vague epigastric fullness, which becomes more distressing after eating and later in the day. Nausea and epigastric pain may occur as the muscles of the stomach contract in attempts to force chyme past the obstruction. These symptoms disappear when the chyme finally moves into the duodenum. As obstruction progresses, anorexia develops, sometimes accompanied by weight loss. Severe obstruction causes gastric distention and atony (lack of muscle tone and gastric motility). Gastric distention stimulates gastric secretion, which increases the feeling of fullness. Rolling or jarring of the abdomen produces a sloshing sound called the *succussion splash*. At this stage, vomiting is a cardinal sign of obstruction. It is usually copious and occurs several hours after eating. The vomitus contains undigested food but no bile. Prolonged vomiting leads to dehydration, which is accompanied by a hypokalemic and hypochloremic metabolic alkalosis caused by loss of potassium and gastric acid. Because food does not enter the intestine, stools are infrequent and small. Prolonged pyloric obstruction causes malnutrition, dehydration, and extreme debilitation.

EVALUATION AND TREATMENT Diagnosis is based on clinical manifestations, a history of ulcer disease, and examination of residual gastric contents. Endoscopy is performed if gastric carcinoma is the suggested cause of pyloric obstruction.

Obstructions resulting from ulceration often resolve with conservative management. A large-bore nasogastric tube is used to aspirate stomach contents and relieve distention. Then nasogastric suction is maintained for 2 to 3 days to decompress the stomach and restore normal motility. Gastric secretions that contribute to inflammation and edema can be suppressed with proton pump inhibitors or histamine 2 (H2) receptor antagonists. Fluids and electrolytes (saline and potassium) are given intravenously to promote rehydration and correct hypokalemia

CAUSE	PATHOPHYSIOLOGY
Hernia	Protrusion of intestine through weakness in abdominal muscles or through inguinal ring
Intussusception	Telescoping of one part of intestine into another; this usually causes strangulation of blood supply; more common in infants 10-15 months of age than in adults (see p. 943)
Torsion (volvulus)	Twisting of intestine on its mesenteric pedicle, with occlusion of blood supply; often associated with fibrous adhesions; occurs most often in middle-aged and elderly men
Diverticulosis	Inflamed saccular herniations (diverticuli) of mucosa and submucosa through tunica muscularis of colon; diverticuli are interspersed between thick, circular, fibrous bands; most common in obese individuals older than 60 years (see p. 910)
Tumor	Tumor growth into intestinal lumen; adenocarcinoma of colon and rectum is most common tumoral obstruction; most common in individuals older than 60 years
Paralytic (adynamic) ileus	Loss of peristaltic motor activity in intestine; associated with abdominal surgery, peritonitis, hypokalemia, ischemic bowel, spinal trauma, or pneumonia
Fibrous adhesions	Peritoneal irritation from surgery, trauma, or Crohn disease leads to formation of fibrin and adhesions that attach to intestine, omentum, or peritoneum and can cause obstruction; most common in small intestine

and alkalosis (see Chapter 4). Severely malnourished individuals may require parenteral hyperalimentation (intravenous nutrition). Surgery or the placement of pyloric stents may be required to treat gastric carcinoma or persistent obstruction caused by fibrosis and scarring.[18]

Intestinal Obstruction and Paralytic Ileus

Intestinal obstruction can be caused by any condition that prevents the normal flow of chyme through the intestinal lumen (Table 34-2). Obstructions can occur in either the small or the large intestine (Table 34-3). The small intestine is more commonly obstructed because of its narrower lumen. Criteria for classifying intestinal obstruction are summarized in Table 34-4. Intestinal obstruction is classified by cause as simple or functional. *Simple obstruction* is mechanical blockage of the lumen by a lesion and it is the most common type of intestinal obstruction. Paralytic ileus, or *functional obstruction*, is a failure of intestinal motility often occurring after abdominal surgery. Acute obstructions usually have mechanical causes, such as adhesions or hernias (Figure 34-4). Chronic or partial obstructions are more often associated with tumors or inflammatory disorders, particularly of the large intestine.

PATHOPHYSIOLOGY The major pathophysiologic alterations are presented in Figure 34-5. Postoperative paralytic ileus results from inhibitory neural reflexes associated with inflammatory mediators, and the influence of exogenous (meperidine) and endogenous opioids (endorphins).[19] If the obstruction is at the pylorus or high in the small intestine, metabolic alkalosis develops initially as a result of excessive loss of hydrogen ions that normally would be reabsorbed from the gastric juice. With prolonged obstruction or obstruction lower in the intestine, metabolic acidosis is more likely to occur because bicarbonate from

TABLE 34-3 LARGE AND SMALL BOWEL OBSTRUCTION

TYPE OF OBSTRUCTION	CAUSE
Small bowel obstruction	Adhesions: secondary to previous abdominal surgeries—75%
	Hernia: inguinal, ventral, or femoral—10%
	Tumors: may be associated with intussusception—10%
	Mesenteric ischemia—3-5%
	Crohn disease—<1%
Large bowel obstruction	Colon/rectal cancer—90%
	Volvulus—4-5%
	Diverticular disease—3-5%
	Other causes (inflammatory bowel disease, adhesions, hernia)

Data from Turnage RH, Heldmann M: Chapter 19, Intestinal obstruction. In Feldman M et al, editors: *Sleisenger & Fordtran's gastrointestinal and liver disease*, ed 9, pp 2105–2117, Philadelphia, 2010, Saunders.

TABLE 34-4 CLASSIFICATIONS OF INTESTINAL OBSTRUCTION

CRITERIA FOR CLASSIFICATION	DEFINITION
Onset	
Acute	Sudden onset; often caused by torsion, intussusception, or herniation
Chronic	Protracted onset; more commonly from tumor growth or progressive formation of strictures
Extent of Obstruction	
Partial	Incomplete obstruction of intestinal lumen
Complete	Complete obstruction of intestinal lumen
Location of Obstructing Lesion	
Intrinsic	Obstruction develops within intestinal lumen; examples: gut wall edema or hemorrhage, foreign bodies (gallstones), tumors, or gut wall fibrosis
Extrinsic	Obstruction originates outside intestine; examples: tumors, torsion, fibrosis, hernia, intussusception
Effects on Intestinal Wall	
Simple	Luminal obstruction without impairment of blood supply
Strangulated	Luminal obstruction with occlusion of blood supply
Closed loop	Obstruction at each end of a segment of intestine
Casual Factors	
Mechanical	Blockage of intestinal lumen by intrinsic or extrinsic lesions; usually treated surgically
Functional (paralytic ileus)	Paralysis of intestinal musculature caused by trauma, peritonitis, electrolyte imbalances, or spasmolytic agents; usually treated by decompression with suction or surgery if death of tissue

pancreatic secretions and bile cannot be reabsorbed. Hypokalemia can be extreme, promoting acidosis and atony of the intestinal wall. Metabolic acidosis also may be accentuated by ketosis, the result of declining carbohydrate stores caused by starvation. Gas from swallowed air, and to a lesser extent from bacterial overgrowth, contribute to the distention. If

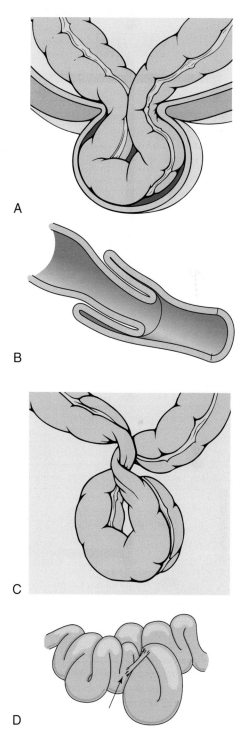

FIGURE 34-4 Intestinal Obstructions. **A,** Hernia. **B,** Intussusception. **C,** Volvulus. **D,** Constriction adhesions. (A, B, and C from Damjanov I: *Pathology for the health professions,* ed 3, Philadelphia, 2006, Saunders. D from Monahan FD et al: *Phipps' medical-surgical nursing: concepts and clinical practice,* ed 8, St Louis, 2007, Mosby.)

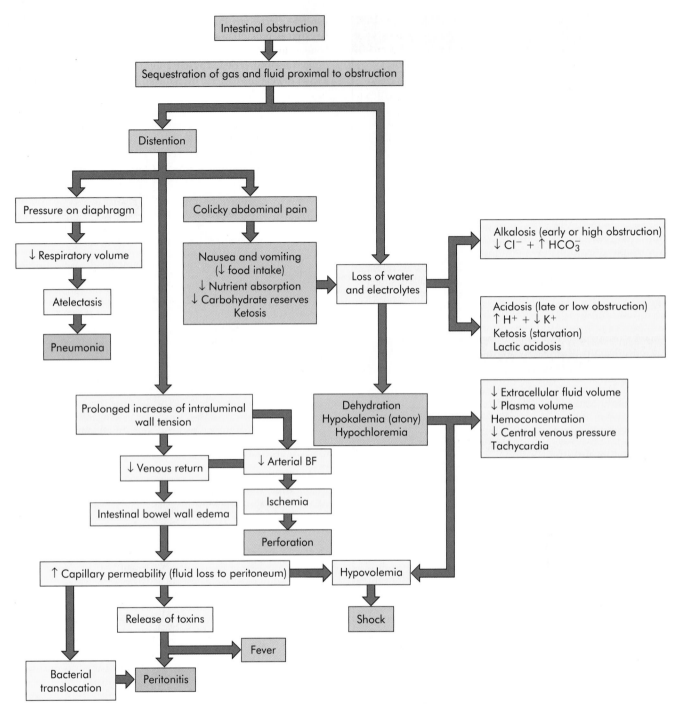

FIGURE 34-5 Pathophysiology of Intestinal Obstruction.

pressure from the distention is severe enough, it occludes the arterial circulation and causes ischemia and necrosis leading to perforation.[20] Continued intestinal secretion and decreased absorption lead to decreased blood volume and elevated hematocrit, decreased central venous pressure, and tachycardia. Severe dehydration leads to hypovolemic shock. Lack of circulation permits the buildup of significant amounts of lactic acid, which worsen the metabolic acidosis. Bacteria also proliferate and may cross the mucosal barrier and cause peritonitis or sepsis.

CLINICAL MANIFESTATIONS Crampy/colicky pains followed by vomiting and distention are the cardinal symptoms of small bowel

obstruction. Colonic obstruction usually presents as hypogastric pain and abdominal distention. Typically the pain occurs intermittently and intensifies for seconds or minutes as a peristaltic wave of muscle contraction meets the obstruction. Sweating, nausea, and hypotension occur as an autonomic response. The passing of the wave is followed by a pain-free interval. With severe distention, the pain may diminish in intensity. If strangulation occurs, the pain loses its colicky character, becoming more constant and severe as ischemia progresses to necrosis, perforation, and peritonitis.

Vomiting and distention vary, depending on the level of the obstruction. Obstruction at the pylorus causes early, profuse vomiting of clear golden-yellow gastric fluid. Obstruction in the proximal small intestine causes mild distention and vomiting of bile-stained (green to brown) fluid. Obstruction lower in the intestine causes more pronounced distention, and vomiting may not occur or may occur later and contain fecal material. Partial obstruction can cause diarrhea or constipation, but complete obstruction usually causes constipation only. Early in the course of complete obstruction, the frequency of bowel sounds increases and they may be tinkly and accompanied by peristaltic rushes and crampy/colicky abdominal pain as the bowel contracts to overcome the obstruction. During advanced stages of bowel obstruction the abdomen will become distended and silent. Distention may be severe enough to push against the diaphragm and decrease lung volume. This can lead to atelectasis and pneumonia, particularly in debilitated individuals. Signs of dehydration, hypovolemia, and metabolic acidosis may be observed as early as 24 hours after the occurrence of complete obstruction.

EVALUATION AND TREATMENT Evaluation is based on clinical manifestations and imaging. Successful management requires early identification of the site and type of obstruction. Preventive approaches to postoperative paralytic ileus include correction of fluid and electrolyte imbalances, early postsurgical ambulation, and use of nonnarcotic analgesics. Persistent ileus requires a multimodal approach, including thoracic epidural blockade with local anesthetic, nasogastric suction, mu opioid receptor blockade, and antisecretory and intestinal motility agents.[21] Immediate surgical intervention is required for complete obstruction, strangulation, or perforation.

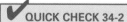

> **QUICK CHECK 34-2**
> 1. Why is heartburn associated with gastroesophageal reflux?
> 2. How does peritonitis develop with bowel obstruction?
> 3. What causes postoperative paralytic ileus?

Gastritis

Gastritis is an inflammatory disorder of the gastric mucosa. It can be acute or chronic and affect the fundus or antrum, or both.

Acute gastritis erodes the surface epithelium in a diffuse or localized pattern. The erosions are typically superficial. Acute gastritis is usually the result of injury of the protective mucosal barrier caused by drugs or chemicals. Nonsteroidal anti-inflammatory drugs (NSAIDs) that inhibit the action of cyclooxygenase-1 (COX-1) cause gastritis, perhaps because they inhibit prostaglandins, which normally stimulate the secretion of mucus. Alcohol, histamine, digitalis, and metabolic disorders such as uremia are contributing factors. The clinical manifestations of acute gastritis can include vague abdominal discomfort, epigastric tenderness, and bleeding. Healing usually occurs spontaneously within a few days. Discontinuing injurious drugs, using antacids, or decreasing acid secretion with H2-receptor antagonists facilitates healing.

Chronic gastritis tends to occur in elderly individuals and causes thinning and degeneration (atrophy) of the gastric mucosa. Chronic gastritis is classified as type A (fundal) or type B (antral), depending on the pathogenesis and location of the lesions. When both types of chronic gastritis occur, it is known as type AB or pangastritis, and the antrum is more severely involved.

Chronic fundal gastritis, also called atrophic or autoimmune gastritis, is the most severe type. The gastric mucosa degenerates extensively in the body and fundus of the stomach, leading to gastric atrophy. Loss of chief cells and parietal cells diminishes acid secretion, so the feedback mechanism that normally inhibits gastrin secretion is impaired, causing elevated plasma levels of gastrin. Pernicious anemia (see Chapter

20) may develop because intrinsic factor is less available to facilitate vitamin B_{12} absorption in the ileum.

A significant number of individuals with chronic fundal gastritis have antibodies to parietal cells, intrinsic factor, and gastric cells in their sera, suggesting that an autoimmune mechanism is involved in pathogenesis of the disease. The fact that chronic fundal gastritis occurs in association with other autoimmune diseases (e.g., rheumatoid arthritis, autoimmune thyroid disease, or type 1 diabetes mellitus) strengthens this association. Chronic fundal gastritis is a risk factor for gastric carcinoma, particularly in individuals who develop pernicious anemia.

Chronic antral gastritis generally involves the antrum only and occurs more often than fundal gastritis. It is caused by H. pylori bacteria and it is also associated with use of alcohol, tobacco, and nonsteroidal anti-inflammatory drugs.[22] There are high levels of hydrochloric acid secretion. H. pylori can also cause autoimmune atrophic gastritis and involve the fundus. In these cases there is greater risk for the development of gastric cancer.

Signs and symptoms of chronic gastritis often include vague symptoms: anorexia, fullness, nausea, vomiting, and epigastric pain. Gastric bleeding may be the only clinical manifestation of gastritis. Gastroscopic examination and biopsy may show a long-standing inflammatory process and gastric atrophy in an individual with no history of abdominal distress. Failure to stimulate acid secretion confirms achlorhydria (diminished secretion of hydrochloric acid). The gastric secretions also can be evaluated for the presence of intrinsic factor. Symptoms can usually be managed by eating smaller meals in conjunction with a soft, bland diet and by avoiding alcohol and aspirin. H. pylori infection is treated with antibiotics, and vitamin B_{12} is administered to correct pernicious anemia.

Peptic Ulcer Disease

A peptic ulcer is a break, or ulceration, in the protective mucosal lining of the lower esophagus, stomach, or duodenum. Ulcers develop when mucosal protective factors are overcome by erosive factors. Risk factors for peptic ulcer disease are summarized in Risk Factors: Peptic Ulcer. The exact mechanism of causation is unknown.[23] Zollinger-Ellison syndrome is a rare syndrome that is also associated with peptic ulcers caused by a gastrin-secreting neuroendocrine tumor or multiple tumors (gastrinoma) of the pancreas or duodenum. Increased secretion of gastrin causes excess secretion of gastric acid, resulting in gastric and duodenal ulcers, gastroesophageal reflux with abdominal pain, and diarrhea.[24]

Peptic ulcers can be single or multiple, acute or chronic, and superficial or deep. Superficial ulcerations are called erosions because they erode the mucosa but do not penetrate the muscularis mucosae (Figure 34-6). True ulcers extend through the muscularis mucosae and

RISK FACTORS

Peptic Ulcer

- Infection of the gastric and duodenal mucosa with *Helicobacter pylori*
- Chronic use of nonsteroidal anti-inflammatory drugs (NSAIDs)
- Alcohol
- Smoking
- Advanced age
- Chronic diseases, such as emphysema, rheumatoid arthritis, cirrhosis, and obesity and diabetes

Data from Garrow D, Delegge MH: Risk factors for gastrointestinal ulcer disease in the US population, *Dig Dis Sci* 55(1):66–72, 2010; Yuan Y, Padol IT, Hunt RH: Peptic ulcer disease today, *Nat Clin Pract Gastroenterol Hepatol* 3(2):80–89, 2006.

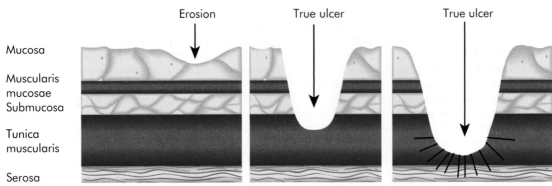

FIGURE 34-6 Lesions Caused by Peptic Ulcer Disease.

damage blood vessels, causing hemorrhage, or perforate the gastrointestinal wall.

Duodenal Ulcers

Duodenal ulcers occur with greater frequency than other types of peptic ulcers and tend to develop in younger persons and perhaps in individuals with type O blood.[25]

PATHOPHYSIOLOGY Infection with *H. pylori* and chronic use of nonsteroidal anti-inflammatory drugs (NSAIDs) that inhibit the action of cyclooxygenase-1 (COX-1) are the major causes of duodenal ulcer.[26] The following factors contribute to ulcer formation:

1. Serum gastrin levels remain high longer than normal after eating and continue to stimulate secretion of hydrochloric acid and pepsin (may be caused by *H. pylori*).
2. There is failure of the feedback mechanism in which acid in the gastric antrum inhibits gastrin release.
3. Rapid gastric emptying overwhelms the buffering capacity of the bicarbonate-rich pancreatic secretions.
4. *H. pylori* is associated with death of mucosal epithelial cells and elevated levels of gastrin and pepsinogen.
5. *H. pylori* releases toxins and enzymes that promote inflammation and ulceration.
6. Use of NSAIDs inhibits the action of cyclooxygenase-1 (COX-1), resulting in inhibition of prostaglandins and consequent reduced maintenance of the mucosal barrier as well as decreased bicarbonate secretion.
7. Cigarette smoking stimulates acid production.
8. The mass of gastric parietal (acid-secreting) cells increases.

All these factors, singly or in combination, cause acid and pepsin concentrations in the duodenum to penetrate the mucosal barrier and cause ulceration (Figure 34-7).

CLINICAL MANIFESTATIONS The characteristic manifestation of a duodenal ulcer is chronic intermittent pain in the epigastric area. The pain begins 2 or 3 hours after eating, when the stomach is empty. It is not unusual for pain to occur in the middle of the night and disappear by morning. Pain is relieved rapidly by ingestion of food or antacids, creating a typical pain-food-relief pattern. Some individuals with duodenal ulcer may have no symptoms; the first manifestation may be hemorrhage or perforation, particularly with a history of NSAID or anticoagulant use.

Complications of duodenal ulcer include bleeding, perforation, and obstruction of the duodenum or outlet of the stomach. Bleeding is the most common cause of mortality, particularly among the elderly. Perforation occurs with destruction of all layers of the duodenal wall and causes sudden, severe epigastric pain. Obstruction may be the result of edema from inflammation or scarring from chronic injury.

Duodenal ulcers often heal spontaneously but recur within months without treatment. Exacerbations tend to develop in the spring and fall. Relief of pain accompanies healing. Constant, unremitting pain may be caused by complications, such as intestinal obstruction or perforation. Bleeding from duodenal ulcers causes hematemesis or melena.

EVALUATION AND TREATMENT Several diagnostic approaches are used to differentiate duodenal ulcers from gastric ulcers or gastric carcinoma. Endoscopic evaluation allows visualization of lesions and biopsy. Radioimmune assays of gastrin levels are evaluated to identify ulcers associated with gastric carcinomas. The urea breath test, *H pylori* specific serum IgG and IgA antibodies, *H. pylori* stool antigen levels, and positive findings from gastric biopsy detect *H. pylori* infection and confirm eradication after treatment.[27]

Management of duodenal ulcers is aimed at (1) relieving the causes and effects of hyperacidity, (2) administering antacids and drugs that suppress acid secretion (omeprazole), and (3) preventing complications. *H. pylori* is treated with a combination of antibiotics and proton pump inhibitors.[28,29] Surgical resection may be required for bleeding or perforating ulcers, obstruction, or peritonitis. Research is in progress for an *H. pylori* vaccine.[30]

Gastric Ulcers

Gastric ulcers are ulcers of the stomach and occur about equally in males and females, usually between the ages of 55 and 65 years. They are about one fourth as common as duodenal ulcers (Table 34-5).

PATHOPHYSIOLOGY Use of NSAIDs and *H. pylori* infection are major causes of gastric ulcer. Generally, gastric ulcers develop in the antral region, adjacent to the acid-secreting mucosa of the body. The primary defect is an abnormality that increases the mucosal barrier's permeability to hydrogen ions. Gastric secretion may be normal or less than normal and there may be a decreased mass of parietal cells.

Chronic gastritis is often associated with development of gastric ulcers and may precipitate ulcer formation by limiting the mucosa's ability to secrete a protective layer of mucus (Figure 34-8). Other factors include the following:

1. Decreased mucosal synthesis of prostaglandins
2. Duodenal reflux of bile and pancreatic enzymes
3. Use of ulcerogenic drugs (e.g., aspirin, ibuprofen, naproxen)

An increased concentration of bile salts disrupts the gastric mucosa and may decrease the electrical potential across the gastric

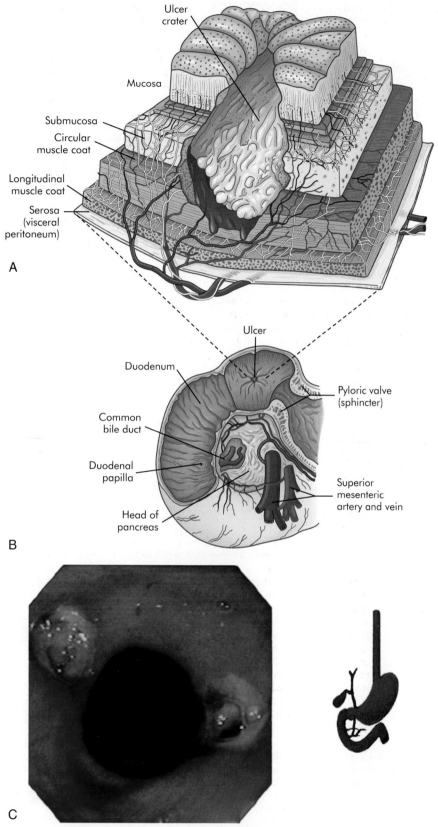

FIGURE 34-7 Duodenal Ulcer. **A,** A deep ulceration in the duodenal wall extending as a crater through the entire mucosa and into the muscle layers. **B,** Sequence of ulcerations from normal mucosa to duodenal ulcer. **C,** Bilateral (kissing) duodenal ulcers in a person using nonsteroidal anti-inflammatory drugs (NSAIDs). (**C** courtesy David Bjorkman, MD, University of Utah School of Medicine, Department of Gastroenterology, Salt Lake City, Utah.)

TABLE 34-5 CHARACTERISTICS OF GASTRIC AND DUODENAL ULCERS

CHARACTERISTICS	GASTRIC ULCER	DUODENAL ULCER	CHARACTERISTICS	GASTRIC ULCER	DUODENAL ULCER
Incidence			**Pathophysiology, cont'd**	Stimulates reduced acid secretion, gastric atrophy, and risk of gastric cancer	Stimulates acid hypersecretion
Age at onset	50-70 years	20-50 years			
Family history	Usually negative	Positive			
Gender (prevalence)	Equal in women and men	Greater in men			
Stress factors	Increased	Average	**Clinical Manifestations**		
Ulcerogenic drugs	Normal use	Increased use	Pain	Located in upper abdomen	Located in upper abdomen
Cancer risk	Increased	Not increased		Intermittent	Intermittent
Pathophysiology				Pain-antacid-relief pattern	Pain-antacid or food-relief pattern
Abnormal mucus	May be present	May be present		Food-pain pattern (when food in stomach)	Pain when stomach empty Nocturnal pain common
Parietal cell mass	Normal or decreased	Increased			
Acid production	Normal or decreased	Increased			
Serum gastrin	Increased	Normal	Clinical course	Chronic ulcer without pattern of remission and exacerbation	Pattern of remissions and exacerbation for years
Serum pepsinogen	Normal	Increased			Heals more quickly
Associated gastritis	More common	Usually not present		Heals more slowly	
Helicobacter pylori	May be present (60-80%)	Often present (95-100%)			

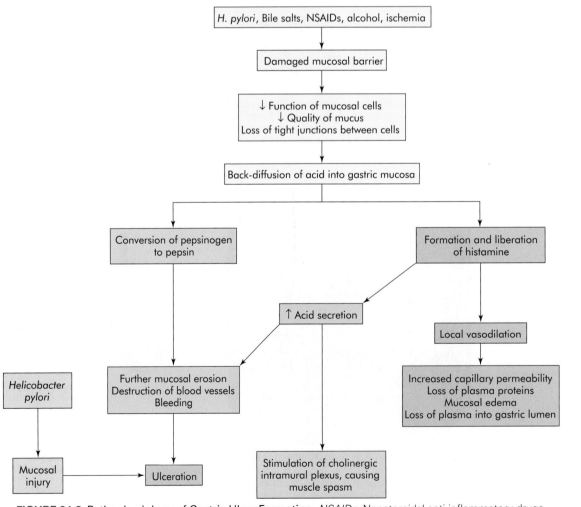

FIGURE 34-8 Pathophysiology of Gastric Ulcer Formation. _NSAIDs,_ Nonsteroidal anti-inflammatory drugs.

mucosal membrane. The break permits hydrogen ions to diffuse into the mucosa, where they disrupt permeability and cellular structure. A vicious cycle can be established as the damaged mucosa liberates histamine, which stimulates the increase of acid and pepsinogen production, blood flow, and capillary permeability. The disrupted mucosa becomes edematous and loses plasma proteins. Destruction of small vessels causes bleeding.

CLINICAL MANIFESTATIONS The clinical manifestations of gastric ulcers are similar to those of duodenal ulcers (see Table 34-5). The pattern of pain is different from that of duodenal ulcers because pain frequently occurs immediately after eating. Gastric ulcers cause more anorexia, vomiting, and weight loss than duodenal ulcers. Gastric ulcers also tend to be chronic rather than alternating between periods of remission and exacerbation. The evaluation and treatment of gastric ulcers are similar to the evaluation and treatment of duodenal ulcers, although duration of treatment is longer than with duodenal ulcers.

Stress-Related Mucosal Disease

A **stress-related mucosal disease (stress ulcer)** is an acute form of peptic ulcer that tends to accompany severe illness, systemic trauma, or neural injury. Emotional stress may also cause peptic ulcer.[31] Usually multiple sites of ulceration are distributed within the stomach or duodenum. Decreased mucosal blood flow, mucosal ischemia, and reperfusion injury are important contributing events in stress ulcer formation.[32] Stress ulcers may be classified as follows:

1. **Ischemic ulcer.** Develops within hours of events such as hemorrhage, multisystem trauma, severe burns, heart failure, or sepsis that causes ischemia of the stomach and duodenal mucosa; those that develop as a result of burn injury are often called *Curling ulcers.*
2. **Cushing ulcer.** Stress ulcer associated with severe head trauma or brain surgery that results from decreased mucosal blood flow and hypersecretion of acid caused by overstimulation of the vagal nuclei.

The primary clinical manifestation of stress-related mucosal disease is bleeding. Acid suppression with H2-receptor antagonists and proton pump inhibitors may provide the best prophylactic treatment.[33] Stress ulcers seldom become chronic.

Surgical Treatment of Ulcer

Advances in the medical treatment of peptic ulcer disease have reduced the number of cases requiring surgery. The most common indications for ulcer surgery are recurrent or uncontrolled bleeding and perforation of the stomach or duodenum. The primary objectives of surgical treatment are to reduce stimuli for acid secretion, decrease the number of acid-secreting cells in the stomach, and correct complications of ulcer disease.

Acute complications of gastrectomy or anastomosis are relatively uncommon except in debilitated persons. Chronic complications, however, are likely to develop if a large portion of the stomach has been removed. These complications and their pathophysiologic mechanisms are described in the next section.

QUICK CHECK 34-3
1. What is the most common cause of chronic gastritis?
2. Compare the three types of peptic ulcers.
3. What is Cushing ulcer?

Postgastrectomy Syndromes

Postgastrectomy syndromes are a group of signs and symptoms that occur after gastric resection for the treatment of peptic ulcer, gastric carcinoma, or bariatric surgery for extreme obesity. They are caused by anatomic and functional changes in the stomach and upper small intestine and include the following:

1. **Dumping syndrome.** Rapid emptying of hypertonic chyme from the surgically residual stomach (the stomach component remaining after surgical resection following gastric or bariatric surgery) into the small intestine 10 to 20 minutes after eating; promoted by loss of gastric capacity, loss of emptying control when pylorus is removed, and loss of feedback control by duodenum when it is removed; responds to dietary management. Symptoms include cramping pain, nausea, vomiting, osmotic diarrhea, weakness, pallor, and hypotension.[34]
2. **Alkaline reflux gastritis.** Stomach inflammation caused by reflux of bile and alkaline pancreatic secretions containing proteolytic enzymes that disrupt the mucosal barrier in the remnant stomach. Symptoms include nausea, bilious vomiting, and sustained epigastric pain that worsens after eating and is not relieved by antacids; responds somewhat to avoidance of aspirin and alcohol,[35] but surgical correction may be required.
3. **Afferent loop obstruction.** Intermittent severe pain and epigastric fullness after eating as a result of volvulus, hernia, adhesion, or stenosis of the duodenal stump on the proximal side of the gastrojejunostomy; vomiting relieves symptoms; management includes low-fat diet, but surgery is required for complete obstruction.[36]
4. **Diarrhea.** Either frequent, persistent elimination of liquid stool or intermittent, precipitous, and unpredictable elimination of a large volume of stool; related to rapid gastric emptying and osmotic attraction of water into the gut, especially after large intake of high-carbohydrate liquids; small, dry meals and anticholinergic drugs are effective control measures.
5. **Weight loss.** Commonly caused by inadequate caloric intake because individual cannot tolerate carbohydrates or a normal-size meal; stomach is also less able to mix, churn, and break down food. In the case of bariatric surgery for extreme obesity, weight loss is the intended outcome.
6. **Anemia.** Iron malabsorption may result from decreased acid secretion or lack of duodenum after Billroth II procedure (gastrojejunostomy); deficiencies of iron and vitamin B_{12} or folate may result.
7. **Bone and mineral disorders.** Related to altered calcium absorption and metabolism with increased risk for fractures and deformity and malabsorption of vitamins and nutrients, such as vitamin D.

Malabsorption Syndromes

Malabsorption syndromes interfere with nutrient absorption in the small intestine. Historically they have been classified as maldigestion or malabsorption. **Maldigestion** is failure of the chemical processes of digestion that take place in the intestinal lumen or at the brush border of the intestinal mucosa. **Malabsorption** is failure of the intestinal mucosa to absorb (transport) the digested nutrients. Often these two are interrelated or occur together, making classification difficult. Generally, however, maldigestion is caused by deficiencies of the enzymes needed for digestion. Inadequate secretion of bile salts and inadequate reabsorption of bile in the ileum also contribute to maldigestion. Malabsorption is the result of mucosal disruption caused by gastric or intestinal resection, vascular disorders, or intestinal disease. Celiac disease, an autoimmune disorder related to cereal grain gluten, is discussed in Chapter 35. Both malabsorption syndromes can cause or aggravate diarrhea.

Pancreatic Exocrine Insufficiency

The pancreatic enzymes (lipase, amylase, trypsin, chymotrypsin) are required for the digestion of proteins, carbohydrates, and fats. Pancreatic insufficiency is the deficient production of these enzymes, particularly lipase, by the pancreas. Causes include chronic pancreatitis, pancreatic carcinoma, pancreatic resection, and cystic fibrosis. Significant damage to or loss of pancreatic tissue must occur before enzyme levels decrease sufficiently to cause maldigestion. Although pancreatic insufficiency causes poor digestion of all nutrients, fat maldigestion is the chief problem. Absence of pancreatic bicarbonate in the duodenum and jejunum causes an acidic pH that worsens maldigestion by precipitating bile salts and preventing activation of the pancreatic enzymes that are present. A large amount of fat in the stool (steatorrhea) is the most common sign of pancreatic insufficiency. There is also a deficit of fat-soluble vitamins (A, D, E, and K).[37]

Lactase Deficiency (Lactose Intolerance)

Deficiency of disaccharidase at the brush border of the small intestine is caused by a genetic defect in which a single enzyme, usually lactase, is lacking. Lactase deficiency inhibits the breakdown of lactose (milk sugar) into monosaccharides and therefore prevents lactose digestion and absorption across the intestinal wall. Lactase deficiency is most common in blacks, Latinos, and Native Americans and usually does not develop until adulthood. Secondary (acquired) lactase deficiency can be caused by several diseases of the intestine, including gluten-sensitive enteropathy, enteritis, and bacterial overgrowth.

The undigested lactose remains in the intestine, where bacterial fermentation causes gases to form. Undigested lactose also increases the osmotic gradient in the intestine, causing irritation and osmotic diarrhea. Clinical manifestations of lactose consumption with lactase deficiency are bloating, crampy pain, diarrhea, and flatulence. The disorder is diagnosed by a lactose-tolerance test. Avoiding more than 1 cup of milk per day and adhering to a lactose-free diet relieve symptoms.[38]

Bile Salt Deficiency

Conjugated bile acids (bile salts) are necessary for the digestion and absorption of fats. Bile salts are conjugated in the bile that is secreted from the liver. When bile enters the duodenum, the bile salts aggregate with fatty acids and monoglycerides to form micelles. Micelle formation makes fat molecules more soluble and allows them to pass through the unstirred layer at the brush border of the small intestinal villi (see Chapter 33). A minimum concentration of bile salts, termed the *critical micelle concentration,* is required to allow micelles to form. Therefore, conditions that decrease the production or secretion of bile result in decreased micelle formation and fat malabsorption. These conditions include advanced liver disease, which decreases the production of bile salts; obstruction of the common bile duct, which decreases flow of bile into the duodenum (cholestasis); intestinal stasis (lack of motility), which permits overgrowth of intestinal bacteria that deconjugate bile salts; and diseases of the ileum, which prevent the reabsorption and recycling of bile salts (enterohepatic circulation).

Clinical manifestations of bile salt deficiency are related to poor intestinal absorption of fat and fat-soluble vitamins (A, D, E, K). Increased fat in the stools (steatorrhea) leads to diarrhea and decreased plasma proteins. The losses of fat-soluble vitamins and their effects include the following:
1. Vitamin A deficiency results in night blindness.
2. Vitamin D deficiency results in decreased calcium absorption with bone demineralization (osteoporosis), bone pain, and fractures.
3. Vitamin K deficiency prolongs prothrombin time, leading to spontaneous development of purpura (bruising) and petechiae.
4. Vitamin E deficiency has uncertain effects but may cause testicular atrophy and neurologic defects in children.

The most effective treatment for fat-soluble vitamin deficiency is to increase medium-chain triglycerides in the diet, for example, by using coconut oil for cooking. Vitamins A, D, and K are given parenterally. Oral bile salts are an effective therapy.

Inflammatory Bowel Disease

Ulcerative colitis (UC) and Crohn disease (CD) are complex, idiopathic chronic inflammatory bowel diseases (IBDs). These diseases have some differences in symptoms and macroscopic and microscopic changes. For example, the lesions of UC are continuous and located in the colon, whereas the lesions of CD may involve the entire GI tract and occur in patches with normal areas in between—"skip lesions." However, the combined effects of environmental changes, multiple genetic variations, mucosal immune dysregulation in response to gut microbes, epithelial barrier dysfunction, and alterations in microbial flora have some role for both in disease pathogenesis (Table 34-6).[39] Psychologic stresses have been associated with acute exacerbations for both UC and CD although the role of stress in inflammatory bowel disease is not clear.[40] Nicotine may be protective in UC but is an aggravating factor in CD.[41] The risk of colon cancer increases significantly after 8 to 10 years of inflammatory bowel disease.[42]

Ulcerative Colitis

Ulcerative colitis (UC) is a chronic inflammatory disease that causes ulceration of the colonic mucosa, most commonly in the rectum and sigmoid colon. The lesions appear in susceptible individuals between 20 and 40 years of age. Risk factors include family history of disease and Jewish descent, and the disease is more prevalent among white populations.[43]

The familial tendency to develop UC and the occurrence of disease in identical twins support a genetic theory of causation. Perhaps most significant are humoral immunologic factors (Th2 response) and activated macrophages associated with the disease. Lymphocytes (T cells) in individuals with UC may have cytotoxic effects on the epithelial cells of the colon. Furthermore, autoimmune disorders, such as systemic lupus erythematosus and erythema nodosum, may accompany UC.

PATHOPHYSIOLOGY The primary lesion of UC begins with inflammation at the base of the crypt of Lieberkühn in the large intestine. The disease begins in the rectum (proctitis) and may extend proximally to the entire colon (pancolitis). The mucosa is hyperemic and may appear dark red and velvety, and is involved in a continuous fashion. Small erosions form and coalesce into ulcers. Abscess formation, necrosis, and ragged ulceration of the mucosa ensue. Edema and thickening of the muscularis mucosae may narrow the lumen of the involved colon. Mucosal destruction and inflammation causes bleeding, cramping pain, and an urge to defecate. Frequent diarrhea, with passage of small amounts of blood and purulent mucus, is common. Loss of the absorptive mucosal surface and rapid colonic transit time cause large volumes of watery diarrhea.

CLINICAL MANIFESTATIONS The course of UC consists of intermittent periods of remission and exacerbation. Mild UC involves less mucosa, so that the frequency of bowel movements, bleeding, and pain is minimal. Severe forms may involve the entire colon and are characterized by fever, elevated pulse rate, frequent diarrhea (10 to 20 stools/day), urgency, obviously bloody stools, and continuous,

TABLE 34-6 FEATURES OF ULCERATIVE COLITIS AND CROHN DISEASE

FEATURE	ULCERATIVE COLITIS	CROHN DISEASE
Incidence		
Age at onset	Any age; 10-40 years most common	Any age; 10-30 years most common
Family history	Less common	More common
Gender	Prevalence equal in women and men	Prevalence about equal in women and men
Cancer risk	Increased	Increased
Nicotine use	Later and less severe disease, nicotine withdrawal may cause exacerbation	Increases disease risk and greater disease severity
Pathophysiology		
Location of lesions	Large intestine, continuous lesions	Mouth to anus, "skip" lesions common
	Left side more common	Right side more common
Inflammation	Mucosal layer involved	Entire intestinal wall involved
Granulomata	Rare	Transmural granulomata common; cobblestone appearance
Ulceration	Friable mucosa, superficial ulcers, crypt abscesses common	Small, superficial (aphthoid) ulcers common
Anal and perianal fistulae	Rare	Common; abscesses
Narrowed lumen and possible obstruction	Rare	Common; obstruction
Clinical Manifestations		
Abdominal pain	Mild to severe	Moderate to severe
Diarrhea	Common; 4 times/day	May or may not be present
Bloody stools	Common	Less common
Weight loss	Less common	Common
Abdominal mass	Rare	Common
Small intestine malabsorption	None	Common
Clinical course	Remissions and exacerbations	Remissions and exacerbations
Comorbidities	Extraintestinal manifestations	Extraintestinal manifestations

crampy pain. Dehydration, weight loss, anemia, and fever result from fluid loss, bleeding, and inflammation. Complications include anal fissures, hemorrhoids, and perirectal abscess. Severe hemorrhage is rare. Edema, strictures, or fibrosis can obstruct the colon. Perforation is an unusual but possible complication. Extraintestinal manifestations include cutaneous lesions, polyarthritis, episcleritis, disorders of the liver, and alterations in coagulation.[44]

EVALUATION AND TREATMENT Diagnosis of UC is based on the medical history and clinical manifestations. Colonoscopy with biopsies is used in addition to laboratory data. Biomarkers are being evaluated for use in determining disease progression and severity.[45] Infectious causes are ruled out by stool culture. The symptoms of UC may be similar to those of Crohn disease, making differential diagnosis challenging.

Treatment is individualized and depends on the severity of symptoms and the extent of mucosal involvement. The disease is often treated with mesalamine products (5-aminosalicylic acid). Steroids and aminosalicylates suppress the inflammatory response and help to alleviate the cramping pain. Immunosuppressants and immunomodulatory agents, including tumor necrosis factor-alpha (TNF-α) blocking agents, may induce and maintain remission.[46] Severe, unremitting disease can require hospital admission for administration of intravenous fluids and steroids. Extreme malnutrition may require total parenteral nutrition (TPN). Surgical resection of the colon may be performed if other forms of therapy are unsuccessful or if there are acute serious complications (sepsis, hemorrhage, perforation, or obstruction). Surgical approaches for severe UC include total proctocolectomy, with end ileostomy or ileorectal anastomosis, or ileal pouch anal anastomosis (IPAA).[47]

Crohn Disease

Crohn disease (CD) is an inflammatory disorder that affects both the large and the small intestine. In a small percentage of cases, CD is difficult to differentiate from ulcerative colitis (see Table 34-6), however, the rectum is seldom involved. Risk factors and theories of causation are the same as those for ulcerative colitis, including genetic predisposition and an altered immune response to intestinal bacteria.[48]

Of affected individuals, 10% to 20% have a positive family history. Increased activity of suppressor T cells, alterations in immunoglobulin A (IgA) production, activation of macrophages, and the presence of antibodies against luminal antigens, luminal flora, and susceptibility genes are factors associated with CD.

PATHOPHYSIOLOGY The inflammation process of CD is thought to be triggered by a cell-mediated (Th1) response and increased levels of interferon-gamma (IFN-γ) and tumor necrosis factor-alpha (TNF-α). Inflammation begins in the intestinal submucosa and spreads inward and outward to involve the mucosa and serosa. Activated neutrophils and macrophages promote inflammation and cause tissue injury. The ascending colon and the transverse colon are the most common sites of the disease, but both the large and small intestines may be involved, particularly the ileum. The inflammation can affect some segments of the intestine but not others, creating "skip lesions." One side of the intestinal wall may be affected and not the other. The ulcerations of CD can produce fissures that extend inflammation into lymphoid tissue. The typical lesion is a granuloma (granulomata are described in Chapter 5) with a cobblestone appearance from projections of inflamed tissue surrounded by ulceration. Fistulae may form in the perianal area between loops of intestine or extend into the bladder, rectum, or vagina. Strictures may develop, promoting obstruction. Smoking increases the risk of developing severe disease, and may cause a poorer response to treatment.[49]

CLINICAL MANIFESTATIONS Individuals with CD may have no specific symptoms for several years. Symptoms vary according to the location of the disease. Diarrhea is one of the most common symptoms and, occasionally, rectal bleeding if the colon is involved. Weight loss and abdominal pain accompany CD. If the ileum is involved, the individual may be anemic as a result of malabsorption of vitamin B$_{12}$. There also may be deficiencies in folic acid and vitamin D absorption.

In addition, proteins may be lost, leading to hypoalbuminemia. Extraintestinal complications are similar to those occurring in ulcerative colitis.

EVALUATION AND TREATMENT The diagnosis and treatment of CD are similar to the diagnosis and treatment of ulcerative colitis; however, imaging of the small intestine is used in the diagnosis of CD, including either a small bowel series or a capsule endoscopy (camera pill). Smoking cessation is a component of therapy. Surgery may be performed to manage complications such as fistula, abscess, or obstruction. Routine colonoscopy for cancer screening should be performed for long-standing colonic disease.

Diverticular Disease of the Colon

Diverticula are herniations or saclike outpouchings of the mucosa and submucosa through the muscle layers, usually in the wall of the sigmoid colon (Figure 34-9). **Diverticulosis** is asymptomatic diverticular disease. **Diverticulitis** represents inflammation. Diverticular disease is most common among elderly women, but the incidence is increasing in younger individuals, particularly when much of the diet consists of refined foods.

PATHOPHYSIOLOGY Diverticula can occur anywhere in the gastrointestinal tract, and the most common sites are the left sigmoid colon in Western countries and the right colon in Asian countries. The exact etiology of diverticular disease remains unknown.[50] The diverticula form from increases in intraluminal pressure, particularly at weak points in the colon wall, usually where arteries penetrate the tunica muscularis. A common associated finding is thickening of the circular muscles and shortening of the longitudinal (teniae coli) muscles surrounding the diverticula. Increased collagen and elastin deposition, not muscle hypertrophy, is associated with muscle thickening and this contributes to increased intraluminal pressure and herniation. Habitual consumption of a low-residue diet reduces fecal bulk, thus reducing the diameter of the colon.[51] According to the law of Laplace (see Chapter 22), wall pressure increases as the diameter of a cylindrical structure decreases. Therefore, pressure within the narrow lumen can increase enough to rupture the diverticula, causing inflammation and diverticulitis. Bacteria and local ischemia also may be contributing factors. Diverticulitis can rarely cause fistula, abscess formation, perforation, bowel obstruction, and peritonitis.[52]

CLINICAL MANIFESTATIONS Symptoms of diverticular disease may be vague or absent. Cramping pain of the lower abdomen can accompany constriction of the thickened colonic muscles. Diarrhea, constipation, distention, or flatulence may occur. If the diverticula become inflamed or abscesses form, the individual develops fever, leukocytosis (increased white blood cell count), and tenderness of the lower left quadrant.

EVALUATION AND TREATMENT Diverticula are often discovered during diagnostic procedures performed for other problems. Sigmoidoscopy or colonoscopy permits direct observation of the lesions. Abdominal computed tomography is used for diagnosis of diverticulitis.

An increase of dietary fiber intake often relieves symptoms and probiotics and mesalazine are being evaluated. Uncomplicated diverticulitis is usually treated with nonabsorbable antibiotics, bowel rest, and analgesia.[53] Laparoscopic resection and other minimally invasive approaches are being implemented for more severe complications.[54,55]

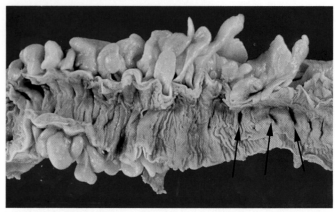

FIGURE 34-9 **Diverticular Disease.** In diverticular disease, the outpouches *(arrows)* of mucosa seen in the sigmoid colon appear as slitlike openings from the mucosal surface of the opened bowel. (Modified from Stevens A, Lowe, J: *Pathology,* ed 2, Edinburgh, 2000, Mosby.)

Appendicitis

Appendicitis is an inflammation of the vermiform appendix, which is a projection from the apex of the cecum. It is the most common surgical emergency of the abdomen and affects 7% to 12% of the population. It generally occurs between 20 and 30 years of age, although it may develop at any age.

PATHOPHYSIOLOGY The exact mechanism of the cause of appendicitis is controversial. Obstruction of the lumen with stool, tumors, or foreign bodies with consequent bacterial infection is the most common theory. The obstructed lumen does not allow drainage of the appendix, and as mucosal secretion continues, intraluminal pressure increases. The increased pressure decreases mucosal blood flow, and the appendix becomes hypoxic. The mucosa ulcerates, promoting bacterial or other microbial invasion with further inflammation and edema. Inflammation may involve the distal or entire appendix. Gangrene develops from thrombosis of the luminal blood vessels, followed by perforation.[56]

CLINICAL MANIFESTATIONS Gastric or periumbilical pain is the typical symptom of an inflamed appendix. The pain may be vague at first, increasing in intensity over 3 to 4 hours. It may subside and then recur in the right lower quadrant, indicating extension of the inflammation to the surrounding tissues. Nausea, vomiting, and anorexia follow the onset of pain, and a low-grade fever is common. Diarrhea occurs in some individuals, particularly children; others have a sensation of constipation. Perforation, peritonitis, and abscess formation are the most serious complications of appendicitis.

EVALUATION AND TREATMENT In addition to clinical manifestations, the clinician can usually locate the painful site with one finger. Rebound tenderness is usually referred to the right lower quadrant. The white blood cell count ranges from 10,000 to 16,000 cells/mm³ with increased neutrophils. Ultrasonography and computed tomography (CT) scans can assist in differentiating appendicitis from perforated ulcer or cholecystitis.

Laparoscopic appendectomy is the treatment for simple or perforated appendicitis.[57] Surgery provides quick recovery for simple appendicitis. Recovery is more complicated in cases of perforation or abscess formation.

Irritable Bowel Syndrome

Irritable bowel syndrome (IBS) is a functional gastrointestinal disorder with no specific structural or biochemical alterations as a cause of disease. It is broadly characterized by recurrent abdominal pain and discomfort associated with altered bowel habits that present as diarrhea or constipation or both. About 7% to 20% of the world's population is estimated to have the disorder, and it is more common in women with a higher prevalence during youth and middle age. Individuals with symptoms of IBS are also more likely to have anxiety, depression, and chronic fatigue syndrome. Symptoms of IBS can negatively affect quality of life and activity and present a significant economic burden.[58]

PATHOPHYSIOLOGY The pathophysiology of IBS is complex, but there is increasing evidence for organic disease. Several mechanisms are proposed to explain the causes for the symptoms listed here.

1. Visceral hypersensitivity or hyperalgesia particularly with distention of the rectum, but also other areas of the gut, may originate in either the peripheral or the central nervous system. The mechanism may be related to dysregulation of the "brain-gut axis" (alterations in gut or central nervous system processing of gut nociceptive information), changes in the role of serotonin in the enteric nervous system of the gut, activation of the gut immune system, or alterations in the autonomic nervous system.[59]
2. Abnormal gastrointestinal motility and secretion are associated with IBS. Individuals with diarrhea-type IBS have more rapid colonic transit times, whereas those with bloating and constipation have delayed transit times. The mechanism may also be related to visceral hypersensitivity as well as dysregulation of the brain-gut axis or alterations in the role of serotonin in the function of the enteric nervous system.[60]
3. Intestinal infection (bacterial enteritis) has been associated with symptoms of IBS, and postinfectious IBS appears to be related to ongoing low-grade inflammation, changes in intestinal permeability, and an abnormal immune response in gut tissues.[61]
4. Overgrowth of small intestinal flora (normal gut bacteria) may precipitate IBS symptoms, and it is proposed that methane gas may slow intestinal transit time, resulting in constipation and bloating.[62]
5. Food allergy or food intolerance is associated with IBS. Food antigens or food-borne pathogens may activate the mucosal immune system, alter intestinal flora, or mediate hypersensitivity reactions and IBS symptoms. Food elimination approaches are helpful in some cases.[63]
6. Psychosocial factors, including emotional stress, influence brain-gut interactions and neuroendocrine, autonomic nervous system, and pain modulatory responses, contributing to the symptoms of IBS.[64]

CLINICAL MANIFESTATIONS IBS is characterized by lower abdominal pain or discomfort (Box 34-1) and can be diarrhea-predominant, constipation-predominant, or alternating diarrhea/constipation. Symptoms including gas, bloating, and nausea are usually relieved with defecation and do not interfere with sleep.

EVALUATION AND TREATMENT The diagnosis of IBS is based on signs and symptoms and includes the exclusion of structural or biochemical causes of disease. Diagnostic procedures to rule out other causes of symptoms may include endoscopic evaluations, computed tomography (CT) scans or abdominal ultrasound, blood tests, and tests for lactose intolerance, celiac disease, or other disorders. The

---

BOX 34-1 ROME III—DIAGNOSTIC CRITERIA FOR IRRITABLE BOWEL SYNDROME (IBS)

Recurrent abdominal pain or discomfort* at least 3 days/month in the last 3 months associated with two or more of the following:
- Improvement with defecation
- Onset associated with a change in frequency of stool
- Onset associated with a change in form (appearance) of stool†

From *Rome III diagnostic criteria for functional gastrointestinal disorders.* Accessed June 2011. Available at www.romecriteria.org/criteria/
*"Discomfort" means an uncomfortable sensation not described as pain.
†Diagnostic criterion.

---

person may be evaluated for food allergies, parasites, or bacterial growth. The Rome III criteria for diagnosing IBS guide evaluation (see Box 34-1).

There is no cure for IBS, and treatment is individualized. Pharmacologic treatment of symptoms may include laxatives and fiber, antidiarrheals, antispasmodics, low-dose antidepressants, visceral analgesics, and serotonin agonists or antagonists. Alternative therapies including probiotics, hypnosis, acupuncture, and psychotherapy are treatment options. Research continues to advance the management of this complex syndrome.[65,66]

Vascular Insufficiency

Three branches of the abdominal aorta supply the stomach and intestines: the celiac axis (stomach, liver, spleen, pancreas), the superior mesenteric artery (small intestine arterial supply), and the inferior mesenteric artery (large intestine arterial supply) (see Figure 33-12). Mesenteric arterial hypoperfusion is less common than occlusive lesions caused by atherosclerosis, thrombi, or emboli. Mesenteric vein thrombosis is the least common cause of mesenteric ischemia with symptoms similar to those for mesenteric arterial insufficiency but with a more prolonged course.[67]

Chronic mesenteric arterial insufficiency (hypoperfusion) is rare but can develop secondary to congestive heart failure, acute myocardial infarction, hemorrhage, stenosis, thrombus formation, or any condition that decreases arterial blood flow. Elderly individuals with arteriosclerosis are particularly susceptible. Chronic occlusion is often accompanied by formation of collateral circulation. The collateral vessels may be able to nourish the resting intestine, but after eating, when the intestine requires more blood, the arterial supply may be insufficient. Ischemia develops, causing cramping abdominal pain (abdominal angina), a cardinal symptom. Some individuals suffer significant weight loss because they stop eating to control the pain. Progressive vascular obstruction eventually causes continuous abdominal pain and necrosis of the intestinal tissue.[68]

Acute mesenteric arterial insufficiency results from dissecting aortic aneurysms, ruptured aortic aneurysms (rare), or emboli. Embolic obstruction is associated with atrial fibrillation, mitral valve disease, and heart valve prostheses. The superior mesenteric artery has a more direct line of flow from the aorta; therefore, emboli enter it more readily than the inferior branch, causing ischemia and necrosis of the small intestine. Initially, there is increased motility. Ischemia and necrosis (intestinal infarction) alter membrane permeability and the damaged intestinal mucosa cannot produce enough mucus to protect itself from digestive enzymes. Bloody diarrhea develops. Fluid moves from the blood vessels into the bowel wall and peritoneum, causing hypovolemia, and further decreases intestinal blood flow. As intestinal infarction progresses, abdominal pain is severe with a rigid distended abdomen, loss of bowel sounds, shock, peritonitis, leukocytosis, fever, and tachycardia.

Diagnosis of mesenteric artery occlusion is based on clinical manifestations, mesenteric artery angiography, and abdominal imaging. Often a bruit can be heard over the occluded artery. Treatment includes aggressive rehydration and the use of antibiotics, anticoagulants, vasodilators, and inhibitors of reperfusion injury. Revascularization surgery is performed for both chronic and acute mesenteric arterial insufficiency when necrosis and infarction are suspected. Mortality is high for individuals with acute occlusion, compromised cardiac output, coexisting systemic disease, or delayed diagnosis.[69]

Disorders of Nutrition
Obesity

Obesity is an increase in body fat mass and a metabolic disorder that has become an epidemic worldwide. The incidence is rapidly increasing among children and adolescents and they tend to become obese adults.[70] Obesity is defined as a body mass index (body mass index [BMI] = kg/m^2) that exceeds 30[71] and generally develops when caloric intake exceeds caloric expenditure. Obesity is a major risk factor for morbidity, death, and increased healthcare costs.[72] Three leading causes of death associated with obesity are coronary artery disease, type 2 diabetes mellitus, and cancer (colon, breast in postmenopausal women, endometrial, prostate, kidney, and esophagus). Obesity also is a risk factor for hypertension, stroke, hepatobiliary disease (gallstones and nonalcoholic steatohepatitis), osteoarthritis, and infectious disease. Pulmonary function can be compromised by a large amount of adipose tissue overlying the chest cage, and obstructive sleep apnea syndrome can occur as a consequence[73] (see Chapter 13).

The causes and consequences of obesity are multiple and complex. Rapidly advancing research regarding risk factors, causal mechanisms, and complications is in progress. Obesity is known to occur in families and genotypes, and gene-environment interactions are important predisposing factors.[74] Environmental factors include culture, socioeconomic status, food intake habits, and physical activity. Metabolic abnormalities associated with obesity include Cushing syndrome, Cushing disease, polycystic ovarian syndrome, hypothyroidism, and hypothalamic injury.

PATHOPHYSIOLOGY The pathophysiology of obesity is complex and involves the interaction of numerous cytokines, hormones, and neurotransmitters. When adipocytes (fat cells) increase in size and number they secrete hormones and cytokines, known as adipocytokines.[75,76] These adipocytokines and other hormones (Box 34-2) participate in regulation of food intake, lipid storage, insulin sensitivity, vascular homeostasis, blood pressure regulation, angiogenesis, inflammatory and immune responses, female reproduction, and regulation of energy metabolism. Visceral fat accumulation causes dysfunction in the regulation and interaction of these cytokines and hormones and contributes to the complications and consequences of obesity.

Neuroendocrine regulation of appetite, eating behavior, energy metabolism, and body fat mass is controlled by a dynamic circuit of signaling molecules from the periphery acting on the hypothalamus.[77] The sources include insulin from the beta cells of the pancreas; ghrelin from the stomach; peptide YY from the intestines; and leptin, adiponectin, and resistin from adipose tissue. These hormones circulate in the blood at concentrations proportional to body fat mass and serve as peripheral signals to the hypothalamus, where appetite and metabolism are regulated. Obesity is associated with increased circulating plasma levels of leptin, insulin, resistin, and ghrelin. There are decreased levels of adiponectin and peptide YY (see Box 34-2). Interaction of these altered levels of hormones and adipocytokines with neuropeptides at the level of the hypothalamus may be an important determinant of excessive fat mass and the complications of obesity. Leptin, adiponectin, and insulin resistance and also inflammation are particularly important in the complications of obesity.[75]

Leptin, a product of the obesity gene (*Ob* gene) and expressed primarily by adipocytes, acts on the hypothalamus to suppress appetite and functions to regulate body weight within a fairly narrow range.[78] Leptin levels increase as the number of adipocytes increases; however, for unknown reasons, high leptin levels are ineffective at decreasing appetite and energy expenditure, a condition known as **leptin resistance.** Leptin resistance disrupts hypothalamic satiety signaling and promotes overeating and excessive weight gain and is a factor in the development of obesity.[79] Leptin resistance is also associated with insulin resistance (hyperinsulinemia/glucose intolerance) and the cardiovascular complications of obesity.[80] Obesity promotes a low-grade systemic inflammation that is related to T lymphocyte and macrophage infiltration of adipocytes with release of proinflammatory mediators. The inflammatory state and accelerated lipolysis contribute to the development of insulin resistance and metabolic syndrome (dyslipidemia, atherosclerosis, hypertension, cardiovascular disease, and type 2 diabetes mellitus).[81,82] Decrease in the level of **adiponectin,** produced primarily by visceral adipose tissue, is associated with insulin

---

BOX 34-2 EXAMPLES OF ADIPOCYTOKINES AND OTHER HORMONES RELATED TO COMPLICATIONS OF OBESITY

Cytokines from Adipose Cells
Adipocytokines

Leptin: Suppresses appetite at hypothalamus; promotes insulin sensitivity

Adiponectin: Insulin sensitizing for regulation of blood glucose level; promotes anti-inflammatory and anti-hypertensive vascular effects; reduces atherosclerosis and oncogenesis; increases metabolic rate

Resistin: Promotes insulin resistance and increases blood glucose levels

Vistatin: Mimics insulin and binds to insulin receptors; role in obesity unclear

Proinflammatory Cytokines

Tumor necrosis factor-alpha (TNF-α): A proinflammatory hormone; suppresses appetite; induces insulin resistance

Interleukins-6, -8, and -10: Proinflammatory mediators; suppress appetite; induce insulin resistance

Plasminogen activator inhibitor-1 (PAI-1): Promotes clot formation by inhibiting plasminogen and urokinase (also released by endothelial cells)

Other Hormones

Insulin: Secreted from pancreatic beta cells; suppresses appetite at hypothalamus; promotes glucose utilization in muscle and fat

Amylin: Secreted from pancreatic beta cells; suppresses appetite and postprandial glucagon secretion

Gherlin: Secreted from stomach; stimulates appetite and controls gastric motility and acid secretion

Peptide YY: Secreted from intestine; reduces appetite and inhibits gastric motility

Incretin: Stimulates insulin release; inhibits glucagon release; slows gastric emptying to reduce postprandial hyperglycemia

Glucagon-like peptide-1 (GLP-1): Gastric inhibitory peptide (glucose-dependent insulinotropic peptide) (GIP)

resistance, coronary artery disease, and hypertension, contributing to the complications of obesity.[83] Figure 34-10 summarizes the pathophysiology and major consequences of obesity.

CLINICAL MANIFESTATIONS   Obesity usually presents with two different forms of adipose tissue distribution. Visceral obesity (also known as intra-abdominal, central, or masculine obesity) occurs when the distribution of body fat is localized around the abdomen and upper body, resulting in an apple shape. Visceral obesity has an increased risk for systemic inflammation, dyslipidemia, and insulin resistance with predisposition to atherosclerosis, hypertension, cardiovascular disease, cancer, and type 2 diabetes mellitus.[81] This combination of traits is also known as *metabolic syndrome*[84] (discussed in Chapter 18). The dyslipidemia of obesity is associated with accelerated lipolysis, particularly from visceral fat, with the elevation in levels of plasma nonesterified fatty acids, triglycerides, and low-density lipoprotein and the reduction

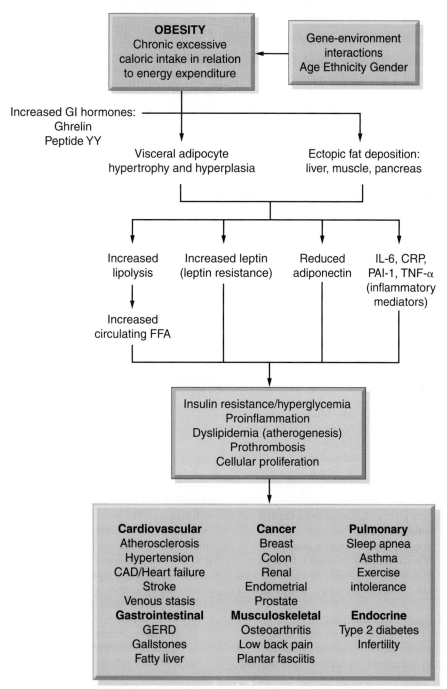

FIGURE 34-10 Pathophysiology and Common Complications of Obesity. *CRP,* C-reactive protein; *FFA,* free fatty acids; *GERD,* gastroesophageal reflux disease; *IL-6,* interleukin-6; *TNF-α,* tumor necrosis factor-alpha; *PAI-1,* plasminogen activator inhibitor-1. (Data from Schelbert KB: Comorbidities of obesity, *Prim Care: Clinics Office Pract* 36[2]:271–285, 2009; Ibrahim MM: Subcutaneous and visceral adipose tissue: structural and functional differences, *Obes Rev* 11[1]:11–18, 2010; Field BC, Chaudhri OB, Bloom SR: Bowels control brain: gut hormones and obesity, *Nat Rev Endocrinol* 6[8]:444–453, 2010.)

in level of high-density lipoprotein increasing the risk for atherosclerosis and cardiovascular disease.

Peripheral obesity (also known as gluteal-femoral or feminine obesity) occurs when the distribution of body fat is extraperitoneal and distributed around the thighs and buttocks, resulting in a pear shape, and is more common in women. Subcutaneous fat is more generally distributed over the body. Peripheral and subcutaneous fat is less metabolically active, is less lipolytic, and releases less adipocytokines (particularly adiponectin) than visceral fat. Risk factors are still present for the complications of obesity but they are less severe than those for visceral obesity.

EVALUATION AND TREATMENT There are several methods for measuring or estimating body fat mass, including computed tomography (CT) and magnetic resonance imaging (MRI) techniques; bioimpedance analysis; underwater weighing; and anthropometric measurements, such as skinfold thickness, circumferences, and various body diameters (i.e., waist-to-hip ratios and waist circumference; body mass index tables).[85] The BMI and waist-to-hip ratios are most commonly used because they are the easiest to measure, and waist measurements are associated with increases in visceral fat. Overweight is defined as a BMI greater than 25 and obesity is a BMI greater than 30. BMI charts are available for children ages 2 to 20 years; these can be used for comparison during adulthood because obese children generally become obese adults.[86] No specific diagnostic criteria for obesity have been established. The complications of obesity affect nearly every body system (see Figure 34-10).

Obesity is a chronic disease for which various approaches to treatment have been used; these include correction of metabolic abnormalities, individually tailored weight reduction diets and exercise programs, psychotherapy, behavioral modification, medications, and weight loss (bariatric) surgery.[87-89] Unraveling the causes of obesity will lead to more specific prevention and pharmacotherapeutic strategies.[90,91]

Anorexia Nervosa and Bulimia Nervosa

Many young adults and adolescents—5 to 10 million young and adult women and 1 million males—are affected by two complex and related eating disorders: anorexia nervosa and bulimia nervosa. Both of these disorders are classified as eating disorders by the American Psychiatric Association.[91a] The conditions have a familial tendency and may be associated with other disorders such as anxiety, depression, and obsessive compulsive disorder.[92]

Anorexia nervosa is a psychologic and physiologic syndrome; it has the highest mortality rate of any psychiatric disease and a familial tendency.[93] It is characterized by the following:

1. Fear of becoming obese despite progressive weight loss
2. Distorted body image: the perception that the body is fat when it is actually underweight
3. Body weight 15% less than normal for age and height because of refusal to eat
4. In women and girls, absence of three consecutive menstrual periods

Persons with anorexia nervosa often deny they have an eating problem. They may engage in vigorous exercise to further promote weight loss. As the disease progresses, muscle and fat depletion give the individual a skeleton-like appearance. Postural hypotension, edema, bradycardia, hypothermia, constipation, and sleep disturbances may ensue. The loss of 25% to 30% of ideal body weight affects multiple organs and can eventually lead to death caused by starvation-induced cardiac failure. Diagnosis of anorexia nervosa involves obtaining a thorough medical history, performing a physical and psychologic examination, and ruling out other causes of anorexia and malnutrition.

Treatment objectives for anorexia nervosa include reversing the compromised physical state, promoting insights and knowledge about the disorder, setting mutual goals, promoting interaction with family members, restoring developmental growth, modifying food habits, and restoring weight. Correction of nutritional status can require hospitalization (see *Health Alert: Refeeding Syndrome*). When the individual demonstrates the willingness to eat food for nourishment, dietary protein, carbohydrate, and fat are introduced in tolerable amounts. Psychotherapy begins as soon as the physical symptoms are stabilized and may continue for several years.[94] Guidelines are available for the early recognition and management of eating disorders.[94a]

HEALTH ALERT
Refeeding Syndrome

Refeeding syndrome occurs in severely malnourished individuals when parenteral or enteral nutritional therapy is initiated. During starvation, loss of body minerals causes the movement of phosphate, magnesium, and potassium out of the cells and into the plasma. When refeeding starts, an increase in insulin levels stimulates the intracellular movement of glucose and these ions and the plasma concentrations can decrease to dangerously low levels, causing hypophosphatemia, hypomagnesemia, and hypokalemia. Rapid expansion of the extracellular fluid volume can also occur with carbohydrate refeeding and may cause fluid overload. Hypophosphatemia contributes to alterations in red blood cell shape and function, causing tissue hypoxia and increased respiratory drive. The consequences of these alterations include life-threatening dysrhythmias, congestive heart failure, muscle weakness (including respiratory muscles), and death. Individuals at greatest risk are those with starvation from any cause including anorexia nervosa, chronic alcoholism, morbid obesity with massive weight loss, and prolonged fasting. Refeeding syndrome is prevented by slowly reinstituting feeding (about 20 kcal/kg/day for the first few days) and monitoring plasma levels of phosphate, potassium, magnesium, and calcium.

Data from Byrnes MC, Stangenes J: Refeeding in the ICU: an adult and pediatric problem, *Curr Opin Clin Nutr Metab Care* 14(2):186–192, 2011; Fuentebella J, Kerner JA: Refeeding syndrome, *Pediatr Clin North Am* 56(5):1201–1210, 2009; Marinella MA: Refeeding syndrome: an important aspect of supportive oncology, *J Support Oncol* 7(1): 11–16, 2009.

Bulimia nervosa is characterized by bingeing—the consumption of normal to large amounts of food, often several thousand calories at a time—followed by self-induced vomiting or purging of the intestines with laxatives. The group at risk is the same as that for anorexia nervosa, except that bulimia nervosa tends to occur in slightly older, less affluent women. Many individuals with anorexia nervosa are bulimic as well.[94] Many young women stimulate vomiting inappropriately to control weight but are not classified as bulimic unless the pattern is obsessional or normal health or activity is interrupted. Diagnosis of bulimia nervosa is based on the following findings:

1. Recurrent episodes of binge eating during which the individual fears not being able to stop
2. Self-induced vomiting, use of laxatives, or fasting to oppose the effect of binge eating
3. Two binge-eating episodes per week for at least 3 months

Although individuals with bulimia nervosa are afraid of gaining weight, their weight usually remains within normal range. Because of negative connotations associated with self-stimulated vomiting and purging, individuals who have bulimia nervosa binge and purge secretly. They may binge and purge as often as 20 times each day. Continual vomiting of acidic chyme can cause pitted teeth, pharyngeal and esophageal inflammation, and tracheoesophageal fistulae. Overuse of laxatives can cause rectal bleeding. Secret bingeing isolates the bulimic individual and leads to depression and anger that is turned inward. A vicious cycle of depression, overeating to try to feel better, vomiting and purging to maintain a normal weight, and returning depression perpetuates this eating disorder.

Because persons with bulimia are usually older than individuals with anorexia nervosa and have usually separated from a family core, individual or group counseling is the treatment focus. Individuals with bulimia nervosa rarely have physical problems requiring hospital care.[95]

Malnutrition and Starvation

Malnutrition is lack of nourishment from inadequate amounts of calories, protein, vitamins, or minerals and is caused by improper diet, alterations in digestion or absorption, chronic disease, or a combination of these factors. Starvation is a state of extreme malnutrition and hunger from lack of nutrients. Short-term starvation (1 to 14 days of fasting) and long-term starvation (14 to 60 days of fasting) have different effects.[96] Therapeutic short-term starvation is part of many weight-reduction programs because it causes an initial rapid weight loss that reinforces the individual's motivation to diet. Therapeutic long-term starvation is used in medically controlled environments to facilitate rapid weight loss in morbidly obese individuals. Pathologic long-term starvation can be caused by poverty (particularly among those living in third world countries); chronic diseases of the cardiovascular, pulmonary, hepatic, renal, and digestive systems; malabsorption syndromes; and cancer. Protein-energy malnutrition in the presence of carbohydrate intake is called kwashiorkor (edematous, severe childhood malnutrition) or marasmus. Cachexia (also known as cytokine-induced malnutrition) is physical wasting with loss of weight and muscle atrophy, fatigue, and weakness. Inflammatory mediators (i.e., TNF-α, interferon-gamma, or interleukin-6) associated with advanced cancer (see Chapter 10), acquired immunodeficiency syndrome (AIDS), tuberculosis, and other major chronic progressive diseases contribute to cachexia. Anorexia and cachexia often occur together. Cachexia is not the same as food deprivation starvation. A healthy person's body can adjust to starvation by slowing metabolism, but in cachexia the body does not make this adjustment.

Short-term starvation, or extended fasting, consists of several days of total dietary abstinence or deprivation. Once all available energy has been absorbed from the intestine, glycogen in the liver is converted to glucose through glycogenolysis, the metabolism of glycogen into glucose. This process peaks within 4 to 8 hours, and gluconeogenesis begins. Gluconeogenesis is the formation of glucose from noncarbohydrate molecules: lactate, pyruvate, amino acids, and the glycerol portion of fats. Like glycogenolysis, gluconeogenesis takes place within the liver. Both of these processes deplete stored nutrients and thus cannot meet the body's energy needs indefinitely. Proteins continue to be catabolized to a minimal degree, providing carbon for the synthesis of glucose. The kidney converts glutamine to glucose, significantly contributing to glucose production. Fatigue decreases physical activity and energy expenditure.

Long-term starvation begins after several days of dietary abstinence and eventually causes death. The major characteristic of long-term starvation is a decreased dependence on gluconeogenesis and an increased use of ketone bodies (products of lipid and pyruvate metabolism) as a cellular energy source. Depressed insulin and glucagon levels promote lipolysis in adipose tissue. Lipolysis liberates fatty acids, which supply energy to cardiac and skeletal muscle cells, as well as ketone bodies, which sustain brain tissue. Fatty acid or ketone body oxidation meets most energy needs of the cells. (Some glucose is still needed as fuel for brain tissue.) Once the supply of adipose tissue is depleted, proteolysis begins. The breakdown of muscle protein is the last process to supply energy for life. Death results from severe alterations in electrolyte balance and loss of renal, pulmonary, and cardiac function.

Adequate ingestion of appropriate nutrients is the obvious treatment for starvation. In medically induced starvation, the body is maintained in a ketotic state until the desired amount of adipose tissue has been lysed. Starvation imposed by chronic disease, long-term illness, or malabsorption is treated with enteral or parenteral nutrition.

> ✓ **QUICK CHECK 34-4**
> 1. Why are Crohn disease and ulcerative colitis called *inflammatory bowel diseases*?
> 2. List the manifestations of anorexia nervosa.
> 3. How is leptin resistance associated with obesity?

DISORDERS OF THE ACCESSORY ORGANS OF DIGESTION

The accessory organs of digestion (liver, gallbladder, pancreas) secrete substances necessary for digestion and, in the case of the liver, carry out metabolic functions needed to maintain life. Disorders of these organs include inflammatory disease, obstruction of ducts, and tumors. (Cancers of the digestive system are described at the end of this chapter.)

Common Complications of Liver Disorders

Of all the accessory organ disorders, acute or chronic liver disease leads to the most significant systemic, life-threatening complications. These complications are common to all liver disorders and include portal hypertension, ascites, hepatic encephalopathy, jaundice, and hepatorenal syndrome.

Portal Hypertension

Portal hypertension is abnormally high blood pressure in the portal venous system. Pressure in this system is normally 3 mm Hg; portal hypertension is an increase to at least 10 mm Hg.

PATHOPHYSIOLOGY Portal hypertension is caused by disorders that obstruct or impede blood flow through any component of the portal venous system or vena cava. *Intrahepatic causes* result from vascular remodeling with shunts, thrombosis, inflammation, or fibrosis of the sinusoids, as occurs in cirrhosis of the liver, biliary cirrhosis, viral hepatitis, or schistosomiasis (a parasitic infection). *Posthepatic causes* occur from hepatic vein thrombosis or cardiac disorders that impair the pumping ability of the right heart. This causes blood to collect and increases pressure in the veins of the portal system. The most common cause of portal hypertension is fibrosis and obstruction caused by cirrhosis of the liver[97] (see p. 921). Long-term portal hypertension causes several pathophysiologic problems that are difficult to treat and can be fatal. These problems include varices, splenomegaly, ascites, hepatic encephalopathy, and hepatopulmonary syndrome.

Varices are distended, tortuous, collateral veins. Prolonged elevation of pressure in the portal vein cause collateral veins to open between the portal vein and systemic veins and their transformation into varices, particularly in the lower esophagus and stomach but also over the abdominal wall (known as the caput medusae [Medusa head]) and rectum (hemorrhoidal varices) (Figure 34-11). Rupture of varices can cause life-threatening hemorrhage.[97]

Splenomegaly is enlargement of the spleen caused by increased pressure in the splenic vein, which branches from the portal vein.

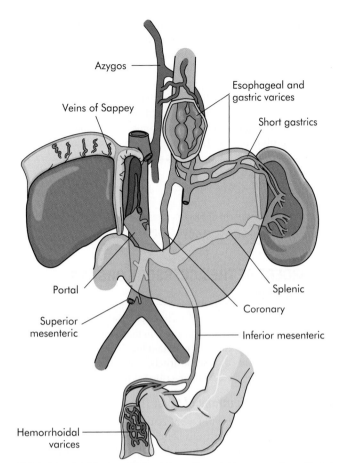

FIGURE 34-11 Varices Related to Portal Hypertension. Portal vein, its major tributaries, and the most important shunts (collateral veins) between the portal and caval systems. The shunted blood returns to the systemic venous system, bypassing the liver. (From Monahan FD et al: *Phipps' medical-surgical nursing: concepts and clinical practice,* ed 8, St Louis, 2007, Mosby.)

Thrombocytopenia is the most common symptom of congestive splenomegaly. The enlarged spleen can be palpated. **Hepatopulmonary syndrome** (vasodilation, intrapulmonary shunting, and hypoxia) and **portopulmonary hypertension** (pulmonary vasoconstriction and vascular remodeling) are complications of liver disease and portal hypertension. The pathophysiology is complex and involves different effects of vasoactive substances. There may be no clinical manifestations, although dyspnea, cyanosis, and clubbing may occur.[98]

CLINICAL MANIFESTATIONS   Vomiting of blood (hematemesis) from bleeding **esophageal varices** is the most common clinical manifestation of portal hypertension. Slow, chronic bleeding from varices causes anemia and the presence of digested blood in the stools. Usually the bleeding is from varices that have developed slowly over a period of years.

Rupture of esophageal varices causes hemorrhage and voluminous vomiting of dark-colored blood. The ruptured varices are usually painless. Rupture is caused by a combination of erosion by gastric acid and elevated venous pressure. Mortality from ruptured esophageal varices ranges from 30% to 60%. Recurrent bleeding of esophageal varices indicates a poor prognosis. Most individuals die within 1 year.

EVALUATION AND TREATMENT   Portal hypertension is often diagnosed at the time of variceal bleeding and confirmed by endoscopy and evaluation of portal venous pressure. The individual usually has a history of jaundice, hepatitis, or alcoholism. Upper gastrointestinal endoscopy is commonly used to diagnose varices.

Emergency management of bleeding varices includes use of vasopressors and compression of the varices with an inflatable tube or balloon, sclerotherapy, variceal ligation or portacaval shunt. Surgical shunts may decompress the varices, but this treatment can precipitate encephalopathy or liver failure and require liver transplant in selected cases.[99,99a]

Ascites

Ascites is the accumulation of fluid in the peritoneal cavity. Ascites traps body fluid in a "third space" (a space where it does not normally collect) from which it cannot escape. The effect is to reduce the amount of fluid available for normal physiologic functions. Cirrhosis is the most common cause of ascites, but other causes include heart failure, constrictive pericarditis, abdominal malignancies, nephrotic syndrome, and malnutrition.[100] Of individuals who develop ascites caused by cirrhosis, 25% die within 1 year. Continued heavy drinking of alcohol is associated with this mortality.

PATHOPHYSIOLOGY   Several factors contribute to the development of ascites, including decreased synthesis of albumin by the liver and fluid retention. Portal hypertension and reduced serum albumin levels cause capillary hydrostatic pressure to exceed capillary osmotic pressure (see Chapter 4). This imbalance pushes water into the peritoneal cavity. Portal hypertension also increases the production of hepatic lymph, which "weeps" into the peritoneal cavity. Bacteria may be translocated from the gut into the peritoneal cavity causing peritonitis. Bacterial peritonitis causes an inflammatory response that increases mesenteric capillary permeability (see Chapter 5) and fluid movement into the peritoneal cavity that promote ascites. Peripheral vasodilation, associated with increased nitric oxide produced by the diseased liver, decreases effective circulating blood volume, activating aldosterone and antidiuretic hormone, which promote renal sodium and water retention. The sodium and water retention expands plasma volume, thereby accelerating portal hypertension and ascites formation.[101] Figure 34-12 summarizes the mechanisms by which cirrhosis of the liver causes ascites.

CLINICAL MANIFESTATIONS   The accumulation of ascitic fluid causes weight gain, abdominal distention, and increased abdominal girth (Figure 34-13). Large volumes of fluid (10 to 20 L) displace the diaphragm and cause dyspnea by decreasing lung capacity. Respiratory rate increases, and the individual assumes a semi-Fowler position to relieve the dyspnea. Approximately 10% of individuals with ascites develop bacterial peritonitis, which causes fever, chills, abdominal pain, decreased bowel sounds, and cloudy ascitic fluid.

EVALUATION AND TREATMENT   Diagnosis is usually based on clinical manifestations and identification of liver disease. Paracentesis is used to aspirate ascitic fluid for bacterial culture, biochemical analysis, and microscopic examination. The goal of treatment is to relieve discomfort. If the restoration of liver function is possible, the ascites diminishes spontaneously. In the meantime, dietary salt restriction and use of potassium-sparing diuretics can reduce ascites. Levels of serum electrolytes are monitored carefully because the individual is at risk for hyponatremia and hypokalemia.

Palliative measures include paracentesis to remove 1 or 2 L of ascitic fluid and relieve respiratory distress. However, the removal of too much fluid relieves pressure on blood vessels and carries the risk of hypotension, shock, or death. Despite repeated paracentesis, ascitic fluid reaccumulates because of the persistent portal hypertension

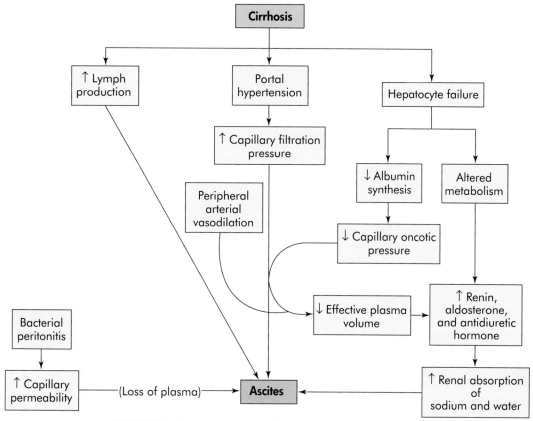

FIGURE 34-12 Mechanisms of Ascites Caused by Cirrhosis.

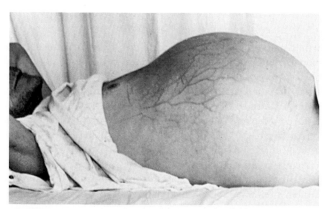

FIGURE 34-13 Massive Ascites in an Individual With Cirrhosis. Distended abdomen, dilated upper abdominal veins, and inverted umbilicus are classic manifestations. (From Prior JA, Silberstein JS, Stang JM: *Physical diagnosis: the history and examination of the patient,* ed 6, St Louis, 1981, Mosby.)

and reduced plasma albumin levels associated with irreversible disease. Paracentesis is also likely to cause peritonitis. Other procedures include peritoneovenous shunt, transjugular intrahepatic portosystemic shunt, and liver transplant.[101] Individuals with ascites and portal hypertension have a poor prognosis.

Hepatic Encephalopathy

Hepatic encephalopathy (portal-systemic encephalopathy) is a complex neurologic syndrome characterized by impaired cerebral function, flapping tremor (asterixis), and electroencephalogram (EEG)

changes. The syndrome may develop rapidly during acute fulminant hepatitis or slowly during the course of chronic liver disease and the development of portal hypertension.

PATHOPHYSIOLOGY Hepatic encephalopathy results from a combination of biochemical alterations that affect neurotransmission. Liver dysfunction and the development of collateral vessels that shunt blood around the liver to the systemic circulation permit toxins absorbed from the gastrointestinal tract to accumulate and circulate freely to the brain. The accumulated toxins alter cerebral energy metabolism, interfere with neurotransmission, and cause edema. The most hazardous substances are end products of intestinal protein digestion, particularly ammonia, which cannot be converted to urea by the diseased liver. Other substances include inflammatory cytokines, short-chain fatty acids, serotonin, tryptophan, and manganese. Infection, hemorrhage, and electrolyte imbalance (including zinc deficiency) as well as the use of sedatives and analgesics can precipitate hepatic encephalopathy in the presence of liver disease.[102]

CLINICAL MANIFESTATIONS Subtle changes in personality, memory loss, irritability, lethargy, and sleep disturbances are common initial manifestations of hepatic encephalopathy. Symptoms then can progress to confusion, flapping tremor of the hands (asterixis), stupor, convulsions, and coma. Coma is usually a sign of liver failure and ultimately results in death.

EVALUATION AND TREATMENT Diagnosis of hepatic encephalopathy is based on a history of liver disease and clinical manifestations. Electroencephalography and blood chemistry tests provide supportive data. Tracking levels of serum ammonia assesses treatment effectiveness and liver function.

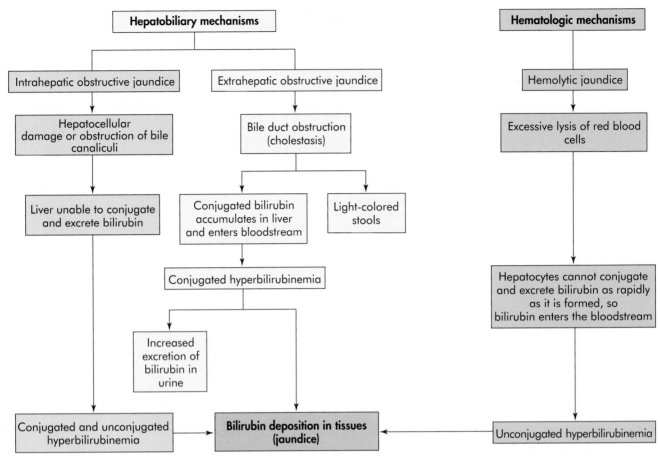

FIGURE 34-14 Mechanisms of Jaundice.

Correction of fluid and electrolyte imbalances and withdrawal of depressant drugs metabolized by the liver are the first steps in the treatment of hepatic encephalopathy. Restricting dietary protein intake and eliminating intestinal bacteria with antibiotics reduce blood ammonia levels. Lactulose or nonabsorbable antibiotics may be administered to prevent ammonia absorption in the colon.[103]

Jaundice

Jaundice, or icterus, is a yellow or greenish pigmentation of the skin caused by hyperbilirubinemia (plasma bilirubin concentrations greater than 2.5 to 3.0 mg/dl). Hyperbilirubinemia and jaundice can result from (1) extrahepatic (posthepatic) obstruction to bile flow, (2) intrahepatic obstruction, or (3) prehepatic excessive production of unconjugated bilirubin (i.e., excessive hemolysis of red blood cells)[104] (Figure 34-14). Jaundice in newborns is caused by impaired bilirubin uptake and conjugation (see Chapter 35).

PATHOPHYSIOLOGY Obstructive jaundice can result from extrahepatic or intrahepatic obstruction.[105] *Extrahepatic obstructive jaundice* develops if the common bile duct is occluded (e.g., by a gallstone, tumor, or inflammation). Bilirubin conjugated by the hepatocytes cannot flow into the duodenum. Therefore, it accumulates in the liver and enters the bloodstream, causing hyperbilirubinemia and jaundice. *Intrahepatic obstructive jaundice* involves disturbances in hepatocyte function and obstruction of bile canaliculi. The uptake, conjugation, or excretion of bilirubin can be affected with elevated levels of both conjugated and unconjugated bilirubin. Obstruction of bile canaliculi diminishes flow of conjugated bilirubin into the common bile duct.

In mild cases, some of the bile canaliculi open. Consequently, the amount of bilirubin in the intestinal tract may be only slightly decreased.

Excessive hemolysis (destruction) of red blood cells can cause hemolytic jaundice *(prehepatic jaundice)*. Increased unconjugated bilirubin is formed through metabolism of the heme component of destroyed red blood cells and exceeds the conjugation ability of the liver, causing blood levels of unconjugated bilirubin to rise. Decreased bilirubin uptake or conjugation also causes unconjugated hyperbilirubinemia, as occurs with reaction to some drugs (e.g., rifampin) and in genetic disorders such as Gilbert syndrome. Because unconjugated bilirubin is not water soluble, it is not excreted in the urine. The causes of jaundice are summarized in Table 34-7.

CLINICAL MANIFESTATIONS Conjugated bilirubin is water soluble and appears in the urine. The urine may darken several days before the onset of jaundice. The complete obstruction of bile flow from the liver to the duodenum causes light-colored stools. With partial obstruction, the stools are normal in color and bilirubin is present in the urine.

Fever, chills, and pain often accompany jaundice resulting from viral or bacterial inflammation of the liver (e.g., viral hepatitis). Yellow discoloration may first occur in the sclera of the eye and then progress to the skin as bilirubin attaches to elastic fibers. Pruritus (itching) often accompanies jaundice because bilirubin accumulates in the skin.

EVALUATION AND TREATMENT Laboratory evaluation of serum establishes whether elevated plasma bilirubin is conjugated or unconjugated, or both. The history and physical examination identify underlying disorders, such as cirrhosis, exposure to hepatitis virus, and

TABLE 34-7 COMMON TYPES OF JAUNDICE

TYPE	MECHANISM	CAUSES
Hemolytic (prehepatic) jaundice (predominantly unconjugated bilirubin)	Destruction of erythrocytes (increased bilirubin production)	Hemolytic anemias (e.g., sickle cell) Severe infection Toxic substances in circulation (e.g., snake venom) Transfusion of incompatible blood
Disorders of bilirubin metabolism (unconjugated bilirubin)	Decreased bilirubin uptake Decreased bilirubin conjugation	Drug induced (e.g., rifampin and cyclosporine) Hereditary disorder (e.g., Gilbert syndrome)
Obstructive (posthepatic) jaundice (predominantly conjugated bilirubin)	Obstruction of passage of conjugated bilirubin from liver to intestine	Obstruction of bile duct by gallstones or tumor (extrahepatic obstructive jaundice) Obstruction of bile flow through liver (intrahepatic obstructive jaundice) Drugs
Hepatocellular (intrahepatic) jaundice (both conjugated and unconjugated bilirubin)	Failure of liver cells (hepatocytes) to conjugate bilirubin and of bilirubin to pass from liver to intestine	Genetic defect of hepatocytes (decreased enzymes), such as occurs in premature infants (see Chapter 35) Severe infections (e.g., hepatitis) Alcoholic liver disease or biliary cirrhosis

gallbladder or pancreatic disease. The treatment for jaundice consists of correcting the cause.

Hepatorenal Syndrome

Hepatorenal syndrome is functional renal failure that develops as a complication of advanced liver disease. The renal failure is not caused by primary renal disease or other extrinsic factors but rather by portal hypertension and other circulatory alterations associated with advanced liver disease, such as alcoholic cirrhosis or fulminant hepatitis with portal hypertension and functional renal failure including oliguria, sodium and water retention (with or without ascites and peripheral edema), hypotension, and peripheral vasodilation.[106] The kidney usually has a normal structure.

PATHOPHYSIOLOGY Hepatorenal syndrome generally accompanies a sudden decrease in blood volume secondary to massive gastrointestinal or variceal bleeding and hypotension caused by bleeding and peripheral vasodilation associated with failing liver function. Hypotension also can be caused by the excessive use of diuretics to treat ascites or decreased cardiac output. The decrease in blood volume and hypotension result in decreased renal perfusion, decreased glomerular filtration, and oliguria (see Chapter 29). A significant number of individuals with advanced liver disease develop oliguria unrelated to any precipitating event. Inappropriate constriction of renal arterioles is proposed as the causative mechanism for decreased glomerular filtration and oliguria. Intrarenal vasoconstriction may result from the selective effects of vasoactive substances that accumulate in the blood because of liver failure. Vasoconstriction also may be a compensatory response to portal hypotension and the pooling of blood in the splanchnic circulation.[107]

CLINICAL MANIFESTATIONS The onset of hepatorenal manifestations may be gradual or acute. Oliguria and complications of advanced liver disease, including jaundice, ascites, and gastrointestinal bleeding, are usually present. Systolic blood pressure is usually below 100 mm Hg. Nonspecific symptoms of hepatorenal syndrome include anorexia, weakness, and fatigue.

EVALUATION AND TREATMENT Despite oliguria, serum potassium levels do not become dangerously elevated until the terminal stages of the hepatorenal syndrome. Blood urea level increases, followed by an increase in creatinine concentration. Urine osmolality increases, but urine sodium concentrations are below normal. Urine specific gravity is greater than 1.015.

The prognosis is usually poor and is related to a failing liver. Renal function improves with improvement in liver function. Secondary complications, including fluid and electrolyte disorders, bleeding, infections, and encephalopathy, also are vigorously treated.[108]

> **✓ QUICK CHECK 34-5**
> 1. How does portal hypertension promote ascites?
> 2. Why is the concentration of unconjugated bilirubin elevated in hemolytic jaundice?
> 3. Describe hepatorenal syndrome.

Disorders of the Liver
Viral Hepatitis

Viral hepatitis is a relatively common systemic disease that affects primarily the liver. Different strains of viruses cause different types of hepatitis: hepatitis A virus (HAV), hepatitis B virus (HBV), hepatitis D virus (HDV) associated with HBV, hepatitis C virus (HCV), and hepatitis E virus (HEV, most common in Asia and Africa). Hepatitis A formerly was known as infectious hepatitis and hepatitis B as serum hepatitis. The first five viruses can cause acute hepatitis, and types B and C also cause chronic liver disease, hepatocellular carcinoma, and liver failure.[109] GB virus C (GBV-C), formerly known as hepatitis G virus (HGV), is a blood-borne virus and is not a significant cause of human liver disease. It may slow the progression of human immunodeficiency virus (HIV) disease when there is co-infection.[109a] Characteristics of the different types of viruses that cause hepatitis are presented in Table 34-8.

PATHOPHYSIOLOGY All five types of viral hepatitis (A, B, C, D, and E) can cause acute, icteric illness. The pathologic lesions of hepatitis include hepatic cell necrosis, scarring (with chronic disease), and Kupffer cell hyperplasia. Infiltration by mononuclear phagocytes occurs with varying severity. Regeneration of hepatic cells begins within 48 hours of injury. The inflammatory process can damage and obstruct bile canaliculi, leading to cholestasis and obstructive jaundice. In milder cases, the liver parenchyma is not damaged. Damage tends to be most severe in cases of hepatitis B and C. Hepatitis B is also associated with acute fulminating hepatitis, a rare form of the disease that is

TABLE 34-8	CHARACTERISTICS OF VIRAL HEPATITIS				
CHARACTERISTIC	**HEPATITIS A**	**HEPATITIS B**	**HEPATITIS D**	**HEPATITIS C**	**HEPATITIS E**
Virus	27-nm RNA virus	42-nm DNA virus	36-nm RNA virus	30-60-nm RNA virus	32-nm RNA virus
Antigens or antibodies	Anti-HAV	HBsAg HBcAg HbeAg	Anti-HDV	Anti-HCV	Anti-HEV
Incubation period	30 days	60-180 days	30-180 days	35-60 days	15-60 days
Route of transmission	Fecal-oral (most common), parenteral, sexual	Parenteral, sexual	Parenteral (?), fecal-oral, sexual	Parenteral, sexual	Fecal-oral
Onset	Nonspecific Acute with fever	Insidious	Insidious	Insidious	Acute
Carrier state	Negative	Positive	Positive	Positive	Negative
Severity	Mild	Severe; may be prolonged or chronic	Severe	Unknown	Severe in pregnant women
Chronic hepatitis	No	Yes Increased risk of HCC	Yes	Yes Increased risk of HCC	No
Age group affected	Children and young adults	Any	Any	Any	Children and young adults
Prophylaxis	Hygiene, immune serum globulin, HAV vaccine	Hygiene, HBV vaccine, blood screening	Hygiene, HBV vaccine	Hygiene, blood screening, interferon-α	Hygiene, safe water
Pathophysiology	Hepatocyte injury caused by cellular immune responses (T cells, NK cells, and cytokines)	Viral replication, co-infection with viral mutation, inflammation, and cellular necrosis	Co-infection with HBV, severe cell injury, inflammation progressing to cirrhosis	Hepatocyte injury caused by immune response, inflammation, and fibrosis leading to cirrhosis	Viral replication, liver is cytotoxic, immune response causes inflammation and cholestasis
Treatment	Symptomatic support	Interferon-α, peginterferon-α, antivirals (lamivudine, adefovir, entecavir, telbivudine, tenofovir)	Interferon-α	Interferon-α, peginterferon-α, antivirals (ribavirin, boceprevir, telaprevir)	Symptomatic support similar to HAV

DNA, Deoxyribonucleic acid; *HAAg,* hepatitis A antigen; *HAV,* hepatitis A virus; *HBcAg,* hepatitis B core antigen; *HBeAg,* hepatitis B e antigen (a fragment derived from the same propeptide for HBcAg); *HBsAg,* hepatitis B surface antigen; *HBV,* hepatitis B virus; *HCC,* hepatocellular carcinoma; *HCV,* hepatitis C virus; *HDV,* hepatitis D virus; *HEV,* hepatitis E virus; *RNA,* ribonucleic acid.

characterized by massive hepatic necrosis. Acute fulminating hepatitis causes severe encephalopathy, which is manifested as confusion, stupor, and coma. Liver failure can occur, leading to intestinal bleeding, cardiorespiratory insufficiency, and renal failure.

Co-infection of hepatitis B virus (HBV), hepatitis C virus (HCV), hepatitis D virus (HDV), and human immunodeficiency virus (HIV) occurs because these viruses share the same route of transmission (contact between infected body fluids and broken skin or mucous membranes or intravenously). Progression of liver disease is more rapid in these cases.[110,111]

CLINICAL MANIFESTATIONS The spectrum of manifestations ranges from absence of symptoms to fulminating hepatitis, with rapid onset of liver failure and coma. Acute viral hepatitis causes abnormal liver function test results. The serum aminotransferase values, aspartate transaminase (AST) and alanine transaminase (ALT), are elevated but not consistent with the extent of cellular damage. The clinical course of hepatitis usually consists of three phases:

1. **Prodromal phase.** Begins about 2 weeks after exposure and ends with the appearance of jaundice; marked by fatigue, anorexia, malaise, nausea, vomiting, headache, hyperalgia, cough, and low-grade fever; infection is highly transmissible during this phase.
2. **Icteric phase.** Begins 1 to 2 weeks after the prodromal phase and lasts 2 to 6 weeks; jaundice, dark urine, and clay-colored stools are common; the liver is enlarged, smooth, and tender, and percussion or palpation of the liver causes pain; this is the actual phase of illness.
3. **Recovery phase.** Begins with resolution of jaundice, about 6 to 8 weeks after exposure; symptoms diminish, but the liver remains enlarged and tender; liver function returns to normal 2 to 12 weeks after the onset of jaundice.

Chronic active hepatitis is the persistence of clinical manifestations and liver inflammation after acute stages of HBV and HCV infection. Liver function tests remain abnormal for longer than 6 months, and hepatitis B surface antigen (HBsAg) persists. Chronic, active HBV and HCV is a predisposition to cirrhosis and primary hepatocellular carcinoma. Extrahepatic manifestations, including arthralgias, fatigue, and neurologic and renal symptoms, occur in some individuals.[112,113]

EVALUATION AND TREATMENT Diagnosis of HAV and HCV is based on the presence of anti-HAV and anti-HCV antibodies. The most specific diagnostic test for HBV is serologic analysis for specific hepatitis virus antigens (i.e., HBsAg, which is the marker for HBV). The assay for HDV is the total antibody to hepatitis D and antigen (anti-HDV). A test for HEV has not been developed. Liver enzyme levels and function tests also can indicate other viral liver diseases, drug toxicity, or alcoholic hepatitis.

Treatments for different types of viral hepatitis are summarized in Table 34-8. Physical activity may be restricted and a low-fat, high-carbohydrate diet is beneficial if bile flow is obstructed. For chronic hepatitis, treatment is directed at suppressing viral replication before irreversible liver cell damage occurs. Antiviral therapies include interferon-α and specific antiviral agents. Cyclic and combination therapy may prevent drug resistance, and new agents are being developed.[114,115]

After ingestion and gastrointestinal uptake, HAV replicates in the liver and is secreted into the bile. To prevent transmission of hepatitis A, handwashing and the use of gloves for disposing of bedpans and fecal matter are imperative. HAV may be shed in the feces for up to 3 months after onset of symptoms. Molecular procedures are available for direct surveillance of HAV in food.[116] Direct contact with blood or body fluids of individuals with HBV or HCV should be avoided. The administration of immune globulin before exposure or early in the incubation period can prevent hepatitis A and hepatitis B. A combined vaccine is available to protect against HAV and HBV infection. A vaccine for HEV has been developed but is not yet commercially available.[117] Preexposure vaccination is recommended for healthcare workers, liver transplant recipients, and others who are at risk for contact with infected body fluids, particularly children.

Fulminant Viral Hepatitis

Fulminant viral hepatitis causing acute liver failure (fulminant liver failure) is a clinical syndrome resulting in severe impairment or necrosis of liver cells and potential liver failure. The disorder rarely occurs with HAV and may occur as a complication of hepatitis C or hepatitis B, particularly HBV infection compounded by infection with the delta virus. Toxic reactions to drugs and congenital metabolic disorders also can cause fulminant hepatitis. Acetaminophen overdose is the leading cause of acute liver failure in the United States (see *Health Alert:* Paracetamol [Acetaminophen] and Acute Liver Failure in Chapter 33). Edematous hepatocytes and patchy areas of necrosis and inflammatory cell infiltrates disrupt the parenchyma. The death of hepatocytes may be caused by viral or immunologic damage.

Acute liver failure usually develops within 6 to 8 weeks after the initial symptoms of viral hepatitis or a metabolic liver disorder. Anorexia, vomiting, abdominal pain, and progressive jaundice are initial signs, followed by ascites and gastrointestinal bleeding. Hepatic encephalopathy is manifested as lethargy, altered motor functions, and coma and is related to cerebral edema, ischemia, and brain stem herniation. Liver function tests show elevations in the levels of both direct and indirect serum bilirubin, serum transaminases, and blood ammonia. Prothrombin time is prolonged. Renal failure and pulmonary distress can occur.[118]

Treatment of acute liver failure is supportive. The hepatic necrosis is irreversible, and 60% to 90% of affected children die. Liver transplantation may be lifesaving. Artificial liver support devices are being evaluated. Survivors usually do not develop cirrhosis or chronic liver disease.[119]

Cirrhosis

Cirrhosis is an irreversible inflammatory, fibrotic liver disease and is a leading cause of death in the United States. Many disorders can cause cirrhosis and are listed in Box 34-3. The process of cellular injury depends on the cause of cirrhosis; however, the pathologic mechanisms are not all clearly understood. Structural changes result from injury (e.g., viruses or toxicity from alcohol) and fibrosis, which is a consequence of infiltration of leukocytes, release of inflammatory mediators, and activation of fibrogenic fibroblasts.[120] Chaotic fibrosis alters or obstructs biliary channels and blood flow, producing jaundice and portal hypertension (see pp. 915 and 918). New vascular channels form shunts, and blood from the portal vein bypasses the liver, contributing to portal hypertension, metabolic alterations, and toxin accumulation. The process of regeneration is replaced by hypoxia, necrosis, atrophy, and (ultimately) liver failure. The fibrosis and regenerating nodules of hepatocytes distort the parenchyma of the liver, and the

---

BOX 34-3   CAUSES OF CIRRHOSIS

Hepatitis virus—B and C (common)
Excessive alcohol intake (common)
Idiopathic (common)
Nonalcoholic fatty liver disease (NAFLD), also known as nonalcoholic steatohepatitis (NASH)
Autoimmune disorders
    Autoimmune hepatitis
    Primary biliary cirrhosis
    Primary sclerosing cholangitis
Hereditary metabolic disorder
    α_1-Antitrypsin deficiency
    Hemachromatosis
    Wilson disease
    Glycogen or lipid storage diseases
Prolonged exposure to drugs or toxins (e.g., carbon tetrachloride, cleaning and industrial solvents, copper salts)
Hepatic venous outflow obstruction
    Budd-Chiari syndrome
    Right-sided heart failure

---

formation of fibrous bands gives the liver a cobblestone appearance. The liver may be larger or smaller than normal, and usually it is firm or hard when palpated.

Cirrhosis develops slowly over a period of years. Its severity and rate of progression depend on the cause. If toxins, such as alcohol, are involved, the rate of cell death and the severity of inflammation depend on the amount of toxin present. Removal of the toxin slows the progression of liver damage and enhances the process of regeneration.[121]

Alcoholic liver disease. Deaths from alcohol-related liver disease have increased over the past decade and the amount and duration of alcohol consumption are positively related to the extent of liver damage. Abuse of any type of alcoholic beverage can cause cirrhosis. Malnutrition may add to the risk of cirrhosis in alcohol abusers. Many alcoholics eat poorly and the liver cannot regenerate without adequate nutrition. The incidence of alcoholic cirrhosis is greatest in middle-age men; however, women develop more severe liver injury than men.[122] Mortality resulting from cirrhosis in the United States is highest among non-whites. Although alcoholic cirrhosis is the most prevalent of the various types of cirrhosis, the occurrence of cirrhosis among persons with alcoholism is relatively low (approximately 25%). The spectrum of alcoholic liver disease includes alcoholic fatty liver, alcoholic steatohepatitis, and alcoholic cirrhosis.

PATHOPHYSIOLOGY   Alcoholic fatty liver (steatosis) is the mildest form of alcoholic liver disease. It can be caused by relatively small amounts of alcohol, may be asymptomatic, and is reversible with cessation of drinking.[123] Fat deposition (deposition of triglycerides) within the liver is caused primarily by increased lipogenesis and decreased fatty acid oxidation by hepatocytes. Lipids mobilized from adipose tissue or dietary fat intake may contribute to fat accumulation.

Alcoholic steatohepatitis is a precursor of cirrhosis characterized by inflammation, degeneration, and necrosis of hepatocytes and infiltration of neutrophils and lymphocytes. The injured hepatocytes contain Mallory bodies (hyaline endoplasmic reticulum), indicating the onset of fibrosis. The mechanism of hepatocyte injury is not clearly understood, but immunologic factors, endotoxins from gut bacteria, and inflammatory mediators are involved. The inflammation and

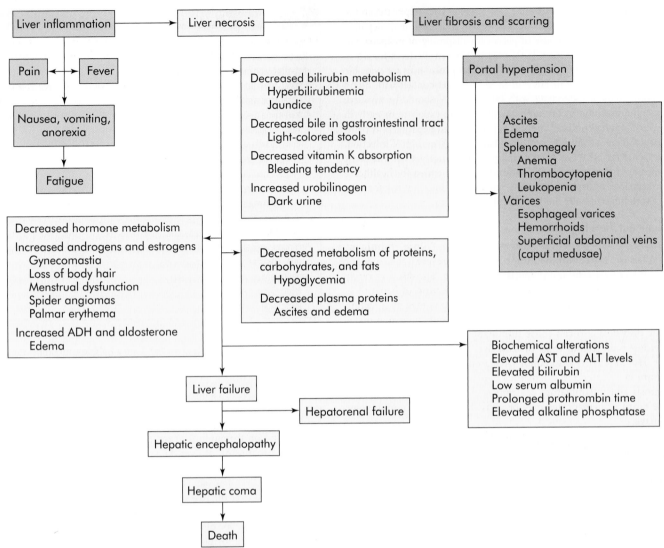

FIGURE 34-15 Clinical Manifestations of Cirrhosis. *ADH,* Antidiuretic hormone; *ALT,* alanine transaminase; *AST,* aspartate transaminase.

necrosis caused by alcoholic steatohepatitis stimulate the irreversible fibrosis characteristic of the cirrhotic stage of disease.[124]

Alcoholic cirrhosis is caused by the toxic effects of alcohol metabolism on the liver, immunologic alterations, inflammatory cytokines, oxidative stress from lipid peroxidation, and malnutrition. Alcohol is transformed to acetaldehyde, and excessive amounts significantly alter hepatocyte function and activate hepatic stellate cells, a primary cell involved in liver fibrosis. Mitochondrial function is impaired, decreasing oxidation of fatty acid. Enzyme and protein synthesis may be depressed or altered, and hormone and ammonia degradation is diminished. Acetaldehyde inhibits export of proteins from the liver, alters metabolism of vitamins and minerals, and induces malnutrition.[125,126] Cellular damage initiates an inflammatory response that, along with necrosis, results in excessive collagen formation. Fibrosis and scarring alter the structure of the liver and obstruct biliary and vascular channels.

CLINICAL MANIFESTATIONS Fatty infiltration causes no specific symptoms or abnormal liver function test results. The liver is usually enlarged, however, and the individual has a history of continuous alcohol intake during the previous weeks or months. Anorexia, nausea,

jaundice, and edema develop with advanced fatty infiltration or the onset of alcoholic steatohepatitis (Figure 34-15).

The clinical manifestations of alcoholic steatohepatitis can be mild or severe. Nonspecific symptoms include fatigue, weight loss, and anorexia. Toxic effects of alcohol also can cause testicular atrophy, reduced libido, azoospermia, and decreased testosterone levels in men. Manifestations of acute illness include nausea, anorexia, fever, abdominal pain, and jaundice. Cirrhosis is a multiple-system disease and causes hepatomegaly, splenomegaly, ascites, gastrointestinal hemorrhage, portal hypertension, hepatic encephalopathy, and esophageal varices. Anemia results from blood loss, malnutrition, and hypersplenism. Renal failure is often a late complication of hepatorenal syndrome. The presence of numerous and severe manifestations increases the risk of death.

EVALUATION AND TREATMENT The diagnosis of alcoholic steatohepatitis or cirrhosis is based on the individual's history and clinical manifestations. The results of liver function tests are abnormal, and serologic studies show elevated levels of serum enzymes and bilirubin, decreased levels of serum albumin, and prolonged prothrombin time that is not easily corrected with vitamin K therapy. Liver biopsy can confirm the diagnosis of cirrhosis, but biopsy is not necessary if clinical manifestations of cirrhosis are evident.

There is no specific treatment for alcoholic steatohepatitis or cirrhosis. Rest, vitamin supplements, a nutritious diet, and management of complications, such as ascites, gastrointestinal bleeding, and encephalopathy, are essential. Cessation of drinking is essential and slows the progression of liver damage, improves clinical symptoms, and prolongs life. Individuals with severe symptoms are treated with a regimen of corticosteroids, and drugs to control fibrosis are being tested. Orthotopic liver transplantation (replacement of the diseased liver with a donor liver [allograft]) can be successful for treatment of end-stage liver disease. Artificial liver support systems are being developed.[127]

Nonalcoholic fatty liver disease and nonalcoholic steatohepatitis. Nonalcoholic fatty liver disease (NAFLD) is infiltration of hepatocytes with fat, primarily in the form of triglycerides, but it occurs in the absence of alcohol intake. It is associated with obesity (including obese children), high levels of cholesterol and triglycerides, metabolic syndrome, and type 2 diabetes mellitus and is the most common chronic liver disease in the United States. Some individuals with NAFLD will develop nonalcoholic steatohepatitis (NASH) with hepatocellular injury, inflammation, and fibrosis; NASH is difficult to distinguish from alcohol-induced liver fibrosis. NAFLD is usually asymptomatic and may remain undetected for years. The most severe forms of NASH progress to cirrhosis and end-stage liver disease.[128,129]

Biliary cirrhosis. Biliary cirrhosis differs from alcoholic cirrhosis in that the damage and inflammation leading to cirrhosis begin in bile canaliculi and bile ducts, rather than in the hepatocytes. The two types of biliary cirrhosis are *primary* and *secondary.* Although both involve bile duct pathologic changes, they differ with respect to cause, risk factors, and mechanisms of obstruction and inflammation as follows:

1. Primary biliary cirrhosis. Caused by autoimmune T lymphocyte and antibody-mediated destruction of the small intrahepatic bile ducts; affects middle-aged women and can be associated with inflammatory bowel disease. It progresses insidiously from pruritus, hyperbilirubinemia, jaundice, and light/clay-colored stools to cirrhosis, portal hypertension, and encephalopathy; life expectancy is 5 to 10 years after onset of symptoms if not treated. Primary biliary cirrhosis can be detected by biochemical evidence of cholestatic liver disease (e.g., presence of anti-mitochondrial antibody [AMA] and elevated alkaline phosphatase level) for at least 6 months' duration, ultrasound imaging of the liver, or biopsy of the liver. Treatment with ursodeoxycholic acid slows disease progression and liver transplant is highly effective.[130]

2. Secondary biliary cirrhosis. Caused by prolonged partial or complete obstruction of the common bile duct or branches by gallstones, tumors, fibrotic strictures, or chronic pancreatitis; biliary atresia and cystic fibrosis are causative in children; necrotic areas develop and lead to proliferation and inflammation of portal ducts, producing edema and fibrosis; surgery or endoscopy relieves obstruction, prolongs survival, and diminishes or resolves symptoms.

✔ **QUICK CHECK 34-6**
1. How are varices and ascites associated with portal hypertension?
2. How does hepatitis A virus (HAV) differ from hepatitis B virus (HBV)?
3. What are the major pathologic differences between alcoholic and biliary cirrhosis?

Disorders of the Gallbladder

Obstruction and inflammation are the most common disorders of the gallbladder. Obstruction is caused by gallstones, which are aggregates of substances in the bile. The gallstones may remain in the gallbladder or be ejected, with bile, into the cystic duct. Gallstones that become lodged in the cystic duct obstruct the flow of bile into and out of the gallbladder and cause inflammation. Gallstone formation is termed cholelithiasis. Inflammation of the gallbladder or cystic duct is known as cholecystitis.

Cholelithiasis (Gallstones)

Cholelithiasis (gallstones) is a prevalent disorder in developed countries, where the incidence is 10% to 15% in white adults and 60% to 70% in Native Americans. Risk factors include obesity, middle age, female gender, use of oral contraceptives, rapid weight loss, Native American ancestry, genetic predisposition, and gallbladder, pancreatic, or ileal disease.[131]

PATHOPHYSIOLOGY Gallstones are commonly of two types: cholesterol (most common) and pigmented. *Cholesterol gallstones* form in bile that is supersaturated with cholesterol produced by the liver. Supersaturation sets the stage for cholesterol crystal formation, or the formation of "microstones." More crystals then aggregate on the microstones, which grow to form "macrostones." This process usually occurs in the gallbladder, which may have decreased motility. The stones may lie dormant or become lodged in the cystic or common duct, causing pain when the gallbladder contracts and cholecystitis. The stones can accumulate and fill the entire gallbladder (Figure 34-16).[132] *Pigmented stones* form from increased levels of unconjugated bilirubin, which binds with calcium. They are associated with chronic liver disease.[133]

CLINICAL MANIFESTATIONS Cholelithiasis is often asymptomatic. Abdominal pain and jaundice are the cardinal manifestations of cholelithiasis. Vague symptoms include heartburn, flatulence, epigastric discomfort, and food intolerances, particularly to fats and cabbage. The pain (biliary colic) occurs 30 minutes to several hours after eating a fatty meal. It is caused by the lodging of one or more gallstones in the cystic or common duct. It can be intermittent or steady and usually occurs in the right upper quadrant, radiating to the mid-upper area of the back. Jaundice indicates that the stone is located in the common bile duct.

EVALUATION AND TREATMENT Diagnosis is based on the history, physical examination, and ultrasound or computed tomography. An

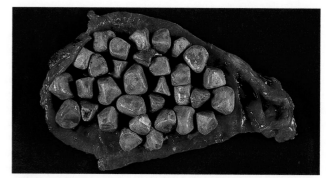

FIGURE 34-16 Resected Gallbladder Containing Mixed Gallstones. (From Kissane JM, editor: *Anderson's pathology,* ed 9, St Louis, 1990, Mosby.)

oral cholecystogram usually outlines the stones. Intravenous cholangiography is used to differentiate cholelithiasis from other causes of extrahepatic biliary obstruction if the cholecystogram is negative. Endoscopic or percutaneous cholangiography is also a diagnostic option. Oral bile acids (ursodeoxycholic acid or chenodeoxycholic acid) may prevent or dissolve cholesterol stones, but the stones may recur when the drug is discontinued. Dietary factors may prevent the development of gallstones, including reducing the intake of polyunsaturated fat, monounsaturated fat, and caffeine and increasing the consumption of fiber.[133a] Endoscopic removal of gallstones by sphincterotomy or endoscopic papillary balloon dilation is the preferred treatment for uncomplicated gallstones causing obstruction of the bile ducts. Lithotripsy may be required.[134]

Cholecystitis

Cholecystitis can be acute or chronic, but both forms are almost always caused by a gallstone lodged in the cystic duct.[135] Acute acalculous cholecystitis has been reported as a complication of surgery, multiple trauma, or burn injury and is treated with cholecystostomy.[136] The gallbladder becomes distended and inflamed, with pain similar to that caused by gallstones. Pressure against the distended wall of the gallbladder decreases blood flow and may result in ischemia, necrosis, and perforation. Fever, leukocytosis, rebound tenderness, and abdominal muscle guarding are common findings. Serum bilirubin and alkaline phosphatase levels may be elevated. The acute abdominal pain of cholecystitis must be differentiated from that caused by pancreatitis, myocardial infarction, and acute pyelonephritis of the right kidney. Cholangiography or radioactive scan can confirm the diagnosis. Narcotics may be required to control pain, and antibiotics (e.g., gentamicin, clindamycin) often are prescribed to manage bacterial infection in severe cases. Persistent symptoms or development of chronic cholecystitis punctuated by recurrent, acute attacks usually requires laparoscopic gallbladder resection (cholecystectomy). Obstruction may also lead to reflux of bile into the pancreatic duct, causing acute pancreatitis.[137]

Disorders of the Pancreas

Pancreatitis, or inflammation of the pancreas, is a relatively rare (17 cases per 100,000 people in the United States)[137a] and potentially serious disorder that occurs equally in men and women usually between 50 and 60 years of age. Risk factors include obstructive biliary tract disease (particularly cholelithiasis), alcoholism, obesity, peptic ulcers, trauma, hyperlipidemia, hypercalcemia, smoking, certain drugs, and genetic factors (hereditary pancreatitis, cystic fibrosis).[138,139] The cause is unknown in 15% to 25% of cases.[140] Pancreatitis can be acute or chronic.

Acute Pancreatitis

PATHOPHYSIOLOGY Acute pancreatitis is usually a mild disease (edematous pancreatitis) and resolves spontaneously, but about 20% of those with the disease develop a severe acute (necrotizing or hemorrhagic) pancreatitis requiring hospitalization. Pancreatitis develops because of obstruction to the outflow of pancreatic digestive enzymes caused by bile and pancreatic duct obstruction (e.g., gallstones). The obstructed ducts result in accumulation of pancreatic secretions and pathologic activation of enzymes (activated trypsin activates chymotrypsin, lipase, and elastase) within the pancreas. The activated intracellular enzymes cause autodigestion of pancreatic cells and tissues, resulting in inflammation and acute pancreatitis. The autodigestion causes vascular damage, coagulation necrosis, fat necrosis (see Chapter 3), and edema within the pancreas. In cases of alcohol abuse,

the pancreatic acinar cell metabolizes ethanol with the generation of toxic metabolites that injure pancreatic acinar cells, causing release of activated enzymes. Chronic alcohol use may also cause formation of protein plugs in pancreatic ducts and spasm of the sphincter of Oddi, resulting in obstruction. The obstruction leads to intrapancreatic release of activated enzymes, autodigestion, inflammation, and pancreatitis.

In severe acute pancreatitis proinflammatory cytokines (e.g., interleukin-6, tumor necrosis factor-alpha, and platelet-activating factor) are released into the bloodstream. Circulating inflammatory cytokines cause activation of leukocytes, injury to vessel walls, and coagulation abnormalities in other organs, such as the lungs and kidneys. Paralytic ileus and gastrointestinal bleeding can occur. Translocation of intestinal bacteria to the bloodstream may cause peritonitis or sepsis. Release of vasoactive peptides can cause vasodilation, hypotension, and shock. These systemic effects can lead to respiratory distress syndrome, renal failure, and the systemic inflammatory response syndrome (see Chapter 23) with increased morbidity and mortality.[141] While the pancreatitis progresses pancreatic stellate cells become activated, causing pancreatic fibrosis, strictures, and duct obstruction and leading to chronic pancreatitis.[142]

CLINICAL MANIFESTATIONS The cardinal manifestation of acute pancreatitis is epigastric or midabdominal constant pain ranging from mild abdominal discomfort to severe, incapacitating pain. The pain may radiate to the back. Pain is caused by (1) edema, which distends the pancreatic ducts and capsule; (2) chemical irritation and inflammation of the peritoneum; and (3) irritation or obstruction of the biliary tract. Nausea and vomiting are caused by paralytic ileus secondary to the pancreatitis or peritonitis. Jaundice can occur from obstruction of the bile duct (e.g., a gallstone) or from pancreatic edema pressing on the duct. Fever and leukocytosis accompany the inflammatory response. Abdominal distention accompanies bowel hypomotility and the accumulation of fluids in the peritoneal cavity. Hypovolemia, hypotension, tachycardia, myocardial insufficiency, and shock occur because plasma volume is lost as inflammatory mediators released into the circulation increase vascular permeability and dilate vessels. With severe pancreatitis, tachypnea and hypoxemia develop secondary to pulmonary edema, atelectasis, or pleural effusions. Hypovolemia can decrease renal blood flow sufficiently to impair renal function and can cause renal failure. Tetany may develop as a result of hypocalcemia when calcium is deposited in areas of fat necrosis or as a decreased response to parathormone. Transient hyperglycemia also can occur if glucagon is released from damaged alpha cells in the pancreatic islets. Multiple organ failure or the systemic inflammatory response syndrome accounts for most deaths in persons who have severe acute pancreatitis.

EVALUATION AND TREATMENT Diagnosis is based on clinical findings, identification of associated disorders, laboratory studies, and CT scan. Elevated serum amylase concentration is characteristic but is not diagnostic of severity or specificity of disease. Elevated serum lipase level is the primary diagnostic marker for acute pancreatitis. Abdominal imaging, particularly CT scan, provides information useful both for differential diagnosis and for grading the severity of pancreatitis.[143]

The goal of treatment for acute pancreatitis is to stop the process of autodigestion and prevent systemic complications. Narcotic medications may be needed to relieve pain. To decrease pancreatic secretions and "rest the gland," oral food and fluids may be withheld initially and continuous gastric suction instituted. Nasogastric suction may not be necessary with mild pancreatitis, but it helps to relieve pain and prevent paralytic ileus in individuals who are nauseated and vomiting. Feeding is usually initiated within 24 to 48 hours if ileus is not present. Parenteral fluids are essential to restore blood volume and prevent hypotension and shock. In severe pancreatitis enteral nutrition with use of jejunal tube feeding usually is well tolerated, may decrease pancreatic enzyme secretion, prevents gut bacterial overgrowth, and maintains gut barrier function.[144] Drugs that decrease gastric acid production (e.g., H2-receptor antagonists) can decrease stimulation of the pancreas by secretin. Antibiotics may control infection. The risk of mortality increases significantly with the development of infection or pulmonary, cardiac, and renal complications.[145]

Chronic Pancreatitis

Irreversible structural or functional impairment of the pancreas leads to chronic pancreatitis. Chronic alcohol abuse is the most common cause; smoking and genetic factors increase the risk of chronic pancreatitis.[146] Chronic exposure to toxic metabolites and release of pro-inflammatory cytokines contribute to cellular destruction including acinar cells and cells in the islets of Langerhans. Fibrosis, strictures, calcification, ductal obstruction, and pancreatic cysts are the common lesions of chronic pancreatitis. The cysts are walled-off areas or pockets of pancreatic juice, necrotic debris, or blood within or adjacent to the pancreas.

Continuous or intermittent abdominal pain and weight loss are common. The pain is difficult to manage and is associated with increased intraductal pressure, increased tissue pressure, ischemia, neuritis, ongoing injury, and changes in central pain perception.[147] Manifestations of pancreatic enzyme deficiency, such as steatorrhea or a malabsorption syndrome, are present in late stages of chronic pancreatitis. To correct enzyme deficiencies and prevent malabsorption, oral enzyme replacements are taken before and during meals. Loss of islet cells can cause insulin-dependent diabetes and requires treatment. Cessation of alcohol intake is essential for the management of both acute and chronic pancreatitis. Endoscopic or surgical drainage or partial resection of the pancreas may be required to relieve pain and to prevent cystic rupture.[148] Chronic pancreatitis is a risk factor for pancreatic cancer.

CANCER OF THE DIGESTIVE SYSTEM

Cancer of the Gastrointestinal Tract

Table 34-9 contains information on the various gastrointestinal cancers by organ, percentage of death compared to all cancer deaths, risk factors, type of cell, and common manifestations.

Cancer of the Esophagus

Carcinoma of the esophagus is a rare type of cancer, but the incidence is increasing in the Western world.[149] The incidence is about 1% of all new cancers (see Table 34-9) in the United States.[150] In the United States, it occurs more in blacks than in whites and peaks at about 60 years of age.

PATHOGENESIS Carcinoma of the esophagus is usually squamous cell carcinoma or, less commonly, adenocarcinoma. The pathogenesis of squamous cell esophageal carcinoma is facilitated by (1) alterations of esophageal structure and function that permit food and drink to remain in the esophagus for prolonged periods; (2) ulceration and metaplasia caused by esophageal reflux; (3) chronic exposure to

---

RISK FACTORS
Esophageal Cancer

- Age greater than 65 years
- Male
- Tobacco use
- Alcoholism
- Dietary factors: deficiencies of trace elements and vitamins
- Malnutrition associated with poor economic conditions or special dietary habits (e.g., very hot drinks, fish preserved in lye; diet deficient in fruits and vegetables)
- Reflux esophagitis with dysplasia
- Sliding hiatal hernia
- Obesity

Data from American Cancer Society: *Esophageal cancer.* Available at www.cancer.org/docroot/CRI/content/CRI_2_4_2X_What_are_the_risk_factors_for_esophagus_ cancer_12.asp?sitearea=.

---

irritants, such as alcohol and tobacco, that cause neoplastic transformation; (4) and obesity.[149] There may be an increased risk associated with long-term use of oral bisphosphonates.[151] Chronic inadequate nutrition can impair esophageal structure and function (see *Risk Factors: Esophageal Cancer*). Adenocarcinomas are often secondary to infiltration by a gastric carcinoma or to the presence of Barrett epithelium, also known as Barrett esophagus (columnar rather than squamous epithelium in the lower esophagus), which is associated with chronic gastroesophageal reflux disease (GERD).[152] Carcinomas can occur at any level of the esophageal tract but are most common at the gastroesophageal junction.

CLINICAL MANIFESTATIONS The two frequent symptoms of esophageal carcinoma are chest pain and dysphagia. The most common type of pain is heartburn (pyrosis). It is initiated by eating spicy or highly seasoned foods and by lying down. Odynophagia (pain on swallowing) may be initiated by the swallowing of cold liquids. Spontaneous chest pain is more difficult to diagnose positively. Some individuals with esophageal cancer complain of a constant retrosternal pain that radiates to the back. Dysphagia (difficulty swallowing) is usually pressure-like and may radiate posteriorly between the scapulae. Dysphagia usually progresses rapidly. Esophageal carcinoma is asymptomatic during the early stages and presents at an advanced stage. Esophageal cancer metastasizes rapidly and, therefore, has a poor prognosis.

EVALUATION AND TREATMENT Individuals with dysphagia undergo endoscopy so that specimens can be obtained and examined for neoplastic change. Endoscopic ultrasound and CT studies of the thorax are used for diagnosis and staging. Prevention of gastroesophageal reflux is essential to the management of Barrett esophagus. It is impossible to remove all lymph nodes with the tumor, but removal of the primary lesion and the local lymph nodes can benefit the individual with esophageal cancer. If the malignancy has not spread beyond these sites, cure is likely. If metastasis has occurred, however, an incomplete resection is of little survival benefit. Treatment is combined radiation and chemotherapy.[153]

Cancer of the Stomach

The incidence of gastric adenocarcinoma has declined in the United States and represents about 2% of all new cancer cases annually. The incidence is greater in males.[150] Other nonenvironmental risk factors

TABLE 34-9 CANCER OF THE GUT, LIVER, AND PANCREAS

ORGAN	DEATHS OUT OF ALL CANCERS COMBINED	RISKS	CELL TYPE	COMMON MANIFESTATIONS
Esophagus	2.5%	Malnutrition Alcohol Tobacco Chronic reflux	Squamous cell Adenocarcinoma	Chest pain Dysphagia
Stomach	1.8%	Salty food Nitrates-nitrosamines	Adenocarcinoma Squamous cell	Anorexia Malaise Weight loss Upper abdominal pain Vomiting Occult blood
Colorectal	9%	Polyps Ulcerative colitis Diverticulitis High-refined carbohydrates, low-fiber, high-fat diets	Adenocarcinoma (left colon grows in ring; right colon grows as mass)	Pain Mass Anemia Bloody stool Obstruction Distention
Liver	3.3%	HBV, HCV, HDV Cirrhosis Intestinal parasite Aflatoxin from moldy peanuts	Hepatomas Cholangiomas	Pain Anorexia Bloating Weight loss Portal hypertension Ascites Jaundice
Pancreas	6.4%	Chronic pancreatitis Cigarette smoking Alcohol (?) Diabetic women	Adenocarcinoma (exocrine part of gland, ductal epithelium)	Weight loss Weakness Nausea Vomiting Abdominal pain Depression ± jaundice May have insulin-secreting tumors with symptoms of hypoglycemia

From American Cancer Society: *Cancer facts & figures 2010,* Atlanta, 2010, Author. Available at www.cancer.org/acs/groups/content/@nho/documents/document/acspc-024113.pdf.
HBV, Hepatitis B virus; *HCV,* hepatitis C virus; *HDV,* hepatitis D virus.

are a family history of gastric adenocarcinoma, blood type A, and pernicious anemia, which results from atrophy of the gastric mucosa in the same locations where gastric tumors arise. Loss of tumor-suppressor genes and other genetic alterations may be important in gastric cancer.[154] The incidence of stomach cancer has remained high consistently in Asian countries, the British Isles, and Iceland. Studies of Japanese immigrants to the United States show that offspring who are born and raised in the United States have an incidence rate comparable with that of other Americans.[155]

The most important environmental causative factors of gastric cancer are (1) infection with *Helicobacter pylori* that carries the *CagA* gene product cytotoxin-associated vacuolating antigen A (*VacA*), (2) consumption of heavily salted and preserved foods (e.g., nitrates in pickled or salted foods such as bacon), (3) low intake of fruits and vegetables, and (4) use of tobacco and alcohol. Dietary salt enhances the conversion of nitrates to carcinogenic nitrosamines in the stomach. Salt is also caustic to the stomach and can cause chronic atrophic gastritis. Finally, hypertonic salt solutions delay gastric emptying. Delayed emptying increases the time during which carcinogenic nitrosamines can exert their effects on the stomach mucosa. Nitrates interact with amino acids in the stomach to form nitrosamines, enhanced at a low pH by iodides and thiocyanates.

Nitrates are thought to be active only when converted to nitrites and to cause stomach cancer once atrophic gastritis has occurred. *H. pylori–*associated gastritis increases the risk for gastric adenocarcinoma and gastric mucosa–associated lymphoid tissue (MALT) lymphoma.[156]

PATHOGENESIS Gastric adenocarcinoma usually begins in the glands of the distal stomach mucosa. Approximately 50% of cancers develop in the prepyloric antrum (Figure 34-17). Inflammation and atrophic gastritis associated with *H. pylori* infection and intestinal metaplasia are strongly linked to the development of gastric cancer. Insufficient acid secretion by the atrophic mucosa creates a relatively alkaline environment that permits bacteria to multiply and act on nitrates. The resulting increase in nitrosamines damages the deoxyribonucleic acid (DNA) of mucosal cells further, promoting metaplasia and neoplasia. Duodenal reflux also may contribute to intestinal metaplasia. The reflux contains caustic bile salts that destroy the mucosal barrier that normally protects the stomach.

CLINICAL MANIFESTATIONS The early stages of gastric cancer are generally asymptomatic or produce vague symptoms such as loss of appetite (especially for meat), malaise, and indigestion. Later

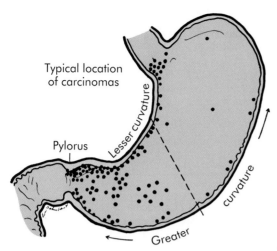

Typical location
of carcinomas

Lesser curvature

Pylorus

Greater curvature

FIGURE 34-17 Typical Sites of Stomach Cancer. (From del Regato JA, Spjut HJ, Cox JD: *Cancer: diagnosis, treatment, and prognosis,* ed 2, St Louis, 1985, Mosby.)

manifestations of gastric cancer include unexplained weight loss, upper abdominal pain, vomiting, change in bowel habits, and anemia caused by persistent occult bleeding. The prognosis is poor because symptoms do not occur until the tumor has spread to surrounding tissues, and entered the draining lymph nodes and veins, causing distant metastases, particularly to the liver and peritoneal structures. Generally the first manifestations of carcinoma are caused by distant metastases, and the disease is already in an advanced stage.

EVALUATION AND TREATMENT Most symptoms suggest a problem in the upper gastrointestinal tract, and a barium x-ray film shows the lesion. Direct endoscopic visualization and biopsy usually establish the diagnosis. Another definitive technique is microscopic examination of exfoliated cells obtained by lavage during endoscopy. Screening and treatment for *H. pylori* infection is the best preventive approach to gastric cancer. Surgery is the usual treatment for gastric cancer. Staging is determined by pathologic findings after resection. Chemotherapy combined with chemoradiation is improving postsurgical outcomes.[157]

 QUICK CHECK 34-7
1. How do gallstones form?
2. Compare acute and chronic pancreatitis.
3. What factors are associated with cancer of the esophagus?
4. What dietary factors are associated with gastric cancer?

Cancer of the Colon and Rectum

Colorectal cancer (CRC) is the third most common cause of cancer and cancer death in the United States for both men and women. CRC accounts for about 9% of estimated new cancers and deaths from all cancers in the United States.[150] CRC tends to occur in individuals older than 50 years and is rare in children. Worldwide, the prevalence of CRC is highest in populations with high socioeconomic standards, possibly because of dietary habits (see *Risk Factors:* Cancer of the Colon and Rectum). **Small intestinal carcinoma** is very rare and represents less than 1% of gastrointestinal cancers.[160]

PATHOGENESIS Most colorectal cancers are sporadic (acquired) or associated with a family history of colorectal cancer. They are caused by

RISK FACTORS

Cancer of the Colon and Rectum

- Advanced age
- High-fat (especially egg consumption), red and processed meat, low-fiber diet
- High consumption of alcohol
- Cigarette smoking
- Obesity
- Familial polyposis or family history of colorectal cancer
- Low levels of physical activity
- Inflammatory bowel disease
- Type 2 diabetes mellitus

Data from American Cancer Society: *Learn about cancer, colorectal cancer, 08/09/2010.* Available at www.cancer.org/Cancer/ColonandRectumCancer/index

complex multiple gene interactions, including gene deletion, mutations of oncogenes, tumor-suppressor genes, and repair genes. Abnormal DNA methylation is also associated with colorectal cancer (see Chapter 9 for mechanisms of oncogenesis). **Familial adenomatous polyposis [FAP]** is a mutation of the *APC* gene (adenomatous polyposis coli), a tumor suppressor gene, and is the most common hereditary cause of colorectal cancer. **Hereditary nonpolyposis colorectal cancer (HNPCC)**, or **Lynch syndrome**, is associated with several DNA repair genes (see Figure 34-18). Both FAP and HNPCC have a rare, family-linked autosomal dominant inheritance trait that accounts for about 3% to 5% of colorectal cancers.[158,159]

Colorectal polyps are closely associated with the development of cancer. A polyp, or papilloma, is a finger-like projection arising from the mucosal epithelium. The most common types of polyps are hyperplastic (a non-neoplastic, or bengin polyp) and adenomatous (a neoplastic). **Neoplastic polyps** are premalignant lesions and are further classified as tubular (the most prevalent), villous, or tubulovillous adenomas[160a] (Figure 34-19).

Adenocarcinomas of the colon and rectum usually arise from adenomatous polyps. Once the malignant cells of an adenoma traverse the muscularis mucosae, the tumor becomes invasive and highly malignant. Adenomas can be detected early, however, and the submucosa may not be penetrated for several years (Figure 34-20). The larger the polyp, the greater the risk of colorectal cancer. Although lesions larger than 1.5 cm occur less often, they are more likely to be malignant than those smaller than 1.0 cm. Thus, screening colonoscopy with polypectomy is important when polyps are found.

Most colorectal cancers are moderately differentiated adenocarcinomas. These tumors have a long preinvasive phase, and when they invade, they tend to grow slowly. Colorectal carcinoma starts in the glands of the mucosal lining. Because the lymphatic channels are located under the muscularis mucosae, the lesions must traverse this layer before metastasis can occur.

CLINICAL MANIFESTATIONS Symptoms of colorectal cancer depend on the location, size, and shape of the lesion. Tumors of the right (ascending) colon and left (descending) colon evolve into two distinct tumor types.[161] On the right side, the lesions are polypoid and extend along one wall of the cecum and ascending colon. These tumors may be silent, evolving to pain, palpable mass in the lower right quadrant, anemia, fatigue, and dark red or mahogany-colored blood mixed with the stool (see Figure 34-19). These tumors can become large and bulky with necrosis and ulceration, contributing to persistent blood loss and anemia. Obstruction is unusual because the growth does not readily encircle the colon.

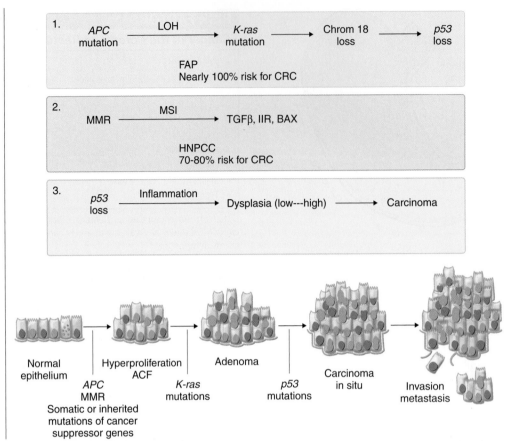

FIGURE 34-18 The Molecular Basis of Colorectal Cancer. Colorectal carcinoma develops from the sequential progression of genetic alterations. **1,** Mutations in the *APC* gene are the earliest known event and inactivation of *APC* accelerates cell cycle progression. *K-ras* over expression leads to loss of *p53*. Loss of *p53* transforms an adenoma into a metastatic carcinoma. **2,** Mutation of mismatch repair genes (MMR) that encode key molecules that repair DNA result in replication errors and deactivation of proteins from other downstream mutations (TGFβ, IIR, BAX). Deletions or mutations in MMR genes exists in 95% of tumors in individuals with hereditary non-polyposis colorectal cancer (HNPCC), but only 10~15% of sporadic tumors. **3,** *p53* loss occur in ~75% of colorectal carcinomas, but infrequently in benign lesions. *APC*, *APC* gene (a tumor suppressor gene); *LOH*, loss of heterozygosity; *K-ras*, a proto oncogene (promotes cell growth); *p53*, protein 53 or tumor protein 53 (a tumor suppressor protein); *FAP*, familial adenomatous polyposis; *MMR*, mutation mismatch repair; *MSI*, microsatellite instability; *TGFβ*, transforming growth factor-β; *IIR*, type II receptor; *BAX*, apoptosis-related protein; *HNPCC*, hereditary nonpolyposis colorectal cancer; *CRC*, colorectal cancer.

Tumors of the left, or descending, colon start as small, elevated, button-like masses. This type grows circumferentially, encircling the entire bowel wall, and eventually ulcerating in the middle as the tumor penetrates the blood supply. Obstruction is common but occurs slowly and stools become narrow and pencil shaped. Manifestations include progressive abdominal distention, pain, vomiting, constipation, need for laxatives, cramps, and bright red blood on the surface of the stool.

Systematic lymphatic distribution occurs along the aorta to the mesenteric and pancreatic lymph nodes. Liver metastasis is common and follows invasion of the mesenteric veins (left colon) or superior veins (right colon), which drain into the portal circulation.

Rectal carcinomas are defined as tumors occurring up to 15 cm from the anal opening. Tumors of the rectum can spread through the rectal wall to nearby structures: the prostate in men and the vagina in women. Penetration occurs more readily in the lower third of the rectum because it has no serosal covering. Systemic and pulmonary metastases occur through the hemorrhoidal plexus, which drains into the vena cava.

EVALUATION AND TREATMENT Individuals with hereditary polyposis should begin screening at an early age (10 to 12 years) using colonoscopy with removal of polyps when they are found.[162] Molecular markers are being developed.[163] Early detection screening procedures for nonhereditary CRC are summarized in Box 34-4. Chemoprophylaxis aspirin and celecoxib may reduce the incidence of CRC in the general population.[164] Dietary modification and other nondietary lifestyle changes can significantly decrease the risk of colorectal cancer.

Treatment for cancer of the colon is always surgical. Resection and anastomosis can be performed for cancer of the ascending, transverse, descending, or sigmoid colon and upper rectum. These surgeries are performed through abdominal incisions and assisted with radiofrequency ablation. Natural defecation is preserved. Growths in the lower portion of the rectum require removal of the entire rectum with the formation of a permanent colostomy. Resection of liver metastases may prolong survival.[165] Prognosis after surgery depends on the stage and location of the tumor.

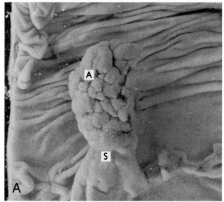

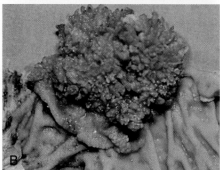

FIGURE 34-19 Neoplastic Polyps. A, Tubular adenomata *(A)* are rounded lesions 0.5 to 2 cm in size that are generally red and sit on a stalk *(S)* of normal mucosa that has been dragged up by traction of the polyp in the bowel lumen. B, Villous adenomata are velvety lesions about 0.6 cm thick that occupy a broad area of mucosa generally 1 to 5 cm in diameter. (From Stevens A, Lowe J: *Pathology*, ed 2, Edinburgh, 2000, Mosby.)

Transverse colon (15%)
Pain, obstruction, change in bowel habits, anemia

Ascending colon (25%)
Pain, mass, change in bowel habits, anemia

Descending colon (15%)
Pain, change in bowel habits, bright red blood in stool, obstruction

Rectum (45%)
Blood in stool, change in bowel habits, rectal discomfort

FIGURE 34-20 Signs and Symptoms of Colorectal Cancer by Location of Primary Lesion. Clinical manifestations are listed in order of frequency for each region (lymphatics of colon also shown).

The staging of colorectal cancer involves endoscopic ultrasonography and operative exploration. Physical examination of the abdomen detects liver enlargement and ascites; appropriate lymph nodes are palpated. Elevated carcinoembryonic antigen (CEA) levels are often detected in the sera of individuals with colorectal carcinoma, but CEA level is not a screening marker for colorectal cancer because it

is elevated with other intestinal diseases. Operative staging consists of careful exploration during surgery and biopsy of possible metastases. The National Cancer Institute[166] classification is widely used for staging of colorectal cancer and is summarized as follows:

Stage 0 (carcinoma in situ): involves only the mucosal lining

Stage I: extension of cancer to middle layers of colon wall

Stage II: extension beyond colon wall to nearby tissues around colon or *rectum*, and/or through *peritoneum*

Stage III: spread beyond colon into lymph nodes and nearby organs and/or through *peritoneum*

Stage IV: spread to nearby *lymph nodes* and spread to other parts of body (*liver* or *lungs*)

A diet rich in fruits and vegetables, grains, folic acid, and calcium and low in fat can modify cancer risk.[167]

Radiation therapy is often given before surgery in the hope that it will shrink the tumor or alter the malignant cells, or both, so that these cells will not survive after surgery. Chemotherapy is used to treat metastatic disease and cases with a high risk of recurrence. New chemotherapeutic agents are improving first-line therapy. Immunotherapy, vaccines, and viral vectors for the treatment of colon cancer are under development.[168,169]

Cancer of the Accessory Organs of Digestion
Cancer of the Liver

Cancer of the liver is the fifth most common cause of cancer and third leading cause of cancer death worldwide, and the incidence is increasing as a result of chronic hepatitis B (HBV) and C viral (HCV) infection.[170] Primary liver cancer is relatively rare in the United States but is common in densely populated parts of southeast Asia and Southern Africa. In the United States, the incidence of primary liver cancer is higher in blacks than in whites and higher in males than in females. Primary liver cancer is rare before the age of 40 years and is most common during the sixth decade. Cancer in the liver is usually caused by metastatic spread from a primary site elsewhere in the body. Together, primary and secondary liver cancers account for about 2% to 3% of all cancer deaths in the United States[150] (see *Risk Factors:* Primary Liver Cancer).

PATHOGENESIS Primary carcinomas of the liver are hepatocellular or cholangiocellular. **Hepatocellular carcinoma (hepatocarcinoma)** develops in the hepatocytes and can be nodular (consisting of multiple, discrete nodules), massive (consisting of a large tumor mass having satellite nodules), or diffuse (consisting of small nodules distributed throughout most of the liver). It is closely associated with chronic hepatitis and cirrhosis. Because carcinoma of the liver invades the hepatic and portal veins, it often spreads to the heart and lungs. Other sites of metastases are the brain, kidney, and spleen.

Cholangiocellular carcinoma (cholangiocarcinoma) develops in the bile ducts and occurs less often than hepatocellular carcinoma in the United States. It is associated with primary sclerosing cholangitis and is geographically associated with areas where liver fluke infestation is prevalent, such as Southeast Asia. Cholangiocellular carcinoma can occur anywhere along the bile duct and extend directly into the liver, usually as a solitary lesion. It is difficult to distinguish an invasion of cholangiocellular carcinoma from a metastatic adenocarcinoma except by neoplastic changes found in nearby ducts.

CLINICAL MANIFESTATIONS The clinical presentation of liver cancer in adults is characterized by vague abdominal symptoms, such as nausea and vomiting, fullness, pressure, and dull ache in the right hypochondrium. Manifestations of hepatocellular carcinoma can occur slowly or abruptly. In individuals with cirrhosis, deepening jaundice or abrupt lack of appetite is a sign of hepatocellular carcinoma. Obstruction by the tumor can cause sudden worsening of portal hypertension and development of ascites. As the tumor enlarges, it causes pain. Cholangiocellular carcinoma more commonly presents insidiously as pain, loss of appetite, weight loss, and gradual onset of jaundice. Some carcinomas of the liver rupture spontaneously, causing hemorrhage. Others are discovered accidentally during evaluation of a bone fracture or surgical exploration.

EVALUATION AND TREATMENT There is no specific test for the diagnosis of liver cancer. For high-risk individuals, α-fetoprotein associated with HBV and abdominal ultrasound are common screening tools. Diagnosis is based on clinical manifestations, laboratory findings, radiologic examination, exploratory laparotomy, and biopsy findings. In individuals without cirrhosis, liver scans can document filling defects. CT or ultrasonography is used to detect solid tumors, but neither can distinguish benign from malignant tumors. Primary prevention may be achieved by vaccinating against hepatitis B, screening all donated blood for the presence of the virus, and reducing contamination of food with aflatoxins.[171]

Surgical resection is possible only if the tumor is localized to a removable lobe of the liver. Surgery is hazardous and usually not undertaken if the individual has cirrhosis. Radiofrequency (thermal) ablation has emerged as the most effective method for local tumor destruction.[172] Most individuals develop metastases after surgical resection, but long-term survival is possible. Chemotherapeutic agents are administered systemically or locally, but their use may be limited to the presence of advanced cirrhosis. Liver transplant offers a cure if the waiting time is short.[173] Gene therapy and immunotherapy are being explored.[174] The prognosis for those with symptomatic liver cancer is poor.

Cancer of the Gallbladder

Cancer of the gallbladder occurs in about 9760 people each year in the United States.[150] It is more common in women than in men by a ratio of about 2 to 1. It occurs rarely before the age of 40 years and is most common between the ages of 50 and 60 years. Most gallbladder cancer is caused by metastasis. Primary carcinoma of the gallbladder is rare and usually is associated with cholelithiasis.

PATHOGENESIS Most primary carcinomas of the gallbladder are adenocarcinomas, and more rarely squamous cell carcinomas. Invasion of the liver occurs early. Spreading to the cystic and periportal lymph nodes occurs with invasion of the pancreas and retroperitoneal lymph nodes. Direct invasion of the stomach and the duodenum can cause pyloric obstruction. Infection often accompanies cancer of the gallbladder. Generalized peritonitis, gangrene, perforation, and liver abscesses are potential complications of infection.

CLINICAL MANIFESTATIONS Early stages of gallbladder carcinoma are asymptomatic. A typical presentation of carcinoma of the gallbladder is steady, upper right quadrant pain for about 2 months. Other manifestations include diarrhea, belching, weakness, loss of appetite, weight loss, and vomiting. Obstructive jaundice can occur if an enlarging tumor presses on the extrahepatic ducts.

EVALUATION AND TREATMENT Early diagnosis of cancer of the gallbladder is rare. Therefore, individuals with gallstones, especially older women, are evaluated carefully. Inflammatory disorders, such as cholangitis (bile duct inflammation) and peritonitis, often obscure an underlying malignancy. Diagnostic procedures include upper gastrointestinal barium study, ultrasonography, cholangiography, and CT scan.

Complete surgical resection of the gallbladder is the only effective treatment. Because advanced malignancies cannot be resected, gallbladders containing stones are removed as a preventive measure. The prognosis of unresectable gallbladder cancer is extremely poor. Molecular therapies are under development.[175]

Cancer of the Pancreas

Pancreatic cancer now ranks fourth as a cause of cancer deaths with 36,800 deaths annually in the United States. The incidence of pancreatic cancer rises steadily with age. Males are affected slightly more often than females, and blacks more often than whites. Mortality is nearly 100%. The cause of pancreatic cancer is not known, but there are modest risks associated with tobacco smoking, certain dietary factors (e.g., high-fat foods and processed meat), obesity, diabetes mellitus, chronic pancreatitis, family history of pancreatic cancer, and hereditary nonpolyposis colon cancer (HNPCC) (Lynch syndrome).[150]

PATHOGENESIS Cancer of the pancreas can arise from exocrine or endocrine cells. Most pancreatic tumors arise from exocrine cells in the ducts and are called *ductal adenocarcinomas.* Tumors arising in small ducts invade nearby glandular tissue, penetrate the covering of the pancreas, and extend into surrounding tissues.[176] Tumors of the head quickly spread to obstruct the common bile duct and portal vein. These tumors can then infiltrate the superior mesenteric artery, the vena cava, and the aorta and form emboli. Tumors of the body and tail infiltrate the posterior abdominal wall. Lymphatic invasion occurs early and rapidly. Venous invasion causes metastases to the liver. Tumor implants on the peritoneal surface can obstruct veins and promote development of ascites.

CLINICAL MANIFESTATIONS   Cancer of the pancreas usually develops with no symptoms. Often there is vague upper abdominal pain that radiates to the back. Jaundice develops in most cases, usually caused by obstruction of the bile duct. Because obstruction impairs enzyme secretion and flow to the duodenum, pancreatic cancer causes fat and protein malabsorption, resulting in weight loss. Distant metastases are found in the cervical lymph nodes, the lungs, and the brain. Most individuals die of hepatic failure, malnutrition, or systemic diseases.

EVALUATION AND TREATMENT   Endoscopic ultrasound and CT are used initially for diagnosis.[177] Laparotomy is often used to establish a definitive diagnosis, evaluate the extent of disease, and determine whether palliative bypass surgery (i.e., cholecystojejunostomy and gastrojejunostomy) is needed. Many surgeons recommend a total pancreatectomy because cancer of the pancreas seldom consists of a single lesion. Molecular markers are under investigation.[178] Adjuvant chemotherapy and new systemic agents are improving survival and radiochemotherapy may produce favorable controls in locally advanced cancer.[179] Five-year survival is less than 6%.

✔ **QUICK CHECK 34-8**
1. What are the primary risk factors for gastric carcinoma?
2. Compare tumors of the right colon with those of the left colon.
3. What is the most common cause of liver cancer?

DID YOU UNDERSTAND?

Disorders of the Gastrointestinal Tract

1. Anorexia is lack of a desire to eat despite physiologic stimuli that would normally produce hunger.
2. Vomiting is the forceful emptying of the stomach effected by gastrointestinal contraction and reverse peristalsis of the esophagus. It is usually preceded by nausea and retching, with the exception of projectile vomiting, which is associated with direct stimulation of the vomiting center in the brain.
3. Constipation is often caused by unhealthy dietary and bowel habits combined with lack of exercise. Constipation also can result from a disorder that impairs intestinal motility or obstructs the intestinal lumen.
4. Diarrhea can be caused by excessive fluid drawn into the intestinal lumen by osmosis (osmotic diarrhea), excessive secretion of fluids by the intestinal mucosa (secretory diarrhea), or excessive gastrointestinal motility (motility diarrhea).
5. Abdominal pain is caused by stretching, inflammation, or ischemia (insufficient blood supply). Abdominal pain originates in the organs themselves (visceral pain) or in the peritoneum (parietal pain) and can be acute or chronic. Visceral pain is often referred to the back.
6. Obvious manifestations of gastrointestinal bleeding are hematemesis (vomiting of blood), melena (dark, tarry stools), and hematochezia (frank bleeding from the rectum). Occult bleeding can be detected only by testing stools or vomitus for the presence of blood.
7. Dysphagia is difficulty swallowing. It can be caused by a mechanical or functional obstruction of the esophagus. Functional obstruction is an impairment of esophageal motility.
8. Achalasia is a form of functional dysphagia caused by loss of esophageal innervation.
9. Gastroesophageal reflux disease is the regurgitation of chyme from the stomach into the esophagus, resulting in an inflammatory response (reflux esophagitis) when the esophageal mucosa is repeatedly exposed to acids and enzymes in the regurgitated chyme.
10. Hiatal hernia is the protrusion of the upper part of the stomach through the hiatus (esophageal opening in the diaphragm) at the gastroesophageal junction. Hiatal hernia can be sliding or paraesophageal.
11. Pyloric obstruction is the narrowing or blockage of the pylorus, which is the opening between the stomach and the duodenum. It can be caused by a congenital defect, inflammation and scarring secondary to a gastric ulcer, or tumor growth.
12. Intestinal obstruction prevents the normal movement of chyme through the intestinal tract. It can be mechanical (i.e., caused by torsion, herniation, or tumor) or functional as a result of paralytic ileus.
13. The most severe consequences of intestinal obstruction are fluid and electrolyte losses, hypovolemia, shock, intestinal necrosis, and perforation of the intestinal wall.
14. Gastritis is an acute or chronic inflammation of the gastric mucosa.
15. Regurgitation of bile, use of anti-inflammatory drugs or alcohol, and some systemic diseases are associated with gastritis.
16. Chronic gastritis of the fundus and body is the most severe form of gastritis. It can result in gastric atrophy and decreased secretion of hydrochloric acid, pepsinogen, and intrinsic factor.
17. Chronic gastritis of the antrum, the most common type, is not usually associated with impaired secretion or gastric atrophy.
18. A peptic ulcer is a circumscribed area of mucosal inflammation and ulceration caused by excessive secretion of gastric acid, disruption of the protective mucosal barrier, or both.
19. There are three types of peptic ulcers: duodenal, gastric, and stress ulcers.
20. Duodenal ulcers, the most common peptic ulcers, are associated with H. pylori infection, chronic use of NSAIDs, increased numbers of parietal (acid-secreting) cells in the stomach, elevated gastrin levels, and rapid gastric emptying. Pain occurs when the stomach is empty, and it is relieved with food or antacids. Duodenal ulcers tend to heal spontaneously and recur frequently.
21. Gastric ulcers develop near parietal cells, generally in the antrum, and tend to become chronic. Gastric secretions may be normal or decreased, and pain may occur after eating.
22. Ischemic stress ulcers develop suddenly after severe illness, systemic trauma, or neural injury. Ulceration follows mucosal damage caused by ischemia (decreased blood flow to the gastric mucosa).
23. Cushing ulcer is a stress ulcer caused by head trauma. Ulceration follows hypersecretion of hydrochloric acid caused by overstimulation of the vagal nuclei.
24. Postgastrectomy syndromes are long-term complications that follow gastrectomy, the resection of all or part of the stomach. The postgastrectomy syndromes include dumping syndrome, alkaline reflux gastritis, afferent loop obstruction, diarrhea, weight loss, and anemia.
25. Dumping syndrome is the rapid emptying of chyme into the small intestine. It causes an osmotic shift of fluid from the vascular compartment to the intestinal lumen, which decreases plasma volume.

26. Alkaline reflux gastritis is stomach inflammation caused by the reflux of bile and pancreatic secretions from the duodenum into the stomach. These substances disrupt the mucosal barrier and cause inflammation.

27. Afferent loop obstruction is an obstruction of the duodenal stump on the proximal side of a gastrojejunostomy. Biliary and pancreatic secretions accumulate in the stump, causing distention, intermittent pain, and vomiting.

28. Malabsorption syndromes result in impaired digestion or absorption of nutrients and usually cause diarrhea.

29. Pancreatic exocrine insufficiency causes malabsorption associated with impaired digestion. The pancreas does not produce sufficient amounts of the enzymes that digest protein, carbohydrates, and fats into components that can be absorbed by the intestine.

30. Deficient lactase production in the brush border of the small intestine inhibits the breakdown of lactose. This prevents lactose absorption and causes osmotic diarrhea.

31. Bile salt deficiency causes fat malabsorption and steatorrhea (fatty stools). Bile salt deficiency can result from inadequate secretion of bile, excessive bacterial deconjugation of bile, or impaired reabsorption of bile salts caused by ileal disease.

32. Ulcerative colitis is a chronic inflammatory bowel disease that causes ulceration, abscess formation, and necrosis of the colonic and rectal mucosa. Cramping pain, bleeding, frequent diarrhea, dehydration, and weight loss accompany severe forms of the disease. A course of frequent remissions and exacerbations is common.

33. Crohn disease is similar to ulcerative colitis, but it affects both the large and small intestines and ulceration tends to involve all the layers of the lumen. "Skip lesion" fissures and granulomata are characteristic of Crohn disease. Abdominal tenderness, diarrhea, and weight loss are the usual symptoms.

34. Diverticula are outpouchings of colonic mucosa through the muscle layers of the colon wall. Diverticulosis is the presence of these outpouchings; diverticulitis is inflammation of the diverticula.

35. Appendicitis is the most common surgical emergency of the abdomen. Obstruction of the lumen leads to increased pressure, ischemia, and inflammation of the appendix. Without surgical resection, inflammation may progress to gangrene, perforation, and peritonitis.

36. Irritable bowel syndrome is a functional disorder with no known structural or biochemical alterations; it can be diarrhea prevalent or constipation prevalent, or may alternate between diarrhea and constipation. Alterations in the brain-gut axis with intestinal hypersensitivity, intestinal infection, and alterations in motility and secretion are associated with the symptoms.

37. Vascular insufficiency in the intestine is most often associated with occlusion or obstruction of the mesenteric vessels or insufficient intestinal arterial blood flow. The resulting ischemia and necrosis produce abdominal pain, fever, bloody diarrhea, hypovolemia, and shock.

38. Obesity is a metabolic disorder with an increase in body fat mass and a BMI greater than 30.

39. The causes of obesity are complex and involve the interaction of adipokines produced by fat cells and other body weight control signals at the level of the hypothalamus. Leptin resistance, insulin resistance, and a proinflammatory state contribute to the complications of obesity.

40. Visceral obesity increases the risk of developing systemic inflammation, dyslipidemia, and insulin resistance with predisposition to atherosclerosis, hypertension, cardiovascular disease, cancer, and type 2 diabetes mellitus.

41. Anorexia nervosa, or self-imposed starvation, is a psychogenic disorder of primarily adolescent and young women. It causes significant weight loss and developmental delays and can be fatal.

42. Bulimia nervosa, or bingeing and purging, involves eating normal or large amounts of food and then purging by inducing vomiting or abusing laxatives. Severe weight loss is rare, but frequent vomiting causes tooth decay, pharyngitis, and esophagitis.

43. Malnutrition is lack of nourishment from inadequate amounts of calories, protein, vitamins, or minerals. Starvation is an extreme state of malnutrition. Cachexia is physical wasting associated with chronic disease.

44. Short-term starvation, or lack of dietary intake for 3 or 4 days, stimulates mobilization of stored glucose by two metabolic processes: glycogenolysis (splitting of glycogen into glucose) and gluconeogenesis (formation of glucose from noncarbohydrate molecules).

45. Long-term starvation triggers the breakdown of ketone bodies and fatty acids. Eventually proteolysis (protein breakdown) begins, and death ensues if nutrition is not restored.

Disorders of the Accessory Organs of Digestion

1. Portal hypertension, ascites, hepatic encephalopathy, jaundice, and hepatorenal syndrome are complications of many liver disorders.

2. Portal hypertension is an elevation of portal venous pressure to at least 10 mm Hg. It is caused by increased resistance to venous flow in the portal vein and its tributaries, including the sinusoids and hepatic vein.

3. Portal hypertension is the most serious complication of liver disease because it can cause potentially fatal complications, such as bleeding varices, ascites, and hepatic encephalopathy.

4. Varices (esophageal, gastric, hemorrhoidal) are distended, tortuous, collateral veins resulting from prolonged elevation of pressure in the portal vein.

5. Hepatopulmonary syndrome and portopulmonary hypertension are complications of portal hypertension caused by release of nitric oxide and carbon monoxide in the presence of liver injury.

6. Ascites is the accumulation and sequestration of fluid in the peritoneal cavity, often as a result of portal hypertension and decreased concentrations of plasma proteins.

7. Hepatic encephalopathy (portal-systemic encephalopathy) is impaired cerebral function caused by blood-borne toxins (particularly ammonia) not metabolized by the liver. Toxin-bearing blood may bypass the liver in collateral vessels opened as a result of portal hypertension, or diseased hepatocytes may be unable to carry out their metabolic functions.

8. Manifestations of hepatic encephalopathy range from confusion and asterixis (flapping tremor of the hands) to loss of consciousness, coma, and death.

9. Jaundice (icterus) is a yellow or greenish pigmentation of the skin or sclera of the eyes caused by increases in plasma bilirubin concentration (hyperbilirubinemia).

10. Obstructive jaundice is caused by obstructed bile canaliculi (intrahepatic obstructive jaundice) or obstructed bile ducts outside the liver (extrahepatic obstructive jaundice). Bilirubin accumulates proximal to the sites of obstruction, enters the bloodstream, and is carried to the skin and deposited.

11. Hemolytic jaundice is caused by destruction of red blood cells at a rate that exceeds the liver's ability to metabolize unconjugated bilirubin.

12. Hepatorenal is functional kidney failure caused by advanced liver disease, particularly cirrhosis with portal hypertension. Renal failure is caused by a sudden decrease in blood flow to the kidneys, usually caused by massive gastrointestinal hemorrhage or liver failure. Its chief clinical manifestation is oliguria.

13. Viral hepatitis is an infection of the liver caused by a strain of the hepatitis virus (i.e., hepatitis A virus [HAV], hepatitis B virus [HBV], or hepatitis C virus [HCV]). Although they differ with respect to modes of transmission and severity of acute illness, all can cause hepatic cell necrosis, Kupffer cell hyperplasia, and infiltration of liver tissue by mononuclear phagocytes. These changes obstruct bile flow and impair hepatocyte function.

Continued

DID YOU UNDERSTAND?—cont'd

14. The clinical manifestations of viral hepatitis depend on the stage of infection. Fever, malaise, anorexia, and liver enlargement and tenderness characterize the prodromal phase (stage 1). Jaundice and hyperbilirubinemia mark the icteric phase (stage 2). During the recovery phase (stage 3), symptoms resolve. Recovery takes several weeks.

15. Fulminant hepatitis is a complication of hepatitis B (with or without hepatitis D infection) or hepatitis C virus. It causes widespread hepatic necrosis and is often fatal.

16. Cirrhosis is an inflammatory disease of the liver that causes disorganization of lobular structure, fibrosis, and nodular regeneration. Cirrhosis can result from hepatitis or exposure to toxins, such as acetaldehyde (a product of alcohol metabolism). The disease causes progressive irreversible liver damage, usually over a period of years.

17. Alcoholic fatty liver and alcoholic steatohepatitis are accumulations of fat in the liver and precursors to alcoholic cirrhosis.

18. Alcoholic cirrhosis impairs the hepatocytes' ability to oxidize fatty acids, synthesize enzymes and proteins, degrade hormones, and clear portal blood of ammonia and toxins. The inflammatory response includes excessive collagen formation, fibrosis, and scarring, which obstruct bile canaliculi and sinusoids. Bile obstruction causes jaundice. Vascular obstruction causes portal hypertension, shunting, and varices.

19. Nonalcoholic fatty liver disease and nonalcoholic steatohepatitis involve accumulation of fat in the liver not associated with alcohol intake and are commonly associated with obesity.

20. Primary biliary cirrhosis is an autoimmune inflammatory destruction of intrahepatic bile ducts. Its cause is unknown.

21. Secondary biliary cirrhosis develops from prolonged obstruction of bile flow with increased pressure in the hepatic bile ducts that causes pooling of bile and necrosis of tissue. Relief of obstruction allays symptoms of jaundice and pruritus. Continued obstruction causes cirrhosis and liver failure.

22. Cholelithiasis (the formation of gallstones) is a common disorder of the gallbladder. Gallstones form in the bile as a result of the aggregation of cholesterol crystals (cholesterol stones) or precipitates of unconjugated bilirubin (pigmented stones). Gallstones that fill the gallbladder or obstruct the cystic or common bile duct cause abdominal pain and jaundice.

23. Cholecystitis is an acute or chronic inflammation of the gallbladder usually associated with obstruction of the cystic duct by gallstones.

24. Acute pancreatitis (pancreatic inflammation) is a serious but relatively rare disorder. Pancreatic duct obstruction and injury permits leakage of digestive enzymes into pancreatic tissue where they become activated and begin the process of autodigestion, inflammation, and destruction of tissues. Release of pancreatic enzymes into the bloodstream or abdominal cavity causes damage to other organs.

25. Chronic pancreatitis results from structural or functional impairment of the pancreas. It causes recurrent abdominal pain and digestive disorders.

Cancer of the Digestive System

1. Cancer of the esophagus is rare and tends to occur in people older than 60 years of age. Alcohol and tobacco use, reflux esophagitis, and nutritional deficiencies are associated with esophageal carcinoma.

2. Dysphagia and chest pain are the primary manifestations of esophageal cancer. Early treatment of tumors that have not spread into the mediastinum or lymph nodes results in a good prognosis.

3. Gastric carcinoma is associated with *Helicobacter pylori* that carries the CagA gene product cytotoxin-associated vacuolating antigen A, a diet high in salt and food preservatives (nitrates, nitrites), and atrophic gastritis.

4. Approximately 50% of all gastric cancers are located in the prepyloric antrum. Clinical manifestations (weight loss, upper abdominal pain, vomiting, hematemesis, anemia) develop only after the tumor has penetrated the wall of the stomach.

5. Cancer of the colon and rectum (colorectal cancer) is the third most common cause of cancer death in the United States. Preexisting polyps are highly associated with adenocarcinoma of the colon. Familial adenomatous polyposis accounts for about 3% to 5% of colorectal cancer cases.

6. Tumors of the right (ascending) colon are usually large and bulky; tumors of the left (descending, sigmoid) colon develop as small, button-like masses. Manifestations of colon tumors include pain, bloody stools, and a change in bowel habits.

7. Rectal carcinoma is located up to 15 cm from the opening of the anus. The tumor spreads transmurally to the vagina in women or prostate in men.

8. Metastatic invasion of the liver is more common than primary cancer of the liver.

9. Primary liver cancers are associated with chronic liver disease (cirrhosis, hepatitis B). Hepatocellular carcinomas arise from the hepatocytes, whereas cholangiocellular carcinomas arise from the bile ducts. Primary liver cancer spreads to the heart, lungs, brain, kidney, and spleen through the circulation.

10. Cancer of the gallbladder is relatively rare and tends to occur in women older than 50 years. Adenocarcinoma is most common. Because clinical manifestations occur late in the disease, metastases to lymph channels have usually occurred by the time of diagnosis and the prognosis is poor.

11. Cancer of the pancreas now ranks fourth as a cause of cancer deaths. Most tumors are adenocarcinomas that arise in the exocrine cells of ducts in the head, body, or tail of the pancreas. Symptoms may not be evident until the tumor has spread to surrounding tissues. Treatment is palliative, and mortality is nearly 100%.

KEY TERMS

- Achalasia 898
- Acute gastritis 903
- Acute liver failure (fulminant liver failure) 921
- Acute pancreatitis 924
- Adiponectin 912
- Afferent loop obstruction 907
- Alcoholic cirrhosis 922
- Alcoholic fatty liver (steatosis) 921
- Alcoholic steatohepatitis 921
- Alkaline reflux gastritis 907
- Anemia 907
- Anorexia 894
- Anorexia nervosa 914
- Appendicitis 910
- Ascites 916
- Barrett esophagus 925
- Biliary cirrhosis 923
- Bone and mineral disorder 907
- Bulimia nervosa 914
- Cachexia 915
- Cholangiocellular carcinoma (cholangiocarcinoma) 930
- Cholecystitis 923
- Cholelithiasis 923
- Chronic active hepatitis 920
- Chronic gastritis 903
- Chronic pancreatitis 925
- Cirrhosis 921
- Colorectal polyp 927

KEY TERMS—cont'd

REFERENCES

1. Meadows N: The central control of vomiting, *J Pediatr Gastroenterol Nutr* 21(suppl 1):S20–S21, 1995.
1a. Rao SS: Constipation: evaluation and treatment of colonic and anorectal motility disorders, *Gastrointest Endosc Clin North Am* 19(1):117–139, 2009. vii.
2. Dinning PG, Smith TK, Scott SM: Pathophysiology of colonic causes of chronic constipation, *Neurogastroenterol Motil* 21(suppl 2):20–30, 2009.
3. Rao SS, Go JT: Update on the management of constipation in the elderly: new treatment options, *Clin Interv Aging* 5:163–171, 2010.
3a. Omotosho TB: Evaluation and treatment of anal incontinence, constipation, and defecatory dysfunction, *Obstet Gynecol Clin North Am* 36(3):673–697, 2009.
4. Bures J, et al: Small intestinal bacterial overgrowth syndrome, *World J Gastroenterol* 16(24):2978–2990, 2010.
5. Sellin JH: A practical approach to treating patients with chronic diarrhea, *Rev Gastroenterol Disord* 7(Suppl 3):S19–S26, 2007.
6. Millham FH: Chapter 10: Acute abdominal pain. In Feldman M, Friedman LS, Brandt LJ, editors: *Sleisenger and Fordtran's gastrointestinal and liver disease: pathophysiology/diagnosis/management*, ed 9, Philadelphia, 2010, Elsevier, pp 151–161.
7. DiMaio CJ, Stevens PD: Nonvariceal upper gastrointestinal bleeding, *Gastrointest Endosc Clin North Am* 17(2):253–272, 2007. v.
8. Kumar R, Mills AM: Gastrointestinal bleeding, *Emerg Med Clin North Am* 29(2):239–252, 2011. viii.
9. Boeckxstaens GE: Achalasia, *Best Pract Res Clin Gastroenterol* 21(4):595–608, 2007.
10. Moawad FJ, Wong RKH: Modern management of achalasia, *Curr Opin Gastroenterol* 26(4):384–388, 2010.
11. Allende DS, Yerian LM: Diagnosing gastroesophageal reflux disease: the pathologist's perspective, *Adv Anat Pathol* 16(3):161–165, 2009.
12. Orlando RC: The integrity of the esophageal mucosa. Balance between offensive and defensive mechanisms, *Best Pract Res Clin Gastroenterol* 24(6):873–882, 2010.
13. Oh DS, Demeester SR: Pathophysiology and treatment of Barrett's esophagus, *World J Gastroenterol* 16(30):3762–3772, 2010.
14. Herbella FA, Patti MG: Gastroesophageal reflux disease: from pathophysiology to treatment, *World J Gastroenterol* 16(30):3745–3749, 2010.
15. Gashi Z, et al: Effectiveness of proton pump inhibitors in the treatment of patients with endoscopic esophagitis, *Med Arh* 64(6):362–364, 2010.
16. van Herwaarden MA, Samsom M, Smout AJ: The role of hiatus hernia in gastro-oesophageal reflux disease, *Eur J Gastroenterol Hepatol* 16(9):831–835, 2004.
17. Schieman C, Grondin SC: Paraesophageal hernia: clinical presentation, evaluation, and management controversies, *Thorac Surg Clin* 19(4):473–484, 2009.
17a. Parkman HP, et al: Gastroparesis and functional dyspepsia: excerpts from the AGA/ANMS meeting, *Neurogastroenterol Motil* 22(2):113–133, 2010.
18. Stawowy M, et al: Endoscopic stenting for malignant gastric outlet obstruction, *Surg Laparosc Endosc Percutan Tech* 17(1):5–9, 2007.
19. Batke M, Cappell MS: Adynamic ileus and acute colonic pseudo-obstruction, *Med Clin North Am* 92(3):649–670, 2008.
20. Romano S, Bartone G, Romano L: Ischemia and infarction of the intestine related to obstruction, *Radiol Clin North Am* 46(5):925–942, 2008. vi.

21. Zeinali F, Stulberg JJ, Delaney CP: Pharmacological management of postoperative ileus, *Can J Surg* 52(2):153–157, 2009.
22. Lahner E, Annibale B: Pernicious anemia: new insights from a gastroenterological point of view, *World J Gastroenterol* 15(41):5121–5128, 2009.
23. Yeomans ND: The ulcer sleuths: the search for the cause of peptic ulcers, *J Gastroenterol Hepatol* 26(Suppl 1):35–41, 2011.
24. Osefo N, Ito T, Jensen RT: Gastric acid hypersecretory states: recent insights and advances, *Curr Gastroenterol Rep* 11(6):433–441, 2009.
25. Edgren G, et al: Risk of gastric cancer and peptic ulcers in relation to ABO blood type: a cohort study, *Am J Epidemiol* 172(11):1280–1285, 2010.
26. Venerito M, Malfertheiner P: Interaction of *Helicobacter pylori* infection and nonsteroidal anti-inflammatory drugs in gastric and duodenal ulcers, *Helicobacter* 15(4):239–250, 2010.
27. Napolitano L: Refractory peptic ulcer disease, *Gastroenterol Clin North Am* 38(2):267–288, 2009.
28. Malfertheiner P, Chan FK, McColl KE: Peptic ulcer disease, 2009, *Lancet* 374(9699):1449–1461, 2009.
29. Pilotto A, et al: Optimal management of peptic ulcer disease in the elderly, *Drugs Aging*(7)545–558, 2010.
30. Dai YC, Tang ZP, Zhang YL: How to assess the severity of atrophic gastritis, *World J Gastroenterol* 17(13):1690–1693, 2011.
31. Fink G: Stress controversies: post-traumatic stress disorder, hippocampal volume, gastroduodenal ulceration, *J Neuroendocrinol* 23(2):107–117, 2011.
32. Ali T, Harty RF: Stress-induced ulcer bleeding in critically ill patients, *Gastroenterol Clin North Am* 38(2):245–265, 2009.
33. Lin PC, et al: The efficacy and safety of proton pump inhibitors vs histamine-2 receptor antagonists for stress ulcer bleeding prophylaxis among critical care patients: a meta-analysis, *Crit Care Med* 38(4):1197–1205, 2010.
34. Tack J, et al: Pathophysiology, diagnosis and management of postoperative dumping syndrome, *Nat Rev Gastroenterol Hepatol* 6(10):583–590, 2009.
35. Ersan Y, et al: Late results of patients undergoing remedial operations for alkaline reflux gastritis syndrome, *Acta Chir Belg* 109(3):364–370, 2009.
36. Aoki M, et al: Afferent loop obstruction after distal gastrectomy with Roux-en-Y reconstruction, *World J Surg* 34(10):2389–2392, 2010.
37. Hammer HF: Pancreatic exocrine insufficiency: diagnostic evaluation and replacement therapy with pancreatic enzymes, *Dig Dis* 28(2): 339–343, 2010.
38. Wilt TJ, et al: Lactose intolerance and health, *Evid Rep Technol Assess (Full Rep)*(192)1–410, 2010.
39. Schirbel A, Fiocchi C: Inflammatory bowel disease: established and evolving considerations on its etiopathogenesis and therapy, *J Dig Dis* 11(5):266–276, 2010.
40. Bernstein CN, et al: A prospective population-based study of triggers of symptomatic flares in IBD, *Am J Gastroenterol* 105(9):1994–2002, 2010.
41. Cosnes J: Smoking, physical activity, nutrition and lifestyle: environmental factors and their impact on IBD, *Dig Dis* 28(3):411–417, 2010.
42. Brackmann S, et al: Widespread but not localized neoplasia in inflammatory bowel disease worsens the prognosis of colorectal cancer, *Inflamm Bowel Dis* 16(3):474–481, 2010.
43. Andrews JM, et al: Un-promoted issues in inflammatory bowel disease: opportunities to optimize care, *Intern Med J* 40(3):173–182, 2010.
44. Larsen S, Bendtzen K, Nielsen OH: Extraintestinal manifestations of inflammatory bowel disease: epidemiology, diagnosis, and management, *Ann Med* 42(2):97–114, 2010.
45. Arai R: Serologic markers: impact on early diagnosis and disease stratification in inflammatory bowel disease, *Postgrad Med* 122(4):177–185, 2010.
46. Burger D, Travis S: Conventional medical management of inflammatory bowel disease, *Gastroenterology* 140(6):1827–1837.e2, 2011.
47. Umanskiy K, Fichera A: Health related quality of life in inflammatory bowel disease: the impact of surgical therapy, *World J Gastroenterol* 16(40):5024–5034, 2010.
48. Sartini A, et al: Update on Crohn's disease: a polymorphic entity, *Minerva Gastroenterol Dietol* 57(1):89–96, 2011.
49. van der Heide F, et al: Effects of active and passive smoking on disease course of Crohn's disease and ulcerative colitis, *Inflamm Bowel Dis* 15(8):1199–1207, 2009.
50. Vermeulen J, van der Harst E, Lange JF: Pathophysiology and prevention of diverticulitis and perforation, *Neth J Med* 68(10):303–309, 2010.
51. Commane DM, et al: Diet, ageing and genetic factors in the pathogenesis of diverticular disease, *World J Gastroenterol* 15(20):2479–2488, 2009.
52. Touzios JG, Dozois EJ: Diverticulosis and acute diverticulitis, *Gastroenterol Clin North Am* 38(3):513–525, 2009.
53. Guslandi M: Medical treatment of uncomplicated diverticular disease of the colon: any progress? *Minerva Gastroenterol Dietol* 56(3):367–370, 2010.
54. Hemming J, Floch M: Features and management of colonic diverticular disease, *Curr Gastroenterol Rep* 12(5):399–407, 2010.
55. Pendlimari R, et al: Short-term outcomes after elective minimally invasive colectomy for diverticulitis, *Br J Surg* 98(3):431–435, 2011.
56. Vissers RJ, Lennarz WB: Pitfalls in appendicitis, *Emerg Med Clin North Am* 28(1):103–118, 2010. viii.
57. Sauerland S, Jaschinski T, Neugebauer EA: Laparoscopic versus open surgery for suspected appendicitis, *Cochrane Database Syst Rev*(10)CD001546, 2010.
58. Bolino CM, Bercik P: Pathogenic factors involved in the development of irritable bowel syndrome: focus on a microbial role, *Infect Dis Clin North Am* 24(4):961–975, 2010. ix.
59. Akbar A, Walters JR, Ghosh S: Review article: visceral hypersensitivity in irritable bowel syndrome: molecular mechanisms and therapeutic agents, *Aliment Pharmacol Ther* 30(5):423–435, 2009.
60. Ohman L, Simrén M: Pathogenesis of IBS: role of inflammation, immunity and neuroimmune interactions, *Nat Rev Gastroenterol Hepatol* 7(3):163–173, 2010.
61. Thabane M, Marshall JK: Post-infectious irritable bowel syndrome, *World J Gastroenterol* 15(29):3591–3596, 2009.
62. Yamini D, Pimentel M: Irritable bowel syndrome and small intestinal bacterial overgrowth, *J Clin Gastroenterol* 44(10):672–675, 2010.
63. Eswaran S, Tack J, Chey WD: Food: the forgotten factor in the irritable bowel syndrome, *Gastroenterol Clin North Am* 40(1):141–162, 2011.
64. Elsenbruch S, et al: Patients with irritable bowel syndrome have altered emotional modulation of neural responses to visceral stimuli, *Gastroenteroloy* 139(4):1310–1319, 2010.
65. Grundmann O, Yoon SL: Irritable bowel syndrome: epidemiology, diagnosis and treatment: an update for health-care practitioners, *J Gastroenterol Hepatol* 25(4):691–699, 2010.
66. Khan S, Chang L: Diagnosis and management of IBS, *Nat Rev Gastroenterol Hepatol* 7(10):565–581, 2010.
67. Bergqvist D, Svensson PJ: Treatment of mesenteric vein thrombosis, *Semin Vasc* 23(1):65–68, 2010.
68. Zeller T, Rastan A, Sixt S: Chronic atherosclerotic mesenteric ischemia (CMI), *Vasc Med* 15(4):333–338, 2010.
69. Wyers MC: Acute mesenteric ischemia: diagnostic approach and surgical treatment, *Semin Vasc Surg* 23(1):9–20, 2010.
70. Nguyen DM, El-Serag HB: The epidemiology of obesity, *Gastroenterol Clin North Am* 39(1):1–7, 2010.
71. World Health Organization: *Obesity and overweight*. Accessed Aug 2011. Available at www.who.int/mediacentre/factsheets/fs311/en/.
72. Wang Y, et al: Will all Americans become overweight or obese? Estimating the progression and cost of the U.S. obesity epidemic, *Obesity (Silver Springs)*(10)2323–2330, 2008.
73. Dixon JB: The effect of obesity on health outcomes, *Mol Cell Endocrinol* 316(2):104–108, 2010.
74. Das UN: Obesity: genes, brain, gut, and environment, *Nutrition* 26(5):459–473, 2010.
75. Galic S, Oakhill JS, Steinberg GR: Adipose tissue as an endocrine organ, *Mol Cell Endocrinol* 316(2):129–139, 2010.
76. Karastergiou K, Mohamed-Ali V: The autocrine and paracrine roles of adipokines, *Mol Cell Endocrinol* 318(1–2):69–78, 2010.
77. Ahima RS, Antwi DA: Brain regulation of appetite and satiety, *Endocrinol Metab Clin North Am* 37(4):811–823, 2008.

78. Cammisotto PG, et al: Cross-talk between adipose and gastric leptins for the control of food intake and energy metabolism, *Prog Histochem Cytochem* 45(3):143–200, 2010.

79. Myers MG Jr, et al: Obesity and leptin resistance: distinguishing cause from effect, *Trends Endocrinol Metab* 21(11):643–651, 2010.

80. Milman S, Crandall JP: Mechanisms of vascular complications in prediabetes, *Med Clin North Am* 95(2):309–325, 2011. vii.

81. Bays HE, et al: Pathogenic potential of adipose tissue and metabolic consequences of adipocyte hypertrophy and increased visceral adiposity, *Exp Rev Cardiovasc Ther* 6(3):343–368, 2008.

82. Gutierrez DA, Puglisi MJ, Hasty AH: Impact of increased adipose tissue mass on inflammation, insulin resistance and dyslipidemia, *Curr Diab Rep* 9(1):26–32, 2009.

83. Matsuzawa Y: Adiponectin: a key player in obesity related disorders, *Curr Pharm Des* 16(17):1896–1901, 2010.

84. Duvnjak L, Duvnjak M: The metabolic syndrome—an ongoing story, *J Physiol Pharmacol* 60(Suppl 7):19–24, 2009.

85. Chan RS, Woo J: Prevention of overweight and obesity: how effective is the current public health approach? *Int J Environ Res Public Health* 7(3):765–783, 2010.

86. Biro FM, Wien M: Childhood obesity and adult morbidities, *Am J Clin Nutr* 91(5):1499S–1505S, 2010.

87. Blackburn GL, Hu FB, Hutter MM: Updated evidence-based recommendations form best practices in weight loss surgery, *Obesity (Silver Springs)* 17(5):839–841, 2009.

88. Kaila B, Raman M: Obesity: a review of pathogenesis and management strategies, *Can J Gastroenterol* 22(1):61–68, 2008.

89. Kloet AD, Woods SC: Molecular neuroendocrine targets for obesity therapy, *Curr Opin Endocrinol Diabetes Obes* 17(5):441–445, 2010.

90. Askie LM, et al: The Early Prevention of Obesity in Children (EPOCH) Collaboration—an individual patient data prospective meta-analysis, *BMC Public Health* 10:728, 2010.

91. Vos MB, Welsh J: Childhood obesity: update on predisposing factors and prevention strategies, *Curr Gastroenterol Rep* 12(4):280–287, 2010.

91a. American Psychiatric Association: *Diagnostic and statistical manual of mental disorders DSM-IV-TR*, ed 4, (text revision), Washington, DC, 2000, Author.

92. Scherag S, Hebebrand J, Hinney A: Eating disorders: the current status of molecular genetic research, *Eur Child Adolesc Psychiatry* 19(3):211–226, 2010.

93. Bulik CM, et al: The genetics of anorexia nervosa, *Annu Rev Nutr* 27:263–275, 2007.

94. Sim LA, et al: Identification and treatment of eating disorders in the primary care setting, *Mayo Clin Proc* 85(8):746–751, 2010.

94a. Academy for Eating Disorders: *Eating disorders: critical points for early recognition and medical risk management in the care of individuals with eating disorders*, ed 2, Deerfield, Ill, 2011. Available at www.aedweb.org/ AM/Template.cfm?Section=Medical_Care_Standards&Template=/CM/ ContentDisplay.cfm&ContentID=24132011.

95. Williams PM, Goodie J, Motsinger CD: Treating eating disorders in primary care, *Am Fam Physician* 77(2):187–195, 2008.

96. Auerbach PS: *Wilderness medicine*, ed 5, Philadelphia, 2008, Mosby.

97. Sass DA, Chopra KB: Portal hypertension and variceal hemorrhage, *Med Clin North Am* 93(4):837–853, 2009. vii–viii.

98. Kochar R, et al: Pulmonary complications of cirrhosis, *Curr Gastroenterol Rep* 13(1):34–39, 2011.

99. Cárdenas A: Management of acute variceal bleeding: emphasis on endoscopic therapy, *Clin Liver Dis* 14(2):251–262, 2010.

99a. Orloff MJ, et al: Liver transplantation in a randomized controlled trial of emergency treatment of acutely bleeding esophageal varices in cirrhosis, *Transplant Proc* 42(10):4101–4108, 2010.

100. Hou W, Sanyal AJ: Ascites: diagnosis and management, *Med Clin North Am* 93(4):801–817, 2009. vii.

101. Salerno F, et al: Refractory ascites: pathogenesis, definition and therapy of a severe complication in patients with cirrhosis, *Liver Int* 30(7): 937–947, 2010.

102. Toris GT, et al: Hepatic encephalopathy: an updated approach from pathogenesis to treatment, *Med Sci Monit* 17(2):RA53–RA63, 2011.

103. Eroglu Y, Byrne WJ: Hepatic encephalopathy, *Emerg Med Clin North Am* 27(3):401–414, 2009.

104. Lidofsky SD: Jaundice. In Feldman M, Friedman LS, Brandt L, editors: *Sleisenger and Fordtran's gastrointestinal and liver disease*, ed 9, Philadelphia, 2010, Saunders, pp 323–325.

105. Roche SP, Kobos R: Jaundice in the adult patient, *Am Fam Physician* 69(2):299–304, 2004.

106. Turban S, Thuluvath PJ, Atta MG: Hepatorenal syndrome, *World J Gastroenterol* 13(30):4046–4055, 2007.

107. Arroyo V, Fernandez J, Ginès P: Pathogenesis and treatment of hepatorenal syndrome, *Semin Liver Dis* 28(1):81–95, 2008.

108. Kiser TH, Maclaren R, Fish DN: Treatment of hepatorenal syndrome, *Pharmacotherapy* 29(10):1196–1211, 2009.

109. Yang JD, Roberts LR: Epidemiology and management of hepatocellular carcinoma, *Infect Dis Clin North Am* 24(4):899–919, 2010. viii.

109a. Alcalde R, et al: Prevalence and distribution of the GBV-C/HGV among HIV-1-infected patients under anti-retroviral therapy, *Virus Res* 151(2):148–152, 2010.

110. Anderson AM, et al: Development of fatal acute liver failure in HIV-HBV coinfected patients, *World J Gastroenterol* 16(32):4107–4111, 2010.

111. Potthoff A, Manns MP, Wedemeyer H: Treatment of HBV/HCV coinfection, *Expert Opin Pharmacother* 11(6):919–928, 2010.

112. Aydeniz A, et al: Rheumatic manifestations of hepatitis B and C and their association with viral load and fibrosis of the liver, *Rheumatol Int* 30(4):515–517, 2010.

113. Chacko EC, et al: Chronic viral hepatitis and chronic kidney disease, *Postgrad Med J* 86(1018):486–492, 2010.

114. Vermehren J, Sarrazin C: New HCV therapies on the horizon, *Clin Microbiol Infect* 17(2):122–134, 2011.

115. Xie YH, et al: Development of novel therapeutics for chronic hepatitis B, *Virol Sin* 25(4):294–300, 2010.

116. Sánchez G, Bosch A, Pintó RM: Hepatitis A virus detection in food: current and future prospects, *Lett Appl Microbiol* 45(1):1–5, 2007.

117. Aggarwal R: Hepatitis E: historical, contemporary and future perspectives, *J Gastroenterol Hepatol* 26(Suppl 1):72–82, 2011.

118. Bernal W, et al: Acute liver failure, *Lancet* 376(9736):190–201, 2010.

119. Stravitz RT, Kramer DJ: Medscape: management of acute liver failure, *Nat Rev Gastroenterol Hepatol* 6(9):542–553, 2009.

120. Wallace K, Burt AD, Wright MC: Liver fibrosis, *Biochem J* 411(1):1–18, 2008.

121. Siegmund SV, Brenner DA: Molecular pathogenesis of alcohol-induced hepatic fibrosis, *Alcohol Clin Exp Res* 29(Suppl 11):S102–S109, 2005.

122. Eagon PK: Alcoholic liver injury: influence of gender and hormones, *World J Gastroenterol* 16(11):1377–1384, 2010.

123. Verrill C, et al: Alcohol-related cirrhosis—early abstinence is a key factor in prognosis, even in the most severe cases, *Addiction* 104(5):768–774, 2009.

124. Stickel F, Seitz HK: Alcoholic steatohepatitis, *Best Pract Res Clin Gastroenterol* 24(5):683–693, 2010.

125. Cubero FJ, Urtasun R, Nieto N: Alcohol and liver fibrosis, *Semin Liver Dis* 29(2):211–221, 2009.

126. Setshedi M, Wands JR, Monte SM: Acetaldehyde adducts in alcoholic liver disease, *Oxid Med Cell Longev* 3(3):178–185, 2010.

127. Lucey MR: Management of alcoholic liver disease, *Clin Liver Dis* 13(2):267–275, 2009.

128. Adams LA, Feldstein AE: Non-invasive diagnosis of nonalcoholic fatty liver and nonalcoholic steatohepatitis, *J Dig Dis* 12(1):10–16, 2011.

129. Rombouts K, Marra F: Molecular mechanisms of hepatic fibrosis in nonalcoholic steatohepatitis, *Dig Dis* 28(1):229–235, 2010.

130. Nguyen DL, Juran BD, Lazaridis KN: Primary biliary cirrhosis, *Best Pract Res Clin Gastroenterol* 24(5):647–654, 2010.

131. Stinton LM, Myers RP, Shaffer EA: Epidemiology of gallstones, *Gastroenterol Clin North Am* 39(2):157–169, 2010. vii.

132. Venneman NG, van Erpecum KJ: Pathogenesis of gallstones, *Gastroenterol Clin North Am* 39(2):171–183, 2010. vii.

133. Silva MA, Wong T: Gallstones in chronic liver disease, *J Gastrointest Surg* 9(5):739–746, 2005.

133a. Gaby AR: Nutritional approaches to prevention and treatment of gall-stones, *Altern Med Rev* 14(3):258–267, 2009.

134. Itoi T, Wang HP: Endoscopic management of bile duct stones, *Dig Endosc* 22(Suppl 1):S69–S75, 2010.

135. Gaby AR: Nutritional approaches to prevention and treatment of gall-stones, *Altern Med Rev* 14(3):258–267, 2009.

136. Barie PS, Eachempati SR: Acute acalculous cholecystitis, *Gastroenterol Clin North Am* 39(2):343–357, 2010. x.

137. Johnson C, Lévy P: Detection of gallstones in acute pancreatitis: when and how? *Pancreatology* 10(1):27–32, 2010.

137a. Brown A, et al: Are health related outcomes in acute pancreatitis improving? An analysis of national trends in the U.S. from 1997 to 2003, *J Pancreas* 9(4):408–414, 2008.

138. Harper SJ, Cheslyn-Curtis S: Acute pancreatitis, *Ann Clin Biochem* 48(Pt 1):23–37, 2011.

139. Thrower EC, Gorelick FS, Husain SZ: Molecular and cellular mechanisms of pancreatic injury, *Curr Opin Gastroenterol* (5)484–489, 2010.

140. Frossard JL, Steer ML, Pastor CM: Acute pancreatitis, *Lancet* 37(9618):1072, 2008.

141. Harper SJ, Cheslyn-Curtis S: Acute pancreatitis, *Ann Clin Biochem* 48 (pt 1):23–37, 2011.

142. Apte MV, Pirola RC, Wilson JS: Mechanisms of alcoholic pancreatitis, *J Gastroenterol Hepatol* 25(12):1816–1826, 2010.

143. Bharwani N, et al: Acute pancreatitis: the role of imaging in diagnosis and management, *Clin Radiol* 66(2):164–175, 2011.

144. Al-Omran M, et al: Enteral versus parenteral nutrition for acute pancreatitis, *Cochrane Database Syst Rev*(1)CD002837, 2010.

145. Lytras D, et al: Persistent early organ failure: defining the high-risk group of patients with severe acute pancreatitis? *Pancreas* 36(3):249–254, 2008.

146. Braganza JM, et al: Chronic pancreatitis, *Lancet* 377(9772):1184–1197, 2011.

147. Vardanyan M, Rilo HL: Pathogenesis of chronic pancreatitis-induced pain, *Discov Med* 9(47):304–310, 2010.

148. Johnson MD, et al: Surgical versus nonsurgical management of pancreatic pseudocysts, *J Clin Gastroenterol* 43(6):586–590, 2009.

149. Holmes RS, Vaughan TL: Epidemiology and pathogenesis of esophageal cancer, *Semin Radiat Oncol* 17(1):2–9, 2007.

150. American Cancer Society: *Cancer facts & figures—2010*, Atlanta, 2010, Author.

151. Green J, et al: Oral bisphosphonates and risk of cancer of oesophagus, stomach, and colorectum: case-control analysis within a UK primary care cohort, *Br J Med* 341:C4444, 2010.

152. Spechler SJ: Barrett's esophagus: clinical issues, *Gastrointest Endosc Clin North Am* 21(1):1–7, 2011.

153. Krasna MJ: Multimodality therapy for esophageal cancer, *Oncology (WillistonPark)* 24(12):1134–1138, 2010.

154. Resende C, Ristimäki A, Machado JC: Genetic and epigenetic alteration in gastric carcinogenesis, *Helicobacter* 15(Suppl 1):3434–3439, 2010.

155. Leung WK, et al: Screening for gastric cancer in Asia: current evidence and practice, *Lancet Oncol* 9(3):279–287, 2008.

156. Compare D, Rocco A, Nardone G: Risk factors in gastric cancer, *Eur Rev Med Pharmacol Sci* 14(4):302–308, 2010.

157. Jiang Y, Ajani JA: Multidisciplinary management of gastric cancer, *Curr Opin Gastroenterol* 26(6):640–646, 2010.

158. Cunningham D, et al: Colorectal cancer, *Lancet* 375(9719):1030–1047, 2010.

159. Jasperson K, et al: Hereditary and familial colon cancer, *Gastroenterology* 138(6):2044–2058, 2010.

160. Will OC, et al: Familial adenomatous polyposis and the small bowel: a loco-regional review and current management strategies, *Pathol Res Pract* 204(7):449–458, 2008.

160a. Up-to-Date, Colon polyps, last updated August 24, 2010.

161. Benedix F, et al: Colon carcinoma—classification into right and left sided cancer or according to colonic subsite? Analysis of 29,568 patients, *Eur J Surg Oncol* 37(2):134–139, 2011.

162. Al-Sukhni W, Aronson M, Gallinger S: Hereditary colorectal cancer syndromes: familial adenomatous polyposis and Lynch syndrome, *Surg Clin North Am* 88(4):819–844, 2008.

163. Winder T, Lenz HJ: Molecular predictive and prognostic markers in colon cancer, *Cancer Treat Rev* 36(7):550–556, 2010.

164. Cooper K, et al: Chemoprevention of colorectal cancer: systematic review and economic evaluation, *Health Technol Assess* 14(32):1–206, 2010.

165. Gallagher DJ, Kemeny N: Metastatic colorectal cancer: from improved survival to potential cure, *Oncology* 78(3–4):237–248, 2010.

166. National Cancer Institute: *Stages of colon cancer.* Available at www.cancer.gov/cancertopics/pdq/treatment/colon/Patient/page1. Accessed June 29 2011.

167. Chan AT, Giovannucci EL: Primary prevention of colorectal cancer, *Gastroenterology* 138(6):2029–2043, 2010.

168. Deschoolmeester V, et al: Tumor infiltrating lymphocytes: an intriguing player in the survival of colorectal cancer patients, *BMC Immunol* 11:19, 2010.

169. Merika E, et al: Review. Colon cancer vaccines: an update, *in vivo* 24(5):607–628, 2010.

170. Thomas MB, et al: Hepatocellular carcinoma: consensus recommendations of the National Cancer Institute Clinical Trials Planning Meeting, *J Clin Oncol* 28(25):3994–4005, 2010.

171. Kew MC: Prevention of hepatocellular carcinoma, *Ann Hepatol* 9(2):120–132, 2010.

172. Sherman M: Modern approach to hepatocellular carcinoma, *Curr Gastroenterol Rep* 13(1):49–55, 2011.

173. Alsina AE: Liver transplantation for hepatocellular carcinoma, *Cancer Control* 17(2):83–86, 2010.

174. Sangro B, Prieto J: Gene therapy for liver cancer: clinical experience and future prospects, *Curr Opin Mol Ther* 12(5):561–569, 2010.

175. Zhu AX, et al: Current management of gallbladder carcinoma, *Oncologist* 15(2):168–181, 2010.

176. Schafer M, Mullhaupt B, Clavien PA: Evidence-based pancreatic head resection for pancreatic cancer and chronic pancreatitis, *Ann Surg* 236(2):137–148, 2002.

177. Simianu VV, et al: Pancreatic cancer: progress made, *Acta Oncol* 49(4):407–417, 2010.

178. Tanase CP, et al: Advances in pancreatic cancer detection, *Adv Clin Chem* 51:145–180, 2010.

179. Brunner TB, Scott-Brown M: The role of radiotherapy in multimodal treatment of pancreatic carcinoma, *Radiat Oncol* 5:64, 2010.

35

Alterations of Digestive Function in Children

Sue E. Huether

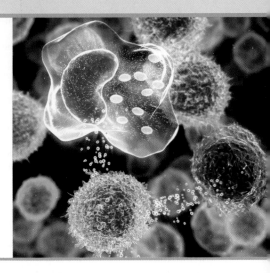

evolve WEBSITE

http://evolve.elsevier.com/Huether/

- Review Questions and Answers
- Animations
- Quick Check Answers

- Key Terms Exercises
- Critical Thinking Questions with Answers
- Algorithm Completion Exercises
- WebLinks

CHAPTER OUTLINE

Disorders of the gastrointestinal tract in children include congenital anomalies with structural and functional alterations, as well as enzyme deficiencies and infections. Structural alterations can occur throughout the gastrointestinal tract and include cleft lip and palate, esophageal atresia, tracheoesophageal fistula, pyloric stenosis, aganglionic megacolon, and imperforate anus. Gastroesophageal reflux, hepatic and pancreatic enzyme deficiencies, and bacterial or viral invasions of the gastrointestinal tract also contribute to the diseases and gastrointestinal clinical manifestations in children.

DISORDERS OF THE GASTROINTESTINAL TRACT

Congenital Impairment of Motility

Cleft Lip and Cleft Palate

Cleft lip (harelip) and cleft palate are developmental anomalies of the first branchial arch (Figure 35-1). These defects, which occur during embryonic development, vary in severity. In whites, the incidence of cleft lip or cleft palate ranges from 1 in 600 to 1 in 1250 births. The incidence of cleft lip, with or without cleft palate, is about 1 in 1000 births, whereas the incidence of cleft palate alone is about 1 in 2500 births. The incidence is lower in black populations and higher in Asian populations. Cleft lip, with or without cleft palate, is more common in males and isolated cleft palate is more common in females. Both anomalies can be unilateral or bilateral, partial or complete.[1]

PATHOPHYSIOLOGY In most cases, cleft lip and cleft palate are caused by multiple gene-environment interactions, including maternal deficiency of B vitamins, maternal tobacco[2] and alcohol use, maternal hyperhomocysteinemia, maternal diabetes mellitus, and genetic variations of several growth factors. The cleft can be part of a syndrome determined by single mutant genes, or part of a chromosomal defect, usually trisomy 13. Cleft lip and cleft palate also may be associated with other malformations (i.e., cardiac, skeletal, and central nervous system malformations). (This phenomenon, called *multifactorial inheritance,* is discussed in Chapter 2.) Together, these factors reduce the amount of neural crest mesenchyme that migrates into the area that will develop into the face of the embryo.[3]

Cleft lip. Cleft lip is caused by the incomplete fusion of the nasomedial or intermaxillary process beginning the fourth week of embryonic development, a period of rapid development. The cleft causes structures of the face and mouth to develop without the normal restraints of encircling lip muscles. The facial cleft may affect not only the lip but also the external nose, nasal cartilages, nasal septum, and alveolar processes. The cleft is usually just beneath the center of one nostril. The defect may occur bilaterally and may be symmetric or asymmetric. The more complete the cleft lip, the greater the chance that teeth in the line of the cleft will be missing or malformed.

Cleft palate. Cleft palate is often associated with cleft lip but may occur without it. The fissure may affect only the uvula and soft palate or may extend forward to the nostril and involve the hard palate and the maxillary alveolar ridge. It may be unilateral or bilateral, with the cleft occupying the midline posteriorly and as far forward as the alveolar process, where it deviates to the involved side. Clefts involving the palate only are usually but not necessarily in the midline. In some cases, the vomer and nasal septum are partly or completely undeveloped. When these facial bones are involved, the nasal cavity may freely communicate with the oral cavity. Teeth in the cleft palate area may be missing or deformed.

CLINICAL MANIFESTATIONS   Feeding difficulty is the most significant clinical manifestation for cleft lip and palate.

EVALUATION AND TREATMENT   Prenatal diagnosis is made by three-dimensional ultrasound.[5] Postnatal facial x-ray films confirm the extent of bone deformity. Soft tissue alterations are evaluated by physical examination. The nature and extent of the cleft, the infant's condition, and the method of surgical correction proposed determine the course of treatment. Surgical correction is planned as soon as possible and may be performed in stages.[6]

Feeding the infant with cleft lip usually presents no difficulty if the cleft lip is simple and the palate intact. A baby with cleft palate usually requires large, soft nipples with cross-cut openings, and a squeezable bottle. Breast-feeding may be impossible for some infants. An orthodontic prosthesis for the roof of the mouth may facilitate sucking for some infants.[4]

Speech training and special attention by a prosthodontist and orthodontist are almost always required.[3] Both before and after surgery, children with cleft palate tend to have repeated infections of the paranasal sinuses. Excessive dental decay is not unusual. Hypertrophy of tonsils and adenoids and otitis media are frequent accompaniments, and the child should be evaluated for hearing loss.[7] Ensuring adequate nutrition (especially B vitamins and folic acid) and reducing tobacco and alcohol use before and during pregnancy may prevent orofacial clefts.[3]

Esophageal Malformations

Congenital malformations of the esophagus occur in 1 of 3000 to 4500 live births. In **esophageal atresia,** the esophagus ends in a blind pouch. It is usually accompanied by a fistula between the esophagus and the trachea (**tracheoesophageal fistula [TEF]**). Either defect can occur alone (Figure 35-2). Many genes have been implicated and other single gene and chromosome anomalies may be present.[8]

PATHOPHYSIOLOGY   The pathogenesis of esophageal abnormalities is unknown. They are thought to arise from defective differentiation as the trachea separates from the esophagus during the fourth to sixth weeks of embryonic development. Defective growth of endodermal cells leads to atresia. Incomplete fusion of the lateral walls of the foregut leads to incomplete closure of the laryngotracheal tube and fistula formation.

CLINICAL MANIFESTATIONS   Polyhydramnios (excessive amniotic fluid) is reported to occur in 14% to 90% of mothers of affected infants because of alterations in fetal swallowing.[9] Swallowed amniotic fluid is usually absorbed into the placental circulation; therefore if the fetus cannot swallow, amniotic fluid accumulates in the uterus. If a fistula connects the trachea with the distal esophagus, the abdomen fills with air and becomes distended, possibly interfering with breathing (see Figure 35-2, *C* to *E*). Intermittent cyanosis may result.

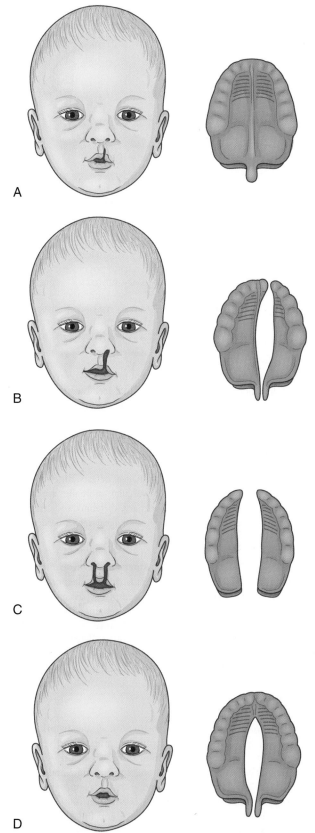

FIGURE 35-1 Variations in Clefts of the Lip and Palate. **A,** Unilateral cleft lip. **B,** Unilateral cleft lip and palate. **C,** Bilateral cleft lip and cleft palate. **D,** Cleft palate.

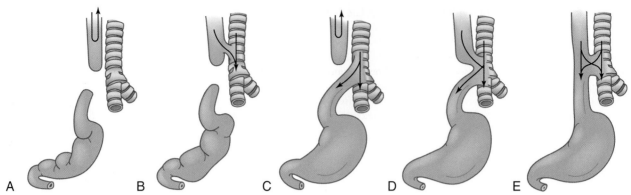

FIGURE 35-2 Five Types of Esophageal Atresia and Tracheoesophageal Fistulae. A, Simple esophageal atresia. Proximal esophagus and distal esophagus end in blind pouches, and there is no tracheal communication. Nothing enters the stomach; regurgitated food and fluid may enter the lungs. **B,** Proximal and distal esophageal segments end in blind pouches, and a fistula connects the proximal esophagus to the trachea. Nothing enters the stomach; food and fluid enter the lungs. **C,** Proximal esophagus ends in a blind pouch, and a fistula connects the trachea to the distal esophagus. Air enters the stomach; regurgitated gastric secretions enter the lungs through the fistula. **D,** Fistula connects both proximal and distal esophageal segments to the trachea. Air, food, and fluid enter the stomach and the lungs. **E,** Simple tracheoesophageal fistula between otherwise normal esophagus and trachea. Air, food, and fluid enter the stomach and the lungs. Between 85% and 90% of esophageal anomalies are type **C;** 6% to 8% are type **A;** 3% to 5% are type **E;** and fewer than 1% are type **B** or **D.**

Pulmonary complications are compounded by reflux of air and gastric secretions into the tracheobronchial tree through the fistula, causing severe chemical irritation. Infants with esophageal atresia but no fistula have scaphoid (boat-shaped), gasless abdomens. In infants with fistula but without atresia (see Figure 35-2, *E*), the usual symptoms are recurrent aspiration, pneumonia, and atelectasis that remains unexpressed for days or even months.

In at least 50% of infants with esophageal defects, other congenital anomalies are present as well. Cardiovascular anomalies are the most common, but other digestive tract, urinary, vertebral, and central nervous system defects can accompany esophageal atresia and tracheoesophageal fistula.

EVALUATION AND TREATMENT Antenatal diagnosis may include ultrasound imaging. Esophageal atresia is usually diagnosed at birth, when the infant is unable to feed and attempts to pass a tube through the esophagus fail. Imaging will show displacement of the tube.

Treatment is surgical. Esophageal continuity is restored, and the fistula is eliminated. The child may continue to have problems with aspiration, gastroesophageal reflux, esophageal strictures, and esophagitis after surgical repair. The overall survival rate for infants with esophageal defects is 95%.[9]

Infantile Pyloric Stenosis

Infantile pyloric stenosis is an obstruction of the pyloric sphincter caused by hypertrophy of the sphincter muscle, and the cause is unknown. One of the most common disorders of early infancy, it affects infants between the ages of 1 and 2 weeks and 3 and 4 months. The incidence of pyloric stenosis among males is approximately 2 to 5 in 1000, whereas that among females is only 1 in 1000.[10] Whites are affected more often than blacks or Asians, and full-term infants are affected more often than premature infants.

PATHOPHYSIOLOGY Individual muscle fibers thicken, so the whole pyloric sphincter becomes enlarged and inelastic. The mucosal lining of the pyloric opening is folded and narrowed by the encroaching muscle. Because of the extra peristaltic effort necessary to force the gastric contents through the narrow pylorus, the muscle layers of the stomach may become hypertrophied as well.

CLINICAL MANIFESTATIONS Between 2 and 3 weeks after birth, an infant who has fed well and gained weight begins to vomit without apparent reason. The vomiting gradually becomes more forceful (projectile). Food is often regurgitated through the nose. The vomiting usually occurs immediately after eating, and the vomitus consists of the bulk of the feeding plus some food retained from previous feedings but is almost always free of bile. Prolonged retention of food in the stomach is characteristic. Constipation occurs because little food reaches the intestine.

In severe, untreated cases, increased gastric peristalsis and vomiting lead to severe fluid and electrolyte imbalances, malnutrition, and weight loss that can be fatal within 4 to 6 weeks. Infants with pyloric stenosis are irritable because of hunger, and they may have esophageal discomfort caused by repeated vomiting and esophagitis. The vomitus may be blood streaked because of rupture of gastric and esophageal vessels.

EVALUATION AND TREATMENT Diagnosis is based on the history, clinical manifestations, and findings on ultrasound.[11] Occasionally, gastric peristalsis is observable over the abdomen. A firm, small, movable mass, approximately the size of an olive, is felt in the right upper quadrant in 70% to 90% of infants with pyloric stenosis. Sonography clearly shows the hypertrophied pyloric muscles and narrowed pyloric channel.

The standard treatment for hypertrophic pyloric stenosis is a pyloromyotomy, in which the muscles of the pylorus are split and separated. Preoperative and postoperative medical management to correct fluid and electrolyte imbalance has been the key to the high success rate and low complication rates associated with this surgery.[12] Some infants may respond to medical and nutritional management or balloon dilation.[13]

Intestinal Malrotation

In **intestinal malrotation of the colon,** there is incomplete rotation around the superior mesenteric artery during fetal development. Additionally, an abnormal membrane (periduodenal band) may press on and obstruct the duodenum. This **periduodenal band (Ladd band)** is one of the most significant findings in malrotation. Associated abnormalities are seen in some children, including duodenal and jejunal atresia.[14]

PATHOPHYSIOLOGY In malrotation, the small intestine lacks a normal posterior fixation because it has only a rudimentary attachment near the origin of the superior mesenteric artery. Therefore, the entire mass can twist when the mobile loops of intestine from the duodenojejunal junction to the middle of the transverse colon twist on themselves. The twisting is known as *volvulus* and leads to symptoms of bowel obstruction (see Figure 34-4). Intestinal twisting around the rudimentary mesentery angulates and obstructs the intestinal lumen and can partly or completely occlude the superior mesenteric artery, causing infarction and necrosis of the entire midgut.

CLINICAL MANIFESTATIONS Although most cases of malrotation-associated volvulus and infarction develop during the neonatal period (50%) or infancy (85% are younger than 1 year), some develop during childhood or even adulthood.[14a] In infants, the obstruction causes intermittent or persistent bile-stained vomiting after feedings. Abdominal distention is limited initially to the epigastrium because only the stomach and duodenum are dilated. Dehydration and electrolyte imbalance may occur rapidly because large amounts of pancreatic juice, bile, and gastric secretions are lost through vomiting (bilious vomiting). Fever usually ensues. Pain, scanty stools, diarrhea, and bloody stools are associated with progressive volvulus, vascular compression, and infarction of the intestine in infants. Intermittent or partial volvulus may be seen in older children and in adults. This condition may be asymptomatic and discovered during unrelated abdominal surgery, or it may cause minor abdominal complaints, such as nausea after meals, vomiting, or abdominal pain.

EVALUATION AND TREATMENT Diagnosis of malrotation with volvulus and infarction is based on a review of the clinical manifestations. Radiographic films of the abdomen and barium studies show gas bubbles and distention proximal to the site of obstruction.

Treatment includes laparoscopic or open surgery to reduce the volvulus (Ladd's procedure).[15] Necrotic bowel may be resected and a primary anastomosis performed. When there is gangrene and question of viability of the bowel ends, an enterostomy may be performed. Follow-up surgery may be done to avoid resection of viable bowel. In cases of malrotation without duodenal obstruction, operative survival is 80%. Operative survival is 40% to 50% in cases of malrotation complicated by obstruction caused by periduodenal bands or other intra-abdominal anomalies. Resection of large segments of the small intestine results in short bowel syndrome and its long-term sequelae.[16]

✓ QUICK CHECK 35-1
1. What structures are affected in cleft palate and cleft lip?
2. What is esophageal atresia?
3. What produces pyloric stenosis?

Meconium Ileus

Meconium is a substance that fills the entire intestine before birth. It consists of intestinal gland secretions and some amniotic fluid. Normally, meconium is passed from the rectum during the first 12 to 72 hours after birth.

Meconium ileus is an intestinal obstruction caused by meconium formed in utero that is abnormally sticky and adheres firmly to the mucosa of the small intestine, resisting passage beyond the terminal ileum. The cause is usually a lack of digestive enzymes during fetal life. This meconium is also found to contain albumin, which is not a normal component of meconium. Meconium ileus is associated with cystic fibrosis (see Chapter 27).[17] In cases *not* associated with cystic fibrosis, the cause usually is unknown. Partial aplasia of the pancreas is an associated factor, however, and one fifth of infants with meconium ileus are premature or have a history of maternal polyhydramnios (excessive amniotic fluid). After intestinal atresia and malrotation with volvulus, meconium ileus is the most common cause of small intestinal obstruction in newborns.

PATHOPHYSIOLOGY The terminal ileum is plugged with thick, viscous meconium resulting from the formation of an insoluble, calcium-glycoprotein compound in abnormal mucus. The segment of the ileum proximal to the obstruction is distended with liquid contents, and its walls may be hypertrophied. The segment distal to the obstruction is collapsed and filled with small pellets of pale-colored stool. Meconium in the obstructed segment has the consistency of thick syrup or glue. Peristalsis fails to propel this viscous material through the ileum, and it becomes impacted. Volvulus, atresia, or perforation of the bowel sometimes accompanies meconium ileus.

CLINICAL MANIFESTATIONS Abdominal distention usually develops during the first few days after birth. The infant begins to vomit within hours or days of birth. Infants with cystic fibrosis may have signs of pulmonary involvement, such as tachypnea, intercostal retractions, and grunting respirations. The distended abdomen shows patterns of dilated intestinal loops that feel doughlike when palpated. Some of the loops contain scattered, firm, movable masses. Despite hyperactive peristalsis, the rectal ampulla is empty.

EVALUATION AND TREATMENT Radiologic examination confirms the presence of meconium ileus. The sweat test, which is accurate in 90% of infants, is performed to detect or rule out cystic fibrosis. In approximately 50% of cases not complicated with volvulus or perforation, a hyperosmolar radiopaque enema done using fluoroscopy evacuates the meconium. If this is not possible, the meconium is removed surgically.[18]

Survival of infants with meconium ileus is improving, with 85% to 100% survival at 1 year.[19] Mortality increases to 70% if the obstruction is complicated by peritonitis.

Distal Intestinal Obstruction Syndrome

Distal intestinal obstruction syndrome (DIOS), formerly called meconium ileus equivalent, affects approximately 15% of older children and adults with cystic fibrosis. Intestinal contents may become abnormally thick and obstruct the intestinal lumen, particularly after episodes of dehydration or insufficient pancreatic enzymes. The child displays signs and symptoms of intestinal obstruction. In most cases, the obstruction is relieved by hypertonic enemas. Meconium ileus and DIOS have been shown to be risk factors for the development of cirrhosis in individuals with cystic fibrosis.[20,21]

Obstructions of the Duodenum, Jejunum, and Ileum

Congenital obstruction of the duodenum can be caused by intrinsic malformations (atresia or stenosis) or external pressure. An annular pancreas—a defect in which the head of the pancreas surrounds part of the duodenum—can obstruct the duodenum. Congenital obstructions of the jejunum and ileum can be attributable to atresia, stenosis, meconium ileus, megacolon (Hirschsprung disease), intussusception, Meckel diverticulum, intestinal duplication, or strangulated hernia.

In **ileal** or **jejunal atresia,** the intestine ends blindly, proximal and distal to an interruption in its continuity, with or without a gap in the mesentery. Stenosis (narrowing of the lumen) causes dilation proximal to the obstruction and luminal collapse distal to it.

Meckel Diverticulum

Meckel diverticulum is an outpouching of all layers of the small intestinal wall (usually in the ileum) and is the most common congenital malformation of the gastrointestinal tract, occurring in about 2% of the population. It develops when there is failure to obliterate the omphalomesenteric duct, which normally leaves a fibrous band that connects the small intestine to the umbilicus during the first months of fetal development. Ectopic gastric mucosal cells are contained in the diverticuli and may cause peptic ulcer and painless bleeding or mimic colonic diverticulitis. Although most Meckel diverticuli are asymptomatic, the most common symptom is painless rectal bleeding. Intestinal obstruction, intussusception, and volvulus can occur, more commonly in adults. Diagnosis is made by symptom presentation and radionucleotide scintigraphy. The scan shows the gastric mucosal cells in the diverticuli. Treatment in those with symptoms is surgical resection.[22]

Congenital Aganglionic Megacolon

Congenital aganglionic megacolon (Hirschsprung disease) is a functional obstruction of the colon. The exact cause is unknown but involves a complex inheritance pattern.[23] It is the most common cause of colon obstruction, accounting for about one third of all gastrointestinal obstructions in infants. The incidence is 1 in 5000, with a predominance in males. There is an increased incidence in children with Down syndrome.[24]

PATHOPHYSIOLOGY   Congenital aganglionic megacolon is caused by the absence of the enteric ganglia (Meissner and Auerbach plexuses) along a variable length of the colon, resulting in inadequate motility (see Figure 33-13 for normal colon structure). In 80% of cases, the aganglionic segment is limited to the rectal end of the sigmoid colon. In rare cases, the entire colon lacks ganglion cells. The abnormally innervated colon obstructs fecal movements, causing the proximal colon to become distended—hence the term *megacolon* (Figure 35-3).

CLINICAL MANIFESTATIONS   Mild to severe constipation is the usual manifestation of congenital aganglionic megacolon with poor feeding, poor weight gain, and progressive abdominal distention. Diarrhea may be the first sign, however, because only water can travel around the impacted feces.

The most serious complication in the neonatal period is enterocolitis related to fecal impaction. Bowel dilation stretches and partly occludes the encircling blood and lymphatic vessels, causing edema, ischemia, infarction of the mucosa, and significant outflow of fluid into the bowel lumen. Copious liquid stools result. Infarction and destruction of the mucosa enable enteric microorganisms to penetrate the bowel wall. Frequently, gram-negative sepsis occurs, accompanied

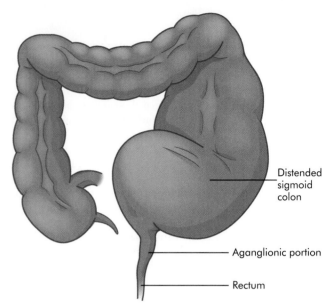

FIGURE 35-3 Congenital Aganglionic Megacolon (Hirschsprung Disease).

by fever and vomiting. Severe and rapid fluid and electrolyte changes may take place, causing hypovolemic or septic shock and death.

EVALUATION AND TREATMENT   Anorectal manometry is a reliable screening tool for the diagnosis of Hirschsprung disease.[25] The definitive diagnosis is made by rectal biopsy showing an absence of ganglion cells in the submucosa of the colon. Radiographic films show dilated loops of colon, and contrast films show aganglionic areas.[26]

The involved segment is resected within the first few months of life. Alternatively, enemas are given until the lumen is clear and then stool softeners are prescribed for life. The child is not treated for diarrhea. In general, the prognosis of congenital megacolon is satisfactory for children who undergo surgical treatment. Bowel training may be prolonged, but most children achieve bowel continence before puberty.[24]

Anorectal Malformations

Several congenital malformations of anorectal structures can obstruct the passage of feces. The incidence of minor abnormalities is approximately 1 in 500, and that of major anomalies is approximately 1 in 5000.

Congenital anorectal malformations range from mild anal stenosis, which is corrected by simple dilation, to complex deformities, such as anal or rectal agenesis, atresia, and fistula (Figure 35-4). Deformities that cause complete obstruction are known collectively as **imperforate anus.**

Approximately 40% of infants with anorectal malformations have other developmental anomalies as well. The most commonly associated major anomalies are Down syndrome, congenital heart disease, renal and urologic abnormalities, esophageal atresia, and malformations of the spine.[27]

Imperforate anus can be detected by gentle insertion of a rectal tube. Radiographic films show dilations throughout the intestinal tract. Anal stenosis can be treated by dilations, but all other anorectal malformations require surgical correction. Overall mortality is approximately 10%. Children with a low (anal) anomaly usually achieve bowel continence but may have some constipation and soiling and require follow up.

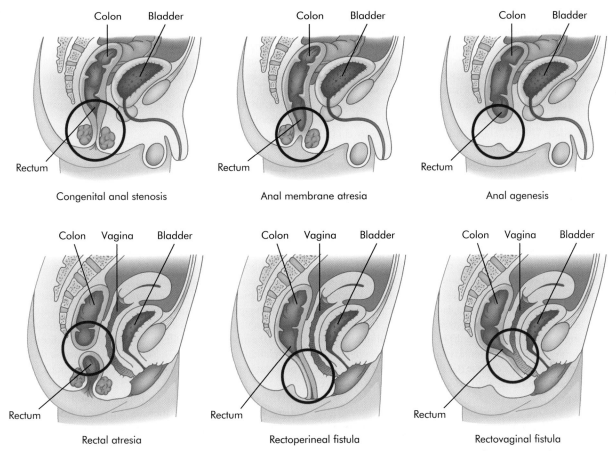

Colon Bladder

Rectum

Congenital anal stenosis

Colon Bladder

Rectum

Anal membrane atresia

Colon Bladder

Rectum

Anal agenesis

Colon Vagina Bladder

Rectum

Rectal atresia

Colon Vagina Bladder

Rectum

Rectoperineal fistula

Colon Vagina Bladder

Rectum

Rectovaginal fistula

FIGURE 35-4 Anorectal Stenosis and Imperforate Anus. **NOTE:** With the exception of the rectovaginal fistula, all of the malformations shown occur in both males and females.

Acquired Impairment of Motility
Intussusception

Intussusception is the telescoping of one portion of the intestine into another. It is the most common cause of acquired intestinal obstruction in infants with most cases occurring between 5 and 7 months of age. Intussusception is more common in males and can occur in children with polyps or tumors, cystic fibrosis, Meckel diverticulum, intestinal adhesions, or immediately after abdominal surgery.[28]

PATHOPHYSIOLOGY In intussusception, the ileum commonly telescopes into the cecum and part of the ascending colon by collapsing through the ileocecal valve, although intussusception can occur anywhere from the duodenum to the rectum. The proximal portion of the intestine (the intussusceptum) collapses into the distal portion (the intussuscipiens) in the direction of peristaltic flow (Figure 35-5). The intussusceptum then drags its mesentery into the enveloping lumen, causing an intussusception. Initially, the mesentery is constricted, obstructing venous return. Compression of the mesenteric vessels between the two layers of intestinal wall and at the U-shaped angle at either end of the intussusceptum leads within hours to venous stasis, engorgement, edema, exudation, and further vascular compression. The tension of the mesentery on the intussusceptum tends to arch the bowel in a curve having its center at the mesenteric root. Edema and compression obstruct the flow of chyme through the intestine. Unless the intussusception is treated, ischemia and necrosis ensue.

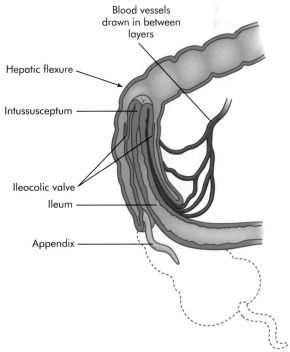

Blood vessels drawn in between layers

Hepatic flexure

Intussusceptum

Ileocolic valve

Ileum

Appendix

FIGURE 35-5 Ileocolic Intussusception.

CLINICAL MANIFESTATIONS The classic symptoms of intussusception include colicky abdominal pain, irritability, knees drawn to the chest, vomiting, and bloody stools. All of these symptoms may not occur and intussusception has been discovered incidentally by computed tomography (CT) or magnetic resonance imaging (MRI) scan for other indications. Abdominal tenderness and distention develop as intestinal obstruction becomes more acute.

EVALUATION AND TREATMENT Diagnosis is based on clinical manifestations, onset of symptoms, and ultrasonographic or radiologic imaging. Reduction is an emergency procedure using an air enema. Surgical reduction is done on children who fail air enema or in the rare case of perforation.[29] Untreated intussusception in infants is nearly always fatal. Most infants recover if the intussusception is reduced within 24 hours.[30]

Gastroesophageal Reflux

Gastroesophageal reflux (GER) is the return of stomach contents into the esophagus because of relaxation or incompetence of the lower esophageal sphincter. In newborns, reflux is normal because neuromuscular control of the gastroesophageal sphincter is not fully developed. The frequency of reflux is highest in premature infants and decreases during the first 6 to 12 months of life. Normal infants and children have been shown to have some reflux but may be asymptomatic. Gastroesophageal reflux disease (GERD) is different from GER and occurs when complications, such as bleeding, dysphagia, or failure to thrive, develop.[31]

PATHOPHYSIOLOGY Delayed maturation of the lower esophageal sphincter or impaired hormonal response mechanisms are possible causes. Factors that maintain lower esophageal sphincter integrity in children include the location of the gastroesophageal junction in a high-pressure zone within the abdomen, mucosal gathering within the sphincter, and the angle at which the esophagus is inserted into the stomach. Reflux persists if any one of these pressure-maintaining factors is altered. Irritation of the mucosa by acidic gastric contents results in inflammation of the esophageal epithelium (esophagitis) and stimulation of the vomiting reflex.

Esophageal inflammation resulting from GERD is differentiated from eosinophilic esophagitis, which can occur in children. It is thought to be an atopic disease involving both immediate and delayed hypersensitivity reactions to food ingestion. An eosinophilic infiltrate is associated with inflammation of the entire esophagus that is nonresponsive to acid-suppression therapy. Dysphagia is a common symptom. Treatment involves food elimination and oral steroids.[32]

CLINICAL MANIFESTATIONS Of affected infants, 85% vomit excessively during the first week of life and usually have other symptoms by 6 weeks. Aspiration pneumonia develops in one third of infants with gastroesophageal reflux. In cases that persist into childhood, chronic cough, wheezing, and recurrent pneumonia are common. Inadequate retention of nutrients can adversely impact growth and weight gain. Esophagitis resulting from exposure of the esophageal mucosa to acidic gastric contents is manifested by pain, bleeding, and eventually stricture formation and abnormal motility. Approximately 25% of affected children have iron deficiency anemia caused by frank or occult blood loss.[33]

EVALUATION AND TREATMENT The clinical manifestations are often adequate to confirm a diagnosis of GERD. Esophageal pH monitoring with a probe for 24 hours and endoscopy are routinely used for diagnosis.[34]

Mild gastroesophageal reflux resolves without treatment. Small, frequent feedings and frequent burping are also accepted strategies for managing infant reflux. Medications to increase motility, to increase lower esophageal sphincter pressure, or to decrease gastric acid production have been used to treat GER. If no improvement is seen with medical management or the child has life-threatening events with reflux, an antireflux surgical procedure, including gastropexy and fundoplication, is performed.[35]

> ✔ **QUICK CHECK 35-2**
> 1. Describe the pathologic defect in meconium ileus.
> 2. Why is there poor bowel motility with Hirschsprung disease?
> 3. Describe the defect in intussusception.

Impairment of Digestion, Absorption, and Nutrition
Cystic Fibrosis

Cystic fibrosis (CF) of the pancreas, also called *mucoviscidosis* or *fibrocystic disease of the pancreas,* is an autosomal recessive disease that involves many organs and systems and leads to death at an earlier age, although new treatments are extending life expectancy. It is the most frequent cause of chronic suppurative lung disease in children and is the most common life-threatening inherited disease in the white population (see Chapter 27). This section focuses on the deficiency of pancreatic enzymes and Chapter 27 discusses pulmonary involvement.

PATHOPHYSIOLOGY The pathophysiologic triad that is the hallmark of CF includes (1) pancreatic enzyme deficiency, which causes maldigestion; (2) overproduction of mucus in the respiratory tract and inability to clear secretions, which cause progressive chronic obstructive pulmonary disease (see Chapter 27); and (3) abnormally elevated sodium and chloride concentrations in sweat. The full spectrum of involvement is evident as shown in Table 35-1.

Approximately 85% of the children have pancreatic insufficiency. Severe problems with maldigestion of proteins, carbohydrates, and fats occur because mucus obstruction of the pancreatic ducts blocks the flow of pancreatic enzymes causing intestinal malabsorption and degenerative and fibrotic changes in the pancreas. Diabetes mellitus may develop from damage to insulin-producing beta cells and insulin resistance.[36]

CLINICAL MANIFESTATIONS Clinical manifestations are summarized in Table 35-1. The child with CF will fail to grow and gain weight related to pancreatic enzyme deficiency and nutrient malabsorption. Steatorrhea and a distended abdomen are common and distal intestinal obstruction syndrome (DIOS) may develop (see p. 941).

EVALUATION AND TREATMENT The extent of pancreatic function is determined by 72-hour stool fat measurements. Stools also may be examined for absence of pancreatic enzymes, including fecal elastase, trypsin, and chymotrypsin.[37] Pancreatic replacement enzymes (i.e., lipase) are administered before or with meals. High-caloric, high-protein diets with frequent snacks and vitamin supplements are used to treat the malnutrition. Nutritional status and growth should be carefully monitored,[38] and growth hormone may be included with nutritional supplements.[39]

Gluten-Sensitive Enteropathy

Gluten-sensitive enteropathy, formerly called celiac sprue or *celiac disease,* is an autoimmune disease that damages small intestinal villous epithelium when there is ingestion of gluten (gliadin), the protein

TABLE 35-1   PATHOPHYSIOLOGY, CLINICAL MANIFESTATIONS, AND COMPLICATIONS OF CYSTIC FIBROSIS

ORGAN INVOLVED	SECRETORY DYSFUNCTION	CLINICAL MANIFESTATIONS	COMPLICATIONS
Sweat glands	Elevated concentration of sodium and chloride in sweat	Hyponatremia; hypochloremia	Heat prostration; shock
Intestine			
Newborn	Viscid meconium	Meconium ileus with intestinal obstruction	Meconium peritonitis
Older child and adult	Inspissated (dried out) mucofecal masses (intestinal sludging)	Partial intestinal obstruction with severe cramping pains	Volvulus (obstruction), intussusception (prolapse)
			Distal intestinal obstruction syndrome
Pancreas (enzyme deficiency)	Inspissation and precipitation of pancreatic secretions, causing obstruction of pancreatic ducts	Absence of pancreatic enzymes, causing malabsorption of food and fatty, bulky stools	Hypoproteinemia; iron deficiency anemia; malnutrition
		Decreased vitamin A, D, E, and K absorption	Vitamins A, D, E, and K deficiency and rectal prolapse
	Insulin deficiency	Glucose intolerance	Diabetes mellitus (see Chapter 18)
Liver	Inspissation and precipitation of bile and biliary system	Focal biliary cirrhosis; shrunken, "hobnail" liver	Portal hypertension with esophageal varices and hematemesis
Salivary glands	Inspissation and precipitation of secretions in small ducts of submaxillary and sublingual salivary glands	Mild patchy fibrosis of salivary glands	None
Respiratory Tract			
Paranasal structures	Viscid mucus	Retention of mucus; clouding seen on sinus roentgenograms	Mucopyoceles (pus accumulations) with nasal deformity or orbital cavity extension
Nose	Nasal polyps	Obstruction of nasal air flow	None
Lungs	Viscid mucus in bronchioles and bronchi	Obstruction of bronchioles causing bronchiolectasis, bronchiectasis, and chronic lung infection	Hemoptysis; pneumothorax; cor pulmonale; respiratory failure
Reproductive Tract			
Male	Viscid genital tract secretions during embryologic development, causing failure of formation of normal vas deferens	Sterility	None
Female	Distention of endocervical epithelial cells with cytoplasmic mucin	Decreased fertility	Polypoid cervicitis (cervical inflammation) while taking oral contraceptives

Data from Egan Marie: Cystic Fibrosis in Kliegman RM et al: *Nelson textbook of pediatrics,* ed 19, Philadelphia, 2011, Saunders.

component of cereal grains. The disease has a prevalence of about 1% worldwide.[40]

Pathogenesis is complex and involves dietary, genetic, and immunologic factors, as well as required exposure of susceptible individuals to environmental agents in addition to gluten. Gluten-sensitive enteropathy has been associated with other immune disorders, including diabetes mellitus, autoimmune thyroiditis, and Addison disease.[41]

PATHOPHYSIOLOGY   The major pathophysiologic characteristic of celiac disease is T cell–mediated autoimmune injury to the intestinal epithelial cells of genetically susceptible individuals. There is atrophy and flattening of villi, crypt hyperplasia in the upper small intestine and malabsorption of most nutrients in the presence of cereal gluten, particularly wheat, rye, and barley (Figure 35-6).[42]

Damage to the mucosa of the duodenum and jejunum exacerbates malabsorption. The secretion of intestinal hormones, such as secretin and cholecystokinin-pancreozymin, may be diminished; consequently, secretion of pancreatic enzymes and expulsion of bile from the gallbladder decrease, contributing to malabsorption.

Destruction of mucosal cells causes inflammation, and water and electrolytes are secreted, leading to watery diarrhea. Potassium loss leads to muscle weakness. Magnesium and calcium malabsorption can cause seizures or tetany. Unabsorbed fatty acids combine with calcium, and secondary hyperparathyroidism increases phosphorus excretion, resulting in bone reabsorption. Calcium is no longer available to bind oxalate in the intestine and is absorbed, which causes hyperoxaluria. Gallbladder function may be abnormal, and bile salt conjugation may decrease.

Fat malabsorption in the jejunum is the major cause of steatorrhea (fatty stools). Deficiencies of fat-soluble vitamins are common in children with gluten-sensitive enteropathy. Vitamin K malabsorption leads to hypoprothrombinemia. In one third of cases, iron and folic acid malabsorption is manifested as cheilosis, anemia, and a smooth red tongue. Vitamin B_{12} absorption is impaired in those with extensive ileal disease, and folate and iron deficiencies are common.

CLINICAL MANIFESTATIONS   The onset of clinical manifestations of gluten-sensitive enteropathy depends on the age of the infant when gluten-containing substances are added to the diet. In 50% of affected children, onset occurs by 18 months of age, with latent intervals varying

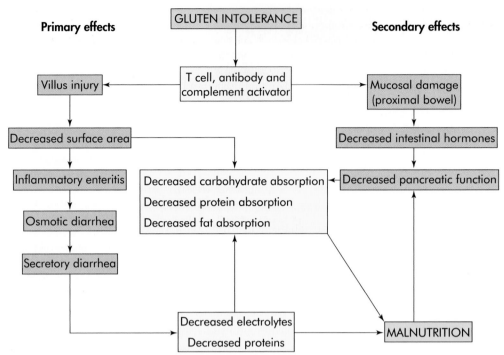

FIGURE 35-6 Pathophysiology of Gluten-Sensitive Enteropathy.

from months to years. Severity of symptoms can vary tremendously and many children older than 3 years of age present with nongastrointestinal symptoms.[43] Diarrhea, failure to thrive, and anemia are early signs in infants. The stools are pale, bulky, greasy, and foul smelling, and they may contain oil droplets. Three to five such movements occur daily. As early as 3 or 4 months of age, growth failure, anorexia, and constipation can begin. In older children, constipation is occasionally seen despite steatorrhea. Vomiting and abdominal pain are prominent in infants but unusual in older children. Anorexia is prevalent. The classic physical manifestations of organic failure to thrive, such as abdominal protuberance, wasted buttocks and limbs, and hypotonia, occur in fewer than 50% of infants with gluten-sensitive enteropathy. Growth is usually diminished and may be related to growth hormone deficiency.[44]

Manifestations of malabsorption, such as rickets, anemia, tetany, frank bleeding, or anemia, may be obvious. Hypomagnesemia and hypocalcemia cause irritability, tremor, convulsions, tetany, bone pain, osteomalacia, and dental abnormalities. If vitamin D deficiency is prolonged, rickets and clubbing of the terminal phalanges are likely. Eighty-six percent of older children have fingerprint changes (ridge atrophy). In older children, delayed puberty and infertility may be manifestations of otherwise subtle gluten-sensitive enteropathy.[45]

An unusual complication of gluten-sensitive enteropathy in infancy is celiac crisis. Celiac crisis is characterized by severe diarrhea, dehydration, and hypoproteinemia as a result of malabsorption and protein loss.

EVALUATION AND TREATMENT Diagnosis includes confirmation with serologic antiendomysial or antitransglutaminase immunoglobulin A (IgA) antibodies, as well as an intestinal biopsy to detect the classic mucosal changes caused by gluten-sensitive enteropathy.[46] A wide variety of screening tests for malabsorption also may be useful, including genetic testing. Many children remain undiagnosed.

Treatment consists of the immediate and permanent institution of a diet free of cereal grains (wheat, rye, barley, malt). Lactose intolerance is presumed because of damage to villi, and lactose (milk sugar) also is excluded from the diet but may be resumed after treatment. Infants are routinely given vitamin D, iron, and folic acid supplements to treat deficiencies. For most children the long-term prognosis is excellent. There is an increased incidence of malignant disease, particularly lymphoma, in individuals who fail to respond to gluten-free diets.[47]

Protein Energy Malnutrition

Kwashiorkor and marasmus are the two most common types of malnutrition in children. These disorders are known collectively as protein energy malnutrition (PEM). Both are states of long-term starvation. Kwashiorkor is a severe protein deficiency, and marasmus is a severe deficiency of all nutrients. Kwashiorkor is a widespread nutritional problem among children in developing countries and economically destitute populations, particularly when associated with human immunodeficiency virus (HIV) infection.[48] The disease usually occurs in infants or children from 1 to 4 years of age who have been weaned from breast milk to a high-starch, protein-deficient diet.

Marasmus can occur at any age, but it is common in children younger than 1 year. In marasmus, starvation is attributable to lack of protein and carbohydrates and, in neglected children, to a psychogenic basis. In developing countries and impoverished populations, early weaning of breast-fed infants to overdiluted commercial formulas is a risk factor for marasmus.

Protein energy malnutrition is also a complication of diseases, such as chronic fever, tuberculosis, malignancy, digestive and malabsorptive disorders, and psychogenic illness. Radiation therapy and chemotherapy can also contribute to protein energy malnutrition.

PATHOPHYSIOLOGY In kwashiorkor, the deficit of dietary amino acids reduces protein synthesis in all tissues. Physical growth and mental growth are stunted and maintenance of minimal life processes is in jeopardy. The lack of sufficient plasma proteins results in generalized edema with a substantial loss of potassium. The liver swells with stored fat because no hepatic proteins are synthesized to form and release lipoproteins. Pancreatic atrophy and fibrosis may be present. Kwashiorkor also causes malabsorption, reduced bone density, and impaired renal function. If the condition is not reversed, the prognosis is very poor.

In marasmus, intake of all dietary nutrients is reduced to a minimum. Metabolic processes, including liver function, are preserved, but growth is severely retarded. Caloric intake is too low to support protein synthesis for growth or the storage of fat. Muscle and fat wasting occur and anemia is common and can be severe.[49]

CLINICAL MANIFESTATIONS Kwashiorkor is characterized by marked generalized edema, dermatoses, hypopigmented hair, distended abdomen, hepatomegaly, and almost normal weight for age (because of edema). Marasmus is characterized by muscle wasting, fatty liver and hepatomegaly, diarrhea, dermatosis, low hemoglobin level, and infection. There is loss of subcutaneous fat and an absence of edema. Both conditions lead to retarded physical, mental, and psychologic development. Severe vitamin A deficiency commonly results in blindness.[50]

EVALUATION AND TREATMENT Evaluation of protein energy malnutrition is based on nutritional history and clinical manifestations. The provision of deficient nutrients will resolve clinical symptoms in 4 to 6 weeks. Physical and mental retardation may not be reversible, however. Nutritional rehabilitation with appropriate environmental stimulation for infants and young children has been shown to resolve or improve cerebral shrinkage, physical growth, and psychomotor development.

Failure to Thrive

Failure to thrive (FTT) is the inadequate physical development of an infant or child. It is manifested as a deceleration in weight gain, a low weight/height ratio, or a low weight/height/head circumference ratio. FTT is a common problem and can present at any time in childhood.[51]

PATHOPHYSIOLOGY **Organic FTT** has a pathophysiologic cause, for example, gastroesophageal reflux, pyloric stenosis, gastroenteritis, infection by intestinal parasites, congenital anomalies, or chronic diseases of major body systems. All these disorders reduce the availability of nutrients for maintenance and growth. **Nonorganic FTT** occurs in the absence of any gastrointestinal or endocrine disorder or other chronic disease. It is usually a syndrome with many psychosocial causes and may be complicated by inadequate economic resources and lack of knowledge. Infants and children are at risk for nonorganic FTT if their parents or primary caregivers are unable to provide nurturance. Various parental stressors may be involved, including the following:

- Lack of nurturance in the parents' own childhood
- Unwanted pregnancy
- Inability to bond with the infant because of health or other problems
- Postpartum or maternal depression
- Family crisis, such as the occurrence of a death or marital problems
- Stress caused by single parenthood or social isolation
- Mental, emotional, or physical illness

CLINICAL MANIFESTATIONS Clinical manifestations of organic FTT are delayed growth accompanied by manifestations of the underlying disease. Manifestations of nonorganic FTT are delayed growth plus reduced energy level, reduced responsiveness and interaction with the environment, social isolation, spasticity and rigidity when held or touched, inability to make eye contact or smile, refusal to eat, and rejection of foods. Weight loss and decelerated growth are accompanied by developmental retardation in many areas. Nonorganic FTT is a complex syndrome involving psychosocial, emotional, and parent-child problems that compound the pathophysiologic abnormalities.[52]

EVALUATION AND TREATMENT FTT is suggested if a child falls below the third percentile on the growth curve or is falling off a previously established growth curve. Organic FTT is manifested in infancy by weight, height, and head circumference growth that may be parallel to but below the normal ranges. If no genetic, endocrine, or other systemic disorder is identified and if the physical and laboratory examinations show no abnormalities other than delayed growth, an environmental cause is indicated.

Hospital admission is recommended if the diagnosis is unclear or the child is in nutritional or emotional jeopardy. Eating patterns, food preferences, caloric intake, and family interactions can be assessed during the hospital stay. If the cause is environmental, the hospitalized child with FTT usually begins to gain weight. Organic and nonorganic FTT can coexist, making the distinction between them more difficult.[51]

If an organic problem has been identified, management of FTT consists of treating the cause. Management of nonorganic FTT involves the immediate total care of the child and measures to address (1) the psychosocial and emotional problems of the caregivers and (2) parent-child interactions. Counseling, parental modeling, and long-term family support are sometimes required.[53]

Necrotizing Enterocolitis

Necrotizing enterocolitis (NEC) is an ischemic, inflammatory condition that causes bowel necrosis and perforation, and infant death if untreated. NEC occurs primarily in premature very-low-birthweight infants. The risk of necrotizing enterocolitis decreases as the gastrointestinal tract matures. The cause is unknown.[54]

PATHOPHYSIOLOGY The exact etiology of NEC is unclear. Factors contributing to the development of NEC include maternal age older than 35 years, infections, abnormal bacterial colonization, intestinal ischemia, immature immunity, immature intestinal motility and barrier function, perinatal stress, the effects of medications and feeding practices, and genetic predisposition. The immature mucosal barrier delays digestion and motility is slower, allowing for the accumulation of noxious substances that damage the intestine, increase permeability, and increase the risk for infection. Translocation of intestinal bacteria and other substances contributes to injury, inflammation, and development of systemic inflammatory disease. Immature intestinal innate immunity and an unfavorable balance between normal and pathogenic bacteria promote intestinal inflammation and release of proinflammatory mediators. Accumulation of gas in the intestine can cause pressure that decreases blood flow, and an imbalance between vasodilator and vasoconstrictor inputs in the immature gut may lead to vasoconstriction promoting ischemia, injury, and necrosis.[55,56]

CLINICAL MANIFESTATIONS Manifestations of NEC usually appear suddenly and usually within 2 weeks of birth. They range from mild abdominal distention to bowel perforation, sepsis, and death. Abdominal pain, unstable temperature, bradycardia, and apnea are nonspecific signs. Affected infants have occult or grossly bloody stools, gastric retention, abdominal distention, and septicemia with elevated white blood cell and falling platelet counts. Premature infants often have more severe disease and other disorders, such as respiratory distress syndrome.

EVALUATION AND TREATMENT   Diagnosis is based on clinical manifestations, laboratory results, and plain films of the abdomen that show gas accumulating in the intestine. Study is in progress to identify predictive biologic markers for early diagnosis.[57] Preventive strategies include encouragement of breast milk feeding, judicious fluid management to prevent vascular fluid overload and patent ductus arteriosus (see Chapter 24), administration of arginine and glutamine supplements to support intestinal epithelial cell growth, and utilization of enteral probiotics to support normal gut bacteria.[58]

Treatments include cessation of feeding, implementation of gastric suction to decompress the intestines, maintenance of fluid and electrolyte balance, and administration of antibiotics to control sepsis. Surgical resection is the treatment of choice for perforation and peritoneal drainage may be used as an adjunct to laparotomy.[59] Overall mortality is high, particularly for infants who have surgery.[54]

> ✔ **QUICK CHECK 35-3**
> 1. Why do individuals with cystic fibrosis have pancreatic insufficiency?
> 2. Why does loss of villi occur with gluten-sensitive enteropathy?
> 3. Compare kwashiorkor and marasmus.

Diarrhea

Diarrhea is an increase in the water content, volume, or frequency of stools and can be acute or chronic. Diarrhea is a common gastrointestinal problem during infancy and early childhood and is the leading cause of death in young children, particularly in developing countries.[60] Severe diarrhea occurs one to three times during the first 3 years of life. Most episodes are self-limiting and resolve within 72 hours. The pathophysiologic mechanisms of diarrhea in children are similar to those described for adults—osmotic diarrhea, secretory diarrhea, or increased motility diarrhea. Prolonged diarrhea is more dangerous in children, however, because they have much smaller fluid reserves than adults. Therefore dehydration can develop rapidly if any disturbance increases fluid secretion into the gastrointestinal lumen (secretory diarrhea), draws fluid into the lumen by osmosis (osmotic diarrhea), or prevents fluid absorption in the intestine (increased motility diarrhea).

Acute or Chronic Diarrhea in Infants and Children

Common causes of diarrhea in infants include infections, congenital aganglionic megacolon, milk protein allergies, and necrotizing enterocolitis. Less common causes are adrenogenital syndrome, impaired chloride-bicarbonate exchange, congenital lactase deficiency, glucose-galactose malabsorption, and sucrase-isomaltase deficiency. Infants have low fluid reserves and relatively rapid peristalsis and metabolism. Therefore the danger of dehydration is great.

Acute infectious diarrhea in infants and young children is usually associated with viral or bacterial gastroenteritis. Viruses include rotaviruses, noroviruses, and adenoviruses. Rotavirus is the most common cause in young children and is associated with a higher death rate in low-income countries. Rotavirus vaccine is an effective preventive strategy.[61] Bacterial contamination of food or water includes *Escherichia coli*, *Klebsiella*, staphylococci, *Salmonella*, *Shigella*, and *Vibrio cholerae*. *Giardia intestinalis*, *Cryptosporidium parvum* or *hominis*, and *Strongyloides stercoralis* are parasites that cause diarrhea in tropical areas. *Clostridium difficile* is often associated with previous antibiotic therapy. Infectious diarrhea has a rapid onset, with watery stools sometimes mixed with blood. Severe dehydration, acidosis, and shock can occur quickly from diarrhea and vomiting.[62] Hemolytic uremic syndrome and renal failure can develop when diarrhea is associated with *Shigella* toxin and *Escherichia coli* infection (see Chapter 30).

Other causes of acute diarrhea in the older child include antibiotic therapy, appendicitis, chemotherapy, inflammatory bowel disease, parasitic infestation, parenteral infections, and ingestion of toxic substances. Causes of diarrhea in young children are unknown in about 40% of cases.[63] Viral gastroenteritis tends to be self-limiting. Bacterial gastroenteritis is treated with antibiotics if the causal pathogen can be identified.

Children with acute gastroenteritis often remain mildly symptomatic for up to 4 weeks; therefore, diarrhea that persists longer than 4 weeks is considered to be chronic. Children with **chronic diarrhea** can be divided into two groups: (1) otherwise well children whose growth is normal and (2) ill children whose growth is retarded. Causes of chronic diarrhea in the first group include abnormal colonic motility, lactose intolerance, encopresis, parasitic infestation, and antibiotic use. Chronic diarrhea in the second group is usually caused by a disease that impairs absorption. Treatment of diarrhea requires rehydration with fluids, electrolytes, and glucose; maintenance of nutrition; and treatment of associated conditions and antibiotics as indicated. Intravenous solutions are used only when oral solutions are not tolerated.[64]

Primary lactose intolerance. Lactose intolerance, the inability to digest milk sugar, is caused by inadequate production of the enzyme lactase. It is a common cause of diarrhea, particularly in nonwhite children under the age of 7 years. The malabsorption of lactose results in osmotic diarrhea accompanied by abdominal pain, bloating, and flatulence. Diagnosis includes elimination of dietary lactose or implementation of hydrogen lactose breath testing. Treatment consists of reducing milk consumption or supplementing the diet with oral lactase. Some children can tolerate lactose in fermented forms, such as cheese and yogurt, or by adding soy food.[65]

DISORDERS OF THE LIVER

Disorders of Biliary Metabolism and Transport
Neonatal Jaundice

Physiologic jaundice (hyperbilirubinemia) of the newborn is usually a transient, benign icterus that occurs during the first week of life in otherwise healthy, full-term infants and is common in preterm infants.[66] It is caused by mild unconjugated (indirect-reacting) hyperbilirubinemia. Jaundice appearing within 24 hours after birth, total serum bilirubin concentration greater than 20 mg/dl, or direct (conjugated) bilirubin concentration greater than 2 mg/dl is considered pathologic jaundice (hyperbilirubinemia). Risk factors include fetal-maternal blood type incompatibility (ABO and Rh incompatibility causing hemolytic disease in the newborn), premature birth, exclusive breast-feeding in some infants, maternal age greater than or equal to 25 years, male gender, delayed meconium passage, glucose-6-phosphate dehydrogenase deficiency, and excessive birth trauma such as bruising or cephalohematomas.[67] Prediction tools for hyperbilirubinemia are available to reduce risk with early hospital discharge (within 48 hours) when hyperbilirubinemia may not yet be evident.[68]

PATHOPHYSIOLOGY   Pathologic jaundice results from the complex interaction of factors that cause (1) increased bilirubin production (e.g., hemolysis), (2) impaired hepatic uptake or excretion of unconjugated bilirubin, or (3) delayed maturation of liver conjugating mechanisms.[69] The most common cause is hemolytic disease of the newborn (ABO blood incompatibility) (see Chapters 7 and 21). Unconjugated bilirubin (indirect bilirubin) is lipid soluble and bound to albumin in the blood, and in the free form it readily crosses the blood-brain barrier in infants. Chronic bilirubin encephalopathy (kernicterus) is caused by the deposition of toxic, unconjugated bilirubin in brain cells and usually does not occur in healthy, full-term infants. Elevated conjugated bilirubin level is a sign of underlying disease.

CLINICAL MANIFESTATIONS Physiologic jaundice develops during the second or third day after birth and usually subsides in 1 to 2 weeks in full-term infants and in 2 to 4 weeks in premature infants. After this, increasing bilirubin values and persistent jaundice indicate pathologic hyperbilirubinemia. Manifestations include yellowing of skin, dark urine, light-colored stools, and weight loss. Premature infants with respiratory distress, acidosis, or sepsis are at greater risk for kernicterus (brain damage related to unconjugated hyperbilirubinemia) and the development of athetoid cerebral palsy and speech and hearing impairment.[70]

EVALUATION AND TREATMENT Both total and direct (conjugated) bilirubin levels are monitored as described previously. Other causes of jaundice must be eliminated to confirm physiologic jaundice. Treatment depends on the degree of hyperbilirubinemia. Physiologic jaundice is commonly treated by phototherapy and several techniques are available.[70a] Pathologic jaundice requires an exchange transfusion and treatment of the underlying disorder.

Biliary Atresia

Biliary atresia is a rare congenital malformation characterized by the absence or obstruction of intrahepatic or extrahepatic bile ducts. The cause of the intrauterine injury to the ducts is not clear but is thought to be related to chromosomal abnormality or a viral-induced, innate immune response. The disease expression is a continuum in which the principal process is one of bile duct destruction.[71] The atresia or obstruction of the bile ducts leads to plugging, inflammation, fibrosis of the bile canaliculi, and cholestasis. Progressive obstruction may lead to biliary cirrhosis (see Chapter 34), portal hypertension, or liver failure.

Jaundice is the primary clinical manifestation of biliary atresia, along with hepatomegaly and acholic (clay-colored) stools. Fat absorption is impaired because of the lack of bile salts, and the infant may fail to gain weight. Cirrhosis and liver failure can lead to death.

Early diagnosis of biliary atresia is essential and is based on clinical manifestations and liver biopsy results. Liver function test results are abnormal. Serum transaminase and alkaline phosphatase levels are elevated, and conjugated (direct) serum bilirubin levels rise progressively.

Extrahepatic atresia can be relieved by the Kasai portoenterostomy. Even with initial restoration of bile flow, however, obliteration of intrahepatic bile ducts continues and cirrhosis results. Liver transplantation is a successful long-term therapy for biliary atresia. Of children with biliary atresia, 80% die before the age of 3 years if not treated.[71]

Inflammatory Disorders
Hepatitis

Hepatitis A virus (HAV). Approximately 30% to 50% of the reported cases of hepatitis A virus (HAV) occur in children,[72] particularly children of nursery school age. Outbreaks tend to occur in day-care centers with large numbers of children who are not toilet trained and staff members who practice poor handwashing techniques.[73] HAV in children is usually mild and asymptomatic, but it may involve nausea, vomiting, and diarrhea. Because jaundice is absent, infected children appear to have the flu. Almost all children recover from hepatitis A

without residual liver damage. Vaccination programs are successfully reducing the incidence of HAV in the United States.[72]

Hepatitis B virus (HBV). Risk factors for hepatitis B virus (HBV) include infants of mothers who are chronic hepatitis B virus (HBV) surface antigen (HBsAg) carriers, children with hemophilia who receive frequent blood transfusions, children who abuse parenteral drugs, and children who live in institutions for mentally retarded persons. Most newborns infected by their mothers (vertical transmission) develop chronic hepatitis and become carriers. Chronic hepatitis may develop because the infant's immune system is immature. Infected infants are at risk for cirrhosis and hepatocellular carcinoma.[74] The most serious consequence of HBV infection is fulminant hepatitis, which occurs in 1% of cases. Hepatitis D virus (HDV) infection depends on active infection with HBV. There is evidence that the risk of fulminant hepatitis is higher in individuals with combined infection of HBV and HDV than in those with HBV infection alone.[75] Most children are treated conservatively and antivirals are used for chronic disease.[76] Aggressive vaccination programs reduce the incidence of HBV. Maternal antiviral therapy during pregnancy and lactation is under investigation.[77]

Hepatitis C virus (HCV). Hepatitis C virus (HCV) in children is most commonly transmitted vertically and is enhanced with maternal co-infection with human immunodeficiency virus (HIV). It also is transmitted with blood transfusions. The disease is usually mild in children, and cirrhosis is rare. Chronic hepatitis C is treated with antiviral drugs.[78]

Chronic hepatitis. Hepatitis B virus (HBV) and hepatitis C virus (HCV) are the main causes of chronic hepatitis in children. Manifestations of chronic hepatitis include malaise, anorexia, fever, gastrointestinal bleeding, hepatomegaly, edema, and transient joint pain. Often there are no symptoms. Serum alanine aminotransferase and bilirubin levels are elevated. There may be evidence of impairment of synthetic functions of the liver: prolonged prothrombin time and hypoalbuminemia. Diagnosis is based on the clinical manifestations and liver biopsy results. There is no curative therapy for chronic HBV or chronic HCV and children are treated with antiviral drugs and should continue to be monitored.[79] There also is an autoimmune form of chronic hepatitis more common in female children that is treated with immunosuppression therapy.[80] Liver transplant may ultimately be required for chronic hepatitis.

More detailed information about viral and fulminant hepatitis is described in Chapter 34 (also see Table 34-8).

Cirrhosis

Cirrhosis is fibrotic scarring of the liver resulting in obstruction to the flow of blood and bile. Most forms of chronic liver diseases in children can progress to cirrhosis, but they seldom do so. The complications of cirrhosis in children are the same as those in adults: portal hypertension, the opening of collateral vessels between the portal and systemic veins, and varices. In addition, children with cirrhosis experience growth failure caused by nutritional deficits, as well as developmental delay, particularly in gross motor function because of ascites and weakness. The cause of cirrhosis may influence its severity and course. Some types of cirrhosis can be stabilized if the cause is identified and treated early.[81] The risk of cirrhosis is increasing in obese children with nonalcoholic fatty liver disease (see *Health Alert:* Childhood Obesity and Nonalcoholic Fatty Liver Disease).

Portal Hypertension

There are two basic causes of portal hypertension in children: (1) increased resistance to blood flow within the portal system and (2) increased volume of portal blood flow. The second cause is rare in children and is not discussed here. Increased resistance to flow can occur anywhere in the

Childhood Obesity and Nonalcoholic Fatty Liver Disease

Nonalcoholic fatty liver disease (NAFLD) is the most common cause of liver disease in children and is associated with obesity and insulin resistance. The rise in childhood obesity worldwide is contributing to the increasing prevalence of NAFLD. The disease usually presents in prepubertal children and is predominant in males and in children of Hispanic origin. Diagnosis is made by exclusion of other disease causes. Liver biopsy is required for definitive diagnosis of steatosis, and there are differences in the extent of fat, inflammation, and fibrosis in children compared to adults. There is no consensus regarding treatment. Exercise and slow, consistent weight loss with a low glycemic index diet have been shown to be more effective than a low-fat diet in lowering body weight. Pharmacologic agents are being evaluated to control insulin resistance and prevent progression of liver disease and cirrhosis. Research is in progress to define the pathophysiology, noninvasive diagnostic procedures, and prevention of this disease.

Data from Alisi A, Locatelli M, Nobili V: Nonalcoholic fatty liver disease in children, *Curr Opin Clin Nutr Metab Care* 13(4):397–402, 2010; Brunt EM: Pathology of nonalcoholic fatty liver disease, *Nat Rev Gastroenterol Hepatol* 7(4):195–203, 2010; Nobili V, Alisi A, Raponi M: Pediatric non-alcoholic fatty liver disease: preventive and therapeutic value of lifestyle intervention, *World J Gastroenterol* 15(48):6017–6022, 2009.

portal circulatory system. Portal hypertension can accompany cirrhosis, intra-abdominal infections, portal vein thrombosis, congenital anomalies of the portal vein, and congenital hepatic fibrosis.

Types of Portal Hypertension

Extrahepatic portal hypertension. Extrahepatic (prehepatic) portal venous obstruction causes 50% to 70% of the cases of extrahepatic portal hypertension in children. In approximately two thirds of these children, no specific cause can be found.[82] Obstruction is almost always in the portal vein and is usually caused by thrombosis as a complication of abdominal trauma, pancreatitis, abdominal infections, and some systemic disorders; however, these causes are rare. Life-threatening bleeding and coagulation disorders can occur. Mesoportal bypass (anastomosis of portal vein to mesenteric vein) restores normal physiologic portal flow to the liver and corrects portal hypertension.[83]

Intrahepatic portal hypertension. Liver fibrosis is the primary cause of intrahepatic portal hypertension. The fibrosis can lead to cirrhosis with increased resistance to portal blood flow by constricting and reducing the compliance of hepatic sinusoids. Chronic hepatitis, biliary atresia, nonalcoholic fatty liver disease, and congenital hepatic fibrosis are causes of liver fibrosis in children.[84-86]

Course of the Disease

The important consequences of portal hypertension in children are the development of collateral circulation, with portal-systemic shunting; hypersplenism; esophageal varices; and ascites.

CLINICAL MANIFESTATIONS The clinical manifestations of portal hypertension are (1) splenomegaly, (2) upper gastrointestinal tract bleeding, (3) ascites, and (4) hepatic encephalopathy (see Chapter 34).

EVALUATION AND TREATMENT The objectives of the clinical investigation are to (1) locate the site of the venous block and (2) identify the disease responsible for the portal hypertension. Thorough physical examination, laboratory tests of liver function, imaging procedures, and biopsy may be included in the diagnostic evaluation. Sclerotherapy is the initial treatment of choice for severe esophageal varices in children. Portosystemic shunts are indicated when bleeding is not controlled with sclerotherapy.[87]

The outcome of portal hypertension depends almost entirely on its cause. Children with extrahepatic disease are expected to recover with

TABLE 35-2	GALACTOSEMIA, FRUCTOSEMIA, AND WILSON DISEASE		
	GALACTOSEMIA	**FRUCTOSEMIA**	**WILSON DISEASE**
Mechanism of disease	Deficiency of galactose-1-phosphate uridyl transferase	Deficiency of fructose-1-phosphate aldolase	Autosomal recessive: defect on chromosome 13 (ATP 7B)
	Autosomal recessive trait	Autosomal recessive trait	Defect in copper excretion by liver
	Cannot convert galactose to glucose	Cannot metabolize fructose, sucrose, or honey; occurs when breast milk is replaced with cow's milk	Impaired transport of copper into bile/blood caused by diminished transport protein (ceruloplasmin)
	Toxic accumulation of galactose in body tissues, liver, and brain	Toxic accumulation of fructose in body tissues	Toxic accumulations of copper in liver, brain, kidney, corneas
Clinical manifestation	High levels of blood galactose	High levels of blood fructose	Intention tremors
	Vomiting	Vomiting	Indistinct speech
	Hypoglycemia	Hypoglycemia	Dystonia
	May have failure to thrive	May have failure to thrive	Greenish yellow rings in cornea
	Symptoms of cirrhosis at 2-6 months—jaundice	Hepatomegaly	Hepatomegaly
	Mental retardation if not treated	Jaundice	Jaundice
	Cataracts if not treated	Seizures	Anorexia
			Renal tubular defects
Evaluation	Newborn screening	Detailed dietary history	Low plasma ceruloplasmin level
	Presence of reducing substances in urine when infant is receiving lactose	Liver or intestinal mucosa biopsy	
Treatment	Galactose-free diet	Fructose, sucrose, honey-free diet	Chelation therapy to remove copper from body
		Vitamin C supplementation	Decreased dietary intake of copper
			Liver transplant

little morbidity. For children with intrahepatic disease, the prognosis varies.

Metabolic Disorders

More than 5000 genetically determined metabolic pathways have been identified in liver tissue. The earliest possible identification of metabolic disorders is essential because (1) early treatment may prevent permanent damage to vital organs, such as the liver or brain; (2) precise genetic counseling may be possible with prenatal diagnosis; and (3) complications can be minimized, even if cure is not possible. Galactosemia, fructosemia, and Wilson disease are treatable metabolic disorders that have hepatic clinical manifestations. The mechanisms of disease, clinical manifestations, evaluation, and treatment of these disorders are presented in Table 35-2.

✓ **QUICK CHECK 35-4**
1. Why is diarrhea such a serious disorder in infants and children?
2. What is biliary atresia?
3. What are the three most common metabolic disorders that cause liver damage in children?

DID YOU UNDERSTAND?

Disorders of the Gastrointestinal Tract

1. Most alterations of digestive function in children include congenital obstructions of the intestinal tract; disorders of digestion, absorption, or nutrition; or liver disease.
2. Cleft lip (harelip) and cleft palate (failure of the bony palate to fuse in the midline) may occur separately or together. The fissure may affect the uvula, soft palate, hard palate, nostril, and maxillary alveolar ridge.
3. Esophageal atresia, a condition in which the esophagus ends in a blind pouch, may occur with or without tracheoesophageal fistula. As the infant swallows oral secretions or ingests milk, the pouch fills, causing either drooling or aspiration into the lungs.
4. Pyloric stenosis is an obstruction of the pyloric outlet caused by hypertrophy of circular muscles in the pyloric sphincter.
5. Intestinal malrotation occurs during fetal development with an obstructing band and volvulus (twisting of the bowel on itself) that may partly or completely occlude the gastrointestinal tract and its blood vessels.
6. Meconium ileus is a newborn condition in which intestinal secretions and amniotic waste products produce a thick, tarry plug that obstructs the intestine. Of children with cystic fibrosis, 10% to 15% present with meconium ileus as a neonate.
7. Duodenal, jejunal, and ileal obstructions can be caused by meconium ileus, atresia, congenital aganglionic megacolon, and acquired obstructive disorders.
8. Meckel diverticulum is a congenital malformation of the gastrointestinal tract involving all layers of the small intestinal wall; it usually occurs in the ileum.
9. Congenital aganglionic megacolon (Hirschsprung disease) is caused by a malformation of the parasympathetic nervous system in a segment of the colon. It is characterized by the absence of nerves needed for peristalsis and causes colon obstruction.
10. Malformations of the anus and rectum range from mild congenital stenosis of the anus to complex deformities, all of which are classified as imperforate anus.
11. Intussusception is a condition in which one portion of the bowel telescopes, or invaginates, into another, most commonly in the area of the ileocecal junction, and causes obstruction.
12. Gastroesophageal reflux is the return of stomach contents into the esophagus caused by relaxation or incompetence of the lower esophageal sphincter that results from immaturity of the gastroesophageal sphincter.
13. Cystic fibrosis is an inherited fibrocystic disease that involves many organs and causes pancreatic enzyme deficiency with maldigestion.
14. Gluten-sensitive enteropathy is caused by hypersensitivity to gluten protein with autoimmune injury and loss of the villous epithelium. It results in malabsorption and growth failure.
15. Protein energy malnutrition is a group of disorders resulting from a severe dietary deficiency of proteins, carbohydrates, or both. Starvation causes stunted mental and physical development.
16. Kwashiorkor is a severe protein deficiency that occurs in children who have stopped breast-feeding and subsist on a high-carbohydrate diet. Marasmus is a deficiency of all dietary nutrients, including carbohydrates.
17. Failure to thrive is inadequate physical growth of a child. Organic failure to thrive is caused by genetic, anatomic, or pathophysiologic factors that retard normal growth and development. Nonorganic failure to thrive is caused by nutritional deficits associated with inadequate nurturing.
18. Necrotizing enterocolitis is an ischemic, inflammatory disorder in neonates, particularly premature infants, thought to result from stress and anoxia of the bowel wall. Bacteria invade the mucosa and submucosa, resulting in colitis, necrosis, and even perforation of the intestinal wall.
19. Acute diarrhea in infants and children can rapidly cause dehydration and electrolyte imbalances because fluid reserves are relatively small.
20. The most common cause of acute diarrhea in children is viral or bacterial enterocolitis (infection of the gastrointestinal tract).
21. Chronic diarrhea (diarrhea persisting longer than 4 weeks) can be caused by a wide variety of underlying conditions and often leads to growth failure and slow development.
22. Primary lactose intolerance is the inability to digest milk sugar because of a lack of the enzyme lactase, resulting in osmotic diarrhea.

Disorders of the Liver

1. Physiologic jaundice of the newborn is caused by mild hyperbilirubinemia that subsides in 1 or 2 weeks. Pathologic jaundice is caused by severe hyperbilirubinemia and can cause brain damage (kernicterus).
2. Biliary atresia is a congenital malformation of the bile ducts that obstructs bile flow. Atresia causes jaundice, cirrhosis, and liver failure.
3. Acute hepatitis is usually caused by a virus, and hepatitis A is the most common form of childhood hepatitis. Chronic hepatitis B or C usually occurs by maternal transmission.
4. Cirrhosis results from fibrotic scarring of the liver and is rare in children, but it can develop from most forms of chronic liver disease.
5. Portal hypertension in children usually is caused by extrahepatic obstruction. Thrombosis of the portal vein is the most common cause of portal hypertension in children, and splenomegaly is the most common sign.
6. The three most common metabolic disorders that cause liver damage in children are galactosemia, fructosemia, and Wilson disease. All three are inherited as genetic traits and allow toxins to accumulate in the liver.

KEY TERMS

- Biliary atresia   949
- Celiac crisis   946
- Chronic diarrhea   948
- Cirrhosis   949
- Cleft lip (harelip)   938
- Cleft palate   938
- Congenital aganglionic megacolon (Hirschsprung disease)   942
- Cystic fibrosis (CF)   944
- Diarrhea   948
- Distal intestinal obstruction syndrome (DIOS)   941
- Eosinophilic esophagitis   944
- Esophageal atresia   939
- Extrahepatic portal hypertension   950
- Failure to thrive (FTT)   947
- Fructosemia   951
- Galactosemia   951
- Gastroesophageal reflux (GER)   944
- Gastroesophageal reflux disease (GERD)   944
- Gluten-sensitive enteropathy (celiac sprue)   944
- Hepatitis A virus (HAV)   949
- Hepatitis B virus (HBV)   949
- Hepatitis C virus (HCV)   949
- Hepatitis D virus (HDV)   949
- Ileal atresia   942
- Imperforate anus   942
- Infantile pyloric stenosis   940
- Intestinal malrotation of the colon   941
- Intrahepatic portal hypertension   950
- Intussusception   943
- Jejunal atresia   942
- Kernicterus   949
- Kwashiorkor   946
- Lactose intolerance   948
- Marasmus   946
- Meckel diverticulum   942
- Meconium   941
- Meconium ileus   941
- Necrotizing enterocolitis (NEC)   947
- Neonatal jaundice   948
- Nonorganic FTT   947
- Organic FTT   947
- Pathologic jaundice (hyperbilirubinemia)   948
- Periduodenal band (Ladd band)   941
- Physiologic jaundice (hyperbilirubinemia) of the newborn   948
- Protein energy malnutrition (PEM)   946
- Rotavirus   948
- Tracheoesophageal fistula (TEF)   939
- Wilson disease   951

REFERENCES

1. Arosarena OA: Cleft lip and palate, *Otolaryngol Clin North Am* 40(1):27–60, 2007.
2. Dixon MJ, et al: Cleft lip and palate: understanding genetic and environmental influences, *Nat Rev Genet* 12(3):167–178, 2011.
3. Mossey PA, et al: Cleft lip and palate, *Lancet* 374(9703):1773–1785, 2009.
4. Karayazgan B, et al: A preoperative appliance for a newborn with cleft palate, *Cleft Palate Craniofac J* 46(1):53–57, 2009.
5. Maarse W, et al: Diagnostic accuracy of transabdominal ultrasound in detecting prenatal cleft lip and palate: a systematic review, *Ultrasound Obstet Gynecol* 35(4):495–502, 2010.
6. Yang IY, Liao YF: The effect of 1-stage versus 2-stage palate repair on facial growth in patients with cleft lip and palate: a review, *Int J Oral Maxillofac Surg* 39(10):945–990, 2010.
7. Szabo C, et al: Treatment of persistent middle ear effusion in cleft palate patients, *Int J Pediatr Otorhinolaryngol* 74(8):874–877, 2010.
8. de Jong EM, et al: Etiology of esophageal atresia and tracheoesophageal fistula: "mind the gap," *Curr Gastroenterol Rep* 12(3):215–222, 2010.
9. Holland AJ, Fitzgerald DA: Oesophageal atresia and tracheo-oesophageal fistula: current management strategies and complications, *Paediatr Respir Rev* 11(2):100–106, 2010.
10. MacMahon B: The continuing enigma of pyloric stenosis of infancy: a review, *Epidemiology* 17(2):195–201, 2006.
11. Boneti C, et al: Ultrasound as a diagnostic tool used by surgeons in pyloric stenosis, *J Pediatr Surg* 43(1):87–91, 2008.
12. Aspelund G, Langer JC: Current management of hypertrophic pyloric stenosis, *Semin Pediatr Surg* 16(1):27–33, 2007.
13. Singh UK, Kumar R, Prasad R: Oral atropine sulfate for infantile hypertrophic pyloric stenosis, *Indian Pediatr* 42(5):473–476, 2005.
14. Sweeney B, Surana R, Puri P: Jejunoileal atresia and associated malformations: correlation with the timing of in utero insult, *J Pediatr Surg* 36(5):774–776, 2001.
14a. Nehra D, Goldstein AM: Intestinal malrotation: varied clinical presentation from infancy through adulthood, *Surgery* 149(3):386–393, 2011.
15. El-Gohary Y, Alagtal M, Gillick J: Long-term complications following operative intervention for intestinal malrotation: a 10-year review, *Pediatr Surg Int* 26(2):203–206, 2010.
16. Murphy FL, Sparnon AL: Long-term complications following intestinal malrotation and the Ladd's procedure: a 15 year review, *Pediatr Surg Int* 22(4):326–329, 2006.
17. Efrati O, et al: Meconium ileus in patients with cystic fibrosis is not a risk factor for clinical deterioration and survival: the Israeli Multicenter Study, *J Pediatr Gastroenterol Nutr* 50(2):173–178, 2010.
18. Copeland DR, et al: Diminishing role of contrast enema in simple meconium ileus, *J Pediatr Surg* 44(11):2130–2132, 2009.
19. Johnson JA, Bush A, Buchdahl R: Does presenting with meconium ileus affect the prognosis of children with cystic fibrosis? *Pediatr Pulmonol* 45(10):951–958, 2010.
20. Speck K, Charles A: Distal intestinal obstructive syndrome in adults with cystic fibrosis: a surgical perspective, *Arch Surg* 143(6):601–603, 2008.
21. Chaudry G, et al: Abdominal manifestations of cystic fibrosis in children, *Pediatr Radiol* 36(3):233–240, 2006.
22. Malik AA, Shams-ul-Bari Wani KA, et al: Meckel's diverticulum—revisited, *Saudi J Gastroenterol* 16(1):3–7, 2010.
23. Mundt E, Bates MD: Genetics of Hirschsprung disease and anorectal malformations, *Semin Pediatr Surg* 19(2):107–117, 2010.
24. Haricharan RN, Georgeson KE: Hirschsprung disease, *Semin Pediatr Surg* 17(4):266–275, 2008.
25. Huang Y, Zheng S, Xiao X: Preliminary evaluation of anorectal manometry in diagnosing Hirschsprung's disease in neonates, *Pediatr Surg* 25(1):41–45, 2009.
26. Kessmann J: Hirschsprung's disease: diagnosis and management, *Am Fam Physician* 74(8):1319–1322, 2006.
27. Levitt MA, Pena A: Anorectal malformations, *Orphanet J Rare Dis* 2:33, 2007.
28. Parikh M, et al: Does all small bowel intussusception need exploration? *Afr J Paediatr Surg* 7(1):30–32, 2010.
29. Shekherdimian S, Lee SL: Management of pediatric intussusception in general hospitals: diagnosis, treatment, and differences based on age, *World J Pediatr* 7(1):70–73, 2011.
30. Blanch AJ, Perel SB, Acworth JP: Paediatric intussusception: epidemiology and outcome, *Emerg Med Australas* 19(1):45–50, 2007.
31. Henry SM: Discerning differences: gastroesophageal reflux and gastroesophageal reflux disease in infants, *Adv Neonatal Care* 4(4):235–247, 2004.
32. Putnam PE: Eosinophilic esophagitis, *Minerva Gastroenterol Dietol* 56(2):139–157, 2010.
33. McGovern MC, Smith MB: Causes of apparent life threatening events in infants: a systematic review, *Arch Dis Child* 89(11):1043–1048, 2004.
34. Dalby K, et al: Reproducibility of 24-hour combined multiple intraluminal impedance (MII) and pH measurements in infants and children. Evaluation of a diagnostic procedure for gastroesophageal reflux disease, *Dig Dis Sci* 52(9):219–265, 2007.

35. Kane TD: Laparoscopic Nissen fundoplication, *Minerva Chir* 64(2): 147–157, 2009.

36. Lek N, Acerini CL: Cystic fibrosis related diabetes mellitus—diagnostic and management challenges, *Curr Diabetes Rev* 6(1):9–16, 2010.

37. Littlewood JM, Wolfe SP, Conway SP: Diagnosis and treatment of intestinal malabsorption in cystic fibrosis, *Pediatr Pulmonol* 41(1):35–49, 2006.

38. Munck A: Nutritional considerations in patients with cystic fibrosis, *Expert Rev Respir Med* 4(1):47–56, 2010.

39. Phung OJ, et al: Recombinant human growth hormone in the treatment of patients with cystic fibrosis, *Pediatrics* 126(5):e1211–e1226, 2010.

40. Rubio-Tapia A, Murray JA: Celiac disease, *Curr Opin Gastroenterol* 26(2):116–122, 2010.

41. Barton SH, Murray JA: Celiac disease and autoimmunity in the gut and elsewhere, *Gastroenterol Clin North Am* 37(2):411–428, 2008:vii.

42. Kaukinen K, et al: Coeliac disease—a diagnostic and therapeutic challenge, *Clin Chem Lab Med* 48(9):1205–1216, 2010.

43. Volta U, Villanacci V: Celiac disease: diagnostic criteria in progress, *Cell Mol Immunol* 8(2):96–102, 2011.

44. Meazza C, et al: Short stature in children with coeliac disease, *Pediatr Endocrinol Rev* 6(4):457–463, 2009.

45. Rossi T: Celiac disease, *Adolesc Med Clin* 15(1):91–103, 2004.

46. Steele R: CRF: Diagnosis and management of coeliac disease in children, *Postgrad Med J* 87(1023):19–25, 2011.

47. Di Sabatino A, Corazza GR: Coeliac disease, *Lancet* 373(9673):1480–1493, 2009.

48. Fergusson P, Tomkins A: HIV prevalence and mortality among children undergoing treatment for severe acute malnutrition in sub-Saharan Africa: a systematic review and meta-analysis, *Trans R Soc Trop Med Hyg* 103(6):541–548, 2009.

49. Grover Z, Ee LC: Protein energy malnutrition, *Pediatr Clin North Am* 56(5):1055–1068, 2009.

50. Maida JM, Mathers K, Alley CL: Pediatric ophthalmology in the developing world, *Curr Opin Ophthalmol* 19(5):403–408, 2008.

51. Cole SZ, Lanham JS: Failure to thrive: an update, *Am Fam Physician* 83(7):829–834, 2011.

52. Levy Y, et al: Diagnostic clues for identification of nonorganic vs. organic causes of food refusal and poor feeding, *J Pediatr Gastroenterol Nutr* 48(3):355–362, 2009.

53. Black MM, et al: Early intervention and recovery among children with failure to thrive: follow-up at age 8, *Pediatrics* 120(1):59–69, 2007.

54. Srinivasan PS, Brandler MD, D'Souza A: Necrotizing enterocolitis, *Clin Perinatol* 35(1):251–272, 2008.

55. Young CM, Kingma SD, Neu J: Ischemia-reperfusion and neonatal intestinal injury, *J Pediatr* 158(2 Suppl):e25–e28, 2011.

56. Petrosyan M, et al: Current concepts regarding the pathogenesis of necrotizing enterocolitis, *Pediatr Surg Int* 25(4):309–318, 2009.

57. Ng PC, Lam HS: Biomarkers for late-onset neonatal sepsis: cytokines and beyond, *Clin Perinatol* 37(3):599–610, 2010.

58. Alfaleh K, et al: Probiotics for prevention of necrotizing enterocolitis in preterm infants, *Cochrane Database Syst Rev* (3): CD005496, 2011.

59. Sola JE, Tepas JJ 3rd, Koniaris LG: Peritoneal drainage versus laparotomy for necrotizing enterocolitis and intestinal perforation: a meta-analysis, *J Surg Res* 161(1):95–100, 2010.

60. Ramani S, Kang G: Viruses causing childhood diarrhoea in the developing world, *Curr Opin Infect Dis* 22(5):477–482, 2009.

61. Soares-Weiser K, et al: Vaccines for preventing rotavirus diarrhea: vaccines in use, *Cochrane Database Syst Rev* (5):CD008521, 2010.

62. Pawlowski SW, Warren CA, Guerrant R: Diagnosis and treatment of acute or persistent diarrhea, *Gastroenterol* 136(6):1874–1886, 2009.

63. Finkbeiner SR, et al: Metagenomic analysis of human diarrhea: vial detection and discovery, *PLoS Pathol* 4(2):e1000011, 2008.

64. Grimwood K, Forbes DA: Acute and persistent diarrhea, *Pediatr Clin North Am* 56(6):1343–1361, 2009.

65. Heyman MB: Committee on Nutrition: Lactose intolerance in infants, children, and adolescents, *Pediatrics* 118(3):1279–1286, 2006.

66. Truman P: Jaundice in the preterm infant, *Pediatr Nurs* 18(5):20–22, 2006.

67. Watchko JF: Identification of neonates at risk for hazardous hyperbilirubinemia: emerging clinical insights, *Pediatr Clin North Am* 56(3):671–687, 2009.

68. De Luca D, Carnielli VP, Paolillo P: Neonatal hyperbilirubinemia and early discharge from the maternity ward, *Eur J Pediatr* 168(9):1025–1030, 2009.

69. Colletti JE, et al: An emergency medicine approach to neonatal hyperbilirubinemia, *Emerg Med Clin North Am* 25(4):1117–1135, 2007:vii.

70. Shapiro SM: Chronic bilirubin encephalopathy: diagnosis and outcome, *Semin Fetal Neonatal Med* 15(3):157–163, 2010.

70a. Watson RL: Hyperbilirubinemia, *Crit Care Nurs Clin North Am* 21(1):97–120, 2009.

71. Hartley JL, Davenport M, Kelly DA: Biliary atresia, *Lancet* 374(9702):1704–1713, 2009.

72. Degertekin B, Lok AS: Update on viral hepatitis, *Curr Opin Gastroenterol* 25(3):180–185, 2008:2009.

73. Klevens RM, et al: The evolving epidemiology of hepatitis A in the United States: incidence and molecular epidemiology from population-based surveillance, 2005-2007, *Arch Intern Med* 170(20):1811–1818, 2010.

74. Slowik MK, Jhaveri R: Hepatitis B and C viruses in infants and young children, *Semin Pediatr Infect Dis* 16(4):296–305, 2005.

75. Grabowski J, Wedemeyer H: Hepatitis delta: immunopathogenesis and clinical challenges, *Dig Dis* 28(1):133–138, 2010.

76. Jonas MM, et al: Hepatitis B Foundation. Treatment of children with chronic hepatitis B virus infection in the United States: patient selection and therapeutic options, *Hepatology* 52(6):2192–2205, 2010.

77. Petrova M, Kamburov V: Breastfeeding and chronic HBV infection: clinical and social implications, *World J Gastroenterol* 16(40):5042–5046, 2010.

78. Jara P, Hierro L: Treatment of hepatitis C in children, *Expert Rev Gastroenterol Hepatol* 4(1):51–61, 2010.

79. Yeung LT, Roberts EA: Current issues in the management of paediatric viral hepatitis, *Liver Int* 30(1):5–18, 2010.

80. Greene MT, Whitington PF: Outcomes in pediatric autoimmune hepatitis, *Curr Gastroenterol Rep* 11(3):248–251, 2009.

81. Badizadegan K, et al: Histopathology of the liver in children with chronic hepatitis C viral infection, *Hepatology* 28(5):1416–1423, 1998.

82. Mack CL, et al: Surgically restoring portal blood flow to the liver in children with primary extrahepatic portal vein thrombosis improves fluid neurocognitive ability, *Pediatrics* 117(3):e405–e412, 2006.

83. Sharif K, McKiernan P, de Ville de Goyet J: Mesoportal bypass for extrahepatic portal vein obstruction in children: close to a cure for most! *J Pediatr Surg* 45(1):272–276, 2010.

84. Brunt EM: Histopathology of non-alcoholic fatty liver disease, *Clin Liver Dis* 13(4):533–544, 2009.

85. Haafiz AB: Liver fibrosis in biliary atresia, *Exp Rev Gastroenterol Hepatol* 4(3):335–343, 2010.

86. Peters L, Rockstroh JK: Biomarkers of fibrosis and impaired liver function in chronic hepatitis C: how well do they predict clinical outcomes? *Curr Opin HIVAIDS* 5(6):517–523, 2010.

87. Maksoud-Filho JG, et al: Long-term follow-up of children with extrahepatic portal vein obstruction: impact of an endoscopic sclerotherapy program on bleeding episodes, hepatic function, hypersplenism, and mortality, *J Pediatr Surg* 44(10):1877–1883, 2009.

Structure and Function of the Musculoskeletal System

Christy L. Crowther-Radulewicz and Kathryn L. McCance

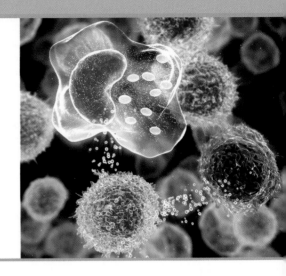

evolve WEBSITE

http://evolve.elsevier.com/Huether/

CHAPTER OUTLINE

The way an individual functions in daily life, moves about, or manipulates objects physically depends on the integrity of the musculoskeletal system. The musculoskeletal system is actually two systems: (1) the skeleton composed of bones and joints and (2) skeletal muscles. Each system contributes to mobility. The skeleton supports the body and provides leverage to the skeletal muscles so that movement of various parts of the body is possible. Contraction of the skeletal muscles and bending or rotation at the joints facilitates movements of the various body parts.

STRUCTURE AND FUNCTION OF BONES

Bones give form to the body, support tissues, and permit movement by providing points of attachment for muscles. Many bones meet in movable joints that determine the type and extent of movement possible. Bones also protect many of the body's vital organs. For example, the bones of the skull, thorax, and pelvis are hard exterior shields that protect the brain, heart and lungs, and reproductive and urinary organs, respectively.

The marrow cavities within certain bones serve as sites of blood cell formation. In adults, blood cells originate exclusively in the marrow cavities of the skull, vertebrae, ribs, sternum, shoulders, and pelvis. The development of blood cells is discussed in Chapter 19. Bones also have a crucial role in mineral homeostasis, storing minerals (i.e., calcium, phosphate, carbonate, magnesium) that are essential for the proper performance of many delicate cellular mechanisms.

Elements of Bone Tissue

Mature bone is a rigid connective tissue consisting of cells, fibers, a gelatinous material termed ground substance, and large amounts of crystallized minerals, mainly calcium, that give bone its rigidity. Ground substance consists of proteoglycans and hyaluronic acid secreted by chondroblasts. The structural elements of bone are summarized in Table 36-1.

Bone cells enable bone to grow, repair itself, change shape, and continuously synthesize new bone tissue and resorb (dissolve or digest) old tissue. The fibers in bone are made of collagen, which gives bone its tensile strength (the ability to hold itself together). Ground substance acts

TABLE 36-1   STRUCTURAL ELEMENTS OF BONE

STRUCTURAL ELEMENTS	FUNCTION
Bone Cells	
Osteoblasts	Synthesize collagen and proteoglycans, mineralize osteoid matrix; produce RANKL, which in turn stimulates osteoclast resorption of bone; also produce osteoprotegerin (OPG), which inhibits osteoclast formation by binding to RANKL
Osteoclasts	Resorb bone; major role in bone homeostasis
Osteocytes	Transform osteoblasts trapped in osteoid; signal both osteoblasts and osteoclasts; maintain bone matrix; mechanosensory receptors to reduce or augment bone mass; produce sclerostin (SOST), which inhibits bone growth
Bone Matrix	
Bone morphogenic proteins (BMPs)	Induce bone and cartilage formation, regulation
BMP-1	Unrelated to other BMPs (is a metalloprotease); key role in extracellular matrix (ECM) formation
BMP-2A	Promotes chondrogenesis
BMP-3 (osteogenin)	Activates TGF-β signaling pathway; inhibits bone formation
BMP-4	Osteoblast differentiation; involved in cartilage repair, enchondral bone formation
BMP-6	Found in osteoblasts; promotes osteoblast differentiation
	Key role in osteoblast differentiation
Collagen fibers	Lend support and tensile strength
Proteoglycans	Control transport of ionized materials through matrix

STRUCTURAL ELEMENTS	FUNCTION
Glycoproteins	
Albumin	Transports essential elements to matrix; maintains osmotic pressure of bone fluid
α-Glycoproteins	Promote calcification
Laminin	Stabilizes basement membranes in bones
Osteocalcin	Vitamin K–dependent protein present in bone; promotes bone resorption; inhibits calcium phosphate precipitation (attracts calcium ions to incorporate into hydroxyapatite crystals); serum osteocalcin is a sensitive marker of bone formation
Osteonectin	Binds calcium in bone
Sialoprotein	Promotes calcification
Minerals	
Calcium	Crystallizes, providing bone rigidity and compressive strength
Phosphate	Balance of organic and inorganic phosphate required for proper bone mineralization; regulates vitamin D, promoting mineralization
Alkaline phosphatase	Promotes mineralization
Vitamins	
Vitamin D	Assists with differentiation, mineralization of osteoblasts
Vitamin K	Increases bone calcification; reduces serum osteocalcin

as a medium for the diffusion of nutrients, oxygen, metabolic wastes, biochemicals, and minerals between bone tissue and blood vessels.

Bone formation begins during fetal life with the growth of cartilage—the precursor of bone tissue. In mature bone, the formation of new tissue begins with the production of an organic matrix by the bone cells. This **bone matrix** consists of ground substance, collagen, and other proteins (see Table 36-1) that take part in bone formation and maintenance.

The next step in bone formation is **calcification,** in which minerals are deposited and then crystallize. Minerals bind tightly to collagen fibers, producing tensile and compressional strength in bone and allowing it to withstand pressure and weight bearing.

Bone Cells

Bone contains three types of cells: osteoblasts, osteocytes, and osteoclasts (Figure 36-1). Osteoblasts are the bone-forming cells. Their primary function is to lay down new bone. Once this function is complete, osteoblasts become osteocytes. Osteocytes are osteoblasts that have become imprisoned within the mineralized bone matrix.

They help maintain bone by synthesizing new bone matrix molecules. Osteoclasts function primarily to resorb (remove) bone during processes of growth and repair.

Osteoblasts. Osteoblasts are multifunctional mononuclear cells derived from osteogenic mesenchymal stromal cells, are the primary bone-producing cells, and are involved in many functions related to the skeletal system (see Table 36-1). Osteoblasts are responsive to parathyroid hormone (PTH) and produce osteocalcin when stimulated by 1,25-dihydroxyvitamin D. Osteoblasts are active on the outer surfaces of bones, where they form a single layer of cells. Osteoblasts initiate new bone formation by their synthesis of osteoid (nonmineralized bone matrix). Osteoblasts also mineralize newly formed bone matrix. Stimulation of new bone formation and orderly mineralization of bone matrix occur by concentrating some of the plasma proteins (growth factors) found in the bone matrix and by facilitating the deposit and exchange of calcium and other ions at the site. Growth factors, including bone morphogenic proteins (BMPs) and other members of the transforming growth factor-beta (TGF-β) superfamily, are critical components of bone formation, maintenance, and remodeling (Table 36-2).

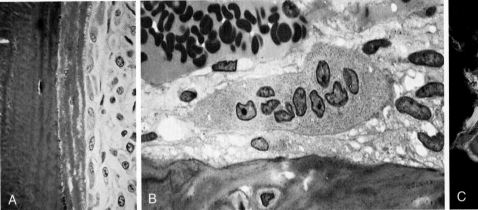

FIGURE 36-1 Bone Cells. A, Osteoblasts are responsible for the production of collagenous and non-collagenous proteins that compose osteoid. Active osteoblasts are lined up on the osteoid. Note the eccentrically located nuclei. **B,** Electron photomicrograph of an osteocyte. Osteocytes reside within the lacunae of compact bone. **C,** Osteoclasts actively resorb mineralized tissue. The scalloped surface in which the multinucleated osteoclasts rest is termed *Howship lacuna.* (**A** and **C** from Damjanov I, Linder J, editors: *Anderson's pathology,* ed 10, St Louis, 1996, Mosby; **B** from Wikimedia Commons, courtesy Robert M. Hunt.)

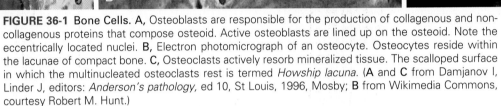

TABLE 36-2	**SELECTED FACTORS AFFECTING BONE FORMATION, MAINTENANCE, AND REMODELING**
FACTOR	**FUNCTION**
Transforming growth factor-beta (TGF-β)	Superfamily of polypeptides; regulates bone formation, many other cellular processes through signaling
Platelet-derived growth factor (PDGF)	Increases number of osteoblasts
Fibroblast growth factor (FGF)	FGF-2 increases osteoblast population, but not function; inhibits alkaline phosphatase activity, osteocalcin, type I collagen, and osteopontin
Insulin-like growth factor (IGF)	
IGF-1	Increases peak bone mass during adolescence; decreases osteoblast apoptosis; maintains bone matrix
IGF-2	Increases BMP-9–induced endochondral ossification
Smad proteins	Mediate signaling cascade of TGF-β, especially in embryonic bone development; play role in cross-talk between BMP/TGF-β and Wnt signaling pathways
Bone morphogenic proteins (BMPs)	Members of TGF-β superfamily of polypeptides; have many functions outside skeletal system; stimulate enchondral bone and cartilage formation and function, promote osteoblast maturation; augment bone remodeling by affecting both osteoblasts and osteoclasts
Tumor necrosis factors (TNFs)	Superfamily of cytokines; play major role in regulating bone metabolism, especially osteoclast function
Osteoprotegerin (OPG)	Inhibits bone remodeling/resorption; produced by several cells, including osteoblasts; is a decoy receptor for RANKL (binds to RANKL, inhibiting RANK/RANKL interactions, suppressing osteoclast formation and bone resorption)
Receptor activator of nuclear factor-κB (RANK)	Stimulates differentiation of osteoclast precursors; activates mature osteoclasts
Receptor activator of nuclear factor-κB ligand (RANKL)	Promotes osteoclast differentiation/activation; inhibits osteoclast apoptosis
Bone morphogenic protein antagonists	Prevent BMP signaling
Noggin	Binds BMP-2 and -4, reducing osteoblast function
Gremlin	Multiple effects in and out of skeletal system, but also binds BMP-2, -4, and -7; may play role in development of osteoporosis
Twisted gastrulation	Acts as either a BMP agonist or a BMP antagonist
Activin (a BMP-related protein)	Affects both osteoblasts and osteoclasts; may promote bone formation and fracture healing; expressed by both osteoblasts and chondrocytes; helps regulate bone mass
Inhibin	Dominant over activin and BMPs; helps regulate bone mass and strength by affecting formation of osteoblasts and osteoclasts
Leptin	Plays role in bone formation and resorption
Wnt (a signaling pathway)	Important in differentiating osteoblasts and bone formation, has overlapping effects with BMPs, helps regulate bone formation and remodeling

TABLE 36-2	SELECTED FACTORS AFFECTING BONE FORMATION, MAINTENANCE, AND REMODELING—cont'd	
FACTOR	**FUNCTION**	
Wnt antagonists		
Dickkopf family (Dkk)	Disrupt Wnt signaling, leading to reduced bone mass	
Sclerostin	A protein secreted by osteocytes, osteoblasts, and osteoclasts; binds to BMP-6 and BMP-7; interferes with Wnt signaling pathway, inhibiting bone formation by osteoblasts	
Transcription factors		
Nuclear factor of activated B cells (NF-κB)	Affects embryonic osteoclastogenesis; plays role in certain osteoclast, osteoblast, and chondroblast functions	
Matrix metalloproteinases (MMPs)		
Family of endopeptidases (enzymes) that includes collagenases, gelatinases, stromelysins, matrilysins	Help maintain equilibrium of extracellular matrix (ECM); breakdown almost all components of ECM	
A disintegrin and metalloproteinase (ADAM)	Proteolytic enzymes; also have cell-signaling functions, usually linked to cell membrane	
A disintegrin and metalloproteinase with thrombospondin motifs (ADAMTS)	Similar to ADAMs but are secreted into circulation, are found around cells; various subgroups affect multiple tissues	
Cysteine protease	Cathepsin K expressed by osteoclasts; assists in bone remodeling by cleaving proteins, such as collagen type I, collagen type II, and osteonectin	
MMP inhibitors		
Tetracyclines (especially doxycycline), bisphosphonates	Block enzymatic function of MMPs	
Tissue inhibitors of metalloproteinases (TIMPs)	Balance effect of MMPs in maintaining ECM equilibrium	

From Boyce BF, Yao Z, Xing L: Functions of NF κB in bone, *Ann N Y Acad Sci* 1192:367–375, 2010; Canalis E: Growth factor control of bone mass, *J Cell Biol* 108(4):769–777, 2009; Kim Y-S et al: Integrative physiology: defined novel metabolic roles of osteocalcin, *J Korean Med Sci* 25:985–991, 2010; Moester MJ et al: Sclerostin: current knowledge and future prospects, *Calcif Tissue Int* 87(2):99–107, 2010; Nicks KN et al: Regulation of osteoblastogenesis and osteoclastogenesis by the other reproductive hormones, activin and inhibin, *Mol Cell Endocrinol* 310(1–2):11–20, 2009; Pasternak B, Aspenberg P: Metalloproteineases and their inhibitors—diagnostic and therapeutic opportunities in orthopedics, *Acta Orthopaedica* 80(6):693–703, 2009; Stewart A, Guan H, Yang K: BBMP-3 mesenchymal stem cell proliferation through the TGF-beta/activin signaling pathway, *J Cell Physiol* 223(3):658–666, 2010; Tat SK et al: New perspectives in osteoarthritis: the OPG and RANKL system as a potential therapeutic target? *Keio Med J* 58(1):29–40, 2009.

Osteoblasts use intercellular calcium signaling to include osteoclastic activity. One of the most important discoveries linking osteoblast and osteoclast function is that of the cytokine **receptor activator nuclear factor kappa-B ligand**, or RANKL (see below). RANKL is expressed on osteoblasts and is necessary for forming osteoclasts (see Osteoclasts). In contact with bone mineral, osteoclasts can be further stimulated by colony-stimulating factor and interleukins-1, -3, and -6 produced by macrophage cells in the presence of PTH.[1] Thus the cells of the osteoblastic lineage (osteoblasts, osteocytes) form a network of cells in bone that sense the shape and structure of bone and determine where it is appropriate that bone be formed or resorbed, according to Wolff law (bone is shaped according to its function).

Originating from mesenchymal stem cells (MSCs), osteoblasts are specialized fibroblasts that have both an active and a resting state. Osteoblasts synthesize and secrete osteoid when active and when in the resting state are termed *satellite cells*. If appropriately stimulated, however, the resting osteoblasts are capable of resuming activity.

Osteoclasts. Osteoclasts are large (typically 20 to 100 μm in diameter), multinucleated cells that develop from the hematopoietic monocyte-macrophage lineage. Osteoclasts are the major resorptive cells of bone. They migrate over bone surfaces to resorption areas that have been prepared and stripped of osteoid by enzymes, such as collagenases produced by osteoblasts in the presence of PTH, which is necessary for the resorptive process. Osteoclasts travel over the prepared bone surfaces, creating irregular, scalloped cavities, known as *Howship lacunae* or *resorption bays,* as they resorb bone areas and then acidify hydroxyapatite in order to dissolve it.

A specific area of the cell membrane forms adjacent to the bone surface and forms multiple infoldings to permit intimate contact with the resorption bay. These infoldings, known as the **ruffled border,** greatly increase the surface areas of cells under their scalloped or ruffled borders. Osteoclasts resorb bone by secretion of hydrochloric acid and acid proteinases (such as cathepsin K) that help digest collagen, along with the action of cytokines (see Table 36-2). Osteoclasts also resorb bone through the action of lysosomes (digestive vacuoles) filled with hydrolytic enzymes in their mitochondria.

Osteoclasts bind to the bone surfaces through attachments called **integrins.**[2] Once resorption is complete, the osteoclasts retract and loosen from the bone surface under the ruffled border through the action of calcitonin. Calcitonin binds to receptor areas of the osteoclasts' cell membranes to effectively loosen the osteoclasts from the bone surfaces. Once resorption is completed, osteoclasts disappear by the process of degeneration, either by reverting to the form of their parent cells or by undergoing cell movements away from the site, in which the osteoclast becomes an inactive or resting osteoclast.

OPG/RANKL/RANK SYSTEM Osteoprotegerin (OPG) inhibits bone remodeling/resorption. It is produced by numerous cells, including osteoblasts. Basically, OPG is key in the interaction between osteoblasts and osteoclasts. Osteoblasts and osteoclasts cooperate to maintain normal bone homeostasis. RANKL is an essential cytokine needed for the formation and activation of osteoclasts (see above). RANKL, like an automobile's accelerator, increases bone loss. OPG, similar to the car brakes, decreases bone loss because when it is activated it promotes bone formation. When RANKL binds to its receptor RANK on osteoclast precursor cells, it triggers their proliferation and increases bone resorption. OPG secreted by the bone matrix serves as a decoy by binding to RANK—preventing RANKL binding to RANK and thus preventing bone resorption. Therefore, the overall balance between RANKL and OPG determines the amount of bone loss. The balance between RANKL and OPG is regulated by cytokines and hormones. Alterations of the RANKL/RANK/OPG system can lead to dysregulation and pathologic conditions, including primary osteoporosis, immune-mediated bone diseases, malignant bone disorders, and inherited skeletal diseases (see Figure 36-5).

Osteocytes. An **osteocyte** is a transformed osteoblast that is trapped or surrounded in osteoid as it hardens as a result of minerals that enter during calcification (see Figure 36-1, *B*). The osteocyte is within a space in the hardened bone matrix called a **lacuna**. Each osteocyte has a high nucleus/cytoplasm ratio with a thin layer of nonmineralized osteoid around it, like the egg white surrounding an egg yolk.

Osteocytes are the most abundant cells found in bone and have numerous functions, including acting as mechanoreceptors and synthesizing certain matrix molecules, playing a major role in controlling osteoblast differentiation and production of growth factors, and maintaining bone homeostasis.[3,4] They also help concentrate nutrients in the matrix. Osteocytes obtain nutrients from capillaries in the canaliculi, which contain nutrient-rich fluids. Through exchanges among these cells, hormone catalysts, and minerals, optimal levels of calcium, phosphorus, and other minerals are maintained in blood plasma. The osteocyte also aids in modifying bone matrix through the release of enzymes to dissolve the mineralized walls of the lacunae to prepare the bone for remodeling. Remodeling is described on p. 962.

Bone Matrix

Bone matrix is made of the *extracellular elements* of bone tissue, specifically collagen fibers, proteins, carbohydrate-protein complexes, ground substance, and minerals.

Collagen fibers. Collagen fibers make up the bulk of bone matrix. They are formed as follows:
1. Osteoblasts synthesize and secrete type I collagen.
2. Collagen molecules assemble into three thin chains (alpha chains) to form **fibrils**.
3. Fibrils organize into the staggered pattern, with each fibril overlapping its nearest neighbor by about one fourth its length. This creates gaps into which mineral crystals are deposited.
4. After mineral deposition, fibrils interlink and twist to form ropelike fibers.
5. The fibers join to form the framework that gives bone its tensile and supportive strength.

Proteoglycans. Proteoglycans are large complexes of numerous polysaccharides attached to a common protein core. They strengthen bone by forming compression-resistant networks between the collagen fibers. Proteoglycans also control the transport and distribution of electrically charged particles (ions), particularly calcium, through the bone matrix, thereby playing a role in bone calcium deposition and calcification.

Glycoproteins. Glycoproteins are carbohydrate-protein complexes that control the collagen interactions that lead to fibril formation. They also may function in calcification. Four glycoproteins are present in bone: **sialoprotein**, which binds easily with calcium; **osteocalcin**, which binds preferentially to crystallized calcium; **bone albumin**, which is identical to serum albumin and possibly transports essential nutrients to and from bone cells and maintains the osmotic pressure of **bone fluid**; and **alpha-glycoprotein** (α-glycoprotein), which probably plays a significant role in calcification and also may facilitate bone resorption by activating osteoclasts (see Table 36-1).

Bone Minerals

After collagen synthesis and fiber formation, **mineralization**, the final step, occurs in areas known as matrix vesicles that "bud" from the surfaces of osteoblasts, chondrocytes (cartilage cells), and odontoblasts

(cells that form dentin in teeth).[5,6] Mineralization has two distinct phases: (1) formation of the initial mineral deposit (initiation) and (2) proliferation or accretion of additional mineral crystals on the initial mineral deposits (growth). The majority of the minerals in the body are an analog of the naturally occurring mineral *hydroxyapatite.* The hydroxyapatite crystals then penetrate the matrix vesicle membrane and enter into the extracellular space.[5,6]

Table 36-3 lists the sequence in which calcium and phosphate form amorphous (fluid) calcium phosphate compounds that are converted, in stages, to solid hexagonal crystals of **hydroxyapatite (HAP)**. As the

TABLE 36-3	SEQUENCE OF CALCIUM AND PHOSPHATE COMPOUND FORMATION AND CRYSTALLIZATION*	
FORMULA	**NAME**	**ABBREVIATION**
$Ca(HPO_4) \cdot 2H_2O$	Dicalcium phosphate dihydrate	DCPD
$Ca_4H(PO_4)_3$	Octacalcium phosphate	OCP
$Ca_9(PO_4)_6$ (var.)	Amorphous calcium phosphate	ACP
$Ca_3(PO_4)_2$	Tricalcium phosphate	TCP
$Ca_5(PO_4)_3OH$	Hydroxyapatite	HAP

*Compounds are listed in the order in which precipitation and crystal formation occur.

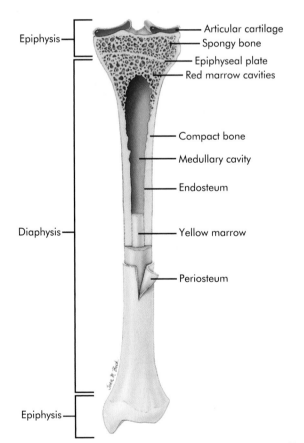

FIGURE 36-2 Cross Section of Bone. Longitudinal section of long bone (tibia) showing spongy (cancellous) and compact bone. (From Thibodeau GA, Patton KT: *Anatomy & physiology,* ed 6, St Louis, 2007, Mosby.)

Labels for Figure 36-2:
- Epiphysis
- Articular cartilage
- Spongy bone
- Epiphyseal plate
- Red marrow cavities
- Compact bone
- Medullary cavity
- Endosteum
- Diaphysis
- Yellow marrow
- Periosteum
- Epiphysis

calcium and phosphorus concentrations increase in the bone matrix, the first precipitate to form is dicalcium phosphate dihydrate (DCPD). Once DCPD precipitation begins, the remaining phases of bone crystal formation proceed until insoluble HAP is produced, with approximately 80% to 90% of the HAP incorporated into the collagen fibers. Amorphous calcium phosphate is distributed throughout the bone matrix.

Types of Bone Tissue

Bone is composed of two types of bony (osseous) tissue: compact bone (cortical bone) and spongy bone (cancellous bone) (Figure 36-2). Cortical bone comprises about 85% of the skeleton; cancellous bone makes up the remaining 15%. Both types of bone tissue contain the same structural elements, with a few exceptions. In addition, both compact

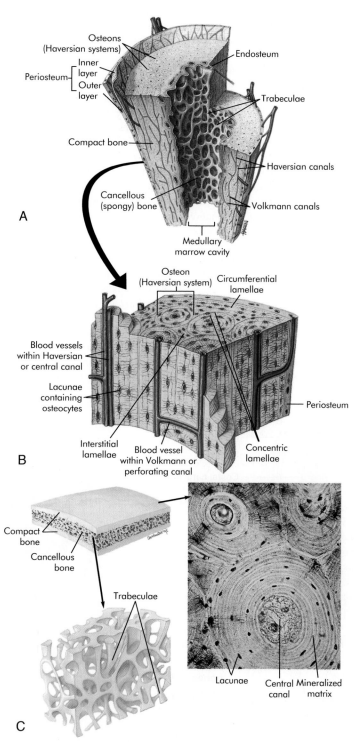

FIGURE 36-3 Structure of Compact and Cancellous Bone. **A,** Longitudinal section of a long bone showing both cancellous and compact bone. **B,** Magnified view of compact bone. **C,** Section of a flat bone. Outer layers of compact bone surround cancellous bone. Fine structure of compact and cancellous bone is shown to the right. (From Thibodeau GA, Patton KT: *Anatomy & physiology,* ed 6, St Louis, 2007, Mosby.)

tissue and spongy tissue are present in every bone. The major difference between the two types of tissue is the organization of the elements.

Compact bone is highly organized, solid, and extremely strong. The basic structural unit in compact bone is the haversian system (Figure 36-3). Each haversian system consists of the following:
1. A central canal called the haversian canal
2. Concentric layers of bone matrix called lamellae (sing., lamella)
3. Tiny spaces (lacunae) between the lamellae
4. Bone cells (osteocytes) within the lacunae
5. Small channels or canals called canaliculi (sing., canaliculus)

Spongy bone is less complex and lacks haversian systems. In spongy bone, the lamellae are not arranged in concentric layers but in plates or bars termed trabeculae (sing., trabecula) that branch and unite with one another to form an irregular meshwork. The pattern of the meshwork is determined by the direction of stress on the particular bone. The spaces between the trabeculae are filled with red bone marrow. The osteocyte-containing lacunae are distributed between the trabeculae and interconnected by canaliculi. Capillaries pass through the marrow to nourish the osteocytes.

All bones are covered with a double-layered connective tissue called the periosteum. The outer layer of the periosteum contains blood vessels and nerves, some of which penetrate to the inner structures of the bone through channels called *Volkmann canals* (see Figure 36-3). The inner layer of the periosteum is anchored to the bone by collagenous fibers (Sharpey fibers) that penetrate the bone. Sharpey fibers also help hold or attach tendons and ligaments to the periosteum of bones.

Characteristics of Bone

The 206 bones of the human skeleton are distributed between the axial skeleton and the appendicular skeleton. The axial skeleton—the skull, vertebral column, and thorax—consists of 80 bones. The other 126 bones of the appendicular skeleton comprise the upper and lower extremities, the shoulder girdle (pectoral girdle), and the pelvic girdle

(os coxae) (Figure 36-4). The skeleton contributes approximately 14% of an adult's body weight.

Bones can be classified by shape as long, flat, short (cuboidal), or irregular. Long bones are longer than they are wide and consist of a narrow tubular midportion (diaphysis) that merges into a broader neck (metaphysis) and a broad end (epiphysis) (see Figure 36-2).

The diaphysis consists of a shaft of thick, rigid compact bone that is able to tolerate bending forces. Contained within the diaphysis is the elongated marrow (medullary) cavity. The marrow cavity of the diaphysis contains primarily fatty tissue, which is referred to as *yellow marrow*. The yellow marrow assists red bone marrow in hematopoiesis only during times of stress. The yellow marrow cavity of the diaphysis is continuous with marrow cavities in the spongy bone of the metaphysis and diaphysis. The marrow contained within the epiphysis is red because it contains primarily blood-forming tissue (see Chapter 19). A layer of connective tissue, the endosteum, lines the outer surfaces of both types of marrow cavity.

The broadness of the epiphysis allows weight bearing to be distributed over a wide area. The epiphysis is made up of spongy bone covered by a thin layer of compact bone. In a child, the epiphysis is separated from the metaphysis by a cartilaginous growth plate (epiphyseal plate). After puberty, the epiphyseal plate calcifies and the epiphysis and metaphysis merge. By adulthood, the line of demarcation between the epiphysis and metaphysis is undetectable.

In flat bones, such as the ribs and scapulae, two plates of compact bone are nearly parallel to each other. Between the compact bone plates is a layer of spongy bone. Short bones, such as the bones of the wrist or ankle, are often cuboidal. They consist of spongy bone covered by a thin layer of compact bone.

Irregular bones, such as the vertebrae, mandibles, or other facial bones, have various shapes that include thin and thick segments. The thin part of an irregular bone consists of two plates of compact bone surrounding spongy bone. The thick part consists of spongy bone surrounded by a layer of compact bone.

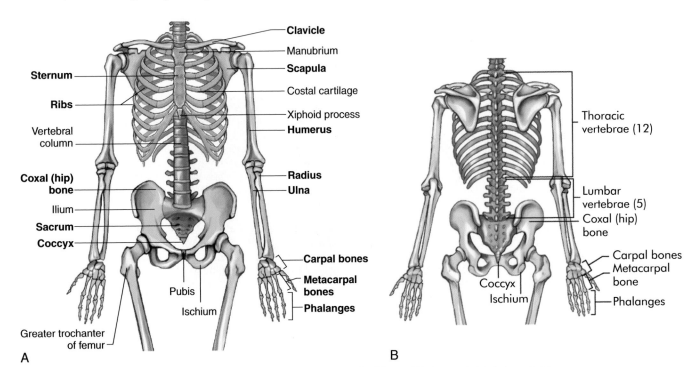

FIGURE 36-4 A, Anterior View of Skeleton. **B,** Posterior View of Skeleton. Axial skeleton in blue; appendicular skeleton in tan. (From Patton KT, Thibodeau GA: *Anatomy & physiology,* ed 7, St Louis, 2010, Mosby.)

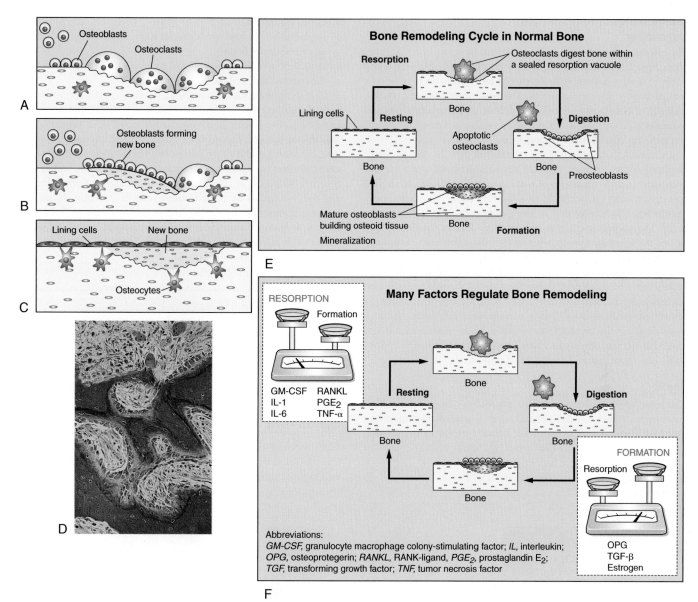

FIGURE 36-5 Bone Remodeling. All bone cells participate in bone remodeling. In the remodeling sequence bone sections are removed by bone-resorbing cells (osteoclasts) and replaced a with new section laid down by bone-forming cells (osteoblasts). Bone remodeling is necessary because it allows the skeleton to respond to mechanical loading, maintains quality control (repair and prevent microdamage), and allows the skeleton to release growth factors and minerals (calcium and phosphate) stored in bone matrix to the circulation. The cells work in response to signals generated in the environment (see **F**). Only the osteoclastic cells mediate the first phase of remodeling. They are activated, scoop out bone (**A**), and resorb it, then the work of the osteoblasts begins (**B**). They form new bone that replaces bone removed by the resorption process (**C**). The sequence takes 4 to 6 months. **D,** Micrograph of active bone remodeling seen in the settings of primary or secondary hyperparathyroidism. Note the active osteoblasts surmounted on red-stained osteoid. Marrow fibrosis is present. **E,** Bone remodeling cycle in normal bone with (**F**). Numerous signaling factors are necessary for remodeling. Factors most important for resorption include granulocyte macrophage-colony stimulating factor (GM-CSF), Interleukins (IL) 1 and 6, receptor activator for nuclear factor κβ ligand (RANKL), prostaglandin E_2 (PGE_2) and tumor necrosis factor alpha (TNF-α). Important factors for bone formation include osteoprotegerin (OPG), transforming growth factor beta (TGF-β) and estrogen. (Adapted nucleus medical art. **D** from Damjananov I, Linder J, ed: *Anderson's pathology*; ed 10, St Louis, 1996, Mosby.)

Maintenance of Bone Integrity

Remodeling

The internal structure of bone is maintained by remodeling, a three-phase process in which existing bone is resorbed and new bone is laid down to replace it. Remodeling is carried out by clusters of bone cells termed basic multicellular units. The basic multicellular units are made up of bone precursor cells that differentiate into osteoclasts and osteoblasts. Precursor cells are located on the free surfaces of bones and along the vascular channels (especially the marrow cavities).

In phase 1 (activation) of the remodeling cycle, a stimulus (e.g., hormone, drug, vitamin, physical stressor) activates the bone cell precursors in a localized area of bone to form osteoclasts. In phase 2 (resorption), the osteoclasts form a "cutting cone," which gradually resorbs bone, leaving behind an elongated cavity termed a *resorption cavity*. The resorption cavity in compact bone follows the longitudinal axis of the haversian system, whereas the resorption cavity in spongy bone parallels the surface of the trabeculae.

Phase 3 (formation) is the laying down of new bone, termed *secondary bone*, by osteoblasts lining the walls of the resorption cavity. Successive layers (lamellae) in compact bone are laid down, until the resorption cavity is reduced to a narrow haversian canal around a blood vessel. In this way, old haversian systems are destroyed and new haversian systems are formed. New trabeculae are formed in spongy bone. The entire process of remodeling takes about 3 to 6 months.

Repair

The remodeling process can repair microscopic bone injuries, but gross injuries, such as fractures and surgical wounds (osteotomies), heal by the same stages as soft tissue injuries, except that new bone, instead of scar tissue, is the final result (see Chapter 5). The stages of bone healing are listed here and shown in Figure 36-5:

1. Inflammation/hematoma formation
2. Procallus formation
3. Callus formation
4. Replacement, by basic multicellular units, of the callus with lamellar or trabecular bone
5. Remodeling of the periosteal and endosteal surfaces of the bone to the size and shape of the bone before injury

The speed with which bone heals depends on the severity of the bone disruption; the type and amount of bone tissue that need to be replaced (spongy bone heals faster); the blood and oxygen supply available at the site; the presence of growth and thyroid hormones, insulin, vitamins, and other nutrients; the existence of systemic disease; the effects of aging (see Chapter 37, "Osteoporosis," on p. 987); and the availability of effective treatment, including immobilization and the prevention of complications such as infection. In general, however, hematoma formation occurs within hours of fracture or surgery, formation of procallus by osteoblasts within days, callus formation within weeks, and replacement and contour modeling within years—up to 4 years in some cases.

> ✓ **QUICK CHECK 36-1**
> 1. Name the different types of bone cells.
> 2. What are the major cells involved in bone resorption?
> 3. What are the stages of bone wound healing?
> 4. Briefly describe the process of remodeling.

STRUCTURE AND FUNCTION OF JOINTS

The site where two or more bones are attached is called a joint, or articulation (Figure 36-6). The primary function of joints is to provide stability and mobility to the skeleton. A joint's function depends on both its location and its structure. Generally, joints that stabilize the

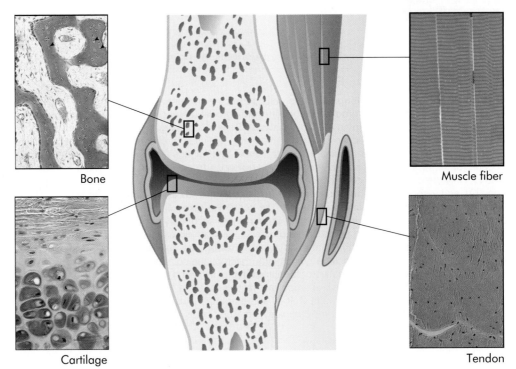

Bone

Cartilage

Muscle fiber

Tendon

FIGURE 36-6 Main Tissues of a Joint. (Micrographs from Gartner LP, Hiatt JL: *Color textbook of histology,* ed 3, Philadelphia, 2007, Saunders.)

skeleton have a simpler structure than those that enable the skeleton to move. Most joints provide both stability and mobility to some degree (Figure 36-7).

Joints are classified based on the degree of movement they permit or on the connecting tissues that hold them together. Based on movement, a joint is classified as a **synarthrosis (immovable joint)**, an **amphiarthrosis (slightly movable joint)**, or a **diarthrosis (freely movable joint)**. On the basis of connective structures, joints are classified broadly as fibrous, cartilaginous, or synovial. Each of these three structural classifications can be subdivided according to the shape and contour of the articulating surfaces (ends) of the bones and the type of motion the joint permits.

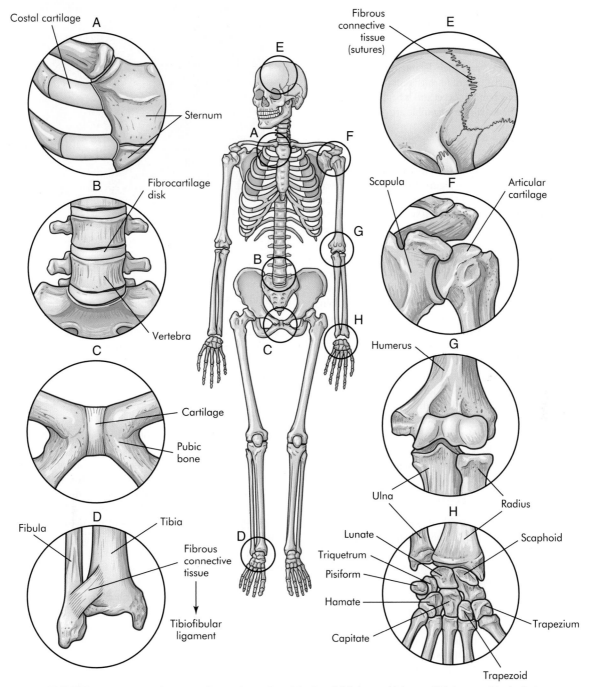

FIGURE 36-7 Types of Joints. Cartilaginous (amphiarthrodial) joints, which are slightly movable, include **(A)** a synchondrosis that attaches ribs to costal cartilage, **(B)** a symphysis that connects vertebrae, and **(C)** the symphysis that connects the two pubic bones. Fibrous (synarthrodial) joints, which are immovable, include **(D)** the syndesmosis between the tibia and fibula and **(E)** sutures that connect the skull bones and the gomphosis (not shown), which holds teeth in their sockets. The synovial joints include **(F)** the spheroid type at the shoulder, **(G)** the hinge type at the elbow, and **(H)** the gliding joints of the hand.

Fibrous Joints

A joint in which bone is united directly to bone by fibrous connective tissue is called a **fibrous joint** (see Figure 36-7, *D*). These joints have no joint cavity and allow little, if any, movement.

Fibrous joints are further subdivided into three types: sutures, syndesmoses, and gomphoses. A **suture** (see Figure 36-7, *E*) has a thin layer of dense fibrous tissue that binds together interlocking flat bones in the skulls of young children. Sutures form an extremely tight union that permits no motion. By adulthood, the fibrous tissue has been replaced by bone. A **syndesmosis** is a joint (see Figure 36-7, *F-H*) in which the two bony surfaces are united by a ligament or membrane. The fibers of ligaments are flexible and stretch, permitting a limited amount of movement. The paired bones of the lower arm (radius and ulna) and the lower leg (tibia and fibula) and their ligaments are syndesmotic joints. A **gomphosis** is a special type of fibrous joint in which a conical projection fits into a complementary socket and is held in place by a ligament. The teeth held in the maxilla or mandible are gomphosis joints.

Cartilaginous Joints

There are two types of cartilaginous joints: symphyses and synchondroses. A **symphysis** is a cartilaginous joint in which bones are united by a pad or disk of fibrocartilage (see Figure 36-7, *B, C*). A thin layer of hyaline cartilage usually covers the articulating surfaces of these two bones, and the thick pad of fibrocartilage acts as a shock absorber and stabilizer. Examples of symphyses are the symphysis pubis, which joins the two pubic bones, and the intervertebral disks, which join the bodies of the vertebrae. A **synchondrosis** is a joint (see Figure 36-7, *A*) in which hyaline cartilage, rather than fibrocartilage, connects the two bones. The joints between the ribs and the sternum are synchondroses. The hyaline cartilage of these joints is called *costal cartilage.* Slight movement at the synchondroses between the ribs and the sternum allows the chest to move outward and upward during breathing.

Joint (Articular) Capsule

The **joint (articular) capsule** is fibrous connective tissue that covers the ends of bones where they meet in a joint; Sharpey fibers firmly attach the proximal and distal capsule to the periosteum, and ligaments and tendons also may reinforce the capsule. It is composed of parallel, interlacing bundles of dense, white fibrous tissue richly supplied with nerves, blood vessels, and lymphatic vessels. Nerves in and around the joint capsule are sensitive to rate and direction of motion, compression, tension, vibration, and pain.

Synovial Membrane

The **synovial membrane** is a smooth, delicate inner lining of joint capsule found in the nonarticular portion of the synovial joint and any ligaments or tendons that traverse this cavity. It is composed of two layers: vascular subintima and thin cellular intima. Vascular intima merges with the fibrous joint capsule and is composed of loose fibrous connective tissue, elastin fibers, fat cells, fibroblasts, macrophages, and mast cells; intima consists of rows of synovial cells embedded in fiber-free intercellular matrix and contains two types of cells—**A** and **B**. **A** cells ingest and remove (phagocytose) bacteria and particles of debris in the joint cavity; **B** cells secrete hyaluronate, which gives synovial fluid its viscous quality. The synovial membrane is richly supplied with blood and lymphatic vessels and is capable of rapid repair and regeneration.

Joint (Synovial) Cavity

The **joint (synovial) cavity** is an enclosed, fluid-filled space between articulating surfaces of two bones, also called *joint space.* It enables two bones to move "against" one another and is surrounded by synovial membrane and filled with synovial fluid.

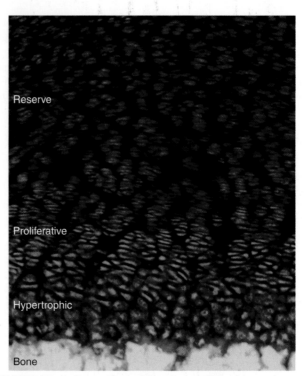

FIGURE 36-8 Collagen Zones. The three collagen zones (reserve, proliferative, and hypertrophic) are distinctly shown in a growth plate. (From Hjorten R et al: *Bone* 41[4]:535, 2007.)

Synovial Fluid

Synovial fluid is superfiltrated plasma from blood vessels that lubricates the joint surfaces, nourishes the pad of the articular cartilage, and covers the ends of the bones. Hyaluronic acid in the synovial fluid gives it important biomechanical properties. It also contains free-floating synovial cells and various leukocytes that phagocytose joint debris and microorganisms.

Articular Cartilage

Articular cartilage is a layer of hyaline cartilage that covers the end of each bone; it may be thick or thin, depending on the size of the joint, the fit of the two bone ends, and the amount of weight and shearing force the joint normally withstands. The function of articular cartilage is to reduce friction in the joint and to distribute the forces of weight bearing. Articular cartilage is composed of **chondrocytes** (cartilage cells) (making up about 2% of the tissue) and an intercellular matrix consisting of type II collagen (making up about 10% to 30% of weight), protein polysaccharides (making up 5% to 10% of weight), and water. The water content ranges from 60% to almost 80% of the net weight of the cartilage, and individual molecules rapidly enter or exit the articular cartilage to contribute to the resiliency of the tissue.

At the surface of articular cartilage, the collagen fibers run parallel to the joint surface and are closely compacted into a dense, protective mat. (Loss of this dense, compacted configuration at the surface subjects the underlying fibers to splitting and thinning, in which case the cartilage is unable to tolerate weight bearing.) In the middle layer (the proliferative zone) of the cartilage, the fibers are arranged tangential to the surface, which allows them to deform and absorb some of the weight bearing (Figure 36-8). In the bottom layer (the hypertrophic zone) of the cartilage, the fibers are perpendicular to the joint surface, allowing them to resist shear forces, and are embedded in a calcified layer of cartilage called the *tidemark.* The **tidemark** anchors the collagen fibers to the underlying (subchondral) bone. Collagen fibers are

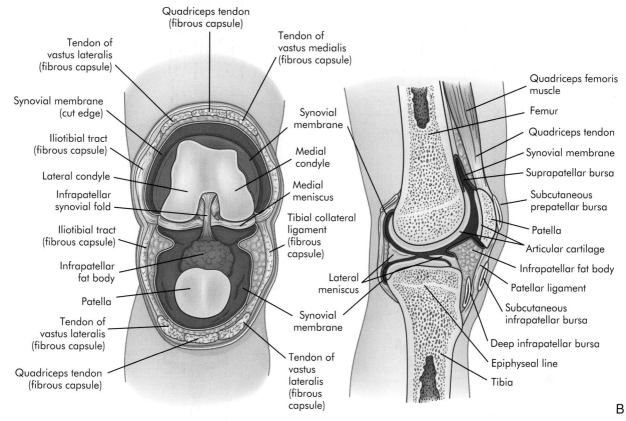

FIGURE 36-9 Knee Joint (Synovial Joint). **A,** Frontal view. **B,** Lateral view.

important components of the cartilage matrix because they account for approximately 60% of the dry weight and because they (1) anchor the cartilage securely to underlying bone, (2) provide a taut framework for the cartilage, (3) control the loss of fluid from the cartilage, and (4) prevent the escape of protein polysaccharides (proteoglycans) from the cartilage. The proteoglycans give articular cartilage its stiff quality and regulate the movement of synovial fluid through the cartilage. The proteoglycans are macromolecules consisting of proteins, carbohydrates (glycosaminoglycans), and hyaluronic acid.

Synovial Joints
Structure of Synovial Joints

Synovial joints (diarthroses) are the most movable and the most complex joints in the body (Figure 36-9).

Movement of Synovial Joints

Synovial joints are described as uniaxial, biaxial, or multiaxial according to the shapes of the bone ends and the type of movement occurring at the joint (Figure 36-10). Usually, one of the bones is stable and serves as an axis for the motion of the other bone. The body movements made possible by various synovial joints are either circular or angular (Figure 36-11).

> **✔ QUICK CHECK 36-2**
> 1. How do the following joints differ from each other: synarthrosis, amphiarthrosis, and diarthrosis?
> 2. Name at least two characteristics of each of the joints in the previous question that either facilitate or hinder movement.
> 3. Name three functions of articular cartilage.

STRUCTURE AND FUNCTION OF SKELETAL MUSCLES

Skeletal muscles arise from mesodermal precursor cells that then form myoblasts. The millions of individual fibers of skeletal muscle contract and relax to perform the work necessary to move the body (Figure 36-12). Muscle constitutes 40% of an adult's body weight and 50% of a child's weight. Muscle is 75% water, 20% protein, and 5% organic and inorganic compounds. Thirty-two percent of all protein stores for energy and metabolism are contained in muscle. Between the ages of 30 and 60, muscle mass decreases by about 0.5 pound of muscle each year. For each 0.5 pound of muscle lost, almost 1 pound of fat is typically gained.

Whole Muscle

There are more than 600 skeletal muscles in the body. The body's muscles vary dramatically in size and shape. They range from 2 to 60 cm in length and are shaped according to function. Fusiform muscles are elongated muscles shaped like straps and can run from one joint to another. The biceps brachii and psoas major are examples of fusiform muscles. Pennate muscles are broad, flat, and slightly fan shaped, with fibers running obliquely to the muscle's long axis. The multipennate deltoid muscle, which flexes and extends the arm, is a good example of a muscle shaped according to its function.

Each skeletal muscle is a separate organ, encased in a three-part connective tissue framework called fascia. The layers of connective tissue protect the muscle fibers, attach the muscle to bony prominences, and provide a structure for a network of nerve fibers, blood vessels, and lymphatic channels. The layers are as follows:

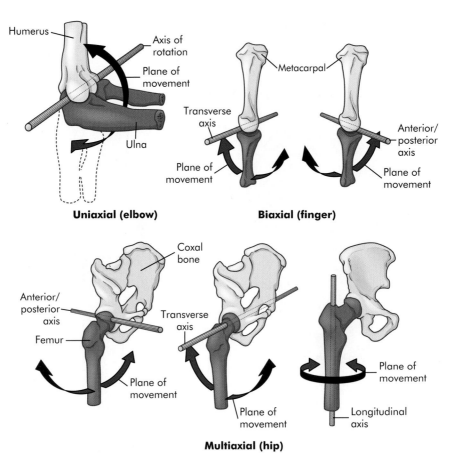

FIGURE 36-10 Movements of Synovial (Diarthrodial) Joints.

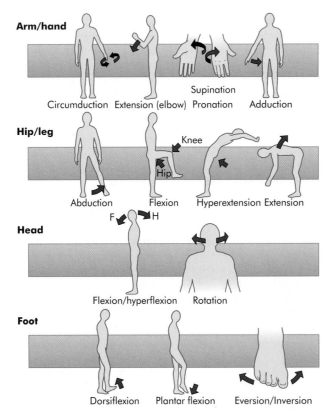

FIGURE 36-11 Body Movements Made Possible by Synovial (Diarthrodial) Joints.

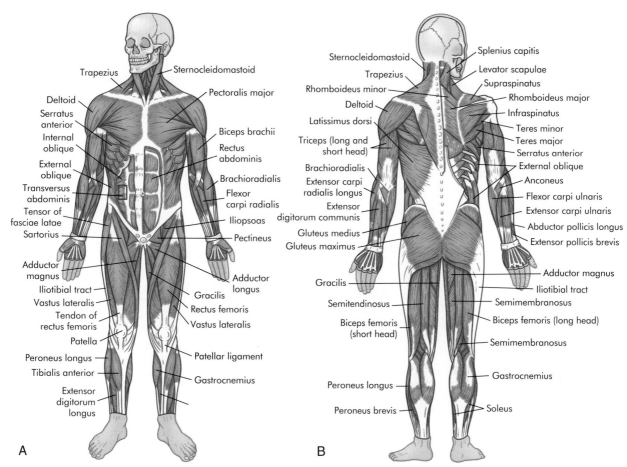

FIGURE 36-12 Skeletal Muscles of Body. **A,** Anterior view. **B,** Posterior view.

1. The outermost layer, the **epimysium,** is located on the surface of the muscle and tapers at each end to form the **tendon** (Figure 36-13, also see p. 973 for a discussion of tendons). Tendons allow short muscles to exert power on a distant joint, whereas a thick muscle would interfere with the joint's mobility.
2. The **perimysium** further subdivides the muscle fibers into bundles of connective tissue, or **fascicles.**
3. The smallest unit of muscle visible without a microscope is the **endomysium,** which surrounds the muscle.

The ligaments, tendons, and fascia are made up of connective tissue that also buffers the limbs from the effects of sudden strains or changes in speed. The rapid recovery necessary for strenuous exercise is supported by the elastic property of muscle and its connective tissue.

Skeletal muscle has been designated as **voluntary** (controlled directly by the nervous system), **striated** (has a striped pattern when viewed under a light microscope), or **extrafusal** (to distinguish from other contractile fibers in the sensory organ of the muscle). Components that are visible on gross inspection of the whole muscle include the motor and sensory nerve fibers. These function together with the muscle, innervating portions of it and providing the electrical impulses needed for motor function.

Motor Unit

From the anterior horn cell of the spinal cord, the axons of motor nerves branch to innervate a specific group of muscle fibers. Each anterior horn cell, its axon (part of the lower motor neuron; see

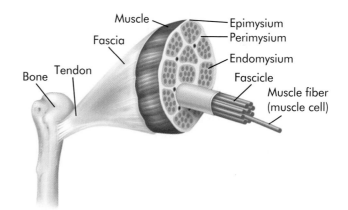

FIGURE 36-13 Cross Section of Skeletal Muscle Showing Muscle Fibers and Their Coverings. (From Thibodeau GA, Patton KT: *Anatomy & physiology,* ed 6, St Louis, 2007, Mosby.)

Chapter 12), and the muscle fibers innervated by it are called a **motor unit** (Figure 36-14). The motor units are composed of lower motor neurons, which extend to skeletal muscles. Often termed the *functional unit* of the neuromuscular system, the motor unit behaves as a single entity and contracts as a whole when it receives an electrical impulse.

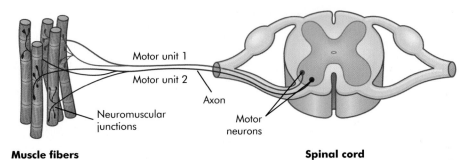

FIGURE 36-14 Motor Units of a Muscle. Each motor unit consists of a motor neuron and all the muscle fibers (cells) supplied by the neuron and its axon branches.

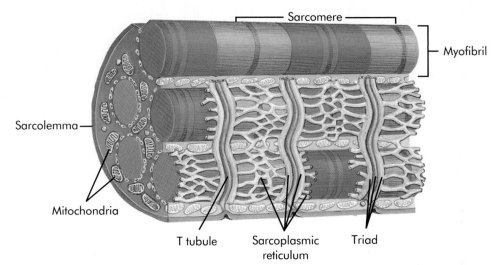

FIGURE 36-15 Myofibrils. Myofibrils of a skeletal muscle fiber (cells) and overall organization of skeletal muscle. (From Thibodeau GA, Patton KT: *Anatomy & physiology,* ed 6, St Louis, 2007, Mosby.)

The whole muscle may be controlled by several motor nerve axons. These branch to innervate many motor units within the muscle. The whole muscle then may be made up of many motor units. The number of motor units per individual muscle varies greatly. In the calf, for example, 1 motor axon innervates approximately 2000 muscle fibers, out of a total of 1,200,000 muscle fibers. This is a high innervation ratio of muscle fibers to axons, and it contrasts markedly with the low innervation ratio found in laryngeal muscles, where two to three muscle fibers constitute each motor unit and the innervation ratio can be of great functional significance. The greater the innervation ratio of a particular organ, the greater its endurance. Higher innervation ratios prevent fatigue, whereas lower innervation ratios allow for precision of movement.

Sensory receptors. Although muscles function as effector organs, they also contain sensory receptors and are involved in sending different signals to the central nervous system. Among these are the muscle spindles and Golgi tendon organs. Spindles are mechanoreceptors that lie parallel to muscle fibers and respond to muscle stretching. Golgi tendon organs are dendrites that terminate and branch to tendons near the neuromuscular junction. The muscle spindles, Golgi tendon organs, and free nerve endings provide a means of reporting changes in length, tension, velocity, and tone in the muscle. This system of afferent signals is responsible for the muscle stretch response and maintenance of normal muscle tone.

Muscle fibers. Each muscle fiber is a single muscle cell, cylindrical in structure and surrounded by a membrane capable of excitation and impulse propagation. The muscle fiber contains bundles of myofibrils, the fiber's functional subunits, in a parallel arrangement along the longitudinal axis of the muscle (Figure 36-15). At birth, the muscle fibers have completed development from precursor cells called myoblasts. All voluntary muscles are derived from the mesodermal layer of the embryo. Genetic transcription factors, most notably MyoD, induce skeletal muscle differentiation. Myoblasts are the main cells responsible for muscle growth and regeneration. Myoblasts are termed *satellite cells* when in a dormant state. Satellite cells are crucial in muscle growth, maintenance, repair, and regeneration. Once muscle is injured, satellite cells become activated and increase the number of transcriptional factors necessary to form myoblasts and assist in repair.[7]

The type of peripheral nerve influences the muscle fiber and motor unit considerably. Whether motor nerves are fast or slow determines the type of muscle fibers in the motor unit. White muscle (type II fibers [white fast-twitch fibers]) is innervated by relatively large type II alpha motor neurons with fast conduction velocities. These fibers rely on a short-term anaerobic glycolytic system for rapid energy transfer. Red muscle (type I fibers [slow-twitch fibers]) depends on aerobic oxidative metabolism. Table 36-4 describes the specific characteristics of type I and type II fibers.

The overlap of muscle fibers that appears with staining gives the checkerboard appearance of muscle biopsy specimens and provides an equal distribution of fiber types throughout the muscle. This overlap also helps to compensate for muscle fiber loss and fatigue of individual

TABLE 36-4 CHARACTERISTICS OF HUMAN SKELETAL MUSCLE FIBERS

CHARACTERISTICS	TYPE I (RED) (OXIDATIVE FIBERS [OFS])	TYPE II (WHITE) TYPE II-1A (OXIDATIVE GLYCOLIC FIBERS [FOGs])
Anatomic location	Deep axial portion of muscle	Surface portion of muscle
Fiber diameter	Small	Large
Motor neuron size	Small	Large
Contraction speed	Slow	Fast
Motor neuron type	Type I, α	Type II-A
Glycogen content	Low	High
Oxidative capacity	High	High (for short periods)
Myosin-ATPase activity	Low	High
Metabolism	Oxidative	Some oxidative pathways, mostly glycolysis
Used for	Maintaining body posture, skeletal support, aerobic activity	Short, intense activity (e.g., sprinting)
Aerobic metabolic capacity	High	Low
Fatigue resistance	High	Intermediate to low
Myoglobin content	High	Low
Capillary supply	Profuse	Intermediate to low
Mitochondria	Many	Few
Intensity of contraction	Low	High
Example (most muscles are mixed)	Soleus muscle	Laryngeal or ocular muscles
Satellite cell content	High	Low

From Spence AP, Mason EE: *Human anatomy and physiology,* ed 4, St Paul, Minn, 1992, West Publishing.

motor units during activity. In spite of this, some muscles contain proportionally more of one fiber type than another. The postural muscles have more type I fibers, allowing them the high resistance to fatigue that is necessary to maintain the same position for extended periods. The ocular muscles have more type II muscle fibers, allowing them to respond rapidly to visual changes.

The number of muscle fibers varies according to location. Large muscles, such as the gastrocnemius, have more fibers (1,200,000) than smaller muscles, such as the lumbrical muscles in the hand (10,000). The diameter of muscle fibers also varies. The closely packed polygons are small (10 to 20 μm) until puberty, when they attain the normal adult diameter of 40 to 80 μm. Women usually have smaller-diameter fibers than men. Small muscles, such as the ocular muscles, are 15 μm in diameter; larger, more proximal muscles are 40 μm in diameter. Fiber size can have functional significance. Studies have shown that larger fiber diameter is associated with generation of greater forces. Fiber diameter can be increased by exercise or occupational overuse, activities that cause hypertrophied muscle.

The major components of the muscle fiber include the muscle membrane, myofibrils, sarcotubular system, sarcoplasm, and mitochondria (see Figure 36-15). The **muscle membrane** is a two-part membrane. It includes the **sarcolemma,** which contains the plasma membrane of the muscle cell, and the cell's **basement membrane.** The sarcolemma is 7.5 μm thick and is capable of propagating electrical impulses to initiate contraction. At the motor nerve end-plate, where the nerve impulse is transmitted, the sarcolemma forms the highly convoluted synaptic cleft. The sarcolemma is made up of lipid molecules and protein systems. The protein systems perform special functions, such as transport of nutrients and protein synthesis. They also provide the sodium-potassium pump and include the cell's cholinergic receptor. The basement membrane is 50 μm thick and is composed primarily of proteins and polysaccharides. It also serves as the cell's microskeleton and maintains the shape of the muscle cell. The basement membrane

also may function in some way to restrict further diffusion of electrolytes once they have crossed the sarcolemma.

The **sarcoplasm** is the cytoplasm of the muscle cell and contains myoglobin plus the intracellular components that are common to all cells (see Chapter 1). **Myoglobin** is a protein found primarily in skeletal and heart muscle. Related to hemoglobin in the blood, myoglobin stores oxygen and iron in the muscle. The sarcoplasm is an aqueous substance that provides a matrix that surrounds the myofibrils. It contains numerous enzymes and proteins that are responsible for the cell's energy production, protein synthesis, and oxygen storage. The mitochondria house enzyme systems for energy production, particularly those that regulate processes such as the citric acid cycle and adenosine triphosphate (ATP) formation. Many other structures are present in the sarcoplasm. The ribosomes are composed of primarily ribonucleic acid (RNA) and participate in the process of protein synthesis. The cell nucleus, satellite cells, glycogen granules, and lipid droplets are suspended in the sarcoplasmic matrix. Blood vessels, nerve endings, muscle spindles, and Golgi tendon organs are also directly located within this structure.

Unique to the muscle is the **sarcotubular system,** a network that includes the transverse tubules and the sarcoplasmic reticulum, which crosses the interior of the cell. The **sarcoplasmic reticulum** is constructed like the endoplasmic reticulum in other cells. In muscle cells, the sarcoplasmic reticulum is involved in calcium transport, which initiates muscle contraction at the **sarcomere,** a portion of the myofibril. The sarcoplasmic reticulum is composed of tubules that run parallel to the myofibrils. The longitudinal tubules are termed **sarcotubules.** The **transverse tubules,** which are closely associated with the sarcotubules, run across the sarcoplasm and communicate with the extracellular space. Together, the tubules of this membrane system allow for uptake and regulation of intracellular calcium, release of calcium during muscle contraction, and storage of calcium during muscle relaxation.

TABLE 36-5	**CONTRACTILE PROTEINS OF SKELETAL MUSCLE SARCOMERE**	
PROTEIN	**LOCATION**	**FUNCTION**
Actinin	Z disk	Attaches actin to Z disks; helps coordinate sarcomere contraction; cross-links thin filaments in adjacent sarcomeres
Actin	I band (thin filaments)	Contraction; activates myosin-ATPase; interacts with myosin
α-Actin	Z disk	Main ligand of titin; links and controls filament length
β-Actin	Z disk	Regulatory and structural function; links filaments, controls filament length
Myosin	A band (thick filament)	Contraction; hydrolyzes ATP and develops tension
Titin* (third most abundant muscle protein)	Half of sarcomere (from Z disk to M band)	Coordinates assembly of proteins that comprise sarcomere; regulates resting length of sarcomere; important for myofibril assembly, stabilization, and maintenance
Nebulin*	I band (with α-actin)	Interacts with myosin to produce contraction; binding site for actin, desmin, titin, other proteins; stabilizes and regulates length of actin filaments; plays role in assembly, structure, and maintenance of Z disks
Obscurin*	Surrounds sarcomere (mainly at Z disk and M band)	May coordinate assembly of sarcoplasmic reticulum and interacts with its components; possibly regulates diameter of myofibrils; plays role in muscle response to injury; has role in formation and stabilization of M bands and A band

Data from Konstantopoulos A et al: Muscle giants: molecular scaffolds in sarcomerogenesis, *Physiol Rev* 89(4):1217–1267, 2009; Luther PK: The vertebrate muscle Z-disc: sarcomere anchor for structure and signaling, *J Muscle Res Cell Motil* 30:171–185, 2009; Pappas CT, Kreig PA, Gregosio CC: Nebulin regulates actin filament lengths by a stabilization mechanism, *J Cell Biol* 189(5):858–870, 2010.
*Also may function as molecular scaffolds for myofibril formation.
ATP, Adenosine triphosphate; *ATPase,* adenosinetriphosphatase.

Myofibrils. The myofibrils are the functional units of muscle contraction. Each myofibril contains sarcomeres, which appear at intervals (see Figure 36-15). The speed with which sarcomeres lengthen and shorten during movement directly influences the strength and function of skeletal muscles. Sprinters tend to have more fast-twitch (FT) fibers than slow-twitch (ST) fibers in their leg muscles, and endurance runners have more ST fibers in their leg muscles. Sarcomeres are composed of several proteins. The two most abundant are actin and myosin, but three other giant, muscle-specific proteins (titin, nebulin, and obscurin) play important roles in myofibril formation and function (see Table 36-5).

The myofibrils are the most abundant subcellular muscle component, equaling 85% to 90% of the total volume. On cross section, they are seen to be irregular polygons with a mean diameter of less than 1 μm. Each myofibril is composed of serially repeating sarcomeres, separated by Z bands, which give the muscle its striped, cross-striated appearance. Each sarcomere has a dark A band and is flanked by two light I bands (Figure 36-16). The A band is 1.5 to 1.6 μm long and contains the thick myosin filaments. Included in the A band is a lighter zone called the *H band,* and in the center of the H band is the dark *M band,* or *M line.* The *I band,* which contains actin, is divided at the midpoint of each sarcomere by the *Z band.* Its length varies with the start of muscle contraction. The *Z disk* (made up of different layers of Z bands, depending on muscle type) marks the boundaries of the sarcomere.[8]

Myofibrils are composed of myofilaments. Each myofilament is structured in a closely packed hexagonal arrangement, with two thin filaments for every thick filament. The thick filament, along with C protein and M line protein, is made up of myosin. Myosin has two subunits—heavy and light meromyosin, which resemble twisted golf club shafts. The thin filaments are twisted double strands consisting of actin, troponin, and tropomyosin (see Chapter 22 and Figure 22-13).

Muscle proteins. A multitude of muscle proteins have been identified and their functions are still being discovered. Table 36-5 summarizes the location and function of some of the important muscle proteins.

Nonprotein constituents of muscle. Substances such as nitrogen, creatine, creatinine, phosphocreatine, purines, uric acid, and amino acids all serve in the complex process of muscle metabolism. Energy is provided by glycogen and its derivatives.

Creatine metabolism and creatinine metabolism have been used to measure muscle mass. Plasma creatine is taken up by muscle and converted into the high-energy phosphate compound phosphocreatine by the enzyme creatine kinase. Creatinine is formed in muscle from creatine at a constant rate of 2% per day. (Tests for plasma creatine are discussed in Chapter 28.) Creatine excretion is increased in muscle wasting. This change reflects the reduction in total body creatine stores and the loss of muscle mass.

Inorganic compounds, anions (phosphate, chloride), and cations (calcium, magnesium, sodium, potassium) are important in the regulation of protein synthesis, muscle contraction, and enzyme systems as well as in the stabilization of cell membranes. Total body potassium (TBK), measured by the K40 method, has been used to measure muscle mass, also called *lean body mass.* Total body potassium levels reflect changes in muscle mass seen during growth, malnutrition, and muscle wasting.

Components of Muscle Function

The ultimate function of muscle is to accomplish work. Although variously expressed in such measures as foot-pounds or kilogram-meters, work usually refers to the amount of energy liberated or force exerted over a distance (work = force × distance). Muscles usually contract or tense while doing work. Muscle contraction occurs on the molecular level and leads to the observable phenomenon of muscle movement.

Muscle Contraction at the Molecular Level

The four steps of muscle contraction are (1) excitation, (2) coupling, (3) contraction, and (4) relaxation. The process involves the electrical properties of all cells and the movement of ions across the plasma membrane (see Chapter 1). The muscle fiber is an excitable tissue. At rest, an electric charge of −90 mV is continually maintained across the sarcolemma. This resting potential, generated by the separation of positive and negative charges on either side of the membrane, creates an electrochemical equilibrium caused by the selective permeability of the sarcolemma to electrolytes in the intracellular and extracellular fluids, particularly potassium and sodium.

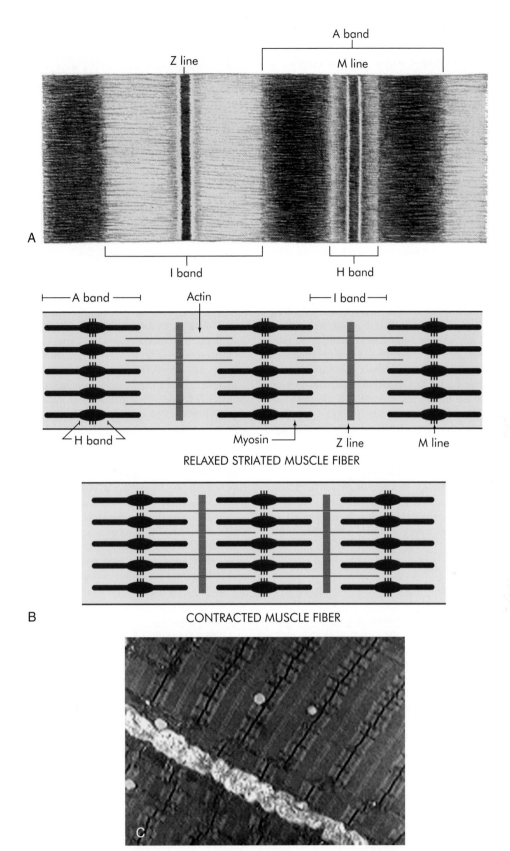

FIGURE 36-16 Muscle Fibers. A, The Z disks define the end of an individual sarcomere. The M line (which lies within the H band) is made of cross-connecting elements of the cytoskeleton. **B,** Actin is the primary protein of the I band (thin filament). Nebulin also extends along the I band and contains binding sites for actin and myosin. Myosin (thick filament) extends through the A band. Titin extends from the Z disk to the M band, binding with myosin; strong titin anchoring within the I band is necessary for proper muscle function. During contraction, the I bands and H bands shorten, moving the Z disks closer together. **C,** Electron photomicrograph of human muscle tissue corresponding to schematics in **A** and **B.** (A modified from Thompson JM et al: *Mosby's clinical nursing,* ed 5, St Louis, 2002, Mosby; C courtesy Louisa Howard.)

Excitation, the first step of muscle contraction, begins with the spread of an action potential from the nerve terminal to the neuromuscular junction. The rapid depolarization of the membrane initiates an electrical impulse in the muscle fiber membrane called the muscle fiber action potential. As the action potential advances along the sarcolemmal membrane, it spreads to the transverse tubules. (The velocity of conduction is much slower in muscle fibers than in myelinated nerve fibers—only 3 to 5 m/sec compared with 54 to 90 m/sec in nerve fibers.)

The second stage, coupling, follows the depolarization of the transverse tubules. This triggers the release of calcium ions from the sarcoplasmic reticulum, exposing binding sites on the actin molecule. Calcium affects troponin and tropomyosin, muscle proteins that bind with actin when the muscle is at rest. In the presence of calcium, however, both these proteins are attracted to calcium ions, leaving the actin free to bind with myosin.

Contraction begins as the calcium ions combine with troponin, a reaction that overcomes the inhibitory function of the troponin-tropomyosin system. Myosin binds to actin, forming cross-bridges. The myosin heads attach to the exposed actin-binding sites, pulling actin (the thin filament) inward. The thin filament, actin, then slides toward the thick filament, myosin. The two ends of the myofibril shorten after contraction when the myosin heads attach to the actin molecules, forming a cross-bridge that constitutes an actin-myosin complex. ATP, located on the actin-myosin complex, is released when the cross-bridges attach. The process of contraction was first described by A.F. Huxley in the 1950s. It is commonly known as the cross-bridge theory because the actin and myosin proteins form cross-bridges as they contract. The useful distance of contraction of a skeletal muscle is approximately 25% to 35% of the muscle's length.

The last step, relaxation, begins as calcium ions are actively transported back into the sarcoplasmic reticulum, removing ions from interaction with troponin. The cross-bridges detach, and the sarcomere lengthens. (The cross-bridge theory of muscle contraction is discussed in Chapter 22.)

Muscle Metabolism

Skeletal muscle requires a constant supply of ATP and phosphocreatine. These substances are necessary to fuel the complex processes of muscle contraction, driving the cross-bridges of actin and myosin together and transporting calcium from the sarcoplasmic reticulum to the myofibril. Other internal processes of the muscular system that require ATP include protein synthesis, which replenishes muscle constituents and accommodates growth and repair. The rate of protein synthesis is related to hormone levels (particularly insulin), the presence of amino acid substrates, and overall nutritional status. At rest, the rate of ATP formation by oxidation of glucose or acetoacetate is sufficient to maintain internal processes, given normal nutritional status. During activity, the need for ATP increases 100-fold. The metabolic pathways for muscle activity in Table 36-6 show reactions to the immediate need for increased ATP caused by contraction. Activity lasting longer than 5 seconds expends the available stored ATP and phosphocreatine.

Stored glycogen and blood glucose are converted anaerobically to sustain brief activity without increasing the demand for oxygen. Anaerobic glycolysis is much less efficient than aerobic glycolysis, using six to eight times more glycogen to produce the same amount of ATP. With increased activity, such as intense exercise, or with ischemia, an increase in the amount of lactic acid occurs because of the breakdown of glycogen, thus causing a shift in muscle pH (see Table 36-6). This short-term mechanism buys time by allowing ATP formation in spite of inadequate energy stores or oxygen supply. When the anaerobic threshold is reached and more oxygen is required, physiologic changes

TABLE 36-6   ENERGY SOURCES FOR MUSCULAR ACTIVITY

SOURCES	REACTIONS
Short-term (anaerobic) sources	Adenosine triphosphate (ATP) → Adenosine diphosphate (ADP) + Inorganic phosphate (P_i) + Energy
	Phosphocreatine + ADP ⇌ Creatine + ATP
	Glycogen/glucose + P_i + ADP → Lactate + ATP
Long-term (aerobic) sources	Glycogen/glucose + ADP + P_i + O_2 → H_2O + CO_2 + ATP
	Free fatty acids + ADP + P_i + O_2 → H_2O + CO_2 + ATP
	Creatine kinase catalyzes reversible reaction of ATP to ADP: Creatine phosphate + ATP $\xrightleftharpoons{\text{Creatine Kinase}}$ Creatine + ATP

From Spence AP, Mason EE: *Human anatomy and physiology,* ed 4, St Paul, Minn, 1992, West Publishing.

occur, including an increase in lactic acid level and increases in oxygen consumption, heart rate, respiratory rate, and muscle blood flow.

Strenuous exercise requires oxygen, which activates the aerobic glycogen pathway for ATP formation. During maximal exercise, free fatty acid mobilization and the aerobic glycogen pathways provide ATP over an extended time. These pathways require oxygen both to maintain maximal activity and to return the muscle to the resting state. Maximal exercise increases oxygen uptake by 15 to 20 times over the resting state. When this system becomes exhausted or inadequate to respond to the need for ATP, fatigue and weakness finally force the muscle to reduce activity with a resultant buildup of lactic acid in muscle fibers. Creatine supplementation may provide some protective effects on muscle in older adult athletes as well as after strenuous physical activity.[9,10]

Sustaining maximal muscular activity accumulates an oxygen debt, which is the amount of oxygen needed to oxidize the residual lactic acid, convert it back to glycogen, and replenish ATP and phosphocreatine stores. For example, after running at maximal speed for 10 seconds, the average person has consumed 1 L of oxygen. At rest, oxygen consumption for the same period is approximately 40 ml. As the person recovers, the measured oxygen debt is 4 L greater than the amount used during activity.

Oxygen consumption is measured to calculate the metabolic cost of activity in normal and diseased muscle. It is an indirect measure of energy expenditure, along with timed tests of activity, heart rate, and respiratory quotient (ratio of carbon dioxide to expired oxygen consumed). Energy expenditure is measured directly by heat production because heat is released whenever work is accomplished.

Another factor that changes energy requirements is muscle fiber type. Type II fibers rely on anaerobic glycolytic metabolism and fatigue readily. Type I fibers can resist fatigue for longer periods because of their capacity for oxidative metabolism.

Muscle Mechanics

Muscle contraction cannot be viewed in isolation. Several factors determine how force is transmitted from the cross-bridges on individual muscle fibers to accomplish whole-muscle contraction. First, when a motor unit responds to a single nerve stimulus, it develops a phasic contraction, also called a *twitch*. Because the motor unit contracts in an all-or-nothing manner, the contraction that is generated will be a maximal contraction. The central nervous system smoothly grades the force generated by recruiting additional motor units and varying the discharge frequency of each active motor unit. This adding of motor units within the muscle is called repetitive discharge.

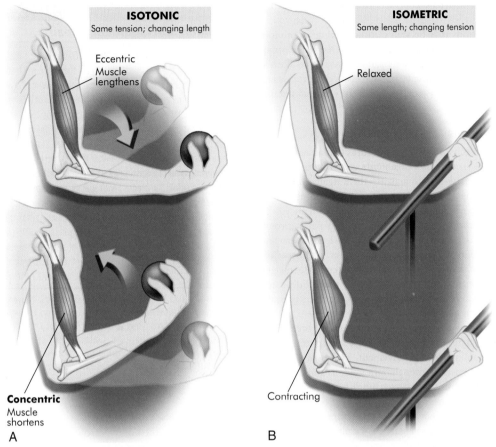

FIGURE 36-17 Isotonic and Isometric Contraction. **A,** In isotonic contraction, the muscle shortens, producing movement. **B,** In isometric contraction, the muscle pulls forcefully against a load but does not shorten. (From Thibodeau GA, Patton KT: *Anatomy & physiology,* ed 6, St Louis, 2007, Mosby.)

Recruitment and repetitive discharge of motor units allow the muscle to activate the number of motor units needed to generate the desired force. The total force developed is the sum of the force generated by each motor unit. If the motor units are stimulated again and the muscle unit has not been able to relax between stimulation and the next contraction, the second contraction will fuse with the first, causing physiologic tetanus (not to be confused with the disease tetanus).

Other variables, such as fiber type, innervation ratio, muscle temperature, and muscle shape, influence the efficiency of muscular contraction. The two muscle fiber types differ in their responses to electrical activity. Tetanus and duration of phasic contractions, which take microseconds to accomplish, are achieved more rapidly in type II (white fast-twitch) than in type I (red slow-twitch) muscle fibers. Low innervation ratios promote control and coordination, whereas high ratios promote strength and endurance. Muscles work best at normal body temperature, 98.6° F (37° C). Finally, muscles with a large cross-sectional area, such as the fan-shaped pennate muscles, develop greater contractile forces than smaller-diameter muscles. The initial length of a muscle and the range of shortening that occur when the muscle contracts also determine the force it can generate. The long fusiform muscles have a greater range of shortening and can contract up to 57% of their resting length. A certain amount of elongation is necessary to generate sufficient tension and muscular force. The elongation that occurs during the swing of a golf club or tennis racket is an example of how stretch improves contractile force.

Types of Muscle Contraction

During isometric contraction, the muscle maintains constant length as tension is increased (Figure 36-17). Isometric contraction occurs, for example, when the arm or leg is pushed against an immovable object. The muscle contracts, but the limb does not move. Isometric contraction is also called static (holding) contraction.

During isotonic contraction, the muscle maintains a constant tension as it moves. Isotonic contractions can be eccentric (lengthening) or concentric (shortening). Positive work is accomplished during concentric contraction, and energy is released to exert force or lift a weight. In contrast, during an eccentric contraction the muscle lengthens and absorbs energy. Negative work is accomplished on the muscle by the load. Eccentric contraction requires less energy to accomplish and has been said to result in the development of pain and stiffness after unaccustomed exercise.

Movement of Muscle Groups

Muscles do not act alone but in groups, often under automatic control. When a muscle contracts and acts as a prime mover, or agonist, its reciprocal muscle, or antagonist, relaxes. This is easily tested by holding the right arm in the horizontal position in front of the body, and then bending the elbow and using the other hand to feel the biceps on the top and the triceps on the bottom of the arm. The biceps is firm, and the triceps is soft. As the arm is extended, the muscles change. When the elbow is completely extended, the biceps is soft and the triceps firm. Completing this movement causes the agonist and antagonist to change automatically; only the movement is commanded, not the alternate contraction and relaxation of the specific muscle groups.

Other associated actions may be seen during walking; as the foot leaves the ground, the paravertebral and gluteal muscles on the opposite sides of the body contract to maintain balance. One notices the loss of the associated muscle's action when paralysis offsets this process and decreases balance. If a person is paralyzed, difficulty in maintaining balance is noticeable.

Tendons and Ligaments

Tendons are important musculoskeletal structures that attach muscle to bone at a site called an enthesis. Ligaments attach bone to bone, helping to form joints as well as stabilizing them against excessive movement. Both tendons and ligaments are primarily composed of types III, IV, V, and VI collagen and fibroblasts (termed tenocytes in tendons).[11] The fibroblasts in tendon are arranged in parallel rows; fibroblasts appear less organized in ligaments. Collagen fibers and fibroblasts form fascicles, with multiple fascicles then forming whole tendon or ligament.[12] In the proteoglycan matrix of tendons, collagen oligomeric matrix protein (COMP) assists in providing gliding and viscoelastic properties. Compared to tendons, ligament fibers typically contain a greater proportion of elastin.

Two main functions of tendons are (1) transferring forces from muscle to bone and (2) acting as a type of biologic spring for muscles to allow additional stability during movement. Ligaments stabilize joints by restricting movement. Although both tendons and ligaments can withstand significant distraction (stretching) force, they tend to buckle when compressive force is applied.

Both tendons and ligaments have complex structures at the attachment site of two dissimilar tissues. Figure 36-18 illustrates the transition of tissue between tendon/ligament and bone. These complex structures and differences in mechanical and structural characteristics (either tendon and bone or ligament and bone) make healing and repair of damaged tissue complicated (see *Health Alert:* Tendon and Ligament Repair).

AGING & THE MUSCULOSKELETAL SYSTEM

Aging of Bones

Aging is accompanied by the loss of bone tissue. Bones become less dense, less strong, and more brittle with aging. The bone remodeling cycle takes longer to complete, and the rate of mineralization also slows. With aging, women experience loss of bone density, accelerated with the rapid bone loss that occurs during early menopause from increased osteoclastic bone resorption. By age 70 years, susceptible women have, on the average, lost 50% of their peripheral cortical bone mass (see Chapter 37). Bone mass losses to such an extent lead to deformity, pain, stiffness, and high risk for fractures. Men experience bone loss also but at later ages and much slower rates than women. Also, initial bone masses in men are approximately 30% higher than those in women; therefore bone loss in men causes less risk of disability than that found in women. Men's peak bone mass is related to their race, heredity, hormonal factors, physical activity, and calcium intake during childhood. Bone loss in both genders is related to smoking, calcium deficiency, alcohol intake, and physical inactivity. Bone mass can be gained in healthy young women up to the third decade through participation in physical activity, intake of dietary calcium and other minerals, and use of oral contraceptives. Height is also lost with aging because of intervertebral disk degeneration and, sometimes, osteoporotic spinal fractures.

HEALTH ALERT
Tendon and Ligament Repair

Injury of tendons and ligaments constitutes one of the greatest challenges in musculoskeletal rehabilitation. When these types of structures are damaged, attempts to engineer suitable tissue replacements have proved disappointing. The structures and intricate protein composition of tendons and ligaments are the basis for their complex biomechanical properties. One reason for poor clinical outcome in synthetic tendon structures has been the inability to replicate any material that can bear the high mechanical stresses that occur at the interface between two dissimilar materials (i.e., either tendon and bone or ligament and bone). One promising area of investigation is finding or engineering a biodegradable material, or "scaffold," implanted with specific cells that would regenerate into normal tendon or ligament. The scaffold must be strong enough to withstand the forces at the tissue/bone interface and then gradually break down as it is completely replaced by new cells. Currently, investigators are using synthetic polymers, silk, and collagen as scaffolds, with tendon or ligament fibroblasts and mesenchymal stem cells as the implanted cells. Once these biochemical hurdles are overcome, the repair of damaged tendons and ligaments will be revolutionized.

Data from Kuo CK, Marturano JE, Tuan RS: Novel strategies in tendon and ligament tissue engineering: advanced biomaterials and regeneration motifs, *Sports Med Arthrosc Rehabil Ther Technol* 2:20, 2010; Thomopoulos S, Genin GM, Galatz LM: The development and morphogenesis of the tendon-to-bone insertion—what development can teach us about healing, *J Musculoskelet Neuronal Interact* 10(1):35–45, 2010; Yang PJ, Temenoff JS: Engineering orthopedic tissue interfaces, *Tissue Eng Part B Rev* 15(2):127–141, 2009.

Stem cells in the bone marrow perform less efficiently with aging, predisposing older persons to acute and chronic illnesses. Such illnesses cause weakness and confusion in older persons and may increase the risk of injury or falling.

Aging of Joints

With aging, cartilage becomes more rigid, fragile, and susceptible to fraying because of increased cross-linking of collagen and elastin, decreased water content in the cartilage ground substance, and reduced concentrations of glycosaminoglycans. Decreased range of motion of the joint is related to the changes in ligaments and muscles. Bones in joints develop evidence of osteoporosis with fewer trabeculae and thinner, less dense bones, making them prone to fractures. Intervertebral disk spaces decrease in height. The rate of loss of height accelerates at age 70 years and beyond. Tendons shrink and harden.

Aging of Muscles

The function of skeletal muscle depends on many influences that are affected by aging, including nervous, vascular, and endocrine systems. In the young child, the development of muscle tissue depends greatly on continuing neurodevelopmental maturation. Muscle loss begins at about age 50; however, muscle function remains trainable even into advanced age. Maintaining musculoskeletal fitness at any age can improve overall health.[13]

Age-related loss in skeletal muscle is referred to as sarcopenia and is a direct cause of the age-related decrease in muscle strength. As the body ages, muscle mass and strength decline slowly; thus, strength is maintained through the fifth decade, with a slow decline in dynamic and isometric strength evident after age 70. The amount of type II fibers also decreases. There is reduced RNA synthesis, loss of mitochondrial function,[14] and reduction in the size of motor units. The regenerative

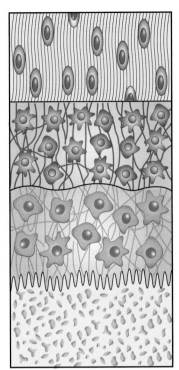

Tendon/ligament
Aligned collagen fibrils (lines)
Fibroblasts embedded throughout (blue oval cells)
Collagen fibrils extend into uncalcified fibrocartilage

Uncalcified fibrocartilage
Larger, less parallel collagen bundles (vertical blue lines)
Collagen types I and II, aggrecan (irregular-shaped cells)
Avascular (yellow background)
Ovoid-shaped, aligned cells (smooth-edged cells)

Wavy tidemark (marks beginning of calcification)

Calcified fibrocartilage
Mineralized tissue
Hypertrophic, more circular chondrocytes
Consists of collagen types I, II, and X

Bone
Interdigitation at surface (zig-zag line)
Calcified tissue

FIGURE 36-18 Cartilage-Bone, Tendon/Ligament-Bone, Meniscus-Bone, and Muscle-Tendon Interfaces. This diagram depicts the cartilage-bone, tendon/ligament-bone, meniscus-bone, and muscle-tendon interfaces and their compositions. Orange indicates levels of aggrecan concentration, light blue indicates collagen fibers, dark blue indicates mineralized tissue, and red indicates muscle fibers. Gradients of matrix composition, interdigitation of tissue zones, and interconnecting collagen fibers all enable load transfer between disparate tissues. (From Yang PJ, Temenoff JS: Engineering orthopedic tissue interfaces, *Tissue Eng Part B Rev* 15[2]:128, 2009.)

function of muscle tissue remains normal in aging persons. As much as 30% to 40% of skeletal muscle mass and strength may be lost from the third to ninth decades. Muscle fatigue also may contribute to loss of function with aging.[14] Sarcopenia is thought to be secondary to progressive neuromuscular changes and diminishing levels of anabolic hormones. There is an age-related decline in the synthesis of mixed proteins, myosin heavy chains, and mitochondrial protein.[15] Changes in these muscle proteins are related to reduced levels of insulin-like growth factor-1 (IGF-1), testosterone, and dehydroepiandrosterone (DHEA) sulfate.

Maximal oxygen intake declines with age. Basal metabolic rate is reduced and lean body mass decreases in the aged population.

> **✓ QUICK CHECK 36-3**
> 1. Name three differences between slow-twitch and fast-twitch muscle fibers.
> 2. Why is adenosine triphosphate (ATP) used for muscle contraction?
> 3. Define the differences between tendons and ligaments.
> 4. Describe significant changes in the musculoskeletal system with aging.

DID YOU UNDERSTAND?

Structure and Function of Bones

1. Bones provide support and protection for the body's tissues and organs and are important sources of minerals and blood cells.
2. Bone formation begins with the production of an inorganic matrix by bone cells. Bone minerals crystallize in and around collagen fibers in the matrix, giving bone its characteristic hardness and strength.
3. Bone tissue is continuously being resorbed and synthesized by basic multicellular units of osteoclasts and osteoblasts, respectively.
4. Bones in the body are made up of compact bone tissue and spongy bone tissue. Compact bone is highly organized into haversian systems that consist of concentric layers of crystallized matrix surrounding a central canal that contains blood vessels and nerves. Dispersed throughout the concentric layers of crystallized matrix are small spaces containing osteocytes. Smaller canals, called *canaliculi,* interconnect the osteocyte-containing

spaces. The crystallized matrix in spongy bone is arranged in bars or plates. Spaces containing *osteocytes* are dispersed between the bars or plates and interconnected by canaliculi.

5. Osteoblasts are multifunctional mononuclear cells derived from osteogenic mesenchymal stromal cells; they are the primary bone-producing cells and are involved in many functions related to the skeletal system.
6. Osteoclasts are large (typically 20 to 100 μm in diameter), multinucleated cells that develop from the hematopoietic monocyte-macrophage lineage. Osteoclasts are the major resorptive cells of bone.
7. There are 206 bones in the body divided into the axial skeleton and the appendicular skeleton. Bones are classified by shape as long, short, flat, or irregular. Long bones have a broad end (epiphysis), broad neck (metaphysis), and narrow midportion (diaphysis) that contains the medullary cavity.

DID YOU UNDERSTAND?—cont'd

8. Bone injuries are repaired in stages. Hematoma formation provides the fibrin framework for formation and organization of granulation tissue. The granulation tissue provides a cartilage model for the formation and crystallization of bone matrix. Remodeling restores the original shape and size to the injured bone.

Structure and Function of Joints

1. A joint is the site where two or more bones attach. Joints provide stability and mobility to the skeleton.
2. Joints are classified as synarthroses, amphiarthroses, or diarthroses, depending on the degree of movement they allow. Joints are also classified by the type of connecting tissue holding them together. Fibrous joints are connected by dense fibrous tissue, ligaments, or membranes. Cartilaginous joints are connected by fibrocartilage or hyaline cartilage. Synovial joints are connected by a fibrous joint capsule. Within the capsule is a small fluid-filled space. The fluid in the space nourishes the articular cartilage that covers the ends of the bones meeting in the synovial joint.
3. Articular cartilage is a highly organized system of collagen fibers and proteoglycans. The fibers firmly anchor the cartilage to the bone, and the proteoglycans control the loss of fluid from the cartilage.
4. Joints help move bones and muscle.

Structure and Function of Skeletal Muscles

1. Skeletal muscle is made up of millions of individual fibers.
2. Whole muscles vary in size (2 to 60 cm) and shape (fusiform, pennate). They are encased in a three-part connective tissue framework. The fundamental concept of muscle function is the motor unit, defined as those muscle fibers innervated by a single motor nerve, its axon, and anterior horn cell.
3. Satellite cells are dormant myoblasts; however, they can regenerate muscle when activated.
4. Muscle fibers contain bundles of myofibrils arranged in parallel along the longitudinal axis and include the muscle membrane, myofibrils, sarcotubular

system, aqueous sarcoplasm, and mitochondria. There are two types of muscle fibers, type I and type II, determined by motor nerve innervation.

5. Myofibrils and myofilaments contain the major muscle proteins actin and myosin, which interact to form cross-bridges during muscle contraction. The nonprotein muscle constituents provide an energy source for contraction and regulate protein synthesis and enzyme systems as well as stabilize cell membranes.
6. Muscle contraction includes excitation, coupling, contraction, and relaxation.
7. Muscle strength is graded by the all-or-nothing phenomenon and recruitment. Speed of contraction is affected by several factors: muscle fiber type, temperature, stretch, and weight of the load.
8. There are two types of muscle contraction: isometric and isotonic. Muscle shortening occurs during contraction but can be seen also during pathologic and physiologic contracture.
9. Skeletal muscle requires a constant supply of adenosine triphosphate (ATP) and phosphocreatine to fuel muscle contraction and for growth and repair. ATP and phosphocreatine can be generated aerobically or anaerobically.
10. Tendon attachment sites of muscle to bone are called entheses.
11. Ligaments attach bone to bone, helping to form joints as well as stabilizing them against excessive movement. Both tendons and ligaments are mostly composed of types III, IV, V, and VI collagen and fibroblasts (termed tenocytes in tendons).

Aging & the Musculoskeletal System

1. Sarcopenia, or age-related loss in skeletal muscle, is a direct cause of decrease in muscle strength. A slow decline in dynamic and isometric strength is evident after age 70 years.
2. The regenerative function of muscle tissue remains normal in elderly persons.
3. On average, people lose about one third of a pound of muscle every year after age 40 years and gain at least as much body fat.
4. Reduced basal metabolic rate and decreased lean body mass are also noted in the elderly population.

KEY TERMS

KEY TERMS—cont'd

- Osteocalcin 958
- Osteoclast 957
- Osteocyte 958
- Osteoid 955
- Osteoprotegerin (OPG) 957
- Oxygen debt 972
- Pennate muscle 965
- Perimysium 967
- Periosteum 960
- Physiologic tetanus 973
- Proteoglycan 958
- Receptor activator nuclear factor kappa-B ligand (RANKL) 957
- Relaxation 972
- Remodeling 962
- Repetitive discharge 972

- Resorb 954
- Ruffled border 957
- Sarcolemma 969
- Sarcomere 969
- Sarcopenia 974
- Sarcoplasm 969
- Sarcoplasmic reticulum 969
- Sarcotubular system 969
- Sarcotubule 969
- Satellite cell 968
- Short bone 960
- Sialoprotein 958
- Skeletal muscle (voluntary, striated, or extrafusal muscle) 967
- Spindle 968
- Spongy bone (cancellous bone) 959

- Suture 964
- Symphysis 964
- Synarthrosis (immovable joint) 963
- Synchondrosis 964
- Syndesmosis 964
- Synovial fluid 964
- Synovial joint 965
- Synovial membrane 964
- Tendon 967
- Tidemark 964
- Trabecula (pl., trabeculae) 960
- Transverse tubule 969
- Type I fiber (slow-twitch fiber) 968
- Type II fiber (white fast-twitch fiber), 968
- Voluntary muscle 968

REFERENCES

1. Boyce BF, Yao Z, Xing L: Functions of NF κB in bone, *Ann N Y Acad Sci* 1192:367–375, 2010.
2. Zou W, Teitelbaum SL: Integrins, growth factors, and the osteoclast cytoskeleton, *Ann N Y Acad Sci* 1192:27–31, 2010.
3. Clark B: Normal bone anatomy and physiology, *Clin J Am Soc Nephrol* 3(suppl 3):S131–S139, 2008.
4. Hughes JM, Petit MA: Biological underpinnings of Frost's mechanostat thresholds: the important role of osteocytes, *J Musculosklet Neuronal Interact* 10(2):128–135, 2010.
5. Golob EE: Role of matrix vesicles in biomineralization, *Biochim Biophys Acta* 1790(12):1592–1598, 2009.
6. Orimo H: The mechanism of mineralization and the role of alkaline phosphatase in health and disease, *J Nippon Med Sch* 77(1):4–12, 2010.
7. Tsivites S: Notch and Wnt signaling, physiological stimuli and postnatal myogenesis, *Int J Biol Sci* 6(3):268–281, 2010.
8. Luther PK: The vertebrate muscle Z-disc: sarcomere anchor for structure and signaling, *J Muscle Res Cell Motil* 30:171–185, 2009.
9. Bassit RA, et al: Effect of short-term creatine supplementation on markers of skeletal muscle damage after strenuous contractile activity, *Eur J Appl Physiol* 108(5):945–955, 2010.
10. Tarnopolsky MA: Nutritional consideration in the aging athlete, *Clin J Sport Med* 18(6):531–538, 2008.
11. Kuo CK, Marturano JE, Tuan RS: Novel strategies in tendon and ligament tissue engineering: advanced biomaterials and regeneration motifs, *Sports Med Arthrosc Rehabil Ther Technol* 2:20, 2010.
12. Yang PJ, Temenoff JS: Engineering orthopedic tissue interfaces, *Tissue Eng Part B Rev* 15(2):127–141, 2009.
13. Waters DL, et al: Advances of dietary, exercise-related, and therapeutic interventions to prevent and treat sarcopenia in adult patients: an update, *Clin Interv Aging* 5:259–270, 2010.
14. Burton LA, Sumukadas D: Optimal management of sarcopenia, *Clin Interv Aging* 5:217–228, 2010.
15. Lang T, et al: Sarcopenia: etiology, clinical consequences, intervention, and assessment, *Osteoporos Int* 21(4):543–559, 2010.

37

Alterations of Musculoskeletal Function

Christy L. Crowther-Radulewicz and Kathryn L. McCance

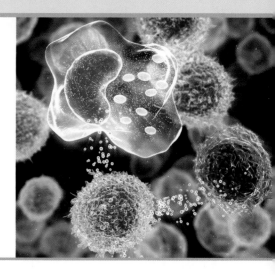

evolve WEBSITE

http://evolve.elsevier.com/Huether/
- Review Questions and Answers
- Animations
- Quick Check Answers

- Key Terms Exercises
- Critical Thinking Questions with Answers
- Algorithm Completion Exercises
- WebLinks

CHAPTER OUTLINE

Musculoskeletal injuries include fractures, dislocations, sprains, and strains. Fractures are the most serious. Alterations in bones, joints, and muscles may be caused by metabolic disorders, infections, inflammatory or noninflammatory diseases, or tumors. The most common disease affecting bone is osteoporosis; much attention and debate has been focused on its risk factors and pathophysiology. Muscle disorders, including inflammatory diseases such as myositis, also are increasing in incidence.

MUSCULOSKELETAL INJURIES

Trauma is referred to as the "neglected disease." It is the leading cause of death of people ages 1 to 44 years of all races and socioeconomic levels. Each year, more than 120,000 persons in the United States die from unintentional injuries.[1]

Musculoskeletal injuries have a major impact on the affected individuals, families, and society in general because of the physical and psychologic effects of limitation on mobility and daily activities, pain, and decreased quality of life; the direct costs of diagnosis and treatments; and the indirect economic costs related to the loss of employment and decreased productivity.

Skeletal Trauma
Fractures

A **fracture** is a break in the continuity of a bone. A break occurs when force is applied that exceeds the tensile or compressive strength of the bone. The incidence of fractures varies for individual bones according to age and gender, with the highest incidence of fractures in young males (between the ages of 15 and 24 years) and older persons (65 years of age and older). Fractures of healthy bones, particularly the tibia, clavicle, and lower humerus, tend to occur in young persons and to be the result of trauma. Fractures of the hands and feet are usually caused by accidents in the workplace. The incidence of fractures of the upper femur, upper humerus, vertebrae, and pelvis is highest in older adults and is often associated with osteoporosis (see p. 987). Hip fractures, the most serious outcome of osteoporosis, are occurring much more often because the world's population is aging.[2]

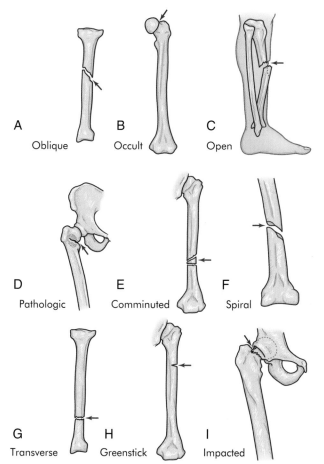

A, Oblique   B, Occult   C, Open

D, Pathologic   E, Comminuted   F, Spiral

G, Transverse   H, Greenstick   I, Impacted

FIGURE 37-1 Examples of Types of Bone Fractures. **A,** Oblique: fracture at oblique angle across both cortices. *Cause:* Direct or indirect energy, with angulation and some compression. **B,** Occult: fracture that is hidden or not readily discernible. *Cause:* Minor force or energy. **C,** Open: skin broken over fracture; possible soft tissue trauma. *Cause:* Moderate to severe energy that is continuous and exceeds tissue tolerance. **D,** Pathologic: transverse, oblique, or spiral fracture of bone weakened by tumor pressure or presence. *Cause:* Minor energy or force, which may be direct or indirect. **E,** Comminuted: fracture with two or more pieces or segments. *Cause:* Direct or indirect moderate to severe force. **F,** Spiral: fracture that curves around cortices and may become displaced by twist. *Cause:* Direct or indirect twisting energy or force with distal part held or unable to move. **G,** Transverse: horizontal break through bone. *Cause:* Direct or indirect energy toward bone. **H,** Greenstick: break in only one cortex of bone. *Cause:* Minor direct or indirect energy. **I,** Impacted: fracture with one end wedged into opposite end of inside fractured fragment. *Cause:* Compressive axial energy or force directly to distal fragment. (Redrawn from Mourad L: Musculoskeletal system. In Thompson JM et al, editors: *Mosby's clinical nursing,* ed 7, St Louis, 2002, Mosby.)

Classification of fractures. Fractures can be classified as complete or incomplete and open or closed (Figure 37-1). In a **complete fracture** the bone is broken entirely, whereas in an **incomplete fracture** the bone is damaged but is still in one piece. Complete and incomplete fractures also can be called **open** (formerly referred to as compound) if the skin is broken and **closed** (formerly called simple) if it is not. A fracture in which a bone breaks into two or more fragments is termed a **comminuted fracture.** Fractures are also classified according to the direction of the fracture line. A **linear fracture** runs parallel to the long

TABLE 37-1	**TYPES OF FRACTURES**
TYPE OF FRACTURE	**DEFINITION**
Typical Complete Fractures	
Closed	Noncommunicating wound between bone and skin
Open	Communicating wound between bone and skin
Comminuted	Multiple bone fragments
Linear	Fracture line parallel to long axis of bone
Oblique	Fracture line at an angle to long axis of bone
Spiral	Fracture line encircling bone (as a spiral staircase)
Transverse	Fracture line perpendicular to long axis of bone
Impacted	Fracture fragments pushed into each other
Pathologic	Fracture at a point where bone has been weakened by disease, for example, by tumors or osteoporosis
Avulsion	Fragment of bone connected to a ligament or tendon detaches from main bone
Compression	Fracture wedged or squeezed together on one side of bone
Displaced	Fracture with one, both, or all fragments out of normal alignment
Extracapsular	Fragment close to joint but remains outside joint capsule
Intracapsular	Fragment within joint capsule
Typical Incomplete Fractures	
Greenstick	Break in one cortex of bone with splintering of inner bone surface; commonly occurs in children and elderly persons
Torus	Buckling of cortex
Bowing	Bending of bone
Stress	Microfracture
Transchondral	Separation of cartilaginous joint surface (articular cartilage) from main shaft of bone

axis of the bone. An **oblique fracture** occurs at an oblique angle to the shaft of the bone. A **spiral fracture** encircles the bone, and a **transverse fracture** occurs straight across the bone.

Incomplete fractures tend to occur in the more flexible, growing bones of children. The three main types of incomplete fractures are greenstick, torus, and bowing fractures. A **greenstick fracture** perforates one cortex and splinters the spongy bone. The name is derived from the damage sustained by a young tree branch (a green stick) when it is bent sharply. The outer surface is disrupted, but the inner surface remains intact. Greenstick fractures typically occur in the proximal metaphysis or diaphysis of the tibia, radius, and ulna. In a **torus fracture,** the cortex buckles but does not break. **Bowing fractures** usually occur when longitudinal force is applied to bone. This type of fracture is common in children and usually involves the paired radius-ulna or the fibula-tibia. A complete diaphyseal fracture occurs in one of the bones of the pair, which disperses the stress sufficiently to prevent a complete fracture of the second bone, which bows rather than breaks. A bowing fracture resists correction (**reduction**) because the force necessary to reduce it must be equal to the force that bowed it. Treatment of bowing fractures is also difficult because the bowed bone interferes with reduction of the fractured bone. Types of fractures are summarized in Table 37-1.

Fractures may be further classified by cause as pathologic, stress, or transchondral fractures. A **pathologic fracture** is a break at the site of a preexisting abnormality, usually by force that would not fracture a normal bone. Any disease process that weakens a bone (especially the cortex) predisposes the bone to pathologic fracture. Pathologic fractures are commonly associated with tumors, osteoporosis, infections, and metabolic bone disorders.

Stress fractures occur in normal or abnormal bone that is subjected to repeated strain, such as occurs during athletics. The stress on the bone is cumulative and eventually causes a fracture. Two types of stress fractures are recognized: fatigue fracture and insufficiency fracture. A fatigue fracture is caused by abnormal stress or torque applied to a bone with normal ability to deform and recover. Fatigue fractures usually occur in individuals who engage in a new or different activity that is both strenuous and repetitive (e.g., joggers, skaters, dancers, military recruits). Because gains in muscle strength occur more rapidly than gains in bone strength, the newly developed muscles place exaggerated stress on the bones that are not yet ready for the additional stress. The imbalance between muscle and bone development causes microfractures to develop in the cortex. If the activity is controlled and increased gradually, new bone formation catches up to the increased demands and microfractures do not occur.

Insufficiency fractures, also known as fragility fractures, are breaks that occur in bones lacking the normal ability to deform and recover; these fractures can occur with normal weight bearing or activity. Rheumatoid arthritis, osteoporosis, Paget disease, osteomalacia, rickets, hyperparathyroidism, and radiation therapy all cause bone to lose its normal ability to deform and recover (i.e., the stress of normal weight bearing or activity fractures the bone). Pathologic fractures are generally a result of bone weakness caused by another disease such as cancer or infection. Although usually considered insufficiency fractures, breaks in the bone attributable to osteoporosis can also be referred to as pathologic fractures.

A transchondral fracture consists of fragmentation and separation of a portion of the articular cartilage that covers the end of a bone at a joint. (Joint structures are defined in Chapter 36.) Single or multiple sites may be fractured, and the fragments may consist of cartilage alone or cartilage and bone. Typical sites of transchondral fracture are the distal femur, the ankle, the patella, the elbow, and the wrist. Transchondral fractures are most prevalent in adolescents.

PATHOPHYSIOLOGY Fracture healing is a complex process that occurs primarily in one of two ways: direct or indirect. Both types of healing require integration of cells, signaling pathways, and various molecules. Direct (or primary) healing is similar to intramembranous bone formation and occurs when adjacent bone cortices are in contact with one another. This most often occurs when surgical fixation is used to repair a broken bone. No callus formation occurs with direct bone healing. Indirect (or secondary) healing is similar to endochondral bone formation and involves formation of callus with eventual remodeling of solid bone.[3] Bone formation that begins with an underlying cartilage scaffold is termed endochondral bone formation. A hallmark of indirect fracture healing is the formation of callus. Indirect fracture healing is most often observed when a fracture is treated with a cast or other nonsurgical method. When a bone is broken, the periosteum and blood vessels in the cortex, marrow, and surrounding soft tissues are disrupted. Bleeding occurs from the damaged ends of the bone and from the neighboring soft tissue. A clot (hematoma) forms within the medullary canal, between the fractured ends of the bone, and beneath the periosteum (Figure 37-2). Bone tissue immediately adjacent to the fracture dies. This dead tissue (along with any debris in the fracture area) stimulates an intense inflammatory response characterized by vasodilation, exudation of plasma and leukocytes, and infiltration by inflammatory leukocytes, growth factors,

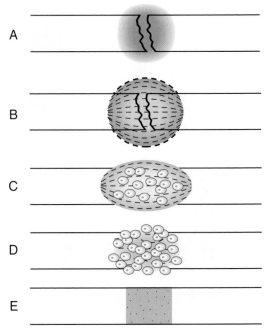

FIGURE 37-2 Bone Healing (Schematic Representation). **A,** Bleeding at broken ends of the bone with subsequent hematoma formation. **B,** Organization of hematoma into fibrous network. **C,** Invasion of osteoblasts, lengthening of collagen strands, and deposition of calcium. **D,** Callus formation; new bone is built while osteoclasts destroy dead bone. **E,** Remodeling is accomplished while excess callus is reabsorbed and trabecular bone is deposited. (From Monahan FD et al: *Phipps' medical-surgical nursing: health and illness perspectives,* ed 8, St Louis, 2007, Mosby.)

and mast cells that simultaneously decalcify the fractured bone ends. Within 48 hours after the injury, vascular tissue from surrounding soft tissue and the marrow cavity invades the fracture area, and blood flow to the entire bone increases. Bone-forming cells in the periosteum, endosteum, and marrow are activated to produce subperiosteal procallus along the outer surface of the shaft and over the broken ends of the bone (see Figure 37-2). Osteoblasts within the procallus synthesize collagen and matrix, which becomes mineralized to form callus. As the repair process continues, remodeling occurs, during which unnecessary callus is resorbed and trabeculae are formed along lines of stress as the repair tissues bring it in line with the tissue cells of the host (Figure 37-3). Except for the liver, bone is unique among all body tissues in that it will form new bone, not scar tissue, when it heals after a fracture.

CLINICAL MANIFESTATIONS The signs and symptoms of a fracture include unnatural alignment (deformity), swelling, muscle spasm, tenderness, pain and impaired sensation, and decreased mobility. The position of the broken bone segments is determined by the pull of attached muscles, gravity, and the direction and magnitude of the force that caused the fracture.

Immediately after a bone is fractured, usually there is numbness at the fracture site because of trauma to the nerve or nerves at the site. The numbness may last up to 20 minutes, during which time the injured person may use the fractured bone. However, once the numbness dissipates, the subsequent pain is quite severe and incapacitating until relieved with medication and treatment of the fractured bones. The pain is related to muscle spasms at the fracture site, overriding of the fracture segments, or damage to adjacent soft tissues.

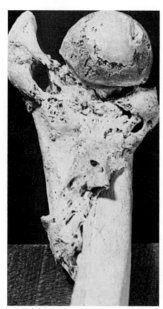

FIGURE 37-3 Exuberant Callus Formation Following Fracture. (From Rosai J: *Ackerman's surgical pathology*, ed 8, St Louis, 1996, Mosby.)

Pathologic fractures usually cause angular deformity, painless swelling, or generalized bone pain. Stress fractures are painful because of accelerated remodeling. The pain occurs during activity and is usually relieved by rest. Stress fractures also cause local tenderness and soft tissue swelling. Transchondral fractures may be entirely asymptomatic or may be painful during movement. Range of motion in the joint is limited, and movement may evoke audible clicking sounds (crepitus).

EVALUATION AND TREATMENT Treatment of a displaced fracture involves realigning the bone fragments (reduction) close to their normal or anatomic position and holding the fragments in place (immobilization) so that bone union can occur. Several methods are available to reduce a fracture: closed manipulation, traction, and open reduction. Adequate immobilization with a splint or cast is often all that is required for healing of fractures that are *not* misaligned. Many displaced fractures can be reduced by closed manipulation and reduction. The bone is moved or manipulated into place without opening the skin. Closed reduction is used when the contour of the bone is in fair alignment and can be maintained well with immobilization. Splints and casts are used to immobilize and hold a reduction in place.

Traction may be used to accomplish or maintain reduction. When bone fragments are displaced (not in their anatomic position), weights may be used to apply firm, steady traction (pull) and countertraction to the long axis of the bone. Traction stretches and fatigues muscles that have pulled the bone fragments out of place, allowing the distal fragment to align with the proximal fragment. Traction can be applied to the skin (skin traction), directly to the involved bone, or distal to the involved bone (skeletal traction). Skin traction is used when only a few pounds of pulling force are needed to realign the fragments or when the traction will be used for brief times only, such as before surgery or, for children with femoral fractures, for 3 to 7 days before applying a cast. In skeletal traction, a pin or wire is drilled through the bone below the fracture site, and a traction bow, rope, and weights are attached to the pin or wire to apply tension and to provide the pulling force required to overcome the muscle spasm and help realign the fracture fragments. More often, surgical repair (open reduction and internal fixation) or external fixation devices are used to realign displaced fractures.

Open reduction is a surgical procedure that exposes the fracture site; the fragments are manipulated into alignment under direct visualization. Some form of prosthesis, such as a screw, plate, nail, or wire, is used most often to maintain the reduction (internal fixation). External fixation, a procedure in which pins or rods are surgically placed into uninjured bone near the fracture site and then stabilized with an external frame of bars, is another method used to treat fractures that would not be adequately stabilized with a cast. Bone grafts, using donor bone from the individual (autograft), cadaver (allograft), or bone substitutes (ceramic composites, bioactive cement), can fill voids in the bone.

Improper reduction or immobilization of a fractured bone may result in nonunion, delayed union, or malunion. Nonunion is failure of the bone ends to grow together. The gap between the broken ends of the bone fills with dense fibrous and fibrocartilaginous tissue instead of new bone. Occasionally, the fibrous tissue contains a fluid-filled space that resembles a joint and is termed a *false joint*, or *pseudoarthrosis*. Delayed union is union that does not occur until approximately 8 to 9 months after a fracture. Malunion is the healing of a bone in an incorrect anatomic position.

Dislocation and Subluxation

Dislocation and subluxation are usually caused by trauma. Dislocation is the displacement of one or more bones in a joint in which the opposing joint surfaces entirely lose contact. If contact between the opposing joint surfaces is only partially lost, the injury is called a subluxation.

Dislocation and subluxation are most common in persons younger than 20 years of age and are generally associated with fractures. However, they may be the result of congenital or acquired disorders that cause (1) muscular imbalance, as occurs with congenital dislocation of the hip or neurologic disorders; (2) incongruities in the articulating surfaces of the bones, as occur with rheumatoid arthritis (see p. 999); or (3) joint instability.

The joints most often dislocated or subluxated are the joints of the shoulder, elbow, wrist, finger, hip, and knee. The shoulder joint most often injured is the glenohumeral joint. Finger dislocations are common injuries in contact sports such as football and rugby, and in basketball.

Traumatic dislocation of the elbow joint is common in the immature skeleton. In adults, an elbow dislocation is usually associated with a fracture of the ulna or head of the radius. Traumatic dislocation of the wrist usually involves the distal ulna and carpal bones. Any one of the eight carpal bones can be dislocated after an injury. Dislocation in the hand usually involves the metacarpophalangeal and interphalangeal joints.

Considerable trauma is needed to dislocate the hip. Anterior hip dislocation is rare in healthy persons; it is caused by forced abduction—for example, when an individual lands on his or her feet after falling from an elevated height. Posterior dislocation of the hip can occur as a result of an automobile accident in which the flexed knee strikes the dashboard, causing the head of the femur to be pushed posteriorly from the hip joint.

The knee is an unstable weight-bearing joint that depends heavily on the soft tissue structures around it for support. It is exposed to many different types of motion (flexion, extension, rotation) and is one of the most commonly injured joints. A knee dislocation can be anterior, posterior, lateral, medial, or rotary. It is usually the result of an injury that occurs during sports activities.

PATHOPHYSIOLOGY Dislocations and subluxations are often accompanied by fracture because stress is placed on areas of bone not usually subjected to stress. In addition, as the bone separates from the joint, it may bruise or tear adjacent nerves, blood vessels, ligaments, supporting structures, and soft tissue. Dislocations of the shoulder may damage the shoulder capsule and the axillary nerve. Damage to axillary nerves can cause anesthesia in the sensory distribution of the nerve and paralysis of the deltoid muscle. Dislocations also may disrupt circulation, leading to ischemia and possibly permanent disability of the affected extremity tissues.

CLINICAL MANIFESTATIONS Signs and symptoms of dislocations or subluxations include pain, swelling, limitation of motion, and joint deformity. Pain may be caused by effusion of inflammatory exudate into the joint or by associated tendon and ligament injury. Joint deformity is usually caused by muscle contractions that exert pull on the dislocated or subluxated joint. Limitation of motion results from effusion into the joint or the displacement of bones.

EVALUATION AND TREATMENT Evaluation of dislocations and subluxations is based on clinical manifestations and radiographic evaluation. Treatment consists of reduction and immobilization for 2 to 6 weeks and exercises to maintain normal range of motion in the joint. Depending on the joint that is injured, healing is usually complete within months to sometimes years.

Support Structures
Sprains and Strains of Tendons and Ligaments

Tendon and ligament injuries can accompany fractures and dislocations. A tendon is a fibrous connective tissue that attaches skeletal muscle to bone. A ligament is a band of fibrous connective tissue that connects bones where they meet in a joint. Tendons and ligaments support the bones and joints and either facilitate or limit motion. Tendons and ligaments can be torn, ruptured, or completely separated from bone at their points of attachment.

Tearing or stretching of a muscle or tendon is commonly known as a strain. Major trauma can tear or rupture a tendon at any site in the body. Most commonly injured are the tendons of the hands and feet, the knee (patellar), the upper arm (biceps and triceps), the thigh (quadriceps), the ankle, and the heel (Achilles).

Ligament tears are commonly known as sprains. Ligament tears and ruptures can occur at any joint but are most common in the wrist, ankle, elbow, and knee joints. A complete separation of a tendon or ligament from its bony attachment site is known as an avulsion and is commonly seen in young athletes, especially sprinters, hurdlers, and distance runners.

Strains and sprains are classified as first degree (least severe), second degree, and third degree (most severe). In first-degree sprains, the fibers are stretched but the muscle (strain) or joint (sprain) remains stable. In second-degree sprains, there is more tearing of the tendon or ligament fibers, with muscle weakness (strain) or some joint instability (sprain) but incomplete tearing of fibers. Third-degree strains result in inability to contract the muscle normally and cause significant joint instability.

PATHOPHYSIOLOGY When a tendon or ligament is torn, an inflammatory exudate develops between the torn ends. Later, granulation tissue containing macrophages, fibroblasts, and capillary buds grows inward from the surrounding soft tissue and cartilage to begin the repair process. Within 4 to 5 days after the injury, collagen formation begins. At first, collagen formation is random and disorganized. As the collagen fibers interweave and connect with preexisting tendon fibers, they become organized parallel to the lines of stress. Eventually vascular fibrous tissue fuses the new and surrounding tissues into a single mass. As reorganization takes place, the healing tendon or ligament separates from the surrounding soft tissue. Usually a healing tendon or ligament lacks sufficient strength to withstand some stress for 4 to 5 weeks after the injury but may take more than 3 months to achieve mechanical stability of a joint.[4] If powerful muscle pull does occur during this time, the tendon or ligament ends may separate again, which causes the tendon or ligament to heal in a lengthened shape with an excessive amount of scar tissue that renders the tendon or ligament functionless.

CLINICAL MANIFESTATIONS Tendon and ligament injuries are painful and are usually accompanied by soft tissue swelling, changes in tendon or ligament contour, and dislocation or subluxation of bones. The pain is generally sharp and localized, and tenderness persists over the distribution of the tendon or ligament. Depending on the tendon or ligament involved, such injuries may result in decreased mobility, instability, and weakness of the affected joints, even with prompt treatment.

EVALUATION AND TREATMENT Evaluation is based on clinical manifestations, stress radiography, arthroscopy, or arthrography. Initial treatment consists of PRICE (*Protection, Rest, Ice, Compression, and Elevation*) for the first 48 to 72 hours. Once swelling and acute pain subside, in most cases, support of the affected tendon or ligament with a compression dressing or brace will provide appropriate support while the tissues heal. In severe (third-degree) injuries, treatment may include suturing the tendon or ligament ends in close approximation. If this is not feasible because of the extent of damage, tendon or ligament grafting may be necessary. Prolonged rehabilitation exercises help ensure return of near-normal functions, but recovery may be complicated by post-traumatic arthritis.

Tendinopathy, Epicondylopathy, and Bursitis

Trauma also can cause painful inflammation of tendons (tendinopathy [tendonitis]) and bursae (bursitis). Other causes, however, of damage to tendons include reduced tissue perfusion, mechanical irritation, crystal deposits, postural misalignment, and hypermobility of a joint. Thus, *tendinopathy* is a more accurate term than *tendonitis* in most cases.

The histopathology of common conditions, such as lateral epicondylopathy ("tennis elbow") or medial epicondylopathy ("golfer's elbow"), is a degenerative process (Figure 37-4). A bony prominence at the end of a bone where tendons or ligaments attach is termed an epicondyle. When force is sufficient to cause microscopic tears (microtears) in tissue, the result is known as tendinopathy or epicondylopathy. Microtears in the tendon, the presence of disorganized collagen fibers, and neovascularization are indicative of incomplete tissue repair.[5,6] Initial inflammatory changes cause thickening of the tendon sheath, limiting movements and causing pain. Microtears cause bleeding, edema, and pain in the involved tendon or tendons. At times, after repeated inflammation, calcium may be deposited in the tendon origin area. The Achilles tendon also can be affected.

Lateral epicondylopathy (tennis elbow) is caused by irritation and overstretching of the extensor carpi radialis brevis (ECRB) tendon and forearm extensor muscles, resulting in tissue degradation.[7] Medial epicondylopathy (golfer's elbow) is the result of similar forces affecting the forearm muscles responsible for forearm flexion and pronation

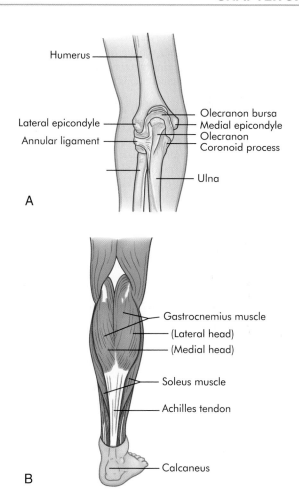

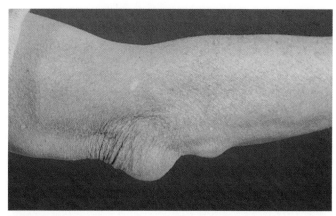

FIGURE 37-5 Olecranon Bursitis. Note swelling at the point of the elbow (olecranon). A smaller, rheumatoid nodule also is present. (From Klippel JH, Deippe PA, editors: *Rheumatology,* ed 2, London, 1998, Mosby.)

FIGURE 37-4 Epicondylopathy and Tendinopathy. **A,** Lateral and medial epicondyles of the distal humerus, sites of tennis elbow (lateral) and golfer's elbow (medial). **B,** Achilles tendon, common site of tendinopathy.

(see Figure 37-4). Load-bearing activities that involve flexion, extension, pronation, or supination of the elbow and forearm can lead to either lateral or medial elbow symptoms. Studies have shown that vascular in-growth in tendinopathy (neovascularization) is accompanied with nerve in-growth, facilitating pain transmission in Achilles and patellar tendinopathy.[8]

Bursae are small sacs lined with synovial membrane and filled with synovial fluid that are located between bony prominences and soft tissues, such as tendons, muscles, and ligaments (Figure 37-5). The primary function of bursa is to separate, lubricate, and cushion these structures. When irritated or injured, these sacs become inflamed and swell. Because most bursae lie outside joints, joint movement is rarely compromised with bursitis. Acute bursitis occurs primarily in middle age and is caused by trauma. Chronic bursitis can result from repeated trauma. Septic bursitis is caused by wound infection or bacterial infection of the skin overlying the bursae. Bursitis commonly occurs in the shoulder, hip, knee, and elbow.

PATHOPHYSIOLOGY   Bursitis usually is an inflammation that is reactive to overuse or excessive pressure but also can be caused by infection or acute trauma. The inflamed bursal sac becomes engorged, and the inflammation can spread to adjacent tissues. The inflammation may decrease with rest, ice, and aspiration of the fluid. (Inflammation is discussed in Chapter 6.)

CLINICAL MANIFESTATIONS   Clinical manifestations of epicondylopathy are usually localized to one side of the joint. Generally there is local tenderness and more pain with active motion than with passive motion. With tendinopathy or tendonitis, the pain is localized over the involved tendon. Stressing the tendon with simple activities, such as lifting even a few pounds of weight, can increase pain. Pain and sometimes weakness limit joint movement.

Joint motion is rarely limited in bursitis, except by pain. Shoulder pain may impair arm abduction. Bursitis in the knee produces pain when climbing stairs, and crossing the legs is painful in bursitis of the hip. Lying on the side of the inflamed trochanteric bursa is also very painful. Signs of infectious bursitis may include the presence of a puncture site, warmth and erythema, prior corticosteroid injection, severe inflammation, or an adjacent source of infection, such as from total joint replacement surgery.

EVALUATION AND TREATMENT   The diagnosis of tendinopathy, epicondylopathy, and bursitis is primarily based on clinical history and physical examination. Other imaging techniques, such as ultrasound or magnetic resonance imaging (MRI), may be used to evaluate the severity of the problem. Treatment (see *Health Alert: Managing Tendinopathy*) may include immobilization of the joint with a sling, splint, or cast; administration of systemic analgesics; application of ice or heat; or local injection of an anesthetic, a corticosteroid, platelet-rich plasma (PRP), or a combination local anesthetic/corticosteroid. Physical therapy to prevent loss of function begins after acute inflammation subsides.

Muscle Strains

Muscle strain is a general term for local muscle damage. Mild injury such as muscle strain is usually seen after traumatic or sports injuries. It is often the result of sudden, forced motion causing the muscle to become stretched beyond normal capacity. Strains often involve the tendon as well. Penetrating injuries, such as knife and gunshot wounds, can cause traumatic rupture (see Chapter 3). Muscles are ruptured more often than tendons in young people; the opposite is true in the older population. Muscle strain may be chronic when the muscle is repeatedly stretched beyond its usual capacity. There is evidence of tissue disruption with subsequent signs of muscle regeneration and connective tissue repair when a biopsy is performed. Hemorrhage into the surrounding tissue and signs of inflammation also may be

Managing Tendinopathy

Tennis and golfer's elbow, Achilles tendinopathy, and other tendon problems account for a large percentage of sports-related overuse injuries. Successful treatment of these conditions is challenging because of inconsistent results with many interventions. Chronic pain is common and may be the result of in-growth of nerves that accompanies in-growth of new blood vessels during the healing process. Recent studies suggest that the traditional approach of corticosteroid injections is helpful only for the short term. Other therapies that show promise include the following:

Prolotherapy: An irritant such as glucose or lidocaine is injected into the affected tendon, inducing an inflammatory response, thereby stimulating growth of new tendon fibers.

Eccentric exercises: The tendon is "prestretched," increasing its resting length and resulting in less strain during movement. The load on the tendon is gradually increased, causing the tendon, itself, to strengthen.

Extracorporeal shockwave therapy (SWT): External acoustic or sonic waves are focused on the affected area. The shockwaves stimulate soft tissue healing and inhibit pain receptors.

Aprotinin: This protease inhibitor may block matrix metalloproteinases (MMPs), thereby reducing the activity of enzymes such as collagenases. A major limitation to its use is the risk of anaphylaxis.

Platelet-rich plasma (PRP): This autologous source of concentrated platelets is obtained by centrifugation of plasma. The resulting solution contains high concentrations of cytokines and growth factors, such as platelet-derived growth factor (PDGF) and transforming growth factor-beta (TGF-β), which are thought to promote the growth of new, healthy tissue.

Whole blood injections: Autologous injection of blood at the site of tendinopathy is thought to provide necessary mediators of tissue healing and collagen regeneration.

To date, a combination of eccentric exercises and SWT has been shown to be both beneficial and safe with few, if any, side effects in treating tendinopathy.

Data from Coombes BK, Bisset L, Vicenzo B: Efficacy and safety of corticosteroid injections and other injections for management of tendinopathy: a systematic review of randomised controlled trials, *Lancet* 376(9754):1751–1767, 2010; de Vos RJ et al: Platelet-rich plasma injection for chronic Achilles tendinopathy: a randomized controlled trial, *J Am Med Assoc* 303(2):144–149, 2010; Hall MP et al: Platelet-rich plasma: current concepts and applications in sports, *J Am Acad Orthop Surg* 17(10):602–608, 2009; Maffulli N, Longo UG, Denaro V: Novel approaches for the management of tendinopathy, *J Bone Jt Surg Am* 92(15):2604–2613, 2010; Mafulli N et al: New options in the management of tendinopathy, *Open Acc J Sports Med* 1:29–37, 2010; Rabago D et al: A systematic review of four injection therapies for lateral epicondylosis: prolotherapy, polidocanol, whole blood and platelet-rich plasma, *Br J Sports Med* 43:471–481, 2009.

present. Regardless of the cause of trauma, muscle cells are usually able to regenerate. Regeneration may take up to 6 weeks, and the affected muscle should be protected during that time. (Degrees of acute muscle strain, together with their manifestations and treatment, are summarized in Table 37-2.)

A late complication of some muscle injuries is myositis ossificans, also known as heterotopic ossification (HO). Its exact pathophysiology remains unknown, but the basic problem seems to be the inability of mesenchymal cells to differentiate into osteoblastic stem cells and inappropriate differentiation of fibroblasts into bone-forming cells. Though uncommon, it is associated with burns, joint surgery, and trauma to the musculoskeletal system or central nervous system. HO may involve the muscle or tendons, ligaments, or bones near the muscle,[9] causing stiffness or deformity of an extremity. Soft tissue calcifications may be seen on plain radiographs.

Rhabdomyolysis

Once used interchangeably with the term *myoglobinuria*, rhabdomyolysis is the rapid breakdown of muscle that causes the release of intracellular contents, including the protein pigment myoglobin, into the extracellular space and bloodstream. Physical interruptions in the sarcolemmal membrane, called delta lesions, suggest that the sarcolemmal membrane is the route by which muscle constituents are released. Myoglobinuria, first described in victims of crush injuries in London during World War II, refers to the presence of the muscle protein myoglobin in the urine.

PATHOPHYSIOLOGY Rhabdomyolysis is sometimes incorrectly used interchangeable with *crush injury* (a description of injuries resulting from crushing of a body part), *compartment syndrome* (the consequences of increased intracompartmental pressures of a muscle), or *crush syndrome* (the pathophysiologic events caused by rhabdomyolysis, primarily involving the kidneys and coagulation syndrome).[10] Although relatively rare, rhabdomyolysis has many causes (Box 37-1) and can result in serious complications, including hyperkalemia (because of the release of intracellular potassium into the circulation), metabolic acidosis (from liberation of intracellular phosphorus and sulfate), acute renal failure (myoglobin precipitates in the tubules, obstructing flow through the nephron and producing injury), and even disseminated intravascular coagulation (DIC) (likely caused by activation of the clotting cascade by sarcolemma damage and release of intracellular components from the damaged muscles).

CLINICAL MANIFESTATIONS A *classic triad* of muscle pain, weakness, and dark urine is considered typical of rhabdomyolysis, but those affected may have no complaint of pain or muscle weakness.[10] Abnormally dark urine caused by myoglobinuria may be the first and only symptom. The renal threshold for myoglobin is low

TABLE 37-2 **MUSCLE STRAIN**		
TYPE	**MANIFESTATIONS**	**TREATMENT**
First degree (example: bench press in untrained athlete)	Muscle overstretched, pain but no muscle deformity	Ice should be applied 5 or 6 times in first 24-48 hr; gradual resumption of full weight bearing after initial rest for up to 2 weeks Exercises individualized to specific injury
Second degree (example: any muscle strain with bruising and pain)	Muscle intact with some tearing of fibers, swelling, pain	Treatment similar to that for first-degree strains
Third degree (example: traumatic injury)	Caused by tearing of fascia, marked weakness, deformity	Surgery to approximate ruptured edges; immobilization and non–weight-bearing status for 6 weeks

(approximately 0.5 mg/dl of urine); therefore only 200 g of muscle need to be damaged to cause visible changes in the urine. Myoglobin is rapidly cleared and levels may return to normal within 24 hours of injury. Along with the release of myoglobin, creatine kinase (CK) and other serum enzymes are released in massive quantities. The CK level may reach 2000 times normal (5 to 25 units/ml for women and 5 to 35 units/ml for men). The efflux of proteins and enzymes also includes loss of potassium, phosphate, nucleotides, creatinine, and creatine. Serum hypocalcemia is seen early in the course of myoglobinuria and is followed by late hypercalcemia. The risk of renal failure increases proportionately to the increase in serum CK, potassium, and phosphorus levels.

EVALUATION AND TREATMENT The most important and clinically useful measurement in rhabdomyolysis is serum creatine kinase (CK) level. A level five times the upper limit of normal (about 1000 units/L) is used to identify rhabdomyolysis. Once CK levels exceed 5000 units/L, acute renal failure is likely. A recent study evaluated the ultrasonographic appearance of rhabdomyolysis in damaged muscle from earthquake victims and found abnormalities in muscle texture and subcutaneous tissue, as well as liquid areas in the damaged tissue.[11]

Maintaining adequate urinary flow and prevention of kidney failure are goals of treatment. Rapid intravenous hydration maintains adequate kidney flow. Other issues, such as hyperkalemia, may require temporary hemodialysis. Treatments such as using mannitol to cause

---

BOX 37-1   SELECTED CAUSES OF RHABDOMYOLYSIS

Direct Trauma
Blunt trauma or crush injury (motor vehicle crashes, collapsed buildings)
Burns (thermal)
Electrical injury
Excessive compression (from immobility attributable to stroke, alcohol or drug intoxication)

Drugs
Alcohol
Amphetamines
Anesthetic and paralytic agents (halothane, propofol, succinylcholine—malignant hyperthermia syndrome)
Antihistamines (diphenhydramine, doxylamine)
Anti-hyperlipidemic agents (statins, clofibrate, bezafibrate)
Antipsychotics and antidepressants (amitriptyline, doxepine, fluoxetine, haloperidol, lithium, protriptyline, perphenazine, promethazine, chlorpromazine, trifluoperazine)
Caffeine
Cocaine
Corticosteroids
HIV integrase inhibitor (raltegravir)
Hypnotics and sedatives (benzodiazepines, barbiturates)
Heroin
LSD (lysergic acid diethylamide)
Methamphetamine
Methadone
Methylenedioxymethamphetamine (MDMA; "ecstasy")
Miscellaneous medications (amphotericin B, azathioprine, ε-aminocaproic acid, quinidine, penicillamine, salicylates, theophylline, terbutaline, thiazides, vasopressin)
Phencyclidine
Protease inhibitors

Excessive Muscular Contraction
Status epilepticus
Delirium tremens
Acute psychosis
Severe dystonia
Sporadic strenuous exercise (e.g., marathons, squats)
Tetanus

Infectious Agents
Bacteria (group B streptococci, *Streptococcus pneumoniae, Staphylococcus epidermidis, Borrelia burgdorferi, Escherichia coli, Clostridium perfringens, Clostridium tetani, Streptococcus viridans; Bacillus, Brucella, Legionella, Listeria, Leptospira, Mycoplasma, Plasmodium, Rickettsia, Salmonella,* and *Vibrio* species)
Fungal organisms (*Aspergillus, Candida* species)
Viruses (influenza types A and B, coxsackievirus, dengue, Epstein-Barr, HIV, cytomegalovirus (CMV), parainfluenza, varicella-zoster, West Nile)

Toxins
Carbon monoxide
Envenomation (black widow spider, Africanized honey bees, vipers)
Hemlock
Methanol
Toluene

Hereditary Enzyme Disorders (Rare)
McArdle disease (myophosphorylase deficiency)
Tarui disease (type VII glycogen storage disease)
Phosphoglycerate mutase deficiency (glycogen storage disease type X)
Carnitine palmitoyltransferase deficiency (CPT-1 deficiency)

Miscellaneous Causes
Diabetic ketoacidosis
Endocrinopathy
Heatstroke
Hypothermia
Nonketotic hyperosmolar coma
Polymyositis
Severe electrolyte disorders (near-drowning or water intoxication, severe vomiting or diarrhea)

Data from: Acharya S et al: Acute dengue myositis with rhabdomyolysis and acute renal failure, *Ann Indian Acad Neurol* 13(3):221–222, 2010; Cervellin G, Comelli I, Lippi G: Rhabdomyolysis: historical background, clinical, diagnostic, and therapeutic features, *Coin Chem Lab Med* 48(6): 749–756, 2010; Croce F et al: Severe raltegravir-associated rhabdomyolysis: a case report and review of the literature, *Int J STD AIDS* 21(11): 783–785, 2010; Halpern P et al: Morbidity associated with MDMA (ecstasy) abuse—a survey of emergency department admissions, *Hum Exp Toxicol* 29(5):259–266, 2010; Mammen AL, Amato AA: Statin myopathy: a review of recent progress, *Curr Opin Rheumatol* 22(6):644–650, 2010.

BOX 37-2 FACTORS AFFECTING DEVELOPMENT OF COMPARTMENT SYNDROME

Increased Intracompartmental Pressure

Fracture (open or closed)
Traction
Crush syndrome
Vigorous exercise
High-energy soft tissue injury (blast injuries, blunt force trauma)
Fluid infusion
Arterial puncture
Ruptured abdominal aortic aneurysm
Ruptured ganglion/other cyst
Envenomation (venomous snakes, black widow spiders)
Nephrotic syndrome
Viral myositis
Acute hematogenous osteomyelitis
Orthopedic procedures (e.g., osteotomy, joint replacement)
Seizures
Tetany

Reduced Compartment Volume

Burns
Repair of muscle herniation
Circumferential dressings
Too-tight casts

Conditions That Disturb Microcirculation

Diabetes
Hypothyroidism
Bleeding disorders (hemophilia, von Willebrand disease, leukemia, vitamin K deficiency, viral hemorrhagic fevers [dengue])
Excessive anticoagulation

Adapted from Shadgan B et al: Current thinking about acute compartment syndrome of the lower extremity, *Can J Surg* 53(5):329–334, 2010.

an osmotic diuresis or bicarbonate to alkalinize the urine have not been shown to consistently improve outcomes.

Compartment Syndrome

Compartment syndrome is the result of increased pressure within a muscle compartment. Skeletal muscles are surrounded by several layers of fibrous fascia that do not expand. Increased pressure on the muscle tissue causes diminished capillary blood flow, resulting in local tissue hypoxia and necrosis. Causes of compartment syndrome include conditions that increase the contents of the compartment, decrease the compartment volume, or disturb the muscle's microvasculature (Box 37-2).[12,13]

PATHOPHYSIOLOGY The weight of a limp extremity can generate enough pressure to produce muscle ischemia (Figures 37-6 and 37-7). This causes edema, rising compartment pressure, and tamponade that lead to muscle infarction and neural injury and eventually result in cell loss. Physical interruptions in the sarcolemmal membrane, called *holes* or *delta lesions,* suggest that the sarcolemmal membrane may be the route by which muscle constituents are released. (The sarcolemmal membrane, the plasma membrane of the muscle cell, is described in Chapter 36.)

CLINICAL MANIFESTATIONS Compartments often affected are the anterior and deep posterior tibial compartments in the leg, the gluteal

compartments in the buttocks, and the abdominal wall. Diagnosis is initiated by clinical examination. The "5 Ps" of compartment syndrome are *Pain* (out of proportion to expected injury), *Pallor,* *Paresthesia,* *Paresis* (of the involved extremity), and *Pulselessness.* None of these signs are truly dependable, although pain and paresthesia are the findings most suggestive of compartment syndrome.

A condition known as Volkmann ischemic contracture can develop when the muscles of the forearm are affected by severe burns, bleeding disorders, crush injury, animal bites, or any other condition that causes increased pressure within the forearm muscle compartments. The resulting contracture deformities of the fingers, hand, and wrist can lead to partial or complete disability of the affected limb.

EVALUATION AND TREATMENT Direct measurement of intracompartmental pressure, using a tonometer, is essential to confirm the diagnosis. Laboratory tests, ultrasonography, and imaging studies may help exclude other conditions but generally are not helpful in diagnosing compartment syndrome. Once intracompartmental pressures reach 30 mm Hg, surgical intervention is warranted to relieve pressure within the compartment.

Surgical intervention consists of performing a fasciotomy of the affected area to decompress the compartment and allow return of normal blood supply. Skin grafts are often required to close the resultant opening, but vacuum-assisted wound closure devices also have been used successfully in accelerating wound closure.

Malignant Hyperthermia

Malignant hyperthermia (MH) is an inherited muscle disorder characterized by a hypermetabolic reaction to certain volatile anesthetics or succinylcholine that activates a prolonged release of intracellular calcium from the sarcoplasmic reticulum. This process can cause hypermetabolism with extremely high body temperature, muscle rigidity, rhabdomyolysis, and death if not quickly treated with dantrolene infusion.[14,15]

Although several potential links between coexisting conditions and MH have been proposed, none have yet been identified as strong predictors of developing the condition.[14-17] Young males tend to be more susceptible to MH. Common signs and symptoms are respiratory acidosis, sinus tachycardia, masseter muscle spasm, and elevated body temperature.[18]

EVALUATION AND TREATMENT Careful and thorough preoperative assessment should alert the anesthesiologist to the possibility of an individual being susceptible to malignant hyperthermia. A family history of anesthetic problems and previous untoward anesthetic experiences (muscle cramping, unexplained fevers, dark urine) are criteria that require further clarification before administration of a volatile anesthetic, such as halothane, or of the muscle relaxant succinylcholine.

Priorities in treatment of myoglobinuria include identifying and treating the underlying disorder and preventing life-threatening renal failure. Malignant hyperthermia and myoglobinuria can be treated by infusing dantrolene sodium (Dantrium). Secondary problems include electrolyte imbalance, volume depletion, acidosis, hyperuricemia, hyperkalemia, and calcium imbalance; these need specific treatment. Short-term dialysis also may be necessary.

> **✓ QUICK CHECK 37-1**
> 1. How are fractures classified?
> 2. What is the primary pathology of epicondylopathy?
> 3. Why is myoglobinuria a dangerous complication of rhabdomyolysis?

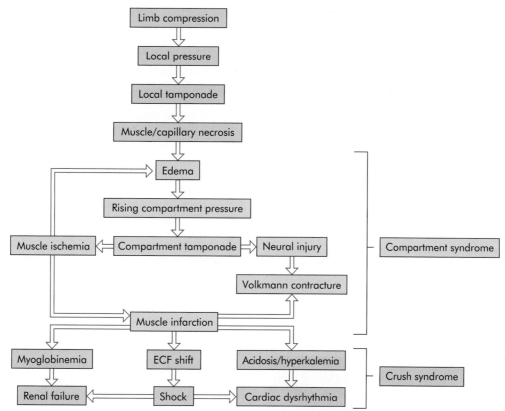

FIGURE 37-6 Pathogenesis of Compartment Syndrome and Crush Syndrome Caused by Prolonged Muscle Compression. *ECF,* Extracellular fluid.

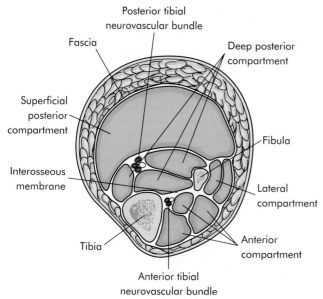

FIGURE 37-7 Muscle Compartments of the Lower Leg. (From Mohahan FD et al: *Phipps' medical-surgical nursing: health and illness perspectives,* ed 8, St Louis, 2007, Mosby.)

DISORDERS OF BONES

Metabolic Bone Diseases

Metabolic bone disease is characterized by abnormal bone structure that is caused by altered or inadequate biochemical reactions, which may be attributable to genetics, diet, or hormones.

Osteoporosis

Osteoporosis, or porous bone, is a complex, multifactorial, chronic disease that often progresses silently for decades until fractures occur. It is the most common disease that affects bone but is not necessarily a consequence of the aging process because some elderly people retain strong, relatively dense bones. In osteoporosis, old bone is being resorbed faster than new bone is being made, causing the bones to lose density, becoming thinner and more porous. A progressive loss of bone mass may continue until the skeleton is no longer strong enough to support itself. Eventually, bones can fracture spontaneously. As bone becomes more fragile, falls or bumps that would not have caused a fracture previously now cause bone to break. Osteoporosis appears to be most severe in the femoral neck, thoracic and lumbar spine,[19] and wrist.

Bone tissue can be normally mineralized in osteoporosis but the mass (density) of bone is decreased and the structural integrity of trabecular bone is impaired. Cortical bone becomes more porous and thinner, making bone weaker and prone to fractures (Figures 37-8 and 37-9). The World Health Organization (WHO) has defined osteoporosis as "…a systematic skeletal disease characterized by low bone density and microarchitectural deterioration of bone tissue with a consequent increase in bone fragility."[20]

Bone density is based on the number of standard deviations away from the mean bone mineral density of a young-adult reference population (a T-score). Table 37-3 lists these categories. Bone density between 1.5 and 2.5 standard deviations below normal is considered osteopenia. A T-score of 2.5 or more standard deviations below normal bone density is considered osteoporotic. Severe or established osteoporosis is identified when there has been a fragility fracture associated with low bone density. The disease can be (1) generalized, involving major portions of the axial skeleton, or (2) regional, involving one segment of the appendicular skeleton.

Skeletal homeostasis depends on a narrow range of plasma calcium and phosphate concentrations, which are maintained by the endocrine system. Therefore, endocrine dysfunction ultimately can cause metabolic bone disease. In addition to declining levels of sex steroids, the hormones most commonly associated with osteoporosis are parathyroid hormone, cortisol, thyroid hormone, and growth hormone. (Endocrine function is discussed in Chapters 17 and 18.)

Throughout a lifetime, old bone is removed (resorption) and new bone is added (formation) to the skeleton. During childhood and teenage years, new bone is added faster than old bone is removed. Consequently, bones become larger, heavier, and denser. Bone formation continues at a pace faster than resorption until peak bone mass or maximum bone density and strength is reached, around age 30. Up to 90% of peak bone mass is obtained by age 20. After age 30, bone resorption slowly exceeds bone formation. In women, bone loss is most rapid in the first years after menopause but persists throughout the postmenopausal years. In 2011, the United States Preventive Services Task Force (USPSTF) issued a new recommendation that women age 65 and older be routinely screened for osteoporosis.[21] Fractures are the major complication of osteoporosis and it has been estimated that nearly one in two American Caucasian

women over the age of 50 will sustain at least one fragility fracture in her lifetime.[22] The estimated costs of direct medical care for osteoporotic fractures was estimated to be between $12.2 to $17.9 billion per year in 2002 U.S. dollars.[23] Hip fractures, in particular, can have devastating effects on an individual's life. In addition to direct medical costs, studies have shown decreased quality of life as well as excess loss of life-years for those experiencing hip or osteoporotic fractures.[24,25] The major risks for persons with osteoporosis are fractures (see *Health Alert: Osteoporosis Facts and Figures at a Glance*). Men lose bone density with aging but because they begin with a higher bone density they reach osteoporotic levels at an older age than do women. The lifetime fracture risk for men is estimated to be 20%, compared to 50% for women.[26]

Vertebral fractures tend to occur in the later years of life; however, they are more difficult to ascertain because people are unaware of the fracture. The degree of compression necessary to define a vertebral fracture is not standardized, although attempts have been made to standardize the definition and diagnosis of vertebral fractures.[27] Thus, the true prevalence is unknown but fractures do increase in frequency by the sixth and seventh decades, and vertebral fracture prevalence in men is close to that in women (see *Health Alert: Osteoporosis Facts and Figures at a Glance*).

Age-related loss of bone density and osteoporosis is most common in Asians and whites but affects all races. Blacks have only about half the fracture rate of whites, but African American women remain at high risk because of factors such as decreased calcium intake, a high percentage of lactose intolerance, and increased prevalence of diseases such as sickle cell disease and lupus that increase the risk of developing

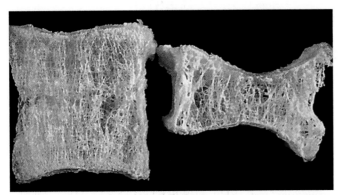

FIGURE 37-8 Vertebral Body. Osteoporotic vertebral body *(right)* shortened by compression fractures compared with a normal vertebral body. Note that the osteoporotic vertebra has a characteristic loss of horizontal trabeculae and thickened vertical trabeculae. (From Kumar V et al: *Robbins and Cotran pathologic basis of disease*, ed 7, Philadelphia, 2005, Saunders.)

TABLE 37-3	**T-SCORE AND WORLD HEALTH ORGANIZATION DIAGNOSIS OF BONE DENSITY**
T-SCORE	**DIAGNOSIS**
0 to −0.99 SD	Normal BMD
−1.0 to −2.49 SD	Low bone density (osteopenia)
≤2.5 SD	Osteoporosis
≤2.5 SD with any fracture	Severe osteoporosis

Adapted from Licata AA: Diagnosing primary osteoporosis: it's more than a T-score, *Clev Clin J Med* 73(5):473–476, 2006.
BMD, Bone mineral density; *SD,* standard deviation.

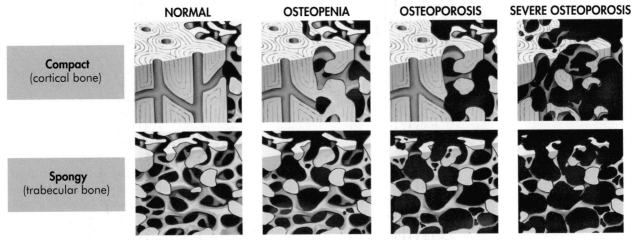

FIGURE 37-9 Osteoporosis in Cortical and Trabecular Bone.

TOOL	STRENGTHS	POTENTIAL LIMITATIONS
TABLE 37-4	**COMPARISON OF STUDY OF FRACTURES (SOF), GARVAN, AND FRAX FRACTURE PREDICTION TOOLS**	
Study of Fractures (SOF)	Based on BMD alone Predicted 10-year hip, major osteoporotic, and clinical fracture risk as well as FRAX in women 65 and older Simple model Does not require Internet access	Validated only for age 65 or older
Garvan	Takes into account previous fractures, history, and number of previous falls Predicts more types of fractures than FRAX Allows 5- and 10-year fracture prediction	Does not include risk factors, such as smoking, glucocorticoid exposure, alcohol intake, rheumatoid arthritis, individual with hip fracture Based on a single population (Australia)
FRAX	Is country-specific (Europe, North America, Asia, Australia) Takes into account prior fracture, parental history of fracture, BMI, use of glucocorticoids or alcohol, current cigarette smoking, and secondary osteoporosis Calculates 10-year absolute fracture risk for individuals with hip, wrist, humerus, and clinical spine fractures Has been well validated in clinical studies Can be used with or without BMD information	Does not take into account single versus multiple fractures Can be used only in individuals untreated for osteoporosis Available only on-line (www.shef.ac.uk); not all practitioners have Internet access Assumes relationship between BMI and mortality is similar in all races, ethnic groups Assumes similar variability in fracture rates across all race and ethnic groups in U.S.

Data from Ensrud KE et al: Study of osteoporotic fractures research group: a comparison of prediction models for fractures in older women: is more better? *Arch Intern Med* 169(22):2087–2094, 2009; Honig S: Osteoporosis—new treatments and updates, *Bull NYU Hosp Jt Dis* 68(3): 166–170, 2010; Silverman SL, Calderon AD: The utility and limitations of FRAX: a US perspective, *Curr Osteoporos Rep* 8:192–197, 2010; Van den Bergh JP et al: Assessment of individual fracture risk: FRAX and beyond, *Curr Osteoporos Rep* 8:131–137, 2010.

HEALTH ALERT

Osteoporosis Facts and Figures at a Glance

- Osteoporosis is the most common bone disease of adults and the foremost cause of fractures in the elderly.
- More than 10 million Americans have osteoporosis (T-score *equal to or more than* 2.5 SD below normal peak bone mass) and nearly 34 million have low bone density (T-score 1.5 to 2.5 SD below normal peak bone mass).
- The National Osteoporosis Foundation (NOF) estimates that 24% of individuals with a hip fracture die within the first year of injury.
- Hip fractures account for only 14% of fractures in osteoporosis, but are responsible for 72% of fracture costs.
- Osteoporosis-related fractures result in approximately 180,000 nursing home admissions, more than 432,000 hospital admissions, and nearly 2.5 million medical office visits annually.
- By 2025, fractures are estimated to increase to $3 million annually, with medical costs escalated to $35 billion.
- It is estimated that 4 in 10 Caucasian women and 1 in 8 Caucasian men will experience a hip, spine, or wrist fracture sometime in their lives.
- By 2025, Hispanics are predicted to account for 20% of fractures in Arizona and California, with Asians and other non-white ethnic groups sustaining 27% of fractures in New York.

Data from Burge R et al: Incidence and economic burden of osteoporosis-related fractures in the United States, 2005-2025, *J Bone Miner Res* 22:465, 2007; King AB et al: Interstate variation in the burden of fragility fractures, *J Bone Miner Res* 24(4):681–692, 2009; National Osteoporosis Foundation: *Clinicians' guide to prevention and treatment of osteoporosis*, Washington DC, 2010, Author.

osteoporosis.[28] Both African American women and men have generally been undertreated for osteoporosis.[29]

Fracture prevention is a primary goal of osteoporosis treatment. Measuring bone mineral density (BMD) by using dual x-ray absorptiometry (DXA) and calculating an individual's T-score continues to be the most common method of evaluating bone health and predicting fracture risk. Predicting future fracture risk has been improved through the development of new instruments, such as the Study of Osteoporosis Fractures (SOF), Garvan, and FRAX™ tools. Table 37-4 compares the strengths and limitations of each tool.

Bone quality is not defined by bone mass alone (as measured by BMD) but also by the microarchitecture of the bone. Thus, other variables include crystal size and shape, brittleness, vitality of bone cells, structure of the bone proteins, integrity of the trabecular network, and the ability to repair tiny cracks. Because bone density relates to *quantity* of bone, *quality* of bone is not accurately identified by bone density testing alone. As a result, bone density testing may not accurately identify those who will eventually be susceptible to fractures.

Postmenopausal osteoporosis is bone loss that occurs in middle-aged and older women. It can occur because of estrogen deficiency as well as from estrogen-independent age-related mechanisms (e.g., secondary causes such as hyperparathyroidism and decreased mechanical stimulation). Estrogen deficiency can also increase with stress, excessive exercise, and low body weight. Postmenopausal changes include a substantial increase in bone turnover—that is, a remodeling imbalance between the activity of osteoclasts (bone destroyers) and osteoblasts (bone formers). Increased formation and activity of osteoclasts causes removal or resorption of bone and results in a cascade of proinflammatory cytokines. Increased cytokine activation, especially tumor necrosis factor (TNF), can occur with declining estrogen levels.[30] In addition, estrogen helps osteoclast apoptosis (programmed cell death) so estrogen level decrease is associated with *survival* of the bone-removing osteoclasts. Biologically, these processes involve the receptor activator nuclear factor κβ ligand (RANKL), osteoprotegerin (OPG) signaling pathways, and insulin-like growth factor (IGF) (see Chapter 36, p. 957 and Figure 36-5). Other causes may include a combination of inadequate dietary calcium intake and lack of vitamin D, possibly decreased magnesium, lack of exercise, low body mass, and family history. IGF is known to help in fracture healing and collagen synthesis and improves conditions for bone mineralization. IGF levels significantly decline by age 60. Excessive phosphorus intake, chiefly through the intake of sodas and junk foods, interferes with the calcium/phosphorus balance.

In clinical studies of women, data have suggested that levels of serum androgens may influence bone density in pre-, peri-, and postmenopausal women.[31,32] Androgens (i.e., testosterone and dihydrotestosterone) have long been recognized as stimulants of bone formation. Increasing age in both men and women is associated with declining levels of estradiol and androgen, leading to losses in BMD. In addition, progesterone deficiency may be related to osteoporosis. Decreases in weight-bearing exercise are associated with osteoporosis as well. Other risk factors are identified in *Risk Factors:* Osteoporosis.

RISK FACTORS
Osteoporosis

Genetic	**Lifestyle**
Family history of osteoporosis	Sedentary
White race	Smoker
Increased age	Alcohol consumption (excessive)
Female gender	Low-impact fractures as an adult
	Inability to rise from a chair without
Anthropometric	using one's arms
Small stature	
Fair or pale skinned	**Concurrent**
Thin build	Hyperparathyroidism
Low bone mineral density	
	Illness and Trauma
Hormonal and Metabolic	Renal insufficiency, hypocalciuria
Early menopause (natural or surgical)	Rheumatoid arthritis
Late menarche	Spinal cord injury
Nulliparity	Systemic lupus
Obesity	
Hypogonadism	**Liver Disease**
Gaucher disease	Marrow disease (myeloma, mastocy-
Cushing syndrome	tosis, thalassemia)
Weight below healthy range	
Acidosis	**Drugs**
	Corticosteroids
Dietary	Dilantin
Low dietary calcium and vitamin D	Gonadotropin-releasing hormone
Low endogenous magnesium	agonists
Excessive protein*	Loop diuretics
Excessive sodium intake	Methotrexate
Anorexia	Thyroid medications
Malabsorption	Heparin
	Cyclosporin
	Medroxyprogesterone acetate
	(Depo-Provera)
	Retinoids

*Low levels of protein intake also have been reported.

Insufficient intake or malabsorption of dietary minerals is a factor in the development of osteoporosis. Calcium absorption from the intestine decreases with age and studies of individuals with osteoporosis show that their calcium intake is lower than that of age-matched controls. Other mineral deficiencies, including magnesium, also may be important. Vitamin deficiencies, particularly vitamins C and D, as well as either deficiencies or excesses of protein also contribute to bone loss. Significant differences in the levels of trace elements (zinc, copper, manganese) were noted in the bones and hair of unaffected individuals compared to those with osteoporosis.[33] Excessive intake of caffeine, phosphorus, alcohol, and nicotine along with low body fat (weight less than 125 pounds) also have been considered risk factors. Secondary osteoporosis is osteoporosis caused by other conditions, including hormonal imbalances (endocrine disease, diabetes, hyperparathyroidism, hyperthyroidism), medications (e.g., heparin, corticosteroids, phenytoin, barbiturates, lithium), and other substances (e.g., tobacco, ethanol). Other conditions, including rheumatoid disease, human immunodeficiency virus (HIV), malignancies, malabsorption syndrome, liver or kidney disease, also increase risk for developing osteoporosis (see *Risk Factors*: Osteoporosis).

Secondary osteoporosis sometimes develops temporarily in individuals receiving large doses of heparin, perhaps because heparin promotes bone resorption by decreasing collagen synthesis or by increasing collagen breakdown. Osteoporosis caused by heparin therapy usually resolves when therapy ceases. Other medications increasing risk of osteoporosis include glucocorticoids and lithium, methotrexate, anticonvulsants, cyclophosphamide, and cyclosporine.

Regional osteoporosis—osteoporosis confined to a segment of the appendicular skeleton—usually has a known cause. Classic regional osteoporosis is associated with disuse or immobilization of a limb because of fractures or bone or joint inflammation.[34] A negative calcium balance develops early and continues throughout the period of immobilization. After 8 weeks of immobilization, significant osteoporosis is present, although it may develop earlier in persons younger than 20 years or older than 50 years. A uniform distribution of osteoporosis also has been observed in astronauts and in individuals treated with air suspension therapy as a result of weightlessness.

Transient regional osteoporosis has no known etiology and is characterized by bone marrow edema and sometimes severe pain. Transient regional osteoporosis is usually self-limiting, and tends to occur in middle-aged men and women in their late second or third trimester of pregnancy.[35] Bone marrow edema can be seen on magnetic resonance imaging (MRI) and areas of localized bone demineralization are seen in plain radiographs. The lower extremity is most often affected but other areas also can be involved.[36] Treatment is primarily symptomatic and the condition usually resolves spontaneously over 3 to 6 months, with no long-term adverse effects.

PATHOPHYSIOLOGY Whatever the cause, osteoporosis develops when the remodeling cycle (coupling)—bone resorption and bone formation—is disrupted, leading to an imbalance in the coupling process. Osteoclasts are differentiated cells that function to resorb bone. The explosion of new information in the field of bone biology has led to new understandings of osteoclast biology and bone pathophysiology. Of primary importance is the osteoclast differentiation pathway that is dependent on various processes including proliferation, maturation, fusion, and activation. These processes, in turn, are dependent on the availability of stem cells to allow differentiation to occur and are controlled by hormones, cytokines, and paracrine stromal-cell interactions. Thus, proper intracellular communication within bone among its molecular regulators is necessary for normal bone homeostasis.

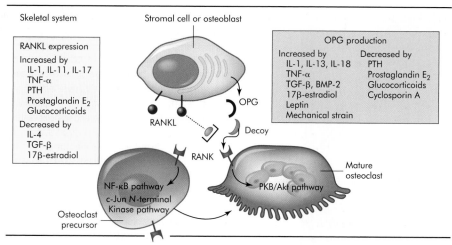

FIGURE 37-10 OPG/RANKL/RANK System. Expression of RANKL, a cytokine and part of the TNF family, and OPG, a glycoprotein receptor antagonist, is modulated by various cytokines, hormones, drugs, and mechanical strains (see inserts). In bone RANKL is expressed by both stromal cells and osteoblasts. RANKL stimulates the receptor RANK on osteoclast precursor cells and mature osteoclasts and activates intracellular signaling pathways to promote osteoclast differentiation and activation as well as cytoskeletal reorganization and survival (PKB/Akt pathway), which increase resorption and bone loss. OPG, secreted by stromal cells and osteoblasts, acts as a "decoy" receptor and blocks RANKL binding to and activation of RANK. *BMP,* Bone morphogenic protein; *IL,* interleukin; *OPG,* osteoprotegerin; *PTH,* parathyroid hormone; *RANK,* receptor activator nuclear factor κβ; *RANKL,* receptor activator nuclear factor κβ ligand; *TGF-β,* transforming growth factor-beta; *TNF-α,* tumor necrosis factor-alpha. (Adapted from Hofbauer LC, Schoppet M: *JAMA* 292[4]:490–495, 2004.)

Numerous interleukins, tumor necrosis factor (TNF), transforming growth factor-beta (TGF-β), prostaglandin E₂, and hormones interact to control osteoclasts (Figure 37-10). Staggering in its importance to understanding osteoclast biology is the cytokine **receptor activator of nuclear factor κβ ligand (RANKL)**; its **receptor activator nuclear factor κβ (RANK)**; and its decoy receptor **osteoprotegerin (OPG)**, a glycoprotein (see Chapter 36 and Figure 36-5).

Glucocorticoid-induced osteoporosis (e.g., cortisone) is characterized by the inhibition of osteoblast formation and function and possibly an increase in osteocyte apoptosis.[37] Glucocorticoids increase RANKL expression and inhibit OPG production by osteoblasts.

Age-related bone loss begins in the fourth decade. The cause remains unclear, but it is known that decreased serum growth hormone (GH) and insulin-like growth factor 1 (IGF-1) levels, along with increased binding of RANKL and decreased OPG production, affect osteoblast and osteoclast function.[38] Loss of trabecular bone in men proceeds in a linear fashion with thinning of trabecular bone rather than complete loss, as is noted in women (Figure 37-11). Men have approximately 30% greater bone mass than women, which may be a factor in their later involvement with osteoporosis (Figure 37-12). In addition, men have a more gradual decrease in the levels of testosterone and estradiol (and possibly progesterone), thereby maintaining their bone mass longer than women. The reduction in physical activity in older persons also may be a factor.

CLINICAL MANIFESTATIONS The specific clinical manifestations of osteoporosis depend on the bones involved. The most common manifestations, however, are pain and bone deformity. Unfortunately, these manifestations occur only in an advanced disease state. Fractures are likely to occur because the trabeculae of spongy bone become thin and sparse, and compact bone becomes porous. As the bones lose volume, they become brittle and weak and may collapse or become misshapen. Vertebral collapse causes **kyphosis** (hunchback) and diminishes height

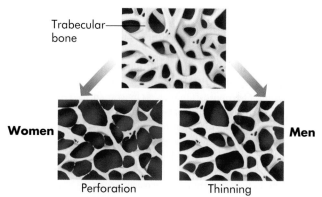

FIGURE 37-11 Mechanism of Loss of Trabecular Bone in Women and Trabecular Thinning in Men. Bone thinning predominates in men because of reduced bone formation. Loss of connectivity and complete trabeculae predominates in women.

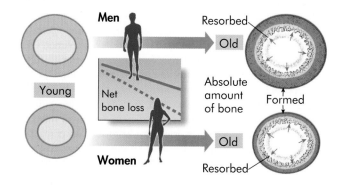

FIGURE 37-12 Bone Loss in Men and Women. Absolute amount of bone resorbed on the inner bone surface and formed on the outer bone surface is more in men than women during aging.

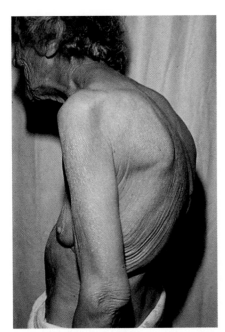

FIGURE 37-13 Kyphosis. This elderly woman's condition was caused by a combination of spinal osteoporotic vertebral collapse and chronic degenerative changes in the vertebral column. (From Kamal A, Brocklehurst JC: *Color atlas of geriatric medicine*, ed 2, St Louis, 1992, Mosby.)

(Figure 37-13). Fractures of the long bones (particularly the femur),[19] distal radius, ribs, and vertebrae are most common. Fracture of the neck of the femur—the so-called broken hip—tends to occur in older or elderly women with osteoporosis. Fatal complications of fractures include fat or pulmonary embolism, pneumonia, hemorrhage, and shock. Approximately 20% of persons may die as a result of surgical complications. Osteoporosis in men, as in women, also may be related to hypogonadism, with estradiol levels being more clinically important than testosterone levels in both genders.[39-41] Adequate dietary intake of calcium, vitamin D, magnesium, and possibly boron (see *Health Alert: Calcium, Vitamin D, and Bone Health*); a regular regimen of weight-bearing exercise; and avoidance of alcoholism, tobacco, and glucocorticoids seem to help prevent primary osteoporosis.

EVALUATION AND TREATMENT   Generally, osteoporosis is detected radiographically as increased radiolucency of bone. By the time abnormalities are detected by radiologic examination, up to 25% to 30% of bone tissue may have been lost.

Dual x-ray absorptiometry (DXA) is the current gold standard for detecting and monitoring osteoporosis; however, bone density is not necessarily indicative of bone quality. New high-resolution imaging techniques, such as quantitative computed tomography (QCT) scans and peripheral quantitative computed tomography (pQCT), offer improved detail of bone microarchitecture. New, high-resolution peripheral computed tomography (CT) imaging, with less radiation exposure that traditional CT scans, has shown changes of trabecular and cortical microarchitecture in osteopenic women.[42] Newer magnetic resonance imaging techniques also show promise for providing more detailed information about cortical and trabecular bone and have the added safety of no radiation exposure.[22,42] Other evaluation procedures include tests for levels of serum calcium, phosphorus, and alkaline phosphatase as well as protein electrophoresis studies. Serum and urinary biochemical markers are useful in monitoring bone turnover (Box 37-3).

HEALTH ALERT
Calcium, Vitamin D, and Bone Health

Adequate calcium intake is essential for developing and maintaining normal bone structure, but the following question remains a topic of discussion and research: "What is adequate calcium intake?" Calcium is the most abundant mineral in the body and plays a role in maintaining muscle function, hormonal secretion, neurotransmission, and vascular health. Recent conflicting evidence about the effect of calcium on heart disease, for example, has been hotly debated in the medical literature. The conflicting reports about extraskeletal health benefits of vitamin D also were reviewed by the Institute of Medicine (IOM) and were found to lack enough evidence to be considered reliable.

The role of vitamin D in bone health is unquestioned; the clinical effects of inadequate vitamin D (osteomalacia, rickets) have been well-known for many years. Vitamin D is essential for absorbing and maintaining calcium homeostasis in the body. Recently, vitamin D has been postulated to be involved in many extraskeletal functions, such as reducing cancer risk, improving cognitive function in the elderly, preventing autoimmune diseases, improving resistance to infection, providing cardiovascular support, stabilizing posture, and inhibiting metabolic syndrome. Some of these potentially beneficial effects are from data gleaned from the National Health and Nutrition Examination Survey III (NHANES III), whereas other descriptions are based on observational or small studies. Vitamin D levels are evaluated by measuring serum 1,25-dihydroxyvitamin D levels. There is still disagreement about what constitutes an "optimal" vitamin D level, but many sources indicate it should be at least 30 to 32 ng/ml. Based on these levels, it has been estimated that nearly three fourths of the adult population in the United States have low vitamin D levels.

The IOM recently evaluated and summarized clinical evidence and literature reviews regarding the roles of calcium and vitamin D in disease reduction and other health outcomes in North America. Review of these findings resulted in updates of the recommended daily intake of both nutrients. In general, daily calcium intakes of 500 mg for ages 1 through 3, 800 mg for ages 4 through 8, 1100 to 1300 mg for ages 9 to 13, and 800 to 1000 mg for ages 14 through adulthood are adequate for maintaining proper bone health. Recommended dietary allowances for vitamin D vary from 400 to 600 international units (IU) a day for all ages. Additionally, the IOM found that once calcium intake exceeds more than 2000 mg a day or vitamin D intake is more than 4000 IU per day, there is increased risk for harm.

Data from Adams JS, Hewison M: Update in vitamin D, *J Clin Endocrinol Metab* 95(2):471–478, 2010; Annweiler C et al: Fall prevention and vitamin D in the elderly: an overview of the key role of the non-bone effects, *J Neuroeng Rehabil* 7:50, 2010; Binkley N, Ramamurthy R, Krueger D: Low vitamin D status: definition, prevalence, consequences, and correction, *Endocrinol Metab Clin North Am* 39(2):287–301, 2010; Bolland MJ et al: Effect of calcium supplements on risk of myocardial infarction and cardiovascular events: meta-analysis, *BMJ* 341:3691, 2010; Dawson-Hughes B: Calcium and heart attacks. The heart of the matter, *BMJ* 341:4993, 2010; Grove ML, Cook D: Calcium and heart attacks. Doesn't apply to most calcium prescriptions, *BMJ* 341:5003, 2010; Heiss G et al: Calcium and heart attacks. No evidence for increased risk, *BMJ* 341:4995, 2010; Holick MF: Sunlight and vitamin D for bone health and prevention of autoimmune diseases, cancers, and cardiovascular disease, *Am J Clin Nutr* 80(suppl): 1678S–1688S, 2004; Hsia J et al: Calcium/vitamin D supplementation and cardiovascular events, *Circulation* 115(7):846–854, 2007; Kidd PM: Vitamins D and K as pleiotropic nutrients: clinical importance to the skeletal and cardiovascular system and preliminary evidence for synergy, *Altern Med Rev* 15(3):199–222, 2010; Nordin BE et al: Calcium and heart attacks. Making too much of a weak case, *BMJ* 341:4997, 2010; Ross AC et al, editors: *Dietary reference intakes for calcium and vitamin D*, Washington, DC, 2010, National Academies Press; Slomski A: IOM endorses vitamin D, calcium only for bone health, dispels deficiency claims, *J Am Med Assoc* 305(5):453–456, 2011; Wang L et al: Systematic review: vitamin D and calcium supplementation in prevention of cardiovascular events, *Ann Intern Med* 152(5):315–323, 2010; Weisman Y: Non-classic unexpected functions of vitamin D, *Pediatr Endocrinol Rev* 8(2):103–107, 2010.

BOX 37-3 BIOCHEMICAL MARKERS OF BONE TURNOVER

Biochemical markers of bone turnover are useful in monitoring osteoporosis treatment. Markers of resorption include urinary N-telopeptide (NTx), C-telopeptide (CTx), and deoxypyridinoline. Markers of bone formation include bone-specific alkaline phosphatase (BSAP) and osteocalcin. However, these tests have diurnal variability within the same individual, so there must be significant changes in levels to indicate a difference in bone turnover.

The goals of osteoporosis treatment are to slow the rate of calcium and bone loss and to stop the disease. Bisphosphonates are first-line medications for treating osteoporosis; they primarily work by inhibiting hydroxyapatite breakdown, reducing bone resorption. New medications formulated to prevent or treat osteoporosis are currently being prescribed and evaluated. There are new treatments that may rebuild the skeleton (see *Health Alert: New Treatments for Osteoporosis*). Other selective steroid agents—for example, raloxifene—also may be prescribed (see Chapter 32). Regular, moderate weight-bearing exercise can slow the rate of bone loss and, in some cases, reverse demineralization because the mechanical stress of exercise stimulates bone formation. An exercise program to enhance strength and balance has the added benefits of reducing the risk of falls and promoting bone quality.

The anabolic or bone-building drug parathyroid hormone (PTH) has been widely studied, and the results are encouraging. PTH directly stimulates bone formation, particularly in trabecular bone[43] (see *Health Alert: New Treatments for Osteoporosis*).

Osteomalacia

Osteomalacia is a metabolic disease characterized by inadequate and delayed mineralization of osteoid in mature compact and spongy bone. In osteomalacia, the remodeling cycle proceeds normally through osteoid formation, but mineral calcification and deposition do not occur. Bone volume remains unchanged, but the replaced bone consists of soft osteoid instead of rigid bone. Rickets is similar to osteomalacia in pathogenesis, but it occurs in the growing bones of children, whereas osteomalacia occurs in adult bone. (Rickets is described in Chapter 38.)

Both osteomalacia and rickets are rare in the United States and Western Europe but are significant health problems in Great Britain, Ethiopia, Pakistan, Iran, and India. In the United States, these diseases are prevalent in elderly persons, in premature infants of very low birth-weight, and in individuals adhering to rigid macrobiotic vegetarian diets. Breast-fed African-American infants who do not receive vitamin D supplementation have been shown to be at risk for developing nutritional rickets.[44,45]

Many factors contribute to the development of osteomalacia, but the most important is a deficiency of vitamin D. The major risk factors in vitamin D deficiency are diets deficient in vitamin D, decreased endogenous production of vitamin D, intestinal malabsorption of vitamin D, renal tubular diseases, certain types of tumors (particularly of mesenchymal origin), and anticonvulsant therapy. Classic vitamin D deficiency is rare in the United States because of the addition of synthetic vitamin D to dairy products and bread.

Disorders of the small bowel, hepatobiliary system, and pancreas are causes of vitamin D deficiency in the United States. In malabsorptive disease of the small bowel, vitamin D and calcium absorption are decreased, so vitamin D is lost in feces. Liver disease interferes with the metabolism of vitamin D to its more active form, and diseases of the

HEALTH ALERT
New Treatments for Osteoporosis

Although bisphosphonates remain the first line of osteoporosis therapy, not all individuals are able to tolerate them and side effects can include bisphosphonate-related osteonecrosis of the jaw (BRONJ), atrial fibrillation, and fractures. Zoledronic acid, a third-generation bisphosphonate, is given as an annual intravenous infusion and has demonstrated efficacy in treating glucocorticoid-associated osteoporosis, in addition to reducing vertebral and nonvertebral fractures in women and men. However, it can cause an acute phase response in recipients and still carries some risk of BRONJ. Several new treatment options promise progress in treating osteoporosis and may be better tolerated than bisphosphonates.

Denosumab is the first commercially available human monoclonal antibody for treatment of osteoporosis. It binds to the receptor activator nuclear factor κβ ligand (RANKL) (see Chapter 36), preventing activation of osteoclasts. By reducing osteoclast activity, bone density is increased and bone resorption is reduced, thus lessening the incidence of fractures. Because denosumab is not cleared by the kidneys (as are bisphosphonates), it has the potential to be useful in those with chronic kidney disease. It is given every 6 months as a 60-mg subcutaneous injection.

Raloxifene, a selective estrogen receptor modulator (SERM), has been in use for several years to treat postmenopausal osteoporosis. It has been effective in reducing vertebral fractures but not hip or other nonspinal fractures. Newer SERMs, including lasofoxifene (which is approved for use in Europe, but not the United States), have been shown to reduce both vertebral and nonvertebral fractures. Bazedoxifene, in combination with estrogen, has been designated as a tissue-selective estrogen complex (TSEC), and is approved for use in Japan and Europe. It has been shown to reduce both vertebral and nonvertebral fractures in postmenopausal women. Neither of these agents, given as daily oral doses, stimulates endometrial or breast tissue.

Other biologic agents for treating osteoporosis include odanacatib, a cathepsin K inhibitor. By affecting this enzyme (produced by osteoclasts), bone density is increased. It is given as a once weekly oral agent. Agents directed at signaling pathways of bone formation and homeostasis are another target of osteoporosis intervention. One of the main signaling targets is the Wnt pathway (see Chapter 36). Wnt stimulates osteoblast function and bone formation but is blocked by sclerostin (which is produced by the osteocyte gene *SOST*). Parathyroid hormone (PTH) inhibits sclerostin expression, which may result in increased numbers of osteoblasts. The development of monoclonal antibodies to sclerostin may provide another means to increase bone formation and density.

Data from Honig S: Osteoporosis—new treatments and updates, *Bull NYU Hosp Jt Dis* 68(3):166–170, 2010; Piper PK Jr, Gruntmanis U: Management of osteoporosis in the aging male: focus on zoledronic acid, *Clin Interv Aging* 4:289–303, 2009; Reid R, Banjerjee SS, Sciot R: Giant cell tumour. In Christopher DM et al, editors: *World Health Organization classification of tumours International Agency for Research on Cancer (IARC) pathology and genetics of tumours of soft tissue and bone*, pp 303–312, Lyon, France, 2002, IARC Press; Sims NA: Building bone with a SOST-PTH partnership, *J Bone Miner Res* 25(2):175–177, 2010.

pancreas and biliary system cause a deficiency of bile salts, which are necessary for normal intestinal absorption of vitamin D.

The mechanism by which anticonvulsant drug therapy results in vitamin D deficiency is not completely understood, but researchers think that the anticonvulsants phenobarbital and phenytoin interfere with calcium absorption and increase degradation of vitamin D metabolism in the liver. Renal osteodystrophy is another cause of osteomalacia.

PATHOPHYSIOLOGY Crystallization of minerals in osteoid requires adequate concentrations of calcium and phosphate. When the concentrations are too low, crystallization (and hence ossification) does not proceed normally.

Vitamin D deficiency disrupts mineralization because vitamin D normally regulates and enhances the absorption of calcium ions from the intestine. A lack of vitamin D causes the plasma calcium concentrations to fall. Low plasma calcium levels stimulate increased synthesis and secretion of PTH. Although the increase in circulating PTH level raises the plasma calcium concentration, it also stimulates increased renal clearance of phosphate. When the concentration of phosphate in the bone decreases below a critical level, mineralization cannot proceed normally. Newer research has identified a complex interplay of matrix proteins, hormones, metallopeptidases, and certain proteins as also being involved in the development of osteomalacia.

Abnormalities occur in both spongy and compact bone. Trabeculae in spongy bone become thinner and fewer, whereas haversian systems in compact bone develop large channels and become irregular. Because osteoid continues to be produced but not mineralized, abnormal quantities of osteoid accumulate, coating the trabeculae and the linings of the haversian canals. Excessive osteoid also can accumulate in areas beneath the periosteum. The excess of osteoid leads to gross deformities of the long bones, spine, pelvis, and skull.

CLINICAL MANIFESTATIONS Osteomalacia causes varying degrees of diffuse muscular and skeletal pain and tenderness. Pain is noted particularly in the hips, and the individual may be hesitant to walk.[46] Muscular weakness is common and may contribute to a waddling gait. Facial deformities and bowed legs or "knock-knees" may be present. Bone fractures and vertebral collapse occur with minimal trauma. Low back pain may be an early complaint, but pain may also involve ribs, feet, other areas of the vertebral column, and other sites. Fragility fractures may occur. Uremia may be present in renal osteodystrophy.

EVALUATION AND TREATMENT Laboratory data may include elevated blood urea nitrogen (BUN) and creatinine levels, normal or low serum calcium levels, and a serum inorganic phosphate level that is usually more than 5.5 mg. Alkaline phosphatase and PTH levels are usually elevated. Radiographic findings may show symmetric bowing deformities and fractures with callus formation, particularly in the lower extremities. These types of fractures, known as pseudofractures, along with radiolucent bands perpendicular to the surface of involved bones can help differentiate osteomalacia from fragility fractures that are seen in osteoporosis. A bone biopsy is used to obtain information on bone structure and remodeling and evaluate the presence of subclinical renal osteodystrophy to determine bone aluminum deposits.[47]

Treatment of osteomalacia may vary, depending on its etiology, but the following general principles are included:

1. Adjustment of serum calcium and phosphorus levels to normal
2. Suppression of secondary hyperthyroidism
3. Chelation of bone aluminum if needed
4. Administration of calcium carbonate to decrease hyperphosphatemia
5. Administration of vitamin D supplements (oral or infusion)
6. Administration of bisphosphonate
7. Implementation of renal dialysis, if indicated

Paget Disease

Paget disease of bone (PDB, or osteitis deformans) is a state of increased metabolic activity in bone characterized by abnormal and excessive bone remodeling, both resorption and formation. Chronic accelerated remodeling eventually enlarges and softens the affected bones.

Paget disease can occur in any bone but most often affects the vertebrae, skull, sacrum, sternum, pelvis, and femur. The disease process may occur in one or more bones without causing significant clinical manifestations.

Paget disease occurs with equal frequency in men more than 55 years of age and women older than 40 years of age. It is often symptomless, and diagnosis is made by x-ray and radioisotope bone scan. Autopsy data from England and Germany indicate that approximately 3% to 4% of the population older than 40 years of age have Paget disease. It is most prevalent in Australia, Great Britain, New Zealand, and the United States. Paget disease affects several members of the same family in 5% to 25% of individuals.

The cause of PDB is not yet fully known, but studies have implicated both genetic and environmental factors. Of individuals diagnosed with PDB, 10% to 30% have mutations of a specific gene, *sequestosome-1*.[48,49]

PATHOPHYSIOLOGY Paget disease begins with excessive resorption of spongy bone and deposition of disorganized bone. The trabeculae diminish, and bone marrow is replaced by extremely vascular fibrous tissue.

The resorption phase of Paget disease is followed by the formation of abnormal new bone at an accelerated rate. The collagen fibers are disorganized, and glycoprotein levels in the matrix decrease. Mineralization may extend into the bone marrow. Bone formation is excessive around partially resorbed trabeculae, causing them to thicken and enlarge. The net result of this accelerated remodeling process is increased bone fragility and an increased risk for bone tumors.[50]

CLINICAL MANIFESTATIONS In the skull, abnormal remodeling is first evident in the frontal or occipital regions; then it encroaches on the outer and inner surfaces of the entire skull. The skull thickens and assumes an asymmetric shape. Thickened segments of the skull may compress areas of the brain, producing altered mentality and dementia. Impingement of new bone on cranial nerves causes sensory abnormalities, impaired motor function, deafness (because of involvement of the middle ear ossicles or compression of the auditory nerve), atrophy of the optic nerve, and obstruction of the lacrimal duct. Headache is commonly noted.

Extensive alterations of the facial bones are rare except in the jaw, where sclerosis and thickening of the maxilla and mandible displace teeth and produce malocclusion. In long bones, resorption begins in the subchondral regions of the epiphysis and extends into the metaphysis and diaphysis. Occasionally, Paget disease affects both ends of a tubular bone. In the femur, Paget disease produces an exaggerated lateral curvature. In the tibia, anterior curvature is also exaggerated. Stress fractures are common in the lower extremities.

Clinical manifestations of Paget disease in the vertebral column depend on the level of involvement and are caused by compression of adjacent structures. In the cervical spine, cord compression can lead to spastic quadriplegia. Approximately 1% of persons with Paget disease develop osteogenic sarcoma.

EVALUATION AND TREATMENT Evaluation of Paget disease is made on the basis of radiographic findings of irregular bone trabeculae with a thickened and disorganized pattern. Early disease is detected by bone scanning that shows increased uptake of bone radionuclides. Alkaline phosphatase and urinary hydroxyproline levels are elevated.

Many individuals require no treatment if the disease is localized and does not cause symptoms. Treatment during active disease is for relief of pain and prevention of deformity or fracture. Bisphosphonates are the treatment of choice; zoledronic acid is considered second-line

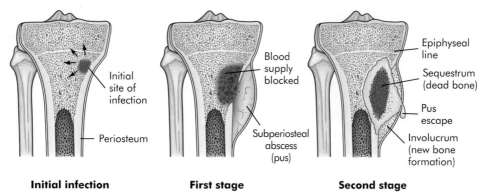

Initial infection **First stage** **Second stage**

FIGURE 37-14 Osteomyelitis Showing Sequestration and Involucrum.

therapy. Newer agents, including denosumab and those that alter the Wnt-signaling pathway, are under study for treatment of PDB.[50-52]

Infectious Bone Disease: Osteomyelitis

Osteomyelitis is a bone infection most often caused by bacteria; however, fungi, parasites, and viruses also can cause bone infection (Figure 37-14). It is further categorized according to the pathogen's mode of entry into bone tissue. The most common type is exogenous osteomyelitis, an infection that enters from outside the body, for example, through open fractures, penetrating wounds, or surgical procedures. In exogenous osteomyelitis, the infection also can spread from soft tissue into adjacent bone. An example of this is a diabetic foot infection. Endogenous osteomyelitis is caused by pathogens carried in the blood from sites of infection elsewhere in the body; the infection can then spread to adjacent soft tissue. Hematogenous osteomyelitis (a common form of osteomyelitis) is usually found in infants, children, and elderly persons. (Osteomyelitis in children is discussed in Chapter 38.) In infants, incidence rates among males and females are approximately equal. In children and older adults, however, males are most commonly affected. Osteomyelitis is a common complication of sickle cell anemia and low oxygen tension.

Staphylococcus aureus remains the primary microorganism responsible for osteomyelitis.[53,54] Other microorganisms include group B streptococcus, *Haemophilus influenzae*, *Salmonella*, and gram-negative bacteria. Group B streptococcus and *H. influenzae* tend to infect young children; *Salmonella* infection is associated with sickle cell anemia; and gram-negative infections are most common in older adults and immunocompromised individuals with impaired immunity. Mycobacterial, viral, and fungal infections occur in immunocompromised individuals.

Cutaneous, sinus, ear, and dental infections are the primary sources of bacteria in hematogenous bone infections. Soft tissue infections, disorders of the gastrointestinal tract, infections of the genitourinary system, and respiratory tract infections are also sources of bacterial contamination. In addition, infections that occur after total joint replacement procedures are sometimes the cause. The vulnerability of specific bone depends on the anatomy of its vascular supply.

In adults, hematogenous osteomyelitis is more common in the spine, pelvis, and small bones. Microorganisms reach the vertebrae through arteries, veins, or lymphatic vessels. The spread of infection from pelvic organs to the vertebrae is well documented. Vaginal, uterine, ovarian, bladder, and intestinal infections can lead to iliac or sacral osteomyelitis.

Exogenous osteomyelitis can be caused by human bites or fist blows to the mouth. Superficial animal or human bites inoculate local soft tissue with bacteria that later spread to underlying bone. Deep bites can introduce microorganisms directly onto bone. The most common infecting organism in human bites is *S. aureus*. In animal bites, the most common infecting organism is *Pasteurella multocida*, which is part of the normal mouth flora of cats and dogs.

Direct contamination of bones with bacteria can also occur in open fractures or dislocations with an overlying skin wound. Intervertebral disk surgery and operative procedures involving implantation of large foreign objects, such as metallic plates or artificial joints, are associated with exogenous osteomyelitis. Local injections and venous punctures are significant causes of exogenous osteomyelitis. Exogenous osteomyelitis of the arm and hand bones tends to occur in persons who abuse drugs. In general, persons who are chronically ill, have diabetes or alcoholism, or are receiving large doses of steroids or immunosuppressive drugs are particularly susceptible to exogenous osteomyelitis or recurring episodes of this disease.

PATHOPHYSIOLOGY Regardless of the source of the pathogen, the pathologic features of bone infection are similar to those in any other body tissue (see Chapter 5). First, the invading pathogen provokes an intense inflammatory response. Primarily through activation of the cytokine pathway, inflammation also can alter the normal balance between osteoblast and osteoclast activity.[54] Inflammation in bone is characterized by vascular engorgement, edema, leukocyte activity, and abscess formation. Once inflammation is initiated, the small terminal vessels thrombose and exudate seals the bone's canaliculi. Inflammatory exudate extends into the metaphysis and the marrow cavity and through small metaphyseal openings into the cortex. In children, exudate that reaches the outer surface of the cortex forms abscesses that lift the periosteum of underlying bone. Lifting of the periosteum disrupts blood vessels that enter bone through the periosteum, which deprives underlying bone of its blood supply; this leads to necrosis and death of the area of bone infected, producing sequestrum, an area of devitalized bone. Lifting of the periosteum also stimulates an intense osteoblastic response. Osteoblasts lay down new bone that can partially or completely surround the infected bone. This layer of new bone surrounding the infected bone is called an involucrum (Figure 37-15). Openings in the involucrum allow the exudate to escape into surrounding soft tissue and ultimately through the skin by way of sinus tracts.

In adults, this complication is rare because the periosteum is firmly attached to the cortex and resists displacement. Instead, infection disrupts and weakens the cortex, which predisposes the bone to pathologic fracture.

CLINICAL MANIFESTATIONS Clinical manifestations of osteomyelitis vary with the age of the individual, the site of involvement, the initiating event, the infecting organism, and the type of infection—acute, subacute, or chronic. Acute osteomyelitis causes abrupt onset of inflammation (see Figure 37-15).

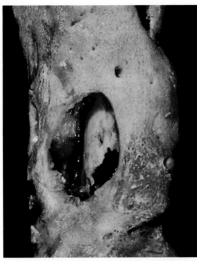

FIGURE 37-15 Resected Femur in a Person With Draining Osteomyelitis. The drainage tract in the subperiosteal shell of viable new bone (involucrum) reveals the inner native necrotic cortex (sequestrum). (From Kumar V et al: *Robbins and Cotran pathologic basis of disease,* ed 7, Philadelphia, 2005, Saunders.)

If an acute infection is not completely eliminated, the disease may become subacute or chronic. In subacute osteomyelitis, signs and symptoms are usually vague. In the chronic stage, infection is indolent or silent between exacerbations. The microorganisms persist in small abscesses or fragments of necrotic bone and produce occasional exacerbations of acute osteomyelitis. The progression from acute to subacute osteomyelitis may be the result of inadequate or inappropriate therapy, or the development of drug-resistant microorganisms.

In the adult, hematogenous osteomyelitis has an insidious onset. The symptoms are usually vague and include fever, malaise, anorexia, weight loss, and pain in and around the infected areas. Edema may or may not be evident. Recent infection (urinary, respiratory, cutaneous) or instrumentation (catheterization, cystoscopy, myelography, diskography) usually precedes onset of symptoms.

Single or multiple abscesses (Brodie abscesses) characterize subacute or chronic osteomyelitis. Brodie abscesses are circumscribed lesions 1 to 4 cm in diameter, usually in the ends of long bones and surrounded by dense ossified bone matrix. The abscesses are thought to develop when the infectious microorganism has become less virulent or the individual's immune system is resisting the infection somewhat successfully.

In exogenous osteomyelitis, signs and symptoms of soft tissue infection predominate. Inflammatory exudate in the soft tissues disrupts muscles and supporting structures and forms abscesses. Low-grade fever, lymphadenopathy, local pain, and swelling usually occur within days of contamination by a puncture wound.

EVALUATION AND TREATMENT Laboratory data show an elevated white cell count and an elevated level of noncardiac C-reactive protein (CRP). Radiographic studies include radionuclide bone scanning, CT, and MRI. MRI scanning with gadolinium contrast shows both bone and soft tissue, providing more accurate assessment of infection. Treatment of osteomyelitis includes bone biopsy to identify the causative organism, use of antimicrobial agents, and débridement of infected bone. Biodegradable antibiotic-impregnated bioabsorbable beads have also benefited many individuals.[55,56] Chronic conditions may require surgical removal of the inflammatory exudate followed by continuous wound irrigation with antibiotic solutions in addition to systemic treatment with antibiotics. The ideal antibiotic regimen for treating osteomyelitis has not yet been developed. Hyperbaric oxygen therapy of 100% oxygen may stimulate healing by suppressing proinflammatory cytokines and prostaglandins. Implants for total joint replacements may be removed to treat the infected joint more thoroughly.

> **✔ QUICK CHECK 37-2**
> 1. What are the causes associated with osteoporosis in women and men?
> 2. How does osteoporosis differ from osteomalacia? Name three differences.
> 3. What are the risk factors for osteomyelitis?

DISORDERS OF JOINTS

The American Rheumatism Association recognizes 13 groups of joint disease (arthropathies). Most of these disorders can be placed into two major categories: noninflammatory joint disease and inflammatory joint disease. With the improvement in detection methods, however, inflammatory pathways are now being identified in conditions previously classified as noninflammatory, such as osteoarthritis.

Osteoarthritis

Osteoarthritis (OA) is a common, age-related disorder of synovial joints. It is characterized by local areas of loss and damage of articular cartilage, new bone formation of joint margins (osteophytosis), subchondral bone changes, variable degrees of mild synovitis, and thickening of the joint capsule (Figure 37-16). Pathology centers on load-bearing areas. Advancing disease shows narrowing of the joint space attributable to cartilage loss, bone spurs (osteophytes), and sometimes changes in the subchondral bone. OA can arise in any synovial joint but is commonly found in the hands, hips, and spine. It is less common in people younger than 40 years of age and its prevalence increases with age. Although the exact causes of OA are unclear, they involve low-grade inflammation, calcification of articular cartilage, genetic alterations, and metabolic disorders.[57,58] OA involves a complex interaction of transcription factors, cytokines, growth factors, matrix molecules, and enzymes[59] (see the Pathophysiology section).

Traditionally, noninflammatory joint disease was differentiated from inflammatory joint disease by (1) the absence of synovial membrane inflammation, (2) the lack of systemic signs and symptoms, and (3) the presence of normal synovial fluid. Degenerative joint disease (osteoarthritis) was the most prevalent noninflammatory joint disease. Because of the use of MRI and arthroscopy, inflammation has been identified and is emerging as an important feature of osteoarthritis.

Although incidence rates are quite similar in men and women, women typically are more severely affected. OA usually occurs in those persons who put exceptional stress on joints (e.g., obese persons, gymnasts, long-distance runners or marathoners); persons participating in such sports as basketball, soccer, or football have been shown to develop osteoarthritis at earlier ages than usual. A previously torn anterior cruciate ligament or meniscectomy increases the risk for accelerated osteoarthritis of the knee.[60-62]

Types of Osteoarthritis

PATHOPHYSIOLOGY The primary defect in OA is loss of articular cartilage.[63] Early in the disease, the articular cartilage loses its glistening appearance, becoming yellow-gray or brownish gray. As the

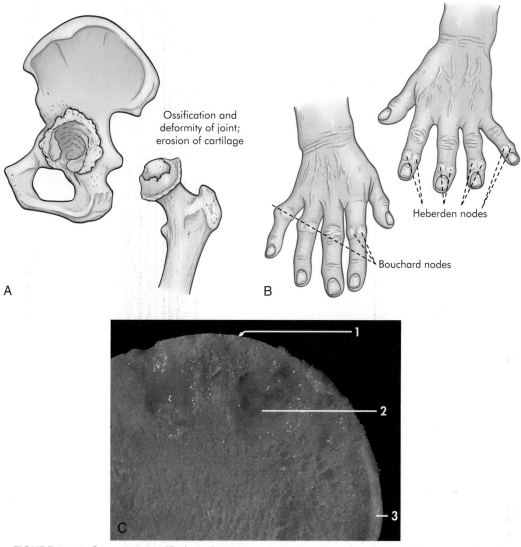

FIGURE 37-16 Osteoarthritis (OA). A, Cartilage and degeneration of the hip joint from osteoarthritis. **B,** Heberden nodes and Bouchard nodes. **C,** Severe osteoarthritis with small islands of residual articular cartilage next to exposed subchondral bone. *1,* Eburnated articular surface. *2,* Subchondral cyst. *3,* Residual articular cartilage. (**C** from Kumar V et al: *Robbins and Cotran pathologic basis of disease,* ed 7, Philadelphia, 2005, Saunders.)

disease progresses, surface areas of the articular cartilage flake off and deeper layers develop longitudinal fissures (fibrillation). The cartilage becomes thin and may be absent over some areas, leaving the underlying bone (subchondral bone) unprotected. Consequently, the unprotected subchondral bone becomes sclerotic (dense and hard). Cysts sometimes develop within the subchondral bone and communicate with the longitudinal fissures in the cartilage. Pressure builds in the cysts until the cystic contents are forced into the synovial cavity, breaking through the articular cartilage on the way. As the articular cartilage erodes, cartilage-coated osteophytes may grow outward from the underlying bone and alter the bone contours and joint anatomy. These spurlike bony projections enlarge until small pieces, called *joint mice,* break off into the synovial cavity. If osteophyte fragments irritate the synovial membrane, synovitis and joint effusion result. The joint capsule also becomes thickened and at times adheres to the deformed underlying bone, which may contribute to the limited range of motion of the joint (see Figure 37-16).

Articular cartilage is lost through a cascade of cytokine and anabolic growth factor pathways.[64] Enzymatic processes (including matrix metalloproteinases) assist in breaking the macromolecules of proteoglycans, glycosaminoglycans, and collagen into large, diffusible fragments. Then the fragments are taken up by the cartilage cells (chondrocytes) and digested by the cell's own lysosomal enzymes. (Processes of cellular uptake and lysosomal digestion are described in Chapter 1.) The loss of proteoglycans from articular cartilage is a hallmark of the osteoarthritic process.

Enzymatic destruction of articular cartilage begins in the matrix, with destruction of proteoglycans and collagen fibers. Enzymes, particularly stromelysin and acid metalloproteinase, affect proteoglycans by interfering with assembly of the proteoglycan subunit or the proteoglycan aggregate (see Chapter 36); levels of these enzymes are markedly elevated in OA. Changes in the conformation of proteoglycans disrupt the pumping action that regulates movement of water and synovial fluid into and out of the cartilage. Without the regulatory action of the proteoglycan pump, cartilage imbibes too much fluid and becomes less able to withstand the stresses of weight bearing. With aging, the proteoglycan content is decreased, and water content in cartilage can be increased by as much as 8%, affecting the strength of the cartilage. Persons with OA, even those with fairly extensive cartilage destruction, have elevated levels of proteoglycans/fragments in their synovial fluid, perhaps indicative of the degree of disease activity. Other studies indicate that cytokines, such as interleukin-1 and tumor necrosis factor (TNF) (see Chapter 6 for discussion of cytokines), play a major role in cartilage degradation[64] as a result of release and activation of proteolytic and collagenolytic enzymes associated with an imbalance of cell responses to growth factor activity.

Enzymes that degrade collagen (i.e., collagenases) probably originate in the chondrocytes or in leukocytes. Collagen breakdown destroys the fibrils that give articular cartilage its tensile strength and exposes the chondrocytes to mechanical stress and enzyme attack. Thus, a cycle of destruction begins that involves all the components of articular cartilage: proteoglycans, collagen fibers, and chondrocytes.

CLINICAL MANIFESTATIONS Clinical manifestations of OA typically appear during the fifth or sixth decade of life, although asymptomatic, articular surface changes are common after the age of 40 years. Pain in one or more joints—usually with weight bearing, use of the joint, or load bearing—is the first and most predominant symptom of the disease. Resting the joint often relieves pain. If present, nocturnal pain is usually not relieved by rest and may be accompanied by paresthesias (numbness, tingling, or prickling sensations). Sometimes pain is referred to another part of the body. For example, osteoarthritis of the lumbosacral spine may mimic sciatica, causing severe pain in the back of the thigh along the course of the sciatic nerve. OA in the lower cervical spine may cause brachial neuralgia (pain in the arm) and is aggravated by movement of the neck. Osteoarthritic conditions in the hip cause pain that may be referred to the lower thigh and knee area. Sleep deprivation adds to the stress of the chronic pain of OA. Physical examination of the person with OA usually shows general involvement of both peripheral and central joints. Peripheral joints most often involved are in the hands, wrists, knees, and feet. Central joints most often afflicted are in the lower cervical spine, lumbosacral spine, shoulders, and hips.

Joint structures are capable of generating a limited number of signs and symptoms. The primary signs and symptoms of osteoarthritic joint disease are pain, stiffness, enlargement or swelling, tenderness, limited range of motion, muscle wasting, partial dislocation, and deformity (see *Risk Factors: Osteoarthritis*).

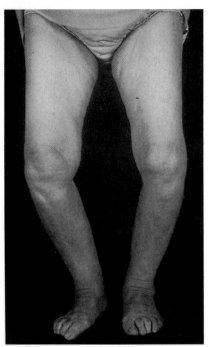

FIGURE 37-17 Typical Varus Deformity of Knee Osteoarthritis. (From Doherty M: *Color atlas and text of osteoarthritis*, London, 1994, Wolfe.)

The origin of joint stiffness is unknown. **Joint stiffness** is generally defined as difficulty initiating joint movement, immobility, or a loss of range of motion. The stiffness usually occurs as joint movement begins, and it dissipates rapidly after a few minutes. Stiffness lasting longer than 30 minutes is uncommon in OA. Enlargement and bulging of joint contour, commonly described as swelling, may be caused by bone enlargement or the proliferation of osteophytes around the margins of the joint. These areas are called Heberden and Bouchard nodes in the hands and are typical features of OA (see Figure 37-16). Swelling also occurs if inflammatory exudate or blood enters the joint cavity, thereby increasing the volume of synovial fluid. This condition, termed **joint effusion,** is caused by (1) the presence of osteophyte fragments in the synovial cavity, (2) drainage of cysts from diseased subchondral bone, or (3) acute trauma to joint structures, resulting in hemorrhage and inflammatory exudation into the synovial cavity (see Figure 37-16, *C*).

Range of motion is limited to some degree, depending on the extent of cartilage degeneration. Frequently, joint motion is accompanied by sounds of crepitus, creaking, or grating. Hypermobility and subluxation of joints occur in OA secondary to a neurologic disorder. Abnormal knee alignment (either varus or valgus of more than 5 degrees) has been shown to increase progression of the disease.[65]

As OA of the lower extremity progresses, the person may begin to limp noticeably (Figure 37-17). Having a limp is distressing because it affects the person's independence and ability to perform usual activities of daily living. The affected joint is also more symptomatic after use, such as at the end of a period of strenuous activity.

EVALUATION AND TREATMENT Evaluation consists primarily of clinical assessment and radiologic studies. More expensive studies, including CT scan, arthroscopy, and MRI, are rarely needed. Treatment is either conservative or surgical. Conservative treatment includes rest of the involved joint until inflammation (if present)

RISK FACTORS
Osteoarthritis

- Trauma, sprains, strains, joint dislocations, and fractures
- Long-term mechanical stress—athletics, ballet dancing, repetitive physical tasks, and obesity
- Inflammation in joint structures
- Joint instability from damage to supporting structures
- Neurologic disorders (e.g., diabetic neuropathy, Charcot neuropathic joint) in which pain and proprioceptive reflexes are diminished or lost
- Congenital or acquired skeletal deformities
- Hematologic or endocrine disorders, such as hemophilia, which causes chronic bleeding into the joints, or hyperparathyroidism, which causes bone to lose calcium
- Drugs (e.g., colchicine, indomethacin, steroids) that stimulate the collagen-digesting enzymes in the synovial membrane

subsides; implementation of range-of-motion exercises to prevent joint capsule contraction; use of a cane, crutches, or walker to decrease weight bearing; loss of body fat if obesity is present (obese persons are five times more likely to have OA of the knees and twice as likely to have OA of the hips as persons of ideal body weight) (see *Health Alert:* Body Weight and Osteoarthritis); and use of analgesic and anti-inflammatory drug therapy to reduce swelling and pain. Glucosamine and possibly chondroitin, so-called nutraceuticals, have shown some success in reducing the pain and progression of OA.[66,67] Intra-articular injection of high-molecular-weight viscose supplements, such as hyaluronic acid, also has been successful in decreasing knee pain with OA. Newer agents, including inhibitors of cytokines, matrix metalloproteinases (MMPs), and leptin, are under investigation and may prove more effective in treating OA. Surgery is used to improve joint movement, correct deformity or malalignment, or create a new joint with artificial implants. It has been estimated by some researchers that one in four individuals has a lifetime risk of developing symptomatic OA of the hip.[68] More than 250,000 total hip replacement surgeries are performed yearly in the United States, most of which are related to OA. It is estimated that by 2015, almost 600,000 hip replacements and 1.4 million knee replacements will be performed in the United States.[69]

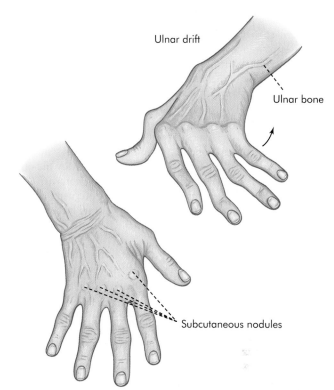

FIGURE 37-18 Rheumatoid Arthritis of the Hand. Note swelling from chronic synovitis of metacarpophalangeal joints, marked ulnar drift, subcutaneous nodules, and subluxation of metacarpophalangeal joints with extension of proximal interphalangeal joints and flexion of distal joints. Note also deformed position of thumb. Hand has wasted appearance. (Redrawn from Mourad LA: *Orthopedic disorders,* St Louis, 1991, Mosby.)

HEALTH ALERT

Body Weight and Osteoarthritis

> Longitudinal studies have shown obesity to be a major risk factor in developing osteoarthritis of the knee. In addition to altered biomechanics, increased weight may make subchondral bone stiffer and thus less capable of handling joint impact loading.

Data from Brennan et al: Does an increase in body mass index over 10 years affect knee structure in a population-based cohort study of adult women? *Arthritis Res Ther* 21(4):R139, 2010; Pallu S et al: Obesity affects the chondrocyte responsiveness to leptin in patients with osteoarthritis, *Arthritis Res Ther* 12(3):R112, 2010.

Classic Inflammatory Joint Disease

Inflammatory joint disease is commonly called arthritis. Inflammatory joint disease is characterized by inflammatory damage or destruction in the synovial membrane or articular cartilage and by systemic signs of inflammation (fever, leukocytosis, malaise, anorexia, hyperfibrinogenemia).

Inflammatory joint disease can be infectious or noninfectious. In infectious inflammatory joint disease, inflammation is caused by invasion of the joint by bacteria, mycoplasmas, viruses, fungi, or protozoa. These agents can invade the joint through a traumatic wound, surgical incision, or contaminated needle, or they can be delivered by the bloodstream from sites of infection elsewhere in the body, typically bones, heart valves, or blood vessels. In noninfectious inflammatory joint disease, which is the most common form, inflammation is caused by immune reactions or the deposition of crystals of monosodium urate in and around the joint. Rheumatoid arthritis and ankylosing spondylitis are noninfectious inflammatory diseases caused by immune reactions and possibly hypersensitivity reactions; gouty arthritis is a noninfectious inflammatory disease caused by crystal deposition.

Rheumatoid Arthritis

Rheumatoid arthritis (RA) is a chronic, systemic, inflammatory autoimmune disease distinguished by joint swelling and tenderness and destruction of synovial joints leading to disability and premature death.[70] (Autoimmune disease is described in Chapter 7.) The first joint tissue

to be affected is the synovial membrane, which lines the joint cavity (see Chapter 36, Figure 36-9). Eventually, inflammation may spread to the articular cartilage, fibrous joint capsule, and surrounding ligaments and tendons, causing pain, joint deformity, and loss of function (Figure 37-18). The joints most commonly affected are in the fingers, feet, wrists, elbows, ankles, and knees, but the shoulders, hips, and cervical spine also may be involved, as well as the tissues of the lungs, heart, kidneys, and skin.

The incidence and prevalence of RA have decreased over the past five decades and now affects between 0.5% and 1% of the adult population in developed countries.[71] The frequency of RA increases with age. Besides inflammation and destruction of the joints, RA can cause fever, malaise, rash, lymph node or spleen enlargement, and Raynaud phenomenon (transient lack of circulation to the fingertips and toes).

Despite intensive research, the exact cause of RA remains obscure. It is likely a combination of genetic factors interacting with inflammatory mediators. There is a strong genetic predisposition to developing RA. The chronic inflammation characteristics of RA result from an intricate interplay of chemokines that are powerful mediators of inflammation. Ligand/receptor chemokines attract T cells and produce inflammatory changes.[72] A key genetic element has been localized to the human leukocyte antigen (HLA) areas of the major histocompatibility complex in all ethnic groups. A surprising new discovery is the presence of T cell abnormalities in individuals with RA indicating a defect in telomere repair that may result in faster aging of telomeres and consequent less efficient immune function.[72] With long-term or intensive exposure to the antigen, normal antibodies (immunoglobulins [Ig]) become autoantibodies—antibodies that attack host tissues (self-antigens). Because they are usually present in individuals with RA, the altered antibodies are termed **rheumatoid factors (RFs)**. The RFs usually consist of two classes of immunoglobulin antibodies (antibodies for IgM and IgG) but occasionally involve antibodies for IgA. Their main antigenic targets are portions of the immunoglobulin molecules. RFs bind with their target self-antigens in blood and synovial membrane, forming immune complexes (antigen-antibody complexes). (See Chapter 5 for a discussion about antigen-antibody binding in the immune response.)

Environmental factors, including geographic area of birth, length of breast-feeding, socioeconomic status, and, especially, smoking, have been identified as risk factors for developing RA.[73] RA and other autoimmune diseases have a higher prevalence among women.[74] Additionnally, because disease symptoms lessen during pregnancy and are increased again in the postpartal period, researchers are including hormonal involvement.

PATHOPHYSIOLOGY   Although no specific events (such as trauma, illness, or environmental conditions) have been identified that would cause immune abnormalities to develop into localized tissue and joint inflammation, the pathology of RA is fairly well understood. During inflammation, arginine (an α-amino acid) can be enzymatically modified into another α-amino acid, citrulline. This process (citrullination) changes the structure and function of the protein. Other proteins, like fibrin and vimentin, become citrullinated during cell death and tissue inflammation.[75] In turn, the citrullinated proteins can be seen as antigens by the body's immune system. Thus both T and B cells play a role in the autoimmune response. T cells express receptor activator of nuclear factor κβ ligand (RANKL), which promotes osteoclast formation and causes bony erosion.[72]

Basically, cartilage damage in RA is the result of at least three processes: (1) neutrophils and other cells in the synovial fluid become activated, degrading the surface layer of articular cartilage; (2) inflammatory cytokines, particularly tumor necrosis factor-alpha (TNF-α), interleukin-1 beta (IL-1β), interleukin-6 (IL-6), interleukin-7 (IL-7), and interleukin-21 (IL-21), induce enzymatic (metalloproteinase) breakdown of cartilage and bone; and (3) T cells also interact with synovial fibroblasts through TNF-α, converting synovium into a thick, abnormal layer of granulation tissue known as **pannus** (see Chapter 6). Macrophages, components of pannus (Figure 37-19), stimulate the release of IL-1, platelet-derived growth factor (PDGF), and fibronectin. The B lymphocytes are stimulated to produce more RFs. The newly targeted self-antigens (immunoglobulins) are in relatively constant supply and can thus perpetuate inflammation and the formation of immune complexes indefinitely (Figure 37-20).

Inflammatory and immune processes have several damaging effects on the synovial membrane. Along with the swelling caused by leukocyte infiltration, the synovial membrane undergoes hyperplastic thickening as its cells proliferate and abnormally enlarge. As synovial inflammation progresses to involve its blood vessels, small venules become occluded by hypertrophied endothelial cells, fibrin, platelets, and inflammatory cells, which decrease vascular flow to the synovial tissue. Compromised circulation, coupled with increased metabolic needs as a result of hypertrophy and hyperplasia, causes hypoxia and metabolic acidosis. Acidosis stimulates the release of hydrolytic enzymes from synovial cells into the surrounding tissue, initiating erosion of the articular cartilage and inflammation in the supporting ligaments and tendons. Pannus formation does not lead to synovial or articular regeneration but rather to formation of scar tissue that immobilizes the joint.

CLINICAL MANIFESTATIONS   The onset of RA is usually insidious, although as many as 15% of cases have an acute onset. RA begins

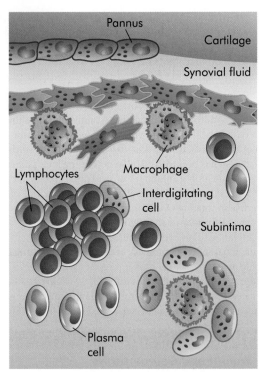

FIGURE 37-19 Synovitis. Inflamed synovium showing typical arrangements of macrophages *(red)* and fibroblastic cells.

with general systemic manifestations of inflammation, including fever, fatigue, weakness, anorexia, weight loss, and generalized aching and stiffness. Local manifestations also appear gradually over a period of weeks or months. Typically, the joints become painful, tender, and stiff. Pain early in the disease is caused by pressure from swelling. Later in the disease, pain is caused by sclerosis of subchondral bone and new bone formation. Stiffness usually lasts for about 1 hour after rising in the morning and is thought to be related to synovitis. Initially the joints most commonly involved are the metacarpophalangeal (MCP) joints, proximal interphalangeal (PIP) joints, and wrists, with later involvement of larger weight-bearing joints.

Joint swelling, which is widespread and symmetric, is caused by increasing amounts of inflammatory exudate (leukocytes, plasma, plasma proteins) in the synovial membrane, hyperplasia of inflamed tissues, and formation of new bone. On palpation, the swollen joint feels warm and the synovial membrane feels boggy. The skin over the joint may have a ruddy, cyanotic hue and may look thin and shiny.

An inflamed joint may lose some of its mobility. Even mild synovitis can lead to reduced range of motion, which becomes evident after inflammation subsides. Extension becomes limited and is eventually lost if flexion contractures develop. Limited range of motion can progress to permanent deformities of the fingers, toes, and limbs, including ulnar deviation of the hands, boutonnière and swan neck deformities of the finger joints, plantar subluxation of the metatarsal heads of the foot, and hallux valgus (angulation of the great toe toward the other toes). Flexion contractures of the knees and hips are also common.

Joint deformities cause the physical limitations experienced by persons with RA (see Figure 37-18). Loss of joint motion is quickly followed by secondary atrophy of the surrounding muscles. With secondary muscle atrophy, the joint becomes unstable, which further aggravates joint pathology.

Two complications of chronic RA are caused by excessive amounts of inflammatory exudate in the synovial cavity. One complication is

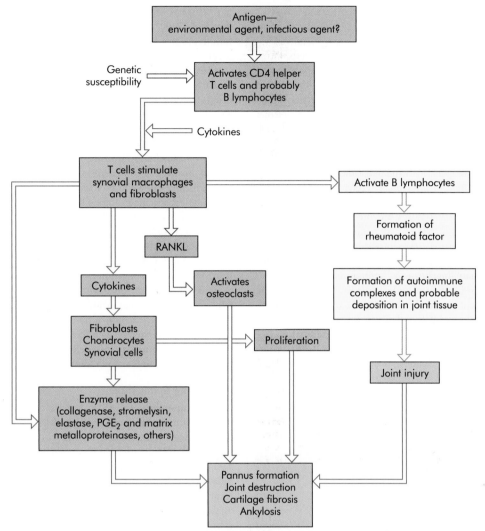

FIGURE 37-20 Emerging Model of Pathogenesis of Rheumatoid Arthritis. Rheumatoid arthritis is an autoimmune disease of a genetically susceptible host triggered by an unknown antigenic agent. Chronic autoimmune reaction with activation of CD4+ helper T cells and possibly other lymphocytes and the local release of inflammatory cytokines and mediators eventually destroy the joint. T cells stimulate cells in the joint to produce cytokines that are key mediators of synovial damage. Apparently, immune complex deposition also plays a role. Tumor necrosis factor (TNF) and interleukin-1 (IL-1), as well as some other cytokines, stimulate synovial cells to proliferate and produce other mediators of inflammation, such as prostaglandin E_2 (PGE$_2$), matrix metalloproteinases, and enzymes that all contribute to destruction of cartilage. Activated T cells and synovial fibroblasts also produce receptor activator of nuclear factor κβ ligand (RANKL), which activates the osteoclasts and promotes bone destruction. Pannus is a mass of synovium and synovial stroma with inflammatory cells, granulation tissue, and fibroblasts that grows over the articular surface and causes its destruction.

the formation of cysts in the articular cartilage or subchondral bone. Occasionally, these cysts communicate with the skin surface (such as in the sole of the foot) and can drain through passages called *fistulae*. The second complication is rupture of a cyst or of the synovial joint itself, usually caused by strenuous physical activity that places excessive pressure on the joint. Rupture releases inflammatory exudate into adjacent tissues, thereby spreading inflammation.

Extrasynovial **rheumatoid nodules,** or swellings, are observed in areas of pressure or trauma in 20% of individuals with RA. Each nodule is a collection of inflammatory cells surrounding a central core of fibrinoid and cellular debris. T lymphocytes are the predominant leukocytes in the nodule. B lymphocytes, plasma cells, and phagocytes are found around the periphery. Nodules are most often found in subcutaneous tissue over the extensor surfaces of elbows and fingers. Less common sites are the scalp, back, feet, hands, buttocks, and knees.

Rheumatoid nodules also may invade the skin, cardiac valves, pericardium, pleura, lung parenchyma, and spleen. These nodules are identical to those encountered in some individuals with rheumatic fever and are characterized by central tissue necrosis surrounded by proliferating connective tissue. Also noted are large numbers of lymphocytes and occasional plasma cells. Acute glaucoma may result with nodules forming on the sclera. Pulmonary involvement may result in diffuse pleuritis or multiple intraparenchymal nodules. Together, the occurrence of pulmonary nodules and pneumoconiosis (chronic inflammation of the lungs from inhalation of dust) creates the syndrome called Caplan syndrome. Diffuse pulmonary fibrosis may occur because of immunologically mediated immune complex deposition.

Rheumatoid nodules within the heart may cause valvular deformities, particularly of the aortic valve leaflets, and pericarditis. Lymphadenopathy of the nodes close to the affected joints may develop. Rheumatoid nodules within the spleen result in splenomegaly. Involvement of blood vessels results in an acute necrotizing vasculitis, characteristic of that noted in other immunologic/inflammatory states. Thromboses of such involved vessels may lead to myocardial infarctions, cerebrovascular occlusions, mesenteric infarction, kidney damage, and vascular insufficiency in the hands and fingers (Raynaud phenomenon). The vascular changes are primarily noted in individuals receiving steroid therapy; thus there is some concern that RA therapy may play a role in initiating these lesions. Changes in skeletal muscle are often noted in the form of nonspecific atrophy secondary to joint dysfunction.

EVALUATION AND TREATMENT The diagnosis of RA relies on clinical evaluation of joint swelling; however, limitation of movement and pain often prevent identification of individuals in early stages of the disease who would benefit from early treatment. Early treatment can be effective in preventing the systemic and joint abnormalities of chronic disease. Research has shown that the autoantibodies rheumatoid factor (RF) and anti-citrullinated protein antibody (ACPA) can be present for years to decades before synovial or radiographic involvement becomes apparent.[70,72,76] ACPA is a much more specific serum marker for RA than RF. The American College of Rheumatology (ACR) and the European League Against Rheumatism (EULAR) revised their RA classification criteria in 2010 in order to better identify the early stage

Data from Reumann MK, Weiser MC, Mayer-Kuckuk P: Musculoskeletal molecular imaging: a comprehensive review, *Trends Biotechnol* 28(2): 93–1001, 2010; Malviya G et al: Molecular imaging of rheumatoid arthritis by radiolabelled monoclonal antibodies: new imaging strategies to guide molecular therapies, *Eur J Med Mol Imaging* 37(2):386–398, 2010.

of RA.[70] These new criteria are shown in Table 37-5. Clinical examination and history are the mainstays of RA diagnosis, but new imaging techniques show promise for earlier diagnosis, leading to earlier treatment with a better chance for avoiding disability and joint destruction (see *Health Alert: Musculoskeletal Molecular Imaging*).

Early treatment of RA begins with disease-modifying antirheumatic drugs (DMARDs), such as methotrexate (MTX), azathioprine, sulfasalazine, hydroxychloroquine, leflunomide, and cyclosporine. These agents have been shown to slow the progression of RA and may prevent complications such as joint deformities and extra-articular complications. MTX remains the first line of treatment. More recently, targeted treatment for RA has involved use of agents aimed at interrupting the pathogenesis of the disease. Known as biologic DMARDs (bDMARDs), these medications affect specific processes in the development of RA and include tumor necrosis factor inhibitors, such as etanercept, adalimumab, and infliximab. They have recently been augmented by the monoclonal antibodies golimumab and certolizumab. Other agents interfere with cytokine function (anakinra inhibits IL-1 function and tocilizumab targets IL-6), inhibit T cell activation (abatacept), or deplete B cells (rituximab).

Education for individuals with RA is fundamental to treatment. Other treatments and therapies include nonsteroidal anti-inflammatory drugs (NSAIDs), glucocorticoids, intra-articular steroid injections, physical and occupational therapy with therapeutic exercise, and use of assistive devices. Surgery is used to treat deformities or mechanical deficiencies of joints and can include synovectomy or joint replacement surgery.

Ankylosing Spondylitis

Ankylosing spondylitis (AS) is the most common of a group of inflammatory arthropathies known as *spondyloarthropathies*. It is a chronic, inflammatory joint disease characterized by stiffening and fusion (ankylosis) of the spine and sacroiliac joints. Like RA, ankylosing spondylitis is a systemic, autoimmune inflammatory disease. Although inflammation is the primary pathologic process in both RA and ankylosing spondylitis, the two diseases differ in the primary site of inflammation and the end result. In RA, the primary site of inflammation is the synovial membrane, resulting in the destruction and instability of synovial joints. In ankylosing spondylitis, excessive bone formation occurs. The primary pathologic site is the enthesis (the point at which ligaments, tendons, and the joint capsule are inserted into bone), and the end result is fibrosis, ossification, and fusion of the joint, primarily the sacroiliac joints and the vertebral column (axial skeleton).

AS primarily affects men of Northern European descent[71] between the ages of 15 and 40. In women, AS may affect the peripheral joints of the appendicular skeleton rather than the axial skeleton, progress less rapidly, and cause less dramatic spinal changes. Primary AS usually develops in late adolescence and young adulthood, with peak incidence at about 20 years of age. Secondary AS affects older age groups and is often associated with other inflammatory diseases (e.g., psoriatic arthropathy, inflammatory bowel disease, Reiter syndrome).

The overall prevalence of AS in the United States is approximately 0.5% to 1%, with certain ethnic groups having a greater incidence. Worldwide, the disease appears to be most prevalent in whites. AS is rare in native, genetically unmixed populations of South America, Australia, and portions of Africa.[71]

The exact cause of AS is unknown, but its high association with histocompatibility antigen human leukocyte antigen (HLA-B27) has been known for decades. New research has shown that misfolding of HLA-B27 in the endoplasmic reticulum (ER) may play a key role in developing AS. As misfolded proteins accumulate, they may cause an unfolded protein response (UPR) that disrupts normal cellular functions and causes a stress response of the ER (also see Chapter 3).

HEALTH ALERT

Musculoskeletal Molecular Imaging

With improved understanding of the molecular and cellular mechanisms responsible for the effects of rheumatoid arthritis (RA), new imaging techniques promise benefits in earlier and more accurate diagnosis and monitoring of cartilage and bone involvement. Imaging on that same molecular level can provide a "biological read-out" of disease progression and response to treatment. Nuclear medicine imaging, positron emission tomography (PET), and magnetic resonance imaging (MRI) all incorporate some element of molecular imaging.

New modalities of molecular imaging use various probes and contrast agents that have an affinity for specific targets, such as cells, hormones, antigens, and enzymes. Certain monoclonal antibodies have already been successfully labeled with various nuclides and could be used to identify disease progression. Bioluminescent and fluorescent imaging techniques have the advantage of being radiation-free tests and are being used to view in vivo activity, osteoblast activity, osteocalcin expression in bone damage, and osteoclast activity and gene expression during inflammation. A significant area of promise for molecular imaging in RA is recognition of the initial molecular events that occur before cartilage and joint damage becomes apparent. Better monitoring of response to medications also may allow more accurate dosing with the potential for fewer side effects. Because certain bioluminescent and fluorescent agents have specific affinities for particular cells, more efficient bone regeneration may be possible by targeted delivery of appropriate growth factors or stem cells to damaged bone and cartilage.

TABLE 37-5	THE 2010 AMERICAN COLLEGE OF RHEUMATOLOGY/EUROPEAN LEAGUE AGAINST RHEUMATISM CLASSIFICATION CRITERIA FOR RHEUMATOID ARTHRITIS

Target population to be tested:
1. Persons who have at least one joint with definite clinical synovitis (swelling)[a]
2. Persons who have synovitis not better explained by another disease[b]

Classification criteria for RA (score-based algorithm: add scores of categories A to D; a score of ≥6/10 is needed for positive RA diagnosis)[c]

CLINICAL FINDING	SCORE
A. Joint involvement[d]	
1 large joint[e]	0
2-10 large joints	1
1-3 small joints (with or without involvement of large joints)[f]	2
4-10 small joints (with or without involvement of large joints)	3
>10 joints (at least 1 small joint)[g]	5
B. Serology (at least 1 test result is needed for classification)[h]	
Negative RF *and* negative ACPA	0
Low-positive RF *or* low-positive ACPA	2
High-positive RF *or* high-positive ACPA	3
C. Acute-phase reactants (at least 1 test result is needed for classification)[i]	
Normal CRP *and* normal CRP	0
Abnormal CRP *or* abnormal ESR	1
D. Duration of symptoms[j]	
<6 weeks	0
≥6 weeks	1

Data from Aletaha D et al: The 2010 American College of Rheumatology/European League Against Rheumatism classification criteria for rheumatoid arthritis: an American College of Rheumatology/European League Against Rheumatism collaborative initiative, *Arthritis Rheum* 62(9):2574, 2010.

[a]The criteria are aimed at classification of newly presenting persons. In addition, persons with erosive disease typical of rheumatoid arthritis (RA) with a history compatible of prior fulfillment of the 2010 criteria should be classified as having RA. Persons with longstanding disease—including those whose disease is inactive (with or without treatment) and who, based on retrospectively available data, have previously fulfilled the 2010 criteria—should be classified as having RA.

[b]Differential diagnoses vary among persons with different presentations, but may include conditions such as systemic lupus erythematosus, psoriatic arthritis, and gout. If it is unclear about the relevant differential diagnoses to consider, an expert rheumatologist should be consulted.

[c]Although persons with a score <6/10 are not classifiable as having RA, their status can be reassessed and the criteria might be fulfilled cumulatively over time.

[d]Joint involvement refers to any *swollen* or *tender* joint on examination, which may be confirmed by imaging evidence of synovitis. Distal interphalangeal joints, first metacarpophalangeal joints, and first metatarsophalangeal joints are *excluded from assessment*. Categories of joint distribution are classified according to the location and number of involved joints, with placement into the highest category possible based on the pattern of joint involvement.

[e]"Large joints" refer to shoulders, elbows, hips, knees, and ankles.

[f]"Small joints" refer to the metacarpophalangeal joints, proximal interphalangeal joints, second through fifth metatarsophalangeal joints, thumb interphalangeal joints, and wrists.

[g]In this category, at least one of the involved joints must be a small joint; the others can include any combination of large and additional small joints, as well as other joints not specifically listed elsewhere (e.g., temporomandibular, acromioclavicular, sternoclavicular).

[h]Negative refers to international unit (IU) values that are less than or equal to the upper limit of normal (ULN) for the laboratory and assay; low-positive refers to values that are higher than the ULN but ≤3 times the ULN for the laboratory and assay; high-positive refers to IU values that are >3 times the ULN for the laboratory and assay. Where rheumatoid factor (RF) information is only available as positive or negative, a positive result should be scored as low-positive for RF. *ACPA,* Anti-citrullinated protein antibody.

[i]Normal/abnormal is determined by local laboratory standards. *CRP,* C-reactive protein; *ESR,* erythrocyte sedimentation rate.

[j]Duration of symptoms refers to individual's self-report of the duration of signs and symptoms of synovitis (e.g., pain, swelling, tenderness) of joints that are clinically involved at the time of assessment, regardless of treatment status.

That stress response increases production of interleukin-23 (IL-23), a potent cytokine that also may act on T-helper 17 (Th17) cells, promoting their survival.[77] Th17 cells are important mediators in human immune diseases.[78]

PATHOPHYSIOLOGY Ankylosing spondylitis begins with inflammation of fibrocartilage in cartilaginous joints. The sacroiliac joint is affected first, usually before any damage can be radiographically detected.[77] Inflammatory cells infiltrate the fibrous tissue of the joint capsule, the cartilage that surrounds intervertebral disks, the entheses, and the periosteum. As inflammatory cells (chiefly macrophages) and lymphocytes infiltrate and erode bone and fibrocartilage in joint structures, repair begins. Repair of cartilaginous structures begins with the proliferation of fibroblasts. Fibroblasts synthesize and secrete collagen. The collagen becomes organized into fibrous scar tissue that eventually undergoes calcification and ossification. With time, all the cartilaginous structures of the joint are replaced by ossified scar tissue, causing the joint to fuse, or lose flexibility.

Repair of eroded bone begins with osteoblast activation and proliferation. Osteoblasts lay down new bone (callus), which is remodeled and replaced by compact, lamellar bone. Bone repair changes the contour of the bone's surface because the new bone grows outward to form a new enthesis with the end of the eroded ligament. The new enthesis, which forms on top of the old one, is called a syndesmophyte. As calcification of the spinal ligaments progresses, the vertebral bodies lose their concave anterior contour and appear square. The spine assumes the classic bamboo spine appearance of ankylosing spondylitis.

CLINICAL MANIFESTATIONS The most common signs and symptoms of early AS are low back pain and stiffness. Typically, the individual with primary disease develops low back pain during the early twenties. The pain is at first insidious but progressively becomes persistent. It is often worse after prolonged rest and is alleviated by physical activity. Early morning stiffness usually accompanies the low back pain, and the individual typically has difficulty sitting up or twisting the spine. Forward flexion, rotation, and lateral flexion of the spine are restricted and painful. Early pain and resultant loss of motion are caused by the underlying inflammation and reflex muscle spasm rather than by soft tissue or bony fusion.

As the disease progresses, the normal convex curve of the lower spine (lumbar lordosis) diminishes and concavity of the upper spine (kyphosis) increases. The individual becomes increasingly stooped. The thoracic spine becomes rounded, the head and neck are held forward on the shoulders, and the hips are flexed (Figure 37-21).

Inflammation in the tendon insertions of the many costosternal and costovertebral muscles can cause pleuritic chest pain and restricted chest movement. The pain is usually worse on inspiration. Movement of the diaphragm is normal and full. Pressure on the anterior chest wall over the sternum, ribs, and costal cartilages may cause tenderness. Tenderness over the pelvic brim may cause discomfort at night and interfere with sleep because turning onto the iliac crests causes pain. Tenderness over the ischial tuberosities may make sitting on hard seats unbearable. Tenderness in the heels may contribute to a limp or cautious placement of the feet during walking.

Along with low back pain and sacroiliac pain, inflammation of the bowels, anterior uveitis, aortic regurgitation, fibrosis of the upper lobes of the lung, Achilles tendonitis, and immune-related (IgA) kidney disease frequently accompany AS.[79] Elevated sedimentation rate (ESR) and elevated level of C-reactive protein (CRP) also are common. The presence of these symptoms aids in the diagnosis of AS.

EVALUATION AND TREATMENT Diagnosis of AS is based on specific criteria. One of the previous problems with diagnosing AS has been a requirement for radiographic (x-ray) evidence of sacroiliitis; MRI can discover sacroiliitis an average of 7.7 years before x-rays.[80] New classification criteria for AS developed in 2009 allowed the inclusion of MRI findings, as well as radiographic findings, for individuals less than 45 years of age with back pain of at least 3 months' duration.[81]

If sacroiliitis is present on imaging, one or more of the following features allow a diagnosis of spondyloarthritis (SpA): inflammatory back pain, arthritis, uveitis, heel pain, dactylitis, psoriasis, Crohn disease or ulcerative colitis, good response to NSAIDs, family history of SpA, positive HLA-B27, or elevated CRP. If the individual has a positive HLA-B27, at least two of the previously mentioned items must

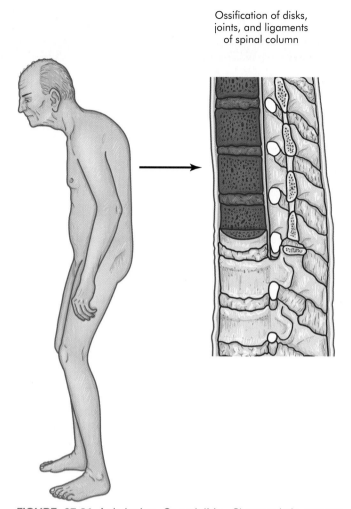

Ossification of disks, joints, and ligaments of spinal column

FIGURE 37-21 Ankylosing Spondylitis. Characteristic posture and primary pathologic sites of inflammation and resulting damage. (Redrawn from Mourad LA: *Orthopedic disorders,* St Louis, 1991, Mosby.)

be present along with sacroiliitis on MRI or radiographic imaging in order to make a diagnosis.[81]

Treatment of individuals with AS consists of education about the disease, as well as physical therapy to maintain skeletal mobility and prevent the natural progression of contractures. Prevention of deformity and maintenance of mobility require a continuous program of physical therapy. Exercises are performed several times each day to maintain chest expansion, full extension of the spine, and complete range of motion in the proximal joints.

Nonsteroidal anti-inflammatory drugs (NSAIDs) will often provide temporary symptom relief within 48 hours. Analgesic medications are prescribed to suppress some of the pain and stiffness and to facilitate exercise. The medications do not prevent disease progression, but they do provide relief from symptoms. Biologic response modifying agents, such as tumor necrosis factor inhibitors (certolizumab, golimumab) or B cell depleting agents (rituximab), are increasingly being used to treat AS. Surgical procedures, such as osteotomy, total hip replacement, and cervical spinal fusion, and radiation therapy are sometimes used to provide relief for individuals with end-stage disease or intolerable deformity. Individuals should stop smoking to lessen pulmonary problems.

TABLE 37-6	MEAN URATE CONCENTRATIONS BY AGE AND GENDER	
CHARACTERISTIC	**MEAN URATE LEVELS (mg/dL)**	
Prepuberty	3.5	
Males (at puberty)	Steep rise to 5.2	
Females (puberty to after premenopause)	Slow rise to ≈4.0	
Females (after menopause)	4.7	
Hyperuricemia		
Males	7.0	
Females	6.0	

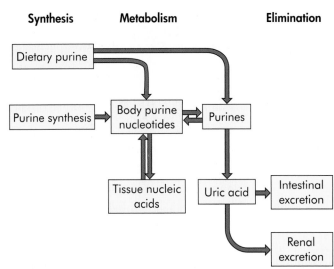

FIGURE 37-22 Uric Acid Synthesis and Elimination. Uric acid is derived from purines ingested or synthesized from ingested foods, as well as being recycled after cell breakdown. Uric acid is then eliminated through the kidneys and gastrointestinal tract. (Redrawn from Klippel JH, Dieppe PA, editors: *Rheumatology*, ed 2, St Louis, 1998, Mosby.)

Gout

Gout is a syndrome caused by incomplete purine metabolism, resulting in excess serum uric acid levels (hyperuricemia). It is characterized by inflammation and pain of the joints. Either excessive uric acid production or underexcretion of uric acid by the kidneys will cause hyperuricemia. Underexcretion of uric acid is responsible for about 90% of the cases of elevated uric acid level.[82] When uric acid reaches a certain concentration in fluids, it crystallizes, forming insoluble precipitates that are deposited in connective tissues throughout the body. Crystallization in synovial fluid causes acute, painful inflammation of the joint, a condition known as gouty arthritis. With time, crystal deposition in subcutaneous tissues causes the formation of small, white nodules, or tophi, that are visible through the skin. Crystal aggregates deposited in the kidneys can form urate renal stones and lead to renal failure.

In classic gouty arthritis, monosodium urate crystals form and are deposited in joints and their surrounding tissues, initiating a powerful inflammatory response.[83] Pseudogout is caused by the formation of calcium *pyrophosphate*-dihydrate crystals. The effect of either crystal is the same—the onset of an acute inflammatory response (see Chapter 5).

Gout is rare in children and premenopausal women and is uncommon in males younger than 30 years. Male gender, increasing age, and high intake of alcohol, red meat, and fructose are all risk factors for gout.[84] The peak age of onset in males is between 40 and 50 years. The risk of developing gouty arthritis is similar in males and females for a particular urate concentration. Females tend to have onset at a later age and have greater use of diuretics, more coexisting diseases (hypertension, renal insufficiency), more frequent involvement of other joints, and fewer recurrent episodes.[85] Plasma urate concentration is the single most important determinant of the risk of developing gout (Table 37-6).

Uric acid is a weak acid that is ionized at normal body pH and thus occurs in the blood or tissues in the form of urate ion. When ionized, uric acid can form salts with various cations, but 98% of extracellular uric acid is in the form of monosodium urate (uric acid salt). At any time the proportion of uric acid or urate is pH dependent, so the ratio of these two forms varies considerably in urine.

The solubility of urate and uric acid is critical to the development of crystals. Urate is more soluble in plasma, synovial fluid, and urine than in aqueous solutions. The solubility of uric acid in urine rises dramatically as the pH increases. There is little change, however, in the solubility of urate within the normal pH range that exists in the plasma, synovial fluid, and other tissues. pH can be 5.0 in the collecting tubules of the kidney, thus favoring formation of uric acid. Decreasing temperatures cause both urate and uric acid solubility to fall. The pathways of production of uric acid are shown in Figure 37-22.

PATHOPHYSIOLOGY The pathophysiology of gout is closely linked to purine metabolism (or cellular metabolism of purines) and kidney function. Most mammals, except humans, have the enzyme uricase, which catalyzes the conversion of uric acid to allantoin, thus preventing overproduction of uric acid. Environmental and genetic factors also play a role in an individual's urate concentration. At the cellular level, purines are synthesized to purine nucleotides, which are used in the synthesis of nucleic acids, adenosine triphosphate (ATP), cyclic adenosine monophosphate (cAMP), and cyclic guanosine monophosphate (cGMP). Uric acid is a breakdown product of purine nucleotides (urate synthesis and elimination are illustrated in Figure 37-23).

Most uric acid is eliminated from the body through the kidneys. Urate is filtered at the glomerulus and undergoes both reabsorption and excretion within the renal tubules. In primary gout, urate excretion by the kidneys is sluggish. The sluggish excretion may be the result of a decrease in glomerular filtration of urate or an acceleration in urate reabsorption. In addition, monosodium urate crystals are deposited in renal interstitial tissues, causing impaired urine flow. (Kidney function is described in Chapter 28.)

The exact process by which crystals of monosodium urate are deposited in joints and induce gouty arthritis is unknown, but several mechanisms may be involved, including the following:

1. Monosodium urate precipitates at the periphery of the body, where lower body temperatures may reduce the solubility of monosodium urate.
2. Albumin or glycosaminoglycan levels decrease, which causes decreased urate solubility.
3. Changes in ion concentration and decreases of pH enhance urate deposition.
4. Trauma promotes urate crystal precipitation.

The monosodium urate crystals may form in the synovial fluid or in the synovial membrane, cartilage, or other connective tissues in joints

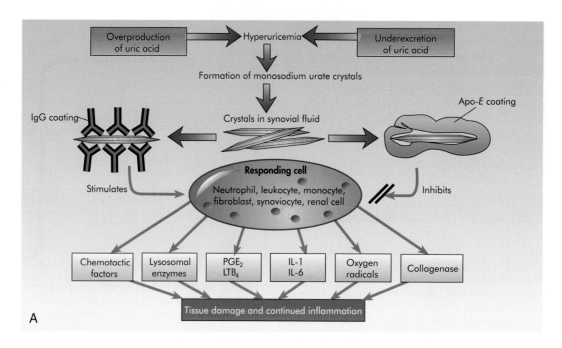

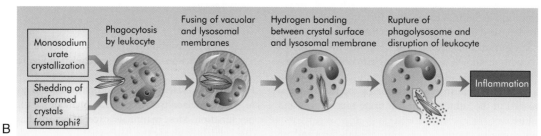

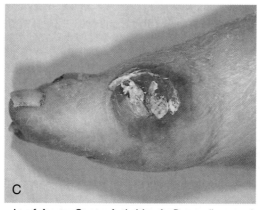

FIGURE 37-23 Pathogenesis of Acute Gouty Arthritis. **A,** Depending on the urate crystal coating, a variety of cells may be stimulated to produce a wide range of inflammatory mediators. *Apo-E,* Apolipoprotein E; *IgG,* immunoglobulin G; *IL,* interleukin; *LTB₄,* leukotriene B₄; *PGE₂,* prostaglandin E₂. **B,** Sequence of events in the production of the inflammatory response to urate crystals. **C,** Gouty tophus on right foot. (**C** from Dieppe PA et al: *Arthritis and rheumatism in practice,* London, 1991, Gower.)

and elsewhere, such as in the heart, earlobes, and kidneys. Evidence suggests that an acute attack of gout is the result of the *formation* of crystals rather than the release of crystals from connective tissues into the synovial fluid.

Monosodium urate crystals can stimulate and perpetuate the inflammatory response (see Figure 37-23, *A* and *B*). The presence of the crystals triggers the acute inflammatory response, releasing pro-inflammatory cytokines and tumor necrosis factors, during which

neutrophils are attracted out of the circulation and begin to phagocytose (ingest) the crystals.

CLINICAL MANIFESTATIONS Gout is manifested by (1) an increase in serum urate concentration (hyperuricemia); (2) recurrent attacks of monoarticular arthritis (inflammation of a single joint); (3) deposits of monosodium urate monohydrate (tophi) in and around the joints; (4) renal disease involving glomerular, tubular, and interstitial tissues and blood vessels; and (5) the formation of renal stones. These manifestations appear in three clinical stages:

1. **Asymptomatic hyperuricemia.** The serum urate level is elevated but arthritic symptoms, tophi, and renal stones are not present; this stage may persist throughout life.
2. **Acute gouty arthritis.** Attacks develop with increased serum urate concentrations; tends to occur with sudden or sustained increases of hyperuricemia but also can be triggered by trauma, drugs, and alcohol.
3. **Tophaceous gout.** The third and chronic stage of the disease; can begin as early as 3 years or as late as 40 years after the initial attack of gouty arthritis. Progressive inability to excrete uric acid expands the urate pool until monosodium urate crystal deposits (tophi) appear in cartilage, synovial membranes, tendons, and soft tissue.

Trauma is the most common aggravating factor of an acute gouty exacerbation. Attacks of gouty arthritis occur abruptly, usually in a peripheral joint (see Figure 37-23, *C*). The primary symptom is severe pain. Approximately 50% of the initial attacks occur in the metatarsophalangeal joint of the great toe (a condition known as podagra). The other 50% involve the heel, ankle, instep of the foot, knee, wrist, or elbow. The pain is usually noted at night. Within a few hours the affected joint becomes hot, red, and extremely tender and may be slightly swollen. Lymphangitis and systemic signs of inflammation (leukocytosis, fever, elevated sedimentation rate) are occasionally present. Untreated, mild attacks usually subside in several hours but may persist for 1 or 2 days. Severe attacks may persist for several days or weeks. When the individual recovers, the symptoms resolve completely.

Tophaceous deposits produce irregular swellings of the fingers, hands, knees, and feet. The helix of the ear is the most common site of tophi, which are the characteristic diagnostic lesions of chronic gout. Tophi also may develop along the ulnar surface of the forearm, the tibial surface of the leg, the Achilles tendon, olecranon bursa, or other areas. Tophi may produce marked limitation of joint movement and eventually cause grotesque deformities of the hands and feet (see Figure 37-23, *C*). Although the tophi themselves are painless, they often cause progressive stiffness and persistent aching of the affected joint. Tophi in the extremities can cause nerve compression—carpal tunnel syndrome in the wrists, tarsal tunnel syndrome in the ankles. Tophi also may erode and drain through the skin.

Renal stones are 1000 times more prevalent in individuals with primary gout than in the general population. The stones can be the size of a grain of sand or a piece of gravel, or they can accumulate in massive deposits called *staghorn calculi.* They range in color from pale yellow to brown to reddish black, depending on their composition. Some stones consist of pure monosodium urate; others consist of calcium oxalate or calcium phosphate. Renal stones can form in the collecting tubules, pelvis, or ureters, causing obstruction, dilation, and atrophy of the more proximal tubules and leading eventually to acute renal failure. Stones deposited directly in renal interstitial tissue initiate an inflammatory reaction that leads to chronic renal disease and progressive renal failure.

TREATMENT   The goals of gout treatment are to terminate the acute gouty attack as promptly as possible, avoid recurring attacks, prevent or reverse complications associated with urate deposits in the joints and kidneys, and block formation of kidney stones. Acute gouty arthritis is treated with anti-inflammatory drugs. The drugs of choice are colchicine, nonsteroidal anti-inflammatory drugs (NSAIDs, especially indomethacin), and corticosteroids. In persons unable to tolerate NSAIDs, colchicine is useful but can be poorly tolerated because of

a number of side effects. Once infection has been ruled out, hydrocortisone may be injected into the joint to relieve pain. Ice also may relieve some of the inflammation of the joint. Weight bearing on the involved joint is avoided until the acute attack subsides. A diet that includes mostly vegetables and fruit with little meat can help alkalinize urine and increase uric acid excretion.[86] High fluid intake, particularly water, can increase urinary output. Long-term use of antihyperuricemic drugs helps reduce serum urate concentrations. Allopurinol and febuxostat are both used to lower serum urate levels by inhibiting the activity of xanthine oxidase.

 QUICK CHECK 37-3

1. How does noninflammatory joint disease differ from inflammatory joint disease? Describe two principal features of each.
2. How does rheumatoid arthritis affect the skin, heart, lungs, and kidneys?
3. How does uric acid (or urates) cause gout to develop?

DISORDERS OF SKELETAL MUSCLE

Muscle diseases (myopathies) encompass many entities. Muscle weakness and fatigue are common symptoms. In many cases, neural, traumatic, and psychogenic causes provide an adequate explanation for the failure to generate force (weakness) or sustain force (fatigue) seen in myopathies. The pathophysiologic mechanisms in some of the metabolic and inflammatory muscle diseases have been explored, but the cause of many of the myopathies remains obscure. The complex interaction between muscles and nerves affects muscular function as well. Only inherited and acquired disorders of skeletal muscles are discussed here.

Secondary Muscular Dysfunction

Muscular symptoms arise from a variety of causes unrelated to the muscle itself. Secondary muscular phenomena (contracture, stress-related muscle tension, immobility) are common disorders that influence muscular function.

Contractures

Contractures can be pathologic or physiologic. A physiologic muscle contracture occurs in the absence of a muscle action potential in the sarcolemma. Muscle shortening is explained on the basis of failure of the calcium pump in the presence of plentiful adenosine triphosphate (ATP). A physiologic contracture is seen in McArdle disease (muscle myophosphorylase deficiency) and malignant hyperthermia. The contracture is usually temporary if the underlying pathology is reversed.

A pathologic contracture is a permanent muscle shortening caused by muscle spasm or weakness. Heel cord (Achilles tendon) contractures are examples of pathologic contractures. They are associated with plentiful ATP and occur in spite of a normal action potential. The most common form of contracture is seen in conditions such as muscular dystrophy and central nervous system (CNS) injury. Contractures also may develop secondary to scar tissue contraction in the flexor tissues of a joint, for example, contracture of burned tissues in the antecubital area of the forearm leading to a flexion contracture.

Stress-Induced Muscle Tension

Abnormally increased muscle tension has been associated with chronic anxiety as well as a variety of stress-related muscular symptoms including neck stiffness, back pain, and headache. Abnormalities in the CNS, reticular activating system, and autonomic nervous system (ANS) have been implicated. For example, as an individual progressively relaxes, the amplitude of the knee jerk reflex diminishes. Conversely, individuals with absent reflexes increase tension by such maneuvers as clenching the teeth or strengthening the handgrip. The underlying pathophysiology may be related to the fact that as a muscle contracts, the muscle spindle is activated. This gamma-feedback system produces a series of impulses that are transmitted to the brain by the sensitive 1A afferent fibers. Unconscious tension is thought to increase the activity of the reticular activating system as well, which stimulates firing of the efferent loop of the gamma fibers, produces further muscle contraction, and increases muscle tension. ANS function that regulates increased blood flow to the muscle during sympathetic activity may be related to increased muscle contraction tension.

Various forms of treatment have been used to reduce the muscle tension associated with stress. Progressive relaxation training, yoga, meditation, and biofeedback are examples of stress reduction therapies. Biofeedback uses an integrated electromyograph (EMG) to make recordings from the skin surface. The goal is to teach the individual to control maladaptive tension. It is particularly useful in individuals who have a connection between skeletal muscle tension and pain. Progressive relaxation training emphasizes the individual's ability to perceive the difference between tension and relaxation. This technique involves sequential tensing and a relaxing environment. The individual is taught to practice this routine daily, often with the use of audiotaped instructions. By teaching the individual to recognize excessive contraction of skeletal muscle, one hopes to enhance the person's ability to relax specific muscle groups to relieve tension and thus reduce CNS arousal as well as ANS arousal.

Disuse Atrophy

The term disuse atrophy describes the pathologic reduction in normal size of muscle fibers after prolonged inactivity from bed rest, trauma (casting), or local nerve damage as can be seen with spinal cord trauma or polio. Decreased muscle activity reduces muscle mass through both decreased muscle protein synthesis and increased muscle protein breakdown. Reduced protein synthesis is primarily responsible for muscle atrophy.[87,88] The effects of muscular deconditioning associated with lack of physical activity may be apparent in a matter of days. The normal individual prescribed bed rest loses muscle strength from baseline levels at a rate of 3% per day. Bed rest also is associated with cardiovascular, skeletal, and other organ system changes. Also, as people age, their muscles atrophy and become weaker (sarcopenia).

Measures to prevent atrophy include frequent forceful isometric muscle contractions and passive lengthening exercises. Artificial gravity (through the use of a "human centrifuge") has shown benefit in maintaining muscle strength.[88] If reuse is not restored within 1 year, regeneration of muscle fibers becomes impaired.

Fibromyalgia

Fibromyalgia (FM) is a chronic musculoskeletal syndrome characterized by diffuse pain, fatigue, increased sensitivity to touch (i.e., tender points), the absence of systemic or localized inflammation, and the presence of fatigue and nonrestorative sleep; anxiety and depression also are frequently present. FM has often been misdiagnosed or completely dismissed by clinicians because there are few objective clinical findings on examination. A common misdiagnosis has been chronic fatigue syndrome. Of affected individuals, 80% to 90% are women, and the peak age is 30 to 50 years. New research indicates a genetic predisposition and environmental factors play a role in development of symptoms.[89,90] FM and its symptoms are viewed as the result of central nervous system dysfunction, where pain transmission and interpretation are amplified, a condition called central sensitization.[91] Although the incidence is unknown, the prevalence is reported to be 2% and increases with age. Certain autoimmune diseases, especially systemic lupus erythematosus (SLE) and irritable bowel syndrome (IBS), are often seen in association with FM and may coexist if not initially present with fibromyalgia.

PATHOPHYSIOLOGY Genetic factors are increasingly being suggested as important in developing FM. Relatives of individuals with FM have an increased risk of developing FM. Studies of genetic factors have implicated alterations in genes affecting serotonin, catecholamines, and dopamine—all of these substances are involved in stress response and sensory processing.[89,91] In spite of these studies, the role of genetic factors has not yet been fully identified in FM. External stressors, such as infection, psychosocial stress, and physical or emotional trauma, may precipitate onset of FM, but no single stressor triggers it.

Functional magnetic resonance imaging (fMRI) and positron emission tomography (PET) scans of the brains of individuals with FM have shown activity in different areas of the brain than normally seen in healthy individuals exposed to painful stimuli.[92-94] These functional abnormalities within the central nervous system (CNS) are shown in Figure 37-24. Other pathophysiologic evidence includes hypothalamic-pituitary-adrenal axis alterations that show abnormal response to stress. Recent investigations suggest cytokines are involved in the pathogenesis of FM.

CLINICAL MANIFESTATIONS The prominent symptom of fibromyalgia is diffuse, chronic pain. Chronic pain is defined as being present more than 3 months. The locations of 9 pairs (18) of tender points for diagnostic classification of fibromyalgia are shown in Figure 37-25. Tenderness in 11 of these 18 points is necessary for diagnosis along with a history of diffuse pain. The only reliable finding on examination is the presence of multiple tender points that include areas on both sides of the spine and both above and below the waist. The pain often begins in one location, especially the neck and shoulders, but then becomes more generalized. People describe the pain as *burning* or *gnawing*. Fatigue is profound. The effect on everyday life is considerable. Fatigue is most notable when arising from sleep and in midafternoon. Headaches and memory loss are common complaints. There is a strong association between fibromyalgia, Raynaud phenomenon, and irritable bowel syndrome. Individuals with fibromyalgia are light sleepers and awake frequently, which may explain why individuals feel nonrefreshed upon waking.

Almost 25% of individuals seek psychologic support for depression. Anxiety, particularly with regard to their diagnosis and future, is almost universal.

EVALUATION AND TREATMENT Because the manifestations of chronic, generalized pain and fatigue are present in many musculoskeletal (e.g., rheumatic) disorders, these disorders should be considered in the diagnosis of FM. In an effort to simplify and more accurately diagnose FM, the American College of Rheumatology (ACR) recently expanded the diagnostic criteria to include a widespread pain index (WPI) definition as "axial pain, left- and right-sided pain, and upper and lower segment pain"[95] and a symptom severity (SS) score. The SS score includes symptoms such as fatigue, waking unrefreshed, and cognitive difficulty. The WPI and SS scores are then tabulated to identify or exclude the diagnosis of FM in individuals who also meet the following criteria:

1. Symptoms have been present at a similar level for at least 3 months.
2. The individual does not have a disorder that would otherwise explain the pain.[95]

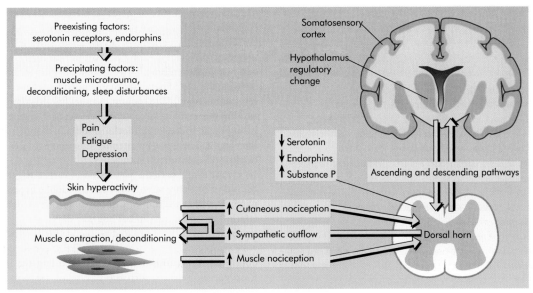

FIGURE 37-24 Theoretic Pathophysiologic Model of Fibromyalgia.

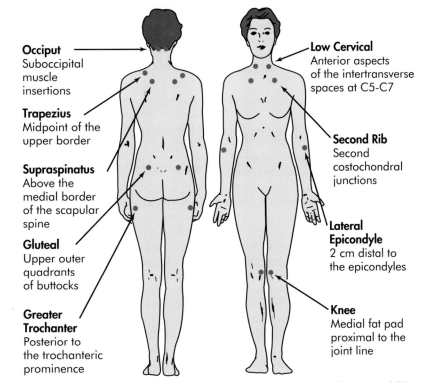

Occiput
Suboccipital
muscle
insertions

Trapezius
Midpoint of the
upper border

Supraspinatus
Above the
medial border
of the scapular
spine

Gluteal
Upper outer
quadrants
of buttocks

**Greater
Trochanter**
Posterior to
the trochanteric
prominence

Low Cervical
Anterior aspects
of the intertransverse
spaces at C5-C7

Second Rib
Second
costochondral
junctions

**Lateral
Epicondyle**
2 cm distal to
the epicondyles

Knee
Medial fat pad
proximal to the
joint line

FIGURE 37-25 Location of Specific Tender Points for Diagnostic Classification of Fibromyalgia. (Redrawn from Freundlich B, Leventhal L: The fibromyalgia syndrome. In Schumacher HR Jr, Klippel JH, Koopman WJ, editors: *Primer on the rheumatic diseases,* ed 11, Atlanta, 1997, Arthritis Foundation.)

Treatment should be highly individualized. No one regimen of medication has proved successful for FM. Exercise regimens are beneficial in reducing symptoms. Recommended exercises for individuals with FM include aerobic activities (including kick boxing and weight lifting), stretching, and gentle strengthening programs. Medications also are helpful. The FDA has currently approved three medications specifically to treat FM: pregabalin, duloxetine, and milnacipran. Pregabalin reduces the release of several neurochemicals, decreasing pain. Duloxetine and milnacipran are norepinephrine and serotonin reuptake inhibitor antidepressants that also improve pain and depression. Milnacipran also improves fatigue, cognition, and other FM symptoms. In addition, tricyclic antidepressants (e.g., amitriptyline) have analgesic properties but have more side effects. Certain CNS-active medications, most notable the tricyclic antidepressants, amitriptyline, and cyclobenzaprine, were significantly better than placebos in controlled trials. Amitriptyline significantly improved pain, morning stiffness, and sleep but not the sensitivity of tender points. One of the most important aspects of treatment is education and reassurance (Box 37-4).

Muscle Membrane Abnormalities

Two defects of the muscle membrane (plasma membrane of the muscle fiber) have been linked to clinical syndromes: the hyperexcitable membrane seen in myotonic disorders and the intermittently unresponsive membrane seen in periodic paralyses. Although these are infrequent disorders, research into the pathologic processes has led to an improved understanding of the cell membrane.

Myotonia

Myotonia is a delayed relaxation after voluntary muscle contraction, such as grip, eye closure, or muscle percussion. The distinctive "dive bomber" noise, audible on needle EMG, is caused by the prolonged depolarization of the muscle membrane. Because the depolarization is not terminated by neuromuscular blocking agents, such as curare, the abnormality has been localized at the muscle membrane; the basic defect is the result of ion channel dysfunction. (These structures are described in Chapter 12.)

Myotonia is seen in several disorders: myotonia congenita, paramyotonia congenita, myotonic muscular dystrophy, and some forms of periodic paralysis. Most are inherited disorders and are mild in symptomatology, with the exception of myotonic muscular dystrophy. Myotonia is treated by drugs that reduce muscle fiber excitability, such as procaine, procainamide, phenytoin, and quinine preparations. Treatments include acetazolamide, a carbonic anhydrase inhibitor, and verapamil, a calcium channel blocker.

Periodic Paralysis

Periodic paralysis encompasses a rare group of muscle diseases characterized by episodes of flaccid weakness. Most are hereditary (autosomal dominant) and caused by potassium or sodium channel abnormalities because of specific genetic mutations. In normal skeletal muscle, potassium channels regulate the duration of the action potential. Sodium channels, in response to nerve stimulation, create the action potentials that initiate muscle contraction.[96] During an attack of periodic paralysis, the resting muscle membrane potential both is unresponsive to neural stimuli and is reduced from −90 to −45 mV.

Thyrotoxic hypokalemic periodic paralysis (TPP) is caused by potassium channelopathy that causes increased flow of potassium into the cell; it does not indicate a potassium deficiency.[97] Most common in Asian males, TPP is increasingly being seen in all ethnic groups.[97,98]

The main consequence of increased intracellular potassium is depolarization of the muscle and resulting weakness.

Hyperkalemic periodic paralysis can be activated by several factors, including pregnancy, eating potassium-rich foods, exposure to cold, and rest after exercising.[96,99] Although the most striking feature of the condition is flaccid paralysis, many individuals have myotonia present on examination.[99] The sodium channel fails to completely inactivate, causing more sodium to enter the cell and forcing potassium into the extracellular space, thus blocking sodium channels from depolarizing. This can be a life-threatening situation because death may occur because of respiratory insufficiency.

Hypokalemic periodic paralysis also can be triggered by exposure to cold or rest after strenuous exercise. Unlike hyperkalemic periodic paralysis, eating sodium- or carbohydrate-rich foods also can cause an attack. This condition can last hours to days.

Treatment consists of avoiding known foods or activities that provoke symptoms. Acute treatment of TPP is careful administration of potassium. Prevention is aimed at correcting the hyperthyroidism. β-Adrenergic blockers, such as propranolol, are sometimes given until thyroid function is normal.[98] In acute hyperkalemic periodic paralysis, inhaled albuterol or glucose/insulin therapy can reduce symptoms. Oral and intravenous administration of potassium can relieve acute hypokalemic attacks. For both hyper- and hypokalemic periodic paralysis, carbonic anhydrase inhibitors, such as acetazolamide and dichlorphenamide, are helpful in preventing episodes.[96]

Metabolic Muscle Diseases

Disorders in muscle metabolism can be caused by endocrine abnormalities or diseases of energy metabolism, such as glycogen storage disease, enzyme deficiencies, and abnormalities in lipid metabolism and mitochondrial function. The term *metabolic myopathies* refers to a group of hereditary muscle disorders caused by defective genes.

Endocrine Disorders

Often the systemic effects of hormonal imbalance overshadow the individual's muscular symptoms. For example, individuals with thyrotoxicosis may have signs of proximal weakness, paresis of the extraocular muscles (exophthalmic ophthalmoplegia), and, rarely, hypokalemic periodic paralysis. Hypothyroidism is often associated with a decrease in muscle mass and strength, with weak, flabby skeletal muscles and sluggish movements.

Thyroid hormone is believed to regulate muscle protein synthesis and electrolyte balance. Changes in muscle protein synthesis and electrolyte balance may therefore explain the changes in muscle mass and contractility seen in endocrine disorders. The muscular symptoms subside with appropriate treatment of the primary hormonal disorder.

Diseases of Energy Metabolism

Muscles rely on carbohydrates (such as glycogen) and lipids (free fatty acids) for energy. When stored glycogen or lipids cannot be metabolized because of lack of enzymes necessary to generate ATP for muscle contraction, the individual experiences cramps, fatigue, and exercise intolerance. Disorders of muscle metabolism can be self-limiting, such as McArdle disease and some lipid disorders, or they can cause widespread irreparable muscle destruction, as in acid maltase deficiency.

McArdle disease. McArdle disease, or myophosphorylase deficiency, is also known as glycogen storage disease type V. It was the first myopathy in which a single enzyme defect was identified. It is now one of nine diseases identified to date that have in common an underlying defect in glycogen synthesis, glycogenolysis, or glycolysis. These diseases are often referred to as glycogen storage diseases (GSDs) because each defect results in the abnormal deposition and accumulation of glycogen in skeletal muscle. Individuals with McArdle disease lack muscle phosphorylase, an enzyme responsible for the breakdown of glycogen in muscle. Normally, after the body uses the short-term ATP and phosphocreatine stores, intramuscular lactic acid accumulates as glycogen is used (see Chapter 17). The individual with McArdle disease is not able to metabolize glycogen or produce lactic acid.

The altered energy production manifests itself in exercise intolerance, fatigue, and painful muscle cramps. When exercise is carried to an extreme, painful muscle contracture and myoglobinuria develop. Some individuals describe a "second wind" phenomenon, in which exercise tolerance increases if they slow their pace once the initial sensation of fatigue commences.[100] This may be caused by the use of free fatty acids as a secondary source of energy. As the disease progresses, some individuals have pronounced muscle weakness and wasting. Other organs are not involved, because the absence of phosphorylase is limited to muscle. Generally, individuals with McArdle disease learn to adapt their daily routine to avoid muscle symptoms.

Acid maltase deficiency. Acid maltase deficiency, or glycogen storage disease type II, is an autosomal recessive disease that causes an accumulation of glycogen in the lysosomes of muscle cells and other tissues.[101] The usual pathways of glycogen degradation are preserved. The absence of the enzyme acid maltase is responsible for the abnormality in glycogen metabolism, although the exact mechanism is unknown.

The infantile form, which is more severe, is called Pompe disease and is recognized shortly after birth by hypotonia, dysreflexia, and an enlarged heart, tongue, and liver. Hypertrophy of these tissues is thought to be the result of glycogen deposition. Children die of cardiac or respiratory failure within 1 year of diagnosis. The adult variety becomes evident subacutely. The muscular symptoms resemble those of muscular dystrophy or polymyositis (see p. 1030). A distinguishing feature in adults may be the presence of severe respiratory muscle weakness.

Myoadenylate deaminase deficiency. An enzyme deficiency that produces changes in skeletal muscle and is associated with exercise intolerance is myoadenylate deaminase deficiency (MDD). Because these individuals lack myoadenylate deaminase, they have a poor capacity for sustained energy production. Myoadenylate deaminase is the catalytic enzyme that forms phosphocreatine and ATP during exercise through a metabolic pathway that binds the purine and phosphate molecules that constitute ATP. Persons with MDD differ from those with McArdle disease in that, during the ischemic exercise test, lactate production is normal when ATP and phosphocreatine are synthesized. The enzyme defect has been reported to be quite common, but in practice it may be rarely recognized as a cause of exercise intolerance.

Lipid deficiencies. Disorders of lipid metabolism are uncommon but account for severe changes in muscle metabolism. These disorders are caused by abnormalities in the transport and processing of fatty acids for energy. The lipid content of muscle cells consists of free fatty acids, which are oxidized in the mitochondria. These acids require carnitine and the enzyme carnitine palmitoyltransferase (CPT) to transport long-chain fatty acids to the mitochondria. There are two types of CPT: CPT1 is found in liver, muscle, and brain tissue; and CPT2 is considered a ubiquitous protein. CPT2 deficiency is an autosomal recessive disorder that invariably causes attacks of severe myalgia and myoglobinuria.[102] Carnitine deficiency causes abnormal lipid deposition in skeletal muscles.

Measuring the CPT and carnitine content in muscle aids in the diagnosis. Cells in the muscle biopsy show vacuoles and lipid deposits. Treatments with riboflavin, medium-chain triglycerides, oral carnitine, prednisone, and propranolol have been beneficial to some

individuals. Bezafibrate, a drug to lower lipid levels, also has shown promise in treating CPT2 deficiency.[102]

Inflammatory Muscle Diseases: Myositis
Viral, Bacterial, and Parasitic Myositis

Viral, bacterial, and parasitic infections of varying severity are known to produce inflammatory changes in skeletal muscle, a group of conditions collectively described by the term myositis. In tuberculosis and sarcoidosis, chronic inflammatory changes and granulomata are found in muscle as well as in other affected tissues. In trichinosis, *Trichinella* larvae reside in infected pork and, after ingestion, migrate to the intestinal mucosa and then to the lymphatics. Symptoms include severe pain, rash, and muscle stiffness. Treatment includes the administration of corticosteroids, immunotherapeutic agents, and the antiparasitic agent thiabendazole. Toxoplasmosis, a common parasitic infection, is also associated with a generalized polymyositis that responds rapidly to therapy.

In the tropics, more prevalent disorders include bacterial infections with *Staphylococcus aureus* and parasites such as cysticercus, the larva of the tapeworm *Taenia solium*. Viral infections can be associated with an acute myositis. Muscle pain, tenderness, signs of inflammation, and creatine kinase (CK) elevation are common manifestations of viral myositis. The self-limiting symptoms of muscle aches and pains during a bout of influenza may actually be a subacute form of viral myopathy.

Polymyositis, Dermatomyositis, and Inclusion-Body Myositis

Idiopathic inflammatory myopathies (IIMs) are a group of autoimmune diseases that target skeletal muscle. Their exact cause is unknown, but IIMs can affect both children and adults. IIMs are characterized by symmetric proximal (shoulder girdle and quadriceps) muscle weakness and myalgia that develops over weeks to months. The three principal types are polymyositis (PM), dermatomyositis (DM), and inclusion-body myositis (IBM). Non-Caucasian women older than age 50 are most often affected by IIM but DM also has a juvenile form, juvenile dermatomyositis (JDM). The incidence of IIM appears to be increasing, although this may simply reflect improved diagnosis.

CLINICAL MANIFESTATIONS   The acute symptoms include many of those seen in any inflammatory process: malaise, fever, muscle swelling, pain and tenderness, lethargy, listlessness, morning stiffness, anorexia, and weight loss. These illnesses are usually associated with a symmetric proximal muscle weakness and can be initially confused with other myopathies. A thorough evaluation is required to exclude other disorders. Clinical features common in both PM and DM are dysphagia, reduced esophageal motility, vasculitis, Raynaud phenomenon, cardiomyopathy, and interstitial pulmonary fibrosis. Reduced mobility with frequent falls is a common symptom in IBM because both proximal and distal muscles are affected. Some individuals have other coexisting collagen vascular disorders, such as rheumatoid arthritis, systemic lupus erythematosus, and progressive systemic sclerosis (formerly called *scleroderma*).

Although PM and DM have similar histories of onset, DM includes cutaneous manifestations. The two most classic signs of skin involvement are rashes: a typical heliotrope (reddish purple) rash that generally covers the eyelids and periorbital tissue (Figure 37-26); and erythematous, scaly lesions that cover joints such as the knees and elbows, known as Gottron lesions. Other differences between PM and DM include their suspected pathology. PM may be caused by T cell invasion of the muscle fibers.[103] DM is associated with immune complex deposition with malignancy. Both PM and DM seem to respond to prednisone, with or without the addition of immunosuppressives, and intravenous immunoglobulin administration.[104,105]

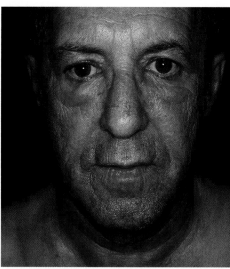

FIGURE 37-26 Dermatomyositis. Heliotrope (violaceous) discoloration around the eyes and periorbital edema. (From Habif TP: *Clinical dermatology*, ed 3, St Louis, 1996, Mosby.)

IBM differs from both PM and DM in several important ways. Muscle biopsy and histopathologic studies of IBM show degenerative changes of muscle, accumulation of multiple proteins within muscle fibers, and evidence of endoplasmic reticular stress with misfolding of proteins.[106,107] Clinical presentation may show earlier onset of asymmetric atrophy and weakness of the quadriceps as well as the wrists and finger flexors.[108] Additionally, IBM generally does not improve with standard immunosuppressants or immune-modifying drugs.

EVALUATION AND TREATMENT Muscle biopsy results are striking in DM, with most individuals showing inflammatory cells grouped around blood vessels and atrophy of cells in muscle fascicles. This change, perifascicular atrophy, is absent in PM. Creatinine kinase (CK) level is often extremely elevated in both disorders and is a helpful indicator of disease activity. Levels of other muscle enzymes, including aldolase, aspartate aminotransferase (AST), alanine aminotransferase (AST), and lactate dehydrogenase (LDH), are also found to be elevated in most individuals. The presence of serum antinuclear antibodies (ANAs) also may be helpful. Muscle biopsy is indispensable for a diagnosis of PM or DM as opposed to other myotonic disease. MRI reveals inflammation and edema of the muscles. Electromyography (EMG) is useful in guiding the site for muscle biopsy.[109]

Treatment primarily includes immunosuppressive drugs, although they are not always successful if uniformly applied. Most clinicians choose corticosteroids initially, usually prednisone on a daily or alternating day schedule, tapering the dosage as the symptoms subside. Successful treatment with azathioprine, methotrexate, and cyclophosphamide also has been reported. High-dose intravenous immunoglobulin administration is sometimes used during active disease. Individuals with muscle weakness require careful physiotherapy to design a regular exercise program that prevents contractures and maximizes functional ability.

Toxic Myopathies

Muscle damage caused by drugs or toxins is also called toxic myopathy. Alcohol, lipid-lowering agents (fibrates and statins), antimalarial drugs, steroids, thiol derivatives, and narcotics (particularly heroin) can all cause symptoms. Many drugs, diseases, and infectious and environmental agents can cause myopathy. The combination of certain

---

BOX 37-5 AGENTS THAT CAN CAUSE TOXIC MYOPATHY

Drug-Induced
- Alcohol
- Amiodarone (and others that inhibit CYP3A4 when combined with simvastatin)
- Amphotericin B
- Azathioprine
- AZT (zidovudine)
- Chloroquine
- Clofibrate
- Cocaine
- Colchicine
- Ethanol
- Ipecac (withdrawn from U.S. markets)
- 3,4-Methylenedioxymethamphetamine (MDMA, "ecstasy")
- Pentachlorophenol (PCP)
- Statins
- Steroids (especially with prolonged high doses; doses >25 mg/day; fluorinated steroids)

Endocrine Disorders
- Adrenal disorders (Addison disease, Cushing disease)
- Hyperparathyroidism
- Hyperthyroidism (CK may be normal)
- Hypothyroidism (CK may be mildly elevated)

Infectious
- Coxsackie A and B viruses
- Human immunodeficiency virus (HIV)
- Influenza
- Lyme disease
- *Staphylococcus aureus* muscle infection (frequent cause of pyomyositis)
- Toxoplasmosis
- Trichinosis

Miscellaneous
- Licorice
- Certain edible wild mushrooms
- Lead poisoning
- Organophosphates
- Red yeast rice
- European migratory quail (quail eat toxic hemlock, hellebore seeds)
- Any medication that alters serum concentrations of sodium, potassium, calcium, phosphorus, or magnesium levels

Data from Hall AP, Henry JA: Acute toxic effects of 'Ecstasy' (MDMA) and related compounds: overview of pathophysiology and clinical management, *Br J Anaesth* 96(6):678–685, 2006; Kuncl RW: Agents and mechanisms of toxic myopathy, *Curr Opin Neurol* 22(5):506–515, 2009; Valiyil VR, Christopher-Stine L: Drug-related myopathies of which the clinician should be aware, *Curr Rheumatol Rep* 12(3):213–220, 2010.

---

medications can sometimes cause muscle injury.[110] Box 37-5 lists some of the causes of toxic myopathy.

Alcohol remains the most common cause of toxic myopathy. Two clinical syndromes are prevalent: (1) an acute attack of muscle weakness, pain, and swelling after a drinking binge; or (2) a more chronic, progressive proximal weakness in a long-term drinker. The incidence of acute alcoholic myopathy has been estimated as being up to 20% of individuals admitted with acute alcoholic withdrawal.

The pathologic abnormalities include necrosis of individual muscle fibers; whole segments can be found in the same stage of degeneration. The mechanism by which alcohol affects the muscle fiber is uncertain, but a direct toxic effect and nutritional deficiency have both received experimental support.

Acute alcoholic myopathy can range from benign cramps and pain resolving in a matter of hours to severe weakness and markedly increased CK level associated with myoglobinuria and renal failure. Individuals are prone to repeated attacks following recovery. The only treatment is abstinence from alcohol and improved nutrition. The individual with chronic alcoholic myopathy often has coexisting peripheral neuropathy that complicates the diagnosis.

The most severe complication of toxic myopathy is rhabdomyolysis (acute muscle fiber necrosis with leakage of muscle protein into the bloodstream) that leads to myoglobinuria and acute renal failure. Most individuals with toxic myopathy present with acute muscle weakness. Pain is an unreliable indicator as many toxic myopathies are painless, but necrotizing toxic myopathies can cause severe pain. Dark-colored urine may indicate rhabdomyolysis, a serious complication that can lead to death (see p. 984). Other serious complications can include involvement of respiratory and cardiac muscles.

Measurement of serum creatine levels is helpful in determining muscle damage. Other tests such as electromyography (EMG) may show characteristics changes in function. Magnetic resonance imaging (MRI) can demonstrate muscle edema. Features of myopathy can be seen on muscle biopsy.

Repeated intramuscular injections have been associated also with changes in muscle fibers. Local necrosis of muscle fibers and elevated CK level have been reported after intramuscular injections of cephalothin, lidocaine, diazepam, and digoxin; these effects were not produced with injections of saline. When drugs are injected over long periods, a chronic focal myopathy develops. Proliferation of connective tissue in both the muscle fiber and overlying skin and subcutaneous tissue has been reported. Over time, segments of the muscles, particularly the deltoid and quadriceps, are converted into fibrotic bands. Pathophysiologic mechanisms for these changes include repeated needle trauma and infection, along with the nonphysiologic acidity or alkalinity of the injected material.

Treatment primarily consists of removing or stopping the offending agent and providing supportive care. Supportive care may include hemodialysis and respiratory or cardiovascular support, depending on severity of symptoms.

> ✓ **QUICK CHECK 37-4**
> 1. What is the main objective clinical finding in fibromyalgia?
> 2. How do metabolic muscle diseases develop? What causes them?
> 3. Name one toxic myopathy, and explain why it develops.

MUSCULOSKELETAL TUMORS

Bone Tumors

Many different types of tumors involve the skeleton. Although the skeleton is the major site for metastatic spread of multiple myeloma, breast, lung, and prostate cancers, primary bone tumors are relatively rare. Bone tumors may originate from bone cells, cartilage, fibrous tissue, marrow, or vascular tissue. Based on the tissue of origin, bone tumors are classified as osteogenic, chondrogenic, collagenic, or myelogenic. Box 37-6 identifies the World Health Organization's (WHO) classification of bone tumors. Each of the types arises from

---

BOX 37-6   WORLD HEALTH ORGANIZATION (WHO) CLASSIFICATION OF BONE TUMORS

Cartilage Tumors
Chondrosarcoma (M)
Chondroma (B)
Osteochondroma (B; but may become malignant)
Chondroblastoma (B)

Osteogenic Tumors
Osteoblastoma (B)
Osteoid osteoma (B)
Osteosarcoma (M)

Fibrogenic Tumors (Often Produce Collagen; Do Not Have a Mineralizing Matrix)
Fibrosarcoma (M)

Fibrohistiocytic Tumors (Comprised of Fibroblasts)
Benign fibrous histiocytoma (B)
Malignant fibrous histiocytoma (M)

Ewing Sarcoma
Ewing sarcoma (M)

Hematopoietic Tumors
Plasma cell myeloma (M)
Malignant lymphoma (M)

Giant Cell Tumor
Giant cell tumor (B, but can grow aggressively)
Malignancy in giant cell tumor (M; very rare tumor)

Smooth Muscle Tumors
Leiomyoma (B)
Leiomyosarcoma (M)

Miscellaneous Tumors
Adamantinoma (M; almost exclusively found in tibia)
Metastatic malignancy (M; most common skeletal malignancy)

Miscellaneous Lesions
Aneurysmal bone cyst (B)
Simple cyst (B)
Fibrous dysplasia (B; rarely can become malignant)
Osteofibrous dysplasia (B)
Langerhans cell histiocytosis (B, but can aggressively grow)
Chest wall hamartoma (B; is excessive growth of mesenchymal tissue [mostly cartilage])

Joint Lesions
Synovial chondromatosis (B; rarely becomes M)

Data from Dorfman HD et al: WHO classification of tumours of bone: introduction. In Christopher DM et al, editors: *World Health Organization classification of tumours International Agency for Research on Cancer (IARC) pathology and genetics of tumours of soft tissue and bone*, p 226, Lyon, France, 2002, IARC Press.
B, Benign; *M*, malignant.

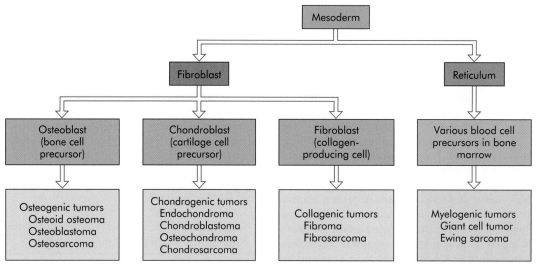

FIGURE 37-27 Derivation of Bone Tumors.

one of the four stem cells that are ultimately derived from the primitive mesoderm (Figure 37-27). In addition, bone tumors may be classified as being of histiocytic, notochordal, lipogenic, or neurogenic origin.

The mesoderm contributes the primitive fibroblast and reticulum cells. The fibroblast is the progenitor of the osteoblast and chondroblast cells. Each cell synthesizes a specific type of intercellular ground substance, and the tumor derived from the cell is generally characterized by the type of ground substance produced by the cell. For example, osteogenic tumors usually contain cells that have the appearance of osteoblasts and produce an intercellular substance that can be recognized as osteoid. Chondrogenic tumors contain chondroblasts and produce an intercellular substance similar to chondroid (cartilage). Collagenic tumors contain fibrous tissue cells and produce an intercellular substance similar to the type of collagen found in fibrous connective tissue.

Tumors are also classified as benign or malignant, based on characteristics of the tumor cells (see Chapter 9). The criteria used to identify tumor cells as malignant are (1) an increased nuclear/cytoplasmic ratio, (2) an irregular nuclear border, (3) an excess of chromatin, (4) a prominent nucleolus, and (5) an increase in the number of cells undergoing mitosis. However, many young, rapidly growing, normal cells and cells subjected to inflammation and change in their blood supply also exhibit many of these same characteristics. (Tumor characteristics in general are described in Chapter 9.)

EPIDEMIOLOGY   The incidence rate of bone tumors varies with age. In children younger than 15 years, the rate of bone tumors is relatively low, constituting approximately 5% of all malignancies. Adolescents have the highest incidence of bone tumors, and adults between the ages of 30 and 35 have the lowest incidence. After age 35 years, the incidence rate slowly increases until at age 60 years it equals the incidence rate in adolescents, primarily related to secondary metastatic tumors.

Patterns of Bone Destruction

The general pathologic features of bone tumors include bone destruction, erosion or expansion of the cortex, and periosteal response to changes in underlying bone. The least amount of pathologic damage occurs with benign bone tumors, which push against neighboring tissue. Because they usually have a symmetric, controlled growth pattern, benign bone tumors tend to compress and displace neighboring

TABLE 37-7	PATTERNS OF BONE DESTRUCTION CAUSED BY BONE TUMORS
TYPE	**FEATURES**
Geographic pattern	Least aggressive type
	Generally indicative of slow-growing or benign tumor
	Well-defined margins on tumor, easily separated from surrounding normal bone
	Uniform and well-defined lytic area in bone
	Margin smooth or irregular, demarcated by short zone of transition between normal and abnormal bone tissue
Moth-eaten pattern	Characteristic of rapidly growing, malignant bone tumors
	More aggressive pattern
	Tumor margin less defined or demarcated; cannot easily be separated from normal bone
	Areas of partially destroyed bone adjacent to completely lytic areas
Permeative pattern	Caused by aggressive malignant tumor with rapid growth potential
	Margins of tumor poorly demarcated
	Abnormal bone merges imperceptibly with normal bone

normal bone tissue, which weakens the bone's structure until it is incapable of withstanding the stress of ordinary use, leading to pathologic fracture. Other tumors invade and destroy adjacent normal bone tissue by producing substances that promote resorption by increasing osteoclast activity or by interfering with a bone's blood supply. Three patterns of bone destruction by bone tumors have been identified: (1) the geographic pattern, (2) the moth-eaten pattern, and (3) the permeative pattern (Table 37-7).

Tumors that erode the cortex of the bone usually stimulate a periosteal response—that is, new bone formation at the interface between the surface of the bone and the periosteum. Slow erosion of the cortex

STAGE	GRADE	SITE (T)	METASTASIS (M)
TABLE 37-8	**SURGICAL STAGING SYSTEM FOR BONE TUMORS**		
IA	Low (G_1)	Intracompartmental (T_1)	None (M_0)
IB	Low (G_1)	Extracompartmental (T_2)	None (M_0)
IIA	High (G_2)	Intracompartmental (T_1)	None (M_0)
IIB	High (G_2)	Extracompartmental (T_2)	None (M_0)
IIIA	Low (G_1)	Intracompartmental or extracompartmental (T_1 or T_2)	Regional or distant (M_1)
IIIB	High (G_2)	Intracompartmental or extracompartmental (T_1 or T_2)	Regional or distant (M_1)

Data from Simon SR, editor: *Orthopaedic basic science,* Chicago, 1994, American Academy of Orthopaedic Surgeons.

usually stimulates a uniform periosteal response. Additional layers of bone are added to the exterior surface of the bone to buttress the cortex. Eventually, the additional layers expand the bone's contour. Aggressive penetration of the cortex usually elevates the periosteum and stimulates erratic patterns of new bone formation. Examples of erratic patterns include concentric layers of new bone; a sunburst pattern, in which delicate rays of new bone radiate toward the periosteum from a single focus on the underlying surface; and rays of new bone that grow perpendicularly, creating a brush or bristle pattern.

EVALUATION A malignant bone tumor must be identified early to allow survival of the individual and preservation of the affected limb. However, individuals often have only vague symptoms that may be attributed to minor trauma, degenerative changes, or inflammatory conditions. In addition, other conditions may obscure the diagnosis.

Thorough diagnostic studies are needed to determine the exact type and extent of bone tumor present, which also helps determine the optimal treatment regimen. Serum alkaline phosphatase levels are elevated in bone lytic tumors and significantly elevated in osteosarcoma. Radiologic studies, including plain radiologic films, CT scan, and MRI, have become the examination of choice for the local staging of bone tumors, especially the staging of peripheral osteosarcomas (Table 37-8). MRI is also used to monitor the response of osteosarcomas to radiation or chemotherapy and to detect recurrent disease. A CT scan can evaluate involvement of osteosarcoma in flat bones when the tumor is not well-defined on a plain film, can assist in differentiating the tumor, and can locate pulmonary metastases. Radionucleotide bone scans show an increased uptake at the tumor site. (Tumor staging is discussed in Chapter 9.)

Additional diagnostic studies done for specific bone tumors include a complete blood count and erythrocyte sedimentation rate (to rule out infection or myeloma) and serum levels of calcium and phosphorus to detect hypercalcemia. Serum glucose levels may be elevated in chondrosarcoma. Acid phosphatase level may be moderately elevated in bone metastases, multiple myeloma, and advanced Paget disease. Serum protein electrophoresis and immunoelectrophoresis are performed to exclude other diseases. Fine needle biopsy is done, usually at the time of surgery, to determine the exact tumor type.

Types
A large number of lesions are classified as bone tumors. The bone tumors most representative of the four derivative types—osteogenic, chondrogenic, collagenic, and myelogenic tumors—are described here (Figure 37-28).

Osteogenic tumors: osteosarcoma. Osteogenic (bone-forming) tumors are characterized by the formation of bone or osteoid tissue with a sarcomatous tissue. The tissue can have the appearance of callus or compact or spongy bone. The most common malignant bone-forming tumor is the osteosarcoma.

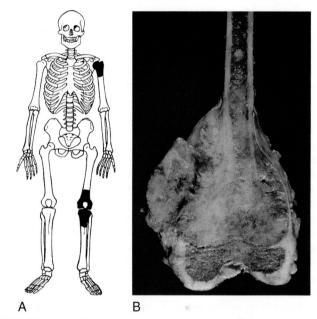

A   **B**

FIGURE 37-28 Osteosarcoma. A, Common locations of osteosarcoma. **B,** Femur has a large mass involving the metaphysis of the bone; the tumor has destroyed the cortex, forming a soft tissue component. (From Damjanov I, Linder J, editors: *Anderson's pathology,* ed 10, St Louis, 1996, Mosby.)

The incidence of osteosarcomas, the most commonly diagnosed primary bone tumor, peaks around puberty in both boys and girls, with a slight preference for males.[111] Sixty percent of osteosarcomas occur in persons younger than 20 years. A secondary peak incidence for osteosarcoma occurs in the 50- to 60-year age group, primarily in individuals with a history of radiation therapy several years previously for pelvic or other malignancies or for Paget disease of bone[111] (see Figure 37-28). Though considered a bone-forming tumor, the radiologic appearance of sarcoma is quite variable and often shows a moth-eaten (lytic) pattern of destruction with the tumor extending into the adjacent soft tissue. Occasionally, the tumor may spread to nonadjacent bone or across a joint with normal-appearing areas of bone between tumors (i.e., "skip lesions"). Radionuclide bone scans are used to find skip lesions. MRI is useful in determining bony changes associated with the tumor.

The borders of the tumor are indistinct and merge into adjacent normal bone. Osteosarcomas contain osteoid produced by anaplastic stromal cells, which are atypical, abnormal cells not seen in normal developing bone; they are neither normal nor embryonal. Many tumors are heterogeneous; for example, the osteosarcoma also may contain chondroid (cartilage) and fibrinoid tissue that may form the bulk of the tumor. The osteoid is deposited as thick masses or "streamers," which infiltrate the normal compact bone, destroy it, and replace it with masses of osteoid. Bone tissue produced by osteosarcomas never matures to compact bone.

Ninety percent of osteosarcomas are located in the metaphyses of long bones, especially the distal femoral metaphysis, with 50% around the knee area. The tumor typically impregnates the cortex, lifts the periosteum, and forms a soft tissue mass that is not covered by a smooth shell of new bone. Lifting of the periosteum stimulates bizarre patterns of new bone formation called a *periosteal reaction*. Distinct osteosarcomas occur on the surface of long bones, called parosteal, periosteal, and high-grade surface osteosarcomas; dedifferentiated parosteal and central osteosarcomas also occur.

The most common initial symptoms are pain and an enlarging mass.[112] Initially, the pain is slight and intermittent, but within a short time the pain increases in severity and duration. Pain is usually worse at night and gradually requires medication. Systemic symptoms are uncommon. Usually, a coincidental history of trauma is noted. Occasionally, the individual may present with a pathologic fracture.

Bone biopsy is critical to diagnosis. Because the most frequent site of metastasis is the lung, a chest CT or MRI of the thorax also should be performed. There are no specific laboratory tests that aid in diagnosing sarcoma but laboratory studies are helpful in assessing overall health before beginning treatment. The best clinical outcomes occur in those who receive both preoperative and postoperative chemotherapy.[113] Surgery is directed at salvaging the affected limb.[112,114]

Surgery is a major treatment of choice, with the tumor's location and size, the extent of malignancy, and evidence of metastasis dictating the type and extent of surgery (see Table 37-8). Preoperative chemotherapy has greatly increased the number of individuals qualifying for limb salvage surgery. Limb-salvaging procedures have been made possible by advances in reconstructive techniques and endoprosthetics. Limb salvage ultimately may be successful in as many as 80% of persons.

If an amputation is done, individuals are monitored closely with chest radiographs and CT. Pulmonary metastases are surgically resected, and chemotherapy is now a common therapy given both before and after surgery, using combinations of chemotherapeutic agents.

Other sarcomas include Ewing sarcoma (the third most common primary bone sarcoma) and synovial sarcoma, each of which has specific genetic alterations.[115] Others include rhabdomyosarcoma (a soft tissue sarcoma that likely originates in the skeleton but with features more like skeletal muscle) and sarcomas that have no definite morphologic pattern, such as leiomyosarcoma and pleomorphic liposarcoma.[116]

Chondrogenic tumors: chondrosarcoma. Chondrogenic (cartilage-forming) tumors produce cartilage or chondroid, a primitive cartilage or cartilage-like substance. The most common chondrogenic tumor is chondrosarcoma.

Chondrosarcoma is the second most common primary malignant bone tumor[117] and is a tumor of middle-aged and older adults. Incidence of chondrosarcoma peaks in the sixth decade of life.[113] Secondary chondrosarcoma (a chondrosarcoma derived from an endochondroma) occurs most often in young adults between 20 and 30 years of age. The tumor is more common in men than in women.

A chondrosarcoma is a large, ill-defined malignant tumor that infiltrates trabeculae in spongy bone. It occurs most often in the metaphysis or diaphysis of long bones, especially the femur, and in the bones of the pelvis. If located near the end of the bone, the tumor will infiltrate into the joint space. The tumor expands and enlarges the contour of the bone, causes extensive erosion of the cortex, and grows into the soft tissues.

Symptoms associated with a chondrosarcoma have an insidious onset. Local swelling and pain are the usual presenting symptoms. At first the pain is dull and intermittent, then gradually intensifies and becomes constant; it may awaken the person at night.

Diagnostic studies include radiographs, which must be reviewed carefully for an accurate diagnosis. MRI is useful in determining the extent of soft tissue involvement. Biopsy is done at the time of surgery. (If biopsy is conducted before scheduled surgical incision, seeding of tumor cells could occur.) Sufficient tumor material must be obtained to facilitate an accurate diagnosis.

Surgical excision is generally regarded as the treatment of choice because chemotherapy generally is ineffective.[113,117] Many surgically treated individuals demonstrate recurrences, however, so amputation is becoming one treatment of choice. Consequently, individuals with tumors located in the limbs may have a better prognosis than those with pelvic lesions.

Collagenic tumors: fibrosarcoma. Collagenic (collagen-forming) tumors originate from mesenchymal cells and produce fibrous connective tissue. Fibrosarcoma is the most common collagenic tumor and can affect bone or soft tissue.

Fibrosarcomas represent 4% of the primary malignant bone tumors, with a broad age distribution. They may occur at any age but are most common in adults between 30 and 50 years of age. The incidence is slightly greater in females.[118] Fibrosarcoma also may be a secondary complication of radiation therapy, Paget disease, and long-standing osteomyelitis.

Fibrosarcoma is a solitary tumor that most often affects the metaphyseal region of the femur or tibia. The tumor is composed of a firm, fibrous mass of tissue that contains collagen, malignant fibroblasts, and occasional osteoclast-like giant cells.

The tumor begins in the marrow cavity of the bone and infiltrates the trabeculae. It demonstrates a permeative growth pattern, destroys the cortex, and extends into the soft tissue. Metastasis to the lung is common.

Symptoms associated with the tumor have an insidious onset, which delays diagnosis. Pain and swelling are the usual presenting symptoms and usually indicate that the tumor has infiltrated the cortex. Local tenderness, a palpable mass, and limitation of motion also may be present. A pathologic fracture in the affected bone is often the reason for seeking medical help. Diagnostic studies include radiographs and MRI.

Radical surgery and amputation are the treatments of choice for fibrosarcoma. There is a high probability of metastases. Radiation therapy is generally considered ineffective treatment for this tumor. Promising investigations of third-generation bisphosphonates, such as zoledronic acid, and newer biologic agents may alter future treatment of fibrosarcoma.[119-121]

Myelogenic tumors. Myelogenic tumors originate from various bone marrow cells. Two types of myelogenic tumors are giant cell tumor and myeloma.

Giant cell tumor. Giant cell tumor is the sixth most common of the primary bone tumors, accounting for 4% to 5% of bone tumors. It is generally benign but can become malignant after radiation treatment. Giant cell tumors have a wide age distribution; however, they are rare in persons younger than 10 years or older than 70 years. Most giant cell tumors are found in persons between 20 and 40 years of age. Unlike most other bone tumors, giant cell tumors affect females more often than males.[122]

The giant cell tumor is a solitary, circumscribed tumor that causes extensive bone resorption because of its osteoclastic origin. The giant cell tumor is located in the center of the epiphysis in the femur, tibia, radius, or humerus. The tumor has a slow, relentless growth rate and is usually contained within the original contour of the affected bone. It may, however, extend into the articular cartilage. When the tumor extends, it is usually covered by periosteum or periosteal bone growth. The tumor also may extend into local soft tissue, but it has a low rate of metastasis to other organs or tissues, although it has a high recurrence rate.

The most common symptoms associated with the giant cell tumor are pain, local swelling, and limitation of movement. Diagnostic studies include radiographs, CT, and MRI. Cryosurgery and resection of the tumor with the use of adjuvant polymethylmethacrylate (PMMA) for bone grafts decrease recurrence and are more successful treatments than curettage and radiation. Depending on the extent of the tumor and its recurrence, amputation may be necessary.

Muscle Tumors

Rhabdomyoma

Rhabdomyoma is an extremely rare benign tumor of muscle that generally occurs in the tongue, neck muscles, larynx, uvula, nasal cavity, axilla, vulva, and heart. These tumors are usually treated by surgical excision and typically do not recur.

Rhabdomyosarcoma

The malignant tumor of striated muscle is called rhabdomyosarcoma. Infants, children, and teenagers account for more than 85% of cases. This tumor is highly malignant with rapid metastasis. Rhabdomyosarcomas are located in the muscle tissue of the head, neck, and genitourinary tract in 75% of cases, with the remainder found in the trunk and extremities.

Three types of rhabdomyosarcoma are differentiated on pathologic section: pleomorphic, embryonal, and alveolar. Each type differs from the other molecularly. Although rare, the pleomorphic, or spindle cell, type is considered to be one of the most highly malignant tumors of the extremities seen in adulthood. Embryonal tumors are most often seen in infancy and childhood and appear to be shaped like a tadpole or tennis racquet. Alveolar-type tumors appear lattice-like and look like lung tissue alveoli; they are typically more resistant to therapy and have a worse prognosis.[123]

The diagnosis of rhabdomyosarcoma is made by incisional biopsy and examination of the specimen by a pathologist. CT scan also helps define the tissue borders. Staging is based on the pathologic grade of the tumor and is helpful in determining prognosis and treatment.

Treatment consists of a combination of surgical excision, radiation therapy, and systemic chemotherapy. Cure is unlikely when distant metastases are present.[124]

Other Tumors

Metastatic tumors in muscles are rare in spite of the extensive vascular supply of skeletal muscles. It is suggested that local pH or metabolic changes within muscles prevent metastatic involvement from other tumors. When adjacent carcinomas do cause muscle damage, it is usually related to the compression of tissue and resultant muscle atrophy.

QUICK CHECK 37-5

1. From what cells do bone tumors originate?
2. Compare five major characteristics of benign bone tumors with those of malignant bone tumors.
3. How does the presence of metastatic tumors affect treatment options and prognosis of persons with osteosarcoma?

DID YOU UNDERSTAND?

Musculoskeletal Injuries

1. The most serious musculoskeletal injury is a fracture. A bone can be completely or incompletely fractured. A closed fracture leaves the skin intact. An open fracture has an overlying skin wound. The direction of the fracture line can be linear, oblique, spiral, or transverse. Greenstick, torus, and bowing fractures are examples of incomplete fractures that occur in children. Stress fractures occur in normal or abnormal bone that is subjected to repeated stress. Fatigue fractures occur in normal bone subjected to abnormal stress. Normal weight bearing can cause an insufficiency fracture in abnormal bone.
2. Dislocation is complete loss of contact between the surfaces of two bones. Subluxation is partial loss of contact between two bones. As a bone separates from a joint, it may damage adjacent nerves, blood vessels, ligaments, tendons, and muscle.
3. Tendon tears are called strains, and ligament tears are called sprains. A complete separation of a tendon or ligament from its attachment is called an avulsion.
4. Rhabdomyolysis, often manifested by the presence of myoglobinuria, can be a life-threatening complication of severe muscle trauma.

Disorders of Bones

1. Metabolic bone diseases are characterized by abnormal bone structure. In osteoporosis the density or mass of bone is reduced because the bone-remodeling cycle is disrupted. Osteomalacia is a metabolic bone disease characterized by inadequate bone mineralization. Excessive and abnormal bone remodeling occurs in Paget disease.

2. Osteomyelitis is a bone infection caused *most often* by bacteria. Bacteria can enter bone from outside the body (exogenous osteomyelitis) or from infection sites within the body (hematogenous osteomyelitis).

Disorders of Joints

1. Because of improved imaging technology, inflammation has been identified as an important feature of osteoarthritis.
2. Osteoarthritis (OA) is a common, age-related disorder of synovial joints. The primary defect in OA is loss of articular cartilage.
3. Rheumatoid arthritis is an inflammatory joint disease characterized by inflammatory destruction of the synovial membrane, articular cartilage, joint capsule, and surrounding ligaments and tendons. Rheumatoid nodules also may invade the skin, lung, and spleen and involve small and large arteries. Rheumatoid arthritis is a systemic disease that affects the heart, lungs, kidneys, and skin, as well as the joints.
4. Ankylosing spondylitis is a chronic, systemic autoimmune disease characterized by stiffening and fusion of the sacroiliac and spine joints.
5. Gout is a syndrome caused by defects in uric acid metabolism with high levels of uric acid in the blood and body fluids. Uric acid crystallizes in the connective tissue of a joint where it initiates inflammatory destruction of the joint.

Disorders of Skeletal Muscle

1. A pathologic contracture is permanent muscle shortening caused by muscle spasticity, as seen in central nervous system (CNS) injury or severe muscle weakness.

DID YOU UNDERSTAND?—cont'd

2. Stress-induced muscle tension is presumably caused by increased activity in the reticular activating system and gamma loop in the muscle fiber. The use of progressive relaxation training and biofeedback has been advocated to reduce muscle tension.

3. Fibromyalgia is a chronic musculoskeletal syndrome characterized by diffuse pain and tender points. Theories have proposed that the muscle is the end organ responsible for the pain and fatigue, although this has not been confirmed. Most cases of FM involve women, and the peak age is 30 to 50 years. Genetic factors are being increasingly recognized as agents in developing fibromyalgia.

4. Atrophy of muscle fibers and overall diminished size of the muscle are seen after prolonged inactivity. Isometric contractions and passive lengthening exercises decrease atrophy to some degree in immobilized persons.

5. Hyperexcitable membranes cause the physical and electrical phenomenon of myotonia. The disorder is treated with drugs that reduce muscle fiber excitability. The biochemical defect is possibly related to changes in the muscle membrane and sarcoplasmic reticulum.

6. Metabolic muscle diseases are caused by endocrine disorders, glycogen storage diseases, enzyme deficiencies, and abnormal lipid function. The muscle depends on a complex system of carbohydrates and fats converted by enzymes to produce energy for the muscle cell. Abnormalities in these pathways can inhibit function or cause damage to the muscle fiber. These illnesses are rare, yet they account for significant functional abnormalities.

7. Viral, bacterial, and parasitic infections of muscles produce the characteristic clinical and pathologic changes associated with inflammation. These are usually treatable and self-limiting disorders.

8. Polymyositis (generalized muscle inflammation) and dermatomyositis (polymyositis accompanied by skin rash) are characterized by inflammation of connective tissue and muscle fibers and muscle fiber necrosis. Cell-mediated and humoral immune factors have been implicated. Treatment with immunosuppressive agents is effective in many cases.

9. The most common cause of toxic myopathy is alcohol abuse. It has been suggested that alcohol use affects muscle fibers both directly (by causing necrosis) and indirectly (by the concomitant nutritional deficiencies typically associated with excessive use of alcohol). Drug administration can also lead to toxic myopathy; muscle fibers can be mechanically damaged by a needle used during an injection, by secondary infection, and by alterations in the acidity and alkalinity of muscle fibers.

Musculoskeletal Tumors

1. Sarcomas of muscle tissue are rare. Rhabdomyosarcoma has a uniformly poor prognosis because of an aggressive invasion and early, widespread dissemination. The usual treatment includes surgical excision, radiation therapy, and systemic chemotherapy.

2. Bone tumors originate from bone cells, cartilage cells, fibrous tissue cells, or vascular marrow cells. Each cell produces a specific type of ground substance that is used to classify the tumor as osteogenic (bone cell), chondrogenic (cartilage cell), collagenic (fibrous tissue cell), or myelogenic (vascular marrow cell). Malignant bone tumors are usually large, aggressively destroy surrounding bone, invade surrounding tissue, and initiate independent growth outside the site of origin. Benign bone tumors are generally less destructive, limit their growth to the anatomic confines of the bone, and have a well-demarcated border. Certain benign tumors can become malignant.

KEY TERMS

- Acid maltase deficiency   1011
- Acute gouty arthritis   1007
- Age-related bone loss   991
- Ankylosing spondylitis (AS)   1002
- Asymptomatic hyperuricemia   1007
- Avulsion   982
- Biofeedback   1008
- Bone tumor   1013
- Bowing fracture   979
- Bursa (pl., bursae)   983
- Caplan syndrome   1002
- Central sensitization   1008
- Chondrogenic (cartilage-forming) tumor   1016
- Chondrosarcoma   1016
- Closed (simple) fracture   979
- Collagenic (collagen-forming) tumor   1016
- Comminuted fracture   979
- Compartment syndrome   986
- Complete fracture   979
- Contracture   1007
- Degenerative joint disease (osteoarthritis)   996
- Delayed union   981
- Direct (primary) healing   980
- Dislocation   981
- Disuse atrophy   1008
- Dual x-ray absorptiometry (DXA)   992
- Endochondral bone formation   980
- Endochondroma   1016
- Endogenous osteomyelitis   995
- Enthesis   1002
- Epicondyle   982
- Epicondylopathy   982
- Exogenous osteomyelitis   995
- External fixation   981
- Fatigue fracture   980
- Fibromyalgia (FM)   1008
- Fibrosarcoma   1016
- Fracture   978
- Giant cell tumor   1016
- Glucocorticoid-induced osteoporosis   991
- Glycogen storage disease (GSD)   1010
- Gout   1005
- Gouty arthritis   1005
- Greenstick fracture   979
- Hematogenous osteomyelitis   995
- Heterotopic ossification (Ho)   984
- Hyperbaric oxygen therapy   996
- Immobilization (of a fracture)   981
- Incomplete fracture   979
- Indirect (secondary) healing   980
- Inflammatory joint disease (arthritis)   999
- Insufficiency fracture (fragility fracture)   980
- Internal fixation   981
- Involucrum   995
- Joint effusion   998
- Joint stiffness   998
- Kyphosis   991
- Lateral epicondylopathy (tennis elbow)   982
- Ligament   982
- Linear fracture   979
- Malignant hyperthermia (MH)   986
- Malunion   981
- McArdle disease   1010
- Medial epicondylopathy (golfer's elbow)   982
- Muscle strain   983
- Myelogenic tumor   1016
- Myoadenylate deaminase deficiency (MDD)   1011
- Myoglobinuria   984
- Myositis   1011
- Myositis ossificans (heterotopic ossification, HO)   984
- Myotonia   1010
- Noninflammatory joint disease   996
- Nonunion   981
- Oblique fracture   979
- Open (compound) fracture   979
- Osteoarthritis (OA)   996
- Osteogenic (bone-forming) tumor   1015

KEY TERMS—cont'd

REFERENCES

1. Office of Statistics and Programming, National Center for Injury Prevention and Control, CDC: 10 leading causes of nonfatal injury, United States 2009. Available at www.cdc.gov/injury/nonfatal.html. Accessed Jan 15, 2011.
2. Shumway-Cook A, et al: Incidence of and risk factors for falls following hip fractures in community-dwelling older adults, *Phys Ther* 85(7): 648–655, 2005.
3. Secreto FJ, Hoeppner LH, Westendorf JJ: Wnt signaling during fracture repair, *Curr Osteoporos Rep* 7(2):64–69, 2009.
4. Hubbard TJ, Hicks-Little CA: Ankle ligament healing after an acute ankle sprain: an evidence-based approach, *J Athl Train* 43(5):523–529, 2008.
5. Rabago D, et al: A systematic review of four injection therapies for lateral epicondylosis: prolotherapy, polidocanol, whole blood and platelet-rich plasma, *Br J Sports Med* 43:471–481, 2009.
6. Rineer CA, Ruch DS: Elbow tendinopathy: epicondylopathy and tendon ruptures: epicondylitis, biceps and triceps ruptures, *J Hand Surg Am* 34(3):566–576, 2009.
7. Flatt AE: Tennis elbow, *Proc (Bayl Univ Med Cent)* 21(4):400–402, 2008.
8. Knobloch K: The role of tendon microcirculation in Achilles and patellar tendinopathy, *J Orthop Surg Res* 3:18, 2008.
9. Baird EO, Kang QK: Prophylaxis of heterotopic ossification—an updated review, *J Orthop Surg Res* 4:12, 2009.
10. Cervellin G, Comelli I, Lippi G: Rhabdomyolysis: historical background, clinical, diagnostic, and therapeutic features, *Coin Chem Lab Med* 48(6):749–756, 2010.
11. Su B-H, et al: Ultrasonic appearance of rhabdomyolysis in patients with crush injury in the Wenchuan earthquake, *Chin Med J* 122(16):1872–1876, 2009.
12. McDonald S, Bearcroft P: Compartment syndromes, *Semin Musculoskelet Radiol* 14(2):236–244, 2010.
13. Shadgan B, et al: Current thinking about acute compartment syndrome of the lower extremity, *Can J Surg* 53(5):329–334, 2010.
14. Parness J, Bandschapp O, Girard T: The myotonias and susceptibility to malignant hyperthermia, *Anesth Analg* 109(4):1054–1064, 2009.
15. Protasi F, Paolini C, Dainese M: Calsequestrin-1: a new candidate gene for malignant hyperthermia and exertional/environmental heat stroke, *J Physiol* 587(13):3095–3100, 2009.
16. Benca J, Hogan K: Malignant hyperthermia, coexisting disorders, and enzymopathies: risks and management options, *Anesth Analg* 109(4):1049–1053, 2009.
17. Carpenter D, et al: The role of CACNA1S in predisposition to malignant hyperthermia, *BMC Med Genet* 13(10):104, 2009.
18. Larach MG, et al: Clinical presentation, treatment, and complications of malignant hyperthermia in North America from 1987 to 2006, *Anesth Analg* 110(2):498–507, 2009.

19. Warriner AH, et al: Which fractures are most attributable to osteoporosis? *J Clin Epidemiol* 64(1):46–53, 2011.
20. World Health Organization (WHO) Scientific Group on the Prevention and Management of Osteoporosis: *WHO technical report series; 921*, Geneva, Switzerland, 2000, Author.
21. U.S. Preventive Services Task Force: Screening for osteoporosis: U.S. Preventive Services Task Force recommendation statement, *Ann Intern Med*, Jan 18, 2011. Accessed Jan 19, 2011. [Epub ahead of print.].
22. Honig S: Osteoporosis—new treatments and updates, *Bull NYU Hosp Jt Dis* 68(3):166–170, 2010.
23. U.S. Department of Health and Human Services (USDHHS): *Bone health and osteoporosis: a report of the surgeon general*, Rockville, Md, 2004, Author.
24. Adachi JD, et al: Impact of prevalent fractures on quality of life: baseline results from the global longitudinal study of osteoporosis in women, *Mayo Clin Proc* 5(9):806–813, 2010.
25. Vestergaard V, et al: Loss of life years after a hip fracture, *Acta Ortho* 80(5):525–530, 2009.
26. Geusens P, Sambrook P, Lems W: Fracture prevention in men, *Nat Rev Rheumatol* 5(9):497–504, 2009.
27. Schousbe JT, et al: Vertebral fracture assessment: the 2007 ISCD official positions, *J Clin Densitom* 11(1):92–108, 2008.
28. NIH Osteoporosis and Related Bone Diseases National Resource Center: Osteoporosis and African American women, June 2010. Available at www.niams.nih.gov/Health_Info/Bone/Osteoporosis/Background/default.asp. Accessed Jan 20, 2011.
29. Curtis JR, et al: Population-based fracture risk assessment and osteoporosis treatment disparities by race and gender, *J Gen Intern Med* 24(8):856–962, 2009.
30. Krum SA, Brown M: Unraveling estrogen action in osteoporosis, *Cell Cycle* 15(7):1348–1352, 2008.
31. Brown M: Skeletal muscle and bone: effect of sex steroids and aging, *Adv Physiol Educ* 32(2):120–126, 2008.
32. van Geel TA, et al: Measures of bioavailable serum testosterone and estradiol and their relationships with muscle mass, muscle strength, and bone mineral density in postmenopausal women: a cross-sectional study, *Eur J Endocrinol* 160(4):681–687, 2009.
33. Vondracek SF, Hansen LB, McDermott MT: Osteoporosis risk in premenopausal women, *Pharmacotherapy* 29(3):305–317, 2009.
34. Bauman WA, et al: Effect of pamidronate administration on bone in patients with acute spinal cord injury, *J Rehab Res Develop* 42:305–314, 2005.
35. Rocchietti March M, et al: Transient osteoporosis of the hip, *Hip Int* 20(3):297–300, 2010.
36. Grey A, Dalbeth N, Doyle A: Clinical images: transient regional osteoporosis, *Arthritis Rheum* 60(10):3145, 2009.
37. Dore RK: How to prevent glucocorticoid-induced osteoporosis, *Clev Clin Med J* 77(8):529–536, 2010.

38. Perrini S, et al: The GH/IGF1 axis and signaling pathways in the muscle and bone: mechanism underlying age-related skeletal muscle wasting and osteoporosis, *J Endocrinol* 205(3):201–210, 2010.

39. Clapauch R, et al: Total estradiol, rather than testosterone levels predicts osteoporosis in aging men, *Arq Bras Endocrinol Metabol* 53(8):1020–1025, 2009.

40. Lapauw B: Anthropometric and skeletal phenotype in men with idiopathic osteoporosis and their sons is consistent with deficient estrogen action during maturation, *J Clin Endocrinol Metab* 94(11):4300–4308, 2009.

41. LeBlanc ES, et al: Osteoporotic fractures in men study group: the effects of serum testosterone, estradiol, and sex hormone binding globulin levels on fracture risk in older men, *J Clin Endocrinol Metab* 94(9):3337–3346, 2009.

42. Link YM: The founder's lecture 2009: advances in imaging of osteoporosis and osteoarthritis, *Skelet Radiol* 39:943–955, 2010.

43. Lane NE, Silverman SL: Anabolic therapies, *Curr Osteoporos Rep* 8:23–27, 2010.

44. Thacher TD, Clarke BL: Vitamin D deficiency, *Mayo Clin Proc* 86(1):50–60, 2011.

45. Unuvar T, Buyukgebiz A: Nutritional rickets and vitamin D deficiency in infants, children and adolescents, *Pediatr Endocrinol Rev* 7(3):283–291, 2011.

46. Bhan A, Rao AD, Rao DS: Osteomalacia as a result of vitamin D deficiency, *Endocrinol Metab Clin North Am* 39(2):321–331, 2010.

47. Kulak CA, Dempster DW: Bone histomorphometry: a concise review for endocrinologists and clinicians, *Arq Bras Endocrinol Metabol* 54(2):87–98, 2010.

48. Roodman GD: Insights into the pathogenesis of Paget's disease, *Ann N Y Acad Sci* 1192:176–180, 2010.

49. Visconti MR, et al: Mutations of SQSTM1 are associated with severity and clinical outcome in Paget disease of bone, *J Bone Miner Res* 25(11):2368–2373, 2010.

50. Brandi ML: Current treatment approaches for Paget's disease of bone, *Discov Med* 10(52):209–212, 2010.

51. McCarthy HS, Marshall MJ: Dickkopf-1 as a potential therapeutic target in Paget's disease of bone, *Expert Opin Ther Targets* 14(2):221–230, 2010.

52. Polyzos SA, et al: The effect of zoledronic acid on serum dickkopf-1, osteoprotegerin, and RANKL in patients with Paget's disease of the bone, *Horm Metab Res* 41(11):846–850, 2009.

53. Jorge LS, Chueire AG, Rossit AR: Osteomyelitis: a current challenge, *Braz J Infect Dis* 14(3):310–315, 2010.

54. Wright JA, Nair SP: Interaction of staphylococci with bone, *Int J Med Microbiol* 300(2–3):193–204, 2010.

55. Neut D, et al: A biodegradable antibiotic delivery system based on poly-(trimethylene carbonate) for the treatment of osteomyelitis, *Acta Orthop* 80(5):514–519, 2009.

56. Rasyid HN, et al: Concepts for increasing gentamicin release from handmade bone cement beads, *Acta Orthop* 80(5):508–513, 2009.

57. Evangelou E, et al: Meta-analysis of genome-wide association studies confirms a susceptibility locus for knee osteoarthritis on chromosome 7q22, *Ann Rheum Dis* 70(2):349–355, 2011.

58. Heinegård D, Saxne T: The role of cartilage matrix in osteoarthritis, *Nat Rev Rheumatol* 7(1):50–56, 2010.

59. Goldring MB, Marcu KB: Cartilage homeostasis in health and rheumatic diseases, *Arthritis Res Ther* 11(3):224, 2009.

60. Brennan SL, et al: Does an increase in body mass index over 10 years affect knee structure in a population-based cohort study of adult women? *Arthritis Res Ther* 12(4):R139, 2010.

61. Lotz MK: New developments in osteoarthritis: posttraumatic osteoarthritis: pathogenesis and pharmacological treatment options, *Arthritis Res Ther* 12(3):211, 2010.

62. Pallu S, et al: Obesity affects the chondrocyte responsiveness to leptin in patients with osteoarthritis, *Arthritis Res Ther* 12(3):R112, 2010.

63. Loeser RF: Aging and osteoarthritis: the role of chondrocyte senescence and aging changes in the cartilage matrix, *Osteoarthritis Cartilage* 17(8):971–979, 2009.

64. Kapoor M, et al: Role of proinflammatory cytokines in the pathophysiology of osteoarthritis, *Nat Rev Rheumatol* 7:33–42, 2011.

65. Tanamas S, et al: Does knee malalignment increase the risk of development and progression of knee osteoarthritis? A systematic review, *Arthritis Rheum* 61(4):459–466, 2009.

66. Black C, et al: The clinical effectiveness of glucosamine and chondroitin supplements in slowing or arresting progression of osteoarthritis of the knee: a systematic review and economic evaluation, *Health Technol Assess* 13(52):1–148, 2009.

67. Kubo M, et al: Chondroitin sulfate for the treatment of hip and knee osteoarthritis: current status and future trends, *Life Sci* 85(13–14):477–483, 2009.

68. Murphy LB, et al: One in four people may develop symptomatic hip osteoarthritis in his or her lifetime, *Osteoarthritis Cartilage* 18(11):1372–1379, 2010.

69. Kim S: Changes in surgical loads and economic burden of hip and knee replacements in the US: 1997–2004, *Arthritis Rheum* 59(4):481–488, 2008.

70. Aletaha D, et al: The 2010 American College of Rheumatology/European League Against Rheumatism classification criteria for rheumatoid arthritis: an American College of Rheumatology/European League Against Rheumatism collaborative initiative, *Arthritis Rheum* 62(9):2569–2581, 2010.

71. Gabriel SE, Michaud K: Epidemiological studies in incidence, prevalence, mortality, and comorbidity of the rheumatic diseases, *Arthrits Res Ther* 11(3):229, 2009.

72. Goronzy JJ, Weyand CM: Developments in the scientific understanding of rheumatoid arthritis, *Arthritis Res Ther* 11(5):249, 2009.

73. Liao KP, Alfredsson L, Karlson EW: Environmental influences on risk for rheumatoid arthritis, *Curr Opin Rheumatol* 21(3):279–283, 2009.

74. Oliver JE, Silman AJ: Why are women predisposed to autoimmune rheumatic diseases? *Arthritis Res Ther* 11(5):252, 2009.

75. Song YW, Kang EH: Autoantibodies in rheumatoid arthritis: rheumatoid factors and anticitrullinated protein antibodies, *Q J Med* 103(3):139–146, 2010.

76. Pruijn GJ, Wiik A, van Venrooij WJ: The use of citrullinated peptides and proteins for the diagnosis of rheumatoid arthritis, *Arthritis Res Ther* 12(1):203, 2010.

77. Colbert RA, et al: From HLA-B27 to spondyloarthritis: a journey through the ER, *Immunol Rev* 233(1):181–202, 2010.

78. Dong C: Genetic controls of Th17 cell differentiation and plasticity, *Exp Mol Med* 43(1):1–6, 2011.

79. Rozin AP, et al: Seronegative polyarthritis as severe systemic disease, *Neth J Med* 68(6):236–241, 2010.

80. Haroon N, Inman RD: Ankylosing spondylitis: new criteria, new treatments, *Bull NYU Hosp Jt Dis* 68(3):171–174, 2010.

81. Rudwaleit M, et al: The development of assessment of SpondyloArthritis International Society classification criteria for axial spondyloarthritis (part II): validation and final selection, *Ann Rheum Dis* 68(6):777–783, 2009.

82. Richette P, Bardin T: Gout, *Lancet* 375(9711):318–328, 2010.

83. VanItallie TB: Gout: epitome of painful arthritis, *Metabolism* 59(Suppl 1):S32–S36, 2010.

84. Doherty M: New insights into the epidemiology of gout, *Rheumatology (Oxford)* 48(Suppl 2), 2009. ii2–ii8.

85. Dirken-Heukensfeldt KJ, et al: Clinical features of women with gout arthritis: a systemic review, *Clin Rheumatol* 29(6):575–582, 2010.

86. Kanbara A, Hakoda M, Seyama I: Urine alkalization facilitates uric acid excretion, *Nutr J* 9:45, 2010.

87. Chen Y-W, et al: Transcriptional pathways associated with skeletal muscle disuse atrophy in humans, *Physiol Genomics* 31:510–520, 2007.

88. Rennie MJ, Phillips SM, Richter EA: Newton's force as countermeasure for disuse atrophy, *J Appl Physiol* 107:6–7, 2009.

89. Branco JC: State-of-the-art on fibromyalgia mechanism, *Acta Rheumatol Port* 35:10–15, 2010.

90. Solitar BM: Fibromyalgia: knowns, unknowns, and current treatment, *Bull NYU Hosp Jt Dis* 68(3):157–161, 2010.

91. Buskila D: Developments in the scientific and clinical understanding of fibromyalgia, *Arthritis Res Ther* 11(5):242, 2009.
92. Cook DB, et al: Functional imaging of pain in patients with primary fibromyalgia, *J Rheumatol* 31:364–378, 2004.
93. Harris RE, et al: Decreased central mu-opioid receptor availability in fibromyalgia, *J Neurosci* 27:10,000–10,006, 2007.
94. Nebel MB, Gracely RH: Neuroimaging of fibromyalgia, *Rheum Dis Clin North Am* 35(2):313–327, 2009.
95. Wolfe F, et al: The American College of Rheumatology preliminary diagnostic criteria for fibromyalgia and measurement of symptom severity, *Arthritis Care Res (Hoboken)* 62(5):600–610, 2010.
96. Platt D, Griggs R: Skeletal muscle channelopathies: new insights into the periodic paralyses and nondystrophic myotonias, *Curr Opin Neurol* 22(5):524–531, 2009.
97. Rolim AL, et al: Ion channelopathies in endocrinology: recent genetic findings and pathophysiological insights, *Arq Bras Endocrinol Metabol* 54(8):673–681, 2010.
98. Barahona MJ, et al: Thyrotoxic periodic paralysis: a case report and literature review, *Clin Med Res* 7(3):96–98, 2009.
99. Jurkat-Rott K, et al: Sodium channelopathies of skeletal muscle result from gain or loss of function, *Pflugers Arch Eur J Physiol* 460:239–248, 2010.
100. Das AM, Steuerwald U, Illsinger S: Inborn errors of energy metabolism associated with myopathies, *J Biomed Biotechnol* 340849, 2010. [Epub 2010 May 26.].
101. de Vries JM, et al: Fatigue in neuromuscular disorders: focus on Guillain-Barré syndrome and Pompe disease, *Cell Mol Life Sci* 67(5):701–713, 2010.
102. Bonnefont JP, et al: Long-term follow-up of bezafibrate treatment in patients with the myopathic form of carnitine palmitoyltransferase 2 deficiency, *Clin Pharmacol Ther* 88(1):101–108, 2010.
103. Dalakas MC: Inflammatory muscle diseases: a critical review on pathogenesis and therapies, *Curr Opin Pharmacol* 10(3):346–352, 2010.
104. Amato AA, Barohn RJ: Evaluation and treatment of inflammatory myopathies, *J Neurol Neurosurg Psychiatry* 80(10):1060–1068, 2009.
105. Dalakas MC: Immunotherapy of myositis: issues, concerns and future prospects, *Nat Rev Rheumatol* 6(3):129–137, 2010.
106. Askanas V, Engel WK, Nogalska A: Inclusion body myositis: a degenerative muscle disease associated with intra-muscle fiber multi-protein aggregates, proteasome inhibition, endoplasmic reticulum stress and decreased lysosomal degradation, *Brain Pathol* 19(3):493–506, 2009.
107. Weihl CC, Pestronk A: Sporadic inclusion body myositis: possible pathogenesis inferred from biomarkers, *Curr Opin Neurol* 23(5):482–488, 2010.
108. Amato AA, Barohn RJ: Inclusion body myositis: old and new concepts, *J Neurol Neurosurg Psychiatry* 80(11):1186–1193, 2009.
109. Prieto S, Grau JM: The geoepidemiology of autoimmune muscle disease, *Autoimmun Rev* 9(5):A330–A334, 2010.
110. Kuncl RW: Agents and mechanisms of toxic myopathy, *Curr Opin Neurol* 22(5):506–515, 2009.
111. Miralbello L, Troisi RJ, Savage SA: International osteosarcoma incidence patterns in children and adolescents, middle aged and elderly persons, *Int J Cancer* 125(1):229–234, 2009.
112. Lietman SA, Joyce MJ: Bone sarcomas: overview of management, with a focus on surgical treatment considerations, *Clev Clin J Med* 77(Suppl 1):S8–S12, 2010.
113. Wesolowski R, Budd GT: Use of chemotherapy for patients with bone and soft-tissue sarcomas, *Clev Clin J Med* 77(Suppl 1):S23–S26, 2010.
114. Bielack S, Carrie D, Casali PG: Osteosarcoma: ESMO clinical recommendations for diagnosis, treatment and follow-up, *Ann Oncol* 20(Suppl 4), 2009. iv137–iv139.
115. Maheshwari AV, Cheng EY: Ewing family of tumors, *J Am Acad Orthop Surg* 18(2):94–107, 2010.
116. Jain S, et al: Molecular classification of soft tissue sarcomas and its clinical applications, *Int J Clin Exp Pathol* 3(4):416–428, 2010.
117. Reidel RF, et al: The clinical management of chondrosarcoma, *Curr Treat Options Oncol* 10(1–2):94–106, 2009.
118. Casillas J, et al: Soft tissue sarcomas. In Bleyer A, et al: Cancer epidemiology in older adolescents and young adults 15 to 29 years of age, including SEER incidence and survival: 1975-2000, Bethesda, Md, 2006, National Cancer Institute, NIH Pub No 06–5767.
119. Adepoju LJ, Geiger JD: Antitumor activity of polyuridylic acid in human soft tissue and bone sarcomas, *J Surg Res* 164(1):E107–E114, 2010.
120. Dong M, et al: Impact of the Src inhibitor saracatinib on the metastatic phenotype of fibrosarcoma (KHT) tumor model, *Anticancer Res* 30(11):4405–4413, 2010.
121. Koto K, et al: Zoledronic acid inhibits proliferation of human fibrosarcoma cells with induction of apoptosis, and shows combined effects with other anticancer agents, *Oncol Rep* 24(1):233–239, 2010.
122. Reid R, Banjerjee SS, Sciot R, et al: Giant cell tumour. In Christopher DM, editor: World Health Organization classification of tumours International Agency for Research on Cancer (IARC) pathology and genetics of tumours of soft tissue and bone, Lyon, France, 2002, IARC Press, pp 303–312.
123. McDonald PC, Dedhar S, Keller C: Integrin-linked kinase: both Jekyll and Hyde in rhabdomyosarcoma, *J Clin Invest* 119(6):1452–1455, 2009.
124. Rodeberg DA, et al: Prognostic significance of tumor response at the end of therapy in group III rhabdomyosarcoma: a report from the children's oncology group, *J Clin Oncol* 27(22):3705–3711, 2009.

Alterations of Musculoskeletal Function in Children

Kristen Lee Carroll, Lynne M. Kerr, and Kathryn L. McCance

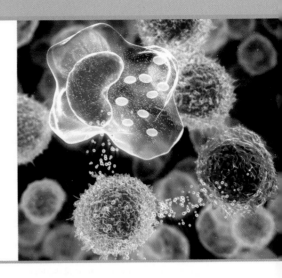

CHAPTER OUTLINE

Musculoskeletal problems in children can be either congenital or acquired. Both pathology and treatment can cause long-term sequelae because of the growing nature of the immature skeleton. In addition, the emotional trauma of an injured or malformed child is substantial and requires that careful attention be paid to the emotional health of both the child and his or her family.

CONGENITAL DEFECTS

Clubfoot

Clubfoot describes a range of foot deformities in which the foot turns inward and downward. It can affect one or both feet. Technically called congenital equinovarus (Table 38-1), the heel is positioned varus (inwardly deviated) and equinus (plantar flexed) (Figures 38-1 and 38-2). The clubfoot deformity can be positional (correctable passively), idiopathic, or teratologic (as a result of

another syndrome, such as spina bifida). The idiopathic clubfoot occurs in 1:1000 live births, with males twice as likely as females to be affected.

In the idiopathic clubfoot, manipulation and casting above the knee as described by Ponseti,[1] begun soon after birth and before the child starts walking, can correct the forefoot deformity in 70% to 90% of feet[2] (see Figure 38-1, *B*). The hindfoot equinus often requires lengthening of the Achilles tendon, which can be performed in a clinic with the use of a local anesthetic. Achilles tenotomy (complete transection of the tendon) can be safely performed with local anesthetic until 8 or 9 months after birth. After this age, a formal lengthening and repair procedure using a general anesthetic is required. Bracing is required until age 3. Idiopathic feet resistant to these procedures require a surgical posteromedial release (PMR). The posteromedial release includes lengthening of the Achilles, posterior tibialis, and flexor tendons, and surgical release of the capsules of the ankle, subtalar, and midfoot

TABLE 38-1	TERMS USED TO DESCRIBE FOOT ABNORMALITIES
TERM	**DEFINITION**
Position*	
Abduction	Lateral deviation away from the midline of the body
Adduction	Lateral deviation toward the midline of the body
Eversion	Twisting of the foot outward along its long axis
Inversion	Twisting of the foot inward on its long axis
Dorsiflexion	Bending of the foot upward and backward
Plantar flexion	Bending of the foot downward and forward
Abnormality	
Talipes	Congenital abnormality of the foot (clubfoot)
Pes	Acquired deformity of the foot
Varus	Inversion and adduction of the heel and forefoot
Valgus	Eversion and abduction of the heel and forefoot
Equinus	Plantar flexion of the foot in which the heel is lower than the toes
Calcaneus	Dorsiflexion of the foot in which the heel is lower than the toes
Planus	Flattening of the medial longitudinal arch of the foot (flatfoot)
Cavus	Elevation of the medial longitudinal arch of the foot (high arch)
Equinovarus	Coexistent equinus and varus deformities
Calcaneovarus	Coexistent calcaneus and varus deformities
Equinovalgus	Coexistent equinus and valgus deformities
Calcaneovalgus	Coexistent calcaneus and valgus deformities

*NOTE: The positions listed can all be achieved by voluntary movement of the normal foot; an abnormality exists if the foot is fixed in one or more of the positions while at rest.

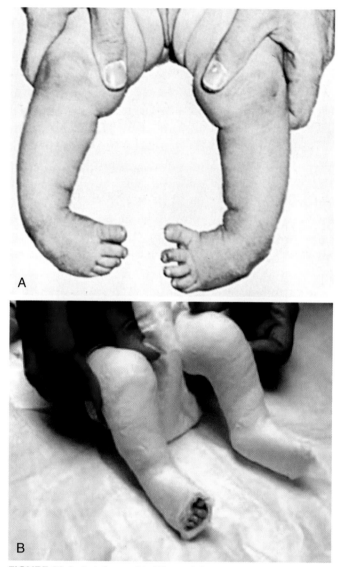

A

B

FIGURE 38-1 A, Infant with Bilateral Congenital Talipes Equinovarus. B, Ponseti Casting. (From Brashear HR, Raney RB: *Shand's handbook of orthopedic surgery*, ed 9, St Louis, 1978, Mosby.)

joints. Teratologic clubfeet are successfully treated by Ponseti casting (see Figure 38-1, *B*) and Achilles tenotomy only 60% of the time. Bracing is required, often through childhood. Secondary procedures are much more common in children with teratologic clubfeet than in those with idiopathic clubfeet.[3]

Developmental Dysplasia of the Hip

Developmental dysplasia of the hip (DDH) describes imperfect development of the hip joint and can affect the femur, the acetabulum, or both (Figure 38-3). Although most often present congenitally, dysplasia may develop later in the newborn or infant period. Like clubfoot, DDH can be idiopathic or teratologic. Teratologic hips (i.e., those attributable to another disorder such as cerebral palsy, spina bifida, or arthrogryposis) are more difficult to treat and often need operative intervention. In idiopathic DDH, 70% of cases involve the left side only, 10% to 15% are bilateral, and girls are four times as likely as boys to be affected. Positive family history, breech presentation, and oligohydramnios (low levels of intrauterine fluid) all predispose children to DDH. Children in these groups are considered high risk and must be carefully evaluated with physical examination and, possibly, ultrasound.[4] Variants of idiopathic DDH are dislocated hip (no contact between femoral head and acetabulum), subluxated hip (partial contact only), and acetabular dysplasia (the femoral head is located properly but the acetabulum is shallow). Idiopathic instability of the hip ranges from 3 to 7 per 1000 live births, but a true dislocation is present in only 1 of 1000 live births.

Clinical examination is the mainstay of diagnosis. The examination must be performed on a relaxed infant for accuracy. Absolute indications for treatment include a positive Barlow sign (hip reduced, but dislocatable) (Figure 38-4, *A*) or Ortolani sign (hip dislocated, but reducible) (Figure 38-4, *B*). Other indicators for further evaluation are limitation of abduction,[5] or apparent shortening of the femur (Galeazzi sign). Asymmetric skin folds at the groin crease also may be observed.

In children younger than 4 months old, bracing with a Pavlik harness is successful in 90% of DDH cases. A Barlow positive hip (hip reduced, but dislocatable) is easier to treat with a Pavlik harness, and success rates approach 95% to 98% (Figure 38-5). An Ortolani positive hip (hip dislocated, but reducible) must be followed closely with ultrasound and exam; the success rate with Pavlik harness is 70% in this situation. If a stable reduction is not attained within 2 to 3 weeks of treatment, the Pavlik harness should be abandoned. A partially reduced hip applies pressure on the rim of the acetabulum by the femoral head and can worsen dysplasia and make treatment more difficult. In older children, or those who failed bracing with a Pavlik harness, closed reduction of the hip and spica (body) casting under general anesthesia is required. The spica cast is worn for 3 months. Children older than 12 months require surgery on the joint, the femur, or the acetabulum, or all three (see Figure 38-3).

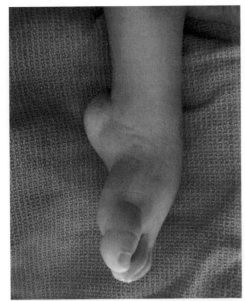

FIGURE 38-2 Idiopathic Clubfoot. Idiopathic clubfoot displaying forefoot adduction (toward midline of body) and supination (upturning) and hindfoot equinus (pointed downward). Note skin creases along arch and back of heel.

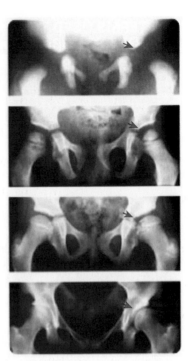

FIGURE 38-3 Hip Dysplasia in Children. Development dysplasia of the hip (DDH) with residual acetabular dysplasia. Radiographs at birth, 3, 10, and 19 years (top to bottom) show persisting dysplasia.

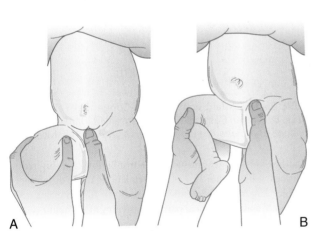

A   B

FIGURE 38-4 Congenital Dislocation of the Hip. A, Barlow maneuver *(left side).* With one hand pressing the symphysis in front and the sacral spine in back, lateral pressure is applied to the thigh with the thumb of the other hand while pressure is applied with the palm to the knee on the side being examined. The hip that has been flexed to 90 degrees is then adducted. A positive sign is a sensation of abnormal movement, indicating dislocation of the femoral head from the acetabulum. The hands are reversed for examining the other hip. This sign and Ortolani sign may be found only in the first weeks of life. **B,** Ortolani maneuver *(right side).* Sign of jerking into correct position. After Barlow maneuver **(A),** the hip should be abducted to about 80 degrees while the femur is lifted anteriorly with the fingers along the thigh. A positive sign is a sensation of a jerk or snap with reduction into the joint socket. (Adapted from Specht EE: Congenital dislocation of the hip, *Am Fam Physician* 9:88–96, 1974.)

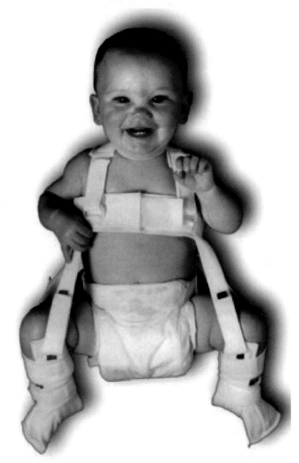

FIGURE 38-5 Pavlik Harness for Bilateral Hip Dislocation. (From Wheaton Brace Co.)

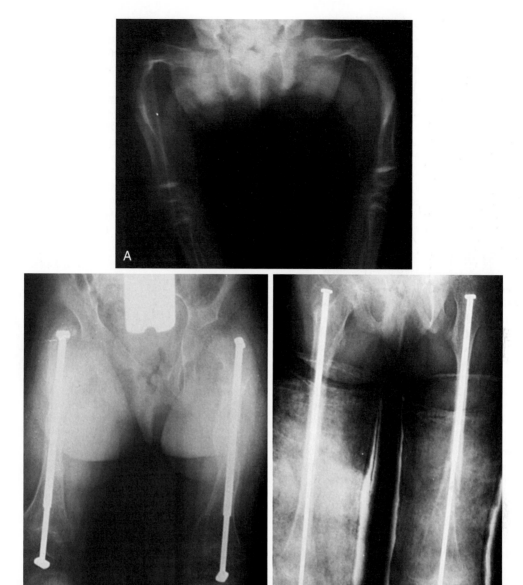

FIGURE 38-6 Osteogenesis Imperfecta Treated with Osteotomies and Telescoping Medullary Rods. **A,** Severe deformity of both femurs. **B,** Same individual after multiple osteotomies with telescoping medullary rod fixation. **C,** Same individual 4 years later demonstrating growth of femurs, no recurrence of deformity, and elongation of rods. (Plaster casts are in place for immobilization of tibial osteotomies.) (From Crenshaw AH, editor: *Campbell's operative orthopaedics,* ed 8, vol 3, St Louis, 1992, Mosby.)

The incidence of good or excellent outcome falls to only 20% by age 4, underscoring the need for early diagnosis and treatment.[6]

Osteogenesis Imperfecta

Osteogenesis imperfecta (OI; brittle bone disease) is a spectrum of disease caused by genetic mutation in the gene that encodes for type I collagen, the main component of bone and blood vessels. The Sillence classification defines four types. Types I and IV are milder forms and are inherited in an autosomal dominant pattern. Types II and III are more severe and are inherited in a recessive pattern. Children with type II often die during infancy because of extreme bone fragility.

The classic clinical manifestations of osteogenesis imperfecta (OI) are osteopenia (decreased bone mass) and an increased rate of fractures.

Children can also have fatigue, pain, hearing loss, and abnormal dentition. With recurrent fractures, bone deformity (bowing) often occurs. In type III OI, the most severe form compatible with life, children have short stature and triangular faces, possibly blue sclera, and poor dentition. Because type I collagen also is the main component of blood vessels, vascular deformity, such as aortic aneurysm, can occur. Type IV OI can be subtle with the child presenting with more normal stature and with fractures often not occurring until the child is older; it can be misdiagnosed as child abuse. Analysis of skin fibroblasts is diagnostic in 85% of children with OI.

Treatment is a combination of medical and surgical approaches (Figure 38-6). For fractures and deformity, intramedullary rodding of the long bones improves position and also splints new fractures.

Telescoping rods, which grow with the child, are improving in efficacy. Unfortunately, these children may have to undergo multiple surgeries and reroddings with growth. The medical treatment, classically involving calcium and vitamin D supplementation, is under intense study. Pamidronate and other bisphosphates, such as alendronate (Fosamax), which decrease bone resorption by inhibiting osteoclasts, are now frequently used. In a multicenter trial,[7] pamidronate was given at 2- to 4-month intervals to children with severe (type III) and mild (type IV) OI. In the 30 children in the study, bone mineral density increased by 41.9%, fractures decreased by 1.7% per year, and mobility increased in 51% of the children. All children claimed their fatigue and chronic bone pain improved.[8] Fracture healing remained unchanged. A large multicenter study is now trying to refine these treatments for all children with OI.

BONE INFECTION

Osteomyelitis

Osteomyelitis, or bone infection, is caused by either bacterial or granulomatous (i.e., tuberculosis) infective processes (Box 38-1, Figures 38-7 and 38-8). Antibiotic drugs and often surgical interventions are used to treat these infections. Morbidity and mortality resulting from osteomyelitis declined drastically until the 1980s. Unfortunately, with the escalation in the development of methicillin-resistant *Staphylococcus aureus* (MRSA) new confrontations have arisen that contribute to changes in morbidity and mortality, as described in the following paragraphs.

Acute hematogenous osteomyelitis is the most common form in children. The infection usually begins as an abscess in the metaphysis of a long bone where blood flow is sluggish and bacteria can collect. With increasing pressure, the infection will rupture out of the periosteum and spread along the diaphysis. A new shell of bone can develop under the elevated periosteum and can become an involucrum. The portion of bone that is separated from adequate blood supply by the infection can die, thereby leading to an involucrum. All three of these changes are apparent on radiograph and signify the need for surgical débridement as well as antibiotic treatment.

These radiographic bone changes take 2 to 3 weeks to develop. Initially, osteomyelitis presents as pain, swelling, and warmth. Children often will have fever, elevated white blood cell count (50% to 70%), elevated C-reactive protein (CRP) (98%) level, and elevated erythrocyte sedimentation rate (ESR) (90%). Blood culture is positive in only 40% of cases. Without changes on plain radiograph, bone scan can help define the location of infection and magnetic resonance imaging (MRI) can clarify the extent of the process. In infants, where osteomyelitis can be multifocal in up to 40% of cases, bone scan identifies other locations of infection that may need surgical intervention.

Treatment of osteomyelitis consists of appropriate antibiotic management for 6 weeks. If blood cultures are negative, bone aspirate must be analyzed to determine the bacterial source of the infection. With MRSA or bone changes on MRI, surgical débridement is required. MRSA often leads to more systemic illness, such as organ failure and infected thrombotic events.[9]

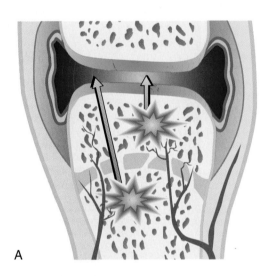

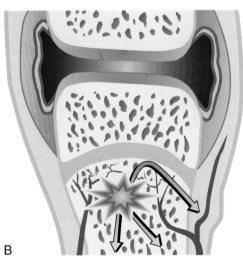

FIGURE 38-7 Pathogenesis of Acute Osteomyelitis Differs With Age. **A,** In infants younger than 1 year the epiphysis is nourished by arteries penetrating through the physis, allowing development of the condition within the epiphysis. **B,** In children up to 15 years of age, the infection is restricted to below the physis because of interruption of the vessels.

BOX 38-1	CAUSATIVE MICROORGANISMS OF OSTEOMYELITIS ACCORDING TO AGE

Newborns
Methicillin-resistant *Staphylococcus aureus* (MRSA)
Group B streptococcus
Gram-negative enteric rods

Infants
Methicillin-resistant *Staphylococcus aureus* (MRSA)
Haemophilus influenzae (decreasingly less common secondary to immunization)

Older Children
Staphylococcus aureus
Pseudomonas
Salmonella
Neisseria gonorrhoeae

Adolescents and Adults
Pseudomonas
Mycobacterium tuberculosis

Septic Arthritis

Septic arthritis is a bacterial or granulomatous infection of the joint space. This is always a surgical emergency. The bacteria, and the lysosomes created by white blood cells fighting the bacteria, can quickly destroy the articular cartilage of the joint and affect the blood supply to the epiphyseal bone nearby. Both of these complications have poor outcomes and can lead to a lifetime of disability.

Septic arthritis can occur primarily or secondary to osteomyelitis that spreads from the metaphysis of the bone into the joint space. The metaphyses of the pediatric hip, shoulder, proximal radius, and distal lateral tibia are all located within the joint capsule, and therefore osteomyelitis in these regions must be carefully monitored for secondary septic arthritis. The most common sites for septic arthritis are knees, hips, ankles, and elbows.

Children with septic arthritis present with severe joint pain, "pseudoparalysis" or marked guarding to motion of the joint, inability to bear weight, and malaise, often with anorexia. Children appear quite ill with this diagnosis. Nonpyogenic arthritis, such as juvenile idiopathic arthritis, can be difficult to distinguish clinically from septic arthritis because both can lead to malaise and elevated ESR. An elevation in CRP, fever, and complete inability to bear weight are more common with septic arthritis. Blood cultures are positive in 30% to 40% of cases. Joint aspirate positive for pus defines the diagnosis and determines bacterial etiology. As in osteomyelitis, *Staphylococcus aureus* is the most common bacteria; however, MRSA is now present in up to 30% of affected children.[9]

After surgical débridement of the joint, antibiotics are required for 2 to 3 weeks. Long-term follow-up to assess articular or physeal damage is required.

JUVENILE IDIOPATHIC ARTHRITIS

Juvenile idiopathic arthritis (JIA) is the childhood form of rheumatoid arthritis (see Chapter 37) and accounts for 5% of all cases of rheumatoid arthritis. Juvenile idiopathic arthritis has three distinct modes of onset: **oligoarthritis** (fewer than three joints), **polyarthritis** (more than three joints), and **Still disease** (severe systemic onset) (Table 38-2). JIA differs from rheumatoid arthritis in several ways:
1. Large joints are most commonly affected.
2. Chronic uveitis (inflammation of the anterior chamber of the eye) is common if the blood test for antinuclear antibody (ANA) is positive; slit lamp examination by a trained ophthalmologist is required every 6 months to avoid vision loss.

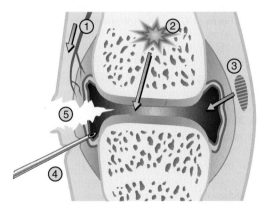

FIGURE 38-8 Routes of Infection to the Joint. *1,* Hematogenous route. *2,* Dissemination from osteomyelitis. *3,* Spread from an adjacent soft tissue infection. *4,* Diagnostic or therapeutic measures. *5,* Penetrating damage by puncture or cutting.

3. Serum tests may be negative for rheumatoid factor (RF); RF-positive children have a worse prognosis.
4. Subluxation and ankylosis may occur in the cervical spine if disease progresses.
5. Rheumatoid arthritis that continues through adolescence can have severe effects on growth and adult morbidity.

Many children with oligoarthritis who are "seronegative" (blood tests negative for RF or ANA) will resolve their symptoms over time. Systemic onset, or "seropositivity," of the disease is more likely consistent with lifelong arthritis. Therefore, treatment is supportive, not curative. Nonsteroidal anti-inflammatory drugs are a mainstay of treatment, and methotrexate is also being used with success. The goals are to minimize inflammation and deformity.

✔ **QUICK CHECK 38-1**
1. Why is an early diagnosis of developmental dysplasia of the hip imperative?
2. How does osteomyelitis develop?
3. How does juvenile idiopathic arthritis differ from the adult form?
4. How has MRSA changed musculoskeletal infections in children?

OSTEOCHONDROSES

The **osteochondroses** are a series of childhood diseases involving areas of significant tensile or compressive stress (i.e., tibial tubercle, Achilles insertion, hip). The pathophysiology is partial loss of blood supply, death of bone (osseous necrosis), progressive bony weakness, and then microfracture. The cause of the decreased blood supply is controversial; trauma, a change in clotting sensitivity, vascular injury, genetic predisposition, or a combination of these factors is presently considered most likely. Additionally, during the years of rapid bone growth, blood supply to the growing ends of bones (epiphyses) may become insufficient, resulting in necrotic bone, usually near joints. Because bone is normally undergoing a continuous rebuilding process, the necrotic areas can self-repair over a period of weeks or months.

Use of anti-inflammatories, modification of activities, immobilization, and rest are recommended during active disease. Reparative correction by revascularization is the rule, although years may be required for full healing, and deformity from compression during the period of osseous necrosis can persist.

Legg-Calvé-Perthes Disease

Legg-Calvé-Perthes (LCP) disease is a common osteochondrosis usually occurring in children between the ages of 3 and 10 years, with a peak incidence at 6 years. The disorder is bilateral in 10% to 20% of children, and boys are affected five times more often than girls. Boys have a more poorly developed blood supply to the femoral head than do girls of the same age, and this is thought to be the reason for male predilection. The role of genetics is unclear, but LCP is more common in northern European and Japanese children and rare in black children; family history is positive in 20% of cases. This self-limited disease of the hip, which runs its natural course in 2 to 5 years, is presumably created by recurrent interruption of the blood supply to the femoral head. The ossification center first becomes necrotic (osteonecrosis) and then is gradually replaced by live bone.

PATHOPHYSIOLOGY Several causative theories have been proposed, including a generalized disorder of epiphyseal cartilage growth, thyroid hormone deficiency, trauma, infection, and blood clotting disorders. However, a Harvard study did not show increases in thrombotic

	SYSTEMIC ONSET	PAUCIARTICULAR (TWO OR THREE SUBTYPES)	POLYARTICULAR (TWO SUBTYPES)
TABLE 38-2		**CHARACTERISTICS OF JUVENILE IDIOPATHIC ARTHRITIS RELATED TO MODE OF ONSET**	
Percentage of patients	30	45	25
Age at onset	Bimodal distribution 1-3 yr of age 8-10 yr of age	Type I: younger than 10 yr Type II: older than 10 yr	Throughout childhood and adolescence
Gender ratio (female/male)	1.5:1	Type I: almost all female Type II: 1:9	Mostly female
Joints involved	Any Only 20% have joint involvement at time of diagnosis	Usually confined to lower extremities—knee, ankle, and eventually sacroiliac; sometimes elbow	Any joint; usually symmetric involvement of small joints Hip involvement in 50% Spine involvement in 50%
Extra-articular manifestations	Fever, malaise, myalgia, rash, pleuritis or pericarditis, adenomegaly, splenomegaly, hepatomegaly Systemic signs minimal	Type I: chronic iridocyclitis; mucocutaneous lesions Type II: acute iridocyclitis; sacroiliitis common; eventual ankylosing spondylitis in many	Possible low-grade fever, malaise, weight loss, rheumatoid nodules, or vasculitis
Laboratory test results	Elevated ESR, CRP levels; RF negative; ANA rarely positive; anemia; leukocytosis	Elevated ESR, CRP levels; ANA positive Type I: HLA-DRW5 positive Type II: HLA-B27 positive Type III: HLA-TMo positive	Elevated ESR, CRP levels Type I: RF positive Type II: RF negative
Long-term prognosis	Mortality: 1-2% of all JIA patients Joint destruction in 40%	Continuous disease; eventual remission in 60% Type I: ocular damage; functional blindness in 10% Type II: ankylosing spondylitis Type III: best outlook for recovery	Longer duration; more crippling; remission in 25% Type I: high incidence of crippling arthritis Type II: outlook good

From Hockenberry MJ, Wilson D: *Wong's nursing care of infants and children,* ed 8, St Louis, 2007, Mosby.
ANA, Antinuclear antibody; *CRP,* C-reactive protein; *ESR,* erythrocyte sedimentation rate; *HLA,* human leukocyte antigen; *JIA,* juvenile idiopathic arthritis; *RF,* rheumatoid factor.

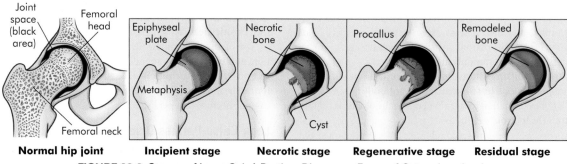

FIGURE 38-9 Stages of Legg-Calvé-Perthes Disease, a Form of Osteochondrosis.

disorders in consecutive children with LCP.[10] Boys with a hypercoagulable state are three times more likely to acquire LCP than girls with the same disorder.[11] Another study has shown the risk of LCP is five times greater in children exposed to passive smoke as opposed to children living in a smoke-free environment.[12]

In the first stage of LCP, the soft tissues of the hip (synovial membrane and joint capsule) are swollen, edematous, and hyperemic, often with fluid present in the joint (Figure 38-9). In the second necrotic stage, the anterior 50% or more of the epiphysis of the femoral head dies because of a lack of blood supply, and the metaphyseal bone at the junction of the femoral neck and capital epiphyseal plate is softened because of increased blood supply and decalcification. Granulation tissue (procallus) and blood vessels then invade the dead bone. The third, or regenerative healing, stage ordinarily lasts 2 to 4 years. The dead bone

in the femoral head is replaced by procallus, and new bone is established (see Figure 38-9). In the fourth, or residual, stage, remodeling takes place and the newly formed bone is organized into a live spongy bone.

CLINICAL MANIFESTATIONS Injury or trauma precedes the onset of LCP in approximately 30% to 50% of children with Legg-Calvé-Perthes disease. For several months the child complains of a limp and pain that can be referred to the knee, inner thigh, and the groin, following the path of the obturator nerve. The pain is usually aggravated by activity and relieved by rest and administration of anti-inflammatories.

The typical physical findings include spasm on rotation of the hip, limitation of internal rotation and abduction, and hip flexion–adduction deformity. If the child is walking, an early abnormal gait termed an antalgic (painful) abductor lurch, or a "Trendelenburg gait" (gluteus

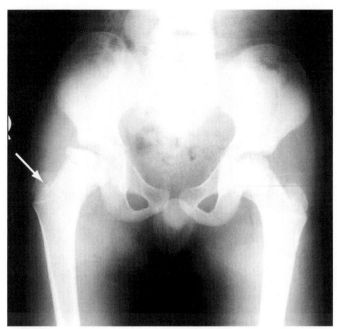

FIGURE 38-10 Pelvis of a 7-Year-Old Boy with Legg-Calvé-Perthes Disease. The femoral head is flat and extruded from the edge of the joint. This hip is at risk for early arthritis if left to revascularize and heal in this position.

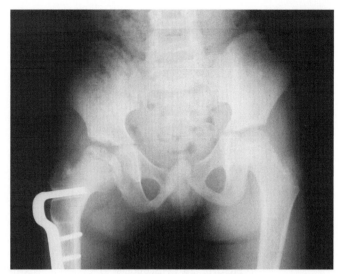

FIGURE 38-11 Surgical Replacement of Femoral Head of a 7-Year-Old Boy with Legg-Calvé-Perthes Disease. As the Perthes heals, the ball has assumed a round shape that matches the socket well.

medius gait pattern), is apparent. If the hip pain or limp has been present for a prolonged period, muscles of the hip and thigh atrophy.

EVALUATION AND TREATMENT The goals of treatment are to preserve normal congruity of the femoral head and acetabulum and maintain spasm-free and pain-free range of motion in the hip joint. Currently, most children can be managed with anti-inflammatory medications and activity modification during periods of synovitis. Serial radiographs are obtained to monitor the progress of the disease and to ensure that the femoral head remains congruent in the acetabulum. Surgery may be necessary if the femoral head becomes subluxated or incongruent with the acetabulum (Figures 38-10 and 38-11).[13-15] Children older than age 6 (by bone age) have a worse prognosis attributable to poorer remodeling potential. Older children require surgery more often to avoid poor congruence of the hip. Poor congruence predisposes to early osteoarthritis, with nearly 50% requiring hip replacement surgery by age 40.

Osgood-Schlatter Disease

Osgood-Schlatter disease consists of osteochondrosis of the tibia tubercle and associated patellar tendonitis. Osgood-Schlatter disease occurs most often in preadolescents and adolescents who participate in sports and is more prevalent in boys than in girls. Osgood-Schlatter disease is one of the most common ailments reported in the 30 million children who are involved in sports.[16]

The severity of the lesion varies from mild tendonitis to a complete separation of the anterior tibial apophysis, a part of the tibial tubercle. The mildest form of Osgood-Schlatter disease causes ischemic (avascular) necrosis in the region of the bony tibial tubercle, with hypertrophic cartilage formation during the stages of repair. In more severe cases, the abnormality involves a true apophyseal separation of the tibial tubercle with avascular necrosis.

The child complains of pain and swelling in the region around the patellar tendon and tibial tubercle, which becomes prominent and is tender to direct pressure. The pain is most severe after physical activity that involves vigorous quadriceps contraction (jumping or running) or direct local trauma to the tibial tubercle area.

The goal of treatment for Osgood-Schlatter disease is to decrease the stress at the tubercle. Often a period of 4 to 8 weeks of restriction from strenuous physical activity is sufficient. Bracing with a tubercle band can be very helpful. If the pain is not relieved, a cast or knee immobilizer is required, a situation that is particularly difficult if the condition is bilateral.

Gradual resumption of activity is permitted after 8 weeks, but return to unrestricted athletic participation requires an additional 8 weeks to allow for revascularization, healing, and ossification of the tibial tubercle.[13,17] With skeletal maturity and closure of the apophysis, Osgood-Schlatter disease resolves.

SCOLIOSIS

Scoliosis is a rotational curvature of the spine most obvious in the anteroposterior plane (Figure 38-12). It can be classified as nonstructural or structural. Nonstructural scoliosis results from a cause other than the spine itself, such as posture, leg length discrepancy, or splinting from pain. Structural scoliosis is a curvature of the spine associated with vertebral rotation. Nonstructural scoliosis can become structural if the underlying cause is not found and treated.

There are three main types of structural scoliosis: idiopathic; congenital (attributable to bony deformity such as hemivertebrae); and teratologic (caused by another systemic syndrome such as cerebral palsy). Eighty percent of all scoliosis is idiopathic, which may have a genetic component. Although girls and boys are equally affected, once the curve becomes more than 20 degrees, girls are five times more likely to be affected. Ninety-eight percent of curves are apex right thoracic. If a left thoracic curve appears in the adolescent with idiopathic scoliosis, MRI is performed to rule out a neurologic etiology. MRI also should be performed in children with kyphoscoliosis (round back) or loss of abdominal reflexes as well as in children who have exertional headaches or a congenital curve.[18]

Idiopathic curves progress while a child is growing, and progression can be very rapid during growth spurts. When idiopathic curves progress to 25 degrees or greater, and the child is skeletally

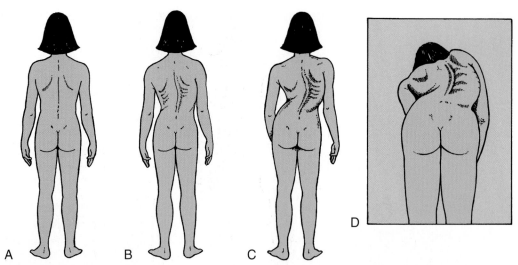

FIGURE 38-12 Scoliosis in Children. Normal spine alignment and abnormal spinal curvatures associated with scoliosis. **A,** Normal. **B,** Mild. **C,** Severe. **D,** Rotation and curvature of scoliosis.

immature, bracing is required. The total number of hours a brace is worn correlates to efficacy of treatment; 82% of children who wore the brace as prescribed had minimal progression.[19] Curves of more than 50 degrees will progress after skeletal maturity, so spinal fusion is required to stop progression. Bracing is the only nonoperative measure known to slow scoliotic progression. Chiropractic manipulation, physical therapy, exercise, and diet regimens have not been shown to alter natural history. Bracing is less successful in teratologic or congenital curves; therefore, these conditions may require surgical intervention more often.

MUSCULAR DYSTROPHY

The muscular dystrophies are a group of inherited disorders that cause progressive muscle fiber loss leading to weakness, mostly of the voluntary muscles. Some dystrophies cause disease in infancy, others in childhood, and others not until adulthood. Muscular dystrophies have different inheritance patterns and different biochemical alterations that cause each specific type. Three are discussed in detail in this chapter. Individuals with Duchenne muscular dystrophy (DMD) have a mutation in a specific gene that leads to alterations in the muscle protein dystrophin. Individuals with facioscapulohumeral (FSH) muscular dystrophy have a genetic defect unassociated with a particular gene that causes the muscle disease. Individuals with myotonic muscular dystrophy (MMD) have a genetic alteration that leads to systemic disease. Although there is no cure for any of the muscular dystrophies, aggressive preventive management has increased the life expectancy and quality of life of children with these disorders. Common forms of muscular dystrophy are described in Table 38-3.

Duchenne Muscular Dystrophy

PATHOPHYSIOLOGY Duchenne muscular dystrophy (DMD) is X-linked, generally occurring in boys, and is present in about 1 in 3500 male births. It is the most common childhood dystrophy. DMD is caused by mutations in the dystrophin gene, which lead to alterations or deletions of the muscle protein dystrophin

The protein dystrophin mediates anchorage of the actin cytoskeleton of skeletal muscle fibers to the basement membrane through a

TABLE 38-3   MAJOR MUSCULAR DYSTROPHY SYNDROMES

DISEASE	MODE OF INHERITANCE	AGE AT CLINICAL ONSET	DISTRIBUTION OF WEAKNESS
Duchenne muscular dystrophy/ Becker muscular dystrophy (DMD/ BMD)	X-linked, sporadic	2-3 years/ 5-7 years	Proximal with pseudohyper-trophy
Facioscapulo-humeral (FSH) muscular dystrophy	Autosomal dominant	Early adolescence	Face, arms, legs
Myotonic muscular dystrophy (MMD)	Autosomal dominant	Variable—birth to adulthood	Distal muscles, face

From Moxley RT 3rd et al: Practice parameter: corticosteroid treatment of Duchenne dystrophy: report of the Quality Standards Subcommittee of the American Academy of Neurology and the Practice Committee of the Child Neurology Society, *Neurology* 64(1):13–20, 2005.

membrane-glycoprotein complex. With lack of dystrophin, the poorly anchored fibers tear themselves apart under the repeated stress of contraction. Free calcium then enters the muscle cells, causing cell death and fiber necrosis (Figure 38-13).

CLINICAL MANIFESTATIONS Boys with DMD will present in the preschool years with muscle weakness, difficulty walking, and large calves (pseudohypertrophy) caused by normal muscle fiber replacement with fat and connective tissue (see Figures 38-13, *B* and *C*). Although the calves are large the muscle is actually weak. Clinical weakness starts in the pelvic girdle, initially causing difficulty rising from the floor (Gower sign) and climbing stairs, and a waddling gait because of weakness in the lumbar and gluteal muscles. Boys with DMD often toe-walk because of weakness of the anterior tibial and

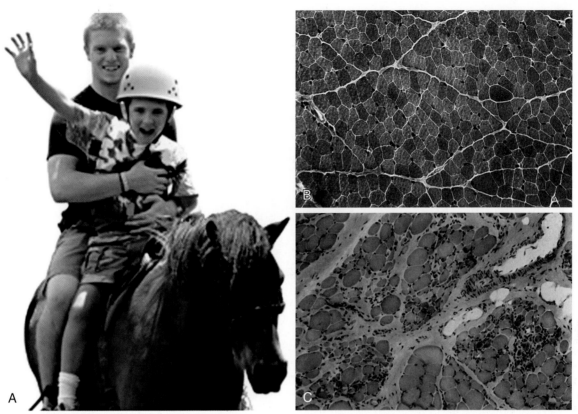

FIGURE 38-13 Duchenne Muscular Dystrophy. A, Young boy with DMD but on horseback. **B,** Transverse section of gastrocnemius muscle from a healthy boy. **C,** Transverse section of gastrocnemius muscle from a boy with Duchenne muscular dystrophy. Normal muscle fiber is replaced with fat and connective tissue. (From Jorde LB et al: *Medical genetics,* ed 3, updated, St Louis, 2006, Mosby.)

peroneal muscles, causing the feet to assume a talipes equinovarus position. The weakness worsens over the subsequent few years, resulting in the loss of ability to ambulate by 8 to 13 years of age. Muscle weakness also leads to contractures of the knees, hips, and other joints, and scoliosis develops in most boys with DMD. Once scoliosis begins, it is relentlessly progressive. Curves of more than 20 degrees are treated surgically to maintain pulmonary function. Muscle weakness and inactivity, particularly once a person is in a wheelchair full time, lead to osteoporosis and pathologic fractures. If fracture occurs, bisphosphonates may be used to strengthen bone, although long-term studies on safety have not been performed in this population.

As children age, muscle weakness progresses and respiratory weakness leads to breathing difficulty, particularly when sleeping. Susceptibility to respiratory tract infections and progressive deterioration of pulmonary function generally lead to premature death, usually in the twenties. Cardiomyopathy also may occur and, despite treatment, is generally progressive. Bowel and bladder function are often mildly affected, with constipation and urinary urgency as frequent symptoms. Mild to moderate cognitive problems are common but not universal.

EVALUATION AND TREATMENT Diagnosis is suggested (a high CK does not confirm the diagnosis because many other alterations can also increase CK) by measuring the blood creatinine kinase level, which can be 100 times the normal level, with confirmation by genetic testing for mutations in the dystrophin gene.

Management involves maintaining function for as long as possible. Treatment with steroids can prolong the ability to walk by several years and improves life expectancy.[20] Prednisone is used in the United States, although many families prefer to use deflazacort, (it is however, not currently approved in the United States but available from the Internet) which is a steroid that may have fewer side effects than prednisone. Treatment also involves range-of-motion exercises, bracing, and surgical release of contracture deformities and scoliosis when necessary. Children with DMD require a multidisciplinary approach to care, including attention to heart and breathing problems, weight loss/gain, constipation, rehabilitative/developmental problems, psychosocial needs, neurologic, and orthopedic problems (Figure 38-14). New guidelines for the evaluation and treatment of Duchenne muscular dystrophy were developed after reviewing thousands of clinical scenarios and are presented as a multisystem, two-part approach. One part is for diagnosis and the other part for management.

If appropriate, families should receive genetic counseling for recurrence risk and prenatal screening. Family support is necessary throughout the lifespan of the child because needs vary depending on the stage of the disease.

Becker Muscular Dystrophy

Although Becker muscular dystrophy (BMD) has been designated historically as a separate muscular dystrophy, it is actually caused by alterations of the same dystrophin gene (i.e., dystrophinopathies) and protein as seen in DMD. Children with BMD present later and have a

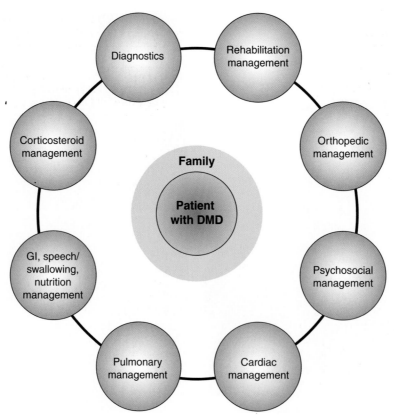

FIGURE 38-14 Multisystem Approach for Evaluation and Treatment of Duchenne Muscular Dystrophy. (Adapted from Bushby K: *Diagnosis and management of Duchenne muscular dystrophy part 1: diagnosis and pharmacological and psychosocial management*, 2009; Bushby K: *Diagnosis and management of Duchenne muscular dystrophy part 2: implementation of multidisciplinary care*, 2009. Available at www.thelancet.com/neurology. Published online Nov 30, 2009 [doi:10.1016/S1474-4422(09)70271].)

longer life expectancy than those with DMD; however, they are part of the same clinical spectrum.

Facioscapulohumeral Muscular Dystrophy

Facioscapulohumeral (FSH) muscular dystrophy, one of the most common muscular dystrophies and is inherited in an autosomal dominant fashion. It is more variable in presentation than Duchenne muscular dystrophy. FSH muscular dystrophy is usually observed in *late* childhood. Progression is usually slow and lifespan is normal or near normal. FSH muscular dystrophy occurs because of a deletion on chromosome 4 that is not associated with any particular gene and causes disease by still unknown mechanisms.

Muscle weakness, which is often asymmetric, usually begins in the face and is then observed in the shoulders and legs. Individuals with FSH muscular dystrophy often have weak eye closure, are not able to whistle or inflate a balloon, and have scapular winging.

Diagnosis is by genetic testing, although sometimes biopsies or electrodiagnostic testing may also be performed as part of the diagnostic evaluation. FSH muscular dystrophy also may be associated with mild hearing loss, retinal abnormalities, and mild cardiac problems. Unlike DMD or BMD, children with FSH muscular dystrophy often have muscle pain, particularly in their arms and shoulders.

Treatment involves administration of nonsteroidal anti-inflammatory drugs to decrease pain and inflammation. Massage and heat treatments also may be helpful. Bracing may be performed for function, for example, dorsiflexion of the feet with ankle-foot orthotics to prevent tripping or to provide support and comfort.

Myotonic Muscular Dystrophy

PATHOPHYSIOLOGY Myotonic muscular dystrophy (MMD) is a multisystem disease that can occur because of mutations in either of two genes resulting in type 1 (*DMPK* gene) and type 2 (*CNBP* gene) MMD. MMD1 may demonstrate a genetic mechanism called *anticipation,* in which children born to a mother with MMD usually have a more severe form of the disease.

CLINICAL MANIFESTATIONS MMD affects the brain, skeletal and smooth muscles, the eyes, the heart, and the endocrine system, manifesting as distal muscle weakness, learning problems or intellectual disability, or both. Additionally, children can have dysphagia, constipation, cardiac dysrhythmias that if untreated may be life-threatening, diabetes, and cataracts. Boys with MMD also may manifest testicular atrophy and early male pattern baldness. A hallmark of the disease is myotonia—individuals have difficulty relaxing muscles; for example, they may have difficulty relaxing their hand grip after a handshake or opening their eyes after closing them tightly.

Children with mild disease do not develop symptoms until adolescence or older and may display mild muscle weakness, usually more pronounced in the distal muscle, cataracts, and myotonia, but have normal lifespans. Children with a more classic form of the disease also have onset of symptoms in the teenage years but have progressive muscle weakness, cataracts, and cardiac conduction abnormalities; they may have a shortened lifespan and require a wheelchair for mobility. The congenital form, the most severe, may be present at birth or become obvious over the first few years of life.

EVALUATION AND TREATMENT Diagnosis is made by genetic testing for the two genes known to cause MMD. In each case, an abnormal segment of DNA, caused by an abnormally large trinucleotide, repeat expansion (CTG) in an untranslated region of a gene, causes abnormal functioning of muscle and other cells. Type 1 is more common and can present in infancy (the congenital form). Infants with MMD may have life-threatening breathing and swallowing problems and developmental delay or intellectual disability, although MMD is not observed until childhood or even adolescence.

Steroids are not useful for the treatment of MMD; however, maintaining muscle function is important, including range-of-motion exercises, bracing, and surgical release of contractures when necessary. Children need to be followed closely by neurologists and primary care providers with treatment for the various aspects of the disease, such as dysphagia, heart dysrhythmias, and constipation, as well as other problems.

> ✔ **QUICK CHECK 38-2**
> 1. What is the pathophysiology of osteochondrosis?
> 2. What is the cause of Duchenne muscular dystrophy?
> 3. Discuss the clinical manifestations of Duchenne muscular dystrophy.
> 4. Which dystrophy is really a systemic disease?
> 5. What is the difference between Becker and Duchenne Muscular Dystrophy?

MUSCULOSKELETAL TUMORS

Benign Bone Tumors

The two most common forms of benign bone tumors are osteochondroma and nonossifying fibroma.

Osteochondroma

Osteochondroma (or exostosis) can occur as a solitary lesion or as an inherited syndrome of hereditary multiple exostoses (HME). HME is an autosomal dominant condition with exostoses occurring throughout the skeleton. Osteochondromas appear as bony protuberances because of *EXT1* and *EXT2* genetic anomalies near active growth plates of the proximal humerus, distal femur, or proximal tibia. The most common presentation is a palpable mass that is painful when traumatized. Rarely, the lesion can cause neurologic or vascular problems, or tendon rupture from local compression. The lesions can lead to growth disturbance and mildly short stature. Knee valgus (knock-knee), ankle valgus, and hip problems are common. Upper extremity lesions can lead to a pronounced deformity in the forearm with a very short ulna bone. These lesions grow until skeletal maturity; growth or pain after skeletal maturity is a sign of possible malignant transformation, especially in the pelvis or scapular region. Transformation to chondrosarcoma is very rare, occurring in less than 1% of children.

Treatment involves minimizing growth disturbance, local tissue compression, and pain by resection of symptomatic lesions. The regrowth rate is 30% when lesions are removed in early childhood; therefore only symptomatic lesions should be surgically addressed in the growing child.[21]

Nonossifying Fibroma

Of all benign bone tumors, 50% are nonossifying fibromas or fibrous cortical defects. Nonossifying fibromas are sharply demarcated, cortically based lesions of fibrocytes that have replaced normal bone.

The lesion can occur in any bone, at any age. Nearly 30% of all children have at least one.

Microscopically, these benign nonmetastasizing lesions appear as whorled bundles of fibroblasts and osteoclast-like giant cells. As the tumor grows, lipids make the fibroblasts foamy in appearance, and they are known as *foam cells*.

Treatment is observational only. If these lesions grow too large, however, they will compromise the biomechanical strength of the bone and lead to pathologic fractures. Curettage and bone grafting is suggested after pathologic fracture or if impending fracture (nonossifying fibroma greater than 50% of the diameter of the bone or greater than 3 or 4 cm) is noted radiographically.

Malignant Bone Tumors

Malignant bone tumors are uncommon tumors in childhood, accounting for fewer than 5% of childhood malignancies and occurring mostly during adolescence. The two main tumors are osteosarcoma and Ewing sarcoma.

Osteosarcoma

Osteosarcoma is the most common malignant bone tumor found during childhood and originates in bone-producing mesenchymal cells. Tumors can be broadly classified as those arising within the bone and those arising on the surface of bone. Approximately 75% of these tumors occur in children between the ages of 10 and 25 years, with most being diagnosed between 15 and 19 years of age during the adolescent growth spurt. Incidence is the same for males and females.

Osteosarcoma may develop as a result of rapid local growth, which increases the likelihood of mutation. It can be induced by ionizing radiation, even with relatively low doses, and can be a tragic consequence of therapeutic radiation for other forms of cancer. The latent period after radiation exposure is 5 to 40 years. There also has been a link to individuals with retinoblastoma (a hereditary eye tumor).

Osteosarcoma has not been linked to chemical carcinogens or viruses. No deoxyribonucleic acid (DNA) or ribonucleic acid (RNA) virus has been isolated.

Molecular analysis has demonstrated deletion of genetic material on the long arm of chromosome 13, which led to the identification of a tumor-suppressor gene as being part of the mechanism for tumor development. The oncogene *src* also has been associated with osteosarcoma.

PATHOPHYSIOLOGY Osteosarcoma occurs mainly in the metaphyses of long bones near sites of active physeal growth. The tumor most commonly occurs at the distal femur, proximal tibia, or proximal humerus. As a tumor of mesenchymal cells, osteosarcoma demonstrates production of osteoid cells.

Osteosarcoma is a bulky tumor that extends beyond the bone into a soft tissue mass. It may encircle the bone and destroy the trabeculae of the diseased area. Osteosarcoma disseminates through the bloodstream, usually to the lung. As many as 25% of children diagnosed with osteosarcoma exhibit lung metastases at diagnosis. Other sites of metastatic spread include other bones and visceral organs.

CLINICAL MANIFESTATIONS The most common presenting complaint is pain. Night pain, awakening a child from sleep, is a particularly foreboding sign. There may be swelling, warmth, and redness caused by the vascularity of the tumor. Symptoms also may include cough, dyspnea, and chest pain if lung metastasis is present. If a lower extremity is involved, a child may limp or suffer a pathologic fracture.

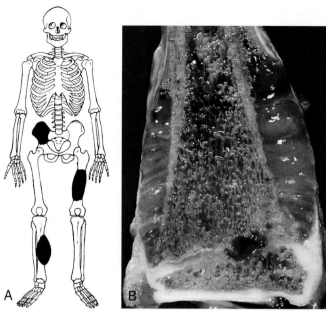

FIGURE 38-15 Ewing Sarcoma. **A,** Most common anatomic sites. **B,** Close-up view of Ewing sarcoma of the distal end of the tibia. Tumor extends into the soft tissue. (From Damjanov I, Linder J, editors: *Anderson's pathology,* ed 10, St Louis, 1996, Mosby.)

Although osteosarcoma is not the result of trauma, trauma may call attention to a preexisting tumor.

EVALUATION AND TREATMENT The five histologic types of osteosarcoma are determined by the predominant cell type. The tumor is graded according to degree of malignancy; the higher the grade, the worse the prognosis.

Surgery and chemotherapy are the primary treatments for osteosarcoma. The tumor is resistant to radiation. Traditionally, surgery includes amputation at the joint above the involved bone; however, more recent limb salvage procedures have gained acceptance, and amputation may be avoided in many children.

Chemotherapy is an important component of treatment. Children routinely receive chemotherapy preoperatively; then the disease is restaged with MRI and surgical biopsy to determine rate of "tumor kill." If more than 90% of tumor cells are killed by chemotherapy, the prognosis is markedly improved. Chemotherapy is then used after surgery for any additional cell spill during surgery. The use of chemotherapy with surgery has increased the 5-year survival rate to 60% or more.[22]

A number of approaches have been used to treat pulmonary metastases. Because pulmonary metastases are generally solitary, thoracotomy with wedge resection has proven to be the most effective treatment.

Ewing Sarcoma

Ewing sarcoma is the second most common and most lethal malignant bone tumor that occurs during childhood. This tumor is named after James Ewing, who first identified it as a separate clinical diagnosis in 1921. The most common period of diagnosis is between 5 and 15 years of age; it is rare after age 30 years. Ewing sarcoma is slightly more common in males than females. Cytogenic studies have shown a translocation of chromosomes 11 and 22 resulting in a fusion protein (EWS-FLI 1) forming at the chromosomal junction.

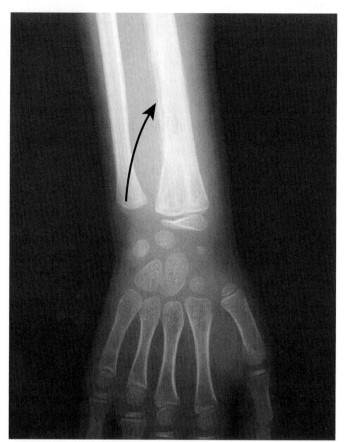

FIGURE 38-16 Ewing Sarcoma of the Distal Radius. Radiograph of an 8-year-old boy showing a permeative lesion of the distal radius. Note the loss of bone cortex on the ulnar border suggesting an aggressive process. Bone biopsy revealed Ewing sarcoma.

PATHOPHYSIOLOGY Ewing sarcoma is most commonly located in the midshaft of long bones or in flat bones. The most common sites include the femur, pelvis, and humerus (Figure 38-15).

Arising from bone marrow, Ewing sarcoma can penetrate the cortex of the bone to form a soft tissue mass. Unlike osteosarcoma, Ewing sarcoma does not make bone and radiographically appears as a permeative, destructive lesion (Figure 38-16). Ewing sarcoma metastasizes to nearly every organ. Metastasis occurs early and is usually apparent at diagnosis or within 1 year. The most common sites are the lung, other bones, lymph nodes, bone marrow, liver, spleen, and central nervous system.

CLINICAL MANIFESTATIONS As with osteosarcoma, the most common complaint is pain that increases in severity. A soft tissue mass is often present. Additional symptoms may include fever, malaise, and anorexia. The radiographic appearance is similar to that of osteomyelitis, and diagnosis is only confirmed with biopsy.

EVALUATION AND TREATMENT Evaluation is determined from genetic testing, elevated sedimentation rate, and lactic acid dehydrogenase (LDH) levels. Biopsy is used to conclusively establish the diagnosis of a small round cell tumor.

Treatment includes radiation, chemotherapy, and, if possible, surgical débridement. Chemotherapy is continued for 12 to 18 months after resection. Present 5-year survival with this tritheuretic approach is 60%; however, tumors of the pelvis have a markedly worse prognosis. Metastasis at diagnosis is another poor prognostic indicator, with 5-year survival rate dropping to under 40%.

NONACCIDENTAL TRAUMA

It is estimated that more than 2.0 million children are abused per year in the United States. Maltreatment may be psychologic, sexual, or physical.[23] Thirty percent of children who have been physically abused are seen by an orthopedist. Accurate and appropriate referrals to child protection agencies not only are legally mandated but also are essential for the well-being of the child. An abused child who is returned to the same situation without intervention has a 10% to 15% chance of subsequent mortality.

Fractures in Nonaccidental Trauma

Children who are not yet ambulatory and present with a long bone fracture have more than a 75% chance of that fracture being caused by nonaccidental trauma.[24] "Corner" metaphyseal fractures are nearly always from abuse but occur only 25% of the time (Figure 38-17). Fractures at multiple stages of healing also suggest abuse; however, osteogenesis imperfecta or other causes of systemic osteomalacia must be ruled out. The most common presentation is a transverse tibia fracture. After walking age, only 2% of long bone fractures are the result of nonaccidental trauma.[25]

EVALUATION Nonaccidental trauma necessitates early consultation with child protective services. The child should undergo skeletal survey (especially if less than 2 years of age) and have a complete physical examination to evaluate for pattern bruising, burns, or multiple soft tissue injuries. A thorough history must be obtained for all identified injuries. It is important to remember that social isolation can lead to an increased likelihood of abuse, but no social status is immune. One study reported that nonwhite children were three times more likely than whites to be reported for nonaccidental trauma; however, it is important to remember that all races are at risk.[26]

When the cause of injury is unclear, bone scan can be helpful in diagnosing subtle injuries, especially rib fractures. Posterior rib fractures are especially likely to be the result of abuse. MRI/CT of the brain to check for subdural hematoma and retinal examination to look for hemorrhages are essential.

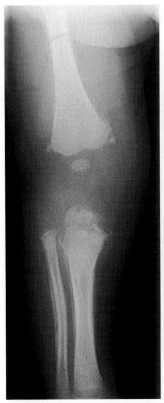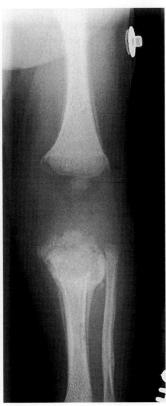

FIGURE 38-17 Corner Fracture. Bilateral knee radiograph showing healing corner fractures of bilateral proximal tibias and distal femurs. Note the varying amount of callus formation signifying fractures at different stages of healing.

TREATMENT The treating healthcare provider must have a nonjudgmental attitude. The child and family involved in nonaccidental trauma are emotionally delicate and require not only physical but also emotional care. Social workers need to be involved early to ensure that the child receives appropriate medical care. Fortunately, fractures tend to heal quickly for those in this age group. Neurologic injury and social disease, however, are much more difficult to cure.

DID YOU UNDERSTAND?

Congenital Defects

1. Clubfoot is a common deformity in which the foot is twisted out of its normal shape or position. Clubfoot can be positional, idiopathic, or teratologic.
2. Developmental dysplasia of the hip (DDH) is an abnormality in the development of the femoral head, acetabulum, or both. Like clubfoot, DDH can be idiopathic or teratologic. It is a serious and disabling condition in children if not diagnosed and treated.
3. Osteogenesis imperfecta (brittle bone disease) is an inherited disorder of collagen that affects primarily bones and results in serious fractures of many bones.

Bone Infection

1. Osteomyelitis is a local or generalized bacterial or granulomatous (e.g., tuberculosis) infection of bone and bone marrow. Bacteria are usually introduced by direct extension from a nearby infection, through the bloodstream, or by trauma.
2. Septic arthritis can occur de novo or secondary to osteomyelitis in very young children in which the metaphysis is still located within the joint capsule of certain joints.

Juvenile Idiopathic Arthritis

1. Juvenile idiopathic arthritis is an inflammatory joint disorder characterized by pain and swelling. Large joints are most commonly affected.

Osteochondroses

1. Avascular diseases of the bone are collectively referred to as osteochondroses and are caused by an insufficient blood supply to growing bones.
2. Legg-Calvé-Perthes disease is one of the most common osteochondroses. This disorder is characterized by epiphyseal necrosis or degeneration of the head of the femur followed by regeneration or recalcification.
3. Osgood-Schlatter disease is characterized by tendonitis of the anterior patellar tendon and inflammation or partial separation of the tibial tubercle caused by chronic irritation, usually as a result of overuse of the quadriceps muscles. The condition is seen primarily in muscular, athletic adolescent males.

Scoliosis

1. Scoliosis is a lateral curvature of the spinal column that can be caused by congenital malformations of the spine, poliomyelitis, skeletal dysplasias, spastic paralysis, and unequal leg length, but it is most often idiopathic.

Muscular Dystrophy

1. The muscular dystrophies are a group of genetically transmitted diseases characterized by progressive atrophy of skeletal muscles. There is an insidious loss of strength in all forms of the disorder with increasing disability and deformity. The most common type in childhood is Duchenne muscular dystrophy.

Musculoskeletal Tumors

1. The two most common forms of benign bone tumors are osteochondroma and nonossifying fibroma.
2. The two main types of malignant childhood bone tumors are osteosarcoma and Ewing sarcoma.
3. Osteosarcoma, the most common malignant childhood bone tumor, originates in bone-producing mesenchymal cells and is most often located near active growth plates, such as distal femur, proximal tibia, or proximal humerus.
4. Most children with osteosarcoma are diagnosed between 15 and 19 years of age, and osteosarcoma occurs equally in males and females.
5. Ewing sarcoma originates from cells within the bone marrow space and is most often located in the midshaft of long bones or in flat bones. The most common sites include the femur, pelvis, and humerus.
6. Ewing sarcoma is more common in males and is diagnosed most often between the ages of 5 and 15 years.
7. Pain is the usual presenting symptom for either osteosarcoma or Ewing sarcoma.
8. The primary treatments for osteosarcoma are surgery and chemotherapy. The primary treatment for Ewing sarcoma is a combination of chemotherapy, radiation, and surgery.

Nonaccidental Trauma

1. Nonaccidental trauma must be considered with any long bone injury in the preambulatory child.
2. The presence of soft tissue injury, corner fractures, and multiple fractures at different stages of healing is extremely helpful for making a diagnosis of nonaccidental trauma.
3. When nonaccidental trauma is suspected, a child must be evaluated radiographically for other fractures, heat trauma, and retinal hemorrhage.
4. All social strata are at risk.
5. The healthcare provider is legally responsible to report suspected nonaccidental trauma.

KEY TERMS

- Acetabular dysplasia 1023
- Acute hematogenous osteomyelitis 1026
- Antalgic abductor lurch 1028
- Becker muscular dystrophy (BMD) 1031
- Clubfoot 1022
- Congenital equinovarus 1022
- Developmental dysplasia of the hip (DDH) 1023
- Dislocated hip 1023
- Duchenne muscular dystrophy (DMD) 1030
- Dystrophin 1030
- Ewing sarcoma 1034

- Facioscapulohumeral (FSH) muscular dystrophy 1032
- Hereditary multiple exostoses (HME) 1033
- Involucrum 1026
- Juvenile idiopathic arthritis (JIA) 1027
- Legg-Calvé-Perthes (LCP) disease 1027
- Malignant bone tumor 1033
- Muscular dystrophy 1030
- Myotonic muscular dystrophy (MMD) 1032
- Nonossifying fibroma 1033
- Nonstructural scoliosis 1029
- Oligoarthritis 1027

- Osgood-Schlatter disease 1029
- Osteochondroma 1033
- Osteochondrosis 1027
- Osteogenesis imperfecta (OI; brittle bone disease) 1025
- Osteomyelitis 1026
- Osteosarcoma 1033
- Polyarthritis 1027
- Scoliosis 1029
- Septic arthritis 1027
- Still disease 1027
- Structural scoliosis 1029
- Subluxated hip 1023

REFERENCES

1. Morcuende JA, et al: Plaster cast treatment of clubfoot: the Ponseti method of manipulation and casting, *J Pediatr Orthop* 3(2):161–167, 1994.

2. Noonan KJ, Richards BS: Nonsurgical management of idiopathic clubfoot, *J Am Acad Orthop Surg* 11(6):392–402, 2003.

3. Janicki JA, et al: Treatment of neuromuscular and syndrome-associated (nonidiopathic) clubfeet using the Ponseti method, *J Pediatr Orthop* 29(4):393–397, 2009.

4. Woolacott NF, et al: Ultrasonography in screening for developmental dysplasia of the hip in newborns: systematic review, *Br Med J* 330(7505):1413, 2005.

5. Jari S, Paton RW, Srinivasan MS: Unilateral limitation of abduction of the hip: a valuable clinical sign for DDH? *J Bone Joint Surg Br* 84(1):104–107, 2002.

6. Halmes J et al: Long term follow-up of open reduction surgery for developmental dysplasia of the hip, *J Pediatr Orthop*, in press.

7. Glorieux FH, et al: Cyclic administration of Pamidronate in children with severe osteogenesis imperfect, *N Engl J Med* 339(14):947–952, 1998.

8. Poyrazoglu S, et al: Successful results of Pamidronate treatment in children with osteogenesis imperfect with emphasis on interpretation of bone mineral density for local standards, *J Pediatr Orthop* 28(4):483–487, 2008.

9. Vaderhave KL, et al: Community-associated methicillin-resistant *Staphylococcus aureus* in acute musculoskeletal infection in children: a game changer, *J Pediatr Orthop* 29(8):927–931, 2009.

10. Hresko MT, et al: Prospective reevaluation of the association between thrombotic diathesis and Legg-Perthes disease, *J Bone Joint Surg Am* 84(9):1613–1618, 2002.

11. Vosmaer A, et al: Coagulation abnormalities in Legg-Calvé-Perthes disease, *J Bone Joint Surg Am* 92(1):121–128, 2010.

12. Mata SG, et al: Legg-Calvé-Perthes disease and passive smoking, *J Pediatr Orthop* 20(3):326–330, 2000.

13. McCullough L, Lyman KS: Musculoskeletal considerations across the life span. In Gates SJ, Mooar PA, editors: *Musculoskeletal primary care*, Philadelphia, 1998, Lippincott.

14. Morrissy R, Weinstein S, editors: *Lovell and Winter's pediatric orthopaedics*, ed 4, Philadelphia, 1996, Lippincott-Raven.

15. Jorde LB, et al: *Medical genetics*, ed 3, St Louis, 2006, Mosby.

16. Cassas KJ, Cassettari-Wayhs A: Childhood and adolescent sports-related overuse injuries, *Am Fam Physician* 73(6):1014–1022, 2006.

17. Kaeding CC, Whitehead R: Musculoskeletal injuries in adolescents, *Prim Care* 25(1):211–223, 1998.

18. Davis JR, Chamberlin E, Blackhurst DW: Indications for magnetic resonance imaging in presumed adolescent idiopathic scoliosis, *J Bone Joint Surg Am* 86:2187–2195, 2004.

19. Katz DE, et al: Brace wear control of curve progression in adolescent idiopathic scoliosis, *J Bone Joint Surg Am* 92:1343–1352, 2010.

20. Moxley RT III, et al: Practice parameter: corticosteroid treatment of Duchenne dystrophy: report of the Quality Standards Subcommittee of the American Academy of Neurology and the Practice Committee of the Child Neurology Society, *Neurology* 64(1):13–20, 2005.

21. Cummings JR, et al: Congenital clubfoot, *Instr Course Lect* 51:385–400, 2002.

22. Heyden JB, Hoang BH: Osteosarcoma: basic science and clinical implications, *Orthop Clin North Am* 37(1):1–7, 2006.

23. Administration for Children and Families Children's Bureau: *Child maltreatment 2009*, Washington DC, 2010, U.S. Department of Health and Human Services. Available at www.acf.hhs.gov; programs/cb/stats_research/index.htm#can.

24. Rex C, Kay PR: Features of femoral fractures in nonaccidental injury, *J Pediatr Orthop* 20(3):411–413, 2000.

25. Thomas SA, et al: Long-bone fractures in young children: distinguishing accident injuries from child abuse, *Pediatrics* 88(3):471–476, 1991.

26. Lane WG, et al: Racial differences in the evaluation of pediatric fractures for physical abuse, *JAMA* 288(13):1603–1609, 2002.

39

Structure, Function, and Disorders of the Integument

Noreen Heer Nicol and Sue E. Huether

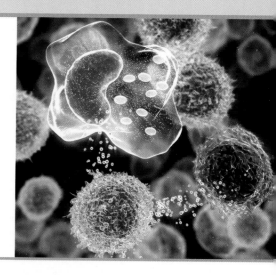

ⓔvolve WEBSITE

http://evolve.elsevier.com/Huether/

- Review Questions and Answers
- Animations
- Quick Check Answers

- Key Terms Exercises
- Critical Thinking Questions with Answers
- Algorithm Completion Exercises
- WebLinks

CHAPTER OUTLINE

The skin is the largest organ of the body. Combined with the accessory structures of hair, nails, and glands, it forms the integumentary system. The skin covers the entire body and accounts for approximately 20% of the body's weight. The primary function of the skin is to protect the body from the environment by serving as a barrier against microorganisms, ultraviolet radiation, loss of body fluids, and the stress of mechanical forces. The skin regulates body temperature and is involved in immune surveillance and the activation of vitamin D. Touch and pressure receptors provide important protective functions and pleasurable sensations. The commensal (normal) microorganisms of the skin protect against pathologic bacteria.

STRUCTURE AND FUNCTION OF THE SKIN

Layers of the Skin

The skin is formed of two major layers: (1) a superficial or outer layer of **epidermis** and (2) a deeper layer of **dermis** (the true skin) (Figure 39-1). The **subcutaneous layer (hypodermis)** is the lowest lying layer

of connective tissue that contains macrophages, fibroblasts, fat cells, nerves, fine muscles, blood vessels, lymphatics, and hair follicle roots. Each skin layer contains cells that represent progressive stages of skin cell differentiation and function as the skin grows. These are summarized in Table 39-1.

Dermal Appendages

The **dermal appendages** include the nails, hair, sebaceous glands, and the eccrine and apocrine sweat glands. The **nails** are protective keratinized plates that appear at the ends of fingers and toes. They have the following structures: (1) the proximal nail fold and cuticle, (2) eponychium, (3) the matrix from which the nail grows and nail root, (4) the hyponychium (nail bed), (5) the nail plate, and (6) paronychia (lateral nail fold) (Figure 39-2). Nail growth continues throughout life at 1 mm or less per day.

Hair color, density, grain, and pattern of distribution vary considerably among people and depend on age, gender, and race. Hair follicles arise from the matrix (or bulb) located deep in the dermis. They

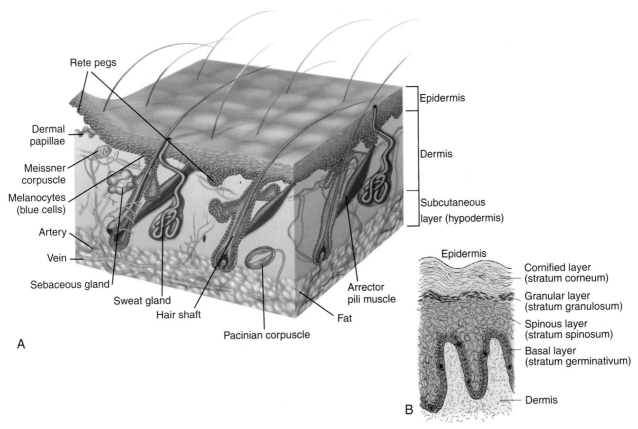

FIGURE 39-1 Structure of the Skin. **A,** Cross section showing major skin structures. **B,** Layers of the epidermis. (**A** from Kumar V, et al: *Robbins and Cotran pathologic basis of disease,* ed 8, St Louis, 2009, Saunders; **B** from Baker S: *Local flaps in facial reconstruction,* ed 2, St Louis, 2007, Mosby.)

TABLE 39-1	LAYERS OF THE SKIN	
STRUCTURE	**CELL TYPES**	**CHARACTERISTICS**
Epidermis	Keratinocytes	Most important layer of skin; normally very thin (0.12 mm) but can thicken and form corns or calluses with constant pressure or friction; includes rete pegs that extend into papillary layer of dermis
	Langerhans cells	Cells with dendrite process and immune functions
Stratum corneum	Keratinocytes	Tough superficial layer covering body
Stratum lucidum	Keratinocytes	Clear layers of cells containing eleidin, which becomes keratin as cells move up to corneum layer
Stratum granulosum	Keratinocytes Melanocytes	Keratohyalin gives granular appearance to this layer
Stratum spinosum	New keratinocytes	Polygonal shaped with spinous processes projecting between adjacent keratinocytes
Stratum basale (germinativum)	Keratinocytes	Basal layer where keratinocytes divide and move upward to replace cells shed from surface
	Melanocytes	Melanocytes synthesize pigment melanin
	Merkel cells	Function of Merkel cells is not clearly known; they are associated with sensory nerve endings
Dermis Papillary layer (thin)	Macrophages Mast cells	Irregular connective tissue layer with rich blood, lymphatic, and nerve supply; contains sensory receptors and sweat glands (apocrine, eccrine, sebaceous), macrophages (phagocytic and important for wound healing), and mast cells (release histamine and have immune functions) (see Chapter 5)
Reticular layer (thick)	Histiocytes	Histiocytes are wandering macrophages that collect pigments and inflammatory debris
Subcutaneous layer (hypodermis)		Subcutaneous tissue or superficial fascia of varying thickness that connects overlying dermis to underlying muscle; contains macrophages, fibroblasts, fat cells, nerves, blood vessels, lymphatics, and hair follicle roots

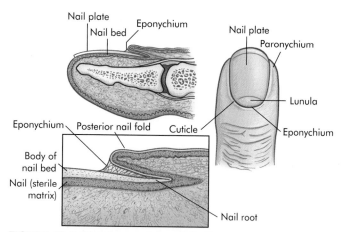

FIGURE 39-2 Structures of the Nail. (Redrawn from Thompson JM et al: *Mosby's clinical nursing*, ed 5, St Louis, 2002, Mosby.)

extend from the dermis at an angle and have an erector pili muscle attached near the mid-dermis that straightens the follicle when contracted, causing the hair to stand up. Hair growth begins in the bulb, with cellular differentiation occurring as the hair progresses up the follicle. Hair is fully hardened, or cornified, by the time it emerges at the skin surface. Hair growth is cyclic, with periods of growth and rest that vary over different body surfaces.

The sebaceous glands open onto the surface of the skin through a canal. They are found in greatest numbers on the face, chest, and back, with modified glands on the eyelids, lips, nipples, glans penis, and prepuce. Sebaceous glands secrete sebum, composed primarily of lipids, which oils the skin and hair and prevents drying. Androgens stimulate the growth of sebaceous glands, and their enlargement is an early sign of puberty.

The eccrine sweat glands are distributed over the body, with the greatest numbers in the palms of the hands, soles of the feet, and forehead. They open onto the surface of the skin and are important in thermoregulation and cooling of the body through evaporation. The apocrine sweat glands are fewer in number but produce significantly more sweat than the eccrine glands. They are located near the bulb of hair follicles in the axillae, scalp, face, abdomen, and genital area. Their ducts open into the hair follicle. The interaction of sweat with commensal (normal) flora bacteria contributes to the odor of perspiration.

Blood Supply and Innervation

The blood supply to the skin is limited to the papillary capillaries, or plexus, of the dermis. These capillary loops are supplied by a deeper arterial plexus. Branches from the deep plexus also supply hair follicles and sweat glands. A subpapillary network of veins drains the capillary loops. Arteriovenous anastomoses in the dermis facilitate the regulation of body temperature. Heat loss can be regulated by varying blood flow through the skin by opening and closing the arteriovenous anastomoses in conjunction with evaporative heat loss of sweat. The sympathetic nervous system regulates both vasoconstriction and vasodilation through α-adrenergic receptors in the skin. The lymphatic vessels of the skin arise in the papillary dermis and drain into larger subcutaneous trunks, removing cells, proteins, and immunologic mediators.

✔ **QUICK CHECK 39-1**
1. Describe the two layers of the skin.
2. How do the skin blood vessels and sweat glands regulate body temperature?
3. What are some changes that occur in skin with aging?

GERIATRIC CONSIDERATIONS
Aging & Changes in Skin Integrity

- Skin becomes thinner, dryer, and more wrinkled.
- DNA repair of damaged skin decreases.
- Epidermal cells contain less moisture and change shape.
- The dermis thins, producing translucent, paper-thin quality that is more susceptible to tearing.
- Dermis becomes more permeable and less able to clear substances, so they accumulate and cause irritation.
- There is a loss of epidermal rete pegs, which weakens the connection to the dermis and gives skin a smooth, shiny, and wrinkled appearance with an increased likelihood to tear from shearing forces.
- There is a loss of elastin, contributing to wrinkling.
- There is a loss of flexibility of collagen fibers, so skin cannot stretch and regain shape as readily.
- The barrier function of the stratum corneum is reduced, increasing risk for injury and infection.
- Significantly decreased number of Langerhans cells reduces the skin's immune response.
- The dermoepidermal border flattens, shortening and decreasing the number of capillary loops.

Other Skin Changes with Aging
- Wound healing decreases as a result of decreased blood flow and slower rate of basal cell turnover.
- There are fewer melanocytes; pigmentation becomes irregular, giving decreased protection from ultraviolet radiation and leading to graying of hair.
- Atrophy of eccrine, apocrine, and sebaceous glands causes dry skin.
- Pressure and touch receptors and free nerve endings decrease in number, causing reduced sensory perception.
- With compromised temperature regulation, loss of cutaneous vasomotion, and decreased eccrine sweat production, there is an increased risk of heat stroke and hypothermia.
- The nail plate thins and nails are more brittle.

Data from Zouboulis CC, Makrantonaki E: Clinical aspects and molecular diagnostics of skin aging, *Clin Dermatol* 29(1):3–14, 2011; Fore J: A review of skin and the effects of aging on skin structure and function, *Ostomy Wound Manage* 52(9):24–35, quiz 36–37, 2006; Holowatz LA et al: Aging and the control of human skin blood flow, *Front Biosci* 15:718–739, 2010; Wickremaratchi MM, Llewelyn JG: Effects of ageing on touch, *Postgrad Med J* 82(967):301–304, 2006.

Clinical Manifestations of Skin Dysfunction
Lesions

Identification of the morphologic structure and appearance of the skin in combination with a health history is necessary to identify underlying pathophysiology. Table 39-2 describes and illustrates the basic lesions of the skin. Clinical manifestations of select skin lesions are described in Table 39-3.

Pressure ulcers. Pressure ulcers are ischemic ulcers resulting from unrelieved pressure, shearing forces, friction, and moisture. The term *decubitus ulcer* refers to ulcers or pressure sores that develop when an individual lies in the recumbent position for a long time. The risks for pressure ulcers are summarized in *Risk Factors:* Pressure Ulcer.[1]

Pressure sores usually develop over bony prominences, such as the sacrum, heels, ischia, and greater trochanters. Continuous pressure on tissue between the bony prominence and a resistant outside surface distorts capillaries and occludes the blood supply. If the pressure is

Text continued on p. 1046

TABLE 39-2   PRIMARY AND SECONDARY SKIN LESIONS

PRIMARY SKIN LESIONS	EXAMPLES		
Macule Flat, circumscribed area that is a change in color of skin; less than 1 cm in diameter	Freckles, flat moles (nevi), petechiae, measles, scarlet fever	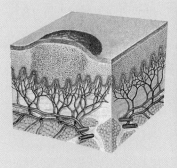	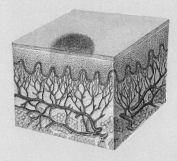Macules[c]
Papule Elevated, firm, circumscribed area less than 1 cm in diameter	Wart (verruca), elevated moles, lichen planus	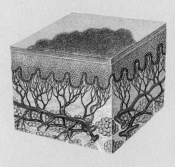	Flat warts[c] (Courtesy Dr. E Sahn.)
Patch Flat, nonpalpable, irregular-shaped macule more than 1 cm in diameter	Vitiligo, port-wine stains, Mongolian spots, café au lait spots	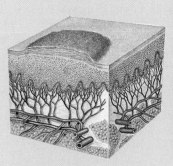	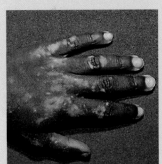Vitiligo[h]
Plaque Elevated, firm, and rough lesion with flat top surface more than 1 cm in diameter	Psoriasis, seborrheic and actinic keratoses	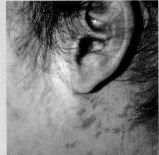	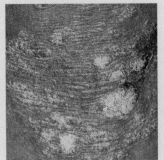Plaque[e]

Continued

TABLE 39-2 PRIMARY AND SECONDARY SKIN LESIONS—cont'd

PRIMARY SKIN LESIONS	EXAMPLES		
Wheal Elevated irregular-shaped area of cutaneous edema; solid, transient; variable diameter	Insect bites, urticaria, allergic reaction	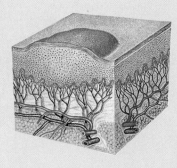	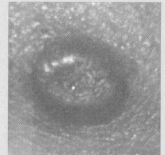Wheal[c]
Nodule Elevated, firm, circumscribed lesion; deeper in dermis than a papule; 1-2 cm in diameter	Erythema nodosum, lipomas	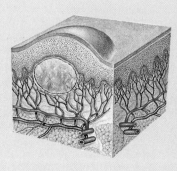	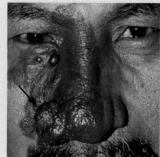Hypertrophic nodule[d]
Tumor Elevated, solid lesion; may be clearly demarcated; deeper in dermis; more than 2 cm in diameter	Neoplasms, benign tumor, lipoma, hemangioma	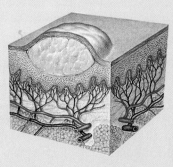	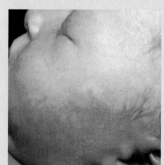Hemangioma[h]
Vesicle Elevated, circumscribed, superficial, not into dermis; filled with serous fluid; less than 1 cm in diameter	Varicella (chickenpox), herpes zoster (shingles)	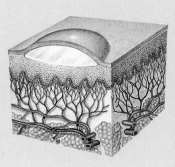	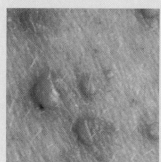Vesicles[c]

TABLE 39-2   PRIMARY AND SECONDARY SKIN LESIONS—cont'd

PRIMARY SKIN LESIONS	EXAMPLES	
Bulla Vesicle more than 1 cm in diameter	Blister, pemphigus vulgaris	Bulla[c] (Courtesy Dr. KA Riley.)
Pustule Elevated, superficial lesion; similar to a vesicle but filled with purulent fluid	Impetigo, acne	Acne[h]
Cyst Elevated, circumscribed, encapsulated lesion; in dermis or subcutaneous layer; filled with liquid or semisolid material	Sebaceous cyst, cystic acne	Sebaceous cyst[h]
Telangiectasia Fine (0.5-1.0 mm), irregular red lines produced by capillary dilation; can be associated with acne rosacea (face), venous hypertension (spider veins in legs), or developmental abnormalities (port-wine birthmarks)	Telangiectasia in rosacea	Telangiectasia[d]

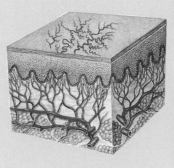

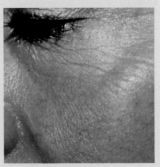

Continued

TABLE 39-2 PRIMARY AND SECONDARY SKIN LESIONS—cont'd

SECONDARY SKIN LESIONS	EXAMPLES		
Scale Heaped-up, keratinized cells; flaky skin; irregular; thick or thin; dry or oily; variation in size	Flaking of skin with seborrheic dermatitis following scarlet fever, or flaking of skin following a drug reaction; dry skin	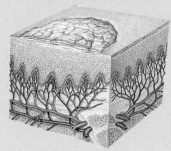	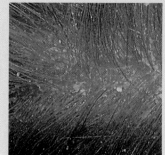 Fine scaling[a]
Lichenification Rough, thickened epidermis secondary to persistent rubbing, pruritus, or skin irritation; often involves flexor surface of extremity	Chronic dermatitis	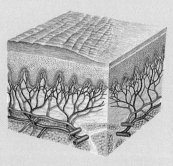	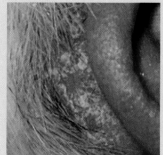 Stasis dermatitis in early stage[f]
Keloid Irregular-shaped, elevated, progressively enlarging scar; grows beyond boundaries of wound; caused by excessive collagen formation during healing	Keloid formation following surgery	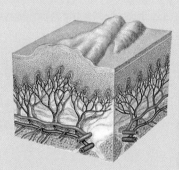	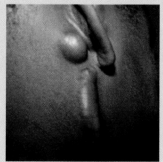 Keloid[h]
Scar Thin to thick fibrous tissue that replaces normal skin following injury or laceration to the dermis	Healed wound or surgical incision	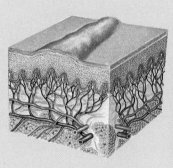	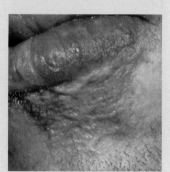 Hypertrophic scar[d]

TABLE 39-2   PRIMARY AND SECONDARY SKIN LESIONS—cont'd

SECONDARY SKIN LESIONS	EXAMPLES		
Excoriation Loss of epidermis; linear, hollowed-out, crusted area	Abrasion or scratch, scabies		 Scabies[h]
Fissure Linear crack or break from epidermis to dermis; may be moist or dry	Athlete's foot, cracks at corner of mouth		 Fissures[d]
Erosion Loss of part of epidermis; depressed, moist, glistening; follows rupture of a vesicle or bulla	Varicella, variola after rupture		 Erosion[b]
Ulcer Loss of epidermis and dermis; concave; varies in size	Decubiti, stasis ulcers		 Stasis ulcer[e]

Continued

TABLE 39-2 PRIMARY AND SECONDARY SKIN LESIONS—cont'd

SECONDARY SKIN LESIONS	EXAMPLES
Atrophy	
Thinning of skin surface and loss of skin markings; skin appears translucent and paper-like	Aged skin, striae

Aged skin[g]

From Thompson JM, Wilson SF: *Health assessment for nursing practice*, ed 2, St Louis, 2002, Mosby.
[a]Baran R, Dawber RR, Levene GM: *Color atlas of the hair, scalp, and nails*, St Louis, 1991, Mosby.
[b]Cohen BA: *Pediatric dermatology*, London, 1993, Wolfe.
[c]Farrar WE et al: *Infectious diseases*, ed 2, London, 1992, Gower.
[d]Goldman MP, Fitzpatrick RE: *Cutaneous laser surgery: the art and science of selective photothermolysis*, ed 2, St Louis, 1998, Mosby.
[e]Habif TP: *Clinical dermatology*, ed 4, St Louis, 2004, Mosby.
[f]Marks JG Jr, DeLeo VA: *Contact and occupational dermatitis*, St Louis, 1991, Mosby.
[g]Seidel HM et al: *Mosby's guide to physical examination*, ed 6, St Louis, 2007, Mosby.
[h]Weston WL, Lane AT: *Color textbook of pediatric dermatology*, ed 3, St Louis, 2002, Mosby.

TABLE 39-3 CLINICAL MANIFESTATIONS OF SELECT SKIN LESIONS

TYPE	CLINICAL MANIFESTATION
Comedone	Plug of sebaceous and keratin material lodged in opening of hair follicle; open comedone has dilated orifice (blackhead) and closed comedone has narrow opening (whitehead)
Burrow	Narrow, raised, irregular channel caused by parasite
Petechiae	Circumscribed area of blood less than 0.5 cm in diameter
Purpura	Circumscribed area of blood greater than 0.5 cm in diameter
Telangiectasia	Dilated, superficial blood vessels

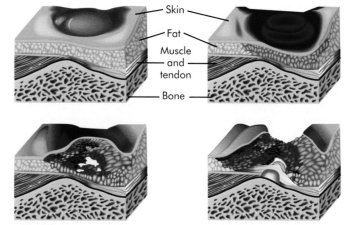

FIGURE 39-3 Progression of Pressure Ulcer. Sustained pressure over a bony prominence compresses the tissue and reduces blood flow, resulting in progressive ischemia and necrosis of tissue.

relieved within a few hours, a brief period of reactive hyperemia (redness) occurs and there may be no lasting tissue damage. If the pressure continues unrelieved, the endothelial cells lining the capillaries become disrupted with platelet aggregation, forming microthrombi that block blood flow and cause anoxic necrosis of surrounding tissues (Figure 39-3). Shearing and friction are mechanical forces moving parallel to the skin (dragging) and can extend to the bony skeleton, causing detachment and injury of tissues. Pressure ulcers are staged or graded and one classification scheme is as follows[2]:

Stage 1—Nonblanchable erythema of intact skin, usually over bony prominence

Stage 2—Partial-thickness skin loss (erosion or blister) involving epidermis or dermis

Stage 3—Full-thickness skin loss involving damage or necrosis of subcutaneous tissue that may extend to, but not through, underlying fascia

Stage 4—Full-thickness tissue loss with exposure of muscle, bone, or supporting structures (tendons or joint capsules); can include undermining and tunneling

A layer of dead tissue forms as an abrasion or blister when there is superficial damage or as a reddish blue discoloration when there is deeper tissue damage. Superficial sores are more common on the sacrum as a result of shearing or friction forces (forces parallel to the skin). Deep sores develop closer to the bone as a result of tissue distortion and vascular occlusion from pressure perpendicular to the tissue (over the heels, trochanter, and ischia).

Bacteria colonize the dead tissue, and infection is usually localized and self-limiting. Individuals who are immunosuppressed or have diabetes mellitus may develop infection and inflammation of adjacent tissues (cellulitis) or septicemia. Proteolytic enzymes from bacteria and macrophages dissolve necrotic tissues and cause a foul-smelling discharge that resembles, but is not, pus.

Pressure sores are painful and cause an inflammatory response with hyperemia, fever, and increased white blood cell count. If the ulceration is large, toxicity and pain lead to loss of appetite, debility,

RISK FACTORS

Pressure Ulcer

External Factors

- Prolonged pressure
- Immobilization
- Lying in bed or sitting in chair or wheelchair without changing position or relieving pressure over an extended period
- Lying for hours on hard x-ray, emergency department and operating tables
- Neurologic disorders (coma, spinal cord injuries, cognitive impairment, or cerebrovascular disease)
- Fractures or contractures
- Debilitation: elderly persons in hospitals and nursing homes
- Pain
- Sedation
- Shearing forces
- Coarse bed sheets used for turning by dragging, which produces a shearing force
- Lack of communication/education regarding pressure ulcer care

Disease/Tissue Factors

- Impaired perfusion; ischemia
- Fecal or urinary incontinence; prolonged exposure to moisture
- Malnutrition, dehydration
- Chronic diseases accompanied by anemia, edema, renal failure, malnutrition, peripheral vascular disease, or sepsis
- Previous history of pressure ulcers
- Thin skin associated with aging or prolonged use of steroids

Data from White-Chu EF et al: Pressure ulcers in long-term care, *Clin Geriatr Med* 27(2):241–258, 2011; Jaul E: Assessment and management of pressure ulcers in the elderly: current strategies, *Drugs Aging* 27(4):311–325, 2010; Jankowski IM, Nadzam DM: Identifying gaps, barriers, and solutions in implementing pressure ulcer prevention programs, *Jt Comm J Qual Patient Saf* 37(6):253–264, 2011; Munro CA: The development of a pressure ulcer risk-assessment scale for perioperative patients, *AORN J* 92(3):272–287, 2010; Willock J, Baharestani MM, Anthony D: The development of the Glamorgan paediatric pressure ulcer risk assessment scale, *J Wound Care* 18(1):17–21, 2009.

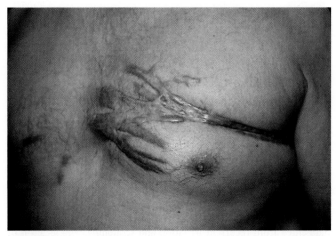

FIGURE 39-4 Keloid Formation. (Courtesy Department of Dermatology, School of Medicine, University of Utah, Salt Lake City, Utah.)

and renal insufficiency. The primary goal for those at risk for pressure ulcers is prevention. Preventive techniques include frequent promotion of movement, pressure avoidance (type of positioning), pressure removal (positioning interval), pressure distribution (positioning aids), and elimination of excessive moisture and drainage. Adequate nutrition, oxygenation, and fluid balance must be maintained.[3-5]

Superficial ulcers should be covered with flat, moisture-retaining dressings (e.g., hydrogel dressings) that cannot wrinkle and cause increased pressure or friction. Successful healing requires continued adequate relief of pressure. Large, deep pressure ulcers may require surgical débridement of necrotic tissue, opening of deep pockets for drainage, and repair with skin flaps. Infection requires treatment with antibiotics and pain should be controlled.[6,7]

Keloids and Hypertrophic Scars

Keloids are elevated, rounded, and firm with irregular clawlike margins that extend beyond the original site of injury. Hypertrophic scars are elevated erythematous fibrous lesions that do not extend beyond the border of injury. Both lesions are caused by abnormal wound healing with excessive fibroblast activity and collagen formation, and loss of control of normal tissue repair and regeneration.[8] Keloids are most common in darkly-pigmented skin types and generally appear within 1 year of trauma. Hypertrophic scars appear within 3 to 4 months and usually regress within 1 year. Genetic susceptibility is likely.[9]

Excessive or poorly aligned tension on a wound, introduction of foreign material into the skin, infection, and certain types of trauma (e.g., burns) are all provocative factors. Those parts of the body at risk include shoulders, back, chin, ears, and lower legs. Individuals 10 to 30 years of age develop lesions much more commonly than do prepubescent children or older adults.

Keloids start as pink or red, firm, well-defined, rubbery plaques that persist for several months after trauma. Later, uncontrolled overgrowth causes extension beyond the site of the original wound, and the overgrowth becomes smoother, irregularly shaped, hyperpigmented, harder, and more symptomatic. The fibrous tissue that accumulates in keloids is associated with increased cellularity and metabolic activity of fibroblasts. The tendency to form clawlike prolongations is typical (Figure 39-4).

Various treatments are available for the management of keloids and hypertrophic scars. There also is a need for research to improve treatment outcome.[10,11]

Pruritus

Pruritus, or itching, is a symptom associated with many primary skin disorders, such as eczema, psoriasis, or insect infestations, or it can be a manifestation of systemic disease (e.g., chronic renal failure, cholestatic liver disease, thyroid disorders, iron deficiency, neuropathies, or malignancy) or the use of opiate drugs. It may be localized or generalized and may move from one location to another.[12] Multiple stimuli can produce itching, and there is interaction between itch and pain sensations. Peripheral itch mediators include histamine, serotonin, prostaglandins, bradykinins, neuropeptides, acetylcholine, and interleukin-31. Small unmyelinated nerve fibers transmit itch sensations and specific spinal pathways may carry itch sensations to the brain.[13]

Management of localized itching depends on the cause, and the primary condition must be treated. Topical therapy, oral histamine H1-receptor antagonists, and phototherapy with ultraviolet (UV) radiation can target pruritus mechanisms in the skin. Antiepileptic drugs, opioid receptor antagonists, and antidepressants can block signal processing in the central nervous system (CNS).[14]

✔ QUICK CHECK 39-2

1. What areas are at greatest risk of pressure ulcers?
2. How does a keloid differ from a normal scar?
3. What stimulates pruritus?

DISORDERS OF THE SKIN

Disorders of the skin may be precipitated by trauma, abnormal cellular function, infection and inflammation, and systemic diseases.

Inflammatory Disorders

The most common inflammatory disorders of the skin are eczema and dermatitis. Eczema and dermatitis are general terms that describe a particular type of inflammatory response in the skin and can be used interchangeably. Eczematous disorders are generally characterized by pruritus, lesions with indistinct borders, and epidermal changes. These lesions can appear as erythema, papules, or scales; they can present in an acute, subacute, or chronic phase. Edema, serous discharge, and crusting occur with continued irritation and scratching. In chronic eczema, the skin becomes thickened, leathery, and hyperpigmented from recurrent irritation and scratching. The location of eczema is related to the underlying cause. Eczematous inflammations need to be differentiated from other rashes and dermatoses, particularly psoriasis.

Allergic Contact Dermatitis

Allergic contact dermatitis is a common form of cell-mediated or delayed hypersensitivity. (See Chapter 6 for different types of allergic responses.) The response is an interaction of skin barrier function, reaction to irritants, and neuronal responses, such as pruritus. Various allergens (e.g., microorganisms, chemicals, foreign proteins, latex, drugs, metals) can form the sensitizing antigen. Contact with poison ivy is a common example (Figure 39-5). As the allergen contacts the skin, the allergen is bound to a carrier protein, forming a sensitizing antigen. The Langerhans cells (dendritic cells) process the antigen and carry it to T cells. T cells then become sensitized to the antigen, inducing the release of inflammatory cytokines and the symptoms of dermatitis.[15]

In latex allergy, there is either a hypersensitivity to chemicals used in latex rubber processing or an increase in immunoglobulin E (IgE) antibodies in response to latex rubber protein.[16]

In delayed hypersensitivity, several hours pass before an immunologic response is apparent. The T cells play an important role because they differentiate and secrete lymphokines that affect macrophage movement and aggregation, coagulation, and other inflammatory responses (see Chapter 6). Sensitization usually develops with first exposure to the antigen, and symptoms of dermatitis occur with reexposure.

The manifestations of allergic contact dermatitis include erythema and swelling with pruritic (itching) vesicular lesions in the areas of allergen contact. The pattern of distribution provides clues to the source of the antigen (e.g., hands exposed to chemical solutions or boundaries from rings and bracelets). The antigen must be removed for the inflammatory response to resolve and tissue repair to begin. Treatment may require topical or systemic steroids.

Irritant Contact Dermatitis

Irritant contact dermatitis is a common nonimmunologically mediated inflammation of the skin that may promote systemic involvement. The severity of the inflammation is related to the concentration of the irritant, length of exposure, and disruption of the skin barrier. Chemical irritation from acids and prolonged exposure to soaps, detergents, and various agents used in industry can cause inflammatory lesions. The skin lesions resemble allergic contact dermatitis. Removing the source of irritation and using topical agents provide effective treatment.[17]

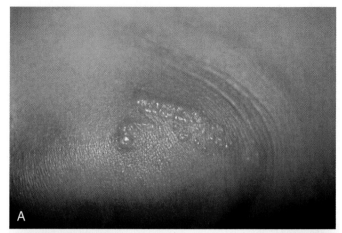
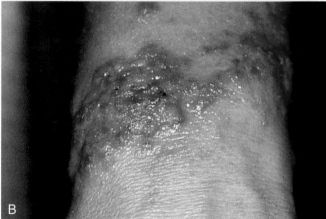

FIGURE 39-5 Poison Ivy. A, Poison ivy on knee. **B,** Poison ivy dermatitis. (Courtesy Department of Dermatology, School of Medicine, University of Utah, Salt Lake City, Utah.)

Atopic Dermatitis

Atopic dermatitis (allergic dermatitis) is common in individuals with a history of hay fever or asthma and is associated with IgE antibodies. It is more common in infancy and childhood; however, some individuals are affected throughout life. Specific details of this disorder are presented in Chapter 40 (p. 1071).

Stasis Dermatitis

Stasis dermatitis usually occurs on the legs as a result of venous stasis and edema and is associated with varicosities, phlebitis, and vascular trauma (see Chapter 23). First, erythema and pruritus develop and then scaling, petechiae, and hyperpigmentation. Progressive lesions become ulcerated, particularly around the ankles and tibia (Figure 39-6).

Treatment includes elevating the legs as often as possible, not wearing tight clothes around the legs, and not standing for long periods. Defined infections are treated with antibiotics. Chronic lesions with ulceration are treated with moist dressings, external compression, and vein ablation surgery.[18]

Seborrheic Dermatitis

Seborrheic dermatitis is a common chronic inflammation of the skin involving the scalp, eyebrows, eyelids, ear canals, nasolabial folds, axillae, chest, and back (Figure 39-7). In infants it is known as *cradle cap*. The cause is unknown, but an inflammatory reaction to *Malassezia* yeasts has been proposed.[19]

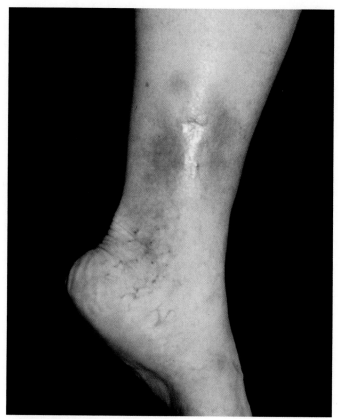

FIGURE 39-6 Stasis Ulcer. (Courtesy Department of Dermatology, School of Medicine, University of Utah, Salt Lake City, Utah.)

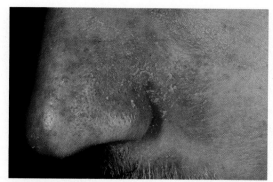

FIGURE 39-7 Seborrheic Dermatitis. (Courtesy Department of Dermatology, School of Medicine, University of Utah, Salt Lake City, Utah.)

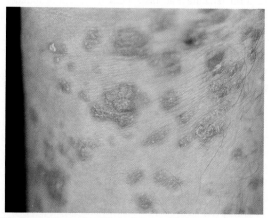

FIGURE 39-8 Psoriasis. Typical oval plaque with well-defined borders and silvery scale. (Courtesy Department of Dermatology, School of Medicine, University of Utah, Salt Lake City, Utah.)

The lesions appear from infancy to old age with periods of remission and exacerbation. The lesions appear as scaly, white or yellowish inflammatory plaques with mild pruritus. Mild cases are treated with shampoos containing sulfur, salicylic acid, or tar. Topical therapy includes antifungals and low-dose steroids. Corticosteroid applications suppress severe symptoms but should not be used for maintenance therapy.

Papulosquamous Disorders

Psoriasis, pityriasis rosea, and lichen planus are characterized by papules, scales, plaques, and erythema. Collectively they are described as papulosquamous disorders.

Psoriasis

Psoriasis is a chronic, relapsing, proliferative, inflammatory disorder that involves the skin, scalp, and nails and can occur at any age. Psoriasis affects 1% to 4% of the population. The onset is generally established by 20 years of age. A family history of psoriasis is often established and the genetic mechanisms are complex.[20] Inflammatory cytokines (i.e., interleukins, tumor necrosis factor-alpha [TNF-α]) from activated Th cells cause the lesions of psoriasis.[21]

Both the dermis and the epidermis are thickened with cellular hyperproliferation, altered keratinocyte differentiation, expanded dermal vasculature, infiltration of neutrophils and lymphocytes, and inflammation. The turnover time for shedding the epidermis is decreased to 3 to 4 days from the normal of 14 to 20 days, with many more germinative cells and increased transit time through the dermis. Cell maturation and keratinization are bypassed, and the epidermis thickens and plaques form. The loosely cohesive keratin gives the lesion a silvery appearance. Capillary dilation and increased vascularization accommodate the increased cell metabolism but also cause erythema. The disease can be mild, moderate, or severe, depending on the size, distribution, and inflammation of the lesions. Psoriasis is marked by remissions and exacerbations.

The types of psoriasis include plaque (psoriasis vulgaris), inverse, guttate, pustular, and erythrodermic. Plaque psoriasis (also called psoriasis vulgaris) is the most common and affects 80% to 90% of individuals with psoriasis. The typical plaque psoriatic lesion is a well-demarcated, thick, silvery, scaly, erythematous plaque surrounded by normal skin (Figure 39-8). Small erythematous papules enlarge and coalesce into larger inflammatory lesions on the face, scalp, elbows, and knees and at sites of trauma.

Inverse psoriasis involves lesions that develop in skin folds (i.e., axilla or groin). In guttate psoriasis, small papules appear suddenly on the trunk and extremities (Figure 39-9) a few weeks after a streptococcal respiratory tract infection. Guttate psoriasis may resolve spontaneously in weeks or months. Pustular psoriasis appears as blisters of noninfectious pus (collections of neutrophils) and erythrodermic (exfoliative) psoriasis is often accompanied by pruritus or pain with widespread red, scaling lesions that cover a large area of the body.

Psoriatic arthritis of hands, feet, knees, and ankle joints develops in 5% to 30% of cases. Psoriatic nail disease can occur in all psoriasis subtypes with pitting, onycholysis, subungual hyperkeratosis, and nail plate dystrophy. A number of comorbidities are associated with the inflammatory mechanisms of psoriasis (see *Health Alert*: Psoriasis and Comorbidities).

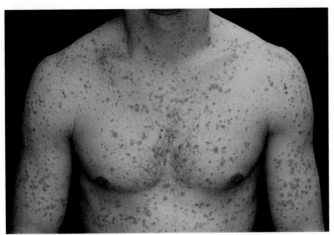

FIGURE 39-9 Guttate Psoriasis Following Streptococcal Infection. Numerous uniformly small lesions may abruptly occur following streptococcal pharyngitis. (Courtesy Department of Dermatology, School of Medicine, University of Utah, Salt Lake City, Utah.)

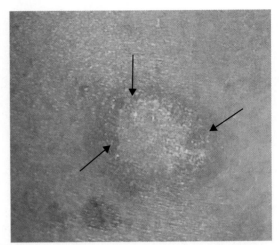

FIGURE 39-10 Pityriasis Rosea Herald Patch. A collarette pattern has formed around the margins *(arrows)*. (Courtesy Department of Dermatology, School of Medicine, University of Utah, Salt Lake City, Utah.)

HEALTH ALERT

Psoriasis and Comorbidities

In addition to skin and joint manifestations including rheumatoid arthritis, severe psoriasis is associated with inflammatory bowel disease metabolic syndrome, which includes hypertension, insulin resistance, dyslipidemias, abdominal obesity, and increased risk for atherosclerosis and myocardial infarction that is independent of traditional risk factors for these diseases. The underlying mechanisms are thought to be related to increased levels of proinflammatory mediators, such as tumor necrosis factor-alpha (TNF-α) and chemokines, which are central to the chronic inflammation, oxidative stress, and angiogenesis of psoriasis. The increased prevalence of cancer, particularly lymphoma, may be related to the pathogenesis of psoriasis or be a consequence of immune modulation therapies. Crohn disease also is associated with psoriasis and there may be a genetic overlap between these two diseases. Treatment considerations need to include screening, monitoring, and management of these comorbidities.

Data from Davidovici BB et al: Psoriasis and systemic inflammatory diseases: potential mechanistic links between skin disease and co-morbid conditions, *J Invest Dermatol* 130(7):1785–1796, 2010; Duarte GV et al: Psoriasis and obesity: literature review and recommendations for management, *Ann Bras Dermatol* 85(3):355–360, 2010; Piérard GE et al: The therapeutic potential of TNF-alpha antagonists for skin psoriasis comorbidities, *Expert Opin Biol Ther* 10(8):1197–1208, 2010; Farley E, Menter A: Psoriasis: comorbidities and associations, *G Ital Dermatol Venereol* 146(1):9-15, 2011.

Treatment is related to maintaining skin moisture, reducing epidermal cell turnover and pruritus, and, ensuring immunomodulation. Mild lesions are usually treated with emollients, keratolytic agents, and corticosteroids. Moderate to severe lesions may respond to ultraviolet light, methotrexate, acitretin, vitamin D analogs, and cyclosporin A. Biologics are used to treat moderate to severe disease including drugs that inhibit the activation and number of T lymphocytes or inhibit or suppress inflammatory cytokines.[22,23]

Pityriasis Rosea

Pityriasis rosea is a self-limiting inflammatory disorder that occurs more often in young adults, usually during the winter months. The cause is thought to be a herpes-like virus.[24] Pityriasis rosea begins as a single lesion (herald patch) that is circular, demarcated, and salmon-pink, approximately 3 to 4 cm in diameter, and usually located on the trunk. Early lesions are macular and papular. Secondary lesions develop within 14 to 21 days and extend over the trunk and upper part of the extremities (Figure 39-10), although rarely on the face. The small erythematous papules expand into characteristic oval lesions. The pattern of distribution follows the skin lines around the trunk and resembles a drooping pine tree. The scales are sloughed from the margin of the lesions, forming a collarette pattern. Itching is the most common symptom. Occasionally headache, fatigue, or sore throat precedes the development of the lesions.

The diagnosis of pityriasis rosea follows the clinical appearance of the lesion. It can be confused with secondary syphilis, psoriasis, or seborrheic dermatitis. The disorder is usually self-limiting and resolves in a few months with symptomatic treatment for pruritus. Ultraviolet light (with some risk for hyperpigmentation) or systemic corticosteroids may be used to control pruritus.[25]

Lichen Planus

Lichen planus is a benign autoimmune inflammatory disorder of the skin and mucous membranes. The age of onset is usually between 30 and 70 years. The cause may be an abnormal T cell–mediated immune response in which epithelial cells are recognized as foreign. Lichen planus also is linked to hepatitis C virus.[26] The disorder begins with nonscaling, violet-colored pruritic papules, 2 to 4 mm in size, usually located on the wrists, ankles, lower legs, and genitalia (Figure 39-11). The papules are flat-topped and have a polygonal shape. New lesions are pale pink and evolve into a dark violet color. Persistent lesions may be thickened and red, forming hypertrophic lichen planus. Oral lesions appear as lacy white rings that must be differentiated from leukoplakia or oral candidiasis.[27] Mucous membrane lesions also can develop on the penis and vulvovaginal area. Usually, oral lesions do not ulcerate, but localized or extensive painful ulcerations can occur, and there may be increased risk for oral cancer. Chronic ulcerated lesions become malignant in 1% of individuals with the disease.[28] Thinning and splitting of nails are common, and part or all of the nail may be shed.

Pruritus is the most distressing symptom. The lesions are self-limiting and may last for months or years, with an average duration of 6 to 18 months. Postinflammatory hyperpigmentation is a common consequence of the lesion. Approximately 20% of individuals have a recurrence.

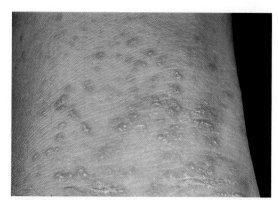

FIGURE 39-11 Hypertrophic Lichen Planus on Arms. (Courtesy Department of Dermatology, School of Medicine, University of Utah, Salt Lake City, Utah.)

Diagnosis is made by the clinical appearance of the lesion. Treatment is individualized. Antihistamines are given for itching and short-term use of topical or systemic corticosteroids may be used to control inflammation. Mucous membrane lesions are treated with topical steroids and topical immunosuppressants (tacrolimus, or pimecrolimus).

> **✔ QUICK CHECK 39-3**
> 1. Why does inflammation occur with contact dermatitis?
> 2. What factors are associated with atopic dermatitis?
> 3. What lesions are associated with papulosquamous disorders?
> 4. Give three examples of papulosquamous disorders.

Acne Vulgaris

Acne vulgaris is an inflammatory disorder of the pilosebaceous follicle (the sebaceous gland contiguous with a hair follicle) that usually occurs during adolescence. It is discussed in Chapter 40 (p. 1070).

Acne Rosacea

Acne rosacea is a chronic inflammation of the skin that develops in middle-aged adults; it has four subtypes: erythematotelangiectatic, papulopustular, phymatous, and ocular (eyelids and ocular surface). The exact cause is unknown but an altered innate immune response is involved.[29] The most common lesions are erythema, papules, pustules, and telangiectasia. They occur in the middle third of the face, including the forehead, nose, cheeks, and chin (Figure 39-12). The lesions are associated with chronic, inappropriate vasodilation resulting in flushing and sun sensitivity. Sebaceous hypertrophy, fibrosis, and telangiectasia may be severe enough to produce an irreversible bulbous appearance of the nose (rhinophyma). Disorders of the eye often accompany rosacea, particularly conjunctivitis and keratitis, which can result in visual impairment. Facial application of fluorinated topical steroids may increase the severity of telangiectasias.

Hot drinks or alcohol should be consumed cautiously because the heat and vasodilation accentuate erythema. Photoprotection, using sunscreens, is essential. Therapeutic options for rosacea include topical agents, oral tetracycline, doxycycline, vitamin D receptor antagonists, and laser and light treatments. Surgical excision of excessive tissue may be required for rhinophyma.[30]

Lupus Erythematosus

Lupus erythematosus is an autoimmune, systemic, inflammatory disease that expresses cutaneous manifestations. Discoid, or cutaneous, lupus erythematosus (DLE) is limited to the skin and can progress to

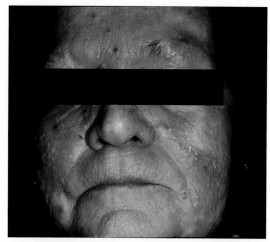

FIGURE 39-12 Granulomatous Rosacea. Pustules and erythema occur on the forehead, cheeks, and nose. (Courtesy Department of Dermatology, School of Medicine, University of Utah, Salt Lake City, Utah.)

systemic lupus erythematosus in about 5% of cases.[31] (Systemic lupus erythematosus [SLE], a diffuse, multisystem disease, is discussed in Chapter 7.)

Discoid (cutaneous) lupus erythematosus. Discoid (cutaneous) lupus erythematosus (DLE) usually occurs in genetically susceptible adults, particularly women in their late thirties or early forties, but people of any age can be affected. The disease can be acute, subacute, or chronic. The lesions may be single or multiple and of various sizes. Often the lesions are located on light-exposed areas of the skin, and photosensitivity is common. The face is the most common site of lesion involvement with a butterfly pattern of distribution found over the nose and cheeks.[32]

The cause is related to both genetic and environmental factors and is thought to be an altered immune response to an unknown antigen or to ultraviolet wavelengths. Autoantibodies and immune complexes cause tissue damage[33] (Figure 39-13). On skin biopsy with immunofluorescent observation, there are lumpy deposits of immunoglobulins, especially IgM.

The early lesion is asymmetric, with a 1- to 2-cm raised red plaque with a brownish scale. The scale penetrates the hair follicle and leaves a visible follicle opening (carpet-tack appearance) when removed. The lesions persist for months and then resolve spontaneously or atrophy. Healing progresses from the center of the lesion, with a residual telangiectasia and hypopigmented scarring. Atrophy of the dermis and epidermis can cause a depressed scar. Other symptoms of cutaneous lupus erythematosus include alopecia (hair loss), telangiectasias, urticaria (i.e., hives), and Raynaud phenomenon. Raynaud phenomenon is characterized by an initial stage of vasospasm that leads to white, numb, and cold digits followed by cyanosis and then a reactive hyperemia as the vasospasm relaxes.[34]

Vesiculobullous Disorders

Vesiculobullous skin disorders share a common characteristic of vesicle, or blister, formation. Two such diseases are pemphigus and erythema multiforme.

Pemphigus

Pemphigus (meaning to blister or bubble) is a rare autoimmune blistering disease of the skin and oral mucous membranes caused by circulating autoantibodies directed against the cell surface adhesion

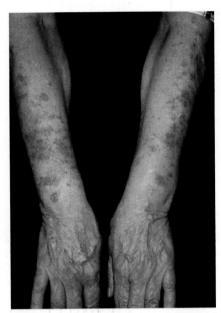

FIGURE 39-13 Subacute Cutaneous Lupus (Discoid Lupus Erythematosus). (Courtesy Department of Dermatology, School of Medicine, University of Utah, Salt Lake City, Utah.)

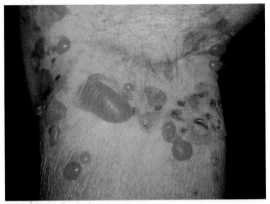

FIGURE 39-14 Bullous Pemphigoid. Generalized eruption with blisters arising from an edematous, erythematous annular base. (Courtesy Department of Dermatology, School of Medicine, University of Utah, Salt Lake City, Utah.)

molecule desmoglein at the desmosomal cell junction in the suprabasal layer in the epidermis. Immunoglobulin G (IgG) autoantibodies and C3 complement bind to the desmoglein adhesion molecules, resulting in the destruction of cell-to-cell adhesion (acantholysis) in the basal layer of the epidermis (see Table 39-1) with fluid accumulation and the resulting symptom of blister formation[35] (Figure 39-14). Pemphigus can occur in all age groups but is more prevalent in persons between 40 and 50 years of age. Pemphigus presents in varying forms:

- **Pemphigus vulgaris** is the most common form. Oral lesions precede the onset of skin blistering, which is more prominent on the face, scalp, and axilla. The blisters rupture easily because of the thin, fragile overlying portion of the epidermis.
- **Pemphigus vegetans** is a variant of pemphigus vulgaris in which large blisters develop in tissue folds of the axilla and groin.
- **Pemphigus foliaceus** is a milder form of the disease and involves acantholysis at the more superficial, subcorneal level of the epidermis (see Table 39-1) with blistering, erosions, scaling, crusting, and erythema usually of the face and chest. Oral mucous membranes are rarely involved.
- **Pemphigus erythematosus** is a subset of pemphigus foliaceus often associated with system lupus erythematosus with positive antinuclear antibodies. The lesions are generally less widely distributed.

The diagnosis of pemphigus is established by the clinical manifestations and by histologic examination of the skin. Immunofluorescence demonstrates the presence of antibodies at the site of blister formation. The clinical course of the disease may range from rapidly fatal to relatively benign. The primary treatment for pemphigus is systemic corticosteroids in combination with adjuvant immunosuppressants. Newer methods of treatment and a clearer understanding of the pathogenesis have improved the prognosis and decreased mortality.[36]

Erythema Multiforme

Erythema multiforme is a syndrome characterized by inflammation of the skin and mucous membranes, often associated with immunologic reactions to a drug or microorganisms. **Bullous erythema multiforme** involves the mucous membranes. It is relatively rare and can occur at any age but occurs more often in individuals between 20 and 40 years of age. Immune complex formation and deposition of C3, IgM, and fibrinogen around the superficial dermal blood vessels, basement membrane, and keratinocytes are found in most individuals with erythema multiforme. Edema develops in the superficial dermis, so vesicles and bullae form. The lesions vary in clinical presentation and may involve the skin or mucous membranes, or both. The characteristic "bull's-eye," or "target," lesions occur on the skin surface with a central erythematous region surrounded by concentric rings of alternating edema and inflammation. The lesions usually occur suddenly in groups over a period of 2 to 3 weeks. Urticarial plaques, 1 to 2 cm in diameter, can develop without the target lesion. A vesiculobullous form is characterized by mucous membrane lesions and erythematous plaques on the extensor surfaces of the extremities. Single or multiple vesicles or bullae may arise on a part of the plaque accompanied by pruritus and burning. The lesions heal within 3 to 4 weeks.

The most common forms of erythema multiforme are usually associated with severe drug reactions and include **Stevens-Johnson syndrome** (severe mucocutaneous bullous form involving 10% of body surface area) and **toxic epidermal necrolysis (TEN)** (severe mucocutaneous bullous form involving 30% of body surface area). An immune mechanism is probably related to drug reactions (see Chapter 40 for pediatric considerations).[37]

Prodromal symptoms of fever, headache, malaise, sore throat, and cough develop in approximately one third of the cases. The bullous lesions form erosions and crusts when they rupture. There is necrosis of the epidermis in TEN. The mouth, air passages, esophagus, urethra, and conjunctiva may be involved. Blindness can result from corneal ulcerations. Difficulty eating, breathing, and urinating may develop with severe manifestations. The disease can involve the kidneys and extend from the upper respiratory passages into the lungs. Severe forms of the disease can be fatal.

Diagnosis follows (1) recognition of the target lesion or by skin biopsy if the target lesion is absent and (2) medication history. Mild acute forms of the disease last 10 to 14 days and require no treatment. Ongoing drug therapy should be reevaluated and underlying infections treated. Topical or oral steroids may be prescribed. Fluid and electrolyte balance should be monitored in severe forms of the disease, and mucous membranes should be carefully managed with a bland diet, warm saline eyewashes, topical anesthetics, or corticosteroids to maintain comfort and prevent infection. Cutaneous blisters can be treated with wet compresses of Burow solution. Ophthalmic, kidney, and lung involvement require special care. Resolution occurs in 8 to 10 days, usually without scarring. Mucosal lesions may take 6 weeks to heal.

> **✔ QUICK CHECK 39-4**
> 1. Describe the inflammatory lesion associated with lupus erythematosus.
> 2. Compare the three forms of pemphigus.
> 3. What is the characteristic lesion of erythema multiforme?

Infections

Cutaneous infections are common forms of skin disease. They generally remain localized, although serious complications can develop with systemic involvement. The types of skin infection include bacterial, viral, and fungal. Most infections occur superficially; however, systemic signs and symptoms occasionally develop and can be life-threatening. The commensal (normal) flora of the skin consists of aerobes, yeast, and anaerobes. These flora often provide protection against pathogens that cause skin infections, including *Staphylococcus* and *Streptococcus*.

Bacterial Infections

Most bacterial infections of the skin are caused by local invasion of pathogens. Coagulase-positive *Staphylococcus aureus* and, less often, β-hemolytic streptococci are the common causative microorganisms.[38] Community-acquired methicillin-resistant *Staphylococcus aureus* (CA-MRSA) also is a cause of serious skin infection, particularly skin abcesses.[39]

Folliculitis. Folliculitis is a bacterial infection of the hair follicle. *S. aureus* commonly causes the infection, which develops from proliferation of the microorganism around the opening of the follicle with distribution into the follicle. Inflammation is caused by the release of chemotactic factors and enzymes from the bacteria. The lesions appear as pustules with a surrounding area of erythema. They are most prominent on the scalp and extremities and rarely cause systemic symptoms. Prolonged skin moisture, skin trauma, and poor hygiene are associated contributing factors. Cleaning with soap and water and topical application of antibiotics are effective treatments.

Furuncles and carbuncles. Furuncles, or "boils," are inflammations of hair follicles (Figure 39-15). They may develop after folliculitis that spreads through the follicular wall into the surrounding dermis. The invading microorganism is usually *S. aureus*. The infecting strain may spread to the skin from the anterior nares. Any skin area with hair can be infected, and one or several lesions may be present. The initial lesion is a deep, firm, red, painful nodule 1 to 5 cm in diameter. Within a few days, the erythematous nodules change to a large, fluctuant, and tender cystic nodule accompanied by cellulitis. No systemic symptoms are present, and the lesion may drain large amounts of pus and necrotic tissue.

Carbuncles are a collection of infected hair follicles and usually occur on the back of the neck, the upper back, and the lateral thighs. The lesion begins in the subcutaneous tissue and lower dermis as a firm mass that evolves into an erythematous, painful, swollen mass that drains through many openings. Abscesses may develop. Chills, fever, and malaise can occur during the early stages of lesion development.

Furuncles and carbuncles are treated with warm compresses to provide comfort and promote localization and spontaneous drainage. Abscess formation requires incision and drainage, and recurrent infections are treated with systemic antibiotics.

Cellulitis. Cellulitis is an infection of the dermis and subcutaneous tissue usually caused by *Staphylococcus aureus*.[40] Cellulitis can occur as an extension of a skin wound, as an ulcer, or from furuncles

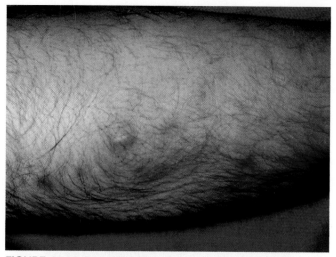

FIGURE 39-15 Furuncle of the Forearm. (Courtesy Department of Dermatology, School of Medicine, University of Utah, Salt Lake City, Utah.)

or carbuncles. The infected area is warm, erythematous, swollen, and painful. The infection is usually in the lower extremities and responds to systemic antibiotics, as well as therapy to relieve pain. Cellulitis also can be associated with other diseases including chronic venous insufficiency and stasis dermatitis.

Erysipelas. Erysipelas is an acute superficial infection of the upper dermis most often caused by group A β-hemolytic streptococci. The face, ears, and lower legs are involved. Chills, fever, and malaise precede the onset of lesions by 4 hours to 20 days. The initial lesions appear as firm, red spots that enlarge and coalesce to form a clearly circumscribed, advancing, bright red, hot lesion with a raised border. Vesicles may appear over the lesion and at the border. Pruritus, burning, and tenderness are present. Cold compresses provide symptomatic relief, and systemic antibiotics are required to arrest the infection.

Impetigo. Impetigo is a superficial lesion of the skin that is caused by coagulase-positive *Staphylococcus* or β-hemolytic streptococci. The disease occurs in adults but is more common in children (see Chapter 40, p. 1072).

Viral Infections

Herpes simplex virus. Skin infections with herpes simplex virus (HSV) are commonly caused by two types of HSV: HSV-1 and HSV-2. Either type can occur in different parts of the body, including oral and genital locations. Their differences are distinguished by laboratory tests. HSV-1 is generally associated with oral infections (cold sore or fever blister) or infection of the cornea (herpes keratitis), mouth (gingivostomatitis), and orolabia (lips/labialis), but it can also cause genital herpes. HSV-1 is transmitted by contact with infected saliva. With initial infection or primary infection, the virus is imbedded in sensory nerve endings and it moves by retrograde axonal transport to the dorsal root ganglion, where the virus develops lifelong latency. During the secondary phase, the lesions occur at the same site from reactivation of the virus. The virus travels down the peripheral nerve to the site of the original infection, where it is shed. Exposure to ultraviolet light, skin irritation, fever, fatigue, or stress may cause reactivation.[41]

The lesions for HSV-1 appear as a rash or clusters of inflamed and painful vesicles (e.g., within the mouth, over the tongue, on the lips, around the nose) (Figure 39-16). Increased sensitivity, paresthesias, and mild burning may occur before onset of the lesions. The vesicles

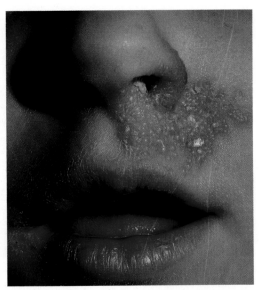

FIGURE 39-16 Herpes Simplex of the Lips (Labialis). Typical presentation with tense vesicles appearing on the lips and extending onto the skin. (From Habif TP: *Clinical dermatology: a color guide to diagnosis and therapy*, ed 4, St Louis, 2004, Mosby.)

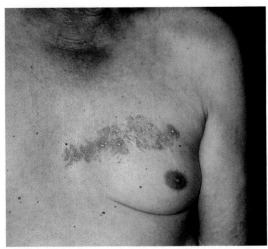

FIGURE 39-17 Herpes Zoster. Diffuse involvement of a dermatome. (Courtesy Department of Dermatology, School of Medicine, University of Utah, Salt Lake City, Utah.)

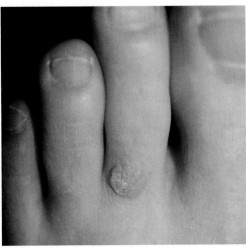

FIGURE 39-18 Verruca Vulgaris (Near Toes). (Courtesy Department of Dermatology, School of Medicine, University of Utah, Salt Lake City, Utah.)

rupture, forming a crust. Lesions may last from 2 to 6 weeks. Treatment is symptomatic and lesions usually resolve within 2 weeks.

Genital infections are more commonly caused by HSV-2. The virus is spread by skin-to-skin mucous membrane contact during viral shedding. Risk of infection is high in immunosuppressed persons or in persons who have sexual contact with infected individuals. Vertical transmission from mother to neonate is associated with significant neonatal morbidity and mortality.[42] The initial infection is asymptomatic. With recurrent exposure, the lesions begin as small vesicles that progress to ulceration within 3 to 4 days with pain, itching, and weeping.

Treatment is symptomatic and includes topical or oral antiviral agents. A vaccine has been effective in controlling recurrent infection, and progress is being made with prophylactic vaccines.[43]

Herpes zoster and varicella. Herpes zoster (shingles) and varicella (chickenpox) are caused by the same herpesvirus—varicella-zoster virus (VZV). Varicella occurs as a primary infection followed years later by activation of the virus to cause herpes zoster (shingles). During this time, the virus remains latent in trigeminal and dorsal root ganglia.

Herpes zoster has initial symptoms of pain and paresthesia localized to the affected dermatome (the cutaneous area innervated by a single spinal nerve; see Chapter 12), followed by vesicular eruptions that follow a facial, cervical, or thoracic lumbar dermatome (Figure 39-17). Local symptoms are alleviated with compresses, calamine lotion, or baking soda. Approximately 20% of individuals experience postherpetic neuralgia (pain) with reactivation of the virus.[44] Antiviral drugs, tricyclic antidepressants, and analgesics are helpful treatments.[45] The varicella vaccine is safe and effective in both children and adults. In children, the vaccine is given to prevent chickenpox and in adults, particularly the elderly, the vaccine is given to prevent herpes zoster (shingles).[46]

Warts. Warts (verrucae) are benign lesions of the skin caused by the many different types of human papillomavirus (HPV) that infect the stratified epithelium of skin and mucous membranes. The lesions are round and elevated with a rough, grayish surface, and they can occur anywhere on the skin. Warts are transmitted by touch. Common warts (verruca vulgaris) occur most often in children and are usually on the fingers, although they may be located on any skin surface or mucous membrane (Figure 39-18). Warts vary in shape, size (flat, round, or fusiform), and location and are commonly treated with cryotherapy or topical salicylic acid.[47] Plantar warts are usually located at pressure points on the bottom of the feet.

Condylomata acuminata (venereal warts) are an epidermal manifestation of subtypes of human papillomavirus (HPV) infection. It is a highly contagious, sexually transmitted disease. The cauliflower-like lesions occur in moist areas, along the glans of the penis, vulva, and anus. Oncogenic types of HPV that are a primary cause of cervical and other types of cancer (see Chapter 32) are not the same types of HPV that cause condylomata acuminata.

Fungal Infections

The fungi causing superficial skin infections are called *dermatophytes*, and they thrive on keratin (stratum corneum, hair, nails). Fungal disorders are known as *mycoses*; when caused by dermatophytes, the mycoses are termed *tinea* (dermatophytosis or ringworm).

Tinea infections. Tinea infections are classified according to their location on the body. The most common sites are summarized in

TABLE 39-4	COMMON SITES OF TINEA INFECTIONS	
SITE	**CLINICAL MANIFESTATIONS**
Tinea capitis (scalp)	Scaly, pruritic scalp with bald areas; hair breaks easily
Tinea corporis (skin areas, excluding scalp, face, hands, feet, groin)	Circular, clearly circumscribed, mildly erythematous scaly patches with slightly elevated ring-like border; some forms are dry and macular, and other forms are moist and vesicular
Tinea cruris (groin, also known as "jock itch")	Small, erythematous, and scaling vesicular patches with well-defined borders that spread over inner and upper surfaces of thighs; occurs with heat and high humidity
Tinea pedis (foot; also known as "athlete's foot")	Occurs between toes and may spread to soles of feet, nails, and skin or toes; slight scaling; macerated, painful skin, occasionally with fissures and vesiculation
Tinea manus (hand)	Dry, scaly, erythematous lesions, or moist, vesicular lesions that begin with clusters of intensely pruritic, clear vesicles; often associated with fungal infection of feet
Tinea unguium or onychomycosis (nails)	Superficial or deep inflammation of nail that develops yellow-brown accumulations of brittle keratin over all or portions of nail

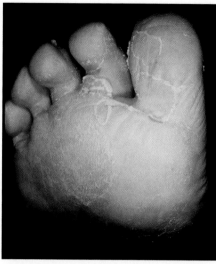

FIGURE 39-19 Tinea Pedis. Inflammation has extended from the web area onto the dorsum of the foot. (Courtesy Department of Dermatology, School of Medicine, University of Utah, Salt Lake City, Utah.)

The accumulation of inflammatory cells and scale produces a whitish yellow curdlike substance over the infected area. The lesion ceases to spread when it reaches dry skin.[50] Treatments include topical or systemic antifungal agents.

Vascular Disorders

Vascular abnormalities are commonly associated with skin diseases; they may be congenital or may involve vascular responses to local or systemic vasoactive substances. Blood vessels may increase in number, dilate, constrict, or become obliterated by disease processes.

Cutaneous Vasculitis

Vasculitis (angiitis) is an inflammation of the blood vessel wall that can result in bleeding aneurysm formation, or occlusion with ischemia or infection. The extensive vascular bed in the skin results in the involvement of vasculitic syndromes that may be localized and self-limiting or generalized with multiorgan involvement. The initiating site may be the blood, the vessel wall, or the adjacent tissue. Small vessels are usually affected.

Cutaneous vasculitis develops from the deposit of immune complexes in small blood vessels as a toxic response to drugs (phenothiazines, barbiturates, sulfonamides) or allergens, as a response to streptococcal or viral infection, or as a component of systemic vasculitic syndromes. The deposits activate complement, which is chemotactic for polymorphonuclear leukocytes.

The disorder is also known as *cutaneous leukocytoclastic angiitis* (from the presence of leukocytes in and around vessel walls). A systemic form (cutaneous systemic vasculitis) can involve other organs, including the kidneys, lungs, and gastrointestinal tract. The pattern of skin involvement includes palpable purpura in the lower legs and feet (from the leakage of blood from damaged vessels) that may progress to hemorrhagic bullae with necrosis and ulceration from occlusion of the vessel. Lesions appear in clusters and persist for 1 to 4 weeks. The disease may be self-limiting and occur as a single episode. Biopsy confirms the diagnosis.

Identifying and removing the antigen (chemical, drug, or source of infection) is the first step of treatment. Corticosteroids and immunosuppressants may be used when symptoms are severe.[51]

Table 39-4. **Tinea unguium** is a fungal infection of the nails. **Tinea pedis (athlete's foot)** is a chronic, superficial fungal infection of the skin of the foot common in adults (Figure 39-19).

Tinea is diagnosed by culture, microscopic examination of skin scrapings prepared with potassium hydroxide wet mount, or observation of the skin with an ultraviolet light (Wood lamp). Cultures establish the particular type of fungus; these are necessary for diagnosis of hair and nail infections. Fungi have characteristic spores and filaments known as *hyphae* that are more prominent when prepared in potassium hydroxide. The spores fluoresce blue-green when exposed to ultraviolet light. Treatment is related to the type of fungi and includes both topical and systemic antifungal medication.[48]

Candidiasis. Candidiasis is caused by the yeastlike fungus *Candida albicans* and normally can be found on mucous membranes, on the skin, in the gastrointestinal tract, and in the vagina. *C. albicans* can, under certain circumstances, change from a commensal (normal) microorganism to a pathogen, particularly in the critically ill and those who are immunosuppressed.[49]

Factors that predispose to infection include (1) local environment of moisture, warmth, maceration, or occlusion; (2) systemic administration of antibiotics; (3) pregnancy; (4) diabetes mellitus; (5) Cushing disease; (6) debilitated states; (7) infants younger than 6 months of age, as a result of decreased immune reactivity; (8) immunosuppressed persons; and (9) certain neoplastic diseases of the blood and monocyte/macrophage system. The commensal (normal) bacteria on the skin, mainly cocci, inhibit proliferation of *C. albicans*. *C. albicans* can activate the complement system by the alternative pathway and produce small abscesses. Candidiasis affects only the outer layers of mucous membranes and skin and occurs in the mouth, vagina, uncircumcised penis, and large skin folds. Table 39-5 lists the points of differentiation of various sites of candidiasis habitation.

The initial lesion is a thin-walled pustule that extends under the stratum corneum with an inflammatory base that may burn or itch.

TABLE 39-5	SITES OF CANDIDIASIS INFECTION		
SITE	**RISK FACTORS**	**CLINICAL MANIFESTATIONS**	**TREATMENT**
Vagina (vulvovaginitis)	Heat, moisture, occlusive clothing Pregnancy Systemic antibiotic therapy Diabetes mellitus Sexual intercourse with infected male	Vaginal itching; white, watery, or creamy discharge Red, swollen vaginal and labial membranes with erosions Lesions may spread to anus and groin	Miconazole cream Clotrimazole tablets or cream Nystatin tablets Ketoconazole cream Loose cotton clothing
Penis (balanitis)	Uncircumcised Sexual intercourse with infected female	Pinpoint, red, tender papules and pustules on glans and shaft of penis	Any of creams listed above Topical steroids for severe inflammation
Mouth	Diabetes mellitus Immunosuppressive therapy Inhaled steroid therapy	Red, swollen, painful tongue and oral mucous membranes Localized erosions and plaques appear with chronic infection	Nystatin oral suspension Clotrimazole troches Ketoconazole

Urticaria

Urticaria (hives) is a circumscribed area of raised erythema and edema of the superficial dermis. Urticarial lesions are most commonly associated with type I hypersensitivity reactions to drugs (penicillin, aspirin), certain foods (strawberries, shellfish), systemic diseases (intestinal parasites, lupus erythematosus), or physical agents (heat or cold) (see Chapter 7). The lesions are mediated by histamine release from sensitized mast cells or basophils, or both, which causes the endothelial cells of skin blood vessels to contract. The leakage of fluid from the vessel appears as wheals, welts, or hives, and there may be few or many that may be distributed over the entire body. Most lesions resolve spontaneously within 24 hours, but new lesions may appear. All possible causes of the reaction should be removed. Antihistamines usually reduce hives and provide relief of itching. Corticosteroids and β-adrenergic agonists may be required for severe attacks. Chronic urticaria (recurrent wheals for more than 6 weeks) is either idiopathic or autoimmune in origin. Angioedema (welts or swelling of the skin) is associated with both groups. The autoimmune group has histamine-releasing autoantibodies and may have antithyroid antibodies.[52]

Scleroderma (Systemic Sclerosis)

Scleroderma means *sclerosis of the skin* and is an autoimmune disease. The disease is associated with vascular, immunologic, and fibrotic processes and is more prominent in women. The etiology is unknown. Genetic predisposition, autoimmunity, and an immune reaction to a toxic substance are possible initiating mechanisms of the disease. Autoantibodies are often recovered from the skin and serum of individuals with scleroderma. Impaired regulation of collagen gene expression by fibroblasts probably underlies the persistent fibrosis.[53]

The systemic form (systemic sclerosis) involves the connective tissues of the skin and many organs, including the kidneys, gastrointestinal tract, and lungs. There are massive deposits of type I collagen with fibrosis, accompanied by inflammatory reactions, vascular changes in the capillary network with a decrease in the number of capillary loops, dilation of the remaining capillaries, perivascular infiltrates, occlusion, and ischemia.[54]

The clinical features of scleroderma can be summarized using the CREST acronym as a guide:

Calcinosis—calcium deposits in the subcutaneous tissue that cause pain

Raynaud phenomenon—episodes of arteriolar vasoconstriction or spasm in response to cold or stress

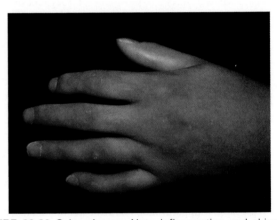

FIGURE 39-20 Scleroderma. Note inflammation and shiny skin resulting from a combination of Raynaud phenomena and scleroderma affecting the fingers (acrosclerosis). (Courtesy Department of Dermatology, School of Medicine, University of Utah, Salt Lake City, Utah.)

Esophageal changes—swallowing difficulty related to acid reflux and increased esophageal fibrosis

Sclerodactyly—tightening of skin over the fingers and toes leading to tapering of the digits with scarring and tissue atrophy

Telangiectasias—dilation of capillaries causing small (0.5 cm) red marks on skin surface

The cutaneous lesions are most often on the face and hands, the neck, and the upper chest, although the entire skin can be involved. The skin is hard, hypopigmented, taut, shiny, and tightly connected to the underlying tissue. The tightness of the facial skin projects an immobile masklike appearance, and the mouth may not open completely. The nose may assume a beaklike appearance. The hands are shiny and sometimes red and edematous (Figure 39-20). Progression to body organs may occur, and death is caused by subsequent respiratory failure, renal failure, cardiac dysrhythmias, or esophageal or intestinal obstruction or perforation.

Suitable clothing and a warm environment are essential for protecting the hands. Trauma and smoking should be avoided. Vasodilator drugs or sympathectomy rarely has lasting effects. There is no specific treatment. Targeted immunomodulatory therapies, tyrosine kinase inhibitors, and agents that promote vascular repair are under investigation.[55] Survival is improving with advances in the understanding of pathogenesis and treatment.[56]

Insect Bites

Insect bites and stings are the cause of local and systemic toxic and allergic hypersensitivity reactions (see Chapter 7). Local reactions include immediate pain, itching, and swelling. Systemic responses include generalized pruritus, hives, or life-threatening anaphylaxis. Bites from scabies mites, lice, fleas, ticks (including Lyme disease), and bedbugs are discussed in Chapter 40. Other bites and stings are discussed next.

Mosquitoes, Flies, Bees, and Ants

There are thousands of species of **mosquitoes** throughout the world. Species from the Culicidae family are responsible for malaria, yellow fever, dengue fever, filariasis, and St. Louis encephalitis. Mosquitoes can bite through thin, loose clothing and are attracted to warmth and sweat. The edema, pruritus, and papular lesions of the mosquito bite are caused by the disruption of the skin that results from the insertion of a blood tube by a female mosquito. Irritating salivary secretions also contain anticoagulants. Reactions vary depending on the sensitivity of the victim.

Several species of **flies** are bloodsuckers. The blackfly (Simuliidae family) is usually found in swarms, near moving bodies of water in the late spring and early summer, and is a vicious biter. The initial bite is painless because the fly injects an anesthetic while biting. Subsequent lesions are painful and accompanied by significant swelling of surrounding tissues. Systemic reactions, such as fever, headache, and nausea, are common.

Very small flies of the Ceratopogonidae family, also known as *no-see-ums, midges, punkies,* or *sand fleas,* also are bloodsuckers. The bite of the female is particularly miserable and produces immediate pain, erythema, and vesicles. Pruritus and vesicular reactions may persist for weeks.

The fiercest blood-sucking flies are the Tabanidae, or horseflies, deerflies, gadflies, greenheads, and clegs. These flies vary in size from 1 to 5 cm and produce painful, bleeding bites because of their large mouthparts. The bites produce urticaria that may be accompanied by weakness, dizziness, and wheezing.

Bees, wasps, hornets, yellow jackets, and ants are stinging insects. The stinger is implanted in the skin with the release of venom. The stinger should be flicked away and not pinched and pulled, which releases more venom. Reactions to venom can be localized or generalized depending on individual sensitivity. Wounds produced by biting insects should be cleansed with soap and water and a local antiseptic applied. Local applications of steroid creams or antihistamine will alleviate symptoms. Systemic reactions may require emergency care and administration of epinephrine.[57]

Benign Tumors

Most benign tumors of the skin are associated with aging. Benign tumors include seborrheic keratosis, keratoacanthoma, actinic keratosis, and moles.

Seborrheic Keratosis

Seborrheic keratosis is a benign proliferation of cutaneous basal cells that produces flat or slightly elevated lesions that may be smooth or warty in appearance. The pathogenesis is unknown. They are usually

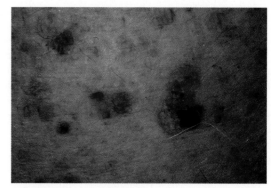

FIGURE 39-21 Seborrheic Keratosis. Typical lesion that is broad, flat, and comparatively smooth surfaced. (Courtesy Department of Dermatology, School of Medicine, University of Utah, Salt Lake City, Utah.)

seen in older people and occur as multiple lesions on the chest, back, and face. The color varies from tan to waxy yellow, flesh colored, or dark brown-black. Lesion size varies from a few millimeters to several centimeters, and they are often oval and greasy appearing with a hyperkeratotic scale (Figure 39-21). Cryotherapy with liquid nitrogen and laser therapy are effective treatments.[58]

Keratoacanthoma

A **keratoacanthoma** is a benign, self-limiting tumor of squamous cell differentiation arising from hair follicles. It usually occurs on sun-damaged skin of elderly individuals and smokers. Incidence is highest among smokers and males. The most commonly affected sites are the face, back of the hands, forearms, neck, and legs. The lesion develops over a period of 1 to 2 months with a histologic pattern resembling squamous cell carcinoma[59]:
1. *Proliferative stage:* Lesion appears as a rapid-growing, dome-shaped nodule with a central crust.
2. *Mature stage:* Lesion fills with whitish-colored keratin and requires differentiation from squamous cell carcinoma.
3. *Involution stage:* Occurs over a 3- to 4-month period with regression of the lesion.

Although the lesions will resolve spontaneously, they can be removed by curettage or excision to improve cosmetic appearance.

Actinic Keratosis

Actinic keratosis is a premalignant lesion composed of aberrant proliferations of epidermal keratinocytes caused by prolonged exposure to ultraviolet radiation. The prevalence is highest in individuals with unprotected, light-colored skin and is rare in those with black skin. The lesions appear as rough, poorly defined papules, which may be felt more than seen. Surrounding areas may have telangiectasias. Freezing with liquid nitrogen provides quick, effective treatment. Topical modulators, such as 5-fluorouracil, diclofenac sodium gel, or imiquimod cream, are prescribed.[60]

Excisions also may be performed, providing tissue for cellular analysis. The lesions should continue to be evaluated for progression to squamous cell carcinoma. Protection from the sun with clothing or a sun-blocking agent to prevent lesions from developing elsewhere is advised.

Nevi (Moles)

Nevi (sing., **nevus**) (also known as moles or birthmarks) are benign pigmented or nonpigmented lesions. Melanocytic nevus, formed from melanocytes, may be congenital or acquired. During the early stages of development, the cells accumulate at the junction of the dermis and epidermis and are macular lesions. Over time, the cells move deeper into the dermis and the nevi become nodular and palpable. Nevi may appear on any part of the skin and vary in size. They occur singly or in groups. Nevi may undergo transition to malignant melanoma (see p. 1060).[61] Nevi irritated by clothing or large lesions may be excised.

✔ **QUICK CHECK 39-6**
1. List two diseases caused by insect bites.
2. Compare keratoacanthoma and actinic keratosis.

Cancer

Skin cancers are the most prevalent form of cancer in the United States. The most common types are basal cell carcinoma and squamous cell carcinoma with 1 million cases occurring annually. An estimated 11,790 people die of skin cancer each year, 8700 from malignant melanoma.[62] Important trends related to skin cancer are described in Box 39-1.

Ultraviolet radiation causes most skin cancers.[63] Protection from the sun, particularly during the childhood years of life, significantly reduces the risk of skin cancer in later years. Areas widely exposed to the sun's rays—the face, neck, and hands—are highly vulnerable for such lesions (see *Health Alert:* Skin Photoprotection from the Inside Out). Outdoor workers (farmers, sailors, fishermen, construction workers) are high-risk skin cancer populations. Box 39-1 summarizes the risk factors for skin cancer.[64]

HEALTH ALERT

Skin Photoprotection from the Inside Out

Chronic exposure to ultraviolet (UV) radiation is associated with basal cell, squamous cell, and melanoma skin cancers; premature skin aging; and actinic keratosis. UV radiation is carcinogenic by suppressing cutaneous antitumor immunity and by causing mutations in skin keratinocytes. Normally, skin keratinocytes have several mechanisms of protection from UV radiation. DNA-damaged keratinocytes can undergo repair or apoptosis (programmed cell death) with elimination by macrophages. The damaged cells also secrete inflammatory cytokines that recruit T cells that recognize and eliminate the damaged cells. Excessive and chronic sun exposure can overcome these mechanisms, leading to elevated levels of inflammatory cytokines, toxic oxygen free radicals, irreversibly damaged cells, and malignancy. The malignant cells usually have mutations in the *p53* tumor-suppressor gene. Exogenous protection against UV radiation includes avoidance of the sun, use of photoprotective clothing, and adequate application of broad-spectrum sunscreens. Endogenous mechanisms of protection from UV radiation include melanin synthesis, epidermal thickening, and establishment of an antioxidant network. Research is in progress to understand how botanical dietary agents inhibit, reverse, or retard the processes of inflammation, oxidative stress, immune suppression, and DNA damage that cause photocarcinogenesis (photochemoprotection). These agents are polyphenols and include green tea polyphenols, grape seed proanthocyanidins, silymarin (a flavonoid of milk thistle), resveratrol (grape skins), genistein (an isoflavone found in soy and fava beans), and catechin (a flavonoid from the acacia catechu tree).

Data from Afaq F: Natural agents: cellular and molecular mechanisms of photoprotection, *Arch Biochem Biophys* 508(2):144–151, 2011; Masnec IS et al: New option in photoprotection, *Coll Antropol* 34(suppl 2):257–262, 2010; Nichols JA, Katiyar SK: Skin photoprotection by natural polyphenols: anti-inflammatory, antioxidant and DNA repair mechanisms, *Arch Dermatol Res* 302(2):71–83, 2010.

BOX 39-1 **IMPORTANT TRENDS FOR SKIN CANCER**

Incidence
- More than 1 million new cases of skin cancer are diagnosed each year with the majority being the highly curable *basal* (90%) or *squamous cell cancers*.
- Malignant melanoma is the most serious form of skin cancer; it is not as common with an estimated 68,130 new cases per year.

Mortality
- Total estimated deaths from skin cancer in 2010 were 11,790: 8700 from malignant melanoma, 3090 from other nonepithelial skin cancers.

Risk Factors
- Excessive exposure to ultraviolet radiation from the sun or tanning salons
- Fair complexion
- Occupational exposure to coal tar, pitch, creosote, arsenic compounds, and radium
- In people of color, skin cancer is less common, is diagnosed at a more advanced stage, and has higher morbidity and mortality than in people with light-colored skin.

Warning Signs
- Any unusual skin condition, especially a change in the size or color of a mole or other darkly pigmented growth or spot

Prevention and Early Detection
- Avoid the sun when ultraviolet light is strongest (e.g., 10 AM to 3 PM), seek shade, use sunscreen preparations, especially those containing ingredients such as PABA (para-aminobenzoic acid), and wear protective clothing.
- Basal and squamous cell skin cancers often form a pale, waxlike pearly nodule or a red, scaly, sharply outlined patch.
- Melanomas usually have dark brown or black pigmentation; they start as small mole-like growths that increase in size, change color, become ulcerated, and bleed easily from slight injury.

Treatment
- Options for treatment include surgery, electrodesiccation (tissue destruction by heat), radiation therapy, or cryosurgery (tissue destruction by freezing).
- Malignant melanomas require wide and often deep excisions and removal of nearby lymph nodes; selective lymphadenectomy or immunotherapy can be used; vaccines and gene therapy are in development.

Survival
- For basal cell and squamous cell cancers, cure is virtually ensured with early detection and treatment; malignant melanoma, however, metastasizes quickly and accounts for a lower 5-year survival rate.

Basal Cell Carcinoma

Basal cell carcinoma of the skin is the most common skin cancer in individuals with light-colored skin, particularly those with intense sunlight (ultraviolet radiation) exposure. Lesions are seen most often on the face and neck, the areas with the most intense sunlight exposure. Although ultraviolet radiation seems to be the primary causative agent, arsenic in food or water and genetic predisposition are contributing factors. There are alterations in both tumor-suppressor genes and DNA repair mechanisms (see Chapter 9).[65]

The lesion starts as a nodule (more than 5 mm in diameter) that is pearly or ivory and slightly elevated above the skin surface with small blood vessels on the surface (Figure 39-22). As the tumor grows it usually

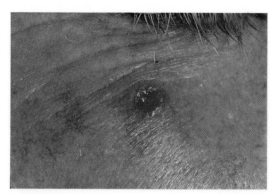

FIGURE 39-22 Basal Cell Carcinoma. Center has ulcerated. (Courtesy Department of Dermatology, School of Medicine, University of Utah, Salt Lake City, Utah.)

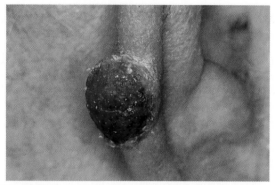

FIGURE 39-23 Squamous Cell Carcinoma. The sun-exposed ear is a common site for squamous cell carcinoma. (Courtesy Department of Dermatology, School of Medicine, University of Utah, Salt Lake City, Utah.)

has a depressed center and rolled border (see Figure 39-22). Early tumors are so small they are not clinically apparent. The lesion grows slowly, often ulcerates, develop crusts, and is firm to the touch. If left untreated, basal cell lesions invade surrounding tissues and, over months or years, can destroy a nose, eyelid, or ear (for treatment, see Box 39-1). Metastasis is rare because these tumors do not invade blood or lymph vessels.

Squamous Cell Carcinoma

Squamous cell carcinoma (SCC) of the skin is a tumor of the epidermis generally characterized by two types: in situ (Bowen disease) and invasive. Because of the invasive nature of some tumors, squamous cell carcinoma is significantly more malignant if left untreated.

Ultraviolet radiation exposure causes SCC and actinic keratosis is a precursor. Other risk factors include arsenic at a higher level in drinking water, exposure to x-rays and gamma rays, immunosuppression, and light-colored skin. It is unclear how ultraviolet light produces SCC. *P53* gene mutations are common in SCC and they produce tumor cells resistant to apoptosis.[66] The most common areas affected are sun exposed: the head and neck and the hands.[67]

Premalignant lesions include actinic keratosis, leukoplakia, or whitish discolored areas; scars; radiation-induced keratosis; tar and oil keratosis; chronic ulcers; and sinuses. In situ SCC is usually confined to the epidermis (intraepidermal) but may extend into the dermis. Bowen disease is a dysplastic epidermal lesion often found on unexposed areas of the body such as the penis and demonstrated by flat, reddish, scaly patches. These lesions rarely invade surrounding tissue and rarely metastasize. Other cellular components of the skin (e.g., sweat glands, hair follicles) can develop into skin cancer, but this is relatively uncommon.

Invasive SCC can arise from premalignant lesions of the skin, rarely develops from normal-appearing skin, and is usually confined to the epidermis (intraepidermal) but may extend into the reticular layer of the dermis (see Table 39-1). Invasive SCC grows more rapidly than basal cell carcinomas and can spread to regional lymph nodes. These tumors are firm and increase in both elevation and diameter. The surface may be granular and bleed easily (Figure 39-23). Treatment includes surgical excision and radiotherapy.[68]

Cutaneous Melanoma

Cutaneous melanoma is a malignant tumor of the skin originating from melanocytes, or cells that synthesize the pigment melanin. Malignant melanoma is the most serious skin cancer with 68,130 new cases per year in the United States and the incidence is increasing worldwide. Risk factors include genetic predisposition, ultraviolet radiation,

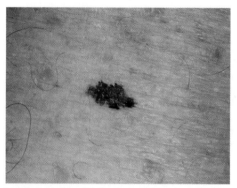

FIGURE 39-24 Lentigo Malignant Melanoma. Lentigo malignant melanoma is most common on the head and neck. (Courtesy Department of Dermatology, School of Medicine, University of Utah, Salt Lake City, Utah.)

steroid hormone activity, fair hair, light skin with a propensity to sunburn, freckles, male gender, geographic location, past pesticide exposure, sunbed use before age 30 years, and three or more clinically atypical (dysplastic) nevi.[69,70]

Melanomas arise as a result of malignant degeneration of melanocytes located either along the basal layer of the epidermis (see Figure 39-1) or in a benign melanocytic nevus. The clinical varieties of cutaneous melanoma include lentigo malignant melanoma (LMM) (Figure 39-24), superficial spreading melanoma (SSM) (the most common), primary nodular melanoma (PNM), and acral lentiginous melanoma (ALM) (occurs on nonhair surfaces and mucous membranes). The pathogenesis of malignant melanoma is complex and a number of proto-oncogenes have been identified.[71] The relationship between nevi and melanoma makes it important for the clinician to understand the various forms of nevi (Table 39-6). Most nevi never become suspicious; however, suspicious pigmented nevi need to be evaluated and removed.[72] Indications for biopsy include color change, size change, irregular notched margin, itching, bleeding or oozing, nodularity, scab formation, and ulceration or an unusual pattern of presentation. The ABCDE rule is used as a guide: **A**symmetry, **B**order irregularity, **C**olor variation, **D**iameter larger than 6 mm, and **E**levation, which includes raised appearance or rapid enlargement. Staging is determined by lesion thickness (presence of **t**umor), lymph **n**ode involvement, and presence of **m**etastasis (TNM staging).[73]

Treatment of melanoma with no evidence of metastatic disease involves surgical excision of the primary lesion site and involved

TABLE 39-6	CLASSIFICATION OF NEVI
TYPE	**COMMON CHARACTERISTICS**
Junctional nevus	Flat, well-circumscribed; vary in size up to 2 cm; dark color hairs may be present; originate in basal layer of epidermis and can eventually reach cutaneous surface; most likely to develop into melanoma
Compound nevus	Most common in adolescents; majority of pigmented lesions in children; rarely does this lesion develop into melanoma; usually 1 cm in size; hairs may be present; surface is elevated and smooth
Intradermal nevus	Small, less than 1 cm, with regular edges and bristle-like hairs; color ranges from fair skin tone to light brown; has slight likelihood of developing into melanoma

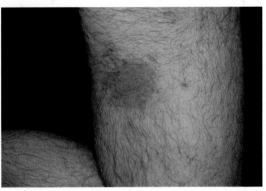

FIGURE 39-25 Kaposi Sarcoma. The purple lesion commonly seen on the skin. (Courtesy Department of Dermatology, School of Medicine, University of Utah, Salt Lake City, Utah.)

regional lymph nodes. Radiation therapy, chemotherapy, and biologic response modifiers may be prescribed. Lesions of the extremities have the best surgical prognosis. Immunotherapy is advancing and vaccines, gene therapy, and biomarkers are under investigation.[74-76] Less than 10% of individuals with regional metastasis are alive after 5 years. Early detection is critical to decreasing mortality from metastatic disease.[77]

Kaposi Sarcoma

Kaposi sarcoma (KS) is a vascular malignancy associated with immunodeficiency states and occurs among transplant recipients taking immunosuppressive drugs. A rapidly progressive form of KS appears with acquired immunodeficiency syndrome (AIDS) and is associated with human herpesvirus-8 (HHV-8) (see Chapter 32). KS is endemic in sub-Saharan Africa. Four forms of the disease have been described: classic, epidemic, post-transplant, and acquired immunodeficient associated virus.[78]

The endothelial cell is thought to be the progenitor of KS. The lesions emerge as purplish brown macules and develop into plaques and nodules with angioproliferation. They tend to be multifocal rather than spreading by metastasis. The lesions initially appear over the lower extremities in the classic form (Figure 39-25). The rapidly progressive form associated with AIDS tends to spread symmetrically over the upper body, particularly the face and oral mucosa. The lesions are often pruritic and painful. About 75% of individuals with epidemic KS have involvement of lymph nodes, particularly in the gastrointestinal tract and lungs. Organ involvement is much less common in the classic form. The rapidly progressive form has a poor prognosis and shorter survival rates than the classic form. (See Chapter 6 for a further discussion of AIDS.)

Diagnosis is by skin biopsy, with a high index of suspicion for those with immunodeficiency. Local lesions can be excised. Multiple disseminated lesions may be treated with a combination of α-interferon, radiotherapy, and cytotoxic drugs. Antiangiogenic agents are being tested. Individuals receiving highly active antiretroviral therapy (HAART) have a markedly reduced incidence of KS.[79]

> ✔ **QUICK CHECK 39-7**
> 1. What is the most common skin cancer?
> 2. What malignancy can arise from melanocytes?
> 3. How is Kaposi sarcoma related to AIDS?

Burns

The incidence of burn injuries has declined in the past several years. About 1 million people are burned in the United States each year, with 450,000 visits to hospital emergency departments, 45,000 hospitalizations, and 3500 burn-related deaths. Most burns occur in the home, and the highest percentage (70%) occur in men.[80] Burns may be caused by thermal or nonthermal sources including chemical, electrical, or radioactive sources. Thermal injuries result from exposure to direct flames, hot liquids, or radiation. Direct contact, inhalation, and ingestion of acids, alkalis, or blistering agents cause chemical burns. Electrical burns occur with the passage of electrical current through the body to the ground. Associated electrical flames or flashes also can burn the skin.

Burn Wound Depth

The depth of injury identifies the level of tissue destruction; the extent of injury determines clinical management, healing, and mortality. The depth of the burn is divided into four categories (Table 39-7).

First-degree burns (superficial burns) involve only the epidermis. The skin maintains water vapor and bacterial barrier functions. There is local pain and erythema, and usually no blisters (e.g., sunburn). An extensive first-degree burn may cause systemic responses, such as chills, headache, localized edema, and nausea or vomiting. No treatment is required unless the person is elderly or an infant, in which case severe nausea and vomiting may lead to inadequate fluid intake and dehydration. Fluid therapy may be required in these cases. First-degree burns heal in 3 to 5 days without scarring.

Second-degree burns include superficial and deep partial-thickness burns. Superficial partial-thickness burns involve thin-walled, fluid-filled blisters that develop within just a few minutes after injury (Figure 39-26). Tactile and pain sensors remain intact throughout the healing process, and wound care can cause extreme pain. Wounds heal in 3 to 4 weeks with adequate nutrition and no wound complications. Scar formation is unusual and is genetically determined.

Deep partial-thickness burns involve the entire dermis, sparing skin appendages such as hair follicles and sweat glands (see Table 39-7 and Figure 39-27). These wounds look waxy white and take weeks to heal. Necrotic tissue is surgically removed followed by an application of the person's own unburned skin from another body area (autograft). Healing commonly results in hypertrophic scarring with poor functional and cosmetic results (Figure 39-28).

Third-degree burns, or full-thickness burns, involve destruction of the entire epidermis, dermis, and often underlying subcutaneous tissue (see Table 39-7). The wound has a dry, leathery appearance from

TABLE 39-7 DEPTH OF BURN INJURY

CHARACTERISTIC	FIRST DEGREE	SECOND DEGREE SUPERFICIAL PARTIAL-THICKNESS	DEEP PARTIAL-THICKNESS	THIRD DEGREE FULL-THICKNESS	FOURTH DEGREE FULL-THICKNESS AND DEEPER TISSUE
Morphology	Destruction of epidermis only	Destruction of epidermis and some dermis	Destruction of epidermis and dermis, leaving only skin appendages	Destruction of epidermis, dermis, and underlying subcutaneous tissue	Destruction of epidermis, dermis, and underlying subcutaneous tissue, tendons, muscle, and bone
Skin function	Intact	Absent	Absent	Absent	Absent
Tactile and pain sensors	Intact	Intact	Intact but diminished	Absent	Absent
Blisters	Present only after first 24 hr	Present within minutes; thin walled and fluid filled	May or may not appear as fluid-filled blisters; often is layer of flat, dehydrated tissue paper–like skin that lifts off in sheets	Blisters rare; usually is layer of flat, dehydrated tissue paper–like skin that lifts off easily	None
Appearance of wound after initial débridement	Skin peels at 24-48 hr; normal or slightly red underneath	Red to pale ivory, moist surface	Mottled with areas of waxy, white, dry surface	White, cherry red, or black; may contain visible thrombosed veins; dry, hard, leathery surface	Black and charred appearing wound
Healing time	3-5 days	21-28 days	30 days to many months	Will not heal; may close from edges as secondary healing if wound is small	Will not heal; requires skin grafting; may require amputation and/or reconstructive surgery
Scarring	None	May be present; low incidence influenced by genetic predisposition	Highest incidence because of slow healing rate promoting scar tissue development; also influenced by genetic predisposition	Skin graft; scarring minimized by early excision and grafting; influenced by genetic predisposition	Degree of scarring associated with reconstruction and grafting success

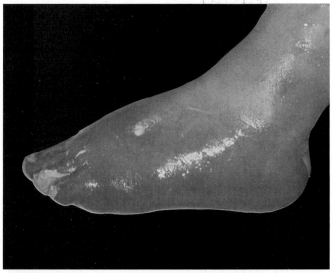

FIGURE 39-26 Superficial Partial-Thickness Burn. Scald injury following débridement of overlying blister and nonadherent epithelium. (Courtesy Intermountain Burn Center, University of Utah, Salt Lake City, Utah.)

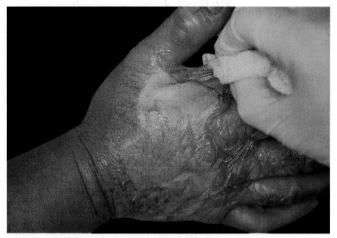

FIGURE 39-27 Deep Partial-Thickness Burn. Note pale appearance and minimal exudates. (Courtesy Intermountain Burn Center, University of Utah, Salt Lake City, Utah.)

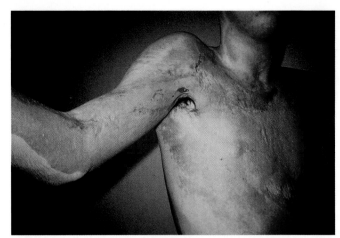

FIGURE 39-28 Axillary Burn Scar Contracture. Note the blanching of the anterior axillary fold and small ulceration from a deep partial-thickness burn, both indicating the diminished range of motion. (Courtesy Intermountain Burn Center, University of Utah, Salt Lake City, Utah.)

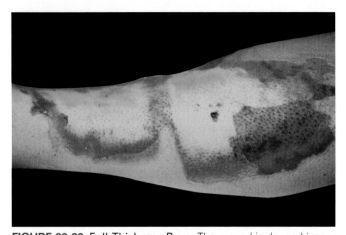

FIGURE 39-29 Full-Thickness Burn. The wound is dry and insensate. (Courtesy Intermountain Burn Center, University of Utah, Salt Lake City, Utah.)

loss of dermal elasticity (Figure 39-29). In areas of circumferential burns, distal circulation may be compromised from pressure caused by edema. **Escharotomies** (tissue decompression by cutting through burned skin) are performed to release pressure and prevent compartment syndrome (the compression of blood vessels, veins, muscles, or abdominal organs resulting in irreversible injury). Full-thickness burns are painless because all nerve endings have been destroyed by the injury. **Fourth-degree burns** destroy all of the skin and underlying subcutaneous tissue, tendons, muscle, and bone.

The extent of **total body surface area (TBSA)** burned is estimated using either the "rule of nines" (Figure 39-30) or the modified Lund and Browder chart.[81] The severity of burn injury also considers many factors, including age, medical history, extent and depth of injury, and body area involved. The American College of Surgeons has defined criteria to assist healthcare professionals in identifying who should be referred to a specialized burn center (Box 39-2).

PATHOPHYSIOLOGY AND CLINICAL MANIFESTATIONS Burn injury results in dramatic changes in most physiologic functions of the body within the first few minutes after the event. The effect of burns depends on two parameters: the extent of body surface affected and the

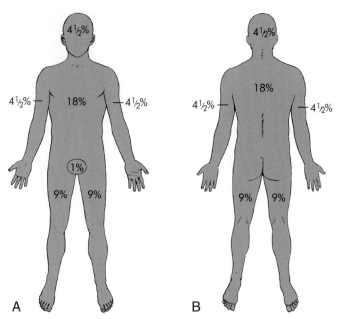

FIGURE 39-30 Estimation of Burn Injury: Rule of Nines. A commonly used assessment tool with estimates of the percentages (in multiples of 9) of the total body surface area burned. **A,** Adults (anterior view). **B,** Adults (posterior view).

BOX 39-2 BURN UNIT REFERRAL CRITERIA

A burn unit may treat adults or children or both. Burn injuries that should be referred to a burn unit include the following:

1. Partial-thickness burns greater than 10% total body surface area (TBSA)
2. Burns that involve the face, hands, feet, genitalia, perineum, or major joints
3. Third-degree burns in any age group
4. Electrical burns, including lightning injury
5. Chemical burns
6. Inhalation injury
7. Burn injury in persons with preexisting medical disorders that could complicate management, prolong recovery, or affect mortality
8. Any person with burns and concomitant trauma (such as fractures) in which the burn injury poses the greatest risk of morbidity or mortality; in such cases, if the trauma poses the greater immediate risk, the person may be initially stabilized in a trauma center before being transferred to a burn unit; physician judgment will be necessary in such situations and should be in concert with the regional medical control plan triage protocols
9. Burned children in hospitals without qualified personnel or equipment for the care of children
10. Burn injury in persons requiring special social, emotional, or long-term rehabilitative intervention

Excerpted from American College of Surgeons: *Guidelines for the operation of burn centers,* pp 79–86, Resources for Optimal Care of the Injured Patient 2006, Committee on Trauma. Available at www.ameriburn.org/BurnCenterReferralCriteria.pdf.

depth of cutaneous injury. Burns exceeding 40% TBSA in most adults are considered to be major burn injuries and are associated with massive evaporative water losses and fluctuations of large amounts of fluid, electrolytes, and plasma proteins into the body tissues, manifested as generalized edema, circulatory hypovolemia, and hypotension.

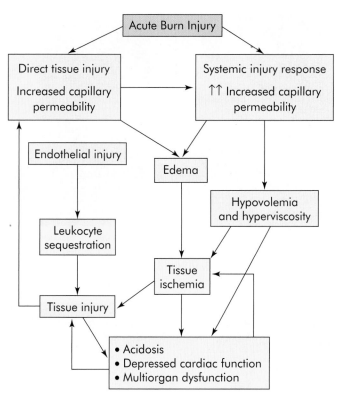

FIGURE 39-31 Immediate Cellular and Immunologic Alterations of Burn Shock.

The immediate (acute) systemic physiologic consequences of major burn injury focus on the profound, life-threatening hypovolemic shock that occurs in conjunction with cellular and immunologic disruption within a few minutes of injury (Figure 39-31). **Burn shock** is a condition consisting of a hypovolemic cardiovascular component and a cellular component.

Hypovolemia associated with burn shock results from massive fluid losses and shifts to the interstitial space from the circulating blood volume. The losses are caused by an increase in capillary permeability that persists for approximately 24 hours after burn injury. There is decreased cardiac contractility and decreased blood volume. Blood is shunted away from the liver, kidney, and gut—known as the "ebb phase" of the burn response. This phase lasts during the first 24 hours after burn injury and most organ systems are affected. Decreased perfusion of the viscera can decrease gut barrier function and result in translocation of bacteria and endotoxemia with sepsis.[82] Intravenous **fluid resuscitation** is critical to restore the circulating blood volume during this phase, often using lactated Ringer solution. The rate of fluid replacement must be carefully monitored to prevent complications associated with fluid overload.

Cellular metabolism is disrupted with onset of the burn wound, resulting in altered cell membrane permeability and loss of normal electrolyte homeostasis. Many cytokines and inflammatory mediators in burn serum play a role in these cellular processes. The cardiovascular and systemic responses to burn injury are integrated with the cellular response but are presented here as discrete entities.

Cardiovascular and Systemic Response to Burn

The clinical manifestations of burn shock are the result of multiple physiologic alterations related to burn injury, in addition to the loss of fluid. The hallmark of burn shock is decreased cardiac contractility and decreased cardiac output with inadequate capillary perfusion in most tissues. Decreased cardiac output is related to myocardial depressant factors, as well as decreased intravascular volume.

Fluid and protein movement out of the vascular compartment results in an elevated hematocrit and white blood cell count, and hypoproteinemia. If not treated immediately, profound hypovolemic shock and inadequate perfusion lead to irreversible shock and death within a few hours. Restoration of capillary integrity and a functional lymphatic system are required for resolution of the edema. Usually this occurs within 24 hours, but in extensive burns, it may take days or weeks. After the individual has reached the end point of burn shock, the term used to describe the person's condition is **capillary seal.**

The liver, with its metabolic, inflammatory, immune, and acute phase functions, plays a pivotal role in burn injury survival and recovery by modulating multiple metabolic pathways. Hepatic changes are common following a major burn, including fatty changes and hepatomegaly, which can influence burn wound recovery.[83] The hepatic response also alters clotting factors, leads to a hypercoagulable state, and can increase the risk for disseminated intravascular coagulation (systemic formation of microthrombi and abnormal bleeding).[84]

Cellular Response to Burn Injury

In addition to capillary endothelial permeability changes resulting in vascular fluid, electrolyte, and protein losses, there are transmembrane potential changes in cells not directly damaged by heat.[85] Cellular dysfunction resulting from burn injury impairs the sodium-potassium pump and results in increased amounts of intracellular sodium and water and decreased potassium level with disruption of the transmembrane potential. Intracellular calcium concentration also may be elevated, thereby influencing myocardial function.[86] Loss of intracellular magnesium and phosphate[87] and elevated serum lactic dehydrogenase (LDH) level occur.[88]

Metabolic Response to Burn Injury

Major burn injury (greater than 40% of total body surface area) initiates a systemic hypermetabolic response with an increase in metabolic rate and a hyperdynamic circulation that begins 24 hours after burn injury—known as the "flow phase."[89] This phase can persist for up to 2 years following a burn.[90] Metabolic responses involve the sympathetic nervous system and other homeostatic regulators. Levels of catecholamines, cortisol, glucagon, and insulin (insulin resistance) are elevated with a corresponding increase in energy expenditure and increased gluconeogenesis, glycogenolysis, lipolysis, proteolysis, and lactic acidosis. Myocardial oxygen consumption is elevated and there is catabolic loss of muscle mass.[91] Hyperglycemia and insulin resistance can be prolonged in severe burns and require management with intensive insulin therapy to improve postburn morbidity and mortality.[92,93]

Burn injury initiates an inflammatory response with local activation and recruitment of inflammatory cells, such as leukocytes and monocytes, at the site of injury. These cells release inflammatory cytokines that contribute to the hypermetabolic state.[90] The metabolic rate increases in proportion to burn size and compensates for the profound water and heat loss associated with the burn. The inflammatory response and the release of cytokines at the wound level are magnified into a generalized systemic inflammatory response syndrome that can lead to multiple organ dysfunction.[94,95] Acute kidney injury is associated with hypovolemia, hypervolemia, and the inflammatory response.[96]

Hypermetabolism also increases the thermal regulatory set point and core and skin temperatures. There is persistent tachycardia, hypercapnia, and body wasting. Wound healing may be impaired, contributing to increased risk for infection and sepsis. Increasing the ambient temperature and early excision and grafting can decrease resting energy expenditure and improve mortality after major burns.[97,98] Inflammatory mediators circulating to the lung result in pulmonary edema that can be life-threatening.[99]

Immunologic Response to Burn Injury

The immunologic/inflammatory response to burn injury is immediate, prolonged, and severe. The end result in individuals surviving burn shock is *immunosuppression* with increased susceptibility to potentially fatal systemic burn wound sepsis. White blood cells are altered at a time when their need to inhibit sepsis is vital.[100] Phagocytosis is impaired, and cellular and humoral immunity is abnormal. Individuals with altered immunocompetence or chronic disease before burn injury are at additional risk for complications, including wound sepsis.[101]

Macrophages, neutrophils, lymphocytes, and platelets release large amounts of inflammatory cytokines and antibodies, with their levels remaining elevated for weeks after burn injury. When combined with bacterial products, they produce peripheral vasodilation, pulmonary vasoconstriction, increased capillary permeability, and local tissue ischemia in the burn wound. There is distant organ dysfunction and multiple organ failure.[95]

Evaporative Water Loss

With major burn injury, there is loss of the skin's barrier function and ability to regulate evaporative water loss. Normally, the skin is the major source of insensible loss (75%), and the lungs are minor sources (25%), with a total loss of only approximately 600 to 800 ml/day. This changes dramatically with burns because both the skin and the lungs have increased loss of water as a result of hypermetabolism and hyperventilation, especially in an intubated individual. Total evaporative losses exceed many liters per day in an adult with large burn wounds. Replacement of the loss is mandatory to prevent volume deficit and shock.

EVALUATION AND TREATMENT Burn recovery is complex and prolonged with complications the rule rather than the exception. Severity of inhalation injury is also a significant morbidity and mortality factor. The goal of burn management is wound débridement and closure in a manner that promotes survival. Scar formation with contractures is often a consequence of healing in deep partial-thickness and third-degree burns (Figure 39-32).

The essential elements of survival of major burn injury are (1) provision of adequate fluids and nutrition, (2) meticulous management of wounds with early surgical excision and grafting (Figure 39-33),[102] (3) aggressive treatment of sepsis, and (4) promotion of thermoregulation. Several drugs are used for the management of severe burns, including β-adrenergic antagonists, β-adrenergic agonists, recombinant human growth hormone, insulin, androgenic steroids, and antibiotics.[89,95] Burn pain is almost always acute and severe, and treatment strategies are aggressive.[103-105]

Nutritional therapy focuses on early enteral therapy to reduce gut-mediated sepsis and to reduce the catabolic state.[82,106] Advancements in skin replacement technology are effective and promising.[107]

Frostbite

Frostbite is injury to the skin caused by exposure to extreme cold. The most common areas affected are fingers, toes, ears, nose, and cheeks. Mild frostbite (frostnip) is cold exposure without tissue freezing. It

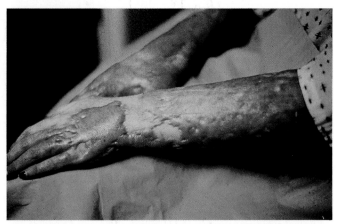

FIGURE 39-32 Hypertrophic Scarring. Deep partial-thickness thermal injury can result in extensive hypertrophic scarring. (Courtesy Intermountain Burn Center, University of Utah, Salt Lake City, Utah.)

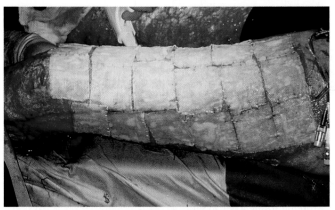

FIGURE 39-33 Application of Cultured Epithelial Autografts. The thin sheets of keratinocytes are attached to gauze backing to allow application onto the clean, excised thigh. (Courtesy Intermountain Burn Center, University of Utah, Salt Lake City, Utah.)

causes pallor and pain followed by redness and discomfort during rewarming, with no tissue damage. Frostbite occurs when tissues freeze slowly with ice crystal formation. Frozen skin becomes white or yellowish and has a waxy texture. There is numbness and no sensation of pain. Frostbite injury is related to direct cold injury to cells, indirect injury from ice crystal formation, and endothelial cell damage. During rewarming, there is progressive microvascular thrombosis followed by reperfusion release of inflammatory mediators, including thromboxanes and prostaglandins, with impaired circulation and anoxia to the exposed area.[108] Cyanosis and mottling develop followed by redness, edema, and burning pain on rewarming in more severe cases. Within 24 to 48 hours, vesicles and bullae appear that resolve into crusts that eventually slough, leaving thin, newly formed skin. Frostbite may be classified by depth of injury: superficial includes partial skin freezing (first degree) and full-thickness skin freezing (second degree); deep includes full-thickness and subcutaneous freezing (third degree) and deep tissue freezing (fourth degree). Third and fourth degree frostbite results in gangrene with loss of tissue.

Immediate treatment of frostbite is to cover affected areas with other body surfaces and warm clothing. The area should not be rubbed or massaged. Rewarming for severe frostbite should occur after emergency transport. Immersion in a warm water bath (40°

to 42° C) until frozen tissue is thawed is the best treatment. Pain is severe and should be treated with potent analgesics. Antibiotics may be given. Vasodilators, thrombolytics, hyperbaric oxygen, and sympathectomy may improve healing responses. Débridement or amputation of necrotic tissue occurs when there is a clear line of demarcation.[108,109]

DISORDERS OF THE HAIR

Alopecia

Alopecia means loss of hair from the head or body. Hair loss occurs when there is disruption in the growth phase of the hair follicle. Hair loss can be associated with systemic disorders such as hypothyroidism and iron deficiency, chemotherapy for cancer, malnutrition, compulsive hair pulling (trichotillomania), traction on hair from braiding and ponytails, use of hair treatment chemicals, hormonal alterations, and immune reactions.

Male-Pattern Alopecia (Androgenic Alopecia)

Male-pattern alopecia (androgenic alopecia) is localized hair loss in men. It is not a disease but a genetically predisposed response to androgens. Within the distribution of hair over the scalp, androgen-sensitive hair follicles are on top and androgen-insensitive follicles are on the sides and back. In genetically predisposed men, the androgen-sensitive follicles are transformed into vellus follicles. Male-pattern baldness begins with frontotemporal recession and progresses to loss of hair over the top of the scalp. Minoxidil and finasteride (a 5α-reductase inhibitor) decrease the effect of androgens on hair follicles and are used to stimulate hair growth.[110]

Female-Pattern Alopecia

Some genetically susceptible women in their twenties and thirties experience progressive thinning and loss of hair over the central part of the scalp, and prevalence increases with advancing age. Contrary to male-pattern baldness, there is usually no loss of hair along the frontal hairline. Many of these women have elevated serum levels of the adrenal androgen dehydroepiandrosterone sulfate (DHEAS) and some women have decreased hair loss when treated with daily doses of spironolactone.[111]

Alopecia Areata

Alopecia areata is an autoimmune T cell–mediated chronic inflammatory disease directed against hair follicles and results in hair loss. There is rapid onset of hair loss in multiple areas of the scalp, usually in round patches. The eyebrows, eyelashes, beard, and other areas of body hair are rarely involved. Stressful events, cell-mediated immune cytokines, genetic susceptibility, and metabolic disorders, such as Addison disease, thyroid disease, and lupus erythematosus, are associated with alopecia areata.[112]

Diagnosis is made by observation of the pattern of hair loss. Biopsy may show a lymphocytic infiltrate around the follicle. There are several treatments for alopecia areata, including corticosteroids and topical immunotherapy, but none are curative or preventive.[113]

Hirsutism

Hirsutism occurs in women and is the abnormal growth and distribution of hair on the face, body, and pubic area in a male pattern. There is also frontotemporal hair recession. These areas of hair growth are androgen sensitive. Variations of hair growth in women are great, and a male pattern may be normal. Women who develop hirsutism may be secreting hormones associated with polycystic ovarian syndrome, adrenal hyperplasia, or adrenal tumors and these disorders require treatment. If no hormonal pathologic conditions exist, treatment may include cosmetic removal of hair, suppression of excessive androgen production, or blockage of peripheral androgen receptors.[114]

DISORDERS OF THE NAIL

Paronychia

Paronychia is an acute or chronic infection of the cuticle. One or more fingers or toes may be involved. Individuals whose hands are frequently exposed to moisture are at greatest risk. The most common causative microorganisms are staphylococci and streptococci. Occasionally *Candida* will be present. Acute paronychia is manifested by the rapid onset of painful inflammation of the cuticle, usually after minor trauma. An abscess may develop requiring incision and drainage for relief of pain. The skin around the nail becomes more edematous and painful with progressive infection. Pus may be expressed from the proximal nail fold and an abscess may develop. The nail plate is usually not affected, although it can become discolored with ridges. Chronic paronychia develops slowly, with tenderness and swelling around the proximal or lateral nail folds.

Treatment includes keeping the hands dry. Oral antifungals are not effective because they do not penetrate the affected tissues. Topical application of thymol is usually effective.[115]

Onychomycosis

Onychomycosis (tinea unguium) is a fungal or dermatophyte infection of the nail plate. The most common pattern is a nail plate that turns yellow or white and becomes elevated with the accumulation of hyperkeratotic debris within the plate. Fungal infections of the nail are differentiated from psoriasis, lichen planus, and trauma by culture and microscopy and the absence of pitting on the nail surface, which is characteristic of psoriasis. Treatment is difficult because topical or systemic antifungal agents do not penetrate the nail plate readily. New antifungal drugs are more effective. Surgical excision of the nail may be required. Education is essential to preventing recurrence.[116]

✔ **QUICK CHECK 39-8**
1. Describe the three degrees of burn injury.
2. What dangers accompany frostbite?
3. What is alopecia? Compare the different types.
4. What disorders of the nail are seen?

DID YOU UNDERSTAND?

Structure and Function of the Skin

1. Skin is the largest organ of the body and equals 20% of body weight. The major functions are to provide a protective barrier and regulate body temperature.
2. The skin has two layers—the dermis and epidermis. The underlying hypodermis contains connective tissue, fat cells, fibroblasts, and macrophages.
3. The epidermis contains basal and spinous layers with melanocytes, Langerhans cells, and Merkel cells.
4. The dermis is composed of connective tissue elements, hair follicles, sweat glands, sebaceous glands, blood vessels, nerves, and lymphatic vessels.
5. The papillary capillaries provide the major blood supply to the skin, arising from deeper arterial plexuses.
6. The dermal appendages include nails, hair, and eccrine and apocrine sweat glands.
7. Heat loss and heat conservation are regulated by arteriovenous anastomoses that lead to the papillary capillaries in the dermis.
8. Pressure ulcers develop from pressure and shearing forces that occlude capillary blood flow with resulting ischemia and necrosis. Areas at greatest risk are pressure points over bony prominences, such as the greater trochanters, sacrum, ischia, and heels.
9. Keloids are sharply elevated scars that extend beyond the border of traumatized skin. Hypertrophic scars do not extend beyond the border of injury.
10. Pruritus is itching and is associated with many skin disorders. Small unmyelinated nerve fibers transmit itch sensation.

Disorders of the Skin

1. Contact dermatitis is a form of delayed hypersensitivity that develops with sensitization to allergens, such as metal, chemicals, or poison ivy.
2. Irritant contact dermatitis develops from prolonged exposure to chemicals, such as acids or soaps, with disruption of the skin barrier.
3. Atopic or allergic dermatitis is associated with a family history of allergies, hay fever, elevated IgE levels, and increased histamine sensitivity. Pruritus and scratching predispose the skin to infection, scaling, and thickening.
4. Stasis dermatitis occurs on the legs and results from venous stasis and edema.
5. Seborrheic dermatitis involves scaly, yellowish, inflammatory plaques of the scalp, eyebrows, eyelids, ear canals, chest, axillae, and back. The cause is unknown but *Malassezia* yeasts have been implicated.
6. Papulosquamous disorders are characterized by papules, scales, plaques, and erythema.
7. Psoriasis is a chronic inflammatory skin disease associated with T cell activation and cellular proliferation of both the epidermis and the dermis; it is characterized by scaly, erythematous, pruritic plaques.
8. Pityriasis rosea is a self-limiting disease characterized by oval lesions with scales around the edges; it is located along skin lines of the trunk and may be caused by a herpes-like virus.
9. Lichen planus is an autoimmune papular, violet-colored inflammatory lesion of unknown origin manifested by severe pruritus.
10. Acne vulgaris is an inflammation of the pilosebaceous follicle.
11. Acne rosacea develops on the middle third of the face with hypertrophy and inflammation of the sebaceous glands.
12. Discoid (cutaneous) lupus erythematosus is an autoimmune disease that can affect only the skin. The systemic form also presents cutaneous lesions. The cutaneous inflammatory lesions usually occur in sun-exposed areas with a butterfly distribution over the nose and cheeks.
13. Pemphigus is a chronic, autoimmune, blistering disease that begins in the mouth or on the scalp and spreads to other parts of the body, often with a fatal outcome.
14. Erythema multiforme is an acute inflammation of the skin and mucous membranes (bullous form) with lesions that appear target-like with alternating rings of edema and inflammation, often associated with allergic reactions to drugs.
15. Folliculitis is a bacterial infection of the hair follicle.
16. A furuncle is an infection of the hair follicle that extends to the surrounding tissue.
17. A carbuncle is a collection of infected hair follicles that forms a draining abscess.
18. Cellulitis is a diffuse infection of the dermis and subcutaneous tissue.
19. Erysipelas is a superficial streptococcal infection of the skin commonly affecting the face, ears, and lower legs.
20. Impetigo may have a bullous or an ulcerative form and is caused by *Staphylococcus* or *Streptococcus.*
21. Herpes simplex virus type 1 (HSV-1) causes cold sores but can infect the cornea, mouth, and labia. HSV-2 causes genital lesions and is usually spread by sexual contact.
22. Herpes zoster (shingles) and varicella (chickenpox) are both caused by the same herpesvirus.
23. Warts are benign, rough, elevated lesions caused by human papillomavirus. Condylomata acuminata, or venereal warts, are spread by sexual contact.
24. Tinea infections (fungal infections) can occur anywhere on the body and are classified by location (i.e., tinea pedis, tinea corporis, tinea capitis).
25. Candidiasis is a yeastlike fungal infection (*Candida albicans*) occurring on skin, mucous membranes, and the gastrointestinal tract.
26. Cutaneous vasculitis is an inflammation of skin blood vessels related to immune complex deposition with purpura, ischemia, and necrosis resulting from vessel necrosis.
27. Urticarial lesions are commonly associated with type I hypersensitivity responses and appear as wheals, welts, or hives.
28. Scleroderma is an autoimmune-mediated sclerosis of the skin that may also affect systemic organs and cause renal failure, bowel obstruction, or cardiac dysrhythmias.
29. Mosquitoes can transmit infectious diseases, and the saliva from their bite produces the characteristic itching and wheal formation.
30. Blood-sucking flies are represented by many species and their bites are usually painful and produce bleeding, and the pruritus and local reactions may last for days with systemic symptoms of fever and malaise.
31. Bee and ant sting venom may produce a local or systemic reaction that can be anaphylactic.
32. Seborrheic keratosis is a proliferation of basal cells that produce elevated, smooth, or warty lesions of varying size. They are most common among the elderly population.
33. Keratoacanthoma arises from hair follicles on sun-exposed areas. Three stages of development characterize the lesion, which results in a dome-shaped, crusty lesion filled with keratin that resolves in 3 to 4 months.
34. Actinic keratosis is a pigmented scaly lesion that develops in sun-exposed individuals with fair skin. The lesion may become malignant in the form of a squamous cell carcinoma.
35. Nevi arise from melanocytes and may be pigmented or fleshy pink. They occur singly or in groups and may undergo transition to malignant melanoma.
36. Basal cell carcinoma is the most common skin cancer and occurs most often on ultraviolet-exposed areas of the skin.
37. Squamous cell carcinoma is a tumor of the epidermis and can be localized (in situ) or invasive.

DID YOU UNDERSTAND?—cont'd

38. Cutaneous malignant melanoma arises from melanocytes, and if not excised early, metastasis occurs through the lymph nodes.
39. Kaposi sarcoma is a vascular malignancy associated with immunodeficiency states and herpesvirus-8.
40. Burns are classified according to depth and extent of injury as first-, second-, third-, or fourth-degree burns.
41. Severe burns cause profound edema and burn shock related to an inflammatory response throughout the cardiovascular system with loss of capillary seal. Fluid resuscitation is critical to prevent shock and death.
42. Burns cause a hypermetabolic response with increased cortisol, glucagon, and insulin levels.
43. Immune suppression associated with inflammatory cytokine release from burned tissue increases risk for infection and can delay wound healing.
44. Frostbite usually occurs on the face and digits, with direct injury to cells and impaired circulation.

Disorders of the Hair

1. Alopecia is loss of hair from the head or body.
2. Male-pattern alopecia is an inherited form of irreversible baldness with hair loss in the central scalp and recession of the temporofrontal hairline.
3. Female-pattern alopecia is a thinning of the central hair of the scalp beginning in women at 20 to 30 years of age.
4. Alopecia areata is an autoimmune-mediated loss of hair and may be associated with stress or metabolic diseases; it is usually reversible.
5. Hirsutism is a male pattern of hair growth in women that may be normal or the result of excessive secretion of androgenic hormones.

Disorders of the Nail

1. Paronychia is an inflammation of the cuticle that can be acute or chronic and is usually caused by staphylococci, streptococci, or fungi.
2. Onychomycosis is a fungal infection of the nail plate.

KEY TERMS

- Acne rosacea   1051
- Acne vulgaris   1051
- Actinic keratosis   1057
- Allergic contact dermatitis   1048
- Alopecia   1065
- Alopecia areata   1065
- Apocrine sweat gland   1040
- Atopic dermatitis (allergic dermatitis)   1048
- Basal cell carcinoma   1058
- Bullous erythema multiforme   1052
- Burn shock   1063
- Candidiasis   1055
- Capillary seal   1063
- Carbuncle   1053
- Cellulitis   1053
- Clawlike prolongation   1047
- Condylomata acuminata (venereal warts)   1054
- Cutaneous melanoma   1059
- Cutaneous vasculitis   1055
- Deep partial-thickness burn   1060
- Dermal appendage   1038
- Dermatitis   1048
- Dermis   1038
- Discoid (cutaneous) lupus erythematosus (DLE)   1051
- Eccrine sweat gland   1040
- Eczema   1048
- Epidermis   1038
- Erysipelas   1053
- Erythema multiforme   1052
- Erythrodermic (exfoliative) psoriasis   1049
- Escharotomy   1062
- First-degree burn   1060
- Fluid resuscitation   1063
- Fly   1057
- Folliculitis   1053
- Fourth-degree burns   1062
- Frostbite   1064
- Furuncle   1053
- Guttate psoriasis   1049
- Herald patch   1050
- Herpes simplex virus (HSV)   1053
- Herpes zoster (shingles)   1054
- Hirsutism   1065
- Human papillomavirus (HPV)   1054
- Impetigo   1053
- Inverse psoriasis   1049
- Irritant contact dermatitis   1048
- Kaposi sarcoma (KS)   1060
- Keratoacanthoma   1057
- Lichen planus   1050
- Lupus erythematosus   1051
- Male-pattern alopecia (androgenic alopecia)   1065
- Mosquito   1057
- Nails   1038
- Nevus (pl., nevi)   1057
- Onychomycosis (tinea unguium)   1065
- Papillary capillary   1040
- Papulosquamous disorder   1049
- Paronychia   1065
- Pemphigus   1051
- Pemphigus erythematosus   1052
- Pemphigus foliaceus   1052
- Pemphigus vegetans   1052
- Pemphigus vulgaris   1052
- Pityriasis rosea   1050
- Plaque psoriasis   1049
- Psoriasis   1049
- Psoriatic arthritis   1049
- Psoriatic nail disease   1049
- Pustular psoriasis   1049
- Scleroderma (systemic sclerosis)   1056
- Sebaceous gland   1040
- Seborrheic dermatitis   1048
- Seborrheic keratosis   1057
- Second-degree burn   1060
- Squamous cell carcinoma (SCC)   1059
- Stasis dermatitis   1048
- Stevens-Johnson syndrome   1052
- Subcutaneous layer (hypodermis)   1038
- Superficial partial-thickness burn   1060
- Systemic sclerosis   1056
- Third-degree burn (full-thickness burn)   1060
- Tinea infection   1054
- Tinea pedis (athlete's foot)   1055
- Tinea unguium   1055
- Total body surface area (TBSA)   1062
- Toxic epidermal necrolysis (TEN)   1052
- Urticaria (hives)   1056
- Urticarial lesion   1056
- Varicella (chickenpox)   1054
- Wart   1054

REFERENCES

1. de Laat EH, et al: Epidemiology, risk and prevention of pressure ulcers in critically ill patients: a literature review, *J Wound Care* 15(6):269–275, 2006.
2. National Pressure Ulcer Advisory Panel: *Pressure ulcer stages revised by NPUAP*, Feb 2007. Accessed March 10, 2011. Available at www.npuap.org/pr2.htm.
3. Anders J, et al: Decubitus ulcers: pathophysiology and primary prevention, *Dtsch Arztebl Int* 107(21):371–381, 2010.
4. Doley J: Nutrition management of pressure ulcers, *Nutr Clin Pract* 25(1):50–60, 2010.
5. Black JM, et al: National Pressure Ulcer Advisory Panel. Pressure ulcers: avoidable or unavoidable? Results of the National Pressure Ulcer Advisory Panel Consensus Conference, *Ostomy Wound Manage* 57(2):24–37, 2011.

6. Keys KA, et al: Multivariate predictors of failure after flap coverage of pressure ulcers, *Plast Reconstr Surg* 125(6):1725–1734, 2010.

7. National Guideline Clearinghouse (NGC): Guideline synthesis: management of pressure ulcers. In *National Guideline Clearinghouse (NGC)* [website], Rockville, Md, 2006 Dec (revised 2011 Jan). Accessed March 15, 2011. Available at www.guideline.gov.

8. Shih B, et al: Molecular dissection of abnormal wound healing processes resulting in keloid disease, *Wound Repair Regen* 18(2):139–153, 2010.

9. Shih B, Bayat A: Genetics of keloid scarring, *Arch Dermatol Res* 302(5):319–339, 2010.

10. Juckett G, Hartman-Adams H: Management of keloids and hypertrophic scars, *Am Fam Physician* 80(3):253–260, 2009.

11. Gupta S, Sharma VK: Standard guidelines of care: keloids and hypertrophic scars, *Indian J Dermatol Venereol Leprol* 77(1):94–100, 2011.

12. Feramisco JD, Berger TG, Steinhoff M: Innovative management of pruritus, *Dermatol Clin* 28(3):467–478, 2010.

13. Metz M, Ständer S: Chronic pruritus—pathogenesis, clinical aspects and treatment, *J Eur Acad Dermatol Venereol* 24(11):1249–1260, 2010.

14. Cassano N, et al: Chronic pruritus in the absence of specific skin disease: an update on pathophysiology, diagnosis, and therapy, *Am J Clin Dermatol* 11(6):399–411, 2010.

15. Cavani A, De Luca A: Allergic contact dermatitis: novel mechanisms and therapeutic perspectives, *Curr Drug Metab* 11(3):228–233, 2010.

16. Rolland JM, O'Hehir RE: Latex allergy: a model for therapy, *Clin Exp Allergy* 38(6):898–912, 2008.

17. Usatine RP, Riojas M: Diagnosis and management of contact dermatitis, *Am Fam Physician* 82(3):249–255, 2010.

18. Raffetto JD, Marston WA: Venous ulcer: what is new? *Plast Reconstr Surg* 127(Suppl 1):279S–288S, 2011.

19. Zisova LG: Malassezia species and seborrheic dermatitis, *Folia Med (Plovdiv)* 51(1):23–33, 2009.

20. Duffin KC, Woodcock J, Krueger GG: Genetic variations associated with psoriasis and psoriatic arthritis found by genome-wide association, *Dermatol Ther* 23(2):101–113, 2010.

21. Nograles KE, Davidovici B, Krueger JG: New insights in the immunologic basis of psoriasis, *Semin Cutan Med Surg* 29(1):3–9, 2010.

22. Weger W: Current status and new developments in the treatment of psoriasis and psoriatic arthritis with biological agents, *Br J Pharmacol* 160(4):810–820, 2010.

23. Rozenblit M, Lebwohl M: New biologics for psoriasis and psoriatic arthritis, *Dermatol Ther* 22(1):56–60, 2009.

24. Rebora A, Drago F, Broccolo F: Pityriasis rosea and herpesviruses: facts and controversies, *Clin Dermatol* 28(5):497–501, 2010.

25. Stulberg DL, Wolfrey J: Pityriasis rosea, *Am Fam Physician* 69(1):87–91, 2004.

26. Shengyuan L, et al: Hepatitis C virus and lichen planus: a reciprocal association determined by a meta-analysis, *Arch Dermatol* 145(9):1040–1047, 2009.

27. Carrozzo M, Thorpe R: Oral lichen planus: a review, *Minerva Stomatol* 58(10):519–537, 2009.

28. Ramos-e-Silva M, Jacques CM, Carneiro SC: Premalignant nature of oral and vulval lichen planus: facts and controversies, *Clin Dermatol* 28(5):563–567, 2010.

29. Yamasaki K, Gallo RL: The molecular pathology of rosacea, *J Dermatol Sci* 55(2):77–81, 2009.

30. Gallo R, et al: Rosacea treatments: what's new and what's on the horizon? *Am J Clin Dermatol* 11(5):299–303, 2010.

31. Obermoser G, Sontheimer RD, Zelger B: Overview of common, rare and atypical manifestations of cutaneous lupus erythematosus and histopathological correlates, *Lupus* 19(9):1050–1070, 2010.

32. Wenzel J, Zahn S, Tüting T: Pathogenesis of cutaneous lupus erythematosus: common and different features in distinct subsets, *Lupus* 19(9):1020–1028, 2010.

33. Rothfield N, Sontheimer RD, Bernstein M: Lupus erythematosus: systemic and cutaneous manifestations, *Clin Dermatol* 24(5):348–362, 2006.

34. Jessop S, Whitelaw DA, Delamere FM: Drugs for discoid lupus erythematosus, *Cochrane Database Syst Rev*(4):CD002954, 2009.

35. Yokoyama T, Amagai M: Immune dysregulation of pemphigus in humans and mice, *J Dermatol* 37(3):205–213, 2010.

36. Strowd LC, et al: Therapeutic ladder for pemphigus vulgaris: emphasis on achieving complete remission, *J Am Acad Dermatol* 64(3):490–494, 2011.

37. Williams PM, Conklin RJ: Erythema multiforme: a review and contrast from Stevens-Johnson syndrome/toxic epidermal necrolysis, *Dent Clin North Am* 49(1):67–76, 2005:viii.

38. Rogers RL, Perkins J: Skin and soft tissue infections, *Prim Care* 33(3):697–710, 2006.

39. Odell CA: Community-associated methicillin-resistant *Staphylococcus aureus* (CA-MRSA) skin infections, *Curr Opin Pediatr* 22(3):273–277, 2010.

40. Chira S, Miller LG: *Staphylococcus aureus* is the most common identified cause of cellulitis: a systematic review, *Epidemiol Infect* 138(3):313–317, 2010.

41. Bloom DC, Giordani NV, Kwiatkowski DL: Epigenetic regulation of latent HSV-1 gene expression, *Biochim Biophys Acta* 1799(3–4):246–256, 2010.

42. Malm G: Neonatal herpes simplex virus infection, *Semin Fetal Neonatal Med* 14(4):204–208, 2009.

43. Dasgupta G, et al: New concepts in herpes simplex virus vaccine development: notes from the battlefield, *Expert Rev Vaccines* 8(8):1023–1035, 2009.

44. Johnson RW: Pain following herpes zoster: implications for management, *Herpes* 11(3):63–65, 2004.

45. Johnson RW: Herpes zoster and postherpetic neuralgia, *Expert Rev Vaccines* 9(suppl 3):21–26, 2010.

46. Willison CB, et al: Shingles vaccine, *Expert Opin Biol Ther* 10(4):631–638, 2010.

47. Bruggink SC, et al: Cryotherapy with liquid nitrogen versus topical salicylic acid application for cutaneous warts in primary care: randomized controlled trial, *CMAJ* 182(15):1624–1630, 2010.

48. Andrews RM, et al: Skin disorders, including pyoderma, scabies, and tinea infections, *Pediatr Clin North Am* 56(6):1421–1440, 2009.

49. Playford EG, Lipman J, Sorrell TC: Prophylaxis, empirical and preemptive treatment of invasive candidiasis, *Curr Opin Crit Care* 16(5):470–474, 2010.

50. Habif TP: *Clinical dermatology*, ed 5, St Louis, 2009, Mosby, p 523.

51. Carlson JA: The histological assessment of cutaneous vasculitis, *Histopathology* 56(1):3–23, 2010.

52. Kaplan AP, Greaves M: Pathogenesis of chronic urticaria, *Clin Exp Allergy* 39(6):777–787, 2009.

53. Jinnin M: Mechanisms of skin fibrosis in systemic sclerosis, *J Dermatol* 37(1):11–25, 2010.

54. Wigley FM: Vascular disease in scleroderma, *Clin Rev Allergy Immunol* 36(2–3):150–175, 2009.

55. Ong VH, Denton CP: Innovative therapies for systemic sclerosis, *Curr Opin Rheumatol* 22(3):264–272, 2010.

56. Al-Dhaher FF, Pope JE, Ouimet JM: Determinants of morbidity and mortality of systemic sclerosis in Canada, *Semin Arthritis Rheum* 39(4):269–277, 2010.

57. Müller UR: Insect venoms, *Chem Immunol Allergy* 95:141–156, 2010.

58. Brodsky J: Management of benign skin lesions commonly affecting the face: actinic keratosis, seborrheic keratosis, and rosacea, *Curr Opin Otolaryngol Head Neck Surg* 17(4):315–320, 2009.

59. Mandrell JC, Santa Cruz D: Keratoacanthoma: hyperplasia, benign neoplasm, or a type of squamous cell carcinoma? *Semin Diagn Pathol* 26(3):150–163, 2009.

60. Shoimer I, Rosen N, Muhn C: Current management of actinic keratoses, *Skin Therapy Lett* 15(5):5–7, 2010.

61. Lyon VB: Congenital melanocytic nevi, *Pediatr Clin North Am* 57(5):1155–1176, 2010.

62. American Cancer Society: *Cancer facts & figures—2010*, Atlanta, 2010, Author. Available at www.cancer.org/research/cancerfactsfigures/cancerfactsfigures/cancer-facts-and-figures-2010.

63. Afaq F: Natural agents: cellular and molecular mechanisms of photoprotection, *Arch Biochem Biophys* 508(2):144–151, 2011.

64. Arora A, Attwood J: Common skin cancers and their precursors, *Surg Clin North Am* 89(3):703–712, 2009.

65. Dessinioti C, et al: Basal cell carcinoma: what's new under the sun, *Photochem Photobiol* 86(3):481–491, 2010.

66. Rodust PM, et al: UV-induced squamous cell carcinoma—a role for antiapoptotic signaling pathways, *Br J Dermatol* 161(suppl 3):107–115, 2009.

67. Youl PH, et al: Body-site distribution of skin cancer, pre-malignant and common benign pigmented lesions excised in general practice, *Br J Dermatol* 165(1):35–43, 2011.

68. Lee DA, Miller SJ: Nonmelanoma skin cancer, *Facial Plast Surg Clin North Am* 17(3):309–324, 2009.

69. Erdei E, Torres SM: A new understanding in the epidemiology of melanoma, *Exp Rev Anticancer Ther* 10(11):1811–1823, 2010.

70. MacKie RM, Hauschild A, Eggermont AM: Epidemiology of invasive cutaneous melanoma, *Ann Oncol* 20(suppl 6):vi1–vi7, 2009.

71. Tímár J, Gyorffy B, Rásó E: Gene signature of the metastatic potential of cutaneous melanoma: too much for too little? *Clin Exp Metastasis* 27(6):371–387, 2010.

72. Psaty EL, et al: Defining the patient at high risk for melanoma, *Int J Dermatol* 49(4):362–376, 2010.

73. American Joint Committee on Cancer: *Melanoma of the skin staging*, ed 7, Atlanta, 2010, American Cancer Society. Also available at www.cancerstaging.org/staging/posters/melanoma8.5x11.pdf.

74. Gasent Blesa JM, et al: Melanoma: from darkness to promise, *Am J Clin Oncol* 34(2):179–187, 2011.

75. Erickson C, Miller SJ: Treatment options in melanoma in situ: topical and radiation therapy, excision and Mohs surgery, *Int J Dermatol* 49(5):482–491, 2010.

76. Nezos A, et al: Methods of detection of circulating melanoma cells: a comparative overview, *Cancer Treat Rev* 37(4):284–290, 2011.

77. Rigel DS, Russak J, Friedman R: The evolution of melanoma diagnosis: 25 years beyond the ABCDs, *CA Cancer J Clin* 60(5):301–316, 2010.

78. Wen KW, Damania B: Kaposi sarcoma-associated herpesvirus (KSHV): molecular biology and oncogenesis, *Cancer Lett* 289(2):140–150, 2010.

79. Uldrick TS, Whitby D: Update on KSHV epidemiology, Kaposi sarcoma pathogenesis, and treatment of Kaposi Sarcoma, *Cancer Lett* 305(2): 150–162, 2011.

80. American Burn Association: *Burn incidence and treatment in the United States: 2011 fact sheet, American Burn Association National Burn Repository (2010 report)*. Available at www.ameriburn.org/resources_factsheet.php.

81. Yu CY, Lin CH, Yang YH: Human body surface area database and estimation formula, *Burns* 36(5):616–629, 2010.

82. Magnotti LJ, Deitch EA: Burns, bacterial translocation, gut barrier function, and failure, *J Burn Care Rehabil* 26(5):383–391, 2005.

83. Jeschke MG: The hepatic response to thermal injury: is the liver important for postburn outcomes? *Mol Med* 15(9–10):337–351, 2009.

84. Lippi G, Ippolito L, Cervellin G: Disseminated intravascular coagulation in burn injury, *Semin Thromb Hemost* 36(4):429–436, 2010.

85. Kramer GC, Lund T, Beckum O: Pathophysiology of burn shock and burn edema. In Herndon DN, editor: *Total burn care*, ed 3, Philadelphia, 2007, Saunders.

86. White DJ, et al: Cardiomyocyte intracellular calcium and cardiac dysfunction after burn trauma, *Crit Care Med* 30(1):14–22, 2002.

87. Klein GL, Herndon DN: Magnesium deficit in major burns: role in hypoparathyroidism and end-organ parathyroid hormone resistance, *Magnes Res* 11(2):103–109, 1998.

88. Liu ZJ, Wang W, He CS: Comparison of serum and plasma lactate dehydrogenase in postburn patients, *Burns* 26(1):46–48, 2000.

89. Pruitt BA Jr, Wolf SE: An historical perspective on advances in burn care over the past 100 years, *Clin Plast Surg* 36(4):527–545, 2009.

90. Williams FN, Herndon DN, Jeschke MG: The hypermetabolic response to burn injury and interventions to modify this response, *Clin Plast Surg* 36(4):583–596, 2009.

91. Mecott GA, et al: The role of hyperglycemia in burned patients: evidence-based studies, *Shock* 33(1):5–13, 2010.

92. Ballian N, et al: Glucose metabolism in burn patients: the role of insulin and other endocrine hormones, *Burns* 36(5):599–605, 2010.

93. Williams FN, et al: What, how, and how much should patients with burns be fed? *Surg Clin North Am* 1(3):609–269, 2011.

94. Dahiya P: Burns as a model of SIRS, *Front Biosci* 14:4962–4967, 2009.

95. Nguyen LN, Nguyen TG: Characteristics and outcomes of multiple organ dysfunction syndrome among severe-burn patients, *Burns* 35(7):937–941, 2009.

96. Mosier MJ, et al: Early acute kidney injury predicts progressive renal dysfunction and higher mortality in severely burned adults, *J Burn Care Res* 231(1):83–92, 2010.

97. Saffle JR: Closure of the excised burn wound: temporary skin substitutes, *Clin Plast Surg* 36(4):627–641, 2009.

98. Wilmore W, et al: Effect of ambient temperature on heat production and heat loss in burn patients, *J Appl Phys* 38(4):593–597, 1975.

99. Turnage RH, et al: Mechanisms of pulmonary microvascular dysfunction during severe burn injury, *World J Surg* 26(7):848–853, 2002.

100. Goebel A, et al: Injury induces deficient interleukin-12 production, but interleukin-12 therapy after injury restores resistance to infection, *Ann Surg* 231(2):253, 2000.

101. Chipp E, Milner CS, Blackburn AV: Sepsis in burns: a review of current practice and future therapies, *Ann Plast Surg* 65(2):228–236, 2010.

102. Ladak A, Tredget EE: Pathophysiology and management of the burn scar, *Clin Plast Surg* 36(4):661–674, 2009.

103. Connor-Ballard PA: Understanding and managing burn pain: part 1, *Am J Nurs* 109(4):48–56, 2009.

104. Connor-Ballard PA: Understanding and managing burn pain: part 2, *Am J Nurs* 109(5):54–62, 2009.

105. Richardson P, Mustard L: The management of pain in the burns unit, *Burns* 35(7):921–936, 2009.

106. Chan MM, Chan GM: Nutritional therapy for burns in children and adults, *Nutrition* 25(3):261–269, 2009.

107. Sheridan R: Closure of the excised burn wound: autografts, semipermanent skin substitutes, and permanent skin substitutes, *Clin Plast Surg* 36(4):643–651, 2009.

108. Mohr WJ, Jenabzadeh K, Ahrenholz DH: Cold injury, *Hand Clin* 25(4):481–496, 2009.

109. Imray C, et al: Cold damage to the extremities: frostbite and non-freezing cold injuries, *Postgrad Med J* 85(1007):481–488, 2009.

110. Rathnayake D, Sinclair R: Male androgenetic alopecia, *Expert Opin Pharmacother* 11(8):1295–1304, 2010.

111. Rathnayake D, Sinclair R: Innovative use of spironolactone as an antiandrogen in the treatment of female pattern hair loss, *Dermatol Clin* 28(3):611–618, 2010.

112. Alkhalifah A, et al: Alopecia areata update: part I. Clinical picture, histopathology, and pathogenesis, *J Am Acad Dermatol* 62(2):177–188, 2010.

113. Alkhalifah A, et al: Alopecia areata update: part II. Treatment, *J Am Acad Dermatol* 62(2):191–202, 2010.

114. Lumachi F, Basso SM: Medical treatment of hirsutism in women, *Curr Med Chem* 17(23):2530–2538, 2010.

115. Rigopoulos D, et al: Acute and chronic paronychia, *Am Fam Physician* 77(3):339–346, 2008.

116. Welsh O, Vera-Cabrera L, Welsh E: Onychomycosis, *Clin Dermatol* 28(2):151–159, 2010.

Alterations of the Integument in Children

Noreen Heer Nicol and Sue E. Huether

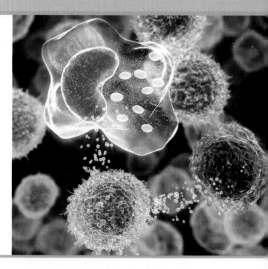

evolve WEBSITE

CHAPTER OUTLINE

Children frequently develop alterations of the skin, which may be minor or severe and localized or generalized. Skin diseases in children may have different forms of expression than those found in adults, although the causative mechanisms may be similar. Some skin diseases resolve spontaneously and require no treatment. Diagnosis is commonly made from the history, appearance, and distribution of the lesion or lesions. Common skin diseases of childhood are presented here.

ACNE VULGARIS

Acne vulgaris is the most common skin disease; it affects 85% of the population between the ages of 12 and 25 years; however, the age of onset is earlier than in the past, which may be associated with the earlier onset of puberty in the United States.[1] Genetic influences also determine an individual's susceptibility and the severity of the disease. The incidence of acne is the same in both genders, although severe disease affects males more often.

Acne develops at distinctive pilosebaceous units, known as *sebaceous follicles*. Located primarily on the face and upper parts of the chest and back, these follicles have many large sebaceous glands, a small vellus hair (very short, nonpigmented, and very thin hair), and a dilated follicular canal that is visible as a pore on the skin surface. Acne lesions may be noninflammatory or inflammatory (cystic) (Figure 40-1). In **noninflammatory acne,** the comedones are open (blackheads) and closed (whiteheads), with the accumulated material causing distention of the follicle and thinning of follicular canal walls. **Inflammatory (cystic) acne** develops in closed comedones when the follicular wall ruptures, expelling sebum into the surrounding dermis and initiating inflammation. Pustules form when the inflammation is close to the surface; papules and cystic nodules can develop when the inflammation is deeper, causing mild to severe scarring. Both types of lesions may exist in the same individual (see *Health Alert:* Hidradenitis Suppurativa [Inverse Acne] for a review of this condition).

The principal causative factors are (1) hyperkeratinization of the follicular epithelium, (2) excessive sebum production, (3) follicular proliferation of *Propionibacterium acnes* with release of inflammatory mediators, (4) increased sebaceous lipogenesis, and (5) inflammation and rupture of a follicle from accumulated debris and bacteria within

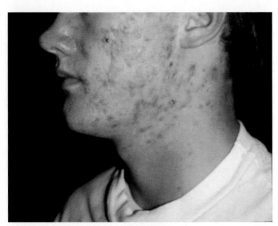

FIGURE 40-1 Inflammatory (Cystic) Acne. Multiple pustules (erythematous papules and pustules) are present, and several have become confluent. Note areas of scarring. (Courtesy Department of Dermatology, School of Medicine, University of Utah, Salt Lake City, Utah.)

HEALTH ALERT

Hidradenitis Suppurativa (Inverse Acne)

Hidradenitis suppurativa (inverse acne) is a chronic, inflammatory, recurring, scarring disease of the pilosebaceous follicular ducts involving areas of skin where there are folds, hair follicles, and apocrine (sweat) glands (i.e., axillary, inguinal, inframammary, genital, buttocks, and perineal areas of the body). The incidence is unknown but estimated at 1% to 4% of the population and is more common in females. The pathogenesis of the disease is complex and includes a combination of genetic, hormonal, immune, and environmental factors. Aggravating factors include tight clothing, heat and perspiration, obesity, stress, and smoking. Follicular occlusion obstructs the pilosebaceous unit, causing perifolliculitis, abscess formation, sinus tracks, and scarring. Bacterial infection is a secondary event. The lesions present as deep, firm, painful subcutaneous nodules that track and rupture horizontally under the skin. They are differentiated from "boils" (carbuncles) because boils extend vertically and discharge onto the skin. Diagnosis can be difficult, delaying effective treatment. Treatment can include systemic medications, incision and drainage of nodules, culture of exudate, and administration of antibiotics, with concern about the presence of methicillin-resistant *Staphylococcus aureus* (MRSA), topical or intralesional corticosteroids, and retinoids. Lesions often require surgical excision and skin grafting. Complete, spontaneous resolution is rare. Deterrence includes avoiding heat and perspiration, losing weight if obese, wearing loose clothing, refraining from shaving affected areas, stopping smoking, and using zinc gluconate supplements to reduce inflammation. The disease can recur for years with negative effects on quality of life.

Data from Alikhan A, Lynch PJ, Eisen DB: Hidradenitis suppurativa: a comprehensive review, *J Am Acad Dermatol* 60(4):539–561, 2009; Bieniek A et al: Surgical treatment of hidradenitis suppurativa: experiences and recommendations, *Dermatol Surg* 36(12):1998–2004, 2010; Danby FW, Margesson LJ: Hidradenitis suppurativa, *Dermatol Clin* 28(4):779–793, 2010; Yazdanyar S, Jemec GB: Hidradenitis suppurativa: a review of cause and treatment, *Curr Opin Infect Dis* 24(2):118–123, 2011.

the follicle (see Figure 40-1). Androgens (dihydrotestosterone and testosterone), synthesized in increasing amounts during puberty, increase the size and productivity of the sebaceous glands and promote *P. acnes*. Recent advances in understanding and treatment are related to the discovery of the interaction of *P. acnes* with Toll-like receptors (TLRs), the development of vaccines targeting *P. acnes* or its components, the function of antimicrobial peptides, and the role of hormones.[2]

The treatment combination of a topical retinoid and antimicrobial agents is preferred. Retinoids are anticomedogenic and comedolytic and have some anti-inflammatory effects. Benzoyl peroxide is antimicrobial with some keratolytic effects. Antibiotics have anti-inflammatory and antimicrobial effects. Use of systemic therapies, including oral antibiotics, sex hormones, corticosteroids, and isotretinoin, may be limited by side effects.[3] Acne surgery, including comedo extraction, intralesional steroids, and cryosurgery, is useful in selected individuals. Severe scarring may be treated with dermabrasion, lasers, and resurfacing techniques.

Acne conglobata is a highly inflammatory form of acne with communicating cysts and abscesses beneath the skin that can cause scarring. Remissions tend to occur during the summer, perhaps from more exposure to sunlight. This type of acne requires the use of systemic and combination therapies to prevent drug resistance.[4]

DERMATITIS

Atopic Dermatitis

Atopic dermatitis (AD) is the most common cause of eczema in children, with a prevalence of about 9% to 18%. The incidence of AD is increasing. The wide range of prevalence suggests that social or environmental factors may influence disease expression.[5]

The etiology is unknown and complex. From 75% to 80% of individuals with atopic dermatitis have a personal or family history of asthma, allergic rhinitis (hay fever), or food allergy. Onset is usually from 2 to 6 months of age, and 85% of cases develop within the first 5 years of life. There are no specific laboratory features of AD that can be used for diagnostic purposes. Most affected individuals show an increased serum immunoglobulin E (IgE) level, elevated interleukin-4 level, elevated levels of eosinophils, and positive skin tests to a variety of common food and inhalant allergens.[6] Similarly, blood eosinophilia is a common finding in AD.

The cause of this chronic relapsing form of pruritic eczema involves an interplay of genetic predisposition; altered skin barrier function associated with filaggrin gene mutations (proteins that bind keratin in the epidermis); reduced ceramide (a stratum corneum lipid [see Figure 39-1]) levels; altered innate immunity; and altered immune responses to allergens, irritants, and microbes. Filaggrin gene mutations also are associated with increased risk for asthma in AD and ichthyosis vulgaris (dry, scaly skin).[7]

AD has a constellation of clinical features that include severe pruritus, a characteristic eczematoid appearance, and an age-dependent distribution of lesions. The skin becomes increasingly dry, itchy, sensitive, and easily irritated because the barrier function of the skin is impaired. In young children, a rash appears primarily on the face, scalp, trunk, and extensor surfaces of the arms and legs (Figure 40-2). In older children and adults, the rash tends to be found on the neck, antecubital and popliteal fossae, and hands and feet. Individuals with AD also tend to develop viral, bacterial, and fungal skin infections in the eczematous areas.

Management of individuals with AD includes accurate diagnosis and comprehensive evaluation of triggers and response to treatment; management of confounding factors, including sleep disruption; and education of individuals and caregivers.[8] Skin hydration is the key to good therapy. Anti-inflammatory agents, such as topical corticosteroids or

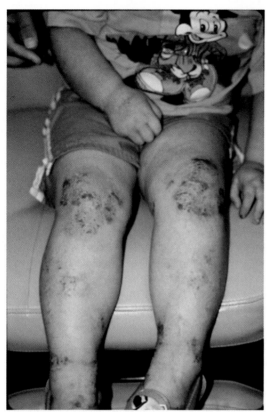

FIGURE 40-2 Atopic Dermatitis. Characteristic lesions with crusting from irritation and scratching over knees and around ankles. (Courtesy Department of Dermatology, School of Medicine, University of Utah, Salt Lake City, Utah.)

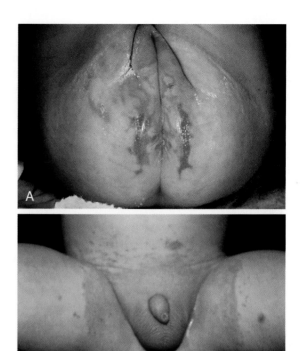

FIGURE 40-3 Diaper Dermatitis. A, Diaper dermatitis with erosions. **B,** Diaper dermatitis with *Candida albicans* secondary infection. (Courtesy Department of Dermatology, School of Medicine, University of Utah, Salt Lake City, Utah.)

tar preparations, are necessary during active flares of eczema. Immunomodulator therapy is used for severe eczema. Systemic therapy includes the use of sedating antihistamines and antibiotics.[9]

Diaper Dermatitis

Diaper dermatitis (diaper rash) is a form of irritant contact dermatitis initiated by a combination of factors including prolonged exposure to and irritation by urine and feces as well as maceration by wet diapers or airtight plastic diaper covers. Often, diaper dermatitis is secondarily infected with *Candida albicans*. The resulting inflammation affects the lower aspect of the abdomen, genitalia, buttock, and upper portion of the thigh.

The lesions vary from mild erythema to erythematous papular lesions. Candidal (monilial) diaper dermatitis is usually very erythematous, with sharp margination and pustulovesicular satellite lesions (Figure 40-3).

Treatment involves frequent diaper changes to keep the affected area clean and dry or regular exposure of the perineal area to air. Topical antifungal medication is used to treat *C. albicans*. Short-term use of low-potency topical steroids alternately with antifungals at each diaper change helps to reduce the inflammation. Use of various topical medications to provide a barrier between the irritating agents and the skin promotes healing.[10]

> ✔ **QUICK CHECK 40-1**
> 1. What causes the inflammation of acne vulgaris?
> 2. What lesions are typical of atopic dermatitis in children?
> 3. What causes diaper dermatitis?

INFECTIONS OF THE SKIN

Infectious diseases caused by bacteria, viruses, and fungi constitute the major forms of skin disease. Skin infections are caused by breaks in the skin or alterations in the protective barrier functions of the skin with resulting introduction of pathogens. Most infections tend to occur superficially; however, systemic signs and symptoms develop occasionally and can be life-threatening, particularly in immunosuppressed children.

Bacterial Infections
Impetigo Contagiosum

Impetigo is a common bacterial skin infection in infants and children. The mode of transmission is by both direct and indirect contact. The disease is more common in midsummer to late summer, with a higher incidence in hot, humid climates. Impetigo is particularly infectious among people living in crowded conditions with poor sanitary facilities or in settings such as day-care facilities. It affects children in good health, but conditions such as anemia and malnutrition are predisposing factors. There are two types of impetigo: vesicular and, more rarely, bullous. *Staphylococcus aureus* (*S. aureus*) is currently the most common overall cause of impetigo, but *Streptococcus pyogenes* remains an important cause in developing nations. Community-acquired methicillin-resistant *S. aureus* (CA-MRSA) poses a challenge because of its enhanced virulence and increasing prevalence in children[11] (Box 40-1). Both forms of impetigo begin as vesicles with a thin vesicular roof composed of stratum corneum (Figure 40-4). Impetigo is clinically characterized by crusted erosions or ulcers that may arise as a primary infection in which bacterial invasion occurs through minor breaks in the cutaneous surface or as a secondary infection of a preexisting dermatosis or infestation.

BOX 40-1   IMPETIGO

Vesicular Impetigo

- Contagious, acute, superficial, vesiculopustular, and most common form
- Caused by group A *Streptococcus pyogenes* (alone or with *S. aureus*)
- Spread by direct physical contact with other infected individuals or through insect bites
- Presents as small vesicles with a honey-colored serum; yellow to white-brown crusts form as vesicles rupture and extend radially
- Untreated lesions last for weeks and cover large area
- Regional lymphadenitis common
- Most significant complication is acute glomerulonephritis
- Treatment is aggressive in light of this complication

Bullous Impetigo

- Caused by Staphylococcus aureus
- Bacterial toxin produced (exfoliative toxin [ET]) causes disruption in cellular adhesion with blister formation
- Occurs in neonates
- Highly contagious
- Source is family member with pustule or asymptomatic carrier with pathogen in anterior nares, perineal region, or fingernails
- Transmitted by contact with individual or contaminated equipment
- Presents with vesicles that enlarge or coalesce to form superficial bullae, few localized lesions or many scattered over the skin surface; as bullae rupture, thin, flat, honey-colored crust appears (hallmark of impetigo)
- Lesions found on face around the nose and mouth; hands and other exposed areas also susceptible

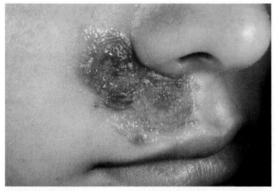

FIGURE 40-4 Impetigo and Herpes Simplex Virus (HSV) of Upper Lip. Note weeping and crusting lesions. (Courtesy Department of Dermatology, School of Medicine, University of Utah, Salt Lake City, Utah.)

The treatment of choice for both types of impetigo is topical mupirocin or fusidic acid for uncomplicated lesions. For extensive or complicated impetigo, systemic antibiotics may be warranted but beta-lactam antibiotics should be avoided if methicillin-resistant *S. aureus* (MRSA) is suspected. Prompt treatment avoids complications, such as glomerulonephritis. Good handwashing techniques and isolation of the infected child's washcloth, towels, drinking glass, and linen are important.[12]

Staphylococcal Scalded-Skin Syndrome

Staphylococcal scalded-skin syndrome (SSSS) is the most serious staphylococcal infection that affects the skin. SSSS is caused by virulent group II strains of staphylococci that produce an exfoliative toxin.

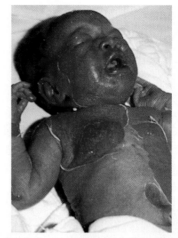

FIGURE 40-5 Staphylococcal Scalded-Skin Syndrome (SSSS). The skin lesions, showing desquamation and wrinkling of the skin margins, appeared 1 day after drainage of a staphylococcal abscess. (From Kliegman R, Stanton B, St. Geme J, Schnor N, and Behrman R: *Nelson textbook of pediatrics,* ed 19, St. Louis, 2011, Saunders.)

The toxin attacks desmoglein and adhesion molecules and causes a separation of the skin just below the granular layer of the epidermis (see Figure 39-1).[13] The toxin is usually produced at body sites other than the skin and arrives at the epidermis through the circulatory system. Staphylococci typically are not found in the skin lesions themselves. Adults have circulating antistaphylococcal antibodies and are better able to metabolize and excrete the toxin. Neonates are at the highest risk because of their lack of immunity, having no prior exposure to the toxin.[14]

The clinical symptoms begin with fever, malaise, rhinorrhea, and irritability followed by generalized erythema with exquisite tenderness of the skin. There may be an associated impetigo, but the infection often begins in the throat or chest. The erythema spreads from the face and trunk to cover the entire body except for the palms, soles, and mucous membranes. Within 48 hours, blisters and bullae may form, giving the child the appearance of being scalded. The pain is severe (Figure 40-5). Fluid loss from ruptured blisters and water evaporation from denuded areas may cause dehydration. Perioral and nasolabial crusting and fissures develop. In severe cases, the skin of the entire body may slough. When secondary infection can be prevented, healing of the involved skin occurs in 10 to 14 days, usually without scarring.

Before medical intervention is initiated, culture and histologic or exfoliative cytologic studies must be performed to differentiate SSSS from *erythema multiforme* and *toxic epidermal necrolysis* (TEN), both of which are usually caused by an immune reaction to drugs.[15] When SSSS infection is confirmed, treatment with oral or intravenous antibiotics begins. The skin should be treated in the same manner as a severe burn, with meticulous aseptic technique. Special care is required when there is involvement of the lips and eyelids.

Fungal Infections
Tinea Capitis

Tinea capitis, a fungal infection of the scalp (scalp ringworm), is the most common fungal infection of childhood. It rarely affects infants and is seen in children between 2 and 10 years of age. Primary organisms responsible for this disease are *Microsporum canis* and *Trichophyton tonsurans* (most common). *M. canis* is found on cats, dogs, and certain rodents. Humans appear to be a terminal host for *M. canis,* and children who handle such animals are possible hosts. Direct transmission between humans does not occur. However, there is direct human

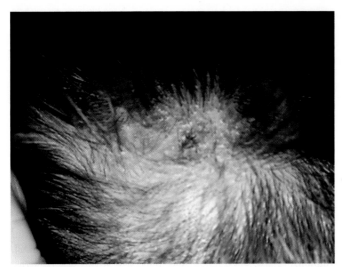

FIGURE 40-6 Tinea Capitis. (Courtesy Department of Dermatology, School of Medicine, University of Utah, Salt Lake City, Utah.)

transmission of *T. tonsurans* in crowded areas, the most prevalent environment of the fungus.[16]

The lesions are often circular and manifested by broken hairs 1 to 3 mm above the scalp, leaving a partial area of alopecia from 1 to 5 cm in diameter (Figure 40-6). A slight erythema and scaling with raised borders can be observed.

Diagnosis is best confirmed by potassium hydroxide (KOH) examination, and fungal culture. Tinea capitis always requires systemic treatment because topical antifungal agents do not penetrate the hair follicle. Several oral antifungal agents, particularly griseofulvin, are available for treatment.[17] Wood's light examination has decreased due to a number of dermatophytes that fluoresce under an ultraviolet light.

Tinea Corporis

Tinea corporis (ringworm) is a common superficial dermatophyte infection in children. The organisms most commonly responsible for this disease are *M. canis* and *Trichophyton mentagrophytes*. As in tinea capitis, contact with young kittens and puppies is a common source of the disorder. Tinea corporis preferentially affects the nonhairy parts of the face, trunk, and limbs. Lesions are often erythematous, round or oval scaling patches that spread peripherally with clearing in the center, creating the ring appearance, which is why this disease is commonly referred to as *ringworm*. The lesions are distributed asymmetrically, and multiple lesions, when present, overlap. Transmission occurs by direct contact with an infected lesion and through indirect contact with personal items used by the infected person. Potassium hydroxide examination of the scale from the border of the lesions confirms the diagnosis. Most lesions respond well to applications of appropriate topical antifungal medications.[18]

Thrush

Thrush is the term used to describe the presence of *Candida* in the mucous membranes of the mouth of infants. It occurs less commonly in adults and they are usually immunocompromised. Thrush is characterized by the formation of white plaques or spots in the mouth that lead to shallow ulcers caused by keratolytic proteases from the microorganism. The tongue may have a dense, white covering. The underlying mucous membrane is red and tender and may bleed when the plaques are removed. The disease is often accompanied by fever and gastrointestinal irritation. The infection commonly spreads to the

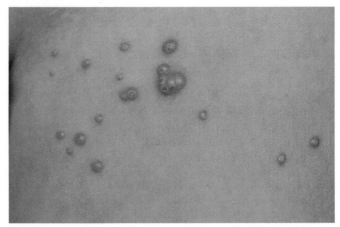

FIGURE 40-7 Molluscum Contagiosum. Waxy pink globules with umbilicated centers. (From Habif TP: *Clinical dermatology: a color guide to diagnosis and therapy*, ed 4, St Louis, 2004, Mosby.)

groin, buttocks, and other parts of the body. Treatment may be difficult and may include oral antifungal washes, such as nystatin oral suspension. Simultaneous treatment of a *Candida* nipple infection or vaginitis in the mother is helpful in reducing the *C. albicans* surface colonization of the infant. Feeding bottles and nipples should be sterilized to prevent reinfection. The diaper area should be kept clean and dry.

Viral Infections

Viral infections of the skin in children are caused by poxvirus, papovavirus, and herpesvirus.

Molluscum Contagiosum

Molluscum contagiosum is a common, highly contagious viral infection of the skin and, occasionally, conjunctiva that affects school-aged children, sexually active young adults, and immunocompromised individuals. The disease can be more severe or prolonged in individuals with atopic dermatitis and a variety of immunodeficient states, including acquired immunodeficiency syndrome.[19]

The poxvirus proliferates within the follicular epithelium and induces epidermal cell proliferation. The epidermis grows down into the dermis to form saccules containing clusters of virus. The characteristic molluscum body is composed of mature, immature, and incomplete viruses and cellular debris.[20] The disease is transmitted by skin-to-skin contact or from contact with contaminated clothing, washcloths, or towels. The incidence is higher among children who swim in public pools.[21]

The lesions of molluscum are discrete, slightly umbilicated, dome-shaped papules 1 to 5 mm in diameter that appear anywhere on the skin or conjunctiva. The lesions are mainly on the trunk, face, and extremities in children (Figure 40-7). There is usually no inflammation surrounding molluscum lesions unless they are traumatized or secondary infection occurs. Scarring may occur with healing.

The three best diagnostic procedures are (1) staining smears of the expressed molluscum body, (2) examining a biopsy specimen, or (3) inoculating a molluscum suspension into cell cultures to demonstrate the cytotoxic reactions. Most lesions are self-limiting and clear in 6 to 9 months if not manipulated.

Therapeutic intervention may be indicated to prevent autoinoculation and transmission, especially in those at risk for severe disease. The three major treatments include physical destruction, immunomodulation, and antiviral agents, which can be used either alone or

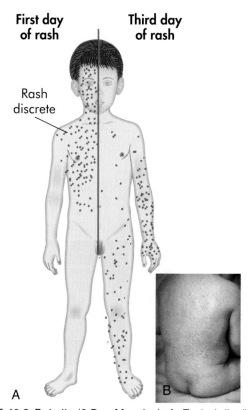

First day of rash

Third day of rash

Rash discrete

A

B

FIGURE 40-8 Rubella (3-Day Measles). **A,** Typical distribution of full-blown maculopapular rash with tendency to coalesce; **B,** Rash of rubella. (From Centers for Disease Control and Prevention Image Bank, Figure #712. Available at http://phil.cdc.gov/phil/home.asp. Accessed June 27, 2011.)

in combination. Benign neglect, curettage, and cryotherapy as well as administration of cantharidin, imiquimod, or retinoids are the most common approaches to treatment.[19,22] However, if multiple lesions are present, these procedures may be too painful for small children and thus are not justified. Therapy may leave pigment alterations and sometimes scars. Measures to prevent spread of infection must be taken. Recurrences are common.

Rubella (German or 3-Day Measles)

Rubella is a common communicable disease of children and young adults caused by a ribonucleic acid (RNA) virus that enters the bloodstream through the respiratory route. This disease is mild in most children. The incubation period ranges from 14 to 21 days. Prodromal symptoms include enlarged cervical and postauricular lymph nodes, low-grade fever, headache, sore throat, rhinorrhea, and cough. A faint-pink to red coalescing maculopapular rash develops on the face with spread to the trunk and extremities 1 to 4 days after the onset of initial symptoms (Figure 40-8). The rash is thought to be the result of virus dissemination to the skin. The rash subsides after 2 to 3 days, usually without complication. Children are usually not contagious after development of the rash (Table 40-1).

Vaccination for rubella is usually combined with vaccines for mumps and measles (rubeola) (MMR). Measles is known to occur in previously immunized children. Rubella has almost been eliminated in the United States because of vaccination campaigns. However, challenges to maintain elimination include large outbreaks of measles in highly traveled developed countries, frequent international travel, and clusters of U.S. residents who remain unvaccinated because of personal belief exemptions.[23]

There is no specific treatment for rubella. Recovery is spontaneous, although lymph nodes may remain enlarged for weeks. Supportive

TABLE 40-1	DIFFERENTIAL PRESENTATION OF VIRAL DISEASES PRODUCING RASHES			
VIRAL DISEASE	**INCUBATION PERIOD**	**PRODROMAL SYMPTOMS**	**DURATION/ CHARACTERISTICS**	**CLINICAL SYMPTOMS**
Rubella (German measles)	14-21 days	1-2 days Mild fever Malaise Respiratory symptoms	1-3 days Pink-red maculopapular Face and trunk	Enlarged and tender occipital and periauricular lymph nodes
Rubeola (red measles)	7-12 days	2-5 days Fever Cough Respiratory symptoms	3-5 days Purple-red to brown maculopapular Face, trunk, extremities	Koplik spots 1-3 days before rash
Roseola (exanthema subitum)	5-15 days	2-5 days High fever	1-3 days Red macular Neck and trunk	Rash develops when fever subsides
Varicella (chickenpox)	11-20 days	1-2 days Low-grade fever Cough May be asymptomatic	7-14 days Red papules, vesicles, pustules in clusters	Eruption of new lesions for 4-5 days Occasional ulcerative lesion in mouth
Fifth disease (human parvovirus B19, Erythrovirus)	4-28 days	May be asymptomatic Low-grade fever, malaise before rash	7-10 days "Slapped-cheek" rash on face; lacy red rash on trunk and limbs; may itch	Rash develops when fever subsides

therapy includes rest, fluids, and use of a vaporizer. In rare cases, a mild encephalitis or peripheral neuritis may follow rubella.

Women of childbearing age are immunized if their rubella hemagglutination-inhibition titer is low. Pregnancy should be avoided for 3 months after vaccination because the attenuated virus in the vaccine may remain viable for this period. Pregnant women who have rubella early in the first trimester may have a fetus that develops congenital defects.

Rubeola (Red Measles)

Rubeola is a highly contagious, acute viral disease of childhood. Transmitted by direct contact with droplets from infected persons, rubeola is caused by an RNA-containing paramyxovirus with an incubation period of 7 to 12 days, during which there are no symptoms. Prodromal symptoms include high fever (up to 40.5° C), malaise, enlarged lymph nodes, rhinorrhea, conjunctivitis, and barking cough. Within 3 to 4 days, an erythematous maculopapular rash develops over the head and spreads distally over the trunk, extremities, hands, and feet. Early lesions blanch with pressure, followed by a brownish hue that does not blanch as the rash fades. Characteristic pinpoint white spots surrounded by an erythematous ring develop over the buccal mucosa and are known as *Koplik spots*. These spots precede the rash by 1 to 2 days. The rash then subsides within 3 to 5 days.

Complications associated with measles may be caused by the primary infection or by a secondary bacterial infection. Measles encephalitis occurs in about 1 of 800 cases, and most children recover completely. Only a small minority of children develop permanent brain damage or die. Bacterial complications include otitis media and pneumonia, usually caused by group A hemolytic streptococcus, *Haemophilus influenzae,* or *S. aureus* infection.

Measles is prevented by vaccination. There is no specific treatment for measles, and supportive therapy is the same as that recommended for rubella. Antibiotic therapy is initiated if secondary bacterial infections develop.

Roseola (Exanthema Subitum)

Roseola is a presumed viral infection of infants between 6 months and 2 years of age and can be seen in children up to 4 years of age. The incubation period is 5 to 15 days, followed by the sudden onset of fever (38.9° to 40.5° C) that lasts 3 to 5 days. Following the fever, an erythematous macular rash that lasts about 24 hours develops primarily over the trunk and neck. Children usually feel well, eat normally, and have few other symptoms. There is usually no treatment.

Chickenpox, Herpes Zoster, and Smallpox

Chickenpox (varicella) and herpes zoster (shingles) are both produced by the varicella-zoster virus (VZV). VZV is a complex deoxyribonucleic acid (DNA) virus of the herpes group. The incubation period is 10 to 27 days, averaging 14 days. Vesicular lesions occur in the epidermis as infection occurs within kerotinocytes. An inflammatory infiltrate is often present. Vesicles eventually rupture, followed by crust formation or the development of transient ulcers on mucous membranes. Varicella occurs in people not previously exposed to VZV, whereas herpes zoster occurs in partially immune individuals who had varicella in the past. Since the introduction of live attenuated varicella-zoster virus (VZV) vaccine in 1995, there has been a significant reduction in varicella incidence and its associated complications.[24]

Chickenpox. Chickenpox (varicella) is a disease of early childhood, with 90% of children contracting the disease during the first decade of life. Being a highly contagious virus, chickenpox is spread by close person-to-person contact and by airborne droplets. Introduction of an

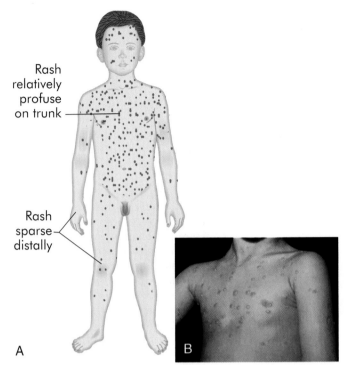

Rash relatively profuse on trunk

Rash sparse distally

A

B

FIGURE 40-9 Chickenpox. A, Pattern of generalized, polymorphous eruption; **B,** Chickenpox lesions on 5th day of illness. (From Centers for Disease Control and Prevention Image Bank, Figure #2882. Available at http://phil.cdc.gov/phil/home.asp. Accessed June 27, 2011.)

infected person into a household results in a 90% possibility of susceptible persons developing the disease within the incubation period, usually 14 days. Children are contagious for at least 1 day before development of the rash. Transmission of the virus may occur until approximately 5 to 6 days after the onset of the first skin lesions in healthy children. In immunocompromised children, the virus is recoverable for a longer period, but infected children must be considered contagious for at least 7 to 10 days. Transmission occurs more readily in temperate climates than in tropical climates.

Normally, children who develop chickenpox have no prodromal symptoms. The first sign of illness may be pruritus or the appearance of vesicles, usually on the trunk, scalp, or face. The rash later spreads to the extremities. Characteristically, lesions can be seen in various stages of maturation with macules, papules, and vesicles present in a particular area at the same time (Figure 40-9). The vesicular lesions are superficial and rupture easily. New lesions will erupt for 4 to 5 days, until there are approximately 100 to 300 in different stages of development. The vesicles become crusted, and over time only the crust remains, although there may be an occasional vesicle on the palm later in the disease. Although uncommon, ulcerative lesions are sometimes seen in the mouth and, less commonly, on the conjunctiva and pharynx. Fever usually lasts 2 to 3 days, with body temperature ranging from 38.5° to 40° C.

Complications are rare in children but more common in adults. They can include transient hematuria (from rupture of vesicles in the bladder), epistaxis, laryngeal edema, and varicella pneumonia. One case of chickenpox produces almost complete immunity against a second attack. The fetus may be malformed (congenital varicella syndrome) if chickenpox develops in the first half of pregnancy. Infants whose mothers have chickenpox at any stage of pregnancy have a higher risk of developing herpes zoster during the first few years of life.[25]

Uncomplicated chickenpox requires no specific therapy. Baths, wet dressings, and oral antihistamines occasionally help to relieve pruritus and to prevent secondary infection from developing as a result of scratching. Oral antistaphylococcal drugs should be given if secondary bacterial infection is present. Zoster immune globulin may be administered to immunodeficient individuals if given within 72 hours after exposure to chickenpox. Oral acyclovir may be valuable in immunosuppressed or other select groups of children. The varicella vaccine protects against both varicella and herpes zoster. However, wild-type (vaccine-resistant) viruses are a continuing threat.[26]

Herpes zoster. Although herpes zoster (shingles) occurs mainly in adults, approximately 5% of cases are in children younger than 15 years. The course of the disease in children with an immune defect is more complicated and requires intravenous treatment with antiviral agents.[27] The most frequent, severe complications are invasive streptococcal and staphylococcal superinfections, especially in children.[28]

The chickenpox virus persists for life in sensory nerve ganglia and can reactivate to cause herpes zoster. The eruption of zoster consists of groups of vesicles situated on an inflammatory base and follows the course of a sensory nerve. Common dermatomal distribution in childhood is thoracic. The base of the lesions often appears hemorrhagic, and some of the lesions may become necrotic and ulcerative. Therapy is similar to that for chickenpox unless the infection is an ophthalmic or disseminated form of zoster, for which systemic antiviral medication is indicated. Varicella vaccine substantially decreases the risk of herpes zoster among vaccinated children and its widespread use will likely reduce the overall herpes zoster burden in the United States.[29]

Smallpox. Smallpox (variola) was a highly contagious and deadly, but also preventable, disease caused by poxvirus variolae. Smallpox was eradicated worldwide in 1977. Routine vaccination in the United States was discontinued in 1972, and a new vaccine, ACAM2000, has been produced for the U.S. Strategic National Stockpile.[30,31]

✔ QUICK CHECK 40-2

1. Compare the cause and presentation of impetigo and staphylococcal scalded-skin syndrome.
2. Describe rubella and rubeola.
3. How are chickenpox and herpes zoster related?

INSECT BITES AND PARASITES

Insect bites and infestations are common causes of skin disorders in children and adults. Skin damage occurs by various mechanisms, including trauma of bites and stings, allergic reactions, transmission of disease, injection of substances that cause local or systemic reactions, and inflammatory reactions resulting from embedded and retained insect mouth parts and scratching of the skin.

Scabies

Scabies is a contagious disease caused by the itch mite, *Sarcoptes scabiei* (Figure 40-10, *A*), that can colonize the human epidermis. Scabies is a common skin infection in tropical settings affecting large numbers of people, particularly children. It is transmitted by close personal contact and by infected clothing and bedding. Scabies is often epidemic in areas of overcrowded housing and poor sanitation. Immunocompromised individuals are at greater risk. Infestation is initiated by a female mite that tunnels into the stratum corneum, depositing eggs and creating a burrow several millimeters to 1 cm long. Over a 3-week period, the eggs mature into adult mites, which sometimes are recognized as tiny dots at the ends of intact burrows.

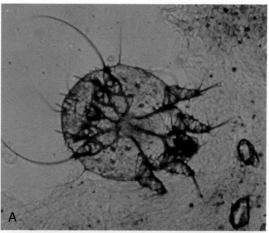

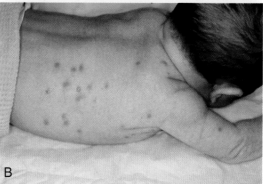

FIGURE 40-10 Scabies. A, Scabies mite, as seen clinically when removed from its burrow. **B,** Characteristic scabies bites. (Courtesy Department of Dermatology, School of Medicine, University of Utah, Salt Lake City, Utah.)

Symptoms appear 3 to 5 weeks after infestation. The primary lesions are burrows, papules, and vesicular lesions, with severe pruritus that worsens at night. Pruritus is thought to be related to sensitization to the larval stages of the parasite. In older children and adults, the lesions occur in the webs of fingers; in the axillae; in creases of the arms and wrists; along the belt line; and around the nipples, genitalia, and lower buttocks. Infants and young children have a different pattern of distribution, with involvement of the palms, soles, head, neck, and face (Figure 40-10, *B*). Secondary infections and crusting develop as a result of scratching and eczematous changes.

Diagnosis of scabies is made by observation of the tunnels and burrows and by microscopic examination of scrapings of the skin to identify the mite or its eggs or feces. Treatment involves the application of a scabicide, which is curative. All clothing and linens should be washed and dried in hot cycles or dry-cleaned.[32]

Pediculosis (Lice Infestation)

The three known types of human lice are (1) the head louse (*Pediculus capitis*), (2) the body louse (*Pediculus corporis*), and (3) the crab or pubic louse (*Phthirus pubis*). They are parasites and survive by sucking blood. The female louse reproduces every 2 weeks, producing hundreds of nits as newly hatched lice mate with older lice. The mouthparts are shaped for piercing and sucking and are attached to the skin of the host while the louse is feeding. When piercing the skin, the louse secretes toxic saliva, and the mechanical trauma and toxin produce a pruritic dermatitis. Head and body lice are acquired by direct personal contact or indirectly by sharing of combs, brushes, or towels or contact with infested clothes, toys, furniture, carpets, or bedding. Crab lice are spread by close body contact, usually with an infected adult. Sharing clothing or headphones are also common sources of transmission.

Pruritus is the major symptom of lice infestation. With head lice, the ova attach to hairs above the ears and in the occipital region. The primary lesion caused by the body louse is a pinpoint red macule, papule, or wheal with a hemorrhagic puncture site. The primary lesion often is not seen, because it is masked by excoriations, wheals, and crusts. The crab louse is found on pubic hairs but also may be found in other body hair, such as eyelashes, mustache, beard, and underarm hair. Young children in particular may become infected with crab lice on their eyebrows or eyelashes.

The live louse, 2 to 3 mm long, is rarely observed. The ova, or nits, can be observed as oval, yellowish, pinpoint specks fastened to a hair shaft. The ova fluoresce under an ultraviolet light (Wood lamp) and are observed best with a microscope. Nits are removed with a nit comb, and pediculicides, such as lindane shampoo or lotion, are the most effective treatment. Success or failure of therapy for ectoparasitic infestation depends much more on proper use of the topical preparation than on the type of scabicide or pediculicide used.[33]

All clothes, towels, bedding, combs, and brushes should be washed and dried in hot air or instead washed in boiling water, or clothes can be ironed to rid them of lice. Individuals who have close personal contact with the infected person also should be treated.

Fleas

Young children are very susceptible to fleabites; bites from cat, dog, and human fleas are most common.[34] Bites occur in clusters along the arms and legs or where clothing is tight fitting, such as near elastic bands that circle the thigh or waist. The bite produces an urticarial wheal with a central hemorrhagic puncture (Figure 40-11). Treatment includes spraying carpets, crevices, and furniture with malathion or lindane powder. Infected animals should be treated, and clothes and bedding should be washed in hot water.

Ticks

Lyme disease is a multisystem (affecting the skin, joints, nervous system, and heart) inflammatory disease caused by the spirochete *Borrelia burgdorferi,* which is transmitted by infected deer tick bites. The highest incidence of this disease is among children, and 50% of infected individuals are symptom free. The incidence is increasing.[35]

The disease occurs in stages with different presentations, and the mechanisms of injury are not well understood:
1. Soon after the tick bite, localized infection (rash—erythema migrans, myalgia, and fatigue)
2. Nine months later, disseminated infection (secondary erythema migrans, arthralgias, meningitis, neuritis, carditis)
3. Late persistent infection continuing for years (arthritis, encephalopathy, polyneuropathy)

The rash of erythema migrans (EM) occurs in 70% to 80% of infected persons. It begins at the tiny tick bite site 3 to 30 days after the bite. It is usually circular and expands (migrates) over a period of several days, reaching up to 12 inches in diameter. The rash clears from the center, leaving a bull's eye appearance. EM rashes can develop at other body sites after several days. The diagnosis of Lyme disease is based on the clinical presentation; history of tick bite, if known; and serologic studies. *Borrelia burgdorferi* is difficult to culture. Diagnosis and treatment can be challenging because of the unique pathophysiology of late Lyme borreliosis, which involves not only bacterial infection but also immunologic response. Because there is no completely reliable method of diagnosis, it is difficult to choose the proper treatment and

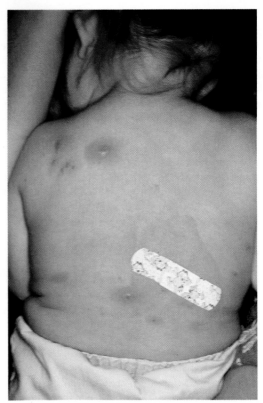

FIGURE 40-11 Fleabites. Fleabite producing an urticarial wheal with central puncture.

to evaluate treatment efficacy. Different types of antibiotics are used to treat the different stages of the disease.[36] Lyme disease should not be treated with steroids. Prevention of tick bites is essential. No vaccine is currently available.

Bedbugs

Bedbugs *(Cimex lectularius)* are blood-sucking parasites that live in the crevices and cracks of floors, walls, and furniture and in bedding or furniture stuffing. They are 3 to 5 mm long and reddish brown. Bedbugs are nocturnal, emerging to feed in darkness by attaching to the skin to suck blood. Feeding occurs for 5 to 15 minutes, and the bedbug then leaves. It will move long distances to search for food and can travel from house to house.

Immunologic reactions to bedbug saliva vary, but bites typically yield erythematous and pruritic papules. The face and distal extremities, areas uncovered by sleeping clothes or blankets, are preferentially involved. If the host has not been previously sensitized, the only symptom is a red macule that develops into a nodule, lasting up to 14 days. In sensitized children and adults, pruritic wheals, papules, and vesicles may form. Most lesions respond to oral antihistamines or topical corticosteroids, or both. Secondary infections require antibiotic treatment.[37]

Until the late 1990s, bedbug infestations in the United States were declining. Resurgence is attributed to increased travel and resistance to insecticides. Bedbugs are eliminated by spraying with chlordane or lindane and by cleaning or disposing of infested bedding, mattresses, and furniture; however, their ability to remain buried in crevices within the bedroom makes eradication difficult. Pest control and eradication also is challenging because of insecticide resistance, lack of effective products, and health concerns about spraying mattresses with pesticides.[38,39]

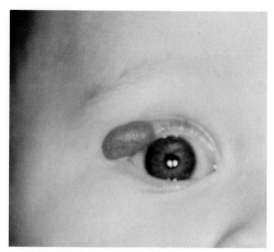

FIGURE 40-12 Capillary Hemangioma. (Courtesy Department of Dermatology, School of Medicine, University of Utah, Salt Lake City, Utah.)

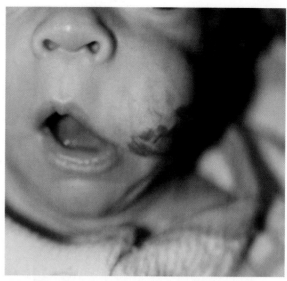

FIGURE 40-13 Cavernous Hemangioma. (Courtesy Department of Dermatology, School of Medicine, University of Utah, Salt Lake City, Utah.)

HEMANGIOMAS AND VASCULAR MALFORMATIONS

Vascular anomalies are frequent tumors of early infancy and are categorized as either hemangiomas or vascular malformations.

Hemangiomas

Hemangiomas are benign tumors that form from the rapid growth of vascular endothelial cells, which results in formation of extra blood vessels. Hemangiomas can be superficial or deep. Superficial hemangiomas are known as strawberry hemangiomas and deep lesions are known as cavernous hemangiomas. The etiology may be related to embolization of fetal placental endothelial cells with placental trauma or loss of placental angiogenic inhibitor of placental and maternal origin. There is proliferation of mast cells, which are thought to promote the angiogenesis. Infiltration of fat cells, fibrosis, and the rich vascular network give the lesions a firm, rubbery feel. Females are affected more often than males. About 30% of hemangiomas are apparent at birth, with most emerging during the first few weeks of life. They grow rapidly during the first few years of life, then shrink or involute during childhood years. With involution the lesions become darker in color and then gradually turn to a flesh color. There may be some residual telangiectasia. Although it depends on their location, most hemangiomas require no treatment. Hemangiomas located over the eye, ear, nose, mouth, urethra, or anus may require treatment because they interfere with function and have a higher risk for infection or injury. Systemic or intralesional steroids are the treatment of choice. Interferons, vincristine, cyclophosphamide, and radiotherapy can suppress angiogenesis. Cryosurgery, laser surgery, sclerotherapy, and embolization are alterative treatment options.[40]

Strawberry (capillary) hemangiomas are distinct, superficial hemangiomas that may be present at birth but usually emerge 3 to 5 weeks after birth. They proliferate and become bright red and elevated with minute capillary projections that give them a strawberry appearance. Only one lesion is usually present and is located on the head and neck area or trunk (Figure 40-12). After the initial growth, the lesion grows at the same rate as the child and then starts to involute at 12 to 16 months of age. Approximately 90% of strawberry hemangiomas involute by 5 to 6 years of age, usually without scarring.

Cavernous hemangiomas are present at birth and have larger and more mature vessels within the lesion than strawberry hemangiomas. Some lesions, however, are composed of a mixture of strawberry and cavernous hemangiomas. They appear primarily on the head and neck area and have a bluish red color with less distinct borders (Figure 40-13). Cavernous hemangiomas grow rapidly up to 6 months of age and mature by 1 year of age. A period of involution begins and proceeds for 6 to 12 months, with complete involution by 2 to 3 years in 30% of children and by 9 years of age in 90% of children.

Vascular Malformations

Vascular malformations are rare congenital anomalies of blood vessels that are present at birth but may not be apparent for several years.[41] They grow proportionately with the child and never regress. The malformations occur equally among males and females. Occasionally they expand rapidly, particularly during the hormonal changes of puberty or pregnancy and in association with trauma. Vascular malformations are classified as low flow or high flow. *Low-flow malformations* involve capillaries, veins, and lymphatics. *High-flow malformations* involve arteries. In addition to locations within the skin, they may involve the gastrointestinal tract, bone (Maffucci syndrome or Sturge-Weber syndrome), facial capillary malformation, skin, eye, or brain (leptomeningeal hemangioma). *Overgrowth syndromes* can occur with either high-flow or low-flow malformations, with overgrowth of the underlying structures (i.e., legs, arms, facial bones). The most common vascular malformations are nevus flammeus (port-wine stains) and salmon patches (stork bite, angel kiss).

Port-wine (nevus flammeus) stains are congenital malformations of the dermal capillaries. The lesions are flat, and their color ranges from pink to dark reddish purple. They are present at birth or within a few days after birth and do not fade with age. Involvement of the face and other body surfaces is common, and the lesions may be large (Figure 40-14). Treatments using cryosurgery or tattooing are not satisfactory. The pulsed dye laser is the treatment of choice to successfully lighten the color and flatten the more nodular and cavernous lesions. Waterproof cosmetics may be used to cover the lesions.

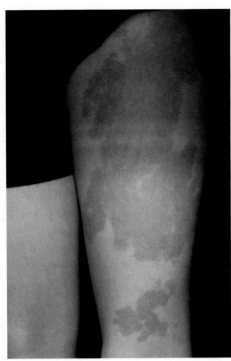

FIGURE 40-14 Port-Wine Hemangioma. Port-wine hemangioma in a child. (Courtesy Department of Dermatology, School of Medicine, University of Utah, Salt Lake City, Utah.)

Salmon patches are macular, pink lesions present at birth and located on the nape of the neck, forehead, upper eyelids, or nasolabial fold region. They are a variant of nevus flammeus, more superficial, and one of the most common congenital malformations in the skin. The pink color results from distended dermal capillaries, and 95% fade by 1 year of age. Those located at the nape of the neck may persist for a lifetime. They generally do not present a cosmetic problem.

OTHER SKIN DISORDERS

Miliaria

Miliaria is a dermatosis commonly seen in infants that is characterized by a vesicular eruption after prolonged exposure to perspiration with subsequent obstruction of the eccrine ducts. There are two forms of miliaria: miliaria crystallina and miliaria rubra. In **miliaria crystallina,** ductal rupture occurs within the stratum corneum and appears as 1- to 2-mm clear vesicles without erythema. They rupture within 24 to 48 hours and leave a white scale. In miliaria rubra, the ductal rupture occurs in the lower epidermis with inflammatory cells attracted to the

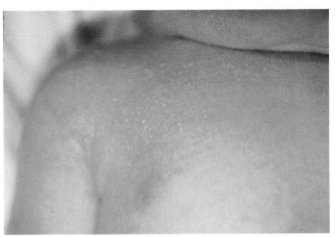

FIGURE 40-15 Miliaria Rubra. Note discrete erythematous papules or papulovesicles. (Courtesy Department of Dermatology, School of Medicine, University of Utah, Salt Lake City, Utah.)

site of the rupture. Miliaria rubra (prickly heat) is characterized by 2- to 4-mm discrete erythematous papules or papulovesicles (Figure 40-15). Both forms may become secondarily infected, requiring systemic antibiotics. The key to management is avoidance of excessive heat and humidity, which cause sweating. Light clothing, cool baths, and air conditioning assist in keeping the skin surface dry and cool.

Erythema Toxicum Neonatorum

Erythema toxicum neonatorum (toxic erythema of the newborn) is a benign, erythematous accumulation of macules, papules, or pustules that appear at birth or 3 to 4 days after birth. The lesions first appear as a blotchy, macular erythematous rash. The macules vary from 1 mm to 1 cm in diameter. When papules or pustules develop, they are light yellow or white and 1 to 3 mm in diameter. There may be a few or several hundred lesions, and any body surface can be affected, with the exception of the palms and soles, where there are no pilosebaceous follicles. The cause of the lesion is unknown but may be related to an innate immune response to the first commensal microflora with release of mast cell mediators. It is self-limiting and resolves spontaneously within a few weeks of birth. No treatment is required.

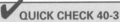

QUICK CHECK 40-3
1. Give two examples of insect bites or parasites that affect children. What features are observed in each?
2. Compare a strawberry hemangioma and a cavernous hemangioma.

DID YOU UNDERSTAND?

Acne Vulgaris

1. Acne vulgaris is a common disorder related to obstruction of pilosebaceous follicles and proliferation of *Propionibacterium acnes,* primarily of the face, neck, and upper trunk. It is characterized by both noninflammatory and inflammatory lesions.

Dermatitis

1. Atopic dermatitis commonly occurs as red, scaly lesions on the face, cheeks, and flexor surfaces of the extremities in infants and young children and is associated with elevated IgE levels and a family history of asthma and hay fever.
2. Diaper dermatitis is a type of irritant contact dermatitis that develops from prolonged exposure to urine and feces and often becomes secondarily infected with *Candida albicans.*

Infections of the Skin

1. Impetigo is a contagious bacterial disease occurring in two forms: bullous and vesicular. The toxins from the bacteria produce a weeping lesion with a honey-colored crust.
2. Staphylococcal scalded-skin syndrome (SSSS) is a staphylococcal skin infection that occurs more commonly in young children with low titers of anti-staphylococcal antibody. Painful blisters and bullae form over large areas of the skin, requiring systemic antibiotics for treatment.
3. Tinea capitis and tinea corporis are fungal infections of the scalp and body caused by dermatophytes.
4. Thrush is a fungal infection of the mouth caused by *Candida albicans.*
5. Molluscum contagiosum is a poxvirus of the skin that produces pale papular lesions filled with viral and cellular debris.
6. Rubella (3-day measles) is a communicable viral disease characterized by fever, sore throat, enlarged cervical and postauricular lymph nodes, and a generalized maculopapular rash that lasts 1 to 4 days.
7. Rubeola is a viral contagious disease with symptoms of high fever, enlarged lymph nodes, conjunctivitis, and a red rash that begins on the head, spreads to the trunk and extremities, and lasts 3 to 5 days. Both bacterial and viral complications may accompany rubeola.
8. Roseola is a benign disease of infants with a sudden onset of fever that lasts 3 to 5 days, followed by a rash that lasts 24 hours.
9. Chickenpox (varicella) is a highly contagious disease caused by the varicella-zoster virus. Vesicular lesions occur on the skin and mucous membranes. Individuals are contagious from 1 day before the development of the rash until about 5 to 6 days after the rash develops.
10. Herpes zoster (shingles) is a viral eruption of vesicles on the skin along the distribution of a sensory nerve caused by chickenpox virus that persists in sensory nerve ganglia.
11. Smallpox (variola) was a highly contagious, deadly viral disease that has been eradicated worldwide by vaccination but may be a bioterrorist threat.

Insect Bites and Parasites

1. Scabies is a pruritic lesion caused by the itch mite, which burrows into the skin and forms papules and vesicles. The mite is very contagious and is transmitted by direct contact.
2. Pediculosis (lice infestation) is caused by blood-sucking parasites that secrete toxic saliva and damage the skin to produce a pruritic dermatitis. Lice are spread by direct contact and are recognized by the ova or nits that attach to the shafts of body hairs.
3. Fleabites produce a pruritic wheal with a central puncture site and occur as clusters in areas of tight-fitting clothing.
4. Lyme disease is caused by the spirochete *Borrelia burgdorferi* transmitted by tick bites with cutaneous and systemic inflammatory symptoms.
5. Bedbugs are blood-sucking parasites that live in cracks of floors, furniture, or bedding and feed at night. They produce pruritic wheals and nodules.

Vascular Disorders

1. Hemangiomas are benign tumors that form from the rapid growth of vascular endothelial cells and result in formation of extra blood vessels.
2. A strawberry hemangioma is a vascular lesion present at birth that proliferates in size and then grows at the same rate as the child. Most lesions resolve spontaneously by 5 years of age.
3. A cavernous hemangioma is present at birth, with larger vessels than a strawberry hemangioma, and is bluish red. Cavernous hemangiomas usually involute by 9 years of age and may require surgical removal if located near the eyes, nares, or genitalia.
4. Salmon patches are macular pink lesions with dilated capillaries that usually resolve by 1 year of age.
5. Port-wine stains are congenital malformations of dermal capillaries that do not fade with age.

Other Skin Disorders

1. Miliaria is small pruritic papules or vesicles that result from obstruction of the sweat duct opening in infants.
2. Erythema toxicum neonatorum is a benign accumulation of macules, papules, and pustules that spontaneously resolves within a few weeks after birth.

KEY TERMS

- Acne conglobata 1071
- Acne vulgaris 1070
- Atopic dermatitis (AD) 1071
- Bedbug 1078
- Cavernous hemangioma 1079
- Chickenpox (varicella) 1076
- Diaper dermatitis (diaper rash) 1072
- Erythema toxicum neonatorum 1080
- Fleabite 1078
- Hemangioma 1079
- Herpes zoster (shingles) 1077
- Impetigo 1072
- Inflammatory acne 1070
- Lyme disease 1078
- Miliaria 1080
- Miliaria crystallina 1080
- Miliaria rubra (prickly heat) 1080
- Molluscum contagiosum 1074
- Noninflammatory acne 1070
- Port-wine (nevus flammeus) stain 1079
- Roseola 1076
- Rubella 1075
- Rubeola 1076
- Salmon patch 1080
- Scabies 1077
- Smallpox (variola) 1077
- Staphylococcal scalded-skin syndrome (SSSS) 1073
- Strawberry (capillary) hemangioma 1079
- Thrush 1074
- Tinea capitis 1073
- Tinea corporis (ringworm) 1074

REFERENCES

1. Friedlander SF, et al: Acne epidemiology and pathophysiology, *Semin Cutan Med Surg* 29(2 suppl 1):2–4, 2010.
2. Bhambri S, Del Rosso JQ, Bhambri A: Pathogenesis of acne vulgaris: recent advances, *J Drugs Dermatol* 8(7):615–618, 2009.
3. Eichenfield LF, et al: Perspectives on therapeutic options for acne: an update, *Semin Cutan Med Surg* 29(2 suppl 1):13–16, 2010.
4. Newman MD, et al: Therapeutic considerations for severe nodular acne, *Am J Clin Dermatol* 12(1):7–14, 2011.
5. Shaw TE, et al: Eczema prevalence in the United States: data from the 2003 National Survey of Children's Health, *J Invest Dermatol* 131(1):67–73, 2011.
6. Caubet JC, Eigenmann PA: Allergic triggers in atopic dermatitis, *Immunol Allergy Clin North Am* 30(3):289–307, 2010.
7. Boguniewicz M, Leung DY: Recent insights into atopic dermatitis and implications for management of infectious complications, *J Allergy Clin Immunol* 125(1):4–13, 2010.
8. Boguniewicz M, et al: A multidisciplinary approach to evaluation and treatment of atopic dermatitis, *Semin Cutan Med Surg* 27(2):115–127, 2008.
9. Nicol NH, Boguniewicz M: Successful strategies in atopic dermatitis management, *Dermatol Nurs* (Suppl):3–18, 2008.
10. Atherton DJ: A review of the pathophysiology, prevention and treatment of irritant diaper dermatitis, *Curr Med Res Opin* 20(5):645–649, 2004.
11. Geria AN, Schwartz RA: Impetigo update: new challenges in the era of methicillin resistance, *Cutis* 85(2):65–70, 2010.
12. Cole C, Gazewood J: Diagnosis and treatment of impetigo, *Am Fam Physician* 75(6):859–864, 2007.
13. Aalfs AS, et al: Staphylococcal scalded skin syndrome: loss of desmoglein 1 in patient skin, *Eur J Dermatol* 20(4):451–456, 2010.
14. Neylon O, et al: Neonatal staphylococcal scalded skin syndrome: clinical and outbreak containment review, *Eur J Pediatr* 169(12):1503–1509, 2010.
15. Williams PM, Conklin RJ: Erythema multiforme: a review and contrast from Stevens-Johnson syndrome/toxic epidermal necrolysis, *Dent Clin North Am* 49(1):67–76, 2005. viii.
16. Abdel-Rahman SM, et al: The prevalence of infections with *Trichophyton tonsurans* in schoolchildren: the CAPITIS study, *Pediatrics* 125(5):966–973, 2010.
17. Kakourou T, Uksal U: European Society for Pediatric Dermatology. Guidelines for the management of tinea capitis in children, *Pediatr Dermatol* 27(3):226–228, 2010.
18. Andrews MD, Burns M: Common tinea infections in children, *Am Fam Physician* 77(10):1415–1420, 2008.
19. Lee R, Schwartz RA: Pediatric molluscum contagiosum: reflections on the last challenging poxvirus infection, Part 1, *Cutis* 86(5):230–236, 2010.
20. Smith KJ, Skelton H: Molluscum contagiosum: recent advances in pathogenic mechanisms, and new therapies, *Am J Clin Dermatol* 3(8):535–545, 2002.
21. Centers for Disease Control and Prevention: *Recommendations: patients with molluscum contagiosum and swimming pool safety*, updated, Jan 13, 2011. Available at www.cdc.gov/ncidod/dvrd/molluscum/swimming/swimming_recommendations.htm.
22. Coloe J, Morrell DS: Cantharidin use among pediatric dermatologists in the treatment of molluscum contagiosum, *Pediatr Dermatol* 26(4):405–408, 2009.
23. Parker Fiebelkorn A, et al: Measles in the United States during the post-elimination era, *J Infect Dis* 202(10):1520–1528, 2010.
24. Pahud BA, et al: Varicella zoster disease of the central nervous system: epidemiological, clinical, and laboratory features 10 years after the introduction of the varicella vaccine, *J Infect Dis* 203(3):316–323, 2011.
25. Smith CK, Arvin AM: Varicella in the fetus and newborn, *Semin Fetal Neonatal Med* 14(4):209–217, 2009.
26. Galea SA, et al: The safety profile of varicella vaccine: a 10-year review, *J Infect Dis* 197(suppl 2):S165–S169, 2008.
27. Whitley RJ, et al: Management of herpes zoster and post-herpetic neuralgia now and in the future, *J Clin Virol* 48(suppl 1):S20–S28, 2010.
28. [No authors listed]: Varicella, herpes zoster and nonsteroidal anti-inflammatory drugs: serious cutaneous complications, *Prescrire Int* 19(106):72–73, 2010.
29. Civen R, et al: The incidence and clinical characteristics of herpes zoster among children and adolescents after implementation of varicella vaccination, *Pediatr Infect Dis J* 28(11):954–959, 2009.
30. Nalca A, Zumbrun EE: ACAM2000: the new smallpox vaccine for United States Strategic National Stockpile, *Drug Des Devel Ther* 4:71–79, 2010.
31. Meseda CA, Weir JP: Third-generation smallpox vaccines: challenges in the absence of clinical smallpox, *Future Microbiol* 5(9):1367–1382, 2010.
32. Hay RJ: Scabies and pyodermas—diagnosis and treatment, *Dermatol Ther* 22(6):466–474, 2009.
33. Wolf R, Davidovici B: Treatment of scabies and pediculosis: facts and controversies, *Clin Dermatol* 28(5):511–518, 2010.
34. Demain JG: Papular urticaria and things that bite in the night, *Curr Allergy Asthma Rep* 3(4):291–303, 2003.
35. O'Connell S: Lyme borreliosis: current issues in diagnosis and management, *Curr Opin Infect Dis* 23(3):231–235, 2010.
36. Bhate C, Schwartz RA: Lyme disease: Part II. Management and prevention, *J Am Acad Dermatol* 64(4):639–653, 2011.
37. Kolb A, et al: Bedbugs, *Dermatol Ther* 22(4):347–352, 2009.
38. Goddard J, deShazo R: Bed bugs (*Cimex lectularius*) and clinical consequences of their bites, *J Am Med Assoc* 301(13):1358–1366, 2009.
39. Krause-Parello CA, Sciscione P: Bedbugs: an equal opportunist and cosmopolitan creature, *J Sch Nurs* 25(2):126–132, 2009.
40. Greene AK: Management of hemangiomas and other vascular tumors, *Clin Plast Surg* 38(1):45–63, 2011.
41. Huang JT, Liang MG: Vascular malformations, *Pediatr Clin North Am* 57(5):1091–1110, 2010.

A

Most Common Laboratory Values

CONSTITUENT	NORMAL MEAN VALUE AND SOME RANGES	NORMAL RANGE IN SI UNITS
Electrolytes	Total, 1% of plasma weight	
Na^+	142 mEq/L (136-145)	136-145 mmol/L
K^+	3.5-5.0 mEq/L	3.5-5.0 mmol/L
Ca^{++}	8.8-10.5 mg/dl	2.25-2.75 mmol/L
Mg^{++}	1.8-3.0 mg/dl	1.25-1.75 mmol/L
Cl^-	95-105 mEq/L	95-105 mmol/L
HCO_3^-	24-28 mEq/L	24-28 mmol/L
Phosphate (mostly HPO_4^-)	2.5-5.0 mg/L	0.5-1.25 mmol/L
SO_4^-	1 mEq/L	0.25-0.75 mmol/L
Proteins	6-8 g/dl	60-80 g/L
Albumins	4-6 g/dl	40-60 g/L
Gamma globulin	0.5-1.6 g/dl	5-16 g/L
Globulins	2-4 g/dl	20-40 g/L
Fibrinogen	200-400 mg/dl	2-4 mmol/L
Blood Gases		
pH	7.35-7.45	
CO_2 content (arterial)	35-45 mm Hg	4.65-5.32 kPa
O_2 content (arterial)	75-100 mm Hg	9.97-13.30 kPa
Bicarbonate	24-28 mEq/L	24-28 mmol/L
Nutrients		
Glucose (fasting)	75-110 mg/dl	3.85-6.05 mmol/L
Total proteins	6-8 g/dl	—
Total lipids	400-800 mg/dl	4.0-8.0 g/L
Cholesterol (total)	<200 mg/dl	<5.20 mmol/L
Triglycerides	<160 mg/dl	0.45-1.81 mmol/L (males)
		0.40-1.52 mmol/L (females)
Phospholipids	150-380 mg/dl	1.50-3.80 mol/L
Free fatty acids	9.0-15.0 mM/L	9.0-15.0 mM/L
Waste Products		
Urea (BUN)	7-18 mg/dl	2.9-8.2 mmol/L
Uric acid	2-6 mg/dl	0.110-0.360 mmol/L
Creatinine	0.6-1.2 mg/dl	53-106 μmol/L
Creatinine clearance	107-139 ml/min	1.78-2.32 mmol/L
Uric acid (from nucleic acids)	2-7 mg/dl	0.120-0.360 mmol/L
Bilirubin (direct)	Up to 0.3 mg/dl	Up to 5.1 μmol/L
Bilirubin (indirect)	0-1.0 mg/dl	1.7-17.1 μmol/L

Continued

CONSTITUENT	NORMAL MEAN VALUE AND SOME RANGES	NORMAL RANGE IN SI UNITS
Individual Hormones		
Prolactin	<20 ng/ml	<869 pmol
Thyroid tests		
Thyroxine (T_4)	4-11 ng/dl	51-142 nmol/L
T_4 expressed as iodine	3.2-7.2 ng/dl	253-569 nmol/L
T_3	75-220 ng/dl	975.00 nmol/L
Free thyroxine (T_4)	0.8-2.4 ng/dl	10.4 nmol/L
T_3 resin uptake	25%-38% relative uptake	0.25%-0.38% relative uptake
TSH*	0.3-3.04 ml U/L	2-11 ml U/L
Hematology Values		
Erythrocyte (red blood cell count)	4.2-6.2 million/mm^3	
Leukocyte (white blood cell count)	5000-10,000/mm^3	
Lymphocyte	25%-33% of leukocyte count (leukocyte differential)	
Monocyte and macrophage	3%-7% of leukocyte differential	
Eosinophil	1%-4% of leukocyte differential	
Neutrophil	57%-67% of leukocyte differential	
Basophil	0-0.75% of leukocyte differential	
Platelet	140,000-340,000/mm^3	
Hematocrit	40%-50%	
Hemoglobin	13.5-18.0 g/dl	
Mean corpuscular volume	80-100 fL	
Other		
Bile acids	0.3-3.0 mg/dl	3.00 mg/L
Bilirubin, direct (conjugated)	Up to 0.3 mg/dl	Up to 5.1 mmol/L
Bilirubin, indirect (unconjugated)	0.1-1.0 mg/dl	1.7-17.1 mmol/L
Creatine (s)	0.1-0.4 mg/dl	7.6-30.5 mmol/L
Iron, total (s)	60-150 µg/dl	11-27 mmol/L
Iron-binding capacity (s)	300-360 µg/dl	54-64 mmol/L
Lactic dehydrogenase	80-120 units at 30° C	38-62 units/L at 30° C
Phosphatase P acid (units/dl)	Cherry-Crandall	0-5.5 units/L
	King-Armstrong	0-5.5 units/L
	Bodansky	0-5.5 units/L
Alkaline (units/dl)	King-Armstrong	30-120 units/L
	Bodansky	30-120 units/L
	Bessey-Lowry-Brock	30-120 units/L
Phosphorus, inorganic (s)	3.0-4.5 mg/dl	0.97-1.45 mmol/L
Prostate specific antigen (PSA)	0-4 ng/mL	—

*Recently changed.
s, Serum.

ABO blood group A system for classifying human blood on the basis of antigenic components of red blood cells and their corresponding antibodies. The ABO blood groups are identified by the presence or absence of two different antigens, A and B, on the surface of the red blood cell. The four blood types in this grouping, A, B, AB, and O, are determined by and named for these antigens.

Achalasia The failure of a sphincter, usually an esophageal sphincter, to relax completely, often because of a neuromuscular disorder of the esophagus that reduces the ability to move food down the esophagus.

Acidosis An excess of acids or a decrease in bases in body fluids.

Acne rosacea A chronic form of dermatitis of the face in which the middle of the face appears red with small red lines that result from dilated capillaries.

Acne vulgaris An inflammatory lesion of sebaceous hair follicles usually occurring on the face, upper back, and chest that consists of blackheads, cysts, papules, and pustules.

Acromegaly A condition of excessive growth hormone that originates from the anterior pituitary; it is manifested by progressive enlargement of the head, face, hands, feet, and chest.

Actinic keratosis A condition in which a premalignant small, reddish, rough lesion appears on skin that has been chronically exposed to the sun.

Active transport An energy-requiring process (e.g., from ATP) in which transport proteins bind with particles and move them through a cell membrane

Acute epiglottitis A bacterial infection that causes inflammation of the epiglottis and surrounding tissues that may lead to upper airway blockage, which increases the work of breathing, the retention of carbon dioxide, and the reduction in oxygen intake; may cause death if left untreated.

Acute kidney injury (AKI) A condition characterized by the rapid loss of renal function resulting in retention of nitrogenous and nonnitrogenous waste products that may lead to metabolic disturbances, altered body fluid balance, or oliguria.

Acute rejection Rejection of a graft within days to months after transplantation or termination of immunosuppressive drugs; caused by a cell-mediated immune response against incompatible antigens.

Acute respiratory distress syndrome (ARDS) A condition in which capillaries or alveoli of the lungs are damaged from infection, injury, blood loss, or inhalation injury, causing fluid to leak from the capillaries into the alveoli and some alveoli to collapse.

Acute tubular necrosis (ATN) A condition in which the kidney tubules undergo ischemic or nephrotoxic injury because of severe hypotension or from administration of aminoglycosides or radiocontrast agents; produces granular and epithelial cell casts in urine.

Adaptive immunity Also known as acquired or specific immunity. Immunity acquired from vaccines or prior infection; involves memory.

Adrenal gland Either of two small endocrine glands located above the kidney that secrete several steroid hormones, epinephrine, and norepinephrine.

Adrenergic transmission Transmission of a nerve impulse using epinephrine or norepinephrine as a neurotransmitter.

Adrenomedullin (ADM) A protein hormone discovered in human pheochromocytoma to function as a vasodilator as well as a regulator of growth cytokines and neurotransmission.

Afterload The tension or pressure that must be generated by a ventricle of the heart in order to eject blood.

Agnosia Loss of comprehension of sensory stimuli, such as sounds or images.

Aldosterone A mineralocorticoid that is synthesized and secreted by the adrenal cortex and that promotes sodium reabsorption and potassium excretion by the kidney.

Alkalosis An increase in bases or a decrease in acids in body fluids.

Allergy Hypersensitivity and immunologic protective reaction caused by exposure to an antigen.

Alloimmunity Also called isoimmunity. An inappropriate immune response directed against beneficial foreign tissues such as organ transplants.

Alveolar ventilation The volume of gas that reaches the alveoli per minute, or the difference between tidal volume and dead space multiplied by ventilation rate.

Alzheimer disease (AD) (dementia of Alzheimer type [DAT], senile disease complex) A condition characterized by progressive mental deterioration, often with confusion, memory failure, disorientation, restlessness, agnosia, speech disturbances, inability to carry out purposeful movement, and hallucinosis. There are amyloid plaques and fibrillary tangles in the cortex and atrophy and widened sulci in the frontal and temporal lobes.

Amyotrophy Atrophy of muscle tissue.

Anabolism A cellular process that uses energy to synthesize complex molecules from simpler molecules.

Anaerobic glycolysis The process of adenosine triphosphate (ATP) formation in the absence of oxygen, during which carbohydrate-derived pyruvate is reduced to form lactic acid.

Anaphase The third phase of mitosis, during which centromeres are separated and sister chromatids are moved to opposite poles.

Anaphylactic shock A severe and sometimes fatal systemic allergic reaction to an allergen, such as a drug, vaccine, specific food, serum, allergen extract, insect venom, or chemical. This condition may occur within seconds to minutes from the time of exposure to the allergen and is commonly marked by respiratory distress and vascular collapse.

Anaphylatoxin Fragments of C3a, C4a, and C5a that degranulate mast cells, resulting in the release of histamine that vasodilates and increases capillary permeability.

Anaphylaxis A potentially life-threatening immediate hypersensitivity response caused by exposure of a sensitized individual to a specific antigen.

Anaplasia The loss of structural differentiation within a cell or groups of cells.

Anemia A reduction in the total number of circulating red blood cells or a decrease in the quality or quantity of hemoglobin.

Aneurysm A localized dilation or ballooning of a blood vessel wall or cardiac chamber. Three fourths of all aneurysms occur in the abdominal aorta and atherosclersosis is the main cause.

Angina pectoris A condition in which myocardial ischemia, resulting from reduced blood flow around the heart's blood vessels, causes chest pain.

Angiogenesis The process of forming new blood vessels that occurs in the development of the embryo and fetus, tumor formation, and wound healing. Inflammation can promote the angiogenic response and is noted in such diseases as atherosclerosis, diabetes, arthritis, and cancer.

Anion gap The difference between the concentrations of serum or plasma cations and anions; determined by measuring the concentrations of sodium cations and chloride and bicarbonate anions. It is helpful in the diagnosis and treatment of acidosis, and it is estimated by subtracting the sum of chloride and bicarbonate concentrations in the plasma from that of sodium.

Ankylosing spondylitis (AS; spondyloarthritis) A condition in which the spine and sacroiliac joints are chronically inflamed, causing pain and stiffness in and around the spine and a gradual fusion of the vertebrae that immobilizes the spine.

Anorexia nervosa A mixed psychologic and physiologic disorder that begins with dieting to lose weight but over time becomes a sign of control and continued restrictive eating; may lead to starvation and eventual death.

Anoxia A lack of oxygen caused by vascular obstruction.

---

*A more extensive Glossary is available at http://evolve.elsevier.com/Huether.

Antimicrobial peptide Protein released by epithelial cells that is toxic to some bacteria, fungi, and viruses and is capable of activating cells involved in innate and acquired immunity.

Aortic stenosis A condition in which the aortic valves do not open completely, thereby increasing afterload so that more pressure must be generated in the left ventricle to eject blood; a condition that results in ventricular hypertrophy.

Aphasia The inability to articulate ideas or comprehend spoken or written language.

Aplastic crisis A condition that occurs when bone marrow temporarily ceases erythropoiesis, resulting in an acute fall in hemoglobin levels and subsequent anemia.

Apoptosis A type of programmed cell death. An active process in which cells self-destruct in normal and pathologic tissues.

Appendicitis A condition in which the appendix becomes inflamed because of a blockage of the opening from the appendix into the cecum; the appendix wall becomes infected and ruptures so that the infection spreads throughout the abdomen and causes pain, anorexia, fever, nausea, vomiting, and diarrhea.

Arteriosclerosis A condition in which the blood vessel walls thicken, harden, lose elasticity, and typically accumulate lipids, resulting in elevated blood pressure and a decrease in the diameter of the coronary arteries as well as pain when walking from decreased perfusion to leg vessels.

Ascites A condition in which fluid accumulates in the peritoneal cavity because of liver disease, portal hypertension, tuberculosis, and nephritic or nephrotic syndrome, resulting in abdominal distention and paraumbilical herniations of the abdominal wall.

Asphyxial injury Classified as intentional/unintentional injury and includes suffocation, strangulation, chemical, or drowning injury that results from oxygen deprivation in cells.

Aspiration The removal of a gas or fluid by suction or the sucking of fluid or a foreign body into the airway when breathing.

Aspiration pneumonitis A condition caused by the abnormal entry of fluids, particulate matter, or secretions into the lower airways; can lead to chemical pneumonitis by materials toxic to lungs such as gastric acid, bacterial infection, or mechanical obstruction of the lower airways.

Astrocyte A neuroglial cell of the central nervous system that branches into many processes and fills spaces between neurons and surrounding blood vessels.

Atelectasis A condition in which part of a lung or a whole lung collapses and the alveoli deflate as a result of surgery, smoking, or blockage of a bronchiole.

Atherosclerosis Most common form of arteriosclerosis in which soft deposits of intra-arterial fat and fibrin in the vessel walls harden over time. It is the leading cause of coronary artery and cerebrovascular disease.

Atopic dermatitis (AD) A chronic hereditary skin disease characterized by intense pruritus and inflamed skin that causes redness, swelling, cracking, crusting, and scaling.

Atrial natriuretic peptide (ANP) or factor A protein hormone that is synthesized and released from the atria in response to high sodium concentration, high extracellular fluid volume, or high blood volume; it promotes sodium excretion and causes vasodilation in the circulatory system.

Atrial septal defect (ASD) Any of a group of congenital heart diseases involving the interatrial septum of the heart separating the right and left atria; results in flow of blood between the two sides of the heart.

Atrioventricular canal (AVC) defect A condition in which a large hole is present in the center of the heart where the wall between the upper chambers joins the wall between the lower chambers; the tricuspid and mitral valves are formed into a single large valve that crosses the defect.

Atrioventricular node (AV node) The tissue between the atria and the ventricles that contains pacemaker cells; capable of setting the heart rate but mainly functions to slowly conduct the normal electrical impulse from the atria to the ventricles.

Autocrine stimulation The ability of a cell to secrete a substance that can produce feedback and provide continued stimulation or inhibition of that cell.

Autonomic hyperreflexia (dysreflexia) A syndrome resulting from a lesion above the splanchnic nerves that is characterized by hypertension, bradycardia, sweating of the forehead, severe headache, and gooseflesh upon distention of the bladder and rectum.

Autoregulation Changes in blood vessel diameter to maintain a constant blood flow despite changes in arterial pressure.

Bacterial pneumonia An acute or chronic disease marked by inflammation of the lungs caused by bacterial infection.

Balanitis Inflammation of the glans penis resulting from irritation by environmental substances, physical trauma, or infection.

Baroreceptor reflex A homeostatic mechanism consisting of baroreceptors that regulate the amount of blood being received by the tissues by altering cardiac output and resistance to maintain mean arterial blood pressure.

Baroreceptors Nerve endings located in the heart, aortic arch, and carotid sinuses that sense changes in blood pressure and volume.

Basopenia A condition in which the number of basophils decreases because of thyrotoxicosis, acute hypersensitivity reactions, or infection.

Benign prostatic hyperplasia (BPH) A condition in which the prostate gland becomes enlarged and may press against the urethra and bladder, interfering with urine flow.

Benign tumor Noncancerous but abnormal overgrowth or mass of cells; nonrecurrence and complete recovery after excision are common.

Biliary atresia A condition found in newborn children in which the biliary tract is blocked or absent, resulting in liver failure because of bile accumulation.

Blood group antigens Antigens present on the surface of erythrocytes that determine blood groups.

Blunt force injuries Tearing, shearing, or crushing of tissues caused by blows, impacts, or a combination of both.

Brain death (brain stem death) Irreversible brain damage that renders an individual unresponsive to all stimuli and lacking in muscle activity, such as that required for respiration and heart activity.

Brain stem The portion of the brain comprising the medulla oblongata, the pons, and the mesencephalon. It performs motor, sensory, and reflex functions and contains the corticospinal and reticulospinal tracts.

Brain stem gliomas A group of tumors located in the brain stem usually classified as high-grade that result in the sudden onset of symptoms including headaches, vomiting, and visual disturbances.

Bronchiectasis A condition in which the bronchi of the lungs become dilated in response to obstruction.

Bronchiolitis Inflammation of the bronchioles usually as a result of viral infection.

Bronchiolitis obliterans A condition in which the bronchioles and possibly some of the bronchi are partly or completely obliterated by granulation and fibrotic tissue masses.

Bronchopulmonary dysplasia (BPD) Inflammation, scarring, and abnormal development of the lung resulting in chronic pulmonary insufficiency and associated with long-term artificial pulmonary ventilation; usually present in premature infants but may also occur in mature infants.

Bulimia nervosa A psychologic disorder in which recurrent binge eating—followed by intentional vomiting; using laxatives, enemas, diuretics, or other medication inappropriately; excessive exercising; and fasting in order to compensate for eating—becomes uncontrollable.

Burkitt lymphoma An undifferentiated malignant lymphoma characterized by a large osteolytic lesion in the facial bones that is associated with the Epstein-Barr virus.

Cachexia A syndrome common in individuals with cancer that includes anorexia, early filling (satiety), weight loss, anemia, weakness, poor performance, and altered metabolism.

Calcification Hardening of tissue by the insertion of calcium or calcium salts.

Calculi An abnormal buildup of substances, usually mineral salts, that most commonly occurs in the gallbladder, kidney, or urinary bladder.

Candidiasis A fungal infection caused by an overgrowth of normal bacteria that usually occurs in the skin and mucous membranes of the mouth, respiratory tract, or vagina but may invade the bloodstream in the immunocompromised person.

Carbuncles A condition in which a bacterial infection of the hair follicle or sebaceous gland ducts becomes painful and discharges pus through various openings.

Carcinoma A cancerous tumor that arises from epithelial tissue and can invade surrounding tissue and metastasize.

Cardiogenic shock Usually results from a decreased cardiac output with evidence of tissue hypoxia despite the presence of adequate intravascular volume. Associated with acute myocardial infarction and congestive heart failure. Cardiogenic shock is fatal in about 80% of cases.

Cardiomyopathy A condition in which the cardiac muscle of the heart wall becomes dysfunctional because of ischemic or nonischemic mechanisms.

Carrier An individual that possesses genes for a disease but does not show phenotypical characteristics of the disease.

Caseous necrosis A combination of coagulative and liquefactive necrosis in which dead cells disintegrate but are not completely digested, resulting in soft, granular, clumped cellular debris.

Catabolism Cellular process that provides energy by breaking down complex molecules into simpler molecules.

Cavernous hemangioma A birthmark that is similar to the strawberry hemangioma but is more deeply rooted and may appear as a red-blue spongy mass of tissue filled with blood.

Cell adhesion molecules (CAMs) Proteins located on the cell surface; they bind with other cells or with the extracellular matrix (ECM) in the process called cell adhesion. When cells no longer adhere to each other, they can become motile, such as with cancer metastases.

Cell cycle Series of events during which the nuclear material of a parent cell is duplicated and divided to form two daughter cells.

Cellular accumulation (infiltration) Accumulation of normal cellular substances in the cytoplasm or nucleus as a result of cellular injury or inefficient cell function.

Cellular immunity Immune protection afforded by the ability of cytotoxic T cells to lyse target cells that contain antigens that bind specific receptors.

Cellular receptor Protein molecule that can be embedded in the membrane or located within the cell in the cytoplasm or on the nucleus; this protein contains binding sites for a specific chemical (ligand) that when bound initiates a particular response.

Cellulitis A condition in which subcutaneous or connective tissue becomes infected and inflamed, causing tenderness, swelling, and redness that spreads to other regions of the body.

Cerebellar astrocytoma Brain tumor in which cancer (malignant) cells begin to grow in the tissues of the brain, resulting in head tilt, limb ataxia, and nystagmus when the eyes are turned toward the tumor.

Cerebral death Irreversible brain damage that renders an individual unresponsive to all stimuli but able to maintain the necessary respiratory and cardiovascular functions of life.

Cerebral palsy A developmental brain injury that occurs before or shortly after birth; causes muscular impairment that affects motor function and also may alter speech and learning abilities.

Cerebrovascular accident (CVA, stroke) A localized brain infarction that may result in facial, arm, or leg numbness and weakness; confusion; difficulty speaking or understanding; visual disturbances; dizziness; loss of balance; difficulty walking; and headache.

Cervicitis Inflammation of the mucous membrane of the uterine cervix because of infection, typically resulting from *Chlamydia,* genital herpes, or gonorrhea.

Chemical asphyxiant Chemical or gas that prevents the delivery of oxygen to tissues or blocks its use.

Chemotaxis Directional movement and attraction of microorganisms or phagocytes to substances released in the environment or tissues.

Cheyne-Stokes respiration An abnormality of the pattern of breathing in which tidal volume gradually increases followed by a gradual decrease and a period of apnea before returning to a normal respiratory pattern.

Chickenpox An infectious viral disease spread by direct contact or through the air by coughing or sneezing; results in a blister-like rash that appears first on the face and trunk and can spread over the entire body, resulting in 250 to 500 itchy blisters; fatigue and fever are also present.

Cholecystitis Inflammation of the gallbladder commonly resulting from impaction of a gallstone that causes right upper quadrant pain and possibly a rupture and abscess in the gallbladder.

Chronic obstructive pulmonary disease (COPD) Any of a group of irreversible respiratory diseases that are characterized by airflow obstruction or limitation, usually caused by smoking.

Chronic rejection Rejection of a graft months to years after transplantation because of a gradual loss of organ function.

Chronic renal failure A slowly developing condition that can result as a complication of a large number of kidney diseases, such as IgA nephritis, glomerulonephritis, chronic pyelonephritis, and urinary retention; leads to end-stage renal failure for which dialysis is generally required while a donor kidney is found.

Cirrhosis Fibrosis and scarring of the liver with loss of liver function commonly associated with chronic liver disease related to alcoholism or viral hepatitis.

Cleft lip (harelip) A deformity of the lip caused by abnormal facial development in utero.

Cluster headache A condition characterized by attacks of intense unilateral pain, occurring most often over the eye and forehead and lasting 15 minutes to 3 hours. It is accompanied by flushing and watering of the eyes and nose. Attacks occur in clusters or cycles over days or weeks with pain-free intervals between clusters.

Coagulative necrosis A type of cell death in which the cells are dense and maintain their shape, usually associated with hypoxia. Hypoxic injury causes protein denaturation, and occurs primarily in kidneys, heart, and adrenal glands.

Coarctation of the aorta (COA) A condition in which the aorta narrows in the area where the ductus arteriosus inserts. Narrowing usually occurs preductal in children and postductal in adults.

Codon A triplet of adjacent nucleotides located in mRNA that specifies the type and sequence of amino acids for protein synthesis; for example, GCC (guanine-cytosine-cytosine) results in alanine.

Communicating (extraventricular) hydrocephalus A disorder in which the cerebrospinal fluid pathways are intact but cerebrospinal fluid absorption is impaired.

Compensation Adjustment of acid or base content by removal or addition in response to changes in pH; for example, in metabolic acidosis there is an increase in carbon dioxide removal by the lungs, thus decreasing carbonic acid formation and causing pH to increase.

Compensatory hyperplasia An increased rate of cell division that compensates for absent or dysfunctional cells of the same tissue.

Compliance A measure of the ease with which a structure, such as the lungs or chest wall, may be deformed or stretched.

Condyloma acuminatum A warty growth in the uterine cervix or anogenital area as a result of a human papillomavirus infection.

Congenital aganglionic megacolon (Hirschsprung disease) A congenital defect in which the nerves that innervate the anus through the wall of the bowel are absent, resulting in enlargement of the bowel above the point where the nerves are missing and a subsequent decrease in peristalsis that results in chronic constipation.

Congestive heart failure (CHF) An abnormal condition that reflects impaired cardiac pumping and the inability to maintain the metabolic needs of the body. Its causes include myocardial infarction, ischemic heart disease, and cardiomyopathy. Failure of the ventricles to eject blood efficiently results in volume overload, ventricular dilation, and elevated intracardiac pressure.

Connexon A channel composed of six protein subunits that form a hollow center through the plasma membrane at a gap junction; when two connexons in adjacent cells are aligned, chemical and electrical communication can occur between the cells.

Contact dermatitis An allergic response to an environmental antigen binding to specific carrier proteins contained in an individual's skin.

Contracture A permanent shortening of muscle or scar tissue that distorts or deforms affected joints.

Contrecoup injury An injury, usually involving the brain, in which the tissue damage is on the side opposite the trauma site, as when a blow to the left side of the head results in brain damage on the right side.

Contusion A bruise produced by bleeding into the skin or underlying tissues from an insult that did not break the skin but did rupture blood vessels.

Cor pulmonale Right-sided heart failure resulting from prolonged pulmonary artery hypertension.

Craniopharyngioma A brain tumor that develops in the pituitary gland and most often affects children, causing headache, seizure, diabetes insipidus, early onset of puberty, and delayed growth.

Craniosynostosis Premature ossification of the skull and closure of the sutures, resulting in abnormal skull expansion and asymmetric skull growth.

Crohn disease Also called regional enteritis; a chronic inflammatory autoimmune disease of the digestive tract that can occur from the mouth to the anus. The ulcerative lesions can involve the entire intestinal wall in a patchy pattern of ulceration with regions of normal tissue between lesions. Anal fissures and abscesses may develop. Symptoms include abdominal pain, chronic diarrhea, disrupted digestion, malnutrition, and dehydration.

Croup An acute viral infection of the vocal cords that occurs primarily in infants and young children 3 months to 3 years of age. It is characterized by inflammation and edema with hoarseness; irritability; fever; a distinctive harsh, barking cough; persistent stridor during inspiration; and dyspnea and tachypnea, resulting from obstruction of the larynx.

Cryoglobulin An immunoglobulin that precipitates at low body temperatures.

Cryptorchidism A condition in which the scrotum of one or both testes is absent because of failure of the testis to descend from the abdominal position during fetal development.

Cushing syndrome A condition caused by increased synthesis and secretion of cortisol from a tumor of the adrenal cortex or from excessive administration of glucocorticoid drugs causing excess production of adrenocorticotropic hormone (ACTH) by the anterior lobe of the pituitary gland. Symptoms include accumulations of fat on the abdomen, chest, upper back, and face and occurrence of edema, hyperglycemia, increased gluconeogenesis, muscle weakness, purplish striae on the skin, decreased immunity to infection, osteoporosis with susceptibility to bone fractures, acne, and facial hair growth in women.

Cutaneous vasculitis A type of vasculitis affecting the skin and other organs that is characterized by a polymorphonuclear infiltrate of the small vessels.

Cyanosis A condition in which the skin, mucous membranes, and nail beds appear blue because of a lack of oxygenated hemoglobin in the blood secondary to congenital heart defects, cardiovascular or pulmonary disease, or possibly poison.

Cyclooxygenase (COX) An enzyme responsible for formation of prostaglandins, prostacyclin, and thromboxane and the subsequent inflammatory response.

Cystic fibrosis (CF) A genetic disorder of the exocrine glands caused by a mutation in the *CF* transmembrane regulator gene causing impairment in chloride transfer across cell membranes and subsequent chloride and water accumulation in organs; thickened secretions block ducts and form cysts.

Cystitis A condition characterized by acute or chronic inflammation of the urinary bladder, usually resulting from bacterial infection of the urethra; results in frequent burning urination, blood in the urine, pain in the pubic area, chills and fever, back pain, and nausea.

Cystocele A condition in which the muscles between a woman's bladder and vagina weaken and the bladder descends into the vagina, causing discomfort, urine leakage, and incomplete emptying of the bladder.

Cytokine Small proteins or biologic factors that are released by cells that have messenger effects on cell-cell interaction, communication, and behavior of other cells. Similar to hormones but the term specifies interleukins, lymphokines, and other related signaling molecules such as interferons.

Cytotoxic (metabolic) edema Cerebral edema resulting from tissue hypoxia and impairment of the Na^+-K^+ ATP pump, causing a loss of intracellular potassium and a gain of intracellular sodium and water.

Cytotoxic T lymphocyte (Tc cell) Killer lymphocyte that binds to and lyses specific cells containing particular antigen receptors.

Deep venous thrombosis (DVT) The formation of one or more thrombi in the deep veins, usually of the lower extremity. DVT is often asymptomatic but carries a high risk of pulmonary embolism; symptoms (principally unilateral) include pain, tenderness, swelling, warmth, and skin discoloration.

Degenerative disk disease A condition in which intervertebral disk tissue is replaced by fibrocartilage during aging; functional capacity is rarely altered.

Dementia A progressive organic mental disorder characterized by chronic personality disintegration, confusion, disorientation, stupor, deterioration of intellectual capacity and function, and impairment of control of memory, judgment, and impulses.

Depolarization The movement of sodium across the membrane, resulting in a change in membrane charge from a negative to a positive potential.

Dermatome An area of skin that is innervated by a specific spinal nerve.

Dermoid cyst A benign tumor resulting from congenital malformation of the skin or ovary.

Desmosome A region of tight adhesion between neighboring cells that provides structural strength to the tissue and allows the cells of the tissue to function as a unit.

Developmental dysplasia of the hip (DDH) A condition in which the hip joint of babies or young children is malformed with the ball being completely out of the socket or the socket being too shallow to support the ball.

Diabetes insipidus A disease caused by antidiuretic hormone deficiency or resistance; characterized by excretion of large amounts of diluted urine because of the inability of the kidneys to conserve water and concentrate urine.

Diabetic ketoacidosis (DKA) A complication of diabetes mellitus caused by the buildup of byproducts of fat metabolism that occurs when glucose is not available as a fuel source for the body because of insulin deficiency.

Diabetic neuropathy Combined sensory and motor disorder often seen in older diabetic patients as a result of microvascular injury involving small blood vessels that supply nerves.

Diabetic retinopathy Damage to the retina caused by an overaccumulation of glucose or fructose that damages the blood vessels in the retina; in advanced stages, lack of oxygen in the retina causes fragile blood vessels to grow along the retina and in the vitreous fluid of the eye that may bleed and cause blurred vision.

Diaper dermatitis A type of contact dermatitis characterized by inflammation of the skin in the diaper area in infants and caused by exposure of the skin to feces and urine.

Diaphysis The shaft of a long bone, consisting of a tube of compact bone enclosing the medullary cavity.

Diarrhea An increase in the frequency of watery bowel movements or a greater looseness of stools as a result of disease, excessive consumption of alcohol or other liquids or foods that irritate the stomach or intestine, allergy to certain food products, poisoning, hyperactivity of the nervous system, or viral or bacterial infection.

Diastole The period of time when the heart relaxes after contraction, resulting in a pressure drop in the relaxed region.

Diastolic heart failure A condition in which heart contractions are normal but the ventricle does not relax completely; therefore less blood enters the heart.

Diffuse brain injury (diffuse axonal injury) Injury to neuronal axons in many areas of the brain caused by stretching and shearing forces received during brain injury.

DiGeorge syndrome A congenital disorder characterized by severe immunodeficiency and structural abnormalities, including hypertelorism; notched, low-set ears; small mouth; downward-slanting eyes; cardiovascular defects; and absence of the thymus and parathyroid glands. Death, often as a result of infection, usually occurs before 2 years of age.

Disseminated intravascular coagulation (DIC) A condition in which the blood coagulates throughout the entire body following the uncontrolled activation of clotting factors and fibrinolytic enzymes throughout small blood vessels, resulting in platelet and coagulation factor depletion and increased bleeding.

Diverticulitis Inflammation of the diverticula in the colon, usually occurring in elderly patients.

Down-regulation The process by which a cell decreases its sensitivity to a hormone or neurotransmitter by decreasing the number of receptors in response to a high concentration of that particular hormone or neurotransmitter.

Drowning Breathing in fluid that causes airway obstruction, thereby decreasing oxygen delivery to tissues.

Duchenne muscular dystrophy A genetic disorder in which fat and fibrous tissue infiltrate and weaken muscle tissues in the legs, pelvis, lungs, and heart.

Dumping syndrome A condition in which the lower end of the small intestine fills too quickly with undigested food from the stomach following stomach surgery, resulting in nausea, vomiting, bloating, diarrhea, and shortness of breath during or immediately following a meal.

Dyspareunia A reversible condition in which sexual intercourse is painful.

Dysphasia Impairment of speech that manifests as the inability to arrange words in logical order.

Dyspnea Shortness of breath and difficulty in breathing; usually the result of lung or heart disease.

Ectopic testis A testis that has descended from the abdominal cavity and settled in the suprapubic area, the thigh, or the perineum instead of the scrotum.

Eisenmenger syndrome A congenital defect in which the abnormal development of circulation causes a reversed right-to-left shunt secondary to increased pressures on the right side of the heart resulting from pulmonary hypertension.

Electron-transport chain A series of transfer reactions that include transferring electrons from a donor to an acceptor, thereby releasing energy during each transfer.

Embolic stroke A stroke caused by blockage of cerebral vessels and usually caused by a blood clot that has broken free and traveled to the brain as an embolus.

Embolus An air bubble, a detached blood clot, or a foreign body that travels in the bloodstream and is wedged in a blood vessel, resulting in obstruction in vessels supplying the lungs, brain, or heart. It is often a medical emergency.

Empyema (infected pleural effusion) A condition in which purulent material is persistently discharged into the pleural space because of complications of bacterial infections.

Encephalitis Inflammation of the brain usually caused by a virus.

Encephalocele A congenital abnormality in which a gap in the skull results in a protrusion of brain material.

Encephalopathy Any of the various diseases or syndromes of the brain.

End-diastolic volume The volume of blood in the left ventricle at the end of diastole, just before systole (contraction).

Endometriosis A condition common in women of reproductive age in which the tissue lining the uterus is found outside of the uterus, resulting in pain and infertility.

Endothelial cell A cell of the endothelial layer that lines the heart, blood vessels, lymph vessels, and the lung cavity.

Endotoxin Lipopolysaccharide released during cell lysis from the bacterial outer membrane that causes fever, leukopenia, and possibly diarrhea and hemorrhagic shock.

Enthesis The site of attachment of a muscle or ligament to bone.

Enuresis A condition in which urination is uncontrolled or involuntary.

Eosinopenia A reduction in the number of eosinophils present in the blood.

Eosinophil A granulocyte that functions as a phagocyte that destroys antigen-antibody complexes, allergens, and inflammatory chemicals and aids in fighting parasitic infections.

Eosinophilia A condition in which the number of eosinophils in the blood elevates because of diseases such as parasitic infections, allergies, cholesterol emboli, chronic myeloid leukemia, and some drug reactions.

Ependymoma An intracranial tumor most commonly found in children that typically arises from the inner lining of the fourth ventricle and the spinal canal.

Epididymitis A painful condition where the epididymis becomes inflamed; usually caused by a secondary bacterial infection resulting from a variety of underlying conditions, such as urinary tract or sexually transmitted infections.

Epidural hematoma A collection of blood between the inner surface of the skull and the dura caused by torn arteries secondary to skull fracture.

Epigenetic Chemical modifications that alter the expression of genes or phenotype without alteration of gene (genotype) sequence.

Epilepsy Any of a group of syndromes characterized by recurring seizures of an unknown cause.

Epiphyseal plate A plate of hyaline cartilage at the end of long bones that provides a site for lengthening of the bone.

Epispadias A birth defect in which the urethra opens on the upper (ventral) penile surface.

Erysipelas A highly contagious bacterial infection that produces shiny, red, swollen areas and fever and can lead to blood poisoning and pneumonia.

Erythema multiforme A skin disease caused by allergies, seasonal changes, or drug sensitivities, resulting in the formation of red macules, papules, or subdermal vesicles on the skin and mucous membranes.

Erythema toxicum neonatorum A temporary eruption of redness of the skin, small papules, and occasionally pustules in newborns accompanied by contact dermatitis or hypersensitivity to milk or other allergens.

Escharotomy A surgical incision into necrotic tissue resulting from a severe burn. The procedure is sometimes necessary to prevent edema from generating sufficient interstitial pressure to impair capillary filling, causing ischemia.

Esophageal varices A complex of longitudinal tortuous veins at the lower end of the esophagus, enlarged and swollen as the result of portal hypertension. These vessels are especially susceptible to hemorrhage. Conditions that can cause portal hypertension include cirrhosis and chronic hepatitis.

Exotoxin A protein synthesized and secreted by a specific species of bacteria.

Exstrophy of the bladder A congenital defect in which the lower abdominal wall is malformed and ruptures, allowing communication between the bladder and the amniotic fluid; results in anomalies of the lower abdominal wall, bladder, anterior bony pelvis, and external genitalia.

Extracellular matrix (basement membrane) Fibrous proteins embedded in a carbohydrate-rich liquid secreted by the cell that functions as a pathway for diffusion of nutrients, wastes, and other substances between the blood and tissues.

Extrinsic allergic alveolitis (hypersensitivity pneumonitis) An inflammation of the lung caused by an immune reaction to small airborne particles such as bacteria, mold, and fungi; causes fever, chills, coughing, shortness of breath, and body aches.

Exudate Fluids or cells that have leaked from blood vessels, usually associated with inflammation.

Fat necrosis A lipase-induced cellular dissolution of triglycerides in breast, pancreas, and other abdominal structures.

Fibromyalgia A condition in which muscles, tendons, and joints are painful, stiff, and tender; frequently accompanied by restless sleep, fatigue, anxiety, depression, and disturbances in bowel function.

Fibrosarcoma A malignant tumor of the fibrous connective tissue usually derived from immature proliferating fibroblasts.

First-degree burn A burn that affects the epidermis only, causing erythema and, in some cases, mild edema, without vesiculation.

Focal segmental glomerulosclerosis (FSGS) A condition in which glomerular capillaries with thickened basement membranes and increased mesangial matrix collapse in segments.

Follicular cyst A cyst caused by the retention of secretions in a follicular space because of obstruction of a duct, resulting in failure of the dominant follicle to rupture or failure of the nondominant follicles to regress.

Folliculitis Inflammation of a hair follicle damaged by friction from clothing, blockage of the follicle, or shaving that becomes infected with bacteria.

Frailty Physiologic and immune changes that waste the body during aging and leave the affected person susceptible to falls, functional decline, disease, and death.

Frank-Starling law of the heart The idea that fluctuations in the volume of blood filling the heart will change the volume ejected by the same amount because the force of the contraction will increase as the heart is filled with more blood.

Free radical Highly reactive and destructive particle with an unpaired electron; is produced from an atom or molecule.

Fulminant hepatitis A type of viral hepatitis that has a high mortality rate and causes fatigue, nausea, jaundice, dark urine, flulike symptoms, hepatomegaly, and eventually encephalopathy.

Furuncles A condition in which staphylococcal infection produces painful, pus-filled, inflamed sites on the skin and subcutaneous tissue.

Fusiform aneurysm (giant aneurysm) A large aneurysm that stretches to affect the entire circumference of the arterial wall.

Galactorrhea (inappropriate lactation) A condition in which milklike fluid is secreted from the breast because of hormonal alterations, but it is not associated with childbirth or nursing.

Ganglia (plexus) A knot or knotlike mass of nervous tissue; one of the nerve cell bodies, chiefly collected in groups outside the central nervous system. Very small groups abound in association with alimentary organs. The two types of ganglia in the body are the sensory ganglia on the dorsal roots of spinal nerves and on the sensory roots of the trigeminal, facial, glossopharyngeal, and vagus nerves and the autonomic ganglia of the sympathetic and parasympathetic systems.

Gangrenous necrosis Tissue death typically found in the lower leg as a result of severe hypoxic injury secondary to arteriosclerosis or blockage of major arteries.

Gap junction Tunnel or connexon that joins two adjacent cells and allows for the passage of molecules and electrical signals between the cells.

Gas gangrene The formation of gas bubbles and subsequent destruction of connective tissue and cell membranes resulting from the hydrolytic enzymes produced by bacteria of the *Clostridium* species.

Gastritis A condition in which the lining of the stomach is inflamed because of bacterial infection, bile reflux, or excessive consumption of alcohol or certain foods or drugs.

Gastroesophageal reflux disease (GERD) A type of injury to the esophagus caused by chronic exposure of the esophagus to stomach liquid reflux made up of acid and pepsin; creates heartburn, inflammation of the esophageal lining, strictures, dysphagia, and chronic chest pain.

Gastroileal reflex A process by which food entering an empty stomach increases ileal motility and causes the ileocecal valve to open.

Gate control theory A proposal that a pain gate is present in the spinal cord that allows or blocks pain signals to the brain depending on whether the impulse is traveling on a large or small afferent fiber.

Gating A calcium-induced decrease in permeability of a junctional complex that may aid in protecting uninjured cells from the increased calcium levels released by injured cells.

Germline mosaicism A mechanism in which the germ cells (egg or sperm cells) have a different genetic composition, or mixture (mosaic), than cells in the rest of the body. A child can inherit a genetic disease even though the parents do not express the disease; the mechanism is believed to involve a mutation during the embryonic development of the parent germ cells.

Giant cell tumor A benign tumor usually near the end of the bone near a joint in arms, legs, knee, and flat bones.

Giantism Severely increased long bone growth caused by excessive growth hormone secretion before and during puberty.

Glomerulonephritis An autoimmune or infectious disease characterized by acute or chronic inflammation of the glomeruli that may not produce symptoms or may present with hematuria and proteinuria.

Glucose-6-phosphate dehydrogenase (G6PD) deficiency An inherited condition that is asymptomatic in the absence of exposure to particular substances, such as certain medicines, mothballs, or severe infections; with exposure, the red blood cells undergo destruction that produces excessive bilirubin, which overloads the liver and causes jaundice.

Gluten-sensitive enteropathy Also known as celiac sprue, this condition is characterized by mucosal lesions in the gastrointestinal tract formed in response to a genetic predisposition for an immune response to gluten and similar proteins.

Goiter A noncancerous enlargement of the thyroid gland that is visible as a swelling at the front of the neck.

Gout A disorder of uric acid metabolism that causes painful inflammation of the joints, commonly the big toe, and arthritic attacks caused by elevated levels of uric acid in the blood and the deposition of urate crystals around the joints.

Granulation tissue Vascularized tissue that replaces the fibrin clot during the reconstructive phase of wound healing.

Granulocytopenia A condition in which the number of granular white blood cells in the blood is decreased.

Granulocytosis A condition in which the number of granulocytes, usually neutrophils, in the blood is increased secondary to bacterial infection, leukemia, or autoimmune disease.

Granuloma A tumor-like mass containing macrophages and fibroblasts that forms as a result of chronic inflammation and isolation of the infected area.

Graves disease An autoimmune disease of the thyroid whereby autoantibodies stimulate the TSH receptor, causing the increased synthesis and secretion of thyroid hormone and hyperthyroidism. Symptoms include an enlarged thyroid gland, protrusion of eyeballs (exophthalmos), a rapid heartbeat, and nervous excitability.

Gynecomastia Abnormal breast tissue development on adolescent boys or men usually because of an imbalance in hormones.

Haploid cell A cell that contains 1 copy of each chromosome, giving each cell 23 chromosomes.

Hematoma A collection of blood in soft tissue or an enclosed space.

Hematopoiesis The normal formation and development of blood cells in the bone marrow. In severe anemia and other hematologic disorders, cells may be produced in organs outside the marrow.

Hemolytic anemia A disorder characterized by chronic premature destruction of red blood cells. Anemia may be minimal or absent, reflecting the ability of the bone marrow to increase production of red blood cells.

Hemolytic disease of the newborn (HDN) An alloimmunity disease also called erythroblastosis fetalis in which the maternal blood and fetal blood are antigenically (ABO or Rh factor) incompatible, causing the mother's immune system to produce antibodies against fetal erythrocytes.

Hemolytic-uremic syndrome A condition in which platelets aggregate within the kidney's small blood vessels, resulting in reduced blood flow to the kidney and subsequent kidney failure and destruction of the red blood cells.

Hemoptysis A period during which blood or blood-stained sputum is spit or coughed from bronchi, larynx, trachea, or lungs.

Hemorrhagic stroke (intracranial hemorrhage) Stroke usually caused by hypertension that results in bleeding in the brain; typically increases intracranial pressure and may lead to death.

Henoch-Schönlein purpura nephritis A condition in which small blood vessels are inflamed, causing bleeding into the skin and mucous membranes (purpura), hematuria, and gastrointestinal bleeding; abdominal pain; inflammation in the joints, kidneys, and testis; subcutaneous edema; and encephalopathy.

Hepatic encephalopathy A condition usually caused by liver cirrhosis and portal hypertension in which toxins produced by the gut and not metabolized by the liver pass into the systemic circulation and damage brain cells, resulting in impaired cognition, tremor, and a decreased level of consciousness.

Hepatorenal syndrome A condition in which progressive renal failure occurs because of a decrease in renal blood flow associated with cirrhosis of the liver.

Herpes simplex virus (HSV) An infection that has an affinity for the skin and nervous system and usually produces small, transient, irritating, and sometimes painful fluid-filled blisters on the skin and mucous membranes. HSV-1 infections tend to occur in the facial area, particularly around the mouth and nose; HSV-2 infections are usually limited to the genital region.

Hiatal hernia An anatomic abnormality in which the esophageal hiatus is larger than normal, causing part of the stomach to protrude through the diaphragm and up into the chest.

Histamine A compound, found in all body tissues. Produced primarily in mast cells and other immune cells by the breakdown of histidine. Mast cells are more numerous in the skin, gastrointestinal tract, pulmonary system, and nervous tissue. It is released in allergic and inflammatory reactions. Cellular receptors of histamine include the H1 receptors, which are responsible for the dilation of blood vessels and the contraction of smooth muscle; the H2 receptors, which are responsible for the stimulation of heart rate and gastric secretion; and the H3 receptors, which are believed to play a role in the regulation of the release of histamine and other neurotransmitters from neurons.

Hodgkin lymphoma (HL) A neoplasm causing a progression from one group of lymph nodes to another group; includes diverse systemic symptoms and the presence of Reed-Sternberg (RS) cells.

Human papillomavirus (HPV) A virus that is the cause of common warts of the hands and feet, as well as lesions of the mucous membranes of the oral, anal, and genital cavities. More than 50 types of HPV have been identified, some of which are associated with cancerous and precancerous conditions. The virus can be transmitted through sexual contact, and specific types of the virus are a precursor to cancer of the cervix.

Humoral immunity Immune protection afforded by the presence of antibodies in blood.

Huntington disease (HD) An autosomal dominant disease causing a progressive increase in involuntary, jerky, dyskinetic movements; mental deterioration; and premature death.

Hydrocele A condition in which serous fluid accumulates in a bodily cavity such as the testis.

Hydrops fetalis Massive edema in the fetus or newborn, usually in association with severe erythroblastosis fetalis. Severe anemia and effusions of the pericardial, pleural, and peritoneal spaces also occur. The condition usually leads to death.

Hyperaldosteronism A disorder marked by excessive secretion of aldosterone, a mineralocorticoid secreted from the adrenal cortex that promotes the retention of sodium (secondarily water) and bicarbonate, and the excretion of potassium and hydrogen ions. It can cause weakness, cardiac irregularities, and abnormally high blood pressure.

Hyperhemolytic crisis A condition in which the rate of destruction of red blood cells is increased, resulting in decreased hemoglobin levels, increased reticulocyte count, elevated bilirubin levels, and elevated lactate dehydrogenase levels; caused by infections, hemolytic transfusion reactions, sickle cell crisis, or a combination of glucose 6-phosphodiesterase deficiency with oxidant stress.

Hyperhomocysteinemia A condition in which plasma homocysteine concentration is elevated because of diet, vitamin B_6 or B_{12} deficiency, congenital enzyme deficiency, or renal failure, increasing the risk of developing atherosclerosis and venous thromboembolism.

Hyperpolarized The state of a membrane when the membrane potential is more negative than the resting membrane potential, thereby increasing the stimulus required to elicit an action potential.

Hypersensitivity A state in which the body undergoes an exaggerated immune response to an antigen.

Hypertonic hyponatremia Decreased sodium concentration caused by increases in levels of plasma lipids and proteins that result in an osmotic shift.

Hypertrophic cardiomyopathy An abnormal condition characterized by gross hypertrophy of the interventricular septum and left ventricular free wall of the heart. Ventricular hypertrophy results in impaired diastolic filling and reduced cardiac output.

Hyperventilation A condition in which overventilation reduces carbon dioxide concentration because of breathing faster or deeper than

necessary, resulting in respiratory alkalosis with numbness or tingling in the hands, feet, and lips; lightheadedness; dizziness; headache; chest pain; and sometimes fainting.

Hypocortisolism Abnormally diminished secretion of corticosteroids by the adrenal cortex, as in Addison disease.

Hypoglycemia A state of low blood glucose level that stimulates epinephrine and glucagon secretion, mobilizing stored glycogen and fat and their conversion into glucose.

Hypoparathyroidism A condition marked by decreased function of the parathyroid glands, resulting in hypocalcemia and associated tremor, tetany, and convulsions.

Hypoplastic anemia A condition in which anemia results from greatly depressed, inadequately functioning bone marrow and smaller-than-normal erythrocytes.

Hypoplastic left heart syndrome (HLHS) A condition in which the left side of the heart (including the aorta, aortic valve, left ventricle, and mitral valve) is underdeveloped so that blood returning from the lungs must flow through an opening in the atrial septum; the right ventricle pumps the blood into the pulmonary artery and then into the aorta.

Hypospadias A birth defect in which the urethral opening is abnormally placed, opening anywhere from the tip of the glans of the penis to the shaft or the junction of the penis and scrotum or perineum in males and usually opening in the vagina in females.

Hypothyroidism A condition caused by insufficient thyroid hormone synthesis and secretion, resulting in impaired memory, increased sensitivity to heat and cold, slow heart rate, depression, weight gain, slowed metabolism, and several other systemic alterations.

Hypoventilation A condition in which ventilation is inadequate for proper gas exchange, causing an increase in carbon dioxide concentration and subsequent respiratory acidosis.

Hypovolemia Decreased blood volume capable of causing hypotension, tachycardia, and decreased urine output.

Hypovolemic shock A state of physical collapse and prostration caused by massive blood loss, about one fifth or more of the total blood volume. The common signs include low blood pressure, thready pulse, clammy skin, tachycardia, rapid breathing, and reduced urinary output. The associated blood losses may stem from GI bleeding, internal or external hemorrhage, or excessive reduction of the intravascular plasma volume and body fluids.

Hypoxemia Insufficient oxygenation of arterial blood.

Hypoxia State in which the oxygen level reaching cells is insufficient, resulting in tissue injury; may be caused by a reduction in oxygen content of inspired air, a decrease in hemoglobin available for oxygen binding, or cardiovascular or respiratory disease.

Icterus neonatorum (neonatal jaundice) Temporary jaundice in newborns caused by functional immaturity of the liver.

Idiopathic thrombocytopenia purpura (ITP) A deficiency of platelets that results in bleeding into the skin and other organs. Acute ITP is a disease of children that may follow a viral infection, lasts a few weeks to a few months, and usually has no residual effects. Chronic ITP is more common in adolescents and adults, begins more insidiously, and lasts longer. Antibodies to platelets are found in patients with ITP.

Imperforate anus A congenital defect in which the anal opening is absent because of the presence of a membranous septum or complete absence of the anal canal.

Impetigo A contagious skin infection caused by hemolytic streptococci or staphylococci that results in small red spots or blisters that rupture, discharge, and become encrusted; can spread over the skin.

Infectious mononucleosis (IM) A disease caused by Epstein-Barr virus or cytomegalovirus that is transmitted by exchanging saliva or blood or by coughing and sneezing; acts by infecting the B cells and atypical T cells, resulting in fever, sore throat, and fatigue.

Inflammatory acne A condition characterized by comedones that appear as red, swollen, and inflamed blemishes and larger, deeper, swollen, tender lesions that become inflamed and rupture under the skin.

Inflammatory joint disease A disease in which inflammation affects joint structures and often leads to structural derangement of the joint, structural joint problems, and pain at rest and with motion.

Inflammatory response A tissue reaction to injury or an antigen that may include pain, swelling, itching, redness, heat, and loss of function. The response may involve dilation of blood vessels and consequent leakage of fluid, causing edema; leukocytic exudation; and release of plasma proteases and vasoactive amines such as histamine.

Innate resistance (immunity) Protection from or resistance to infection by nonimmune mechanisms such as natural, physical, mechanical, and biochemical barriers.

Inotropic agent A substance that influences the force of muscular contractions. An agent that increases the force of muscular contractions of the heart.

Insulin Protein hormone secreted by the beta cells of the islets of Langerhans that functions in carbohydrate and fat metabolism by increasing glucose uptake into muscle and by activating adipose cells to form glycogen and fat.

Insulin resistance A cause of type 2 diabetes mellitus characterized by a need for an increased amount of insulin per day to control hyperglycemia and ketosis. It is associated with decreased or ineffective glucose transporter proteins with insulin-sensitive cells or insulin binding by high levels of antibody.

Interstitial edema Cerebral edema in which interstitial fluid accumulates in conjunction with hydrocephalus, usually containing no protein.

Intrarenal acute renal injury A type of acute renal injury characterized by renal parenchymal damage that disrupts glomerular filtration and eventually destroys the glomeruli.

Intrinsic factor A small protein secreted by the parietal cells of gastric glands required for adequate absorption of vitamin B_{12}.

Intrinsic pathway A sequence of reactions leading to fibrin formation, beginning with the contact activation of factor XII, followed by the sequential activation of factors XI and IX, and resulting in the activation of factor X, which in activated form initiates the common pathway of coagulation.

Intussusception An infolding or prolapse of a segment of the small intestine into the adjacent but more distal segment of the intestine.

Ion Positively or negatively charged molecule.

Iron deficiency anemia (IDA) A condition caused by insufficient dietary intake or absorption of iron, resulting in decreased incorporation of hemoglobin into red blood cells and subsequent feelings of fatigue, weakness, and shortness of breath, as well as pale earlobes, palms, and conjunctivae.

Ischemia Insufficient blood flow to tissues that may result in hypoxia and subsequent cell injury or death.

Islets of Langerhans The endocrine region of the pancreas that contains four cell types: alpha cells that secrete glucagon, beta cells that secrete insulin, delta cells that secrete somatostatin, and PP cells that secrete pancreatic polypeptide.

Isohemagglutinin An antibody that causes agglutination of erythrocytes in other members of the same species that carry an isoagglutinogen on their erythrocytes.

Isolated systolic hypertension A condition caused by loss of elasticity of the arteries, resulting in an increase in cardiac output or stroke volume, a systolic blood pressure consistently above 160 mm Hg, and a diastolic pressure below 90 mm Hg.

Isthmus A narrow passage connecting two larger parts of an anatomic structure.

Jaundice (icterus) A yellowish brown staining of the skin and the whites of the eyes caused by high bilirubin levels in blood secondary to excessive erythrocyte breakdown, obstruction in or around the liver, or liver disease.

Juvenile rheumatoid arthritis (JRA) A condition in which children under the age of 16 develop rheumatoid arthritis and experience swelling, tenderness, and pain in one or more joints and lymph nodes and splenic enlargement.

Kaposi sarcoma (KS) A type of fatal cancer caused by the herpesvirus in which many bluish red nodules appear on the skin, especially skin of the lower extremities; occurs in a particularly virulent form in individuals with AIDS.

Kawasaki disease A vascular disease characterized by inflamed heart and vessels; coronary artery aneurysm, thickening, and stenosis; a fever that lasts at least 5 days; and at least four of the following: inflammation with reddening of the whites of the eyes; red, swollen hands or feet; peeling skin; rash; swollen lymph glands in the neck; inflamed lips, throat, or red "strawberry" tongue.

Keloid A red, raised, overgrown fibrous scar formed by excessive cell growth during tissue repair following trauma or surgical incision.

Keratoacanthoma A benign, rapidly growing, flesh-colored papule or nodule of the skin with a central plug of keratin. The lesion is most common on the face or the back of the hands and arms. It disappears spontaneously in 4 to 6 months, leaving a slightly depressed scar.

Kernicterus A form of jaundice in the newborn caused by elevated levels of unconjugated bilirubin in the blood secondary to an increase in red blood cell number and breakdown, and by jaundice-induced lesions in the cerebral gray matter that cause neurologic disorders.

Kussmaul respiration (hyperpnea) Deep, rapid respiration commonly seen in conditions causing acidosis.

Kwashiorkor A condition in which children do not receive enough protein in their diet, resulting in a swollen and severely bloated abdomen and generalized edema secondary to decreased albumin in the blood, skin changes resulting in a reddish discoloration of the hair and skin in black children, severe diarrhea, fatty liver, muscle atrophy, and retarded development.

Lactase deficiency A condition in which not enough lactase is present in the small intestine to digest lactose, resulting in lactose intolerance characterized by diarrhea, bloating, and gas in response to exposure to lactose.

Lactose intolerance A condition caused by lactase deficiency in which lactose is not metabolized, making it impossible for the small intestine to absorb it, and causing excessive gas production and osmotic diarrhea when exposed to lactose-containing foods.

Legg-Calvé-Perthes disease A condition in which the blood supply to the head of the femur near the hip joint is interrupted, resulting in osteonecrosis of the corresponding epiphysis.

Leiomyoma A benign smooth muscle mass that can occur in any organ but most commonly occurs in the myometrium of the uterus or in the esophagus.

Leptin A protein hormone produced by adipose tissue that provides the brain with an assessment of adipose mass and regulates appetite and metabolism by altering the actions of neuropeptide Y.

Leukemia An acute or chronic disease of the bone marrow in which excessive proliferation of white blood cells occurs and is usually accompanied by anemia, impaired blood clotting, and enlargement of the lymph nodes, liver, and spleen.

Leukocytosis An increase in the number of leukocytes in the blood as a result of fever, inflammation, hemorrhage, or infection.

Leukopenia A condition in which the number of white blood cells in the blood decreases, increasing the risk for infection.

Leukotriene A mediator of the prolonged inflammatory response that acts to contract smooth muscle, increase vascular permeability, and attract neutrophils.

Lichen planus A condition in which a recurrent rash of small, flat-topped bumps and rough scaly patches appears on the skin, in the lining of the mouth, and in the vagina in response to inflammation or an allergy to a specific medication.

Ligand Substance that binds to a specific cellular receptor, initiating cellular events specific to that receptor.

Lipofuscin A yellow-brown pigment produced by the breakdown of damaged blood cells in heart and smooth muscle.

Liquefactive necrosis Liquefaction of neurons and glial cells in the brain as a result of ischemic injury or bacterial infection.

Loss of heterozygosity Loss of a region on one chromosome that corresponds to a mutated region on the other chromosome; loss of the same loci on both chromosomes inactivates the affected gene.

Lupus erythematosus Any of a group of chronic autoimmune connective tissue disorders that commonly produce red, scaly lesions and a facial "butterfly" pattern rash and are accompanied by fever, malaise, myalgias, fatigue, and weight loss. It is more common in women.

Lyme disease An infection caused by the spirochete *Borrelia burgdorferi* and transmitted by the bite of the tiny infected deer tick living in wooded grassy areas. In the first few weeks symptoms include an expanding bull's eye rash at the bite site, erythema migrans, myalgia, and fatigue. Months later arthralgias, neuritis, meningitis, or carditis may develop. Symptoms can be vague and mimic other diseases. Serologic tests to detect *Borrelia burgdorferi* antibodies assist diagnosis.

Lymphocyte A nonphagocytic leukocyte of the adaptive immune response that is immunologically competent and serves as the precursor for B and T lymphocytes.

Lymphocytopenia A condition in which the number of lymphocytes in the blood decreases because of diseases and conditions such as human immunodeficiency virus or because of severe stress, administration of corticosteroids, chemotherapy, or radiation therapy.

Lymphocytosis A condition in which the number of lymphocytes in the blood increases because of infection, inflammation, or leukemia.

Lymphoma Cancer arising from cell proliferation in lymphoid tissue.

Lysosomal storage diseases A group of more than 50 disorders that result from genetic defects causing impaired lysosomal function with lack of enzymes that normally digest and recycle intracellular macromolecules. Examples include mucopolysaccharidoses, lipid storage disorders, mucolipidoses, leukodystrophies, and glycoprotein storage disorders.

Macrocytic anemia (megaloblastic anemia) A condition characterized by a deficiency of vitamin B_{12} or folic acid caused by inadequate intake or insufficient absorption secondary to alcoholism or drugs that inhibit DNA replication.

Macrophage A large white blood cell, highly phagocytic, derived from monocytes that occur in the walls of blood vessels (adventitial cells) and in loose connective tissue (histiocytes). They become mobile when stimulated by inflammation. The phenotypes of macrophages include the M1 phenotype that is proinflammatory and produces reactive oxygen species (ROS) and the M2 phenotype that is involved in resolution of inflammation.

Major histocompatibility complex (MHC) A cluster or complex of genes located on chromosome 6 important for antigen production and critical to the success of transplantation. The MHC includes the human leukocyte antigen (HLA) genes.

Malignant hypertension A sudden and rapid elevation of blood pressure. The lower (diastolic) blood pressure reading is often >130 mm Hg. It is considered a medical emergency.

Malignant hyperthermia A rare genetic hypermetabolic condition characterized by severe hyperthermia and rigidity of the skeletal muscles, occurring in affected people exposed to inhalation anesthetics and succinylcholine, a nondepolarizing muscle relaxant.

Malignant tumor A tumor that tends to spread (metastasize) to other parts of the body.

Marasmus Childhood disorder characterized by protein and energy malnutrition, resulting in dry skin, loss of adipose tissue from normal areas of fat deposits like buttocks and thighs, and fretful, irritable behavior.

Margination (pavementing) A process by which leukocytes adhere better to endothelial cells of the capillary walls and venules by the reciprocal change in adhesion molecules on leukocytes.

Mast cell A large granular cell of the connective tissue that produces substances that cause activation of the inflammatory response, vasoconstriction, and muscle contraction.

McArdle disease A metabolic disorder in which a deficiency in the enzyme that helps metabolize glycogen (i.e., muscle phosphorylase) causes an energy deficit in the muscles, resulting in muscle pain and cramping.

Meconium A dark green fecal material that accumulates in the fetal intestines and is discharged at or near the time of birth.

Meconium ileus A condition in which the intestine of a newborn is obstructed with thickened meconium resulting from a lack of trypsin; associated with cystic fibrosis of the pancreas.

Mediated transport The transport of inorganic ions and some organic compounds across the cell membrane by way of integral membrane or transmembrane proteins that contain specific receptors.

Medulloblastoma A malignant cerebellar tumor near the fourth ventricle most often found in children that consists of neoplastic cells that resemble the undifferentiated cells of the neural tube.

Memory cell A T or B lymphocyte that remembers a specific antigen after the initial exposure and initiates a more efficient immunologic response in subsequent exposures to the same antigen.

Meningioma A slow-growing mass of the meninges that is usually benign but increases intracranial pressure.

Meningocele A neural tube defect in the skull or spinal column that forms a cyst filled with cerebrospinal fluid through which the meninges of the brain protrude.

Mesodermal germ layer A tissue located between the ectoderm and endoderm that gives rise to an epithelial component of genital and urinary structures, striated muscle, connective tissue, cartilage, bone, smooth muscle, and blood cells.

Metabolic acidosis A decrease in pH caused by an increase in noncarbonic acids or a decrease in bicarbonate.

Metabolic alkalosis An increase in pH caused by an increase in bicarbonate ions secondary to an increase in metabolic acid loss.

Metabolic syndrome A group of symptoms including insulin resistance, obesity, hypertension, dyslipidemia, and systemic inflammation that increases risk for type 2 diabetes mellitus, coronary artery disease, and stroke.

Metastasis An active process by which tumor cells move from the primary location of a cancer by severing connections from the original cell group and establishing remote colonies. Because malignant tumors have a nonenclosing capsule, cells may escape, become emboli, and be transported by the lymphatic circulation or the bloodstream to implant in lymph nodes and other organs far from the primary tumor.

Microcephaly A defect in which failure of normal brain growth causes delayed skull growth and production of a small head.

Microcytic-hypochromic anemia A condition in which red blood cells are smaller than normal.

Microglia A neuroglial cell that migrates and functions as a phagocyte for nerve tissue waste products.

Microtubule A hollow cylindrical structure that occurs widely within plant and animal cells. Microtubules increase in number during cell division and are associated with the movement of deoxyribonucleic acid material.

Migraine headache A recurring headache characterized by unilateral onset, severe throbbing pain, photophobia, phonophobia, nausea and vomiting, light sensitivity, and autonomic disturbances during the acute phase, which may last for hours or days. It may be preceded by a visual, motor, or sensory aura. A predisposition to migraine may be inherited. The exact mechanism responsible for the disorder is not known, but the head pain may be related to dilation of extracranial blood vessels, or cortical spreading depression (a wave of spreading cortical depolarization) with release of pain-generating substances.

Miliaria A skin disease caused by partially obstructed sweat glands that results in small and itchy rashes usually located in skin folds and on areas of the body that may rub against clothing, such as the back, chest, and stomach.

Minimal change nephropathy (MCN) A condition in which the foot processes of the renal capillary basement membrane are fused and deformed because of a T cell disorder that reduces the anion component of the basement membrane and allows proteins to leak into the renal tubule.

Mitosis The process of nuclear division during which two identical nuclei are produced from one parent cell after chromosomal replication.

Mitral valve A valve in the heart that lies between the left atrium and left ventricle; allows blood to flow into the left ventricle during ventricular diastole and prevents regurgitation from the ventricle to the left atrium during systole.

Mitral valve prolapse syndrome The ballooning of the support structures of the mitral valve into the left atrium during systole. Severe cases can cause mitral regurgitation, infective endocarditis, and congestive heart failure.

Molluscum contagiosum A disease of the skin and mucous membranes caused by a poxvirus, which occurs worldwide. It is characterized by scattered flesh-toned or white papules. Palms of the hands and soles of the feet are not affected. The disease most frequently occurs in children and in adults with an impaired immune response. It is transmitted from person to person by direct or indirect contact and lasts up to 3 years, although individual lesions persist for only 6 to 8 weeks.

Monocyte A white blood cell; a cell of the immune system. It has several roles and can differentiate into macrophages and dendritic cells to cause an immune response.

Monocytopenia A condition in which the number of monocytes in the blood decreases because of the release of toxins into the blood by bacteria or by administration of chemotherapy or corticosteroids.

Monocytosis A condition in which the number of monocytes in the blood increases because of a chronic infection, autoimmune disorder, blood disorder, or cancer.

Mononuclear phagocyte system (MPS) Part of the immune system consisting mostly of monocytes and macrophages. The macrophages are located in the reticular connective tissue previously called the reticuloendothelial system. Monocytes emigrate from circulation and differentiate into mononuclear macrophages. The functions on the MPS include the formation of new red blood cells (RBCs) and white blood cells (WBCs), destruction of old RBCs and WBCs, formation of antibody, formation of plasma proteins, and formation of bile pigments.

Moyamoya disease A cerebrovascular disorder in which the main cerebral arteries at the base of the brain are replaced by a fine network of vessels. It is caused by progressive stenosis of the large-caliber vessels and development of a collateral network. It tends mainly to affect Japanese children and young adults and is characterized by convulsions, hemiplegia, mental retardation, and subarachnoid hemorrhage.

Mucopurulent cervicitis (MPC) Inflammation of the cervix with purulent endocervical exudate that may be asymptomatic or cause abnormal vaginal discharge and vaginal bleeding.

Multiple sclerosis A chronic demyelinating disease of the central nervous system that causes inflammation and scarring of myelin sheaths.

Myasthenia gravis A neuromuscular disorder caused by an autoimmune response in which antibodies to acetylcholine receptors impair neuromuscular transmission.

Myelodysplasia An abnormal formation of the spinal cord.

Myelodysplastic syndrome A group of hematologic conditions characterized by ineffective production of blood cells, resulting in anemia that requires chronic blood transfusion.

Myoadenylate deaminase deficiency (MDD) A genetic disorder in which an enzyme deficiency prevents the conversion of adenosine monophosphate (AMP) to inosine monophosphate, resulting in increased AMP loss and the inability to synthesize adenosine triphosphate for energy.

Myocardial infarction A heart condition of sudden onset in which muscle tissue dies because of a lack of blood flow, resulting in varying degrees of chest pain or discomfort, weakness, sweating, nausea, vomiting, and possibly loss of consciousness.

Myositis A condition in which a muscle, usually a voluntary muscle, is inflamed, resulting in pain, tenderness, and sometimes spasm in the affected area.

Myositis ossificans A condition in which bone is deposited in muscle tissue, causing pain and swelling.

Myotonia A neuromuscular disorder in which muscle relaxation following voluntary contraction is delayed.

Myxedema A disease caused by hypothyroidism in adults characterized by thickened, nonpitting edematous changes in the skin usually in the pretibial area caused by increased deposition of connective tissue (e.g., hyaluronic acid). There may also be swelling around the lips and nose, mental deterioration, and a decrease in basal metabolic rate.

Natural killer (NK) cell A lymphocyte capable of killing target cells by binding specific receptors with or without the aid of antibodies and by releasing chemicals toxic to the targeted cells.

Necrosis The death of cells. The sum of all changes after local cell death includes cellular lysis and provokes an inflammatory reaction in surrounding tissue.

Necrotizing enterocolitis A condition of extensive ulceration and necrosis of the ileum and colon in premature infants during the neonatal period.

Neovascularization New blood vessel formation in abnormal tissue or in abnormal positions; revascularization or angiogenesis.

Nephritic syndrome A group of signs and symptoms of a urinary tract disorder including hematuria, hypertension, and renal failure.

Nephroblastoma Also known as Wilms tumor, this condition is characterized by a malignant renal tumor that compresses the normal kidney parenchyma, causing abdominal mass, blood in the urine, and fever; may be associated with anorexia, vomiting, and malaise occurring in children.

Nephrotic syndrome A condition in which there is increased permeability of the glomerular filtration membrane with the passage of protein into the urine, resulting in proteinuria greater than 50 mg/kg per day and resulting in hypoalbuminemia, edema, hyperlipidemia, and in some cases anemia when transferrin is lost.

Neuroblastoma A malignant tumor containing neuroblast cells that originates in the autonomic nervous system or the adrenal medulla; is most common in infants and young children.

Neurofibrillary tangle An intracellular clump of neurofibrils made of insoluble protein (tau protein) in the brain of a patient with Alzheimer disease.

Neurogenic bladder The underactivity or overactivity of the bladder caused by nervous system damage that prevents the bladder muscles from contracting to empty completely or that causes rapid bladder contraction resulting in too rapid or frequent emptying.

Neurogenic shock (vasogenic shock) Widespread and massive vasodilation that results from parasympathetic overstimulation and sympathetic understimulation.

Neuroglia The supporting or nonneuronal tissue cells of the central and peripheral nervous system. They perform the less specialized functions of the nerve network.

Nissl substances Structures, also known as *Nissl bodies,* located in the cell bodies of neurons that are involved in protein synthesis.

Nonbacterial prostatitis A condition in which prostatitis causes chronic pain that dissipates and returns without warning, but the prostatic fluid does not show signs of bacterial infection even though the semen and other fluids from the prostate contain immune cells that the body produces in response to infection.

Nonbacterial thrombotic endocarditis A condition in which fibrin is deposited on the valve leaflets of the heart, especially on the left side, because of cancer, rheumatic fever, or arteriosclerosis.

Noncommunicating hydrocephalus Cerebrospinal fluid accumulation within the skull caused by obstruction of the cerebrospinal fluid pathways.

Non-Hodgkin lymphoma (NHL) B cell neoplasm or cancer of the lymphoid tissue that mimics Hodgkin disease but does not produce the cells characteristic of Hodgkin disease; does not have a definitive cause but the risk factors include latent Epstein-Barr virus, HIV, human herpesvirus-8, HTLV-1, hepatitis C, certain mutagenic chemicals, irradiation, and immune suppression related to organ transplantation. Gastric infection with *Helicobacter pylori* increases the risk for gastric lymphoma.

Noninflammatory acne A common skin disease characterized by areas of skin seborrhea (scaly red skin), open comedones (blackheads and whiteheads), papules (pinheads), pustules (pimples), nodules (large papules), and sometimes scarring.

Noninflammatory joint disease A disease in which alterations in the structure or mechanics of the joint result in pain during motion. Traditionally, osteoarthritis was classified as noninflammatory joint disease but because of newer imaging technologies inflammation has emerged as an important feature of osteoarthritis.

Nonossifying fibroma (fibrous cortical deficit) A condition found in children and adolescents in which a benign fibrous tissue tumor forms in the metaphysis of any of the long bones; but usually occurs in the thigh and shin bones.

Non-REM (slow wave) sleep A period of sleep during which dreams do not occur and brain waves are slow and high voltage.

Nonvolatile A substance that does not have a vapor form.

Nucleolus A small structure in the nucleus that contains the DNA of the cell and the associated binding proteins and where RNA subunits of ribosomes are assembled.

Nucleotide A DNA subunit containing one deoxyribose molecule, one phosphate group, and one nitrogenous base.

Nucleus A large membrane-bound organelle that contains the cellular DNA and is located mostly in the center of the cell.

Nystagmus Involuntary, rapid, rhythmic movements of the eyeball in the horizontal, vertical, or rotational direction.

Obstructive sleep apnea syndrome (OSAS) Airway obstruction resulting in disruption of sleep or arousal that is accompanied by snoring.

Obstructive uropathy A condition in which the flow of urine is blocked, frequently by ureteral or kidney stones, resulting in the reflux of urine and subsequent injury to kidneys.

Occult bleeding Blood that is not obvious on examination and is from a nonspecific source, with obscure signs and symptoms. It may be detected by means of a chemical test or by microscopic or spectroscopic examination. Occult blood is often present in the stools of patients with GI lesions.

Oligodendroglioma A slow-growing mass of the oligodendrocytes that is usually benign.

Oncogene A tumor-causing gene or mutated proto-oncogene that helps turn a normal cell into a tumor cell. Increases the rate of cell proliferation.

Oncotic pressure (colloid osmotic pressure) Pressure created by large molecules in blood plasma, such as plasma proteins, that cannot penetrate the membrane and tend to pull water into the circulation.

Onychomycosis A fungal infection of the fingernails or toenails that causes thickening, roughness, and splitting of the nails.

Opsonin A molecule such as C3b fragment or antibody that attaches antigens to phagocytes, thereby tagging the antigens for phagocytosis.

Orchitis Swelling of the testicles that can result in ejaculation of blood, blood in the urine, and pain and visible swelling of a testicle or testicles.

Orthostatic (postural) hypotension A condition in which blood pressure suddenly falls when assuming a standing position, resulting in dizziness, lightheadedness, blurred vision, and temporary loss of consciousness.

Osmotic pressure The amount of hydrostatic pressure (force of water pushing against membranes) to oppose the osmotic movement of water.

Osteoarthritis (OA) Now understood to involve inflammation; a degenerative synovial joint disease resulting in local areas of loss and damage of cartilage.

Osteochondrosis A disease affecting the ossification centers of bone in children. It is initially characterized by degeneration and necrosis, followed by regeneration and recalcification.

Osteocyte A bone cell; a mature osteoblast that has become embedded in the bone matrix. It occupies a small cavity and sends out protoplasmic projections that anastomose with those of other osteocytes to form a system of minute canals within the bone matrix.

Osteogenesis imperfecta (brittle bone disease) A genetic disease in which collagen production is deficient, making the bones abnormally fragile and causing recurring fractures with minimal trauma, deformity of long bones, a bluish coloration of the sclerae, and often the development of otosclerosis.

Osteomalacia A disease in which vitamin D or calcium deficiency or excessive renal phosphate loss causes a softening of the bones with accompanying pain and weakness.

Osteomyelitis A bacterial infection of the bone and bone marrow that occurs through open fractures, penetrating wounds, surgical operations, or any means in which bacteria enter the bloodstream; causes pain, high fever, and formation of an abscess at the site of infection.

Osteoporosis A disease in which bone becomes porous and weakened, making it easily fractured and slow to heal.

Ovarian torsion A condition in which an ovary twists or turns on its supporting ligament to the point that its blood supply is compromised.

Oxidative stress Pathologic changes or tissue injury in response to excessive levels of cell-injuring oxidants and free radicals in the environment. Antioxidants can counter the oxidant damage.

Oxyhemoglobin dissociation curve A sigmoid plot of the percentage of hemoglobin-binding sites occupied by oxygen versus the partial pressure of oxygen, which illustrates the affinity of hemoglobin for oxygen.

Paget disease (osteitis deformans) A bone disorder in which excessive bone remodeling causes enlarged, weakened, and deformed bones that can result in bone pain, arthritis, deformities, or fractures.

Pancreatic insufficiency A condition in which the pancreas does not secrete enough hormones and digestive enzymes for normal digestion to occur, resulting in malabsorption, malnutrition, vitamin deficiencies, and weight loss.

Pancreatitis Inflammation of the pancreas, usually resulting in abdominal pain.

Papilloma A benign nodular breast lesion consisting of hyperplastic distorted ductal cells.

Paraneoplastic syndrome A collective term used to describe disorders arising from the metabolic effects of cancer on tissues remote from the tumor or metastatic site. They may result from the production of active proteins, polypeptides, or inactive hormones by the tumor.

Paraphimosis A condition in which the foreskin becomes trapped behind the glans penis and cannot return to its normal flaccid position covering the glans penis.

Parathyroid hormone (PTH) A protein hormone, secreted by the parathyroid glands, that regulates calcium and phosphate levels in the body by promoting the absorption of calcium by the intestine, encouraging mobilization of calcium and phosphate from bones, and increasing the tendency of the kidney to reabsorb calcium and excrete phosphate.

Parkinson disease Degeneration of the basal ganglia dopaminergic nigrostriatal pathway that causes hypokinesia, tremor, and muscular rigidity.

Paronychia A condition in which the tissue surrounding a fingernail or toenail is inflamed.

Passive acquired immunity (passive immunity) A form of acquired immunity in which the antibody or lymphocyte is provided by a donor.

Pathogen-associated molecular pattern (PAMP) Molecular patterns on infectious agents or their products that allow recognition by specific receptors.

Pattern recognition receptor (PRR) A receptor involved in innate resistance that recognizes cellular damage or specific patterns on infectious agents.

Pelvic inflammatory disease (PID) Inflammation of the female genital tract because of microorganisms, typically those that are sexually transmitted, such as *Chlamydia* and gonococci; characterized by severe abdominal pain, high fever, vaginal discharge, and possibly infertility.

Pemphigus Any of a group of autoimmune skin diseases marked by groups of itching blisters and open sores on the skin and mucous membranes.

Peptic ulcer A nonmalignant stomach or duodenal wall ulceration; commonly caused by the bacterium *Helicobacter pylori* that thrives in the acidic environment of the stomach.

Periodic paralysis One of a group of diseases in which muscular weakness or flaccid paralysis occurs without loss of consciousness, speech, or sensation.

Peripheral artery disease (PAD) Also known as peripheral vascular disease (PVD); all diseases caused by the obstruction of large peripheral arteries secondary to atherosclerosis, inflammatory processes, embolism, or thrombus formation.

Pernicious anemia An autoimmune disorder that causes a deficiency in intrinsic factor, resulting in the inability to absorb vitamin B_{12} and a subsequent increase in the production of abnormal erythrocytes.

Peyronie disease (bent nail syndrome) A condition in which fibrous plaques grow in the soft tissue of the penis because of injury of the internal cavity of the penis; accompanied by bleeding and scar tissue formation at the tunica albuginea of the corpora cavernosa.

Phagocytosis A type of endocytosis sometimes referred to as cell eating in which substances such as bacteria and cell particulates are incorporated into large vesicles or vacuoles and digested.

Phenylketonuria (PKU) A genetic disorder in which the body lacks the enzyme necessary to metabolize the amino acid phenylalanine to tyrosine, resulting in accumulation of phenylalanine and subsequent brain damage and progressive mental retardation.

Pheochromocytoma A tumor of the adrenal medulla that causes the chromaffin cells to secrete increased amounts of epinephrine or norepinephrine.

Phimosis A condition in which the foreskin of the penis of an uncircumcised male cannot be fully retracted.

Pityriasis rosea A skin disorder in which patches of ovular pink rash appear primarily on the trunk and extremities; thought to be caused by a virus.

Plasma cell A B lymphocyte that secretes antibodies in response to local cytokines released during the primary immune response.

Plasmin A degrading enzyme associated with fibrinolysis of many proteins of blood but primarily of fibrin clots.

Platelet-activating factor A mast cell–derived substance that increases vascular permeability, leukocyte adhesion to endothelial cells, and platelet activation.

Pleural effusion An abnormal accumulation of fluid in the intrapleural spaces of the lungs. It is characterized by chest pain, dyspnea, adventitious lung sounds, and nonproductive cough. The fluid is an exudate or a transudate from inflamed pleural surfaces and may be aspirated or surgically drained.

Pneumoconiosis A chronic disease of the lungs typically seen in miners, sandblasters, and metal grinders caused by repeated inhalation of dusts, including iron oxides, silicates, and carbonates, that collect in the lungs and become sites for the formation of fibrous nodules that eventually replace lung tissue.

Pneumonia An infection of one or both lungs caused by a bacterium, virus, fungus, or other microorganism that enters the body through respiratory passages and causes high fever, chills, pain in the chest, difficulty breathing, cough with sputum, and possibly bluish skin from insufficiently oxygenated blood.

Pneumothorax The collapse of a lung and escape of air into the pleural cavity between the lung and the chest wall that is caused by trauma, environmental factors, or spontaneous occurrence; results in a sudden pain in the chest.

Polycystic kidney disease A condition in which several fluid-filled cysts grow in the kidneys that may reduce kidney function and result in kidney failure as well as damage to the liver, pancreas, and possibly the heart and brain.

Polycystic ovary syndrome (PCOS) A hormonal condition in which multiple ovarian cysts form because of elevated androgens, resulting in hirsutism, obesity, menstrual abnormalities, infertility, and enlarged ovaries.

Polycythemia A condition characterized by an increase in the production of red blood cells in the blood.

Polycythemia vera A chronic, progressive disease that is characterized by overgrowth of the bone marrow, excessive red blood cell production, and an enlarged spleen; causes headache, inability to concentrate, and pain in the fingers and toes.

Port-wine (nevus flammeus) stain A birthmark caused by superficial and deep dilated capillaries in the skin that produce a reddish to purplish discoloration of the skin.

Postmortem change Diffuse physiologic changes that occur within minutes after death.

Postobstructive diuresis Elevated urine output following removal of an obstruction that causes the renal tubules to be unable to reabsorb water and electrolytes normally.

Postrenal acute renal injury A condition characterized by an obstruction that affects the normal flow of urine out of both kidneys and causes pressure to build in the nephrons that eventually causes them to fail.

Precocious puberty Occurs when a boy or girl undergoes the changes associated with puberty at an unexpectedly early age; often caused by a pathologic process that increases the secretion of estrogens or androgens.

Preload The volume of blood in the ventricle after atrial contraction and ventricular filling.

Premenstrual dysphoric disorder (PMDD) A mental health condition in women that begins 1 or 2 weeks before menstrual flow. Symptoms include depression, tension, mood swings, irritability, decreased interest, difficulty in concentrating, fatigue, changes in appetite or sleep, physical symptoms, and a sense of being overwhelmed.

Premenstrual syndrome (PMS) A group of symptoms that occur in many women from 2 to 14 days before menstruation begins, such as abdominal bloating, breast tenderness, headache, fatigue, irritability, depression, and emotional distress.

Prerenal acute renal injury A condition characterized by azotemia that results from a reduction in effective arterial blood volume, which causes the kidney to behave as though renal perfusion is impaired.

Presbyopia A form of farsightedness usually accompanying advanced age in which the lens loses elasticity and becomes unable to accommodate and focus light for near vision.

Priapism A painful condition in which the erect penis maintains an erection in the absence of physical or psychologic stimulation.

Primary dysmenorrhea A condition in which menstruation is painful because of a functional disturbance rather than as a result of inflammation, growths, or anatomic factors.

Primary hyperparathyroidism Usually the result of a benign parathyroid tumor that loses its sensitivity to circulating calcium levels; this condition is accompanied by hypercalcemia, nausea, vomiting, lethargy, depression, muscular weakness, and an altered mental state.

Primary hypertension A condition of elevated blood pressure of unknown etiology that is accompanied by increased total peripheral vascular resistance produced by vasoconstriction, increased cardiac output, or both.

Primary immune response The time interval between the first and second exposures to an antigen, during which antibodies against the antigen are produced.

Prolactinoma The most common type of anterior pituitary tumor; produces visual disturbances and prolactin excess, which results in infertility and changes in menstruation in females and impotence, loss of libido, and infertility in males.

Protopathic The sensation of pain, heat, cold, or pressure without the ability to localize the stimulus.

Psammoma bodies Calcium salt layers present in calcified tissues.

Psoriasis A chronic T cell mediated inflammatory skin disorder in which the skin becomes scaly and inflamed when cells in the outer layer of skin reproduce faster than normal and accumulate on the skin surface (form plaques).

Pulmonary embolism A condition in which a blood clot dislodges from its site of origin and embolizes to the arterial blood supply of one of the lungs, resulting in shortness of breath and difficulty breathing, rapid breathing that is painful, cough, and, in severe cases, hypotension, shock, loss of consciousness, and death.

Pulmonary fibrosis Scarring of the lungs caused by any of several conditions such as sarcoidosis, hypersensitivity pneumonitis, rheumatoid arthritis, lupus, asbestosis, and certain medications; causes shortness of breath, coughing, and diminished exercise tolerance.

Pulmonary thromboembolism A condition in which the pulmonary artery or one of its branches is obstructed by a blood clot that originated in the deep venous system.

Pyloric stenosis A congenital abnormality or acquired defect in which the pylorus is narrowed by a hypertrophic pyloric sphincter muscle or scar tissue, resulting in poor feeding, weight loss, and progressively worsening vomiting.

Rapid eye movement (REM) sleep A period of sleep during which dreams occur, autonomic activities are irregular, and brain waves are fast and of low voltage.

Raynaud disease A condition in which the blood vessels spasm, which results in inadequate blood supply and discoloration of the fingers or the toes, after exposure to changes in temperature or emotional events.

Reactive response The secretion of stress hormones in response to a psychologic stressor.

Recombination A physical exchange of genetic information between homologous chromosomes that results in the creation of new genotypes.

Relative polycythemia A relative increase in the number of red blood cells resulting from a loss of the fluid portion of the blood.

Remodeling A constant process in which bone is resorbed and then replaced without changing shape in order to release calcium and repair mildly damaged bones. Ventricular remodeling after a myocardial infarction includes ventricular dilation, hypertrophy, and geometric distortion.

Renal adenoma A benign tumor originating in the renal tubules of the cortex that is similar in appearance to a renal cell carcinoma.

Renal agenesis A failure of fetal formation of one or both kidneys.

Renal cell carcinoma (RCC) A malignancy arising from the renal tubule that produces hematuria, flank pain, and an abdominal mass.

Renal colic A condition in which a tiny stone passing through the ureter produces intermittent but severe abdominal pain that begins in the side or upper abdomen and travels down to the lower abdomen and possibly radiating into the pubic region or into the penis or testis in men.

Renal dysplasia A condition in which tissue development in one or both kidneys is abnormal.

Renin An enzyme secreted by the juxtaglomerular cells of the kidney that is released in response to decreased blood pressure in the kidney and sympathetic nerve stimulation.

Renin-angiotensin-aldosterone system A mechanism by which sodium and water levels are regulated in the body, including the release of renin, conversion of angiotensinogen into angiotensin I, conversion of angiotensin I into angiotensin II, and the release of aldosterone and its actions on the kidney that increase water and sodium reabsorption.

Reperfusion (reoxygenation) injury Tissue injury resulting from the restoration of oxygen after an interval of hypoxia or anoxia.

Respiratory acidosis A decrease in pH caused by elevated levels of carbon dioxide (hypercapnia), which forms carbonic acid secondary to depressed alveolar ventilation.

Respiratory alkalosis An increase in pH caused by alveolar hyperventilation and reduced levels of carbon dioxide (hypocapnia).

Respiratory distress syndrome (RDS) of the newborn Also known as hyaline membrane disease (HMD), this condition is a type of respiratory distress in newborns, most often in prematurely born infants, those born by cesarean section, or those who have a diabetic mother; the immature lungs do not produce enough surfactant to retain air so the air spaces empty completely and collapse after exhalation.

Resting membrane potential The difference in electrical charge across the membrane of an unstimulated cell that is accomplished by the unequal distribution of charged ions.

Reye syndrome A type of encephalopathy that occurs primarily in children after a viral infection, such as chickenpox or influenza, and is characterized by fever, vomiting, fatty liver, disorientation, and coma. It is associated with aspirin use in children.

Rhabdomyolysis A potentially fatal condition in which skeletal muscle breaks down because of injury such as physical damage to the muscle, high fever, metabolic disorders, excessive exertion, convulsions, or anoxia of the muscle for several hours; large amounts of myoglobin are usually excreted. Sometimes secondary to drugs such as statins.

Rhabdomyosarcoma A highly malignant tumor derived from primitive striated muscle cells that occurs most frequently in the head and neck and is also found in the genitourinary tract, extremities, body wall, and retroperitoneum. In some cases the onset is associated trauma. The initial symptoms depend on the site of tumor development and indicate local tissue or organ destruction, such as dysphagia, vaginal bleeding, hematuria, or obstructed flow of urine.

Rheumatic fever An inflammatory disease associated with a recent streptococcal infection that causes inflammation of the joints, fever, chorea (jerky movements), nodules under the skin, and skin rash. It is frequently followed by rheumatic heart disease and serious heart damage.

Rheumatoid arthritis An autoimmune disease that causes chronic inflammation of the joints and the tissue around the joints and other organs.

Right heart failure A condition in which the right side of the heart loses its ability to pump blood efficiently because of left-sided heart failure, lung disease, congenital heart disease, clots in pulmonary arteries, pulmonary hypertension, or heart valve disease.

Roseola A viral disease in infants and young children that causes fever and a spotty rash that appears shortly after the fever has subsided.

Rotavirus A viral infection seen in young children that causes diarrhea by attacking the lining of the small intestine, resulting in the inability to absorb fluid and electrolytes and their subsequent loss.

Rubella (German measles) An infectious viral disease of children and young adults spread by a droplet spray from the respiratory tract of an infected individual that causes a rash (which lasts about 3 days) and tender and swollen lymph nodes behind the ears.

Rubeola (red measles) An infectious viral disease of young children spread by a droplet spray from the nose, mouth, and throat of individuals

in the infective stage; causes white spots in the mouth, a rash on the face that spreads to the rest of the body, and fever.

Saccular aneurysm (berry aneurysm) A localized, progressively growing sac that affects only a portion of the circumference of the arterial wall and may be the result of congenital anomalies or degeneration.

Salmon patches Also known as stork bites, these small, pink, flat spots are small blood vessels that are visible through the skin; usually found on the forehead, eyelids, upper lip, between the eyebrows, and the back of the neck.

Salpingitis Inflammation of one of the two fallopian tubes because of infection spreading from the vagina or uterus.

Sarcopenia A condition in which muscle mass and strength is lost because of advanced age and decreased activity, resulting in impaired sense of balance.

Scabies A contagious disease caused by *Sarcoptes scabiei,* the human itch mite, characterized by intense itching of the skin and excoriation from scratching. The mite, transmitted by close contact with infected humans or domestic animals, burrows into outer layers of the skin, where the female lays eggs. About 2 to 4 months after the first infection, sensitization to the mites and their products begins, resulting in a pruritic papular rash most common on the webs of fingers, flexor surfaces of wrists, and thighs.

Sclerosing adenosis A condition in which the number of acini per terminal duct is more than twice the number of normal terminal ducts; associated with a significantly increased risk of subsequent breast carcinoma.

Scoliosis A condition in which the spine is curved laterally to varying degrees.

Seborrheic dermatitis Condition in which the skin of the scalp, face, and trunk becomes scaly, flaky, itchy, and red, possibly because of a yeast infection.

Secondary amenorrhea A condition in which menstruation begins at puberty but then is subsequently suppressed for three or more cycles or 6 months in women who previously menstruated.

Secondary dysmenorrhea A condition in which menstruation is altered as a result of inflammation, infection, tumor, or anatomic factors.

Secondary hyperparathyroidism A condition of elevated parathyroid hormone resulting from disease, such as renal failure, in which parathyroid hormone level is elevated in response to vitamin D deficiency.

Secondary hypertension A condition of elevated blood pressure that is associated primarily with renal disease by a renin-dependent mechanism or a fluid volume–dependent mechanism.

Second-degree burn A burn that affects the epidermis and the dermis, classified as superficial or deep according to the depth of injury. The superficial type involves the epidermis and the papillary dermis and is characterized by pain, edema, and the formation of blisters; it

heals without scarring. The deep type extends into the reticular dermis, is pale and anesthetic, and results in scarring.

Seizure A transient event of excessive, disorderly neurologic activity that results in disturbances of motor, sensory, and autonomic function and alters behavior and the state of consciousness.

Sentinel nodes Lymph nodes that are the first to receive drainage and are the first targets during cancer metastasis.

Sequestration crisis A condition in which the cardiovascular system collapses, causing blood to pool in the spleen and liver.

Serum sickness A form of hypersensitivity caused by injection of soluble antigen, such as antiserum, that results in complement activation.

Shock An abnormal condition of inadequate blood flow to the body's tissues, with life-threatening cellular dysfunction. The condition is usually associated with inadequate cardiac output, hypotension, oliguria, changes in peripheral blood flow resistance and distribution, and tissue damage. Causal factors include hemorrhage, vomiting, diarrhea, inadequate fluid intake, or excessive fluid loss, resulting in hypovolemia.

Sialoprotein (osteopontin) A glycoprotein that may play a role in maintaining or reconfiguring tissues during the inflammatory process; required for stress-induced bone remodeling and cell-mediated immunity.

Sickle cell anemia An inherited disorder of the blood caused by abnormal hemoglobin that distorts red blood cells and makes them fragile and prone to rupture. When an excessive number of red blood cells rupture, anemia occurs, as well as pain in the joints, fever, leg ulcers, and jaundice.

Sickle cell trait An inherited condition in which an individual carries only one gene for sickle cell disease and is without symptoms.

Sideroblastic anemia (SA) A refractory anemia of varying severity caused by altered mitochondrial metabolism that is marked by sideroblasts in the bone marrow.

Signal transduction The transmission of signals from an extracellular chemical to the intracellular region where cellular activity is affected. Signal transduction occurs when environmental stimuli are translated into electrical signals in the body, as well as when a signal is transmitted between extracellular and intracellular domains.

Silencing Epigenetic process of gene regulation by "switching off" of a gene. Genes may be silenced by DNA methylation.

Smallpox (variola) An infectious viral disease caused by a poxvirus that results in high fever and aches, as well as the widespread eruption of large sores that leave scars.

Spermatocele A cyst of the rete testis or the head of the epididymis distended with a milky fluid that contains spermatozoa.

Spina bifida A congenital defect in which the spinal column is not closed correctly causing protrusion of that part of the meninges or spinal cord.

Spinal stenosis Narrowing of the vertebral canal, nerve root canals, or intervertebral foramina of the lumbar and cervical spine, caused by encroachment of bone on the space. Symptoms are caused by compression of the cauda equina and include pain, paresthesias, and neurogenic claudication. The condition either may be congenital or may be caused by spinal degeneration.

Stable angina A condition in which ischemic attacks occur at predictable frequencies and duration following activities that increase myocardial oxygen demands, such as exercise and stress.

Staphylococcal scalded-skin syndrome (SSSS) A disease in infants caused by an upper respiratory tract staphylococcal infection that results in the release of bacterial toxins that cause intraepidermal splitting of the skin with blistering of large skin regions.

Stasis dermatitis A condition in which the skin appears brown and ulcerates because of blood pooling in the leg secondary to insufficient venous return.

Stevens-Johnson syndrome An inflammatory eruption of circular erythematous lesions of the skin (usually less than 10% of the body surface) and mucous membranes; usually occurs following a respiratory tract infection or as an allergic reaction to drugs or other substances.

Strangulation Cerebral hypoxia or anoxia caused by compression and closure of the blood vessels and air passages by applying external pressure on the neck.

Strawberry hemangioma A birthmark caused by densely packed blood vessels that is red in color, and usually appears on the face, scalp, back, and chest.

Stress ulcer An acute peptic ulcer occurring in association with various other pathologic conditions, including burns, cor pulmonale, intracranial lesions, and surgical operations.

Struvite stone Also called an infection stone, this urinary stone develops when a urinary tract infection neutralizes the urine, enabling the bacteria to grow more rapidly and a jagged ammonium magnesium phosphate stone to develop.

Subdural hematoma A collection of blood between the inner surface of the dura mater and the surface of the brain caused by rupture of bridging veins of the subdural region.

Sudden infant death syndrome (SIDS) Also known as crib death, this syndrome is characterized by the sudden, unexpected, and unexplained death of an apparently healthy infant under 1 year of age.

Suffocation The failure of oxygen to reach the blood because of a lack of oxygen in the environment or the blockage of external airways.

Syndrome of inappropriate secretion of ADH (SIADH) A condition in which the release of ADH is elevated relative to sodium levels, resulting in increased water reabsorption in the kidneys.

Systole The period of time when the chambers of the heart contract and force blood out of the chambers.

Systolic heart failure A condition in which the heart muscle contracts weakly so that there is not enough oxygenated blood being pumped throughout the body.

Tamponade The blockage or compression of a body part, such as heart compression because of a collection of blood or fluid.

Tay-Sachs disease An autosomal recessive disorder in which an enzyme deficiency leads to the accumulation of gangliosides in the brain and nerve tissue, resulting in mental retardation, convulsions, blindness, and premature death.

Telomere Regions of repetitive DNA at the end of a chromosome are shortened during each cycle of DNA replication; this shortening of the telomere is believed to be a component of cellular aging because it deletes vital genetic information over time. Telomeres protect a cell's chromosome from fusing with each other or rearranging and alterations can lead to cancer.

Tetralogy of Fallot A congenital condition that is characterized by four malformations including ventricular septal defect, misplacement of the origin of the aorta, narrowing of the pulmonary artery, and enlargement of the right ventricle.

Thalassemia An inherited autosomal recessive blood disease results in a reduced rate of synthesis or no production of the globin chains that form hemoglobin The disorder can result in severe anemia; enlarged heart, liver, and spleen; and skeletal deformation.

Therapeutic index A ratio of the median lethal dose to the median effective dose for a drug.

Third-degree burn (full-thickness burn) A burn that destroys both the epidermis and the dermis, often also involving the subcutaneous tissue. Also called full-thickness burn.

Thromboangiitis obliterans (Buerger disease) A condition in which the medium-sized arteries and veins are inflamed because of thrombotic occlusion, resulting in ischemia and gangrene.

Thrombocythemia A condition in which the number of platelets in the blood increases, resulting in clot formation.

Thrombotic stroke (cerebral thrombosis) Stroke symptoms caused by thrombosis; typically secondary to atherosclerosis.

Thrombotic thrombocytopenic purpura (TTP) A disorder of blood coagulation caused by an enzymatic deficiency that is characterized by a reduced number of platelets in the blood, the formation of blood clots in tissue arterioles and capillaries, and neurologic damage.

Thrombus A fibrinous blood clot formed in a vessel or in a chamber of the heart that remains attached at its site of origin.

Thrush A yeast infection of the mouth and throat that presents as creamy white, curdlike patches on the tongue, inside the mouth, and on the back of the throat; commonly associated with yeast infection of the esophagus.

Tinea infection One of a group of fungal skin infections that include athlete's foot, folliculitis, jock itch, ringworm, and pityriasis versicolor.

Toll-like receptor (TLR) A receptor expressed on the surface of many cells that interacts with many pathogens to increase resistance and bridges innate resistance and acquired immune response through cytokine production.

Toxic epidermal necrolysis A condition associated with drug reactions in which a large portion of the skin (30% or more) and mucous membranes becomes intensely erythematous and can progress to full-thickness epidermal necrosis with bullous formation and peeling similar to a burn injury.

Tracheoesophageal fistula (TEF) A condition in which a connection is formed between the esophagus and the trachea because of esophageal atresia or laryngostomy.

Transferrin An iron-binding plasma protein that transports iron into the cell by binding a transferrin surface receptor and entering the cell where it releases iron ions.

Transposition of the great arteries (TGA) A condition in which the aorta arises from the right ventricle and the pulmonary artery arises from the left ventricle.

Transudate The passage of extravascular fluid through a membrane. The fluid is low in protein and without cells and develops as a result of changes in tissue hydrostatic or oncotic pressure and usually is not due to an inflammatory process.

Truncus arteriosus A congenital defect in which a large great vessel arises from a ventricular septal defect and does not divide into the aorta and pulmonary artery, resulting in one vessel carrying blood both to the body and to the lungs.

Tuberculosis (TB) An infectious disease of humans caused by a tubercle bacillus that results in the formation of tubercles on the lungs and other tissues of the body.

Tumor A growth of tissue caused by the uncontrolled replication of cells.

Tumor marker A biochemical marker sensitive to specific types of tumors that is used to screen, diagnose, assess prognosis and treatment, and monitor recurrence.

Tumor-suppressor gene A gene whose protein product terminates cell proliferation, thereby inhibiting tumor formation.

Type 1 diabetes mellitus A disorder of carbohydrate metabolism characterized by a decrease in insulin production, resulting in hyperglycemia and eventually renal failure and coronary artery disease. It usually develops in childhood but can occur at any age. The cause is unknown but probably related to a gene-environment interaction and autoimmunity. There is destruction of pancreatic beta cells causing insulin deficiency and glucagon level is elevated. Ketosis is common with insulin deficiency.

Type I fibers Slow-twitch fibers that are used primarily during aerobic metabolism and function during activities that require high endurance.

Type 2 diabetes mellitus A condition of glucose intolerance that normally appears first in adulthood and is exacerbated by obesity and an inactive lifestyle.

Ulcerative colitis A chronic inflammatory bowel disease in which the mucosal and submucosal lining of the large intestine is chronically inflamed and ulcerated, resulting in abdominal pain, diarrhea, and rectal bleeding. Genetic, immune, and environmental factors contribute to the disease.

Ultrafiltration The process of filtering blood across a barrier between the capillary of the glomerulus and the Bowman capsule of the nephron at a rate that is determined by hydrostatic and oncotic pressures.

Unstable angina A condition in which unprovoked ischemic attacks occur at unpredictable frequencies and may increase in severity, causing chest pain that is not relieved by rest.

Upper airway obstruction Any abnormal condition of the mouth, nose, or larynx that interferes with breathing when the rest of the respiratory system is functioning normally.

Up-regulation The process by which a cell increases the number of receptors for a given hormone or neurotransmitter to improve sensitivity in response to low hormone concentration.

Urethritis Inflammation of the urethra usually caused by a sexually transmitted microorganism that results in painful urination.

Uric acid stone A condition in which uric acid levels in urine are elevated, preventing the uric acid from dissolving and causing uric acid stones to form.

Urinary tract infection An infection of the urinary tract that may occur anywhere from the kidneys to the urethra; much more common in females because of a decreased distance between the urethra and the anus.

Uterine prolapse The descent or herniation of the uterus into or beyond the vagina because of weakness of the pelvic musculature, ligaments, and fascia or obstetric trauma and lacerations sustained during labor and delivery.

Vacuolar myelopathy HIV-induced loss of myelin and spongy degeneration of the spinal cord that may cause spastic paraparesis, sensory ataxia in lower limbs, and unsteady gait.

Vaginismus A form of sexual dysfunction caused by a psychologic disorder or vaginal inflammation in which the muscles at the entrance to the vagina contract and prevent sexual intercourse.

Vaginitis An infection of the vagina usually caused by a fungus that may cause itching or burning and a discharge.

Valvular regurgitation A condition in which one or more of the heart's valves does not close properly, producing a backflow of blood.

Valvular stenosis A condition in which one or more of the heart's valves becomes narrow, stiff, thickened, fused, or blocked, and blood does not flow through it smoothly.

Varicocele A painful condition in which the veins in the scrotum that develop in the spermatic cord enlarge; if the valves that regulate blood flow from these veins become dysfunctional, blood does not leave the testis, causing swelling in the veins above and behind the testis.

Vasogenic edema An accumulation of fluid in the cerebrum that is typically caused by an increase in capillary endothelial cell permeability and usually occurs near a tumor.

Vasomotor flush A sudden, brief sensation of heat, typically occurring over the entire body, that is caused by a transient dilation of the blood vessels of the skin and possibly alterations in the temperature-regulating center of the hypothalamus secondary to decreased estrogen levels.

Vaso-occlusive crisis (thrombotic crisis) A condition that occurs when the microcirculation is obstructed by sickled red blood cells, resulting in ischemic injury to the organ supplied, pain, and possibly irreversible organ damage.

Vegetative state (VS) A physical condition in which a previously comatose patient continues to be unable to communicate or respond to stimuli, despite at times giving the appearance of wakefulness. The eyes may be open, but, because of senile brain disease, cerebral arteriosclerosis, or injury to the cerebral cortex, the patient remains immobile and all physical needs of the patient must be performed for them (e.g., feeding, toileting).

Venous stasis ulcer A condition affecting the lower leg in which leaky valves, obstructions, or regurgitation in veins impairs blood flow back to the heart, resulting in pooling of blood in the lower leg and subsequent tissue damage.

Ventricular septal defect (VSD) A congenital malformation in which the wall between the left and right ventricles has a hole that allows blood to travel between them, potentially leading to congestive heart failure.

Volatile A substance such as carbonic acid that can evaporate rapidly.

Volkmann ischemic contracture A condition in which the distal humerus is fractured and disrupts the radial artery and median nerve, resulting in necrosis of the extensor muscles, contracture of elbow flexion, and a claw hand.

von Willebrand factor (vWF) A glycoprotein synthesized in endothelial cells and megakaryocytes that circulates complexed to factor VIII; it mediates adhesion of platelets to damaged epithelial surfaces and may participate in platelet aggregation. Deficiency results in the prolonged bleeding time seen in von Willebrand disease.

Wart An outgrowth of the skin caused by a virus that is easily transmitted by close contact and that may persist for years.

Wheal-and-flare reaction A condition caused by an allergic reaction in which the area of skin around the site of antigen contact becomes flattened and red with fluid-filled blisters.

Page numbers followed by *b*, indicate box; *f*, figure, *t*, table. Syndromes and disorders appear in boldface.

PREFIXES AND SUFFIXES USED IN MEDICAL TERMINOLOGY

Prefix	Meaning	Suffix	Meaning
a-	Without, not	-al, -ac	Pertaining to
af-	Toward	-algia	Pain
an-	Without, not	-aps, -apt	Fit; fasten
ante-	Before	-arche	Beginning; origin
anti-	Against; resisting	-ase	Signifies an enzyme
auto-	Self	-blast	Sprout; make
bi-	Two; double	-centesis	A piercing
circum-	Around	-cide	To kill
co-, con-	With; together	-clast	Break; destroy
contra-	Against	-crine	Release; secrete
de-	Down from, undoing	-ectomy	A cutting out
dia-	Across; through	-emesis	Vomiting
dipl-	Twofold, double	-emia	Refers to blood condition
dys-	Bad; disordered; difficult	-flux	Flow
ectop-	Displaced	-gen	Creates; forms
ef-	Away from	-genesis	Creation, production
em-, en-	In, into	-gram	Something written
endo-	Within	-graph(y)	To write, draw
epi-	Upon	-hydrate	Containing H_2O (water)
eu-	Good	-ia, -sia	Condition; process
ex-, exo-	Out of, out from	-iasis	Abnormal condition
extra-	Outside of	-ic, -ac	Pertaining to
hapl-	Single	-in	Signifies a protein
hem-, hemat-	Blood	-ism	Signifies "condition of"
hemi-	Half	-itis	Signifies "inflammation of"
hom(e)o-	Same; equal	-lemma	Rind; peel
hyper-	Over; above	-lepsy	Seizure
hypo-	Under; below	-lith	Stone; rock
infra-	Below, beneath	-logy	Study of
inter-	Between	-lunar	Moon; moonlike
intra-	Within	-malacia	Softening
iso-	Same, equal	-megaly	Enlargement
macro-	Large	-metric, -metry	Measurement, length
mega-	Large; million(th)	-oid	Like; in the shape of
mes-	Middle	-oma	Tumor
meta-	Beyond, after	-opia	Vision, vision condition
micro-	Small; millionth	-oscopy	Viewing
milli-	Thousandth	-ose	Signifies a carbohydrate (especially sugar)
mono-	One (single)		
neo-	New	-osis	Condition, process
non-	Not	-ostomy	Formation of an opening
oligo-	Few, scanty	-otomy	Cut
ortho-	Straight; correct, normal	-penia	Lack
para-	By the side of; near	-philic	Loving
per-	Through	-phobic	Fearing
peri-	Around; surrounding	-phragm	Partition
poly-	Many	-plasia	Growth, formation
post-	After	-plasm	Substance, matter
pre-	Before	-plasty	Shape; make
pro-	First; promoting	-plegia	Paralysis
quadr-	Four	-pnea	Breath, breathing
re-	Back again	-(r)rhage, -(r)rhagia	Breaking out, discharge
retro-	Behind	-(r)rhaphy	Sew, suture
semi-	Half	-(r)rhea	Flow
sub-	Under	-some	Body
super-, supra-	Over, above, excessive	-tensin, -tension	Pressure
trans-	Across; through	-tonic	Pressure, tension
tri-	Three; triple	-tripsy	Crushing
		-ule	Small, little
		-uria	Refers to urine condition